# Clinical Medicine

# Clinical Medicine

## A TEXTBOOK FOR MEDICAL STUDENTS AND DOCTORS

EDITED BY

### Parveen Kumar
BSc, MD, FRCP
*Senior Lecturer,*
*Medical College of St Bartholomew's Hospital, London*
*and Honorary Consultant Physician,*
*St Bartholomew's and Homerton Hospitals, London*

AND

### Michael Clark
MD, FRCP
*Honorary Senior Lecturer,*
*Medical College of St Bartholomew's Hospital, London*

## Third Edition

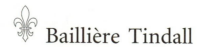
Baillière Tindall

Baillière Tindall    24–28 Oval Road
W. B. Saunders    London NW1 7DX

The Curtis Center
Independence Square West
Philadelphia, PA 19106–3399, USA

Harcourt Brace & Company
55 Horner Avenue
Toronto, Ontario, M8Z 4X6, Canada

Harcourt Brace & Company, Australia
30–52 Smidmore Street
Marrickville
NSW 2204, Australia

Harcourt Brace & Company, Japan
Ichibancho Central Building
22–1 Ichibancho
Chiyoda-ku, Tokyo 102, Japan

First published 1987
Second edition 1990
Third edition 1994
Second printing 1995

**British Library Cataloguing in Publication Data**
Clinical Medicine. 3rd Edn.
  1. Pathology  2. Medicine
  I. Kumar, PJ  II. Clark, ML
  616  RB 111

ISBN 0–7020–1739–6

Typeset by Photo·graphics, Honiton, Devon
Printed and bound in Great Britain
by Butler & Tanner Ltd, Frome and London

# Contents

# Contributors

**Jane Anderson** PhD MRCP
*Senior Lecturer*
*Medical College of St Bartholomew's Hospital;*
*Honorary Consultant Physician*
*St Bartholomew's and Homerton Hospitals*
*London*
SEXUALLY TRANSMITTED DISEASES

**John V Anderson** MD MA MBBS MRCP
*Consultant Physician*
*St Bartholomew's and Homerton Hospitals*
*London*
DIABETES MELLITUS AND LIPIDS

**Larry R I Baker** MA MD FRCP
*Consultant Physician*
*Department of Nephrology*
*St Bartholomew's Hospital*
*London*
RENAL DISEASE

**A John Camm** BSc MD FRCP FACC
*Professor of Clinical Cardiology*
*St George's Hospital Medical School*
*London*
CARDIOVASCULAR DISEASE

**Anthony W Clare** MD, FRCPsych, FRCPI
*Professor of Clinical Psychiatry*
*Trinity College Dublin;*
*Medical Director*
*St Patrick's Hospital*
*Dublin*
PSYCHOLOGICAL MEDICINE

**Michael L Clark** MD FRCP
*Honorary Senior Lecturer*
*Medical College of St Bartholomew's Hospital*
*London*
NUTRITION; GASTROENTEROLOGY; LIVER, BILIARY TRACT
AND PANCREATIC DISEASES; ENVIRONMENTAL MEDICINE

**Charles R A Clarke** MB BChir FRCP
*Consultant Neurologist*
*St Bartholomew's and Whipps Cross Hospitals*
*London*
ENVIRONMENTAL MEDICINE; NEUROLOGY AND MUSCLE
DISEASE

**Robert J Davies** MA MD FRCP
*Professor of Respiratory Medicine*
*Department of Respiratory Medicine and Allergy*
*Medical College of St Bartholomew's Hospital*
*London*
RESPIRATORY DISEASE

**Paul L Drury** MA FRCP
*Medical Director*
*Auckland Diabetes Centre;*
*Physician*
*Auckland Hospital*
*New Zealand*
ENDOCRINOLOGY; BONE DISEASE

**Michael J G Farthing** MD FRCP
*Professor of Gastroenterology*
*Medical College of St Bartholomew's Hospital*
*London*
INFECTIOUS DISEASES AND TROPICAL MEDICINE

**Elizabeth Fisher** BA PhD
*Senior Research Fellow*
*Department of Biochemistry and Molecular Genetics*
*St Mary's Hospital Medical School, Imperial College*
*London*
GENETICS AND MOLECULAR BIOLOGY

**Edwin A M Gale** MA FRCP
*Professor of Diabetes*
*Department of Diabetes and Metabolism*
*Medical College of St Bartholomew's Hospital*
*London*
DIABETES AND OTHER DISORDERS OF METABOLISM

**Charles J Hinds** FRCP FFARCS
*Consultant and Senior Lecturer*
*Department of Anaesthesia and Intensive Care*
*St Bartholomew's Hospital*
*London*
INTENSIVE CARE

**Edward C Huskisson** MD FRCP
*Rheumatologist*
*King Edward VII Hospital for Officers*
*London*
RHEUMATOLOGY AND BONE DISEASE

**Donald J Jeffries** BSc MB FRCPath
*Professor of Virology*
*Medical College of St Bartholomew's Hospital*
*London*
VIROLOGY

**John D T Kirby** FRCP
*Consultant Physician*
*Department of Dermatology*
*St Bartholomew's Hospital*
*London*
DERMATOLOGY

**Parveen J Kumar** BSc MD FRCP
*Senior Lecturer*
*Medical College of St Bartholomew's Hospital;*
*Honorary Consultant Physician*
*St Bartholomew's and Homerton Hospitals*
*London*
GENETICS AND MOLECULAR BIOLOGY;
GASTROENTEROLOGY; LIVER, BILIARY TRACT AND
PANCREATIC DISEASES

**W John W Morrow** BSc PhD
*Senior Lecturer*
*Department of Immunology*
*St Bartholomew's Hospital*
*London*
IMMUNOLOGY

**Michael F Murphy** MD FRCP FRCPath
*Senior Lecturer and Honorary Consultant in Haematology*
*Department of Haematology*
*Medical College of St Bartholomew's Hospital*
*London*
DISEASES OF THE BLOOD

**Jacqueline M Parkin** MB PhD MRCP
*Senior Lecturer and Honorary Consultant in Clinical*
*Immunology*
*Department of Immunology*
*Medical College of St Bartholomew's Hospital*
*London*
IMMUNOLOGY

**Richard M Pearson** MA MB MRCP
*Consultant Physician (Clinical Pharmacology)*
*Harold Wood Hospital;*
*Senior Lecturer*
*Department of Clinical Pharmacology*
*Medical College of St Bartholomew's Hospital*
*London*
POISONING

**Anthony J Pinching** DPhil FRCP
*Professor of Immunology*
*Medical College of St Bartholomew's Hospital*
*London*
IMMUNOLOGY

**Ama Z S Rohatiner** MD FRCP
*Senior Lecturer and Consultant Physician*
*Department of Medical Oncology*
*Medical College of St Bartholomew's Hospital*
*London*
MEDICAL ONCOLOGY

**Maurice L Slevin** MD FRCP
*Consultant Physician and Medical Oncologist*
*Department of Medical Oncology*
*Medical College of St Bartholomew's Hospital*
*London*
MEDICAL ONCOLOGY

**Theresa Tate** FRCR
*Senior Lecturer and Honorary Consultant in Palliative*
*Medicine*
*Medical College of St Bartholomew's Hospital;*
*Consultant*
*Whipps Cross Hospital*
*London*
PALLIATIVE CARE

**Charles R V Tomson** MA BM BCh DM MRCP
*Consultant Nephrologist*
*Southmead Hospital*
*Bristol*
WATER AND ELECTROLYTES AND ACID−BASE HOMEOSTASIS
RENAL DISEASE

**Paul Turner** CBE MD FRCP FFPM
*Emeritus Professor of Clinical Pharmacology*
*Medical College of St Bartholomew's Hospital*
*London*
ADVERSE DRUG REACTIONS

# Preface to the First Edition

There must be a good reason to write a new textbook of medicine when there are already a number on the market. It seemed to us that none of those currently available adequately conveyed the detail and background needed for medical practice in the late 1980s and 1990s. We have tried to strike a balance between exciting new developments in medical research and the vast quantity of established fact that needs to be absorbed by today's student. For this reason each chapter attempts to link scientific advances with clinical practice so that the management of disease can be based on sound physiological concepts.

This book is designed for both medical students and practising doctors and we have tried to produce a detailed but comprehensible text that bridges the gap between the purely introductory and the larger reference works. Tropical diseases have been included, and because the book will have a worldwide distribution we have discussed the presentation of disease as seen in developing countries. Disorders seen only in childhood have been excluded as these are well covered in other texts and would make this book too large. However, there are chapters on intensive care, nutrition, adverse drug reactions, poisoning and environmental medicine, which are often neglected yet play an important role in modern medical practice. There is inevitably an enormous chapter on infectious diseases but we felt that a description of all infectious agents should be included for quick reference; this chapter also contains basic information on antibiotic chemotherapy and a section on epidemiology and host resistance. A short chapter on genetics, molecular biology and immunology provides the basic principles of these subjects.

Today's clinical students will have covered much of this in their preclinical course, but we hope that established practitioners will find it a useful introduction. Specific genetic and immunological disorders are covered in appropriate chapters.

We have concentrated on the management of disease but, within the text, have highlighted details of practical procedures and emergency therapy so that this book will be an invaluable companion in clinical practice. The practising clinician can use the book for reference or as a quick and easy guide to the management of an individual patient. Each chapter contains many tables and figures as an aid to learning. There are many cross-references, so that it is easy to move through different parts of the book to pursue different aspects of a particular topic and repetition has been minimized.

The contributors are all actively engaged in both clinical and research work, so the text has been written by clinicians who are not only in the forefront of medical advance but who also do ward rounds and outpatient clinics. At the time of writing all the contributors were working at St Bartholomew's Hospital, London, and thus combine a unified teaching approach with high academic standards.

We would like to thank all our colleagues for their hard work and cooperation and also our families and the many friends who have supported us during the preparation of this book.

*Parveen Kumar*
*Michael Clark*

# Preface to the Third Edition

This edition, after an interval of four years, has become necessary because of the enormous advances in clinical medicine. New molecular biological tools have become available, increasing the understanding of the mechanisms of disease. In addition these and other techniques are revolutionizing therapy for many common conditions. We have, therefore, reviewed every chapter in great detail to incorporate all these changes so that medical practice is updated.

The previous editions of this book have been used by undergraduate and post-graduate medical students as well as doctors both in primary care and hospital environments. To accommodate all these groups, we have kept the original format which ties in scientific knowledge and clinical practice. In addition we have provided boxes for emergency treatments as well as practical procedures so that the book can be used for day-to-day management of patients.

We welcome new authors who have brought fresh ideas to keep the book alive and at the forefront of medical texts. We would like to thank all of our previous contributors who helped us in the earlier editions.

All figures have been redesigned and more colour has been added to make the text even more user friendly. Some of the chapters have been re-arranged with enlarged sections, for example, on bone, the control of pain and sexually transmitted disease (including HIV infection). We have placed a greater emphasis on care both inside and outside the hospital emphasizing the role of all professionals allied to medicine. Care of the elderly has, once again, been emphasized throughout the book, thus avoiding the artificial separation between general and geriatric medicine.

This book remains a standard medical textbook in many hospitals and medical colleges throughout the world, and we welcome the views of colleagues who regularly write in to us offering suggestions and new ideas. Arising from these we have developed two handy companions based on the main text: *Baillière's Pocket Essentials of Clinical Medicine* by A. Ballinger and S. Patchett and *MCQs in Clinical Medicine*. These books can now be used in conjunction with *Clinical Medicine*, providing a comprehensive package designed to cater for study and reference as well as for examination needs.

Finally, we would like to thank our families and friends for their enormous support and who have made it possible for us to complete this edition.

*Parveen Kumar*
*Michael Clark*

# Acknowledgements

We would like to thank all our colleagues who have helped us in the preparation of this edition. These include Alison McLean, Susan Davis, John Garrow, David Leaver, David Silk, Neil Rothnie, Anne Ballinger, Steve Patchett, William Cattell, James Malpas, Rodney Reznik, David Rolston, Shoba Char, Neville Wathen, Paul Kelly, Peter Fairclough, Andrew Norton, David Lowe and Pamela Todd.

We would particularly like to acknowledge the invaluable help of our two secretaries, Wendy Draper and Victoria Hollings. The Medical Illustration Department of St Bartholomew's Hospital prepared the illustrations for dermatology.

We are deeply indebted for the skill and support of our publishers. In particular, Rachael Stock's single minded and good humoured enthusiasm has been enormously appreciated. Seán Duggan and Carol Parr have now taken us through two editions with continuing professionalism. Jan Ross prepared the index.

# Important notice

Every effort has been made to check the drug dosages given in this book. However, as it is possible that dosage schedules have been revised, the reader is strongly urged to consult the drug companies' literature before administering any of the drugs listed.

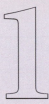

# 1

# Infectious diseases, tropical medicine and sexually transmitted diseases

## Global impact

Infectious diseases are the commonest afflictions of humans and are a major source of morbidity and mortality in both developed and developing countries. Table 1.1 shows estimated morbidity and mortality figures for the common infectious diseases.

Increase in world travel in the past 30–40 years has brought Westerners into contact with a number of diseases unusual in the West, such as malaria and schistosomiasis. New infective agents continue to be identified including *Helicobacter pylori*, the new hepatitis viruses C and E, the agent of Whipple's disease, *Tropheryma whippeii*, and new diarrhoea-producing enteropathogens such as *Cyclospora cayatenensis*. Human immunodeficiency virus (HIV) infection continues to increase. There is an increasing problem of infections in the immunosuppressed, not only in those with HIV but also in organ transplant recipients and those receiving anticancer chemotherapy.

The control of infectious diseases worldwide has been vastly improved by the use of effective vaccines and antimicrobial agents. Technological advances in molecular biology have also improved diagnosis, treatment and the development of new vaccines.

## Epidemiology

The prevalence of infectious diseases varies markedly throughout the world and depends on climatic conditions, sanitation, the quality of the water supply, and to some extent the specific disease resistance of the indigenous population at risk. The continuance of infectious diseases in a human population requires:

- Reservoirs of infection
- Effective modes of transmission

### Reservoirs

HUMAN RESERVOIRS are necessary for the agents of those diseases that (under natural conditions) exclusively afflict humans. Specific examples of such diseases are hepatitis A and B, cholera and shigellosis. Many sites in the body act as permanent reservoirs for microorganisms:

- Skin, e.g. *Staphylococcus epidermidis*
- Nasopharynx, e.g. meningococci
- Intestinal tract, e.g. *Giardia, Entamoeba histolytica*— both can continue to colonize after clinical recovery

Viruses may remain in the body for many months or years, notable examples being hepatitis B virus and the neurotropic herpesviruses.

Helminths may remain in the circulation (e.g. schistosomes in the portal vein) or lymphatic system (e.g. filarial worms) for many years, the former constantly producing millions of ova, a high proportion of which are deposited back into the environment.

ANIMAL RESERVOIRS of human disease are also important both in the developed and developing worlds. The following are common examples of zoonoses (infections that can be transmitted from animals, except arthropods, to man):

- From battery-farmed chickens—*Salmonella* or *Campylobacter jejuni* infection
- From domestic cats—*Toxoplasma gondii* infection

| Disease | Estimated morbidity (No. of cases in thousands per year) | Estimated mortality (No. of deaths in thousands per year) |
|---|---|---|
| Diarrhoeal disease | 3 000 000– 5 000 000 | 10 000 |
| Respiratory infection | ? | 5 000 |
| Malaria | 270 000 | 1 500 |
| Measles | 80 000 | 1 000 |
| Schistosomiasis | 20 000 | 1 000 |
| Whooping cough | 20 000 | 400 |
| Neonatal tetanus | ? | 150 |

**Table 1.1**  League table of infectious diseases worldwide.

- From domestic and wild animals—*Giardia* infection
- From cattle—*Cryptosporidium parvum* infection

Diseases that rely on arthropods for their transmission include malaria, yellow fever, Dengue fever and rickettsial infections.

ENVIRONMENT RESERVOIRS may also act as a temporary lodging place for some bacteria, viruses and parasites.

Water contaminated with enteropathogens is a constant cause of concern in the tropics; water may also be a reservoir of hepatitis A virus. Cysts of some protozoa, notably *Giardia*, may remain viable despite apparently effective water-purification procedures.

Soil is also a source of the agents of human disease, particularly spore-forming bacteria such as *Clostridium* spp. and *Bacillus anthracis*, whose spores can remain viable under suitable climatic conditions for many months.

### Transmission

AIRBORNE SPREAD. Some viruses, bacteria and bacterial spores can be carried directly by the wind. Some are generally spread by droplets in the air, e.g. influenza viruses, and other microorganisms such as *Legionella* are spread by aerosol, characteristically from air-conditioning units.

SPREAD BY DIRECT CONTACT. This includes:
- Person-to-person spread, e.g. skin infections (impetigo, ringworm and scabies) and sexually transmitted diseases
- Faecal–oral spread, particularly amongst children in residential institutions, e.g. shigellosis, giardiasis and hepatitis A
- Inoculation of infection, e.g. transfusion of blood or blood products containing hepatitis B, C or HIV or by contaminated needles (drug abusers, medical and paramedical personnel)
- Insect bites, e.g. mosquitoes (malaria), sandfly (leishmaniasis), ticks (babesiosis) and bugs (Chagas' disease)
- Entry through the skin, which occurs with the larval forms of some helminths that can survive in soil or water, e.g. *Schistosoma*, *Strongyloides* and hookworm

SPREAD BY FOOD AND WATER. Contaminated food and water is the usual mode of transmission of enteropathogens. Some bacteria, such as *Shigella*, require as few as $10^2$ organisms to initiate infection, whereas others like *Vibrio cholerae* require approximately $10^8$ organisms. Cysts of parasites such as *Giardia* and *Entamoeba histolytica* can survive in water for many months and are relatively resistant to water-treatment procedures. Swimming pools are also recognized to be a source of these parasites.

SPREAD BY FOMITES. Transmission of infection can occur between persons via an inanimate object, e.g. bed linen, books.

## Principles and basic mechanisms

Figure 1.1 summarizes the important steps that occur during the pathogenesis of infection.

### Specificity

Some infectious agents are strictly species selective. Amoebiasis, for example, only naturally affects humans. Even within a species, relative resistance is apparent, such as the decreased susceptibility of Duffy blood group negative individuals to *Plasmodium vivax* malaria.

Microorganisms are also highly specific with respect to the organ or tissue that they infect. This predilection for specific sites in the body relates partly to the *milieu exterieur*, i.e. the immediate environment in which the organism finds itself; for example, anaerobic organisms colonize the highly anaerobic colon, whereas aerobic organisms are generally found in the mouth, pharynx and proximal intestinal tract. Other organisms that clearly show selectivity are:
- *Streptococcus pneumoniae* (respiratory tract)
- *Escherichia coli* (urinary and alimentary tract)

Even within a species of bacterium such as *E. coli*, different strains will show selectivity towards a particular organ, e.g. the enterotoxigenic *E. coli* causes acute diarrhoeal disease, whereas the uropathogenic *E. coli* is responsible for urinary tract infection.

Even within an organ a pathogen may show selectivity for a particular cell type. In the intestine, for example, rotavirus predominantly invades and destroys intestinal epithelial cells on the upper portion of the villus, whereas reovirus selectively enters the body through the specialized epithelial cells, known as M cells, that cover the Peyer's patches.

### Epithelial attachment

Many bacteria attach to the epithelial substratum by specific organelles called pili (or fimbriae) that contain a surface lectin(s): a protein or glycoprotein that recognizes specific sugar residues on the host cell. Such is the specificity of this attachment mechanism that it limits enterotoxigenic *E. coli* infection, for example, to certain species. Some viruses and protozoa (*Plasmodium*, *Entamoeba histolytica*) also interact with their target-cell surface membrane by a similar mechanism. Other parasites such as hookworm have specific attachment organelles (buccal plates) that firmly grip the intestinal epithelium.

### Multiplication and colonization

These follow epithelial attachment. Pathogens may then either remain within the lumen of the organ that they have colonized or may invade the tissues.

### Invasion

Invasion may result in:
1 An intracellular location for the pathogen (e.g. viruses,

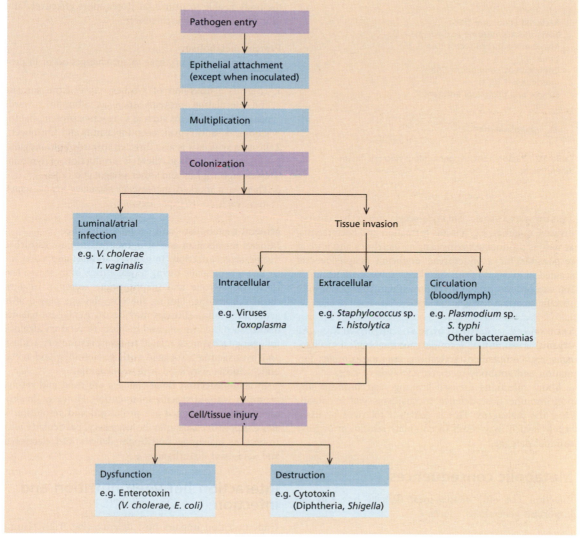

**Fig. 1.1** The pathogenesis of infection.

*Toxoplasma, Leishmania, Plasmodium*)
2 An extracellular location for the pathogen (e.g. mycobacteria, staphylococci and *Entamoeba histolytica*)
3 Invasion directly into the blood or lymph circulation (e.g. schistosome larvae, trypanosomes, *Leishmania* and *Plasmodium*)
Once the pathogen is firmly established in its target tissue, a series of events follow that usually culminates in damage to the host.

### Tissue dysfunction or damage
The mechanism by which microorganisms produce disease has been the subject of intensive investigation and a number of well-defined mechanisms have now been described.

EXOTOXINS AND ENDOTOXINS. Microorganisms may secrete exotoxins. These have many diverse activities, including inhibition of protein synthesis (diphtheria

toxin), neurotoxicity (*Clostridium perfringens, C. tetani* and *C. botulinum*) and enterotoxicity, which results in intestinal secretion of water and electrolytes (*E. coli, V. cholerae*).

Endotoxin is a lipopolysaccharide (LPS) in the cell wall of Gram-negative bacteria. It is responsible for many of the features of shock, namely hypotension, fever, intravascular coagulation and, at high doses, death.

TUMOUR NECROSIS FACTOR (TNF). This is released from a variety of phagocytic cells (macrophages/monocytes) and non-phagocytic cells (lymphocytes, natural killer cells) in response to infections and inflammatory stimuli (Table 1.2). TNF itself then stimulates the release of a cascade of other mediators involved in inflammation and tissue remodelling, e.g. interleukin (IL-1 and IL-6), prostaglandins, leukotrienes, corticotrophin. TNF is therefore responsible for many of the effects of an infection.

Bacterial endotoxin (LPS)
Toxic shock syndrome toxin-1 (TSST-1)
Mycobacterial cord factor (see p. 36)
Virus
Complement component C5a
Interleukin-1 (IL-1)
Fungal and protozoal antigens

———

LPS, lipopolysaccharide.

**Table 1.2** Factors that trigger tumour necrosis factor biosynthesis.

TISSUE INVASION. *Staphylococcus aureus* has tissue-invasive qualities, e.g. abscess formation and bacteraemia, as well as producing toxins causing diarrhoea and a toxin responsible for a widespread erythema (staphylococcal scalded skin syndrome). Similarly, some pathogenic *E. coli* can produce tissue invasion without production of a specific toxin.

SECONDARY IMMUNOLOGICAL PHENOMENA. All organisms can initiate secondary immunological mechanisms, e.g. complement activation, immune complex formation and antibody-mediated cytolysis of cells.

Many infections are self-limiting, and immune and non-immune host defence mechanisms will eventually clear the pathogens. This is generally followed by tissue repair, which may result in complete resolution or leave residual damage.

## Metabolic consequences

Infection not only causes local damage but also has important generalized effects.

### Fever
Body temperature is controlled by the thermoregulatory centre in the anterior hypothalamus in the floor of the third ventricle. This centre is sensitive to endogenous pyrogen (IL-1) which is released from a variety of cells involved in host defence, primarily blood monocytes and phagocytes, under the influence of microbial exogenous pyrogens. IL-1 is thought to act on the thermoregulatory centre by increasing prostaglandin synthesis. The antipyretic effect of salicylates is brought about, at least in part, through its inhibitory effects on prostaglandin synthetase.

Fever production is thought to have a positive effect on the course of infection. However, for every 1°C rise in temperature, there is a 13% increase in basal metabolic rate and oxygen consumption. Fever therefore leads to increased energy requirements at a time when anorexia leads to decreased food intake. The normal compensatory mechanisms in starvation, e.g. mobilization of fat stores, are inhibited in acute infections. This leads to an increase in skeletal muscle breakdown, releasing amino acids, which, via gluconeogenesis, are used to provide energy.

In chronic infection there is time for adaptation and the body is able to utilize fat stores more effectively and thus weight loss is much slower.

### Protein metabolism
During acute infection three major changes occur in protein metabolism:
1 There is a diversion of synthesis away from somatic and circulating proteins such as albumin towards acute-phase proteins such as C-reactive protein, haptoglobin, $\alpha_1$-antitrypsin, caeruloplasmin and fibrinogen.
2 Protein synthesis is also directed towards immunoglobulin production and there is production of lymphocytes, neutrophils and other phagocytic cells.
3 There is a marked increase in nitrogen losses, which may reach 10–15 g per day.

### Mineral metabolism and acid–base balance
Mineral metabolism and acid–base balance are disturbed during acute infection. In general, sodium and water are retained, principally owing to the effects of increased levels of aldosterone and inappropriate secretion of antidiuretic hormone. During the convalescent period after acute infection, a diuresis may occur. Acid–base balance disturbance is common, and includes respiratory alkalosis following tachypnoea related to fever, respiratory acidosis and hypoxaemia associated with pneumonia, and metabolic acidosis associated with septicaemia.

In acute infection these changes are mild and resolve promptly without specific intervention. However, in situations where infections are prolonged and resolution is slow, supportive care may be necessary, particularly with respect to managing nutritional deficits and electrolyte and acid–base disturbances.

## Interaction between nutrition and infection

Undernutrition impairs host defence (Fig. 1.2). Natural resistance to infection is lowered by alterations in the integrity of body surfaces, the reduced ability to repair epithelia, and the reduction in gastric acid production. In addition, immunological abnormalities are found:

MACROPHAGE FUNCTION. Tissue and circulating macrophage function is impaired.

T LYMPHOCYTE FUNCTION is depressed.

TOTAL LYMPHOCYTE COUNT is below $1 \times 10^9$ cells/litre, which is indicative of a relatively immunocompromised host.

CELL-MEDIATED IMMUNITY is in a state of anergy, i.e. the body fails to respond to a recall antigen such as the Mantoux test.

ANTIBODY PRODUCTION is less sensitive to undernutrition, but in severe malnutrition depression in both circulating and secretory immunity are detectable. This is of importance clinically in that vaccination (e.g. against polio) may have to be more aggressive in malnutrition before protective immunity is achieved.

COMPLEMENT LEVELS fall rapidly in severe acute malnutrition and remain low during long periods of established suboptimal nutritional status. Complement

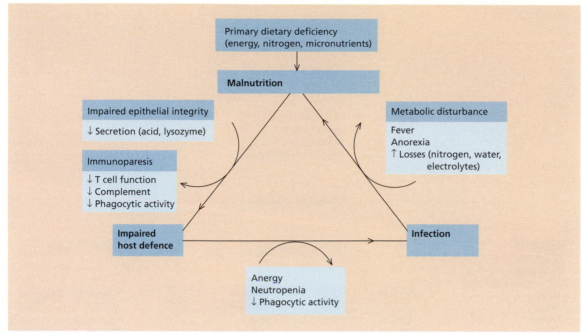

**Fig. 1.2** Nutrition–infection–host defence: a complex interaction.

levels have been used as a biochemical marker of nutritional status.

## Host defence and susceptibility

See Chapter 2.

## *Diagnosis* (Fig. 1.3)

### HISTORY

Particular attention should be paid to the following:
1 Age of the patient
2 Foreign travel—remembering that certain diseases can exist both in the tropics and Europe, e.g. leishmaniasis, giardiasis
3 Immigrants—country of origin
4 Food and water—food poisoning is extremely common
5 Occupation, e.g.
  (a) Sheep farmers—hydatid disease
  (b) Sewer workers—leptospirosis
  (c) Leather workers—anthrax
6 Domestic pets, e.g.
  (a) Budgerigars—psittacosis
  (b) Cats—toxoplasmosis
  (c) Dogs—*Toxocara canis* infection, rabies
7 Sexual activity—hepatitis B, mixed enteric infections and HIV should be particularly considered in male homosexuals
8 Drug addiction—consider hepatitis B and C, HIV and pyogenic infections, e.g. staphylococcal

9 Tattooing—consider hepatitis B and C, HIV
10 Injections and transfusions—may act as a route of transmission for infections
11 Immunization history, e.g. BCG

### CLINICAL EXAMINATION

A general examination should be performed with particular attention to skin rashes, lymphadenopathy and hepatosplenomegaly. In cases of sexually transmitted diseases the perineum, rectum and vagina should be inspected. The presence of a fever is helpful, but less emphasis is now placed on fever patterns because of improved laboratory diagnosis. High swinging fevers are characteristically seen with localized pus.

### INVESTIGATION

Tests should be performed as appropriate. If the diagnosis is obvious, e.g. a measles rash is present, no tests are necessary. The list below gives examples of situations in which tests are useful.
1 Full blood count and film are usually performed and often give a guide to the type of infection, although the changes are not invariable:
  (a) Polymorphonuclear leucocytosis—bacterial infections
  (b) Neutropenia—viral infections, brucellosis, typhoid, overwhelming septicaemia
  (c) Lymphocytosis—viral infections, whooping cough
  (d) Atypical lymphocytes—infectious mononucleosis
  (e) Eosinophilia—parasitic infections, helminths
The erythrocyte sedimentation rate (ESR) and C-reactive protein are usually raised.
2 Liver biochemistry is often slightly abnormal in

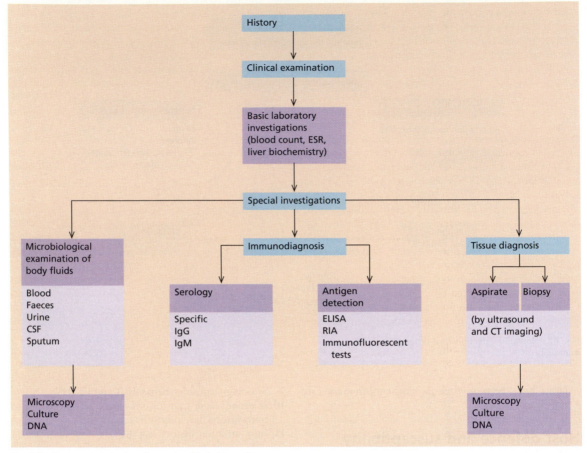

**Fig. 1.3**  An approach to the diagnosis of infectious diseases.

infections but this is a non-specific sign. The serum transferases are also raised in hepatitis and other liver infections.

3  Urine analysis   ⎫  These should also be
4  Chest X-ray    ⎬  performed, even in
              ⎭  the absence of
                symptoms and signs.

Further investigations are often required to make the specific diagnosis:

1  Blood culture.
2  Microscopic examination and culture of appropriate body fluids, e.g. urine, faeces, CSF, sputum.
3  Viruses can be identified in the above body fluids by:
(a)  Electron microscopy.
(b)  Tissue culture (cytomegalovirus).
(c)  Immunological antigen capture techniques (rotavirus).
4  Immunodiagnosis—immunological techniques are now available for the identification of:
(a)  *Pathogen-specific antigens* which can be detected in body fluids using polyvalent antisera or monoclonal antibodies.
(b)  *Specific serological responses* to infection using immunodiffusion, complement fixation, indirect haemagglutination, indirect immunofluorescence

or enzyme-linked immunosorbent assay (ELISA). A high titre of IgM specific to a pathogen (e.g. hepatitis A or B virus, cytomegalovirus) is diagnostic of a recent infection. In infection a single raised IgG is unhelpful as this only indicates a previous rather than a current infection. However, a rising titre can confirm the diagnosis (e.g. in brucellosis or *Mycoplasma* infection).

These immunological techniques are particularly useful in the identification of pathogens that are difficult to culture by standard microbiological techniques or intracellular pathogens that require tissue culture.

5  Tissue diagnosis—biopsy/aspiration with isolation of pathogen:
(a)  Bone marrow/liver biopsy for generalized infections such as tuberculosis, leishmaniasis.
(b)  Rarely, if the above technique is negative, splenic aspiration for leishmaniasis.
(c)  Transbronchial biopsy for *Pneumocystis carinii*.
6  DNA/RNA-based techniques. Many genes encoding virulence factors and other specific proteins of pathogenic microorganisms have been cloned and sequenced. From this information DNA probes have been constructed and used for the detection of pathogen-specific DNA in body fluids or tissue. The use of amplification techniques like the polymerase chain

reaction has increased the sensitivity of this approach which has already been introduced into practice.

7 Imaging procedures—ultrasound and CT scan (with needle aspiration) for abscesses in liver, lung, brain or abdomen.

# Pyrexia of unknown origin (PUO)

A major diagnostic problem is the patient who has a pyrexia, either intermittent or continuous, that lasts for 2 weeks or more and in whom routine investigations have failed to reveal a cause. PUO may merely be an unusual presentation of a common disease. Information box 1.1 shows some of the common causes of PUO.

Age is an important pointer, since cancer and the connective tissue diseases are more common in the elderly.

Immunocompromised individuals are at particular risk of infectious disease and often present with a particularly unusual spectrum of infections (see p. 100).

An aggressive approach to the diagnosis of PUO is justified since there is a good chance that determination of a specific diagnosis will influence management and result in curative treatment. It is always worth repeating the history and examination since new signs may have evolved since the patient's initial admission to hospital. All drug therapy should be reassessed and, if possible, stopped.

---

*Infection (40%)*
Pyogenic abscess, e.g. liver
Tuberculosis
Urinary infection
Biliary infection
Subacute infective endocarditis
EBV infection
CMV infection
Q fever
Toxoplasmosis
Brucellosis

*Cancer (30%)*
Lymphomas
Leukaemia
Solid tumours, e.g.
   Renal carcinoma
   Hepatocellular carcinoma
   Pancreatic carcinoma

*Immunogenic (20%)*
Drugs
Connective tissue and autoimmune diseases, e.g.
   Rheumatoid disease
   Systemic lupus erythematosus
   Polyarteritis nodosa
   Polymyalgia/cranial arteritis
Sarcoidosis

*Factitious (1–5%)*
Switching thermometers
Injection of pyrogenic material

*Remain unknown (5–9%)*

**Information box 1.1** Some causes of pyrexia of unknown origin (PUO).

---

## INVESTIGATION

First-line investigations such as a full blood count, blood culture, urinalysis, routine blood chemistry and chest X-ray should be repeated.

### Other investigations

CT AND ULTRASOUND SCANNING are particularly valuable in revealing primary and secondary neoplastic diseases and also for showing occult abscesses. MRI is occasionally useful.

ASPIRATION OR NEEDLE BIOPSY under imaging control provides a histological diagnosis.

LAPAROSCOPY may be required to confirm a gynaecological cause, e.g. pelvic inflammatory disease, multiple peritoneal metastases or tuberculous peritonitis.

NEEDLE BIOPSY OF THE LIVER (histology and culture) may be required to confirm granulomatous hepatitis, tuberculosis or metastatic cancer.

SCANNING WITH $^{59}$GALLIUM, which is taken up by polymorphs, or indium-111 or technetium-labelled leucocytes, can localize an abscess.

## Septicaemia

The term *bacteraemia* refers to the transient presence of organisms in the blood (generally without causing symptoms) as a result of local infection or penetrating injury.

The term *septicaemia*, on the other hand, is usually reserved for when bacteria or fungi are actually multiplying in the blood, usually with the production of severe systemic symptoms such as fever and hypotension.

*Pyaemia* describes the serious situation when, in a septicaemia, organisms and neutrophil polymorphs embolize to many sites in the body causing abscesses, notably in the lungs, liver and brain.

Septicaemia has an extremely high mortality and demands immediate attention. Septic shock is discussed on p. 713.

### CAUSES

The term *primary septicaemia* is used to describe the situation when the focus of infection is not apparent. Such patients are generally elderly, undernourished or suffering from chronic disease, particularly alcoholic cirrhosis and diabetes.

The common sites of infection and infective agents responsible for *secondary septicaemia* are shown in Tables 1.3 and 1.4. Pneumococcus and *Haemophilus influenzae* are common causes of septicaemia in children, whereas in neonates Gram-negative rods and group B streptococci are the most likely aetiological agents. *Neisseria gonorrhoeae* is a common cause of septicaemia in young adults, but it is usually mild without serious effects. Intravenous drug abusers frequently suffer bacteraemia and septicaemia often caused by *Staph. aureus*, *Pseudomonas* and *Serratia*.

| Site of origin | Usual pathogen(s) |
|---|---|
| Skin | *Staphylococcus aureus* and other Gram-positive cocci |
| Urinary tract | *Escherichia coli* and other aerobic Gram-negative rods |
| Respiratory tract | *Streptococcus pneumoniae* |
| Gallbladder or bowel | *Streptococcus faecalis, Escherichia coli* and other Gram-negative rods *Bacteroides fragilis* |
| Pelvic organs | *Neisseria gonorrhoeae*, anaerobes |

**Table 1.3**  Septicaemia in a previously healthy adult.

## CLINICAL FEATURES

Fever, rigors and hypotension are the cardinal features of severe septicaemia. However, the illness may be preceded by less specific symptoms such as headache, lethargy, apprehension and subtle changes in conscious level. Other clinical features and their pathogenesis are shown in Table 1.5.

## INVESTIGATION

Septicaemia is almost always treated initially on the basis of a clinical diagnosis after appropriate specimens have been sent to the laboratory. Probable origins of infection and likely pathogens must be sought on the basis of a careful history and examination. The type of infection

will clearly differ in hospitalized and otherwise previously healthy adults (see Tables 1.3 and 1.4). Body fluids or other specimens (blood, urine, CSF, tissue or abscess aspirates) should be submitted to full microbiological examination. Imaging investigations such as ultrasonography and CT scan may be required.

Catheters or cannulae, which might be sources of infection, should be removed and sent for culture.

## TREATMENT

Management of septic shock is discussed on p. 720. Antibiotic therapy should be commenced immediately. If the organism and its antibiotic sensitivities are unknown, a combination of drugs should be chosen to cover the likely pathogens. If there is an obvious site of skin sepsis, drugs such as flucloxacillin (1 g 6-hourly i.v.) plus benzylpenicillin (to cover $\beta$-haemolytic streptococci) should be used. In severe sepsis with osteomyelitis or endocarditis, an aminoglycoside to cover *Staph. aureus* should be used. If bowel sepsis is suspected, then a broaderspectrum drug of the cephalosporin group (e.g. cefuroxime/cefotaxime/ceftazidime) would be advisable. In the absence of any helpful clinical guidelines, a combination of a penicillin drug that is active against *Pseudomonas* such as piperacillin (200–300 mg kg$^{-1}$ daily) with an aminoglycoside such as gentamicin (3–5 mg kg$^{-1}$ daily in divided doses every 8 hours) should be given. Metronidazole (1 g every 8 hours by rectum) is often added to provide additional cover against anaerobic organisms. Steroids should not be used for the treatment of septicaemia or septicaemic shock.

| Clinical problem | Usual pathogen(s) |
|---|---|
| Urinary catheter | *Escherichia coli, Klebsiella, Proteus, Serratia, Pseudomonas* |
| Intravenous catheter | *Staphylococcus aureus* and *Staphylococcus epidermidis, Klebsiella, Pseudomonas, Candida albicans* |
| Peritoneal catheter | *Staphylococcus epidermidis* |
| Post surgery: | |
| Wound infection | *Staphylococcus aureus, Escherichia coli*, anaerobes (depending on site) |
| Deep infection | Depends on anatomical location |
| Burns | Gram-positive cocci, *Pseudomonas, Candida albicans* |
| Immunocompromised patients | Any of the above |

**Table 1.4**  Septicaemia in hospitalized patients.

| Clinical feature | Cause and effect |
|---|---|
| Hypotension | Liberation of bacterial endotoxin (cell-wall lipopolysaccharide) that reduces vascular tone and increases permeability |
| Pulmonary oedema and adult respiratory distress syndrome (ARDS) | Increased permeability of the alveolar capillary endothelium, impaired gas exchange and hypoxia |
| Disseminated intravascular coagulation (DIC) | Activation of blood coagulation by endothelial damage, endotoxins and immune complexes |

**Table 1.5**  Special clinical features of septicaemia.

# Antimicrobial chemotherapy

Widespread and often inappropriate use of antibiotics has led to increasing numbers of organisms with multiple drug resistance. Antibiotics are not required for minor infections.

Although the majority of antibiotics are relatively safe drugs, important toxic effects do occur when used in the incorrect dosage and in the presence of other disease states, notably renal disease. In addition, antibacterial therapy may result in secondary yeast or fungal infection or may facilitate the growth of a second bacterial pathogen, such as *Clostridium difficile*, an important cause of antibiotic-associated colitis.

## Choice of drug

BLIND THERAPY. Antimicrobial therapy is often begun before the organism is identified and its antibiotic sensitivities known. The choice of drug(s) is therefore dependent on a clinical diagnosis and a knowledge of the organisms likely to be involved in a given situation. Before beginning 'blind' therapy it is essential to obtain appropriate body fluids or other specimens for microbiological examination. Adjustments to the antibiotic regimen can then be made, if necessary, when antibiotic sensitivities are available.

SPECTRUM OF ACTIVITY. The spectrum of antibacterial activity of the drug chosen should ideally be as narrow as possible, as it will then have fewer detrimental effects on the normal bacterial flora of the host. 'Blind' therapy, however, by necessity generally covers a broader spectrum than required.

BACTERICIDAL VS. BACTERIOSTATIC. In the majority of infections there is no firm evidence that bactericidal drugs (penicillins, cephalosporins, aminoglycosides) are more effective than bacteriostatic drugs, but it is generally considered important to use the former in the treatment of bacterial endocarditis and in patients in whom host defence mechanisms are compromised.

PATIENT FACTORS. In addition to age and pregnancy, the following factors should be considered.
1 The site of infection. The chosen drug must be able to gain access to the part of the body involved. The brain, eye, biliary tract, prostate and loculated abscesses are inaccessible to many drugs.
2 Renal and hepatic function. Impaired renal or hepatic function necessitates a major modification of the dose regimen or even complete avoidance of certain drugs. Care should be taken when using aminoglycosides, ticarcillin, flucytosine and some antimycobacterial agents in patients with renal impairment. Other drugs, such as nalidixic acid and tetracycline, should be avoided altogether.

## Dose

This is influenced by the type of infection to be treated and the age of the patient. Bacterial endocarditis and deep-seated abscesses (e.g. in brain or lung) generally require high-dose therapy for several weeks.

## Route of administration

Some drugs (e.g. some of the cephalosporins) are only available as intravenous preparations, but many antibiotics are well absorbed by the oral route and in the absence of severe infection such as septicaemia there is no advantage to the patient for therapy to be administered by the more expensive parenteral route. Patient compliance must, however, be taken into account.

## Duration of therapy

With more potent drugs, only short courses or even single doses may be required, e.g. uncomplicated urinary tract infection, gonorrhoea.

## Monitoring

In serious infections (e.g. infective endocarditis), monitoring of circulating drug concentrations is routinely performed for assessing efficacy of treatment. Drug concentrations can be measured directly in serum, but the efficacy of therapy is usually determined by serum bactericidal assay just before and at a standard time after administration of antibiotics. The highest dilution of serum that completely kills the causative organism can then be determined. The clinical value of serum bactericidal assays is still debated.

Monitoring for toxicity is particularly important with the aminoglycoside antibiotics. Concentrations are determined immediately before ('trough' levels) and usually 1 hour after ('peak' levels) of the drug. High 'trough' levels of $>2$ mg ml$^{-1}$ are considered to be the most important factor in causing the ototoxicity and nephrotoxicity commonly seen with these agents. The 'peak' level should be 5–10 mg ml$^{-1}$ to be therapeutically effective.

## Combination antibiotic therapy

Combinations of antibiotics are commonly used in the empirical treatment of many serious infections such as septicaemia, meningitis, tuberculosis and endocarditis, but some care must be taken in the choice of drugs within such combinations. There is still some concern that a combination of a bactericidal and a bacteriostatic antibiotic may impair their therapeutic efficacy. However, this concept is by no means universally applicable, since the bacteriostatic drug tetracycline and the bactericidal drug rifampicin are thought to be synergistic. Generally, combinations of bactericidal drugs are at least additive and in some situations are synergistic, whereas combinations of bacteriostatic drugs are generally only additive.

## Antibiotic chemoprophylaxis

This is required in certain disease states (Table 1.6).

## MECHANISMS OF RESISTANCE TO ANTIMICROBIAL AGENTS

The development or acquisition of resistance to an antibiotic by bacteria invariably involves a mutation at a

| Clinical problem | Aim | Drug regimen |
|---|---|---|
| Rheumatic fever | To prevent recurrence and further cardiac damage | Phenoxymethylpenicillin 250 mg twice daily or sulphadiazine 1g if penicillin-allergic |
| Infective endocarditis | To prevent infection on abnormal, prosthetic or homograft heart valves, patent ductus or septal defect | *Dental/oropharyngeal procedures* Oral amoxycillin 3 g 1 hour before procedure For penicillin-allergic individuals clindamycin 600 mg 1 hour before procedure, chlorhexidine mouthwash may also be used |
| | | *For genito urinary instrumentation* Amoxycillin 1 g i.m. + gentamicin 1.5 mg kg$^{-1}$ i.m. before and oral amoxycillin 500 mg 6 hours after procedure (vancomycin for penicillin allergic patient) |
| | 'Special' risk patients only (prosthetic valves and/or previous endocarditis) | *Gastrointestinal, obstetric or gynaecological and dental (GA) procedures* Amoxycillin 1 g i.m. plus gentamicin 1.5 mg kg$^{-1}$ i.m. before, oral amoxycillin 500 mg 6 hours after procedure (vancomycin for penicillin-allergic patient) |
| Splenectomy/spleen malfunction | To prevent serious pneumococcal sepsis | As for rheumatic fever |
| Meningitis: Due to meningococci | To prevent infection in close contacts | Adults: rifampicin 600 mg twice daily for 2 days Children: <1 month 5 mg kg$^{-1}$ >1 month 10 mg kg$^{-1}$ |
| Due to *Haemophilus influenzae* | To reduce nasopharyngeal carriage and prevent infection in close contacts | Rifampicin 20 mg kg$^{-1}$ daily for 4 days (max. dose 600 mg) |
| Tuberculosis | To prevent infection in exposed (close contacts) tuberculin-negative individuals, infants of infected mothers and immunosuppressed patients | Oral isoniazid 5 mg kg$^{-1}$ daily for 6–12 months |
| Malaria | To prevent infection | Oral chloroquine 400–500 mg as a single dose each week, and/or proguanil 200 mg daily 2 weeks before and for 4 weeks after leaving endemic area. Where chloroquine resistance occurs mefloquine 250 mg once a week but get advice (and see p. 72) |

**Table 1.6**  Antibiotic chemoprophylaxis.

single point in a gene or transfer of genetic material from another organism (Fig. 1.4). Single-point mutations occur in *E. coli*, for example, at the rate of approximately 1 per $10^5$–$10^7$ cell divisions. A mutation resulting in antibiotic resistance by this mechanism would involve alteration of a single nucleotide base.

Larger fragments of DNA may be introduced into a bacterium either by transfer of 'naked' DNA or via a bacteriophage (a virus) DNA vector. Both the former (transformation) and the latter (transduction) are dependent on integration of this new DNA into the recipient chromosomal DNA. This requires a high degree of homology between the donor and recipient chromosomal DNA.

Finally, antibiotic resistance can be transferred from one bacterium to another by conjugation, when extrachromosomal DNA (a plasmid) containing the resistance factor (R factor) is passed from one cell into another during direct contact. Transfer of such R factor plasmids can occur between unrelated bacterial strains and involve large amounts of DNA.

Transformation is probably the least clinically important mechanism, whereas transduction and R factor transfer are probably the most important for the sudden emergence of multiple antibiotic resistance in a single bacterium. Increasing resistance to many antibiotics has developed (Table 1.7)

# Antibacterial drugs

## PENICILLINS

STRUCTURE. Penicillins, like cephalosporins, have a beta-lactam ring fused to a thiazolidine ring (Fig. 1.5).

Relatively minor changes to the side-chain of benzylpenicillin render the phenoxymethyl derivative acid resistant and allow it to be absorbed well when given orally. The presence of an amino group in the phenyl radical of benzylpenicillin increases the antimicrobial spectrum of the native penicillin and makes it active against both Gram-negative and Gram-positive organisms. More extensive modification of the side-chain (e.g. as in cloxacillin) renders the drug insensitive to bacterial

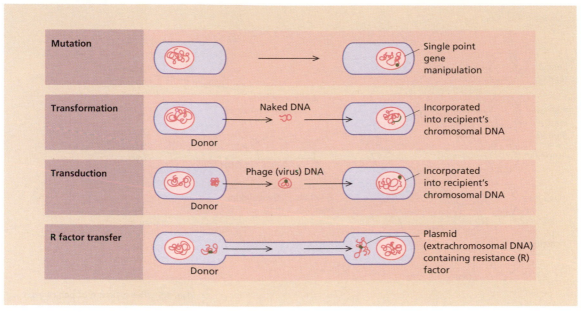

**Fig. 1.4**  Mechanisms of resistance to antimicrobial drugs.

| | |
|---|---|
| *Streptococcus pneumoniae* | Penicillin, erythromycin, tetracycline |
| *Streptococcus pyogenes* | Erythromycin, tetracycline |
| *Staphylococcus aureus* | Penicillin, ciprofloxacin |
| *Neisseria gonorrhoeae* | Penicillin, ciprofloxacin |
| *Haemophilus influenzae* | Amoxycillin |
| Enterobacteria | Amoxycillin, trimethoprim |
| *Salmonella* spp. | Amoxycillin, sulphonamides |
| *Shigella* spp. | Amoxycillin, trimethoprim |

**Table 1.7**  Some bacteria that have recently developed resistance to common antibiotics.

penicillinase, a major advance in treating infections caused by penicillinase (β-lactamase)-producing staphylococci.

MECHANISMS OF ACTION. Penicillins block the terminal cross-linking reaction (between alanine and glycine) of bacterial cell-wall mucopeptide formation. Penicillins and other β-lactam antibiotics bind to and inactivate specific penicillin-binding proteins (PBPs) which are peptidases involved in the final stages of cell wall assembly and remodelling during growth and division.

INDICATIONS FOR USE. Benzylpenicillin can only be given parenterally and is often the drug of choice for serious infections, notably infective endocarditis, pneumococcal, meningococcal, streptococcal and gonococcal infections, clostridial infections (tetanus, gas gangrene), actinomycosis, anthrax, and spirochaetal infections (syphilis, yaws).

Phenoxymethylpenicillin (penicillin V) is an oral preparation that is chiefly used as maintenance therapy for rheumatic fever prophylaxis.

Flucloxacillin is used in infections caused by penicillinase-producing staphylococci. Methicillin is also effective but must be given by injection.

Ampicillin is susceptible to penicillinase, but its antimicrobial activity includes Gram-negative organisms such as *Salmonella*, *Shigella*, *E. coli*, *H. influenzae* and *Proteus*. It is useful in the treatment of urinary tract and upper respiratory tract infections. Amoxycillin has a similar sphere of activity to ampicillin, but is better absorbed when given by mouth.

Clavulanic acid is a powerful inhibitor of many bacterial β-lactamases and when given in combination with an otherwise susceptible agent such as amoxycillin or ticarcillin can broaden the spectrum of activity of the drug.

The extended-spectrum penicillins carbenicillin and ticarcillin are active against *Pseudomonas* infection and the acylureidopenicillin derivatives (azlocillin and piperacillin) have increased activity against Gram-negative organisms, including *Pseudomonas*, compared with other penicillins. However, they are susceptible to staphylococcal β-lactamases and are therefore not reliable for treating staphylococcal disease. Oral pivmecillinam (a mecillinam) is active against many Gram-negative bacteria including salmonellae but excluding *Pseudomonas*.

RESISTANCE. Bacteria producing penicillinase are resistant to some penicillins.

INTERACTIONS. Penicillins inactivate aminoglycosides when mixed in the same solution.

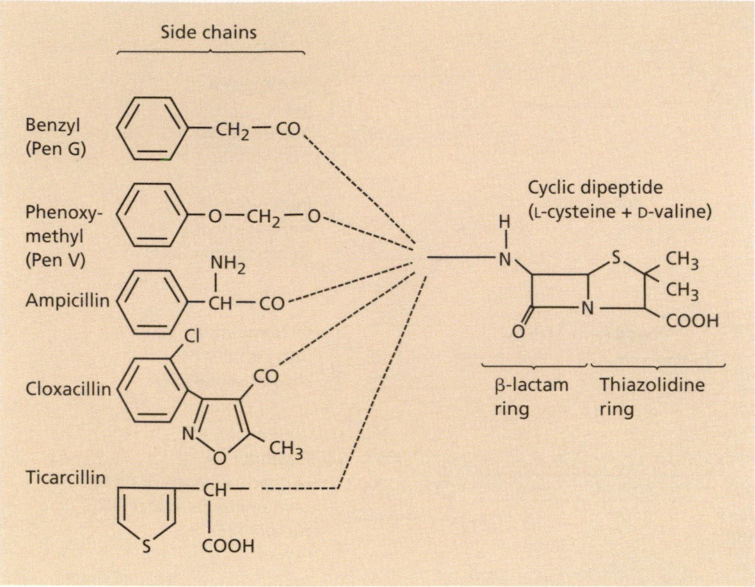

**Fig. 1.5** The structure of penicillins.

TOXICITY. Hypersensitivity (skin rash, urticaria, anaphylaxis), encephalopathy and tubulo-interstitial nephritis can occur. Ampicillin also produces a hypersensitivity rash in approximately 90% of patients with infectious mononucleosis who receive this drug. Generally, the penicillins are very safe.

## CEPHALOSPORINS

The cephalosporins have major advantages over the penicillins in that they are innately resistant to staphylococcal penicillinases and have a broader range of activity that includes both Gram-negative and Gram-positive organisms. Like the penicillins they have a $\beta$-lactam ring, but this is associated with a dihydrothiazine ring in place of the thiazolidine ring found in penicillins (Fig. 1.6). Sidechain modifications increase their potency and range of activity. Structural modifications have produced orally active drugs such as cephalexin and cephradine and a variety of highly potent parenteral preparations such as cefuroxime, cefotaxime and ceftazidime (Table 1.8).

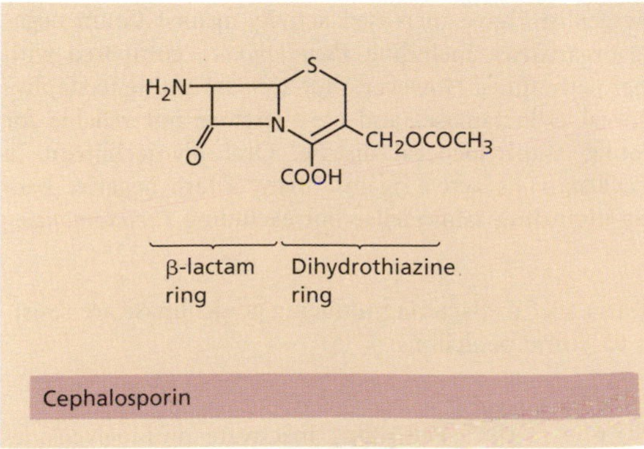

MECHANISM OF ACTION. Like penicillins, cephalosporins inhibit bacterial cell-wall synthesis.

INDICATIONS FOR USE. These potent broad-spectrum antibiotics are useful for the treatment of serious systemic infections, particularly when the precise nature of the infection is unknown. They are commonly used for serious postoperative sepsis and in immunocompromised patients, particularly during treatment of leukaemia and other malignancies.

RESISTANCE. Cephalosporins generally resist the action of $\beta$-lactamase-producing bacteria. They are inactive against enterococci and *Pseudomonas aeruginosa* (except ceftazidime).

INTERACTIONS. Increased nephrotoxicity is seen when cephalosporins are used in conjunction with other nephrotoxic antibiotics such as aminoglycosides and some diuretics.

TOXICITY. This is as for penicillin; some patients (about 10%) are allergic to both groups of drugs. The early cephalosporins caused proximal tubule damage, although the newer derivatives have less nephrotoxic effects.

## MONOBACTAMS
Aztreonam is the only member of this class currently available.

STRUCTURE. Aztreonam is a synthetic analogue of an antibiotic found in soil bacteria (Fig. 1.7), with a novel structure containing $\beta$-lactam ring in core configuration.

Cephalosporin

**Fig. 1.6** The structure of a cephalosporin.

| | Activity | Use |
|---|---|---|
| *First generation*<br>Cephazolin<br>Cephalothin<br>Cephalexin (oral)<br>Cephradine (oral) | Broad spectrum<br>Gram-positive cocci and Gram-negative<br>   organisms | Surgical prophylaxis<br>Urinary tract infections<br>Penicillin allergy |
| *Second generation*<br>Cefuroxime<br>Cephamandole<br>Cefoxitin<br>Cefaclor (oral)<br>Cefuroxime axetil (oral) | Extended spectrum. More effective than<br>   first generation against *Escherichia*<br>   *coli*, *Klebsiella* spp. and *Proteus*<br>   *mirabilis* but less effective against<br>   Gram-positive organisms | Prophylaxis and treatment of Gram-<br>   negative infections, mixed aerobic–<br>   anaerobic infections |
| *Third generation*<br>Cefotaxime<br>Ceftazidime<br>Ceftizoxime<br>Cefodizime<br>Ceftriaxone | Broad spectrum; more potent against<br>   aerobic Gram-negative bacteria than<br>   first or second generation | Especially severe infection with<br>   Enterobacteriaceae, *Pseudomonas*<br>   *aeruginosa* (ceftazidime) and *Neisseria*<br>   *gonorrhoeae*, Lyme disease (ceftriaxone) |

**Table 1.8** Cephalosporins—some examples.

MECHANISM OF ACTION is inhibition of bacterial cell-wall synthesis. It is resistant to most $\beta$-lactamases and does not induce $\beta$-lactamase production.

INDICATIONS FOR USE. Aztreonam's spectrum of activity is limited to aerobic Gram-negative bacilli, thus to some extent resembling aminoglycosides. With the exception of urinary tract infections, aztreonam should be used in combination with metronidazole (for anaerobes) and an agent active against Gram-positive cocci (a penicillin or erythromycin). It is a useful alternative to aminoglycosides in combination therapy.

TOXICITY is as for $\beta$-lactam antibiotics.

## CARBAPENEMS
*N*-Formimidoyl thienamycin (imipenem) is the only drug of this class available.

STRUCTURE. Imipenem has a novel structure with a carbon replacing the sulphur in the five-membered ring (Fig.

1.8). It is highly resistant to $\beta$-lactamases.

MECHANISM OF ACTION. Inhibition of bacterial cell-wall synthesis. Imipenem is partially inactivated in the kidney by enzymatic inactivation and is therefore administered in combination with cilastatin.

INDICATIONS FOR USE. Imipenem has the broadest spectrum of activity of all known antibiotics. It is active against Gram-positive cocci (similar potency to penicillins), Gram-negative organisms and anaerobes (similar potency to metronidazole and clindamycin). It should only rarely be used for community-acquired infection, its main indications being nosocomial infections when multiple-resistant Gram-negative bacilli or mixed aerobe and anaerobe infections are suspected.

TOXICITY is similar to that of other $\beta$-lactam antibiotics. Nausea, vomiting and diarrhoea occur in less than 5%. There is no evidence of nephrotoxicity or coagulation abnormalities.

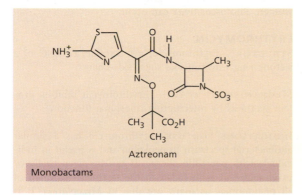

Monobactams

Aztreonam

*N*-formimidoyl thienamycin (imipenem)

**Fig. 1.7** The structure of monobactams.

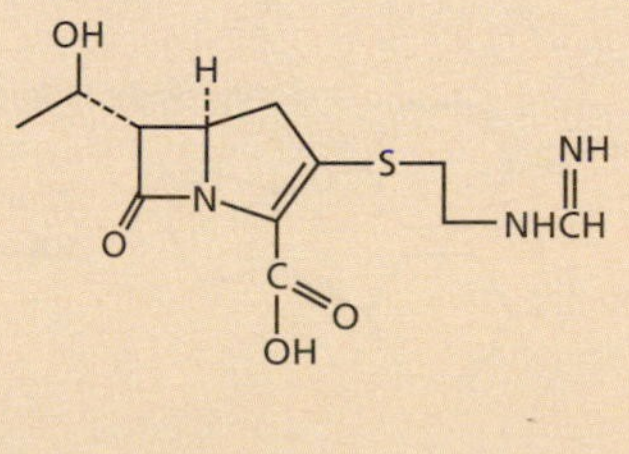

**Fig. 1.8** The structure of imipenem.

## AMINOGLYCOSIDES

STRUCTURE. These antibiotics are derived from *Streptomyces* spp. and are polycationic compounds of amino sugars (Fig. 1.9).

MECHANISMS OF ACTION. Aminoglycosides interrupt bacterial protein synthesis by inhibiting ribosomal function (messenger and transfer RNA).

INDICATIONS FOR USE. Streptomycin is bactericidal for susceptible organisms but is not often used. Neomycin is only used for the topical treatment of eye and skin infections and orally for preoperative 'bowel sterilization' and in the management of portosystemic encephalopathy. Even though it is poorly absorbed, prolonged oral administration can produce toxic effects such as ototoxicity.

Gentamicin and tobramycin are given parenterally. They are highly effective against many Gram-negative organisms including *Pseudomonas*. They are synergistic with a penicillin against *Streptococcus faecalis*. The newer aminoglycosides, netilmicin and amikacin, have a similar spectrum of antibacterial activity and are generally resistant to the aminoglycoside-inactivating enzymes produced by some bacteria. Their use should be restricted to gentamicin-resistant organisms.

RESISTANCE. Some bacteria produce phosphorylating, adenylating or acetylating enzymes that inactivate aminoglycoside antibiotics. These enzymes are coded for and transferred by R factors (extrachromosomal DNA, see p. 10).

INTERACTIONS. Enhanced nephrotoxicity occurs with other nephrotoxic drugs, ototoxicity with some diuretics, and neuromuscular blockade with curariform drugs.

TOXICITY. Aminoglycosides are nephrotoxic and ototoxic (vestibular and auditory), particularly in the elderly. Blood levels must be checked (see p. 747).

## TETRACYCLINES

STRUCTURE. These are bacteriostatic drugs possessing a four-ring hydronaphthacene nucleus (Fig. 1.10). Variation of the native compound is obtained by different

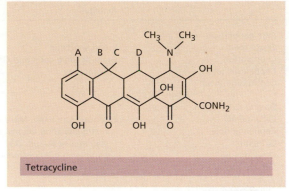

Tetracycline

**Fig. 1.10** The structure of tetracycline. Substitution of $CH_3$, OH or H at positions A to D produces variants of tetracycline.

substitutions to give, for example, oxytetracycline and chlortetracycline, or doxycycline.

MECHANISM OF ACTION. Tetracyclines inhibit bacterial protein synthesis by interrupting ribosomal function (transfer RNA).

INDICATIONS FOR USE. Tetracyclines are active against Gram-positive and Gram-negative bacteria but their use is now limited. Tetracycline is used for the treatment of acne and rosacea. Tetracyclines are also active against *V. cholerae*, *Rickettsia*, *Mycoplasma*, *Coxiella burnetii*, *Chlamydia* and *Brucella*.

RESISTANCE. Some bacteria possess reduced cell permeability to tetracycline, which is coded for by an R factor. Resistance is particularly important in infections with pneumococci and *H. influenzae*.

INTERACTIONS. The efficacy of tetracyclines is reduced by antacids, barbiturates and oral iron-replacement therapy.

TOXICITY. Tetracyclines are generally safe drugs, but they may enhance established or incipient renal failure, although doxycycline is safer than others in this group. They cause brown discoloration of growing teeth, and thus these drugs are not given to children or pregnant women. Photosensitivity can occur.

## ERYTHROMYCIN

STRUCTURE. Erythromycin, a macrolide, consists of a lactone ring with unusual sugar side-chains.

MECHANISM OF ACTION. Erythromycin inhibits protein synthesis by interrupting ribosomal function.

INDICATIONS FOR USE. Erythromycin has a similar antibacterial spectrum to penicillin and is useful in individuals with penicillin allergy. It can be given orally or parenterally. It is included in the treatment regimen of all pneumonias as many are due to *Mycoplasma*. It is effective in the treatment of infections due to *Bordetella*

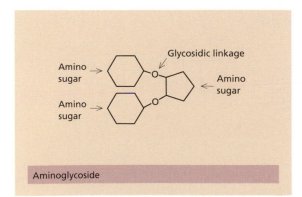

Aminoglycoside

**Fig. 1.9** The structure of an aminoglycoside.

*pertussis* (whooping cough), *Legionella*, *Campylobacter*, *Chlamydia*, *Coxiella* and *Listeria*.

The newer macrolides (erythromycin derivatives), azithromycin, clarithromycin and roxithromycin, have a broader spectrum of activity that includes Gram-negative organisms, mycobacteria and *Toxoplasma gondii*, and superior pharmacokinetic properties with enhanced tissue and intracellular penetration and longer half-life that allows once or twice daily dosage.

TOXICITY. Erythromycin estolate may produce cholestatic jaundice after prolonged treatment.

## CHLORAMPHENICOL
STRUCTURE. Chloramphenicol is the only naturally occurring antibiotic containing nitrobenzene (Fig. 1.11). This structure is probably important for its toxicity in humans and for its activity against bacteria.

MECHANISM OF ACTION. Chloramphenicol is structurally similar to uridine-5-phosphate and competes with messenger RNA for ribosomal binding. It also inhibits peptidyl transferase.

INDICATIONS FOR USE. Despite its toxicity, chloramphenicol is indicated for the treatment of severe infection due to *Salmonella typhi* and *S. paratyphi* (enteric fevers) and severe infections due to *H. influenzae* (meningitis and acute epiglottitis). It is also active against *Yersinia pestis* (plague) and is used topically for purulent conjunctivitis.

RESISTANCE. Bacterial R factors code for acetylating enzymes that can inactivate chloramphenicol and also reduce bacterial cell permeability to this agent.

INTERACTIONS. Chloramphenicol enhances the activity of anticoagulants, phenytoin and oral hypoglycaemic agents.

TOXICITY. Severe irreversible bone marrow suppression is rare but nevertheless restricts the usage of this drug to the indications above and for ill patients. Chloramphenicol should not be given to premature infants or neonates because of their inability to conjugate and excrete this drug; high blood levels lead to circulatory collapse and the often fatal 'grey baby syndrome'.

## FUSIDIC ACID
STRUCTURE. Fusidic acid has a structure resembling that of bile salts.

MECHANISM OF ACTION. It is a potent inhibitor of bacterial protein synthesis. Its entry into cells is facilitated by the detergent properties inherent in its structure.

INDICATIONS FOR USE. Fusidic acid is mainly used for penicillinase-producing *Staph. aureus* infections such as osteomyelitis or endocarditis, and for other staphylococcal infections associated with bacteraemia or septicaemia. The drug is well absorbed orally but is relatively expensive. It is well concentrated in bone.

RESISTANCE may occur rapidly and is the reason why fusidic acid is given in combination with another antibiotic.

TOXICITY. Fusidic acid may occasionally be hepatotoxic but is generally a safe drug and if necessary can be given during pregnancy.

## SULPHONAMIDES
STRUCTURE. The sulphonamides are all derivatives of the prototype sulphanilamide (Fig. 1.12).

MECHANISM OF ACTION. Sulphonamides block thymidine and purine synthesis by inhibiting microbial folic acid synthesis. Trimethoprim also inhibits folic acid synthesis.

INDICATIONS FOR USE. Sulphamethoxazole is mainly used in combination with trimethoprim (as co-trimoxazole) for treatment of *P. carinii* infection. Trimethoprim alone is now used for other infections such as urinary tract infections and acute-on-chronic bronchitis, as the side-effects of co-trimoxazole are most commonly due to the sulphonamide component. Sulphapyridine in combination with 5-aminosalicylic acid (i.e. sulphasalazine) is used in inflammatory bowel disease.

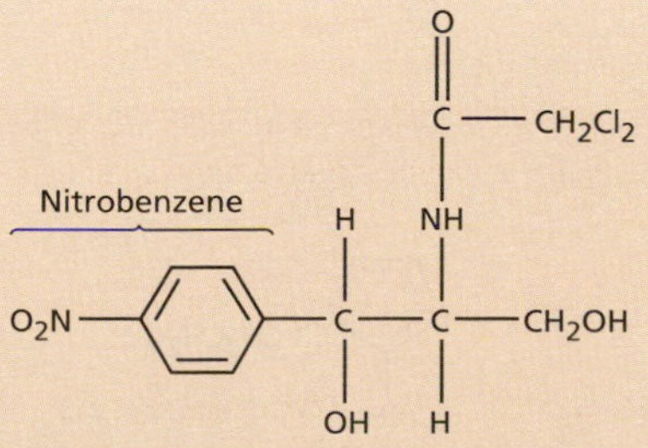

Fig. 1.11 The structure of chloramphenicol.

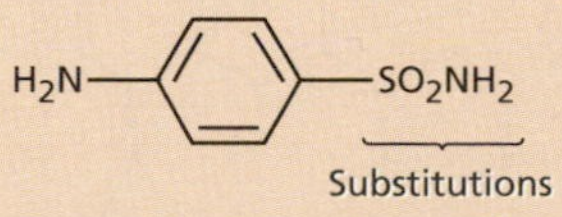

Fig. 1.12 The structure of a sulphonamide.

RESISTANCE. Bacteria may become resistant to sulphonamides by production of sulphonamide-resistant dihydropteroate synthetase and by altering bacterial cell permeability to these agents.

INTERACTIONS. Sulphonamides potentiate oral anticoagulants and hypoglycaemic agents.

TOXICITY. Sulphonamides cause thrombocytopenia, folate deficiency and megaloblastic anaemia and haemolysis in individuals with glucose-6-phosphate dehydrogenase deficiency, and therefore should not be used in such people. Co-trimoxazole should be avoided in the elderly if possible, as deaths have been recorded, probably due to the sulphonamide component.

### QUINOLONES

The new quinolone antibiotics, such as ciprofloxacin, norfloxacin and olfloxacin are useful oral broad-spectrum antibiotics, related structurally to nalidixic acid. The latter achieves only low serum concentrations after oral administration and its use has been limited to the urinary tract where it is concentrated.

STRUCTURE—see Fig. 1.13.

MECHANISM OF ACTION. This group of bactericidal drugs inhibits bacterial DNA synthesis by inhibiting DNA gyrase, the enzyme responsible for maintaining the superhelical twists in DNA.

INDICATIONS FOR USE. The 4-fluoroquinolones should be reserved for infections caused by organisms resistant to standard drugs. The extended spectrum quinolones such as ciprofloxacin have activity against Gram-negative and some Gram-positive bacteria. Useful in Gram-negative septicaemia, skin and bone infections, gastrointestinal, urinary and respiratory tract infections, meningococcal carriage and in some sexually transmitted diseases such as gonorrhoea and non-specific urethritis due to *Chlamydia trachomatis*. The newer quinolones are the only orally effective anti-pseudomonal antibiotics currently available. They are probably the drugs of choice for treatment of traveller's diarrhoea (see Table 1.18).

TOXICITY. Gastrointestinal disturbances, photosensitive rashes and occasional neurotoxicity can occur.

### NITROIMIDAZOLES

STRUCTURE. These agents are active against anaerobic organisms, notably anaerobic bacteria and some pathogenic protozoa. The most widely used drug is metronidazole (Fig. 1.14). Minor modifications in the structure of nitroimidazole have produced other related compounds such as tinidazole and nimorazole.

MECHANISM OF ACTION. After reduction of their nitro group to a nitrosohydroxyl amino group by microbial enzymes, nitroimidazoles cause strand breaks in microbial DNA.

INDICATIONS FOR USE. Metronidazole is of major importance in the treatment of anaerobic bacterial infection, particularly that due to *Bacteroides*. It is also used prophylactically in colonic surgery. It may be given orally, by suppository (entirely satisfactory blood levels can be obtained by this route) or intravenously (very expensive). It is also the treatment of choice for amoebiasis, giardiasis and infection with *Trichomonas vaginalis*.

INTERACTIONS. Nitroimidazoles can produce a disulfiram-like reaction with ethanol.

TOXICITY. Nitroimidazoles are tumorigenic in animals and mutagenic for bacteria, although carcinogenicity has not been described in humans. They cause a metallic taste, and peripheral neuropathy with prolonged use. They should be avoided in pregnancy.

### Vancomycin

Vancomycin is produced by *Streptomyces orientalis*.

STRUCTURE. Vancomycin is a complex and unusual glycopeptide active against Gram-positive bacteria.

MECHANISM OF ACTION. Vancomycin inhibits cell-wall synthesis and is bactericidal.

INDICATIONS FOR USE. Vancomycin is given orally for *Clostridium difficile*-related pseudomembranous enterocolitis and intravenously for methicillin-resistant *Staph.*

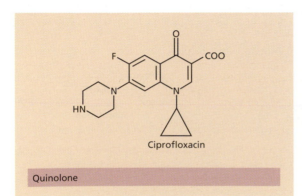

Quinolone

**Fig. 1.13**  The structure of a quinolone.

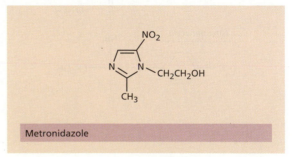

Metronidazole

**Fig. 1.14**  The structure of metronidazole, a nitroimidazole.

*aureus* and other multiresistant Gram-positive organisms. Also used for treatment and prophylaxis against Gram-positive infections in penicillin-allergic patients.

TOXICITY. Vancomycin can cause ototoxicity and nephrotoxicity and thus serum levels should be monitored. Care must be taken to avoid extravasation at the injection site as this causes necrosis and thrombophlebitis.

### Teicoplanin

This is another glycopeptide antibiotic which is less nephrotoxic. More favourable pharmacokinetic properties, allowing once daily dosing.

## Antifungal drugs

### NATURALLY OCCURRING COMPOUNDS
#### Polyenes

The most potent of these is amphotericin B, which is used intravenously in severe systemic fungal infections. Nephrotoxicity is a major problem and dosage levels must take background renal function into account. Liposomal amphotericin B is less toxic but very expensive. Nystatin is not absorbed through mucous membranes and is therefore useful for the treatment of oral and enteric candidiasis and for vaginal infection. It can only be given orally or as pessaries. Polyenes react with the sterols in fungal membranes, increasing permeability and thus damaging the organism.

#### Griseofulvin

This naturally occurring antifungal is concentrated in keratin and is therefore useful for chronic fungal infection of nails, although treatment may be required for many months. It is also widely used for the treatment of ringworm.

### SYNTHETIC DRUGS

Imidazoles such as miconazole (Fig. 1.15), ketoconazole and clotrimazole are broad-spectrum antifungal drugs.
CLOTRIMAZOLE is used topically for the treatment of ringworm.
MICONAZOLE is a potent systemic antifungal and is active both orally and parenterally. It is not as effective as amphotericin B and has been superseded by the triazoles, fluconazole and itraconazole.

KETOCONAZOLE is active orally but can produce liver damage. It is effective in candidiasis and deep mycoses including histoplasmosis and blastomycosis but not in aspergillosis and cryptococcosis.

FLUCONAZOLE is noted for its ability to enter CSF and is used for treatment of central nervous system (CNS) infection with *Cryptococcus neoformans* and candidiasis.

ITRACONAZOLE fails to penetrate CSF. The indications are as for ketoconazole but may also be effective in cryptococcosis and aspergillosis. Toxicity is mild.

The fluorinated pyridine derivative, flucytosine, is usually used in combination with amphotericin B for systemic fungal infection. Side-effects are uncommon, although it may cause bone marrow suppression. It is active when given both orally and parenterally.

## Antiviral drugs

### Idoxuridine

This agent is active against herpes simplex virus (HSV) as a 5% solution with dimethyl sulphoxide (DMSO), but to be effective it must be applied to the skin before the appearance of vesicles. It is also effective as a 0.1% solution when instilled into the eye for HSV keratitis. Similar topical use in herpes zoster probably alters the clinical course of the illness if given early.

### Vidarabine (adenine arabinoside)

This agent may be given intravenously and is active against HSV and varicella zoster virus (VZV). It is also used in severe varicella infection (chickenpox). Its major effects include bone marrow suppression and renal impairment.

### Acyclovir

This agent, which inhibits viral DNA synthesis, is relatively free from side-effects and is effective against many herpes virus infections. Oral and topical preparations are available for the treatment of herpes simplex and zoster viral infections. An intravenous preparation can be used for the treatment of systemic virus infection in the immunocompromised host, particularly VZV infections, and also for primary HSV infection, e.g. encephalitis.

### Ribavirin (Tribavirin)

Given during the first week of Lassa fever this drug reduces mortality from about 50% to 5%. Oral prophylaxis for 10 days is indicated for contacts.

### Azidodeoxythymidine (AZT)

AZT (zidovudine) (Fig. 1.16), a thymidine analogue, inhibits HIV reverse transcriptase and thereby impairs viral replication. It is strongly recommended for HIV patients in Group IV (see p. 99), particularly those with opportunistic infection and neurological disease. Bone marrow toxicity is frequent (*c.* 30%) and serious.

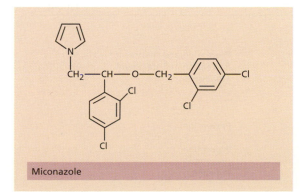

Miconazole

**Fig. 1.15** The structure of miconazole, an imidazole.

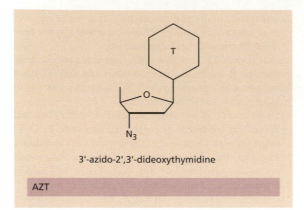

3'-azido-2',3'-dideoxythymidine

**AZT**

**Fig. 1.16**  The structure of AZT.

Polymyositis and an encephalitis-like syndrome may also occur.

### Ganciclovir
This guanine analogue is used for cytomegalovirus retinitis and gastrointestinal disease in patients with HIV. The major complication is neutropenia.

### Foscarnet
This is a simple phosphonate analogue. It inhibits both viral DNA polymerase and reverse transcriptase but at different loci to acyclovir and AZT. It is active against herpes virus including cytomegalovirus and is used for this in patients with HIV infection. Side-effects are reduced renal function and anaemia.

### Interferon (see p. 139)
This is a naturally occurring substance produced by T lymphocytes during virus infection. Interferon production occurs in response to many different viruses and production stimulated by one virus may confer protection against a second viral invader. It is currently being used as a treatment for acute and chronic hepatitis B and C as well as in certain malignancies.

## Prevention

Although effective antimicrobial chemotherapy is available for many diseases, the ultimate aim of any infectious disease control programme is to prevent infection occurring. This may be achieved either by:
1  Eliminating the source or mode of transmission of an infection, or
2  Reducing host susceptibility to environmental pathogens.

### CONTROL OF SOURCES AND TRANSMISSION
Water and food supplies constitute a major reservoir of infection and careful surveillance of supplies reduces the incidence of many diseases e.g. acute diarrhoeal disease, bovine tuberculosis. For many diseases vector control, e.g. mosquitoes, is essential to control disease.

Screening of blood donors has proved essential to control the spread of hepatitis and HIV. Defining high-risk carrier populations, such as male homosexuals and immigrants from endemic areas of infectious disease, is also important.

### REDUCTION OF HOST SUSCEPTIBILITY
Immunization has changed the course and natural history of many infectious diseases. Passive immunization by administering preformed antibody, either in the form of immune serum or purified gamma globulin, provides short-term immunity and has been effective in both the prevention and treatment of a number of bacterial and viral diseases (Table 1.9). Long-lasting immunity is, however, only achieved by active immunization with a live attenuated organism, a dead organism or an antigen preparation of part of an organism, ideally produced by recombinant DNA technology. Active immunization may also be performed with microbial toxin (either native or modified), in which case the immunogen is called a toxoid. Important preparations available for active immunization are shown in Table 1.10. The active immunization schedule currently recommended is summarized in Infor-

| Infection | Antibody | Indication | Efficacy |
|---|---|---|---|
| *Bacterial* | | | |
| Tetanus | Human tetanus immune globulin | Prevention and treatment | + |
| Diphtheria | Horse serum | Prevention and treatment | ± |
| Botulism | Horse serum | Treatment | + |
| *Viral* | | | |
| Hepatitis A | | | |
| Measles | Human normal immune globulin | Prevention | + |
| Rubella | | | |
| Hepatitis B | Human hepatitis B immune globulin | Prevention | + |
| Varicella zoster | Human varicella zoster immune globulin | Prevention | + |
| Rabies | Human rabies immune globulin | Prevention | + |

**Table 1.9**  Examples of passive immunization available.

*Live vaccines*
Oral polio (Sabin)
Measles
Mumps
Rubella
Yellow fever
BCG
Typhoid (TY 21a)

*Dead organisms, crude or purified extracts*
Hepatitis A
Pertussis
Typhoid—whole cell and Vi antigen
Polio (Salk)
Influenza
Cholera
Meningococci (group A and C)
Rabies
Pneumococcal
Haemophilus influenza B

*Toxoids*
Diphtheria
Tetanus

*Recombinant vaccines*
Hepatitis B

———

BCG, bacille Calmette–Guérin.

**Table 1.10**   Preparations available for active immunization.

| Year of life | Vaccines | Dose schedule |
|---|---|---|
| 1 | DTP plus OPV plus Hib or DT Hib (if P contraindicated) | At 2, 3 and 4 months |
| 1–2 | MMR | Single dose[a] |
| 4–5 | Booster DT plus OPV | Single dose |
| 10–14 (females) | Rubella | Single dose |
| 10–14 | BCG (tuberculin-negative individuals) | Single dose[b] |
| 15–18 | T plus OPV | Single dose |
| *Developing countries* Birth or first contact | BCG + OPV | |
| 6, 10, 14 weeks | DPT, OPV | |
| 9 months | Measles | |

———

BCG, bacille Calmette–Guérin; DTP, diphtheria (D)/tetanus (T)/pertussis (P) (triple vaccine); Hib, *Haemophilus influenzae* b; MMR, measles, mumps and rubella (single antigen measles vaccine still available if MMR refused); OPV, oral polio vaccine.
[a]Can be given at any age >1 year.
[b]Interval of 3 weeks between rubella and BCG.

**Information box 1.2**   Immunization schedule recommended in the UK and developing countries (WHO).

mation box 1.2. Immunization should be kept up to date with booster doses throughout life. Travellers to developing countries, especially if visiting rural areas, should in addition enquire about further specific immunizations.

# Bacterial infections

# Gram-positive cocci

## STAPHYLOCOCCAL INFECTIONS

Staphylococci are aerobic, facultatively anaerobic, Gram-positive cocci. They contain a number of cellular antigens and produce enzymes such as coagulase as well as toxins such as enterotoxin. Their pathogenicity correlates most closely with the production of the coagulase enzymes. Three pathogenic species are recognized. *Staph. aureus* is coagulase positive and *Staph. epidermidis* and *Staph. saprophyticus* are coagulase negative. Staphylococci are part of the normal microflora of the human skin, the upper respiratory tract, especially the nasopharynx, and the intestinal tract. Twenty-five per cent of the population are permanent carriers of *Staph. aureus*.

Approximately 20% of all human staphylococcal infections are autogenous. Transmission is most frequently by direct contact with an infected individual but may be airborne or via fomites. Several predisposing host factors have been identified (Table 1.11).

The organism can cause a wide clinical spectrum of diseases. These are usually localized, but infection may spread, resulting in bacteraemia or metastatic infection. Table 1.12 shows a list of conditions due to *Staph. aureus*; a few of these will be considered below.

### Skin infections

These are discussed on p. 1011.

### Osteomyelitis

Acute osteomyelitis is almost always due to staphylococcal infection. It occurs predominantly in males between the ages of 3 and 12 years, usually affecting the lower limbs. A history of trauma is often present. The diaphysis is initially involved, with subsequent spread of the infection to the periosteum and the subcutaneous tissues. Signs of inflammation are present. The child is usually irritable and febrile. There is leucocytosis and blood cultures are positive in about 75% of patients.

Osteomyelitis involving the vertebrae occurs in adults

Injury to skin or mucous membranes, e.g.
   Abrasions
   Trauma (accidental or surgical)
   Burns
   Insect bites

Metabolic abnormalities, e.g.
   Diabetes mellitus
   Uraemia

Foreign bodies[a], e.g.
   Intravenous and other indwelling catheters
   Cardiac and orthopaedic prostheses
   Tracheostomies

Abnormal leucocyte function, e.g.
   Job's syndrome
   Chediak–Higashi syndrome
   Steroid therapy
   Drug-induced leucopenia

Postviral infections, e.g.
   Influenza

Miscellaneous conditions, e.g.
   Excess alcohol consumption
   Malnutrition
   Malignancies
   Old age

———

[a]Often *Staphylococcus epidermidis*.

**Table 1.11**   Host factors that increase susceptibility to staphylococcal infections (predominantly *Staphylococcus aureus*).

*Due to invasion*

Skin
   Furuncles
   Cellulitis
   Impetigo
   Carbuncles

Lungs
   Pneumonia
   Lung abscesses

Heart
   Endocarditis
   Pericarditis

Central nervous system
   Meningitis
   Brain abscesses

Bones and joints
   Osteomyelitis, arthritis

Miscellaneous
   Parotitis
   Pyomyositis
   Septicaemia
   Enterocolitis

*Due to toxin*

Staphylococcal food poisoning

Scalded-skin syndrome
Bullous impetigo
Staphylococcal scarlet fever

Toxic shock syndrome

**Table 1.12**   Clinical conditions produced by *Staphylococcus aureus*.

over 50 years of age. The onset is insidious, with pain; often there are no other features of infection.

Radiographs are usually normal in the first week after onset in both varieties of osteomyelitis.

## Food poisoning (see Table 1.19)

This results from ingestion of food contaminated with preformed heat-stable enterotoxins A, B, C, D and E in varying combinations. *Staph. aureus* accounts for approximately 5% of all food poisoning in the UK. Contamination is usually from an infected individual.

Foods such as canned foods, processed meats, milk and cheese favour the growth of *Staph. aureus*. The illness is manifest within 6 hours of ingestion of contaminated foods and affects close to 100% of individuals who have eaten such foods. In contrast to food poisoning due to other organisms, staphylococcal food poisoning is characterized by the presence of persistent vomiting. Fever, when present, is usually below 38°C. Abdominal discomfort, diarrhoea or dysentery may be present. No specific treatment is necessary as the illness is short-lived (12–24 hours); however, supportive treatment with fluids and electrolytes is occasionally indicated.

### Acute staphylococcal enterocolitis

This presents as a more severe fulminant clinical syndrome, typically following broad-spectrum antibiotics. Pseudomembranes may be seen at sigmoidoscopy.

## Toxic shock syndrome (TSS)

Staphylococci that produce the toxic shock syndrome toxin-1 (TSST-1) are responsible for this syndrome. TSS is seen most frequently in menstruating women below the age of 30 years who use high absorbancy polyacrylate-containing tampons. However, it can occur in other situations including the use of female barrier contraceptives and men and children are not exempt. It is characterized by the abrupt onset of fever, a diffuse macular erythema, vomiting, diarrhoea, severe myalgia and shock. Blood cultures are negative and anti-TSST-1 antibodies are present in low concentrations in serum. Treatment is supportive. Antibiotics are usually given, although the syndrome is produced by the exotoxin. Mortality is about 10%.

## Scalded skin syndrome (SSS)

Scalded skin syndrome is caused by staphylococci which elaborate the toxin exfoliatin. It is seen in children under 5 years of age and is characterized by a painful macular skin rash followed by bullae and generalized shedding of the epidermis.

# Treatment of staphylococcal infections

Any local lesion, e.g. an abscess, should be drained. Systemic infection is treated with antibiotics. Hospital-acquired infections are usually penicillin resistant and therefore treatment is with flucloxacillin often together with fusidic acid. Of infections acquired outside the hospital 75% are penicillin sensitive and a penicillin is the drug of choice. Increasing antibiotic resistance is still a problem and most hospitals have restrictions on the use of single antibiotics. The control of staphylococcal cross-infection as discussed below is important.

Methicillin-resistant *Staph. aureus* (MRSA) were detected in 1961 soon after methicillin was introduced. Such strains were only resistant to β-lactam antibiotics and never caused serious problems. The MRSA strains that emerged first in Australia in the late 1970s and have spread worldwide are resistant to many other antibiotics, including aminoglycosides. These are now referred to as MARSA (methicillin-aminoglycoside-resistant *Staph. aureus*). There have been many outbreaks of infection, particularly in patients in tertiary referral centres, in the seriously ill and in those with surgical wounds and venous access sites. Origin of infection is often 'another hospital' or from healthy staff carriers. Control is essential and involves:

- Close and constant microbiological surveillance both before and during attacks
- Immediate isolation of infected individuals
- Appropriate management of the carrier state

Although topical antibiotics have been used to eradicate nasal colonization their efficacy is now in doubt. Careful handwashing with chlorhexidine solution is still widely recommended. MARSA can be treated with vancomycin but teichoplanin and the quinolones are effective.

# STREPTOCOCCAL INFECTIONS

Streptococci are round or ovoid Gram-positive bacteria. Virulence is attributed to the cell-wall M protein and the production by some streptococci of hyaluronidase, DNAses or streptokinase. The spread of streptococci is mediated by direct contact, fomites or airborne droplet infection. Group A β-haemolytic streptococci (*Strep. pyogenes*) are responsible for over 95% of human infections (Table 1.13). Group B streptococci frequently produce neonatal sepsis and meningitis, group C, F and G organisms occasionally cause pharyngitis and group D endocarditis and septicaemia. α-Haemolytic streptococci (known collectively as *Strep. viridans*) found commonly in the mouth, e.g. *Strep. sanguis* and *Strep. mitior* as well as *Strep. mutans*, a non-haemolytic streptococcus, cause three-quarters of all streptococcal endocarditis.

*Strep. pneumoniae* is the commonest cause of pneumonia (see p. 676).

# Scarlet fever

Scarlet fever occurs when the infectious organism (usually a group A streptococcus) produces erythrogenic toxin in

*Suppurative*

**Skin**
Impetigo
Pyoderma
Erysipelas
Cellulitis

**Pharyngeal**
Pharyngitis
Tonsillitis
Peritonsillar abscess

**Pulmonary**
Pneumonia
Empyema

**Others**
Osteomyelitis
Infective endocarditis
Meningitis
Peritonitis
Lymphangitis
Bacteraemia

**Infections confined to women**
Puerperal sepsis
Endometritis

*Non-suppurative*

Rheumatic fever
Glomerulonephritis
Scarlet fever

**Table 1.13**  Diseases caused by streptococci.

an individual who does not possess neutralizing antitoxin antibodies. This is a notifiable disease in the UK.

### CLINICAL FEATURES

The incubation period of this relatively mild disease of childhood is 2–4 days following a streptococcal infection, usually in the pharynx. Regional lymphadenopathy, fever, rigors, headache and vomiting are present. The rash, which usually appears on the second day of illness, initially occurs on the neck but rapidly becomes punctate, erythematous and generalized. It is typically absent from the face, palms and soles, and is prominent in the flexures. The rash usually lasts about 5 days and is followed by extensive desquamation of the skin. The face is flushed with characteristic circumoral pallor. Early in the disease the tongue has a white coating through which prominent bright red papillae can be seen ('strawberry tongue'). Later the white coating disappears, leaving a raw-looking, bright red colour ('raspberry tongue').

Scarlet fever may be complicated by the development of peritonsillar or retropharyngeal abscesses and otitis media.

### DIAGNOSIS

The diagnosis is established by the typical clinical features and culture of throat swabs, where the organisms are usually found in abundance, or more rapidly by latex agglutination of throat swab extracts. Elevated antistreptolysin

O and anti-DNAse B levels in the serum are indicative of streptococcal infection.

## TREATMENT OF STREPTOCOCCAL INFECTIONS

Treatment is directed at preventing the non-suppurative complications of streptococcal infections (see Table 1.13).

Penicillin is the drug of choice and may be given orally as phenoxymethylpenicillin 125 mg four times daily for 10 days or as a single intramuscular injection of benzathine penicillin 916 mg in adults. Individuals allergic to penicillin can be treated effectively with erythromycin 250 mg four times daily for 10 days.

The role of tonsillectomy in preventing further attacks of pharyngitis remains controversial.

### PREVENTION

Chemoprophylaxis with penicillin or erythromycin should be given in epidemics.

## Erysipelas

Erysipelas is an acute, rapidly progressive infection of the skin that is almost always due to group A streptococci. It usually occurs in the very young, the elderly, the debilitated or the immunosuppressed. The onset is abrupt; fever, headache and vomiting are common. The erythematous skin lesion, which is usually on the face, enlarges rapidly and has a sharply demarcated raised edge. Vesicles and bullae appear within this lesion, which then rupture, leaving crusts on the surface. Regional lymphadenopathy is common. Bacteraemia, when present, is associated with a high mortality rate. Treatment with penicillin is rapidly effective.

## Rheumatic fever

This is discussed on p. 590.

## Acute glomerulonephritis

This is discussed on p. 449.

# *Gram-negative cocci*

## NEISSERIAL INFECTIONS

*Neisseria* are Gram-negative diplococci. *N. meningitidis* and *N. gonorrhoeae* are the only two bacteria in this group that are commonly pathogenic to humans.

## Meningococcal infection

Meningococci (*N. meningitidis*) are ubiquitous. However, group A is commonly found in Africa and group B on the European and American continents. The incidence of groups C, Y and W135 infections is steadily rising worldwide. Group A is responsible for epidemics of meningitis and group B and C for sporadic infections. Its virulence is attributed to the polysaccharide capsule (which resists phagocytosis) and the lipopolysaccharide–endotoxin complex (which is responsible for its clinical toxicity). Transmission is by droplet infection or direct contact. Humans are the only known reservoirs. Following transmission, *N. meningitidis* colonize the nasopharynx preferentially because of the humidity, increased carbon dioxide tension and specific receptor substances synthesized by the nasopharynx to which they adhere. Invasiveness of the organism appears to be almost solely dependent on the amount of specific antimeningococcal bactericidal antibody in the host. A history of a recent viral respiratory infection is common.

### CLINICAL FEATURES

Four major clinical syndromes due to meningococci are recognized:

MENINGOCOCCAEMIA may occur alone or in association with meningitis. It is characterized by the presence of headache, fever, malaise and myalgia. The patient looks toxic, and has tachycardia and tachypnoea. Skin manifestations occur early and consist of a purpuric rash and/or petechiae that also affect the conjunctivae.

FULMINANT MENINGOCOCCAEMIA (Waterhouse–Friderichsen syndrome) occurs in about 10% of patients. It is characterized by an extremely rapid downhill clinical course, with extensive haemorrhage into the skin, hypotension, shock, confusion, coma and death within a few hours of the onset of symptoms. Disseminated intravascular coagulation (DIC), due to activation of the complement system, may further complicate the clinical picture. Haemorrhage into the adrenal glands may or may not be present. Without prompt treatment, the mortality rate approaches 100%.

MENINGOCOCCAL MENINGITIS presents with fever, nausea, vomiting, headache, photophobia, altered consciousness and neck rigidity. The clinical presentation is indistinguishable from other acute bacterial meningitides (see p. 925).

CHRONIC MENINGOCOCCAEMIA is rare. It is characterized by intermittent fever, a maculopapular rash, arthralgia and splenomegaly. Blood cultures are positive during bacteraemic episodes.

*N. meningitidis* may also rarely result in polyarthritis, pericarditis and nephritis.

### DIAGNOSIS

This is established by demonstrating meningococci in body fluids such as blood, CSF, petechial or joint aspirates. The CSF is turbid with an increase in neutrophils and protein. Counterimmunoelectrophoresis and latex agglutination to the polysaccharide antigen of group A, C, D and Y have recently been found useful.

### TREATMENT

Benzylpenicillin is the treatment of choice, the dose being 1.2–2.4 g i.v. 4-hourly for adults started immediately on suspicion of diagnosis. Cefotaxime is equally effective.

Chloramphenicol (75–100 mg kg$^{-1}$) is the drug of choice in individuals allergic to penicillin. Resistance to penicillin has been reported. Treatment for shock (see p. 720) and DIC (see p. 345) should be instituted. Steroids should be used in children with meningococcal meningitis (see p.926). On discharge from hospital, rifampicin should be given—see below.

### PREVENTION AND CONTROL

Penicillin does not affect the carrier state. Family contacts of patients are protected effectively by rifampicin 600 mg two times daily for 2 days. Immunoprophylaxis with a quadrivalent vaccine against group A, C, Y and W135 organisms is effective and is recommended when travelling to high-risk places—Africa, Asia, South America, Middle and Far East.

## Gonorrhoea

Gonorrhoea is caused by *N. gonorrhoeae*. It is discussed further on p. 89.

---

# Gram-positive bacilli

## CORYNEBACTERIA INFECTION

*Corynebacterium diphtheriae* is a Gram-positive, club-shaped bacillus. Three morphological varieties are recognized—*mitis*, *intermedius* and *gravis*. Of these, *mitis* is generally associated with mild infections. Only corynebacteria exposed to the bacteriophage β, which carries the *tox*$^+$ gene are capable of toxin production. The toxin has two subunits, A and B. Subunit A is responsible for clinical toxicity. Subunit B serves only to transport the toxin component to specific receptors, present chiefly on the myocardium and in the peripheral nervous system. Humans are the only natural hosts.

## Diphtheria

Diphtheria caused by *C. diphtheriae* occurs worldwide. Its incidence in the West has fallen dramatically following widespread active immunization. Transmission is mainly through airborne droplet infection and rarely through fomites.

### CLINICAL FEATURES

The incubation period varies from 2 to 7 days. Diphtheria is essentially a disease of childhood. The manifestations may be regarded as local (due to the membrane) or systemic (due to exotoxin). The presence of a membrane, however, is not essential to the diagnosis. The illness is insidious in onset and is associated with tachycardia and low-grade fever. If complicated by infection with other bacteria such as *Strep. pyogenes*, fever is high and spiking.

NASAL DIPHTHERIA is characterized by the presence of a unilateral, serosanguinous nasal discharge that crusts around the external nares.

PHARYNGEAL DIPHTHERIA is associated with the greatest toxicity and is characterized by marked tonsillar and pharyngeal inflammation and the presence of a membrane. This tough greyish-white membrane is formed by fibrin, bacteria, epithelial cells, mononuclear cells and polymorphs, and is firmly adherent to the underlying tissue. Regional lymphadenopathy is prominent and produces the so-called 'bull-neck'.

LARYNGEAL DIPHTHERIA is usually a result of extension of the membrane from the pharynx. A husky voice, a brassy cough, and later dyspnoea and cyanosis due to respiratory obstruction are common features.

Clinically evident myocarditis occurs, often weeks later, in patients with pharyngeal or laryngeal diphtheria. Acute circulatory failure due to myocarditis may occur in convalescent individuals around the tenth day of illness and is usually fatal. Neurological manifestations may occur either early in the disease (palatal and pharyngeal wall paralysis) or several weeks after its onset (cranial nerve palsies, paraesthesiae, peripheral neuropathy or, rarely, encephalitis).

CUTANEOUS DIPHTHERIA is increasingly being seen in association with burns and in individuals with poor personal hygiene. Typically the ulcer is punched-out with undermined edges and is covered with a greyish-white to brownish adherent membrane. Constitutional symptoms are uncommon.

### DIAGNOSIS

This must be made on clinical grounds since therapy is usually urgent and bacteriological results of culture studies and toxin production cannot be awaited.

### TREATMENT

The patient should be isolated and bed rest advised. Antitoxin therapy is the only specific treatment. It must be instituted rapidly to prevent further fixation of toxin to tissue receptors, since fixed toxin is not neutralized by antitoxin. Depending on the severity, 20 000–120 000 units of horse-serum antitoxin should be administered intravenously after an initial test dose to exclude any allergic reaction. There is a risk of anaphylaxis immediately after antitoxin administration and of serum sickness 2–3 weeks later. Antibiotics should be administered concurrently to eliminate the organisms and thereby remove the source of toxin production. Penicillin is given for 1 week.

The cardiac and neurological complications need intensive therapy, as described on p. 709.

### PREVENTION

Diphtheria can be effectively prevented by active immunization in childhood (see p. 21).

All contacts of the patient should have throat swabs sent for culture; those with a positive result should be treated with penicillin or erythromycin and active immunization or a booster dose of toxoid given.

## LISTERIAL INFECTION

*Listeria monocytogenes* is a non-spore-forming, facultatively anaerobic bacillus that is motile at 20–25°C. It grows optimally at 30–37°C but can multiply at 4°C and survive heating to 60°C. It is found worldwide and is widely disseminated in the environment. Listeriosis predominantly occurs perinatally but may occasionally occur in adults, particularly the immunocompromised and elderly. It causes abortions, septicaemia and meningitis (see p. 925). The mortality rate is high. Concern has arisen because of the increasing number of food-borne outbreaks in the past 10 years. Foods most commonly implicated are raw vegetables, coleslaw, milk, non-pasteurized soft cheeses, chicken and paté. Cook–chill catering has come under scrutiny, the implication being that the organism can survive if reheating is inadequate. The organism can multiply in the refrigerator if temperatures are not kept below 4°C

Diagnosis is established by blood or CSF culture. Treatment is with ampicillin and gentamicin. Erythromycin, co-trimoxazole or rifampicin are alternatives.

## CLOSTRIDIAL INFECTIONS

*Clostridium* is a Gram-positive, spore-forming, obligatory anaerobic bacillus. Some species, such as *C. botulinum* and *C. tetani*, produce potent neurotoxins, whereas *C. perfringens* produces numerous enzymes and only occasionally an enterotoxin (see Table 1.19). All clostridia that are pathogenic to humans produce exotoxins and require a low redox potential for growth. They are normal commensals of human and animal gastrointestinal tracts, and are widely distributed in soil, where, as spores, they may survive for many years in adverse conditions.

## Tetanus

Tetanus occurs when a wound is contaminated by *C. tetani* in unimmunized individuals. The wound may be trivial and disregarded by the patient. The clinical manifestations of the disease are due to the potent neurotoxin, tetanospasmin. Tetanospasmin acts on both the $\alpha$ and $\gamma$ motor systems at synapses, resulting in disinhibition. It also produces neuromuscular blockade and skeletal muscle spasm, and acts on the sympathetic nervous system. The end result is marked flexor muscle spasm and autonomic dysfunction. The organism is not invasive.

### CLINICAL FEATURES

The incubation period varies from a few days to several weeks. Four clinical varieties are recognized.

GENERALIZED TETANUS is the commonest form. Initially the patient complains of feeling unwell. This is followed by trismus (lockjaw) due to masseter muscle spasm. Spasm of the facial muscles produces the characteristic grinning expression known as risus sardonicus. If the disease is severe, painful reflex spasms develop, usually within 24–72 hours of the initial symptoms. The

interval between the first symptom and the first spasm is referred to as the 'onset time'. The spasms may occur spontaneously but are easily precipitated by noise, handling of the patient or by light. The frequency of spasms usually increases and respiration becomes impaired due to laryngeal spasm. Oesophageal and urethral spasm lead to dysphagia and urinary retention, respectively. Arching of the neck and back muscles (opisthotonus) occurs. Autonomic dysfunction is evidenced by tachycardia, a labile blood pressure, sweating and cardiac arrhythmias. Patients with tetanus are mentally alert.

Death results from aspiration, hypoxia, respiratory failure, cardiac arrest or exhaustion. Mild cases with rigidity usually recover. Poor prognostic indicators are:

- Short incubation period
- Short onset time
- Cephalic tetanus
- Extremes of age
- 'Skin poppers' (narcotic addicts who inject drugs subcutaneously)

LOCALIZED TETANUS. Pain and stiffness is confined to the site of the wound. The tone of the surrounding muscles is increased. Recovery usually occurs.

CEPHALIC TETANUS is an uncommon form and invariably fatal. It usually occurs when the portal of entry of *C. tetani* is the middle ear. Cranial nerve abnormalities, particularly of the seventh nerve, are usual. Generalized tetanus may or may not develop.

TETANUS NEONATORUM occurs in neonates owing to infection of the umbilical stump. Failure to thrive, poor sucking, grimacing and irritability are followed by rapid development of intense rigidity and spasms. Mortality approaches 100%.

### DIAGNOSIS

Few diseases resemble tetanus in its fully developed form. The diagnosis is therefore a clinical one. Rarely, *C. tetani* may be isolated from wounds.

Phenothiazine overdosage, strychnine poisoning, meningitis and tetany can mimic tetanus.

### TREATMENT

NURSING CARE. Improvement in nursing-care techniques has contributed more than any other single measure to the decrease in the mortality rate from 60% to nearer 20%. Patients are nursed in a quiet, isolated, well-ventilated, darkened room. Intragastric feeds may be necessary; bladder and bowel care are also important.

WOUND DEBRIDEMENT should be carried out where indicated.

ANTIBIOTICS AND ANTITOXIN. Both antibiotics and antitoxin should be administered, even in the absence of an obvious wound (Information box 1.3). Intravenous penicillin is the drug of choice. Human antitetanus immunoglobulin 2000–3000 units i.m. should be given to

**Information box 1.3** Antitoxin administration.

neutralize any circulating toxin; it has no effect on fixed toxin. If human antitetanus immunoglobulin is not available, immune equine tetanus immunoglobulin 10 000–20 000 units i.m. should be given, after excluding allergy to this product.

CONTROL OF SPASMS. Diazepam is the drug of choice. Up to 120 mg per 24 hours may be required to control spasm and rigidity in adults. β-Blocking drugs may be useful to control autonomic dysfunction.

The role of corticosteroids is controversial. Curarization and artificial respiratory support is best left to specialist units. The judicious use of a tracheostomy may be helpful in averting death.

ACTIVE IMMUNIZATION. Once recovery has occurred, active immunization should be instituted, as immunity following tetanus is incomplete.

### PREVENTION

Tetanus is an eminently preventable disease and all persons should be immunized regardless of age. Those who work in a contaminated environment, such as farmers, are particularly at risk. Active immunization with either plain toxoid or the alum-adsorbed toxoid can be given. Of these, the latter is superior. Initially two doses of 0.5 ml of the toxoid are given intramuscularly at 8-week intervals. The third dose is given 6–12 months later as a booster. Subsequent boosters are required at 5-year intervals. Infant immunization schedules in the UK include tetanus (see Information box 1.2, p. 19).

Protection by passive immunization with either the equine or human antitetanus toxin is short-lived, lasting only about 2 weeks.

## Botulism

Botulism is caused by *C. botulinum*. This organism is found in the soil and food is easily contaminated with the spores, which can survive heating to 100°C. The organisms proliferate in preserved canned foods and produce toxins. Only three types of neurotoxin—A, B and E—have been shown consistently to produce disease in humans. The toxins, which are the most potent known to man, result in marked neuromuscular blockade. They are heat-labile and are inactivated by heating at 80°C for 30 min or at 100°C for 10 min.

Three clinical forms are recognized:
1 Food-borne: ingestion of preformed toxin usually in home canned or bottled food
2 Infant botulism: toxin production *in vivo*
3 Wound botulism

### CLINICAL FEATURES

Nausea, vomiting and diarrhoea are early symptoms and usually occur 18–20 hours after ingesting contaminated food. Neurological symptoms dominate the clinical picture and include blurred vision and diplopia. Laryngeal and pharyngeal paralysis occur, and later generalized paralysis; consciousness is not altered. Respiratory insufficiency may occur. The marked cholinergic blockade results in urinary retention and constipation. Fever is unusual.

A strabismus occurs due to lateral rectus weakness and the pupil is fixed mid position or dilated and unresponsive to light or accommodation.

### DIAGNOSIS

The presence of toxin in faeces, serum or suspected food items is demonstrated by injecting the material into mice. The differential diagnosis includes the Guillain–Barré syndrome and myasthenia gravis.

### TREATMENT

Treatment is supportive and should be directed at maintaining adequate respiration, with assisted ventilation if necessary. Intravenous administration of 20 ml of antitoxin is followed by 10 ml 2–4 hours later and then every 12–24 hours as necessary. The role of antibiotics has not been adequately evaluated. Guanidine hydrochloride in doses of 15–40 mg kg$^{-1}$ improves botulism-induced paralysis by reversing the intramuscular blockage.

### PROGNOSIS

The overall mortality rate for botulism is high (50–70%) but patients who survive the acute paralysis can recover completely.

## Gas gangrene

Gas gangrene (clostridial myonecrosis) is commonly caused by *C. perfringens*; *C. novyi* and *C. septicum* are less frequently implicated. Gas gangrene occurs in lacerated wounds associated with fractures or retained foreign bodies. It is characterized by the onset of inordinately severe pain, with thickened induration and oedema at the injury site. When gas gangrene occurs in a limb, the part distal to the injury becomes cold and pulseless. Blebs occur and discharge a watery fluid, which later becomes haemorrhagic. The involved muscles at first appear pale and oedematous, but later they become beefy-red in colour and then brownish-black and frankly gangrenous. The characteristic crepitus of gas gangrene is a late feature. Systemic signs of toxicity are prominent. The patient is febrile, tachypnoeic and has a marked tachycardia. Hypotension, renal failure and hepatic failure develop as terminal events. Consciousness remains unaltered.

### TREATMENT
Treatment consists of adequate surgical debridement, with parenteral penicillin or chloramphenicol combined with another antibiotic to cover aerobic and anaerobic organisms that are frequent wound contaminants. The role of anti-gas gangrene toxin and hyperbaric oxygen is controversial.

## Pseudomembranous colitis

Pseudomembranous colitis is caused by the A and B toxins produced by *C. difficile*. It usually occurs a few days after institution of antibiotic therapy, although it has been known to occur even a month after discontinuing antibiotics. Clindamycin has been most frequently implicated, but ampicillin, tetracycline and the cephalosporins have also been causally related to some cases. Fever, diarrhoea (rarely with blood) and abdominal cramps are usual. Sigmoidoscopic examination may reveal a markedly erythematous, ulcerated mucosa covered by a membrane-like material, although in about 20% of patients only the ascending colon is involved. A normal sigmoidoscopy therefore does not exclude infection. The presence of this membrane is not essential to the diagnosis.

### DIAGNOSIS
Identification of the toxin (by observing its cytopathic effect on cells in tissue culture or by ELISA) in stool specimens is usually diagnostic but the test can be unreliable. Culture of the organism alone is insufficient as 5% of healthy adults carry *C. difficile*. Both the organism and its toxin are commonly found in healthy neonates in whom it has no pathological significance.

### TREATMENT
All suspected antibiotics should be discontinued and this alone may result in the diarrhoea stopping. Vancomycin 125 mg orally, four times daily, for 10 days is often used but metronidazole is also effective and considerably less expensive. Relapses are common. There is no evidence that changing chemotherapy helps. Patients should be isolated to try and prevent spread to other susceptible individuals.

## *BACILLUS* INFECTIONS

## Anthrax

Anthrax is caused by *Bacillus anthracis*. Its spores are extremely hardy and withstand extremes of temperature and humidity. The organism is capable of toxin production and this property correlates most closely with its virulence. The disease occurs worldwide. Epidemics have been reported in The Gambia, in both North and South America and in southern Europe. Transmission is through direct contact with an infected animal and is seen in farmers, butchers and dealers in wool and animal hides. Spores can also be ingested or inhaled.

### CLINICAL FEATURES
The incubation period varies from 1 to 5 days.

THE CUTANEOUS FORM is the commonest mode of presentation and is seen most frequently in the tropics. It is self-limiting in the majority of patients. Typically, a small erythematous, maculopapular lesion is present that subsequently vesiculates and undergoes ulceration, with formation of a central black eschar. Occasionally the perivesicular oedema is marked and toxaemia may be present.

RESPIRATORY INVOLVEMENT (woolsorter's disease) due to inhalation of spores results in a non-productive cough, fever and retrosternal discomfort. Pleural effusions are common. In some patients there is apparent clinical improvement followed by the abrupt onset of dyspnoea, marked cyanosis and death.

GASTROINTESTINAL ANTHRAX presents as severe gastroenteritis. Haematemesis and bloody diarrhoea may occur.

### DIAGNOSIS
Diagnosis is established by demonstrating the organism in smears or by culture. Detection of a fourfold increase in antibodies measured by indirect microhaemagglutination or ELISA in paired sera (i.e. acute and convalescent samples) is diagnostic.

### TREATMENT
Penicillin is the drug of choice. In mild cutaneous infections, phenoxymethylpenicillin 500 mg four times daily for 2 weeks is adequate. In more severe infections, e.g. when septicaemia is present, up to 24 g of intravenous penicillin is required daily. Sulphonamides, chloramphenicol and tetracycline have also been used successfully. The role of steroids in fulminant anthrax infections is questionable.

Any infected animal that dies should be burned and the area in which it was housed disinfected. Where animal husbandry is poor, mass vaccination of animals may prevent widespread contamination.

Vaccination of exposed workers is effective.

## *Bacillus cereus* infection

This Gram-positive, aerobic, spore-forming bacillus can cause food poisoning (see Table 1.19) often from contaminated rice. It also causes wound sepsis.

## OTHER INFECTIONS
## Cat-scratch disease

Between 7 and 14 days after a scratch or bite, a small red papule appears at the site associated with regional lymph-node enlargement. Lymphadenopathy may persist for several weeks and suppurate in up to 40%. The disease may progress systemically with encephalitis, neuroretinitis, arthritis, hepatitis, osteolytic bone lesions and pleurisy. A cell wall defective Gram-positive bacilli has been tentatively identified as the cause and serologically there is a humoral response to *Rochalimaea henselae* suggesting that this or a closely related organism is the aetiologic agent. The organism is sensitive to some cephalosporins (cefoxitin, cefotaxime) and aminoglycosides (gentamicin, tobramycin).

# Gram-negative bacilli

## Brucellosis (Malta fever, undulant fever)

*Brucella* is a Gram-negative coccobacillus. Three species are recognized — *B. abortus*, *B. melitensis* and *B. suis*. Brucellosis is a zoonosis and has a worldwide distribution (Table 1.14), although it has been virtually eliminated from cattle in the UK. The organism does not withstand pasteurization. The *Brucella* endotoxin (a cell-wall lipopolysaccharide) is responsible for systemic symptoms and host hypersensitivity accounts for formation of granulomas. The organisms usually gain entry into the human body via the mouth, though less frequently they may enter via the respiratory tract, genital tract or abraded skin. The bacilli travel in the lymphatics and infect lymph nodes. This is followed by haematogenous spread with ultimate localization of the bacilli in the reticuloendothelial system. Spread is largely by the ingestion of raw milk from infected cattle or goats. The disease often occurs in workers in close contact with animals or carcasses.

### CLINICAL FEATURES

The incubation period varies from 1 to 3 weeks.

| Organism | Geographical distribution | Natural host |
|---|---|---|
| B. abortus | Worldwide, except northern Europe, Japan, former Yugoslavia | Cattle |
| B. melitensis | Mediterranean region (especially Malta), Middle East | Goats, sheep and camels |
| B. suis | Far East, USA | Pigs |
| B. canis[a] | | Beagles |

[a]Rarely causes disease in humans.

**Table 1.14** Main geographical distribution and natural hosts of the *Brucella* species.

ACUTE BRUCELLOSIS. The onset is insidious, with malaise, headache, weakness, generalized myalgia and night sweats. The fever pattern is classically undulant, although continuous and intermittent patterns are frequent. Lymphadenopathy, hepatomegaly and spinal tenderness may also be present. The presence of splenomegaly is indicative of severe infection. Arthritis, spondylitis, bursitis, osteomyelitis, orchitis, epididymitis, meningoencephalitis and endocarditis have all been described, especially in infections with *B. melitensis* or *B. suis*.

CHRONIC BRUCELLOSIS is characterized by easy fatiguability, myalgia, occasional bouts of fever and depression, which may persist for several months. Splenomegaly is present. It needs to be distinguished from other causes of prolonged fever (see p. 7).

LOCALIZED BRUCELLOSIS is uncommon. Bones and joints, spleen, endocardium, lungs, urinary tract and nervous system may be involved. Systemic symptoms occur in less than one-third. Antibody titres are low. Diagnosis is established by culturing the organisms from the involved site.

### DIAGNOSIS

Blood cultures are positive during the acute phase of illness in 50% of patients. Serological tests are of greater value. The *Brucella* agglutination test, which demonstrates a fourfold or greater rise in titre over a 4-week period, is highly suggestive of brucellosis. A single titre greater than 1 in 60 is also suggestive of brucellosis in the appropriate clinical setting. An elevated serum IgG level detected by extraction with 2-mercaptoethanol (2-ME) is evidence of current or recent infection. A negative 2-ME test excludes chronic brucellosis. Specific *Brucella* antibodies can be detected by ELISA.

### TREATMENT

Tetracycline 500 mg orally four times daily is given combined with rifampicin 800 mg once daily for 6 weeks, but relapses occur. Alternatively, tetracycline can be combined with streptomycin, which is usually only given for the first 2 weeks of treatment. Co-trimoxazole 960 mg two times daily is also effective.

### PREVENTION AND CONTROL

Prevention and control involves careful attention to hygiene when handling infected animals, eradication of infection in infected animals, and pasteurization of milk. No vaccine is available for use in humans.

## *BORDETELLA* INFECTIONS

*Bordetella* is a Gram-negative coccobacillus. *B. pertussis* causes pertussis (whooping cough). *B. parapertussis* and *B. bronchiseptica* produce milder infections.

## Pertussis

Pertussis occurs worldwide. Humans are both the natural hosts and reservoirs of infection. Pertussis is highly contagious and is spread by droplet infection. In its early stages it is indistinguishable from other types of upper respiratory tract infection and hence spread occurs easily. Epidemics are common and have increased in the UK since the safety of the whooping cough vaccine was questioned.

## CLINICAL FEATURES

The incubation period varies from 7 to 14 days. It is a disease of childhood, with 90% of cases occurring below 5 years of age. However, no age is exempt. During the *catarrhal stage* the patient is highly infectious, and cultures from respiratory secretions are positive in over 90% of patients. Malaise, anorexia, mucoid rhinorrhoea and conjunctivitis are present. The *paroxysmal stage*, so called because of the characteristic paroxysms of coughing, begins about a week later. Paroxysms with the classic inspiratory whoop are seen only in younger individuals in whom the lumen of the respiratory tract is compromised by mucus secretion and mucosal oedema. The whoop results from air being forcefully drawn through the narrowed tract. These paroxysms usually terminate in vomiting. Conjunctival suffusion and petechiae and ulceration of the frenulum of the tongue are usual. Lymphocytosis due to the elaboration of lymphocyte-promoting factor by *B. pertussis* is characteristic; lymphocytes may account for over 90% of the total white blood cell count. This stage lasts approximately 2 weeks and may be associated with several complications, including bronchitis, lobar pneumonia, atelectasis, rectal prolapse and inguinal hernia. Cerebral anoxia may occur, especially in younger children, resulting in convulsions. Bronchiectasis is a late sequel.

## DIAGNOSIS

The diagnosis is suggested clinically by the characteristic whoop and a history of contact with an infected individual. It is confirmed by growing the organism in culture. Cultures of swabs of nasopharyngeal secretions result in a higher positive yield than cultures of 'cough plates'.

## TREATMENT

If the disease is recognized in the catarrhal stage, erythromycin will abort or decrease the severity of the infection. In the paroxysmal stage antibiotics have little role to play in altering the course of the illness.

## PREVENTION AND CONTROL

Affected individuals should be isolated to prevent contact with others. This is particularly important in hostels and boarding schools. Pertussis is an easily preventable disease and effective active immunization is available (see Table 1.10). Convulsions and encephalopathy have been reported as rare complications of vaccination but they are probably less frequent than after whooping cough itself. An acellular vaccine that is less reactogenic than the currently used whole-cell vaccine is being evaluated. Any exposed susceptible infant should receive prophylactic erythromycin.

# HAEMOPHILUS INFECTIONS

*Haemophilus* is a Gram-negative, pleomorphic, coccobacillus. Those pathogenic to humans include *H. influenzae*, *H. ducreyi* and *H. parainfluenzae*. In general, non-encapsulated forms produce luminal infections, e.g. bronchitis, and encapsulated organisms produce invasive disease, e.g. meningitis. *Haemophilus* is a normal commensal of the upper respiratory tract and is found in about 80% of healthy individuals.

Of the six antigenic types of *H. influenzae* identified, type b is the most important in humans and demonstrates the greatest pathogenicity, especially in children below 5 years of age. It can produce disease in several human organs (Table 1.15). Infection is generally autogenous and hence sporadic cases are common.

High risk factors include:
- Children, 6–48 months
- Sickle cell disease
- Splenectomy
- Hypogammaglobulinaemia
- Treated Hodgkin's disease
- Alcohol abuse

There is evidence of increasing immunity to *Haemophilus* with age. This is related to the presence of anticapsular and specific bactericidal antibodies. Cross-reacting antibodies to other Gram-negative bacteria can also contribute to immunity. Adults with impaired host defence mechanisms, e.g. alcohol abusers, appear to have an increased risk of infection. A history suggestive of an antecedent viral fever is usual.

## Infections with *Haemophilus influenzae*

*H. influenzae* infections have a worldwide distribution.

### Meningitis

*H. influenzae* is the commonest cause of meningitis in the second year of life. The clinical features are described on p. 925.

---

*Respiratory system*
Sinusitis
Bronchitis
Pneumonia

*Central nervous system*
Meningitis
Brain abscess

*Cardiac system*
Endocarditis
Pericarditis

*Miscellaneous*
Septic arthritis
Cellulitis
Epiglottitis
Otitis media

**Table 1.15** Major clinical syndromes associated with *Haemophilus influenzae*.

Generally the response to treatment is slow. About 25% of children have permanent residual neurological deficits such as deafness.

### Epiglottitis
This is characterized by a dramatically rapid course and fatal outcome in children if appropriate treatment is not instituted. The onset is acute with high fever, pooling of oropharyngeal secretions, dysphagia and marked respiratory distress. Examination reveals a markedly swollen and inflamed epiglottis.

### Pneumonia
*H. influenzae* type b accounts for about 30% of all childhood bacterial pneumonias and 3–6% of pneumonias in adults.

### DIAGNOSIS
This is made by isolation and culture of the organism. Counterimmunoelectrophoresis can be used to detect type b capsular antigen in 75% of patients.

### TREATMENT
Treatment is urgent, as delay may result in a high mortality, especially in patients with meningitis and epiglottitis. In these conditions the drug of choice is chloramphenicol 50–100 mg kg$^{-1}$ per day i.v. for children and 4 g per day i.v. for 7–10 days for adults. Cefuroxime can be given orally or, for meningitis 3 g 8 hourly. Ampicillin can be used for less severe cases, but resistance to this drug is increasing.

### PREVENTION
Children in close contact with an infected individual are at an increased risk of developing the disease. Rifampicin 20 mg kg$^{-1}$ for 4 days is helpful. Recently, conjugate vaccines have been developed in which a purified capsular polysaccharide is linked to a protein to improve immunogenicity. Primary vaccination is now recommended in the UK in the first year of life (see Information box 1.2).

## CHOLERA

Cholera is caused by the curved, actively motile, flagellated Gram-negative bacillus, *Vibrio cholerae*. The organism is killed by temperatures of 100°C in a few seconds but can survive in ice for up to 6 weeks. The El Tor biotype has replaced the classical biotype as the major cause of cholera. This is because the El Tor *V. cholerae* is a hardier organism. Infection with the El Tor biotype is frequently unrecognized because it produces milder clinical symptoms; a chronic gall-bladder carrier state can result in about 3% of all infected adults. All three strains (Inaba, Ogawa and Hikojima) are pathogenic. The fertile, humid Gangetic plains of West Bengal have traditionally been regarded as 'the home of cholera'. However, the seventh pandemic of cholera, which was caused by the El Tor biotype, affected large areas of Asia, North Africa and southern Europe. The pandemic has spread to South and Central America in recent years claiming thousands of lives. It has recently been suggested that the eighth cholera pandemic has begun and is due to a non-O1 *V. cholerae* which may be an El Tor mutant. Humans are the only known natural hosts. Transmission is by the faecal–oral route. Contaminated water plays a major role in the dissemination of cholera, although contaminated foods and contact carriers may contribute in epidemics.

Achlorhydria or hypochlorhydria facilitates passage of the cholera bacilli into the small intestine, where they proliferate and elaborate an exotoxin with A and B subunits. The B subunit binds to specific GM1 ganglioside receptors and the A subunit activates the intracellular enzyme adenylate cyclase (Fig 4.34). This produces elevation of 3′,5′-cyclic-AMP, which in turn produces massive secretion of isotonic fluid into the intestinal lumen (see p. 227).

*V. cholerae* has recently been shown to produce a second toxin known as zonula occludens toxin (ZOT). This impairs the integrity of the 'tight junctions' between enterocytes allowing escape of water and electrolytes. A third toxin, accessory cholera toxin (ACE), which also produces intestinal secretion, has recently been identified.

### CLINICAL FEATURES
The incubation period varies from a few hours to 6 days. The majority of patients with cholera have a mild illness that cannot be distinguished clinically from diarrhoea due to other infective causes. Classically, however, three phases are recognized in the untreated disease. The *evacuation phase* is characterized by the abrupt onset of painless, profuse, watery diarrhoea, associated with vomiting in the severe forms. 'Rice water' stools, so called because of mucus flecks floating in the watery stools, are characteristic of this stage. If appropriate supportive treatment is not given, the patient passes on to the *collapse phase*. This is characterized by features of circulatory shock (cold clammy skin, tachycardia, hypotension and peripheral cyanosis) and dehydration (sunken eyes, hollow cheeks and a diminished urine output). The patient, though apathetic, is usually lucid. Muscle cramps may be severe. Children may, in addition, present with convulsions due to hypoglycaemia. At this stage renal failure and aspiration of vomitus present major problems. Should the patient survive this stage, then the *recovery phase* starts, with a gradual return to normal of clinical and biochemical parameters in 1–3 days.

*Cholera sicca* is an uncommon but severe form of cholera. It presents with massive outpouring of fluid and electrolytes into dilated intestinal loops. Diarrhoea and vomiting do not occur and hence the disease is frequently not recognized. The mortality rate is high.

### DIAGNOSIS
Diagnosis is largely clinical. Examination of freshly passed stools may demonstrate rapidly motile organisms. This is not diagnostic, as *Campylobacter jejuni* may also give a similar appearance. However, demonstration of the rapidly motile vibrios by dark-field illumination and

subsequent inhibition of their movement with type-specific antisera is diagnostic.

Stool and rectal swabs should be taken for culture.

## TREATMENT

With appropriate and effective rehydration therapy, mortality has decreased to less than 1%. Rehydration is mainly oral, but intravenous therapy is occasionally required.

ORAL REHYDRATION, for maintenance therapy or for correction of mild to moderate dehydration, is best carried out by giving a glucose–electrolyte solution. The World Health Organization (WHO) oral rehydration solution (ORS) is shown in Table 1.16. Mildly dehydrated individuals are given ORS 50 ml kg$^{-1}$ in the first 4 hours followed by a maintenance solution of 100 ml kg$^{-1}$ daily until the diarrhoea stops. For moderate dehydration, ORS 100 ml kg$^{-1}$ is given within the first 4 hours followed by 10–15 ml kg$^{-1}$ per hour. Rice- and other cereal-based electrolyte solutions (Table 1.16) have been found to be as effective and actually reduce stool volume as well as rehydrating, so that they are replacing WHO ORS.

INTRAVENOUS REHYDRATION is required only for severely dehydrated individuals with features of collapse. Intravenous solutions recommended by WHO include Ringer's lactate solution and the 'Diarrhoea Treatment Solution' (sodium chloride 4.0 g, sodium acetate 6.5 g, potassium chloride 1.0 g, and glucose 9.0 g, per litre). Several litres of intravenous fluid are usually required to overcome the features of shock. Maintenance of hydration is effectively carried out by oral rehydration solutions.

Antibiotics such as tetracycline 250 mg four times daily for 3 days or doxycycline help to eradicate the infection, decrease stool output and shorten the duration of the illness dramatically. Drug resistance is becoming an increasing problem.

## PREVENTION AND CONTROL

Immunization with currently available parenteral vaccines results in poor immunity and is no longer recommended. Attenuated live oral cholera vaccines are under intensive evaluation. Chemoprophylaxis with tetracycline 500 mg two times daily for 3 days for adults and 125 mg daily for children is effective. The most effective preventive measures, however, are good hygiene and sanitary living conditions.

Table 1.17 compares the pattern of infection caused by *V. cholerae* with the patterns of infection caused by other gut organisms.

# ENTEROBACTERIACEAE INFECTIONS

The Enterobacteriaceae is a diverse group of aerobic Gram-negative organisms. Included in this category are *E. coli*, *Salmonella* and *Shigella*.

## *Escherichia coli* infection

*E. coli* is commonly responsible for urinary tract infections, bacteraemia, neonatal meningitis, and peritoneal and biliary infections. Such infections are indistinguishable from similar clinical conditions caused by other bacteria.

*E. coli* responsible for enteric disease have different serotype characteristics from those that cause disease elsewhere in the body. Four main categories of *E. coli* capable of producing human diarrhoeal disease are recognized.

1 *Enterotoxigenic E. coli* (ETEC) produces a diarrhoeal illness that is mediated through a heat-labile toxin (LT) and/or a heat-stable toxin (ST). Toxin production is genetically encoded by transferable DNA plasmids. LT resembles cholera toxin in its mode of action since it also acts via cyclic AMP and is associated with massive secretion of water and electrolytes into the intestinal lumen. ST activates guanylate cyclase with elevation of cyclic GMP levels and subsequent secretion of water and electrolytes (see Fig. 4.34). Clinically ETEC produces three syndromes:
  (a) An illness indistinguishable from severe cholera.
  (b) 'Traveller's diarrhoea', a milder disease (other causes are shown in Table 1.18).
  (c) Diarrhoea of varying severity in children, especially in developing countries.
2 *Enteroinvasive E. coli* (EIEC) produces an illness similar to that produced by *Shigella* (see below).
3 *Enteropathogenic E. coli* (EPEC) attaches to and damages intestinal epithelium, producing diarrhoea, primarily in children below 2 years of age. Toxins are

| | Sodium (mmol litre$^{-1}$) | Potassium (mmol litre$^{-1}$) | Chloride (mmol litre$^{-1}$) | Bicarbonate (mmol litre$^{-1}$) | Glucose (mmol litre$^{-1}$) | Citrate (mmol litre$^{-1}$) | Rice (g litre$^{-1}$) |
|---|---|---|---|---|---|---|---|
| WHO/UNICEF[a] | 90 | 20 | 80 | — | 111 | 10 | — |
| Cereal based ORS[a] | 90 | 20 | 80 | — | — | 10 | 50–80 |
| UK/Europe ORS[b] | 35–60 | 20 | 37 | 18–30 | 90–200 | 10 | — |

[a]Used in cholera.
[b]ORS composition currently recommended for children in UK and Europe.

**Table 1.16**  Oral rehydration solutions.

| | Non-inflammatory | Inflammatory | Penetrating |
|---|---|---|---|
| Major location | Jejunum | Colon | Ileum |
| Clinical presentation: | Watery diarrhoea | Dysentery | Enteric fever |
| Common pathogens: | *Vibrio cholerae* Enterotoxigenic *Escherichia coli* | *Shigella* sp. Enteroinvasive *Escherichia coli* *Salmonella* sp. *Clostridium difficile* *Campylobacter jejuni* *Entamoeba histolytica* (see p. 72) | *Salmonella typhi* *Yersinia enterocolitica* |
| Pathogenetic mechanisms: | Enterotoxin (CT, LT, ST) production causing intestinal secretion of water and electrolytes | Invasion of gut epithelium ± cytotoxin release | Invasion and bacteraemia |

CT, cholera toxin; LT and ST, *Escherichia coli* heat-labile and heat-stable toxins.

**Table 1.17** Patterns of gut infection.

| Pathogen | Proportion of cases (%) |
|---|---|
| Enterotoxigenic *Escherichia coli* | 40–75 |
| *Shigella* sp. | 0–15 |
| *Salmonella* sp. | 0–10 |
| Rotavirus, Norwalk family of viruses | 0–10 |
| *Giardia lamblia, Entamoeba histolytica* | 0–3 |
| Unknown | 22–25 |

**Table 1.18** Causes of traveller's diarrhoea.

thought to be involved in the production of diarrhoea. Epidemics are common, especially in nurseries.

4 *Enterohaemorrhagic E. coli* (EHEC) produce a shiga-like cytotoxin that causes bloody diarrhoea and colitis. Fever is unusual. Outbreaks have been linked with contaminated food, particularly hamburgers.

### TREATMENT

Oral administration of fluids and electrolytes is the mainstay of therapy for *E. coli* gut infections as many are self-limiting and require no specific antimicrobial therapy. For severe infection, particularly with colitis and a systemic illness, ciprofloxacin 500 mg twice daily is often used as resistance to ampicillin and co-trimoxazole is widespread. Gentamicin 2–5 mg kg$^{-1}$ daily or tobramycin 3–5 mg kg$^{-1}$ daily in divided 8-hourly doses are used in severe illness with septicaemia. Urinary tract infection is discussed on p. 456.

Trimethoprim and doxycycline have been used in the prophylaxis of ETEC Traveller's diarrhoea, but early treatment rather than prophylaxis is now recommended.

## Salmonellosis

*Salmonella* is a Gram-negative, generally motile bacillus. Biochemically three species are recognized—*S. typhi* and *S. paratyphi, S. choleraesuis* and *S. enteritidis*. Their thermal death point is 60°C but they can withstand freezing and dry conditions for prolonged periods of time. Although salmonellae have a worldwide distribution, they usually result in disease only where there is poor hygiene and overcrowding. Transmission occurs by ingestion of contaminated foods (particularly eggs and poultry products) or water. In the past few years there has been a dramatic increase in *S. enteritidis* phage type 4 illnesses owing to widespread contamination of battery chickens. The organism is found in the alimentary tract, the oviducts and within the egg itself. In the UK, spread is often by carriers, usually food handlers, who contaminate the food. Following ingestion, the salmonellae colonize the small intestine and proliferate in Peyer's patches. They are then carried through the lymphatics, enter the bloodstream, and are thereby transported to the reticuloendothelial system.

A spectrum of clinical syndromes due to *Salmonella* is recognized:

- Enteric fever (typhoid or paratyphoid fever)
- Enterocolitis
- Extra-intestinal focal infections, e.g. osteomyelitis
- Food poisoning
- Carriers

### TYPHOID FEVER

This is caused by *S. typhi*. Humans are the only known reservoirs. The incubation period is usually 10–14 days. The onset is insidious, with headache being a prominent symptom. The fever is remittent and gradually increases in severity in a step-ladder fashion over 3–4 days. Cough, sore throat and altered behaviour may also be present. Constipation is usually present initially and diarrhoea only occurs late in the disease. Physical examination during the first week reveals a toxic individual with a relative bradycardia. During the second week several physical signs can be elicited. An erythematous maculopapular rash that blanches on pressure and is referred to as 'rose spots' appears, chiefly on the upper abdomen and thorax, and lasts for only 2–3 days. These spots are not easily visible on dark-skinned patients. A soft splenomegaly occurs in about 75% of patients. Cervical lymphadenopathy, hepatomegaly (present in about 30% of patients) and right iliac fossa tenderness are other physical signs that may be present. The third week of illness, aptly referred to as 'the week of complications', is the time when the majority of complications occur. These include lobar pneumonia, haemolytic anaemia, meningitis, peripheral neuropathy, acute cholecystitis, urinary tract infection and osteomyelitis. Intestinal perforation occurs in 2–3% and intestinal haemorrhage in 2–8%. The fourth week of illness ('the week of convalescence') is characterized by a gradual return to health.

## DIAGNOSIS

Leucopenia is present. Blood cultures are positive in about 80% during the first week and 30% in the third week. Urine cultures are helpful during the second week and stool cultures during the second to fourth week. Marrow cultures are occasionally helpful. Of the serological tests, the Widal test, which measures serum agglutinins against the O and H antigens, is most helpful; a fourfold increase in titre in sequential blood samples is suggestive of *Salmonella* infection.

### Carriers

Carriers can be divided into chronic carriers, defined as individuals who excrete *Salmonella* for at least 1 year, and convalescent carriers. The presence of Vi agglutinin in the serum in a dilution greater than 1 : 10 is suggestive of a carrier state. Since the gallbladder is frequently the focus of infection, duodenal aspirates for culture of the bile-containing duodenal juice may yield useful information.

## TREATMENTS

Chloramphenicol is effective but increasing resistance is developing. Ciprofloxacin 500 mg twice daily is therefore being used but is expensive. The temperature may take 4–6 days before settling, although subjective improvement is noted earlier. Treatment should be continued for 2 weeks. Co-trimoxazole 960 mg daily and ampicillin 6 g daily are also effective. Complications such as intestinal perforation or haemorrhage may occur despite adequate treatment. These complications can often be managed conservatively.

Eradication of a carrier state can be difficult, but ciprofloxacin for 4 weeks may be effective. Chemotherapy does not effect a cure in about 40%. In such individuals cholecystectomy remains the only mode of treatment.

### Prevention and control

This includes provision of safe drinking water, sanitary disposal of excreta and proper attention to hygiene by those who handle food. The parenteral monovalent typhoid vaccine is used as it is less likely to produce local and systemic reactions, but protection is incomplete and relatively short-lived (1 year). An improved parenteral vaccine based on the Vi polysaccharide antigen gives protection for about 3 years. An attenuated strain of *S. typhi* (Ty 21a) is available as a live oral vaccine and appears to confer moderately good protection for 3 years.

## PARATYPHOID FEVER

Paratyphoid fever is due to *S. paratyphi* A, B or C. They result in an illness clinically indistinguishable from typhoid fever. However, paratyphoid fever is a milder illness. Treatment is with co-trimoxazole 960 mg daily for 2 weeks.

## ENTEROCOLITIS

This is an acute, short-lived infection, and is usually due to *S. enteritidis* serotype *typhimurium*. It is generally mild, lasting 2–3 days, and presents with fever, malaise, cramping abdominal pain, bloody diarrhoea and vomiting. Occasionally a cholera-like picture may be present. Treatment is symptomatic. This *Salmonella* is an important cause of food poisoning; other organisms responsible are shown in Table 1.19 and are notifiable in the UK.

As with typhoid fever, a chronic carrier state may develop. Treatment is as described for *S. typhi* carriers.

# Shigellosis (bacillary dysentery)

Shigellosis is an acute self-limiting intestinal infection caused by one of four species of Gram-negative non-spore-forming bacilli. These include *Shigella dysenteriae*, *S. flexneri*, *S. boydii* and *S. sonnei*. While all of them are enteroinvasive, *S. dysenteriae* type 1 and some strains of *S. flexneri* and *S. sonnei* have been demonstrated to elaborate a toxin that is enterotoxic, neurotoxic and cytotoxic. Like salmonellosis, shigellosis is found worldwide and is more prevalent in areas with poor hygiene and overcrowding. Transmission is by the faecal–oral route.

## CLINICAL FEATURES

The incubation period is short, usually 2 days. The onset is acute, with fever, malaise, abdominal pain and watery diarrhoea. As the disease increases in intensity, bloody diarrhoea with mucus, tenesmus, faecal urgency and severe cramping abdominal pain becomes prominent. Nausea, vomiting, headache and convulsions (in children) may occur and have been attributed to the neurotoxin. When the disease is due to *S. dysenteriae*, which is responsible for the more fulminant forms of shigellosis, a cholera-like picture is occasionally seen. Sigmoidoscopy shows the presence of a markedly hyperaemic and inflamed mucosa, with transversely distributed ulcers with ragged undermined edges. The appearances are often indistinguishable from other dysenteric infections and from non-specific inflammatory bowel disease. Complications may be mild (arthritis, conjunctivitis, morbilliform rash) or life-threatening, such as colonic perforation, septicaemia and the haemolytic uraemic syndrome.

## DIAGNOSIS

The diagnosis is made on the basis of a stool culture.

| Organism | Source | Incubation period | Symptoms | Diagnosis | Recovery |
|---|---|---|---|---|---|
| Staphylococcus aureus | Contaminated food, usually by humans | 2–6 h | Diarrhoea, vomiting and dehydration | Culture organism in vomitus or remaining food | Rapid (few hours) |
| Bacillus cereus | Spores in food (often rice) survive boiling | 1–6 h | Diarrhoea, vomiting and dehydration | Culture organism in faeces and food | Rapid |
| Clostridium perfringens | Spores in food survive boiling | 8–22 h | Watery diarrhoea and cramping pain | Culture organism in faeces and food | 2–3 days |
| Clostridium botulinum | Spores survive cooking but only germinate in anaerobic conditions, e.g. canned or bottled food | 18–36 h | Brief diarrhoea and paralysis due to neuromuscular blockade | Demonstrate toxin in food or faeces | 10–14 days |
| Salmonella eneritidis[a] | Bowels of animals especially fowl | 12–24 h | Abrupt diarrhoea, fever and vomiting | Culture organism in stool | Usually 2–5 days, but may be up to 2 weeks |
| Campylobacter jejuni | Bowels of animals especially fowl; also milk | 48–96 h | Diarrhoea ± blood, fever, malaise and abdominal pain | Culture organism in stool | 3–5 days |

Non-microbial toxins such as dinoflagellate plankton toxin in shellfish ('red tide'), scrombotoxin from some varieties of spoiled fish (see p. 758) and red kidney bean toxin (haemagglutinin) from partially cooked beans also cause acute diarrhoea.
[a]Many strains, including Salmonella typhimurium.

**Table 1.19** Bacterial causes of food poisoning.

## TREATMENT

Treatment is symptomatic. In severe cases, trimethoprim 200 mg twice daily or ciprofloxacin 500 mg twice daily are used.

Public health measures, particularly the disposal of excreta and the provision of potable water, prevent infection. Outbreaks in schools can only be controlled by good hygiene.

## *CAMPYLOBACTER* INFECTION

*Campylobacter jejuni* is a Gram-negative, motile, curved spiral rod that is microaerophilic and thus fails to multiply under aerobic or strict anaerobic conditions. *C. jejuni* causes acute diarrhoea, sometimes with blood, and is now one of the most common causes of acute gastroenteritis in the UK. In developing countries asymptomatic carriers occur in young children.

## CLINICAL FEATURES

Symptoms begin 2–5 days after eating infected material (usually chicken or milk), the commonest being fever, headache and malaise. These are followed rapidly by diarrhoea, often with blood, and quite severe cramping abdominal pain. The patient generally appears unwell. Sigmoidoscopy can show the changes of acute colitis, which may be indistinguishable from those of ulcerative colitis. Complications include cholecystitis, pancreatitis, a reactive arthritis, the Guillain–Barré syndrome and the haemolytic uraemic syndrome.

## DIAGNOSIS

Direct phase microscopy of a wet mount of stool may reveal the motile curved rods resembling 'flying birds'. The organism may be cultured on special media within 48 hours. In severe infections the organism may be cultured from the blood.

## TREATMENT

In the majority of cases, *Campylobacter* enteritis is a self-limiting illness, resolving in 5–7 days. Although the organism is sensitive to erythromycin, there is no evidence that treatment with this antibiotic alters the natural history of the infection. However, if systemic symptoms continue in association with persistent bacteraemia, antibiotics are usually administered.

## *HELICOBACTER* INFECTION (see p. 190)

*Helicobacter pylori*, a curved Gram-negative organism, colonizes the gastric epithelium beneath the mucus layer and in areas of gastric metaplasia such as occur in the duodenum. *H. pylori* is noted for its ability to produce urease, which is thought to be involved in the pathogenesis of disease.

## *YERSINIA* INFECTIONS

The only three major human pathogens are *Y. pseudotuberculosis* and *Y. enterocolitica*, which cause mesenteric lymphadenitis and enterocolitis, respectively, and *Yersinia pestis*, which causes plague.

## *Yersinia enterocolitica* and *Yersinia pseudotuberculosis* infections

These result in a number of clinical syndromes depending on the host's age and immune status. Patients may present with enterocolitis, acute mesenteric lymphadenitis or terminal ileitis. Enterocolitis is characterized by the presence of fever, diarrhoea and severe abdominal pain, which may lead to a mistaken diagnosis of appendicitis. Arthritis (sometimes with Reiter's syndrome—see p. 836) and erythema nodosum are seen and are immunologically mediated.

This is usually a self-limiting disease and no treatment is required. In very severe cases, tetracycline 1 g daily may be given.

## Plague

Plague is caused by *Y. pestis*, a Gram-negative, pleomorphic bacterium. Nowadays it is mainly limited to animals, but sporadic cases of plague, as well as occasional epidemics, occur worldwide in humans. The major reservoirs are woodland rodents, which transmit infection to domestic rats (*Rattus rattus*). The vector is the rat flea, *Xenopsylla cheopis*. These fleas bite humans when there is a sudden decline in the rat population. Occasionally, spread of the organisms may be through infected faeces being rubbed into skin wounds or through inhalation of droplets.

Virulence is attributed to the presence of the endotoxin, exotoxin and fraction I (a soluble protein that prevents phagocytosis of the organism). Clinical manifestations are attributed to the lipopolysaccharide endotoxin.

### CLINICAL FEATURES
Four clinical forms are recognized—bubonic, pneumonic, septicaemic and cutaneous plague.

BUBONIC PLAGUE is the commonest form and occurs in about 90% of infected individuals. The incubation period is about 1 week. The onset of illness is acute, with high fever, chills, headache, myalgia, nausea, vomiting and, when severe, prostration. This is rapidly followed by the development of lymphadenopathy, most commonly involving the inguinal lymph nodes (buboes). Characteristically these are matted and tender, and suppurate in 1–2 weeks. Petechiae, ecchymoses and bleeding from the gastrointestinal tract, the respiratory tract and the genitourinary tract may occur. Mental confusion follows the development of toxaemia.

PNEUMONIC PLAGUE is characterized by the abrupt onset of features of a fulminant pneumonia with bloody sputum, marked respiratory distress, cyanosis and death in almost all affected patients.

SEPTICAEMIC PLAGUE presents as an acute fulminant infection with evidence of shock and DIC. If left untreated, death usually occurs in 2–5 days. Lymphadenopathy is unusual.

CUTANEOUS PLAGUE presents either as a pustule, eschar or papule or an extensive purpura, which can become necrotic and gangrenous.

### DIAGNOSIS
The diagnosis is easily established by demonstrating the organism in lymph node aspirates, in blood cultures or on examination of sputum.

### TREATMENT
Treatment is urgent and should be instituted before the results of culture studies are available. Several antimicrobial drugs are effective, including streptomycin 0.5 g i.m. every 4 hours for 48 hours followed by 0.5 g every 6 hours for 5 days, or tetracycline 2–3 g daily for 14 days.

### PREVENTION AND CONTROL
Prevention of plague is largely dependent on the control of the flea population and the use of potent antiflea agents such as 2% aldrin. Outhouses, or huts, should be sprayed with insecticides that are effective against the local flea. Rodents should not be killed until the fleas are under control as the fleas will leave dead rodents to bite humans. Tetracycline 500 mg four times daily or sulphonamides 2–4 g daily for 7 days are effective chemoprophylactic agents. Patients themselves can be infective when the buboes break down; patients with pneumonic plague can spread the organism by droplets. A partially effective formalin-killed vaccine is available for use by travellers to plague-endemic areas.

## TULARAEMIA

Tularaemia is due to infection by *Francisella tularensis*, a Gram-negative organism. It is primarily a zoonosis, affecting mainly rodents, including rabbits and squirrels. Vectors are ticks, flies and mosquitoes. Humans are infected by handling infected animals or from vector bites. The microorganisms enter through the skin or through minor abrasions in the mouth or conjunctivae. Occasionally infection occurs from contaminated water or from eating uncooked meat. The disease occurs worldwide and is frequently seen in the USA, particularly in hunters and butchers.

### CLINICAL FEATURES
The incubation period of 2–7 days is followed by a generalized illness. A number of clinical syndromes can be seen:

THE ULCEROGLANDULAR FORM is the commonest. A papule occurs at the site of inoculation. This ulcerates and is followed by tender, suppurative lymphadenopathy. Infected material entering the eye is followed by a purulent conjunctivitis with periauricular lymphadenopathy.

PNEUMONIC FORMS present with cough, chest pain and eventually a pneumonia, sometimes accompanied by a pericarditis.

THE SEPTICAEMIC FORM presents with the sudden onset of a fever, myalgia, headache and shock.

## DIAGNOSIS

Diagnosis is by culture of the organism or by a rising titre seen on a bacterial agglutination test.

## TREATMENT

Treatment is with streptomycin or more usually gentamicin. The patient should be isolated.

## PREVENTION

In endemic areas all wild animals should be handled using gloves. Infected meat and water should be adequately cooked. A vaccine is available for laboratory staff handling possibly infected animals.

## GLANDERS

Glanders is caused by a Gram-negative bacillus, *Pseudomonas mallei*. It affects mainly horses but can very rarely be transmitted to humans, mainly horse handlers. The disease is acquired by inhalation or inoculation of infected material. In the acute state, the patient is toxic with a high fever and delirium. There is an ulceration of the upper respiratory tract with eventual pneumonia, empyema and lung abscess. Septicaemia develops. Treatment is with i.v. broad spectrum antibiotics.

## MELIOIDOSIS

Melioidosis is due to the Gram-negative bacillus, *Pseudomonas pseudomallei*, which is a soil saprophyte. It infects humans (particularly diabetics or traumatized patients) by penetrating through skin abrasions, occasionally by inhalation, or via ingestion of contaminated water. It is found worldwide, but occurs mainly in South East Asia.

Septicaemia with abscesses in the lung, kidney, liver and spleen may occur. The CNS may be involved. The prognosis is poor. A chronic form, usually presenting with an unresolved pneumonia, also occurs.

Diagnosis is by culture of the organism. An indirect haemagglutination test is positive after 1 week.

## TREATMENT

The patient should be barrier-nursed and treated with ceftazidime.

## PASTEURELLOSIS

Pasteurelloses are infections primarily of animals. Three species are known to infect humans, the commonest being *Pasteurella multocida*, which is also the most virulent. All these organisms are commensal in the nasopharynx and gastrointestinal tract of a number of domestic and wild mammals. Transmission to humans may occur through a bite or scratch.

## CLINICAL FEATURES

Focal soft tissue infection with marked erythema, severe tenderness and regional lymphadenopathy may be present. These organisms are also responsible for chronic respiratory infections, bacteraemia, and brain and renal abscesses.

## TREATMENT

Penicillin is the drug of choice and should be given parenterally as benzylpenicillin 1–2 g every 4 hours.

## BARTONELLOSIS (CARRIÓN'S DISEASE)

This is caused by *Bartonella bacilliformis*, a Gram-negative bacillus. It is mainly restricted to the habitat of its main vector, sandfly, in the river valleys of the Andes mountains at an altitude of 500–3000 m. Two to six weeks following the bite, the patient develops 'oroya fever' with myalgia, arthralgia, severe headache and confusion followed by a haemolytic anaemia. Four to five weeks later reddish-purple haemangiomatous nodules develop and persist for 3–4 months. Superinfection can occur particularly with *Salmonella*.

## DIAGNOSIS

Diagnosis is by finding bacilli in erythrocytes or blood culture.

## TREATMENT

Treatment is with chloramphenicol, tetracycline or penicillin.

## LEGIONNAIRES' DISEASE

This is caused by the fastidious *Legionella pneumophila*, a weakly Gram-negative, catalase-positive bacillus. It is described on p. 679.

## *BACTEROIDES* INFECTION

*Bacteroides* is an obligate anaerobic, Gram-negative bacillus. *B. fragilis* is the most important anaerobic human pathogen and is a normal commensal in the human large gut. It does not produce an endotoxin and because of its polysaccharide capsule it resists phagocytosis. *B. fragilis* also produces heparinase, which may be involved in the development of thrombophlebitis, and β-lactamases, which inhibit the action of penicillin. It is not a highly invasive organism and grows best in necrotic tissues.

## CLINICAL FEATURES

Seventy-five per cent of all intra-abdominal infections, particularly postoperative infections, are caused by anaerobes. *Bacteroides* is a frequent cause of hepatic, subhepatic, pelvic and splenic abscesses. The pus has a characteristic putrid smell. *Bacteroides* also causes pelvic infections and may result in endometritis, Bartholin's abscess and pelvic peritonitis. Bacteraemia and Fournier's gangrene are also caused by *B. fragilis*.

### DIAGNOSIS
This depends on strict anaerobic culture with special media. Gas–liquid chromatography has been used to detect the volatile fatty acids produced by anaerobic bacteria.

### TREATMENT
Surgery is usually required as well as chemotherapy. Metronidazole (1–2 g daily by mouth or 1 g 8-hourly by rectum) is the drug of choice; it is also used prophylactically in colorectal surgery, with a dramatic reduction in postoperative infections.

# Actinomycetes

Actinomycetes are Gram-positive, branching higher bacteria (not fungi) and include *Actinomyces israelii*, *Nocardia asteroides* and *N. brasiliensis*.

Actinomyces is a normal mouth and intestine commensal, but *Nocardia* is a soil saprophyte. *Actinomyces* produces an illness characterized by chronicity and poor infectivity. It has a worldwide distribution. Disease due to *N. asteroides* is frequently seen in the USA and Europe, whereas *N. brasiliensis* gives rise to disease more commonly in southern Asia.

## Actinomycosis

In actinomycosis, characteristic clusters of organisms referred to as 'sulphur granules' are formed. *Actinomyces* is a rare cause of disease in the Western World. Three clinical forms of disease are recognized:
1 The *cervicofacial variety* usually occurs following dental extraction. It is often indolent and slowly progressive, associated with little pain, and results in induration and localized swelling of the lower part of the mandible ('lumpy jaw'). Lymphadenopathy is uncommon. Occasionally acute inflammation occurs.
2 The *thoracic variety* follows inhalation of these organisms into a previously damaged lung. The clinical picture is not distinctive and is often mistaken for malignancy or tuberculosis. Symptoms such as fever, malaise, chest pain and haemoptysis are present. Empyema occurs in 25% of patients and local extension produces chest-wall sinuses with discharge of sulphur granules.
3 *Abdominal actinomycosis* most frequently affects the caecum. Characteristically, a hard indurated mass is felt in the right iliac fossa. Later, sinuses develop. The differential diagnosis includes malignancy, tuberculosis, Crohn's disease and amoeboma. Pelvic actinomycosis

appears to be increasing with wider use of intrauterine contraceptive devices.

### TREATMENT
Treatment involves surgery, and penicillin is the drug of choice. High-dose i.v. penicillin is given for 4–6 weeks followed by oral penicillin for some weeks after clinical resolution. Tetracyclines are also effective.

## Nocardiosis

### CLINICAL FEATURES
*Nocardia* gives rise to two distinct clinical entities:
1 *Pulmonary disease* presents with cough, fever, and haemoptysis. Pleural involvement and empyema may occur.
2 *Mycetoma* is the result of local invasion by *Nocardia* and presents as a painless swelling, usually on the sole of the foot (madura foot). The swelling of the affected part of the body continues inexorably. Nodules gradually appear from which purulent fluid containing characteristic 'grains' of the organisms are discharged. Systemic symptoms and regional lymphadenopathy are distinctly uncommon. Sinuses may occur several years after the onset of the first symptom.

Mycetoma may also be produced by several other members of actinomycetes, including *Actinomadura* and *Streptomyces*. It is then referred to as an actinomycetoma. When caused by true fungi belonging to Eumycetes, e.g. *Madurella mycetomi* or *Petriellidium boydii*, it is referred to as eumycetoma. The clinical presentation, with the exception of differently coloured 'grains', is similar to that of mycetoma.

### DIAGNOSIS
This is often difficult to establish, as *Nocardia* is not easily detected in sputum cultures or on histological section.

### TREATMENT
Treatment consists of adequate surgical drainage of the pus combined with prolonged chemotherapy. The drug of choice is sulphadiazine in doses of up to 9 g daily. Co-trimoxazole may also be used.

# Mycobacteria

Mycobacteria are acid-fast, aerobic bacilli that grow extremely slowly. The cell wall contains complex lipids and glycolipids, one of which—the cord factor—is responsible for producing granulomas. No extracellular enzyme or toxins have been identified. The capacity of mycobacteria to produce disease is therefore attributed to their ability to multiply within phagocytic cells and to withstand intracellular enzymatic digestion.

A clinical classification of mycobacteria is shown in Table 1.20.

| Species | Disease produced |
|---|---|
| **Obligate intracellular bacteria:** | |
| *M. leprae* | Leprosy |
| **Facultative intracellular bacteria:** | |
| *M. tuberculosis* | Most cases of human tuberculosis |
| *M. bovis* | Cattle and rarely human tuberculosis |
| **Other forms:** | |
| *M. avium intracellulare* | Fowl and human tuberculosis particularly in HIV infection |
| *M. paratuberculosis* | Johne's disease (chronic granulomatous enteritis) in cattle |
| *M. scrofulaceum* | Lymph node infection |
| *M. kansasii* | Human tuberculosis (occasionally) |

**Table 1.20** Classification of *Mycobacterium* species based on their capacity to produce disease.

# Tuberculosis

Tuberculosis is largely due to *Mycobacterium tuberculosis*.

### EPIDEMIOLOGY
Tuberculosis is present worldwide with an extremely high prevalence in Asian countries, where 60–80% of children below the age of 14 years are infected. Tuberculosis is spread predominantly by droplet infection.

The prevalence of tuberculosis increases with poor social conditions, inadequate nutrition and overcrowding.

### PATHOLOGY
The characteristic lesion is a granuloma with central caseation and Langhans' giant cells.

The primary infection usually involves the lungs, but can involve other areas such as the ileocaecal region of the gastrointestinal tract. It is almost always accompanied by lymph node involvement.

In most people the primary infection heals leaving some surviving tubercle bacilli. With a lowering of host resistance these are reactivated producing local spread as well as haematogenous spread to all organs of the body, including the lungs, bones and kidneys. This particularly occurs in the elderly, in alcohol abusers, in patients with diabetes mellitus, lung disease, or after gastrectomy, as well as in patients who are on corticosteroids or are immunosuppressed. There is a high incidence in patients infected with HIV.

Occasionally the primary infection progresses locally to a more widespread lesion; haematogenous spread can also occur.

Tuberculosis in the adult is therefore usually the result of reactivation of old disease, occasionally a primary infection or, more rarely, reinfection.

### CLINICAL FEATURES
Pulmonary tuberculosis is the commonest form; this is described on p. 683, along with the chemotherapeutic regimens.

Tuberculosis also affects other organs, including:
GASTROINTESTINAL TRACT—mainly the ileocaecal area, but occasionally the peritoneum is affected, producing ascites (see p. 212)
GENITOURINARY SYSTEM—the kidney is mainly involved, but tuberculosis is also the cause of painless, craggy swellings in the epididymis and salpingitis, tubal abscesses and infertility in females
CENTRAL NERVOUS SYSTEM—tuberculous meningitis and tuberculomas
SKELETAL SYSTEM—arthritis and osteomyelitis with cold abscess formation can occur
SKIN—producing lupus vulgaris
EYE—producing choroiditis, iridocyclitis or phlyctenular keratoconjunctivitis
PERICARDIUM—producing constrictive pericarditis
ADRENAL GLANDS—causing destruction and producing Addison's disease
LYMPH NODES—this is a common mode of presentation, especially in young adults and children. Any group of lymph nodes may be involved but hilar and paratracheal lymph nodes are the commonest. Initially the nodes are firm and discrete but later they become matted and can suppurate and form sinuses.

SCROFULA is the term used to describe massive cervical lymph node enlargement with discharging sinuses (Fig 1.17). It is most often due to *M. tuberculosis*, and rarely to *M. scrofulaceum* or *M. kansasi*. Signs of acute inflammation are absent.

# Leprosy (Hansen's disease)

The causative organism is the acid-fast bacillus *M. leprae*. Unlike other mycobacteria, it does not grow in artificial media or even in tissue culture. While inability to culture the organism obtained from lesions and secretions is suggestive of *M. leprae*, it is not diagnostic. The following additional properties have been found to be useful in its identification:

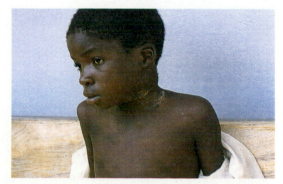

**Fig. 1.17** Scrofula—showing enlarged cervical lymph nodes.

- Loss of acid fastness following pyridine extraction.
- The ability of the organism to grow slowly in the foot-pad of mice. Other mycobacteria also grow in the foot-pad of mice, but these produce distinct histological changes.
- The ability of *M. leprae* to oxidize 3,4-dihydroxy-phenylalanine to pigmented products.
- The ability of this organism to invade peripheral nerves, a property not demonstrated by other mycobacteria.

Leprosy is found primarily in Asia and Africa (Fig. 1.18). Endemic foci are still present in the former USSR and parts of the USA. Of the 15 million people with leprosy worldwide, about two-thirds are in Asia. The precise mode of transmission is still uncertain but it is likely that nasal secretions play an important role.

Once an individual has been infected, subsequent progression to clinical disease appears to be dependent on several factors:

SEX—males appear to be more susceptible than females. In India, the ratio of affected males to females is 2 : 1.

GENETIC SUSCEPTIBILITY—studies in twins have shown a concordance in identical but not in non-identical twins.

IMMUNOLOGICAL RESPONSE of the individual to the bacillus.

## CLASSIFICATION

Two polar types of leprosy are recognized:

1 *Tuberculoid leprosy*—a localized disease that occurs in individuals who exhibit a marked immunological resistance to the organism.

2 *Lepromatous leprosy*—a generalized disease that occurs in individuals with impaired cell-mediated immunity (CMI).

Two subdivisions of lepromatous leprosy are included in the classification. The patient is said to have the 'subpolar' lepromatous ($LL_s$) form when he has passed through a borderline phase before becoming lepromatous, and the polar lepromatous ($LL_p$) form when the patient is lepromatous throughout.

The following types are also recognized:

BORDERLINE LEPROSY has features of both the polar varieties and is subdivided into borderline-tuberculoid, borderline and borderline-lepromatous. Borderline leprosy is an unstable state characterized by increasing numbers of *M. leprae* bacilli and decreasing numbers of lymphocytes.

INDETERMINATE LEPROSY is characterized by one or more hypopigmented, sometimes erythematous, ill-defined macules of variable size. Sensation, sweating and hair growth over the macules are usually normal.

NEURITIC LEPROSY is not associated with skin lesions. The affected nerve is enlarged and firm and sensory loss in the area of the nerve's distribution is present.

Two indices are currently in use to evaluate the response to treatment of patients in whom the skin-smear test for acid-fast bacilli is positive:

1 Bacteriological index (BI). This index is an objective way of evaluating the response to treatment. The skin-

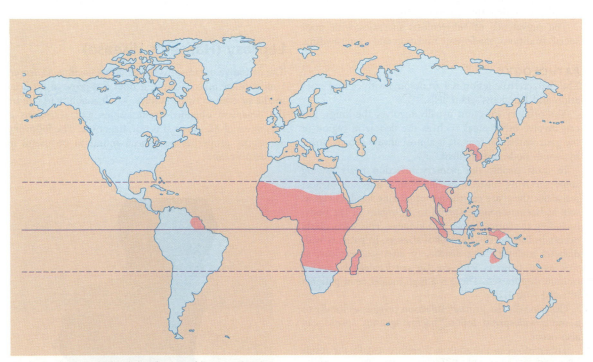

**Fig. 1.18** The geographical distribution of leprosy, showing areas where the prevalance is 5 in 1000 or greater.

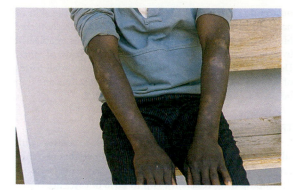

**Fig. 1.19** Multiple asymmetrical hypopigmented anaesthetic patches.

smear is graded from 1+ to 6+ depending upon the number of bacilli present per high-power field. The BI is calculated by taking the mean result of four slide examinations. For example, a decrease in BI from 6 to 3.5 on therapy indicates a good response to treatment.
2  Morphological index (MI). This is the percentage of solid staining acid-fast bacilli on smears (solid bacilli represent viable bacteria). A patient with an MI of 0% is not infectious.

## CLINICAL FEATURES
The incubation period varies from 2 to 6 years, although it may be as short as a few months or as long as 20 years. Leprosy should be considered in any individual who presents with hypopigmented skin patches (Fig. 1.19) associated with loss of sensation, especially to touch or temperature, and evidence of nerve involvement (thickening or tenderness), in whom non-cultivable acid-fast bacilli have been identified in skin smears.

The onset of leprosy is generally insidious. However, acute onset is known to occur and patients may present with a transient rash, with features of an acute febrile illness, with evidence of nerve involvement, or with any combination of these.

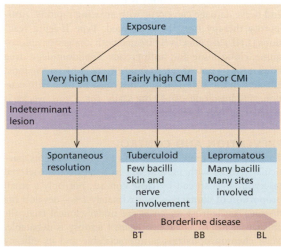

**Fig. 1.20** Clinical spectrum of leprosy.

## CLINICAL SPECTRUM (Fig. 1.20)
### Tuberculoid leprosy (TT)
In tuberculoid leprosy the infection is localized because the patient has unimpaired cell-mediated immunity. The characteristic, usually single, skin lesion is a hypopigmented, anaesthetic patch with thickened, clearly demarcated edges, central healing and atrophy. The face, gluteal region and extremities are most commonly affected. Frequently the nerve leading to this hypopigmented patch and the regional nerve trunk are thickened and tender. Unlike other parts of the body, a tuberculoid patch on the face is not anaesthetic. Nerve involvement leads to marked muscle atrophy. Tuberculoid lesions are known to heal spontaneously.

### Borderline-tuberculoid (BT) leprosy
Resembles TT but skin lesions are usually more numerous, smaller and may be present as small 'satellite' lesions around larger ones. Peripheral but not cutaneous nerves are thickened, leading to deformity of hands and feet.

### Borderline (BB) leprosy
Skin lesions are numerous varying in size and form (macules, papules, plaques). The annular, rimmed lesion with punched out, hypopigmented anaesthetic centre is characteristic. There is widespread nerve involvement and limb deformity (Fig 1.21).

### Borderline-lepromatous (BL) leprosy
There are a large number of florid asymmetrical skin lesions of variable form, which are strongly positive for acid-fast bacilli. Skin between the lesions is normal and often negative for bacilli.

### Lepromatous leprosy (LL)
Although practically every organ can be involved, the changes in the skin are the earliest and most obvious manifestation. Peripheral oedema and rhinitis are the earliest symptoms. The skin lesions predominantly occur on the face, the gluteal region and the upper and lower limbs. They may be macules, papules, nodules or plaques. Of these, the macule is the earliest lesion. Infiltration is most noticeable in the ear lobes. Thinning of the lateral margins of the eyebrows is characteristic. The mucous membranes are frequently involved, resulting in nasal stuffiness, laryngitis and hoarseness of the voice. Nasal

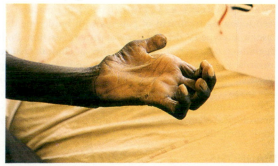

**Fig. 1.21** Leprosy—claw hand due to median and ulnar nerve damage.

septal perforation with collapse of the nasal cartilages produces a saddle-nose deformity. With progression of the disease, the typical leonine facies due to infiltration of the skin becomes apparent. Glove and stocking anaesthesia, gynaecomastia, testicular atrophy, ichthyosis and nerve palsies (facial, ulnar, median and radial) develop late in the disease. Neurotrophic atrophy affecting the phalanges leads to the gradual disappearance of fingers. Nerve involvement is less pronounced than in TT.

LUCIO'S PHENOMENON is seen only in Mexico and Central America, where LL is associated with an endarteritis which results in skin ulceration. The ulcers are large, with undermined edges and markedly necrotic bases. Smears from the base generally reveal numerous acid-fast bacilli. Healing is by scar formation. Treatment is wide surgical excision with skin grafts. Chemotherapy alone is ineffective in healing ulcers.

### The lepromin test

This is a measure of host resistance to leprosy and not a test for detecting leprosy: 0.1 ml of a suspension of dead bacilli (either Mitsuda lepromin or the Dharmendra lepromin) is injected intradermally. Two reactions are observed:
1 The early Fernandez reaction becomes positive in 48 hours and reflects the *sensitivity* of the tissue to the leprosy bacilli protein.
2 The late (Mitsuda) reaction develops in 4–5 weeks and reflects the resistance of the host to the bacteria. This reaction is strongly positive in TT and is negative in LL.

### Lepra reactions

Lepra reactions are immunologically mediated acute reactions that occur in patients with the borderline or lepromatous spectrum of disease. Two forms are recognized.

ERYTHEMA NODOSUM LEPROSUM (ENL; type II lepra reaction) is a humoral antibody response to an antigen–antibody complex (i.e. a type III hypersensitivity reaction). It is seen in 50% of patients with treated LL. It is characterized by fever, arthralgia and crops of painful, subcutaneous erythematous nodules, iridocyclitis and other systemic manifestations. It may last from a few days to several weeks.

THE BORDERLINE REACTION (type I lepra reaction) is seen following treatment of patients with borderline disease; it is a type IV delayed hypersensitivity reaction. Both upgrading or reversal reactions (i.e. a clinical change towards a more tuberculoid form) and downgrading reactions (i.e. a change towards the lepromatous form) can occur. The borderline reaction is characterized by acute inflammation of pre-existing borderline lesions. Neurological deficits such as an ulnar nerve palsy may occur abruptly.

### DIAGNOSIS

The diagnosis of leprosy is essentially clinical. Patients should be examined in adequate natural light. The demonstration of acid-fast bacilli in smears from the skin or nasal mucosa is highly suggestive. Occasionally nerve biopsies are helpful. The definitive diagnosis is established by cultivating the organisms in the foot-pads of mice. Detection of *M. leprae* DNA is now possible in all forms of leprosy using the polymerase chain reaction and can be used to assess the efficacy of treatment.

### TREATMENT

Leprosy should be treated in specialist centres with adequate physiotherapy and occupational therapy support. Multidrug therapy is now essential because of developing drug resistance (up to 20% of cases are resistant to dapsone).

Dapsone (di-amino-di-phenyl sulphone, DDS), a folate synthetase inhibitor, is bacteriostatic. It has the advantage of being cheap and well tolerated. Side-effects are few and include haemolytic anaemia and sulphaemoglobinaemia. In 1982 the World Health Organization recommended that for multi-bacillary forms of leprosy (BB, BL and LL types) it should be taken on a daily basis (100 mg) along with rifampicin 600 mg once monthly and clofazimine 50 mg daily with an extra dose of 300 mg monthly. The monthly doses are given under supervision. This triple therapy should be given for a minimum of 2 years or continued until a patient's skin smears become negative for acid-fast bacilli. However, in paucibacillary forms (TT or BT) 6 months' therapy with DDS 100 mg daily and rifampicin 600 mg monthly is recommended.

The major disadvantage with clofazimine is that it is a dye and causes a generalized reddish-brown pigmentation in light-skinned individuals and a slate grey pigmentation in dark-skinned individuals. Ethionamide is a suitable alternative. Acedapsone (DADDS), a depot sulphone, has been used with some success.

Surgery and physiotherapy play an important role in the management of trophic ulcers and deformities of the hands, feet and face.

### Treatment of lepra reactions

Treatment of lepra reactions is urgent, as irreversible eye and nerve damage can occur with amazing rapidity. Antileprosy therapy must be continued. Type II lepra reactions (ENL) are effectively treated with analgesics, chloroquine, clofazimine and antipyretics. Thalidomide, a drug known for its potent teratogenic effects, is by far the most effective in the ENL reaction, but must be used with caution. Prednisolone 30–40 mg daily for a few weeks is effective in type I reactions.

### PREVENTION AND CONTROL

This depends on rapid treatment of infected patients, particularly those with LL and BL, to decrease the bacterial reservoir. It is spread by close contact, but only a small proportion of contacts—approximately 1%—develop the disease. Antileprosy vaccines are under clinical trial; the efficacy of the BCG vaccine against leprosy is debatable. Mass chemoprophylaxis is impracticable and its efficacy in household contacts has not been established.

## Mycobacterial ulcer

Also known as Buruli ulcer, after the Buruli region in Uganda, this condition occurs in tropical, rural areas near rivers, e.g. in Zaire, Nigeria and Malaysia. It is caused by *M. ulcerans*. The disease is contracted by swimming in infected water. Initially a small subcutaneous nodule develops. This undergoes ulceration that involves the subcutaneous tissue, muscle and fascial planes. The ulcers are usually large, with undermined edges and markedly necrotic bases. Smears taken from necrotic tissue generally reveal numerous acid-fast bacilli. Treatment is wide surgical excision with skin grafts. Antituberculous therapy is ineffective.

# Mycoplasma

*Mycoplasma* is a small, free-living, motile bacterium that lacks a cell wall. *Mycoplasma pneumoniae* is found worldwide and may cause up to 20% of pneumonias. Infection is endemic but epidemics also occur, the infection being spread by airborne droplets between close contacts. *M. pneumoniae* infection is found most commonly in childhood, adolescence and early adulthood.

The oropharynx, trachea and bronchi are commonly involved, but there is frequently infiltration into the lung, causing pneumonia.

The clinical features and treatment are described on p. 677.

*M. hominis* and *Ureaplasma urealyticum* cause non-specific urethritis and cervicitis.

| Disease | Organism |
| --- | --- |
| Syphilis | *Treponema pallidum* |
| Yaws | *Treponema pertenue* |
| Bejel (endemic non-venereal syphilis) | *Treponema pallidum* variant |
| Pinta | *Treponema carateum* |
| Leptospirosis | *Leptospira interrogans icterohaemorrhagiae, canicola, hardjo, pomona* |
| Louse-borne relapsing fever | *Borrelia recurrentis* |
| Tick-borne relapsing fever | *Borrelia duttonii* and others |
| Cancrum oris | *Borrelia vincenti* |
| Lyme disease | *Borrelia burgdorferi* |
| Rat-bite fever | *Spirillum minus Streptobacillus moniliformis* |

**Table 1.21** Spirochaetal infections.

# Spirochaetes

Spirochaetal infections include those due to *Treponema, Leptospira* and *Borrelia* (Table 1.21).

## Syphilis

This is described on p. 91.

## Bejel (endemic non-venereal syphilis), yaws and pinta

These diseases are endemic throughout the tropical and subtropical regions of the world (Fig. 1.22). WHO have treated over 50 million cases, thus reducing the prevalence of these diseases, but improvements in sanitation and an increase in living standards will be required to eradicate the diseases completely.

**Yaws**

Apart from syphilis, yaws is the most widespread of the treponemal diseases. It is spread by direct contact often in overcrowded huts at night, usually in children; the organism enters through damaged skin. After an incubation period of weeks or months, a primary inflammatory reaction occurs at the inoculation site, from which organisms can be isolated. Dissemination of the organism leads to multiple papular lesions containing treponemes; these skin lesions usually involve the palms and soles. There may also be bone involvement, particularly the long bones and those of the hand.

In late yaws bony lesions may progress to cause gross destruction and disfigurement, particularly of the skull and facial bones, the interphalangeal joints and the long bones. Plantar hyperkeratosis is characteristic. Like syphilis, there may be a latent period between the early and late phases of the disease, but visceral, neurological and cardiovascular problems do not occur. Serological tests for syphilis are positive. Treatment is with long-acting penicillin.

**Bejel (endemic syphilis)**

A variant strain of *Treponema pallidum*, sometimes referred to as *T. pallidum endemicum*, is responsible for this infection and is spread by non-venereal routes in situations where hygiene is poor. The organism enters through abrasions in the skin. The disease is also found in children and differs from venereal syphilis in that a primary lesion is not commonly seen, although the late stages are indistinguishable from syphilis. Specific treponemal serology tests cannot differentiate these conditions and treatment is the same as for syphilis.

**Pinta**

Pinta is restricted mainly to Central and South America but otherwise closely resembles endemic syphilis. The primary lesion is a pruritic red papule, usually on the hand

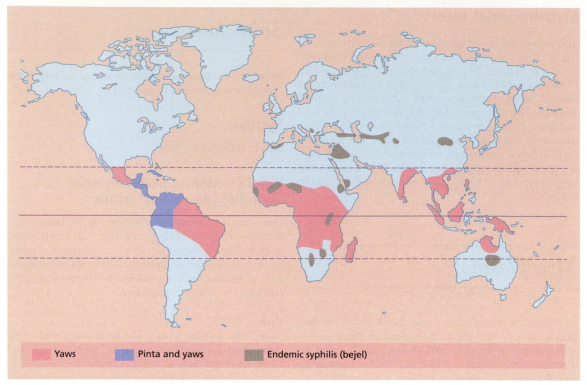

| Yaws | Pinta and yaws | Endemic syphilis (bejel) |

**Fig. 1.22**  The geographical distribution of bejel, yaws and pinta.

or foot. It may become scaly but never ulcerates and is generally associated with regional lymphadenopathy. In the later stages similar lesions can continue to occur for up to 1 year associated with generalized lymphadenopathy. Eventually the lesions heal, leaving hyperpigmented or depigmented patches. Syphilis serology is positive and treatment is as for other treponemal infections by long-acting penicillin.

## Leptospirosis

This zoonosis is caused by the Gram-negative organism *Leptospira interrogans*. There are over 200 serotypes; the main types affecting humans are *L. interrogans icterohaemorrhagiae* (from rodents and other wild animals), *L. interrogans canicola* (from dogs and pigs) and *L. interrogans hardjo* and *L. interrogans pomona* from cattle. Leptospires are excreted in the animal urine and enter the host through a skin abrasion or through intact mucous membranes. Certain occupational groups are particularly at risk, namely veterinarians, those involved in animal husbandry, abattoir workers and, in the past, miners and sewer workers. Pet owners and those who take part in water sports in inland waters are also exposed to the infection and now make up over 50% of all reported cases. Weil described a disease that consisted of jaundice, haemorrhage and renal impairment due to *L. icterohaemorrhagiae* but, fortunately, only 10–15% of patients suffer such a severe illness. The majority of infections are subclinical or cause a mild non-specific fever often undiagnosed.

### CLINICAL FEATURES

The incubation period is usually 10 days (range 2–20 days). More severe leptospirosis has two phases: a leptospiraemic phase lasting up to 1 week, followed by an immune phase, which is generally separated from the former phase by an asymptomatic period of 1–3 days.

The leptospiraemic phase, which lasts 4–9 days, is similar to many acute systemic infections and is characterized by severe headache, fever, malaise, anorexia and myalgia. The majority of patients have suffusion of the conjunctivae. Infrequently there is arthralgia, hepatosplenomegaly, lymphadenopathy and various skin rashes.

During the immune phase of the illness 50% of patients have meningism, about one-third of whom have CSF lymphocytosis and a modest elevation of CSF protein concentration. The majority recover uneventfully at this stage. However, a small proportion go on to develop tender hepatomegaly, jaundice, haemolytic anaemia and oliguric renal failure with microscopic haematuria. Occasionally cardiac involvement develops, characterized by atrial and ventricular dysrhythmias and congestive cardiac failure occurs. The mortality of leptospirosis is very variable but with a severe infection in the elderly it can be as high as 15–20%.

## DIAGNOSIS

Although diagnosis is most often made clinically:

CULTURE. Leptospires can be cultured from blood or CSF during the first week of the illness. A minority of patients excrete the organism in the urine during the second week of the illness and may continue to do so for a further 2–4 weeks.

SPECIFIC IgM LEPTOSPIRAL ANTIBODIES appear by the end of the first week.

BLOOD TESTS show a polymorpholeucocytosis and a raised ESR.

OTHER LABORATORY INVESTIGATIONS may be abnormal, depending on the organs involved.

## TREATMENT

Leptospires are sensitive to penicillins, erythromycin, tetracycline and chloramphenicol. Penicillin is most commonly used (2.4 g daily for 1 week) and should be given at any stage of the illness. Complications, e.g. renal or liver failure, are treated appropriately.

## PREVENTION

Avoid direct contact with rats, avoid immersion in natural waters and shower after canoeing, windsurfing, waterskiing or swimming.

# The relapsing fevers

These conditions are so named because, after apparent recovery from the initial infection, one or more recurrences may occur after a week or more without fever. The disease is caused by members of the genus *Borrelia*. *B. recurrentis* is spread by body lice and only humans are affected. This louse-borne variety occurs in epidemics when humans live in close contact in impoverished conditions; the infected louse is crushed by scratching allowing the spirochaete to penetrate through the skin. *B duttoni* and other *Borrelia* species are spread by soft (Argasid) ticks. Rodents are also infected and humans are incidental hosts acquiring the spirochaete from the saliva of the infected tick. This disease is found where traditional mud huts are the form of shelter but is also found in old houses and in camp sites in the USA.

These diseases are however found mainly in Africa, India, the Middle East, Mediterranean Europe and South America.

## CLINICAL FEATURES

Symptoms begin 7–10 days after infection and consist of a high fever of abrupt onset with rigors, generalized myalgia and headache. A petechial or ecchymotic rash may be seen. The general condition then deteriorates, with delirium, hepatosplenomegaly, jaundice, haemorrhagic problems and circulatory collapse. Although complete recovery may occur at this time, the majority experience one or more relapses of diminishing severity approximately 1 week after the initial illness. Without specific treatment, approximately one-third of patients will die.

Louse- and tick-borne relapsing fevers are clinically similar, although louse-borne fever tends to have a shorter initial illness with more frequent relapses.

## DIAGNOSIS

Spirochaetes can be demonstrated microscopically in the blood during febrile episodes.

## TREATMENT

Tetracycline or erythromycin are most commonly used. A severe Jarisch–Herxheimer reaction (see p. 92) occurs in many patients often requiring intensive nursing care and intravenous fluids.

## PREVENTION

Ticks live for years and remain infected, passing the infection to their progeny. These reservoirs of infection should be controlled by spraying houses with insecticides such as 2% benzene hexachloride and by reducing the number of rodents. In contrast, patients infested with lice should be deloused by washing with 1% Lysol or dusting with 10% dicophane (DDT); all clothes must be thoroughly disinfected.

# Cancrum oris

Cancrum oris is caused by *Borrelia vincenti* in association with anaerobic bacteria, commonly a member of the fusobacteria. The disease occurs in deprived and undernourished individuals with poor hygiene.

Cancrum oris usually occurs in children who are recovering from a debilitating illness, commonly measles. Rapidly progressive gangrenous destruction of the inner aspect of the mouth and cheek occurs, which may continue to progress even after treatment with penicillin. The mortality is high, probably reflecting the underlying poor physical state of the patient.

# Lyme disease

This disease is caused by *Borrelia burgdorferi*. The disease is transmitted by *Ixodes dammini* or related ixodid ticks (*Ixodes ricinus* in Europe). It was originally described in Lyme, Connecticut, but is now known to occur in many parts of the USA, in Europe and in Australia. Ticks (on deer and sheep) are widespread in the UK, particularly in forests and woodland. Prompt removal of any tick is essential as infection is unlikely to take place until the tick begins to engorge. Ticks should be removed by grasping them with forceps near to the point of attachment to the skin and then withdrawn by gentle traction.

## CLINICAL FEATURES

The first stage of the illness (within 7–10 days) consists of the unique and characteristic skin lesion—erythema chronicum migrans, often accompanied by headache, fever, malaise, myalgia, arthralgia and lymphadenopathy. The second stage follows weeks or months later, when some patients develop neurological (meningo-encephalitis, cranial or peripheral neuropathies) or cardiac (myocarditis) problems. Finally, the third stage of the disease consists of arthritis (see p. 398), which recurs in attacks for several years, often with associated erosion of cartilage and bone.

### DIAGNOSIS

The clinical features and epidemiological considerations are usually strongly suggestive of infection with this spirochaete. The diagnosis can only rarely be confirmed by isolation of the organisms from blood, skin lesions or CSF. IgM antibodies are detected in the first month; IgG antibodies are invariably present late in the disease. IgM antibodies can also be found in CSF.

### TREATMENT

Penicillin or tetracycline given early in the course of the disease shortens the duration of the illness in approximately 50% of patients. High-dose parenteral penicillin (benzathine penicillin, 2.4 g weekly for 3 weeks) or intravenous benzylpenicillin (2 g daily for 10 days) should be given for the later stages. Ceftriaxone can also be used.

## Rat bite fevers

Two spirochaetes, *Spirillum minus* and *Streptobacillus moniliformis*, produce similar febrile illnesses following rat bites. With *S. minus*, the bite usually heals but a local inflammatory response occurs 1–3 weeks later and is associated with swelling, ulceration (sodoku) and lymphadenopathy. A dark maculopapular rash is present during the febrile period and arthralgia occurs.

*S. moniliformis* infection can also occur after drinking infected milk (Haverhill fever). The incubation period is short (1–3 days), the rash is morbilliform and petechial and arthritis is common.

Systemic sequelae of generalized infection occurs with both conditions and periodic fever may continue for several weeks. *S. minus* usually causes a milder illness with a shorter incubation period and has less prolonged sequelae.

### DIAGNOSIS

Spirochaetes can be identified in aspirates from the inflammatory site, from a regional lymph node (*S. minus*), or from the blood (*S. moniliformis*). Serological tests are available and may be helpful in diagnosis.

Remember that rat bites can also cause other illness, e.g. leptospirosis, murine typhus.

### TREATMENT

Both organisms are sensitive to penicillin and tetracycline. Rodent control is vital.

# Rickettsiae and similar organisms

Rickettsiae are small bacteria that are spread to humans by arthropod vectors, namely human body lice, fleas, ticks and larval mites. Rickettsiae inhabit the alimentary tract of these arthropods and the disease is spread to the human host by inoculation of their faeces through human skin, generally by irritation and scratching. Rickettsiae multiply intracellularly and can enter most mammalian cells, although the main lesion produced is a vasculitis due to invasion of endothelial cells of small blood vessels. Thus multisystem involvement is usual. The causative organisms and arthropod vectors for rickettsial infections are shown in Table 1.22.

### CLINICAL FEATURES

#### Epidemic typhus

This is the most important rickettsial infection. Major outbreaks of typhus fever have occurred, mainly during famines and wars. It is found in Africa, Mexico, South America and Asia.

The incubation period is 1–3 weeks followed by an abrupt febrile illness associated with profound malaise and generalized myalgia. After 2 or 3 days the fever remains constant at around 40°C. Headache is severe and there may be conjunctivitis with orbital pain. A measles-like eruption appears around the fifth day, the macules increasing in size and eventually becoming purpuric in character. At the end of the first week, signs of meningo-encephalitis are evident and CNS involvement may progress to stupor or coma, sometimes with extrapyramidal involvement. At the height of the illness, splenomegaly, pneumonia, myocarditis and gangrene at the peripheries

| Disease | Organism | Reservoir | Vector |
|---|---|---|---|
| Typhus fevers: | | | |
|   Epidemic typhus | *Rickettsia prowazekii* | Man | Human lice |
|   Endemic (murine) typhus | *Rickettsia typhi (R. mooseri)* | Rat | Flea |
|   Rocky Mountain spotted fever | *Rickettsia rickettsii* | Rodents, dog | Tick |
|   Tick typhus (*fièvre boutonneuse*) | *Rickettsia conori* | Rodents, dog | Tick |
|   Scrub typhus | *Rickettsia tsutsugamushi* | Rodents | Larval mite |
| Rickettsial pox | *Rickettsia akari* | House mice | Mite |
| Trench fever | *Rochalimaea quintana* | Man | Human lice |
| Q fever | *Coxiella burnetii* | Domestic animals | None (airborne) |

**Table 1.22** Infections due to Rickettsia and Rickettsia-like organisms.

may be evident. Oliguric renal failure occurs in fulminating disease, which is usually fatal. Recovery begins in the third week but is generally slow.

The disease may recur many years after the initial attack owing to rickettsiae that lie dormant in lymph nodes. The recrudescence is known as Brill–Zinsser disease. The factors that precipitate recurrence are not clearly defined, although other infections may be important.

### Endemic (murine) typhus

This is a rat infection that is inadvertently spread to humans by a rickettsiae-carrying rat flea. The disease closely resembles epidemic typhus but is much milder and rarely fatal.

### Rocky Mountain spotted fever and other tick-borne typhus fevers

Infected hard ticks transmit this infection to humans, the same arthropod vector being responsible for other tick-borne typhus fevers in Africa, India and the Mediterranean (*Rickettsia conori* causing '*fièvre boutonneuse*'), in Central Asia and the Far East (*Rickettsia siberica*), and in Australia (*Rickettsia australis*).

Rocky Mountain spotted fever is limited to North and South America. As in other tick-borne typhus fevers, many patients will be able to give an account of tick bites or exposure to ticks. Clinical features closely resemble those of epidemic typhus, although the incubation period may be shorter and an eschar (crusted necrotic papule) may develop at the site of the bite in association with regional lymphadenopathy. The typical, generalized maculopapular rash occurs, which includes the palms and soles of the feet. The rash eventually becomes petechial. Neurological, haematological and cardiovascular complications occur as in epidemic typhus.

### Scrub typhus

Found throughout Asia and the Western Pacific, this disease is spread by larval trombiculid mites (chiggers). Like tick-borne typhus, an eschar can often be found. Again the clinical illness resembles that of epidemic typhus, with an abrupt-onset febrile illness, rash and severe toxaemia. Bronchitis and interstitial pneumonia occur commonly but physical findings in the chest are minimal. The infection may recur despite treatment with antibiotics.

### Rickettsial pox and trench fever

*Rickettsial pox* is an urban disease described initially in New York City in 1946. A rodent mite was responsible for the spread of the infection to humans, the epidemic being related to massive expansion of the mouse community in large apartment buildings. The disease is mild, but similar in character to other rickettsial infections. *Trench fever* is also a relatively mild illness but multiple relapses are common. Although the causative agent of this disease, *Rochalimaea quintana*, was originally classified with the rickettsiae, it is now known that the organism does not demand an intracellular existence and may be cultured on bacteriological media. Both of these diseases are now rare.

## DIAGNOSIS

The diagnosis is generally made on the basis of the history and clinical course of the illness. Although the causative organisms can be isolated by inoculation of infected blood into laboratory animals, this is laborious and may take several weeks.

Serodiagnosis using the Weil–Felix *Proteus* agglutination test, which relies on the fact that *Rickettsia* and *Proteus* OX strains have common antigens, has been used for more than 50 years. The Weil–Felix test is now being replaced by complement fixation, indirect fluorescent antibody or indirect haemagglutination tests which are more sensitive and specific. The polymerase chain reaction (PCR) is established for the diagnosis of scrub typhus.

## TREATMENT

Tetracycline 500 mg four times daily for 7 days is given and improvement generally occurs in 48 hours. Ciprofloxacin is also effective. Doxycycline 200 mg weekly protects against scrub typhus; it is reserved for highly endemic areas.

## CONTROL

This is achieved by control of vectors, namely lice, fleas, mites and ticks. Lice and fleas can be eradicated from clothing by insecticides (0.5% malathion or DDT). Chemical repellants are also useful. Control of rodents is vital.

Bites from ticks and mites should be avoided by wearing protective clothing on exposed areas of the body, especially in high-risk regions. Mites can also be destroyed by chemical spraying from the air.

# Q fever

Q fever is a zoonosis due to the rickettsial-like organism *Coxiella burnetii*. This organism is smaller than true rickettsiae, more resistant to physical and chemical injury and has a negative Weil–Felix reaction, since it does not share common antigens with *Proteus*. Clinically, Q fever differs from rickettsial illnesses as the rash is not a major feature and transmission of the disease to humans is independent of an arthropod vector. Important modes of spread to humans are thought to be dust, aerosols and unpasteurized milk from infected cows. *C. burnetii* is widespread in domestic and farm animals. It is spread between them by ticks, which constitute an important arthropod reservoir of the disease.

## CLINICAL FEATURES

Fever begins insidiously, together with other symptoms of an influenza-like illness, 1–2 weeks after exposure. The acute illness may resolve spontaneously without treatment, but with persisting infection, symptoms and signs of pneumonia may develop, followed by endocarditis. A petechial rash may be apparent at this stage. Occasionally epididymo-orchitis, uveitis and osteomyelitis may be present. Untreated chronic infection is usually fatal.

## DIAGNOSIS

Serodiagnosis by complement fixation tests is important since *C. burnetii* is an obligate intracellular organism and does not grow on standard microbiological culture media. The organism possesses two classes of antigens, phase I and phase II. Antibodies to the phase I antigens appear later in the illness than antibodies to the phase II antigens; high titres are diagnostic in endocarditis. Persistently high titres of both antibodies confirm chronic infection.

## TREATMENT

Tetracycline is the treatment of choice for acute infection. For endocarditis a prolonged course of treatment is required, clindamycin often being given in association with tetracycline. Co-trimoxazole and rifampicin may also be useful.

# Chlamydiae

Chlamydiae are obligate intracellular bacteria. They are ubiquitous and found in almost every avian and mammalian species and it has been estimated that up to 20% of the human population is infected with this organism. They are highly infectious, but rarely kill their host. There are three species—*Chlamydia trachomatis*, *C. psittaci* and the recently discovered *C. pneumoniae*; Table 1.23 shows the diseases produced.

## Trachoma

This is the commonest cause of blindness in the world and is found in the tropics and the Middle East. It is entirely preventable. It commonly occurs in children and is probably spread by direct transmission or possibly by flies.

Infection is bilateral and begins in the conjunctiva, with marked inflammation and scarring. Scarring of the upper eyelid causes entropion, leaving the cornea exposed to further damage. The corneal scarring that eventually occurs leads to blindness. The changes in the eye are sometimes accompanied by an upper respiratory tract infection.

Trachoma may also occur as an acute ophthalmic infection in the neonate.

## DIAGNOSIS

The diagnosis is generally established by:
- The typical clinical picture
- The presence of intracytoplasmic inclusion bodies in conjunctival cells

## TREATMENT

Tetracycline ointment applied locally each day for 2–3 months is effective, as is systemic therapy with oral tetracycline or sulphonamide. In endemic areas repeated courses of therapy are necessary. Recent data suggest that eradication of the disease may be possible with azithromycin. Once infection has been controlled, surgery may be required for eyelid reconstruction and for treatment of corneal opacities. Community health education with respect to hygiene and earlier case reporting could make a substantial impact on disease prevalence.

## Genital infections

Lymphogranuloma venereum is caused by *C. trachomatis* serotypes L 1, 2 and 3 and is described on p. 93.

Genital infections are also caused by other strains of *C. trachomatis* (see p. 89).

## Psittacosis (ornithosis)

Although originally thought to be limited to the psittacine birds (parrots, parakeets and macaws), it is now known that the disease is widely spread amongst many species of birds, including pigeons, turkeys, ducks and chickens, hence the broader term 'ornithosis'. Human infection is related to exposure to infected birds and is therefore a true zoonosis. The causative organism, *C. psittaci*, is excreted in avian secretions; it can be isolated for prolonged periods from birds who have apparently recovered from infection. The organism gains entry to the human host by inhalation.

## CLINICAL FEATURES AND TREATMENT

These are discussed on p. 679.

## Respiratory infection (see p. 679)

*C. pneumoniae* strain TWAR causes relatively mild pneumonias in young adults, clinically resembling *Mycoplasma* pneumonia. Infection occurs in outbreaks. Diagnosis can be confirmed by specific IgM serology. Treatment is with erythromycin or tetracycline.

# Viral infections

| Disease | Organism |
|---------|----------|
| Trachoma | *C. trachomatis* |
| Lymphogranuloma venereum | *C. trachomatis* (serotypes L 1, 2 and 3) |
| Urethritis, cervicitis, proctitis | *C. trachomatis* |
| Psittacosis | *C. psittaci* |
| Respiratory | *C. pneumoniae* |

**Table 1.23** *Chlamydia* infections.

Viruses are much smaller than other infectious agents (viruses are not, by definition, microorganisms), and con-

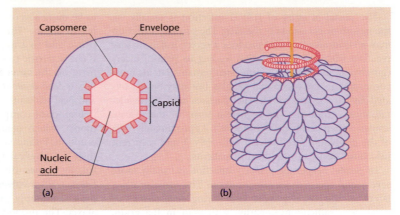

**Fig. 1.23** Viruses. (a) Schematic diagram of a virus structure (icosahedral). (b) Helical symmetry, showing capsomers arranged along the helical nucleic acid molecule.

tain either DNA or RNA. Since they are metabolically inert, they must live intracellularly, using the host cell for synthesis of viral proteins and nucleic acid. Viruses have a central nucleic acid core surrounded by a protein coat that is antigenically unique for a particular virus. The protein coat (capsid) imparts a helical or icosahedral structure to the virus. Some viruses also possess an envelope consisting of lipid and protein (Fig. 1.23).

Hepatitis viruses are discussed on p. 249.

# DNA viruses

Details of the structure, size and classification of DNA viruses are shown in Table 1.24.

## ADENOVIRUSES

Adenovirus infection commonly presents as an acute pharyngitis and extension of infection to the larynx and trachea in infants may lead to croup. By school age the

majority of children show serological evidence of previous infection. Certain subtypes produce an acute conjunctivitis associated with pharyngitis. In adults, adenovirus causes acute follicular conjunctivitis and rarely pneumonia that is clinically similar to that produced by *Mycoplasma* (see p. 677). Adenoviruses have also been implicated as a cause of gastroenteritis (see p. 52) without respiratory disease and may be responsible for acute mesenteric lymphadenitis in children and young adults. Mesenteric adenitis due to adenoviruses may lead to intussusception in infants.

## HERPESVIRUSES

### Herpes simplex virus infection

Two types of HSV have been identified: HSV-1 is the major cause of herpetic stomatitis, herpes labialis ('cold sore'), keratoconjunctivitis and encephalitis, whereas HSV-2 causes genital herpes and may also be responsible for systemic infection in the immunocompromised host. These divisions, however, are not rigid, for HSV-1 can give rise to genital herpes and HSV-2 can cause pharyngitis.

| Structure | | | | |
|---|---|---|---|---|
| Symmetry | Envelope | Approximate size | Family | Viruses |
| Icosahedral | – | 80 nm | Adenovirus | Adenoviruses |
| Icosahedral | + | 100 nm (160 nm with envelope) | Herpesvirus | Herpes simplex virus types 1 and 2 Varicella zoster virus Cytomegalovirus Epstein–Barr virus Human herpes virus type 6 (HHV6) |
| Icosahedral | – | 50 nm | Papovavirus | Human papillomavirus Polyomavirus |
| Icosahedral | – | 23 nm | Parvovirus | Parvovirus B19 |
| Complex | + | 300 nm × 200 nm | Poxvirus | Variola virus Vaccinia virus Orf Molluscum contagiosum |

**Table 1.24** Human DNA viruses.

The portal of entry of HSV-1 infection is usually via the mouth or occasionally the skin. The primary infection may go unnoticed or may produce a severe inflammatory reaction with vesicle formation leading to painful ulcers (gingivo-stomatitis). The virus then remains latent, most commonly in the trigeminal ganglia, but may be reactivated by stress, trauma, febrile illnesses and ultraviolet radiation, producing the recurrent form of the disease known as herpes labialis ('cold sore'). Approximately 70% of the population are infected with HSV-1 and recurrent infections occur in one-third of patients.

In genital herpes the primary infection is usually more severe and recurrences are common. The virus remains latent in the sacral ganglia and during recurrence can produce a radiculomyelopathy, with pain in the groin, buttocks and upper thighs. Primary anorectal herpes infection is now common in male homosexuals (see p. 93).

Immunocompromised patients such as those receiving intensive cancer chemotherapy or those with the acquired immunodeficiency syndrome (AIDS) may develop disseminated HSV infection involving many of the viscera. In severe cases death may result from severe hepatitis and encephalitis.

Neonates may develop primary HSV infection following vaginal delivery in the presence of active genital HSV infection in the mother. Caesarean section should therefore be considered in the presence of active genital HSV infection.

Humoral antibody develops following primary infection, but mononuclear cell responses are probably more important in preventing dissemination of disease.

The clinical picture, diagnosis and treatment are described on p. 1014.

# Varicella zoster virus infection

VZV produces two distinct diseases—varicella (chickenpox) and herpes zoster (shingles). The primary infection is chickenpox. It usually occurs in childhood, the virus entering through the mucosa of the upper respiratory tract. Chickenpox almost never occurs twice in the same individual. The virus then remains latent in dorsal root and cranial nerve ganglia. It may recur as localized disease limited to a dermatome innervated by a single spinal or cranial sensory ganglion (shingles) and/or may affect a motor nerve such as the facial nerve, causing facial palsy (see p. 889). Shingles is never the direct result of a primary infection. Patients with chickenpox or shingles are infective, the virus being spread from fresh skin lesions by direct contact or airborne transmission and causing chickenpox in susceptible individuals.

## CLINICAL FEATURES

Fourteen to twenty-one days after exposure to VZV, a brief prodromal illness of fever, headache and malaise heralds the eruption of chickenpox, characterized by the rapid progression of macules to papules to vesicles to pustules in a matter of hours. In young children the prodromal illness may be very mild or absent. The illness tends to be more severe in older children and can be debilitating in adults. The lesions occur on the face, scalp and trunk, and to a much lesser extent on the extremities. It is characteristic to see skin lesions at all stages of development on the same area of skin. Fever subsides as soon as new lesions cease to appear. Eventually the pustules crust and heal without scarring.

Important complications of chickenpox include pneumonia, which generally begins 1–6 days after the skin eruption. Pulmonary symptoms are usually more striking than the physical findings, although a chest radiograph usually shows diffuse changes throughout both lung fields. CNS involvement occurs in about 1 per 1000 and most commonly presents as an acute truncal cerebellar ataxia. The immunocompromised are susceptible to disseminated infection with multi-organ involvement.

Shingles (see p. 1015) occurs in adults, particularly the elderly, producing an identical skin lesion to chickenpox, although classically it is unilateral and restricted to a sensory nerve (dermatomal) distribution.

## DIAGNOSIS

The diseases are usually recognized clinically but can be confirmed by electron microscopy, immunofluorescence or culture of vesicular fluid and by serology.

## TREATMENT

Chickenpox requires no treatment in healthy children and infection results in life-long immunity. However, the disease may be fatal in the immunodeficient or the immunosuppressed, when it is reasonable to use passive immunization, with zoster immune immunoglobulin (ZIG). In the immunocompromised host it is also reasonable to give acyclovir 10 mg kg$^{-1}$ three times daily i.v. for 7 days or vidarabine 10 mg kg$^{-1}$ daily i.v. for 7 days. Treatment for shingles is discussed on p. 1015.

# Cytomegalovirus (CMV) infection

Infection with CMV is found worldwide and has its most profound effects as an opportunistic infection in the immunocompromised, particularly in recipients of bone-marrow and solid organ transplants and in patients with AIDS—90% of patients with AIDS are infected with CMV and 95% of this population have disseminated CMV at autopsy. A large proportion (50% +) of the adult population has serological evidence of latent infection with the virus, although infection is generally symptomless.

## CLINICAL FEATURES

In healthy adults CMV infection is usually asymptomatic but may cause an illness similar to infectious mononucleosis, with fever, occasionally lymphocytosis with atypical lymphocytes, and hepatitis with or without jaundice. Infection may be spread by kissing, sexual intercourse and blood transfusion. Disseminated fatal infection with widespread visceral involvement occurs in the immunocompromised including encephalitis, retinitis, pneumonitis and diffuse involvement of the gastrointestinal tract.

Intrauterine infection may have serious consequences on the fetus; CNS involvement may cause microcephaly and motor disorders. Jaundice and hepatosplenomegaly are common and thrombocytopenia and haemolytic anaemia also occur.

### DIAGNOSIS
Serological tests can identify latent (IgG) or primary (IgM) infection. The virus can also be identified in tissues by the presence of characteristic intranuclear 'owl's eye' inclusions and by direct immunofluorescence. Culture in human embryo fibroblasts is usually slow but diagnosis can be accelerated by immunofluorescent detection of antigen in the cultures.

### TREATMENT
In the immunocompetent, infection is usually self-limiting and no specific treatment is required. In the immunosuppressed, ganciclovir (5 mg kg$^{-1}$ daily for 14–21 days) reduces retinitis and gastrointestinal damage and can eliminate CMV from blood, urine and respiratory secretions. It is less effective against pneumonitis and encephalitis. Drug resistance has been reported and bone marrow toxicity is common.

## Epstein–Barr virus (EBV) infection

This virus causes an acute febrile illness known as infectious mononucleosis (glandular fever), which occurs worldwide in adolescents and young adults. EBV is probably transmitted in saliva and by aerosol.

### CLINICAL FEATURES
The predominant symptoms are fever, headache, malaise and sore throat. Palatal petechiae and a transient macular rash are common, the latter occurring in 90% of patients who have received ampicillin for the sore throat. Cervical lymphadenopathy, particularly of the posterior cervical nodes, and splenomegaly are characteristic. Mild hepatitis is common, but other complications such as myocarditis, meningitis, mesenteric adenitis and splenic rupture are rare. Although some young adults remain debilitated and depressed for some months after infection, the evidence for reactivation of latent virus in healthy individuals is controversial, although this is thought to occur in immunocompromised patients.

### DIAGNOSIS
EBV infection should be strongly suspected if atypical mononuclear cells (glandular fever cells) are found in the peripheral blood. It can be confirmed during the second week of infection by a positive Paul–Bunnell reaction, which detects heterophile antibodies (IgM) that agglutinate sheep erythrocytes. False-positives can occur in other conditions such as hepatitis, Hodgkin's disease and acute leukaemia. Specific EBV IgM antibodies indicate recent infection by the virus. The Monospot test is a sensitive and easily performed screening test. Clinically similar illnesses are produced by CMV and toxoplasmosis but these can be distinguished serologically.

### TREATMENT
The majority of cases require no specific treatment and recovery is rapid. Corticosteroid therapy is advised when there is neurological involvement, e.g. encephalitis, meningitis, Guillain–Barré syndrome or when there is marked thrombocytopenia or haemolysis. Corticosteroid therapy has also been used when malaise and intermittent fever are prolonged but this is not recommended.

EBV is also considered to be the major aetiological agent responsible for Burkitt's lymphoma and nasopharyngeal carcinoma.

## Human herpesvirus type 6

This recently discovered human herpesvirus infects T lymphocytes, occurs worldwide, and exists as a latent infection in over 90% of the adult population. The virus causes roseola infantum (exanthem subitum) which presents as a high fever followed by generalized macular rash in infants. Reactivation in the immunocompromised may lead to severe pneumonia.

### TREATMENT
Supportive management only is recommended for the common infantile disease. Ganciclovir can be used in the immunocompromised.

## PAPOVAVIRUSES

These small viruses tend to produce chronic infections, often with evidence of latency. They are capable of inducing neoplasia in some animal species and were among the first viruses to be implicated in tumorigenesis. Human papillomaviruses, of which there are many types, are responsible for the common wart and have been implicated in the aetiology of carcinoma of the cervix (types 16 and 18). The human BK virus, a polyomavirus, is generally found in immunosuppressed individuals and may be detected in the urine of between 15 and 40% of renal transplant patients, in patients receiving cytotoxic chemotherapy and in those with immunodeficiency states. A related virus, JC, is the cause of progressive multifocal leukoencephalopathy (PML) which presents as dementia in the immunocompromised and is due to progressive cerebral destruction resulting from accumulation of the virus in brain tissue.

For genital warts see p. 94.

## PARVOVIRUSES

Human parvovirus B19 produces:
- Erythema infectiosum (fifth disease), a common infection in schoolchildren. The rash is typically on the face (slapped-cheek appearance). The patient is well and the rash can recur over weeks or months.
- Asymptomatic infection occurs in 20% of children.

- Moderately severe self-limiting arthropathy (see p. 399).
- Aplastic crises in patients with chronic haemolysis, e.g. sickle cell disease.
- Chronic infection with anaemia in immunocompromised subjects.

## POXVIRUSES

### Smallpox (variola)

This disease has been eradicated following an aggressive vaccination policy and careful detection of new cases.

### Vaccinia virus

This is a laboratory virus and does not occur in nature in either humans or animals. Its origins are uncertain but it is thought to be a derivative of the cowpox virus used by Jenner for vaccination against smallpox. Vaccination is now not recommended except for laboratory personnel handling certain poxviruses for experimental purposes.

### Orf

This poxvirus causes contagious pustular dermatitis in sheep and hand lesions in humans (see p. 1015).

## Molluscum contagiosum

See p. 1015.

## RNA viruses (Table 1.25)

## PICORNAVIRUSES

### Poliovirus infection (poliomyelitis)

Poliomyelitis occurs when a susceptible individual is infected with poliovirus type 1, 2 or 3. These viruses have a propensity for the nervous system, especially the anterior horn cells of the spinal cord and cranial nerve motor neurones. Poliomyelitis is found worldwide but its incidence has decreased dramatically following improvements in sanitation, hygiene and the widespread use of polio vaccines. Spread is usually via the faecal–oral route, as the virus is excreted in the faeces.

#### CLINICAL FEATURES

The incubation period varies from 7 to 14 days. Although polio is essentially a disease of childhood, no age is exempt. The clinical manifestations vary considerably:

| Structure | | | | |
|---|---|---|---|---|
| Symmetry | Envelope | Approximate size | Group | Viruses |
| Icosahedral | – | 30 nm | Picornavirus | Poliovirus, Coxsackievirus, Echovirus, Enterovirus } Enteroviruses, Rhinovirus |
| Icosahedral | – | 80 nm | Reovirus | Reovirus, Rotavirus |
| Icosahedral | + | 50–80 nm | Togavirus | Rubella virus, Alphaviruses, Flaviviruses |
| Spherical | + | 80–100 nm | Bunyavirus | Congo–Crimean haemorrhagic fever, Hantavirus |
| Helical | + | 80–120 nm | Orthomyxovirus | Influenza viruses A, B and C |
| Helical | + | 100–300 nm | Paramyxovirus | Measles virus, Mumps virus, Respiratory syncytial virus |
| Helical | + | 60–175 nm | Rhabdovirus | Rabies virus |
| Helical | + | 100 nm | Retrovirus | Human immunodeficiency virus (HIV) |
| Helical | + | 100–300 nm | Arenavirus | Lassa virus, Lymphocytic choriomeningitis virus |
| Pleomorphic | + | Filaments or circular forms; 100 × 130–2600 nm | — | Marburg virus, Ebola virus |

**Table 1.25**  Human RNA viruses.

INAPPARENT INFECTION is common and occurs in 95% of infected individuals.

ABORTIVE POLIOMYELITIS occurs in approximately 4–5% and is characterized by the presence of fever, sore throat and myalgia. The illness is self-limiting and of short duration.

NON-PARALYTIC POLIOMYELITIS has features of abortive poliomyelitis as well as signs of meningeal irritation, but recovery is complete.

PARALYTIC POLIOMYELITIS occurs in approximately 0.1% of infected children (1.3 % of adults). Several factors predispose to the development of paralysis:
- male sex,
- exercise early in the illness,
- trauma, surgery or intramuscular injection which localize the paralysis,
- recent tonsillectomy (bulbar poliomyelitis)

This form of the disease is characterized initially by features simulating abortive poliomyelitis. Symptoms subside for 4–5 days, only to recur in greater severity with signs of meningeal irritation and muscle pain, which is most prominent in the neck and lumbar region. These symptoms persist for a few days and are followed by the onset of asymmetric paralysis without sensory involvement. The paralysis is usually confined to the lower limbs in children under 5 years of age and the upper limbs in older children, whereas in adults it manifests as paraplegia or quadriplegia.

BULBAR POLIOMYELITIS occurs in 5–30% and is characterized by the presence of cranial nerve involvement. Soft palate, pharyngeal and laryngeal muscle palsies are common.

Aspiration pneumonia, myocarditis, paralytic ileus and urinary calculi are late complications of poliomyelitis.

POST-POLIO SYNDROME refers to an increase in the degree of muscle atrophy of an affected limb many years after the primary attack.

## DIAGNOSIS

The diagnosis is a clinical one. Distinction from the Guillain–Barré syndrome is easily made by the absence of sensory involvement and the asymmetrical nature of the paralysis in poliomyelitis. Laboratory confirmation and distinction between the wild virus and vaccine strains is achieved by virus culture, neutralization and temperature marker tests.

## TREATMENT

Treatment is symptomatic. Bed rest is essential during the early course of the illness. Respiratory support with intermittent positive pressure respiration is required if the muscles of respiration are involved. Once the acute phase of the illness has subsided, occupational therapy, physiotherapy and occasionally surgery play an important role in patient rehabilitation.

## PREVENTION AND CONTROL

Immunization has dramatically decreased the prevalence of this disease worldwide. Trivalent oral poliovaccine (OPV) (active virus) is used (see Information box 1.2); occasionally, inactivated poliovirus vaccine is used intramuscularly.

# Coxsackievirus, echovirus and enterovirus infection

These viruses are spread by the faecal–oral route. They each have a number of different types and are responsible for a broad spectrum of disease involving the skin and mucous membranes, muscles, nerves, the heart (Table 1.26), and rarely other organs, such as the liver and pancreas.

## Skin and oropharyngeal disease

There is a vesicular eruption on the fauces, palate and uvula (herpangina). The lesions eventually evolve into

| Disease | Coxsackievirus A (types A$_1$–A$_{22}$, A$_{24}$) | Coxsackievirus B (types B$_1$–B$_6$) | Echovirus (types 1–9, 11–27, 29–33) | Enterovirus (types 68–71) |
|---|---|---|---|---|
| *Cutaneous and oropharyngeal* | | | | |
| Herpangina | +++ | + | + | |
| Hand, foot and mouth | +++ | + | | + |
| Erythematous rashes | + | + | +++ | |
| *Neurological* | | | | |
| Paralytic | + | | ± | + |
| Meningitis | ++ | ++ | +++ | + |
| Encephalitis | ++ | ++ | ± | + |
| *Cardiac* | | | | |
| Myocarditis and pericarditis | + | +++ | + | |
| *Muscle* | | | | |
| Myositis (Bornholm disease) | + | +++ | + | |

+++, often causes; ++, sometimes causes; +, rarely causes; ±, possibly causes.

**Table 1.26** Picornavirus infections (excluding poliovirus and rhinovirus).

aphthous ulcers. The illness is usually associated with fever and headache but is short-lived, recovery occurring within a few days.

### Hand, foot and mouth disease

Oral lesions are similar to those seen in herpangina but may be more extensive in the oropharynx. Vesicles and a maculopapular eruption also appear, typically on the palms of the hands and the soles of the feet, but also on other parts of the body. This infection commonly affects children; recovery occurs within a week.

### Neurological disease

Other enteroviruses in addition to poliovirus can cause a broad range of neurological disease, including meningitis, encephalitis, and a paralytic disease characteristic of poliomyelitis.

### Heart and muscle disease

Enteroviruses are an important cause of acute myocarditis and pericarditis, from which, in general, there is complete recovery. However, these viruses can also cause chronic congestive cardiomyopathy and, rarely, constrictive pericarditis.

Skeletal muscle involvement, particularly of the intercostal muscles, is an important feature of Bornholm disease, a febrile illness usually due to Coxsackievirus B. The pain may be of such an intensity as to mimic pleurisy or an acute abdomen. The infection affects both children and adults and may be complicated by meningitis or cardiac involvement.

## Rhinovirus infection

Rhinoviruses are responsible for the common cold (p. 652); peak incidence rates occur in the colder months, especially spring and autumn. There are multiple rhinovirus immunotypes, which makes vaccine control impracticable. In contrast to enteroviruses which replicate at 37°C, rhinoviruses grow at 33°C, the temperature of the upper respiratory tract, which explains the localized disease characteristic of common colds.

## REOVIRUS

## Reovirus infection

Reovirus infection occurs mainly in children, causing mild respiratory symptoms and diarrhoea. A few deaths have been reported following disseminated infection of brain, liver, heart and lungs.

## Rotavirus infection

Rotavirus (Latin *rota* = wheel) is so named because of its characteristic circular outline with radiating spokes. It is responsible worldwide for both sporadic cases and epidemics of diarrhoea, and is presently one of the most important causes of childhood diarrhoea. The prevalence

is higher during the winter months.

Other viruses associated with gastroenteritis are shown in Table 1.27.

Clinically the illness is characterized by vomiting, fever, diarrhoea, and the metabolic consequences of water and electrolyte loss. Histology of the jejunal mucosa in children shows shortening of the villi, with crypt hyperplasia and mononuclear cell infiltration of the lamina propria. Diagnosis can be established by ELISA for the detection of rotavirus antigen in faeces but this is rarely indicated clinically, since infection is self-limiting and there is no specific treatment.

Treatment is directed at overcoming the effects of water and electrolyte imbalance with adequate oral rehydration therapy and, when indicated, intravenous fluids. Antibiotics should not be prescribed.

Adults may become infected with rotavirus but symptoms are usually mild or absent. The virus may, however, cause outbreaks of diarrhoea in patients on geriatric wards.

Rotavirus vaccines are under evaluation. Live, attenuated, oral bovine rotavirus vaccines (RIT 4237 and WC3) are moderately effective in the industrialized world but less so in the developing world. Reassortant rotaviruses are being constructed by recombinant DNA technology that have an attenuated animal rotavirus 'backbone' but contain RNA inserts from human rotavirus in an attempt to improve immunogenicity.

## TOGAVIRUSES

These can be divided into the rubella virus and the arboviruses.

## Rubella

Rubella ('German measles') is caused by a spherical, enveloped fragile RNA virus that is easily killed by heat and ultraviolet light. While the disease can occur sporadically, epidemics are not uncommon. It has a worldwide distribution. Spread of the virus is via droplets; maximum infectivity occurs before and during the time the rash is present.

### CLINICAL FEATURES

The incubation period varies from 14 to 21 days, averaging 18 days. The clinical features are largely determined by age, with symptoms being mild or absent in children under 5 years of age. The peak incidence of the disease is at 15 years.

| Rotavirus (Groups A, B, C, D and E) |
| Enteric adenovirus (types 40 and 41) |
| Norwalk and related viruses |
| Calicivirus |
| Astrovirus |
| Parvovirus |
| Other small round viruses |

**Table 1.27**  Viruses associated with gastroenteritis.

During the prodrome the patient complains of malaise and fever. Mild conjunctivitis and lymphadenopathy may be present. The distribution of the lymphadenopathy is characteristic and involves the suboccipital, postauricular and posterior cervical groups of lymph nodes. Small petechial lesions on the soft palate (Forchheimer spots) are suggestive but not diagnostic. Splenomegaly may be present.

The eruptive or exanthematous phase usually occurs within the first 7 days of the initial symptoms. The rash first appears on the forehead and then spreads to involve the trunk and the limbs. It is pinkish-red, macular and discrete, although some of these lesions may coalesce. It usually fades by the second day and rarely persists beyond the third day after its appearance.

## COMPLICATIONS

Complications are rare; they include superadded pulmonary bacterial infection, arthralgia, haemorrhagic manifestations due to thrombocytopenia, encephalitis and the *congenital rubella syndrome*. Rubella affects the fetuses of 15–30% of all women who contract the infection during the first trimester of pregnancy. The incidence of congenital abnormalities diminishes in the second trimester and no ill-effects result from infection in the third trimester. Congenital rubella syndrome is characterized by the presence of fetal cardiac malformations, especially patent ductus arteriosus and ventricular septal defect, eye lesions, especially cataracts, microcephaly, mental retardation and deafness. The *expanded rubella syndrome* consists of the manifestations of the congenital rubella syndrome plus hepatosplenomegaly, myocarditis, interstitial pneumonia and metaphyseal bone lesions.

## DIAGNOSIS

The diagnosis may be suspected clinically but the laboratory diagnosis is essential to distinguish the illness from other virus infections (e.g. echovirus) and drug rashes. This is achieved by demonstrating a rising antibody titre (measured using the sensitive haemagglutination inhibition test) in two successive blood samples taken 14 days apart or by the detection of rubella-specific IgM. The virus can be cultured from throat swabs, urine and, in the case of intrauterine infection, the products of conception.

## TREATMENT

Treatment is symptomatic.

## PREVENTION

Prevention of rubella is important. Human immunoglobulin can decrease the symptoms of this already mild illness, but does not prevent the teratogenic effects. Several live attenuated rubella vaccines have been used with great success in preventing this illness and these have been successfully combined with the measles and mumps vaccine. The side-effects of vaccination have been dramatically decreased by using vaccines prepared in human embryonic fibroblast cultures (RA 27/3 vaccine). Use of the vaccine is contraindicated during pregnancy or if there is a likelihood of pregnancy within 3 months of immunization. Inadvertent use of the vaccine during pregnancy has not, however, revealed a risk af teratogenicity.

# Arbovirus (arthropod-borne) infection

Arboviruses are zoonotic viruses, with the possible exception of the O'nyong-nyong fever virus of which humans are the only known vertebrate hosts. They are transmitted through the bites of insects, especially mosquitoes and ticks. Over 385 viruses are classified as arboviruses. *Culex*, *Aedes* and *Anopheles* mosquitoes account for the transmission of the majority of these viruses.

Although most arbovirus diseases are generally mild, epidemics are frequent and when these occur the mortality is high. In general, the incubation period is less than 10 days. The illness tends to be biphasic and, as in other viral fevers, pyrexia, conjunctival suffusion, a rash, retro-orbital pain, myalgia and arthralgia are common. Lymphadenopathy is seen in dengue. Lifelong immunity to a particular virus is usual. In some of these viral fevers, haemorrhage is a feature (Table 1.28), although its pathogenesis is speculative. Increased vascular permeability, capillary fragility and DIC have been implicated. Encephalitis due to cerebral invasion may be prominent in some fevers.

### Alphaviruses

The 24 viruses of this group are all transmitted by mosquitoes; eight result in human disease. These viruses are globally distributed and tend to acquire their names from the location where they were first isolated (such as Ross River, Eastern Venezuelan, and Western encephalitis viruses) or by the local expression for a major symptom caused by the virus (such as chikungunya meaning 'chronic bleeding'). Infection is characterized by fever, skin rash, arthralgia, myalgia and sometimes encephalitis.

*Flavivirus*
Yellow fever (urban and sylvan)
Dengue haemorrhagic fever
Kyasanur Forest disease
Omsk haemorrhagic fever
Rift Valley fever

*Bunyavirus*
Congo–Crimean haemorrhagic fevers
Hantavirus infections

*Arenavirus*
Argentinian haemorrhagic fever
Bolivian haemorrhagic fever
Lassa fever
Epidemic haemorrhagic fever

*Picornavirus*
Acute haemorrhagic conjunctivitis (localized)

*Alphavirus*
Chikungunya

**Table 1.28** Viral infections associated with haemorrhagic manifestations.

**Flaviviruses**

There are 60 viruses in this group, some of which are transmitted by ticks and others by mosquitoes.

# Yellow fever

Yellow fever, caused by a flavivirus, results in an illness of widely varying severity. It is a disease confined to Africa and South America between latitudes 15°N and 15°S of the equator. For poorly understood reasons, yellow fever has not been reported from Asia, despite the fact that climatic conditions are suitable and the vector, *Aedes aegypti*, is common. The infection is transmitted in the wild by *A. africanus* in Africa and the *Haemagogus* species in South and Central America. These mosquitoes are responsible for maintaining infection in monkeys, which form the sylvan reservoir. *A. aegypti* and the *Haemagogus* species are responsible for transmission of this disease from monkeys to humans in Africa and South and Central America, respectively. Once infected, a mosquito remains so for its whole life.

## CLINICAL FEATURES

The incubation period varies from 3 to 6 days. When the infection is mild, the disease is indistinguishable from other viral fevers such as influenza or dengue. Classically, however, jaundice, proteinuria and haemorrhage occur.

Three phases in the illness are recognized. Initially the patient presents with a high fever of acute onset, usually 39–40°C, which then returns to normal in 4–5 days. During this time, headache is prominent. Retrobulbar pain, myalgia, arthralgia, a flushed face and suffused conjunctivae are common. Epigastric discomfort and vomiting are present when the illness is severe. Relative bradycardia (Faget's sign) is present from the second day of illness. The patient then makes an apparent recovery and feels well for several days. Following this 'phase of calm' the patient again develops increasing fever, deepening jaundice and hepatomegaly. Ecchymosis, bleeding from the gums, haematemesis and melaena may occur. Coma, which is usually a result of uraemia or haemorrhagic shock, occurs for a few hours preceding death. The mortality rate is up to 40% in severe cases.

## DIAGNOSIS

The diagnosis is established by isolating the virus (when possible) from blood during the first 3 days of illness, by demonstrating increasing neutralizing antibody titres, or by finding the typical histological lesions on liver biopsy. These include mid-zone necrosis, fatty degeneration and intracellular hyaline necrosis (Councilman bodies).

## TREATMENT

Treatment is supportive. Bed rest, analgesics, and maintenance of fluid and electrolyte balance are important.

## PREVENTION AND CONTROL

Yellow fever is an internationally notifiable disease. It is easily prevented using either the 17 d chick embryo vaccine, which is more popular, or the Dakar vaccine. Eradication of the breeding places of the vectors will help in decreasing the prevalence of the disease.

# Dengue

Dengue is caused by a flavivirus and is found mainly in Asia and Africa, although it has been reported from the USA as well. Four different antigenic varieties of the dengue virus are recognized and all are transmitted by the daytime-biting *A. aegypti*. Humans are infective during the first 3 days of the illness (viraemic stage). Mosquitoes become infective about 2 weeks after feeding on an infected individual, and remain so for the rest of their lives. The disease is usually endemic, but epidemics have been recorded. Immunity after the illness is partial.

## CLINICAL FEATURES

The incubation period varies from 5 to 6 days. Two clinical forms are recognized.

CLASSIC DENGUE FEVER is characterized by the abrupt onset of fever, malaise, headache, retrobulbar pain which worsens on eye movements, conjunctival suffusion and severe backache, which is a prominent symptom. Lymphadenopathy, petechiae on the soft palate and skin rashes may also occur. The rash is transient and morbilliform. It appears on the limbs and then spreads to involve the trunk. Desquamation occurs subsequently. Cough is uncommon. The fever subsides after 3–4 days, the temperature returns to normal for a couple of days, and then the fever returns, together with the features already mentioned, but milder. This biphasic or saddleback pattern is considered characteristic. Severe fatigue, a feeling of being unwell and depression are common for several weeks after the fever has subsided.

DENGUE HAEMORRHAGIC FEVER is a severe form of dengue fever and is believed to be the result of two or more sequential infections with different dengue serotypes. It is a disease of children and has been described almost exclusively in South East Asia. The disease has a mild start, often with symptoms of an upper respiratory tract infection. This is then followed by the abrupt onset of shock and haemorrhage into the skin and ear, epistaxis, haematemesis and melaena known as the dengue shock syndrome. Serum complement levels are depressed and there is laboratory evidence of a consumptive coagulopathy.

## DIAGNOSIS

Isolation of the dengue virus by tissue culture in sera obtained during the first few days of illness is diagnostic. Demonstration of rising antibody titres by neutralization (most specific), haemagglutination inhibition or complement-fixing antibodies in sequential serum samples is evidence of dengue virus infection.

**TREATMENT**
Treatment is symptomatic.

# Rift Valley fever

Rift Valley fever is primarily an acute febrile illness of livestock—sheep, goats and camels. It is found in southern and eastern Africa. The vector in East Africa is *Culex pipiens* and in southern Africa, *Aedes caballus*. Following an incubation period of 3–6 days, the patient has an acute febrile illness that is difficult to distinguish clinically from other viral fevers. The temperature pattern is usually biphasic. The initial febrile illness lasts 2–4 days and is followed by a remission and a second febrile episode. Complications are indicative of severe infection and include retinopathy, meningo-encephalitis, haemorrhagic manifestations and hepatic necrosis. Mortality approaches 50% in severe forms of the illness. Treatment is symptomatic.

# Japanese encephalitis

Japanese encephalitis is a mosquito-borne encephalitis caused by a flavivirus. It has been reported most frequently from the rice-growing countries of South East Asia and the Far East. *Culex tritaeniorhynchus* is the most important vector and feeds mainly on pigs as well as birds such as herons and sparrows. Humans are accidental hosts.

As with other viral infections, the clinical manifestations are variable. The onset is heralded by severe rigors. Fever, headache and malaise last from 1 to 6 days. Weight loss is prominent. In the acute encephalitic stage the fever is high (38–41°C), neck rigidity occurs and neurological signs such as altered consciousness, hemiparesis and convulsions develop. Mental deterioration occurs over a period of 3–4 days and culminates in coma. Mortality varies from 7 to 40% and is higher in children. Residual neurological defects such as deafness, emotional lability and hemiparesis occur in about 70% of patients who have had CNS involvement. Convalescence is prolonged. Antibody detection in serum and CSF by IgM capture ELISA is a useful rapid diagnostic test. An inactivated mouse brain vaccine is effective and available. Treatment is symptomatic.

# BUNYAVIRUSES

Bunyaviruses belong to a large family of more than 200 viruses, most of which are arthropod-borne.

## Congo-Crimean haemorrhagic fever

This is found mainly in Asia and Africa. The primary hosts are cattle and hare and the vectors are the Hyalomma ticks. Following an incubation period of 3–6 days there is an influenza-like illness with fever and haemorrhagic manifestations. The mortality is 10–50%.

# Hantaviruses

Hantaviruses are enzootic viruses of wild rodents which are spread by aerosolized excreta and not by insect vectors. The disease was first recognized in 1951 in United Nations soldiers in Korea. The most severe form of this infection is Korean haemorrhagic fever (or haemorrhagic fever with renal syndrome HFRS). This condition has a mortality of 5–10% and is characterized by fever, shock and haemorrhage followed by an oliguric phase. Milder forms of the disease are associated with related viruses e.g. Puumala virus, and may present as Nephropathia epidemica, an acute fever with renal involvement. This has been recognized for many years in Scandinavia (and recently in other European countries in people who have been in contact with bank voles). In the United States, a new Hantavirus (transmitted by the deer mouse) causes the acute respiratory distress syndromes (ARDS).

Diagnosis is made by an ELISA technique.

# ORTHOMYXOVIRUSES

## Influenza

Three types of influenza virus are recognized—A, B and C. The influenza A virus is a spherical or filamentous enveloped virus. Haemagglutinin, a surface glycopeptide, aids attachment of the virus to the wall of susceptible host cells at specific receptor sites. Cell penetration, probably by pinocytosis, and release of replicated viruses from the cell surface is effected by budding through the cell membrane or by the action of viral neuraminidase.

INFLUENZA A is generally responsible for pandemics and epidemics.

INFLUENZA B often causes smaller or localized and milder outbreaks, e.g. in camps or schools.

INFLUENZA C rarely produces disease in humans.

Antigenic shift (major antigenic change within an influenza A subtype) usually heralds the onset of a pandemic. This results from genetic recombination of the virus with an animal virus. Antigenic drift (minor changes in influenza A and B viruses) results from point mutations leading to amino acid changes in haemagglutinin and neuraminidase.

Sporadic cases of influenza and outbreaks among groups of people living in a confined environment are frequent. The incidence increases during the winter months, when crowding is common. Spread is mainly by droplet infection but fomites and direct contact have also been implicated.

The clinical features, diagnosis, treatment and prophylaxis of influenza are discussed on p. 656.

# PARAMYXOVIRUSES

These are a heterogeneous group of enveloped viruses of varying size that are responsible for parainfluenza, mumps, measles and other respiratory infections.

# Parainfluenza

Parainfluenza is caused by the parainfluenza viruses types I to IV, which have a worldwide distribution. Type IV has been identified only in the USA.

Parainfluenza is essentially a disease of children and presents with features similar to the common cold. When severe, a brassy cough with inspiratory stridor and features of laryngotracheobronchitis (croup) are present. Treatment is symptomatic with oxygen, humidification and sedation when required. The role of steroids is controversial.

# Measles (rubeola)

Measles is a highly communicable disease that occurs worldwide. With the introduction of aggressive immunization policies, the incidence of measles has fallen dramatically in the West, but it still remains one of the commonest childhood infections in the developing countries, where it is associated with a high morbidity and mortality. It is spread by droplet infection.

### CLINICAL FEATURES

The incubation period varies from 8 to 14 days. Two distinct phases of the disease can be recognized.

#### Typical measles

1 *The infectious pre-eruptive and catarrhal stage.* This is the stage of viraemia and viral dissemination. Malaise, fever, rhinorrhoea, cough, conjunctival suffusion and the pathognomonic Koplik's spots are present during this stage. Koplik's spots are small, greyish, irregular lesions surrounded by an erythematous base and are found in greatest numbers on the mucous membrane opposite the second molar tooth. They occur a day or two before the onset of the rash.
2 *The non-infectious eruptive or exanthematous stage.* This is characterized by the presence of a maculopapular rash that initially occurs on the face, chiefly the forehead, and then spreads rapidly to involve the rest of the body. At first the rash is discrete but later it may become confluent and patchy, especially on the face and neck. It fades in about 1 week and leaves behind a brownish discoloration with desquamation.

Although measles is a relatively mild disease in the healthy child, it carries a high mortality in the malnourished and in those who have other diseases. Complications are common in such individuals and include bacterial pneumonia, bronchitis, otitis media and gastroenteritis. Less commonly, myocarditis, hepatitis and encephalomyelitis may occur. The virus has also been implicated in the rare condition subacute sclerosing panencephalitis.

Maternal measles, unlike rubella, does not cause congenital fetal abnormalities. It is, however, associated with spontaneous abortions and premature delivery.

#### Atypical measles

Atypical measles is a severe illness that usually occurs in individuals who have previously received an inactivated vaccine (now withdrawn) and are exposed to wild measles virus. The high fever (>40°C), myalgia, abdominal pain and cough are followed by vesicles, petechiae and purpura. Skin lesions may be mistaken for scarlet fever, meningococcaemia or varicella. Pneumonia invariably occurs and the pulmonary infiltrates may persist for years.

### DIAGNOSIS

Immunofluorescence, virus culture and serological tests (complement fixation test (CFT), haemagglutination inhibition tests) are used to confirm the diagnosis.

### TREATMENT

Treatment is symptomatic. Antibiotics are indicated only if secondary bacterial infection occurs.

### PREVENTION

A previous attack of measles confers a high degree of immunity and second attacks are uncommon.

Human immunoglobulin 0.25 ml kg$^{-1}$ given within 5 days of exposure effectively aborts an attack of measles. It is indicated for previously unimmunized children below 3 years of age, during pregnancy, and in those with debilitating disease.

Active immunization involves a single dose of 0.5 ml live attenuated measles vaccine given subcutaneously (see Information box 1.2). Children are now immunized with the combined mumps, measles, rubella vaccine (MMR).

# Mumps

Mumps is the result of infection with a paramyxovirus. It is spread by droplet infection, by direct contact or through fomites. Humans are the only known natural hosts. The peak period of infectivity is 2–3 days before the onset of the parotitis and for 3 days afterwards.

### CLINICAL FEATURES

The incubation period averages 18 days. Although no age is exempt, it is primarily a disease of school-aged children and young adults; it is uncommon before the age of 2 years. The prodromal symptoms are non-specific and include fever, malaise, headache and anorexia. This is usually followed by severe pain over the parotid glands, with either unilateral or bilateral parotid swelling. The enlarged parotid glands obscure the angle of the mandible and may elevate the ear lobe, which does not occur in cervical lymph node enlargement. Trismus due to pain is common at this stage. Submandibular gland involvement occurs less frequently.

### COMPLICATIONS

CNS involvement is the commonest extra-salivary-gland manifestation of mumps. Clinical meningitis occurs in 5% of all infected patients, and 30% of patients with CNS involvement have no evidence of parotid gland involvement.

Epididymo-orchitis develops in about one-third of

patients who develop mumps after puberty. Bilateral testicular involvement results in sterility in only a small percentage of these patients.

Pancreatitis, oophoritis, myocarditis, mastitis, hepatitis and polyarthritis may also occur.

### DIAGNOSIS

The diagnosis of mumps is on the basis of the clinical features. In doubtful cases, serological demonstration of a fourfold rise in antibodies detected by complement fixation or indirect haemagglutination or neutralization tests on acute and convalescent sera is diagnostic. Virus can be isolated in cell culture from saliva, throat swab, urine and CSF and identified by immunofluorescence or haemadsorption.

### TREATMENT

Treatment is symptomatic. Attention should be given to adequate nutrition and mouth care. Analgesics should be used to relieve pain. The role of steroids in the treatment of mumps orchitis is controversial.

### PREVENTION

Live attenuated mumps virus vaccine given as a single 0.5 ml intramuscular dose can prevent the disease in children over the age of 1 year. This vaccine should not be used in children below this age as it may be inhibited by maternally acquired antibodies. Vaccination is contraindicated in immunosuppressed individuals, during pregnancy, or in those with severe febrile illnesses, because the live attenuated vaccine may cause disease.

## Respiratory syncytial virus infection

Respiratory syncytial virus is a paramyxovirus that causes many respiratory infections in epidemics each winter. It is a common cause of bronchiolitis in infants, which is complicated by pneumonia in approximately 10% of cases. Immunity is short-lived and consequently reinfection can occur throughout life.

### DIAGNOSIS

Immunofluorescence, virus culture and serology are the usual ways of confirming the diagnosis.

### TREATMENT

Generally supportive, but aerosolized ribavirin can be given to severe cases. No vaccine is available.

## RHABDOVIRUSES

## Rabies

Rabies is a major problem in some countries and carries a high mortality.

The rabies virus is bullet-shaped and has spike-like structures arising from its surface containing glycoproteins that cause the host to produce neutralizing, haemagglutination-inhibiting antibodies. The virus has a marked affinity for nervous tissue and the salivary glands. It exists in two major epidemiological settings:

1 *Urban rabies*, which is most frequently transmitted to humans through rabid dogs and, less frequently, cats.
2 *Sylvan (wild) rabies*, which is maintained in the wild by a host of animal reservoirs such as foxes, skunks, jackals, mongooses and bats.

With the exception of Australia, New Zealand and the Antarctic, human rabies has been reported from all continents. Transmission is through the bite of an infected animal. However, the percentage of rabid bites leading to clinical disease ranges from 10% (on the legs) to 80% (on the head). Rabies has been transferred by corneal grafting but anecdotal reports of human-to-human spread by kissing, biting and sexual intercourse have not been confirmed. Rabid animals can also transmit the disease by licking abraded skin or mucosa. Rarely, airborne droplet infection occurs from exposure to infected bats in caves or in laboratory workers handling concentrated virus.

Having entered the human body, the virus replicates in the muscle cells near the entry wound. It penetrates the nerve endings and travels in the axoplasm to the spinal cord and brain. In the CNS the virus again proliferates before spreading to the salivary glands, lungs, kidneys and other organs via the autonomic nerves.

### CLINICAL FEATURES

The incubation period is variable and may range from a few weeks to several years; on average it is 1–3 months. In general, bites on the head, face and neck have a shorter incubation period than those elsewhere. In humans, two distinct clinical varieties of rabies are recognized:

1 'Furious rabies'—the classical variety
2 'Dumb rabies'—the paralytic variety

**Furious rabies**

The only characteristic feature in the prodromal period is the presence of pain and tingling at the site of the initial wound. Fever, malaise and headache are also present. About 10 days later, marked anxiety and agitation or depressive features develop. Hallucinations, bizarre behaviour and paralysis may also occur. Hyperexcitability, the hallmark of this form of rabies, is precipitated by auditory or visual stimuli. Hydrophobia (fear of water) is present in 50% of patients and is due to severe pharyngeal spasms on attempting to eat or drink. Aerophobia (fear of air) is considered pathognomonic of rabies. Examination reveals hyperreflexia, spasticity, and evidence of sympathetic overactivity indicated by pupillary dilatation and diaphoresis.

The patient goes on to develop convulsions, respiratory paralysis and cardiac arrhythmias. Death usually occurs in 10–14 days.

**Dumb rabies**

Dumb rabies, or paralytic rabies, presents with a symmetrical ascending paralysis resembling the Guillain–Barré syndrome. This variety of rabies commonly occurs after bites from rabid bats.

There have been only two recorded cases of survival

from clinical rabies; with these exceptions, the disease has been uniformly fatal.

### DIAGNOSIS

The diagnosis of rabies is generally made clinically. Recently, fluorescent antibody has been used to detect rabies antigen in corneal impressions or in salivary secretions; this is a useful test. The classical Negri bodies are detected at post mortem in 90% of all patients with rabies; these are eosinophilic, cytoplasmic, ovoid bodies, 2–10 nm in diameter, seen in greatest numbers in the cells of the hippocampus and the cerebellum.

### TREATMENT

Once the disease is established, therapy is symptomatic. The patient should be nursed in a quiet, darkened room. Nutritional, respiratory and cardiovascular support may be necessary.

Drugs such as morphine, diazepam and chlorpromazine should be used liberally in patients who are excitable.

### PREVENTION

The vaccine is the human diploid cell strain vaccine (HDCSV).

#### Postexposure prophylaxis

Five 1.0 ml doses of HDCSV should be given intramuscularly: the first dose is given on day 0 and is followed by injections on days 3, 7, 14 and 28. Reactions to the vaccine is uncommon. The wound should be carefully cleaned with soap and water, adequately debrided and left open. Antirabies serum injected locally around the site of the wound may be helpful.

#### Pre-exposure prophylaxis

This is given to individuals with a high risk of contracting rabies, e.g. laboratory workers, animal handlers and veterinarians. HDCSV 1.0 ml intramuscularly on days 0, 7 and 21 should provide effective immunity. Vaccines of nervous-tissue origin are still used in some parts of the world. These, however, are associated with significant side-effects and are best avoided if HDCSV is available.

## RETROVIRUSES

Retroviruses (Table 1.29) are distinguished from other RNA viruses by their ability to replicate through a DNA

| Subfamily | Virus | Disease |
|-----------|-------|---------|
| Lentivirus | HIV-1 | AIDS |
|  | HIV-2 | AIDS |
| *Oncovirus* | HTLV-1[a] | Adult T-cell leukaemic lymphoma |
|  |  | Tropical spastic paraparesis |
|  | HTLV-2 | None known |

[a]HTLV, human T-cell leukaemia virus.

**Table 1.29** Human lymphotropic retroviruses.

intermediate using an enzyme, reverse transcriptase. HIV-1 and the related virus HIV-2 are further classified as lentiviruses ('slow' viruses) because of their slowly progressive clinical effects.

HIV-1 and HIV-2 are discussed on p. 97.

HTLV-1 causes tropical spastic paraparesis (see p. 894).

## ARENAVIRUSES

Arenaviruses are pleomorphic, round or oval viruses with diameters ranging from 50 to 300 nm. The virion surface has club-shaped projections, and the virus itself contains a variable number of characteristic electron-dense granules that represent residual, non-functional host ribosomes. The prototype virus of this group is lymphocytic choriomeningitis viruses, which is a natural infection of mice. Arenaviruses are also responsible for Argentinian and Bolivian haemorrhagic fevers and Lassa fever.

## Lassa fever

This illness was first documented in the town of Lassa, Nigeria, in 1969 and is confined to sub-Saharan West Africa (Nigeria, Liberia and Sierra Leone). The multimammate rat, *Mastomys natalensis*, is known to be the reservoir. Humans are infected by ingesting foods contaminated by rat urine or saliva containing the virus. Direct inoculation is also a common mode of spread of this disease.

### CLINICAL FEATURES

The incubation period varies from 7 to 18 days. The disease is insidious in onset and is characterized by fever, myalgia, severe backache, malaise and headache. A transient maculopapular rash may be present. Sore throat and lymphadenopathy occur in over 50% of patients. In severe cases epistaxis and gastrointestinal bleeding may occur, hence the classification of Lassa fever as a viral haemorrhagic fever. The fever usually lasts from 1 to 3 weeks and recovery within 1 month of the onset of illness is usual. However, death occurs in 15–20% of hospitalized patients, usually from irreversible hypovolaemic shock.

### DIAGNOSIS

The diagnosis is established by serial serological tests (including the Lassa-specific IgM titre) or by culturing the virus from the throat, serum or urine.

### TREATMENT

Treatment is supportive and, in addition, clinical benefit and reduction in mortality can be achieved with ribavirin therapy.

In non-endemic countries, strict isolation procedures should be used, the patient ideally being nursed in a flexible-film isolator. Specialized units for the management of Lassa fever and other haemorrhagic fevers have been established in the UK.

## Lymphocytic choriomeningitis (LCM)

This infection is a zoonosis, the natural reservoir of the LCM virus being the house mouse. Infection is characterized by:

NON-NERVOUS SYSTEM ILLNESS, with fever, malaise, myalgia, headache, arthralgia and vomiting.

ASEPTIC MENINGITIS in addition to the above symptoms. Occasionally, a more severe form occurs, with encephalitis leading to disturbance of consciousness.

This illness is generally self-limiting and requires no specific treatment.

## MARBURG VIRUS DISEASE AND EBOLA VIRUS DISEASE

These severe, haemorrhagic, febrile illnesses are discussed together because their clinical manifestations are similar. The diseases are named after Marburg in Germany and the Ebola river region in the Sudan and Zaire where these viruses were first isolated. The natural reservoir for these viruses has not been identified and the precise mode of spread from one individual to another has not been elucidated.

The illness is characterized by the acute onset of severe headache, severe myalgia and high fever, followed by prostration. On about the fifth day of illness a non-pruritic maculopapular rash develops on the face and then spreads to the rest of the body. Diarrhoea is profuse and is associated with abdominal cramps and vomiting. Haematemesis, melaena or haemoptysis may occur between the seventh and sixteenth day. Hepatosplenomegaly and facial oedema are usually present. In Ebola virus disease, chest pain and a dry cough are prominent symptoms.

Treatment is symptomatic. Convalescent human serum appears to decrease the severity of the attack.

## POSTVIRAL/CHRONIC FATIGUE SYNDROME (see p. 963)

Viral illnesses have been implicated aetiologically, including those due to EBV, Coxsackie B viruses, echoviruses, CMV and hepatitis A virus. Non-viral causes such as allergy to Candida spp. have also been proposed.

The proportion of patients with 'organic' diagnoses remains uncertain. Recent studies suggest that two-thirds of patients with a symptom duration of more than 6 months have an underlying psychiatric disorder.

# Fungal infections

Morphologically, fungi can be grouped into two major categories:
1 Yeasts, which reproduce by budding
2 Moulds, which grow by branching and longitudinal extensions of hyphae

Dimorphic fungi are those that behave as yeasts in the host but as moulds *in vitro*, e.g. *Histoplasma* and *Sporothrix*. Despite the fact that fungi are ubiquitous, systemic fungal infections are uncommon. Fungal infections are transmitted by inhalation of spores or by contact with the skin.

Diseases are usually divided into:
- Systemic
- Subcutaneous
- Superficial

Systemic mycoses are unusual, but opportunistic mycoses can cause disease in immunocompromised patients. Fungi do not produce endotoxin, but exotoxin, e.g. aflatoxin, production has been documented *in vitro*. Fungi may also produce allergic pulmonary disease (see p. 691).

In general, human fungal infections are indolent and respond poorly to treatment. Some fungi such as *Candida albicans* are human commensals.

# Systemic fungal infections

## Histoplasmosis

Histoplasmosis is caused by *Histoplasma capsulatum*, a non-encapsulated, dimorphic fungus. Spores can survive in moist soil for several years, particularly when it is enriched by bird and bat droppings. Histoplasmosis occurs worldwide and is commonly seen in Ohio and the Mississippi river valley. Transmission is mainly by inhalation of the spores.

### CLINICAL FEATURES
Figure 1.24 summarizes the pathogenesis, main clinical forms and sequelae of *Histoplasma* infection.

PRIMARY PULMONARY HISTOPLASMOSIS is usually asymptomatic. The only evidence of infection is conversion of a histoplasmin skin test from negative to positive, and radiological features similar to those seen with the Ghon primary complex of tuberculosis (see p. 683). Calcification in the lungs, spleen and liver occurs in patients from areas of high endemicity. When symptomatic, primary pulmonary histoplasmosis generally presents as a mild influenza-like illness, with fever, chills, myalgia and cough. The systemic symptoms are pronounced in severe disease.

Complications such as atelectasis, secondary bacterial pneumonia, pleural effusions, erythema nodosum and erythema multiforme may also occur.

CHRONIC PULMONARY HISTOPLASMOSIS is clinically indistinguishable from pulmonary tuberculosis (see p. 683). It is usually seen in white males over the age of 50 years. Radiologically, pulmonary cavities, infiltrates and characteristic fibrous streaking from the periphery towards the hilum are seen.

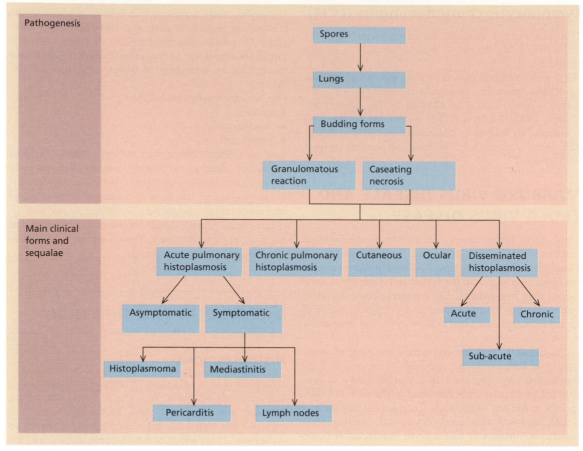

**Fig. 1.24**  Histoplasma infection—summary of pathogenesis, main clinical forms and sequelae.

DISSEMINATED HISTOPLASMOSIS resembles disseminated tuberculosis clinically. Fever, lymphadenopathy, hepatosplenomegaly, weight loss, leucopenia and thrombocytopenia are common. Rarely, features of meningitis, hepatitis, Addison's disease, endocarditis and peritonitis may dominate the clinical picture.

### DIAGNOSIS

Definitive diagnosis is possible only by culturing the fungi or by demonstrating them on histological sections. The histoplasmin skin test is usually positive.

Antibodies usually develop within 3 weeks of the onset of illness and are best detected by the complement-fixation test. Titres above 1 : 32 are suggestive of *Histoplasma* infection. Agar gel diffusion and latex agglutination antibody tests may also be helpful.

### TREATMENT

Only severe acute pulmonary histoplasmosis, chronic histoplasmosis and acute disseminated histoplasmosis require therapy. Intravenous amphotericin 0.5–0.6 mg kg$^{-1}$ daily or 1.0–1.2 mg kg$^{-1}$ on alternate days for 10 weeks is the mainstay of therapy. The less toxic antifungal agent ketoconazole is effective, as are the newer agents itraconazole and fluconazole. Surgical excision of histoplasmomas (pulmonary granuloma due to *H. capsulatum*) or chronic cavitatory lung lesions and release of adhesions following mediastinitis is often required.

## African histoplasmosis

African histoplasmosis is caused by *Histoplasma duboisii*, the spores of which are larger than those of *H. capsulatum*. Skin lesions, e.g. abscesses, nodules, lymph node involvement and lytic bone lesions are prominent. Pulmonary lesions do not occur. Treatment is similar to that for *H. capsulatum* infection.

## Aspergillosis

Aspergillosis is caused by several species of dimorphic fungi of the genus *Aspergillus*. Of these, *A. fumigatus* is the commonest cause of disease in humans, although *A. flavus* and *A. niger* have also been implicated as pathogens. These fungi are ubiquitous in the environment and are commonly found on decaying leaves and trees. Humans are infected by inhalation of the spores. Disease manifestation depends on the dose of the spores inhaled as well as the immune response of the host. Three major forms of the disease are recognized:

1 *Bronchopulmonary allergic aspergillosis* (see p. 691), with symptoms suggestive of bronchial asthma.
2 *Aspergilloma* (see p. 692), sometimes referred to as a pulmonary mycetoma.
3 *Fulminant disease*, which occurs in immunosuppressed patients, presenting as acute pneumonia, meningitis or an intracerebral abscess, lytic bone lesions, and granulomatous lesions in the liver; less commonly endocarditis, paranasal *Aspergillus* granuloma or keratitis may occur. Urgent treatment with intravenous amphotericin is required.

The diagnosis and treatment are described in more detail on p. 692.

# Cryptococcosis

Cryptococcosis is caused by the yeast-like fungus, *Cryptococcus neoformans*. It has a worldwide distribution and appears to be spread by birds, especially pigeons, in their droppings. The spores gain entry into the body through the respiratory tract, where they elicit a granulomatous reaction. Pulmonary symptoms are, however, uncommon and meningitis, which is clinically indistinguishable from bacterial meningitis, is the usual mode of presentation.

Lung cavitation, hilar lymphadenopathy, pleural effusions and occasionally pulmonary fibrosis occur. Less commonly, the skin and bones are involved.

## DIAGNOSIS

This is established by demonstrating the organisms in appropriately stained tissue sections. A positive latex cryptococcal agglutinin test performed on the CSF is diagnostic of cryptococcosis.

## TREATMENT

Amphotericin (0.3–0.5 mg kg$^{-1}$ daily i.v.) alone or in combination with flucytosine (100–200 mg kg$^{-1}$ daily) has reduced the mortality of this once always fatal condition. Therapy should be continued for 3 months if meningitis is present. Fluconazole has greater CSF penetration and is likely to become the treatment of choice.

# Coccidioidomycosis

Coccidioidomycosis is caused by the non-budding spherical form (spherule) of *Coccidioides immitis*. This is a soil saprophyte and is found in the southern USA, Central America and parts of South America.

Humans are infected by inhalation of the thick-walled barrel-shaped spores called arthrospores. Occasionally epidemics of coccidioidomycosis have been documented following dust storms.

## CLINICAL FEATURES

The majority of patients are asymptomatic. Infection is detected by the conversion of a skin test using either coccidioidin (extract from a culture of mycelial growth of *C. immitis*) or spherulin (the soluble fraction from a culture of *C. immitis* spherules) from negative to positive.

Acute pulmonary coccidioidomycosis presents, after an incubation period of about 10 days, with fever, malaise, cough and expectoration. Erythema nodosum, erythema multiforme, phlyctenular conjunctivitis and, less commonly, pleural effusions may occur. Complete recovery is usual.

Pulmonary cavitation with haemoptysis, pulmonary fibrosis, meningitis, lytic bone lesions, hepatosplenomegaly, and skin ulcers and abscesses may occur in severe disease.

## DIAGNOSIS

Because of the high infectivity of this fungus, and consequent risk to laboratory personnel, serological tests (rather than culture of the organism) are widely used for diagnosis. These include the highly specific latex agglutination and precipitin tests. A positive complement-fixation test performed on the CSF is diagnostic of coccidioidomycosis meningitis.

## TREATMENT

Mild pulmonary infections are self-limiting and require no treatment, but progressive and disseminated disease requires urgent therapy. Amphotericin is the drug of choice. Surgical excision of cavitatory pulmonary lesions or localized bone lesions may be necessary. For meningitis, intrathecal amphotericin may be required; the role of steroids remains controversial. Ketoconazole or miconazole can be of value.

# Blastomycosis

Blastomycosis is a systemic infection caused by the biphasic fungus *Blastomyces dermatitidis*. Although initially believed to be confined to certain parts of North America, it has recently been reported in Canada, Africa, Israel, Eastern Europe and Saudi Arabia.

## CLINICAL FEATURES

Blastomycosis primarily involves the skin, where it presents as non-itchy papular lesions that later develop into ulcers with red verrucous margins. The ulcers are initially confined to the exposed parts of the body but later involve the unexposed parts as well. Atrophy and scarring may occur. Pulmonary involvement presents as a solitary lesion resembling a malignancy or gives rise to radiological features similar to the primary complex of tuberculosis. Systemic symptoms such as fever, malaise, cough and weight loss are usually present. Bone lesions are common and present as painful swellings.

## DIAGNOSIS

The diagnosis is confirmed by demonstrating the organism in histological sections or by culture. Serology is not useful because of the marked cross-reactivity of antibodies to *Blastomyces* with *Histoplasma*.

**TREATMENT**
The drug of choice is amphotericin.

## Invasive zygomycosis

Invasive zygomycosis, mucormycosis, is rare and is caused by several fungi, including *Mucor*, *Rhizopus* and *Absidia*. It occurs in ill patients. The hallmark of the disease is vascular invasion with marked haemorrhagic necrosis.

Rhinocerebral mucormycosis is the commonest form. Nasal stuffiness, facial pain and oedema, and necrotic, black nasal turbinates are characteristic. It is rare and is mainly seen in diabetics with ketoacidosis. Other forms include pulmonary and disseminated infection (immunosuppressed), gastrointestinal infection (in malnutrition) and cutaneous involvement (in burns). Treatment is with amphotericin. This condition is invariably fatal if left untreated.

## CANDIDIASIS

Candidiasis is the most common fungal infection in humans and is caused by *Candida albicans*. *Candida* are small asexual fungi. All the species that are pathogenic to humans are normal oropharyngeal and gastrointestinal commensals. Candidiasis is found worldwide.

**CLINICAL FEATURES**
Practically any organ in the body can be invaded by *Candida*, but vaginal infection and oral thrush (see p. 180) are the commonest forms. This latter is seen in the very young, in the elderly, following antibiotic therapy and in those who are immunosuppressed. Candidal oesophagitis may present with painful dysphagia. Cutaneous candidiasis (see p. 1017) typically occurs in intertriginous areas. It is also an important cause of paronychia. Balanitis and vaginal infection are also common (see p. 95).

CHRONIC MUCOCUTANEOUS CANDIDIASIS is a rare manifestation, usually occurring in children, and is associated with a T-cell defect. It presents with hyperkeratotic plaque-like lesions on the skin, especially the face, and on the finger-nails. It is associated with several endocrinopathies, including hypothyroidism and hypoparathyroidism. Less commonly dissemination of candidiasis may lead to haematogenous spread, with meningitis, pulmonary involvement, endocarditis or osteomyelitis.

**DIAGNOSIS**
The fungi can be demonstrated in scrapings from infected lesions or in tissue secretions.

**TREATMENT**
This varies depending on the site and severity of infection. Oral lesions respond to nystatin, oral amphotericin or miconazole. For more severe systemic infections, parenteral therapy with amphotericin or ketoconazole, or oral therapy with flucytosine 50–75 mg kg$^{-1}$ daily for 2–3 weeks may be required.

# Local fungal infections

## Dermatophytosis

Dermatophytoses are chronic fungal infections of keratinous structures such as the skin, hair or nails (see p. 1017). *Trichophyton*, *Microsporum* and *Epidermophyton* are traditionally referred to as dermatophytes, although other fungi such as *Candida* can also infect keratinous structures.

## Sporotrichosis

Sporotrichosis is due to the saprophytic fungus *Sporothrix schenckii*, which is found worldwide. Infection usually follows cutaneous inoculation, at the site of which a reddish, non-tender, maculopapular lesion, referred to as 'plaque sporotrichosis' develops. Pulmonary involvement and disseminated disease rarely occur.

**TREATMENT**
Treatment with saturated potassium iodide (10–12 ml daily orally for adults) is curative in the cutaneous form. Amphotericin or miconazole is required for systemic infection.

## Subcutaneous zygomycosis

Subcutaneous zygomycosis is caused by several filamentous fungi of the *Basidiobolus* genus. The disease usually remains confined to the subcutaneous tissues and muscle fascia. It presents as a brawny, woody infiltration involving the limbs, neck and trunk. Less commonly, the pharyngeal and orbital regions may be affected.

Treatment is with saturated potassium iodide solution given orally.

## Chromomycosis

Chromomycosis (chromoblastomycosis) is caused by fungi of the genus *Philalophora* and *Cladosporium carrionii*. It presents initially as a small papule, usually at the site of a previous injury. This persists for several months before ulcerating. The lesion later becomes warty and encrusted and gradually spreads. Satellite lesions may be present. Itching is frequent. The drug of choice is flucytosine in combination with amphotericin in small doses.

## Rhinosporidiosis

Rhinosporidiosis is caused by *Rhinosporidium seeberi*. This organism has not been cultured. Although recognized worldwide, it is seen mainly in South India and Sri Lanka. Mucosal lesions present as polyps that are friable and vascular; the nose, nasopharynx and soft palate are most frequently involved. Haematogenous dissemination may occur. Treatment is surgical excision and cautery.

## Protozoal infections

## Blood and tissue infection

### LEISHMANIASIS

Three clinical entities caused by *Leishmania* have been described:

1 Visceral leishmaniasis (kala-azar)
2 Cutaneous leishmaniasis of the New World
3 Cutaneous leishmaniasis of the Old World

The geographical distribution is shown in Fig. 1.25.

The life-cycle of the parasite involves two stages:

1 The *amastigote* (Leishman–Donovan body) occurs in vertebrate hosts such as humans, dogs or rodents. The parasites infect macrophages and reticuloendothelial cells and multiply until the cells rupture, releasing the organisms into the circulation. When the female sandfly (*Phlebotomus* or *Lutzomyia*) bites an infected host, it draws blood containing the amastigotes.

2 In the sandfly the parasites develop into the infective *promastigotes*, which move to the salivary glands in about 10 days.

The cycle is completed by the sandfly biting another vertebrate.

The presentation in humans is dependent on the patient's cellular immunity as well as the parasite species.

In the *kala-azar syndrome* there is little or no immune response and the reticuloendothelial system is laden with amastigote-laden histiocytes. In subjects with an increased immune response, hepatic and lymph node granulomas are found and either there are no clinical symptoms or a localized lesion is seen.

*Inapparent infection* is common in endemic areas and is recognized by the high incidence of leishmanin-positive skin tests. There is usually no previous history of skin ulceration or systemic disease. Infection is eradicated by the immune system and the subject is left with permanent immunity to that species of *Leishmania*.

### Visceral leishmaniasis (kala-azar)

Visceral leishmaniasis is caused by *L. donovani* and occurs in Asia, the Mediterranean, South America and Africa. Dogs, foxes, jackals and wild rodents can be reservoirs, but in India humans are the only known reservoir. Primary skin lesions (leishmaniomas) are usually small, but can be found at the site of the sandfly bite.

The disease usually affects young people. The incubation period may be months or years. The onset is abrupt or insidious. The patient feels remarkably well despite many symptoms and signs. Fever occurs and may

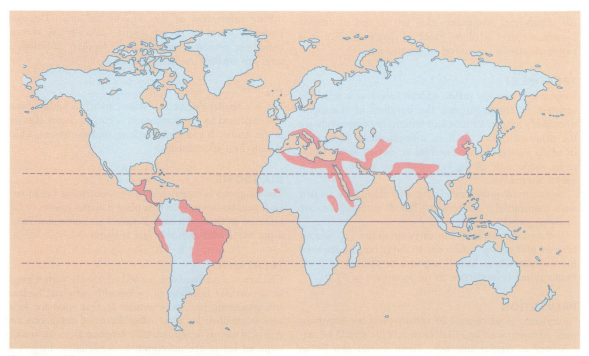

**Fig. 1.25** Leishmaniasis—geographical distribution.

exhibit a characteristic biphasic pattern. Cough is frequent and diarrhoea may occur. The skin is dry and rough and with time becomes pigmented. Splenic enlargement may be massive and hypersplenism is chiefly responsible for the pancytopenia seen. Epistaxis may occur due to thrombocytopenia. Hepatomegaly is less prominent than the splenomegaly. In African kala-azar, warty skin eruptions and lymphadenopathy also occur. If left untreated, death occurs within 3 years in the majority of patients and is due to pulmonary or gastrointestinal superinfection, to which these patients are predisposed.

INFANTILE KALA-AZAR is seen chiefly in the Mediterranean region and is a disease of children below the age of 5 years.

POST-KALA-AZAR DERMAL LEISHMANIASIS (PKDL) occurs 1–2 years after successful treatment for visceral leishmaniasis in a small proportion of patients in India and less often in Africa. It is characterized by macular, erythematous lesions and pale pink nodules on the face.

### INVESTIGATION AND DIAGNOSIS

CHARACTERISTIC LEISHMAN–DONOVAN BODIES may be demonstrated in buffy coat preparations of blood or in bone-marrow smears or lymph node, liver or spleen aspirates.

CULTURE. The organism can be cultured in the Nicolle–Novy–McNeal culture medium.

COMPLEMENT-FIXING ANTIBODIES may be detected by indirect immunofluorescence, ELISA and haemagglutination.

FORMOL GEL TEST is positive owing to hyperglobulinaemia.

An intradermal leishmanin skin test (a test of delayed hypersensitivity) is of no value in diagnosis since it is negative early in the course of the disease.

### TREATMENT

Response to therapy varies. African kala-azar is relatively resistant to treatment and the duration of therapy is necessarily longer. Pentavalent antimony compounds are the drugs of choice. Sodium stibogluconate 30 mg kg$^{-1}$ in adults should be continued for at least 40 days. Meglumine antimonate 50 mg kg$^{-1}$ daily for 10–30 days is a useful alternative.

Intercurrent pulmonary infections should be treated with appropriate antibiotics. Blood transfusions are rarely required.

Intravenous amphotericin or pentamidine (up to four courses of 3 mg kg$^{-1}$ daily for 10 days) may be required for patients whose initial response to therapy is poor. Pentamidine is ineffective in the treatment of PKDL.

### PREVENTION

In endemic areas control of vectors plays an important part. Spraying with an effective insecticide should be carried out at regular intervals. There should also be an attempt to decrease the reservoir of infection by destroying infected animals and treating infected humans early.

# Cutaneous leishmaniasis of the New World (American cutaneous leishmaniasis)

Four forms are recognized.

### Chiclero's ulcer

This is caused by *L. mexicana* and is found in Mexico, Guatemala, Brazil, Venezuela and Panama. It occurs on the exposed parts of the body, and runs a benign course with spontaneous healing within 6 months. However, infection of the pinna (chiclero's ear) results in gross destruction of the external ear. A lesion at this site may persist for over 20 years.

### Espundia (mucocutaneous leishmaniasis)

This is caused by *L. braziliensis* and is found in Brazil, Ecuador, Bolivia, Uruguay and northern Argentina. Initially painful, itchy nodules appear on the lower limbs, and then ulcerate. Lymphangitis is usual. Healing occurs spontaneously in 6 months.

Several years later, secondary lesions develop at mucocutaneous junctions such as the nasopharynx. There is evidence of nasal obstruction, ulceration, septal perforation and destruction of the nasal cartilages. Death usually occurs from secondary bacterial infection or aspiration.

### Diffuse cutaneous leishmaniasis

This is caused by *L. amazonensis* and is characterized by diffuse infiltration of the skin by Leishman–Donovan bodies. Visceral lesions are absent. Clinically this chronic condition resembles lepromatous leprosy, although it does not involve the nasal septum.

### Uta

Uta is a similar disease to diffuse cutaneous leishmaniasis and is caused by *L. peruviana*. It occurs in cooler climates in the Andes. It produces single or multiple ulcers, which usually heal spontaneously.

### DIAGNOSIS

The diagnosis is established by demonstrating Leishman–Donovan bodies in spleen or bone marrow smears or histological sections of tissues. Parasites are scanty and hence a positive leishmanin skin test is useful.

### TREATMENT

Chiclero's ulcer has been treated effectively with a single intramuscular injection of cycloguanil pamoate. Sodium stibogluconate in a dose similar to that used for kala-azar is effective for most other forms of cutaneous and mucocutaneous leishmaniasis. Amphotericin is usually required for severe infections. Reconstructive surgery of any deformity is an important part of therapy.

## Cutaneous leishmaniasis of the Old World

*L. major* and *L. tropica* are found in the former USSR, the Middle East, around the Mediterranean and sub-Sahara and west Africa. The reservoir for *L. major* is infected desert rodents whilst *L. tropica* has an urban distribution with dogs and humans as reservoirs. *L. aethiopica* is found in the highlands of Ethiopia and Kenya and the animal reservoir is often the hyrax. The vectors are usually the phlebotomus sandfly.

### CLINICAL FEATURES

Single or multiple papules occur on exposed areas within 2 weeks to 3 months of infection. These enlarge and ulcerate, often with an overlying crust. The lesions heal spontaneously with scarring but may take years. *Leishmaniasis recidivans*, which is characterized by features resembling lupus vulgaris, describes the lesions seen many years after the healing of the primary lesions.

### TREATMENT

Cutaneous lesions respond to application of direct heat (40°C). Pentavalent antimony compounds provide the mainstay of therapy. In patients with indolent lesions, levamisole has been used with some success.

## TRYPANOSOMIASIS

## African trypanosomiasis

*African trypanosomiasis* (sleeping sickness) follows the bite of the tsetse fly and is caused by *Trypanosoma brucei*.

*T. brucei* is found in West and Central Africa between latitudes 20°N and 20°S (Fig. 1.26). Two clinical forms are recognized (Table 1.30):

GAMBIAN SLEEPING SICKNESS is found mainly in West Africa, but also in southern Sudan and Uganda. Gambian sleeping sickness is caused by *T. b. gambiense* and transmitted to humans by the tsetse fly species *Glossina palpalis* and *G. tachinoides*. Humans are the only important reservoirs although domestic and wild animals may carry the infection. Transmission occurs most frequently at river banks where the flies lie under trees.

RHODESIAN SLEEPING SICKNESS is found from Ethiopia in the north to Botswana in the south. *T. b. rhodesiense*, the causative agent of Rhodesian sleeping sickness, is a zoonosis and is transmitted by *G. morsitans*, *G. swynnertoni*, *G. pallidipes*, and *G. palpalis*. Antelopes and other wild animals as well as domestic animals are reservoirs.

Tsetse flies are daylight biting and both male and female flies can be infected. Following the bite, metacyclic forms (the infective forms of trypomastigotes) are deposited into the subcutaneous tissue, where a marked perivascular reaction occurs. Lymphatics are then invaded, followed by spread to the lymph nodes. Invasion of the bloodstream occurs in 2 or 3 weeks, at which time the organisms reach all parts of the body, especially the CNS. In the CNS they elicit a marked perivascular mononuclear infiltration that results in leptomeningitis or encephalomyelitis.

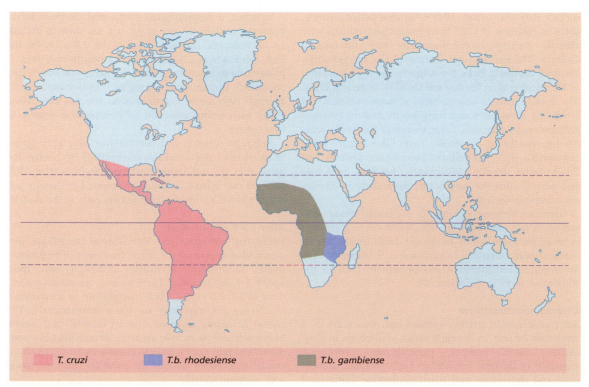

| T. cruzi | T.b. rhodesiense | T.b. gambiense |

**Fig. 1.26** Trypanosomiasis—geographical distribution.

| | Gambian | Rhodesian |
|---|---|---|
| Causative agent: | *Trypanosoma brucei gambiense* | *Trypanosoma brucei rhodesiense* |
| Main insect vector: | *Glossina palpalis* | *Glossina morsitans* |
| Reservoir: | Humans (pigs, goats, cattle, ? dogs) | Wild animals (antelopes and hogs), cattle and humans |
| Geographical distribution: | West Africa (Gambia to Congo), Central Africa, scattered areas in East Africa | East Africa |
| *Clinical features* | | |
| Duration: | Chronic | Acute |
| Severity: | Mild | Severe |
| Trypanosoma chancre: | Uncommon | Common |
| Fever: | Insidious and low grade | Acute and with large variations |
| Lymphadenopathy: | Prominent, especially posterior cervical group (Winterbottom's sign) | Less prominent |
| Hepatosplenomegaly: | Present | Present |
| CNS abnormalities: | Marked | Less marked |
| Other organs involved | Uncommon | Common |
| Chemoprophylaxis: | Effective | Less effective |

**Table 1.30** Comparison between Gambian and Rhodesian sleeping sickness.

## CLINICAL FEATURES

A tender nodule appears at the site of the bite. This is referred to as a trypanosoma chancre and is seen more commonly in Rhodesian sleeping sickness and in Caucasians. Tachycardia and persistent headache are common. Spontaneous healing of the chancre occurs at about 3 weeks and this is followed by haematogenous dissemination.

The lymph glands are discrete, non-tender and have a peculiar rubbery consistency. Splenomegaly and hepatomegaly may also occur. After a variable period of time, there is evidence of CNS involvement and features of a chronic meningo-encephalomyelitis with behavioural changes. The patient loses interest in the surroundings, becomes apathetic, has a mask-like facies, and a tendency to fall asleep during the day and inability to sleep at night. The eyelids tend to droop, there is facial puffiness, the lower lips are swollen and hang loosely and the patient's attention span decreases. Later, tremor of the hands, areas of hyperaesthesia, especially over the ulnar nerve (Kerandel's sign), choreiform movements, seizures and finally coma develop. Myocarditis, hepatitis, petechiae and pleural effusions may occur, particularly in Rhodesian sleeping sickness.

Gambian sleeping sickness is a chronic illness with symptom-free periods, while Rhodesian sleeping sickness is an acute, more severe form, and death usually occurs within 1 year, often due to myocarditis. Features of CNS involvement are therefore less prominent than in the Rhodesian form (see Table 1.30).

### Unusual manifestations

An erythematous, patchy, annular rash that fades in a week may be seen in the early stages of infection in Caucasians. Facial oedema, paraesthesiae, periosteitis, especially of the tibia resulting in hyperaesthesia, iridocyclitis and choroiditis may occur. Endocrine dysfunction may develop, manifesting as amenorrhoea or impotence.

## DIAGNOSIS

The definitive diagnosis depends on demonstrating trypomastigotes in the peripheral blood, lymph node aspirates or CSF. If the organism is not easily demonstrated, concentration techniques should be utilized. IgM levels in the serum and CSF are markedly elevated.

## TREATMENT

Therapy is usually effective if commenced *before CNS symptoms develop.*

Suramin, a polysulphated compound, is given intravenously; initially 0.1 g is given as a test dose to exclude an idiosyncratic reaction, followed by 1.0 g i.v. on the first, third, seventh, fourteenth and twenty-first days. If proteinuria or haematuria develop, therapy should be discontinued. Pentamidine 3–4 mg kg$^{-1}$ intramuscularly on alternate days for 10 injections is an effective alternative. Rapid intravenous injection of pentamidine results in hypotension.

Although suramin and pentamidine have been found to be effective and should be used initially to control the fever, they do not cross the blood–brain barrier. It is believed that relapse or failure to respond to therapy will occur when CNS involvement occurs early in the disease.

### After CNS involvement

Drugs that penetrate the blood–brain barrier are recommended as part of the initial treatment of trypanosomiasis. Melarsoprol, a trivalent arsenic, is used most widely for this purpose. Three to four consecutive injections of 2.0–3.6 mg kg$^{-1}$ body weight (up to a maximum of 250 mg per injection) are given intravenously. The course is usually repeated after an interval of 2 weeks. Major side-effects include an acute encephalitis-like condition and skin rashes. Jarisch–Herxheimer-type reactions can be reduced by clearing the parasites from the blood with suramin initially.

Oral nitrofurazone 10 mg kg$^{-1}$ in divided doses three

times daily for 10 days has also been found to be useful in cerebral trypanosomiasis. Peripheral neuropathy and haemolytic anaemia may be troublesome side-effects in patients with glucose-6-phosphate dehydrogenase deficiency.

Difluoromethylornithine is also used for Gambian sleeping sickness.

## PREVENTION AND CONTROL

Elimination of the vector—the tsetse fly—by insecticides or by making environmental conditions unsuitable for its inhabitation would effectively eradicate trypanosomiasis. Both these approaches require formidable mobilization of manpower and money. Insect repellents and protective, light-coloured clothing should be used when visiting endemic areas.

A single intramuscular prophylactic injection of pentamidine 4 mg kg$^{-1}$ body weight (up to a maximum dose of 300 mg) gives effective protection against Gambian sleeping sickness, but is less effective against Rhodesian sleeping sickness.

# African trypanosomiasis in children

In children the early manifestations and CNS symptoms overlap. Lymphadenopathy and neurological abnormalities may occur together. Seizures and choreiform movements are not uncommon. Treatment is as for the adult form.

# American trypanosomiasis (Chagas' disease)

This is a zoonotic disease caused by *T. cruzi* that is transmitted by various reduviid insects. The principal vectors are *Triatoma infestans* and *Rhodnius prolixus* (Latin America) and *Panstrongylus megistus* (Venezuela). Once infected, these insects remain infective for at least 2 years. Domestic and wild animals are important reservoirs. Humans are infected usually at night when the insect feeds and infected faeces are rubbed into a skin abrasion or mucosal surface such as the conjunctiva. Less commonly the infection may spread via blood transfusions or transplacentally.

Chagas' disease is confined to South and Central America. Occasional cases have also been reported from southern Texas.

## CLINICAL FEATURES

The incubation period varies from 1 to 2 weeks. Two clinically distinct presentations are recognized.

### Acute Chagas' disease

Acute Chagas' disease predominantly affects children. In 50% of cases an erythematous, indurated papule (chagoma) develops at the site of bite, and is associated with regional lymphadenopathy. This resolves spontaneously. If the portal of entry is the conjunctiva, unilateral periorbital and palpebral oedema (Romana's sign),

conjunctivitis and preauricular lymphadenopathy develop. Systemic findings such as fever, a transient morbilliform or urticarial rash, a peculiar gelatinous oedema of the face and trunk, tender lymphadenopathy and hepatosplenomegaly may be present. Death may occur in a small proportion of patients owing to myocarditis or meningo-encephalitis. More commonly the patient recovers completely in a few weeks.

### Chronic Chagas' disease

Chronic Chagas' disease occurs after a latent period of many years. It is due to an autoimmune reaction mediated by cytotoxic T cells and antibodies against the endocardium, vascular tissue and striated muscle, together with myenteric plexus damage by amastigotes. The heart is invariably involved. The patient may complain of chest pain, dyspnoea or syncope. Cardiac abnormalities and arrhythmias are usual. Signs of right-sided cardiac failure may be present. Thromboembolic phenomena may occur.

With gastrointestinal involvement, megaoesophagus, leading to dysphagia and aspiration pneumonia, and megacolon, giving constipation and progressive abdominal distension, may occur. Dilatation of the biliary tree and of the bronchi have also been documented.

## DIAGNOSIS

In acute Chagas' disease trypomastigotes may be demonstrated in peripheral blood. If parasites are not demonstrated in the blood, xenodiagnosis may be used: a parasite-free laboratory-reared vector feeds on a patient or the patient's blood suspected to have the disease and 2–3 weeks later the intestinal contents of the vector are examined for parasites.

In chronic Chagas' disease complement fixation (Machado–Guerreiro reaction), indirect fluorescent antibody or haemagglutination tests may be used. Radiological assessment of gastrointestinal abnormalities is helpful.

## TREATMENT

Nifurtimox, a nitrofurazone derivative, has been found to be useful in acute disease. The dose is 20 mg kg$^{-1}$ daily for children below the age of 2 years and 8–10 mg kg$^{-1}$ daily for 3–4 months in older children and adults. Side-effects are few and include transient leucopenia, vomiting, sleeplessness and paraesthesiae. Benzimidazole is a useful alternative drug.

Over 80% of patients with the acute form of the disease and slightly more with the chronic form are cured of the infection.

## PREVENTION AND CONTROL

No vaccine or chemoprophylactic agent is available. Prevention therefore involves the regular spraying of houses with benzene hexachloride in order to decrease the vector population.

# TOXOPLASMOSIS

Toxoplasmosis is caused by *Toxoplasma gondii*, an intracellular protozoon, which requires for completion of its life-cycle a definitive host, e.g. a cat, sheep or pig, and an intermediate host, e.g. a human. Infection of humans occurs either congenitally or by ingestion of foodstuffs contaminated by infected cat faeces or lamb or pork contaminated with *T. gondii* cysts. Toxoplasmosis is rare in the UK.

### CLINICAL FEATURES

Five major clinical forms of toxoplasmosis are recognized:
1 *Asymptomatic lymphadenopathy* is the commonest mode of presentation.
2 *Lymphadenopathy* usually involves the cervical lymph nodes and is associated with a febrile illness. This may be clinically indistinguishable from infectious mononucleosis but the Paul–Bunnell test is negative.
3 *Neurological abnormalities* include neck stiffness and headache, associated with sore throat and maculopapular rashes. The CSF is under pressure and the level of protein is elevated.
4 An *acute febrile illness* occurs, with a maculopapular rash, hepatosplenomegaly and reactive lymphocytes in the peripheral blood. Uveitis, chorioretinitis, myocarditis and hepatitis may occur.
5 *Congenital toxoplasmosis* exhibits symptoms and signs are indicative of CNS involvement. The characteristic 'syndrome of Savin', which comprises internal hydrocephalus, chorioretinitis, convulsions and cerebral calcification, may be seen. Tremors, nystagmus, microophthalmia and pneumonitis are also present. The prognosis is usually poor, the survivors generally exhibiting mental retardation, epilepsy and spastic paraplegia.

In the immunocompromised host, features present in the acute febrile and neurological forms are prominent.

### DIAGNOSIS

Serological tests are the mainstay of diagnosis of acquired infection. The Sabin–Feldman dye test, a measure of IgG antibodies, has been widely used. Antibodies can also be detected by indirect fluorescence or indirect haemagglutination. Raised antibody levels are common in the general population and only a rising antibody titre is highly suggestive of toxoplasmosis. The IgM-immunofluorescent antibody (IgM-IFA) test is particularly useful for detecting acute infection since titres rise early and fall rapidly.

*T. gondii* can be isolated by injecting the peritoneum of mice with tissue extracts, e.g. bone marrow, body fluids or CSF when available, and examining the peritoneal fluid 6–10 days later for the organism.

### TREATMENT

Most patients require no therapy as the disease is mild. Pyrimethamine (25–50 mg three times daily) and sulphadiazine (4–5 g daily) are used in combination for severe disease since they are synergistic. Therapy should be continued for at least 1 month. Since pyrimethamine is teratogenic, spiramycin is a useful alternative during pregnancy. Steroids are probably useful in ocular toxoplasmosis.

### PREVENTION

Domestic cats that kill mice and birds are the chief source of infection and care should be taken in handling their faeces.

## *Pneumocystis carinii* infection (see also p. 101 and p. 680)

Although genetic analysis has shown this organism to be homologous with fungi, its morphological characteristics are more similar to protozoa. The organism exists as a trophozoite, which is probably motile and reproduces by binary fission. After the trophozoite invades the lung parenchyma, its wall thickens and forms a cyst. On maturation, further division takes place to yield eight merozoites which, after cyst wall rupture, develop into trophozoites.

### CLINICAL FEATURES

Infection is probably common in infancy but most infections in otherwise healthy infants remain undetected. Outbreaks in infant nurseries have been reported but are now less common. Infection in adults is associated with a major defect in cell-mediated immune mechanisms. Thus, infection with *P. carinii* is one of the most common opportunistic infections in AIDS.

## BABESIOSIS

This is a tick-borne disease, found chiefly in North America and Europe, and is occasionally transmitted to humans, especially those who are immunosuppressed. The causative organism is the plasmodium-like *Babesia microti*. The incubation period averages 10 days. In patients with normal splenic function, the symptoms are mild and usually comprise fever, nausea, myalgia, chills, vomiting and abdominal pain. Hepatosplenomegaly and mild to moderate haemolytic anaemia may also be present. In splenectomized individuals, systemic symptoms are more pronounced and haemolysis is associated with haemoglobinuria, jaundice and renal failure. Examination of a peripheral blood smear may reveal the characteristic plasmodium-like organisms.

### TREATMENT

The treatment of choice is a combination of quinine 650 mg and clindamycin 600 mg orally three times daily for 7 days. This reduces the fever and parasitaemia but is not curative.

## MALARIA

Malaria affects 270 million people each year and has a mortality rate of 1%.

Endemic and epidemic malaria are found in all countries between latitudes 30°S and 40°N (Fig. 1.27). Malaria is primarily a disease of hot, humid countries at altitudes

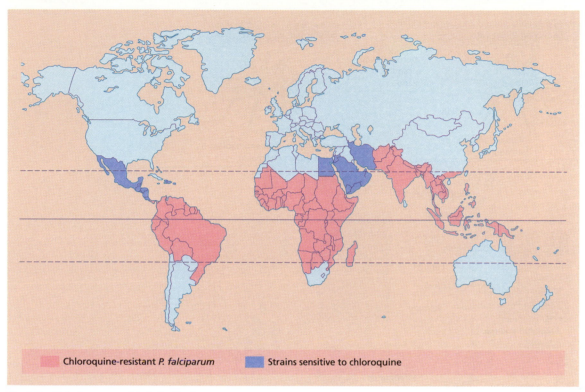

Chloroquine-resistant *P. falciparum*    Strains sensitive to chloroquine

**Fig. 1.27**   Malaria—geographical distribution.

less than 2200 m above mean sea level, where conditions are ideal for prolific breeding of the mosquito vector, *Anopheles*. It is endemic in India, in parts of Africa and parts of South and Central America. Malaria may also be transmitted by the importation of infected mosquitoes by air, so-called airport malaria.

In humans, malaria is caused by four species of *Plasmodium*: *P. vivax, P. ovale, P. falciparum* and *P. malariae*. The four species are distinguishable from each other on examination of peripheral blood smears.

*P. ovale* has been reported predominantly from East and West Africa. *P. vivax* is the major species in temperate zones, whereas in the tropics all forms of malaria are seen. With present-day ease and speed of travel, sporadic cases of malaria are being increasingly recognized. Unfortunately, the initial impact of the WHO eradication programme lost its impetus in several countries in the early 1970s and malaria has once more become a major cause of morbidity and mortality in tropical and subtropical countries. In addition, the emergence of drug (chloroquine) and insecticide (DDT) resistance has also become a major problem.

Humans, the intermediate hosts, are infected following the bite of an infected female *Anopheles* mosquito, the definitive host. The parasite can also be transmitted by blood transfusion, transplacentally, and, increasingly, between drug addicts who use improperly cleaned syringes.

The introduction of sporozoites, the infective form of the parasite, through the skin by the *Anopheles* mosquito heralds the commencement of the human cycle (Fig. 1.28). The following stages occur.

### Pre-erythrocytic schizogony

During this phase clinical symptoms are absent and humans are not infective. Those sporozoites that are not removed by the body's defence mechanisms undergo development within the liver. A variable number of days later, micromerozoites are liberated (primary attack). Other sporozoites (*P. vivax* and probably *P. ovale*) remain in a latent form in the liver as hypnozoites.

### Erythrocytic schizogony

This is the phase when red blood cells (RBCs) become infected by the micromerozoites. In the RBCs they pass through several stages of development, namely trophozoites, schizonts and finally merozoites. These asexual parasitic forms are found in peripheral blood about 12 days after inoculation of the sporozoites in *P. vivax* infection and 9 days in *P. falciparum* infection. The different *Plasmodium* species differ in their ability to invade RBCs. *P. falciparum* is capable of invading all RBCs, especially young RBCs. It therefore has the potential to produce the most severe form of malaria. *P. vivax* and *P. ovale* preferentially invade reticulocytes and young RBCs, whereas *P. malariae* invades senescent RBCs. Each cycle in the RBCs terminates with rupture of the cell and release of merozoites into the circulation. This occurs

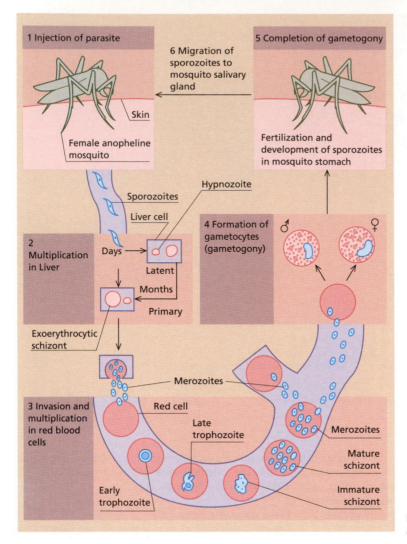

**Fig. 1.28** A schematic life-cycle of *Plasmodium vivax*.

every 48 hours in *P. falciparum* infection, every 48–72 hours in *P. vivax* and *P. ovale* infection, and approximately every 72 hours in *P. malariae*.

### Gametogony

The erythrocytic phase may continue for a considerable period of time before the stage of gametogony occurs. In this stage a few merozoites develop into the sexual form of the parasites known as gametocytes. Of these only the mature forms are found in peripheral blood. At this stage the patient is infective.

### Exoerythrocytic schizogony

This fourth stage, which occurs in the liver, is found only with *P. vivax*, probably *P. ovale* and possibly *P. malariae* infections. It does not occur with *P. falciparum* infection and is believed to be responsible for the relapses in *P. vivax* and *P. ovale* infections. The parasites in this phase are referred to as hypnozoites.

When an *Anopheles* mosquito ingests human blood containing gametocytes it marks the commencement of

the sexual cycle in the mosquito. The external incubation period varies from 7 to 20 days.

### Pathogenesis

The severity of malaria can be explained partly on the magnitude of the parasitaemia, with *P. falciparum* causing severe disease as it can invade RBCs of any age.

### IMMUNITY

Immunity may be natural or acquired. Natural immunity is present in individuals of West African extraction who are blood group Duffy-negative (FyFy) and therefore lack the specific receptor on the RBC surface to which the merozoites attach. They cannot develop *P. vivax* malaria. The presence of haemoglobin S, glucose-6-phosphate dehydrogenase deficiency, thalassaemia and pyruvate kinase deficiency also offer resistance against *P. falciparum*. The presence of abnormal haemoglobins or altered RBC metabolism retards *P. falciparum* maturation and reduces the severity of the disease. Certain HLA antigens have been shown to be protective against *P. falciparum* in Gambian children.

The spleen plays an important role in natural immunity, since splenectomized individuals are highly susceptible to the malarial parasite.

Infants are protected by the transfer of maternal IgG antibodies across the placenta.

Partial immunity may be acquired following an attack of malaria, and is attributed to macrophage stimulation by T cells.

CYTOKINES. Tumour necrosis factor-$\alpha$ (TNF-$\alpha$) blood levels correlate with the severity of the disease but a cause-and-effect relationship has not been shown.

## CLINICAL FEATURES

The incubation period varies, being:
- 10–14 days in *P. vivax*, *P. ovale* and *P. falciparum*
- 18 days to 6 weeks in *P. malariae* infection

Although individual variations in clinical presentation are noted, febrile paroxysms, anaemia, splenomegaly and hepatomegaly are usually present. Malarial febrile paroxysms typically have three stages:

1 The '*cold stage*' is characterized by marked vasoconstriction and lasts from 30 min to 1 hour. The patient feels intensely cold and uncomfortable. There is marked shivering. The temperature rises rapidly, often to as high as 41°C.

2 The '*hot stage*' abruptly follows and lasts for 2–6 hours. The patient feels intensely hot and uncomfortable. Delirium may be present.

3 The '*sweating stage*' then occurs, during which the bedclothes are drenched. The patient feels fatigued and exhausted but otherwise well and often sleeps. The fever is due to schizont rupture and the release of pyrogens.

Herpes labialis frequently occurs in established malaria. Anaemia is usually present and is largely a result of haemolysis.

### P. vivax and P. ovale

The fever occurs every other day when established. These species of *Plasmodium* give rise to a clinically mild infection. The presence of an exoerythrocytic stage is responsible for relapses and makes eradication of the organisms difficult.

### P. malariae

This is usually a mild disease with a fever, but tends to run a more chronic course. The nephrotic syndrome can complicate this type of malaria and may be fatal between the ages of 4 and 5 years. Because of its chronicity, the patient develops a sallow complexion, marked muscle wasting, mild icterus and massive splenomegaly. Growth retardation may occur in children.

### P. falciparum

This is the most severe form of malaria (pernicious malaria), with high levels of parasitaemia. Infected RBCs develop peculiar knob-like surface projections that facilitate adhesion of these RBCs to the endothelium of blood vessels via I CAM-1. The consequent vascular occlusion causes severe organ damage, chiefly in the kidneys, liver, brain and gastrointestinal tract. The prodrome tends to be severe. The fever follows no particular pattern. Splenomegaly tends to occur late and the characteristic cold, hot and sweating stages are not prominent. The following clinical forms of falciparum malaria are recognized and are likely to occur when more than 2% of RBCs are parasitized (Information box 1.4).

CEREBRAL MALARIA is characterized by a marked elevation in body temperature, a rapid deterioration in consciousness, convulsions, coma and death.

BLACKWATER FEVER, so called because of the production of dark brown-black urine owing to intravascular haemolysis, is seen only in falciparum malaria. It can be precipitated by very small amounts of quinine in quinine-sensitive cases. This is a rapidly progressive illness characterized by the abrupt onset of fever, marked haemolysis, haemoglobinuria, hyperbilirubinaemia, vomiting, circulatory collapse and acute renal failure. Malarial parasites cannot usually be detected in peripheral blood smears after the onset of intravascular haemolysis.

### Tropical splenomegaly syndrome

Tropical splenomegaly syndrome is seen in areas where malaria is hyperendemic. It is uncommon before 10 years of age. Characteristic features are massive splenomegaly, marked elevation in serum IgM levels, and IgM aggregates (detected by immunofluorescence) in Kupffer cells in the liver. The splenomegaly responds to antimalarial therapy. However, malarial parasites are not detected in the spleen or peripheral blood smears.

---

*CNS*
Cerebral malaria (coma, convulsion)

*Renal*
Haemoglobinuria (blackwater fever)
Oliguria
Uraemia (acute tubular necrosis)

*Blood*
Severe anaemia
DIC (haemorrhage)

*Respiratory*
Adult respiratory distress syndrome

*Metabolic*
Hypoglycaemia (particularly in children)
Metabolic acidosis

*Gastrointestinal/Liver*
Diarrhoea
Jaundice
Splenic rupture

*Other*
Shock—hypotensive
Hyperpyrexia

**Information box 1.4**  Some features of severe falciparum malaria.

## PREVALENCE

The following indices are used to measure the prevalence of malaria:

SPLEEN RATE, defined as the percentage of children between 2 and 10 years of age with splenomegaly, is used as a measure of the endemicity of malaria in a community.

INFANT PARASITE RATE, defined as the percentage of infants below 1 year of age in whom malarial parasites are demonstrable in peripheral blood smears, is regarded as the most sensitive index of transmission of malaria to a locality.

## DIAGNOSIS

The parasite can be demonstrated in either thin or thick peripheral blood smears stained with Giemsa, Wright or Leishman stains. Two to three blood smears taken each day for 3 or 4 days and found to be negative are necessary before a patient is declared malaria-free.

Serological methods are not widely used but include indirect immunofluorescence, indirect haemagglutination and gel diffusion techniques.

ELISA for antigen detection and probes for parasite DNA are currently being evaluated.

## TREATMENT

### General

Analgesics and antipyretics such as aspirin and paracetamol are given as necessary. Intravenous fluids may be required to combat dehydration and shock.

### Treatment of an acute attack

The 4-aminoquinolines are the drugs of choice. Chloroquine-sensitive malaria is treated with chloroquine 600 mg of the base followed by 300 mg in 6 hours and then 150 mg twice daily for 3 days, or amodiaquine hydrochloride 600 mg of the base followed by 400–600 mg daily for 2 days up to a total maximum dose of 2400 mg.

Chloroquine-resistant malaria is treated with quinine sulphate 650 mg three times daily for 5 days given in combination with pyrimethamine 25 mg twice daily for 3 days and sulphadiazine 500 mg twice daily for 5 days. Mefloquine is a synthesized quinolone which is useful in chloroquine- and some quinine-resistant cases; again resistance to this is developing. Halofantrine, an amino alcohol, is another drug for resistant cases. Both these last two drugs are too expensive for widespread use.

DRUG SIDE-EFFECTS. These drugs are potentially toxic. With quinine, tinnitus, haemolytic anaemia and drug fever may occur. Chloroquine may cause vomiting, abdominal pain, agranulocytosis or convulsions.

### Eradication

1 *P. falciparum.* Chloroquine alone or in combination with either pyrimethamine 25 mg or primaquine 45 mg as a single dose effects a radical cure because there is no exoerythrocytic stage in falciparum malaria.
2 *P. vivax, P. malariae* and *P. ovale.* Primaquine, an 8-aminoquinoline, is essential for eliminating the exoer-

ythrocytic cycle and effecting a radical cure. A course of one of the 4-aminoquinolines should be followed by primaquine 7.5 mg daily for 14 days. Alternatively, 300 mg chloroquine combined with 45 mg primaquine once a week for 8 weeks is also effective.

### Treatment of severe malaria

Severe malaria (more than 1% of RBCs infected) or any of the pernicious forms of falciparum malaria constitutes a medical emergency. Quinine, given by a slow intravenous infusion, is the drug of choice: Quinine dihydrochloride 20 mg kg$^{-1}$ intravenously over 4 hours followed by 100 mg kg$^{-1}$ infused over 4 hours at 8-hourly intervals until the patient is able to tolerate oral therapy.

## PREVENTION AND CONTROL

Owing to changing patterns of resistance, advice about chemoprophylaxis should be sought prior to leaving for a malaria-endemic area. Chemoprophylaxis is essential for those visiting endemic areas—generally chloroquine 300 mg once a week in areas where there is no chloroquine resistance, but where there is resistance it should be combined with proguanil 200 mg daily or in South East Asia or Papua New Guinea dapsone/pyrimethamine (Maloprim) one tablet (100 mg and 125 mg respectively) each week as above. Mefloquine 250 mg weekly (adults) can be used where falciparum malaria is highly resistant to chloroquine (East and Central Africa) for periods up to 6 months. Doxycycline has also been used apparently successfully in South East Asia. Prophylaxis should be continued for 6 weeks after leaving a high-risk area.

On the basis of the 1979 WHO Expert Committee report on malaria, the following preventive measures have been suggested. Measures to be applied to the community include prevention of man–vector contact, destruction of adult mosquitoes and mosquito larvae, and active elimination of human infection by presumptive treatment (i.e. treatment of all fevers in endemic areas with antimalarials) and radical treatment. Measures to be applied to individuals include use of mosquito repellents, impregnated bed nets, protective clothing, chemoprophylaxis and chemotherapy where indicated.

# Intestinal and genital infections

## Amoebiasis

The most important human disease due to amoebae is amoebiasis, which is caused by *Entamoeba histolytica*. This intestinal pathogen can be differentiated from other enteric amoebae such as *Entamoeba hartmani, Entamoeba coli* and *Endolimax nana*, since *E. histolytica* is the only amoeba found in the intestine that phagocytoses RBCs. It occurs worldwide, although much higher incidence rates are found in the tropics and subtropics. It can be found in active male homosexuals who carry the pathogen (usually strains of low virulence) and between whom it is spread by sexual contact.

## LIFE-CYCLE AND PATHOGENESIS
The organism exists both as a motile trophozoite and as a cyst that can survive outside the body. Cysts are transmitted chiefly by ingestion of contaminated food or water or spread directly by person-to-person contact. Trophozoites emerge from the cyst in the small intestine and then pass on to the colon, where they multiply (Fig. 1.29). Many individuals can carry the pathogen without obvious evidence of clinical disease (asymptomatic cyst passers). However, under certain conditions, *E. histolytica* trophozoites invade the colonic epithelium, probably with the aid of their own cytotoxins and proteolytic enzymes. The parasites continue to multiply and finally frank ulceration of the mucosa occurs. If penetration continues trophozoites may enter the portal vein, via which they reach the liver and cause hepatitis and intrahepatic abscesses. This invasive form of the disease is particularly serious and unless treated promptly is often fatal.

## CLINICAL FEATURES
The incubation period is highly variable and may be as short as a few days or as long as several months or even a year. The presentation of amoebic colitis may be:
GRADUAL ONSET with mild intermittent diarrhoea and abdominal discomfort, usually progressing to bloody diarrhoea with mucus. Systemic manifestations such as headache, nausea and anorexia are often present.
SEVERE ACUTE (AMOEBIC) DYSENTERY, closely resembling that due to *Shigella* (bacillary dysentery).
A FULMINATING COLITIS. Typically, patients with amoebic colitis appear less unwell than those with bacillary dysentery, fever is low-grade or absent, and dehydration is unusual.

## COMPLICATIONS
Complications are unusual, but include:
PROGRESSION OF FULMINANT COLITIS to toxic dilatation of the colon with perforation and peritonitis.
CHRONIC INFECTION leading to stricture formation.

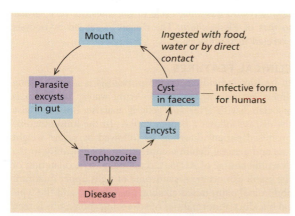

**Fig. 1.29** A schematic life-cycle of intestinal protozoa.

SEVERE HAEMORRHAGE.
AMOEBOMA, i.e. a mass of fibrotic granulation tissue, develops most commonly in the caecum or rectosigmoid region. Amoebomas occur in 10% of patients and may bleed, cause obstruction, intussuscept and are sometimes mistaken for a carcinoma.
AMOEBIC LIVER ABSCESS, which often develops in the absence of a recent episode of colitis. Tender hepatomegaly, a high swinging fever and profound malaise are characteristic, although early in the course of the disease both symptoms and signs may be minimal. The clinical features are described in more detail on p. 275.

## DIAGNOSIS
### Serodiagnosis
The amoebic fluorescent antibody titre (FAT) is positive in at least 90% of patients with liver abscess and 75% with active colitis. Seropositivity is low in asymptomatic cyst passers.

### Colonic disease
Direct examination of colonic exudate obtained at sigmoidoscopy or of freshly passed stool as a saline-wet mount is the most rapid and least expensive way of confirming amoebic infection. *E. histolytica* trophozoites must be distinguished from non-pathogenic amoebae and from polymorphonuclear leucocytes, with which they are sometimes confused. Cysts may also be present in the stool. Sigmoidoscopy and barium enema examination may show colonic ulceration but are rarely diagnostic.

### Liver disease
Liver abscess should be suspected if the serum alkaline phosphatase is elevated, even when clinical signs are absent. Hepatic ultrasound scan should confirm the presence of an abscess, which may be either single or multiple. Pus from an amoebic abscess has a classic 'anchovy sauce' appearance and may contain trophozoites.

## TREATMENT
Metronidazole 800 mg three times daily for 5 days is given in amoebic colitis and a more prolonged course for 10–14 days in liver abscess or other extra-intestinal spread.

An alternative drug is the other nitroimidazole derivative, tinidazole. Dehydroemetine is used when nitroimidazoles fail (rarely). Diloxanide furoate is a luminal amoebicide and may be a helpful adjunct in clearing cysts.

Large, tense abscesses in the liver may require percutaneous drainage, using an ultrasound scan to localize accurately the abscess and to position the drainage needle.

## CONTROL AND PREVENTION
This disease will be difficult to eradicate because of the substantial human reservoir of asymptomatic cases. There is no immediate hope of vaccine development, particularly as the same individual may experience several episodes of amoebic infection, indicating that only partial protective immunity develops after exposure to the pathogen. Improved standards of personal hygiene and water quality are important. Cysts are destroyed by boil-

ing water for at least 10 min, but the effects of chlorination are variable.

## Balantidiasis

*Balantidium coli* is the only ciliate that produces clinically
significant infection in humans. It is found throughout
the tropics, particularly in Central and South America,
Iran, Papua New Guinea and the Philippines. It is usually
carried by pigs and infection is most common in those
communities that live in close association with swine. Its
life-cycle is identical to that of *E. histolytica*.

*B. coli* produces a dysenteric illness owing to invasion
of the distal ileal and colonic mucosa. The colitis may
be acute and fulminant and if untreated may be fatal.
Trophozoites rather than cysts are found in the stool.
Treatment is with tetracycline, ampicillin or metronidazole.

## Giardiasis

*Giardia lamblia* is a flagellate (Fig. 1.30) that is found
worldwide. It causes small-intestinal disease, with diarrhoea and malabsorption. Prevalence is high throughout
the tropics. It is an important cause of traveller's diarrhoea worldwide usually occurring on return from travel.
In certain parts of Europe, the former USSR, and in some
rural and mountainous areas of North America, large
water-borne epidemics have been reported. Person-to-
person spread is common in day nurseries and residential
institutions and between male homosexuals. Like *E. histolytica*, the organism exists both as a trophozoite and a
cyst, the latter being the form in which the protozoon
is transmitted.

The organism colonizes and multiplies within the small
intestine and may remain there without causing detri-
ment to the host. Severe malabsorption may occur and
is thought to be related to morphological damage to the
small intestine; changes in villous architecture vary from
mild partial villous atrophy to rarely subtotal villous atrophy. The mechanism by which *Giardia* causes alteration
in mucosal architecture and produces diarrhoea and

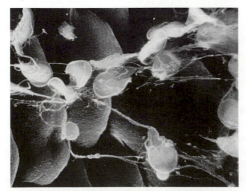

**Fig. 1.30**  *Giardia lamblia*. Courtesy of Dr A. Phillips,
Department of Electron Microscopy, Queen Elizabeth Hospital
for Children, London.

intestinal malabsorption is unknown. There is evidence
that the morphological damage may be immune
mediated. Bacterial overgrowth has also been found in
association with giardiasis and may contribute to fat malabsorption.

### CLINICAL FEATURES

Many individuals excreting *Giardia* cysts have no symptoms and are therefore carriers. Others develop symptoms
within 1 or 2 weeks of ingesting cysts. These include diarrhoea, often watery in the early stage of the illness, nausea, anorexia, abdominal discomfort and distension.
Stools may then become paler, with the characteristic features of steatorrhoea. If the illness is prolonged, weight
loss ensues, which, even in previously healthy adults, can
be marked. Chronic giardiasis can result in growth retardation in children.

### DIAGNOSIS

Both cysts and trophozoites can be found in the stool, but
negative stool examination does not exclude the diagnosis
since the parasite may be excreted at irregular intervals.
The parasite can also be seen in duodenal aspirates and
in histological sections of jejunal mucosa. Raised specific
anti-*Giardia* IgG and, in acute infections, IgM antibodies
are found.

### TREATMENT

Metronidazole 2 g as a single dose on three successive
days will cure the majority of infections, although sometimes a second or third course is necessary. Preventive
measures are similar to those outlined for *E. histolytica*.
Alternative drugs include mepacrine, furazolidone and
albendazole.

## *Cryptosporidium parvum*

This organism is found worldwide, cattle being a major
natural reservoir. It has also been demonstrated in drinking water supplies. It produces a devastating diarrhoeal
illness in patients with immunodeficiency, particularly
those with AIDS. It has recently become a recognized
cause of gastroenteritis, particularly in children.

The parasite is able to reproduce both sexually and
asexually and has a life-cycle in the intestine very similar
to that of *Plasmodium*. The disease is spread by oocysts
excreted in the faeces.

### CLINICAL FEATURES

In healthy individuals cryptosporidiosis is a self-limiting
illness lasting for 7–10 days. Acute watery diarrhoea is
associated with fever and general malaise, but otherwise
the disease follows a benign course. In the immunocompromised patient diarrhoea is followed by severe weight
loss and general debility, contributing significantly to the
downhill course of AIDS. Occasionally toxic dilatation of
the colon can occur. A syndrome of right upper quadrant
abdominal pain, raised alkaline phosphatase and the typical bile duct abnormalities of sclerosing cholangitis is seen
in AIDS patients.

## DIAGNOSIS

The parasite can be detected in intestinal biopsies but is now most commonly found in faeces (as oocysts) using concentration techniques and a modified Ziehl–Nielsen stain.

## TREATMENT

As yet there is no effective antimicrobial treatment for this infection. AZT can reduce diarrhoea temporarily in AIDS as can paromomycin, although the agent does not affect the cryptospiridiosis itself. Good hygiene, especially hand washing, prevents spread of organism.

## *Blastocystis hominis*

*B. hominis* is a strictly anaerobic protozoan pathogen that inhabits the colon. For decades, its pathogenicity for humans was questioned but there is increasing evidence that it may cause diarrhoea. It is sensitive to metronidazole.

## *Cyclospora cayatenensis*

Recently cyanobacterium-like bodies were detected in the stools of travellers returning from Nepal with diarrhoea. This coccidian parasite, which has not been detected within enterocytes, is thought to cause diarrhoea and has tentatively been named *Cyclospora cayatenensis*.

## Microsporidiosis

This is now a common cause of diarrhoea in patients with HIV infection. Spores can be detected with high accuracy in the stools. Albendazole is effective in eradication.

## Trichomoniasis

*Trichomonas vaginalis* is a flagellate that causes vaginitis and urethritis (see p. 95).

# *Helminthic infections*

# *Nematode (roundworm) infections*

## FILARIASIS

Several nematodes belonging to the superfamily Filarioidea are responsible for filariasis (Table 1.31). The adult worms are thread-like. Females are larger than males. The viviparous females give birth to larvae known as microfilariae. The microfilariae of various species can be easily differentiated from each other by the presence or absence of a sheath and the pattern of nuclear distribution in the tail. These nematodes require two hosts to complete their life-cycle.

## Bancroftian and Malayan (lymphatic) filariasis

*Wuchereria bancrofti* is found mainly in the tropics and subtropics—in northern Australia, the Pacific Islands, West and Central Africa, South America and India. *Brugia malayi* infection is less widespread than Bancroftian filariasis and is found in India, southern China, Malaysia, Indonesia and Borneo (Fig. 1.31). Humans are the definitive hosts and mosquitoes of various types are the intermediate hosts. Humans are the only known reservoirs of Bancroftian filariasis, whereas, in addition to humans, animals such as cats are reservoirs of Malayan filariasis. *Culex fatigans*, which bites at night, is the main vector of Bancroftian filariasis. *Aedes* and *Anopheles* spp. have also been implicated. The major vector for Malayan filariasis is *Mansonia annulifera*.

Following the bite of an infected mosquito, the larvae

| Organism | Habitat of adult worms in humans | Vector | Clinical manifestations |
|---|---|---|---|
| *Wuchereria bancrofti* | Lymphatics, lymph nodes | *Culex, Aedes, Anopheles* | Fever, lymphangitis, elephantiasis of limbs, breasts and scrotum |
| *Brugia malayi* | Lymphatics | *Mansonia* | Fever, lymphangitis, elephantiasis (scrotal involvement is uncommon) |
| *Loa loa* | Subcutaneous tissue, subconjunctiva | *Chrysops* | 'Calabar swellings', urticaria |
| *Onchocerca volvulus* | Subcutaneous tissue | *Simulium* | Subcutaneous nodules, elephantiasis, ocular lesions |
| *Dipetalonema* | Body cavities | *Culicoides* | Occasionally dermatitis |

**Table 1.31**   Habitat, vectors and major clinical manifestations of some nematodes of the superfamily Filarioidea.

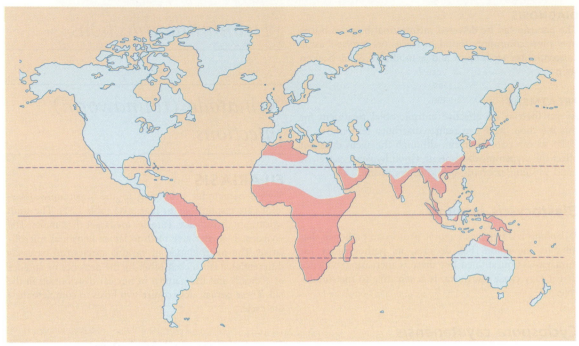

**Fig. 1.31** Filariasis—geographical distribution.

penetrate the skin, enter the lymphatics and are carried to the regional lymph nodes. Here they grow and mature for up to 18 months. After fertilization the microfilariae produced are carried from the lymphatics into the blood; they do not produce any symptoms or signs. Adult worms produce lymphangitis, which is believed to be a hypersensitivity reaction. The lymphangitis is followed by fibrosis, a granulomatous reaction and later irreversible lymphatic blockade. Secondary bacterial infection may add considerably to the inflammatory response and resultant fibrosis.

### CLINICAL FEATURES
Following an incubation period that averages 10–12 months, the patient presents with fever ranging from 39 to 41°C accompanied by lymphangitis, both of which usually subside in 3–5 days. Lymphangitis typically involves the lymphatics of the lower or upper limbs or of the abdomen. Involvement of the lymphatics of the epididymis, testis and spermatic cord occurs almost exclusively in Bancroftian filariasis. The involved superficial lymphatics appear as red streaks on the skin, and are tender and cord-like. The inflammation may subside either with treatment or spontaneously but there is a tendency for recurrences. The inflammatory phase is usually followed by the obstructive phase, which is characterized by features of lymphatic blockade. Many sites may be affected, but lower limb and scrotal oedema occur frequently. Long-standing obstruction produces thick, rough skin, which occasionally ulcerates. Less frequently chyluria, chylous ascites and pleural effusions occur. The obstructive phase may be punctuated by episodes of acute lymphangitis.

### DIAGNOSIS
The clinical presentation is characteristic. Eosinophilia and the presence of microfilariae in thin or thick peripheral blood smears is diagnostic. Since *W. bancrofti* and *B. malayi* are released into the peripheral circulation at night coinciding with the time of the mosquito bite, blood for examination should be taken between 9 p.m. and 1 a.m. If, despite repeated examination, microfilariae cannot be demonstrated in thick or thin blood smears, diethylcarbamazine 100 mg given as a single dose followed by blood removal 30 min later for examination may give a positive yield. Various parasite-concentration techniques such as Knott's concentration or membrane filtration techniques have resulted in a higher positive yield. Serological tests are available but not highly specific.

### TREATMENT
Diethylcarbamazine (DEC) 3–9 mg kg$^{-1}$ daily in three divided doses for 2–3 weeks is recommended. A second course after 6 weeks increases the cure rate. The WHO Expert Committee has recommended that a total of 72 mg kg$^{-1}$ be given for eradication of Bancroftian filariasis and 30–40 mg kg$^{-1}$ for Malayan filariasis. DEC is filaricidal. Following initiation of therapy, marked allergic reactions can occur and require concomitant administration of antihistamines or steroids.

Associated bacterial infections should be appropriately treated. Reconstructive surgery plays an important role in removing unsightly tissue.

### PREVENTION AND CONTROL
Mass chemotherapy with DEC (often added to table salt) has been effective in decreasing the *microfilariae rate* (the

percentage of individuals who have microfilariae in a unit volume of their blood in a given population) and the *microfilariae density* (the number of microfilariae per unit volume of blood in individual patients). Primary prophylaxis should be aimed at vector control and protection of humans from mosquitoes, particularly at night with impregnated nets and repellant creams and sprays.

## Tropical eosinophilia

Tropical eosinophilia has been attributed to microfilariae such as *Dirofilaria* and more recently to *W. bancrofti* and *B. malayi*. Two forms are recognized, one characterized by lymphadenopathy and splenomegaly, and the other by cough, bronchospasm and an asthma-like picture (see p. 62).

## Loiasis

Loiasis is caused by *Loa loa*. As in Bancroftian and Malayan filariasis, the microfilariae of *L. loa* do not produce any symptoms. Unlike Bancroftian filariasis, the microfilariae are found in the peripheral circulation mainly during the day. The disease is confined to the hot, humid, swampy areas of West and Central Africa, in which environment the deerfly vectors *Chrysops silacea* and *Chrysops dimidiata* thrive. Following the bite of a female *Chrysops*, the microfilariae are introduced into the skin of the human host and tend to migrate in the subcutaneous tissues. They have a predilection for subconjunctival and periorbital tissues.

### CLINICAL FEATURES
The main feature of loiasis is *Calabar swellings*, which are painless, localized, transient, hot, soft-tissue swellings, often near joints. They persist for periods varying from a few hours to several weeks. They occur more commonly during the hotter months and may be preceded by numbness and tingling. They are produced by toxin released from the adult worm.

Urticaria, pruritus, lymphoedema, arthritis and chorioretinitis may occur.

A picture resembling meningo-encephalitis that occurs only during treatment is thought to be an allergic reaction.

### DIAGNOSIS
The worm can be seen in subcutaneous tissues or crossing the conjunctivae.

The characteristic microfilariae may be demonstrable in peripheral blood smears. Eosinophilia is present. Serological tests such as the complement-fixation test are also useful.

### TREATMENT
DEC 2–6 mg kg$^{-1}$ in gradually increasing dosage is effective against both adult worms and microfilariae although multiple courses may be necessary. Treatment should be continued for 2–3 weeks. Side-effects of treatment

(caused by death of parasites) are fever, headache, urticaria and encephalitis; steroids may be necessary for these effects.

### PREVENTION AND CONTROL
Prevention is best effected by adequate personal protection. In addition, houses should be sprayed with dieldrin. Mass treatment of all the inhabitants of villages with DEC 2 mg kg$^{-1}$ daily for 3 days has reduced the incidence of this disease.

## Onchocerciasis

Onchocerciasis (river blindness) is produced by the filarial worm *Onchocerca volvulus*. The gravid female has a life-expectancy of 15 years. The microfilariae are found in the skin and subcutaneous tissue. Humans are the only known definitive host and the day-biting female blackfly of the genus *Simulium* is the vector. The flies breed in rapidly flowing water both in the rain forest and savannah. The species involved are *S. damnosum* and *S. neavei* in Africa and *S. metallicum* in Venezuela. The disease is confined to West, Central and East Africa, Central and South America, and southern parts of Saudi Arabia.

### CLINICAL FEATURES
The incubation period averages 1 year. Initially a papular, reddish, itchy rash develops. With repeated infections, characteristic subcutaneous nodules of various sizes appear. Usually they number fewer than 10 and are unevenly distributed over the body. In chronic disease, lichenification, xeroderma, pseudoichthyosis and atrophy of the skin occur. The nodules may be associated with the development of genital elephantiasis, hydrocele and the so-called 'hanging groin', in which large folds of wrinkled and thickened skin develop in the groin.

Ocular lesions represent the most serious manifestation of this disease and in some communities 40% of people are blind by 50 years of age. Eye disease is commoner in the savannah. Initially the patient complains of lacrimation, photophobia and a foreign-body sensation in the eye. Conjunctivitis, iridocyclitis, chorioretinitis, secondary glaucoma and optic atrophy may occur. The eye lesions have been attributed to toxin production by the microfilariae and adult worms, mechanical irritation and hypersensitivity.

### DIAGNOSIS
This is established by demonstrating microfilariae in snips of bloodless tissue obtained from the nodules and kept in saline for 30 min to 1 hour before microscopic examination. The organism may also be identified in the anterior chamber of the eye by slit-lamp examination. Serological tests are not helpful in the indigenous population as the positivity rate is high. Eosinophilia occurs.

### TREATMENT
Ivermectin, a broad-spectrum antiparasitic drug, is effective in filariasis and is now the drug of choice. A single

dose of $150 \mu g \, kg^{-1}$ orally produces a prolonged reduction in microfilarial levels. Six- to twelve-monthly therapy must be given in endemic areas as ivermectin is not curative and re-infection occurs. DEC is still sometimes used when ivermectin is unavailable but reactions (pruritus and a rash) occur and were used for diagnosis (Mazzotti's test).

### PREVENTION AND CONTROL

Prevention and control depends partly on personal protection to avoid bites and attempts at destroying the vector. Eradication of blackfly is expensive and mass treatment with ivermectin (provided free by the pharmaceutical industry) once a year is being used in endemic areas with good success.

## DRACUNCULIASIS

Dracunculiasis (Guinea worm infection) results from infection with *Dracunculus medinensis*. It is found sporadically throughout the tropics but is common in certain parts of India, Central, East and West Africa, Pakistan, the Middle East, parts of South America and the eastern regions of the former USSR.

Humans are the definitive host and are infected by ingestion of water containing infected *Cyclops*. The larvae are liberated in the human stomach by the action of acid. These penetrate the intestinal wall, where the male dies after fertilizing the female. The gravid female then wanders in connective tissue for several months before emerging through the skin. On reaching the skin, the parasite elicits an allergic reaction with blister formation and later protrusion of the worm associated with the discharge of motile larvae. The larvae are then taken up by *Cyclops*, which once again are infective to humans.

### CLINICAL FEATURES

A generalized reaction can occur that is associated with nausea, vomiting, generalized urticaria and diarrhoea. These symptoms abate with rupture of the blister. Secondary bacterial infection, especially with streptococci, is common and results in cellulitis and abscess formation. In Nigeria, tetanus is a frequent complication. If attempts at extraction of the worm result in damage to it, intense cellulitis may occur. Arthritis, synovitis, ankylosis of joints and epididymitis are rare sequelae.

### DIAGNOSIS

Keeping the appropriate part of the body immersed in water may induce the worm to wriggle out. Fluorescent antibody tests are useful. Radiography may reveal the presence of the worm.

### TREATMENT

Gradual physical extraction of the worm by winding it carefully around a stick is the treatment of choice. It may take several days before the entire worm is extruded. Niridazole and thiabendazole are of questionable value in facilitating worm extrusion.

### PREVENTION AND CONTROL

Prevention of this parasitosis is easily effected by chemically treating infected sources of water.

## ANIMAL NEMATODES

## Toxocariasis

Toxocariasis (visceral larva migrans) occurs worldwide and is caused by *Toxocara canis* or *T. cati*. The adult worm is found in the intestine of dogs and cats. The infective ova are passed in animal faeces and may be accidentally ingested by humans. The liberated larvae penetrate the intestinal wall and reach the liver and lung via the circulation. Epidemiologically, puppies are the most important natural hosts and the infection is most commonly seen in children between 1 and 4 years of age. Several viscera may be involved and the clinical manifestations are dependent on the organ involved and the intensity of infection. Eosinophilia is common. Urticaria and dermatitis may occur. With pulmonary involvement the presentation is that of bronchial asthma. Chest radiographs may reveal transient pulmonary infiltrates. Splenomegaly and hepatomegaly may occur. Rarely involvement of the myocardium and CNS may result in death. Eye involvement (ocular larva migrans) produces a retinoblastoma-like picture; other organs are usually spared.

### DIAGNOSIS

The presence of marked eosinophilia, hepatomegaly, and elevated plasma IgG, IgM and IgE is suggestive, as is the identification of foreign-body eosinophilic granulomas in histological sections. Recently detection of specific antibodies by ELISA has been found to be useful.

### TREATMENT

Treatment is difficult to evaluate in view of the mild nature of the illness and the tendency for spontaneous cure. DEC $2-6 \, mg \, kg^{-1}$ daily in divided doses for 3 weeks or thiabendazole $25 \, mg \, kg^{-1}$ twice daily for 5 days is probably effective.

## Cutaneous larva migrans

Cutaneous larva migrans (creeping eruption) is a disease of the hot, humid areas of tropical and subtropical countries. It is caused by the dog and cat hookworms *Ancylostoma braziliense* and *A. caninum* and, occasionally, the human parasites *A. duodenale*, *Necator americanus* and *Strongyloides stercoralis*. The adult forms of these worms are found in the intestine of the host (see p. 79). The filariform larva emerges from the ova passed in the faeces and penetrates intact human skin. An itchy papule develops at the site of larval entry. Two to three days later a markedly itchy, erythematous, serpiginous skin lesion develops. This is due to the larva, which migrates at approximately 1 cm per day. The skin over the lesion may vesiculate. Healing occurs by crusting. Although the lesions are more frequent on the lower limbs, any part of the body may be affected. Secondary bacterial infection may result in a mistaken diagnosis of pyoderma. The only systemic manifestations are transient pulmonary infiltrates and occasional breathlessness. Eosinophilia is seen.

### TREATMENT

Thiabendazole applied locally as a 10% solution or given systemically (25 mg kg$^{-1}$ for 5 days) is effective.

## Anisakiasis

Anisakiasis (herring worm disease) is caused by the larval stage of several species of *Anisakis*, and possibly of the related nematode *Phocanema*, which are found in abundance in herring, and dolphins, whales and other large sea mammals. The disease is prevalent in Japan and northern Europe, where raw herring and other raw fish are considered a delicacy. In Japan the illness is characterized by an acute gastric syndrome that presents as epigastric pain, nausea and vomiting. Upper gastrointestinal endoscopy may reveal the presence of larvae in the gastric mucosa. In contrast, in Europe the small intestine is predominantly involved and the patient presents with colicky, generalized abdominal pain and fever. Eosinophilia is unusual.

## Trichinosis

This is caused by the intestinal nematode *Trichinella spiralis*. The larval form is found in rats, hares, pigs, dogs and cats. Although cases of trichinosis have been reported from all parts of the world, it is found predominantly in the USA and Europe. It is uncommon in India. Transmission to humans occurs when improperly cooked meats, contaminated with infective larvae, are eaten.

### CLINICAL FEATURES

Vomiting, diarrhoea, abdominal pain and headache occur 24–72 hours after ingestion of contaminated meat. The severity of the clinical manifestations depends on the number of infecting larvae.

The larvae mature into the adult form in the intestine, where they reproduce and discharge larvae into the circulation. When these larvae migrate into the bloodstream and striated muscles (a stage that lasts 10–21 days), periorbital oedema, conjunctivitis, photophobia, fever with chills, and muscle pain and spasm occur. An urticarial rash, diarrhoea, dyspnoea and pleurisy may also occur. Myocardial and CNS involvement is unusual and, if it occurs, may result in death. In the next stage of development, larvae encyst in striated muscle. During encystment symptoms gradually subside, although weakness, muscle pain and cramps may persist for several months.

### DIAGNOSIS

A firm diagnosis can be made on the clinical presentation, marked eosinophilia, and positive serology using ELISA. If necessary the diagnosis can be established by a biopsy of the deltoid or gastrocnemius muscle 3 weeks after the onset of illness and demonstrating the presence of the larvae.

### TREATMENT

Analgesics, sedatives and bed rest are the mainstays of treatment. Steroids are indicated only in the presence of myocarditis, CNS involvement or marked allergic phenomena. Thiabendazole 25 mg kg$^{-1}$ body weight twice daily for 7 days is effective against intestinal worms and larvae.

## INTESTINAL NEMATODE INFECTION   (Table 1.32)

Some adult nematodes live within the intestinal lumen. The disease is spread to humans (Fig. 1.32):
PASSIVELY by ingesting infective eggs, as occurs with *Ascaris lumbricoides* ('roundworm'), *Trichuris trichiura* (whipworm) and *Enterobius vermicularis* (threadworm)
ACTIVELY by percutaneous spread of filariform larvae that penetrate the skin (hookworm and *Strongyloides*)
*Ascaris* deviates from the simplified life-cycle shown in Fig. 1.32 in that it invades the duodenum and enters the venous system, via which it reaches the lungs. The worm is eventually expectorated and swallowed, entering the intestine where it completes its maturation. *Strongyloides* is the only nematode that is able to complete its life-cycle in humans; its rhabditiform larvae, which hatch in the intestine, are able to reinfect the host by penetrating the intestinal wall and entering the venous system.

| Organism | Site | Clinical manifestations |
|---|---|---|
| *Strongyloides stercoralis* | Small intestine | Malabsorption |
| Hookworm: *Ancylostoma duodenale* and *Necator americanus* | Small intestine | Iron deficiency anaemia |
| *Capillaria philippinensis* | Small intestine | Malabsorption |
| *Ascaris lumbricoides* ('roundworm') | Small intestine | ?Undernutrition, intestinal obstruction |
| *Trichuris trichiura* (whipworm) | Large intestine | Usually nil, colitis, rectal prolapse |
| *Enterobius vermicularis* (threadworm) | Large intestine | Usually nil, pruritus ani |

**Table 1.32**  Intestinal nematode (roundworm) infections.

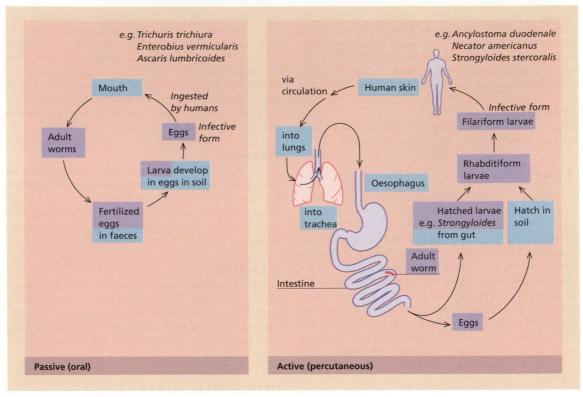

**Fig. 1.32**   Intestinal nematodes—schematic life-cycle.

## Strongyloidiasis

*Strongyloides stercoralis* is found worldwide but is particularly common in warm, wet regions such as parts of Central America and South-East Asia. Infection can persist for decades and is still being discovered in war veterans, particularly prisoners of war who worked on the Burma–Thailand railway and veterans from Vietnam. Adult worms inhabit the crypts of the small intestine, causing little damage, but in heavy infection worms are embedded in the mucosa, and cause an inflammatory response with mucosal injury. The worms are passed in the stools and autoinfection is common.

### CLINICAL FEATURES

After penetration of the skin by the filariform larvae, a local reaction occurs characterized by itching, erythema, oedema and urticaria. This subsides within 2 days. A week later, migration of the adolescent worms causes irritation of the upper airways, producing cough and occasionally more severe respiratory symptoms. After about 3 weeks, intestinal colonization occurs, often leading to abdominal discomfort, intermittent diarrhoea and constipation. These symptoms can be mild and may pass unnoticed. However, in some individuals, heavy infection may lead to persistent diarrhoea, nausea, anorexia and evidence of intestinal malabsorption, notably steatorrhoea. Hypoalbuminaemia and weight loss also occur. Disseminated strongyloidiasis is a very serious and often fatal condition and has been described in patients receiving cortico-

steroid or other immunosuppressive therapy or in those who are immunocompromised for other reasons.

### DIAGNOSIS

Motile rhabditiform larvae can be detected in fresh stool or in duodenal aspirate. Eosinophilia is common. In heavy infection, anaemia and biochemical evidence of malabsorption are found.

### TREATMENT

Treatment consists of thiabendazole 1.5 g twice daily for 2 days. Therapy should be given for at least 5 days (often longer) in the hyperinfected patient with disseminated disease. Albendazole 400 mg kg$^{-1}$ for 3 days is also effective. Repeated therapy may be required. The mortality is high in the hyperinfected group owing to an accompanying Gram-negative septicaemia and treatment should include i.v. broad-spectrum antibiotics.

## Hookworm infection

Hookworm is seen worldwide and affects approximately 25% of the world's population. *Ancylostoma duodenale* is found in Europe, the Middle East and North Africa, whereas *Necator americanus* is found in the Western Hemisphere, sub-Saharan Africa, South-East Asia and the Far East.

Adult worms inhabit the small intestine and attach firmly to the intestinal mucosa by the teeth or cutting

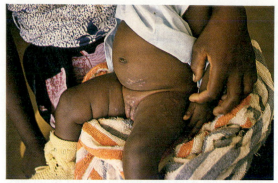

**Fig. 1.33** *Ancylostoma braziliensis* (dog hookworm) causes this characteristic cutaneous lesion.

plates in their large buccal capsule. Blood loss is approximately 0.2 ml daily in *A. duodenale* infection (five- to tenfold less with *N. americanus*); in heavy infection it has been estimated that up to 100 ml of blood is lost daily.

### CLINICAL FEATURES

Local irritation at the site of larval entry in the skin is known as 'ground itch', but this rapidly disappears to be followed some 2 weeks later by mild and transitory pulmonary symptoms. Most patients are asymptomatic once the larvae have reached the small intestine. Some patients experience ulcer-like symptoms and those with heavy chronic infection eventually develop symptoms and signs of anaemia. Hookworm infection is the commonest cause of iron deficiency anaemia worldwide. *A. braziliensis* (dog hookworm) causes characteristic patterns of subcutaneous infection in children (Fig 1.33).

### DIAGNOSIS

Hookworm ova appear in the stool, the number of eggs present giving a guide to the severity of the infection. Early in the infection, eosinophilia may be found in the peripheral blood. This is followed later by the appearance of iron deficiency anaemia.

### TREATMENT

Mebendazole 100 mg twice daily for 3 days is effective in both types of hookworm, although the infection may not be cleared with a single course of treatment.

## *Ascaris lumbricoides* ('roundworm') infection

*A. lumbricoides* is a large worm (Fig. 1.34) that is found worldwide but is particularly common in poor rural com-

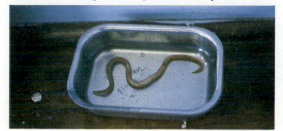

**Fig. 1.34** *Ascaris lumbricoides,* approximately 20 cm long.

munities where there is heavy faecal contamination of the immediate environment. Infection may be entirely asymptomatic, although heavy infections are associated with nausea, vomiting, abdominal discomfort and anorexia. Worms may obstruct the small intestine, the commonest site being at the ileocaecal valve. Worms occasionally invade the appendix, causing acute appendicitis, or the bile duct, resulting in biliary obstruction and suppurative cholangitis. Larvae in the lung may produce pulmonary eosinophila (p. 691). The nutritional impact of *Ascaris* infection in children is controversial, although it is very likely that heavy infection in malnourished children compounds the situation, largely by competition for host nutrients.

### DIAGNOSIS

*Ascaris* eggs may be identified in the stool and occasionally adult worms emerge from the mouth or the anus.

### TREATMENT

Mebendazole 100 mg twice daily for 3 days or a single dose of piperazine 100 mg kg$^{-1}$ or pyrantel pamoate 10 mg kg$^{-1}$ are effective. Surgical or endoscopic intervention may be required for intestinal or biliary obstruction.

## *Trichuris trichiura* (whipworm) infection

*T. trichiura* is a common parasite and is found worldwide. Prevalence varies from 1% to 90%, being highest in poor communities with inadequate sanitation. Adult worms are most commonly found in the distal ileum and caecum, although in heavy infection no part of the colon is spared. The adult worm embeds its cephalic region into the intestinal mucosa, leaving the distal tail free within the lumen. Such invasion damages the intestinal mucosa and in heavy infection overt colonic and rectal ulceration may result, leading to significant blood and protein loss.

### CLINICAL FEATURES

Most infections are asymptomatic and haematological or biochemical deficits do not occur provided nutritional intake is adequate. Heavy infection is associated with diarrhoea with blood and mucus, often associated with abdominal discomfort, tenesmus, anorexia and weight loss. Involvement of the appendix can cause appendicitis, and rectal prolapse has been reported in children.

### DIAGNOSIS

Stool examination confirms the presence of typical barrel-shaped eggs. Proctosigmoidoscopy may reveal adult worms firmly attached to the rectal mucosa.

### TREATMENT

Mebendazole 100 mg twice daily for 3 days or a single dose of pyrantel pamoate 10 mg kg$^{-1}$ are effective therapies.

## *Enterobius vermicularis* (threadworm) infection

This parasite occurs worldwide but is more prevalent in temperate and cold climates. Children are most commonly infected, but it may affect whole families, inhabitants of residential institutions, and any group of people living in overcrowded circumstances. Adult worms reside largely in the colon, the female migrating to the anus to deposit embryonated eggs on the perianal and perineal areas. Superficial damage to the colonic mucosa occurs during heavy infection and secondary bacterial infection of these lesions may rarely result in submucosal abscesses.

### CLINICAL FEATURES

Intense pruritus ani is usually the only symptom of threadworm infection. This is usually nocturnal and related to egg-laying in the perianal region by the female worms. Scratching results in dissemination of eggs and autoinfection. Infection has little significance while the parasite remains within the intestinal lumen, although on occasions migration occurs to the peritoneum and the viscera may be involved.

### DIAGNOSIS

Diagnosis is best achieved by applying a piece of clear adhesive tape to the perianal region; this tape may then be examined microscopically for the presence of adherent eggs. Adult worms may be observed leaving the anus by the child's parents.

### TREATMENT

A single dose of mebendazole 100 mg followed by a second dose 2 weeks later is usually effective. Alternatives include pyrantel pamoate or piperazine. Family members should also be treated.

---

# Trematode (fluke) infections

(Table 1.33)

---

## BLOOD INFECTIONS

## Schistosomiasis (bilharzia)

Three major species of schistosomes produce human dis-
ease. These have marked differences in geographical distribution (Fig. 1.35). Prevalence is dependent on the presence of a susceptible intermediate snail host and faecal contamination of water supplies. The size of snail populations varies with the season and availability of freshwater breeding grounds. An increase in the world prevalence of schistosomiasis is partly due to dam construction and irrigation programmes.

### LIFE-CYCLE AND PATHOGENESIS

Human infection occurs after penetration of the skin or mucous membranes by cercariae, the infective form of the parasite that is liberated into fresh water by the specific intermediate snail host (Fig. 1.36). Cercariae penetrate unbroken skin and migrate as schistosomules through the venous circulation to the liver, where the adult worms mature. Eventually pairs of male and female worms migrate upstream along the portal vein to the mesenteric venules, until the calibre of the vessels halts their progress. They remain in this location for many years copulating continuously and producing enormous numbers of eggs. To complete the life-cycle, eggs must leave the body, either by penetrating the intestinal wall (*Schistosoma mansoni* and *S. japonicum*) or the bladder wall (*S. haematobium*) and returning to the environment via faeces or urine, respectively. The larvae (miracidia) develop inside the eggs but do not hatch until they arrive in fresh water, when they search actively for the specific snail host to invade. Once inside the snail, multiplication occurs—a single miracidium produces up to 100 000 cercariae, released at the rate of 5000 per day.

Eggs retained in host tissues, particularly the liver, urinary bladder and intestine, are responsible for the clinical manifestations of schistosomiasis. Egg antigens initiate both immediate and delayed-type hypersensitivity reactions with granuloma formation. Humoral substances such as lymphokines, macrophage migration inhibitory factor and fibroblast stimulating factors are found at the site of these granulomas and presumably support the cellular inflammatory response. Healing eventually occurs by fibrosis.

### CLINICAL FEATURES

The first clinical sign of an acute infection is a local inflammatory response at the site of the invading cercariae known as 'swimmer's itch'. Within a week or more there is a generalized allergic response characterized by fever, urticaria, eosinophilia, myalgia and malaise. Nau-

| Organism | Location | Major disease site(s) |
|---|---|---|
| *Schistosoma mansoni* | Mesenteric veins | Liver, colon |
| *Schistosoma japonicum* | Mesenteric veins | Liver, colon, small intestine |
| *Schistosoma haematobium* | Pelvic veins, vesical plexus | Bladder, distal colon, rectum |
| *Fasciola hepatica* | Bile ducts | Bile ducts, liver |
| *Clonorchis sinensis* | Bile ducts | Bile ducts, liver |
| *Fasciolopsis buski* | Small intestine | Small intestine |
| *Paragonimus westermani* | Lung | Lung |

**Table 1.33** Trematode (fluke) infection.

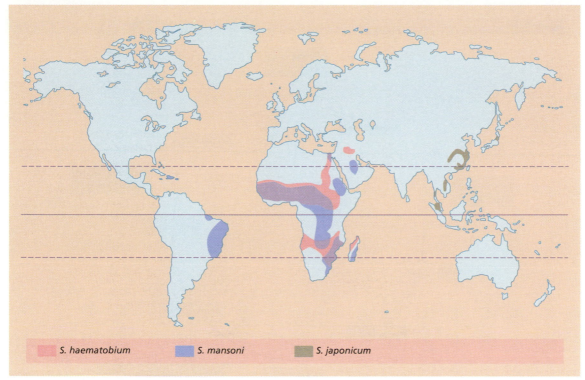

S. haematobium    S. mansoni    S. japonicum

**Fig. 1.35** Schistosomiasis—geographical distribution.

sea, vomiting and profuse diarrhoea are common, as are respiratory symptoms, particularly cough. Clinical findings at this time include generalized lymphadenopathy, hepatosplenomegaly and signs of patchy pneumonia. In Asia the acute disease is called Katayama fever. It is most pronounced in infection with *S. japonicum* and *S. mansoni*.

Chronic schistosomiasis varies in its clinical presentation depending on the type of schistosome involved.

### Schistosoma mansoni and Schistosoma japonicum

*S. mansoni* is found predominantly in Africa, South America and the West Indies, whereas *S. japonicum* is common in China and other specific sites in South East Asia.

*S. mansoni* predominantly affects the colon, where the presence of ova produces macroscopic lesions such as mucosal granularity, erythema and superficial ulceration. However, a particularly severe form of colonic disease is seen in Egyptians, with gross ulceration and polyp formation, particularly in the rectosigmoid; extensive polyposis results in significant blood and protein loss from the colon. Progressive fibrosis in the intestinal wall leads to rigidity and stricture formation, although intestinal obstruction is rare. A localized granulomatous reaction in the intestine (pseudotumour or bilharzioma) may be mistaken for a colonic cancer.

The development of granulomatous hepatitis, followed by progressive periportal fibrosis and portal hypertension, is signified by marked hepatosplenomegaly, often associated with oesophageal varices. In advanced cases death is due to the complications of portal hypertension, as hepatocellular function remains remarkably good.

*S. japonicum* affects the small intestine and proximal colon in addition to causing fibrotic liver disease. *S. japonicum* produces larger numbers of eggs than *S. mansoni*, which accounts for the more extensive pattern of disease and the frequency of ectopic deposition of ova, particularly in the lungs, spinal cord and brain. The latter may result in fits or hemiplegia.

Epithelial dysplasia in the colon has been reported in patients with chronic *S. japonicum* colitis, and it is now clear that this condition has premalignant potential in endemic areas.

### Schistosoma haematobium

This is mainly a urinary tract schistosome found predominantly in Egypt, East Africa and the Middle East. Chronic inflammation is found in the bladder, ureters and urethra, causing urinary frequency, dysuria and haematuria. Chronic infection leads to obstructive uropathy, chronic pyelonephritis and renal failure, and contraction of the bladder. Epidemiological studies confirm an association between bladder carcinoma and this infection. The internal genitalia may be involved and rectal inflammation and ulceration may be found in up to 70% of patients.

### DIAGNOSIS

In endemic areas a confident diagnosis can often be obtained on clinical grounds. Confirmation is achieved

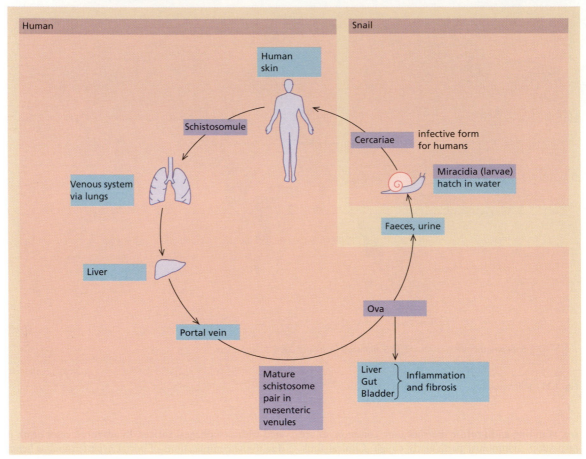

**Fig. 1.36** *Schistosoma*—schematic life-cycle.

by detecting the characteristic eggs in the stools, the urine or in a rectal biopsy. Different species of *Schistosoma* can be distinguished not only by the clinical pattern but also by egg morphology.

A plain abdominal radiograph may reveal intramural calcification in the wall of the bladder or the colon. Barium contrast studies of the colon show spiculating mucosal ulceration, polyposis, strictures, and possibly a mass lesion that could either be a bilharzioma or, in the case of *S. japonicum* infection, a carcinoma.

Intravenous urography may confirm an obstructive uropathy and demonstrate bladder contraction.

Immunodiagnostic tests are available, the most sensitive of which detect antibodies against a gut-associated polysaccharide antigen by either ELISA or indirect immunofluorescence.

### TREATMENT

The two major objectives of treatment of schistosomiasis are:

1 Reduction in egg production
2 Prevention or reduction of tissue damage by eggs already *in situ*

In endemic and hyperendemic areas, curative therapy is usually inappropriate, since reinfection occurs rapidly, whereas infected individuals who are no longer exposed to the parasite can be effectively treated. Suppressive non-curative chemotherapeutic approaches have been used in mass treatment programmes in Egypt with good clinical improvement following a reduction in the 'worm burden'. All antischistosomal drugs have the same effect: they cause worms to leave the mesenteric and vesical veins and to enter the liver and lungs where they are eventually destroyed by host tissue responses.

Praziquantel is active against all species of schistosome and is probably the drug of choice as it is well tolerated and relatively free from serious side-effects. A single dose (40 mg kg$^{-1}$) cures more than 90% of patients with *S. haematobium*, with slightly lower rates against *S. mansoni*. *S. japonicum* is best treated with a total dose of 60 mg kg$^{-1}$ given in divided doses over 1 or 2 days.

Oxamniquine is active against *S. mansoni* and metriphonate against *S. haematobium*.

Colonscopic polypectomy can control the number of colonic polyps, but surgery may be required to relieve obstructive uropathy and for inflammatory masses in the CNS.

## PREVENTION

Personal protection is to avoid infected water. General control is difficult but depends on the provision of good sanitation, which is largely an economic problem.

# LIVER AND BILIARY TRACT INFECTIONS

## Fascioliasis

*Fasciola hepatica* infects sheep, goats and cattle, in which it produces liver disease, and is only accidentally transmitted to humans via consumption of wild watercress grown on the grazing land of infected animals. The disease is found worldwide, including the UK. Animals excrete eggs in their faeces, from which ciliated miracidia emerge. These enter the freshwater snail (the intermediate host) in which larval development takes place. Eventually cercaria are released and these encyst on aquatic or surface vegetation.

After ingestion by a mammalian host, the parasites excyst, migrate through the intestinal wall and penetrate the liver capsule after traversing the peritoneal cavity. Immature flukes reach the bile duct by passing through liver parenchyma and after maturation begin to produce eggs. Adult flukes remain within the biliary tract for many years.

### CLINICAL FEATURES

Early symptoms of intermittent fever, malaise, weight loss, right upper quadrant pain and urticaria relate to migration of flukes through the liver and generally occur 2–3 months after infection.

A second phase of the illness relates to the presence of flukes in the biliary tract, where they can cause obstruction with jaundice and cholangitis, although infection may remain asymptomatic. Flukes have been found in many ectopic sites, including lung, brain and skin.

### DIAGNOSIS

Eosinophilia is common in the early phase of the illness and is often associated with liver biochemical abnormalities and a positive complement fixation test. Ova are not found in the stool until the second phase of the illness when the mature flukes are established in the biliary tract. However, in up to 30% of cases, stools remain negative; the diagnosis can then be confirmed either by identifying ova in duodenal aspirate or by serological tests. Treatment is with bithionol 30–50 mg kg$^{-1}$ for 10–15 doses given either daily or on alternate days.

## Clonorchiasis

*Clonorchis sinensis* is a common fluke of the dog, cat and pig that affects millions of animals in the Far East, particularly Indo-China, Japan, Korea, Hong Kong and Vietnam. A related fluke, *Opisthorchis felineus*, also affects foxes and is found predominantly in India, the Philippines, Korea and Japan. The life-cycles of both these flukes are similar to that of *F. hepatica*, except that freshwater fish become infected by the cercaria and thereby function as a second intermediate host. Human infection occurs by ingestion of infected raw fish.

### CLINICAL FEATURES

Infected individuals may remain symptom-free, although prolonged exposure with heavy infection results in recurrent cholestatic jaundice, suppurative cholangitis, liver abscess and cholangiocarcinoma.

### DIAGNOSIS

The diagnosis is made on microscopic examination of faeces or duodenal aspirate.

### TREATMENT

Praziquantel 25 mg kg$^{-1}$ as a single dose is the treatment of choice.

# INTESTINAL INFECTIONS

## Fasciolopsiasis

*Fasciolopsis buski* causes intestinal infection in humans and pigs. There are two intermediate hosts—freshwater snails and water plants. Human infection is initiated by oral contact with contaminated water plants. These large flukes, which are several centimetres in length, are common in China, Vietnam, Thailand and Taiwan.

Mucosal ulceration and inflammation are apparent at the site of attachment in the intestine; abscess formation, haemorrhage and occasionally bowel obstruction may result. The symptoms are usually non-specific. Heavy infection in children may simulate or precipitate protein–energy malnutrition. Anaemia and eosinophilia are common.

### DIAGNOSIS

The diagnosis may be simple if the patient is vomiting or passing flukes per rectum, but may be confirmed by identifying ova in the stools.

### TREATMENT

Treatment is with tetrachloroethylene 0.12 ml kg$^{-1}$ as a single dose (maximum dose of 5 ml) or dichlorophen 100 mg kg$^{-1}$ as a single dose (which may be repeated 1 week later).

# Helminthic (cestode) infections

Tapeworms belong to the subclass Cestoda. These are flat worms measuring a few millimetres (*Echinococcus granulosus*) to several metres (*Taenia saginata*) in length. Structurally they consist of a head that is adorned with suckers and hooks (*Taenia solium*) or suckers alone (*T. saginata*). The head is attached via a short slender neck to several segments or proglottids that form a chain-like structure or strobila. The terminal proglottide is the most mature. The entire worm is covered with a continuous elastic cuticle. Tapeworms are devoid of a gastrointestinal tract or vascular system; nutrients are absorbed directly through the cuticle. They are hermaphrodites and cross-fertilization between proglottids is frequent.

Adults live in the intestinal tract of vertebrates, whereas the larvae (oncospheres) exist in the tissues of vertebrates and invertebrates. Infection is transmitted to humans by ingestion of meats infected with larval forms. Four tapeworms commonly infect humans: *T. saginata*, *T. solium*, *Diphyllobothrium latum* and *Hymenolepsis nana*.

## *Taenia saginata* (beef tapeworm) infection

*T. saginata* measures up to 10 m in length, inhabits the upper jejunum, and is prevalent in humans in all beef-eating countries. The majority of patients are asymptomatic. Symptoms are mild, with vague epigastric and abdominal pain, and occasional diarrhoea and vomiting. Weight loss is unusual. Rarely, appendicitis and pancrea-

titis due to obstruction of the appendix and pancreatic ducts, respectively, by the adult worms may occur. The commonest symptom is the presence of proglottids in the faeces, bed or underclothing.

### DIAGNOSIS
The presence of proglottids, which are visible macroscopically, or the eggs, which are seen microscopically, in the faeces or perianal region is diagnostic. A higher positive yield is obtained by examining perianal clear adhesive tape swabs for ova, in which case the scolex (the head) or proglottids are required to establish the species.

### TREATMENT
Niclosamide 2 g as a single chewed dose is effective. Praziquantel 10 mg kg$^{-1}$ as a single dose is effective but is not available on the UK market.

### PREVENTION
Prevention is easily effected by careful inspection of beef for cysticerci (encysted larval forms). Refrigeration of beef at 0°C for 5 days or cooking it at 57°C for a few minutes destroys the cysticerci.

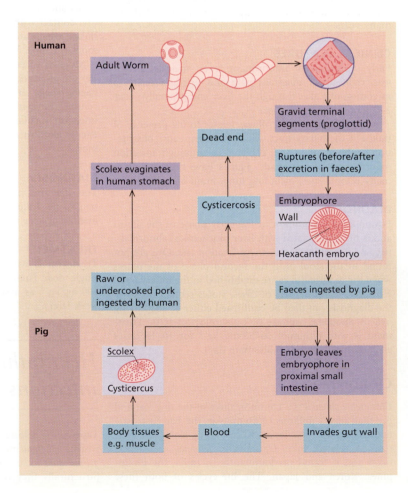

**Fig. 1.37**  *Taenia solium*—schematic life-cycle.

## *Taenia solium* infection and cysticercosis

*T. solium* (the pork tapeworm) measures up to 6 m in length. It has a worldwide distribution but is seen most frequently in Eastern Europe, South East Asia and Africa. In the adult form it lives in the human upper jejunum. The clinical features are similar to those caused by *T. saginata*.

Treatment is similar to that for *T. saginata*. However, because release of ova can occur during treatment and, theoretically, could be carried back into the stomach, releasing the intermediate larval stage, treatment for *T. solium* should be followed by a saline purge.

### Human cysticercosis

Cysticercosis occurs after autoinfection or heteroinfection by eggs of *T. solium* and invasion of tissues by the intermediate larval form—cysticercus cellulosae (Fig. 1.37). Cysticercosis is most commonly seen in parts of Asia, Africa and South America. Cysticerci may develop in any tissue in the body. Most commonly, however, three clinical forms are recognized:

1 *Cerebral cysticercosis* may present as various forms of epilepsy, as a space-occupying lesion or as focal neurological deficits including hemiplegia and behavioural changes.
2 *Ocular cysticercosis* may present as retinitis, uveitis, conjunctivitis or choroidal atrophy. Blindness may ensue.
3 *Subcutaneous cysticercosis* presents as small, pea-sized, hard nodules in the subcutaneous tissue.

The diagnosis is established by biopsy of a subcutaneous nodule and demonstrating the characteristic translucent membrane. Radiography may demonstrate calcified degenerating cysticerci. CT brain scan should be performed when subcutaneous cysticercosis has been diagnosed. Indirect haemagglutination tests are useful.

Treatment involves surgical excision of the cysticerci if possible. Praziquantel is the drug of choice for cysticercosis; steroids are given during therapy to avoid reactions. Antiepileptic drugs are usually necessary for cerebral cysticercosis.

## *Diphyllobothrium latum* infection

Diphyllobothriasis is particularly prevalent in Scandinavian countries, the Baltic region, Japan and the lake region of Switzerland. Infection in humans, the definitive host, results from ingestion of fish that contain the infected plerocercoid form. The adult tapeworm measures several metres in length. The proglottids differ from those of *Taenia* in that they are more wide than long. The adult worm usually attaches itself to the jejunum.

The clinical features are usually mild and consist of vague abdominal discomfort, anorexia, nausea and vomiting. Megaloblastic anaemia, due to competitive utilization of ingested vitamin $B_{12}$ by the parasite, may occur in a small percentage of patients. Rarely, intestinal obstruction occurs.

Treatment is similar to that described for *T. saginata*.

## Hydatid disease

Hydatid disease occurs when humans ingest the hexacanth embryos of the dog tapeworm *Echinococcus granulosus* or of *E. multilocularis*.

Human infection with *E. granulosus* frequently occurs in early childhood by direct contact with infected dogs, or by eating uncooked, improperly washed vegetables contaminated with infected canine faeces. In the duodenum the hexacanth embryos hatch, penetrate the intestinal wall, enter the portal system and are then carried to the liver. Further dissemination of embryos to the lung and to almost every organ in the body may occur, where they form hydatid cysts (Fig. 1.38). The disease is seen in all parts of the world particularly in those countries where sheep and cattle-raising constitutes an important means of livelihood. It is rare in the UK but is seen in the Middle East, North and East Africa, Australia and Argentina. These animals perpetuate the life-cycle of the parasite.

Symptoms largely depend upon the site of the unilocular hydatid cyst. The liver is the commonest site for cyst formation (60%), followed by the lung (20%), kidneys (3%) and brain (1%). In the liver the majority of cysts are situated in the right lobe. The symptoms are those of a slowly growing benign tumour. Pressure on the bile ducts may cause jaundice. Rupture into the abdominal cavity, pleural cavity or biliary tree may occur. In the latter instance, intermittent jaundice, abdominal pain and fever associated with eosinophilia result. A cyst rupturing into a bronchus may result in its expectoration and spontaneous cure, but if secondary infection supervenes a

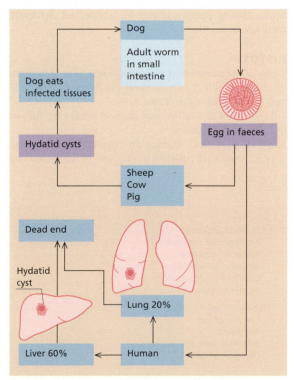

**Fig. 1.38** *Echinococcus granulosus*—schematic life-cycle.

chronic pulmonary abscess will form. Haemoptysis, dyspnoea and chest pain may lead to a mistaken diagnosis of malignancy. Focal seizures may occur if cysts are present in the brain. Renal involvement produces lumbar pain and haematuria. Calcification of the cyst occurs in about 40% of cases.

The alveolar hydatid cyst caused by *E. multilocularis* results from its larval stage. *E. multilocularis* is seen in parts of Canada, the former USSR and Alaska. Foxes and small rodents constitute the intermediate hosts; humans are accidental hosts. The majority of the lesions are in the liver and metastasis may occur.

The diagnosis and treatment of hydatid disease are described on p. 275.

# Sexually transmitted diseases

Sexually transmitted diseases (STDs) remain epidemic in all societies and the range of pathogens that are known to be spread by sex continues to increase. In 1990 over 578 000 new cases were seen in genitourinary medicine (GUM) clinics in the UK. In the last 50 years there has been an increase in viral conditions, particularly Herpes simplex virus (HSV) and human papillomavirus, but a decrease in cases of syphilis and gonorrhoea. The recognition of AIDS and human immunodeficiency virus (HIV) has heightened awareness of STDs. In GUM clinics up to 25% of patients attend for advice and checks on their sexual health.

## HISTORY

Three of the commonest presenting symptoms are vaginal discharge (Table 1.34), urethral discharge (Table 1.35) and genital ulceration (Table 1.36).

In addition to a full general medical history the following should be obtained:

SEXUAL HISTORY: number and types of sexual contact (e.g. orogenital), partner's sex, use of condoms and other forms of contraception, previous history of STDs including dates and treatment received, HIV testing and results and hepatitis B vaccination

TRAVEL ABROAD to areas where antibiotic resistance is known or where particular pathogens are endemic

DRUG MISUSE

IN WOMEN, menstrual and obstetric history

## EXAMINATION

General examination must include a review of the mouth, throat, skin and lymph nodes in all patients. Signs of HIV infection are covered on p. 98.

The inguinal, genital and perianal areas should be examined with a good light source. The groins should be palpated for lymphadenopathy and hernias. The pubic hair must be examined for nits and lice. The external genitalia must be examined for signs of erythema, fissures, ulcers, chancres, pigmented or hypopigmented areas and condylomata. Signs of trauma may be seen.

In *men*, the penile skin should be examined and the foreskin retracted to look for balanitis, ulceration, condylomata or tumours. The urethral meatus is located and the presence of discharge noted. Scrotal contents are pal-

---

Infective
  *Neisseria gonorrhoeae*
  *Chlamydia trachomatis*
  *Ureaplasma urealyticum*
  *Mycoplasma* spp.
  *Trichomonas vaginalis*
  Herpes simplex
  Urethral warts
  Urinary tract infection (rare)
  *Treponema pallidum*

Non-infective
  Physical or chemical trauma
  Non-specific (aetiology unknown)

**Table 1.35**  Causes of urethral discharge.

---

Infective
  Syphilis
    Primary chancre
    Secondary mucous patches
    Tertiary gumma
  Chancroid
  Lymphogranuloma venereum
  Granuloma inguinale
  Herpes simplex
    Primary
    Recurrent
  Herpes zoster

Non-infective
  Behçet's syndrome
  Stevens–Johnson syndrome
  Carcinoma
  Trauma

**Table 1.36**  Causes of genital ulceration.

---

Infective
  *Candida albicans*
  *Trichomonas vaginalis*
  Bacterial vaginosis
  *Neisseria gonorrhoeae*
  *Chlamydia trachomatis*
  Herpes simplex

Non-infective
  Cervical polyps
  Neoplasia
  Retained products, e.g. tampons
  Chemical irritation

**Table 1.34**  Causes of vaginal discharge.

pated and the consistency of the testes and epididymis noted. A rectal examination/proctoscopy should be performed in patients with rectal symptoms, those who practise anoreceptive intercourse and patients with prostatic symptoms. A search for rectal condylomata is indicated in patients with perianal lesions.

In *women*, Bartholin's glands must be identified and examined. The cervix should be inspected for ulceration, discharge, bleeding and ectopy and the walls of the vagina for condylomata. A bimanual pelvic examination is performed to elicit adnexal tenderness or masses, cervical tenderness and to assess the position, size and mobility of the uterus. Rectal examination and proctoscopy are performed if the patient has symptoms or practises anoreceptive intercourse.

## INVESTIGATIONS

Although history and examination will guide investigation it must be remembered that multiple infections may coexist, some being asymptomatic.

1 In men:
   (a) Urethral smears for Gram staining
   (b) Urethral swabs for gonococcal culture and *Chlamydia* testing
   (c) Two glass urine test and urinalysis
   (d) Rectal swabs for Gram staining and culture
   (e) Throat swab for culture
   (f) Blood for syphilis serology
2 In women:
   (a) Smears from the lateral vaginal wall for Gram staining
   (b) Vaginal swab for culture of *Candida* and *Trichomonas*
   (c) A wet preparation is made from the posterior fornix for *Trichomonas* and for the potassium hydroxide test for bacterial vaginosis
   (d) The pH of vaginal secretions using narrow range indicator paper
   (e) Endocervical smears and swabs for Gram staining, gonococcal culture and *Chlamydia* tests
   (f) Urethral smears and swabs for Gram staining and gonococcal culture
   (g) Rectal and throat swabs, if indicated
   (h) Urinalysis
   (i) Cervical cytology
   (j) Blood syphilis serology
3 Additional investigations when appropriate include:
   (a) Blood for hepatitis B and C serology, HIV antibody testing (with full counselling)
   (b) Swabs for HSV and *Haemophilus ducreyi* from clinically suspicious lesions in special media
   (c) Smears and swabs from subpreputial area in men with balanoposthitis (inflammation of glans penis and prepuce)
   (d) Scrapings from lesions suspicious of early syphilis for immediate dark-ground microscopy
   (e) Pregnancy testing
   (f) Stools for *Giardia*, *Shigella* or *Salmonella* from homosexual men

## TREATMENT, PREVENTION AND CONTROL

The treatment of specific conditions is considered in the appropriate section. Many GUM clinics keep basic stocks of medication and dispense directly to the patient.

Tracing the sexual partners of patients is crucial in controlling spread of STDs. The aims are to prevent the spread of infection within the community and to ensure that people with asymptomatic infection are properly treated. Interviewing people about their sexual partners requires considerable tact and sensitivity and specialist health advisors are available in GUM clinics.

Prevention starts with education and information. People begin sexual activity at ever younger ages and education programmes need to include school pupils as well as young adults. Education of health professionals is also crucial. Appropriate and accessible services must be well advertised. The risks of acquiring an STD may be reduced by avoiding multiple partners, correct and consistent use of condoms and avoiding sex with people who have symptoms of infection. For those who change their sexual partners frequently regular check-ups (approximately 3-monthly) are advisable. Once people develop symptoms they should be encouraged to seek medical advice as soon as possible to reduce complications and spread to others.

# CLINICAL SYNDROMES

## Gonorrhoea

The incidence of gonorrhoea (GC) in developing countries has fallen dramatically since the early 1970s but in Asia and Africa it still remains high. In 1990 WHO estimated 35 million cases worldwide, second to *Chlamydia trachomatis* amongst STDs. The causative organism, *Neisseria gonorrhoeae* (gonococcus), is a Gram-negative intracellular diplococcus which infects epithelium particularly of the urogenital tract, rectum, pharynx and conjunctivae. Humans are the only host and the organism is spread by intimate physical contact. It is very intolerant to drying and although occasional reports of spread by fomites exist this route of infection is extremely rare.

### CLINICAL FEATURES

Forty per cent of women and some men are asymptomatic. The incubation period ranges from 2 to 14 days with most symptoms occurring between days 2 and 5. In *men* the commonest syndrome is one of anterior urethritis causing dysuria and/or urethral discharge. Complications include ascending infection involving the epididymis, testes or prostate leading to acute or chronic infection. In homosexual men rectal infection may produce proctitis with pain, discharge and itch.

In *women* the primary site of infection is usually the endocervical canal and symptoms consist of a vaginal discharge, dysuria and intermenstrual bleeding. Complications include ascending infection leading to salpingitis with associated pelvic pain and fever. In rare cases a perihepatitis may develop (Fitz-Hugh–Curtis syndrome). Bartholin's abscesses may develop. On a global basis GC is one of the commonest causes of female infertility.

Rectal infection, due to local spread, may occur in women and is usually asymptomatic as in pharyngeal infection. Conjunctival infection is seen in neonates born to infected mothers and is one cause of ophthalmia neonatorum.

Disseminated GC leads to arthritis (usually monoarticular or pauciarticular)(see p. 398) and a characteristic purplish macular rash in association with fever and malaise.

### DIAGNOSIS

The organism is identified from infected areas by Gram stain and culture on special media. Blood culture and synovial fluid investigations should be performed in cases of disseminated GC. Coexisting pathogens such as *Chlamydia*, *Trichomonas* and syphilis must be sought.

### TREATMENT

The gonococcus is sensitive to a wide range of antimicrobial agents but an increase in antibiotic resistance has been seen over the past two decades. Therapy initiated in the clinic on the basis of Gram-stained slides prior to culture results is influenced by travel history or details known from contacts.

Therapy with single-dose amoxycillin 3 g with probenecid 1 g is given in uncomplicated cases. Spectinomycin 2 g i.m. or ciprofloxacin 250 mg are used in penicillin-resistant or allergic cases. Longer courses of antibiotics are required for complicated infections. Patients must be followed up to ensure that the organism has been eradicated and all sexual contacts should be examined and treated as necessary.

## Chlamydia

*Chlamydia trachomatis* (see p. 46) is an obligate intracellular bacterial parasite which cannot be grown on artificial culture media. Cell culture systems are not universally available and indirect diagnostic methods are still being perfected. The organism has a worldwide distribution and silent infection is common. In men 30–40% of non-gonococcal and postgonococcal urethritis is due to *Chlamydia*. It is frequently found in association with other pathogens: 20% of men and 40% of women with gonorrhoea have been found to have coexisting chlamydial infections.

### CLINICAL FEATURES

In *men Chlamydia* gives rise to an anterior urethritis with dysuria and discharge; infection is often asymptomatic and detected by contact tracing. Ascending infection leads to epididymitis. Rectal infection leading to proctitis may occur in men practising anoreceptive intercourse. In *women* the commonest site of infection is the endocervix where it may go unnoticed; ascending infection causes acute salpingitis. In women subfertility may be the first problem encountered. Reiter's syndrome (see p. 395) has been related to infection with *C. trachomatis*. Neonatal infection, acquired from the birth canal, can result in mucopurulent conjunctivitis and pneumonia.

### DIAGNOSIS

Cell culture systems are still considered the definitive method of diagnosis but are costly and not suitable for routine use.

Antigen detection systems depending on either direct fluorescent antibody or enzyme immunoassay are increasingly available. In view of the intracellular nature of the organism care must be taken to obtain adequate specimens and it is essential that cells are collected. Wooden swabs may interfere with assay techniques. Special transport media are required.

### MANAGEMENT

Tetracyclines or macrolide antibiotics are most commonly used to treat *Chlamydia*. Oxytetracycline 500 mg 6-hourly or doxycycline 100 mg 12-hourly for 7 days are effective. Tetracyclines are contraindicated in pregnancy and erythromycin 500 mg 6-hourly for 7–14 days can be given. Contacts must be traced and treated.

## Urethritis

Urethritis is usually characterized in men by a discharge from the urethra, dysuria and varying degrees of discomfort within the penis. In 10–15% of cases there may be no symptoms. A wide array of aetiologies can give rise to the clinical picture, but may be divided into two broad bands: gonococcal or non-gonococcal urethritis (NGU). NGU occurring shortly after infection with gonorrhoea is known as postgonococcal urethritis (PGU). Gonococcal urethritis and chlamydial urethritis (a major cause of NGU) are discussed above.

In *Chlamydia*-negative NGU, *Ureaplasma urealyticum* is the next most frequent organism. *Bacteroides* sp. and *Mycoplasma* are responsible for a minority of cases. HSV can cause urethritis in about 30% of cases of primary infection, considerably fewer in recurrent episodes. Other causes include syphilitic chancres and warts within the urethra. Non-sexually transmitted NGU may be due to urinary tract infections, prostatic infection, foreign bodies and strictures.

### CLINICAL FEATURES

The urethral discharge is often mucoid and worse in the mornings. It may be noted as crusting at the meatus or stains on underwear. Dysuria is common but not universal. Discomfort or itch within the penis may be present. The incubation is from 1 to 5 weeks with a mean of 2–3 weeks. The importance of asymptomatic urethritis must be recognized as a major reservoir of infection. Associated features of conjunctivitis and/or arthritis may occur, particularly in HLA B27-positive individuals.

### DIAGNOSIS

Smears should be taken from the urethra when the patient has not voided urine for at least 4 hours and should be Gram stained and examined under a high power (×1000) oil immersion lens. The presence of five or more polymorphonucleocytes per high power field is diagnostic. Men who are symptomatic but have no objective evidence of urethritis should be re-examined and tested after holding urine overnight. Cultures for gonorrhoea must be taken together with swabs for *Chlamydia* testing.

## MANAGEMENT

Therapy is with tetracyclines initially, using either oxytetracycline 500 mg 6-hourly or doxycycline 100 mg 12-hourly for 7 days. Sexual intercourse should be avoided. The vast majority of patients will show partial or total response. For those left with objective evidence of urethritis, erythromycin 500 mg 6-hourly for 1–2 weeks should be prescribed. Sexual partners must be traced and treated; *C. trachomatis* can be isolated from the cervix in 50–60% of the female partners of men with gonorrhoea or NGU, many of whom are asymptomatic. This causes long-term morbidity in such women, acts as a reservoir of infection for the community and may lead to reinfection in the index case if not treated.

## RECURRENT/PERSISTENT NGU

This is a common and difficult clinical problem. The usual time for patients to re-present is 2–3 weeks following treatment. Tests for *Chlamydia* and *Ureaplasma* are usually negative. It is important to document objective evidence of urethritis, check compliance and establish any possible contact with untreated sexual partners. Investigations should include wet preparation and culture of a urethral smear for *Trichomonas vaginalis* and fungi. Cultures should be taken for HSV. A mid-stream urine sample should be examined and cultured. A further 2 weeks' treatment with erythromycin may be given and any specific additional infection treated appropriately. If symptoms are mild and all partners have been treated patients should be reassured and further antibiotic therapy avoided. In cases of frequent recurrence and/or florid unresponsive urethritis the prostate should be investigated and urethroscopy or cystoscopy performed to investigate possible strictures, periurethral fistulae or foreign bodies.

# Syphilis

The causative organism, *Treponema pallidum* (TP), is a motile spirochaete that is generally acquired by close sexual contact and transplacentally from mother to fetus. The organism enters the new host through breaches in squamous or columnar epithelium. Primary infection of non-genital sites may occasionally occur but is rare. Syphilis is a chronic systemic disease which can be quiescent or show protean manifestations.

Both congenital and acquired syphilis have early and late stages, each of which has classical clinical features (Table 1.37).

## Primary

Between 10 and 90 days (mean 21 days) after exposure to the pathogen a papule develops at the site of inoculation. This ulcerates to become a painless, firm chancre. There is usually painless regional lymphadenopathy in

| Clinical features | |
|---|---|
| **Acquired** | |
| *Early stages* | |
| Primary | Hard chancre |
| | Painless, regional lymphadenopathy |
| Secondary | *General*: Fever, malaise, arthralgia, sore throat and generalized lymphadenopathy |
| | *Skin*: Red/brown maculopapular non-itchy, sometimes scaly rash; condylomata lata |
| | *Mucous membranes*: Mucous patches, 'snail-track' ulcers in oropharynx and on genitalia |
| *Late stages* | |
| Tertiary | *Late benign*: Gummas (bone and viscera) |
| | *Cardiovascular*: Aortitis and aortic regurgitation |
| | *Neurosyphilis*: Meningovascular involvement, general paralysis of the insane (GPI) and tabes dorsalis |
| **Congenital** | |
| *Early stages* | Stillbirth or failure to thrive |
| | 'Snuffles' (nasal infection with discharge) |
| | Skin and mucous membrane lesions as in secondary syphilis |
| *Late stages* | *'Stigmata'*: Hutchinson's teeth, 'sabre' tibia and abnormalities of long bones |
| | Keratitis, uveitis, facial gummas and CNS disease |

Table 1.37 Classification and clinical features of syphilis.

association. The primary lesion may go unnoticed especially if it is on the cervix or within the rectum. Healing occurs spontaneously within 2–3 weeks.

## Secondary

Between 4 and 10 weeks after the appearance of the primary lesion constitutional symptoms with fever, sore throat, malaise and arthralgia appear. Signs include:

GENERALIZED LYMPHADENOPATHY (50%)

GENERALIZED SKIN RASHES involving the whole body including the palms and soles but excluding the face (75%)

CONDYLOMATA LATA—warty, plaque-like lesions found in the perianal area and other moist body sites

SUPERFICIAL CONFLUENT ULCERATION OF MUCOSAL SURFACES—found in the mouth and on the genitalia

ACUTE NEUROLOGICAL SIGNS (less than 10%)

Without treatment, symptoms and signs abate over 3–12 weeks, but in up to 20% of individuals may recur during a period known as early latency, a 2-year period in the UK (1 year in USA). Late latency is based on reactive syphilis serology with no clinical manifestations for at least 2 years. This may continue for many years before the late stages of syphilis become apparent.

### Tertiary

Late benign syphilis, so called because of its response to therapy rather than its clinical manifestations, generally involves the skin and the bones. The characteristic lesion, the gumma (granulomatous, sometimes ulcerating, lesions), can occur anywhere in the skin, frequently at sites of trauma. Gummas are commonly found in the skull, tibia, fibula and clavicle, although any bone may be involved. Visceral gummas occur mainly in the liver (hepar lobatum) and the testes.

Cardiovascular and neurosyphilis are discussed on p. 628 and p. 928.

### Congenital syphilis

Congenital syphilis usually becomes apparent between the second and sixth week after birth, early signs being nasal discharge, skin and mucous membrane lesions, and failure to thrive. Signs of late syphilis generally do not appear until after 2 years of age and take the form of 'stigmata' relating to early damage to developing structures, particularly teeth and long bones. Other late manifestations parallel those of adult tertiary syphilis.

### DIAGNOSIS

TP is not amenable to *in vitro* culture—the most sensitive and specific method is identification by dark-ground microscopy. Organisms may be found in variable numbers from primary chancres and the mucous patches of secondary lesions. Individuals with either primary or secondary disease are highly infectious.

Serological tests used in diagnosis are either treponemal specific or non-specific. Three main tests are used routinely (Table 1.38):

1 The VDRL (Venereal Disease Reference Laboratory) is non-specific but is a useful screening test, becoming positive within 3–4 weeks of the primary infection. It generally becomes negative by 6 months after treatment. It is a quantifiable test which can be used to monitor treatment efficacy and is helpful in assessing disease activity. The VDRL may also become negative

| Stage of infection | Results | | |
|---|---|---|---|
| | FTA-ABS | TPHA | VDRL |
| Very early primary | – | – | – |
| Early primary | + | – | – |
| Primary | + | ± | + |
| Secondary or latent | + | + | + |
| Late latent | + | + | – |
| Treated | + | + | – |
| Biological false-positive | – | – | + |

FTA–ABS, fluorescent treponema antibodies absorbed; TPHA, *Treponema pallidum* haemagglutination assay; VDRL, Venereal Disease Reference Laboratory.

**Table 1.38**  Syphilis serology.

in untreated patients (50% of patients with late stage syphilis). False-positive results may occur in other conditions particularly: infectious mononucleosis, hepatitis, *Mycoplasma* infections, some protozoal infections, cirrhosis, malignancy, autoimmune disease and chronic infections.

2 *T. pallidum* haemagglutination assay (TPHA) and fluorescent treponema antibodies absorbed (FTA-ABS) test are both highly specific for treponemal disease but will not differentiate between syphilis and other conditions such as yaws.

3 The FTA-ABS test is positive in more than 90% of patients with primary infection and in all patients with latent and late syphilis. It remains positive for life, even after treatment.

All serological investigations may be negative in early primary syphilis. The diagnosis will then hinge on positive dark-ground microscopy and treatment should not be delayed if serological tests are negative in such situations.

In certain cases examination of the CSF for evidence of neurosyphilis and a chest X-ray to determine the extent of cardiovascular disease will be indicated.

### TREATMENT

Early syphilis (primary or secondary) should be treated with long-acting procaine penicillin 1.2 g daily by intramuscular injection for 10 days. When compliance is in doubt, a single injection of benzathine penicillin 2.4 g will maintain adequate levels of drug for approximately 2 weeks. For late stage syphilis, particularly when there is cardiovascular or neurological involvement, the treatment course should be extended to 4 weeks. For patients sensitive to penicillin, either tetracycline or erythromycin may be given. Tetracycline is contraindicated in pregnancy.

The Jarisch–Herxheimer reaction, which is due to release of endotoxin when large numbers of organisms are killed by antibiotics, is seen in 50% of patients with primary syphilis and up to 90% of patients with secondary syphilis. It occurs about 8 hours after the first injection and usually consists of mild fever, malaise and headache lasting several hours. In cardiovascular or neurosyphilis the reaction, although rare, may be severe and exacerbate the clinical manifestations. Prednisolone given for 24 hours prior to therapy ameliorates the reaction. Penicillin should not be withheld because of the Jarisch–Herxheimer reaction; since it is not a dose-related phenomenon, there is no value in giving a smaller dose. The prognosis depends on the stage at which the infection is treated. Early and early latent syphilis have an excellent outlook but once extensive tissue damage has occurred in the later stages the damage will not be reversed although the process may be halted. Symptoms in cardiovascular and neurosyphilis may therefore persist.

The sexual partners of all patients with early syphilis must be contacted and screened.

## Chancroid

Chancroid or soft chancre is an acute STD caused by *Haemophilus ducreyi*. It is common in tropical areas of the world and is endemic in parts of Africa and Asia. Epidemiological studies in Africa have shown an association between genital ulcer disease, frequently chancroid, and the acquisition of HIV infection. A new urgency to control chancroid has resulted from these observations.

**CLINICAL FEATURES**

The incubation period is 4–7 days. An initial erythematous papular lesion forms which then breaks down into an ulcer. Several ulcers may merge to form giant serpiginous lesions. Ulcers appear most commonly on the prepuce and frenulum in men and may erode through tissues. In women the most commonly affected site is the vaginal entrance and the perineum. The lesions in women may go unnoticed.

At the same time inguinal lymphadenopathy develops (usually unilateral) and may progress to form large buboes which can suppurate.

**DIAGNOSIS**

Chancroid must be differentiated from other genital ulcer diseases (see Table 1.36). Isolation of *H. ducreyi* in specialized culture media is definitive but difficult. Swabs should be taken from the ulcer and material aspirated from the local lymph nodes for culture.

**TREATMENT**

Increasing evidence is appearing of clinically significant plasmid-mediated antibiotic resistance of *H. ducreyi*. Co-trimoxazole and tetracyclines are the most commonly used agents but newer cephalosporins and quinolones are effective. All sexual partners should be seen and treated.

## Lymphogranuloma venereum (LGV)

*Chlamydia trachomatis* types 1, 2 and 3 (see p. 46) is responsible for this sexually transmitted infection. It is endemic in the tropics, with the highest incidences in Africa, India and South East Asia.

**CLINICAL FEATURES**

The primary lesion is a painless ulcerating papule on the genitalia and only occurs in one-quarter of the patients. A few days after this heals, regional lymphadenopathy develops. The lymph nodes are painful and fixed and the overlying skin develops a dusky erythematous appearance. Finally, nodes may become fluctuant (buboes) and may rupture. Acute LGV may present as proctitis with perirectal abscesses, the appearances sometimes resembling anorectal Crohn's disease.

**DIAGNOSIS**

The diagnosis is made on the basis of:
- The characteristic clinical picture
- Isolation of an LGV strain of *C. trachomatis* (only possible in specialized laboratories)
- Immunofluorescence using specific monoclonal antibodies for identifying organisms in pus from a bubo
- A rising titre in a complement-fixation test

The intradermal Frei test is non-specific and unreliable. Great care must be taken to exclude syphilis and genital herpes.

**TREATMENT**

Early treatment with oxytetracycline 500 mg four times daily for at least 2 weeks is generally necessary. Chronic infection may result in extensive scarring and abscess and sinus formation. Surgical drainage may be required. Sexual partners should also be treated.

## Granuloma inguinale

Granuloma inguinale is the least common of all STDs in North America and Europe, but is endemic in the tropics and subtropics, particularly the Caribbean, South-East Asia and South India. Infection is caused by *Calymmatobacterium granulomatis*, a short, encapsulated Gram-negative bacillus. The infection was also known as Donovanosis, the organism originally being known as Donovan's body. Although sexual contact appears to be the most important mode of transmission, the infection rates are low, even between sexual partners of many years' standing.

**CLINICAL FEATURES**

In the vast majority of patients, the characteristic, heaped-up ulcerating lesion with prolific red granulation tissue appears on the external genitalia, perianal skin or the inguinal region within 1–4 weeks of exposure. However, almost any cutaneous or mucous membrane site can be involved, including the mouth and anorectal regions. Extension of the primary infection from the external genitalia to the inguinal regions produces the characteristic lesion, the 'pseudo-bubo'.

**DIAGNOSIS**

The clinical appearance usually strongly suggests the diagnosis but *C. granulomatis* (Donovan bodies) may be identified intracellularly in scrapings or biopsies of an ulcer. Culture or serological methods of diagnosis are not available.

**TREATMENT**

Antibiotic treatment should be given for at least 10–14 days. Tetracycline 500 mg four times daily, streptomycin 1 g twice daily i.m. or ampicillin 500 mg four times daily are the three most commonly used drugs. Alternatives include erythromycin and chloramphenicol.

## Herpes simplex

Genital herpes is one of the commonest STDs worldwide—in 1990 in the UK 20 000 new cases were seen in GUM clinics. Transmission occurs during close contact with a person who is shedding virus. Genital contact with oral lesions caused by HSV-1 can produce genital infection.

HSV can be divided into types 1 and 2. Both can cause

genital infection although type 1 is typically associated with sores on the lips. Susceptible mucous membranes include the genital tract, rectum, mouth and oropharynx. The virus has the ability to establish latency in the dorsal root ganglia by ascending peripheral sensory nerves from the area of inoculation. It is this ability which allows for recurrent attacks.

### CLINICAL FEATURES

Asymptomatic infection has been reported but is rare. Primary genital herpes is usually accompanied by systemic symptoms of varying severity including fever, myalgia and headache. Multiple painful shallow ulcers develop which may coalesce. Tender inguinal lymphadenopathy is usual. Over a period of 10–14 days the lesions develop crusts and dry. In women with vulval lesions the cervix is almost always involved. Rectal infection may lead to a florid proctitis. Neurological complications can include aseptic meningitis and/or involvement of the sacral autonomic plexus leading to retention of urine.

Recurrent attacks may be expected in a significant proportion of people following the initial episode. Precipitating factors vary amongst individuals as does the frequency of recurrence. Recurrent attacks are usually less severe. A symptom prodrome may be present in some people prior to the appearance of lesions. Systemic symptoms are rare in recurrent attacks.

The clinical manifestations in immunosuppressed patients (including those with HIV) may be more severe and recurrences may occur with greater frequency. Systemic spread has been documented (see p. 48).

### DIAGNOSIS

Although the history and examination may be highly suggestive of HSV infection a firm diagnosis can only be made on the basis of isolation of virus from lesions. Swabs should be taken and placed in viral transport medium. Virus is most easily isolated from new lesions.

### MANAGEMENT

#### Primary

Salt water bathing or sitting in a warm bath is soothing and may allow the patient to pass urine with some degree of comfort. Oral acyclovir (200 mg five times daily initially for 5 days) is useful if patients are seen whilst lesions are still moist. If lesions are already crusting acyclovir will do little to change the clinical course. Secondary bacterial infection may occasionally be present and should be treated. Rest, analgesia and antipyretics should be advised. In rare instances patients may need to be admitted to hospital and acyclovir given intravenously, particularly if HSV encephalitis is suspected.

#### Recurrence

Recurrent attacks tend to be much less severe and can be managed with simple measures such as salt water bathing. Psychological morbidity may be associated with recurrent genital herpes and frequent recurrences impose strains on relationships; patients need considerable support. Long-term suppressive acyclovir therapy can be given in patients with frequent recurrences. An initial course of 200 mg three to four times daily for 6 months usually reduces the frequency of attacks although there may still be some breakthrough.

#### Pregnancy

If HSV is acquired for the first time during pregnancy transplacental infection of the fetus may occur. For women with previous infection or primary infection at the time of labour concern focuses on the baby acquiring HSV from the birth canal. The risk is very low in recurrent attacks but rather greater in a primary episode. Obstetric opinion is divided but if the woman has an attack around the time of labour Caesarian section may be performed. Acyclovir is not licensed for use in pregnancy but studies are being carried out to evaluate its use in the last few weeks of pregnancy in women with recurrent HSV.

### PREVENTION AND CONTROL

Patients must be advised that they are infectious when lesions are present; sexual intercourse should be avoided during this time or during prodromal stages. Condoms may not be effective as lesions may occur outside the areas covered. Sexual partners should be examined and may need information on avoiding infection.

## Warts

Anogenital warts are amongst the commonest sexually acquired infections with ever growing numbers of people seeking treatment. The causative agent is human papillomavirus (HPV) especially types 6 and 11. HPV is acquired by direct sexual contact with a person with either clinical or subclinical infection. Neonates may acquire HPV from an infected birth canal which may result either in anogenital warts or in laryngeal papillomas. The incubation period may range from 2 weeks to 8 months or even longer.

### CLINICAL FEATURES

Warts may develop around the external genitalia in women, usually starting at the fourchette and may involve the perianal region. The vagina may be infected. Flat warts may develop on the cervix that may not be easily visible on routine examination. Such lesions may have an association with cervical intraepithelial neoplasia and may be diagnosed on cervical cytology or at colposcopy. In men the penile shaft and subpreputial space are the commonest sites although warts may involve the urethra and meatus. Perianal lesions are more common in men who practise anoreceptive intercourse but may be found in any patient. The rectum may become involved. Warts may become more florid during pregnancy or in immunosuppressed patients.

### DIAGNOSIS

The diagnosis is essentially clinical. It is important to differentiate condylomata lata of secondary syphilis.

Unusual lesions should be biopsied if the diagnosis is in doubt. Up to 30% of patients may have coexisting infections with other STDs and a full screen is important.

### TREATMENT
Local agents include podophyllin extract 10–25%, podophyllotoxin and trichloroacetic acid. In extensive or recalcitrant infection cryotherapy, electrocautery or laser ablation is indicated. Podophyllin is contraindicated in pregnancy.

Sexual contacts should be examined and treated if necessary. In view of the difficulties of diagnosing subclinical HPV, condoms should be used for up to 8 months after treatment. Because of the association of HPV with cervical intraepithelial neoplasia women with warts and female partners of men with warts are advised to have cervical cytology carried out annually. Some clinics advocate colposcopy for all women with HPV infection.

## Hepatitis B

This is discussed in Chapter 5.

Sexual contacts should be screened and offered vaccine if they are not immune (see p. 255).

## Trichomoniasis

*Trichomonas vaginalis* (TV) is a flagellated protozoon which is predominantly sexually transmitted. It is able to attach to squamous epithelium and can infect the vagina and urethra.

Infected women may, unusually, be asymptomatic. Commonly the major complaints are of vaginal discharge which may be offensive and of local irritation.

Examination often reveals a frothy yellowish vaginal discharge and erythematous vaginal walls. The cervix may have multiple small haemorrhagic areas which lead to the description 'strawberry cervix'.

In men the infection is usually asymptomatic but may be a cause of NGU.

### DIAGNOSIS
Phase-contrast microscopy of a drop of vaginal discharge shows TV swimming with a characteristic motion. Many polymorphonuclearleucocytes are also seen. Culture techniques are good and confirm the diagnosis.

### TREATMENT
Metronidazole 400 mg twice daily for 7 days is the treatment of choice. There is some evidence of resistance although a single dose of 2 g can be given. Nimorazole may be effective in these cases. Topical therapy with clotrimazole may be effective but if extra-vaginal infection exists this may not be eradicated and vaginal infection reoccurs. It is important that male partners are followed up especially as they are likely to be asymptomatic.

## Candidiasis

Vulvovaginal infection with *Candida albicans* is extremely common. The organism is also responsible for balanitis in men. *Candida* may be isolated from the vagina in a high proportion of women of childbearing age, many of whom will have no symptoms.

The role of *Candida* as pathogen or commensal is difficult to disentangle and it may be changes in host environment which allow the organism to produce pathological effects. Predisposing factors include pregnancy, the oral contraceptive pill, diabetes and broadspectrum antibiotics. Immunosuppression can produce more florid infection.

### CLINICAL FEATURES
In women pruritus vulvae is the dominant symptom. Vaginal discharge is present in varying degree. Many women have only one or occasional isolated episodes but in a minority of patients the symptoms may be recurrent or chronic. Examination reveals erythema and swelling of the vulva with broken skin in severe cases. The vagina may contain adherent curdy discharge. Men may have a florid balanoposthitis. More commonly self-limiting burning penile irritation immediately after sexual intercourse with an infected partner is described. Diabetes must be excluded in men with balanoposthitis.

### DIAGNOSIS
Microscopic examination of a smear from the vaginal wall reveals the presence of spores and mycelia. Culture of swabs should be undertaken but may be positive in women with no symptoms. It is important to exclude *Trichomonas* and bacterial vaginosis in women with itch and discharge.

### TREATMENT
Pessaries or creams containing one of the imidazole antifungals such as clotrimazole used intravaginally are usually effective.

Nystatin is also useful. The triazole drugs such as fluconazole 150 mg single dose or itraconazole 200 mg twice in 1 day may be used systemically in circumstances where topical therapy has failed or is inappropriate.

Although the evidence for sexual transmission of *Candida* is slight, male partners of women with frequent recurrent episodes should be reviewed and possibly treated.

## Bacterial vaginosis

Bacterial vaginosis (BV) or non-specific vaginosis is a disorder characterized by an offensive vaginal discharge. The aetiology and pathogenesis is unclear but the normal lactobacilli of the vagina are replaced by a mixed flora of *Gardnerella vaginalis*, anaerobes including *Bacteroides*, and *Mycoplasma hominis*. Amines and their breakdown products from the abnormal vaginal flora are thought to be responsible for the characteristic odour associated with the condition. As vaginal inflammation is not part of the syndrome the term vaginosis is used rather than vaginitis. It is not clear to what extent BV is a sexually transmitted condition.

## CLINICAL FEATURES

Vaginal discharge and odour are the commonest complaints although a proportion of women are asymptomatic. A homogeneous, greyish white, adherent discharge is present in the vagina, the pH of which is raised (greater than 5). Associated complications are ill-defined but may include chorioamnionitis and an increased incidence of premature labour in pregnant women. Whether BV disposes non-pregnant women to upper genital tract infection is unclear.

## DIAGNOSIS

Different authors have differing criteria for making the diagnosis of BV. In general it is accepted that three of the following should be present for the diagnosis to be made:
1 Characteristic vaginal discharge.
2 A raised vaginal pH using narrow range indicator paper ($>4.7$).
3 A fishy odour on mixing a drop of discharge with 10% potassium hydroxide.
4 The presence of clue cells on microscopic examination of the vaginal fluid. Clue cells are squamous epithelial cells from the vagina which have bacteria adherent to their surface giving a granular appearance to the cell. A Gram stain gives a typical mixed reaction.

Additional laboratory tests include cultures for *G. vaginalis* but this is non-specific as the organism can be recovered in over 50% of women who do not meet the clinical diagnostic criteria for BV. Metabolic by-products of the altered vaginal flora may be detected using gas or thin layer chromatography.

## MANAGEMENT

Metronidazole given orally in doses of 800–1200 mg daily for 5–7 days is usually recommended. A single dose of 2 g metronidazole is less effective. Penicillins and other $\beta$-lactam antibiotics are much less useful presumably because of $\beta$-lactamase production by anaerobes. Topical clindamycin is being evaluated in the UK and is available in the USA where it seems efficacious. Topical acetic acid gel has been used with mixed results.

The rate of recurrence is high with some studies giving a recurrence rate of 80% within 9 months of completing metronidazole therapy. There is debate over the treatment of asymptomatic women who fulfil the diagnostic criteria for BV. The diagnosis should be fully discussed and treatment offered if the woman wishes. Until the relevance of BV to other pelvic infections is elucidated the routine treatment of all women with BV is not to be recommended. There is no convincing evidence that simultaneous treatment of the male partner influences the rate of recurrence of BV and routine treatment of male partners is not indicated.

## INFESTATIONS (see p. 1019)

## Pediculosis pubis

The pubic louse (*Phthirius pubis*) is a blood-sucking insect which attaches tightly to the pubic hair. It is rela-

tively host specific and is transferred only by close bodily contact. Eggs (nits) are laid at hair bases and hatch within a week. Although infestation may be asymptomatic the commonest complaint is of itch.

## DIAGNOSIS

Lice may be seen on the skin at the base of pubic hairs. They may resemble small scabs or freckles but if they are picked up with forceps and placed on a microscope slide will move and walk away. Nits are usually closely adherent to hairs. Both are highly characteristic under the low power microscope.

As with all sexually transmitted infections the patient must be screened for coexisting pathogens.

## TREATMENT

It is important that both lice and eggs are killed. This is achieved with 1% γ-benzene hexachloride or 0.5% malathion. The preparation should be applied to all areas of the body from the neck down and washed off after 24 hours. In a few cases a further application at 1 week may be necessary. In severe infestations antipruritics may be indicated for the first 48 hours. All sexual partners should be seen and screened.

## Scabies

This is discussed on p. 1019.

# HIV and AIDS

## Introduction

HIV was identified as the causative organism of AIDS in 1983. Current WHO estimates are of 13 million adults infected worldwide, of whom 2.5 million have died. By the year 2000 WHO estimates that there will be up to 80 million infections worldwide. In the UK, women currently account for 15% of known HIV infections and 6% of AIDS cases reported.

## Epidemiology

Despite the fact that HIV can be isolated from a wide range of body fluids and tissues the majority of infections are transmitted via semen, cervical secretions and blood. Transmission is via the following routes.

### Sexual intercourse (vaginal and anal)

Worldwide, heterosexual intercourse accounts for the vast majority of infections, and coexistent STDs, especially those causing genital ulceration, enhance transmission. Passage of HIV appears to be more efficient from men to women than vice versa.

There is a geographical variation in the epidemiology. In Europe, USA and Australasia the initial wave of infection was amongst homosexual men with a second wave developing amongst intravenous drug users and their sexual partners. The incidence of HIV in heterosexuals is rising and is likely to form a further epidemic wave over the next 20–30 years.

In central and sub-Saharan Africa the ratio of women to men is at least 1 : 1, the predominant mode of spread being heterosexual intercourse. Similar patterns are seen in South-East Asia, the Indian subcontinent and Latin America.

**Mother to child** (prenatally, perinatally, breastfeeding)
As more women in their reproductive years are infected the numbers of babies acquiring HIV vertically will increase. European studies suggest that 14% of babies born to HIV-infected women are likely to be infected although rates of up to 40% have been reported from Africa and USA. Transmission can occur *in utero*, during childbirth or via breast milk.

**Contaminated blood, blood products and organ donations**
Screening of blood and blood products was introduced in 1985 in Europe and North America. Prior to this HIV infection was associated with the use of clotting factors (for haemophilia) and with blood transfusions. Clotting factors are now heat treated and the risk of transfusion-related HIV infection in developed countries is tiny. In some countries where this is not possible or in areas of the world where the rate of new HIV infections is very high the risk of transfusion-associated transmission remains significant.

**Contaminated needles** (intravenous drug misuse, injections, needlestick injuries)
The practice of sharing needles and syringes for intravenous drug use continues to be a major route of transmission of HIV. Iatrogenic transmission from needles and syringes in developing countries is reported. Health care workers have a risk of approximately 0.3% following a single needlestick injury with known HIV-infected blood.

There is no evidence that HIV is spread by social or household contact nor by blood-sucking insects such as mosquitoes and bed bugs.

## The virus

HIV belongs to the lentivirus group of the retrovirus family. There are at least two types, HIV-1 and HIV-2. HIV-2 is almost entirely confined to West Africa where it is associated with an AIDS-type illness. Retroviruses are characterized by the possession of the enzyme reverse transcriptase, which allows viral RNA to be transcribed into DNA, and thence incorporated into the host cell genome. The structure of the virus is illustrated in Fig. 1.39.

Glycoproteins on the surface of the virus bind to target cells. Multiple regulatory proteins are encoded by the virus which controls the life-cycle and viral expression. Figure 1.40 shows the sequence of events in the reproductive cycle of the virus within infected cells.

**IMMUNOPATHOGENESIS** (see p. 145)
The cellular receptor for HIV is the CD4 molecule, which defines the cells that are susceptible to infection. Many cells within the immune system bear this molecule and include CD4+ T lymphocytes (which are most affected). A number of pathogenic mechanisms have been described (see p. 145) to account for the profound cellular immunodeficiency. There is a progressive and severe depletion of CD4 'helper' lymphocytes and it is this that leads to the clinical manifestation of HIV infection.

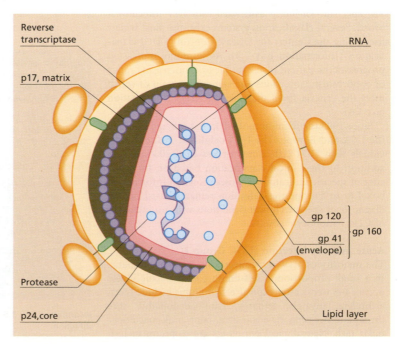

**Fig. 1.39**  Structure of HIV.

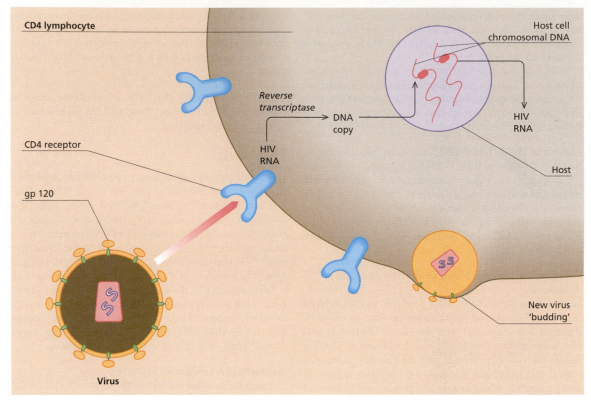

**Fig. 1.40** HIV entry and replication in CD4 T lymphocytes. The virus replicates by making a DNA copy (provirus) of its diploid RNA (using reverse transcriptase) which then becomes inserted into the host cell chromosomal DNA. This then provides RNA genomes for a progeny of new viruses.

## Clinical features

The spectrum of illness associated with HIV infection is broad. Several classification systems exist, the most widely used being the Centers for Disease Control (CDC) classification (Information box 1.5). As immunosuppression progresses the patient is susceptible to an increasing range of opportunistic infections and tumours, certain of which meet the criteria for a diagnosis of AIDS (Information box 1.6).

Since 1993 the definition of AIDS has differed between the USA and Europe. The USA definition includes individuals with CD4 cell counts of less than 200 mm$^{-3}$ in addition to the clinical classification based on the presence of specific indicator diagnoses shown in Information box 1.6. In Europe the definition remains based on the diagnosis of specific clinical conditions with no inclusion of CD4 lymphocyte counts.

### Acute primary infection (CDC Group I)

The majority of HIV seroconversions are asymptomatic. In a small proportion, a self-limiting non-specific illness occurs 4–8 weeks after exposure. Symptoms include fever, arthralgia, myalgia, lethargy, lymphadenopathy, sore throat and occasionally a transient, faint, pink maculopapular rash. Neurological symptoms are common includ-

Group I    Acute infection
Group II   Asymptomatic infection
Group III  Persistent generalized lymphadenopathy
Group IV   Symptomatic infection

Subgroup A   Constitutional disease (fever >1 month, weight loss >10% baseline, diarrhoea >1 month)
Subgroup B   Neurological disease (dementia, peripheral neuropathy, myelopathy)
Subgroup C   Secondary infectious diseases

C1   As specified in the AIDS surveillance definition of the Centers for Disease Control
C2   Others—oral hairy leucoplakia, multidermatomal herpes zoster, oral *Candida*, recurrent *Salmonella* bacteraemia, nocardiasis

Subgroup D   Specified secondary cancers—Kaposi's sarcoma, non-Hodgkin's lymphoma, primary cerebral lymphoma
Subgroup E   Other conditions, e.g. lymphoid interstitial pneumonia, thrombocytopenia

**Information box 1.5**  Summary of classification system for HIV infection.

The following can be used as indicator diseases for AIDS providing other causes of immunodeficiency have been excluded (congenital immune deficiency, lymphoma leukaemia, recent use of steroids or other immunosuppressive drugs).

Bacterial chest infection (recurrent in 12 month period)
Candidiasis, trachea, bronchi or lungs
Cervical carcinoma, invasive
Coccidioidomycosis, disseminated or extrapulmonary
*Cryptococcus*, extrapulmonary
Cryptosporidiosis, with diarrhoea for >1 month
Cytomegalovirus disease (onset after age 1 month) not in liver, spleen or nodes
Encephalopathy (dementia) due to HIV
Herpes simplex ulcers for 1 month or bronchitis, pneumonitis or oesophagitis (onset in infants > 1 month old)
Histoplasmosis, disseminated or extrapulmonary
Isosporiasis, with diarrhoea for >1 month
Kaposi's sarcoma
Lymphoid interstitial pneumonitis and/or pulmonary lymphoid hyperplasia in a child aged <13 years
Mycobacteriosis (including extrapulmonary tuberculosis), disseminated
Mycobacteriosis, pulmonary tuberculosis
*Pneumocystis carinii* pneumonia
Progressive multifocal leucoencephalopathy
*Salmonella* (non-typhoid) septicaemia, recurrent
Toxoplasmosis of brain, onset after 1 month age
Wasting syndrome due to HIV (weight loss >10% baseline, with no other cause identified)

[a]USA definition also includes those with a CD4 count <200/mm³

**Information box 1.6** AIDS-defining diagnoses (1993 classification, Europe[a]).

ing headache, photophobia, myelopathy, neuropathy and in rare cases encephalopathy. The illness lasts up to 3 weeks and recovery is usually complete.

Laboratory abnormalities include lymphopenia with atypical reactive lymphocytes noted on the blood film, thrombocytopenia and raised liver transaminases. CD4 lymphocytes may be markedly depleted and the CD4 : CD8 ratio reversed. Antibodies to HIV may be absent during this early stage of infection although the viral core protein P24 antigen may be present. There is evidence to suggest that patients experiencing a severe seroconversion illness may progress more quickly to AIDS.

## Asymptomatic infection (CDC Group II)
The majority of people with HIV infection are asymptomatic, but the virus continues to replicate and the person remains infectious. The duration of an asymptomatic carrier state is variable but studies suggest a mean of 10 years from infection to development of AIDS. The natural history of HIV infection has yet to be studied for long enough to know whether all those with asymptomatic infection progress to AIDS.

Various laboratory markers of progression are used to monitor asymptomatic patients and to guide therapeutic

intervention. The most commonly used are:
- Depletion of CD4 lymphocyte counts and percentages
- Raised CD8 lymphocyte counts and percentages
- Reversed CD4 : CD8 ratios
- Raised serum $\beta_2$-microglobulin
- Raised serum and urinary neopterin
- Raised p24 antigen titre
- Falling p24 antibody titre

## Persistent generalized lymphadenopathy (PGL) (CDC Group III)
A subgroup of patients with asymptomatic HIV infection have PGL, defined as lymphadenopathy (>1 cm) at two or more extra-inguinal sites for more than 3 months in the absence of causes other than HIV infection. The nodes are usually symmetrical, firm, mobile and non-tender. There may be associated splenomegaly. The architecture of the nodes shows hyperplasia of the follicles and proliferation of the capillary endothelium. Biopsy is rarely indicated. Similar disease progression has been noted in asymptomatic patients with or without PGL. Nodes may disappear with disease progression. The same laboratory markers as above are used to monitor patients.

## Symptomatic HIV infection (CDC Group IV)
Clinical evidence of progression of HIV infection is manifested by an array of symptoms and signs and CD4 cell counts decrease. Susceptibility to a range of opportunistic and conventional pathogens and tumours is increased as immunosuppression becomes more profound. Immunodeficiency leads to the following problems in clinical practice:
- Susceptibility to opportunistic infections and tumours
- Presence of multiple infections at one time
- Lack of typical signs and symptoms due to failure of the inflammatory response, e.g. cryptococcal meningitis commonly presents without signs of meningism and there may be no white cells present in the CSF

These features mean that tissue or body fluid is required to directly identify infecting organisms.

CONSTITUTIONAL SYMPTOMS include general lassitude, weight loss, night sweats (often soaking the sheets) and diarrhoea. Such symptoms may be the earliest signs of major infections or malignancies or can be a direct result of HIV infection.

SKIN AND MUCOUS MEMBRANES are frequently the site of bacterial, fungal and viral infections (Table 1.39). An intensely pruritic, papular eruption favouring the extremities may be found, particularly in patients from sub-Saharan Africa. Generalized dry, itchy, flaky skin is typical and hair may become thin and dry. Seborrhoeic dermatitis occurs on the face and trunk. Folliculitis, usually bacterial and often generalized, is common. Stomatitis, recurrent aphthous ulcers and gum disease may impair the patient's ability to eat. Oral candidiasis is frequently extensive with associated angular cheilitis. In female patients recurrent severe vulvovaginal candidiasis may occur. Oral hairy leucoplakia is a sign of immuno-

*Skin*
Dry skin and scalp
Onychomycosis
Seborrhoeic dermatitis
Tinea
  cruris
  pedis
Pityriasis
  vesicolor
  rosea
Folliculitis
Acne
Molluscum contagiosum
Warts
Herpes zoster
  multidermatomal
  disseminated
Papular pruritic eruption
Scabies
Ichthyosis

*Mucous membranes*
Candidiasis
  oral
  vulvovaginal
Hairy oral leucoplakia
Aphthous ulcers
Herpes simplex
  genital
  oral
  labial
Periodontal disease
Warts
  oral
  genital

**Table 1.39** Mucocutaneous manifestations of HIV infection.

suppression first noted in HIV but now also recognized in other conditions. It appears intermittently on the lateral borders of the tongue or the buccal mucosa as a pale, ridged lesion. It is usually asymptomatic although patients may find it unsightly and occasionally painful. It shows a variable response to acyclovir. Aetiology is not clear but Epstein Barr virus (EBV) particles can be identified histologically. Labial and genital Herpes simplex virus (HSV) occur with increasing frequency and severity. Herpes zoster may occur in an atypical pattern, affecting more than one dermatome or becoming disseminated. Human papillomavirus (HPV) infection produces genital, planar and occasionally oral warts which may be slow to respond to therapy and recur repeatedly. The association of HPV with cervical and anal intraepithelial neoplasia in HIV-infected patients is still subject to scrutiny; however female patients should have cervical cytology on at least an annual basis. Molluscum contagiosum is very common appearing in atypical sites particularly on the face and around the eyes.

NEUROLOGICAL DISEASE (CDC Group IVB). The mechanism for the causation of neurological dysfunction is not well understood but may result from direct infection of the glial cells and/or the effects of viral products on neurones. Loss of neurones and vacuolization occur

in advanced infection. Direct HIV pathology must be differentiated from opportunistic infections and tumours as the management strategies differ.

There may be a sensory polyneuropathy, ranging from mild paraesthesia to severe pain usually in the lower limbs. A progressive myelopathy can occur producing motor signs in the legs and sphincter disturbance. Autonomic neuropathy may be seen.

Intellectual and cognitive impairment can occur, usually in the later stages of disease. The onset is usually insidious, with decrease in memory, poor concentration and personality change. Changes in affect are common and depressive or psychotic features can be present. Functional psychiatric disorders must be differentiated from organic disease. CT scan reveals varying degrees of atrophic change and EEG may give an encephalopathic picture.

GASTROINTESTINAL MANIFESTATIONS (see p. 230). Weight loss, diarrhoea and malabsorption are all common problems in chronic HIV infection. Anorexia, nausea and vomiting frequently complicate acute episodes of opportunistic infection and their therapy. An HIV enteropathy has been described but the exact role of HIV in the pathogenesis of diarrhoea and malabsorption is not clear. Table 4.17 shows the major conditions affecting the gastrointestinal tract in HIV infection.

HAEMATOLOGICAL COMPLICATIONS OF HIV INFECTION. Anaemia, neutropenia and thrombocytopenia are all common in advanced HIV infection and may indicate underlying opportunistic infection or tumour, particularly if the patient is pancytopenic. All may be exacerbated iatrogenically.

1 Anaemia of chronic HIV infection is usually mild, normocytic and normochromic.

2 Neutropenia is common and usually mild.

3 Thrombocytopenia may be the only manifestation of HIV infection. Platelet counts are often moderately reduced, but may fall dramatically ($10–20 \times 10^9$/litre) producing easy bruising and bleeding. The aetiology is unclear. Megakaryocytes are increased in the bone marrow but function may be impaired. Circulating antiplatelet antibodies may lead to peripheral destruction.

## Opportunistic disease in HIV infection

As immunosuppression increases patients are susceptible to a wide range of infections and tumours. In an individual patient the clinical consequences of HIV-related immune dysfunction will depend on:

THE MICROBIAL EXPOSURE OF THE PATIENT THROUGHOUT LIFE. Many of the clinical episodes represent reactivation of previously acquired infection which has been latent. Geographical factors are important in determining the microbial repertoire of an individual patient. Those organisms requiring intact cell-mediated immunity for their control are most likely to cause clinical problems.

THE PATHOGENICITY OF ORGANISMS ENCOUN-
TERED. High-grade pathogens such as *M. tuberculosis,
Candida* and herpes viruses are clinically relevant even
when immunosuppression is mild and will thus occur
earlier in the course of disease. Susceptiblity to infections such as *Pneumocystis carinii* occur at later stages
of immunodeficiency (usually when the CD4 cell count
is less than 200/mm³)

THE DEGREE OF IMMUNOSUPPRESSION OF THE
HOST. When patients are severely immunocompromised (CD4 cell count <100/mm³), disseminated
infections with organisms of very low pathogenicity,
such as atypical mycobacteria and cryptosporidia
occur. These infections are very resistant to treatment,
not only because there are no good antimicrobial treatments available, but also because there is no functioning immune response. This hierarchy of infection
allows for appropriate intervention with prophylactic
drugs.

A summary of the infections in AIDS is given in Table
1.40. The most important are described below.

## PROTOZOA

### Pneumocystis carinii (see p. 68 and p. 680)

This organism most commonly causes pneumonia (PCP)
but can cause disseminated infection. The characteristic
presenting features are persistent, non-productive cough,
increasing shortness of breath, hypoxia and fever.

The clinical features and investigation are discussed on
p. 680. Typically the chest X-ray shows a diffuse interstitial shadowing extending through the mid-zones bilaterally. In mild cases both the clinical examination and the
chest X-ray may be within normal limits.

Treatment should be instituted as early as possible. The
first line therapy is with high doses of co-trimoxazole or
intravenous pentamidine for 21 days. In severe cases the
addition of systemic corticosteroids has been shown to
reduce mortality.

Recurrence is frequent but can be largely prevented by
the use of low-dose co-trimoxazole (960 mg thrice
weekly) or nebulized pentamidine (300 mg monthly).
Prevention of PCP with the use of primary prophylaxis
in HIV-infected patients known to be at risk of PCP
(those with CD4 cell counts <200/mm³) has led to a
marked reduction in incidence from around 50% to 5%
in the UK. Although systemic prophylaxis is associated
with a greater incidence of side-effects, nebulized pentamidine only protects the lungs and extrapulmonary pneu-
mocystosis may occur in patients on this therapy.

### Toxoplasmosis  (see p. 67)

*Toxoplasma gondii* most commonly causes encephalitis
and cerebral abscesses in the context of AIDS, due usually
to reactivation of previously acquired infection. Up to
45% of AIDS patients who have antibodies to *T. gondii*
may still develop cerebral toxoplasmosis. Features of cerebral toxoplasmosis include focal neurological signs, convulsions, headache, multiple ring-enhancing lesions on
CT scan, and positive IgG anti-*Toxoplasma* serology.

The diagnosis is usually made on the basis of the CT
or MRI brain scan. If there is doubt stereotactic brain
biopsy can be performed.

Treatment is with pyrimethamine in combination with
sulphonamide. Clindamycin and pyrimethamine may be
used in sulphonamide-sensitive patients. These regimens
will control but not eradicate infection and thus lifelong
maintenance is required to prevent relapse. Newer drugs
are undergoing evaluation to eradicate the cysts of toxoplasmosis and potentially cure the infection.

### Cryptosporidiosis  (see p. 74)

*Cryptosporidium parvum* can cause a self-limiting acute
diarrhoea in an immunocompetent individual. In HIV
infection it can cause a severe and progressive watery
diarrhoea which may be associated with anorexia,
abdominal pain, nausea and vomiting. Cysts attach to the
epithelium of the wall of small bowel causing secretion
of fluid into the gut lumen and leading to failure of
absorption. It is associated with sclerosing cholangitis.

The cysts may be seen on stool specimens stained with
Kinyoun acid fast stain. The organism can be easily seen
on small bowel biopsy specimens.

Treatment is largely supportive as there are no effective
antimicrobial agents available other than a non-
absorbable aminoglycoside, paromamycin, which may
have a limited effect on diarrhoea.

### Microsporidiosis

This is a frequent cause of diarrhoea. Spores can be
detected with great accuracy in the stools using a tri-

---

Protozoa
  *Pneumocystis carinii*
  *Toxoplasma gondii*
  *Cryptosporidium parvum*
  *Isospora belli*
  *Microsporidia* spp.

Fungi and yeasts
  *Candida* spp.
  *Cryptococcus neoformans*
  *Histoplasma capsulatum*
  *Coccidioides immitis*

Viruses
  Herpes simplex
  Varicella zoster
  Cytomegalovirus
  Papovavirus
  Human papilloma virus

Bacteria
  *Streptococcus pneumoniae*
  *Haemophilus influenzae*
  *Moraxella catarrhalis*
  *Salmonella* spp.
  *Rhodococcus equi*
  *Rochalimaea quintana*
  *Nocardia*
  *Mycobacterium tuberculosis*
  *Mycobacterium avium intracellulare*
  *Penicillium marfenii*

**Table 1.40**  Major pathogens in HIV infection.

chrome or a fluorescent stain that attaches to the chitin of the spore surface. Albendazole is effective in eradicating the organism.

## FUNGI

### *Cryptococcus*

In the context of HIV with AIDS the commonest presentation is with meningitis, although it can cause pulmonary and disseminated infection.

Clinical features of cryptococcal meningitis include headache, fever, impaired conscious level and abnormal affect. Neck stiffness and photophobia are rarely seen.

The diagnosis is made on examination of the CSF (a CT scan must be performed first to exclude space-occupying lesions). India ink staining may show the organisms directly and cryptococcal antigen is positive at variable titre. Cryptococci may be cultured from the CSF and/or blood.

Signs associated with a poor prognosis include high organism count in the CSF, low white cell count in the CSF, and impaired conscious level at presentation.

Treatment is with intravenous amphotericin B or fluconazole. Infection is not eradicated and lifelong maintenance therapy (usually with fluconazole) is needed to suppress infection.

### *Candida* (see p. 1016)

Mucosal infection with *C. albicans* is extremely frequent in HIV-infected patients. Oropharyngeal involvement is common and oesophageal *Candida* causes dysphagia. HIV-infected women may have severe recurrent vulvovaginal *Candida* infection. Disseminated *Candida* is relatively uncommon in the context of HIV infection. Treatment is usually with systemic antifungal agents such as fluconazole and ketoconazole.

## VIRUSES

### Cytomegalovirus (CMV)

CMV is the cause of considerable morbidity in HIV-infected individuals, especially in the later stages of disease. The major problems encountered are retinitis, colitis, oesophagitis, encephalitis and pneumonitis. Polyradiculitis and adrenalitis may also be caused by CMV. The first two are the most common.

CMV RETINITIS. This occurs in up to 30% of AIDS cases and is the commonest cause of eye disease and blindness. Although usually unilateral to begin with, the infection frequently progresses to involve both eyes. Presenting features depend on the area of the retina involved (loss of vision being most common with macular involvement) and include:
- Floaters
- Loss of visual acuity and scotoma
- Orbital pain and headache

Examination reveals haemorrhages and exudate which follow the vasculature of the retina (so-called pizza pie appearances). The features are highly characteristic and the diagnosis is made clinically. If untreated, retinitis spreads within the eye destroying the retina within its path. Routine fundoscopy should be carried out regularly on all HIV-infected patients to look for evidence of early infection. Treatment should be started as soon as possible with either ganciclovir or foscarnet. These agents halt disease but do not eradicate it. Reactivation occurs in a majority of cases and may lead to blindness in one or both eyes. Patients thus need long-term maintenance therapy but as these two agents are available only as intravenous preparations insertion of an indwelling line is necessary for long-term self-administered therapy.

CMV COLITIS. This is a cause of abdominal symptoms in AIDS. The usual presenting features include:
- Abdominal pain, often left iliac
- Diarrhoea which may be bloody
- Tenderness
- Low grade fever

Toxic dilatation of the colon may occur in severe cases. Sigmoidoscopy and biopsy may be performed safely if there is no evidence of toxic dilatation on the abdominal radiograph. Histology shows characteristic 'owl's eye' cytoplasmic inclusion bodies. Treatment with ganciclovir or foscarnet is effective.

CMV may affect any site along the gastrointestinal tract giving rise to:
- Oesophageal ulcers, usually solitary in the lower third
- Small bowel ulceration
- An association with sclerosing cholangitis
- Hepatitis

### Herpes

HSV types 1 and 2 cause frequent, severe, recurrent infections in people with HIV. There may be extensive ulceration and viral shedding may be prolonged in comparison to immunocompetent individuals. Genital, oral and occasionally disseminated infection are seen.

Therapy with acyclovir is effective but frequent recurrences may need suppressive therapy. Acyclovir-resistant HSV (usually due to thymidine kinase-deficient mutations) in HIV-infected patients has become more common. Such strains may respond to foscarnet.

### Papovavirus

Progressive multifocal leukencephalopathy (PML) is a demyelinating disease of cerebral white matter caused by papovavirus. The features are of progressive neurological and/or intellectual impairment. MRI scanning is the most sensitive and reveals characteristic multiple white matter lesions. Definitive diagnosis is made on histological and viral examination of brain tissue. There is no specific treatment for the condition.

## BACTERIAL INFECTIONS

Encapsulated bacteria such as *Strep. pneumoniae*, *H. influenzae* and *Moraxella catarrhalis* show an increased incidence in HIV infection and may result in pneumonia or disseminated disease. Recurrent episodes are common. The response to standard antibiotic therapy is usually good, but long-term prophylaxis may be required if recurrent infection is frequent.

Non-typhoidal *Salmonella* spp. are frequent pathogens in HIV infection as intact cell-mediated immunity is a crucial part of host defence. Organisms are usually acquired orally and frequently result in disseminated infection. Gastrointestinal disturbance may be minimal, and once in the bloodstream any organ may be infected. Response to standard antibiotic therapy, depending on laboratory sensitivities, is usually good in the acute phase but recurrent infection is common and long-term suppressive therapy may be necessary.

### Mycobacterial infections

An association between HIV infection and *M. tuberculosis* was recognized early in the epidemic. TB can cause disease when there is only minimal immunosuppression and thus often appears early in the course of HIV infection. In many countries where HIV is spreading and tuberculosis is endemic there is a substantial increase in the incidence of tuberculosis. Cases of HIV-related tuberculosis frequently represent reactivation of latent TB. There is also evidence for newly acquired infection and nosocomial spread in HIV-infected populations.

The pattern of disease differs from that in the immunocompetent host in that extrapulmonary and disseminated infection is more common. The response to tuberculin testing is blunted in HIV-positive individuals and is unreliable. Sputum examination may be negative even in pulmonary infection and culture techniques are the best diagnostic tool.

TB usually responds well to standard treatment regimens, although there are increasing numbers of cases of multidrug resistance occurring in HIV-infected individuals, particularly in the USA (see p. 686). Increasing numbers of drugs are used in combination. Treatment is not curative and lifelong maintenance, usually with isoniazid, is required. HIV-infected individuals have shown a high frequency of severe adverse reactions to thioacetazone and this drug, although widely used for tuberculosis in developing countries, should be avoided in this group of patients if possible.

Atypical mycobacteria, particularly *M. avium intracellulare* complex (MAI) generally appear only in the later stages of AIDS when patients are profoundly immunosuppressed. It is a saprophytic organism of low pathogenicity that is ubiquitous in soil and water. Entry may be via the gastrointestinal tract or lungs with dissemination via infected macrophages.

The major features are of fevers, weight loss and anorexia. Dissemination to the bone marrow causes anaemia. Gastrointestinal symptoms may be prominent with diarrhoea and malabsorption. At this stage of disease patients may have other concurrent infections and differentiating MAI on clinical grounds is difficult. Direct examination and culture of bone marrow, liver, blood or lymph node give the diagnosis most reliably.

MAI is typically resistant to standard antituberculous therapies. Newer drugs such as rifabutin in combination with clarithromycin and clofazimine have shown some promise in reducing the burden of organisms and ameliorating systemic symptoms but on the whole therapy is disappointing.

Primary prophylaxis with rifabutin in profoundly immunosuppressed patients (CD counts $< 100$ mm$^{-1}$) may reduce the incidence of frank MAI infection.

### TUMOURS

#### Kaposi's sarcoma (KS)

This multifocal disease is caused by a proliferation of vascular endothelial cells, which form slit-like spaces similar to blood vessels that trap red blood cells and cause the characteristic purple hue of the tumour. KS commonly involves:

- Skin
- Lymphatics and lymph nodes
- Lung
- Gut

Treatment depends on the site and extent of the lesions. Localized or cutaneous disease may respond to radiotherapy. Disseminated or visceral KS generally requires systemic chemotherapy.

KS is particularly common in homosexual men and is rare in those who have acquired HIV via blood products or intravenous drug use. The possible existence of a sexually transmitted cofactor in the aetiology of the condition is being explored.

#### Lymphoma

Non-Hodgkin's lymphoma (NHL) of B-cell origin occurs particularly in immunosuppressed individuals. In late stages of AIDS primary CNS NHL is common and responds poorly to therapy. However primary NHL outside the CNS (e.g. gastrointestinal tract or lung) may occur at earlier stages of immunosuppression and is more responsive to therapy.

## Diagnosis

Detection of IgG antibody to envelope components (gp120 and its subunits) is the most commonly used marker of infection with HIV. The routine tests are based on ELISA techniques which may be confirmed with Western blot assays. Up to 3 months may elapse from initial infection to antibody production (the window period). These antibodies have no protective function. As with all IgG antibodies they cross the placenta. All babies born to HIV-infected women will thus have the antibody at birth. In this situation HIV antibody is not a reliable marker of active infection and in uninfected babies will be lost gradually over the first 18 months of life.

HIV antibody testing should be carried out only after full discussion of the implications with the patient and with the patient's express consent.

Additional viral antigens and host antibodies can be detected in blood.

VIRAL p24 ANTIGEN (p24 Ag) is detectable shortly after infection but has usually disappeared by 8–10 weeks after exposure. It can be a useful marker in individuals who have recently been infected and have not yet had time to mount an antibody response. It may reappear at low levels intermittently during the asymptomatic phase and also as infection progresses in some people, in whom it can be used as a surrogate marker of viral activity.

IgG ANTIBODY TO P24 can be detected from the earliest weeks of infection and through the asymptomatic phase. It is often lost as disease progresses.

ISOLATION OF VIRUS IN CULTURE AND DETECTION BY POLYMERASE CHAIN REACTION are specialized techniques available in some laboratories which may aid diagnosis.

## Investigation and management

### Initial assessment
History and examination will provide a basis for the clinical staging of infection and give insight into the patient's approach and particular circumstances. Baseline investigations will depend on the clinical setting but for an asymptomatic person are shown in Practical box 1.1.

The aims of management are to maintain health, avoid transmission of HIV and provide appropriate palliative support. Confidentiality must be strictly adhered to and psychological support must be readily available for the patient, family, friends and carers. Dietary assessment and advice should be freely accessible.

Clear advice on reducing the risk of transmission must be provided and future sexual practices discussed. Information needs to be available for people to make informed choices about childbearing. The implications for existing family members should be considered. General health promotion advice on smoking, drug misuse and exercise is important.

## Therapy

Treatment strategies for specific conditions are discussed in the appropriate sections above.

Various events in the HIV life-cycle have been identified as potential targets for antiretroviral therapy. Antagonists of reverse transcriptase are so far the most developed.

ZIDOVUDINE (3-AZIDO-3-DEOXYTHYMIDINE, AZT) is an analogue of thymidine which inhibits reverse transcriptase and also acts as a DNA chain terminator. It is now widely used in the developed world in patients with symptomatic HIV disease (CDC Group IV). Studies have shown a survival advantage in people with AIDS taking AZT and a reduction in opportunistic infections. Constitutional symptoms may be ameliorated. Neurological disease may improve. A transient rise in CD4 lymphocytes and a fall in P24 antigen levels are seen on treatment. Clinical and survival benefits of AZT in HIV-positive asymptomatic patients still have to be conclusively demonstrated. Side-effects include headache, nausea, abdominal discomfort and insomnia, all of which may resolve after several weeks on AZT. The most common toxicity is bone marrow suppression, particularly megaloblastic change and suppression of the red cell line. Neutropenia also occurs. Myopathy may occur after long-term use. Adverse reactions are more frequent and severe in patients with more advanced disease and are to some extent dose dependent. *In vitro* resistance of HIV to AZT may be seen after 6 months on treatment but its clinical significance is not clear. Dose regimens range from 500 to 1000 mg daily in divided doses.

DIDEOXYINOSINE (DDI) AND DIDEOXYCYTIDINE (DDC) are also inhibitors of reverse transcriptase. They are less well evaluated than AZT. Side-effects include acute pancreatitis and peripheral neuropathy, but bone marrow toxicity is rare. As a result they may be used as second line therapy in patients who cannot tolerate AZT.

OTHER DRUGS include non-nucleoside reverse transcriptase inhibitors and agents that act at other sites in the HIV replication cycle, e.g. protease inhibitors. These compounds are currently undergoing therapeutic trials but are not yet commercially available. Drugs used in combinations are also being evaluated.

## Prevention and control

The development of an effective vaccine against HIV is being pursued but is not a realistic prospect in the near future. Changing behaviour is notoriously difficult, especially in areas that carry as many taboos as HIV and AIDS. It is however the main tool available for prevention of infection. Education programmes providing factual

---

Microbiology
  Syphilis serology
  Toxoplasmosis serology
  Cryptococcal antigen
  Screen for other sexually transmitted diseases

Virology
  HIV antibody (confirmatory)
  P24 antigen/antibody
  Hepatitis serology (B and C)
  Cytomegalovirus antibody

Haematology
  Full blood count, differential and film
  Erythrocyte sedimentation rate

Biochemistry
  Liver and renal function tests

Immunology
  Lymphocyte subsets
  Neopterin
  $\beta_2$-Microglobulin

Other
  Chest X-ray
  Lung function tests
  Cervical cytology

**Practical box 1.1**  Baseline investigations for HIV infection.

knowledge and strategies to avoid infection are fundamental to the process. The use of condoms has been shown to reduce the spread of HIV infection in discordant couples and their use has been strongly promoted. Control of other STDs is crucial in view of their potential role in enhancing HIV transmission. Access to clean needles and syringes to prevent sharing amongst drug users is important, as are programmes to reduce injecting drug use. Screening of blood products has reduced iatrogenic infection in developed countries but is expensive and not globally available. The need for blood transfusion in developing countries could be reduced by improved control of conditions such as malaria and hookworm, which lead to anaemia. Partner notification schemes are in various stages of development worldwide but are controversial. Availability and accessibility of confidential HIV testing is important and provides an opportunity for individual health education and risk reduction to be discussed.

## Further Reading

Adler M (1990) *The ABC of Sexually Transmitted Diseases*, 2nd edn. London: BMA Publications.

Adler M (1993) *The ABC of AIDS*, 3rd edn. London: BMA Publications.

Arnold E (1990) *Modern vaccines*. London: Lancet Publications.

Bannister B (1983) *Infectious Diseases*. London: Baillière Tindall.

Braude AI (1985) *Infectious Diseases and Medical Microbiology*, 2nd edn. Philadelphia: WB Saunders

Collier L & Oxford J (1993) *Human Virology*. Oxford: Oxford University Press.

Cook GC (1988) *Communicable and Tropical Diseases*. London: (Mainstream Medicine series). Heinemann Medical Books.

Department of Health Welsh Office, Scottish Office Home and Health Department, DHSS (Northern Ireland) (1992) *Immunisation against Infectious Disease*. London: HMSO.

Farthing MJG (1990) *Ballière's Clinical Gastroenterology. Virus Infections of the gut and liver*. London: Baillière Tindall.

Farthing MJG & Keusch GT (1989) *Enteric Infection: Mechanisms, Manifestations and Management*. London: Chapman and Hall.

*Fields Virology* (1990) London: Raven Press.

Field M (1991) *Diarrheal Diseases*. New York: Elsevier.

Gracey M & IAD Bouchier (1993) *Baillière's Clinical Gastroenterology. Infectious diarrhoea*. London: Baillière Tindall.

Mandel GL, Douglas RG & Bennett JE (1985) *Principles and Practice of Infectious Diseases*, 2nd edn. London: Baillière Tindall.

Mimms C, Playfair J, Roitt I, Wakelin D, Williams R & Anderson R (1993) *Medical Microbiology*. London: Mosby.

Peters W, Gilles HM (1989) *A Colour Atlas of Tropical Medicine & Parasitology*, 3rd edn. Netherlands: Wolfe Medical Publications Ltd.

Youmans GP, Paterson PY & Sommers HM (eds) (1985) *The Biologic and Clinical Basis of Infectious Diseases*, 3rd edn. Philadelphia: WB Saunders.

Zuckerman AJ, Banntvala JE & Pattison JR (1990) *Clinical Virology*. London: Wiley.

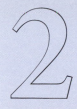

# Molecular biology, genetic disorders and immunology

# MOLECULAR BIOLOGY AND GENETIC DISORDERS

## Introduction

The impact of molecular biology on genetic disorders has been enormous. Over 200 single-gene disorders have now been identified; these include the determination of the molecular genetic defects in cystic fibrosis, sickle cell anaemia and thalassaemia. This understanding of the basic modes of inheritance is fundamental to genetic counselling and prenatal diagnosis.

A glossary of terms commonly used in genetics is on p. 150.

## Molecular basis of genetics

Genetic information is stored in deoxyribonucleic acid (DNA). DNA is a polymer which consists of two strands wound around each other to form a double helix. Each of the single strands is made of basic units called nucleotides. Nucleotides themselves are made up of three components: (i) a pentose sugar molecule called 2-deoxyribose, (ii) a phosphate group, and (iii) a nitrogenous base. DNA has four different types of nitrogenous base, which fall into two classes: the pyrimidines (cytosine (C) and thymine (T)) and the purines (adenine (A) and guanine (G)).

The nucleotides are joined together by phosphodiester bonds into a polynucleotide strand and it is two of these strands wound around each other that make up the double helix of DNA. Phosphodiester bonds are formed between the phosphate group of one nucleotide (which is itself attached to the 3′ carbon of deoxyribose) and the 5′ carbon of deoxyribose on the next nucleotide—so the polynucleotide chain has a 'sugar–phosphate backbone', which has a 5′ end and a 3′ end (Fig. 2.1a). Hydrogen bonds between the bases hold the two strands of DNA together with A always pairing with T and C with G. The two strands run in opposite directions so the 5′ end of one is opposite the 3′ end of the other strand (Fig. 2.1b).

For practical purposes the length of DNA is generally measured by molecular geneticists in numbers of base pairs (bp); a piece of DNA 1000 bp long is 1 kilobase pair (kb) in length.

## Genes

A gene is part of a DNA molecule that codes for a sequence of nucleotides. Genes give instructions for the synthesis of specific proteins. Humans are estimated to have between 30 000 and 100 000 genes. Only an estimated 10–25% of DNA encodes genes, the function (if any) of the remainder being largely unknown.

The enzymatic machinery of the cell can read along one of the polynucleotide chains of DNA and can recognize the specific sequence of base pairs that comprise a gene. Genes vary greatly in size: most extend over 20–40 kb, but a few, such as the gene for the muscle protein called dystrophin, can extend over millions of base pairs.

## Transcription

Moving along one of the polynucleotide strands in a 5′ to 3′ direction, short DNA sequences of As, Cs, Gs and Ts are recognized in a particular order. This sequence is 'upstream' of the gene and is called a promoter sequence. Different genes have different promoters. An enzyme called RNA polymerase recognizes the DNA sequences in

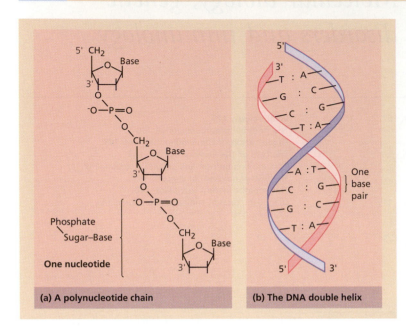

**(a) A polynucleotide chain**

Phosphate
Sugar–Base
**One nucleotide**

**(b) The DNA double helix**

One base pair

**Fig. 2.1** Deoxyribonucleic acid (DNA).
(a) A polynucleotide chain. The chain has the 'sugar–phosphate' backbone and a 5' and 3' end. The bases (A, C, G or T) are attached to the sugar.
(b) The double helix. Two polynucleotide strands are wound around each other. The bases are inside the helix.

the promoter region and then binds onto the DNA when it sees the sequence TATAAAT. This sequence is known as the TATA box and usually it lies about 35 bp upstream of where the process of transcription begins. At this site the RNA polymerase starts transcribing a copy of the DNA sequence (which acts as a template) into a single-stranded molecule called ribonucleic acid (RNA) (Fig. 2.2). The RNA polymerase works along the strand until it reaches the end of the gene where it stops transcribing. The 5' end of the new RNA molecule is 'capped' (or blocked) in that the molecule begins with a complex nucleotide called 7-methylguanine. At the 3' end of the molecule a long run of up to several hundred As is added on, probably to give the RNA stability. This 'poly (A) tail' is added on to the RNA by an enzyme which attaches the tail a few nucleotides downstream of the polyadenylation signal (AAUAAA) at the end of the RNA. RNA is similar to DNA except that it is single stranded, has a slightly different sugar molecule (ribose) and contains a base called uracil (U), rather than the thymine found in DNA.

## RNA splicing

Transcription takes place in the nucleus of the cell, as does the next process called splicing, in which the RNA transcript is 'cut and pasted'. In this process the coding sequences (called exons) are cut by enzymes and spliced together leaving out the intervening, non-coding introns (Fig. 2.2). The final 'messenger RNA' (mRNA) is thus assembled and passes into the cytoplasm.

## Translation

In the cytoplasm organelles called ribosomes read the RNA sequence and build amino acids into the polypeptide chain that is encoded by the spliced mRNA. The

sequence of nucleotides in the mRNA is 'translated' into a polypeptide (Fig. 2.2).

A ribosome attaches to the mRNA and reads along from the 5' end to the 3' end of the molecule. The first nucleotides do not code for amino acids, but are likely to be regulatory sequences. These nucleotides make up the 5' untranslated region (5' UTR). The nucleotides in the middle of the mRNA (which may extend over several thousands of base pairs) code for the amino acids in the polypeptide chain. This region of the mRNA is the 'coding region'. The nucleotides at the end of the mRNA do not code for amino acids, but make up the 3' untranslated region (3' UTR) of the mRNA, and these are also likely to be regulatory sequences of some sort.

The ribosome reads the nucleotides in the coding region as sets of three. Three contiguous nucleotides are called a codon. Each codon is a specific instruction for either an amino acid to be added into a peptide chain, or for the chain to stop. The instructions are encoded by the codons and this is the '*genetic code*'. There are only 20 common amino acids but 64 possible codon combinations that make up the genetic code. This means that some amino acids are coded by more than one codon. The codon AUG initiates the translation of the polypeptide chain; this specifies the amino acid methionine.

The amino acids for the polypeptide chain are carried on small RNA molecules in the cytoplasm called transfer RNA (tRNA). Each tRNA is specific for one amino acid and has three unpaired nucleotide bases (the anticodon) that correspond to the appropriate codons of the mRNA. So every anticodon recognizes its complementary codon in the mRNA. For example, the codon UGC in the mRNA is recognized by the anticodon ACG within a tRNA carrying the amino acid cysteine (Fig. 2.2). The ribosome allows the tRNAs carrying their individual amino acids to recognize the codons in the mRNA. Each

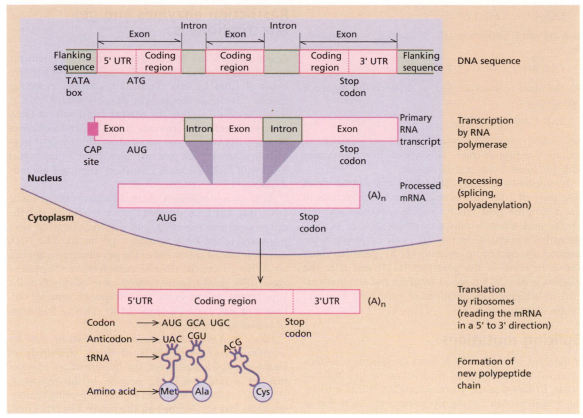

**Fig. 2.2**  From DNA to RNA to protein. Ala, alanine; (A)$_n$, poly (A) or AAAA. . .; AUG, 'start' coding sequence; Cys, cysteine; Met, methionine; mRNA, messenger RNA; UTR, untranslated region.

tRNA deposits its amino acid which is covalently bound by a peptide bond to the previous amino acid in the polypeptide chain. Three condons in mRNA (UAA, UAG and UGA) do not code for amino acids, but are 'stop' codons. If the ribosome reads one of these codons then translation stops and no further amino acids are added to the polypeptide chain and the ribosome and mRNA part company.

# Mutation

Although DNA replication is a very accurate process occasionally mistakes occur producing changes or mutations. These changes can also occur due to other factors such as radiation, ultraviolet light or chemicals. Mutations in gene sequences or in the sequences which regulate gene expression (transcription and translation) may alter the amino acid sequence in the protein encoded by that gene. In some cases protein function will be maintained; in other cases it will change or cease, perhaps producing a clinical disorder.

Many different types of mutation occur.

## Point mutation

This is the simplest type of change and involves the substitution of one nucleotide for another, so changing the codon in a coding sequence. For example, the triplet AAA, which codes for lysine, may be mutated to AGA, which codes for arginine.

Whether a substitution produces a clinical disorder or not depends on whether it changes a critical part of the protein molecule produced. Fortunately, many substitutions have no effect on the function or stability of the proteins produced as several codons code for the same amino acid. However, some mutations may have a severe effect; for example, in sickle cell disease a mutation in the β-globin gene changes one codon from GAG to GTG so that instead of glutamic acid, valine is incorporated into the polypeptide chain, which radically alters its properties.

## Insertion or deletion

Insertion or deletion of one or more bases is a more serious change, as it results in the alteration of the rest of the following sequence to give a frame-shift mutation. For example, if the original code was:

TAA GGA GAG TTT

and an extra nucleotide (A) is inserted, the sequence becomes:

TAA AGG AGA GTT T

or the third nucleotide (A) is deleted, the sequence becomes:

TAG GAG AGT TT

and in both cases different amino acids are incorporated into the polypeptide chain. This type of change is responsible for some forms of thalassaemia.

Insertions and deletions can involve many hundreds of base pairs of DNA; for example some large deletions in the dystrophin gene remove coding sequences and this results in Duchenne muscular dystrophy (see p. 953). Recently an insertion/deletion (ID) polymorphism in the angiotensin converting enzyme (ACE) gene has been shown to result in the genotypes II, ID and DD. The deletion is of a 287 bp repeat sequence and DD is associated with higher concentrations of circulating ACE and cardiac disease (see p. 579).

## Splicing mutations

If the DNA sequences which direct the splicing of introns from mRNA are mutated then abnormal splicing may occur. In this case the processed mRNA which is translated into protein by the ribosomes may carry intron sequences, so altering which amino acids are incorporated into the polypeptide chain.

## Termination mutations

Normal polypeptide chain termination occurs when the ribosomes processing the mRNA reach one of the chain termination or 'stop' codons (see above). Mutations involving these codons will result in either late or premature termination. For example in haemoglobin Constant Spring—a haemoglobin variant—instead of the 'stop' sequence, a single base change allows the insertion of an extra amino acid.

# *Techniques for DNA analysis and isolation of genes*

Modern techniques using recombinant DNA allow great insights into the functioning of genes and the molecular pathology of genetic diseases. Often the first step in studying the DNA of an individual involves preparation of genomic DNA. This is a simple procedure in which 20 ml of blood is taken, the lymphocytes are treated to gently break open their cell and nuclear membranes, and chromosomal DNA is chemically extracted. DNA is stable and can be stored frozen for years.

# Restriction enzymes and gel electrophoresis

Genomic DNA can be cut into a number of fragments by enzymes called restriction enzymes, which are obtained from bacteria. Restriction enzymes recognize specific DNA sequences and cut double-stranded DNA at these sites. For example, the enzyme *Eco*RI will cut DNA wherever it reads the sequence GAATTC, and so human genomic DNA is cut into hundreds of thousands of fragments. Whenever the genomic DNA from an individual is cut with *Eco*RI the same 'restriction fragments' are produced.

As DNA is a negatively charged molecule the genomic DNA that has been digested with a restriction enzyme can be separated according to its size and charge, by electrophoresing the DNA through a gel matrix. The DNA sample is loaded at one end of the gel, a voltage is applied across the gel and the DNA migrates towards the positive anode. The small fragments move more quickly than the large fragments and so the DNA fragments separate out. Fragment size can be determined by running fragments of known size on the same gel.

*Pulsed field gel electrophoresis* (PFGE) can be used for separating very long pieces of DNA (hundreds of kilobases) which have been cut by restriction enzymes that cut at rare sites in the genome. In this technique, DNA molecules are subjected to two perpendicular electric fields that are switched on alternately. The DNA molecules are separated on the basis of molecular size and this technique can be used for long-range mapping of the genome to detect major deletions and rearrangements.

# Southern blotting and DNA probes

This technique allows the visualization of individual DNA fragments (Fig. 2.3).

A DNA probe is used to indicate where the fragment of interest lies. DNA probes are useful because a fundamental property of DNA is that when two strands are separated, for example by heating, they will always reassociate and stick together again because of their complementary base sequences. Therefore the presence or position of a particular gene can be identified using a gene 'probe' consisting of DNA with a base sequence that is complementary to that of the sequence of interest. A DNA probe is thus a piece of single-stranded DNA that can be labelled with a radioactive isotope (usually $^{32}$P) or a fluorescent signal. The probe is added to a hybridization solution into which the membrane with the DNA is also placed. The single-stranded probe will locate and bind to its complementary sequence on the blot and can be identified by autoradiography or fluorescence.

A similar technique for blotting RNA fragments (which are not cut by restriction enzymes, but which are blotted as full length mRNAs) onto membranes is called Northern blotting and one for blotting proteins is called Western blotting.

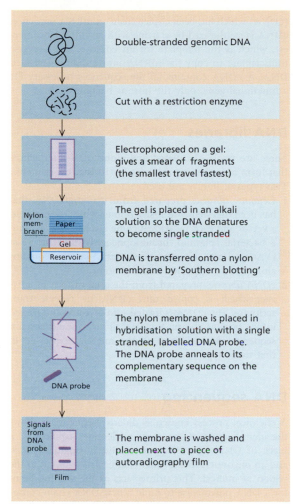

**Fig. 2.3** Southern blotting and DNA probes.

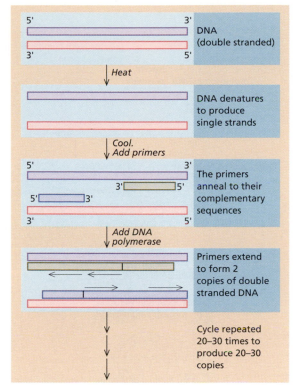

**Fig. 2.4** Polymerase chain reaction.

# The polymerase chain reaction

Minute amounts of DNA can be amplified over a million times within a few hours using this *in vitro* technique (Fig. 2.4). The exact DNA sequence to be amplified needs to be known because the DNA is amplified between two short (generally 17–25 bp) single-stranded DNA fragments ('oligonucleotide primers') which are complementary to the sequences at either end of the DNA of interest. The technique has three steps: the double-stranded genomic DNA is denatured by heat into single-stranded DNA; the reaction is cooled to favour DNA annealing and the primers bind to their target DNA; then a DNA polymerase is used to extend the primers in opposite directions using the target DNA as a template. After one cycle there are two copies of double-stranded DNA; after two cycles there are four copies and this number rises exponentially with the number of cycles. Typically a polymerase chain reaction is set for 25–30 cycles, allowing millions of amplifications.

This technique has revolutionized genetic research as minute amounts of DNA not previously amenable to analysis can be amplified, for example from buccal cell scrapings, blood spots, or single embryonic cells.

# DNA cloning

A particular DNA fragment of interest can be isolated and inserted into a 'vector' so that it can be cloned and prepared in large quantities independent of other sequences. Vectors include small circular DNA molecules called plasmids, which are derived from naturally occurring sequences in bacteria; bacteriophages, which are derived from bacterial viruses; or 'yeast artificial chromosomes' (YACs), which are derived from DNA sequences found in yeast. Each vector takes an optimum size of DNA insert. Small sequences of a few kilobases can be inserted into a plasmid. Large sequences of several hundred kilobases can be inserted into a YAC.

The DNA fragment of interest is inserted into the vector DNA sequence using an enzyme called a ligase. This takes place *in vitro*. The next step, cloning, creates many copies of the 'recombinant DNA molecule' and takes place *in vivo* when the plasmid or other vector is placed back into the bacterial (or yeast) host. Bacteria that have successfully taken up the recombinant plasmid can be selected if the plasmid also carries an antibiotic resistance gene (so bacteria without the plasmid die in the presence of antibiotic) (Fig. 2.5).

The DNA fragment of interest to be cloned may be a restriction fragment. Alternatively it could be DNA

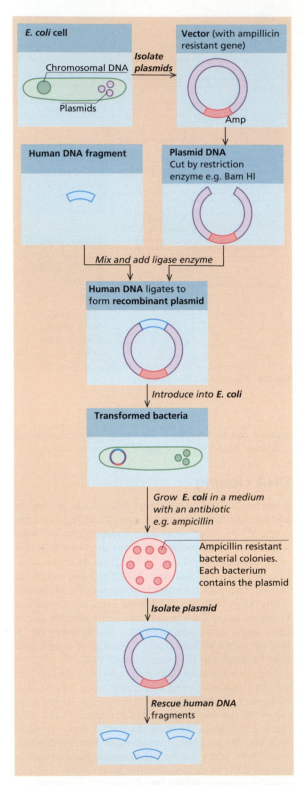

**Fig. 2.5**   DNA cloning. Recombinant DNA technique showing incorporation of foreign DNA into a plasmid. The ampicillin-resistant genes can be used to distinguish transformed *Escherichia coli* cells.

(cDNA) which has been copied from an mRNA sequence. cDNA is synthesized by starting with an mRNA of interest, which is the template for an enzyme called reverse transcriptase to copy the mRNA into a double-stranded DNA. A cDNA contains all the sequences necessary for a functional gene, only the introns being absent.

## DNA libraries

These are pools of isolated and cloned DNA sequences that form a permanent resource for further experiments. Two types of library are used:

1 *Genomic libraries* prepared from genomic DNA that has been digested with restriction enzymes, ligated into a vector and each individual clone has been passed into a bacterial (plasmid, bacteriophage, cosmid) or yeast (YACs) host. A genomic library usually contains almost every sequence in the genome.

2 *cDNA libraries* prepared from the total mRNA of a tissue, which is copied into cDNA by reverse transcriptase. The cDNA is ligated into a vector and passed into a host as above. A cDNA library should contain sequences derived from all the mRNAs expressed in that tissue type.

## DNA sequencing

A chemical process known as dideoxy sequencing allows the identification of the exact nucleotide sequence of a piece of DNA. The DNA of interest is single stranded and an oligonucleotide primer is annealed adjacent to the region of interest. This primer acts as the starting point for a DNA polymerase to build a new DNA chain complementary to the sequence under investigation. The reaction is carried out in four tubes to each of which a mixture of nucleotides is added, one of which is radioactive. To each tube one dideoxy triphosphate of either adenine, guanine, cytosine or thymine is also added at a low level. These are incorporated into the growing chain and stop enzymatic synthesis (because they lack the necessary 3-hydroxyl group). As the dideoxynucleotides are present at a low concentration, not all the chains in a reaction tube will incorporate a dideoxynucleotide in the same place, so the tubes contain sequences of different lengths but which all terminate with a particular dideoxynucleotide. These fragments are electrophoresed in four columns and a sequence of DNA is deduced by autoradiography.

# Chromosomes

The nucleus of each diploid cell contains $6 \times 10^9$ bp of DNA in long molecules called chromosomes. Chromosomes are massive structures containing one molecule of DNA that is wound around histone proteins into small units called nucleosomes and these are further wound to make up the structure of the chromosome itself. Diploid human cells have 46 chromosomes, 23 inherited from each parent; thus there are 23 'homologous' pairs of chromosomes (22 pairs of 'autosomes' and two 'sex chromosomes'). The sex chromosomes, called the X and Y chromosomes, are not homologous but are different in size and shape. Males have an X and a Y chromosome, females have two X chromosomes. (Primary male sexual characteristics are determined by the *SRY* gene on the Y chromosome.) The chromosomes can be classified according to their size and shape, the largest being chromosome 1. The constriction in the chromosome is the centromere, which can be in the middle of the chromosome (metacentric) or at one extreme end (acrocentric). The centromere divides the chromosome into a short arm and a long arm, which are referred to as the p arm and the q arm respectively (Fig. 2.6). In addition chromosomes can be stained when they are in the metaphase stage of the cell cycle and are very condensed. The stain gives a different pattern of light and dark bands that is diagnostic for each chromosome. Each band is given a number and gene mapping techniques allow genes to be positioned within a band within an arm of a chromosome. For example, the *CFTR* gene (in which a defect gives rise to cystic fibrosis) maps to 7q21, that is on chromosome 7 in the long arm in band 21.

During cell division (mitosis), each chromosome divides into two so that each daughter nucleus has the same number of chromosomes as its parent cell. During gametogenesis, however, the number of chromosomes is halved by meiosis so that after conception the number of chromosomes remains the same and is not doubled. In the female, each ovum contains one or other X chromosome but, in the male, the sperm bears either an X or a Y chromosome.

Chromosomes can only be seen easily in actively dividing cells. Typically lymphocytes from the peripheral blood are stimulated to divide and are processed to allow the chromosomes to be examined. Cells from other tissues can also be used, for example amniotic fluid, placental cells from chorionic villus sampling, bone marrow and skin (Information box 2.1).

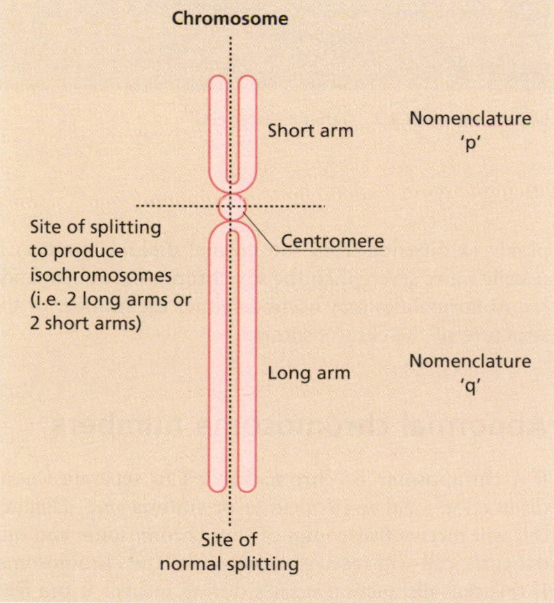

### The X chromosome and inactivation

Although female chromosomes are XX, females do not have two doses of X-linked genes (compared to just one dose for a male XY), because of the phenomenon of X inactivation or Lyonization (after its discoverer, Dr Mary Lyon). In this process one of the two X chromosomes in the cells of females becomes transcriptionally inactive, so the cell has only one dose of the X-linked genes. Inactivation is random and can affect either X chromosome.

**Fig. 2.6** Structure of a chromosome. The sites at which the chromosome can be split are shown. Nomenclature for describing *loci* on chromosome is as follows. Number of chromosome or X or Y plus short arm (p) or long arm (q). The region or subregion is defined by transverse light and dark bands stained with quinacrine or Giemsa and numbered from the centromere outwards.

*Chromosome constitution* = chromosome number + sex chromosome + abnormality

*Examples:*

46 XX = normal female
47 XX + 21 = trisomy 21 (Down's syndrome)
46 XYt (2;19) (p21; p12) = translocation between chromosome 2 and 19 with breaking at band p21 and p12 on the short arm.

Chromosome studies may be indicated in the following circumstances:

*Antenatal*
(a) Pregnancies in women over 35 years
(b) Positive maternal serum screening test for trisomy 21
(c) Ultrasound markers of chromosomal abnormalities
(d) Severe fetal growth retardation
(e) Sexing of fetus in X-linked disorders

*In the neonate*
(a) Congenital malformations
(b) Suspicion of trisomy or monosomy
(c) Ambiguous genitalia

*In the adolescent*
(a) Primary amenorrhoea or failure of pubertal development
(b) Growth retardation

*In the adult*
(a) Screening parents of a child with a chromosomal abnormality for further genetic counselling
(b) Infertility or recurrent miscarriages
(c) Mental handicap
(d) Certain malignant disorders, e.g. leukaemias

**Information box 2.1** Indications for chromosomal analysis.

## THE MITOCHONDRIAL CHROMOSOME

In addition to the 23 pairs of chromosomes in the nucleus of every diploid cell, the mitochondria in the cytoplasm of the cell also have their own chromosomes. The mitochondrial chromosome is a circular DNA molecule of approximately 16 500 bp and every base pair makes up part of the coding sequence. These genes encode proteins or RNA molecules involved in mitochondrial function. These proteins are all components of the mitochondrial respiratory chain involved in oxidative phosphorylation. Every cell contains several hundred mitochondria and therefore several hundred mitochondrial chromosomes. All mitochondria are inherited from the mother as sperm contains no (or very few) mitochondria.

## *Human genetic disorders*

The spectrum of inherited or congenital genetic disorders can be classified as the chromosomal disorders, including mitochondrial chromosome disorders, the Mendelian and sex-linked single gene disorders, a variety of non-Mendelian disorders and the multifactorial and polygenic disorders (Table 2.1 and Information box 2.2).

## CHROMOSOMAL DISORDERS

Chromosomal abnormalities are much more common than generally appreciated. Over half of spontaneous abortions have chromosomal abnormalities, as compared with only 4–6 abnormalities per 1000 live births. Specific chromosomal abnormalities can lead to well-recognized and severe clinical syndromes, although autosomal aneu-

Mendelian (single gene defects)

Inherited or new mutation
Mutant allele or pair of mutant alleles at single locus
Clear pattern of inheritance (autosomal or sex-linked)
    dominant or recessive
High risk to relatives

Chromosomal

Loss, gain or abnormal rearrangement of one or more of
    46 chromosomes in diploid cell
No clear pattern of inheritance
Low risk to relatives

Multifactorial

Common
Interaction between genes and environmental factors
Low risk to relatives

Mitochondrial

Due to mutations in mitochondrial genome
Transmitted through maternal line
Different pattern of inheritance from Mendelian
    disorders

Somatic cell

Mutations in somatic cells
Somatic event is not inherited
Often give rise to tumours

**Information box 2.2**   Genetic disorders.

| Type | Estimated prevalence per 1000 population |
|---|---|
| **Single gene disorders** | |
| Autosomal dominant | 2–10 |
| Autosomal recessive | 2 |
| X-linked recessive | 1–2 |
| Chromosomal abnormalities | 6–7 |
| Common disorders with a genetic component | 7–10 |
| Congenital malformation | 20 |
| Total | 38–51 |

[a]From Kingston H (1989) Clinical genetic services. *British Medical Journal* **298**, 306–307. With permission.

**Table 2.1**   Prevalence of genetic disease[a].

ploidy (a differing from the normal diploid number) is usually more severe than the sex chromosome aneuploidies. Abnormalities may occur in either the number or the structure of the chromosomes.

## Abnormal chromosome numbers

If a chromosome or chromatids fail to separate ('non-disjunction') either in meiosis or mitosis one daughter cell will receive two copies of that chromosome and one daughter cell will receive no copies of the chromosome. If this non-disjunction occurs during meiosis it can lead to an ovum or sperm having either (i) an extra chromosome, so resulting in a fetus that is 'trisomic' and has three instead of two copies of the chromosome; or (ii) no chromosome, so the fetus is 'monosomic' and has one instead of two copies of the chromosome. Non-disjunction can occur with autosomes or sex chromosomes. However, only individuals with trisomy 13, 18 and 21 survive to birth, and most children with trisomy 13 and trisomy 18 die in early childhood. Trisomy 21 (Down's syndrome) is observed with a frequency of 1 in 700 live births regardless of geography or ethnic background. Full autosomal monosomies are extremely rare and very deleterious. Sex chromosome trisomies (for example Klinefelter's syndrome, XXY) are relatively common. The sex chromosome monosomy in which the individual has an X chromosome only and no second X or Y chromosome is known as Turner's syndrome and is estimated to occur in 1 in 2500 live born girls (Table 2.2).

Occasionally, non-disjunction can occur during mitosis shortly after two gametes have fused. It will then result in the formation of two cell lines, each with a different chromosome complement. This occurs more often with the sex chromosome, and results in a 'mosaic' individual.

Very rarely the entire chromosome set will be present in more than two copies, so the individual may be triploid rather than diploid and have a chromosome number of 69. Triploidy and tetraploidy (four sets) result in spontaneous abortion.

## Abnormal chromosome structures

As well as abnormal numbers of chromosomes, chromosomes can have abnormal structures, and the disruption to the DNA and gene sequences may give rise to a genetic disease.

### Deletions

Deletions of a portion of a chromosome may give rise to a disease syndrome if two copies of the genes in the deleted region are necessary, and the individual will not be normal with just the one copy remaining on the non-deleted homologous chromosome. Many deletion syndromes have been well described, for example a deletion of chromosome 22 gives rise to DiGeorge syndrome.

### Duplications

Duplications occur when a portion of the chromosome is present on the chromosome in two copies, so the genes in that chromosome portion are present in an extra dose. A form of the neuropathy Charcot–Marie–Tooth disease is due to a small duplication of a region of chromosome 17.

### Inversion

Inversions involve an end-to-end reversal of a segment within a chromosome, e.g. abcdefgh becomes abcfedgh.

### Translocations

Translocations occur when two chromosome regions join together, when they would not normally. Chromosome translocations in somatic cells may be associated with tumorigenesis (see p. 355). Translocations can be very complex involving more than two chromosomes, but most are simple and fall into two categories:

1 *Reciprocal translocations.* These occur when any two non-homologous chromosomes break simultaneously and rejoin, swapping ends. In this case the cell still has 46 chromosomes but two of them are rearranged. Someone with a balanced translocation is likely to be normal (unless a translocation breakpoint interrupts a gene) but at meiosis, when the chromosomes separate into different daughter cells, the translocated chromosomes will enter the gametes and any resulting fetus may inherit one abnormal chromosome and have an unbalanced translocation with physical manifestations.

2 *Robertsonian translocations.* These are clinically important and occur when two acrocentric chromosomes join and the short arm is lost leaving only 45 chromosomes. This translocation is balanced as no genetic material is lost and the individual is healthy. However any offspring have a risk of inheriting an unbalanced arrangement. This risk depends on which acrocentric chromosome is involved. Clinically important is the 14/21 Robertsonian translocation and a woman with this karyotype has a 1 : 8 risk of a Down's baby (a male carrier has a 1 : 50 risk). However, they have a 50% risk of producing a carrier like themselves, hence the importance of genetic family studies. Relatives should be alerted about the risk of a Down's offspring and should have their chromosomes checked.

Table 2.3 shows some of the syndromes resulting from chromosomal abnormalities.

# MITOCHONDRIAL CHROMOSOME DISORDERS

The mitochondrial chromosome carries its genetic information in a very compact form, for example there are no introns in the genes. Therefore any mutation has a high chance of having an effect. However as every cell contains hundreds of mitochondria, a single altered mitochondrial genome will not be noticed. As mitochondria divide there is a statistical likelihood that there will be more mutated mitochondria and at some point this will give rise to a mitochondrial disease. Most mitochondrial diseases are myopathies and neuropathies with a maternal pattern of inheritance. Many syndromes have been described, including myoclonic epilepsy with ragged red fibres (MERRF) and mitochondrial encephalomyopathy, lactic acidosis and stroke-like episodes (MELAS), Leber's optic atrophy, with late onset bilateral loss of central vision and

| Abnormal chromosome numbers | |
|---|---|
| Autosomal disorders: | |
| Trisomy 21 (Down's syndrome) | 1 in 700 |
| Trisomy 18 (Edwards' syndrome) | 1 in 3000 |
| Trisomy 13 (Patau's syndrome) | 1 in 15 000 |
| Sex chromosome disorders: | |
| 47, XXY (Klinefelter's syndrome) | 1 in 1000 males |
| 47, XYY | 1 in 1100 males |
| 47, XXX | 1 in 1200 females |
| 45, X (Turner's syndrome) | 1 in 2500 females |
| Abnormal chromosome structures | |
| Balanced translocations | 1 in 500 |
| Unbalanced translocations | 1 in 2000 |

Table 2.2 Examples of chromosomal disorders in live births.

| Syndrome | Chromosome karyotype | Incidence and risks | Clinical features | Mortality |
|---|---|---|---|---|
| **Autosomal abnormalities** | | | | |
| Trisomy 21 (Down's syndrome) | 47, + 21 (95%) Mosaicism Translocation 5% | 1 : 650 (Risk with 20–29 year old mother 1 : 1000; >45 year old mother 1 : 30) | Flat facies, slanting eyes, epicanthic folds, small ears, simian crease, short stubby fingers, hypotonia, variable mental retardation, congenital heart disease (up to 50%) | High in first year, but some survive to adulthood |
| Trisomy 13 (Patau's syndrome) | 47, +13 | 1 : 5000 | Low-set ears, cleft lip and palate, polydactyly, micro-ophthalmia, mental retardation | Rarely survive for more than a few weeks |
| Trisomy 18 (Edwards' syndrome) | 47, +18 | 1 : 3000 | Low-set ears, micrognathia, rocker-bottom feet, mental retardation | Rarely survive for more than a few weeks |
| **Sex chromosome abnormalities** | | | | |
| Fragile X syndrome | 46, XX, fra (X) 46, XY, fra (X) | 1 : 2000 | Most common inherited cause of mental retardation predominantly in males. Macro-orchidism | |
| *Female* Turner's syndrome | 45, XO | 1 : 2500 | Infantilism, primary amenorrhoea, short stature, webbed neck, cubitus valgus, normal IQ | |
| Triple X syndrome | 47, XXX | 1 : 1000 | No distinctive somatic features, mental retardation | |
| Others | 48, XXXX 49, XXXXX | Rare | Amenorrhoea, infertility, mental retardation | |
| *Male* Klinefelter's syndrome | 47, XXY (or XXYY) | 1 : 1000 (more in sons of older mothers) | Decreased crown–pubis : pubis–heel ratio, eunuchoid, testicular atrophy, infertility, gynaecomastia, mental retardation (20%; related to number of X chromosomes) | |
| Double Y syndrome | 47, XYY | 1 : 800 | Tall, fertile, minor mental and psychiatric illness, high incidence in tall criminals | |
| Others | 48, XXXY 49, XXXXY | | Mental retardation, testicular atrophy | |

**Table 2.3** Chromosomal abnormalities—examples of a few syndromes.

cardiac arrhythmias, is an example of a mitochondrial disease caused by a point mutation in one gene.

## SINGLE GENE DEFECTS

## Mendelian and sex-linked single gene disorders

Monogenetic disorders involving single genes can be inherited as dominant, recessive or sex-linked characteristics. Inheritance occurs according to simple Mendelian laws making predictions of disease in offspring and therefore genetic counselling more straightforward.

**Autosomal dominant disorders** (Fig 2.7a and Table 2.4)

Each diploid cell contains two copies of all the autosomes. An autosomal dominant disorder occurs when one of the two copies has a mutation and the protein produced by the normal form of the gene cannot compensate. In this case a 'heterozygote' individual who has two different forms (or 'alleles') of the same gene will manifest the disease. The offspring of a heterozygote have a 50% chance of inheriting the chromosome carrying the disease allele and therefore also having the disease. However estimation of risk to offspring for counselling families can be difficult because of three factors:

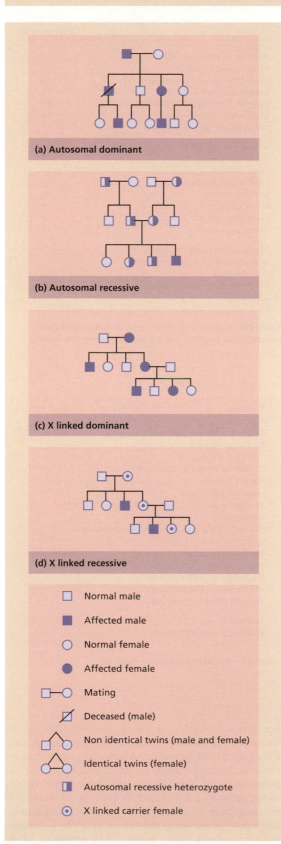

(a) Autosomal dominant

(b) Autosomal recessive

(c) X linked dominant

(d) X linked recessive

☐ Normal male

■ Affected male

○ Normal female

● Affected female

☐—○ Mating

⊘ Deceased (male)

Non identical twins (male and female)

Identical twins (female)

◧ Autosomal recessive heterozygote

⊙ X linked carrier female

**Fig. 2.7** Modes of inheritance of simple gene disorders (a, b, c and d) with a key to the standard pedigree symbols.

Achondroplasia
Acute intermittent porphyria
Adult polycystic disease
Alzheimer's disease (familial)
$\alpha_1$-Antitrypsin deficiency
$C_1$ esterase inhibitor deficiency
Crigler–Najjar syndrome type II
Epidermolysis bullosa (some forms)
Familial adenomatous polyposis
Familial hypercholesterolaemia
Facio-scapulohumeral dystrophy
Hereditary angio-oedema
Hereditary elliptocytosis
Hereditary haemorrhagic telangiectasia
Hereditary spherocytosis
Huntington's chorea
Marfan's syndrome
Dystrophia myotonica
Neurofibromatosis
Osteogenesis imperfecta (some forms)
Peutz–Jegher's syndrome
Rotor syndrome
Tuberose sclerosis
Von Willebrand's disease

**Table 2.4** Autosomal dominant disorders—examples.

1 These disorders have a great variability in their manifestation. 'Incomplete penetrance' may occur if patients have a dominant disorder but it does not manifest itself clinically in them. This gives the appearance of the gene having 'skipped' a generation.
2 Dominant traits are extremely variable in severity (variable expression) and a mildly affected parent may have a severely affected child.
3 New cases in a previously unaffected family may be the result of a new mutation. If it is a mutation, the risk of a further affected child is negligible. Most cases of achondroplasia are due to new mutations.
The overall incidence of autosomal dominant disorders is 7 per 1000 live births.

**Autosomal recessive disorders** (Fig 2.7b; Table 2.5)
These disorders manifest only when an individual is homozygous for the disease allele, i.e. both chromosomes carry the mutated gene. In this case the parents are generally unaffected healthy carriers (heterozygous for the disease allele). There is usually no family history, although the defective gene is passed from generation to generation. The offspring of an affected person will be healthy heterozygotes unless the other parent is also a carrier. If carriers marry, the offspring have a 1 : 4 chance of being homozygous and affected; a 1 : 2 chance of being a carrier; and a 1 : 4 chance of being genetically normal. Consanguinity increases the risk of two carriers having a child who has a 25% chance of being affected. The clinical features of autosomal recessive disorders are usually severe; patients often present in the first few years of life and have a high mortality.

Many inborn errors of metabolism are recessive diseases. The commonest recessive disease in the UK is cystic fibrosis (see pp. 125 and 665) . The overall incidence of

Albinism (oculocutaneous)
Ataxia telangiectasia
Crigler–Najjar syndrome type I
Congenital adrenal hyperplasia
Cystic fibrosis
Deafness (some forms)
Dubin–Johnson syndrome
Epidermolysis bullosa (some forms)
Fanconi syndrome
Friedreich's ataxia
Galactosaemia
Gaucher's disease
Glycogen storage disease
Haemochromatosis
Homocystinuria
Hurler's syndrome (mucopolysaccharidosis I)
Infantile polycystic kidney disease
Laurence–Moon–Biedl syndrome
Phenylketonuria
Sickle cell disease
Tay–Sachs disease
β-Thalassaemia
Wilson's disease

**Table 2.5**  Autosomal recessive disorders—examples.

| | Chromosome |
|---|---|
| *Autosomal dominant disorders* | |
| Familial adenomatous polyposis | 5 |
| Hypertrophic cardiomyopathy | 14 |
| Neurofibromatosis type I | 17 |
| Familial hypercholesterolaemia | 19 |
| Malignant hyperpyrexia | 19 |
| Amyotrophic lateral sclerosis | 21 |
| *Autosomal recessive disorders* | |
| Haemochromatosis | 6 |
| Cystic fibrosis | 7 |
| Friedreich's ataxia | 9 |
| β-Thalassaemia | 11 |
| Sickle cell disease | 11 |
| Phenylketonuria | 12 |
| α-Thalassaemia | 16 |
| *Triplet repeat expansion disorders* | |
| Huntington's disease (autosomal dominant) | 4 |
| Myotonic dystrophy (autosomal dominant) | 19 |

**Table 2.6**  Examples of single gene disorders and their chromosomal location. For X-linked disorders see Table 2.7.

autosomal recessive disorders is about 2.5 per 1000 live births in the UK. Worldwide, diseases such as thalassaemia and sickle cell disease are very common; the frequency of these diseases may be as high as 20 per 1000 births in some populations. Prenatal diagnosis for recessive disorders may be possible by analysing the DNA of the fetus for mutations known in the parents.

Table 2.6 lists some autosomal dominant and autosomal recessive genetic diseases with their chromosomal localization. Some diseases show a racial or geographical prevalence. Thalassaemia is seen mainly in Greeks, South East Asians and Italians, porphyria variegata occurs more frequently in the South African white population, and Tay–Sachs disease particularly occurs in Ashkenazi Jews.

**Sex-linked disorders** (Fig. 2.7c, d)
Genes carried on the X chromosome are said to be X-linked and can be dominant or recessive in the same way as autosomal genes (Table 2.7). As females have two X chromosomes they will be unaffected carriers of X-linked recessive diseases. However as males have just one X chromosome, any deleterious mutation in an X-linked gene will manifest itself as no second copy of the gene is present.

*Recessive*
Albinism (ocular)
Becker's muscular dystrophy
Christmas disease
Colour blindness
Duchenne muscular dystrophy
Fabry's disease
Fragile X syndrome
Glucose-6-phosphate dehydrogenase deficiency
Haemophilia A
Hunter's syndrome (mucopolysaccharidosis II)
Lesch–Nyhan syndrome
Menkes syndrome
Mental retardation (with or without fragile site)
Nephrogenic diabetes insipidus
Red–green colour blindness
Wiskott–Aldrich syndrome

*Dominant*
Vitamin D-resistant rickets

**Table 2.7**  X-linked disorders—examples.

X-LINKED DOMINANT DISORDERS. These are rare. Vitamin D-resistant rickets is the best known example. Females who are heterozygous for the mutant gene and males who have one copy of the mutant gene on their single X chromosome will manifest the disease. Half the male or female offspring of an affected mother and all the female offspring of an affected man will have the disease. Affected males tend to have the disease more severely than the heterozygous female.

X-LINKED RECESSIVE DISORDERS. These disorders always present in males and only present in (usually rare) homozygous females. X-linked recessive diseases are transmitted by healthy female carriers or affected males if they survive to reproduce. An example of an X-linked recessive disorder is haemophilia A, which is caused by a mutation in the X-linked gene for the essential clotting factor, factor VIII. It has recently been shown that in 50% of cases there is an intrachromosomal rearrangement (inversion) of the tip of the long arm of the X chromosome (one break point being within intron 22 of the factor VIII gene).

Of the offspring from a carrier female and a normal male, 50% of the girls will be carriers as they inherit a mutant allele from their mother and the normal allele from their father; 50% of the girls inherit two normal alleles and are themselves normal; 50% of the boys will have haemophilia as they inherit the mutant allele from their mother (and the Y chromosome from their father); 50% of the boys will be normal as they inherit the normal allele from their mother (and the Y chromosome from their father).

The male offspring of a male with haemophilia and a normal female will not have the disease as they do not inherit his X chromosome. However all the female offspring will be carriers as they all inherit his X chromosome.

Genes carried on the Y chromosome are said to be Y-linked and only males can be affected. However, there are no known examples of Y-linked single-gene disorders which are transmitted.

### Sex-limited inheritance

Occasionally a gene can be carried on an autosome but manifests itself only in one sex. For example, frontal baldness is an autosomal dominant disorder in males but behaves as a recessive disorder in females.

## Other single gene disorders

These are disorders which may be due to mutations in single genes but which do not manifest as simple monogenic disorders. They can arise from a variety of mechanisms including:

TRIPLET REPEAT MUTATIONS: in some genetic diseases, for example myotonic dystrophy, the severity of the disease (such as age of onset) increases down through the generations. This phenomenon is known as 'anticipation'. In the allele which is mutated and gives rise to myotonic dystrophy it was found that in the 3′ UTR of the gene was a region in which three nucleotides, GCT, were repeated up to about 35 times. In families with myotonic dystrophy, people with the late onset form of the disease had 20–40 copies of the repeat, but their children and grandchildren who presented with the disease from birth have vast increases in the number of repeats, up to 2000 copies. It is thought that some mechanism during meiosis causes this 'triplet repeat expansion' so that the offspring inherit an increased number of triplets. The number of triplets affects mRNA and protein function (although these repeats are not in the coding region of the gene). Diseases such as Huntington's disease are due to massive triplet repeat expansions which are inherited through the generations.

IMPRINTING: it is known that normal humans need a diploid number of chromosomes, 46. However the maternal and paternal contributions are different and, in some way which is not yet clear, the fetus can distinguish between the chromosomes inherited from the mother and the chromosomes inherited from the father, although both give 23 chromosomes. In some

way the chromosomes are 'imprinted' so that the maternal and paternal contributions are different. Imprinting is relevant to human genetic disease because different phenotypes may result depending on whether the mutant chromosome is maternally or paternally inherited. A deletion of part of the long arm of chromosome 15 will give rise to the Prader–Willi syndrome (PWS) if it is paternally inherited. A deletion of a similar region of the chromosome gives rise to Angelman syndrome (AS) if it is maternally inherited. (Probably two different genes are involved in PWS and AS.)

## COMPLEX TRAITS

## Multifactorial and polygenic inheritance

Characteristics resulting from a combination of genetic and environmental factors are said to be multifactorial; those involving multiple genes can also be said to be polygenic.

Measurements of most biological traits, for example height, show a variation between individuals in a population and a unimodal, symmetrical (Gaussian) frequency distribution curve can be drawn. This variability is due to variation in genetic factors and environmental factors. Environmental factors may play an important part in determining some characteristics, such as weight, whilst other characteristics such as height may be largely genetically determined. This genetic component is thought to be due to the additive effects of a number of alleles at a number of loci, many of which can be individually identified using molecular biological techniques, for example studying identical twins in different environments. One such condition that has been studied is congenital pyloric stenosis. This is more common in boys but if it occurs in girls the latter have a larger number of affected relatives. This difference suggests that a larger number of the relevant genes are required to produce the disease in girls than in boys. Most of the important human diseases, such as heart disease, diabetes, and common mental disorders are multifactorial traits (Table 2.8).

## Analysis of mutations and genetic disease

The first step in the analysis of a genetic disease is to study the pattern of inheritance. This may provide valuable clues about whether a single gene is affected, and whether this gene is likely to be autosomal or on the sex chromosomes or the mitochondrial chromosome. Next, chromosome analysis can be useful and geneticists look

| Disorder | Frequency % | Heritability[a] (%) |
|---|---|---|
| Hypertension | 5 | 62 |
| Asthma | 4 | 80 |
| Schizophrenia | 1 | 85 |
| Congenital heart disease | 0.5 | 35 |
| Neural tube defects | 0.5 | 60 |
| Pyloric stenosis | 0.3 | 75 |
| Ankylosing spondylitis | 0.2 | 70 |
| Cleft palate | 0.1 | 76 |

[a]Percentage of the total variation of a trait which can be attributed to genetic factors.

**Table 2.8**  Examples of disorders that may have a polygenic inheritance.

for chromosomal aberrations (for example deletions) which are present at an unusually high frequency in individuals affected with the disease, compared to the normal population. If there are no further clues often the next stage in locating the gene that is mutated in the disease is to carry out an exercise in 'positional cloning' and this usually involves 'linkage analysis'.

## Positional cloning and linkage analysis

Positional cloning is used to isolate genes whose protein products are not known, but whose existence can be inferred from a disease phenotype. The process involves narrowing the search to a chromosome, then to a region of the chromosome, and finally to a gene in which a mutation is always present in affected individuals and absent in normal individuals. Often the first step in a positional cloning study is linkage analysis.

### Linkage analysis
If two pieces of DNA are very close together on a chromosome then it is less likely that they will be separated by the crossing-over process during meiosis than genes which are far apart. Therefore closely 'linked' pieces of DNA are more likely to be transmitted together into the same gamete. Linkage analysis is a complex process based on probabilities, but the principle is relatively simple: if a disease allele is very near to a region of DNA that can be detected and which is polymorphic in different individuals, then the inheritance of this piece of DNA can be followed and therefore the inheritance of the disease allele which is close by. A large number of polymorphic pieces of DNA are studied and if one always segregates with the disease then it is likely the disease gene is near on the chromosome. The first problem is to find a range of polymorphic pieces of DNA or 'markers' so that segregation

of these loci through generations of one family can be followed.

Polymorphic markers commonly used are:

RESTRICTION FRAGMENT LENGTH POLYMORPHISMS (RFLPs). When variations in the DNA sequences in different individuals affect restriction enzyme cleavage sites then digestion will produce differently sized restriction fragments from the same regions of the genome in different people. These different sizes are the RFLPs. A DNA probe for the piece of DNA will detect differently sized fragments on a Southern blot of digested DNAs from different people. If a person is heterozygous for an RFLP, there will be two different fragment patterns in the Southern blot, one fragment from each chromosome. Thus, a single chromosome region can be tracked through a family to see if any particular fragment segregates with the disease allele.

SIMPLE SEQUENCE REPEATS. More common and more polymorphic (i.e. having greater variability) than RFLPs are simple sequence repeats. These are short di-, tri-, tetra- or penta-nucleotide repeats (such as $(CA)_n$) which are present throughout the genome and have highly variable lengths. By designing primers to the sequence either side of one of these repeats the repeat can be amplified by the polymerase chain reaction. The amplified product is electrophoresed on a gel and different sized products are produced from different people. If the mutant gene is close by then a particular size repeat in that region will always segregate with the disease allele.

Once polymorphic markers from across the genome have been tested it should be possible by linkage analysis to see if any segregate with the disease allele in a family. If the position of the polymorphic marker is known, then the affected gene is likely to be close by and is therefore mapped to a region of the genome.

It is necessary to consider the likelihood of recombination between the marker under study and the disease allele and take into account other factors: for example if the marker is on one chromosome and the disease gene is on another, by chance an affected individual may receive both. In small families statistical variation may make it difficult to distinguish between this and real linkage between a marker and a disease gene on the same chromosome. As most human families are relatively small it has been necessary to consider linkage in terms of the *probability* that the disease gene and the polymorphic marker are linked. This measure of likelihood is known as the 'Lod score' (the logarithm of the odds) and is a measure of the statistical significance of the observed co-segregation of the marker and the disease gene, compared to what would be expected by chance alone. Positive lod scores make linkage more likely, negative lod scores make it less likely. By convention a lod score of +3 is taken to be definite evidence of linkage because this indicates 1000 to 1 odds that the co-segregation of the DNA marker and the disease did not occur by chance alone.

Linkage analysis has provided many breakthroughs in mapping the positions of genes that cause genetic diseases, such as the gene for cystic fibrosis which was found to be tightly linked to a marker on chromosome 7, or the gene for Friedreich's ataxia which is tightly linked to a marker on chromosome 9.

## Isolating the gene

Once linkage analysis has established which chromosome and which region of the chromosome contains the disease gene, the next step is to identify the gene. The region of DNA which contains the gene may span several million base pairs and a variety of techniques exist for cloning cDNAs and gene sequences from such regions. Genes which have been cloned and are very tightly linked to a genetic disease may be 'candidate genes' for that disease and researchers have to show that a mutation in the gene is likely to give rise to the disease. One criteria for candidacy is that the gene is expressed in the affected tissues. It is unlikely that a gene giving rise to a liver disease might give the instructions for making protein purely in neuronal tissue. Probably the most important criteria is to find a mutation in the gene in affected and not unaffected individuals. This is likely to involve DNA sequencing.

# Genetic basis of cancer

All cancers involve changes to the normal cellular genes. In some very rare cancers these changes can be inherited as a single gene defect. With some cancers, such as forms of breast cancer, the mode of inheritance is much more complex. In these cases close relatives may have an increased susceptibility to cancer (Table 2.9), but the genetics are more those of a multifactorial trait, and not a single gene defect. However in the vast majority of cancer cases (especially those in older people) the genetic changes occur in the somatic tissue of the individual and do not enter the germline, so even close relatives do not have an increased risk. Cancer tissues are clonal and

tumours arise from changes in only one cell which then proliferates in the body.

The genes that are primarily damaged by the genetic changes which lead to cancer fall into two categories: oncogenes and tumour suppressor genes.

## Oncogenes

Oncogenes encode proteins that are known to participate in the regulation of normal cellular proliferation. Alteration in structure or control of these genes could promote abnormal cell proliferation. The oncogenes that have been described encode proteins with a variety of functions related to cell growth. Some are known to be receptor molecules that lie in the cell membrane waiting for growth signals. If these receptors become constitutively active due to mutation the cell starts dividing in an uncontrolled fashion. Other molecules lie downstream of the receptors in the signal transduction pathways that carry information from the cell surface to the nucleus. Mutations in these signal transduction molecules can also lead to cellular proliferation.

Well-known examples of oncogenes include:

*SIS* and *INT*-2 which are localized on chromosomes 22q13.1 and 11q13 respectively and encode secreted growth factors to stimulate growth of certain types of cells

*FMS* (5q34) and *ERB* B (7p11–13) encode the receptors for colony stimulating factor and epidermal growth factor

*SRC* and *ABL* which encode non-receptor tyrosine kinases and are proteins involved in signal transduction

H-*RAS* (11p14.1) and K-*RAS* (12p12.1) which encode membrane-associated proteins that relay growth factor and receptor interactions to other proteins in the cell

N-*MYC* and *FOS* which encode nuclear proteins that have DNA-binding properties and may mediate DNA transcription

| | Chromosome localization | Tumour suppressor gene | Neoplasms |
|---|---|---|---|
| Familial adenomatous polyposis | 5q 21 | APC | Colon |
| Familial non-polyposis colon cancer | 2 | MSH2 | Colon |
| Wilms' tumour | 11p13p15 | WT1 | Kidney |
| Retinoblastoma | 13q14.1 | RB1 | Retina |
| Li–Fraumeni syndrome | 17p13.1 | p53 | Breast adrenal cortex, sarcomas, leukaemia, brain tumours |
| Neurofibromatosis type 1 | 17q11 | NF1 | Neural tumours |
| Neurofibromatosis type 2 | 22q | NF2 | Central schwannomas and meningiomas |
| Von Hippel–Lindau disease | 3p25 | VHL | Haemangioblastoma and renal cell carcinoma |
| Multiple endocrine neoplasia (MEN 2a) | 10p11–q11 | RET | Thyroid C cells Adrenal medulla |

**Table 2.9**  Inherited cancer syndromes.

If genetic damage to an oncogene gives rise to signals for uncontrolled growth, the oncogene is said to be 'activated' (Fig. 2.8). Oncogenes can be activated by:

MUTATION. Oncogenes, like other genes, contain structural and control regions and changes in either region can produce an activated oncogene. (Non-activated oncogenes which are functioning normally have been referred to as 'proto-oncogenes'.) Carcinogens such as those found in cigarette smoke can cause point mutations in genomic DNA. By chance some of these point mutations will occur in regions of the oncogene which lead to activation of that gene. Not all bases in an oncogene cause cancer if mutated, but some (for example those in the coding region) are particularly important.

CHROMOSOMAL TRANSLOCATION. If during cell division an error occurs and two chromosomes translocate, so that a portion swaps over, the translocation breakpoint may occur in the middle of two genes. If this happens then the end of one gene is translocated onto the beginning of another gene, giving rise to a 'fusion gene'. Therefore sequences of one part of the fusion gene are inappropriately expressed because they are under the control of the other part of the gene. An example of such a fusion gene occurs in chronic myelogenous leukaemia (CML). In patients with CML a translocated chromosome (the Philadelphia chromosome, see p. 361) is seen in the leukaemic cells. This chromosome is a translocation between chromosomes 9 and 22 in which they exchange a portion of their long arms. This causes the *ABL* gene on chromosome 9 to join onto the *BCR* gene on chromosome 22. The resulting fusion protein is thought to cause the changes which lead to CML. Similarly in Burkitt's lymphoma a translocation causes the regulatory segment of the *MYC* oncogene to be replaced by a regulatory segment of an unrelated immunoglobulin.

VIRAL STIMULATION. Some viruses, such as retroviruses, can cause cancerous changes by activating oncogenes when they infect a cell. When the viral RNA is transcribed by reverse transcriptase into viral DNA and this integrates into the cellular DNA, the viral DNA may integrate within an oncogene and activate it. Alternatively the virus may pick up cellular oncogene DNA, incorporate it into its own viral genome and go on to infect another host cell; an example of this occurs with the Rous sarcoma virus in chickens.

After the initial activation event other changes occur in the DNA. A striking example of this is amplification of gene sequences, which can affect the *MYC* gene for example. Instead of the normal two copies of a gene, multiple copies of the gene appear either within the chromosomes (these can be seen on stained chromosomes as homogeneously staining regions, HSRs) or as extra-chromosomal particles (double minutes). N-*MYC* sequences are amplified in neuroblastomas as are N-*MYC* or L-*MYC* in some lung small-cell carcinomas.

## Tumour suppressor genes

These genes have a role in restricting undue cell proliferation, as opposed to oncogenes which enhance signals for cell growth. Therefore mutations in these genes also lead to uncontrolled cell growth.

The first tumour suppressor gene to be described was the *RB* gene. Mutations in *RB* lead to retinoblastoma which occurs in 1 in 20 000 young children and can be sporadic or familial. In the familial variety the first mutation is inherited and by chance a second somatic mutation occurs with the formation of a tumour. In the

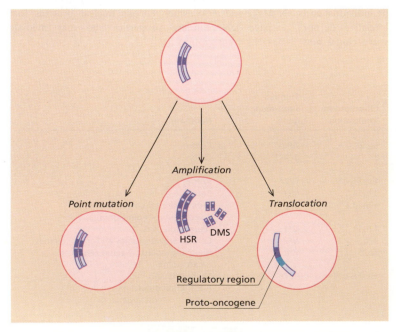

**Fig. 2.8** Activation of cellular oncogenes. DMS, double minutes; HSR, homogeneous staining region.

sporadic variety by chance both mutations occur in both the *rb* genes in a single cell.

Since the finding of *RB*, other tumour suppressor genes have been described, including the gene *p53*. Mutations in *p53* have been found in almost 50% of human tumours, including sporadic colorectal carcinomas, carcinomas of breast and lung, brain tumours, osteosarcomas and leukaemias. The protein, encoded by *p53*, is a cellular 53-kDa nuclear phosphoprotein that plays a role in DNA repair and synthesis, in the control of the cell cycle and cell differentiation and programmed cell death. In some cancers there is a loss of *p53* from both chromosomes in a cell whilst in other tumours, particularly colorectal carcinomas, there is a mutant *p53* allele; this means mutation in a single copy of the gene can promote tumour formation.

# Population genetics

The genetic constitution of a population depends on many factors. The Hardy–Weinberg equilibrium is a concept, based on a mathematical equation, that describes the outcome of random mating within populations. It states that 'in the absence of mutation, non-random mating, selection and genetic drift, *the genetic constitution of the population remains the same from one generation to the next*'.

This genetic principle has clinical significance in terms of the number of abnormal genes in the total gene pool of a population. The Hardy–Weinberg equation states that:

$$p^2 + 2pq + q^2 = 1$$

where *p* is the frequency of the normal gene in the population, *q* is the frequency of the abnormal gene, $p^2$ is the frequency of the normal homozygote, $q^2$ is the frequency of the affected abnormal homozygote, $2pq$ is the carrier frequency, and $p + q = 1$.

This equation can be used, for example, to find the frequency of heterozygous carriers in cystic fibrosis: the incidence of cystic fibrosis is 1 in 2000 live births. Thus,

$$q^2 = 1/2000$$

therefore

$$q = 1/44$$

and as $p = 1 - q$ therefore

$$p = 43/44$$

The carrier frequency is represented by $2pq$, thus, 1 in every 22 persons in the population is a heterozygous carrier for cystic fibrosis.

# Clinical genetics and genetic counselling

Genetic disorders pose considerable health and economic problems because often there is no effective therapy. In any pregnancy the risk of a serious developmental abnormality is approximately 1 in 30 pregnancies; approximately 15% of paediatric inpatients have a multifactorial disorder with a predominantly genetic element.

People with a history of a congenital abnormality in a member of their family often seek advice as to why it happened and about the risks of producing further abnormal offspring. Interviews must be conducted with great sensitivity and psychological insight, as parents may feel a sense of guilt and blame themselves for the abnormality in their child.

The aims of genetic counselling should include:

ESTABLISHING AN ACCURATE DIAGNOSIS. Examination of the child may help in diagnosing a genetically abnormal child with characteristic features, e.g. trisomy 21, or whether a genetically normal fetus was damaged *in utero*.

A FULL AND CAREFUL HISTORY should be taken. The pregnancy history, drug, alcohol ingestion during pregnancy and maternal illnesses, e.g. diabetes, should be detailed.

DRAWING A FAMILY TREE is essential. Questions should be asked about abortions, stillbirths, deaths, marriages, consanguinity and medical history of family members. Diagnoses may need verification from other hospital reports.

ESTIMATION OF THE RISK OF A FUTURE PREGNANCY BEING AFFECTED OR CARRYING A DISORDER. Estimation of risk should be based on the pattern of inheritance. Mendelian disorders (see earlier) carry a high risk; chromosomal abnormalities a low risk. Empirical risks may be obtained from population or family studies.

INFORMATION on prognosis and management.

CONTINUED SUPPORT AND FOLLOW-UP.

EXPLANATION of the implications for other siblings and family members.

GENETIC SCREENING, which includes prenatal diagnosis if requested, carrier detection and data storage in genetic registers.

## Carrier detection

Carrier detection is offered in autosomal recessive disorders for conditions that are relatively common such as thalassaemias (Asian and Mediterranean populations), cystic fibrosis (Caucasian populations), sickle cell disease (African origin) and Tay–Sachs disease (Ashkenazi Jews). Families segregating the severe form of haemophilia A can now have more accurate genetic counselling to detect the inversion of the X chromosome (flip-tip inversion) using Southern blotting.

## Prenatal diagnosis (Information box 2.3)

For families at risk of genetic disease an intrauterine diagnosis is important either to reassure parents if the fetus is unaffected or to allow termination of the pregnancy if requested. Prenatal diagnosis might be carried out if there is a high genetic risk of a severe disorder and if no treatment is available for the particular disorder.

High resolution ultrasonography has replaced amniocentesis in some centres for the diagnosis of neural tube defects. However for diagnosing gene defects in which it is necessary to study fetal DNA, amniocentesis (sampling of fluid from the amniotic sac) gives access to fetal cells. Chorionic villus sampling (transcervical or transabdominal under ultrasound guidance) can be performed at an earlier time (from 10 weeks' gestation), which has the advantage of earlier and easier termination if requested. With embryos produced by *in vitro* fertilization, DNA analysis of one or two embryonic cells at 8–16 cell stage can be undertaken and if normal the embryo is implanted.

Maternal serum is widely used in the second trimester (16–22 weeks) for screening for neural tube defects and trisomy 21. High levels of maternal serum α-fetoprotein are associated with neural tube defects and some other fetal abnormalities. Altered levels of maternal serum α-fetoprotein, unconjugated oestriol and human chorionic gonadotrophin are associated with trisomy 21 affected pregnancies. First trimester maternal serum screening for trisomy 21 using pregnancy-associated plasma protein-A is under evaluation.

Genetic counselling should be non-directive, with the couple making their own decisions on the basis of an accurate presentation of the facts and risks in a way they can understand.

# Applications of molecular genetics

The use of molecular biological techniques in genetics is having a massive impact on the investigation, diagnosis, treatment and control of genetic disorders.

## The avoidance and control of genetic disease

Some genetic disorders, for example phenylketonuria or haemophilia, can be managed by diet or replacement therapy, but most have no effective treatment. By under-

| Technique | Risk and gestation for performing test | Comment |
|---|---|---|
| **Prenatal diagnosis** | | |
| Ultrasound | 1st trimester | Increased nuchal translucency for major chromosomal abnormalities, e.g. trisomies and Turner's* |
| | 2nd trimester | Structural abnormalities, e.g. neural tube defects, congenital heart defects and chromosomal markers, e.g. abnormal digits |
| Amniocentesis | Risk <1% | Chromosomal analysis |
| | From 14 weeks | Measurement of α fetoprotein (AFP) or acetylcholine esterase (AChE). Biochemical analysis. Widely available |
| Chorionic villus sampling | Risk 1–2% | Chromosomal and DNA analysis. Biochemical analysis. Highly specialized |
| | From 10 weeks | |
| Cordocentesis | Risk 1–2% | Fetal blood sampling for chromosomal and DNA analysis. Highly specialized |
| | From 19 weeks | |
| *Maternal blood* | *Test* | *Abnormality in fetus* |
| **Screening** | | |
| 2nd trimester | α Fetoprotein—high | Neural tube defects |
| | *Triple test* | |
| | α Feto protein (low) | |
| | Unconjugated oestradiol (low) | Trisomy 21 |
| | Human chorionic gonadotrophin (high) | |

\*Sensitivity for Trisomy 21 = 85%; Trisomy 13, 18 = 90%

**Information box 2.3**   Methods available for prenatal diagnosis and screening.

standing what causes genetic damage potential mutagens, such as radiation, environmental chemicals, viruses or drugs (such as thalidomide), can be avoided.

# Treatment of genetic disorders— gene therapy

Conventional therapy consists of controlling rather than curing the genetic defect. In some conditions gene product replacement may ameliorate the symptoms, e.g. the production of insulin (from recombinant DNA) for the treatment of diabetes and factor VIII replacement in haemophilia A.

Current research suggests that for many defects 'gene therapy' may be an option in the future. Gene therapy entails placing a normal copy of a gene into the cells of a patient who has a defective copy of the gene. For example it might be possible to remove bone marrow cells from a patient with β-thalassaemia, culture the cells *in vitro* and infect them with a retrovirus carrying a human β-globin gene; cells with normal β-globin would then be selected and replaced into the patient's bone marrow. These sorts of experiments involve somatic tissue only, not the germline, so altered DNA would not be inherited from the offspring of a person who has undergone gene therapy.

Current experiments are concentrated on the recessive disorders, such as cystic fibrosis where the disease is due to absence of a normal gene product. In these cases it is sufficient to introduce one functional normal allele of the relevant gene in order to overcome the genetic deficiency. However in dominant disorders the pathogenic potential of the mutant allele is normally expressed in the presence of a normal allele. This requires gene correction where the mutant sequence is replaced by an equivalent sequence from a normal allele or the mutant allele is inactivated. Such procedures are more difficult and, therefore, attempts have concentrated on recessive disorders focusing on gene insertion into somatic cells.

Suitable diseases for current gene therapy experiments include the following:

## Cystic fibrosis (see p. 665)

The gene responsible for cystic fibrosis was first localized to chromosome 7 by linkage analysis. The cystic fibrosis transmembrane regulator gene (*CFTR*) was then isolated by chromosome-mediated gene transfer, chromosome walking and jumping. The *CFTR* gene spans about 250 kb and contains 27 exons. The DNA sequence analysis predicts a polypeptide sequence of 1480 amino acids. The *CFTR* gene also encodes a simple chloride ion channel within the *CFTR* (Fig 2.9). In most patients there is a single mutation with a 3 bp deletion in exon 10 resulting in the removal of a codon specifying phenylalanine. There are also over 100 different minor mutations of the *CFTR* gene with most mapping to the ATP-binding domains. This has led to the improved diagnosis of cystic fibrosis as well as new strategies for conventional drug-based

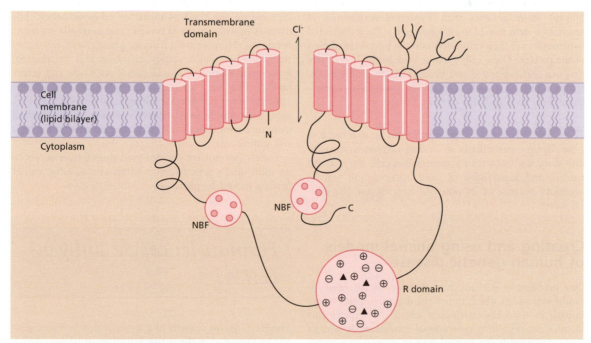

**Fig. 2.9** Model of cystic fibrosis transmembrane conductor regulator (CFTR). This is an integral membrane glycoprotein, consisting of two repeated elements. The cylindrical structures represent 6 membrane-spanning helices in each half of the molecule. The nucleotide-binding folds (NBFs) are in the cytoplasm, and the dots in these hatched areas represent the means of entry by the nucleotide. The regulatory (R) domain links the two halves and contains charged individual amino acids and protein kinase phosphorylation sites (black triangles). N and C are the N and C terminals. The branched structure on the right half represents potential glycosylation sites. The chloride channel is shown.

therapies. Gene therapy experiments are underway that take two different routes to putting a normal version of the *CFTR* gene into the lung epithelial cells of a patient who is homozygous for a defect in this gene. One route entails placing the *CFTR* gene in an adenovirus vector, and infecting the epithelial cells of the patient with the virus. Infection causes the *CFTR* gene to be taken into the cell where it may start functioning normally. A second route entails placing the DNA for the *CFTR* gene into a liposome. Liposomes are then conveyed to the lung using an aerosol spray and the fatty surface of the liposome fuses with the cell membrane to deliver the *CFTR* DNA into the cell, where again the gene should function normally. Ultimately this type of gene therapy should give cystic fibrosis patients a normal life without the need for drugs and intensive physiotherapy.

### Adenosine deaminase (ADA) deficiency

Gene therapy for this rare immunodeficiency disease entails the patient's lymphocytes receiving a normal human *ADA* gene to reconstitute the function of the cellular and humoral immune system in severe combined immunodeficiency (SCID). Currently it is being tried using lymphocytes for short-term therapy, but for longer term treatment bone marrow transplantation would be the definitive approach. See p. 146.

### Familial hypercholesterolaemia

In this disorder a low-density lipoprotein (LDL) receptor gene is inserted into hepatocytes (removed by liver biopsy) from patients with hypercholesterolaemia (a result of a defective LDL receptor gene). Gene-corrected hepatocytes are then reinjected into the portal circulation of the patient. These cells migrate back to the liver where they are reincorporated and should start to produce LDL receptor protein, which dramatically lowers the patient's cholesterol level and risk of heart failure.

There are still many technical problems to overcome in gene therapy, particularly in finding delivery systems to introduce the DNA into a mammalian cell. Very careful control and supervision of gene manipulation will be necessary because of its potential hazards and the ethical issues.

### Creating and using animal models of human genetic disease

One problem in devising new therapies is the need for model systems in which to test the therapies, prior to use in patients. To some extent gene 'knock-out' experiments in mice are providing new animal models of disease. In these experiments the normal gene of interest in a mouse is targeted using recombinant DNA techniques so that gene function is impaired in analogy to the situation in the particular gene of a human patient. However mice and humans are different and it will not be possible to mimic some human genetic diseases in mice.

Transgenic mice are created when exogenous DNA carrying a gene of interest is injected into a mouse egg. If this egg is fertilized then all the cells of the resulting animal will carry the extra gene sequences. Transgenic mice have also been used as animal models of human diseases in which new therapies may be tested.

Other animal models have paved the way for gene therapy techniques. For example, some of the first experiments in the transfer of globin genes (which will be useful for gene therapy for sickle cell disease and thalassaemia) have taken place in mice. These include transplanting normal donor cells with normal genes into lethally irradiated mice, which results in engraftment of the donor cells.

## The human genome mapping project

An international effort is underway to sequence the entire human genome, all $3 \times 10^9$ bp on the 24 different chromosomes. This enormous enterprise has provided resources for many other projects that are trying to increase our understanding of human genetic disease.

## ETHICAL CONSIDERATIONS

Ethical considerations must be taken into account in any discussion of clinical genetics. Options such as prenatal diagnosis with the option of termination may be unacceptable on the basis of moral or religious beliefs. For diseases in which there is no cure and currently no treatment, e.g. Huntington's disease, genetic tests can accurately predict which family members will be affected; however most people would rather not know this information. One very serious outcome of the new genetic information is that disease susceptibility may be predictable, for example in Alzheimer's disease, so the medical insurance companies can decline to give policies for high risk individuals.

Society has not yet decided who should have access to an individual's genetic information and to what extent privacy should be preserved.

## *Human leucocyte antigens (HLA)*

The HLA system consists of a series of closely linked genetic loci situated in the major histocompatibility complex (MHC) on the short arm of chromosome 6. Figure 2.10 shows the classification of these antigens. All loci are highly polymorphic, i.e. a large number of different alleles occur; more than 20 HLA-A, 50 HLA-B, 10 HLA-C, 15 HLA-DR, 3 HLA-DQ and 6 HLA-DP antigens have been

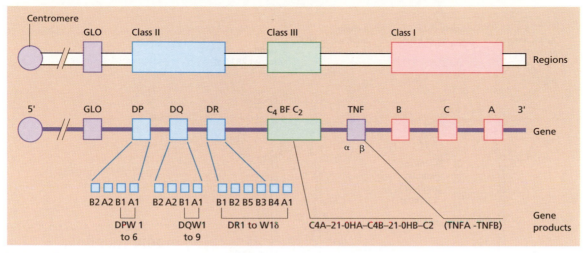

**Fig. 2.10** The major histocompatibility complex, showing the regions, genes and gene products on the short arm of chromosome 6. GLO, glyoxylase; TNF, tumour necrosis factor.

identified so far. The class III series of genes express complement.

## Genetic linkage

The genes at a given locus are inherited as co-dominants, so that each individual expresses both alleles, one transmitted from the mother and the other from the father. Because of the close linkage between the loci, all the genes in the MHC tend to be inherited together. The term 'haplotype' is used to indicate the particular set of HLA genes an individual carries on each chromosome 6. 'Crossing over' can occur within the HLA region. However, certain alleles occur more frequently in the same haplotype than expected by chance and this is known as 'linkage disequilibrium'; for example, the haplotype A1 B8 occurs more frequently than would be expected from the individual gene frequencies of A1 or B8.

There is a wide inter-racial variation in HLA antigens; for example, the HLA haplotype A1,B8 is found mainly in Caucasians, while the antigen B42 is seen only in Africans.

## Products of the HLA genes

The HLA genes code for cell-surface glycoproteins that extend from the plasma membrane to the cytoplasm and are known as class I and class II molecules. These glycoproteins consist of two chains of unequal size ($\alpha$ and $\beta$ chains), and are antigenic.

### Class I molecules (Fig. 2.11)
Class I antigens are expressed on all cell types except erythrocytes and trophoblasts. Striated muscle cells and liver parenchymal cells are normally negative but become strongly positive in inflammatory reactions.

HLA-A, -B and -C antigens can be distinguished serologically by the microlymphocytotoxic test. Lymphocytes from the peripheral blood are incubated with a range of antibodies of known specificity (obtained from parous women or immunized individuals) in the presence of complement and trypan blue dye (which penetrates and stains cells with a damaged cell membrane). If the antibody does not react with the antigen, the lymphocytes survive and exclude the dye; in a positive reaction the dye enters the dead cells, indicating the presence of the specific antigen on that cell.

### Class II molecules (Fig. 2.11)
Class II antigens are expressed on B cells, monocytes, dendritic cells and activated T cells. Inflammation causes aberrant class II expression in many other tissues. They are important in presenting antigens to certain subpopulations of T cells.

HLA-D antigens are recognized by the mixed lymphocyte culture (MLC) technique, which requires a panel of different HLA-D homozygous standard typing cells. The homozygous typing cell (HTC) is treated with mitomycin or irradiation to prevent it dividing when it is cultured with the test responder lymphocytes. The latter will not proliferate (measured by incorporation of tritiated thymidine) if it possesses the same D antigen as the HTC, but it will proliferate if it lacks this antigen. The DR (D-related) antigens are very closely related to D antigens and are also detected on B cells (B cell alloantigens) using a cytotoxic antibody test. These antigens are probably the counterpart of the 'immune-associated' (Ia) antigens on the surface of B cells and macrophages in the mouse.

## Immunoregulatory function of HLA molecules

In the mouse, the *Ir* gene controls the magnitude of the immune response by helping T-cell recognition of the macrophage-bound antigen. Thus, T cells use HLA antigens as recognition molecules (Fig. 2.12). Helper T ($T_H$) cells (identified by monoclonal antibody CD4) usually use

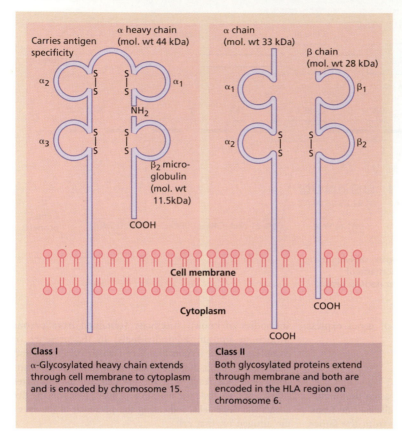

**Class I**
α-Glycosylated heavy chain extends through cell membrane to cytoplasm and is encoded by chromosome 15.

**Class II**
Both glycosylated proteins extend through membrane and both are encoded in the HLA region on chromosome 6.

**Fig. 2.11** Histocompatibility antigens—class I and class II.

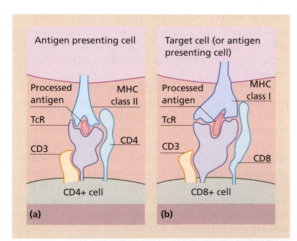

**Fig. 2.12** Schematic representation of antigen processing. The antigen is presented by an antigen-presenting cell, e.g. a macrophage. The T cells (CD4 (a) or CD8 (b)) recognize the antigen via the HLA glycoprotein. TCR, T-cell receptor.

class II antigens, whilst cytotoxic T cells (identified with monoclonal antibody CD8) generally use class I antigens. Thus:

T$_H$ CELLS only cooperate with B cells if they share the same Ia (HLA-DR) antigens.

MACROPHAGES presenting an antigen to a T$_H$ cell must also share the same Ia (DR) antigen in order to stimulate it.

CYTOTOXIC T CELLS also require the same class I HLA molecules to be present on the target cell for cytotoxicity. For example, cytotoxic lymphocytes lyse target cells that have been infected with a specific virus and carry one or more of the same class I antigens, but do not lyse target cells infected with a different virus and/or which do not share the same class I antigens.

## Transplantation requirements

Tissue typing for organ grafting requires HLA typing for A, B, C and DR antigens. The match should be as close as possible, as this increases graft survival. Requirements for matching in bone marrow transplantation are much more stringent, as the rejection process can be either host-versus-graft or graft-versus-host.

## Genetic markers and disease associations

The susceptibility to certain diseases appears to be associated with certain HLA alleles (Table 2.10). In some disorders more than one allele is required to produce the disease; for example, the highest relative risk for developing type I diabetes mellitus is the presence of both DR3 and DR4.

| A3, B14 | Haemochromatosis |
|---|---|
| A28 | Schizophrenia |
| B5 | Behçet's syndrome |
| | Polycystic kidney disease |
| | Ulcerative colitis |
| B8 | Tuberculoid leprosy (Asians) |
| B8, DR3 | Chronic active hepatitis (autoimmune) |
| | Dermatitis herpetiformis |
| | Graves' disease |
| | Idiopathic membranous glomerulonephritis |
| | Myasthenia gravis (without thymoma) |
| | Addison's disease |
| | Sjögren's syndrome |
| | Systemic lupus erythematosus |
| B8, DR3, DR7, DQw2 | Coeliac disease |
| B18 | Hodgkin's disease |
| B27 | Acute anterior uveitis |
| | Ankylosing spondylitis |
| | Psoriatic arthropathy |
| | Reactive arthritis |
| | Reiter's syndrome |
| | Rheumatoid arthritis (juvenile) |
| Bw47 | Congenital adrenal hyperplasia |
| CW6, B13, 17, | Psoriasis vulgaris |
| DR7, DR2 | Goodpasture's syndrome (anti-GBM) |
| | Multiple sclerosis |
| | Narcolepsy (100% association) |
| DR4 | Rheumatoid arthritis |
| DR4, DR3 | Diabetes mellitus (insulin-dependent) |
| (B8, 15 [62] 18) | |
| DR5 | Hashimoto's thyroiditis |
| DR7 | Minimal change disease (nephrotic) |

GBM, glomerular basement membrane.

**Table 2.10** HLA-associated diseases.

Coeliac disease was originally thought to be associated with HLA-DR3 and HLA-DR7 but it has now been shown that the association is much stronger with HLA-DQw2 which is in linkage disequilibrium with HLA-DR3 and HLA-DR7. One or two diseases are linked to specific HLA haplotypes, suggesting that there is a single abnormal gene on chromosome 6, e.g. haemochromatosis is an autosomal recessive disease associated with the A3 B14 haplotype; congenital adrenal hyperplasia is also an autosomal recessive with a defect of steroid 21-hydroxylase, resulting in failure to synthesize cortisol and an increased production of androgenic hormones (see p. 817).

## HLA alleles and adverse drug reactions

There are associations between HLA antigens and adverse drug reactions. For example, HLA-DR4 is present in 75% of patients with systemic lupus erythematosus (SLE) due to hydralazine, compared with 25% of idiopathic SLE patients and slow acetylators who do not develop SLE on hydralazine. Autosomal genes also control the acetylator

status, with the 'rapid' allele being dominant to the 'slow' allele. Homozygotes for the 'slow' allele have reduced levels of N-acetyltransferase in the liver. Acetylation is the controlling factor for the rate of drug metabolism. The percentage of rapid acetylators varies in different ethnic populations—50% in the West, 90% of Japanese and 100% in Eskimos.

# IMMUNOLOGY

## Introduction

Clinical immunology involves the investigation, diagnosis and management of diseases associated with abnormalities in the immune system. The most common problems are overactivity of the immune response leading to allergic and autoimmune disease, or underactivity resulting in immunodeficiency.

## Host defence mechanisms

The immune system is made up of a complex network of cells, humoral factors and soluble messengers or cytokines, which confer protection against disease. However, other mechanisms are also important in defence (Table 2.11).

Several factors can reduce the effectiveness of this 'first line' of defence:
1 Breach of skin/mucous membrane integrity due to trauma, burns, eczema
2 Suppression of cough reflex due to opiates, neurological disease
3 Failure of respiratory mucus clearance
  (a) Smoking (ciliary paralysis)
  (b) Primary ciliary dyskinesis syndromes
  (c) Increased mucus production (asthma)
  (d) Abnormally viscid secretions (cystic fibrosis)

*Physical or chemical barriers*
Skin, mucous membranes
Gastric acid, lysozyme, lactoferrin in secretions

*Mechanical removal*
Sneezing, coughing
Secretions (washing)
Ciliary escalator of respiratory tract
Cough reflex to clear secretions

*Colonization resistance*
Normal flora preventing colonization with pathogenic organisms

*Immune response*
Innate
Specific

**Table 2.11** Host defence mechanisms.

**4** Loss of *colonization resistance*—use of broad-spectrum antibiotics

In these situations pathogenic organisms may gain access and cause disease, despite a normal immune system.

## The normal immune response—the immune system in health

The system is usefully divided into the *innate* and *specific* responses, although there is considerable interaction between these components (Fig. 2.13).

## INNATE IMMUNITY

This comprises the elements of the immune system that can mount a non-specific, 'immediate' response. These are directly activated by infectious agents, inflammation or tumours. The innate response has the advantage of speed, but lacks specificity, and may cause host tissue damage. The main components are:
**1** Phagocytes (neutrophils, monocytes and macrophages)
**2** Other inflammatory cells
  (a) Eosinophils
  (b) Basophils
**3** Complement
**4** Acute phase reactants such as fibronectin, C-reactive protein

## Phagocytes

The neutrophil (polymorphonuclear, or PMN cell) is the most specialized microbicidal phagocyte. The human body contains over $10^{11}$ cells/kg, most of which are in the bone marrow. These cells are released in large numbers during acute infection, and new cells are produced by the action of granulocyte and granulocyte-macrophage colony stimulating factors (G-CSF and GM-CSF, see p. 294) to cause the characteristic neutrophil leukocytosis.

In premature infants, or others with poorly functioning bone marrow, *storage pool exhaustion* can occur and results in peripheral blood neutropenia during severe infections.

### Microbicidal function of neutrophils

RECRUITMENT. Powerful chemoattractants (chemicals which attract phagocytes) are released at sites of infection or inflammation. The main ones are the complement activation products C5a and C3a (see p. 132) and the macrophage-derived leukotriene B₄. These substances cause migration of neutrophils to the site by two mechanisms:
**1** Up-regulation of *adhesion molecules* (see p. 133) on neutrophils, which increases *margination* and adhesion of neutrophils to the vascular endothelium.
**2** Stimulating neutrophil *chemotaxis* (movement towards the stimulus). Cells pass between endothelial cells into the tissues by *diapedesis*.

PHAGOCYTOSIS AND INTRACELLULAR KILLING. Phagocytosis occurs by the formation of pseudopodia around the organism or particle to be ingested. Due to the fluidity of the cell membrane, the tips eventually fuse to form a membrane-bound vesicle. The *phagosome* fuses with the neutrophil cytoplasmic granules (Table 2.12) to form a *phagolysosome*. Within this localized environment killing occurs. There are two major mechanisms:
**1** $O_2$-*dependent response* or *respiratory burst*, in which there is production of reactive oxygen metabolites, such as hydrogen peroxide, hydroxyl radicals and singlet oxygen, via the reduction of oxygen by an NADPH oxidase
**2** $O_2$-*independent response*, due to the toxic action of preformed cationic proteins and enzymes contained within the neutrophil cytoplasmic granules

Ingestion and killing of organisms is much more effective if the particle is first coated or *opsonized* ('made ready to eat') with specific antibody and complement. This is

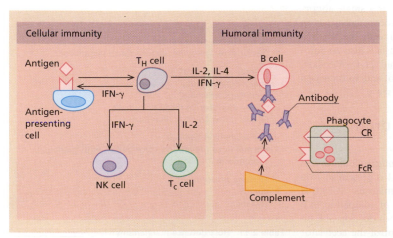

**Fig. 2.13** Components of the immune response. Antigen is presented to T-helper cells ($T_H$ cell) by an antigen-presenting cell. $T_H$ cells secrete lymphokines, which activate cytotoxic T cells ($T_c$ cells) that are involved in antiviral activity. The lymphokines also activate NK cells, which are involved in tumour surveillance. B cells are activated when the antigen binds to the surface immunoglobulins in the presence of lymphokines. This leads to secretion of antibodies. Antibody and complement coat the antigen (opsonize) leading to phagocytosis by phagocytes via binding to the complement receptor (CR) and Fc receptor (FcR).

| Primary granule (azurophilic) | Secondary granule (specific) |
|---|---|
| Defensins | Lysozyme |
| Lysozyme | Lactoferrin |
| Elastase | Collagenase |
| Bactericidal/permeability- | Cytochrome B |
| increasing factor | Vitamin B$_{12}$-binding |
| Cathepsin G | protein |
| Myeloperoxidase | |
| Acid glycolases | |
| Collagenase | |

**Table 2.12** Neutrophil granule proteins. There are two types distinguished by staining characteristics.

because neutrophils have Fc receptors (FcR) for immunoglobulin, and complement receptors (CR), which bind to the coated particle. Binding of the receptors:

- Increases the force of adhesion between particle and phagocyte
- Causes transduction of intracellular signals and activation of the cell to increased phagocytic and killing activity

The role of antibody in this situation demonstrates the interaction of the innate and specific immune responses.

Neutrophils can only ingest particles smaller than themselves and are therefore mainly active against extracellular infections, particularly bacteria and fungi. They provide the major immune response protecting the blood and viscera from these types of organisms.

## Eosinophils

These cells comprise up to 5% of white blood cells in healthy individuals and appear to be used selectively for fighting parasitic (particularly nematode) infections. They have low-affinity surface receptors for IgE. Unlike neutrophils, they do not appear to be phagocytic, but they contain many large granules, which are cytotoxic when released onto the surface of organisms.

MAJOR BASIC PROTEIN (MBP) is the major protein component of eosinophil granules and directly damages helminths, producing ballooning and detachment of the tegumental membrane.

EOSINOPHIL CATIONIC PROTEIN (ECP) is present in the matrix of eosinophil granules and its deposition has been seen in the kidneys of patients with renal disease, certain types of myocardial infarction and allergic gastroenteritis. It is highly toxic to parasites, being eight to ten times more active than MBP, producing complete fragmentation and disruption of the organisms. ECP is a potent neurotoxin.

EOSINOPHIL-DERIVED NEUROTOXIN (EDN) is released from the matrix of eosinophil granules and can damage myelinated neurones in experimental animals.

EOSINOPHIL PEROXIDASE (EPO) is localized in the granule matrix of the eosinophil and in combination with a halide and hydrogen peroxide can kill bacteria, helminths and tumour cells; it inactivates leukotrienes C$_4$ and D$_4$ and causes mast cell degranulation. Eosinophils also participate in immediate hypersensitivity reactions (see p. 147).

## Basophils and mast cells

Mast cells consist of at least two distinct populations, which are distinguished by their enzymic content. The T mast cells contain trypsin alone and were formerly termed mucosal mast cells owing to their location near mucosal surfaces. The TC mast cells contain both trypsin and chymotrypsin and were formerly described as connective tissue mast cells, owing to their location. The TC mast cells contain more histamine, which is released following stimulation with basic amines. Conversely, only T mast cells contain cytoplasmic IgE.

Basophils and the morphologically similar mast cells make up only a very small proportion of the granulocytic white blood cell population. Basophils are involved in inflammation although their role is rather obscure. The cytoplasmic granules of basophils and mast cells contains *histamine* and other *vasoactive amines*. These cells also bear high affinity IgE Fc receptors and participate in immediate hypersensitivity reactions.

## Complement

Complement is involved in the eradication of organisms and immune complexes, as well as inflammation and immunoregulation. The complement system comprises a series of at least 20 serum glycoproteins that are activated in a cascade sequence, with proenzymes that undergo sequential proteolytic cleavage, similar to the coagulation pathway.

Two pathways of activation exist, termed the *classical* and *alternative* pathways (Fig. 2.14). These converge in the activation of C3, both forming individual C3 convertases. This leads into the final common pathway with the assembly of C5–C9 into the *membrane attack complex* (MAC), which forms a 'doughnut-like' transmembrane channel leading to cell lysis by osmotic shock.

### Activation of the classical pathway
Activation of the classical pathway is calcium and magnesium dependent and occurs by the binding of C1q (a subcomponent of the C1 molecule) with:

- IgG-containing antigen–antibody immune complexes
- IgM

### Activation of the alternative pathway
The main components of this pathway are:

- Factor B
- Factor D
- Properdin

In the presence of factor D, factor B is cleaved (to Bb) and combines with C3b to form the alternative pathway C3 convertase, C3bBb. This convertase is stabilized by properdin. The alternative pathway is continually turning

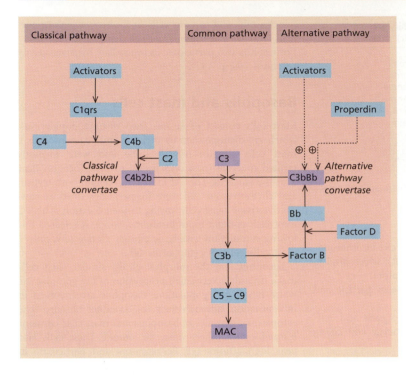

**Fig. 2.14** Complement activation pathways.

In the classical pathway, activated C1 causes cleavage of C4 to C4a (a soluble factor which is released) and C4b, which in turn cleaves C2 to C2a (soluble and released) and C2b. C2b combines with C4b to become C4b2b (classical pathway convertase).

The alternative pathway convertase is formed by the combination of C3b with the cleavage product of factor B (Bb). This is catalysed by factor D and the convertase is stabilized by properdin and alternative pathway activators (see text). The final common pathway leads to the formation of membrane activation complex (MAC) and lysis of the cell.

over at a low rate. This is markedly accelerated by alternative pathway activators which provide a 'protected' site for the C3bBb convertase, by enhancing the binding of properdin and preventing degradation of the complex.

Activators of the alternative pathway include:
- Yeast cell walls
- IgA
- Endotoxin (Gram-negative bacterial cell walls)
- C3 nephritic factor (an autoantibody that stabilizes the convertase), found in patients with membrano-proliferative glomerulonephritis.

### Regulation of complement activation

Complement activation does not occur in the fluid phase, but is localized on the surface of the organism, cell or immune complex that triggered the reaction. This is essential, as many of the by-products of complement activation are potent mediators of inflammation, and would cause extensive tissue damage if not controlled. In addition to the activation sequences described, there are regulatory proteins (factors H and I) that suppress the activation.

### Effector function of complement

The most important effects of complement activation are:

DESTRUCTION OF PATHOGENS AND TUMOUR CELLS by the lytic process described above and by opsonizing them for phagocytosis

RECRUITMENT OF CELLS AND PROTEINS to inflammatory sites, by the chemoattractant activity of the proteolytic products C5a and C3a, and the increase in vascular permeability also produced by these factors (sometimes called anaphylatoxins)

REMOVAL OF IMMUNE COMPLEXES by: opsonization,

solubilization (alternative pathway) and prevention of precipitation (classical pathway)

IMMUNOMODULATION, especially B-cell responses

## Acute phase proteins

Acute phase reactants are proteins that are synthesized in response to trauma, infection, necrosis, tumours or other inflammatory events (Table 2.13). Although of secondary importance, these substances play a part in non-specific defence mechanisms and also appear to be involved in immunopathological processes. The measurement of *C-reactive protein* in the serum is used to monitor disease activity.

## Heat shock proteins (HSPs)

HSPs are a family of highly conserved proteins which act as immunodominant antigens in many infections. They act as molecular chaperones, housekeeping proteins within cells, preserving the cell's protein structure. They are involved in immunity. They are similar in configuration to antigens found on certain microorganisms and may induce autoimmunity through molecular mimicry.

---

C-reactive protein
Serum amyloid protein
Complement components
Fibrinogen
Haptoglobulin
Caeruloplasmin
$\alpha_1$-Antitrypsin

**Table 2.13** Acute phase proteins.

# SPECIFIC (ADAPTIVE) IMMUNITY

Specific immunity is the hallmark of the immune system. This is produced by a mechanism involving multiple rearrangements of original (germline) DNA in T and B lymphocytes. The altered DNA codes for proteins with hypervariable regions and creates the specific antigen-binding T-cell receptor and antibody molecules. This genetic diversity allows the production, for example, of over $10^8$ different antibodies, enough to cover the spectrum of antigens encountered by humans.

# Organization of the lymphoid system

The immune system comprises several masses of lymphoid tissue or organs located throughout the body as well as circulating leucocytes. The circulating cells originate from the bone marrow and are 'programmed' to carry out specific functions by certain lymphoid organs. The principal lymphoid organs are as follows.

## Bone marrow

The bone marrow is the primary site of haematopoiesis in mammals. All blood cells are derived from a *pluripotent stem cell* (see p. 293). Stem cells are primitive cell types that have no specific function, divide rapidly and, under the influence of various *cytokine* signals, will differentiate into myeloid or leucocytic cells.

## Thymus

The thymus is formed from the third and fourth branchial pouches, and contains cells that originate from bone marrow. Lymphocytes derived from the thymus are called *T cells* and comprise about 75% of the lymphoid population. In the passage through this organ, the immature T cells are converted into mature CD4+ or CD8+ cells by the influence of thymic epithelial hormones. Cells that are potentially reactive with the body's own tissues undergo *clonal deletion* here.

## MALT, GALT, BALT and SALT

Lymphoid tissue is frequently found distributed in mucosal surfaces in non-encapsulated patches. This is termed mucosa-associated lymphoid tissue (MALT), gut-associated lymphoid tissue (GALT, or primarily *Peyer's patches*), bronchus-associated lymphoid tissue (BALT, found in the lobes of the lungs along the main bronchi) and skin-associated lymphoid tissue (SALT).

## Tonsils

Tonsils function rather similarly to lymph nodes. They are located in the nasopharyngeal tract and are thus well placed to combat airborne antigens. B cells predominate in these follicles.

Other major sites of lymphoid tissue are the *spleen* (see p. 329) and *lymph nodes.*

# The cells of the immune system

Circulating leucocytes can be subdivided into several groups characterized on morphology, cell surface markers and biological function. There are two families of molecular structures on the cell surface called *clusters of differentiation* (CD; Table 2.14) and *adhesion molecules* (Table 2.15). The biological function of many of the CD molecules is now known and knowledge of their presence is very useful in identifying specific leucocyte subpopulations. Adhesion molecules facilitate many biological activities, particularly those involved in cell–cell recognition. Their functions include cellular activation, cytokine release, capture and 'rolling' of leucocytes along the endothelial cell lining of blood vessels and extravasation. There is an overlap between these two families and certain adhesion molecules have also been assigned CD numbers.

## LYMPHOCYTES

Lymphocytes are spherical cells, approximately 10 μm in diameter with a prominent nucleus of densely packed nuclear chromatin (Fig. 2.15a). There are two main populations, the T and B lymphocytes.

### T cells

T cells have two principal functions, and are divided into:

HELPER/INDUCER CELLS enhance certain immune responses. They receive antigen from specialized presenting cells and initiate or reinforce antibody production, natural killer cell and cytotoxic responses, mainly by the production of the lymphokines interferon-γ, interleukin-2 and interleukin-4. T-helper cells can be distinguished by the presence of the CD4 protein on their surface.

CYTOTOXIC/SUPPRESSOR CELLS which can kill another cell. This kind of response is used in dealing with virus infections and cancer cells. The suppressor cell can down-regulate immune responses at an appropriate time. It may function by releasing soluble factors or messenger molecules which act on the B lymphocytes to reduce their output of antibodies. The cytotoxic/suppressor lymphocyte can be recognized by the presence of the CD8 cell surface molecule.

### B cells

These cells produce *antibody* and comprise approximately 25% of the lymphocyte population. B lymphocytes

| Cluster designation | Tissue distribution | Function |
|---|---|---|
| CD1 | Cortical thymocytes | |
| CD2 | All T cells and NK cells | Ligand for CD58; forms an adhesion pair, e.g. between T cell and antigen-presenting cell |
| CD3 | Found on all mature T cells; intimately associated with the T-cell receptor | Signal transduction following antigen presentation |
| CD4 | T-helper/inducer lymphocytes; comprise 2/3 circulating T cells | Ligand for class II MHC molecules associated with processed antigen fragments |
| CD5 | T cells, also B cells | Ligand for CD72 |
| CD8 | Cytotoxic/suppressor T cells | Ligand for class I MHC molecules associated with processed antigen fragments |
| CD11a | Lymphocytes (especially memory T cells), granulocytes, monocytes and macrophages | Part of adhesion molecule LFA-1 |
| CD16 | NK cells and macrophages | CD16 is a low affinity Fc receptor involved in signal transduction |
| CD19 | All mature B cells | Signal transduction |
| CD20 | All mature B cells | Involved in cell activation; may be a calcium channel |
| CD21 | Mature B cells, follicular dendritic cells, pharyngeal and cervical epithelial cells | Complement C3d receptor |
| CD45 | All cells of hematopoietic origin; also called *leucocyte common antigen* | Cell signalling through the T-cell receptor |
| CD56 | NK cell marker | Mediates cell adhesion |
| CD72 | All mature B cells | Ligand for CD5; involved in signalling |

*Note.* This list is far from exhaustive and has been confined to CD types most commonly encountered in a clinical immunology setting.
NK, natural killer.

**Table 2.14** CD antigens and their cellular distribution.

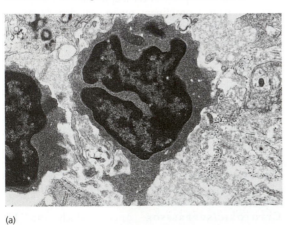

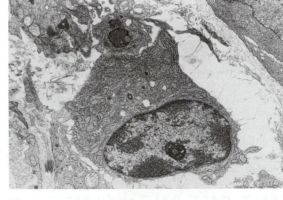

(a)                                                                                    (b)

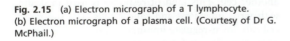

**Fig. 2.15** (a) Electron micrograph of a T lymphocyte. (b) Electron micrograph of a plasma cell. (Courtesy of Dr G. McPhail.)

capable of producing a specific antibody to a given antigen are rapidly encouraged to multiply by a mechanism called *clonal expansion* (Fig. 2.16). In this process, once a B cell has been exposed to a specific antigen (which it recognizes through immunoglobulin molecules located in the cell membrane), and in the presence of cytokines (interleukins 1–6 and B-cell growth factors), it is activated and divides. Following this expansion step, B lymphocytes

differentiate to become *plasma cells* which produce large amounts of antibody. Morphologically, plasma cells are distinguished by a cytoplasm containing large amounts of endoplasmic reticulum (Fig. 2.15b). The plasma cell has a relatively short half-life and is 'terminally differentiated', i.e. after it has fulfilled its antibody producing function it dies. Following the death of these cells, the expanded B cell population shrinks back to its original

| Adhesion molecule | Tissue distribution | Ligand |
|---|---|---|
| **Immunoglobulin superfamily** | | |
| ICAM-1 | Endothelial cells, monocytes, T and B cells, dendritic cells, keratinocytes, chondrocytes, epithelial cells | LFA-1 |
| ICAM-2 | Endothelial cells, monocytes, dendritic cells, subpopulations of lymphocytes | LFA-1 |
| ICAM-3 | Lymphocytes | LFA-1, Mac-1 |
| VCAM-1 | Endothelial cells, kidney epithelium, macrophages, dendritic cells, myoblasts, bone marrow fibroblasts | VLA-4 |
| PECAM-1 | Platelets, T cells, endothelial cells, monocytes, granulocytes | ? |
| **Selectin family** | | |
| E-SELECTIN/ELAM-1 | Endothelial cells | ? |
| L-SELECTIN | Lymphocytes, neutrophils, monocytes | ? |
| P-SELECTIN | Megakaryocytes, platelets and endothelial cells | ? |
| **Integrin family** | | |
| *VLA subfamily* | | |
| VLA-1 to VLA-4 | Endothelial cells, resting T cells, monocytes, platelets and epithelial cells | Various molecules including laminin, fibronectin, collagen and VCAM-1 |
| VLA-5 (fibronectin receptor) | Endothelial cells, monocytes and platelets | Laminin |
| VLA-6 (laminin receptor) | Endothelial cells, monocytes and platelets | Laminin |
| $\beta1\alpha7$ | Endothelial cells, ? | Laminin |
| $\beta1\alpha8$ | Endothelial cells, ? | ? |
| $\beta1\alpha_v$ | Platelets and megakaryocytes | Fibronectin |
| *Leucam subfamily* | | |
| LFA-1 | Leucocytes | ICAM-1–3 |
| Mac-1 | Endothelial cells, ? | ICAM-1, Fibrinogen, C3bi |
| *Cytoadhesin subfamily* | | |
| Vitronectin receptor | Platelets and megakaryocytes | Vitronectin, fibrinogen, laminin, fibronectin, von Willebrand factor, thrombospondin |
| $\beta4\alpha6$ | Endothelial cells, thymocytes and platelets | Laminin |
| $\beta5\alpha_v$ | Platelets and megakaryocytes, ? | Vitronectin, fibronectin |
| $\beta6\alpha_v$ | Platelets and megakaryocytes, ? | Fibronectin |
| $\beta7\alpha4$/LPAM-1 | Endothelial cells, thymocytes, monocytes | Fibronectin, Vcam-1 |
| $\beta8\alpha_v$ | Platelets and megakaryocytes, ? | ? |

ELAM, endothelial leucocyte adhesion molecule (E-SELECTIN); ICAM, intercellular adhesion molecule; LPAM, lymphocyte Peyer's patch adhesion molecule; PECAM, platelet/endothelial cell adhesion molecule; VCAM, vascular cell adhesion molecule; VLA, very late antigen.

**Table 2.15** Adhesion molecules.

size, although some remain as *memory* cells. As well as surface immunoglobulin, B lymphocytes can be distinguished by the presence of the CD19 and CD20 molecules.

## ANTIBODY MOLECULES (IMMUNOGLOBULINS)

Antibodies are serum glycoproteins that are produced as a highly specific response to an antigenic challenge. They consist of (Fig. 2.17):

TWO HEAVY CHAINS (each with four domains).

TWO LIGHT CHAINS (either $\kappa$ or $\lambda$ polypeptides, each with two domains).

VARIABLE 'V' DOMAINS which have great variation in amino acid sequence between immunoglobulins, and have short segments of *hypervariable regions*.

FAB (FRAGMENT ANTIGEN BINDING). Antigen binding occurs where the loops bearing the hypervariable regions of the light and heavy chains come together in space. The conformational structure of the binding site determines the 'goodness of fit' or *affinity/avidity* of any particular antibody for an antigen.

CONSTANT 'C' DOMAINS in which the amino acid sequences are relatively conserved.

FC (FRAGMENT CRYSTALLINE) is formed from constant domains and regulates the *effector* functions (including binding to cell surface receptors and complement fixation), leading to elimination of the bound antigen.

ISOTYPES. These are determined by the type of heavy chain and define the immunoglobulin class (IgG, A, M, D or E).

ALLOTYPES are a result of different allelic forms of $\kappa$ and $\lambda$ light chains, and $\gamma$ and $\alpha$ heavy chains. These are inherited as autosomal co-dominants, and have disease associations.

IDIOTYPES are markers found in the hypervariable region and are associated with the antigen-binding site. The idiotype is antigenic and can be defined by serological techniques.

THE HINGE REGION gives flexibility to the antibody molecule, allowing ease of binding to antigen and cell-surface receptors.

## GENETICS OF ANTIBODY PRODUCTION

Antibody production is unusual in the following ways:

1 The molecule is encoded within three separate chromosomes:
  (a) Chromosome 14 for heavy chain
  (b) Chromosome 2 for $\kappa$ light chain
  (c) Chromosome 22 for $\lambda$ light chain
2 Rearrangement of the multiple elements of germline DNA leads to production of antibodies with many different antigen-binding sites (clonal diversity of Fab, Fig. 2.18).
3 Successive recombinations of VDJ to C$\mu$ (IgM), C$\delta$ (IgD), C$\gamma_3$ (IgG), C$\gamma_1$, C$\alpha_1$ (IgA), C$\gamma_2$, C$\gamma_4$, C$\epsilon$ (IgE), or C$\alpha_2$ cause progressive switching in the isotype of the antibody but as the Fab gene is not altered the same antigen-binding region is maintained.

This explains why the primary immune response is of the IgM isotype, as this is the first to be translocated. Switching to subsequent isotype requires T lymphocyte help. IgG and other isotype responses therefore develop later. However, once the switch has occurred, memory B cells remain. These react rapidly to any further challenge and the IgG of the secondary response is produced.

The extensive variability of antibody molecules is explained by the following factors:

MULTIPLICITY OF V (there are 25–100 genes), D (10 genes) and J (5–6 genes) within the DNA.

COMBINATIONAL FREEDOM of VJ and VDJ genes and light and heavy genes, i.e. any of the multiple genes above can join each other.

JUNCTIONAL DIVERSITY. Splicing of the genes together is frequently inaccurate and 'frame-shift' in base-pairs leads to misreading and production of the 'wrong' amino acid.

SOMATIC MUTATION in V genes.

## IMMUNOGLOBULIN ISOTYPES AND THEIR FUNCTIONS

The main biological features of the human isotypes are summarized in Table 2.16. Different classes of antibody tend to predominate at different sites. The major effector functions of antibody are:

1 Antigen elimination

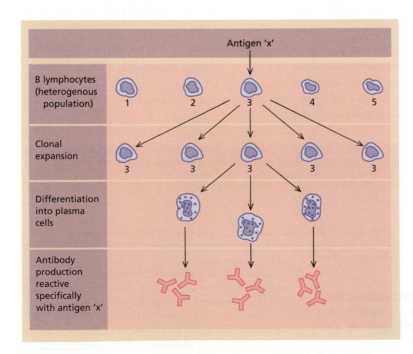

**Fig. 2.16** Clonal expansion of B-cell population in response to specific antigenic stimulus.

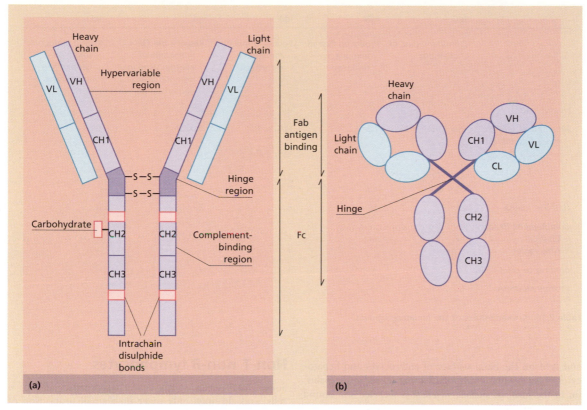

**Fig. 2.17** Immunoglobulin structure: (a) basic subunit structure; (b) schematic structure of the same molecule. C and V, constant and variable domains; H and L, heavy and light chains; Fab, fragment antigen binding; Fc, fragment crystalline.

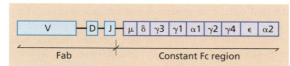

**Fig. 2.18** Schematic diagram showing genes on the Fab and Fc regions of an immunoglobulin. The chain is made up of a 'V' variable gene which is translocated to the 'J' joining chain. The VJ segment is then spliced to the C (constant) gene. Heavy chains have an additional D (diversity) segment which forms the VDJ segment that bears the antigen-binding site determinants.

(a) Binding to prevent adhesion and invasion of organisms
(b) Opsonization of particles for phagocytosis
(c) Lysis
2 Antitoxin activity
3 Immune regulation, acting as the antigen receptor on B cells
4 Sensitization of cells for antibody-dependent cell cytotoxicity (ADCC)

### IgG

This is the most abundant immunoglobulin in serum, present as a monomer. IgG is the antibody of secondary response, but has high antigen affinity. It is the only antibody to cross the placenta in significant quantities. There are four subclasses: $IgG_1$, $IgG_2$, $IgG_3$ and $IgG_4$. $IgG_1$ and $IgG_3$ are produced mainly in response to protein antigens, such as tetanus toxin and many viruses. These subclasses are good opsonins, binding Fc receptors on neutrophils, and having some complement activating activity. $IgG_2$ and $IgG_4$ are produced in response to polysaccharide antigen, for example the capsule of bacteria such as pneumococcus and *Haemophilus*.

### IgM

This antibody is mainly confined to the intravascular pool. It is a pentameric molecule, the single IgM molecules being bound together by the joining 'J' chain. It is the major antibody of the primary immune response. It does not cross the placenta, and is not normally produced until after birth. Therefore antigen-specific IgM is a good marker for intrauterine infection, if present in the newborn infant.

### IgA

There are two subclasses, $IgA_1$ and $IgA_2$, and their functions appear to be similar. $IgA_1$ predominates in the serum, but the subclasses are present in equal amounts in secretions. IgA is mainly monomeric in the serum, but dimeric in secretions, the two molecules complexed by a J chain. IgA in serum binds to a *poly Fc* receptor for IgA

| | IgG | IgM | IgA | IgE | IgD |
|---|---|---|---|---|---|
| | Dominant class of antibody | Produced first in immune response | Found in mucous membrane secretions | Responsible for symptoms of allergy. Used in defence against nematode parasites | Found almost solely on lymphocyte membrane |
| Heavy chain: | $\gamma$ | $\mu$ | $\alpha$ | $\epsilon$ | $\delta$ |
| Mean adult serum levels (mg ml$^{-1}$): | IgG (total) = 12 | 1.5 | IgA$_1$ = 1.5 | 0.0002 | 0.03 |
| | G$_1$ = 6.5 | | IgA$_2$ = 0.2 | | |
| | G$_2$ = 2.5 | | | | |
| | G$_3$ = 0.7 | | | | |
| | G$_4$ = 0.3 | | | | |
| Half-life (days): | 21 | 10 | 6 | 2 | 3 |
| Complement fixation: | | | | | |
| Classical | ++ | +++ | − | − | − |
| Alternative | − | − | + | − | − |
| Binding to mast cells: | − | − | − | + | − |
| Crosses placenta: | + | − | − | − | − |

**Table 2.16**  Characteristics of the immunoglobulins.

and IgM on the basal surface of enterocytes and hepatocytes. Transcellular transport delivers the immunoglobulin to the luminal surface where it is secreted still bound to the receptor which is termed the *secretory component* (SC). The most important function of IgA appears to be in the protection of mucosal surfaces (gut, respiratory tract, urinary tract). Within GALT or BALT there are specialized cells that transport antigen from the lumen to the follicle. IgA precursor B cells in the follicle journey to local, e.g. mesenteric, lymph nodes and to the systemic circulation via the thoracic duct. They then circulate back to settle in the lamina propria of the gut. This *homing* is a generalized phenomenon to all the mucosal surfaces of the body. Therefore localized antigen exposure gives rise to generalized mucosal immunity, which is of importance in vaccination.

IgA in secretions may be important in binding enterotoxins such as that of cholera, preventing the attachment of viruses such as polio and other enteroviruses, and in prevention of invasion by bacteria.

### IgD
Serum levels are very low and its function at this site is uncertain. IgD is present on the surface of B lymphocytes, and may have an immunoregulatory role. Levels are high in conditions with B-cell activation such as systemic lupus erythematosus (SLE), AIDS and Hodgkin's disease.

### IgE
IgE is a monomer that is normally present in very low levels in serum as most is membrane bound on mast cells. Its main physiological role is its anti-nematode activity, but its most common clinical relevance is in the pathogenesis of type 1 hypersensitivity, atopic or allergic disease.

## Non-T non-B lymphocytes

Some lymphocytes do not have characteristics of T or B cells, and although only make up a small proportion of cells, may play an important role in immunity.

## Natural killer (NK) cells

The role of NK cells is to eliminate tumour and virus-infected cells. This process is not antigen-specific. Many of the cells appear as large granular lymphocytes with an indented nucleus. The granules, which contain acid hydrolases including acid phosphatase, $\alpha$-naphthyl acetate esterase and $\beta$-glucuronidase, are thought to be involved in the cytotoxic events. NK cells are non-phagocytic, and most are CD4$^-$, CD8$^-$ and surface immunoglobulin negative but carry the CD56$^+$ CD2$^+$ marker on their surface.

## Antibody-dependent cytotoxic cells and lymphokine-activated killer (LAK) cells

These are populations of lymphocytes that are not characterized by their surface molecules, but by function.

ADCC bear Fc receptors on their surface, and recognize target cells coated with immunoglobulin. They may have a role in eradicating virally infected cells and tumour cells.

Incubation of lymphocytes with interleukin-2 (IL-2) causes them to become highly cytotoxic (hence 'lymphokine activated'), particularly to tumour cells. These have been used in the treatment of malignancies, where patients' blood lymphocytes have been harvested, cultured with IL-2 and then reinfused to target tumours.

# Immune recognition and cellular function

The hallmark of the immune response is its ability to react specifically to given antigen. The mechanism at the heart of this reaction is the way in which antigen is trapped, processed and recognized as foreign (see below).

## Accessory cells

Several cell types, sometimes termed accessory cells, facilitate the antigen-presenting process.

### Macrophages and monocytes (mononuclear phagocytes)

These cells are distributed throughout the body, in the tissues (as macrophages) and in the blood (as monocytes). Macrophages are equipped with various features that make them particularly effective at removing foreign antigens, ready for presentation. They are phagocytic and have, on their surface, receptors that recognize the Fc region of antibody molecules as well as biologically active fragments of complement (C3b). The presence of these structures on cells in the macrophage–monocyte family makes it easy for them to intercept and dispose of antigen–antibody complexes.

### Follicular dendritic cells

Follicular dendritic cells are non-phagocytic and are located in the germinal centres of lymph nodes (follicles). They are surrounded by B lymphocytes to which they present antigen, usually complexed with antibody, on the surface of their dendrites. Their surfaces are rich in Fc and C3b receptors to facilitate antigen trapping.

### Langerhans' cells and dendritic cells

The Langerhans' cell is found primarily in the skin. The dendritic (or veiled) cell is present in the blood (and is different to the follicular dendritic cell described above). They are of macrophage/monocyte lineage.

## Antigen presentation

Antigen fragments are presented to T cells in association with either class I or class II major histocompatibility complex (MHC) molecules (see p. 128). Antigens that are presented with class II molecules are recognized by CD4+, T helper cells. Antigens that associate with class I molecules are presented to CD8+ T cells and a cytotoxic response results (see also Fig 2.12). The responding population of T cells thus recognize the combined shape of the antigen and the MHC molecule. The combination of T-cell receptor, MHC molecule and antigen fragment is known as the *trimolecular complex*. As there are differences in the three-dimensional shape of the MHC molecules due to genetic variation, some antigens may be more effective than others in inducing immune responses because they present an optimum shape or conformation to the T cells. Immune responses that only occur with certain antigen–MHC combinations are called *MHC restricted*.

## HLA (human leucocyte antigens) (see p. 126)

The HLA molecules are distributed throughout the body tissues and it is through differences in this system that cells are classified as *self* or *non-self*. The possibility of two different individuals having the same combination of HLA molecules is very remote. It is this particular aspect of the immune system that presents problems for organ transplantation. Unless the HLA type of the donor and the recipient are virtually identical the organ graft will be recognized as non-self and rejected by the immune system of the host. The process of tissue typing involves the identification of the set of HLA antigens in the tissues of a given individual using specific antisera.

## Cytokine production

Much of the immune system's ability to communicate between its different compartments is achieved through the use of soluble messenger molecules called *lymphokines* (produced by lymphocytes) or cytokines (a generic term meaning made by any cell). Once the cytokine reaches its destination cell it then induces a biological effect, which will of course vary according to the cytokine and the cell involved, but typically these molecules will signal certain cell populations to activate, divide or home in on a particular site in the body.

*Interferons* (a group of cytokines) were discovered in the 1960s and can be divided into $\alpha$, $\beta$ and $\gamma$ varieties. Their main actions are:

- Antiproliferative
- Antiviral
- Immunomodulation

Many cytokines have been isolated, cloned and characterized by the use of recombinant DNA technology (Table 2.17). Some are now being used in clinical practice. For example, IL-2 is used to combat kidney tumours and G-CSF (a substance that cause bone marrow cells to divide and mature) has found application in bone marrow transplantation and treatment of neutropenia.

# The immune system in concert

Following an antigenic stimulus, the components of the immune system cooperate to meet and eliminate the challenge. The foreign antigen is picked up by a cell of the monocyte/macrophage series and the antigen is degraded or processed and presented to both the B and T

| Cytokine | Source | Mode of action |
|---|---|---|
| IL-1 | Macrophages | Immune activation: induces an inflammatory response |
| IL-2 | Primarily T cells | Activates T (and NK) cells and supports their growth. Formerly called *T cell growth factor* |
| IL-3 | T cells | Primarily promotes growth of haematopoietic cells |
| IL-4 | T-helper cells | Lymphocyte growth factor; involved in IgE responses |
| IL-5 | T-helper cells | Promotes growth of B cells and eosinophils |
| IL-6 | Fibroblasts | Promotes B-cell growth and antibody production |
| IL-7 | Stromal cells | Lymphocyte growth factor important in the development of immature cells |
| IL-8 | Primarily macrophages | Chemoattractant |
| G-CSF | Primarily monocytes | Promotes growth of myeloid cells |
| M-CSF | Primarily monocytes | Promotes growth of macrophages |
| GM-CSF | Primarily T cells | Promotes growth of monomyelocytic cells |
| IFN-$\alpha$ | Leucocytes | Immune activation and modulation |
| IFN-$\beta$ | Fibroblasts | Immune activation and modulation |
| IFN-$\gamma$ | T cells and NK cells | Immune activation and modulation |
| TNF-$\alpha$ | Macrophages | Stimulates generalized immune activation as well as tumour necrosis. Also known as *cachectin* |
| TNF-$\beta$ | T cells | Stimulates immune activation and generalized vascular effects. Also known as *lymphotoxin* |

G-CSF, granulocyte colony-stimulating factor; GM-CSF, granulocyte-macrophage colony-stimulating factor; IL, interleukin; IFN; interferon; M-CSF, macrophage colony-stimulating factor; TNF, tumour necrosis factor.

**Table 2.17** Cytokines: origin and biological function.

lymphocytes. T-helper cells are generated which enhance the antibody response made by B cells. Some of this augmentation is due to secreted lymphokines or cytokines from the T-helper population. It should be noted that cytotoxic T cells may be generated if foreign antigens, typically viruses, are presented directly to this cell population. Bacteria are most likely to be processed through the MHC class II pathway and thus generate, primarily, antibody responses. The B cells, once triggered, will differentiate into plasma cells producing specific antibody which binds to the antigen and further triggers the complement system. The complement system, in turn, recruits neutrophils which together eliminate the antigen, perhaps with additional help from lymphokine-activated macrophages. Once the immune system has detected 'foreign antigens' it can communicate this information to other systems, particularly to the brain and neuroendocrine systems. For example, following infection, there is an increase in both pituitary and adrenal gland secretion. Figure 2.19 indicates the complex nature of these relationships.

# The immune system in disease

Some diseases due to immunological abnormalities are common in clinical practice, for example rheumatoid arthritis, thyroid disease and allergy. Immunodeficiency is relatively rare, but the occurrence of certain infections in the context of specific immune defects can illuminate the physiological role of those parts of immune defence in control of infection.

# Immunodeficiency

## General principles

Infection is the result of microbial virulence on the one hand and host defence on the other. Pathogenic organisms have mechanisms of evading normal defence mechanisms. Organisms of low virulence can only cause disease if the host defence mechanisms that normally control them are defective.

## Opportunist infections

Organisms taking advantage of the opportunity of impaired host defence mechanisms are called *opportunists*. Different host defence defects cause increased susceptibility to different groups of organisms. Therefore, recognizing a pattern of infections can provide the best clinical clue to the type of underlying defence defect.

### Patterns of opportunist infection

Examples of opportunist organisms in the setting of non-immunological defence defects include: staphylococci and

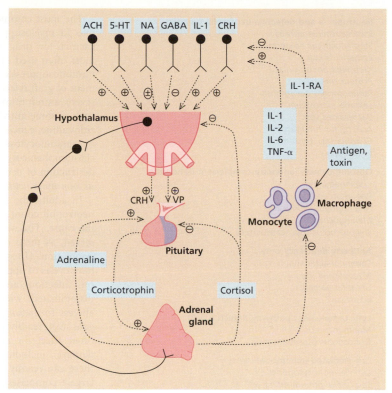

**Fig. 2.19** Interaction of the immune system with the hypothalamo-pituitary axis regulating adrenocortical secretion. In response to infection, activated T cells release cytokines which induce the hypothalamic release of corticotrophin-releasing hormone (CRH) and vasopressin (VP). This overrides the normal negative feedback relationship between corticotrophin and cortisol. Circulating cortisol also acts on peripheral immunocompetent cells to inhibit their activation and secretion of cytokines and other mediators of inflammation. ACH, acetylcholine; NA, noradrenaline; TNF, tumour necrosis factor. (From Reichlim S (1993) *New England Journal of Medicine*, **329**, 1246. With permission.)

*Pseudomonas* in burns patients; *Haemophilus influenzae* and pneumococci in smokers; *Pseudomonas* in cystic fibrosis patients; Gram-negative infections where there is urinary obstruction; staphylococcal and candidal infections with indwelling venous catheters and other foreign bodies; *Candida* and pathogenic *Escherichia coli* following elimination of gut flora after antibiotic therapy.

Table 2.18 shows the main infecting organisms for the principal classes of immunodeficiency. In broad terms, the following principles apply:

NEUTROPHIL DEFECTS lead to staphylococcal, Gram-negative enteric and systemic fungal infections

OPSONIC DEFECTS, due to antibody deficiencies or defects of the main complement pathways, and splenectomy lead to infection with capsulated organisms

DEFECTS OF THE LYTIC PATHWAY OF COMPLEMENT cause susceptibility to disseminated infections with Gram-negative cocci (*Neisseria*)

CELL-MEDIATED IMMUNE DEFECTS, affecting the co-operation between CD4 T cells and macrophages, lead to susceptibility to infection with facultative intracellular pathogens and herpesviruses

## Congenital immunodeficiencies

Congenital defects of specific metabolic or developmental disorders can lead to characteristic deficiencies and are rare.

The main categories of immunodeficiency by host mechanism are as follows:

REDUCED NEUTROPHIL NUMBER AND FUNCTION, with or without accompanying defects in the related phagocytes of the monocyte/macrophage lineage

DEFICIENCIES OF INDIVIDUAL COMPLEMENT COMPONENTS

B-CELL DEFECTS, causing various types of antibody deficiency

T-CELL DEFECTS, impairing cell-mediated immunity

COMBINED T AND B CELL DEFECTS, which cause some of the most severe immunodeficiencies.

Table 2.19 shows the more important examples.

## Acquired immunodeficiencies

Acquired immunodeficiencies are much more common but are often less precisely defined in terms of immunological mechanisms. They can in many cases be best understood against the background of the more specific defects. They include:

IATROGENIC DEFECTS resulting from deliberate immunosuppression or unwanted complications of certain therapies; malnutrition; splenectomy

IMMUNOSUPPRESSION resulting from specific diseases that affect immune competence, such as tumours of the immune system and autoimmune disorders; and transient or progressive immunosuppression caused by certain infections

The most important of the latter is of course the acquired immunodeficiency syndrome (AIDS) resulting from HIV

**Neutropenia and defective neutrophil function**
*Staphylococcus aureus*
*Staphylococcus epidermidis*
*Escherichia coli*
*Klebsiella pneumoniae*
*Proteus mirabilis*
*Pseudomonas aeruginosa*
*Serratia marcescens*
*Bacteroides* spp.
*Aspergillus fumigatus*
*Candida* spp. (systemic)
*Mucor* spp.

**Opsonin defects (antibody/complement deficiency, splenectomy)**
*Pneumococcus*
*Haemophilus influenzae*
*Meningococcus*
*Streptococcus* spp. (capsulated)

**Antibody deficiency only**
*Campylobacter* spp.
*Mycoplasma* spp.
*Ureaplasma* spp.
Echovirus

**Lytic complement pathway defects (C5–9)**
*Meningococcus*
Gonococcus (disseminated)

**Cell-mediated immunodeficiency**
*Listeria monocytogenes*
*Legionella pneumophila*
*Salmonella* spp. (non-typhi)
*Nocardia asteroides*
*Mycobacterium tuberculosis*
Atypical mycobacteria, especially *M. avium-intracellulare*
*Candida* spp. (mucocutaneous)
*Cryptococcus neoformans*
*Histoplasma capsulatum*
*Pneumocystis carinii*
*Toxoplasma gondii*
Herpes simplex
Herpes zoster
Cytomegalovirus
Epstein–Barr virus
Measles virus
Papovaviruses

**Table 2.18**  Immune defects and opportunist organisms.

infection, which is to be covered in some detail (see p. 145). See Table 2.20 for the main categories.

# PHAGOCYTE DEFICIENCY

## Neutropenia

*Congenital neutropenias* are rare and, if severe, are often fatal at an early age. Most however are relatively benign and may even be incidental findings. They generally reflect defects of maturation and release of neutrophils from marrow. Staphylococcal skin infections are common manifestations. A particular variant is *cyclical neutropenia* with cycles of 3–5 weeks, but this disorder is typically benign.

The most common causes of *acquired neutropenia* are due to myelosuppression by disease, such as the leukaemias or drug therapy. Myelosuppressive drugs are most often used in the treatment of tumours; deliberate immunosuppression is also used for prevention or treatment of graft rejection in transplantation and for treating severe autoimmune disease. A number of other drugs such as some antivirals are also immunosuppressive (e.g. zidovudine, ganciclovir) and some can cause neutropenia or agranulocytosis as an idiosyncratic side-effect (e.g. chloramphenicol). Neutropenia due to increased rate of destruction of neutrophils is seen in *hypersplenism* and in *autoimmune neutropenia*.

In adults, the risk of infection rises steeply once the neutrophil count falls below $1.5 \times 10^9$/litre, regardless of the cause. The risk is less if the monocyte count is preserved, as these cells can serve as a back-up phagocyte population. (In cyclical neutropenia, monocytes usually have cycles of opposite phase, which is probably why serious infections are uncommon.) Infections are typically disseminated with septicaemia, fungaemia and deep abscess formation. Colonization of the gut with pathogens can readily lead to septicaemia. Local infections often affect the mouth, perianal area and sites of skin damage, including indwelling vascular catheters, and these can readily lead to systemic infection. Pus, which largely comprises neutrophils, may be scanty and may appear serous.

If myelosuppressive therapy is being used, the dose should be reduced or the drug stopped. Neutropenic episodes can be reduced by the use of G-CSF or GM-CSF, which appear to reduce infective episodes and duration of neutropenia. Antibiotic or antifungal prophylaxis are sometimes of value. Otherwise prompt antimicrobial therapy for febrile episodes during neutropenia is essential, using agents with broad cover for the common organisms encountered (see p. 9).

# Defects of neutrophil function

Defects of neutrophil function (some of which also affect monocyte/macrophage function) interfere with migration into the tissues through vascular endothelium, locomotion in tissues, phagocytosis or intracellular killing.

### CLINICAL FEATURES
Mucocutaneous sepsis in the mouth and perianal areas is common and local infections often lead to chronic abscess formation in the tissues or draining lymph nodes. Granulomas may be seen, because of failure of neutrophils to degrade microbes effectively. Systemic spread is less common than with neutropenia. Congenital causes may first present with infection or delayed separation of the umbilical stump.

## Leucocyte adhesion defect

This is an autosomal recessive disorder caused by abnormal synthesis of the β-chain CD18 that is shared by the

| Congenital | Acquired |
|---|---|
| *Phagocytes* | |
| Congenital neutropenia | Neutropenia due to myelosuppression |
| Cyclical neutropenia | Hypersplenism |
| Leucocyte adhesion defects | Autoimmune neutropenia |
| Hyper-IgE syndrome | Corticosteroid therapy |
| Shwachman's syndrome | Diabetes |
| Chronic granulomatous disease | Hypophosphataemia |
| Other intrinsic killing defects | Myeloid leukaemias |
| Storage diseases | Influenza |
| Chediak–Higashi syndrome | |
| | |
| *Complement deficiency* | |
| C3, Clq, I, H deficiencies | |
| C5, 6, 7, 8, 9, deficiencies | |
| Mannan-binding protein deficiency | |
| Complement-dependent opsonization defects | |
| | |
| *Antibody deficiency (B cell defects)* | |
| X-linked hypogammaglobulinaemia | Myeloma, lymphoma |
| Common variable immunodeficiency | Splenectomy |
| IgA (±IgG$_2$) deficiency | Congenital rubella |
| Specific antibody deficiencies | |
| | |
| *T-cell deficiencies* | |
| DiGeorge anomaly | Measles |
| IL-2 deficiency | Corticosteroid therapy |
| Signal transduction defect | Cyclosporin, FK506 |
| | |
| *Combined immunodeficiencies* | |
| Severe combined immunodeficiency | AIDS |
|    Adenosine deaminase deficiency | Protein–calorie malnutrition |
|    Purine nucleoside phosphorylase deficiency | |
|    Non-expression of MHC class II | |
|    Reticular dysgenesis | |
| Wiskott–Aldrich syndrome | |
| Ataxia telangiectasia | |
| EBV-associated immunodeficiency | |

**Table 2.19**   Main types of immunodeficiency.

CD11a,b and c molecules to form leukocyte function antigen (LFA) LFA-1, the C3bi (inactivated C3b) receptor and the C3dg receptor (p150/95). There is impaired leucocyte tissue localization, locomotion and endocytosis. Bone marrow transplantation has been successful in a few cases.

## Hyper-IgE syndrome

The syndrome is characterized by very high levels of IgE (much of it antistaphylococcal), impaired neutrophil locomotion and severe eczema, with frequent staphylococcal secondary infections and abscesses. Other immune defects may be seen causing a wider spectrum of pyogenic and other infections.

## Shwachman's syndrome

This may resemble cystic fibrosis clinically, with exocrine pancreatic insufficiency and pyogenic infections, in which mild neutropenia is associated with a defect of neutrophil migration.

## Chronic granulomatous disease (CGD)

This is the prototype congenital defect of neutrophil (and monocyte) killing.

### PATHOGENESIS

In this disorder, the oxidative pathway of microbial killing is severely impaired, either due to a defective cytochrome b558 (X-linked CGD) or components of the associated NADPH oxidase (autosomal recessive CGD). Production of superoxide is abnormal, this being the first of a cascade of microbicidal oxygen radicals, including hydrogen peroxide, hypohalites, hydroxyl radicals and singlet oxygen. Impaired production of oxygen radicals can also affect the efficiency of non-oxidative killing.

### CLINICAL FEATURES

Patients have chronic suppurative granulomas or abscesses affecting skin, lymph nodes and sometimes lung and liver, as well as osteomyelitis. They may present during early or late childhood years, depending on the severity of the defect. Most of the typical infections associated with neutrophil defects can be seen, particularly those that produce catalase, which inactivates any endogenous microbial peroxide that can kill organisms inside the phagocytic vacuole. Because macrophages are also affected, cell-mediated opportunist infections may also be seen such as atypical mycobacteria, *Nocardia* and salmonellae.

### DIAGNOSIS

Diagnosis is made with the nitroblue tetrazolium (NBT) test, which uses a coloured dye reaction to assay the oxidative pathway; it can also be used to screen carriers.

### TREATMENT

Infections respond to appropriate antimicrobial therapy and surgical measures as needed; in some patients prophylaxis may be merited. Recent studies have shown that regular interferon-γ can reduce the frequency of infections, probably through enhanced monocyte/ macrophage killing.

A wide variety of other rare disorders can impair microbial killing including other inborn errors in microbicidal mechanisms, such as *leucocyte G6PD deficiency* (much less common than that affecting red cells) and *myeloperoxidase deficiency*. Various storage diseases, such as *Gaucher's* and *glycogen storage diseases*, impair function of phagocytes, particularly macrophages, because of the accumulated material within them.

## Chediak–Higashi syndrome

This, an autosomal recessive disorder, is characterized by giant granules in myeloid cells and large granular lymphocytes; abnormal microbial killing is due to defective fusion with the phagosome in phagocytes; NK cell activity is similarly impaired. Similar fusion abnormalities in melanocytes causes partial oculocutaneous albinism, in addition to recurrent infections.

## Acquired neutrophil function disorders

The most important defect is caused by *corticosteroid therapy*, which also affects T cell–macrophage cooperation causing cell-mediated immunodeficiency. The main effect of corticosteroids on neutrophils is to impair leucocyte–endothelial adhesion. This reduces the marginated pool of leucocytes and impairs their attachment to endothelium at the site of tissue injury or infection. Corticosteroids thus prevent neutrophils reaching the tissues. The corollary of reduced margination is a rise in the neutrophil count; this can be deceptive if its significance is not appreciated.

The effect of corticosteroid therapy on neutrophil function is reflected by increased focal and systemic infections with staphylococci and Gram-negative bacteria. The effect is usually apparent above doses of 15 or 20 mg prednisolone daily or equivalent and can be substantially reduced (as can other side-effects) by alternate-day therapy.

An important infective cause of acquired neutrophil dysfunction is *influenza*, which causes a specific transient impairment of phagosome–lysosome fusion. This is the main reason for the high risk of staphylococcal pneumonia in influenza epidemics.

*Myeloid leukaemias* can cause defective neutrophil function as well as effectively causing neutropenia of normal cells. Neutrophil and macrophage function can also be impaired in abnormal metabolic states such as uncontrolled *diabetes mellitus* and *hypophosphataemia*. The latter may be seen during intravenous feeding of critically ill patients. Inhibitors of endogenous chemotactic factors for neutrophils may be seen in *Hodgkin's disease* and *alcoholic cirrhosis* and may be responsible for increased pyogenic infections in such patients.

## COMPLEMENT DEFICIENCIES

There are two major patterns of infection associated with complement deficiencies:
1 Deficiencies of C3, C1q or of Factors H or I cause increased susceptibility to capsulated bacteria. These patients may also develop immune complex disorders and SLE-like disorders, as do patients with deficiencies of other classical pathway components of complement.
2 Deficiencies of the lytic complement pathway, C5–9, causes susceptibility to disseminated neisserial infections, meningococcaemia and gonococcaemia; the latter has also been seen in association with disorders of complement function.

These complement deficiencies are rare, but functional defects of complement deposition on microbial surfaces are common, as seen in *mannan-binding protein deficiency* (*Saccharomyces* opsonin deficiency) and other less well-characterized *complement-dependent opsonization defects*. These are responsible for increased infections with *Haemophilus* and pneumococcal infections, especially in the early childhood years—before a sufficiently wide specific antibody repertoire is acquired. The C3 depletion caused by C3nef, an autoantibody that stabilizes the alternative pathway convertase, and seen in association with partial lipodystrophy may also increase the risk of pyogenic infection.

*C1 esterase inhibitor deficiency* (see p. 1005) is not associated with infection but with hereditary angio-oedema, with episodes of localised oedema in skin of limbs or face, and the mucosa of the larynx or gut; the latter can cause life-threatening respiratory obstruction or severe episodes of abdominal pain.

## ANTIBODY DEFICIENCIES

### X-linked hypogammaglobulinaemia

There is a profound reduction in all immunoglobulin classes; B cells and plasma cells are reduced. The defect is in the differentiation of pre-B cells into B cells; T cells are normal. It typically presents with infections, e.g. meningococcal meningitis, mycoplasmal infections, after the first 3–6 months of life, when the protection from passively transferred maternal antibody has largely been lost. Immunoglobulin replacement therapy is very successful and is now generally given intravenously. Many patients treat themselves at home.

## Common variable immunodeficiency (CVI)

This is a late onset antibody deficiency, which may present in childhood or adult life. IgG levels are especially low. B-cell numbers are usually normal; the defect appears to result from failure of their further differentiation. Some tests of T-cell function may be abnormal but few clinical manifestations of T-cell immunodeficiency are documented.

### CLINICAL FEATURES
The patients have similar infections to those with the X-linked variety. However, a particular feature is follicular hyperplasia of lymph nodes, which in the gut takes the form of nodular lymphoid hyperplasia, and there may be splenomegaly. CVI patients may develop autoimmune disease and there is also an increased risk of lymphoreticular malignancy.

### DIAGNOSIS
The finding of reduced immunoglobulin levels and normal B-cell numbers indicates the diagnosis.

### TREATMENT
Most of the manifestations are satisfactorily prevented by regular immunoglobulin replacement therapy.

## IgA deficiency

This is an extremely common disorder but is often symptomless. Only a small proportion have an increased risk of pyogenic infection and many of these have another defect, such as $IgG_2$ subclass deficiency. Some have allergic disorders or gluten hypersensitivity, and autoimmune disorders may also occur.

### Isolated $IgG_2$ subclass deficiency
This is a rare cause of increased infection with capsulated organisms, for which it is the main immunoglobulin subclass; intravenous immunoglobulin replacement provides effective restoration.

A variety of other rare immunoglobulin deficiencies exist, including *hypogammaglobulinaemia with raised IgM*, in which there is a defect in isotype switching. Some patients with increased bacterial infections have apparently normal levels of immunoglobulin but fail to produce specific antibodies to certain organisms.

## Acquired hypogammaglobulinaemia

This is seen in the immune paresis of patients with *myeloma* and *chronic lymphatic leukaemia* or *lymphoma*. Infection with capsulated bacteria may be seen, especially with myeloma. *Splenectomy* causes impairment of defence against capsulated bacteria, especially pneumococcus, partly because T-independent antibody responses are largely made in the spleen and partly because of its role as part of the fixed reticuloendothelial system. Hyposplenism associated with severe sickle cell disease is responsible for the increased risk of infection in such patients. Pneumococcal vaccination (see p. 330) before elective splenectomy and the use of penicillin prophylaxis can largely eliminate risk of serious infection. Hypogammaglobulinaemia can be seen in *congenital rubella*.

# T-CELL IMMUNODEFICIENCIES
## Congenital T-cell defects

### DiGeorge anomaly
A defect of branchial arch development leads to abnormal thymic development. This is of varying severity and is associated with other branchial arch defects: dysmorphic facies, hypoparathyroidism and cardiac defects. Patients present with infections including mucocutaneous candidiasis and *Pneumocystis carinii* pneumonia, together with chronic diarrhoea, due to a variety of pathogens. The absent thymus can be documented radiologically. CD3 T cells are variably reduced in number, but the CD4 subset is usually reduced and T-cell proliferative responses are impaired. Immunoglobulin production is typically normal. Thymic transplants and thymic hormone have been reported to have reconstituted some patients with severe disease and bone marrow transplants have also had some success.

### Other causes of cellular immunodeficiency
Various other rare congenital defects have been reported that predominantly affect T-cell responses, including:
- Isolated CD4 lymphopenia
- IL-2 deficiency
- Defects in signal transduction via the T-cell receptor.

## Acquired T-cell defects

### THE ACQUIRED IMMUNODEFICIENCY SYNDROME (AIDS)
By far the most common immunodeficiency encountered in clinical practice is that due to infection with the human immunodeficiency virus (HIV), the cause of AIDS.

### Pathogenesis
The cellular receptor for HIV is the CD4 molecule, which defines the cells that are susceptible and includes the following cells within the immune system:
1 $CD4^+$ T lymphocytes (which are most affected)
2 Monocytes
3 Macrophages and other antigen-presenting cells
    (a) Dendritic cells in the blood
    (b) Langerhans' cells of the skin
    (c) Follicular dendritic cells of the lymph nodes, where much of the early infection and replication of HIV takes place.

Direct cytopathic effects of HIV
Lysis of infected cells by HIV-specific cytotoxic T cells
Tc-mediated lysis of uninfected CD4+ T cells that have
    bound gp120 to the CD4 molecule
Immunosuppressive effects of soluble HIV proteins on
    uninfected cells, e.g. gp120 envelope protein leading
    to decreased proliferation
Molecular mimicry between gp120/160 and MHC class I,
    inducing autoimmune destruction
Signal transduction defects and induction of
    programmed cell death (apoptosis) by unknown
    mechanisms

**Table 2.20**  Mechanisms of the immunopathogenesis of HIV.

A number of pathogenic mechanisms have been described to account for the profound cellular immunodeficiency of HIV infection (Table 2.20).

### Immunological abnormalities

The major defects are shown in Table 2.21. The central and most characteristic is the progressive and severe depletion of CD4+ 'helper' lymphocytes. These cells orchestrate the immune response, responding to antigen presented to them via antigen-presenting cells in the context of class II MHC. They proliferate and release cytokines, in particular IL-2 which leads to proliferation of other reactive T-cell clones, including cytotoxic T cells to eradicate viral infections, and interferon-γ and interleukin which activates B cells to antibody production, NK cells to cytotoxicity and macrophages to microbicidal activity against intracellular pathogens. Loss of this single cell type can therefore explain nearly all the immunological abnormalities of AIDS as other cells' function is so dependent on it. In addition other cells are also affected, if not infected by HIV. Antigen-presenting cells are directly and productively infected; B cells are polyclonally activated by the envelope proteins of HIV. For the presentation and management of HIV infection and AIDS, see p. 96.

### MEASLES

Measles can cause a transient T-cell immunodeficiency, but it is rarely long-lasting enough for severe clinical problems to ensue.

*CD4 lymphocytes*
CD4+-lymphocyte depletion (late)
Decreased CD4+-lymphocyte function (early)
    Decreased proliferation to soluble antigens
    Defective cytokine production

*B lymphocytes*
Polyclonal B-cell activation
    Increased spontaneous antibody production
    Failure of neoantigen production
    Hypergammaglobulinaemia

*Antigen-presenting cells*
Reduced expression of surface class II antigen

**Table 2.21**  Major immunological abnormalities of HIV infection.

### IMMUNOSUPPRESSIVE THERAPY

Immunosuppressive therapy with cytotoxic agents such as cyclophosphamide and azathioprine tends to cause predominant T-cell immunosuppression. *Cyclosporin* and *FK506* are potent immunosuppressive agents which interfere with T-cell activation mechanisms at an intracellular level. Surprisingly, they are associated with only modest increases in infection, unless combined with corticosteroids or other agents. In such combinations, increased risk of Epstein–Barr virus (EBV)-associated lymphoma has been reported. *Antilymphocyte immunoglobulin* or *monoclonal anti-CD3 antibody therapy* also suppress T-cell responses transiently.

### CORTICOSTEROID THERAPY

This interferes with cell-mediated immunity, in particular T cell–macrophage cooperation. This is due to effects on T-cell traffic and impairment of macrophage responses to cytokines, together with impaired antigen presentation. Mucocutaneous candidiasis. *Pneumocystis carinii* pneumonia, cytomegalovirus infection, mycobacterial infection, *Nocardia*, non-typhi *Salmonella* septicaemia and cryptococcosis are some of the very many infections seen with prolonged high-dose steroid therapy.

# COMBINED IMMUNODEFICIENCIES

The most severe immunodeficiencies are those that affect both B and T cell responses. These can stem from a variety of defective mechanisms in lymphocyte function, but tend to have rather similar clinical features, combining the opportunist infections of cell-mediated immunodeficiency with those of antibody deficiency.

## Severe combined immunodeficiency (SCID)

This typically presents in the first weeks of life. Failure to thrive, absent lymphoid tissue, lymphopenia and hypogammaglobulinaemia with multiple severe infections are characteristic.

There are primary X-linked and autosomal recessive variants of SCID. Other causes include adenosine deaminase (ADA) deficiency, in which a defective purine salvage enzyme that is expressed in all cells, has a particular effect on lymphocytes due to the accumulation of substrates and metabolites that interfere with lymphocyte function. An analogous disorder is seen in *purine nucleoside phosphorylase deficiency. Non-expression of MHC class II* and *reticular dysgenesis* cause similar syndromes. Milder expressions of these defects exist, some presenting in later life, and are sometimes termed benign combined immunodeficiency or *Nezeloff's syndrome.*

Even with supportive and antimicrobial therapy, most of these conditions have a very poor prognosis without reconstitutive therapy. Immunoglobulin therapy is effective for the antibody deficiency, but the cell-mediated opportunists are the main determinant of outcome. Bone marrow transplantation is the definitive approach and has had significant success, especially if undertaken before extensive infection has set in. Recent approaches have included attempts to restore the defective enzymes in ADA deficiency and gene therapy is now being attempted.

## Others

Other combined immune deficiencies include the following.

WISKOTT–ALDRICH SYNDROME is an X-linked defect with associated eczema and thrombocytopenia; a mainly cell-mediated defect with falling immunoglobulins is seen and autoimmune manifestations and lymphoreticular malignancy may develop.

ATAXIA TELANGIECTASIA patients have defective DNA repair mechanisms and have cell-mediated defects with low IgA and $IgG_2$; lymphoid malignancy is again common.

EBV-ASSOCIATED IMMUNODEFICIENCY. Apparently normal, but genetically predisposed (usually X-linked) individuals develop overwhelming EBV infection, polyclonal EBV-driven lymphoproliferation, combined immunodeficiency, aplastic anaemia and lymphoid malignancy. EBV appears to act as a trigger for the expression of a hitherto silent immunodeficiency.

PROTEIN–CALORIE MALNUTRITION is a very common cause of acquired combined immunodeficiency, with predominantly cell-mediated defects. Mechanisms are not fully established. Measles is a major cause of morbidity and mortality among children and *Pneumocystis carinii* pneumonia is also a major pathogen; indeed, it was in this setting that *Pneumocystis* was first seen in the Warsaw ghettos.

### Problems of prematurity

An immune response is not essential for normal fetal development and growth, but is necessary for survival after birth. Premature infants of 28 weeks' gestation and under are now surviving and have several immunological deficiencies and problems:

REDUCED ANTIBODY PRODUCTION. IgM synthesis does not occur before 30 weeks' gestation; IgG production does not occur until several weeks after birth.

LOW LEVELS OF MATERNAL ANTIBODY, as active placental transfer of IgG does not occur until the third trimester. Antibody levels continue to drop after birth due to loss of maternal IgG.

NEUTROPENIA AND IMPAIRED CHEMOTAXIS.

INVASION OF FOREIGN BODIES, such as indwelling catheters.

ANTIBIOTIC THERAPY, reducing colonization resistance.

Breast milk has several protective properties including secretory IgA, lysozyme, lactoferrin, leucocytes and small amounts of IgG, IgM and IgD. Colostrum is particularly high in antibody, and provides IgA to protect the gastrointestinal tract.

# Hypersensitivity diseases

Hypersensitivity reactions underlie a number of autoimmune and allergic conditions. The classification of these reactions is shown in Table 2.22.

## Type I reaction (reaginic/anaphylactic/immediate hypersensitivity reaction)

This is an allergic reaction produced within 30 min of exposure to a specific allergen. Allergens, e.g. house dust, pollens, animal danders or moulds, only elicit reactions in certain genetically predisposed individuals, who are said to be atopic. Atopy is diagnosed on skin-prick testing when a reaction is elicited by sensitizing allergens. Type I reactions can be passively transferred by injection of serum containing IgE antibody into the skin (passive cutaneous anaphylaxis). The antibody will remain fixed to the mast cells in the skin for up to 4–5 days and an injection of the antigen will produce a wheal and flare reaction (Prausnitz–Küstner reaction).

Type I reactions are mediated via allergen-specific antibodies of the IgE class and occur as follows.

ALLERGEN INHALATION OR INGESTION results in local generation of specific IgE via the interaction of macrophages and receptive B and T-helper cells.

LOCALLY PRODUCED ALLERGEN-SPECIFIC IgE then binds to the Fc receptors of mast cells and, to a lesser extent, eosinophils and macrophages sensitizing them. IgE also enters the circulation, where it sensitizes basophils.

SUBSEQUENT EXPOSURE TO ALLERGEN results in the cross-linking of the IgE antibodies on the cells and to mediator release.

Binding of allergen to sensitized cells results in the *de novo* synthesis and/or release of several inflammatory mediators:

HISTAMINE. Present as a preformed mediator in sensitized mast cells and basophils, histamine produces vasodilation and bronchial smooth-muscle constriction.

ARACHIDONIC ACID METABOLITES (see p. 670). Arachidonic acid is generated in sensitized cells from membrane lipids following the binding of specific allergen. It is subsequently metabolized to produce prostaglandins (cyclooxygenase pathway), leukotrienes (lipoxygenase pathway) or platelet-activating factor (PAF acetylation), depending on which cell type is being activated.

Leukotrienes and prostaglandins are together termed *eicosanoids*. The arachidonic acid metabolites involved in Type 1 hypersensitivity reactions are PAF, leukotrienes

| | I (immediate) | II (cytotoxin) | III (immune complex) | IV (delayed) | V (stimulating) | VI (antibody-dependent cell-mediated cytotoxicity)[a] |
|---|---|---|---|---|---|---|
| Antigens | Pollens, moulds, mites, drugs, food and parasites | Cell surface or tissue bound | Exogenous (bacteria, fungi, parasites) Autoantigens | Cell/tissue bound | Cell surface | Antibody complexed on cell surface of target cells |
| Mediators | IgE and mast cells | IgG, IgM and complement | IgG, IgM, IgA and complement | $T_D$, $T_C$, activated macrophages and lymphokines | IgG | K cells |
| Diagnostic tests | Skin-prick tests–wheal and flare RAST | Coombs' test Indirect immuno-fluorescence (antibodies) Red cell agglutination Precipitating antibodies | Skin test—oedema, erythema (Arthus reaction) Immune complexes | Skin test—erythema induration (e.g. tuberculin test) | Indirect immuno-fluorescence | As for type II |
| Time taken for reaction to develop | 15–30 min | Rapid | 4–12 hours | 12–48 hours | Variable | Variable |
| Histology | Oedema, vasodilatation, mast cell degranulation, eosinophils | Damage to target cells | Acute inflammatory reaction, neutrophils, vasculitis | Perivascular inflammation, mononuclear cells, fibrin Caseation and necrosis in TB | Hypertrophy | Damage to target cells |
| Diseases and conditions produced | Asthma (extrinsic) Eczema (atopic) urticaria Allergic rhinitis Anaphylaxis | Autoimmune haemolytic anaemia Transfusion reactions Haemolytic disease of newborn Goodpasture's syndrome Addisonian pernicious anaemia Myasthenia gravis | Autoimmune, e.g. SLE, glomerulo-nephritis, rheumatoid arthritis Low-grade persistent infections, e.g. viral hepatitis Disease caused by environmental antigens, e.g. farmer's lung | Pulmonary TB Contact dermatitis Graft-versus-host disease Insect bites Leprosy | Neonatal hyper-thyroidism Graves' disease | Autoimmune tumour rejection Defence against helminthic infection |
| Treatment | Antigen avoidance Antihistamines Corticosteroids (usually topical) Sodium cromoglycate | Exchange transfusion Plasmapheresis | Corticosteroids Immuno-suppressives Plasmapheresis | Immuno-suppressives Corticosteroids | Treatment of individual disease | Treat symptomatically |

[a]Type VI hypersensitivity may also be classified with type II reactions.
RAST, radioallergosorbent test; SLE, systemic lupus erythematosus; TB, tuberculosis; $T_c$, T cytotoxic; $T_D$, T delayed hypersensitivity.

**Table 2.22** Summary of hypersensitivity reactions.

(LT) $B_4$, $C_4$, $D_4$ and $E_4$ and prostaglandins (PG) $D_2$, $E_2$ and $F_{2\alpha}$. They have four main actions:

1 *Inflammatory cell mucosal infiltration.* This is mediated by $LTB_4$ and PAF, which attract and activate neutrophils, eosinophils and monocytes/macrophages. $LTB_4$ is released by activated mast cells and macrophages and PAF is released by mast cells, neutrophils and eosinophils.

2 *Bronchoconstriction.* This is mediated by several metabolites including PAF, $LTC_4$, $LTD_4$ and $LTE_4$ and $PGD_2$

and $PGF_{2\alpha}$. $LTC_4$ and $PGD_2$ are the major arachidonic acid metabolites released by mast cells. The remaining eicosanoids are generated by human lung tissue and/or alveolar macrophages.

3 *Bronchial mucosal oedema* is mediated by $LTC_4$ and $LTD_4$ and $PGE_2$. $PGE_2$ is released from alveolar macrophages and human lung tissue.

4 *Mucus hypersecretion* is mediated by $LTC_4$ and $LTD_4$.

# Autoimmunity

An autoimmune disease occurs when the immune system fails to recognize the body's own tissues as 'self' and mounts an attack on them. Disorders include rheumatoid arthritis, juvenile (insulin-dependent) diabetes, thyroiditis and multiple sclerosis. Illnesses are divided into those that affect just one organ (*organ-specific*) and those which affect many systems (*organ non-specific or multi-systemic*, Table 2.23). Autoimmune diseases are mostly of unknown aetiology although genetic, hormonal, microbiological and environmental factors are known to be implicated in their manifestation and severity.

## Immunopathology of autoimmune disease

Formation of autoantibodies may be a normal physiological process. However, excessive production of such antibodies can be harmful. The way in which autoantibodies cause structural damage to the body's tissues are varied. Antibodies may directly react with a specific tissue resulting in inflammation and tissue damage, such as antiglomerular basement membrane antibodies in Goodpasture's syndrome, or directly affect function, for example acetylcholine receptor antibodies in myasthenia gravis (type II hypersensitivity).

Alternatively, circulating immune complexes may be formed. Immune complexes are biologically active entities which in themselves have certain characteristics. These properties determine whether immune complexes become harmful and cause extensive tissue damage. Some of these features are detailed in Table 2.24. Inflammation or autoimmune conditions resulting from the formation of immune complexes are classified as *type III hypersensitivity reactions*. The complexes are often deposited in the kidney, skin, joint and nervous system. This results in complement activation, accumulation and activation of neutrophils with the release of proteolytic enzymes and further damage. It should also be noted that mononuclear cells are also implicated in tissue destruction. Both $CD4^+$ and $CD8^+$ lymphocytes are observed routinely as infiltrates in inflammatory lesions. While there is little doubt these cells contribute to tissue destruction their precise role in the pathological processes is uncertain. The complexity of the autoimmune diseases is quite formidable, largely because there is so much variation in the interplay of different factors that can influence the reactivity of the immune system to the body's tissues.

# Diagnostic tests in clinical immunology

The major investigations in the diagnosis and monitoring of disorders of the immune system are described below.

## Autoantibodies

A characteristic feature of many autoimmune disorders is the presence of specific autoantibodies. These may be useful markers of disease activity, and in monitoring response to therapeutic inventions.

| Disease | Organ specificity |
|---|---|
| Graves' disease | Single organ involvement |
| Hashimoto's thyroiditis | (organ-specific |
| Pernicious anaemia | autoimmunity) |
| Addison's disease | |
| Diabetes mellitus (insulin-dependent) | |
| Goodpasture's syndrome | |
| Myasthenia gravis | |
| Pemphigus vulgaris | |
| Pemphigoid | |
| Multiple sclerosis | |
| Haemolytic anaemia | |
| Thrombocytopenic purpura | |
| Primary biliary cirrhosis | |
| Crohn's disease (?) | |
| Ulcerative colitis (?) | |
| Wegener's granulomatosis | |
| Psoriatic arthritis (?) | |
| Sjögren's syndrome | |
| Rheumatoid arthritis | |
| Polymyositis/dermatomyositis | |
| Scleroderma | |
| Mixed connective tissue disease | Multiple organ involvement |
| Systemic lupus erythematosus | (non-organ specific autoimmunity) |

**Table 2.23**  Autoimmune diseases as classified by organ specificity.

Size
Nature of the antigen
Class of antibodies
Subclasses of antibodies
Affinity of antibodies
Complement-fixing ability
Ability of patient's complement to solubilize complex

**Table 2.24**  Factors influencing the pathogenicity of immune complexes.

### Indirect immunofluorescence (IIF) (Fig. 2.20)

This technique is used to detect organ- and tissue-specific antibodies, e.g. thyroid, adrenal, smooth muscle, gastric parietal cell, mitochondrial, acetylcholine receptor, antinuclear, antineutrophil cytoplasm, glomerular basement membrane (see p. 382 for methodology).

### Particle agglutination (see Figure 8.2)

This technique is used for the detection or *rheumatoid factors* (RF), in the rheumatoid arthritis haemagglutination assay (RAHA). Sheep red blood cells are coated with rabbit antibody. The results are usually expressed as a titre of the highest serum dilution that gives a positive result. These techniques are therefore only semi-quantitative.

### Enzyme-linked immunosorbent test (ELISA)

ELISA is a commonly used technique for the detection of a wide range of proteins. Wells of microtitre plates are coated with the antigen (e.g. neutrophil cytoplasm proteins, or double-stranded DNA) and the patient's serum applied. Any antibody present will bind to the antigen. A second layer of anti-human antibody conjugated with an enzyme (often alkaline phosphatase) is added, as a 'developing antibody'. A substrate that changes colour if the enzyme is present is added, and the colour intensity is measured spectrophotometrically. The intensity is proportional to the concentration of antibody present. The test is quantitative as the intensity of the reaction of the patient's serum is compared to a standard curve plotted using a serum with known concentration of antibody.

## Cellular tests

The major immunodeficiencies involve abnormalities in the cells of the immune system, for example T and B cells in SCID, DiGeorge syndrome, HIV infection, X-linked agammaglobulinaemia; phagocytes in chronic granulomatous disease.

### Lymphocyte subset phenotypes

Fluorescent-labelled monoclonal antibodies to the surface protein of interest are applied to the cells. The cells can

then be analysed by a flow cytometer. Commonly used antibodies are CD3 (all mature T lymphocytes), CD4 (CD4⁺ or 'helper' T-cells), CD8 (CD8⁺ or 'suppressor' T cells), CD19 or CD20 (mature B cells).

Since the emergence of AIDS, T-cell subset counts have been done on many thousands of individuals, and it is clear that many factors outside of immunodeficiency affect the numbers:

- Age (higher in infancy)
- Exercise (increase)
- Smoking (increase)
- Diurnal variation
- Pregnancy (decrease)
- Splenectomy (increase)

Therefore, results have to be interpreted cautiously. Also, although AIDS characteristically causes CD4-cell depletion, it is important to realize that other conditions, such as tuberculosis and sarcoidosis, can cause similar findings, and that CD4 lymphopenia is not itself diagnostic of HIV infection.

### Functional lymphocyte tests

In addition to the phenotypic studies above, functional tests of lymphocytes may also need to be performed. Peripheral blood lymphocytes are stimulated with:

- Mitogens such as phytohaemagglutinin (T cells), concanavalin A (T cells), poke weed mitogen (B and T cells)
- Recall antigens such as purified protein derivative (ppd) and *Candida*.

The resulting *proliferation* is detected by the uptake of the radiolabelled thymidine into the DNA of the lymphocytes.

### Neutrophil function tests

Tests of phagocytosis and intracellular killing/oxidative burst, random locomotion and chemotaxis are available in specialist centres.

## Glossary

**Acrocentric**. Term used to describe a chromosome in which the centromere lies close to one end, producing one long and one short arm.

**Allele (allelomorph)**. Alternative form of a gene occupying the same locus on a particular chromosome.

**Aneuploid**. Any chromosomal number that is not the exact multiple of the normal haploid number.

**Autosome**. Any chromosome that is not a sex chromosome or mitochondrial chromosome; there are 22 pairs of autosomes in humans.

**Bacteriophage**. A bacterial virus. These are modified and used as vectors for DNA cloning.

**cDNA**. DNA synthesized from an mRNA template by the enzyme reverse transcriptase.

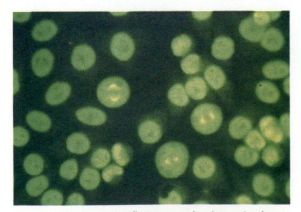

**Fig. 2.20** Indirect immunofluorescence showing antinuclear antibodies.

**Centromere**. The point at which two chromatids of a chromosome are joined and also where the spindle fibres become attached during mitosis and meiosis.

**Character (trait)**. An observable phenotypic feature of an individual.

**Chromatid**. One of the two strands, held together by the centromere, that make up the chromosome as seen during cell division.

**Chromosomal aberration**. An abnormality in the number or structure of a chromosome.

**Chromosome**. A thread-like body containing DNA and protein, situated in the nucleus, and carrying genetic information.

**Clone**. Cells having the same genetic constitution and derived from a single cell by repeated mitoses.

**Codon**. Three adjacent nucleotides in a nucleic acid that code for one amino acid.

**Concordance**. The occurrence of the same trait in both members of a pair of twins.

**Deletion**. Loss of a part of a chromosome.

**Diploid**. The number of chromosomes found in somatic cells, i.e. two sets.

**DNA ligase**. The enzyme that joins two DNA ends together.

**DNA polymerase**. The enzyme that replicates DNA.

**Dominant**. Term used to describe a trait expressed in individuals who are heterozygous for a particular gene.

**Exon**. A segment of a gene that is represented in the final spliced mRNA product.

**Expressivity**. The degree to which the effect of a gene is expressed.

**Gene**. Part of a DNA molecule that directs the synthesis of a specific polypeptide chain.

**Gene pool**. The total genetic information contained in all the genes in a breeding population at a given time.

**Genetic marker**. A genetically controlled phenotypic feature used in inheritance studies.

**Genetics**. The science of heredity and variation.

**Genome**. The total amount of genetic material in the cell.

**Genotype**. The genetic constitution of an individual.

**Haploid**. The number of chromosomes found in germ cells, i.e. one set.

**Heterozygote**. An individual possessing two different alleles at the corresponding loci on a pair of homologous chromosomes.

**Homozygote**. An individual possessing identical alleles at the corresponding loci on a pair of homologous chromosomes.

**Hybridization**. The pairing of complementary DNA or RNA strands to give DNA–DNA or DNA–RNA strands; for example, it is used to search for particular DNA fragments after Southern blotting.

**Intron**. A segment of a gene not represented in the final mRNA product because it has been removed through splicing together of exons on either side of it.

**Karyotype**. The number, size and shape of the chromosomes in a cell.

**Linkage**. The co-segregation of two unrelated DNA sequences which are physically close together on the chromosome.

**Linkage disequilibrium**. The association of particular alleles at two linked loci more frequently than expected by chance.

**Locus**. The site of a gene on a chromosome.

**Metacentric**. Term used to describe a chromosome in which the centromere lies in the middle.

**Monosomy**. A state in which one chromosome of a pair is missing.

**Mosaics**. Patients with two different cell lines in their constitution.

**Non-disjunction**. Failure of a chromosome pair to separate during cell division, resulting in both chromosomes passing to the same daughter cell.

**Nucleotide**. The basic unit of nucleic acids, which is made up of a pyrimidine or purine base, a pentose sugar and a phosphate group.

**Oncogenes**. Genes which when altered in their structure or expression contribute to the abnormal growth of cancer cells.

**Penetrance**. The proportion of individuals with a particular genotype who also have the corresponding phenotype. Full penetrance occurs when a dominant trait is always seen in an individual with one such allele, or when a recessive trait is seen in all individuals possessing two such alleles.

**Phenotype**. The appearance of an individual, resulting from the effects of both environment and genes.

**Plasmid**. A simple circular DNA molecule derived from bacteria which can be modified and used as a vector for DNA cloning.

**Ploidy**. Term that describes the number of chromosome sets, namely 23 = haploid (1 set), 46 = diploid (2 sets).

**Polymerase chain reaction (PCR)**. Technique for rapid analysis of DNA. Oligonucleotide primers corresponding to each end of DNA of interest are synthesized and amplified in genomic DNA using DNA polymerase.

**Positioned cloning (or reverse genetics)**. Methodology used to isolate genes whose protein products are not known but whose existence can be inferred from the disease phenotype.

**Pulsed field gel electrophoresis**. Technique for separation of large fragments of DNA.

**Recessive**. Term used to describe a trait expressed in individuals who are homozygous for a particular gene but not seen in the heterozygote.

**Restriction fragment length polymorphisms (RFLPs)**. When variations in non-coding DNA sequences affect restriction enzyme cleavage sites, DNA fragments of different sizes (RFLPs) will result from enzyme digestion.

**RNA polymerase**. The enzyme that synthesizes RNA, based on a DNA template.

**Sex linkage**. Genes carried on the sex chromosomes.

**'Somy'**. Term referring to the number of copies of an individual chromosome per cell, e.g. 'trisomy' = three copies.

**Splicing**. Removing the introns from an unprocessed RNA molecule.

**Synteny**. Term used to describe genes on the same chromosome.

**Transcription**. The process by which an RNA molecule is synthesized from a DNA template.

**Translation**. The process by which genetic information from mRNA is 'translated' into protein synthesis.

**Translocation**. The transfer of a piece of one chromosome to another non-homologous chromosome.

**Trisomy**. Representation of a chromosome three times rather than twice, giving a total of 47 chromosomes.

**tRNA**. Transfer RNA, a molecule which carries a single amino acid (depending on its anticodon) and which brings the amino acid to the ribosome.

**Vector**. A DNA molecule used to carry DNA regions of interest.

# Further reading

Brock DJH (1993) *Molecular Genetics for the Clinician*. Cambridge: Cambridge University Press.

Brostoff J, Scadding GK, Male D & Roitt IM (1991) *Clinical Immunology*. London: Gower Medical Publishing.

Brown TA (1990) *Gene Cloning: An Introduction*, 2nd edn. London: Chapman and Hall.

Chapel H & Heaney M (eds) (1993) *Essentials of Clinical Immunology*. Oxford: Blackwell Scientific Publishers.

Conner JM & Ferguson-Smith MA (1991) *Essential Medical Genetics*, 3rd edn. Oxford: Blackwell Scientific Publishers.

Gelehrter TD & Collins FS (1990) *The Principles of Medical Genetics*. Baltimore: Williams & Wilkins.

Weatherall DJ (1991) *The New Genetics in Clinical Practice*, 3rd edn. Oxford: Oxford University Press

## Introduction

In developed countries, excess food is available and the commonest nutritional problem is obesity. In the developing countries, lack of food and poor usage of the available food results in protein–energy malnutrition (PEM).

Diet and disease are interrelated in many ways. Excess energy intake, particularly when high in animal (saturated) fat content, is thought to be responsible for a number of diseases, including ischaemic heart disease and diabetes. A relationship between nutrition and cancer has been found in large epidemiological studies. There is evidence that vitamin A deficiency may be associated with certain tumours and a high fat intake is thought to be of importance in producing cancer. Numerous carcinogens, either intentionally added to food (e.g. nitrates for preserving foods) or accidental contaminants (e.g. moulds producing aflatoxin and fungi) may also be involved in the development of cancer.

The proportion of processed foods eaten may affect the development of disease. A number of processed convenience foods have a high sugar and fat content and therefore predispose to dental caries and obesity respectively. They also have a low fibre content, and dietary fibre is possibly important in the prevention of a number of diseases (see p. 156).

Long-term effects of undernutrition are becoming apparent. Low growth rates *in utero* are associated with high death rates from cardiovascular disease in adult life. This is thought to be due to fetal adaptation to undernutrition leading to changes in concentration of a fetal placental hormone.

In 1991 the Department of Health published the dietary reference values for food and energy and nutrients for the UK. Recommended daily amounts (RDAs) are no longer used, but have been replaced by the reference nutrient intake (RNI) and two other values to provide more help in interpreting dietary surveys.

The RNI is roughly equivalent to the previous RDA, i.e. sufficient or more than sufficient to meet the nutritional needs of practically all (97%) of healthy people in a population and therefore exceeds the requirements of most. Most people's daily requirements are less than this and an estimated average requirement (EAR) is also given, which will certainly be adequate for most. A

lower reference nutrient intake (LRNI) which fails to meet the requirement of 97% of the population is also given. The RNI figures quoted in this chapter are for the age group 19–50 years.

# Water and electrolyte balance

Water and electrolyte balance is dealt with fully in Chapter 10. Approximately 1 litre of water per day is required in the diet to balance insensible losses, but much more is usually drunk, the kidneys being able to excrete large quantities. The daily RNI for sodium is 70 mmol (1.6 g) but daily sodium intake varies in the range of 90–440 mmol (2–10 g). These are needlessly high intakes which are thought by some workers to play a role in causing hypertension.

# Dietary requirements

## ENERGY

Food is necessary to provide the body with energy (Fig. 3.1). The oxidation of carbohydrate, fat and protein eventually leads to the generation of high energy bonds in ATP, which is then used for all energy requirements. In addition to providing energy, some of these oxidative products are utilized to generate the carbohydrates, fats and proteins of which the body is composed (Table 3.1).

**Energy balance**
Energy balance is the difference between energy intake and energy expenditure.

ENERGY INTAKE can be estimated from dietary information and in the past has been used to decide daily energy requirements.

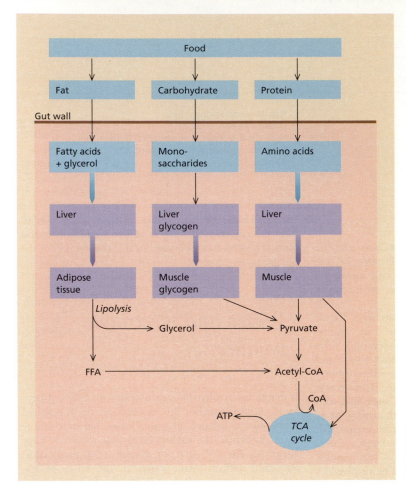

**Fig. 3.1** The production of energy from the main constituents of food. Alcohol produces up to 5% of total calories. One mole of ATP produces 36 moles of glucose.

ENERGY EXPENDITURE gives a more accurate assessment of energy requirements. Daily energy expenditure (Fig. 3.2) is the sum of the

- Basal metabolic rate (BMR)
- Thermic effect of food eaten
- Occupational activities
- Non-occupational activities

Total energy expenditure can be measured using a double-labelled water method measuring decay of body water concentration of the stable isotopes $^2$H and $^{18}$O measured over 7–10 days.

The BMR can be calculated by measuring oxygen consumption, but is more usually taken from standardized tables that require knowledge of the subject's age, weight and sex. The resting metabolic rate (RMR) is 5–10% higher than the BMR and is also used.

The physical activity ratio (PAR) is expressed as multiples of the BMR for both occupational and non-occupational activity of varying intensities (Table 3.2).

Total daily energy expenditure = [BMR × time in bed + (time at work × PAR) + (non-occupational time × PAR)]

To determine the daily energy expenditure of a 50-year-old, 50 kg female doctor, spending 0.3 of a day sleeping, working or on non-occupational activities, the latter at a PAR of 2.1:

[BMR (3240 kJ day$^{-1}$) × 0.3] + [(0.3 × 1.7) + (0.3 × 2.10)] = 7550 kJ day$^{-1}$ or 1806 kcal day$^{-1}$

Remember:

1 kcal = 4.18 kJ

Thus, the estimated average daily requirement for dietary energy in the UK for:

- a 50-year-old female = 8100 kJ (1940 kcal)
- a 50-year-old male = 10 600 kJ (2550 kcal)

This is made up of 50% carbohydrate, 35% fat, 15% protein plus or minus 5% alcohol.

|  | kg | Per cent of body weight |
|---|---|---|
| Water | 42 | 60 |
| Fat | 13 | 18 |
| Protein | 11 | 16 |
| Carbohydrate | 0.5 | 0.7 |
| Minerals | 3.5 | 5.2 |

**Table 3.1** Normal composition of a 70 kg man.

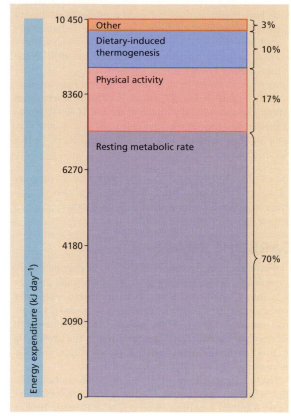

Fig. 3.2   Daily energy expenditure in a sedentary adult.

fasting state. Carbohydrate provides 4 kcal (17 kJ) per gram; however stores are small, consisting of glycogen in the liver and a small amount of circulating glucose.

BODY WEIGHT depends on energy balance. Intake depends partly on food availability but also on a number of complex interrelationships that include the stimulus of good food, the role of hunger, metabolic changes, e.g. hypoglycaemia, and the pleasure and habit of eating. Some people are able to keep their body weight constant within a few kilograms for many years, but most gradually increase their weight owing to a small but continuous increase of intake over expenditure. A gain or loss of energy of 25 000–29 000 kJ (6000–7000 kcal) would respectively increase or decrease body weight by 1 kg.

## PROTEIN

The adult daily RNI for protein is 0.75 g kg$^{-1}$, with protein representing at least 10% of the total energy intake. Most affluent people eat more than this, consuming 80–100 g of protein per day. The total amount of nitrogen excreted in the urine represents the balance between protein breakdown and synthesis. In order to maintain nitrogen balance, at least 40–50 g of protein are needed. The amount of protein required to maintain nitrogen balance in a particular individual can be calculated from the amount of nitrogen excreted in the urine using the following equation:

Urinary nitrogen × 6.25 = grams of protein required

In practice, urinary urea is easily measured and forms 80–90% of the total urinary nitrogen.

Protein contains many amino acids, of which at least eight (probably nine) are essential amino acids necessary for protein synthesis and for maintenance of nitrogen balance. The biological value of a protein is defined as the amount of absorbed protein retained by the body, and this primarily depends on the essential amino acids present. Egg and milk have high biological values, whereas plant proteins have low biological values because at least one essential amino acid is low in concentration.

In developing countries, adequate protein intake is only achieved by increasing the amount of cereal eaten making the diet very bulky. Also, by combining foodstuffs with different low concentrations of amino acids, e.g. maize and beans, protein intake can be adequate providing enough is available.

Adequate energy is required in addition to protein for the normal diet, otherwise protein will be directed towards oxidative pathways and eventually gluconeogen-

In developing countries:
- Carbohydrate may be more than 75% of the total energy
- Fat less than 15% of the total energy

Energy requirements also increase during the growing period, with pregnancy and lactation, and following infection or trauma.

*In the basal state*, energy demands for resting muscle are 20% of the total energy required, abdominal viscera 50%, brain 20% and heart 10%. There is a 10-fold increase in muscle energy demands during exercise.

Energy is derived from various body stores. One-third of protein (e.g. in bone) is unavailable as an energy source, muscle being the main available protein source. Protein breakdown provides only 4 kcal (17 kJ) of energy per gram compared with fat which provides 9 kcal (37 kJ) of energy per gram. Adipose tissue is therefore an efficient way of storing energy and is the only major source of fuel available, apart from muscle protein, in the long-term

| Occupational activity | | Non-occupational activity | |
|---|---|---|---|
| Professional/Housewife | 1.7 | Reading/eating | 1.2 |
| Domestic Helpers/Salesmen | 2.7 | Household/cooking | 2.1 |
| Labourers | 3.0 | Gardening/golf | 3.7 |
| | | Jogging, swimming, football | 6.9 |

Table 3.2   Physical activity ratio (PAR) for various activities.

esis for energy. Alanine is the primary amino acid released from muscle; it is deaminated and converted into pyruvic acid before entering the citric acid cycle.

## FAT

Dietary fat is chiefly in the form of triglycerides which are esters of glycerol and free fatty acids. Fatty acids vary in chain length from medium chain $C_{8-12}$ to long chain $C_{16-20}$. They also vary in saturation from saturated, which is a hard fat, to monounsaturated or to polyunsaturated, which are liquid, depending on the number of double bonds which are found at position C-3, C-6 or C-9 (designated $\omega$ or n) in the fatty acid chain. The hydrogen related to these double bonds can be in the *cis* or the *trans* positions, most natural fatty acids in food being *cis* (Information box 3.1).

The essential fatty acids (EFAs) are linoleic ($C_{18:2}$ n-6, i.e. 18 carbon atoms, 2 double bonds in position 6) and α-linolenic ($C_{18:3}$ n-3). There are several long chain fatty acids of which arachidonic ($C_{20:4}$ n-6), eicosapentaenoic ($C_{20:5}$ n-3) and docosahexaenoic ($C_{22:6}$ n-3) are physiologically important, but can be made to a limited extent in the tissues from linoleic and linolenic acids.

Syntheses of triglycerides, sterols and phospholipids are very efficient and even with low-fat diets subcutaneous fat stores can be normal.

Dietary fat intake has been implicated in the causation of:
- Cardiovascular disease
- Cancer (particularly breast, colonic and prostatic)
- Obesity
- Non-insulin-dependent diabetes

The data on causation are largely epidemiological and disputed by many. Nevertheless, it is often suggested that the consumption of saturated fatty acids should be reduced with an increase in monounsaturated fatty acids ('Mediterranean diet') or polyunsaturated fatty acids. Any increase in polyunsaturated fats should not, however, exceed 10% of the total food energy, particularly as this requires a big dietary change.

Increased consumption of hydrogenated vegetable and fish oils in margarines has led to an increased *trans* fatty acid consumption and their intake should not, on present evidence, increase more than the current estimated average of 2% of the dietary energy. The current recommendations for fat intake for the UK are:
- Saturated fatty acids should provide approximately 10% of the dietary energy.
- *cis*-Monounsaturated acids (mainly oleic acid) should continue to provide approximately 12% of the dietary energy.

---

Saturated fatty acids—mainly animal fat

n-6 Fatty acids—vegetable oils and other plant foods

n-3 Fatty acids—vegetable foods, rapeseed oil, fish oils

*trans* Fatty acids—hydrogenated, often margarine

**Information box 3.1**  Dietary source of fatty acids.

---

- *cis*-Polyunsaturated acids should provide 6% of dietary energy being derived from n-6 and n-3 polyunsaturated fatty acids.
- Total fat intake should be no more than 35% of the total dietary energy.

Cholesterol is found in all animal products. Eggs are particularly rich in cholesterol, which is virtually absent from plants. The average daily intake in the UK is 300–500 mg. Cholesterol is also synthesized (see p. 239) and only very high or low dietary intakes will significantly affect blood levels.

ESSENTIAL FATTY ACID DEFICIENCY may accompany PEM, but it has only been clearly defined as a clinical entity in patients on long-term parenteral nutrition given glucose, protein and no fat.

## CARBOHYDRATE

Carbohydrate intake comprises the polysaccharide starch, some disaccharides (mainly sucrose) and a small amount of lactose. Carbohydrates are cheap compared with other foodstuffs; a great deal is therefore eaten, usually more than required. Dietary fibre, which is largely non-starch polysaccharide (NSP), is often removed in the processing of food, leaving highly refined carbohydrate such as sucrose.

The principal classes of NSP are cellulose, hemicelluloses, lignins, pectins and gums—none of which are digested by gut enzymes. However, NSP is partly broken down in the gastrointestinal tract, mainly by colonic bacteria, producing gas and volatile fatty acids.

All plant food, when unprocessed, contains NSP, so that all unprocessed food eaten will increase the NSP content of the diet. Bran, the fibre from wheat, provides an easy way of adding additional fibre to the diet. It increases faecal bulk and is helpful in the treatment of constipation. NSP deficiency is now accepted as an entity by many workers in the UK. It is suggested that the total NSP be increased to 25–30 g daily. This could be achieved by increased consumption of bread, potatoes, fruit and vegetables, with a reduction in sugar intake. Each extra gram of fibre daily adds approximately 5 g to the daily stool weight.

Refined carbohydrate, with little or no fibre, is less filling and therefore can be eaten in larger quantities, contributing to obesity.

Pectins and gums have been added to food to slow down monosaccharide absorption, particularly in diabetes.

---

# Protein–energy malnutrition

## IN DEVELOPED COUNTRIES

Starvation is unusual in developed countries, although some degree of undernourishment is seen in very poor

Sepsis
Trauma
Surgery, particularly of gastrointestinal tract with
    complications
Gastrointestinal disease, particularly involving the small
    bowel
Psychological—anorexia nervosa, depression
Dementia
Malignancy
Metabolic disease—renal failure
Any very ill patient

**Table 3.3** Common conditions associated with protein–energy malnutrition.

areas. Most nutritional problems occurring in the population at large are due to eating wrong combinations of food, e.g. excess of refined carbohydrate or diets low in fresh vegetables.

## COMMON CAUSES OF PROTEIN–ENERGY MALNUTRITION

Table 3.3 gives a list of conditions in which malnutrition is commonly seen. Surgical complications, with sepsis, are the commonest cause in most hospitals.

The majority of the weight loss, leading to malnutrition, is due to poor intake secondary to the anorexia associated with the underlying condition. Other factors, such as:

● Increased catabolism in the septic patient
● A cachexia factor in cancer patients
● Malabsorption in patients with gastrointestinal disease only contributes a small amount to the weight loss.

## PATHOPHYSIOLOGY OF STARVATION (Fig. 3.3)

In the first 24 hours following low dietary intake, the body relies on the breakdown of hepatic glycogen to glucose for energy. Hepatic glycogen stores are small and

therefore gluconeogenesis is soon necessary to maintain glucose levels. Gluconeogenesis takes place mainly from lactate, glycerol and amino acids. All endogenous proteins can be utilized to provide amino acids for gluconeogenesis and loss of muscle bulk eventually occurs.

Lipolysis, the breakdown of the body's fat stores, also occurs. It is inhibited by insulin, but the level of this hormone falls off as starvation continues. The stored triglyceride is hydrolysed by lipase to glycerol, which is used for gluconeogenesis, and non-esterified fatty acids that can be used directly as a fuel or oxidized in the liver to ketone bodies. As starvation continues, adaptive processes take place lest the body's protein be completely utilized.

There is a decrease in metabolic rate and total body energy expenditure. Central nervous metabolism changes from glucose as a substrate to ketone bodies, which now become the main source of energy. Gluconeogenesis in the liver decreases with a consequent reduction of protein breakdown, both being inhibited directly by ketone bodies. Most of the energy at this stage comes from adipose tissue, with some gluconeogenesis from amino acids, particularly glutamine, occurring in the kidney.

Following trauma or surgery adaptation does not take place and there is in addition a rise in glucocorticoid and catecholamine levels. In addition, energy requirements are often increased. These changes all result in continuing gluconeogenesis with massive muscle breakdown.

## REGULATION OF METABOLISM

The unavailability of the various substrates in starvation produces dramatic changes in hormone levels, these hormones being the main factors in controlling intracellular metabolism.

In the fed state, insulin/glucagon ratios are high. Insulin promotes synthesis of glycogen, protein and fat, and inhibits lipolysis and gluconeogenesis.

In the fasted state, the insulin/glucagon ratios are low.

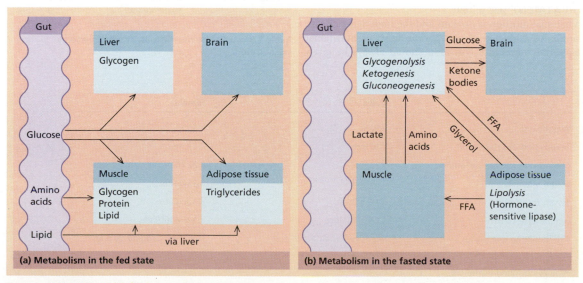

**Fig. 3.3** Metabolism in (a) the fed and (b) the fasted state. FFA, free fatty acids.

Glucagon acts mainly on the liver and has no action on muscle. It increases glycogenolysis and gluconeogenesis, as well as increasing ketone body production from fatty acids. It also stimulates lipolysis in adipose tissue. Catecholamines have a similar action to glucagon but also affect muscle metabolism. These agents both act via cyclic AMP to stimulate lipolysis, producing free fatty acids that can then act as a major source of energy.

Cytokines, such as interleukin 1, interleukin 6 and tumour necrosis factor (TNF) have also been shown to play a role in regulating metabolism. TNF, which inhibits lipoprotein lipase, has been identified as the cachexia factor in cancer patients.

### CLINICAL FEATURES
Patients are sometimes seen with loss of weight or malnutrition (failure to thrive in children) as the primary symptom. Mostly, however, malnourishment is only seen as an accompaniment of some other disease process, e.g. malignancy. The major cause of the weight loss is failure to eat due to anorexia. A careful history may indicate the cause of the weight loss but, if nothing obvious is found, hyperthyroidism must be considered.

Anorexia nervosa commonly occurs in young adolescent females (see p. 987). Patients who have lost more than 10% of their body weight (unless dieting) suffer from malnutrition. Indicators of malnutrition are given in Table 3.4. The clinician can usually decide whether the patient is malnourished by the patient's general appearance. Retrospective dietary evaluation is not helpful, unfortunately, because of the degree of error in patients' recollection of their intake.

Severe malnutrition is mainly seen with advanced organic disease or after surgical procedures followed by complications. PEM leads to a depression of the immunological defence mechanism, leading to decreased resistance to infection (see p. 4).

### TREATMENT (see p. 169)
When malnutrition is obvious and the underlying disease cannot be corrected at once, some form of nutritional support is necessary. Nutrition should always be given enterally if the gastrointestinal tract is functioning adequately. This can most easily be done by encouraging the patient to eat more often and by giving a high-calorie supplement. If this is not possible, a liquefied diet may be given intragastrically via a fine-bore tube. If both of these measures fail, parenteral nutrition is given.

## IN DEVELOPING COUNTRIES

In many areas of the world, many people border on malnutrition. In addition, if events such as drought, war or changes in political climate occur, millions suffer from starvation. Although the basic condition of PEM is the same in all parts of the world from whatever cause, malnutrition due to long periods of near-total starvation produces unique clinical appearances in children virtually never seen in the Western World.

The term PEM covers all the clinical conditions seen in adults and children; a clinical classification is shown in Table 3.5. Marasmus is the childhood form of starvation. Kwashiorkor occurs in a young child displaced from breastfeeding by a new baby and fed a diet with a very low protein content, such as cassava.

This diet, in which energy is not limiting, results in a high plasma insulin and a low plasma cortisol. This hormonal pattern leads to an uptake of amino acids in the muscle (diverting these from the liver) leading to reduced albumin synthesis and, therefore, oedema (i.e. kwashiorkor). Conversely, when energy is limiting, there is an opposite hormonal pattern (i.e. low insulin and high

| Weight (per cent of standard for age) | Oedema | |
| --- | --- | --- |
| | **Present** | **Absent** |
| 60–80 | Kwashiorkor | Undernutrition |
| <60 | Marasmic kwashiorkor | Marasmus |

**Table 3.5**  Wellcome classification of protein–energy malnutrition.

| | **Males** | **Females** |
| --- | --- | --- |
| Weight loss | >10% | >10% |
| Triceps skinfold thickness[a] | <10 mm | <13 mm |
| Mid arm muscle circumference[a] | <23 cm | <22 cm |
| Serum albumin | <35 g litre$^{-1}$ | <35 g litre$^{-1}$ |
| Serum transferrin | <1.5 g litre$^{-1}$ | <1.5 g litre$^{-1}$ |
| Lymphocyte count | <1.5 × 10$^9$/litre | <1.5 × 10$^9$/litre |
| Cell-mediated immunity | Negative *Candida* skin test | Negative *Candida* skin test |

[a]Values obtained in the UK.

**Table 3.4**  Hallmarks of protein–energy malnutrition.

cortisol). Amino acids are now released from the muscles, albumin is synthesized and this results in marasmus rather than kwashiorkor. This classical hypothesis of protein deficiency with adequate carbohydrates as the aetiology of kwashiorkor is difficult to substantiate as most infants will have deficiency of total calorie intake and also other unspecified nutrients. Alternatively, it has been suggested that kwashiorkor results from an imbalance of free radicals and their safe disposal, causing cell membrane damage and oedema.

In addition to the above, infection and diarrhoea with protein loss can affect the clinical picture.

## CLINICAL FEATURES
### Adults
Starvation in adults leads to extreme loss of weight depending upon the severity and duration. They crave for food, complain of cold and weakness with a loss of subcutaneous fat and muscle wasting. In starvation, there is apathy. Infections, i.e. gastrointestinal or bronchopneumonia, are common.

### Children under the age of 5 years (Fig. 3.4)
MARASMUS is the commonest type of severe PEM seen. A child looks emaciated, there is obvious muscle wasting and loss of body fat. There is no oedema. The hair is thin and dry. The child is not so apathetic or anorexic as with

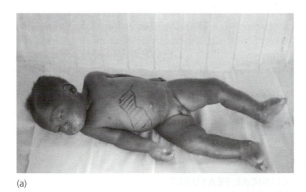

(a)

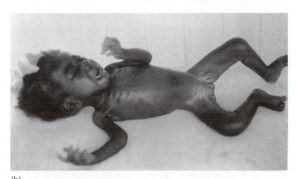

(b)

**Fig. 3.4** Malnourished children. (a) Kwashiorkor; (b) marasmus. (By courtesy of Professor J. Garrow.)

kwashiorkor. Diarrhoea is frequently present and signs of infection must be looked for carefully.

KWASHIORKOR shows the child to be apathetic and lethargic with severe anorexia. There is generalized oedema with skin pigmentation and thickening. The hair is dry, sparse and may become reddish or yellow in colour. The abdomen is distended due to hepatomegaly and/or ascites. The serum albumin is always low.

## INVESTIGATION
This is not always practicable.

ANAEMIA due to folate, iron and copper deficiency is often present, but the haematocrit may be high owing to dehydration.

ELECTROLYTE DISTURBANCES are common.

BLOOD should be examined for malarial parasites and the stools for pathogens.

CHEST X-RAY. Tuberculosis is common and is easily missed if a chest X-ray is not performed.

## TREATMENT
Treatment must involve the provision of protein and energy supplements and the control of infection.

### Resuscitation
The severely ill child will require correction of fluid and electrolyte abnormalities, but intravenous therapy should be avoided if possible because of the danger of fluid overload.

### Refeeding
This needs to be carefully planned and during the initial treatment of the acute case only enough energy and protein should be given to maintain a steady state. Large increases in energy lead to heart failure, circulatory collapse and death. A child requires approximately 100 kcal kg$^{-1}$ (450 kJ kg$^{-1}$) daily, which is provided by 0.6 g kg$^{-1}$ of protein. This is often given as milk with additional water, flour, maize or whatever is available locally. Sugar mixed with dried skimmed milk and small amounts of cottonseed oil (DISCO) is frequently used. Attempts should be made to give the feeds as slowly and as often as possible, although anorexia is often a problem and can be exacerbated by excess feeding. If necessary, fluids and food should be given by nasogastric tube. The child is then gradually weaned to liquids and then solids by mouth.

Hypothermia and hypoglycaemia occur in severely ill children, often with an accompanying infection, and need to be treated urgently. Because of the cold temperatures at night, blankets and sometimes additional heat are necessary.

### Rehabilitation
Gradually, as the child improves, more energy can be given and during rehabilitation maximum weight gain is achieved in the shortest time by extra calories ('catch-up weight gain'). Children who have been severely ill need

constant attention right through the convalescent period, as often home conditions are poor and feeds are refused.

Supplements of vitamins (A, D, B and C) should always be given, together with folic acid and iron. Many children are deficient in minerals such as zinc, copper and selenium, and supplements should be given if deficiency is suspected.

Diarrhoea can lead to potassium deficiency, and glucose electrolyte mixtures (such as the WHO formulation, p. 30) are sometimes necessary. Diarrhoea is often due to bacterial or protozoal overgrowth and metronidazole is very effective and is often given routinely. Parasites are also common and, as facilities for stool examination are usually not available, mebendazole 100 mg twice daily for 3 days should be given. In high-risk areas, antimalarial therapy is given. Adults do not usually suffer such severe malnutrition, but the same principles of treatment should be followed.

### PROGNOSIS

Children with extreme malnutrition have a mortality of over 50%. By careful management this can be significantly reduced to 1–2%. This largely depends on the availability of facilities. Brain development takes place in the first years of life, a time when severe PEM frequently occurs. There is evidence that intellectual impairment and behavioural abnormalities occur in severely affected children. Physical growth is also impaired. Probably both of these effects can be alleviated if it is possible to maintain a high standard of living with a good diet and freedom from infection over a long period.

### PREVENTION

Prevention of PEM depends not only on adequate nutrients being available but also on education of both governments and individuals of the importance of good nutrition (Information box 3.2). Short-term programmes are useful for acute shortages of food, but long-term programmes involving improved agriculture are equally important. Bad feeding practices and infections are more important than actual shortage of food in many areas of the world. However, good surveillance is necessary to avoid periods of famine.

Food supplements (and additional vitamins) should be given to 'at-risk' groups by adding high-energy food, e.g. milk powder, meat concentrates, to the diet. Pregnancy and lactation are times of high energy requirement and supplements have been shown to be beneficial.

# Vitamins

Deficiencies due to inadequate intake (Table 3.6) are commonly seen in the developing countries accompanying PEM. This is not, however, invariable, e.g. vitamin A deficiency is never seen in Jamaica, but is common in PEM in Hyderabad. In the Western World, deficiency of vitamins is rare except in the specific groups shown in Table 3.7. The widespread use of vitamins as 'tonics' is unnecessary and should be discouraged. Toxicity from excess fat-soluble vitamins is occasionally seen.

# Fat-soluble vitamins

## VITAMIN A

Vitamin A (retinol) is found in dairy products, liver and fish, but is also formed in the intestinal wall from its precursor β-carotene found in green leafy vegetables. This is the main source.

## Vitamin A deficiency

Since vitamin A is absorbed in a similar way to all lipids (see p. 202), deficiency can be seen in all chronic conditions where there is fat malabsorption. Nevertheless, the clinical features of vitamin A deficiency are rare in most of these malabsorptive conditions. They are normally only seen associated with severe PEM and other multiple deficiencies in developing countries. As a result of multiple deficiencies being present, it is not always clear which nutrient deficiency is responsible for any one clinical syndrome.

### CLINICAL FEATURES

The clinical features of vitamin A deficiency are impaired dark adaptation followed by night blindness. Later, dryness of the conjunctiva and the cornea (xerophthalmia) occurs as a result of keratinization. Bitot's spots—white plaques of keratinized epithelial cells—are found on the conjunctiva of young children with vitamin A deficiency. These spots can, however, be seen without vitamin A deficiency, possibly due to exposure.

Corneal ulceration and dissolution keratomalacia eventually occur; superimposed infection is a frequent accompaniment. Both may lead to blindness. Vitamin A deficiency is a common cause of blindness in developing countries, affecting 250 000 children per year. Follicular hyperkeratosis, in which there is thickening and dryness of the skin, is also seen with vitamin A deficiency. It is also sometimes seen without vitamin A deficiency.

---

Growth monitoring—**WHO** have a simple growth chart that the mother keeps

Oral rehydration, particularly for diarrhoea (see p. 30)

Breastfeeding supplemented by food after 6 months

Immunization—against measles, tetanus, pertussis, diphtheria, polio and tuberculosis

Family planning

**Information box 3.2**   Prevention of protein–energy malnutrition (a WHO priority programme).

| Vitamin | Daily RNI | Daily LRNI | Major clinical features of deficiency |
|---|---|---|---|
| *Fat-soluble* | | | |
| A (retinol) | 700 μg | 300 μg | Xerophthalmia, night blindness, keratomalacia, follicular hyperkeratosis |
| D (cholecalciferol) | No dietary intake required | 10 μg (living indoors) | Rickets, osteomalacia |
| K | 1 μg kg$^{-1}$ body weight | | Coagulation defects |
| E (α-tocopherol) | $^a$ | | Neurological disorders, e.g. ataxia |
| *Water-soluble* | | | |
| B$_1$ (thiamine) | 0.4 mg per 1000 kcal$^b$ | 0.23 mg per 1000 kcal$^b$ | Beriberi, Wernicke–Korsakoff syndrome |
| B$_2$ (riboflavin) | 1.3 mg | 0.8 mg | Angular stomatitis |
| Niacin (equivalents) | 6.6 mg per 1000 kcal | 4.4 mg per 1000 kcal | Pellagra |
| B$_6$ (pyridoxine) | 15 μg g$^{-1}$ protein | 11 μg g$^{-1}$ protein | Peripheral neuropathy |
| B$_{12}$ (cobalamin) | 1.5 μg | 1.0 μg | Megaloblastic anaemia, neurological disorders |
| Folate | 200 μg | 100 μg | Megaloblastic anaemia |
| C (ascorbic acid) | 40 mg | 10 mg | Scurvy |

$^a$No official RNI because amount varies depending upon polyunsaturated fatty acid content of diet.
$^b$Thiamine requirements are related to energy metabolism.

**Table 3.6**  Fat-soluble and water-soluble vitamins—reference nutrient intake (RNI) and lower reference nutrient intake (LRNI).

*Decreased intake*
Alcohol dependency—chiefly B vitamins, e.g. thiamine
Small bowel disease—chiefly folate, occasionally fat-soluble vitamins
Vegans—vitamin D (if no exposure to sunlight), vitamin B$_{12}$
Elderly with poor diet—chiefly vitamin D (if no exposure to sunlight), folate
Anorexia for any other cause—chiefly folate

*Decreased absorption*
Ileal disease/resection—only vitamin B$_{12}$
Liver and biliary tract disease—fat-soluble vitamins
Intestinal bacterial overgrowth—vitamin B$_{12}$
Oral antibiotics—vitamin K

*Miscellaneous*
Long-term enteral or parenteral nutrition—usually vitamin supplements are given
Renal disease—vitamin D
Drug antagonists, e.g. methotrexate interfering with folate metabolism

**Table 3.7**  Some causes of vitamin deficiency in the Western World.

## DIAGNOSIS

In parts of the world where the deficiency is common, diagnosis is made on the basis of the clinical features and deficiency should always be suspected if any degree of malnutrition is present. Blood levels of vitamin A will usually be low, but the best guide to the diagnosis is a response to replacement therapy.

## TREATMENT

Urgent treatment with retinol palmitate 50 000 i.u. orally should be given on two successive days. In the presence of vomiting and diarrhoea, vitamin A 50 000 i.u. i.m. is given. Associated malnutrition must be treated and superadded bacterial infection should be treated with antibiotics. Referral for specialist ophthalmic treatment is necessary in severe cases.

## PREVENTION

Most Western diets contain enough dairy products and green vegetables but vitamin A is added to foodstuffs, e.g. margarine, in some countries. Vitamin A is not destroyed by cooking. Education of the population is important; in particular, pregnant women and children should be encouraged to eat green vegetables. Vitamin A, but not β-carotene, in excess is teratogenic and can possibly cause liver and CNS damage.

# VITAMIN D

See p. 422.

# VITAMIN K

Vitamin K is present in many plant foods as phylloquinone (vitamin K$_1$). Intestinal bacteria can synthesize menaquinone (vitamin K$_2$), which may make up an important component of daily requirements. Synthesized vitamin K or that derived from the diet (leafy vegetables) is absorbed in a similar manner to other fat-soluble substances and therefore deficiency occurs with malabsorption of fat. Deficiency is most commonly seen in biliary obstruction, when no bile salts are available to facilitate absorption. Antibacterial drugs also interfere with bacterial synthesis of vitamin K.

Vitamin K is a cofactor necessary for the synthesis of clotting factors (see p. 238) and deficiency will increase the prothrombin time. Vitamin K injection (phytomenadione 10 mg i.m.) is effective treatment for vitamin K malabsorption. (NB An increased prothrombin time due to liver disease does not respond to vitamin K, there being no shortage of vitamin K, just poor liver function.) Phytomenadione (1 mg) was always given to all newborn babies but in the UK this practice is not now universal.

# VITAMIN E

Vitamin E occurs mainly in vegetable oils but is also found in fish. Its role in human nutrition is uncertain but severe deficiency leads to anaemia, haemolysis and muscle disorders as well as central nervous lesions. Deficiency is only seen in patients who are virtually unable to absorb any fat or fat-soluble vitamins, e.g. in biliary atresia. In children with abetalipoproteinaemia the severe neurological deficit (gross ataxia) can be prevented by vitamin E injection. Large doses may prevent coronary artery disease.

# *Water-soluble vitamins*

Water-soluble vitamins are non-toxic and relatively cheap and can therefore always be given in excess if a deficiency is possible. The daily requirements of water-soluble vitamins are given in Table 3.6.

## THIAMINE

Thiamine is a co-factor of many enzyme reactions, particularly in the glycolytic pathway. Body stores are small and signs of deficiency will quickly develop with an inadequate intake. Thiamine is found in many foodstuffs and deficiency is only seen:
- As beriberi, where the only food consumed is polished rice
- In chronic alcohol-dependent patients who are consuming virtually no food at all
- Rarely in starved patients, e.g. with carcinoma of the stomach; severe prolonged hyperemesis gravidarum, especially when treated by i.v. fluids alone

## Beriberi

This is now confined to the poorest areas of South East Asia. It can be prevented by eating undermilled or par-

boiled rice, or by fortification of rice with thiamine. Probably the most important factor in the reduction of beriberi is the general increase in overall food consumption so that the staple diet is varied and contains legumes and pulses, which contain a large amount of thiamine. There are two main clinical types of beriberi, which, surprisingly, only rarely occur together.

DRY BERIBERI usually presents insidiously with a symmetrical polyneuropathy. The initial symptoms are heaviness and stiffness of the legs, followed by weakness, numbness, and pins and needles. The ankle jerk reflexes are lost and eventually all the signs of polyneuropathy that may involve the trunk and arms are found (p. 947). Cerebral involvement occurs, producing the picture of the Wernicke–Korsakoff syndrome (p. 947). In endemic areas mild symptoms and signs may be present for years without unduly affecting the patient.

WET BERIBERI causes oedema. Initially this is of the legs, but it can extend to involve the whole body, with ascites and pleural effusions. The peripheral oedema may mask the accompanying features of dry beriberi.

Thiamine deficiency results in inadequate metabolism of glucose and the accumulation of lactate and pyruvate, producing peripheral vasodilatation and eventually oedema. The heart muscle is also affected and heart failure occurs, causing a further increase in the oedema. Initially there are warm extremities, a full, fast, bounding pulse and a raised venous pressure ('high output state') but eventually heart failure advances and a poor cardiac output ensues. The electrocardiogram may show conduction defects.

INFANTILE BERIBERI occurs, usually acutely, in breast-fed babies at approximately 3 months old. The mothers show no signs of thiamine deficiency but presumably their body stores must be virtually nil. The infant becomes anorexic, develops oedema and has some degree of aphonia. Tachycardia and tachypnoea develop and, unless treatment is instituted, death occurs quickly.

### DIAGNOSIS

In endemic areas the diagnosis of beriberi should always be suspected and if in doubt treatment with thiamine should be instituted. A rapid disappearance of oedema after thiamine (50 mg i.m.) is diagnostic. Other causes of oedema must be considered, e.g. renal or liver disease, and the polyneuropathy is indistinguishable from that due to other causes. The diagnosis is confirmed by measurement of transketolase activity in red cells. This enzyme is dependent on thiamine pyrophosphate (TPP). The assay is performed with and without added TPP; an increase in activity of 30% with TPP indicates deficiency.

### TREATMENT

Thiamine 50 mg i.m. is given for 3 days, followed by 20 mg of thiamine daily by mouth. The response in wet beriberi occurs in hours, giving dramatic improvement, but in dry beriberi improvement is often slow to occur. In most cases all the B vitamins are given because of multiple deficiency. Infantile beriberi is treated by giving thiamine to the mother, which is then passed on to the infant via the breast milk.

## Thiamine deficiency in patients with alcohol dependence

In the western hemisphere, this is the only major group to suffer from thiamine deficiency. Rarely they develop wet beriberi, which must be distinguished from alcoholic cardiomyopathy. More usually, however, thiamine deficiency presents with polyneuropathy or with the Wernicke–Korsakoff syndrome. This syndrome, which consists of dementia, ataxia, varying ophthalmoplegia and nystagmus (see p. 947), presents acutely and should be suspected in all heavy drinkers. If treated promptly, it is reversible, but if left, it becomes irreversible; it is a major cause of dementia in the USA.

Urgent treatment with thiamine 50–100 mg i.m. or i.v. is given for 3 days, often combined with other vitamin B complex vitamins. Thiamine must always be given before any intravenous glucose infusion.

## RIBOFLAVIN

Riboflavin is widely distributed throughout all plant and animal cells. Good sources are dairy products, offal and leafy vegetables. Riboflavin is not destroyed appreciably by cooking, but is destroyed by sunlight. Riboflavin is a flavoprotein that is a cofactor for many oxidative reactions in the cell.

Riboflavin deficiency, which is rare in developed countries, is virtually always accompanied by other deficiencies and many features previously attributed to riboflavin deficiency are probably due to multiple deficiencies:

● Angular stomatitis or cheilosis (fissuring at the corners of the mouth)
● A red, inflamed tongue
● Seborrhoeic dermatitis, particularly involving the face (around the nose) and the scrotum or vulva

Riboflavin (5 mg) daily can be tried for the above conditions, usually given as vitamin B complex.

## NIACIN

This is the generic name for the two chemical forms: nicotinic acid and nicotinamide, the latter being found in the two pyridine nucleotides, nicotinamide adenine dinucleotide (NAD) and nicotinamide adenine dinucleotide phosphate (NADP). Both act as hydrogen acceptors in many oxidative reactions and in their reduced forms (NADH and NADPH) act as hydrogen donors in reductive reactions. Many oxidative steps in the production of energy require NAD, and NADP is equally important in the hexose monophosphate shunt for the generation of NADPH, which is necessary for fatty-acid synthesis.

Niacin is found in many foodstuffs, including plants, meat (particularly offal) and fish. Niacin is lost by removing bran from cereals but is added to processed cereals and white bread in many countries.

Niacin can be synthesized in humans from tryptophan, 60 mg of tryptophan being converted to 1 mg of niacin (Fig. 3.5). The amount of niacin in food is given as the niacin equivalent which is equal to the amount of niacin plus one-sixtieth of the tryptophan content.

## Pellagra

This is now rare and is found in people who virtually only eat maize, e.g. in parts of Africa. Maize contains niacin in the form of niacytin, which is biologically unavailable, and has a low content of tryptophan. Many of the features of pellagra can be explained purely by niacin deficiency; some, however, are probably due to multiple deficiencies, including proteins and other vitamins.

### CLINICAL FEATURES

The classical features are of dermatitis, diarrhoea and dementia. Although this is an easily remembered triad, not all are always present and the mental changes are not a true dementia.

### Dermatitis

Initially there is a redness of the skin in the areas exposed to sunlight. This is followed by cracks in the skin, with occasional ulceration. Chronic thickening, dryness and pigmentation develop. The lesions are always symmetrical and often affect the dorsal surfaces of the hands. The perianal skin and vulva are frequently involved. Casal's necklace or collar is the term given to the skin lesion around the neck, which is confined to this area by the clothes worn.

### Diarrhoea

This is often a feature but constipation is occasionally seen. Other gastrointestinal manifestations include painful red raw tongue, glossitis and angular stomatitis. Recurring mouth infections occur.

### Dementia

This occurs in chronic disease. In milder cases there are symptoms of depression, apathy and sometimes thought disorders. Tremor and an encephalopathy frequently occur. Hallucinations and acute psychosis are seen with more severe cases.

Pellagra may also occur in (Fig. 3.5):

THERAPY WITH ISONIAZID, as this can lead to a deficiency of vitamin $B_6$, which is needed for the synthesis of nicotinamide from tryptophan; vitamin $B_6$ is now given concomitantly with isoniazid

HARTNUP DISEASE, a rare inborn error whereby basic amino acids including tryptophan are not absorbed by the gut and there is also loss of this amino acid in the urine

GENERALIZED MALABSORPTION (rare)

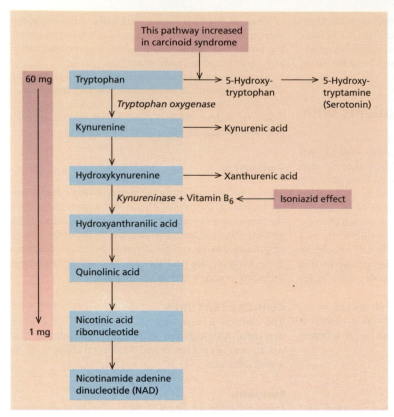

**Fig. 3.5** The oxidative pathway of tryptophan metabolism.

Alcohol-dependent patients who do not eat

Very low protein diets given for renal disease or taken as a food fad

Carcinoid syndrome and phaeochromocytoma, in which tryptophan metabolism is diverted away from the formation of nicotinamide to form amines

### DIAGNOSIS

In endemic areas this is based on the clinical features, remembering that other vitamin deficiencies can produce similar changes, e.g. angular stomatitis. Nicotinamide (approximately 300 mg daily by mouth) with a maintenance dose of 50 mg daily is given. Mostly, however, vitamin B complex is given, as other deficiencies are often present.

An increase in the protein content of the diet and treatment of malnutrition and other vitamin deficiencies is essential. Mild cases respond well but dementia is often permanent.

## VITAMIN B₆

Vitamin B₆ exists as pyridoxine, pyridoxal and pyridoxamine, and is found in plant and animal foodstuffs. Pyridoxal phosphate is involved in the metabolism of amino acids. Dietary deficiency is extremely rare. Some drugs are antagonistic to B₆, e.g. isoniazid, hydralazine and penicillamine. The polyneuropathy occurring after isoniazid usually responds to vitamin B₆. Sideroblastic anaemia occasionally responds to vitamin B₆ (see p. 303).

## BIOTIN AND PANTOTHENIC ACID

Biotin is involved in a number of carboxylase reactions. It occurs in many foodstuffs and the dietary requirement is small. Deficiency is extremely rare and is confined to a few people who consume raw eggs, which contain an antagonist (avidin) to biotin. It causes a dermatitis that responds to biotin replacements.

Pantothenic acid is widely distributed in all foods and deficiency in humans has not been described.

## VITAMIN C

Ascorbic acid is a simple sugar and a powerful reducing agent, its main role being to control the redox potential within cells. It is involved in the hydroxylation of proline to hydroxyproline, which is necessary for the formation of collagen. The failure of this biochemical pathway in vitamin C deficiency accounts for virtually all of the clinical effects found.

Humans, along with a few other animals (e.g. primates and the guinea-pig) are unusual in not being able to synthesize ascorbic acid from glucose.

Vitamin C is present in all fresh fruit and vegetables. Unfortunately, ascorbic acid is easily leached out of vegetables when they are placed in water and it is also oxidized during cooking. Potatoes are a good source as many people eat a lot, but vitamin C is lost during storage.

Vitamin C deficiency is mainly seen in infants fed boiled milk and elderly and single people who cannot be

Keratosis of hair follicles with 'corkscrew' hair
Perifollicular haemorrhages
Swollen, spongy gums with bleeding and superadded
    infection, loosening of teeth
Spontaneous bruising
Spontaneous haemorrhage
Anaemia
Failure of wound healing

Table 3.8  Clinical features of vitamin C deficiency.

bothered to eat vegetables. In the UK it is also seen in Asians eating only rice and chapatis, and in food faddists.

## Scurvy

In adults the early symptoms may be non-specific, with weakness and muscle pain. Other features are shown in Table 3.8. In infantile scurvy there are irritability, painful legs, anaemia and characteristic subperiosteal haemorrhages, particularly into the ends of long bones.

### DIAGNOSIS
The anaemia is usually hypochromic but occasionally a normochromic or megaloblastic anaemia is seen. The type of anaemia depends on whether iron deficiency (due to decreased absorption and loss due to haemorrhage) or folate deficiency (folate is largely found in green vegetables) is present.

Plasma ascorbic acid is very low in obvious deficiency and a vitamin C level of less than 15 μg per $10^8$ cells in the leucocyte–platelet layer (buffy coat) of centrifuged blood indicates deficiency.

### TREATMENT
Ascorbic acid should be given in doses of up to 1 g a day initially and patients should be encouraged to eat fresh fruit and vegetables.

### PREVENTION
Orange juice should be given to bottle-fed infants. The intake of breast-fed infants depends on the mother's diet. In the elderly, eating adequate fruit and vegetables is the best way to avoid scurvy. Careful surveillance of the elderly, particularly those who live alone, is necessary. Ascorbic acid supplements should only be necessary occasionally.

Ascorbic acid in high dosage has been suggested as a treatment of cancer and the common cold. There is some scientific support for its value; however, clinical trials in the common cold have shown that it is of no help.

## VITAMIN B₁₂ AND FOLATE

These are dealt with on p. 304 and in Table 3.6.

## Minerals

A number of minerals have been shown to be essential in animals and an increasing number of deficiency syndromes are becoming recognized in humans. Long-term total parenteral nutrition allowed trace-element deficiency to be studied in controlled conditions; now trace elements are always added to long-term parenteral nutrition regimens. It is highly probable (but difficult to study because of multiple deficiencies) that trace-element deficiency is also an important accompaniment of all PEM states. Sodium, potassium, magnesium and chloride are discussed in Chapter 10.

## IRON (see also p. 300)

The daily RNI for men is 160 μmol (8.7 mg) and for women 260 μmol (14.8 mg).

Iron deficiency is common worldwide, affecting both developing and developed countries alike. It is particularly prevalent in women of a reproductive age.

Dietary iron overload is seen in the South African Bantu men who cook and brew in iron pots.

## COPPER

The daily RNI is 1.2 mg (19 μmol).

## Deficiency

Menkes' kinky hair syndrome is a rare condition due to malabsorption of copper. Infants with this sex-linked abnormality develop growth failure, mental retardation, bone lesions and brittle hair. Anaemia and neutropenia also occur. This condition, which serves as a model for copper deficiency, supports the idea that some of the clinical features seen in PEM are due to copper deficiency. Breast and cows' milk are low in copper and supplementation is occasionally necessary when first treating PEM.

## Toxicity

Copper toxicity occurs in Wilson's disease—see p. 270.

## ZINC

The daily RNI is 9 mg (140 μmol).

Zinc is involved in many metabolic pathways, often acting as a coenzyme; it is essential for the synthesis of RNA and DNA. It is widely available in food.

## Deficiency

Acrodermatitis enteropathica is an inherited disorder due to malabsorption of zinc. Infants develop growth retardation, severe diarrhoea, hair loss and associated *Candida* and bacterial infection. Zinc supplement results in a complete cure.

This condition provides a model for zinc deficiency. Deficiency probably plays a role in PEM.

Zinc levels have also been shown to be low in some patients with malabsorption, skin disease and AIDS, but the exact role of zinc in these situations is disputed. High zinc levels from water stored in galvanized containers interfere with iron and copper metabolism.

## IODINE

The daily RNI is 140 µg (1.1 µmol).

Iodine exists in foods as inorganic iodines which are efficiently absorbed.

Many mountainous areas throughout the world lack iodine in the soil and iodine deficiency is a WHO priority. Endemic goitre occurs in areas where the daily intake is below 70 µg (p. 803) and here 1–5% of babies are born with cretinism. In these areas iodized oil should be given intramuscularly to all reproductive women. In developed countries, salt is iodized and endemic goitre has disappeared.

## FLUORIDE

In areas where the level of fluoride is less than 1 p.p.m. in drinking water, dental caries is more prevalent. Fluoridation of the water reduces this.

Excessive fluorine intake can result in fluorosis, in which there is infiltration of the enamel of the teeth with fluorine, producing pitting and discoloration.

## SELENIUM

The daily RNI is 60 µg (0.8 µmol).

Keshan disease is a selenium-responsive cardiomyopathy found in areas of China.

## CALCIUM (see p. 422)

The daily RNI is 700 mg (17.5 mmol).

This is found in many foods but particularly in milk. Its absorption from the gastrointestinal tract is vitamin D-dependent. Ninety-nine per cent of body calcium is in the skeleton. Increased calcium is required in pregnancy and lactation, when dietary intake must be increased. Calcium deficiency is usually due to vitamin D deficiency.

## PHOSPHATE

The daily RNI is equivalent to calcium, i.e. 17.5 mmol.

Phosphates are present in all natural foods and dietary deficiency has not been described. Patients taking large amounts of aluminium hydroxide can, however, develop phosphate deficiency owing to binding in the gut lumen. It can also be seen in total parenteral nutrition.

Symptoms include anorexia, weakness and osteoporosis.

Other trace elements of possible significance are shown in Table 3.9.

## Nutrition and ageing

Many animal studies have shown that life expectancy can be extended by restricting food intake. It is, however, not

| Element | Deficiency |
|---|---|
| Cadmium | ? |
| Chromium | Glucose intolerance |
| Cobalt | Anaemia |
| Manganese | Growth retardation, skeletal abnormalities, glucose intolerance |
| Molybdenum | ? Animals only |
| Nickel | ? Animals only |
| Vanadium | ? Nutritional oedema |

**Table 3.9** Other trace elements.

known in humans whether the ageing process can be altered by nutrition.

## THE AGEING PROCESS

While wear and tear may play a role in ageing, it does not appear to be a sufficient explanation for the occurrence of ageing. A number of theories have been postulated.

PROGRAMMED AGEING. This theory suggests a predetermined, presumably genetic, age-related alteration in cellular function that leads to susceptibility to disease and death.

THE GENOMIC INSTABILITY THEORY suggests errors in genetic transcription and translation resulting in impaired protein synthesis and deterioration in cell function as age increases.

THE FREE RADICAL THEORY OF AGEING suggests that these highly reactive molecules are no longer metabolized rapidly so that accumulation occurs leading to irreversible cell damage.

RANDOM GENETIC ERRORS have also been implicated and an accumulation of errors over time is said to result in impaired protein synthesis.

Several other mechanisms have been suggested, but it is still unclear whether there is one universal or several independent mechanisms involved.

NUTRITIONAL REQUIREMENTS IN THE ELDERLY. These are qualitatively similar to younger adults, but as energy expenditure is less, there is a lower energy requirement. However, maintaining physical activity is required for the overall health of the elderly.

The daily energy requirements of the elderly have recently been set to be approximately 1.5 × BMR (age 60 and above, irrespective of age). The BMR is reduced due to a fall in the fat-free mass from an average of 60 to 50 kg in men and from 40 to 35 kg in women. The diet should contain the same proportion of nutrients and essential nutrients are still required.

NUTRITIONAL PROBLEMS are due to many factors, such as dental problems, lack of cooking skills, particularly in elderly widowers, depression and sometimes lack of motivation. Significant malnourishment in developed countries is usually secondary to social problems or disease.

In the elderly who are institutionalized, vitamin D supplements may be required as often patients do not go into the sunlight.

Due to the high prevalence of osteoporosis in elderly people, daily calcium intake should be between 1 and 1.5 g.

# Obesity

Some degree of obesity is almost invariable in the Western World and almost all people develop some obesity as they get older. Obesity implies the excess storage of fat and this can most easily be detected by looking at the undressed patient.

|  | Men | Women |
| --- | --- | --- |
| Acceptable weight range | 20.1–25.0 | 18.7–23.8 |
| Obesity | 30+ | 28.6+ |

**Information box 3.3**  BMI values for men and women.

Tables of desirable weights for a given height can be found in the Appendices: 10% greater than these desirable weights is described as overweight; 20% or more than the ideal weight as morbid obesity. Another way of classifying grades of obesity is the body mass index (BMI) (Information box 3.3):

$$BMI = weight\ (kg)/(height\ in\ metres)^2$$

## CAUSES OF OBESITY

Most patients suffer from simple obesity, but in certain conditions obesity is an associated feature (Table 3.10); even in these situations, intake of calories must exceed expenditure. Hormonal imbalance is often incriminated in women, e.g. postmenopause or when taking contraceptive pills, but most weight gain in such cases is usually small and due to water retention.

## SIMPLE OBESITY

Not all obese people eat more than the average, but all obviously eat more than they need.

Genetic syndromes associated with hypogonadism, e.g. Prader–Willi syndrome, Laurence–Moon–Biedl syndrome
Hypothyroidism
Cushing's syndrome
Stein–Leventhal syndrome
Drug-induced, e.g. corticosteroids
Hypothalamic damage, e.g. due to trauma, tumour

**Table 3.10**  Conditions in which obesity is an associated feature.

## Suggested mechanisms

GENETIC AND ENVIRONMENTAL FACTORS. These have always been difficult to separate. However, refeeding experiments in both monozygotic and dizygotic twins, reared together or apart, suggest that genetic influences account for 70% of the differences in BMI later in life and that the childhood environment has little or no influence.

These overfeeding experiments also showed that weight gain did not occur in all pairs of twins, suggesting that in some a facultative increase in thermogenesis occurred so that part of their extra dietary energy was expended inefficiently.

FOOD INTAKE. Many factors related to the home environment, e.g. finance and the availability of sweets and snacks, will affect food intake. Some patients eat more during periods of heavy exercise or during pregnancy and are unable to get back to their former eating habits. The increase in obesity in social class 5 can usually be related to the type of food consumed, i.e. food containing sugar and fat. The underlying mechanisms for controlling satiety are ill-understood; psychological factors and how food is presented may override complex biochemical interactions.

It has been shown that obese patients eat more than they admit to eating and over the years a very small daily excess can lead to a large accumulation of fat.

CONTROL OF APPETITE. This is complex and partially depends on external stimuli, such as the company, the type of food, the surroundings and the usual habitual behaviour.

Appetite is the desire to eat and this usually initiates food intake. Following a meal, satiation occurs. This depends on gastric and duodenal distension and the release of many substances peripherally and centrally.

Cholecystokinin (CCK), bombesin and somatostatin are released from the small intestine and glucagon and insulin from the pancreas following a meal. All of these hormones have been implicated in the control of satiety.

Centrally the hypothalamus, particularly the paraventricular nucleus, and the ventromedial wall of the hypothalamus are thought to be the main satiety centres. Numerous neurotransmitters, e.g. CCK, opioids, serotonin and corticotrophin-releasing hormone, play a role in the central control of satiation.

In obesity, no single abnormality involving appetite control has been identified although the obese eat more than the non-obese.

ENERGY EXPENDITURE. Obese patients tend to expend more energy during physical activity as they have a larger mass to move. On the other hand, many obese patients decrease their amount of physical activity. The energy expended on walking at 3 miles per hour is only 15.5 kJ min$^{-1}$ (3.7 kcal min$^{-1}$) and therefore increasing exercise plays only a small part in losing weight. Nevertheless, as increased body fat develops insidiously over many years, any discrepancy in energy balance is important.

THERMOGENESIS. Brown adipose tissue in animals when stimulated by cold or food dissipates the energy derived from ingested food as heat. This can be a major component of overall energy balance and it has been suggested that this may also apply to humans. A defect in thermogenesis would explain why some obese patients require a very low calorie intake to maintain any weight loss achieved and gain weight easily after only small calorie increases. This mechanism may play some role in the development of obesity.

## CLINICAL FEATURES

Most patients recognize their own problems, although often they are unaware of the main foods that cause obesity. Many symptoms are related to psychological problems, e.g. in women who cannot find fashionable clothes to wear. Social pressures are also important.

The degree of obesity is assessed by comparison with tables of ideal weight for height (see Appendices), the BMI and also by measuring skinfold thickness. This should be measured over the middle of the triceps muscle; normal values are 20 mm in a man and 30 mm in a woman.

Table 3.11 shows the conditions and complications that are associated with obesity. The relationship between cardiovascular disease (hypertension or ischaemic heart disease), hyperlipidaemia, smoking, physical exercise and obesity is complex. Difficulties arise in interpreting mortality figures because of the number of factors involved. Many studies of obesity do not, for instance, differentiate between smokers and non-smokers or between the types of physical exercise that are taken. Many do not take into account the cuff-size artefact in the measurement of blood pressure; an artefact will occur if a large cuff is not used in patients with a large arm. Nevertheless, obesity almost certainly plays a part in all of these diseases and should be treated. The only exception is that stopping smoking, even if accompanied by weight gain, is more important than any of the other factors.

## TREATMENT

This largely depends on a reduction in calorie intake. The commonest diets allow an intake of approximately

---

Psychological
Osteoarthritis
Varicose veins
Hiatus hernia
Gallstones
Postoperative problems
Back strain
Accident proneness
Hypertension
Breathlessness
Ischaemic heart disease
Stroke
Diabetes mellitus
Hyperlipidaemia
Menstrual abnormalities

**Table 3.11**  Conditions and complications associated with obesity.

---

1000 kcal (4200 kJ) per day, although this may need to be nearer 1500 kcal (6300 kJ) per day for someone engaged in physical work. A diet that is too low in total calories will usually result in the patient cheating and keeping to the diet only for short periods. Patients must realize that prolonged dieting is necessary for large amounts of fat to be lost. Furthermore, a permanent change in eating habits is required to maintain the new low weight. It is relatively easy for most patients to lose the first few kilograms, but long-term success in moderate obesity is poor, with an overall success rate of no more than 10–20%.

The aim of any dietary regimen is to lose approximately 1 kg per week. Weight loss will be greater initially owing to accompanying protein and glycogen breakdown and consequent water loss. After 3–4 weeks, weight loss may be very small as only adipose tissue is broken down and there is no accompanying water loss.

Patients must understand the principles of energy intake and expenditure and the best results are obtained in educated, well-motivated patients. Constant supervision, either by a doctor, close relatives or through slimming societies (e.g. WeightWatchers) helps to encourage compliance.

An increase in exercise will increase energy expenditure and should be encouraged, as long as there is no contraindication such as cardiovascular disease. Weight cannot be lost by exercise alone, as even a 15-min brisk daily walk will use less energy than is contained in a small slice of bread and butter.

The diet should contain adequate amounts of each nutrient; a diet of 1000 kcal (4200 kJ) per day should be made up of approximately 100 g of carbohydrate, 50 g of protein and 40 g of fat. The carbohydrate should be in the form of complex carbohydrates such as vegetables and fruit rather than simple sugars. Alcohol contains 7 kcal g$^{-1}$ and should be discouraged. It can be substituted for other foods in the diet, but it often reduces the willpower. With a varied diet, vitamins and minerals will be adequate and supplements are not necessary. A balanced diet, attractively presented, is of much greater value and safer than any of the slimming regimens often advertised in women's magazines.

Most obese people oscillate in weight; they often regain the lost weight, but many manage to lose weight again. This 'cycling' in body weight may play a role in the development of coronary artery disease.

### Drug therapy

Drugs can be used as an adjunct to the dietary regimen but they do not substitute for strict dieting. Amphetamine is addictive, although some less-stimulating derivatives are now available that produce anorexia. However, their use should be discouraged as they cause dependency and psychotic states. The most commonly used drugs are diethylproprion (75 mg daily) and fenfluramine. The latter differs in that it acts on the serotoninergic system rather than the catecholaminergic pathway, which is affected by the amphetamine derivatives. It can be given in doses up to 100 mg daily, but side-effects are frequent.

None of the drugs should be given long-term; they should be withdrawn slowly.

### Surgical treatment

Operations involving bypass of parts of the small intestine have fallen out of favour because of their side-effects and cannot now be recommended. Jejunoileal bypass was the commonest operation and involved the anastomosis of approximately 18 cm of jejunum to the terminal 18 cm of the ileum. Complications are chiefly those of intestinal resection (see p. 210). A fatty liver often occurs and in a few patients cirrhosis is seen.

Three procedures are still performed in cases of severe morbid obesity:

WIRING THE JAWS to prevent eating and allow liquid feeds only. This can be used as a temporary measure but good dental hygiene is essential. Weight gain usually occurs after the wires have been removed, but this can be controlled by the use of a tight waist cord.

GASTRIC PLICATION, in which a small gastric pouch is created by stapling across the wall of the stomach. Good results are claimed without the side-effects of bypass operations.

GASTRIC BALLOON. Here a balloon is placed endoscopically inside the stomach and inflated. Its value has been over-exaggerated and complications include intestinal obstruction.

### MORBIDITY AND MORTALITY

There is an increase in death in obese patients, mainly from diabetes, coronary heart disease and cerebrovascular disease. The greater the obesity the higher the morbidity and mortality figures. For example, men who are 10% overweight have a 13% increased risk of death, whilst the increase in mortality for those 20% overweight is 25%. The rise is less in women. Weight reduction reduces this mortality and therefore should be strongly encouraged.

## Nutritional support in the hospital patient

Nutritional support is now recognized as being necessary in many hospitalized patients. The pathophysiology and hallmarks of malnutrition have been described earlier (p. 157); here the forms of nutritional support that are available are discussed.

### PRINCIPLES

Some form of nutritional supplementation is required in those patients who cannot eat, should not eat, will not eat or cannot eat enough. It is necessary to provide nutritional support for:

- All severely malnourished patients on admission to hospital
- Moderately malnourished patients who, because of

---

*Procedure.*
Fine bore tube with wire stylet inserted intranasally
Confirm position of tube in stomach by aspiration of gastric contents and auscultation of the epigastrium
Check by X-ray if aspiration or auscultation unsuccessful

*Problems*
No satisfactory way of keeping nasogastric tubes in place (up to 60% come out)

*Main complications*
Regurgitation and aspiration into bronchus
Blockage of the nasogastric tube
Gastrointestinal side-effects, the most common being diarrhoea
Metabolic complications including hyperglycaemia and hyperkalaemia, as well as low levels of potassium, magnesium, calcium and phosphate

**Practical box 3.1**   Enteral feeding.

---

their physical illness, are not expected to eat for 3–5 days
- Normally nourished patients not expected to eat for 7–10 days

Enteral rather than parenteral nutrition should always be used if the gastrointestinal tract is functioning normally.

### ENTERAL FEEDING (Practical box 3.1)

Feeds can be given by:
- Mouth.
- Fine-bore nasogastric tube (commonest method).
- Percutaneous endoscopic gastrostomy; this is useful for patients who need enteral nutrition for a prolonged period, e.g. following a head injury with swallowing problems. A catheter is placed percutaneously into the stomach, which has been dilated with air via a gastroscope.
- Needle catheter jejunostomy. A fine catheter is inserted into the jejunum at laparotomy and brought out through the abdominal wall.

### DIET FORMULATION (Table 3.12)

A polymeric diet with whole-protein and fat can be used except in patients with severely impaired gastrointestinal function who may require predigested, i.e. elemental diet.

---

*Energy*
Carbohydrate as glucose polymers (49–53% of total energy)
Fat as triglycerides (30–35% of total energy)

*Nitrogen*
Whole protein (6–7 g of nitrogen per litre)
Ratio of energy to nitrogen (kcal : g) = 150 : 1

Osmolality = 285–300 mosmol kg$^{-1}$

Additional electrolytes, vitamins and trace elements

**Table 3.12**   Standard enteric diet (2000–3000 kcal, approx. 12 000 kJ, per day).

In these patients, the nitrogen source is purified low molecular weight peptides or amino acid mixtures with sometimes the fat being given partly as medium chain triglycerides.

## MANAGEMENT

The aim of any regimen is to achieve a positive nitrogen balance, which can usually be obtained by giving 3–5 g of nitrogen in excess of output. Nitrogen loss can be calculated using the formula:

$N_2$ loss (g per 24 hours)
= urinary urea (mmol per 24 hours) $- 0.028 + 2$

(the 2 representing non-urinary nitrogen excretion).

Daily amounts of diet vary between 2 and 2.5 litres and the full amount can be started immediately.

Hypercatabolic patients require a high supply of nitrogen (15 g per day) and often will not achieve positive nitrogen balance until the primary injury is resolved.

The success of enteral feeding depends on careful supervision of the patient with monitoring of weight, biochemistry and diet charts.

## TOTAL PARENTERAL NUTRITION (TPN)

There are two approaches:

PLACEMENT OF CENTRAL VENOUS CATHETER. This has been the standard approach for many years because of the high incidence of thrombophlebitis in peripheral veins.

PERIPHERAL PARENTERAL NUTRITION. This is now being used with the realization that lower total energy requirements are adequate, i.e. 2000 kcal in 24 hours. Specially formulated mixtures for peripheral use are now available with a low osmolality and containing lipid emulsions. Heparin and corticosteroids are added to the infusion and local application of glyceryl trinitrate patches reduces the occurrence of thrombophlebitis and prolong catheter usage. Initially, peripheral parenteral nutrition is used (each catheter will last for about 5 days) allowing more time to consider the necessity for having to insert a central venous catheter.

TPN is much more complicated and potentially more dangerous than enteral nutrition. It should therefore not be used unless absolutely necessary. It is seldom necessary for periods of less than 10 days.

### Central venous catheter placement (see Practical box 3.2)

A silicone catheter is placed into a central vein, usually using the infraclavicular approach to the subclavian vein. The skin-entry site should be dressed carefully and not disturbed unless there is a suggestion of catheter-related sepsis.

Complications of catheter placement include central vein thrombosis, pneumothorax and embolism, but the major problem is catheter-related sepsis. Organisms, mainly staphylococci, enter along the side of the catheter, leading to septicaemia. Sepsis can be prevented by careful

and sterile placement of the catheter, by not removing the dressing over the catheter entry site, and by not giving other substances (e.g. blood products, antibiotics) via the central vein catheter.

Sepsis should be suspected if the patient develops fever and leucocytosis. In two-thirds of cases, organisms can be grown from the catheter tip. Treatment involves removal of the catheter and appropriate systemic antibiotics.

### Nutrition

With TPN it is possible to provide sufficient nitrogen for protein synthesis and calories to meet energy requirements. Electrolytes, vitamins and trace elements are also necessary. All of these substances are infused simultaneously.

NITROGEN SOURCE. Synthetic L-amino acid solutions are used, which contain between 9 and 17 g of nitrogen per litre. Most patients require at least 14 g of nitrogen per day.

ENERGY SOURCE. This is mainly provided by glucose with additional calories provided by a fat emulsion. Fat infusions provide a greater number of calories in a smaller volume than can be provided by carbohydrate. They are not hypertonic and they also prevent essential fatty acid deficiency.

Essential fatty acid deficiency has been reported in long-term parenteral nutritional regimens without fat emulsions. It causes a scaly skin, hair loss and a delay in healing.

The calorie-to-nitrogen ratio should be approximately (kcal : g) 150:1 (0.6 MJ per gram of protein).

ELECTROLYTES AND TRACE ELEMENTS (Table 3.13) The electrolyte status should be monitored on a daily basis and electrolyte solutions given as appropriate. Water-soluble vitamins can be given daily but fat-soluble vitamins should be given weekly, as overdose can occur. A trace-metal solution is available for patients on long-term parenteral nutrition, but if the patient requires blood transfusions trace-metal supplements are not needed.

### Administration

CENTRAL VENOUS TPN REGIMEN. Most hospitals now use 3-litre bags with the constituents being premixed under sterile conditions by the pharmacy. A standard parenteral nutrition regimen is given in Table 3.14.

PERIPHERAL PARENTERAL NUTRITION. This is administered via 5-litre bags over 48 hours. Table 3.14 shows the composition which provides 12 g of nitrogen and 1500 non-protein calories in 24 hours.

### Complications
- Catheter-related (see above)
- Metabolic, e.g. hyperglycaemia—insulin therapy is usually necessary

This should be performed only by experienced clinicians under aseptic conditions in an operating theatre.

1  The patient is placed supine with 5° of head down tilt to avoid air embolism
2  The skin below the midpoint of the left clavicle is infiltrated with 1–2% lignocaine and a 1 cm skin incision made
3  A 20-gauge needle on a syringe is inserted beneath the clavicle and first rib and angled towards the tip of finger held in the suprasternal notch
4  When blood is aspirated freely, the needle is used as a guide to insert the cannula through the skin incision and into the subclavian vein
5  The catheter is advanced so that its tip lies in the distal part of the superior vena cava
6  A skin tunnel is created under local anaesthetic using an introducer inserted through a point about 10 cm below and medial to the incision and passed upwards to the incision
7  The proximal end of the catheter (with hub removed) is passed backwards through the introducer to emerge 10 cm below the clavicle, where it is sutured to the chest wall
8  The original infraclavicular entry incision is now sutured

**Practical box 3.2**  Central catheter placement for parenteral nutrition.

| | |
|---|---|
| $Na^+$ | 70–220 mmol |
| $K^+$ | 60–120 mmol |
| $Mg^{2+}$ | 5–20 mmol |
| $Ca^{2+}$ | 15–25 mmol |
| $Zn^{2+}$ | 50–100 μmol |
| $Mn^{2+}$ | 120 μmol |
| $Fe^{3+}$ | 70 μmol |
| $Cu^{2+}$ | 20 μmol |
| $Cl^-$ | 70–220 μmol |
| $PO_4^{3-}$ | 15–25 mmol |
| $F^-$ | 50 μmol |
| $I^-$ | 1 μmol |

**Table 3.13**  Daily dietary electrolytes and trace elements required for long-term maintenance.

- Electrolyte disturbances
- Hypercalcaemia
- Liver dysfunction

MONITORING OF PATIENTS ON PARENTERAL NU-TRITION. Essential monitoring includes daily plasma electrolytes and weekly assessments of nutritional status (weight and skinfold thickness). Nitrogen balance should also be measured on a weekly basis. Home parenteral nutrition is occasionally required for patients with virtually no small bowel.

# Food allergy and food intolerance

Many patients ascribe their symptoms to food allergy or food sensitivity and there are a number of clinics in the UK where such sufferers are seen and started on exclusion diets. The scientific evidence that food does harm in most instances is incomplete, but certainly some evidence supports the following disease 'entities':

ACUTE HYPERSENSITIVITY. Some patients develop acute reactions to a particular food, e.g. urticaria, vomiting or diarrhoea after eating strawberries or shellfish. These reactions are presumably immunological hyper-

| | | |
|---|---|---|
| *Central*: all mixed in 3-litre bags; infused over 24 hours | | |
| Nitrogen | Synthamin 14 | 1 litre |
| Energy | Glucose 50% | 0.5 litre |
| | Glucose 20% | 0.5 litre |
| | Lipid 10% | 0.5 litre |
| | e.g. Intralipid | Fractionated soya oil 100 g litre$^{-1}$ |
| | Lipofundin | Soya oil 50 g, medium chain triglycerides 50 g litre$^{-1}$ |
| Electrolytes, water-soluble vitamins, fat-soluble vitamins, trace elements, heparin 2500 u litre$^{-1}$ and insulin 20 u litre$^{-1}$ | | |
| *Peripheral*: all mixed in 5-litre bags; infused over 48 hours | | |
| Nitrogen | Nitrogen 16 g litre$^{-1}$ | 1.5 litres |
| Energy | Glucose 24% | 1 litre |
| | Lipid 20% | 1 litre |
| | Water for injection | 1.5 litres |
| plus | Trace elements, electrolytes and insulin 40 u litre$^{-1}$ | |
| Osmolality 687 mosmol litre$^{-1}$ | | |

**Table 3.14**  Examples of total parenteral nutrition regimens.

sensitivity reactions mediated by IgE. This is usually not a clinical problem as the patients have already learned to avoid the suspected food.

Eczema and asthma—particularly in children—has been successfully treated by removal of eggs from the diet suggesting some form of food allergy.

Rhinitis and asthma have been produced by foods such as milk and chocolate, mainly in atopic subjects; again suggesting some food allergy.

Chronic urticaria. This has been successfully treated by exclusion diet.

Migraine. In some subjects this seems to be triggered by foods such as chocolate, cheese and alcohol suggesting a trigger mechanism, although probably not a true allergic phenomenon.

In addition, some people suffer reactions due to:
- A constituent of food, e.g. the histamine in mackerel or canned food, or the tyramine in cheeses
- Chemical mediators released by food, e.g. histamine may be released by tomatoes or strawberries
- Toxic chemicals found in food, e.g. the food additive tartrazine
- An enzyme deficiency, e.g. milk-induced diarrhoea in alactasia or favabean-induced haemolytic anaemia in glucose-6-phosphate dehydrogenase deficiency

Many other additives and compounds with certain E numbers have been implicated as causing reactions, but here the evidence is less than complete.

There is little or no evidence to suggest that diseases such as arthritis, behaviour and affective disorders, irritable bowel syndrome and Crohn's disease are due to food ingestion.

Multiple vague symptoms such as tiredness or malaise are also not due to food allergy. Most of the patients in this group are suffering from a psychiatric disorder.

## MANAGEMENT

A careful history may help to delineate the causative agent, particularly when the effects are immediate.

Skin-prick testing with allergen and measurement in the serum of antigen or antibodies have not correlated with symptoms and are usually misleading. 'Fringe' techniques such as hair analysis, although widely advertised, are valueless and possibly fraudulent.

Diagnostic exclusion diets are sometimes used, but these are time consuming, although can occasionally be of value in identifying a particular food causing problems.

Dietary challenge is used when the food and the test is given sublingually or by inhalation to try and reproduce the symptoms. Again this may be helpful in a few cases.

Most people who have acute reactions to food realize it and stop the food, and do not require medical attention. In the remainder of patients, a small minority seem to be helped by modifying their diet, but good scientific evidence to support these exclusion diets is non-existent.

# Alcohol

Alcohol is a popular 'nutrient' consumed in large quantities all over the world. In many countries, alcohol consumption is becoming a major problem (see p. 982).

Ethanol (ethyl alcohol) is oxidized in the following steps (Information box 3.4) to acetaldehyde.

1 Acetaldehyde is then converted to acetate mainly in the liver mitochondria.

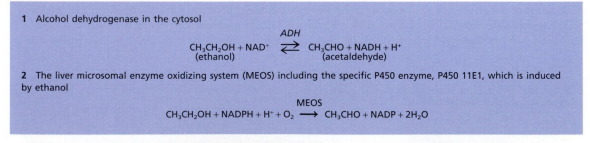

**1** Alcohol dehydrogenase in the cytosol

$$CH_3CH_2OH + NAD^+ \underset{}{\overset{ADH}{\rightleftharpoons}} CH_3CHO + NADH + H^+$$
(ethanol)                              (acetaldehyde)

**2** The liver microsomal enzyme oxidizing system (MEOS) including the specific P450 enzyme, P450 11E1, which is induced by ethanol

$$CH_3CH_2OH + NADPH + H^+ + O_2 \xrightarrow{MEOS} CH_3CHO + NADP + 2H_2O$$

**Information box 3.4**   The main pathways of ethanol oxidization to acetaldehyde.

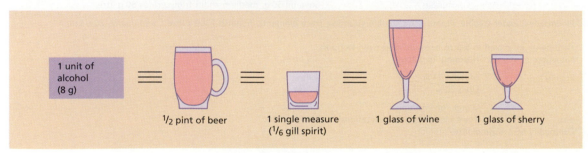

1 unit of alcohol (8 g)  =  ½ pint of beer  =  1 single measure (⅙ gill spirit)  =  1 glass of wine  =  1 glass of sherry

**Fig. 3.6**   Measures of alcohol.

**2** Acetate is released into the blood and oxidized by peripheral tissues to carbon dioxide, fatty acids and water. Alcohol dehydrogenases are found in many tissues and it has been recently suggested that enzymes present in the gastric mucosa may contribute substantially to ethanol metabolism.

Ethanol itself produces $7\,kcal\,g^{-1}$ ($29.3\,kJ\,g^{-1}$), but many alcoholic drinks also contain sugar, which increases their calorific value. For example, one pint of beer provides 250 kcal (1045 kJ). Therefore, the heavy drinker will be unable to lose weight if he or she continues to drink.

## Effects of excess alcohol consumption

Excess consumption of alcohol leads to two major problems, both of which can be present in the same patient:
- Alcohol dependence syndrome—see p. 983
- Physical damage to various tissues

Each unit of alcohol, e.g. half a pint of beer, one single spirit, one small glass of wine, contains 8 g of ethanol (Fig. 3.6). All the long-term effects of excess alcohol consumption are due to excess ethanol, irrespective of the type of alcoholic beverage, i.e. beer and spirits are no different in their long-term effects.

Short-term effects, such as hangovers, depend on additional substances, particularly other alcohols such as isoamyl alcohol, which are known as congeners. Brandy and bourbon contain the highest percentage of congeners.

The amount of alcohol that produces damage varies and not everyone who drinks heavily will suffer physical damage. For example, only 20% of people who drink heavily develop cirrhosis of the liver.

The effect of alcohol on different organs of the body is not the same; in some patients the liver is affected, in others the brain or muscle. The differences may be genetically determined.

In general the effects of a given intake of alcohol seem to be worse in women. The following figures are for men and should be reduced by 50% for women.

### For liver disease
- 160 g ethanol per day (20 single drinks) carries a high risk
- 80 g ethanol per day (10 single drinks) carries a medium risk
- 40 g ethanol per day (five single drinks) carries little risk

Heavy *persistent* drinkers for many years are at greater risk than heavy *sporadic* drinkers.

Susceptibility to damage of different organs is variable and the figures in Information box 3.5 are only a guide.

---

Daily maximum:
  3 units for men
  2 units for women
To help achieve this:
  Use a standard measure
  Do not drink during the day
Have alcohol-free days each week

Remember:
  Health can be damaged without being 'drunk'
  Regular heavy intake is more harmful than occasional binges
  Do not drink to 'drown your problems'

The drinking and driving limit in the UK is a blood level of 800 mg litre$^{-1}$ (80 mg%)
One unit of alcohol is eliminated per hour, therefore spread drinking time
Food decreases absorption and therefore results in a lower blood alcohol level
4–5 units are sufficient to put the blood alcohol level over the legal driving limit in a 70 kg man (less in a lighter person)

**Information box 3.5**  Guide to sensible drinking.

---

*Central nervous system* (see Table 18.54)
e.g. Epilepsy
Wernicke–Korsakoff syndrome
Polyneuropathy

*Muscles*
Acute or chronic myopathy

*Cardiovascular system*
Cardiomyopathy
Beriberi heart disease
Cardiac arrhythmias
Hypertension

*Metabolism*
Hyperuricaemia (gout)
Hyperlipidaemia
Hypoglycaemia
Obesity

*Endocrine system*
Pseudo-Cushing's syndrome

*Respiratory system*
Chest infections

*Gastrointestinal system*
Acute gastritis
Carcinoma of the oesophagus or rectum
Pancreatic disease
Liver disease

*Haemopoiesis*
Macrocytosis (due to direct toxic effect on bone marrow or folate deficiency)
Thrombocytopenia
Leucopenia

*Bone*
Osteoporosis
Osteomalacia

**Table 3.15**  Physical effects of excess alcohol consumption.

**Alcohol consumption in pregnancy**

Women are advised not to drink alcohol at all during pregnancy as even small amounts of alcohol consumed can lead to 'small babies'.

The fetal alcohol syndrome is characterized by mental retardation, dysmorphic features and growth impairment; it occurs in fetuses of alcohol-dependent women.

**Summary**

A summary of the physical effects of alcohol is given in Table 3.15. Details of these diseases are discussed in the relevant chapters. The effects of alcohol withdrawal are discussed on p. 984.

# Further reading

Dietary Reference Values for Food Energy and Nutrients for the United Kingdom. 41 DOH 1991. Report of the Panel on Dietary Reference Values of the Committee on Medical Aspects of Food Policy. London: HMSO.

Garrow GS (1988) *Obesity and Related Disorders*. Edinburgh: Churchill Livingstone.

Truswell AS (1990) *ABC of Nutrition*, 2nd edn. London: British Medical Association.

Shilo ME, Young BR (1988) *Modern Nutrition in Health and Disease*, 7th edn. Philadelphia: Lea & Febiger.

# *Gastroenterology*

## Introduction

Gastrointestinal disease is a major cause of ill-health worldwide. In developing countries infection and malnutrition are common. For example, over a billion people are infested with roundworms and hookworms, and amoebiasis affects over 10% of the world's population. Poor hygiene and malnutrition allows the spread of infective organisms and many infections could be prevented by improved sanitation and education.

In developed countries, much of the work-load is due to non-organic disorders, which are also becoming a worldwide problem. Nevertheless approximately 20% of all cancers occur in the gastrointestinal tract (Fig 4.1).

# *Common symptoms*

## Dysphagia

Dysphagia is difficulty in swallowing (see p. 182).

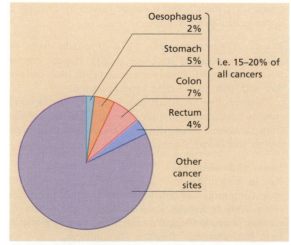

**Fig. 4.1** Incidence (approximate) of cancers at various sites of the gastrointestinal tract.

Oesophagus
2%

Stomach
5%

Colon
7%

Rectum
4%

i.e. 15–20% of all cancers

Other
cancer
sites

## Heartburn

Heartburn is a retrosternal or epigastric burning sensation that spreads upwards to the throat.

## Dyspepsia and indigestion

These are terms often used by lay people to describe any symptom, e.g. nausea, heartburn, acidity, pain or distension, that occurs as a result of eating or drinking. They may also be used to describe an inability to digest food. Careful questioning is required to elicit the exact nature of the patient's complaint. 'Indigestion' is common; 80% of the general population will have had indigestion at some time.

## Flatulence

Flatulence is the term used to describe excessive wind. It indicates belching, abdominal distension (see below) or the passage of flatus per rectum. Excessive belching is not usually associated with organic disease and is a common functional disorder. It is due to air swallowing (aerophagy), which many people do subconsciously. Some of the swallowed air is passed into the intestines, where most is absorbed. Intestinal bacterial breakdown of food, particularly high-fibre legumes, also produces a small amount of gas. Flatus consists of nitrogen, carbon dioxide, hydrogen and methane. On average, flatus is passed 10–20 times per day.

## Hiccups

Hiccups are due to involuntary diaphragmatic contractions with closure of the glottis and are extremely common. Rarely they become continuous, when treatment with chlorpromazine 50 mg three times a day or diazepam 5 mg three times daily may be effective.

## Vomiting

The vomiting centres are located in the lateral reticular formation of the medulla and are stimulated by the chemoreceptor trigger zones (CTZ) in the floor of the fourth ventricle, and also by vagal afferents from the gut. The CTZ are directly stimulated by drugs, motion sickness and metabolic causes. There are three stages:

- Nausea—a feeling of wanting to vomit often associated with autonomic effects including hypersalivation, pallor and sweating
- Retching—a strong involuntary effort to vomit
- Vomiting—the expulsion of gastric contents through the mouth

Many gastrointestinal conditions are associated with vomiting, but nausea and vomiting without pain is frequently non-gastrointestinal in origin (Table 4.1).

CHRONIC NAUSEA AND VOMITING with no other abdominal symptoms are usually due to psychological causes. Early morning vomiting is seen in pregnancy, alcohol dependence and some metabolic disorders, e.g. uraemia.

## Constipation

Constipation is difficult to define in terms of frequency of bowel action because there is considerable individual and geographical variation. Patients usually consider themselves constipated if their bowels are not opened on most days. The difficult passage of hard stools is also regarded as constipation, irrespective of stool frequency.

Normal daily stool weight in the UK is only 50–300 g, whereas in developing countries with a high fibre intake stool weight is 500 g or more with bowel actions two to three times per day.

## Diarrhoea

Diarrhoea is extremely common; a single episode is usually due to dietary indiscretion. True diarrhoea implies the passing of increased amounts (>300 g per 24 hours) of loose stool and is different from the frequent passage of small amounts of stool, which is commonly seen in functional bowel disease. The consistency of the stools is important; watery stools of large volume are always due to an organic cause. Bloody diarrhoea usually implies colonic disease.

Diarrhoea can be either acute or chronic. If it is acute, infective causes must be looked for.

## Steatorrhoea

Steatorrhoea is the passage of pale, bulky stools that contain fat, sometimes float in the lavatory pan and are difficult to flush away. These stools float because of the increased air content. Normally people with steatorrhoea complain of diarrhoea, but occasionally they may pass only one motion per day.

## Abdominal pain

Pain is stimulated mainly by the stretching of smooth muscle or organ capsules. Severe acute abdominal pain can be due to a large number of gastrointestinal conditions, and normally presents as an emergency. An 'acute abdomen' can occasionally be due to referred pain from the chest, as in pneumonia, or to metabolic causes, such as diabetic ketoacidosis.

In patients with abdominal pain the following should be ascertained:

- The site, intensity, character, duration and frequency of the pain
- The aggravating and relieving factors
- Associated symptoms, including non-gastrointestinal symptoms

Localized abdominal pain with tenderness can very rarely arise from the abdominal wall itself. The cause is unknown, but may possibly be due to nerve entrapment; a local anaesthetic injection may help.

### Upper abdominal pain

EPIGASTRIC PAIN. This is very common, often a dull ache, but can be sharp and severe. Its relationship to food intake should be ascertained. It is a common feature of peptic ulcer disease, but it can be caused by a variety of upper gastrointestinal diseases.

RIGHT HYPOCHONDRIAL PAIN is usually from the gallbladder or biliary tract (see p. 281). Hepatic congestion, e.g. in hepatitis, and sometimes peptic ulcer can present with pain in the right hypochondrium.

*Chronic*, often persistent, pain in the right hypochondrium is a frequent symptom in healthy females suffering from functional bowel disease. This chronic pain is not due to gallbladder disease.

### Lower abdominal pain

Pain in the left iliac fossa is usually colonic in origin. It is most commonly associated with functional bowel disease (see p. 230). In females, lower abdominal pain occurs in a number of gynaecological disorders and the differentiation from gastrointestinal disease is often difficult.

Persistent pain in the right iliac fossa over a long period is not due to chronic appendicitis.

---

Any gastrointestinal disease
Acute infections, e.g.
   Influenza
   Pertussis
Central nervous disease, e.g.
   Raised intracranial pressure
   Meningitis
   Vestibular disturbances
   Migraine
Metabolic causes, e.g.
   Uraemia
   Diabetes: ketoacidosis or gastroparesis
   Hypercalcaemia
Drugs, e.g.
   Digitalis toxicity
   Opiates
   Cytotoxics
Reflex, e.g.
   Severe pain—myocardial infarction
Psychogenic
Pregnancy
Alcohol excess

**Table 4.1**  Causes of vomiting.

PROCTALGIA. Proctalgia is a severe pain deep in the rectum that comes on suddenly but lasts only for a short time. It is not due to organic disease.

## Abdominal distension

Abdominal distension or bloating is a common complaint often erroneously attributed to wind. In the absence of physical signs, the symptom is due to functional bowel disease.

## Weight loss

This is due to anorexia (loss of appetite) and is a frequent accompaniment of all gastrointestinal disease. Anorexia is also common in systemic disease and may be seen in psychiatric disorders, particularly anorexia nervosa (see p. 987). Anorexia often accompanies carcinoma but it is a late symptom and not of diagnostic help. Weight loss with a normal or increased dietary intake occurs with hyperthyroidism. Malabsorption is never so severe as to cause weight loss without anorexia. Weight loss should be assessed objectively as patients often 'think' they have lost weight. For a discussion of appetite see p. 167.

## Rectal bleeding (p. 199)

Bright red blood on the toilet paper on wiping the anus is a common symptom of piles (p. 223). There are many other causes (see p. 199).

# Clinical examination

A general examination is performed, with particular emphasis on the examination of all lymph nodes and noting the presence of anaemia or jaundice. Detailed examination of the gastrointestinal tract starts with the mouth and tongue before examining the abdomen.

## Examination of the abdomen (Acute abdomen, see p. 232; Liver disease, see p. 246)

### Inspection
The organs found in a normal abdomen are shown in Fig. 4.2. Fig. 4.3 shows a normal CT scan.

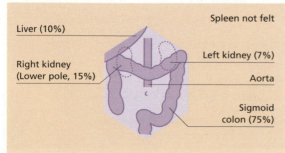

**Fig. 4.2** Organs sometimes palpable (%) in thin subjects.

Liver (10%)

Spleen not felt

Right kidney (Lower pole, 15%)

Left kidney (7%)

Aorta

Sigmoid colon (75%)

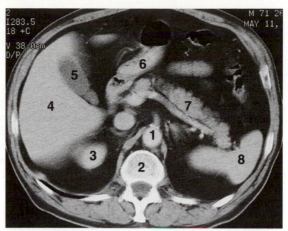

**Fig. 4.3**  CT scan of the normal abdomen at the level of the liver. 1, aorta; 2, spine; 3, top of right kidney; 4, liver; 5, gall bladder; 6, stomach; 7, pancreas; 8, spleen.

Abdominal distension, whether due to flatus, fat, fetus, fluid or faeces, must be looked for. Lordosis may give the appearance of a distended abdomen; it is a common feature of the 'abdominal distension' seen in functional bowel disease.

**Palpation**
The abdominal organs may be felt in some normal subjects (see Fig. 4.2) but this is not common and such organs are usually only just palpable.

Any palpable mass is carefully felt to decide which organs are involved and also to evaluate its size, shape and consistency and whether it moves with respiration.

The hernial orifices should be examined if intestinal obstruction is suspected.

A succussion splash suggests gastric outlet obstruction if the patient has not drunk for 2–3 hours; the splash of fluid in the stomach can be heard with a stethoscope laid on the abdomen when the patient is moved.

**Percussion**
This is performed in the usual way to detect the area of dullness caused by the liver and spleen, and possibly bladder enlargement. The presence of fluid in the peritoneal cavity, i.e. ascites, is detected by shifting dullness. The percussion note changes from resonance to dullness when the patient is moved from one side to the other. It is a good physical sign if performed carefully but 1–2 litres of fluid must be present to elicit it. A fluid 'thrill' can be elicited, but is not always helpful. A large ovarian cyst can sometimes produce an enlarged abdomen, but the dullness is more centrally placed than in ascites.

**Auscultation**
Auscultation is not of great value in gastrointestinal disease, apart from in the evaluation of the acute abdomen. Abdominal bruits are often present in normal subjects,

but these are not clinically significant. Intestinal sounds do not help in diagnosis.

## Examination of the rectum and sigmoid

Digital examination of the rectum should be performed in most patients with gastrointestinal symptoms and in all patients with a change in bowel habit. The anus should be inspected for anal tags, external haemorrhoids, fissures or fistulas. In males, the prostate projects into the rectum anteriorly and its size and consistency should be noted. In women the cervix or uterus may be felt anteriorly.

SIGMOIDOSCOPY (Practical box 4.1) should, in hospital, be part of the routine examination in all cases of diarrhoea and in patients with lower abdominal symptoms such as a change in bowel habit or bleeding.

PROCTOSCOPY (Practical box 4.1) is performed in all patients with a history of bright red blood per rectum; the narrow sigmoidoscope does not distend the lumen and haemorrhoids can be missed.

### Flexible-fibre sigmoidoscopy

The rigid sigmoidoscope allows inspection of only the lower 20–25 cm of the bowel, but a 70 cm flexible fibreoptic sigmoidoscope allows much more bowel to be visualized. It also can be readily used in the outpatient department after minimal bowel preparation (a disposable enema). Seventy per cent of colonic neoplasms occur within the range of the flexible sigmoidoscope.

### Stool examination

This can be occasionally useful to confirm the patient's symptoms, e.g. passing of blood or steatorrhoea. The shape and size may be helpful, e.g. rabbity stools in the irritable bowel syndrome. Stool charts for recording frequency and volume of defecation are useful in inpatients to follow the progress of diarrhoea.

## *Investigation*

Radiology and endoscopy are the principal investigations. These are usually preceded by routine haematology and biochemistry.

## Plain X-rays

Plain X-rays of the abdomen are chiefly used in the investigation of acute abdomen (see p. 233). Areas of calcification can be seen in chronic pancreatitis (see p. 289). Routine abdominal X-rays are of little use in the management of most gastrointestinal disease.

## Barium contrast studies (Practical box 4.2)

### Barium swallow

The oesophagus is visualized as barium is swallowed in the upright and prone positions. Motility abnormalities

---

1  Upper gastrointestinal series—patients are fasted overnight.
2  Barium enema patients are given a low-fibre diet for 3 days and laxatives 24 hours before the procedure.
3  The radiologist should be given correct clinical information so that the particular area under suspicion can be scrutinized.
4  The radiologist screens the patient so that any suspicious area can be re-examined immediately.
5  X-rays should be reviewed by the clinician with the radiologist.

**Practical box 4.2**   Barium contrast studies—useful facts.

---

**Sigmoidoscopy**

The technique is easy to learn, provides valuable information and is safe in competent hands.

1  The patient is placed in the left lateral position with the knees drawn up, and the buttocks over the edge of the couch.
2  No bowel preparation is required.
3  Rectal examination is initially performed.
4  The sigmoidoscope is pointed towards the symphysis pubis and passed into the anus. The obturator is removed and the instrument passed under direct vision to the rectosigmoid junction and beyond if possible (using air insufflation).
5  The mucosa of the anus and rectum is inspected. The normal mucosa is shiny, superficial vessels can be seen and no contact bleeding should occur.
6  Biopsies can be taken of any lesions seen or from apparently normal-looking mucosa which may show histological evidence of inflammation.
7  The technique is relatively painless. In the irritable bowel syndrome, the patient's pain is often reproduced by air insufflation.

**Proctoscopy**

1  The proctoscope is passed into the anus directed towards the symphysis pubis and the obturator is removed.
2  The patient strains down as the proctoscope is removed.
3  Haemorrhoids are seen as purplish veins in the left lateral, right posterior or right anterior positions.
4  Fissures may also be seen.

**Practical box 4.1**   Sigmoidoscopy and proctoscopy.

as well as anatomical lesions can then be observed. Reflux of barium from the stomach into the oesophagus is demonstrated with the patient tipped head down, but minimal reflux under these conditions may well have no clinical significance.

Swallowing bread with the barium (to add bulk) is sometimes useful in a difficult case of dysphagia.

### Barium meal

This is performed to examine the stomach and duodenum. A small amount of barium is given together with effervescent granules or tablets to produce carbon dioxide so that a double contrast between air and barium is obtained. This technique has a high accuracy rate when performed carefully. Single-contrast studies are not recommended.

### Small bowel follow-through

This is used to examine the small bowel and ideally should be performed separately from a barium meal as a different technique is employed. Barium is swallowed and allowed to pass into the small intestine through the jejunum and into the ileum. This technique is the only way of demonstrating the gross anatomy of the small intestine. Views of the terminal ileum should be obtained with the use of a compression pad.

### Small bowel enema (enteroclysis)

A tube is passed through the duodenum and a large volume of dilute barium is introduced. This technique is useful for visualizing suspicious areas seen on the follow-through, particularly strictures.

### Barium enema

Barium and air are insufflated into the rectum via a retained catheter. A double-contrast view is then obtained of the whole colon, often with views of the terminal ileum as well. The patient must be prepared well with laxatives and wash-outs so that the colon is empty. Rectal examination and sigmoidoscopy usually precede this examination.

## Abdominal ultrasound, computed tomography (CT) and magnetic resonance imaging (MRI)

These techniques are being increasingly used for detecting thickened bowel, masses, abscesses and fistulas in, for example, Crohn's disease or tuberculosis. CT, endoscopic ultrasound and MRI are also being used for evaluating tumour size and spread.

## Endoscopy (Practical box 4.3)

Video endoscopes producing images of high quality are now available. This technical advance allows easy data collection.

OESOPHAGOGASTRODUODENOSCOPY (OGD) is often used as the investigation of choice for upper gastrointestinal disorders by gastroenterologists because of easy access, the possibility of interventional therapy and obtaining mucosal biopsies.

COLONOSCOPY allows good visualization of the whole colon and terminal ileum. Biopsies can be obtained and polyps removed. The success rate for reaching the terminal ileum is approximately 80% and the mortality is 1 : 100 000. The major complication is perforation.

Barium studies and endoscopy are frequently complementary and the technique chosen often depends on

---

**Gastroscopy**

1 The patient is fasted overnight and the procedure is carried out as an outpatient.
2 The throat is sprayed with lignocaine.
3 Intravenous sedation is given for the very anxious patient or for additional procedures.
4 $O_2$ via nasal prongs is given to elderly patients.
5 The instrument is passed into the pharynx under direct vision, then down the oesophagus into the stomach and duodenum.
6 The forward-viewing instrument is used for visualization of the oesophagus, stomach and duodenal cap.
7 The side-viewing instrument is needed to visualize certain areas, e.g. the ampulla of Vater.
8 The patient must be 'nil by mouth' for approximately $1\frac{1}{2}$ hours following the procedure.

**Colonoscopy**

1 Two days before procedure—low-residue diet started.
2 One day before procedure—clear fluids only.
3 Afternoon before procedure—71 ml extract of senna with one pint of water is given.
4 Three hours later—one sachet of sodium picosulphate with one pint of water is given.
5 Day of procedure—one sachet of sodium picosulphate with one pint of water is given.
6 Alternative preparation consists of giving large volumes of balanced electrolyte solution by mouth on the day of the test.
7 The instrument is passed under direct vision, and manoeuvred around to the caecum and terminal ileum. Sedation, along with pethidine and hyoscine butyl bromide, is required. Observation is required of sedated patients for 2 hours following procedure.

**Practical box 4.3** Gastroscopy and colonoscopy.

local expertise and work-load. Radiology is better than endoscopy for assessing motility disorders, extrinsic lesions and gastro-oesophageal reflux. Endoscopy is preferable in gastric ulcer disease (as biopsies can be obtained) and in the detection of oesophagitis. Colonoscopy is used in the sick immobile patient, in inflammatory bowel disease, for polyp follow-up and in the investigation of rectal bleeding. Barium enema is usually performed for the investigation of change in bowel habit.

## Radionuclide imaging

Radionuclides are used to a varying degree depending on local enthusiasm and expertise.

Indications are:

- To demonstrate oesophageal reflux using [$^{99m}$Tc]sulphur colloid
- To determine the rate of gastric emptying using [$^{99m}$Tc]-sulphur colloid
- To demonstrate a Meckel's diverticulum using [$^{99m}$Tc]-pertechnetate which has an affinity for gastric mucosa
- To show inflammation and an inflammatory mass in inflammatory bowel disease using $^{111}$In-labelled white cells
- Isotopic techniques can also be used to assess gastrointestinal loss of red cells, albumin and bile acids, and the retention of vitamin B$_{12}$

## The mouth

Mastication of the food takes place in the mouth. The food then passes into the pharynx. Problems in the mouth are extremely common and although they may be trivial they can produce severe symptoms. Poor dental hygiene is often a factor. A bad taste in the mouth and offensive breath (halitosis), particularly if only noticed by the patient, are psychogenic symptoms. Patients with gastric outflow obstruction rarely have halitosis.

Stomatitis is inflammation in the mouth from any cause, such as ill-fitting dentures. Angular stomatitis is inflammation of the corners of the mouth.

## Common mouth lesions

### Ulceration

#### Infective

HERPES SIMPLEX VIRUS type 1, or rarely type 2, presents with fever and widespread confluent painful oral ulcers. After spontaneous resolution, the virus remains latent and recurs as herpes labialis (cold sores) (see p. 1014).

HAND, FOOT AND MOUTH DISEASE due to Coxsackie A virus produces mouth vesicles, usually in children. No

treatment is required. *Herpes zoster* involving the fifth cranial nerve can produce unilateral vesicular lesions (see p. 889).

#### Non-infective

RECURRENT APHTHOUS ULCERATION of unknown aetiology affects approximately 20% of the population and is characterized by recurrent episodes of painful oral ulcers. There are three main clinical types:

- Minor aphthae are 2–4 mm ulcers which heal in 4–14 days without scarring
- Major aphthae are larger and take longer to heal (2–10 weeks), sometimes with scarring
- Herpetiform ulcers in which many (10–100) tiny ulcers coalesce to form large ulcers

The term 'herpetiform' is purely descriptive and does not imply an infective aetiology. The ulcers are sometimes associated with gastrointestinal disease, notably Crohn's disease, ulcerative colitis and coeliac disease. Other diseases associated with oral ulcers include Behçet's disease, Reiter's disease and systemic lupus erythematosus. Deficiencies of iron, folic acid and vitamin B$_{12}$ have been noted in some patients, but in most no cause is found.

Topical corticosteroids may lessen the duration and severity of an attack. The natural history is for the attacks to occur less frequently as the patient ages.

Trauma, sharp teeth or ill-fitting dentures are common causes of all ulcers. Ulcers due to syphilis and tuberculosis are seen in developing countries and rarely in the UK.

SQUAMOUS CELL CARCINOMA. This presents as an indolent ulcer with surrounding induration mainly seen on the tongue and the floor of the mouth. Aetiological factors include tobacco and alcohol, particularly spirits. It used to affect men, mainly in the 50–70 age bracket, but now younger patients or women without obvious risk factors are seen. Biopsy should be undertaken and treatment is with surgery and radiotherapy.

## Vesiculo-bullous disorders

Pemphigus, bullous pemphigoid and benign mucous membrane pemphigoid all cause oral bullae. A severe form of erythema multiforme, known as the Stevens–Johnson syndrome, also has bullae affecting the oral mucosa and conjunctiva.

## Oral white patches

White lesions may be transient or persistent. Transient white patches are either due to *Candida* infection or are very occasionally seen in *systemic lupus erythematosus*. Oral candidiasis in adults is seen in seriously ill or immunocompromised patients, or following therapy with broad spectrum antibiotics or inhaled steroids. Local causes include mechanical, irritative or chemical trauma from drugs, e.g. aspirin. *Leucoplakia* describes white patches for which no local cause can be found. It is associated with alcohol, and particularly smoking, and is regarded as a premalignant condition. A biopsy should always be undertaken, histology showing alteration in the keratinization and dysplasia of the epithelium. Treatment with isotretinoin reduces disease progression. Oral *lichen planus* presents as white striae.

## The tongue

The tongue may be ulcerated in association with more general oral mucosal ulceration. A single ulcer may be malignant and this must be considered in any ulcer which persists for more than 3 weeks (see above).

Loss of filliform papillae producing a smooth sore tongue (atrophic glossitis) can occur in patients with iron, vitamin $B_{12}$ or vitamin folate deficiency. A painful tongue without any evidence of abnormality is often psychological in nature, although deficiency states must be excluded.

Geographic tongue affects 10% of the population. There are discrete areas of depapillation on the dorsum of the tongue which change over a few days or even hours. Geographic tongue may be asymptomatic or the patient may complain of a sore tongue. The aetiology is unknown and there is no treatment other than reassurance.

## The gums

The gum or gingiva is the tissue covering the alveolar process of the mandible and maxilla, and surrounds the necks of the teeth. Bleeding of the gums affects most of the adult population at some time and is due to gingivitis. This is an inflammatory process caused by failure to remove bacteria in the form of plaque from the tooth–gingival junction. Less commonly, bleeding may be associated with a general bleeding disorder. Patients with acute leukaemia, as well as immunocompromised patients often have severe gingivitis with bleeding.

Acute ulcerative gingivitis (Vincent's infection) occurs in the malnourished patient with poor dentition and in the immunosuppressed. It is characterized by ulceration and is usually restricted to the gingiva, particularly the interdental papillae. Smears of affected areas show a mixed infection of fusobacteria and spirochaetes.

Treatment is with oral metronidazole, 200 mg three times daily, for 1 week with accompanying good mouth and oral hygiene. Failure to treat this condition properly may predispose to a more widespread infection, particularly in the immunosuppressed, termed cancrum oris.

Ulceration of the gums may occur in association with more generalized oral ulceration as described above. Generalized gum swelling is a feature of chronic gingivitis and may be a side-effect of pregnancy, various systemic diseases and some drugs, e.g. cyclosporin, phenytoin and nifedipine.

## AIDS and the mouth

Oral lesions are frequently seen in patients with AIDS. Some of these lesions, e.g. *Candida*, aphthous ulceration and acute ulcerative gingivitis, simply reflect immuno-suppression and are not specific for AIDS. The other lesions described are more specific for AIDS. *Kaposi's sarcoma* presents as red/blue or purple patches which may be perioral or in the mouth usually on the palate at the junction of the hard and soft palate. Hairy leucoplakia is characterized by white patches which cannot be removed, usually affecting the lateral surface of the tongue. There is intense epithelial hyperplasia giving rise to a hairy appearance. Hairy leucoplakia is an indicator of a poor prognosis in these patients.

# The salivary glands

## Xerostomia

Xerostomia means dryness of the mouth. Causes include:
- Psychogenic—anxiety
- Pyrexia
- Drugs—anticholinergics, antihistamines, and tricyclic and related antidepressants
- Sjögren's syndrome (see p. 405)
- Diabetic ketoacidosis and dehydration

The sensation of excess salivation (ptyalism) is chiefly psychogenic. It occurs before vomiting and with lesions of the mouth.

## Bacterial and viral infections

These can affect any of the salivary glands, the commonest condition being acute parotitis due to the mumps virus. Acute parotitis due to an ascending infection with staphylococci or streptococci occurs in alcohol-dependent patients and in elderly patients, usually associated with dehydration and poor oral hygiene. Treatment consists of antibiotic and drainage of any abscess that is demonstrated.

## Sarcoidosis

This can produce parotid gland enlargement. When combined with lacrimal gland enlargement it is known as Mikulicz syndrome.

## Salivary duct obstruction due to calculus

Obstruction due to calculus usually involves the submandibular gland. There is painful swelling of the gland after eating. The stones can sometimes be felt in the floor of the mouth and their removal is usually followed by complete relief of symptoms.

## Tumours

Salivary gland tumours are usually of a mixed type. They may involve any of the salivary glands but usually affect the parotid. The gland becomes swollen but not tender and treatment is by removal, although local recurrences occur.

# The pharynx and oesophagus

## STRUCTURE

The oesophagus is a muscular tube, approximately 25 cm long, connecting the pharynx to the stomach. The muscle coat has two layers—an outer longitudinal layer and an inner circular layer of fibres. In the upper portion both muscle layers are striated. They gradually change to smooth muscle in the lower oesophagus, where they are continuous with the muscle layer of the stomach. The oesophagus is lined by stratified squamous epithelium, except near the gastro-oesophageal junction where columnar epithelium is found.

## FUNCTION

The oesophagus is separated from the pharynx by the *upper oesophageal sphincter*, which is normally closed by the continuous contraction of cricopharyngeus muscle.

The *lower oesophageal sphincter* (LOS) consists of an area of the distal end of the oesophagus that has a high resting tone and is largely responsible for the prevention of reflux. The reduction in tone and relaxation that occurs with swallowing is under the control of nervous (vagal) and hormonal mechanisms.

During swallowing, the bolus of food is moved from the mouth to the pharynx voluntarily. Immediately, the upper sphincter relaxes and food enters the oesophagus. A primary peristaltic wave starts in the pharynx at the onset of swallowing and sweeps down the whole oesophagus (Fig. 4.4). Secondary peristalsis occurs locally in response to direct stimulation (e.g. distension by the bolus) and helps to clear food residue from the oesophagus. Non-peristaltic, non-propulsive tertiary waves are frequent in the elderly. The LOS relaxes when swallowing is initiated, before the arrival of the peristaltic wave.

## SYMPTOMS OF OESOPHAGEAL DISORDERS

Major oesophageal symptoms are:
- Dysphagia
- Heartburn
- Painful swallowing

### Dysphagia

This is either due to a local lesion or is part of a generalized disease. Patients will complain of something

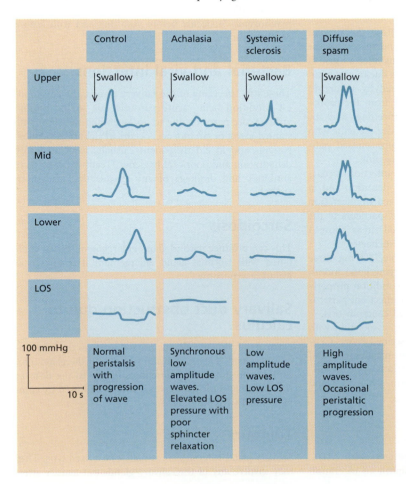

**Fig. 4.4** Oesophageal manometric patterns in normal and diseased states. **LOS**, lower oesophageal sphincter.

sticking in their throat or chest during swallowing or immediately afterwards. It is always a serious symptom and the cause must be found. The causes are shown in Table 4.2; benign and malignant oesophageal strictures are the commonest causes seen in hospital practice. Globus hystericus is the name given to apparent dysphagia—the sensation of a 'lump in the throat' in patients who do not have true dysphagia and can therefore swallow. It has no organic cause and the treatment is reassurance.

### Heartburn

Heartburn is a common symptom of acid reflux. The pain can spread to the neck, across the chest, and can be difficult to distinguish from the pain of ischaemic heart disease. It can also occur at night when the patient lies flat or after bending or stooping. Hot drinks and alcohol often precipitate the pain.

### Painful swallowing

Painful swallowing without real difficulty is a symptom of candidiasis and herpes simplex infection. Both these conditions are seen in AIDS patients. Ingestion of tablets such as emepronium and potassium (slow release) will produce local ulceration if they lodge in the gullet when swallowed lying down and without water.

### SIGNS OF OESOPHAGEAL DISORDERS

There are very few signs associated with oesophageal disease, the main one being of weight loss as a consequence of dysphagia.

### INVESTIGATION OF OESOPHAGEAL DISORDERS

BARIUM SWALLOW AND MEAL
OESOPHAGOSCOPY

Disease of mouth and tongue, e.g. tonsillitis

Neuromuscular disorders
  Pharyngeal disorders
  Bulbar palsy
  Myasthenia gravis
  Oesophageal motility disorders
  Achalasia
  Scleroderma
  Diffuse oesophageal spasm
  Presbyoesophagus
  Diabetes
  Chagas' disease

Extrinsic pressure
  Mediastinal glands
  Goitre
  Enlarged left atrium

Intrinsic lesion
  Foreign body
  Stricture
    Benign—peptic, corrosive
    Malignant—carcinoma
  Lower oesophageal rings
    Oesophageal web
    Pharyngeal pouch

**Table 4.2** Causes of dysphagia.

MANOMETRY, which is performed by passing a fluid-filled catheter through the nose into the oesophagus. Changes in pressure are transmitted up the fluid column and recorded. These studies are useful in motility disorders.

BERNSTEIN TEST—alternate dilute acid and alkali is infused into the oesophagus via a nasal tube to try to reproduce or relieve oesophageal pain. A positive test suggests oesophagitis but there are many false negatives.

pH MONITORING—24-hour monitoring using a pH-sensitive probe positioned in the lower oesophagus is being used increasingly for the identification of reflux episodes (pH <4). Brief episodes can, however, occur in normal subjects.

RADIOISOTOPE STUDIES with technetium–sulphur colloid incorporated into food can also be used to study reflux. It is not widely used in the UK.

## MOTILITY DISORDERS

### Achalasia

Achalasia is a disease of unknown aetiology which is characterized by aperistalsis in the body of the oesophagus and failure of relaxation of the LOS on initiation of swallowing.

#### PATHOLOGY
Degenerative lesions are found in the vagus as well as a decrease in ganglionic cells in the nerve plexus of the oesophageal wall.

#### CLINICAL FEATURES
The disease can present at any age but is rare in childhood. The incidence is about 1 : 100 000 per year. Patients usually have a long history of intermittent dysphagia for both liquids and solids. Regurgitation of food from the dilated oesophagus may be induced by the patient or may occur spontaneously, particularly at night, and aspiration pneumonia may result. Occasionally food gets stuck but patients often learn to overcome this by drinking large quantities, thereby increasing the head of pressure in the oesophagus and forcing the food through. Severe retrosternal chest pain occurs particularly in younger patients with vigorous non-peristaltic contraction of the oesophagus. The dysphagia in these patients can be mild and the pain misdiagnosed as cardiac in origin. Weight loss is usually not marked.

#### INVESTIGATION
A CHEST X-RAY may show a dilated oesophagus, with an occasional fluid level, behind the heart. The fundal gas shadow is not present.

A BARIUM SWALLOW will show dilatation of the oesophagus, lack of peristalsis and often synchronous contractions. The lower end gradually narrows (beak deformity); this appearance is due to failure of the sphincter to relax (Fig. 4.5).

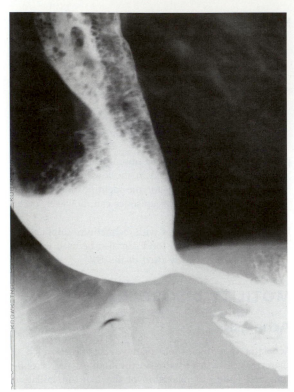

**Fig. 4.5** Barium swallow showing achalasia with atonic body of the oesophagus and a narrowed distal end. Note food residue in dilated oesophagus.

OESOPHAGOSCOPY is necessary to exclude a carcinoma at the lower end of the oesophagus, as this can produce a similar X-ray appearance. When there is marked dilatation, extensive cleansing is necessary to remove food debris in order to obtain a clear view. In achalasia the oesophagoscope easily flops through the apparent narrowing without resistance.

MANOMETRY is used to measure oesophageal motility. It shows aperistalsis of the oesophagus as well as the failure of relaxation of the LOS (see Fig. 4.4).

Chagas' disease (American trypanosomiasis, see p. 67) damages the neural plexus of the gut and produces a similar clinical picture.

### TREATMENT

The LOS is dilated forcibly using a pneumatic bag (passed under X-ray control) so as to weaken the sphincter. This is successful in 80% of cases. Surgical division of the muscle at the lower end of the oesophagus (cardiomyotomy or Heller's operation) is now being performed laparoscopically. Reflux oesophagitis complicates both procedures and the aperistalsis of the oesophagus remains. In older patients, nifedipine (20 mg sublingually) can be tried initially.

### COMPLICATIONS

There is an increased incidence of 5–10% of carcinoma of the oesophagus in both treated and untreated cases.

## Systemic sclerosis (see p. 402)

In 90% or more of patients with this disease there is oesophageal involvement, with diminished peristalsis detected manometrically (see Fig. 4.4) or by barium swallow. This is due to replacement of the smooth muscle layers by fibrous tissue. The LOS pressure is also decreased, allowing reflux; mucosal damage may occur as a consequence. Strictures may develop. Initially there are no symptoms, but dysphagia and heartburn occur as the oesophagus becomes severely involved.

Similar motility abnormalities may be found in other connective-tissue disorders, particularly if Raynaud's phenomenon is present. Treatment is as for reflux (see p. 187) and stricture formation (see below).

## Diffuse oesophageal spasm

This is a severe form of abnormal oesophageal motility that can sometimes produce retrosternal chest pain and dysphagia. Swallowing is accompanied by bizarre and marked contractions of the oesophagus without progression of the waves (see Fig. 4.4). On barium swallow the appearance may be of a 'corkscrew'. However, asymptomatic changes in oesophageal motility are not infrequent, particularly in patients over the age of 60 years (presbyoesophagus). Care must therefore be taken that the symptoms, the manometry and X-ray findings of oesophageal spasm are not falsely attributed.

A variant of diffuse oesophageal spasm is the *nutcracker oesophagus*, which is characterized by finding very high-amplitude peristalsis (pressures >200 mmHg) within the oesophagus. Chest pain and dysphagia occur.

### TREATMENT

True oesophageal spasm producing severe symptoms is rare and treatment is often unhelpful. Antispasmodics, nitrates, or calcium channel blockers such as sublingual nifedipine 10 mg three times daily may be tried. Occasionally, balloon dilatation or even myotomy is necessary.

## Miscellaneous motility disorders

Abnormalities of motility that are mostly asymptomatic but occasionally produce dysphagia are found in the elderly in diabetes mellitus, myotonica dystrophica and myasthenia gravis, as well as in any neurological disorder involving the brain stem.

## OTHER OESOPHAGEAL DISORDERS

## Oesophageal diverticulum

This is a pouch lined with epithelium that can produce dysphagia and regurgitation. It is usually asymptomatic and often detected accidentally on a barium swallow performed for other reasons. Diverticula can occur:

- Immediately above the upper oesophageal sphincter (pharyngeal pouch). If large, it may cause dysphagia as well as spillage of contents into the trachea.
- Near the middle of the oesophagus (traction diverticulum produced by extrinsic inflammation).
- Just above the LOS (epiphrenic diverticulum).

Only when symptoms are severe should surgery be undertaken.

## Rings and webs

A number of rings and webs have been described throughout the oesophagus.

### Lower oesophageal or Schatzki ring

This is a narrowing of the lower end of the oesophagus due to a ridge of mucosa or a fibrous membrane. The ring may be asymptomatic, but it can very occasionally produce dysphagia after swallowing a large bolus of bread or meat. The narrowing or ring is seen on a barium swallow, with the oesophagus well distended with barium. The treatment is reassurance and dietary advice.

### Upper oesophageal web

This is a constriction near the upper oesophageal sphincter in the postcricoid region and appears radiologically as a web. The web may be asymptomatic or may produce dysphagia. In the Plummer–Vinson syndrome (Paterson–Brown–Kelly syndrome) this web is associated with iron-deficiency anaemia, glossitis and angular stomatitis. This rare syndrome affects mainly women and its aetiology is not understood. At oesophagoscopy the web may be difficult to see. Dilatation of the web is rarely necessary. Iron is given for the iron deficiency.

## Benign oesophageal stricture

Peptic stricture secondary to reflux is the commonest cause of benign strictures. They also occur after the ingestion of corrosives, after radiotherapy, after sclerosis of varices and following prolonged nasogastric intubation. All strictures give rise to dysphagia. They are usually treated by dilatation, but occasionally surgery is necessary.

## Oesophageal infections

Infection is becoming increasingly recognized as a cause of painful swallowing, particularly in immunosuppressed debilitated patients and patients with AIDS. Infection can occur with:

- *Candida*
- Herpes simplex
- Cytomegalovirus

It is occasionally difficult to distinguish between these either on barium swallow or oesophagoscopy, as only widespread ulceration is seen. In candidiasis the characteristic white plaques on top of friable mucosa are frequently found, but oral candidiasis is not always present. The diagnosis of *Candida* can be confirmed by examining a direct smear taken at endoscopy, but often infections are mixed and cultures and biopsies must be performed.

### TREATMENT

Most patients on large doses of immunosuppressive agents are treated prophylactically with nystatin or amphotericin. Other antifungal or antiviral treatment is given appropriately (Chapter 1).

## Mallory–Weiss syndrome

This is described on p. 199.

## Oesophageal rupture

This can occur with violent vomiting producing severe chest pain and collapse. It may follow alcohol ingestion and a chest X-ray shows a hydropneumothorax.

# HIATUS HERNIA

In a sliding hiatus hernia, the gastro-oesophageal junction 'slides' through the hiatus so that it lies above the diaphragm. This type of hernia occurs in approximately 30% of people of 50 years of age and by itself is of no diagnostic significance. It does not produce symptoms on its own; symptoms occur because of the presence of associated reflux (see below).

A para-oesophageal or rolling hernia is when a small part of the stomach rolls up through the hernia alongside the oesophagus. The sphincter stays below the diaphragm and remains competent. Occasionally a rolling para-oesophageal hernia will produce pain and require surgical treatment.

# GASTRO-OESOPHAGEAL REFLUX DISEASE (GORD)

Gastro-oesophageal reflux occurs as a normal event, and the clinical features of GORD only occur when the antireflux mechanisms fail sufficiently to allow gastric contents to make prolonged contact with the lower oesophageal mucosa.

ANTIREFLUX MECHANISMS (Fig 4.6). The most important is the LOS which is formed by the distal 4 cm

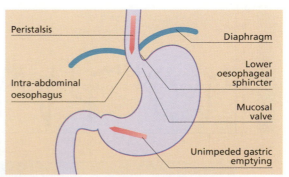

**Fig. 4.6** The main antireflux mechanisms.

Peristalsis

Intra-abdominal oesophagus

Diaphragm

Lower oesophageal sphincter

Mucosal valve

Unimpeded gastric emptying

| Pregnancy or obesity |
| --- |
| Fat, chocolate, coffee or alcohol ingestion |
| Cigarette smoking |
| Anticholinergic drugs |
| Systemic sclerosis |
| After treatment for achalasia |

**Table 4.3**  Factors associated with increased gastro-oesophageal reflux.

| Gastro-oesophageal reflux | Myocardial ischaemia |
| --- | --- |
| Burning pain produced by bending, stooping or lying down | Gripping or crushing pain Radiates into neck, shoulders and both arms |
| Relieved by antacids | Produced by exercise Accompanied by dyspnoea |

**Information box 4.1**  Symptoms of gastro-oesophageal reflux and myocardial ischaemia.

of oesophageal smooth muscle. It rapidly regains its normal tone after relaxation to allow a bolus to enter the stomach and thereby prevent reflux. It is capable of increasing tone in response to rises in intra-abdominal and intragastric pressure.

Other antireflux measures involve the intra-abdominal segment of the oesophagus which acts as a flap valve and the mucosal rosette formed by folds of the gastric mucosa also help to occlude the gastro-oesophageal junctional lumen.

The oesophagus is normally rapidly cleared of any reflux contents by secondary peristalsis.

### PATHOGENESIS OF GORD
The following mechanisms have been implicated:
- The resting LOS tone is low and LOS tone fails to increase, as occurs in normal patients, when lying flat.
- LOS tone fails to increase when intra-abdominal pressure increases.
- Oesophageal mucosal resistance to acid is reduced.
- There is relatively poor oesophageal peristalsis which leads to poor clearance of gastric contents.
- Delayed gastric emptying occurs and this may increase the chance of reflux.
- Prolonged episodes of gastro-oesophageal reflux occur at night and postprandially.

Factors associated with increased gastro-oesophageal reflux are shown in Table 4.3.

All or some of these features play a role in the individual patient and can occur whether or not a hiatus hernia is present. GORD can undoubtedly occur without a hiatus hernia.

### CLINICAL FEATURES
Heartburn is the major feature of GORD. Pain is mainly due to direct stimulation of the hypersensitive oesophageal mucosa, but is also partly due to spasm of the distal oesophageal muscle. The burning is aggravated by bending, stooping or lying down and may be relieved by antacids. The patient may complain of pain on drinking hot liquids or alcohol. The correlation between heartburn and minor degrees of oesophagitis is poor. Some patients have mild oesophagitis, but severe heartburn; others have severe oesophagitis without symptoms and present with a haematemesis or an iron deficiency anaemia from chronic blood loss. Regurgitation of food and acid into the mouth can occur, particularly when the patient is bending or lying flat. Aspiration into the lungs, producing pneumonia, is unusual without an accompanying stricture, but cough and nocturnal asthma from regurgitation and aspiration can occur. The differential diagnosis from angina can be difficult; 20% of cases admitted to a coronary care unit have GORD (Information box 4.1).

### INVESTIGATION
BARIUM SWALLOW is still the most widely used investigation. A hiatus hernia by itself is of no diagnostic significance and free reflux of barium must be demonstrated. Reflux can also be demonstrated with radiolabelled technetium.

24 HOUR INTRALUMINAL pH MONITORING (p. 183). The number of reflux episodes (below pH 4) occurring over 24 hours is noted (Fig. 4.7). This is now considered the most accurate test available, there being a

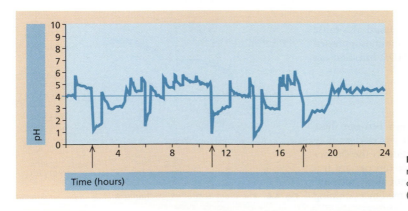

**Fig. 4.7**  24-Hour intraluminal pH monitoring. Five reflux episodes (pH < 4) occurred, but only three gave symptoms (arrows).

reasonable correlation between frequency of reflux and symptoms.

OESOPHAGOSCOPY is used to show the presence of oesophagitis with a red friable mucosa and, in more severe cases, linear ulceration. The mucosa can be normal in GORD.

BERNSTEIN TEST may be helpful in investigating retrosternal chest pain to differentiate oesophageal pain from angina (see p. 183).

## TREATMENT

Many patients (approximately 50%) can be treated successfully with simple antacids, loss of weight, and raising the head of the bed at night. Precipitating factors should be avoided with a reduction in alcohol consumption and cessation of smoking. These measures are simple to say, difficult to carry out, but are useful in mild cases. The chief antacids are magnesium trisilicate and aluminium hydroxide; the former often causes diarrhoea whilst the latter causes constipation. Many antacids contain sodium which may exacerbate fluid retention; aluminium hydroxide has less sodium than magnesium trisilicate.

ALGINATE-CONTAINING ANTACIDS (10 ml three times daily) are the most frequently prescribed agents for GORD. They form a gel or 'foam raft' with gastric contents and thereby prevent reflux.

H$_2$-RECEPTOR ANTAGONISTS are frequently used (see p. 193), to be taken at 6 p.m., doubling the normal dosages if necessary.

PROTON PUMP INHIBITORS, such as *omeprazole*, a substituted benzimidazole which inhibits the H$^+$, K$^+$ proton pump. This produces almost complete reduction of gastric acidity, is extremely effective, and is the drug of choice for all but mild cases. Patients with severe symptoms need prolonged treatment, often for years.

METOCLOPRAMIDE, a dopamine antagonist, is occasionally helpful as it enhances peristalsis and speeds gastric emptying.

CISAPRIDE, a prokinetic agent devoid of dopaminergic activity, increases oesophageal peristalsis, increases LOS pressure and is of value, particularly for maintenance therapy.

Surgery should never be performed for a hiatus hernia alone. The properly selected case with severe reflux and oesophagitis responds well to surgery. Repair of the hernia and some sort of additional antireflux surgery, e.g. Nissen fundoplication, is required. Surgery can now be performed laparoscopically.

## COMPLICATIONS

The major complication of reflux is peptic stricture, which usually occurs in patients over the age of 60. The symptoms are those of intermittent dysphagia over a long period. Treatment is by dilatation of the stricture and management of the reflux usually medical, with omeprazole, but very occasionally surgery is required. There is no increased incidence of carcinoma in hiatus hernia *per se*. However, long-standing acid reflux causes columnization of the oesophageal mucosa (Barrett's oesophagus) which is premalignant, but can be reversed with antireflux therapy.

# Oesophageal Tumours

## Benign

Leiomyomas are the commonest benign tumours. They are usually discovered accidentally and they do not often produce symptoms.

## Malignant

These occur in the middle of the oesophagus and are squamous carcinomas. Adenocarcinomas occur in the lower third of the oesophagus and at the cardia.

Kaposi's sarcoma is frequently found in the mouth and hypopharynx in patients with AIDS (see p. 181). These tumours rarely lead to symptoms and consequently do not require treatment.

### EPIDEMIOLOGY AND AETIOLOGICAL FACTORS

SQUAMOUS CARCINOMA. The incidence of carcinoma varies throughout the world, being high in China, parts of Africa and in the Caspian regions of Iran (where the incidence is the highest observed for any type of cancer anywhere in the world). In the UK it is 5–10 per 100 000 and represents 2.5% of all malignant disease. The variation in incidence throughout the world is greater than for any other carcinoma and is unusual in that sharp differences occur in regions very close to one another. Dietary and other environmental causes have been looked for and it is probable that different causative agents are involved in different parts of the world. Carcinoma of the oesophagus is commoner in men and there is an increased incidence in heavy drinkers of alcohol as well as heavy smokers. Predisposing factors include Plummer–Vinson syndrome, achalasia, coeliac disease and the familial condition of tylosis (hyperkeratosis of palms and soles).

ADENOCARCINOMA. These arise in the columnar lined epithelium of the lower oesophagus (Barrett's oesophagus). This columnization results from long-standing reflux, although one-third of patients will have no preceding symptoms. This premalignant lesion increases the chances of adenocarcinoma 30–40 times. Extension of adenocarcinoma of the gastric cardia can cause oesophageal obstruction.

### CLINICAL FEATURES

Carcinoma of the oesophagus occurs mainly in those aged 60–70 years. Dysphagia is the commonest single symptom and is progressive and unrelenting. Initially there is difficulty in swallowing solids, but eventually dysphagia for liquids also occurs. Benign strictures, on the other hand, initially produce intermittent dysphagia. Impaction of food causes pain, but more persistent pain implies infiltration.

The lesion is usually ulcerative, extending around the wall of the oesophagus to produce a stricture. Direct invasion of the surrounding structures rather than widespread metastases occurs, and at presentation 50% have regional lymph node involvement. Weight loss, due to the dysphagia as well as to anorexia, frequently occurs. The oesophageal obstruction eventually causes difficulty in swallowing saliva, and coughing and aspiration into the lungs is common. Signs are often absent. Weight loss, anorexia and lymphadenopathy are occasionally found.

### INVESTIGATION
BARIUM SWALLOW is often the initial investigation (Fig. 4.8) although many gastroenterologists like to go directly to oesophagoscopy which provides histological or cytological proof of the carcinoma; 90% of oesophageal carcinomas can be confirmed with this technique.

CT SCAN will show the volume of the tumour and also possible spread outside the oesophagus. It has been used to attempt to stage tumours prior to surgery, but results are disappointing.

ENDOSCOPIC ULTRASOUND has an accuracy rate of nearly 90% for assessing depth of tumour infiltration and 80% for staging lymph node involvement and is being increasingly used.

### TREATMENT
The overall results are poor (2% 5-year survival) and only symptomatic and palliative treatment is a realistic possibility in most cases. Dilatation of the stricture and the placing of a tube to keep the oesophagus open is the usual therapy and can be performed via an endoscope. Tumours can be photocoagulated using a laser beam

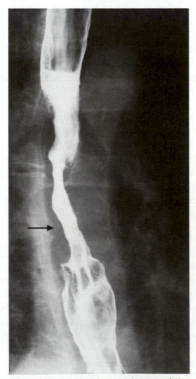

**Fig. 4.8** Barium swallow showing carcinoma of the oesophagus. There is an irregular narrowed area (arrow) at the lower end of the oesophagus.

directed through an endoscope or sloughed using alcohol injections. Both are useful to improve dysphagia.

Surgery carries a high morbidity and mortality, but in some series in which preoperative staging shows no spread outside the wall a 5-year survival rate of 25% has been achieved. Radiotherapy and chemotherapy can be used for squamous carcinoma with limited success. Good palliative care with support for the patient and family is vital in this distressing disease.

# The stomach and duodenum

### STRUCTURE
The *stomach*, which varies considerably in size, is divided into the upper portion (the fundus), the mid-region or body, and the antrum, which extends into the pyloric region.

There are two sphincters, the gastro-oesophageal sphincter and the pyloric sphincter; the latter is largely made up of a thickening of the circular muscle layer. The muscle wall of the stomach has three layers—an outer longitudinal, an inner circular, and an innermost oblique layer of smooth muscle.

The *duodenum* has outer longitudinal and inner smooth muscle layers. It is C-shaped and the pancreas sits in the concavity. It terminates in the jejunum at the duodenojejunal flexure.

The mucosal lining of the stomach, particularly in the greater curvature, is thrown into thick folds or rugae. The upper two-thirds of the stomach contains parietal cells, which secrete hydrochloric acid, and chief cells, which secrete pepsinogen. The junction between the body and the antrum of the stomach can often be seen macroscopically, but can be confirmed by measuring surface pH. The antrum contains only mucus-secreting and G cells, which secrete gastrin. There are two major forms of gastrin, G17 and G34, depending on the number of amino-acid residues. G17 is the major form found in the antrum.

The duodenal mucosa contains Brunner's glands, which secrete alkaline mucus. This, along with the pancreatic and biliary secretions, helps to neutralize the acid secretion from the stomach when it reaches the duodenum.

### FUNCTION
**Acid secretion**
The factors controlling acid secretion are shown in Fig. 4.9. Secretion is under neural and hormonal control. Both stimulate acid secretion through the release of histamine, which acts on the parietal cells either directly or via immunocytes.

**Other major gastric functions**
● Reservoir for food

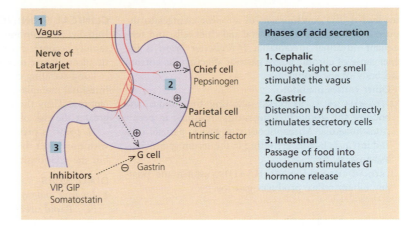

**Fig. 4.9** Control of acid secretion.

- Emulsification of fat and mixing of gastric contents
- Secretion of intrinsic factor
- Absorption (of only minimal importance)

Gastric emptying depends on many factors. There are osmoreceptors in the duodenal mucosa that control gastric emptying by local reflexes and the release of gut hormones. In particular, intraduodenal fat delays gastric emptying by negative feedback through duodenal receptors.

# GASTRITIS

There is no universally accepted classification of this condition partly because there is a poor correlation between clinical, pathological and endoscopic findings.

## Acute gastritis, acute ulceration and erosions

In *acute gastritis* there is an acute inflammatory infiltrate in the superficial gastric mucosa predominantly with neutrophils. This is sometimes accompanied by mucosal erosions. Multiple small erosions, often with an oedematous mucosa, are described as acute erosive gastritis.

*Acute gastric ulceration* occurs in the same setting as erosions, but are larger and less superficial. Gastritis can be commonly produced by drugs such as aspirin and other non-steroidal anti-inflammatory drugs (NSAIDs) (Information box 4.2), and occasionally by infections, e.g. cytomegalovirus and herpes simplex, particularly in the immunocompromised. Aspirin and other NSAIDs deplete mucosal prostaglandins which leads to mucosal damage. Alcohol in high concentrations damages the gastric mucosal barrier and is associated with acute gastric mucosal lesions and upper gastrointestinal bleeding.

Acute ulcers are also seen after severe stress (stress ulcer) and secondary to burns (Curling's ulcer), trauma, shock, renal or liver disease. The underlying mechanism for these ulcers is unknown but may be related to an alteration in mucosal flow.

### CLINICAL FEATURES
The correlation between the pathological changes and symptoms is poor, but some patients with acute gastritis may suffer from indigestion and vomiting, usually short-lived. Gastrointestinal haemorrhage can occur (see p. 197).

### DIAGNOSIS
In many patients symptoms settle without diagnosis, but endoscopy is necessary in patients with a gastrointestinal haemorrhage to confirm the presence of acute ulcers or erosions.

### TREATMENT
No specific therapy is required apart from removal of the offending cause, if possible.

## Chronic gastritis

*Chronic active gastritis* consists of an infiltration of the lamina propria with lymphocytes and plasma cells. This

---

NSAIDs cause gastric erosions and ulcers (10–25% of patients on long-term NSAIDs).

NSAIDs *do not* cause duodenal ulcers.

NSAIDs increase the incidence of complications in patients with both duodenal ulcers and gastric ulcers (20 000 hospitalizations per year in USA).

Rectal administration does not prevent upper gastrointestinal adverse effects.

Misoprostol is the best drug to prevent gastric ulceration, but has not been shown to reduce complications.

All NSAIDs, including aspirin, have been implicated—some more than others.

**Information box 4.2** NSAIDs and the upper gastrointestinal tract.

can lead to the development of atrophic changes in the mucosa including loss of parietal and chief cells, and subsequent intestinal metaplasia. *Helicobacter pylori* is the chief cause of chronic active gastritis affecting the antrum and body of the stomach.

Other causes include:

AUTOIMMUNE GASTRITIS; affecting the fundus and body of the stomach (pangastritis) resulting in pernicious anaemia. Autoantibodies to gastric parietal cells and intrinsic factors are found in the serum (pernicious anaemia, p. 305).

CHRONIC INGESTION OF NSAIDS, aspirin and possibly biliary reflux produces gastritis.

### CLINICAL FEATURES

A consistent relationship between upper gut symptoms and histological chronic gastritis has not been established. There may be a subset of patients in whom the gastritis may account for the symptoms.

Most chronic gastritis is asymptomatic and requires no treatment.

## *Helicobacter pylori* and the upper gastrointestinal tract

This spiral-shaped urease-producing bacterium (Fig. 4.10) is found in the stomach and in areas of gastric metaplasia in the duodenum. *H. pylori* is found in greatest numbers under the mucus layers in gastric pits in close apposition to gastric epithelial cells. Intrafamilial clustering suggests person-to-person spread, but the exact mode of transmission is unclear. Childhood acquisition of *H. pylori* is very prevalent in developing countries. There is a clear relationship between the age of acquisition and lower socio-economic status worldwide. A relationship between *H. pylori* infection and crowded domestic living conditions in childhood has been established.

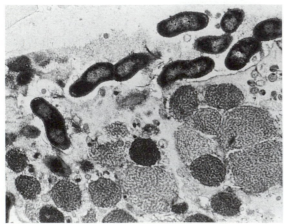

**Fig. 4.10** *Helicobacter pylori* Courtesy of Brocades (GB) Ltd.

### CLINICAL SIGNIFICANCE

Initially, *H. pylori* infection produces acute gastritis which rapidly becomes chronic active gastritis and in some peptic ulcer disease may develop.

Long-standing chronic active gastritis leads to atrophy, intestinal metaplasia and increases the risk of gastric carcinoma. Thus the earlier the *H. pylori* is acquired, the greater the risk of atrophy and metaplasia.

*H. pylori* is present in a greater proportion of patients with non-ulcer dyspepsia than in asymptomatic controls, but the relationship with symptoms is poor.

### DIAGNOSIS

1  *Invasive endoscopy*
   (a) Rapid urease test: biopsies are added to a urea solution containing phenol red. If *H. pylori* is present, the urease enzyme splits the urea to release ammonia which raises the pH of the solution and causes a rapid colour change.
   (b) *H. pylori* can be Gram stained or cultured on special medium and sensitivities to antibodies can be ascertained.
   (c) *H. pylori* can also be detected histologically with routine stained sections.
2  *Non-invasive*
   (a) Urea breath test with $^{13}C$ or $^{14}C$ (see p. 207, but using urea as the substrate). This is a quick and easy way of detecting the presence of *H. pylori* and is used as a screening test and also to demonstrate eradication of the organism following treatment.
   (b) Serum antibodies. Reasonably sensitive and specific serological tests are available and are used mainly for epidemiological studies.

### TREATMENT AND ERADICATION

In patients with peptic ulcer disease, it is necessary to eradicate the organism as this leads to a 'cure' with very low recurrence of ulceration unless reinfection occurs; this is, however, uncommon. The best regimen for eradication is not yet clear, but all regimens must take into account the following factors:

- A good compliance with treatment regimens is required
- The high incidence of antibiotic resistance to metronidazole (25%+)
- That oral metronidazole, when given, increases the side-effects of treatment
- That bismuth chelate is unpleasant to take even as tablets.

Two regimens are currently used, but these will undoubtedly change over the years:

1 Triple therapy—*bismuth chelate*, 2 tablets four times daily for 4 weeks, 30 min before a meal, *metronidazole* 400 mg three times daily for the first week, *tetracycline*, 500 mg three times daily for the first week.
2 An alternative therapy is omeprazole 40 mg daily, together with amoxycillin, or possibly clarithromycin, 500 mg three times per day for 1–2 weeks.

All these treatments give eradication figures of approximately 80%.

Patients with gastritis without peptic ulceration should not be treated, but this is an area which is increasingly changing as more is discovered about the organism and better eradication therapy is found.

# PEPTIC ULCER DISEASE

This is an ulcer of the mucosa in, or adjacent to, an acid-bearing area. Most ulcers occur in the stomach or proximal duodenum but they can occur in the oesophagus (with oesophageal reflux), in the jejunum in the Zollinger–Ellison syndrome or after a gastroenterostomy, and finally in a Meckel's diverticulum, which contains ectopic gastric mucosa.

## EPIDEMIOLOGY

Duodenal ulceration is common; 15% of the population will suffer from a duodenal ulcer at some time. They are two to three times commoner than gastric ulcers. Duodenal ulcers are commoner in men than women (4:1) and both gastric and duodenal ulcers are more common in elderly people, i.e. an age-related incidence. There is considerable geographical variation. Duodenal ulcer is commoner in northern England and Scotland than in other parts of the UK. Much of the previous epidemiological data can be explained on the prevalence of *H. pylori* infection.

## AETIOLOGY

Peptic ulceration is caused by an imbalance between:
- Acid and pepsin, and
- Mucosal defences: mucus, bicarbonate and prostaglandins.

*H. pylori* plays a central role in both gastric and duodenal ulceration, although the mechanisms are unclear. Genetic susceptibility may also play a role, particularly in patients who do not secrete blood group O antigen into gastric secretions.

Possible pathogenetic factors of *H. pylori* infection are:
- An increase in fasting and meal-stimulated gastrin release
- A decrease in somatostatin (D cells) in the antrum
- An increase in parietal cell mass
- An increase in pepsinogen I
- An alteration in the mucus protective layer
- Cytotoxin release

All of these affect acid secretion or the mucosal barrier.

The only other important cause of gastric ulceration is NSAIDs. Peptic ulceration is also seen in hyperparathyroidism (since calcium stimulates acid secretion) and in the Zollinger–Ellison syndrome.

## PATHOLOGY

Gastric ulcer can occur in any part of the stomach, but is most commonly found on the lesser curve. Most duodenal ulcers are found in the duodenal cap with the surrounding mucosa appearing inflamed, haemorrhagic and friable (duodenitis).

Histologically there is a break in the superficial epithelium penetrating down to the muscularis mucosa with a fibrous base and an increase in inflammatory cells. The ulcer may heal with fibrosis.

## CLINICAL FEATURES
### Symptoms

Indigestion is a frequent symptom, but epigastric pain is the characteristic feature of ulcer disease. If the patient points directly to the epigastrium as the site of the pain, this has a high discriminatory value for diagnosis. The pain of a duodenal ulcer classically occurs at night as well as during the day. In both types of ulcer, pain is helped by antacids. The relationship of the pain to food is variable and on the whole is not helpful in diagnosis. However, patients with a duodenal ulcer may complain of pains when they are hungry.

Nausea may accompany the pain, but vomiting is not frequent and when it occurs it may relieve the pain. Another symptom is heartburn, which is due to acid regurgitation. Anorexia and weight loss may occur, particularly with gastric ulcers.

The symptoms of a duodenal ulcer are periodic with spontaneous relapses and remissions. Eighty per cent of patients will have a recurrence of symptoms within 1 year of the first episode. The natural history appears to be for the disease to remit over many years with the onset of gastritis with atrophy and decrease in acid secretion. Fifty per cent of patients with a gastric ulcer will have a recurrence within 2 years. If the patient complains of persistent and severe pain, complications such as penetration into other organs should be considered. Back pain may suggest a penetrating posterior duodenal ulcer.

Patients can present for the first time with either a haematemesis or melaena or with a perforation.

### Signs

The only signs are those of epigastric tenderness but this is a poor discriminating sign. Tenderness does not necessarily imply disease and is frequently found in non-ulcer dyspepsia.

## INVESTIGATION

Many patients, particularly the young presenting with indigestion, can be treated symptomatically for 4–5 weeks without investigation.

ENDOSCOPY is often the first investigation, with biopsy of all gastric ulcers, *or*

BARIUM MEAL (double-contrast technique). A gastric ulcer is shown in Fig. 4.11 and a duodenal ulcer is shown in Fig. 4.12.

ACID SECRETION STATUS. This is not useful to measure in most cases of peptic ulcer disease. The main use of this test is in the Zollinger–Ellison syndrome, but a serum gastrin is more useful. Secretions from the stomach are collected via a nasogastric tube before (basal secretion) and following stimulation by an injection of pentagastrin. This is a synthetic peptide containing the terminal five peptides of gastrin.

BLOOD TESTS are unhelpful in uncomplicated cases.

## TREATMENT
### Duodenal ulcer

There are two main approaches.

1 *Eradication of H. pylori.* This therapy is now thought

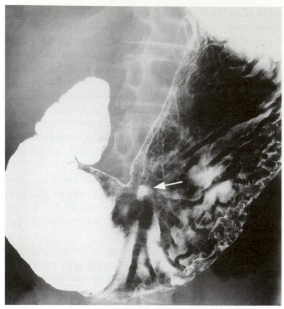

**Fig. 4.11**  Barium meal showing a gastric ulcer (arrow).

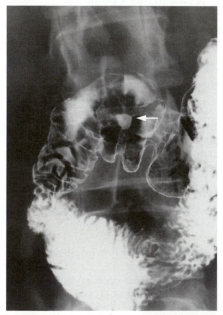

**Fig. 4.12**  Barium meal showing a large chronic duodenal ulcer (arrow).

to 'cure' duodenal ulcers providing the organism is successfully eradicated. Eradication therapy is being given increasingly more frequently and may become the first-line therapy in all patients.

2 *Acid suppression* (Fig 4.13):

  (a)  Omeprazole, a protein pump inhibitor, 20 mg daily produces an 80–90% inhibition of 24 hour intragastric acidity and healing rates of 90% after 4 weeks' treatment. It is being increasingly used for treatment of ulcers as it produces good symptom relief.

  (b)  *H₂ receptor antagonists* (Fig 4.14) have been the first choice of therapy. They have molecular structures that fit the $H_2$ receptors on the parietal cells. A single therapeutic dose in the evening produces, at least, an 80% reduction of nocturnal acid production until the following morning. Over 80% of duodenal ulcers will heal with a 2-month course of this group of drugs and symptoms are relieved quickly. There is little difference between the different $H_2$ antagonists, but cimetidine is not usually given to young males because of the incidence of impotence which is low.

3 *Other drugs.* A number of other drugs have been shown to be effective, but are rarely used compared with the above.

  (a)  *Misoprostol.* A synthetic analogue of prostaglandin $E_1$ inhibits gastric acid secretion and does promote gastric and duodenal ulcer healing. It is mainly used as a cytoprotective agent against NSAID-associated gastric ulcers. Prophylaxis is 200 $\mu$g, two to four times per day. Treatment is 800 $\mu$g daily in divided doses, the main side-effect being diarrhoea.

  (b)  *Sucralfate* possibly acts by protecting the mucosa from acid pepsin attack. It is a complex of aluminium hydroxide and sulphated sucrose, but it has minimal antacid properties. It is also used in the treatment of benign gastric ulceration and sometimes as a cytoprotective agent at a dose of 2 g daily in divided doses.

4 *Miscellaneous.* Stopping smoking should be strongly encouraged as smoking slows healing. Special diets, together with avoidance of coffee, alcohol or acid substances, are not required.

The effectiveness of treatment should be assessed symptomatically. There is no need for follow-up endoscopy. If the patient fails to respond, the diagnosis should be reviewed. Duodenal ulcers are common and care must be taken not to falsely attribute abdominal symptoms to the finding of an ulcer.

**Gastric ulcer**

Treatment is given to ensure ulcer healing which must be checked with follow-up endoscopy and biopsies at 6 weeks. Failure to heal raises the question of malignancy and further treatment and follow-up endoscopy is required.

There are a number of approaches to treatment

1 *H₂-receptor antagonists* have been the most common agents used for treatment, but omeprazole is being increasingly used as the initial therapy as symptom relief is rapid; follow-up with endoscopy and biopsies at 6 weeks.

2 *Eradication of H. pylori.* Eradication treatment should be given to all patients with a gastric ulcer; usually the presence of *H. pylori* has been documented at endoscopy. If the patient is taking an NSAID when the ulcer is discovered, eradication therapy should still be given if *H. pylori* is demonstrated.

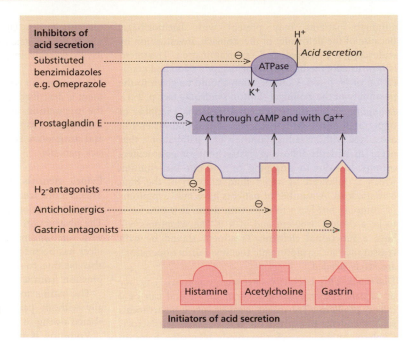

**Fig. 4.13** Diagrammatic representation of the mechanisms involved in acid secretion.

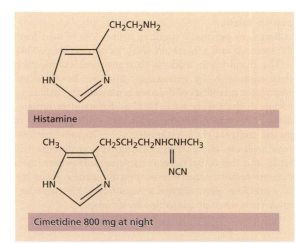

**Fig. 4.14** The chemical formula of the first available $H_2$-receptor antagonist showing the similarity to histamine. Other $H_2$-receptor antagonists include ranitidine, famotidine and nizatidine.

**3** Smoking should be strongly discouraged. Dietary changes are unnecessary.

**4** Attempts should be made to stop NSAIDs in patients with peptic ulceration. This may be difficult in those with severe arthritis and if it is essential to continue NSAIDs either misoprostol or ranitidine should be prescribed concurrently.

## SURGICAL MANAGEMENT

Since the introduction of $H_2$-receptor antagonists, surgery for peptic ulceration is rarely performed. In the past, two types of operation were performed:

**1** *Partial gastrectomy.* The principle in both types of gastrectomy performed for peptic ulcer disease is to remove the antral area that secretes gastrin, since this in turn stimulates acid production.

(a) Billroth I partial gastrectomy. The lower part of the stomach is removed and the stomach remnant is connected to the duodenum.

(b) Billroth II (Polya gastrectomy). The stomach remnant is connected to the first loop of jejunum (a gastroenterostomy) and the duodenum is closed.

**2** *Vagotomy.*

(a) Truncal vagotomy plus gastroenterostomy/ pyloroplasty

(b) Selective vagotomy (preserving the hepatic and coeliac branch of the vagus) plus gastroenterostomy/pyloroplasty.

(c) Highly selective vagotomy or proximal gastric vagotomy, in which only the nerves supplying the parietal cells are transected, and therefore no drainage is required. With this type of operation there is little diarrhoea but the recurrence rate is still 5–10%.

Currently, surgery is reserved for complications:

• Recurrent uncontrolled haemorrhage when the bleeding vessel is ligated

• Perforation which is oversown

(For both of these conditions no other procedure such as a gastrectomy or vagotomy is required.)

• Outflow obstruction which requires gastric resection

LONG-TERM COMPLICATIONS OF SURGERY are still occasionally seen. A recurrent ulcer, which can appear in the stomach, duodenum or jejunum, often occurs at the stoma. The symptoms are similar to those seen in the unoperated stomach, with pain invariably being present, although patients may present with haemorrhage. Because of the deformity of the stomach, investigation by endoscopy is preferred to X-ray examination. Treatment is now usually medical, using acid suppression and eradication of *H. pylori*. Consideration should be given to the possibility of the Zollinger–Ellison syndrome (see p. 291).

*Dumping.* This is the term used to describe a number of upper abdominal symptoms, e.g. nausea and distension associated with sweating, faintness and palpitations, that occur in patients following gastrectomy or gastroenterostomy. It is due to 'dumping' of food into the jejunum, which is followed by rapid fluid dilution of the high osmotic load. A number of patients have mild symptoms of dumping but learn to cope with them. It is rare for it to be a clinical problem and, if it is, the symptoms will have a functional element. Treatment should be with reassurance and symptomatic therapy. Further operations are rarely needed.

*Diarrhoea.* This is chiefly seen after vagotomy. Urgency or recurrent severe episodes occur in 1% and can be a major problem. Treatment consists of antidiarrhoeals such as codeine phosphate but is not entirely satisfactory. Cholestyramine, a resin that binds bile salts, helps in some cases. Very occasionally the diarrhoea or steatorrhoea can be due to bacterial overgrowth in the blind loop of a Polya gastrectomy (see p. 210).

*Vomiting (afferent loop syndrome/bilious vomiting).* The incidence of vomiting has decreased with the introduction of the more conservative operations. Vomiting occurs because food gets trapped owing to the altered anatomy. Treatment is symptomatic, except on the rare occasions when reconstructive surgery is required.

*Nutritional complications.* Anaemia is most commonly due to iron deficiency caused by poor absorption. Treatment is with oral iron, which may be needed long-term. Megaloblastic anaemia is uncommon, but can be due to either folate deficiency (due to poor intake) or vitamin $B_{12}$ deficiency (due to long-term gastritis with atrophy resulting in intrinsic factor deficiency). Osteomalacia is an uncommon late complication (see p. 425). Patients often fail to gain weight owing to anorexia after gastric surgery and a few suffer from severe protein–energy malnutrition as a result.

## COMPLICATIONS OF PEPTIC ULCER

In all patients with any complications of peptic ulcer disease *H. pylori* eradication is imperative. If the patient has been given eradication therapy previously a further course of eradication therapy is necessary.

### Haemorrhage

This is dealt with below.

### Perforation (see also p. 233) (Information box 4.3)

The frequency of perforation of peptic ulcer is decreasing; this is partly attributable to the introduction of $H_2$-recep-

tor antagonists. Duodenal ulcers perforate more commonly than gastric ulcers, usually into the peritoneal cavity. Perforation into the lesser sac may occur.

MANAGEMENT OF PERFORATION. Detailed management is described on p. 233. Surgery is performed to close the perforation and drain the abdomen. Conservative management using nasogastric suction, intravenous fluids and antibiotics is occasionally used in elderly and very sick patients.

### Pyloric stenosis or obstruction

This is more accurately called gastric outflow obstruction, as the obstruction may be prepyloric or in the duodenum. The obstruction occurs either because of an active ulcer with surrounding oedema or because the healing of an ulcer has been followed by scarring. The obstruction can also be due to a gastric malignancy or external compression from a pancreatic carcinoma.

The main symptom of this condition is vomiting, usually without pain as the characteristic ulcer pain has abated owing to healing.

Vomiting is projectile and huge in volume, and the vomitus contains particles of the previous day's food. On examination of the abdomen the patient may have a succussion splash.

Severe or persistent vomiting causes loss of acid from the stomach and a metabolic alkalosis occurs (see p. 519).

The diagnosis is made by barium meal examination (less commonly by endoscopy) but can be suspected when large quantities of fluid are removed by gastric intubation in the fasting state. Fluid and electrolyte replacement is necessary, together with the regular removal of gastric contents via a nasogastric tube. In some patients with oedema rather than scarring, the symptoms will settle with this conservative management. However, most patients require surgery. Postoperative gastric stasis can be a problem, particularly if a vagotomy has been performed, even when accompanied by drainage.

---

*Look for:*

Other acute gastrointestinal conditions, e.g. cholecystitis, pancreatitis (check serum amylase)

Non gastrointestinal conditions, e.g. myocardial infarction

Silent perforations in the elderly or patients on steroids

*Remember*

There *is* harm in leaving an undiagnosed perforation.

There is no real harm in operating even if the perforation has occurred at a different site from that expected clinically.

Avoid laparotomy if pancreatitis is diagnosed.

**Information box 4.3**  Perforation of peptic ulcer.

# MÉNÉTRIER'S DISEASE

Ménétrier's disease is a rare condition in which there is thickening and enlargement of the gastric mucosal folds. Histologically there is hyperplasia of the mucin-producing cells with glandular proliferation and loss of the parietal and chief cells.

The patient may complain of epigastric pain and occasionally peripheral oedema may occur due to hypoalbuminaemia resulting from protein loss through the gastric mucosa. Symptomatic treatment is all that is required for this condition. It is possibly premalignant.

# GASTRIC TUMOURS

### Benign
The commonest benign tumour is a leiomyoma. This tumour is usually discovered by chance but it can occasionally ulcerate and produce haematemesis. Treatment is surgical removal.

Gastric polyps are uncommon and are again found usually by chance. They produce no symptoms. The commonest are regenerative or hyperplastic polyps, which are often multiple and require no treatment. Rarely, adenomatous polyps are found and endoscopic removal is recommended because of possible malignant potential. Most gastric cancers appear not to arise from pre-existing adenomas (in contrast to colonic carcinomas).

### Malignant
Carcinoma of the stomach is one of the commonest malignant tumours of the gastrointestinal tract and is the sixth most common fatal cancer in the UK. The frequency varies throughout the world, being high in Japan and Chile and relatively low in the USA.

In the UK, 15 per 100 000 males are affected per year. The worldwide incidence of gastric carcinoma appears to be falling, even in Japan, for no obvious reason. The incidence increases with age and more men than women are affected.

## EPIDEMIOLOGY
There is a strong link between *H. pylori* infection and gastric cancer. It is suggested that *H. pylori* infection results in chronic active gastritis which eventually leads to gastritis with atrophy and intestinal metaplasia—a premalignant pathological change (Fig. 4.15). Much of the previous epidemiological data, i.e. the increase of cancer in lower socio-economic groups, can be explained by the intrafamilial spread of *H. pylori*.

Dietary factors may still be important as both initiators and promoters may have separate roles in carcinogenesis. These include alcohol, spiced, salted or pickled foods and nitrate ingestion. Nitrates can be converted into nitrosamines by bacteria at neutral pH and nitrosamines are

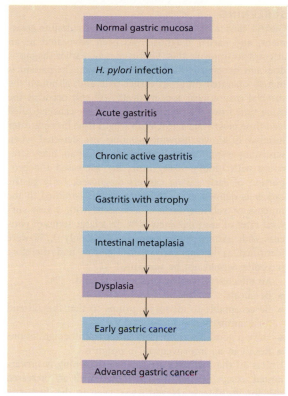

**Fig. 4.15**  Flow diagram showing the development of gastric cancer associated with *H. pylori* infection.

known to be carcinogenic in animals. Nitrosamines are also present in the stomach of patients with achlorhydria who have an increased cancer risk. Smoking is also associated with an increased incidence of stomach cancer.

Genes underlying the inherited susceptibility to gastric cancer have not yet been identified, but certain patterns are emerging as seen in colonic cancer. There is a higher incidence of gastric cancer in blood group A patients.

### Possible precancerous conditions
*Benign gastric ulcers* do not develop into gastric cancer. It can, however, be difficult to differentiate a benign ulcer from a malignant ulcer, as even malignant ulcers can partially heal on medical treatment. For these reasons it was originally thought that gastric ulcers could become malignant.

*Pernicious anaemia* carries a small increased risk of developing gastric carcinoma. Gastritis with atrophy present in the body and fundus of the stomach of these patients may be a precancerous lesion.

*Gastritis with atrophy* and also areas of *intestinal metaplasia* are areas where many gastric cancers develop. Intestinal metaplasia and chronic gastritis are also found in the resected stomach and there is an increased incidence of gastric cancer after *partial gastrectomy* (especially with a gastrojejunostomy). This increased incidence is the same whether the gastric resection was for a gastric or duodenal ulcer and may all be a reflection of *H. pylori* infection.

## SCREENING

Gastric cancer has an appalling prognosis despite treatment, and earlier diagnosis has been advocated in an attempt to improve this. Unfortunately, earlier diagnosis does not necessarily mean longer survival. The patient is merely operated on at an earlier date and, although the survival may appear longer, death will still occur at the same time from the point of genesis of the cancer (called lead time bias) (Fig. 4.16). With length time bias a greater number of slowly growing tumours are detected when screening asymptomatic individuals. In Japan, mass screening with mobile X-ray units has increased the proportion of early gastric cancers diagnosed. Early gastric cancer is defined as a carcinoma that is confined to the mucosa or submucosa. It is associated with 5-year survival rates of approximately 90%. In a large series of patients with gastric cancer from the UK, only 0.7% were identified as having early gastric cancer and therefore screening would not be warranted.

An effective screening procedure should:
- Be cheap
- Be acceptable to all social groups so that they attend for examination
- Have a good discriminatory index from benign lesions
- Result in an improvement in prognosis

Unless all these criteria are fulfilled, screening is unwarranted except possibly in individuals with an increased risk for the disease. Nevertheless, even in this high-risk group, screening asymptomatic subjects is not justified as the overall benefit is minimal.

An alternative approach to screening asymptomatic patients is to investigate symptomatic patients as quickly as possible. At the present time the mean interval between the onset of symptoms and attendance at hospital is approximately 6–9 months. However, dyspepsia is very common in the general population without any gastric lesions and it would obviously be impractical for every dyspeptic member of the general population to consult a physician. Even if they did, most primary physicians would think it unjustified to arrange a complicated series of investigations on the first visit. Thus, the detection of early gastric cancer in symptomatic patients is not a feasible proposition at present.

## PATHOLOGY

Most gastric cancers occur in the antrum and are almost invariably adenocarcinomas. The common type is 'intestinal' and the tumours are polypoid or ulcerating lesions with heaped-up, rolled edges. Intestinal metaplasia is often seen in the surrounding mucosa, along with *H. pylori*. The diffuse type is composed of scattered or small clusters of cells, often with extensive submucosal spread which may result in the picture of 'linitis plastica', where the stomach appears rigid on X-ray.

## CLINICAL FEATURES

### Symptoms

The commonest symptom is epigastric pain, which is indistinguishable from the pain of peptic ulcer disease, both being relieved by food and antacids. The pain can vary in intensity, but may be constant and severe. Most patients with carcinoma of the stomach have advanced disease at the time of presentation, and also have nausea, anorexia and weight loss. Vomiting is frequent and can be severe if the tumour is near the pylorus. Dysphagia can occur with tumours involving the fundus. Gross haematemesis is unusual, but anaemia from occult blood loss is frequent.

Patients can present with metastases causing abdominal swelling due to ascites or jaundice due to liver involvement. Metastases also occur in bone, brain and lung, producing appropriate symptoms.

### Signs

Nearly 50% of patients have a palpable epigastric mass with abdominal tenderness. Often weight loss is the only feature. A palpable lymph node is sometimes found in the supraclavicular fossa (Virchow's node) and signs of metastases are present in up to one-third of patients. Carcinoma of the stomach is the cancer most frequently associated with dermatomyositis and acanthosis nigricans.

## INVESTIGATION

ROUTINE FULL BLOOD COUNT AND LIVER BIOCHEMISTRY. This is necessary to look for anaemia and possible liver metastases.

BARIUM MEAL. A good quality, double-contrast barium meal has a diagnostic accuracy of up to 90%. The carcinoma is usually seen as a filling defect or an irregular ulcer with rolled edges. With the infiltrating type, the X-ray may show a rigid stomach.

GASTROSCOPY (FIG. 4.17). Gastroscopy is usually performed as the primary procedure and has the advantage that biopsies can be performed for histological assessment and to exclude lymphoma. Positive biopsies can be obtained in almost all cases of obvious carcinoma, but a negative biopsy does not necessarily rule out the diagnosis. For this reason, eight to ten biopsies should be taken from around the ulcer margin and its base. Superficial brushings for cytology will further improve the diagnostic rate.

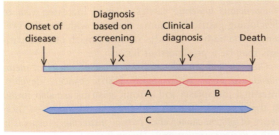

**Fig. 4.16** Lead time bias. Earlier diagnosis, at X, made by screening tests before the clinical diagnosis, at Y, suggests an increased survival time of A + B compared to B. The actual survival time (C) remains unchanged.

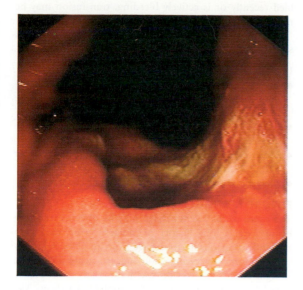

**Fig. 4.17** Carcinoma of the stomach. Endoscopic picture showing a large irregular ulcer.

CT, MRI AND ULTRASOUND. These are used to stage for operability, but have been disappointing in detecting nodular and peritoneal metastases. Endoscopic ultrasound is now being used to stage the depth of the primary tumour invasion.

### TREATMENT

The 5-year survival rate of patients operated on for early gastric cancer (EGC) in Japan is 90%, but outside Japan EGC is rare. Surgery remains the best form of treatment if the patient is operable. Better preoperative staging has reduced the numbers undergoing operation and has improved the 5-year survival rates to around 30%. In curative operations, 5-year survival rates are as high as 50%. Despite these improved figures, the overall survival rate for a patient with gastric carcinoma has not dramatically advanced, with a 10% 5-year survival.

Treatment with chemotherapy has made little impact and is currently not justifiable apart from in clinical trials. Survival may be prolonged by a few months but the toxicity of the drugs limits their use. Cimetidine has been used with some success in trials. Palliative care with relief of pain and counselling is essential (see p. 376).

## Primary lymphoma

Lymphoma of the stomach can account for 10% of all gastric malignancies in the developed world. It is a non-Hodgkin's lymphoma of the B cell type arising from mucosal-associated lymphoid tissue. *H. pylori* is thought to play an aetiological role. Clinical presentation is the same as gastric carcinoma. Treatment is surgical with postoperative radiotherapy and chemotherapy. Eradication of *H. pylori* is strongly recommended. Prognosis is good with a 75% 5-year survival depending on the type of lymphoma.

This section should be read in conjunction with the descriptions of the specific conditions mentioned.

## Acute upper gastrointestinal bleeding

Haematemesis is the vomiting of blood. Melaena is the passage of black tarry stools; the black colour is due to altered blood by acid—50 ml or more is required to produce this. Melaena can occur with bleeding from any lesion from areas proximal to and including the caecum. Following a massive bleed from the upper gastrointestinal tract, unaltered blood (owing to rapid transit) can appear per rectum, but this is rare. The colour of the blood appearing per rectum is dependent not only on the site of bleeding but also on the time of transit in the gut.

### AETIOLOGY

Chronic peptic ulceration still accounts for approximately half of all cases of upper gastrointestinal haemorrhage. This and other causes are shown in Fig. 4.18. The relative

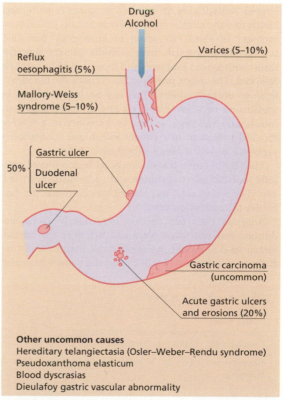

**Other uncommon causes**
Hereditary telangiectasia (Osler–Weber–Rendu syndrome)
Pseudoxanthoma elasticum
Blood dyscrasias
Dieulafoy gastric vascular abnormality

**Fig. 4.18** Causes of upper gastrointestinal haemorrhage. The approximate frequency is also given.

incidences of these causes vary depending on the patient population.

DRUGS. Aspirin and other NSAIDs can undoubtedly produce gastric lesions. These agents are also responsible for gastrointestinal haemorrhage from both duodenal and gastric ulcers, particularly in the elderly. Corticosteroids in the usual therapeutic doses probably have no influence on gastrointestinal haemorrhage.

### IMMEDIATE MANAGEMENT

All cases with a recent (i.e. within 48 hours) significant gastrointestinal bleed should be admitted to hospital. In many, no further immediate treatment is required as the patient's cardiovascular system can compensate for the blood loss. Approximately 85% of patients stop bleeding spontaneously within 48 hours.

*Factors affecting management* are:
- Age (see below).
- The amount of blood lost, which may give some guide to the severity.
- Continuing visible blood loss.
- Signs of chronic liver disease on examination, as the bleeding is often severe and recurrent if it is from varices; liver failure can develop.
- Presence of the classical clinical features of shock (i.e. pallor, cold nose, tachycardia and low blood pressure) (Emergency box 4.1); remember that the peripheral constriction that occurs may keep the blood pressure falsely high.

Urgent resuscitation is required in patients with large bleeds and the clinical signs of shock. Details of the management of shock are given in Emergency box 13.1, p. 721. Many hospitals have multidisciplinary specialist teams with agreed protocols and these should be carefully followed. The major principle is to restore the blood volume to normal rapidly. This can be best achieved by transfusion of whole blood via one or more large bore intravenous cannulae. It may be necessary in a severely shocked patient or in a patient with blood compatibility problems to give a blood substitute initially.

The rate of blood transfusion must be monitored carefully to avoid overtransfusion and consequent heart failure. The pulse rate and venous pressure are the best guides to transfusion rates.

Anaemia does not develop immediately as haemodilution has not taken place and therefore the haemoglobin level is a poor indicator of the need to transfuse. If the level is low ($<10$ g dl$^{-1}$) and the patient has either bled recently or is actively bleeding, transfusion may be necessary.

In most patients the bleeding stops, albeit temporarily, so that further assessment can be made.

### Important factors in reassessment
- Age—below the age of 60 years mortality from gastrointestinal bleeding is small. Above the age of 80 the mortality is greater than 20%.
- Recurrent haemorrhage—these patients have an increased mortality.
- Most re-bleeds (approximately 25% of all cases) occur within 48 hours.
- Melaena is usually less hazardous than haematemesis.

### FUTURE MANAGEMENT

The cause of the haemorrhage may be obvious from the history, e.g. a long history of indigestion or, more significantly, previous haemorrhage from an ulcer. A history of aspirin or NSAID ingestion suggests acute ulceration.

Signs of chronic liver disease, particularly with splenomegaly, suggest bleeding from oesophageal varices. The source of haemorrhage in most patients with chronic liver disease is their varices, but occasionally they may bleed from an accompanying peptic ulcer. The absence of splenomegaly does not rule out oesophageal varices.

ENDOSCOPY should be performed as soon as practically possible, but urgently in patients with suspected liver disease or with continued bleeding. Endoscopy can detect the cause of the haemorrhage in 80% or more of cases. In patients with a peptic ulcer, if the stigmata of a recent bleed are seen, i.e. a visible vessel or adherent clot, the patient is more likely to re-bleed.

At endoscopy:
- Varices should be injected—see p. 264 for management of varices.
- All bleeding ulcers should be either injected with adrenaline and a sclerosant or the vessel coagulated either with a heater probe or with laser therapy. These methods reduce the incidence of re-bleeding, although they do not significantly improve mortality.

MOST CONDITIONS require no specific therapy after resuscitation. There is little evidence that H$_2$-receptor antagonists affect the mortality rate of gastrointestinal haemorrhage, but these agents are usually given to patients with ulcers because of their longer term benefits.

RE-BLEEDS. Endoscopy should be repeated to reassess the bleeding site and to treat, if possible. Surgery is only necessary if bleeding is persistent or recurrent, and if it cannot be controlled.

DISCHARGE POLICY. Patients under the age of 60 years with duodenal ulceration, who are haemodynamically stable and have no stigmata of recent haemorrhage on endoscopy can be discharged from hospital within 24 hours.

### Specific conditions

CHRONIC PEPTIC ULCER. Since the advent of H$_2$-receptor antagonists, omeprazole and the role of *H. pylori*

---

The main indicator is *shock*, i.e.
  pallor
  cold nose
  low blood pressure (systolic <100 mmHg)
  tachycardia (pulse >100 beats min$^{-1}$)

Haemoglobin <10 g dl$^{-1}$ in patients with recent or active bleeding

**Emergency box 4.1** Indications for blood transfusion (see also p. 722).

in aetiology, every effort should be made to avoid surgery. If necessary to control haemorrhage the bleeding vessel is ligated, but no other surgical procedure is undertaken. Eradication of *H. pylori* is mandatory following a bleed.

GASTRIC CARCINOMA. Most patients do not have large bleeds with this condition but surgery may be performed for the lesion *per se*.

OESOPHAGEAL VARICES. These are discussed on p. 264.

MALLORY–WEISS TEAR. This is a linear mucosal tear occurring at the oesophagogastric junction and produced by a sudden increase in intra-abdominal pressure. It often occurs after a bout of coughing or retching and is classically seen after an alcohol binge. There may, however, be no antecedent history of retching. The haemorrhage may be large but most patients stop spontaneously. Rarely, surgery with over-sewing of the tear will be required.

## PROGNOSIS

The mortality of gastrointestinal haemorrhage has not changed over the years, despite many changes in management (see above) partly owing to more patients being elderly. Early endoscopy has not so far reduced the mortality, although bleeding episodes are reduced.

## Acute lower gastrointestinal bleeding

Massive bleeding from the lower gastrointestinal tract is rare. On the other hand, small bleeds from haemorrhoids occur very commonly. Massive bleeding is usually due to diverticular disease or ischaemic colitis and may require urgent resuscitation. Surgery is rarely required as bleeding usually stops spontaneously. The causes of lower gastrointestinal bleeding are shown in Fig. 4.19.

## MANAGEMENT

*Resuscitation* when required.

*Make diagnosis* using the following investigations as appropriate:
- Rectal examination, e.g. carcinoma
- Proctoscopy, e.g. haemorrhoids
- Sigmoidoscopy, e.g. inflammatory bowel disease
- Barium enema—any mucosal lesion
- Colonoscopy—diagnosis and removal of polyps
- Angiography—vascular abnormality, e.g. angiodysplasia

*Treatment.* Individual lesions are treated as appropriate.

## Chronic gastrointestinal bleeding

Patients with chronic bleeding usually present with iron deficiency anaemia (see Chapter 6).

Chronic blood loss producing anaemia in all men and all women after the menopause is always due to bleeding from the gastrointestinal tract. Occult blood tests are not, therefore, necessary (Information box 4.4).

This is frequently performed *unnecessarily*. It is *only* of value in:

Premenopausal women: if a history of menorrhagia is uncertain and the cause of iron deficiency is unclear
As a mass population screening test for large bowel malignancy (see p. 226)

*Advantages*: cheap and easy to perform

*Disadvantages*: high false-positive rate, leading to unnecessary investigations.

**Information box 4.4**   Measurement of faecal occult blood.

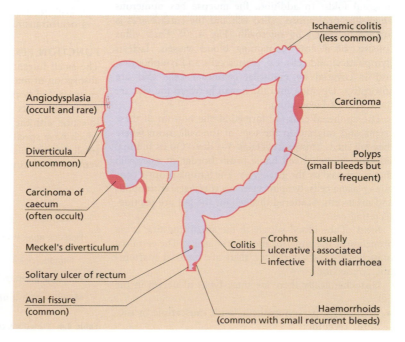

**Fig. 4.19**   Causes of lower gastrointestinal bleeding. The sites shown are illustrative—many of the lesions can be seen in other parts of the colon.

Ischaemic colitis (less common)

Carcinoma

Angiodysplasia (occult and rare)

Diverticula (uncommon)

Carcinoma of caecum (often occult)

Meckel's diverticulum

Solitary ulcer of rectum

Anal fissure (common)

Polyps (small bleeds but frequent)

Colitis — Crohns / ulcerative / infective — usually associated with diarrhoea

Haemorrhoids (common with small recurrent bleeds)

## DIAGNOSIS

Chronic blood loss can occur with any lesion of the gastrointestinal tract that produces acute bleeding (see Figs 4.18 and 4.19). In addition a Meckel's diverticulum and carcinoma of the caecum may present with an iron deficiency anaemia. It should be remembered that, worldwide, hookworm is the commonest cause of chronic gastrointestinal blood loss.

Careful history and examination may indicate the most likely site of the bleeding, but if no clue is available it is usual to investigate both the upper and lower gastrointestinal tract endoscopically at the same session ('top and tail').

For practical reasons an upper gastrointestinal endoscopy is performed first as this takes minutes only. If no lesion is found this is followed by a colonoscopy as a possible lesion can be removed or biopsied. A barium enema is performed if colonoscopy is unavailable.

A small bowel follow-through is the next investigation but the diagnostic yield is very low. Following a negative investigation, an angiogram may show up the site of bleeding, particularly when acute bleeding is occurring. Occasionally intravenous technetium-labelled colloid may be used to demonstrate the bleeding site in a Meckel's diverticulum. Endoscopes to visualize the whole of the small bowel (enteroscopy) are available at specialist centres.

# The small intestine

## STRUCTURE

The small intestine extends from the duodenum to the ileum. Its surface area is enormously increased by mucosal folds. In addition, the mucosa has numerous finger-like projections called villi and the surface area is further increased by microvilli (Fig. 4.20). Each villus consists of a core containing blood vessels, lacteals (lymphatics) and cells, e.g. plasma cells and lymphocytes, and is covered by epithelial columnar cells that are absorptive. Opening into the lumen between the villi are the crypts of Lieberkühn.

The epithelial cells are formed at the bottom of these crypts and migrate to the tops of the villi, from where they are shed. This process takes 3–4 days. On its luminal side the epithelial cell has a brush border of microvilli that is covered by the glycocalyx. The lamina propria contains plasma cells, lymphocytes, macrophages, eosinophils and mast cells. Scattered throughout the gut are peptide-secreting cells.

Most of the blood supply to the small intestine is via branches of the superior mesenteric artery. The terminal branches are end arteries, i.e. there are no local anastomotic connections.

Histochemically there are three types of nerves in the gut:
- Cholinergic parasympathetic (with muscarinic or nicotinic receptors)

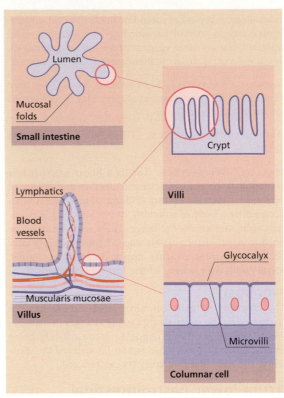

**Fig. 4.20** The structure of the small intestine.

- Adrenergic sympathetic (with both $\alpha$ and $\beta$ receptors)
- Non-cholinergic, non-adrenergic. The transmitters here are thought to be either cyclic nucleotides and ATP (the purinergic system) or intestinal hormones, e.g. vasoactive intestinal peptide (VIP) (peptidergic system) or nitric oxide which is now thought to act as a neurotransmitter.

## FUNCTION (Table 4.4)

The small intestine is concerned with the digestion and absorption of nutrients, salt and water. It produces many enzymes and hormones in order to carry out these processes. Nutrients can be absorbed throughout the small intestine with the exception of vitamin $B_{12}$ and bile salts, which have specific receptors in the terminal ileum. The small intestine also has local defence mechanisms to prevent antigens from entering the body.

Absorption

Defence against antigen entry
   Structural
   Immunological

Hormone production

Motility—transit of nutrients

**Table 4.4** Functions of the small intestine.

## General principles of absorption

SIMPLE DIFFUSION. This process requires no energy and takes place if there is a concentration gradient from the intestinal lumen (high concentration) to the bloodstream (low concentration).

ACTIVE TRANSPORT. This requires energy and can work against a concentration gradient. A carrier protein is required and the process is sodium dependent. For example, glucose enters the enterocyte on the luminal side via a sodium-dependent carrier molecule and leaves on the serosal side via a sodium-independent carrier that is found in the basolateral membrane. A gradient is maintained across the membrane by an energy-dependent sodium pump (Na$^+$, K$^+$ ATPase) that keeps the intracellular sodium concentration low (Fig. 4.21).

FACILITATED DIFFUSION. This is an energy-independent carrier-mediated transport system that allows a faster absorption rate than simple diffusion, e.g. fructose absorption.

## Absorption in the small intestine

CARBOHYDRATE. Dietary carbohydrate consists mainly of starch with some sucrose and a small amount of lactose. Starch is a polysaccharide made up of numerous glucose units. Its hydrolysis begins in the mouth by salivary amylase. The majority of hydrolysis takes place in the upper intestinal lumen by pancreatic amylase. This

hydrolysis is limited by the fact that amylases have no specificity for some glucose/glucose branching links.

$$\text{Starch} \xrightarrow{\text{AMYLASE}} \begin{cases} \alpha\text{-limit dextrins} \\ (5+ \text{ glucose units}) \\ \text{maltotriose} \\ (3 \text{ glucose units}) \\ \text{maltose} \\ (2 \text{ glucose units}) \end{cases}$$

These breakdown products, together with sucrose and lactose, are hydrolysed on the brush border membrane by their appropriate oligo- and di-saccharidases to form the monosaccharides glucose, galactose and fructose. These monosaccharides are transported into the cells, largely by sodium-dependent active transport systems.

PROTEIN. Dietary and endogenous proteins (desquamated cells, intestinal secretions) are mainly digested by pancreatic enzymes prior to absorption. These proteolytic enzymes are secreted as proenzymes and transformed to active enzymes in the lumen. The presence of protein in the lumen stimulates the release of enterokinase, which activates trypsinogen to trypsin, and this in turn activates the other proenzymes, chymotrypsin and elastase. These enzymes break down protein into oligopeptides. Some di- and tri-peptides are absorbed intact by a carrier-mediated process, while the remainder are broken down into free amino acids by peptidases on the microvillus membranes

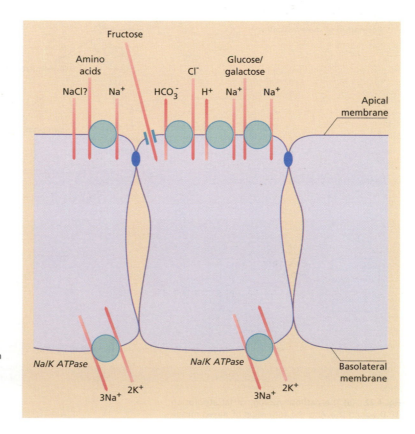

**Fig. 4.21** Diagrammatic representation of solute transport across the apical membrane showing glucose/galactose sodium-linked transport. The Na$^+$, K$^+$ ATPase pump is located in the basolateral membrane.

of the cell, prior to absorption in a similar way to disaccharides. These amino acids are transported into the cell by a number of different carrier systems.

FAT (Fig. 4.22). Dietary fat mainly consists of triglycerides with some cholesterol and fat-soluble vitamins. Emulsification of fat occurs in the stomach and is followed by hydrolysis of triglycerides in the duodenum by pancreatic lipase to yield fatty acids and monoglycerides.

Bile enters the duodenum following gal'bladder contraction. Bile contains phospholipids and bile salts, both of which are partially water soluble and act as detergents. They aggregate together to form micelles with their hydrophilic ends on the outside. Trapped in the hydrophobic centre of this micelle are the monoglycerides, fatty acids and cholesterol; these are then transported to the intestinal cell membrane. At the cell membrane the lipid contents of the micelle are absorbed, while the bile salts remain in the lumen. Inside the cell the monoglycerides and fatty acids are re-esterified to triglycerides. The triglycerides and other fat-soluble molecules (e.g. cholesterol, phospholipids) are then incorporated into chylomicrons to be transported into the lymph.

Medium-chain triglycerides (which contain fatty acids of chain length 6–12) as well as a small amount of long-chain fatty acids are transported via the portal vein.

Bile salts are not absorbed in the jejunum, so that the intraluminal concentration in the upper gut is high. They pass down the intestine to be absorbed in the terminal ileum and are transported back to the liver. This enterohepatic circulation prevents excess loss of bile salts (see p. 239).

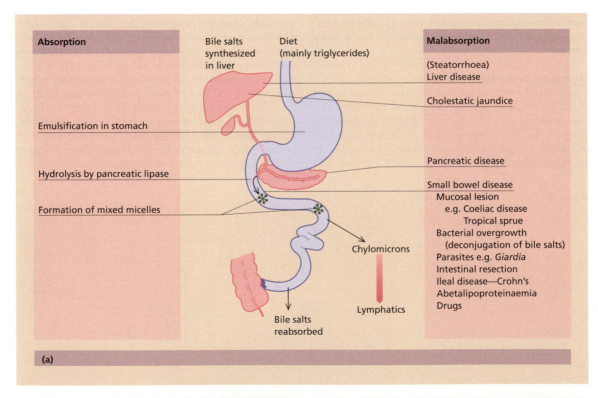

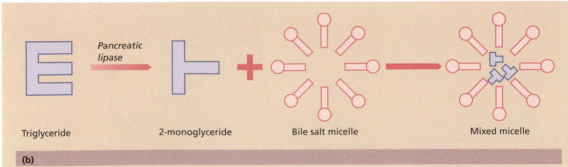

**Fig. 4.22**   (a) The pathophysiology of fat absorption.
(b) Diagram showing the formation of mixed micelles.

The pathophysiology of fat absorption is shown in Fig. 4.22. Interference with absorption can occur at all stages, as indicated, giving rise to steatorrhoea.

WATER AND ELECTROLYTES. A large amount of water and electrolytes, partly dietary, but mainly from intestinal secretions, are absorbed coupled with monosaccharides and amino acids in the upper jejunum. Some water and electrolytes are absorbed in the ileum and right side of the colon, where active sodium transport occurs but which is not coupled to solute absorption. Intestinal secretion also takes place and abnormalities of this mechanism cause secretory diarrhoea (see p. 227).

WATER-SOLUBLE VITAMINS, ESSENTIAL METALS AND TRACE ELEMENTS. These all have to be absorbed in the small intestine. It must be remembered that vitamin $B_{12}$ (see p. 304) is the only substance other than bile salts that is specifically absorbed in the terminal ileum alone and malabsorption of both these substances will always occur following ileal resection.

CALCIUM. See p. 422.

IRON. See p. 300.

## Defence against antigens (see also p. 139)

The normal intestinal mucosa forms an intrinsic barrier to the absorption of many antigens such as bacteria, viruses or dietary proteins. The mucosa contains scattered lymphoid cells as well as lymphoid aggregates, e.g. the tonsils and Peyer's patches, to form the gut-associated lymphoid tissue (GALT) (Fig 4.23).

Antigenic priming of the GALT can give rise to specific secretory immunity, not only in the gut but also in other mucosal-associated lymphoid tissue (MALT), e.g. respiratory tract, lacrimal, salivary and mammary glands. This is because of the migration of specifically primed T and B cells from the GALT via the local mesenteric lymph nodes, and the thoracic duct and peripheral circulation back to the lamina propria (of gut or other mucosal tissue) where they become immunoglobulin (Ig)-producing plasma cells.

Local mucosal immunity is provided by the secretory immunoglobulin (sIg) system. There are approximately $10^{10}$ Ig-producing immunocytes (plasma cells and plasmoblasts) per metre of human small bowel of which 70–90% are IgA immunocytes. Dimeric and polymeric IgA (pIgA) and IgM, containing a disulphide-linked polypeptide called 'J' (or 'joining') chain, are transported through the glandular epithelium via the transmembrane pIg receptor called 'secretory component' (SC) into the gut lumen. These antibodies are the first line of defence against antigens in the lumen and may take part in the immunological homeostasis within the mucosa, e.g. dampening T-cell-mediated hypersensitivity responses against harmless absorbed luminal antigens. SC expression can be up-regulated by lymphokines, e.g. interferon-$\gamma$ (IFN-$\gamma$) and tumour necrosis factor-$\alpha$ (TNF-$\alpha$) secreted by activated T cells and macrophages respectively, thus promoting the transport of IgA and IgM into the lumen.

A specialized epithelial cell above the Peyer's patches, called the 'M' or 'membrane' cell, lacks SC and HLA-DR expression; these cells allow non-selective inward transport of luminal antigens. Antigens may also be taken up by other epithelial cells (expressing HLA-DR) on a genetically restricted basis and may subsequently be

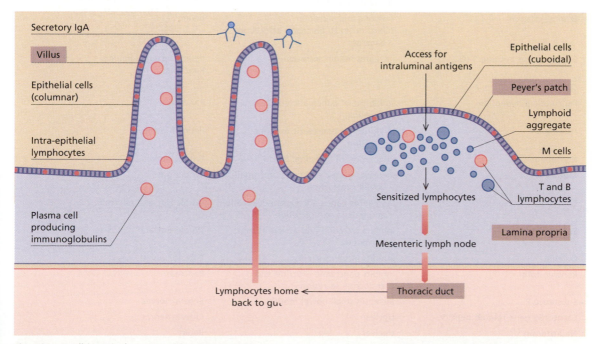

**Fig. 4.23** Small intestinal mucosa with a Peyer's patch showing the gut-associated lymphoid tissue.

presented directly by antigen-presenting cells (macrophages) to primed (memory) T lymphocytes.

Intraepithelial lymphocytes (IEL) are mainly T cells with a predominance of T8 (CD8+) cells, whereas the lamina propria contains mainly T4 (CD4+) subsets. Most human IELs express the T cell receptor $\alpha/\beta$ (TCR$\alpha/\beta$) which, along with considerable CD45RO expression, suggest that they are traditional memory T cells. Few cells express TCR$\gamma/\delta$.

### Peptide production

The hormone-producing cells of the gut are scattered diffusely throughout its length and also occur in the pancreas. The cells that synthesize these hormones are derived from neural ectoderm and are known as APUD (amine precursor uptake and decarboxylation) cells. Many of these hormones have very similar structures. Although they can be detected by radioimmunoassay in the circulation, their action is often local.

Table 4.5 shows some gut hormones and their possible physiological actions. Many are also found in other tissues, particularly the brain. A number do not act as true hormones but act as neurotransmitters or have local effects on adjacent cells only (paracrine effects).

The exact physiological role of these peptides is still being evaluated. Their importance clinically is that they may be secreted in excess, particularly in endocrine tumours of the pancreas (see p. 291).

Growth factors, like transforming growth factor $\alpha$, are also produced by intestinal cells.

| Hormone | Physiological action | Main gut localization |
|---|---|---|
| *Peptides with similar structure* | | |
| Cholecystokinin (CCK) | Stimulates gallbladder contraction and colonic motility. Pancreatic secretion (minor role) ?Role in satiety | Duodenum and jejunum Enteric nerves |
| Gastrin | Stimulates acid secretion. Stimulates growth of gut mucosa | Gastric antrum, duodenum |
| *Secretin and related peptides (all possess structural homology with secretin)* | | |
| Secretin | Pancreatic bicarbonate secretion | Duodenum and jejunum |
| Vasoactive intestinal polypeptide (VIP) | Intestinal secretion. Splanchnic vasodilation | Enteric nerves |
| Peptide histidine, methionine | As for VIP | Enteric nerves |
| Gastric inhibitory polypeptide (GIP) | Facilitates insulin release by islets ?Inhibits acid secretion | Duodenum |
| Enteroglucagon | ?Inhibits acid secretion ?Contributes to glucagon effects on pancreas | Ileum |
| Glucagon-like peptide 1 (GLP-1) | Increases insulin secretion | Ileum. Terminal ileum Pancreas |
| *Other* | | |
| Pancreatic polypeptide | ?Inhibitor of pancreatic and biliary secretion | Pancreas |
| Peptide YY | Inhibition of pancreatic exocrine secretion | Ileum and colon |
| Neuropeptide Y | Regulation of intestinal blood flow | Enteric nerves |
| Motilin | Increases gastric emptying and small bowel contraction | Whole gut |
| Bombesin | Stimulates pancreatic exocrine secretion and gastric acid secretion | Whole gut and pancreas |
| Somatostatin | Inhibits secretion and action of most hormones | Whole gut and pancreas |
| Galanin | Inhibits insulin secretion | Enteric nerves |
| Pancreastatin | Inhibits pancreatic exocrine and endocrine secretion | Pancreas |
| Substance P | Increases small bowel motility | Enteric nerves |
| Calcitonin gene-related peptide | Unclear | Enteric nerves |
| Neurotensin | Unclear | Ileum |

**Table 4.5** Gastrointestinal peptides.

## Gut motility

The contractile patterns of small intestinal muscles are primarily determined by integrated neural circuits within the gut wall—the enteric nervous system. The central nervous system and gut hormones also have a modulatory role on motility. During fasting, a distally migrating sequence of motor events termed the migrating motor complex (MMC) occurs in a cyclical fashion. The MMC consists of a period of motor quiescence (phase I) followed by a period of irregular contractile activity (phase II), culminating in a short (5–10 min) burst of regular phasic contractions (phase III). Each MMC cycle lasts for approximately 90 min. In the duodenum, phase III is associated with increased gastric, pancreatic and biliary secretions. The role of the MMC is unclear, but the strong phase III contractions propel secretions, residual food and desquamated cells towards the colon, acting as an 'intestinal housekeeper'.

After a meal, the MMC pattern is disrupted and replaced by irregular contractions. This seemingly chaotic fed pattern lasts typically for 2–5 hours, depending on the size and nutrient content of the meal. The irregular contractions of the fed pattern have a mixing function, moving intraluminal contents to and fro, aiding the digestive process.

## PRESENTING FEATURES OF SMALL BOWEL DISEASE

Regardless of the cause, the common presenting features of small bowel disease are:

DIARRHOEA. This is a common feature of small bowel disease but approximately 10–20% of patients will have no diarrhoea or any other gastrointestinal symptoms. Steatorrhoea is occasionally present.

ABDOMINAL PAIN AND DISCOMFORT. Abdominal distension can cause discomfort and flatulence. The pain has no specific character or periodicity and is not usually severe.

WEIGHT LOSS. Weight loss is due to the anorexia that invariably accompanies small bowel disease. Although malabsorption occurs, the amount is small relative to intake.

NUTRITIONAL DEFICIENCIES. Deficiencies of iron, vitamin $B_{12}$, folate or all of these, leading to anaemia, are the only common deficiencies. Occasionally malabsorption of other vitamins or minerals occurs, causing bruising (vitamin K deficiency), tetany (calcium deficiency), osteomalacia (vitamin D deficiency), or stomatitis, sore tongue and aphthous ulceration (multiple vitamin deficiencies).

Ankle oedema may be seen and is partly nutritional and partly due to intestinal loss of albumin.

## PHYSICAL SIGNS OF SMALL BOWEL DISEASE

These are few and non-specific. If present they are associated with anaemia and the nutritional deficiencies described above.

Abdominal examination is often normal, but sometimes distension and, rarely, hepatomegaly or an abdominal mass are found. In the severely ill patient gross malnutrition with muscle wasting is seen. A neuropathy, not always due to vitamin $B_{12}$ deficiency, can be present.

## INVESTIGATION OF SMALL BOWEL DISEASE
(Fig. 4.24)

### Blood tests

FULL BLOOD COUNT and film. Anaemia can be microcytic (low mean corpuscular volume [MCV]) or macrocytic (high MCV). The blood film may also show other abnormal cells, e.g. Howell–Jolly bodies, which are seen in splenic atrophy associated with coeliac disease.

SERUM IRON. If the MCV is low, serum iron and total iron-binding capacity or serum ferritin are determined.

SERUM VITAMIN $B_{12}$/FOLATE. If the MCV is high, serum vitamin $B_{12}$, serum and red cell folate are determined. However, with mixed deficiencies, the MCV may be normal. The red cell folate is a good indicator of the presence of small bowel disease. It is frequently low in both coeliac disease and Crohn's disease which are the two commonest causes of small bowel disease in developed countries.

SERUM ALBUMIN gives some indication of the nutritional status.

LOW SERUM CALCIUM and raised alkaline phosphatase may indicate the presence of osteomalacia.

AUTOANTIBODIES. In countries with a high incidence of coeliac disease, measurement in the serum of anti-reticulin and/or endomysial antibodies are a useful adjunct for the diagnosis of coeliac disease.

If the clinical suspicion of malabsorption is high, the structure of the small bowel should be studied next.

### Small bowel anatomy

SMALL BOWEL FOLLOW-THROUGH (see p. 179). This detects gross anatomical defects such as diverticula, strictures and Crohn's disease. Dilatation of the folds and a changed fold pattern may suggest malabsorption but, as these are not specific findings, the diagnosis should not be based on these alone. Gross dilatation is seen in pseudo-obstruction.

JEJUNAL BIOPSY (Practical box 4.4). This is used to assess the microanatomy of the small bowel. Biopsies can be obtained via an endoscope passed into the duodenum either with a Crosby–Kugler capsule inserted retrogradely up the endoscope or with a grab biopsy using large forceps. Alternatively, specimens can be obtained by swallowing a Crosby–Kugler capsule. With either technique, an adequate piece of tissue, well orientated, is necessary for correct evaluation initially under a dissecting microscope. The histological appearances will be described in the sections on individual diseases.

A smear of the jejunal juice or a mucosal impression can also be made and is helpful in the diagnosis of *Giardia lamblia* (see p. 74).

### Tests of absorption

These are only required in complicated cases.

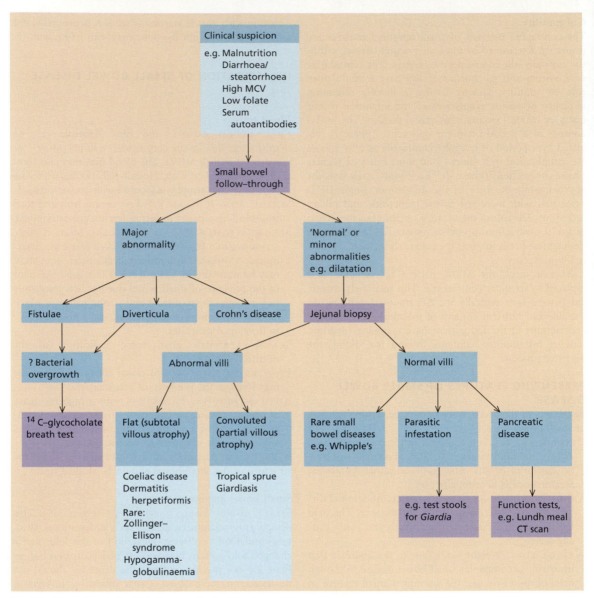

**Fig. 4.24**  Flow diagram for investigation of patients with suspected small bowel disease. MCV; mean corpuscular volume.

FAT MALABSORPTION. The confirmation of the presence of steatorrhoea is occasionally necessary. The fat content of stools is measured using a 3-day collection of faeces with the patient on a diet containing 100 g of fat daily. Normal faecal fat excretion is less than 17 mmol (6 g) per day.

To avoid faecal collections, fat absorption can also be measured using breath analysis. Following oral administration of a radiolabelled fat load, the amount of $^{14}CO_2$ in the expired breath gives an indication of the amount of fat malabsorption. Comparison between a labelled triglyceride ([$^{14}C$]triolein) and a labelled fatty acid ([$^3H$]oleic acid) is used to diagnose pancreatic disease, when fatty acid absorption will be normal.

D-XYLOSE TOLERANCE TEST. Xylose is a sugar which is absorbed from the proximal small intestine. The urinary xylose excretion and the blood xylose level following an oral dose reflect its absorption. This test tends to produce many false-positives and although still used in some centres it should be phased out.

LACTOSE TOLERANCE TEST. This involves the oral ingestion of 50 g of lactose and the measurement of blood glucose. The test is of little use in adults as lactose intolerance is not a clinical problem since these patients avoid milk by choice. There is a high incidence of lactase deficiency in many parts of the world, e.g. the Mediterranean countries, and parts of Africa and Asia. It should be remembered that a glass of milk only contains approximately 11 g of lactose.

A glucose tolerance test should not be performed, as it is influenced by many factors other than absorption.

1  The patient is fasted overnight.
2  A Crosby–Kugler capsule is swallowed, guided through the pylorus with screening, and then allowed to pass to just beyond the duodenojejunal junction.
3  A small piece of mucosa is sucked into the capsule; additional suction triggers the knife to remove a mucosal specimen.
4  The capsule is immediately withdrawn.
5  The specimen is examined immediately under a dissecting microscope.
6  The specimen is then placed in 10% formalin for histological examination.
7  Alternatively, biopsies can be obtained via an endoscope.

*Complications*

Haemorrhage or perforation (very rare).

**Practical box 4.4**   Jejunal biopsy.

SCHILLING TEST. This is performed to look for vitamin $B_{12}$ malabsorption. It is described in detail on p. 306. In gastrointestinal disease it is used to detect:
● Pernicious anaemia
● Ileal disease (when oral vitamin $B_{12}$ is given with intrinsic factor)
● Bacterial overgrowth (measurement of vitamin $B_{12}$ plus intrinsic factor absorption is repeated after antibiotics)

### Other tests

[$^{14}$C]GLYCOCHOLIC ACID BREATH TEST (Fig. 4.25). This is performed to look for bacterial overgrowth (see below). The patient is given $^{14}$C-labelled bile salts by mouth. Bacteria deconjugate the bile salts, releasing [$^{14}$C]glycine, which is metabolized and appears in the breath as $^{14}CO_2$. This radioactivity in the breath can easily be measured. An early rise indicates either bacterial overgrowth in the upper small intestine or rapid transit to the colon where, of course, bacteria are normally present.

HYDROGEN BREATH TEST. This is frequently used as a screening test to detect bacterial overgrowth. Oral lactulose or glucose is metabolized by bacteria with the production of hydrogen. An early rise in the breath hydrogen will indicate bacterial breakdown in the small intestine. Rapid transit of the lactulose to the large intestine will also produce a rise in breath hydrogen. As bacteria are present in the oral cavity, the mouth should be rinsed out with an antiseptic mouthwash prior to the test being performed. This test is simple to perform and it does not involve radioisotopes. However, interpretation is often difficult.

DIRECT INTUBATION. Aspiration of intestinal juices is another method by which bacterial contamination can be detected. Bacterial counts are performed on aerobic and anaerobic cultures. Chromatography of bile salts can also be performed on the aspirate to detect evidence of deconjugation by bacteria.

PANCREATIC TESTS (see p. 286). These are used in the differential diagnosis of steatorrhoea.

OTHER BLOOD TESTS. Serum immunoglobulins are measured to exclude immune deficiencies. Hormones, e.g. VIP, are measured in high-volume secretory diarrhoea.

TEST FOR PROTEIN-LOSING ENTEROPATHY. Intravenous radioactive chromium chloride ($^{51}CrCl_3$) is used to label circulating albumin. In excess gastrointestinal protein loss, the faeces will contain radioactivity. This test is rarely required unless a low serum albumin is a major clinical feature.

BILE SALT LOSS. This can be demonstrated by giving oral 23-selena H,25-homotaurocholate (Se HCAT, a synthetic taurine conjugate) and measuring the retention of the bile acid by whole body counting at 7 days.

INTESTINAL PERMEABILITY TESTS. These tests can be used for the detection of small bowel disease but are not in general use. They are based on the fact that the abnormal intestinal mucosa is permeable to large molecules such as lactulose and cellobiose. An oral load of these sugars is given and the sugars are then measured in the urine. A radiolabelled sodium-EDTA solution has been used in a similar way and is said to be a more accurate investigation.

## MALABSORPTION

In many small bowel diseases, malabsorption of specific substances occurs, but these deficiencies do not dominate the clinical picture. An example is Crohn's disease, in which malabsorption of vitamin $B_{12}$ can be demonstrated,

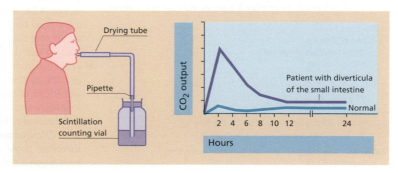

**Fig. 4.25**   The [$^{14}$C]glycocholic acid breath test. The apparatus is shown on the left. The graph shows the amount of $^{14}CO_2$ expired in the breath after an oral dose of [$^{14}$C]glycocholic acid in a normal subject and in a patient with diverticula of the small intestine.

but this is not usually a problem and diarrhoea and general ill-health are the major features.

Steatorrhoea—malabsorption of fat—is discussed on p. 202.

The major disorders of the small intestine that cause malabsorption are shown in Table 4.6.

# COELIAC DISEASE (GLUTEN-SENSITIVE ENTEROPATHY)

Coeliac disease is a condition in which there is an abnormal jejunal mucosa that improves morphologically when the patient is treated with a gluten-free diet and relapses when gluten is reintroduced. Gluten is contained in the cereals wheat, rye, barley and possibly oats.

Dermatitis herpetiformis is a skin disorder that is associated with a gluten-sensitive enteropathy (see below).

## INCIDENCE

Coeliac disease is common in Europe, with an incidence in the UK of approximately 1 in 2000. In Ireland, however, this is 1 in 300. It occurs throughout the world but is rare in the Black African.

## INHERITANCE

There is an increased incidence of coeliac disease within families but the exact mode of inheritance is unknown; 10–15% of first-degree relatives will have the condition, although it may be asymptomatic. Over 90% of patients have the haplotype HLA-A1, B8, DR3, DR7, DQW2 as compared to 20–30% of the general population. However, the fact that not all patients have this haplotype and that as many as 30% of identical twins are discordant for the condition suggests an additional factor such as a B-cell antigen, immunoglobulin heavy-chain allotype or an environmental factor.

## AETIOLOGY

Gluten is a high-molecular-weight, heterogeneous compound that can be fractionated to produce $\alpha$, $\beta$, $\gamma$ and $\omega$ gliadin peptides. $\alpha$-Gliadin is injurious to the small intestinal mucosa although there is some disagreement about the toxicity of other peptides. The exact mechanism of how the damage is produced is still not understood. There are many immunological abnormalities that revert to normal on treatment. An immunogenetic mechanism may be possible in view of the increased incidence of a particular HLA haplotype. An environmental factor, such as a viral infection, may play a role in view of the amino

acid sequence homology between gliadin and adenovirus 12.

## PATHOLOGY

The mucosa of the proximal small bowel is predominantly affected, the mucosal damage decreasing in severity towards the ileum as the gluten is digested into smaller non-toxic fragments. Under the dissecting microscope there is an absence of villi, making the mucosal surface flat. Histological examination shows that the crypts are elongated, with chronic inflammatory cells in the lamina propria (Fig. 4.26). The lesion is described as *subtotal villous atrophy*, although true atrophy of the mucosa is not present because the crypt hyperplasia compensates for villous atrophy and the total mucosal thickness is normal.

The surface cells become cuboidal. There is an increase in the number of IELs (per 100 epithelial cells) which show an increased expression of the $\gamma/\delta$ TCR, instead of the $\alpha/\beta$ receptor (see p. 204), and this appears to be specific to coeliac disease. In the lamina propria there is an increase in lymphocytes and plasma cells.

## CLINICAL FEATURES

Coeliac disease can present at any age. In infancy it appears after weaning on to gluten-containing foods. The peak incidence in adults is in the third and fourth decades, with a female preponderance. The symptoms are very variable and often non-specific with tiredness and malaise. Common gastrointestinal symptoms include diarrhoea or steatorrhoea, abdominal discomfort or pain and weight loss.

Mouth ulcers and angular stomatitis are frequent and can be intermittent. Rare complications include tetany, osteomalacia, neurological symptoms such as paraesthesia, muscle weakness or peripheral neuropathy, or gross malnutrition with peripheral oedema.

There is an increased incidence of atopy and autoimmune disease, including thyroid disease and insulin-dependent diabetes. Other associated diseases include inflammatory bowel disease, chronic liver disease and fibrosing allergic alveolitis.

Physical signs are usually few and non-specific and are related to anaemia and malnutrition.

## INVESTIGATION

JEJUNAL BIOPSY. The mucosal appearance of a jejunal biopsy specimen is diagnostic and this investigation should always be performed in suspected cases. Other causes of a flat mucosa in adults are rare and are shown in Fig. 4.24. If the biopsy is performed endoscopically, a dye can be injected on to the duodenal mucosa to accentuate the smoothness of the mucosa (positive dye test) before the biopsy is taken.

HAEMATOLOGY. A mild or moderate anaemia is present in 50% of cases. Folate deficiency is almost invariably present in coeliac disease, giving rise in most instances to a high MCV. Vitamin $B_{12}$ deficiency is rare but iron deficiency due to malabsorption of iron and increased loss of desquamated cells is common. A blood film may therefore show microcytes and macrocytes as well as hypersegmented polymorphonuclear leucocytes and

Coeliac disease
Dermatitis herpetiformis
Tropical sprue
Bacterial overgrowth
Intestinal resection
Whipple's disease
Radiation enteritis
Parasite infestation, e.g. *Giardia lamblia*

**Table 4.6** Disorders of the small intestine causing malabsorption.

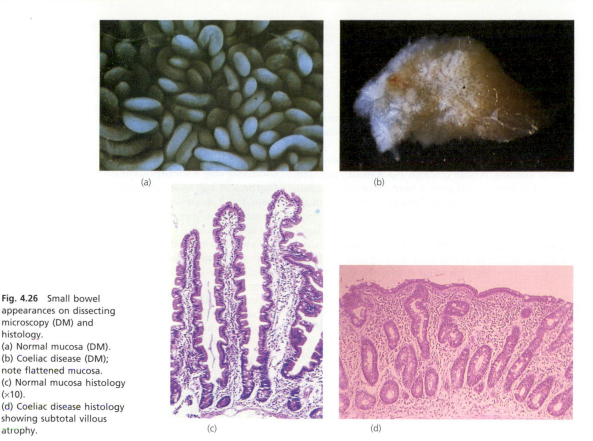

**Fig. 4.26** Small bowel appearances on dissecting microscopy (DM) and histology.
(a) Normal mucosa (DM).
(b) Coeliac disease (DM); note flattened mucosa.
(c) Normal mucosa histology (×10).
(d) Coeliac disease histology showing subtotal villous atrophy.

(a)

(b)

(c)

(d)

Howell–Jolly bodies (due to splenic atrophy).

ANTIRETICULIN ANTIBODIES and endomysial antibodies (IgA) are found in the serum of the majority of cases.

ABSORPTION TESTS are often abnormal (see p. 206) but are seldom performed.

SMALL BOWEL FOLLOW-THROUGH may show dilatation of the small bowel with a change in fold pattern; folds become thicker and in the severer forms total effacement is seen.

OTHER BIOCHEMICAL ABNORMALITIES are seen in the severely ill patient, e.g. hypoalbuminaemia.

### TREATMENT AND MANAGEMENT

A gluten-free diet usually produces a rapid clinical and morphological improvement. Replacement haematinics are given initially to replace body stores. The usual cause for failure to respond to the diet is poor compliance. A gluten challenge, i.e. reintroduction of gluten with evidence of jejunal morphological change, confirms the diagnosis. In the straightforward cases this is not necessary, although transient gluten intolerance has been described in early childhood. Many patients do not keep to a strict diet but nevertheless maintain good health. The long-term effects of this low gluten intake are uncertain.

### COMPLICATIONS

A few patients do not improve on a strict diet (unresponsive 'coeliac disease'). Often no cause for this is found, but intestinal lymphoma, ulcerative jejunitis or carcinoma are sometimes responsible. The incidence of small intestinal T-cell lymphoma (see p. 214) is increased in coeliac disease. Carcinoma of the small bowel and oesophagus as well as extra-gastrointestinal cancers are also seen. Table 4.7 shows the incidence of malignancy compared to the incidence in other gastrointestinal disorders. Malignancy seems to be unrelated to the duration of the disease but the incidence may be reduced by a gluten-free diet.

## Dermatitis herpetiformis (see p. 1010)

This is an uncommon blistering subepidermal eruption of the skin associated with a gluten-sensitive enteropathy. Rarely there may be gross malabsorption, but usually the jejunal morphological abnormalities are not as severe as

| Disorders | % |
|---|---|
| Familial adenomatous polyposis | 100 |
| Barrett's oesophagus | 15 |
| Chronic ulcerative colitis | 13 |
| Coeliac disease | 13 |
| Pernicious anaemia | <5 |
| Postgastrectomy stomach | <5 |

**Table 4.7** Incidence of malignancy in various gastrointestinal disorders, compared to familial adenomatous polyposis.

in coeliac disease. The inheritance and immunological abnormalities are the same as for coeliac disease. The skin condition responds to dapsone but both the gut and the skin will improve on a gluten-free diet.

# Tropical sprue

This is a condition presenting with malabsorption that occurs in residents or visitors to a tropical area where the disease is endemic.

Malabsorption of a mild degree, sometimes following an enteric infection, is quite common and is usually asymptomatic. The term *tropical sprue* is reserved for severe malabsorption (of two or more substances) that is usually accompanied by diarrhoea and malnutrition. Tropical sprue is endemic in most of Asia, some Caribbean islands, Puerto Rico and parts of South America. Epidemics occur, lasting up to 2 years, and in some areas repeated epidemics occur at varying intervals of up to 10 years.

## AETIOLOGY

The aetiology is unknown, but is likely to be infective because the disease occurs in epidemics and patients improve on antibiotics. A number of agents have been suggested but none has been shown to be unequivocally responsible. Different agents could be involved in different parts of the world. An overgrowth of coliforms that produce an enterotoxin has been reported.

## CLINICAL FEATURES

These vary in intensity and consist of diarrhoea, anorexia, abdominal distension and weight loss. The onset is sometimes acute and occurs either a few days or many years after being in the tropics. Epidemics can break out in villages, affecting thousands of people at the same time. The onset can also be insidious, with chronic diarrhoea and evidence of nutritional deficiency. The clinical features of tropical sprue vary in different parts of the world, particularly as different criteria are used for diagnosis.

## DIAGNOSIS

ACUTE INFECTIVE causes of diarrhoea must be excluded (see p. 228), particularly *Giardia*, which can produce a syndrome very similar to tropical sprue.

MALABSORPTION should be demonstrated, particularly fat and vitamin $B_{12}$ malabsorption.

THE JEJUNAL MUCOSA is abnormal, showing some villous atrophy (partial villous atrophy). In most cases the lesion is less severe than that found in coeliac disease, although it affects the whole small bowel. Mild changes can be seen in asymptomatic individuals in the tropics, so jejunal mucosal changes must be interpreted carefully.

## TREATMENT

Many patients improve when they leave the sprue area and take folic acid (5 mg daily). Most patients also require an antibiotic (usually tetracycline 1 g daily) to ensure a complete recovery; it may be necessary to give this for up to 6 months.

The severely ill patient requires resuscitation with fluids and electrolytes for dehydration; any nutritional deficiencies should be corrected. Vitamin $B_{12}$ (1000 $\mu$g) is also given to all acute cases.

## PROGNOSIS

The prognosis is excellent. Mortality is usually associated with water and electrolyte depletion, particularly in epidemics.

# Bacterial overgrowth

The upper part of the small intestine is almost sterile, containing only a few organisms derived from the mouth. Gastric acid kills most organisms and intestinal motility keeps the jejunum empty. The normal terminal ileum contains faecal-type organisms, mainly *Escherichia coli* and anaerobes.

Bacterial overgrowth is normally only found associated with a structural abnormality of the small intestine, although it can occur alone in the elderly. Aspiration of the upper jejunum will reveal the presence of *E. coli* and/or *Bacteroides*, both in concentrations greater than $10^6$/ml as part of a mixed flora. These bacteria are capable of deconjugating and dehydroxylating bile salts, so that unconjugated and dehydroxylated bile salts can be detected in aspirates by chromatography. Steatorrhoea (see p. 202) occurs as a result of conjugated bile salt deficiency.

The bacteria are able to metabolize vitamin $B_{12}$ and interfere with its binding to intrinsic factor, thereby leading to vitamin $B_{12}$ deficiency; this can be demonstrated using the Schilling test. Conversely some bacteria produce folic acid.

Bacterial overgrowth has only minimal effects on other substances absorbed from the small intestine. The clinical features are chiefly diarrhoea, steatorrhoea and vitamin $B_{12}$ deficiency, although this is not so severe as to produce a neurological deficit.

Although bacterial overgrowth may be responsible for the presenting symptoms, it must be remembered that many of the symptoms may be due to the underlying small bowel pathology.

## TREATMENT

If possible, the underlying lesion should be corrected, e.g. a stricture should be resected. With multiple diverticula, grossly dilated bowel, or in Crohn's disease, this may not be possible and rotating courses of antibiotics are necessary, such as metronidazole and tetracycline, or ciprofloxacin.

# Intestinal resection (Fig. 4.27)

Intestinal resection is usually well tolerated, but massive resection is followed by the short-gut syndrome. The effects of resection depend on the extent and the areas involved.

EXTENT. Because the gut is long, a 30–50% resection can usually be tolerated without undue problems.

### Ileal resection

The ileum has specific receptors for the absorption of bile salts and vitamin $B_{12}$, so that relatively small resections

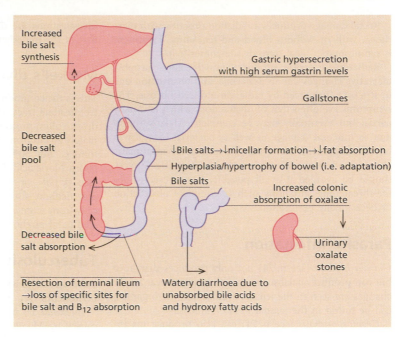

**Fig. 4.27**  The effects of resection of distal small bowel.

will lead to malabsorption of these substances. Removal of the ileocaecal valve increases the incidence of diarrhoea. In ileal resection:

- Bile salts and fatty acids enter the colon and interfere with water and electrolyte absorption, causing diarrhoea.
- Increased bile salt synthesis can compensate for loss of approximately one-third of the bile salts in the faeces. Greater loss than this results in decreased micellar formation and steatorrhoea, and lithogenic bile and gallstone formation.
- Increased oxalate absorption is caused by the presence of bile salts in the colon. This gives rise to renal oxalate stones.
- There is a low serum vitamin $B_{12}$ and macrocytosis.

INVESTIGATION. This includes a small bowel follow-through, measurement of vitamin $B_{12}$, bile salt and occasionally fat absorption (see p. 206).

MANAGEMENT. Many patients require vitamin $B_{12}$ replacement and some need a low-fat diet if there is steatorrhoea. If diarrhoea is a problem, cholestyramine or aluminium hydroxide mixture to bind bile salts sometimes helps.

**Jejunal resection**
Here the ileum can take over jejunal absorptive function. Jejunal resection may lead to gastric hypersecretion with high gastrin levels; the exact mechanism of this is unclear. Intestinal adaptation takes place, with an increase in absorption per unit length of bowel.

**Massive resection (short-gut syndrome)**
This can occur following resection in Crohn's disease, mesenteric occlusion or trauma. Diarrhoea with severe loss of water and electrolytes occurs together with malnutrition. Parenteral nutrition (sometimes long term) is necessary. With intestinal adaptation most will eventually recover, although they continue to have diarrhoea and little functional reserve should another gastrointestinal problem occur.

## Whipple's disease

This is a rare disease usually affecting males. It presents with steatorrhoea and abdominal pain along with systemic symptoms of fever and weight loss. Peripheral lymphadenopathy, arthritis and involvement of the heart, lung and brain may occur. Histologically, the villi are stunted and contain diagnostic periodic acid–Schiff (PAS)-positive macrophages. On electron microscopy, bacilli can be seen 'within' the macrophages. The organism has been identified by the polymerase chain reaction and is similar to actinomycetes and has been given the name *Tropheryma whippeii*.

A dramatic improvement occurs with antibiotic therapy, which should include an antibiotic that crosses the blood–brain barrier, e.g. chloramphenicol.

## RADIATION ENTERITIS

Radiation of more than 50 Gy will damage the intestine. The ileum and rectum are the areas most often involved, as pelvic irradiation is the common cause. There may be diarrhoea and abdominal pain at the time of the irradiation. These symptoms usually improve within 6 weeks after completion of therapy. Chronic radiation enteritis is diagnosed if symptoms persist for 3 months or more. The prevalence is more than 15%, although many more patients suffer from an increased bowel frequency.

Rectal damage produces a radiation proctitis with diarrhoea, with or without blood and tenesmus. Treatment is symptomatic; local steroids sometimes help.

Radiation enteritis produces muscle fibre atrophy, ulcerative changes due to ischaemia, and obstruction due to strictures produced by radiation-induced fibrosis. The symptoms are often that of obstruction, which is usually partial but eventually may be complete. Malabsorption due to mucosal damage as well as bacterial overgrowth in dilated segments can occur. Treatment is symptomatic although often unsuccessful in chronic enteritis. Surgery should be avoided if at all possible, being reserved for life-threatening situations such as complete obstruction or occasionally perforation.

## Parasite infestation

*Giardia lamblia* (see p. 74) not only produces diarrhoea but can produce malabsorption with steatorrhoea. Minor changes are seen in the jejunal mucosa and the organism can be found in the jejunal fluid or mucosa.

*Cryptosporidiosis* (see p. 74) can also produce malabsorption.

## Other causes of malabsorption

DRUGS that bind bile salts, e.g. cholestyramine, and some antibiotics, e.g. neomycin, produce steatorrhoea.

THYROTOXICOSIS. Diarrhoea, rarely with steatorrhoea, occurs in thyrotoxicosis owing to increased gastric emptying and motility. Steatorrhoea occurs in the *Zollinger–Ellison* syndrome (see p. 291).

INTESTINAL LYMPHANGIECTASIA produces diarrhoea and rarely steatorrhoea.

LYMPHOMA that has infiltrated the small bowel mucosa.

IN DIABETES MELLITUS, diarrhoea, malabsorption and steatorrhoea occur in some patients, sometimes due to bacterial overgrowth from stasis.

HYPOGAMMAGLOBULINAEMIA, which is seen in a number of conditions including lymphoid nodular hyperplasia, causes steatorrhoea owing either to an abnormal jejunal mucosa or to secondary infestation with *G. lamblia*.

## MISCELLANEOUS INTESTINAL DISEASES

### Protein-losing enteropathy

Protein-losing enteropathy is seen in many gastrointestinal and systemic conditions. Increased protein loss across an abnormal mucosa causes hypoalbuminaemia. Causes include inflammatory or ulcerative lesions, e.g. Crohn's disease, tumours, Ménétrier's disease, coeliac disease and lymphatic disorders, e.g. lymphangiectasia. Usually it forms a minor part of the generalized disorder, but occasionally hepatic synthesis of albumin cannot compensate for the hypoalbuminaemia, and the peripheral oedema produced may dominate the clinical picture. The investigations are described on p. 207 and treatment is that of the underlying disorder.

## Meckel's diverticulum

This is the commonest congenital abnormality of the gastrointestinal tract, affecting 2–3% of the population. The diverticulum projects from the wall of the ileum approximately 60 cm from the ileocaecal valve. It is usually symptomless, but 50% contain gastric mucosa that secretes hydrochloric acid. Peptic ulcers can occur and may bleed (see p. 199) or perforate. Acute inflammation of the diverticulum also occurs and is indistinguishable clinically from acute appendicitis. Obstruction from an associated band rarely occurs. Treatment is surgical removal.

## Tuberculosis

Tuberculosis (TB) can affect the intestine as well as the peritoneum (see p. 266).

*Intestinal* TB is due to reactivation of primary disease caused by *Mycobacterium tuberculosis*. Bovine TB occurs in areas where milk is unpasteurized and is very rare in the UK. The ileocaecal area is most commonly affected, but the colon, and rarely other parts of the gastrointestinal tract, can also be involved. TB is being seen more frequently in patients with HIV infection.

### CLINICAL FEATURES

These are chiefly diarrhoea and abdominal pain with generalized systemic manifestations, including anorexia and weight loss. Intestinal obstruction may develop.

On examination, a mass may be palpable and 50% have X-ray evidence of pulmonary TB; this is an important aid to the diagnosis.

### DIAGNOSIS

In the western hemisphere TB must be differentiated from Crohn's disease and should always be considered as a possible diagnosis in Asian immigrants. A caecal carcinoma can present with similar symptoms. An ultrasound of the abdomen may show mesenteric thickening and lymph node enlargement. Histological verification and culture of tissue is highly desirable, but it is not always possible to obtain bacteriological confirmation and treatment should be started if there is a high degree of suspicion. Specimens can be obtained by colonoscopy but laparotomy is required in some cases.

### TREATMENT

Drug treatment is similar to pulmonary TB, i.e. rifampicin, isoniazid and pyrazinamide (see p. 686), but treatment should last 1 year.

## Amyloid (see p. 866)

In systemic amyloidosis there is usually a diffuse involvement that may affect any part of the gastrointestinal tract. Occasionally amyloid deposits occur as polypoid lesions.

The symptoms depend on the site of involvement; amyloidosis in the small intestine gives rise to diarrhoea.

## Connective-tissue disorders

SYSTEMIC SCLEROSIS (see p. 402) most commonly affects the oesophagus (see p. 184), although the small bowel and colon are often found to be involved if the appropriate radiological studies are performed. Frequently there are no symptoms of this involvement, but diarrhoea and steatorrhoea can occur. This is usually due to bacterial overgrowth of the small bowel as a result of reduced motility, dilatation and the presence of diverticula.

In *rheumatoid arthritis* (see p. 387) and *systemic lupus erythematosus* (see p. 400), gastrointestinal symptoms may occur, but rarely predominate.

## Chronic intestinal ischaemia

This is due to atheromatous occlusion of mesenteric vessels in the elderly, although such occlusion often does not produce clinical effects because of the collateral circulation. The characteristic symptom is abdominal pain occurring after food. This may be followed by acute mesenteric vascular occlusion (see p. 234). Loud bruits may be heard but, as these are heard in normal subjects, they are of doubtful significance. The diagnosis is made using angiography.

The term 'coeliac axis compression syndrome' has been used in young patients with chronic abdominal pain, bruits and minor angiographic changes. Despite its plausible title, it is not an organic syndrome. Its suggested existence results from the false correlation of pain and bruits.

## Eosinophilic gastroenteritis

This is a condition of unknown aetiology in which there may be eosinophilic infiltration and oedema of any part of the gastrointestinal mucosa. It usually involves the gastric antrum and proximal small intestine either as a localized lesion (eosinophilic granuloma) or diffusely with sheets of eosinophils seen in the serosal and submucosal layers. An association with asthma, eczema and urticaria has been described.

The condition may occur at any age, but mainly in the third decade. Males are affected twice as often as females. The clinical presentation depends on the site of involvement. Abdominal pain, nausea and vomiting occur. An increased number of eosinophils in the blood is present in only 20% of patients. Radiology or endoscopy will demonstrate the lesion. Steroids are used for the widespread infiltration, particularly if peripheral eosinophilia is present.

In some adults the condition appears to be allergic (allergic gastroenteritis) and is associated with peripheral eosinophilia and high levels of blood and tissue IgE.

## Intestinal lymphangiectasia

Dilatation of the lymphatics may be primary or secondary to lymphatic obstruction, such as that occurring in malignancy or constrictive pericarditis. In the rare primary form it may be detected incidentally as dilated lacteals on a jejunal biopsy or it can produce steatorrhoea of varying degrees. Hypoproteinaemia with ankle oedema is the other main feature. Serum immunoglobulin levels are reduced with low circulating lymphocytes. Treatment is with a low-fat diet.

## Abetalipoproteinaemia

In this rare condition, there is failure of apo B100 synthesis in the liver and apo B48 in the intestinal cell, so that chylomicrons are not formed. This leads to fat accumulation in the intestinal cells, giving a characteristic histological appearance of the jejunal mucosa. Clinical features include acanthocytosis (spiky red cells due to membrane abnormalities), a form of retinitis pigmentosa, and mental and neurological abnormalities. The latter can be prevented by vitamin E injections.

## Gastrointestinal problems in patients with HIV infection (see Table 4.17)

# TUMOURS OF THE SMALL INTESTINE

The small intestine is relatively resistant to the development of neoplasia and only 3–6% of all gastrointestinal tumours and fewer than 1% of all malignant lesions occur in the small bowel. The reasons for the rarity of tumours are unknown. Explanations include the fluidity and relative sterility of small bowel contents and the rapid transit time, reducing the time of exposure to potential carcinogens. It is also possible that the high population of lymphoid tissue and secretion of IgA in the small intestine protects against malignancy.

### Benign

Adenomas, leiomyomas or lipomas are rarely found and are usually asymptomatic and picked up incidentally. In familial adenomatous polyposis the upper gut, particularly the duodenum, is affected in one-third of patients. *Peutz–Jegher syndrome* consists of mucocutaneous pigmentation (circumoral, hands and feet) and gastrointestinal polyps and has a Mendelian dominant inheritance. The brown buccal pigment is characteristic of this condition. The polyps, which are hamartomas, can occur anywhere in the gastrointestinal tract but are most frequent in the small bowel. They may bleed or cause intussusception. They virtually never become malignant. Treatment is by individual polypectomy. Multiple polypectomies may have to be performed, but bowel resection should be avoided.

### Malignant

Adenocarcinoma of the small intestine is rare and found most frequently in the duodenum in the periampullary region and in the jejunum. Lymphomas are most frequently found in the ileum. These are of the non-Hodgkin's type and must be distinguished from peripheral or nodal lymphoma involving the gut secondarily.

In developed countries, the commonest type of lymphoma is the B-cell type arising from MALT. These lymphomas tend to be annular or polypoid masses in the distal or terminal ileum, whilst most T-cell lymphomas are ulcerated plaques or strictures in the proximal small bowel.

A tumour similar to Burkitt's lymphoma also occurs and commonly affects the terminal ileum of children in North Africa and the Middle East.

Adenocarcinoma is the commonest malignancy of the small intestine accounting for up to 50% of primary tumours. Carcinoid tumours form the next major group with lymphoma and small muscle tumours making up the remainder.

### Predisposing factors

COELIAC DISEASE. There is an increased incidence of lymphoma of the T-cell type and adenocarcinoma of the small bowel in coeliac disease (see Table 4.7). There is also an increase in other malignancies both of the gastrointestinal tract and elsewhere. The reason for the local development of malignancy is unknown. It is now accepted that coeliac disease is a premalignant condition, but there is no association with a poor response to a gluten-free diet or to the chronicity of symptoms. There is some evidence that treatment of coeliac disease with a gluten-free diet protects against the development of either lymphoma or carcinoma.

CROHN'S DISEASE. There is a small increase in the incidence of adenocarcinoma of the small bowel in Crohn's disease.

IMMUNOPROLIFERATIVE SMALL INTESTINAL DISEASE (IPSID) is a B-lymphocyte disorder in which there is proliferation of plasma cells in the lamina propria of the upper small bowel. These cells produce truncated monoclonal heavy chains, but lack associated light chains. The $\alpha$-chains are found in the gut mucosa on immunofluorescence and these can also be detected in the serum. IPSID occurs usually in countries surrounding the Mediterranean, but it has also been found in other developing countries in South America and the Far East. Recently the condition has been documented in the developed world. IPSID predominantly affects people in lower socio-economic groups in areas with poor hygiene and a high incidence of bacterial and parasitic infection of the gut. IPSID presents itself as a malabsorptive syndrome associated with diffuse lymphoid infiltration of the small bowel and neighbouring lymph nodes. This then progresses in some cases to an immunoblastic lymphoma.

### CLINICAL FEATURES

Patients present with abdominal pain, diarrhoea, anorexia, weight loss and symptoms of anaemia.

### INVESTIGATION

There may be a palpable mass and a small bowel follow-through will detect most lesions. Ultrasound and CT will show bowel wall thickening and the involvement of lymph nodes which is common with lymphoma. Biopsies, to determine histological type, are helpful to decide treatment.

### TREATMENT

Treatment is often with resection, radiotherapy and chemotherapy.

The 5-year survival rate for T-cell lymphomas is 25%, but is better for B-cell lymphomas, varying from 50 to 75%, depending on the grade of lymphoma.

## Carcinoid tumours

These originate from the enterochromaffin cells (APUD cells, see p. 204) of the intestine. They make up 10% of all small-bowel neoplasms, the commonest sites being in the appendix, terminal ileum and the rectum. It is often difficult to be certain histologically whether a particular tumour is benign or malignant. Clinically most carcinoid tumours are asymptomatic until metastases are present. Ten per cent of carcinoid tumours in the appendix present as acute appendicitis, the inflammation being secondary to obstruction. Surgery is sometimes necessary for localized tumours.

CARCINOID SYNDROME. This syndrome occurs in only 5% of patients with carcinoid tumours and only when there are liver metastases. Patients complain of spontaneous or induced bluish-red flushing, predominantly on the face and neck. This can lead to permanent changes with telangiectasis. Gastrointestinal symptoms consist of abdominal pain and recurrent watery diarrhoea. Cardiac abnormalities are found in 50% of patients and consist of tricuspid incompetence or pulmonary stenosis.

Examination of the abdomen reveals hepatomegaly.

BIOCHEMICAL ABNORMALITIES. The tumours secrete a variety of biologically active amines and peptides, including serotonin (5-hydroxytryptamine; 5HT), bradykinin, histamine and tachykinins as well as prostaglandins.

The diarrhoea and cardiac complications are probably caused by 5HT itself but the cutaneous flushing is thought to be produced by one of the kinins, such as bradykinin, which is known to cause vasodilatation, bronchospasm and increased intestinal motility.

### DIAGNOSIS

Ultrasound examination confirms the presence of secondary deposits and the major metabolite of 5HT, 5-hydroxyindoleacetic acid (5HIAA), is found in high concentration in the urine.

### TREATMENT

Octreotide is an octapeptide somatostatin analogue that has been shown to inhibit the release of many gut hormones. It alleviates the flushing and diarrhoea and can control a carcinoid crisis. It is given subcutaneously in doses up to 200 µg three times daily.

Octreotide sometimes inhibits tumour growth and, since its introduction, other therapy is usually unnecessary. Interferon and other chemotherapeutic regimens occasionally reduce tumour growth, but have not been shown to increase survival. Most patients survive for 5–10 years after diagnosis.

# Inflammatory bowel disease

Two major forms of *non-specific* inflammatory bowel disease are recognized: Crohn's disease, which can affect any part of the gastrointestinal tract, and ulcerative colitis, which affects only the large bowel.

There is overlap between these two conditions in their clinical features, and histological and radiological abnormalities; in 10% of cases of colitis a definitive diagnosis of either ulcerative colitis or Crohn's disease is not possible. Currently, it is necessary to distinguish between these two conditions because of certain differences in their management. However, it is possible that these conditions represent two aspects of the same disease. The *incidence* of Crohn's disease varies from country to country but is approximately 5–6 per 100 000 with a prevalence of 50–60 per 100 000. The incidence of ulcerative colitis is 5–10 per 100 000 per year with a prevalence of 80–120 per 100 000.

## EPIDEMIOLOGY AND AETIOLOGY

The aetiology is unknown, but the racial differences and geographical clustering suggest both genetic and environmental causes. A cluster of patients with Crohn's disease has been found in a Cotswold village in England.

Both conditions have a worldwide distribution but are more common in the Western World. The incidence is lower in the non-White races. Jews are more prone to inflammatory bowel disease than non-Jews; the Ashkenazi Jews have a higher risk than the Sephardic Jews.

1 *Familial.* Both conditions are more common amongst relatives of patients than in the general population. There is a high rate of disease concordance in monozygotic twins.
2 *Genetic.* There are no HLA markers but HLA-B27 is increased in patients with inflammatory bowel disease and ankylosing spondylitis.
3 *Smoking.* Patients with Crohn's disease are more likely to be tobacco smokers, and there is an increased risk of ulcerative colitis amongst non-smokers or ex-smokers.
4 *Infective agent.* In Crohn's disease the most attractive hypothesis is that of a transmissible agent. No bacterium, virus or parasite has been definitely identified; recently the measles virus has been implicated.
   (a) *Mycobacterium.* In cattle and sheep, Johne's disease, which is a chronic inflammatory disorder of the distal ileum, is caused by *M. paratuberculosis.* A mycobacterium has been isolated from Crohn's disease tissue, but current evidence is against this being an aetiological agent. Granulomas are characteristic of Crohn's disease, but are also seen in TB and sarcoidosis suggesting a common pathogenetic link, although none has been found.
   (b) *Cell wall deficient organisms,* L-forms, plasmids may be the transmissible agent but this theory lacks any evidence.
   (c) *Viruses* have been reported in tissue from ulcerative colitis and Crohn's disease patients, but there are no compelling data.
5 *Multifocal gastrointestinal infarction* due to granulomatous angiitis has been suggested as a primary event in Crohn's disease.
6 Serum antineutrophil cytoplasmic antibody (ANCA) is increased in ulcerative colitis, but not Crohn's disease; it is distinct from the ANCA seen in Wegener's granulomatosis.
7 Many immunological abnormalities have been described in inflammatory bowel disease. It is unclear whether they are the primary or secondary event in the pathogenesis.

A suggested mechanism is that a specific or generalized luminal antigen can cause stimulation of immune (antigen specific) or inflammatory (antigen non-specific) responses. It is possible that these responses are abnormal or exaggerated in inflammatory bowel disease. Activation of T lymphocytes, tissue macrophages, eosinophils, mast cells, neutrophils and fibroblasts produce a wide variety of cytokines (e.g. interleukin IL-1, IL-6, TNF), eicosanoids (e.g. prostaglandins, thromboxane, LTB4), cell adhesion markers (e.g. E-selectins and endothelial cell leucocyte adhesion molecule (ELAM)) and free oxygen radicals, all of which can lead to tissue damage.

## PATHOLOGY

Crohn's disease is a chronic inflammatory condition that may affect any part of the gastrointestinal tract from the mouth to the anus but has a particular tendency to affect the terminal ileum. The disease can involve one small area of the gut such as the terminal ileum, or multiple areas with relatively normal bowel in between ('skip lesions'). It may also be extensive, involving the whole of the colon and/or small bowel.

Ulcerative colitis can affect the rectum alone (proctitis), can extend proximally to involve the sigmoid and descending colon ('left-sided colitis'), or may involve the whole colon ('total colitis'). In a few of these patients there is also inflammation of the distal terminal ileum ('backwash ileitis').

### Macroscopic changes

In Crohn's disease the involved bowel is usually thickened and narrowed. There are deep ulcers and fissures in the mucosa, producing a cobblestone appearance. Fistulas and abscesses may be seen. An early sign is aphthoid ulceration that can be seen endoscopically.

In ulcerative colitis the mucosa looks reddened,

inflamed and bleeds easily. In severe disease there is extensive ulceration, with the adjacent mucosa appearing as inflammatory polyps. In fulminant disease most of the mucosa is lost, leaving a few islands of oedematous mucosa (mucosal islands) and toxic dilatation occurs. On healing, the mucosa can return to normal, although there is usually some residual glandular distortion.

### Microscopic changes

In Crohn's disease the inflammation extends through all layers of the bowel, whereas in ulcerative colitis a superficial inflammation is seen.

In Crohn's disease there is an increase in chronic inflammatory cells and lymphoid hyperplasia, and in 50–60% of patients granulomas are present. These granulomas are non-caseating epithelioid cell aggregates with Langhans' giant cells.

In ulcerative colitis the mucosa shows a chronic inflammatory cell infiltrate in the lamina propria. Crypt abscesses and goblet cell depletion are also seen.

The differentiation between these two diseases is made not only on the basis of clinical and radiological data but also on the histological differences seen in the rectal and colonic mucosa obtained by biopsy (Table 4.8).

### CLINICAL FEATURES

#### Crohn's disease

This can present at any age; it is uncommon before the age of 10 years and has a peak incidence between 20 and 40 years. A late peak affecting mainly the colon has been reported in women aged over 60 years. Both sexes are equally affected.

The major symptoms are of diarrhoea, abdominal pain and weight loss. Constitutional symptoms of malaise, lethargy, anorexia, nausea, vomiting and low-grade fever may be present. Despite the recurrent nature of this condition, many patients remain well and have an almost normal life-style. However, patients with extensive disease may have frequent recurrences necessitating multiple hospital admissions.

The clinical features are very variable and depend partly on the region of the bowel that is affected. The disease may present insidiously or acutely. The abdominal pain may be colicky, suggesting obstruction but it usually has no special characteristics and sometimes in colonic disease only minimal discomfort is present. Diarrhoea is present in 80% of all cases and in colonic disease usually contains blood, making it difficult to differentiate from ulcerative colitis. Steatorrhoea can be present in small

bowel disease. Some patients (15%) present with only anorexia, weight loss and general ill-health, with an absence of any other gastrointestinal symptoms.

Crohn's disease may present as an emergency with acute right iliac fossa pain mimicking appendicitis. If laparotomy is undertaken, an oedematous, reddened terminal ileum is found. There are many other causes of an acute ileitis, e.g. infections such as *Yersinia*. Crohn's disease is the cause of approximately 10% of acute ileitis.

EXAMINATION. Physical signs are few, apart from loss of weight and general ill-health. Aphthous ulceration of the mouth is often seen. Abdominal examination is often normal, although tenderness and a right iliac fossa mass are occasionally found. This mass is due either to inflamed loops of bowel that are matted together or to an abscess. A careful examination of the anus should always be made to look for oedematous anal tags, fissures or perianal abscesses. These abnormalities are particularly common (80%) in colonic involvement.

Other extra-gastrointestinal features of inflammatory bowel disease should be looked for, e.g. erythema nodosum, arthritis, iritis (see below).

Sigmoidoscopy should always be performed in a patient with Crohn's disease. With small bowel involvement the rectum may appear normal, but a biopsy must be taken as non-specific histological changes may sometimes be found in the mucosa. Even with extensive colonic Crohn's disease the rectum may be spared and be relatively normal, but patchy involvement with an oedematous haemorrhagic mucosa can be present.

#### Ulcerative colitis

This also occurs at any age, but most frequently between 20 and 40 years with women affected more than men.

The major symptom in ulcerative colitis is diarrhoea with blood and mucus, sometimes accompanied by lower abdominal discomfort. General features include malaise, lethargy and anorexia. Aphthous ulceration is seen. The disease can be mild, moderate or severe, and runs a course of remissions and exacerbations. Ten per cent of patients have persistent chronic symptoms, although some patients may have only a single attack.

When the disease is confined to the rectum, blood mixed with the stool, urgency and tenesmus are common. In this group, there are normally very few constitutional symptoms but patients are nevertheless greatly inconvenienced by the frequency of defecation.

In an acute attack patients have bloody diarrhoea, passing 10–20 liquid stools per day. Diarrhoea also occurs at night, with urgency and incontinence that is severely disabling for the patient. Occasionally blood and mucus alone are passed.

The definition of a severe attack is given in Table 4.9. The patient may be very ill and needs careful monitoring in hospital with prompt treatment to avoid the development of complications, such as septicaemia, toxic dilatation and perforation.

EXAMINATION. In general there are no specific signs in ulcerative colitis. The abdomen may be slightly distended

| | Crohn's disease | Ulcerative colitis |
|---|---|---|
| Inflammation | Deep (transmural) Patchy | Superficial Continuous |
| Granulomas | ++ | Rare |
| Goblet cells | Present | Depleted |
| Crypt abscesses | + | ++ |

**Table 4.8** Histological differences between Crohn's disease and ulcerative colitis.

| Stool frequency | >6 stools per day with blood |
|---|---|
| Fever | >37.5°C |
| Tachycardia | >90 min$^{-1}$ |
| ESR | >30 mm hour$^{-1}$ |
| Anaemia | Haemoglobin <10 g dl$^{-1}$ |
| Albumin | <30 g litre$^{-1}$ |

**Table 4.9** Markers of a severe attack of ulcerative colitis.

or tender to palpation. The anus is usually normal. Rectal examination will show the presence of blood. Sigmoidoscopy is always abnormal and shows an inflamed, bleeding, friable mucosa. A biopsy should be taken for histological diagnosis.

### Extra-gastrointestinal manifestations

These occur with both diseases and some are related to the intestinal disease activity (Table 4.10). Patients with Crohn's colitis have more extra-gastrointestinal complications than those with small bowel lesions alone.

## INVESTIGATIONS
### Blood tests

Anaemia is common and is usually the normocytic, normochromic anaemia of chronic disease. Deficiency of iron and/or folate also occurs. Despite terminal ileal involvement in Crohn's disease, megaloblastic anaemia due to vitamin $B_{12}$ deficiency is unusual, although the vitamin $B_{12}$ level can be low. There is often a raised erythrocyte sedimentation rate (ESR) and C-reactive protein (CRP) and a raised white cell count. Hypoalbuminaemia is present in severe disease. Liver biochemistry may be abnormal. Blood cultures are required if septicaemia is suspected.

### Stool cultures

These should always be performed on presentation if diarrhoea is present.

### Radiology

CROHN'S DISEASE. A small bowel follow-through is usually performed first unless the disease is predominantly Crohn's colitis (see below).

A small bowel follow-through shows an asymmetrical alteration in the mucosal pattern with deep ulceration and areas of narrowing (string sign) largely confined to the ileum (Fig. 4.28). Skip lesions with normal bowel between are also seen.

Barium enema has been superseded by colonoscopy, if this is available, for colonic disease. Early changes on barium enema consist of aphthous ulceration; this involvement is again usually patchy with deep ulceration developing later.

*Ultrasound and CT scanning* are helpful in delineating abscesses, masses, thickened bowel wall and mesentery, or other extraluminal problems in Crohn's disease.

ULCERATIVE COLITIS. A plain X-ray of the abdomen is performed in severe colitis cases to look for colonic dilatation. The extent of the disease can be judged by the air distribution in the colon.

|  | Crohn's disease | Ulcerative colitis |
|---|---|---|
| **Eyes** | | |
| Uveitis | | |
| Episcleritis | 4 | 4 |
| Conjunctivitis | | |
| **Joints** | | |
| Monoarticular arthritis | 14 | 11 |
| Ankylosing spondylitis | 2–6 | |
| Sacroiliitis | 15–18 | |
| **Skin** | | |
| Erythema nodosum | 5–10 | 2 |
| Pyoderma gangrenosum | 1 | 3 |
| Vasculitis | | |
| **Liver[a,b] and Biliary Tree** | | |
| Fatty change | Common | Common |
| Pericholangitis | 19 | 25 |
| Sclerosing cholangitis | <1 | 12 |
| Chronic active hepatitis | Uncommon | Uncommon |
| Cirrhosis | 7 | 19 |
| Cholangiocarcinoma | Uncommon | Uncommon |
| **Kidney[a]** | | |
| Stones | 30 | — |
| **Gallbladder[a]** | | |
| Stones | 30 | 5 (as in normal population) |

[a]These manifestations are not related to disease activity.
[b]Biochemical abnormalities are common, but clinically overt disease is uncommon.

**Table 4.10** Extra-gastrointestinal manifestations of inflammatory bowel disease (as per cent of cases).

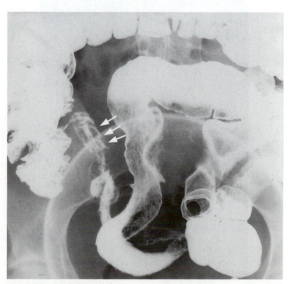

**Fig. 4.28** Small bowel follow-through showing narrowing and ulceration of the terminal ileum (arrow) in Crohn's disease.

In an *instant, unprepared barium enema*, barium is run into the rectum without pressure and a single film taken. This is a good investigation to show the extent of the disease.

Barium enema is again being superseded by colonoscopy. If performed, there may be ulceration and in long-standing disease the colon is shortened and narrowed (Fig. 4.29). The disease is usually continuous.

### Colonoscopy

In Crohn's disease, this is performed if colonic involvement is suspected when biopsies of the whole colon can be taken.

In ulcerative colitis, colonoscopy shows the exact extent of the disease and, again, biopsies from the whole colon and ileum can be taken to differentiate between Crohn's disease and ulcerative colitis.

### Small bowel function tests (see p. 205)

When Crohn's disease involves the small bowel, other tests may be necessary, e.g. a breath test for bacterial overgrowth or a test for vitamin $B_{12}$ absorption.

## ACTIVITY OF DISEASE

A rough estimate of the activity can be made on the clinical picture and laboratory tests of ESR, serum albumin and acute-phase protein (e.g. CRP or orosomucoids). In some centres scans to localize areas of inflammation are performed using radiolabelled leucocytes injected intravenously; these may help in localizing abscesses.

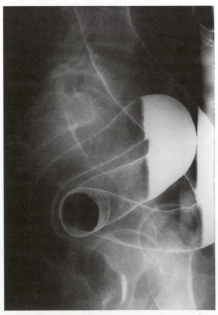

**Fig. 4.29** Double-contrast barium enema showing fine ulceration in ulcerative colitis.

## DIFFERENTIAL DIAGNOSIS

Crohn's disease has to be considered in the differential diagnosis of all chronic diarrhoeas, malabsorption and malnutrition. It is also a differential diagnosis of small stature in children (see p. 797). A small bowel follow-through usually differentiates it from other forms of small bowel disease.

Ileocaecal TB is common in Asia and Africa and in Asian immigrants in the UK. Acute ileitis due to *Yersinia* can be distinguished serologically. Lymphomas occasionally cause a major diagnostic difficulty.

Colitis, both ulcerative and Crohn's, must be differentiated from amoebic and ischaemic colitis as well as infective causes of diarrhoea. The latter are becoming commoner in homosexuals and should be suspected if multiple or unusual organisms are found. A rare cause of colitis is Behçet's disease, which also gives orogenital ulceration.

In a few patients the mucosal appearance on colonoscopy and sigmoidoscopy is macroscopically normal and the inflammation is only detected histologically. This 'microscopic colitis' presents with chronic diarrhoea and is treated as a non-specific colitis. Collagenous colitis also presents as chronic diarrhoea; there is a thick subepithelial deposit of collagen in the macroscopically normal colonic mucosa.

## TREATMENT

### Crohn's disease

MEDICAL MANAGEMENT. Some patients require only symptomatic treatment. Diarrhoea can be controlled with agents such as loperamide 2–4 mg three times daily, codeine phosphate 30–60 mg three times daily, or diphenoxylate with atropine 1–2 tablets four times daily. Patients with more severe disease require specific medical therapy and acute attacks often require admission to hospital. Medical therapy relies mainly on anti-inflammatory and immunosuppressive drugs. The mechanism of action of these drugs in inflammatory bowel disease is unknown and treatment is largely empirical.

Anaemia will improve as the patient gets better, but appropriate haematinics, e.g. ferrous sulphate 400 mg daily or folic acid 5 mg daily, may be required.

*Acute* attacks require oral corticosteroids 30–60 mg daily, and any dehydration and electrolyte loss should be corrected with i.v. fluids. On this regimen patients usually improve quickly and the steroid dosage can then be reduced. Azathioprine ($2 \, \text{mg kg}^{-1}$ daily) is an immunosuppressive agent that has been shown to be helpful in maintaining the steroid-induced remission, although it has not gained universal acceptance. It is often started in an acute attack as it takes a few weeks to be effective. Many other anti-inflammatory and immunosuppressive drugs, e.g. cyclosporin, have been tried with variable success. Mesalazine or sulphasalazine (see below) is used in patients with colonic involvement who can also be given rectal steroids (see below). Metronidazole (800 mg three times daily) and co-trimoxazole (two tablets twice daily) are useful in severe perianal disease owing to their antibacterial action.

Elemental diets (see p. 169) can induce remissions, particularly in small bowel disease. They improve nutrition, allow the bowel to 'rest' and reduce antigen load to the bowel, but their precise mode of action is unclear. Unfortunately, the diets are unpalatable and expensive, and many patients relapse on restarting a normal diet. The treatment is useful in some patients who refuse steroids or who have marked side-effects.

*Remission.* Some patients can come off all therapy. Others require a small dose of steroids and/or azathioprine long term.

SURGICAL MANAGEMENT. Approximately 80% of patients will require an operation at some time during the course of their disease. Nevertheless, surgery should be avoided if possible and only minimal resections undertaken, as recurrence (15% per year) is almost inevitable. The indications for surgery are:

- Failure of medical therapy, with acute or chronic symptoms producing ill-health
- Complications, e.g. toxic dilatation, obstruction, perforation, abscesses, enterocutaneous fistula
- Failure to grow in children

In most patients with small bowel disease, surgical treatment consists of resection and end-to-end anastomosis. The surgery of colonic disease is discussed below.

## Ulcerative colitis

MEDICAL MANAGEMENT. Severe attacks require careful management in hospital as the mortality of this condition is still high. All patients with ulcerative colitis are treated with a 5-aminosalicylic acid (5-ASA) compound. Sulphasalazine consists of 5-ASA attached to sulphapyridine as a carrier. This combination is broken down in the colon by bacteria to release the active agent, 5-ASA. Sulphasalazine is started at a dose of 3–4 g daily, reducing to a maintenance dose of 2 g daily. In mild cases it may induce a remission. Its main role, however, is to reduce the number of relapses when taken long term. Sulphasalazine may induce nausea and has some reversible side-effects, including haemolytic anaemia, skin rashes and infertility in men. These are produced by the sulphapyridine and preparations of slow-release 5-ASA without sulphapyridine have been developed and are superseding sulphasalazine for new patients. Mesalazine consists of 5-ASA itself in a delay-release tablet that dissolves at pH 7 or greater. A dose of 400–800 mg three times daily is used. Olsalazine consists of two molecules of 5-ASA linked by an azo bond that separates in the large bowel and is also used.

*Mild attacks* and proctitis can be treated with local rectal steroids in the form of enemas (prednisolone-21-phosphate 20 mg) or a 10% hydrocortisone foam. 5-ASA retention enemas are also useful.

*Moderate attacks* are treated with oral prednisolone 30–40 mg daily. Patients with their first attack or those who do not respond quickly should be admitted to hospital.

*Severe attacks* (see also toxic dilatation for management) should be treated with high-dose corticosteroids in the form of prednisolone 60 mg, hydrocortisone 100 mg i.v. 6-hourly or corticotrophin (synthetic

ACTH) 1–2 mg i.m. In addition, dehydration and electrolyte disturbances should be corrected by intravenous therapy. Accompanying septicaemia, which is usually due to Gram-negative bacteria, should be treated with antibiotics.

Azathioprine, 2 mg kg$^{-1}$, has been shown to induce a remission (see Crohn's treatment) in some patients who do not respond to treatment.

Intravenous cyclosporin has been shown in some studies to induce a remission, and probably should be tried before advocating colectomy. Surgical treatment is necessary if there is then no improvement.

*Remission.* All patients are maintained on a 5-ASA compound for many years.

SURGICAL MANAGEMENT (INCLUDING CROHN'S COLITIS). Ulcerative colitis is confined to the colon and therefore colectomy is curative.

The main indication for surgery is usually a severe attack which does not respond to medical therapy. A prophylactic colectomy is sometimes performed in patients who have a high cancer risk.

*Protocolectomy with an ileostomy* is the standard operation, in which the colon and rectum are removed and the ileum is brought out through an opening in the right iliac fossa and attached to the skin. The patient wears an ileostomy bag, which is stuck on to the skin over the ileostomy spout. This bag requires to be emptied once or twice daily, adaptation decreasing the initial high output. This is compatible with a near-normal life-style. Stoma-care therapists are readily available with help and advice.

Problems associated with ileostomies include:

- Mechanical problems
- Dehydration, particularly in hot climates
- Psychosexual problems
- Infertility in men
- Recurrence of Crohn's disease

In ulcerative colitis, but *not* in Crohn's disease, *colectomy with an ileorectal or ileoanal anastomosis* is used to avoid ileostomy.

Ileorectal anastomoses leave a diseased rectum *in situ* and frequent diarrhoea still occurs. With an ileoanal anastomosis (Fig. 4.30) a pouch of ileum is formed that acts

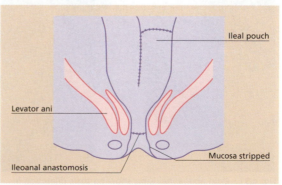

**Fig. 4.30** Diagram of an ileoanal pouch for ulcerative colitis.

as a reservoir and the patient is continent with only a few bowel motions per day. The ileoanal operation is being increasingly used but inflammation of the pouch, 'pouchitis', can be a problem. It is not used for Crohn's disease because of the high recurrence rate.

## COMPLICATIONS

These are similar in both conditions, but vary in frequency. Crohn's disease, with its transmural inflammation, has a higher incidence of fistulas, fissures and abscess formation.

### Perforation

This is a rare but serious complication that occurs in association with toxic megacolon. In Crohn's disease local perforations may occur, forming walled-off abscesses, and occasionally small bowel perforation gives rise to peritonitis.

### Haemorrhage

Massive haemorrhage is rare.

### Toxic dilatation

Toxic dilatation may occur during an acute severe attack of colitis. The diagnosis should be suspected in a patient with a severe episode (see above) who develops abdominal distension. A plain abdominal X-ray (Fig. 4.31) will show a dilated thin-walled colon with a diameter greater than 5 cm that is gas-filled and contains mucosal islands. Treatment is as for a severe attack of colitis plus daily abdominal X-rays and measurements of abdominal girth. If the patient does not settle in 48 hours with high-dose corticosteroids, emergency surgery should be performed. When mucosal islands are present, the risk of perforation is high, as is the mortality, and many favour immediate surgery without medical therapy.

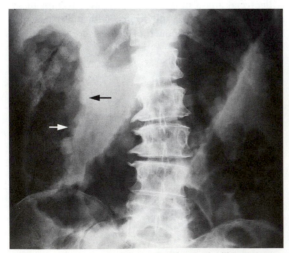

**Fig. 4.31** Plain abdominal X-ray showing toxic dilatation in ulcerative colitis. The arrows indicate mucosal islands.

### Carcinoma

The incidence is increased in both conditions (3–5%). In Crohn's disease the incidence of carcinoma is only marginally increased and does not influence management. In ulcerative colitis the risk of carcinoma of the colon in a patient who has had total colitis for more than 10 years is much greater than it is for the general population. It was suggested that regular sigmoidoscopy and colonoscopy with biopsies might detect early premalignant changes, but this is now not recommended as repeated studies, not surprisingly, have shown no benefit.

A cholangiocarcinoma is also found in increased frequency.

### Amyloid

This is a rare complication and can affect the bowel or other organs; the kidneys may be affected with a deterioration of renal function.

## COURSE AND PROGNOSIS

### Crohn's disease

These patients have recurrent relapses and virtually all have a significant relapse over a 20-year period. The mortality rate is variable but generally appears to be at least twice as high as that seen in the normal population. Most deaths are associated with surgery. Despite this, many patients lead a normal life. Crohn's disease in childhood causes growth retardation.

Self-help groups provide patient information and a number of booklets that are invaluable for health staff and patients with inflammatory bowel disease.

### Ulcerative colitis

The course and prognosis is variable. In proctitis it is very good; only 10% of these cases go on to develop more extensive disease. On the other hand, severe fulminant disease still carries a 15–25% mortality. The mortality is reduced if the acute attack is treated promptly and surgery is performed if no improvement occurs in the first 2–3 days.

Overall, because many cases are mild, the mortality of this disease is not much greater than the mortality rates for the general population, in contrast to Crohn's disease.

There is no particular risk to mother or child during pregnancy in either form of inflammatory bowel disease, but relapses should be treated urgently.

# The colon and rectum

## STRUCTURE

The large intestine starts at the caecum, on the posterior medial wall of which is the appendix. The colon is made up of ascending, transverse, descending and sigmoid parts, which join the rectum at the rectosigmoid junction.

The muscle wall consists of an inner circular layer and an outer longitudinal layer. The outer layer is incomplete, coming together to form the taenia coli, which produce the haustral pattern seen in the normal colon.

The mucosa of the colon is lined with epithelial cells with crypts but no villi, so that the surface is flat. The mucosa is full of goblet cells. A variety of cells, mainly lymphocytes and macrophages, are found in the lamina propria.

The blood supply to the colon is from the superior and inferior mesenteric vessels. Generally there are good anastomotic channels, but the caecum and splenic flexure are areas where ischaemia can occur.

The rectum is about 12 cm long. Its interior is divided by three crescentic circular muscles producing shelf-like folds. These are the rectal valves and can be seen at sigmoidoscopy. The anal canal has an internal and an external sphincter.

### PHYSIOLOGY

The main role of the colon is the absorption of water and electrolytes (Table 4.11). Approximately 2 litres of fluid passes the ileocaecal valve each day. The absorption of fluid and electrolytes takes place mainly in the right side of the colon, and only about 150 ml is passed in the faeces.

The role of the rectum and anus in defecation is complex. The rectum is usually empty and collapsed; the entry of faeces from the colon produces relaxation of the internal sphincter and the puborectalis muscle. This decreases the acute angle between the rectum and the anal canal. When the rectum contains approximately 100 ml of faeces the urge to defecate is experienced. The rectum is emptied by relaxation of the external anal sphincter (under voluntary control) and an increase in intra-abdominal pressure.

## Diverticular disease

Diverticula are frequently found in the colon and occur in 50% of patients over the age of 50 years. They are most frequent in the sigmoid, but can be present over the whole colon.

The term *diverticulosis* indicates the presence of diverticula; *diverticulitis* implies that these diverticula are inflamed. It is perhaps better to use the more general term *diverticular disease*, as it is often difficult to be sure whether the diverticula are inflamed. The precise mechanism of diverticula formation is not known. There is thickening of the muscle layer and, because of high intra-luminal pressures, pouches of mucosa extrude through the muscular wall through weakened areas near blood vessels to form diverticula. Diverticular disease seems to be related to the low-fibre diet eaten in the western hemisphere.

Diverticulitis occurs when faeces obstruct the neck of the diverticulum causing stagnation and allowing bacteria to multiply and produce inflammation. This can then lead to bowel perforation (peridiverticulitis), abscess formation, fistulas into adjacent organs, or even generalized peritonitis.

### CLINICAL FEATURES AND MANAGEMENT

Diverticular disease is asymptomatic in 90% and is usually discovered incidentally on a barium enema examination (Fig. 4.32); no treatment is required.

Left iliac fossa pain, constipation and diarrhoea are often attributed to diverticular disease, but as these symptoms are very similar to those seen in the irritable bowel syndrome, it is debatable whether they are due to diverticular disease. In practice, both conditions are treated symptomatically with a high-fibre diet, antispasmodic drugs (e.g. mebeverine 135 mg three times daily) and agents to regulate the bowel. A barium enema is often performed to exclude colonic carcinoma. Diverticular disease can produce rectal bleeding, which is sometimes massive, particularly from right-sided diverticula. In most

| | Water (ml) | Sodium (mmol) | Potassium (mmol) |
|---|---|---|---|
| *Input* | | | |
| Diet | 1500 | 150 | 80 |
| GI secretions | 7500 | 1000 | 40 |
| Total | 9000 | 1150 | 120 |
| *Output* | | | |
| Faeces | 150 | 5 | 12 |
| Ileostomy (adapted) | 500–1500 | 60–120 | 4 |

**Table 4.11** Input and output of water and electrolytes in the gastrointestinal tract over 24 hours.

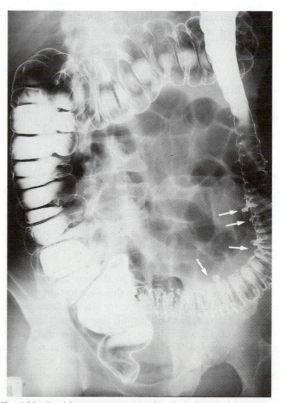

**Fig. 4.32** Double-contrast enema showing diverticular disease (the diverticulae are narrowed). Note the mucosal hypertrophy.

cases the bleeding stops and the cause of the bleeding can be established by X-ray, colonoscopy and sometimes angiography. In rare cases emergency colectomy is necessary. It is unwise to ascribe an iron deficiency anaemia to a bleeding diverticulum unless all other causes, e.g. piles or carcinoma, have been excluded.

ACUTE DIVERTICULITIS almost always affects diverticula in the sigmoid colon. It presents with severe pain in the left iliac fossa, often accompanied by fever and constipation. These symptoms and signs are similar to appendicitis but on the left side. On examination there is tenderness, guarding and rigidity on the left side of the abdomen. Tachycardia and pyrexia are present and the white cell count shows a leucocytosis. Chest and abdominal X-rays are necessary to exclude free air under the diaphragm and an ultrasound is performed to detect an abscess following localized perforation.

### Complications of acute diverticulitis

ABSCESS FORMATION, causing pain, pyrexia and a palpable tender mass in the left iliac fossa. Ultrasound or CT scanning can show the mass. Surgical drainage with or without a defunctioning colostomy may be required. Antibiotics are always given.

PERFORATION, leading to generalized peritonitis (see p. 233).

FISTULA FORMATION into the bladder, causing dysuria or pneumaturia, or into the vagina, causing discharge; the diverticular disease is often chronic, without evidence of acute inflammation. Surgery is usually required.

INTESTINAL OBSTRUCTION (see p. 234).

### TREATMENT

Acute attacks are treated with bowel rest, intravenous fluids and antibiotics, e.g. gentamicin (or a cephalosporin) and metronidazole. Most attacks settle on this regimen, but a few require emergency surgery, which usually consists of a defunctioning colostomy to be followed later by resection.

Acute episodes do not necessarily recur and elective surgery is mainly reserved for patients with intestinal obstruction or fistulae.

## CONSTIPATION (see p. 176)

This is such a major problem in the general population that it need not be considered a disease. Most people simply require reassurance and dietary advice. Constipation is common in the elderly, possibly due to immobility and a poor diet. Constipation in young women is common and in some slow transit through the colon has been identified as the cause, whilst some women after childbirth have pelvic floor abnormalities preventing defecation. A list of the causes of constipation is given in Table 4.12. Most have simple constipation, often due to a low fibre intake. Drugs are a common cause and may need to be stopped. A rectal examination should always

| |
|---|
| Simple |
| Intestinal obstruction |
| Colonic disease, e.g. carcinoma |
| Painful anal conditions |
| Drugs, e.g. opiates, aluminium antacids, antidepressants, codeine, iron |
| Hypothyroidism, hypercalcaemia |
| Depression |
| Immobility |
| Hirschsprung's disease (very occasionally seen in adults) |

**Table 4.12**  Causes of constipation.

be performed. Long-standing constipation does not require investigation, but a change in bowel habit in the middle-aged or elderly requires a barium enema examination.

### TREATMENT

Laxatives should be avoided if at all possible and patients encouraged to take a high-fibre diet. Glycerol suppositories, which can be used by the patient, are often useful. The types of laxatives available are shown in Table 4.13. Bulking agents should be tried first. Stimulant laxatives often cause cramp and their long-term use should be avoided as they cause an atonic non-functioning colon. Magnesium sulphate is useful in very severe constipation.

| Substance | Mechanisms of action |
|---|---|
| *Bulking agents*<br>Dietary fibre<br>Bran<br>Ispaghula husks<br>Sterculia<br>Methylcellulose | Increased faecal mass due to fibre and water |
| *Stimulant laxatives*<br>Anthraquinones, e.g.<br>    Senna<br>    Sodium picosulphate<br>Dioctyl sodium<br>    sulphosuccinate<br>Danthron[a]<br>Bisacodyl | Stimulate intestinal secretion |
| *Osmotic laxatives*<br>Magnesium sulphate<br>Lactulose | Osmotic effect |
| *Suppositories*<br>Bisacodyl<br>Glycerol | |
| *Enemas*<br>Phosphate | |

[a]For elderly patients or for opiate-induced constipation in the terminally ill.

**Table 4.13**  Laxatives and enemas.

# Megacolon

The term megacolon is used to describe a number of congenital and acquired conditions in which the colon is dilated. In many instances it is secondary to chronic constipation and in some parts of the world Chagas' disease is a common cause.

All young patients with megacolon should have Hirschsprung's disease excluded. In this disease, which presents in the first years of life, an aganglionic segment of the rectum gives rise to constipation and subacute obstruction. Occasionally Hirschsprung's disease affecting only a short segment of the rectum can be missed in childhood and a rectal biopsy, using special stains for ganglion cells in the submucosal plexus, should be performed in adult patients with megacolon to exclude it; frozen rectal mucosa should be stained for acetylcholinesterase. Pressure studies show failure of relaxation of the internal sphincter, which is diagnostic of Hirschsprung's disease. This disease can be successfully treated surgically.

Treatment of megacolon is similar to simple constipation, but saline wash-outs and manual removal of faeces are sometimes required.

# Pneumatosis cystoides intestinalis

This is a rare condition in which multiple gas-filled cysts are found in the submucosa of the intestine, chiefly the colon. The cause is unknown, but many cases are associated with chronic bronchitis and some with peptic ulceration. Patients are usually asymptomatic but abdominal pain and diarrhoea do occur and occasionally the cysts rupture to produce a pneumoperitoneum. This condition is diagnosed on X-ray of the abdomen, barium enema or at sigmoidoscopy when cysts are seen.

Treatment is often unnecessary but continuous oxygen therapy will help to disperse the largely nitrogen-containing cysts. Metronidazole may help.

# Ischaemic disease of the colon (ischaemic colitis)

This commonly presents in the older age group (over 50 years) with sudden onset of abdominal pain and the passage of bright red blood with or without diarrhoea. There may be signs of shock and there is sometimes evidence of other cardiovascular disease. This condition has also been described in young women taking the contraceptive pill.

On examination, the abdomen is distended and tender. Sigmoidoscopy is normal apart from the presence of blood. Investigations include an abdominal X-ray to exclude perforation. Thumbprinting—a characteristic sign for ischaemic disease—can be seen on a barium enema performed when the patient is well; strictures can also be seen.

The differential diagnosis is of other causes of acute colitis, but these can usually be excluded on the basis of the sigmoidoscopy findings.

## TREATMENT

Most patients with this condition settle on symptomatic treatment. A few develop gangrene and perforation and require urgent surgery. Some develop strictures.

# Anorectal conditions

These important conditions largely present to surgeons. The major conditions presenting initially to the physician include the following.

### Pruritus ani

Pruritus ani, or an itchy bottom, is common and often no cause is found. Treatment consists of good personal hygiene and keeping the area dry. Secondary causes include any local anal lesions such as haemorrhoids, infestation, e.g. with threadworm (*Enterobius vermicularis*), or fungal infection, e.g. candidiasis. The latter condition often occurs secondary to the use of hydrocortisone creams, which should be avoided.

### Haemorrhoids

Haemorrhoids usually produce rectal bleeding and pruritus ani. Patients may notice red blood on the toilet paper on wiping. They are the commonest cause of rectal bleeding (see Fig. 4.19) and if minor, require no treatment. Diagnosis is made on proctoscopy.

### Anal fissures

Anal fissures cause painful defecation and minor rectal bleeding and can often be seen in the anal margin on inspection. Treatment is by application of a local anaesthetic gel. Dilatation is not required.

### Faecal incontinence

This can be a major problem in the elderly, infirm or demented patient. It is often secondary to impaction. Some of the major factors responsible are rectal prolapse, carcinoma of the rectum and diarrhoea from any cause. The patient should be carefully examined and investigation and treatment instituted as appropriate.

### Faecal impaction

This occurs in the elderly with constipation. It can lead to overflow incontinence. It usually requires manual removal of faeces, and care to prevent recurrences (see constipation).

### Solitary rectal ulcer

These ulcers occur in young adults and produce bowel irregularity and rectal bleeding with the passage of mucus. The cause is unclear, but many seem to be due to excess straining at stool with prolapse of the rectal mucosa (descending perineal syndrome).

Rectal examination is usually normal but sigmoidoscopy reveals redness or an ulcer approximately 10 cm from the anal margin on the anterior rectal wall. It often has an appearance not unlike that of a carcinoma.

Histology is diagnostic; there are non-specific inflammatory changes with bands of smooth muscle extending into the lamina propria.

Treatment is unsatisfactory and many cases run an indolent chronic course with continuation of symptoms. Local steroids may help and surgical excision should be avoided. Patients should be advised to stop straining on defecation.

### Rectal prolapse

In this common condition affecting children and the elderly the rectal mucosa prolapses through the anus owing to excessive straining. Initially prolapse occurs only during defecation but later ulceration, mucosal discharge and faecal incontinence can occur. Surgical treatment is required in complete prolapse.

## COLONIC TUMOURS

## Colon polyps and polyposis syndromes (Table 4.14)

A polyp is an elevation above the mucosal surface. The majority of colorectal polyps are adenomas with malignant potential. Polyps range in size from a few millimetres to 10 cm in diameter. They may be single or multiple and in the polyposis syndromes hundreds may be found. Not all colorectal polyps are adenomas.

In adults, 2–5 mm polyps in the rectum are often found: 90% of these will be of the innocent metaplastic type. Larger polyps in the rectum and 70–80% of all polyps in the colon are adenomas and 5% (20% of those 2 cm or greater in diameter) will contain invasive carcinoma at discovery. Most polyps are asymptomatic and found by chance when patients are investigated for pain, altered bowel habit, bleeding haemorrhoids or some other cause.

HAMARTOMATOUS POLYPS are commonly large and stalked and are either juvenile or Peutz–Jegher in type.

JUVENILE POLYPS (occurring in children and teenagers) are confined mainly to the colon and histologically show mucus-retention cysts. They are inherited as an autosomal dominant and are a cause of bleeding and intussusception, often in the first year of life. In juvenile polyposis (more than 10 colonic polyps) there is an increased risk of colonic cancer and surveillance and removal of polyps must be undertaken.

PEUTZ–JEGHER POLYPS (see p. 213) are usually multiple and histologically have characteristic fibromuscular fronds radiating between disorganized mucosal crypts. They can occur in the large intestine, producing chronic anaemia.

Other non-neoplastic polyps are less common and are shown in Table 4.14.

In the Cronkhite–Canada syndrome, polyps similar to Peutz–Jegher, are associated with ectodermal abnormalities such as alopecia, nail dystrophy and skin hyperpigmentation.

NEOPLASTIC POLYPS Adenomas occur in about 10% of the population in the Western World but are rare elsewhere in the world. Genetic and environmental factors have been implicated but no definite aetiological factors have been identified.

Polyps rarely produce symptoms and most are diagnosed on X-ray or on colonoscopy performed for other reasons. Large polyps may bleed intermittently and cause anaemia. Large sessile villous adenomas of the rectum can present with profuse diarrhoea and hypokalaemia.

The frequency with which invasive carcinoma occurs in adenomas increases with the size of the polyp and most, if not all, colonic carcinomas originate as adenomas. Once a polyp has been found on X-ray or endoscopy it is usually removed endoscopically. Further polyps may develop (30–50% probability) and continuous surveillance in patients under 75 years of age is necessary. An initial colonoscopy examination is made at 3 years, followed by 3–5 yearly colonoscopies thereafter.

| Type | Solitary | Multiple polyposis syndrome |
|---|---|---|
| Hamartomas | Peutz–Jegher polyp<br>Juvenile polyps | Peutz–Jegher syndrome<br>Juvenile polyposis<br>Cronkhite–Canada syndrome |
| Inflammatory | Inflammatory polyps, e.g.<br>    Ulcerative colitis<br>    Crohn's colitis<br>    Schistosomiasis | Inflammatory polyposis |
| Neoplastic | Adenomas—tubular<br>tubulovillous, villous | Familial adenomatous polyposis |
| Miscellaneous | Metaplastic (hyperplastic)<br>    polyps<br>Lymphoid polyps | Benign lymphoid polyposis |

**Table 4.14** Classification of colorectal polyps.

FAMILIAL ADENOMATOUS POLYPOSIS (FAP) is inherited as an autosomal dominant trait. Linkage studies in families have shown that the gene involved (*apc*) is on the long arm of chromosome 5 (between q21–22).

In FAP, multiple polyps are found throughout the gastrointestinal tract, the colon and duodenum being particularly involved. Constant endoscopic surveillance is necessary as all patients with FAP eventually develop cancer if followed long enough. An attempt should be made to remove all colonic polyps, but this is often impossible and, therefore, in this high-risk group and in any relative found to have polyps (relatives must be screened after 12 years of age) a colectomy with an ileorectal anastomosis is performed with long-term surveillance of the rectal stump. A new test using lymphocytes isolated from peripheral blood that can identify APC mutations in approximately 7% of patients may become generally available.

Congenital hypertrophy of the retinal pigment epithelium (CHRPE) can be seen in two-thirds of FAP patients and is useful for screening in young patients.

*Gardner's syndrome* is a variant of this condition in which, in addition to adenomatosis, there are mesodermal tumours (e.g. dermoid tumours, osteomas of the skull) and pigmented ocular fundal lesions.

## Colorectal carcinoma

Adenocarcinoma of the large bowel is the second commonest tumour in the UK with a lifetime incidence of about 1 in 50 (both male and female). The incidence increases with age, the average age at diagnosis being 60–65 years. The disease is rare in Africa and Asia and this difference is thought to be largely environmental rather than racial. There is a correlation between the consumption of meat and animal fat and colonic cancer. Western diets are low in fibre and the resulting intestinal stasis increases the time for which any potential carcinogen is in contact with the bowel wall. The bacterial flora in the colon is also affected by different diets, particularly in amount of fibre present, and it is speculated that certain bacteria convert bile acids

to potential carcinogens. Ulcerative colitis (see p. 220) and FAP are predisposing factors.

### GENETIC INHERITANCE

The development of colon cancer is now felt to involve multiple genetic alterations which occur in a stepwise fashion.

The widespread recognition of the adenoma–carcinoma sequence and the identification of many molecular genetic abnormalities has led to the development of a molecular model for colon cancer tumorigenesis (Fig 4.33). The changes include the activation of dominantly acting proto-oncogenes and the inactivation of recessive tumour suppressive genes. Oncogenes, many of which have a physiological role in the regulation of normal cell division and differentiation, may result in inappropriate stimulation signals. Those most commonly associated with colon cancer are c-*KRAS* and c-*MYC* which are overexpressed in up to 50% and 70% of colon tumours respectively. Other less frequently altered oncogenes include c-*SRC*, c-*MYB* and c-*ERB*-2. Tumour suppressor genes conversely inhibit cell proliferation and tumorigenesis. Mutations of the *apc* gene located on the long arm of chromosome 5 is responsible for the FAP syndrome, but also plays a role in sporadic colon cancer. It appears, however, that the accumulation rather than the order of changes is most important in tumour development.

### Cancer families

There is a two to three times increased lifetime risk of developing colon cancer with one first-degree affected family member. Hereditary non-polyposis colon cancer (HNPCC) occurs in 5–10% of colorectal cancers. The putative gene responsible has recently been localized on chromosome 2. These patients have tumours at an early age and, more commonly, in the right colon. Many of these patients also have a high risk of endometrial and other non-gastrointestinal cancers (Lynch type II) whilst others are colon specific (Lynch type I).

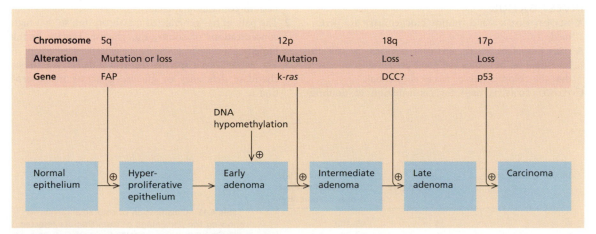

**Fig. 4.33**  A genetic model for colorectal tumorigenesis. FAP, familial adenomatous polyposis (or adenomatous polyposis coli—APC); DCC, deleted in colon cancer. (From E. R. Fearon and B. Vogelstein (1990) *Cell* **61**, 759. With permission.)

### Screening

The case for universal faecal occult blood screening has been made with a reduction of the 13-year cumulative mortality by 33%. It is not yet recommended in the UK. A single, flexible sigmoidoscopy at the age of 55 years or over is being recommended by some as another screening method. Universal colonoscopic screening has not shown any benefit, but colonoscopy should be performed in anyone with a history of cancer in their first- and second-degree relatives. Measurement of DNA in the stools is also being developed for screening.

### PATHOLOGY

Two-thirds of carcinomas occur in the rectosigmoid area. The tumour, which is usually a polypoid mass with ulceration, spreads by direct infiltration through the bowel wall. It then invades the lymphatics and blood vessels with early spread to the liver. Widespread metastases, e.g. to the lung, can occur. Synchronous tumours are present in 2% of cases.

### CLINICAL FEATURES

Alteration in bowel habit, with or without abdominal pain, is a common symptom of left-sided colonic lesions. Rectum and sigmoid carcinomas usually bleed, blood being mixed in with the stool. Carcinoma of the caecum may become large and still remain asymptomatic. It can present simply as an iron deficiency anaemia. The elderly often present with intestinal obstruction. Any change in bowel habit or bleeding per rectum must be investigated, particularly in the older age group.

Clinical examination is usually unhelpful, but a mass may be palpable. With liver metastases, hepatomegaly is found. Digital examination of the rectum is essential and sigmoidoscopy should be performed in all cases. Fibre-optic sigmoidoscopy can be performed on an outpatient basis after a single enema and increases, by three to four times, the extent of the colon seen covering the area with the highest risk of carcinoma.

### INVESTIGATION

A BLOOD COUNT and routine biochemistry are performed.

A DOUBLE-CONTRAST BARIUM ENEMA is still the investigation of choice but good preparation to ensure that the colon is free of faeces is essential.

COLONOSCOPY is used for confirmation of doubtful lesions and to obtain specimens for histological examination.

OCCULT BLOOD TESTS have been used for mass screening but are of no value in hospital practice (see p. 199).

ULTRASOUND. Evaluation of secondary spread is performed prior to surgery with abdominal ultrasound and rectal ultrasound, which is valuable to indicate tumour size and local spread.

### TREATMENT

This is surgical, with resection and end-to-end anastomosis if possible. Anastomosis is now possible with all but the most distal rectal carcinomas, when colostomy is necessary. The 5-year survival rate is 30% overall, but in tumours confined to the bowel wall (i.e. not reaching the serosa—Dukes' grade A), the 5-year survival is over 95% (Table 4.15). Adjuvant chemotherapy increases survival in Dukes' grade B and C. Adjuvant chemotherapy and radiotherapy increase survival in grade C rectal carcinoma. Chemotherapy is sometimes used when metastases are present, but results are poor.

# Diarrhoea

With true diarrhoea there is an increase in stool weight to greater than 300 g per day. This is usually accompanied by increased stool frequency. Patients often interpret the word 'diarrhoea' in different ways (see p. 176).

### Mechanisms

OSMOTIC DIARRHOEA. The gut mucosa acts as a semi-permeable membrane and fluid enters the bowel if there are large quantities of non-absorbed hypertonic substances in the lumen. This occurs because:

1 The patient has ingested a non-absorbable substance, e.g. a purgative such as magnesium sulphate or magnesium-containing antacid.
2 The patient has generalized malabsorption so that high concentrations of solute, e.g. glucose, remain in the lumen.
3 The patient has a specific absorptive defect, e.g. disaccharidase deficiency or glucose–galactose malabsorption.

| Dukes' classification | Cases resected (%) | 5-year survival (%) (corrected for other causes of mortality) |
|---|---|---|
| A | 15 | 95–100 |
| B | 40 | 65–75 |
| $C_1$ (adjacent nodes) | 35 | 30–40 |
| $C_2$ (apical nodes) | 10 | 10–20 |

Table 4.15 Classification of colorectal carcinoma showing the percentage of cases that are resected and their life prognosis. NB. Approximately 20% of the cases at presentation of colorectal carcinoma are inoperable. Of those submitted to surgery the findings are shown in the table.

The volume of diarrhoea produced by these mechanisms is reduced by the absorption of fluid by the ileum and colon. The diarrhoea stops when the patient stops eating or the malabsorptive substance is discontinued.

SECRETORY DIARRHOEA. In this disorder there is both active intestinal secretion of fluid and electrolytes as well as decreased absorption. The mechanism of intestinal secretion is shown in Fig. 4.34(a). Common causes of secretory diarrhoea are:

- Enterotoxins, e.g. cholera, *E. coli* (thermolabile or thermostable toxin).
- Hormones, e.g. VIP in the Verner–Morrison syndrome (p. 292)
- Bile salts (in the colon) following ileal resection
- Fatty acids (in the colon) following ileal resection
- Some laxatives, e.g. dioctyl sodium sulphosuccinate

With secretory diarrhoea, the stool volumes may be very high. Food does not affect the diarrhoea and it therefore continues during fasting.

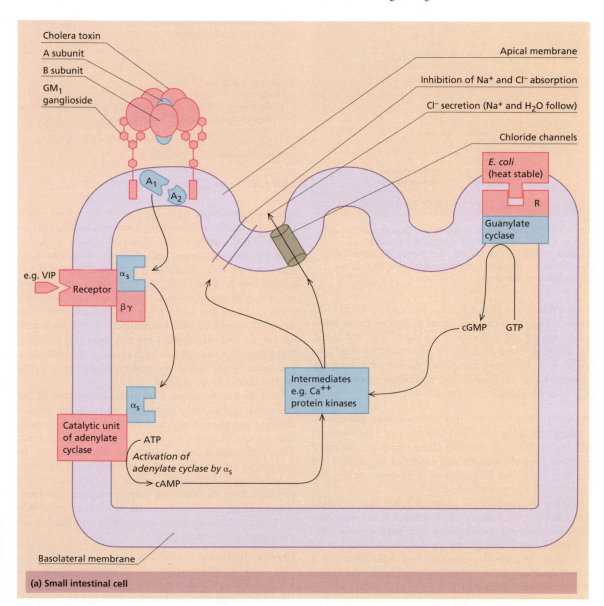

**Fig. 4.34**   (a) Mechanisms of diarrhoea. *Small intestinal cell.* Cholera toxin binds to its receptor (monosialoganglioside $GM_1$) via its B subunits. The enzymatically active $A_1$ subunit activates $G_s$ (G-stimulated) protein shown as its three subunits $\gamma$, $\beta$ and $\alpha_s$. $\alpha_s$ dissociates from $G_s$ protein and activates the catalytic unit of adenylate cyclase on the basolateral membrane. The resulting increase in cAMP activates intermediates, e.g. protein kinases and $Ca^{2+}$, which act on the apical microvillous membrane to cause $Cl^-$ secretion and inhibition of $Na^+$ and $Cl^-$ absorption. Heat-labile *E. coli* shares the same receptor as cholera toxin. Heat-stable *E. coli* (ST) binds to its receptor protein R and this complex activates guanylate cyclase which produces the same effect. The ST receptor is specific for the intestine. In both mechanisms, stimulation occurs without invasion.

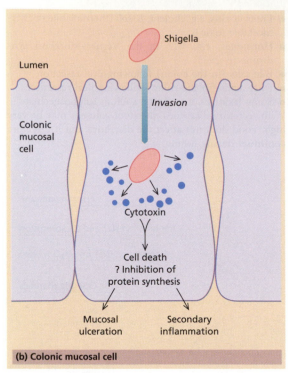

**(b) Colonic mucosal cell**

**Fig. 4.34** (b) Mechanisms of diarrhoea. *Colonic mucosal cell.* This demonstrates one of the mechanisms by which an invasive pathogen, e.g. *Shigella*, acts. Following penetration, the pathogens generate cytotoxins which lead to mucosal ulceration and cell death.

INFLAMMATORY DIARRHOEA (MUCOSAL DESTRUCTION). Diarrhoea occurs because of damage to the intestinal mucosal cell so that there is a loss of fluid and blood. In addition, there is defective absorption of fluid and electrolytes. Common causes are infective conditions, e.g. dysentery due to *Shigella*, and inflammatory conditions, e.g. ulcerative colitis (see Fig. 4.34(b)).

ABNORMAL MOTILITY (usually not true diarrhoea). Diabetic, postvagotomy and hyperthyroid diarrhoea are all due to abnormal motility of the upper gut. In many of these cases the volume and weight of the stool is not all that high, but frequency of defecation occurs; this therefore is not true diarrhoea.

Causes of diarrhoea are shown in Table 4.16. It should be noted that the irritable bowel syndrome and diverticular disease are not mentioned as they do not cause 'true' diarrhoea, even though the patients may complain of diarrhoea. Worldwide, infection and infestation are a major problem and these are discussed under the causative organisms in Chapter 1.

ACUTE DIARRHOEA (excluding cholera, which is discussed on p. 29). Diarrhoea of sudden onset is very common, often short-lived and requires no investigation or treatment. This type of diarrhoea is seen after dietary indiscretions, but diarrhoea due to viral agents also lasts 24–48 hours (see p. 52). The causes of other infective diarrhoeas are shown on p. 31. Traveller's diarrhoea,

*Acute*
Dietary indiscretion
Infective
    Food poisoning, see p. 33
    Viral gastroenteritis, see p. 52
Traveller's diarrhoea, see p. 31, e.g.
    *E. coli*
    *G. lamblia*
    *Shigella*
    *Entamoeba histolytica*

*Chronic*
Inflammatory bowel disease
Parasitic/fungal infections
Malabsorption
Gut resection
Drugs
Colonic neoplasia
Endocrine
    Pancreatic tumours, e.g. gastrinoma
    Medullary carcinoma of the thyroid
    Thyrotoxicosis
    Diabetic neuropathy
Faecal impaction—in the elderly

**Table 4.16** Causes of diarrhoea (see text).

which affects people travelling outside their own countries, particularly to developing countries, usually lasts 2–5 days; it is discussed on p. 31. Clinical features associated with the acute diarrhoeas include fever, abdominal pain and vomiting. If the diarrhoea is particularly severe, dehydration can be a problem; the very young and very old are at special risk from this. Investigations are necessary if the diarrhoea has lasted more than 1 week. Stools (up to three) should be sent immediately to the laboratory for culture and examination for ova, cysts and parasites. If the diagnosis has still not been made, a sigmoidoscopy and rectal biopsy should be performed and radiological studies should be considered.

Oral fluid replacement is of prime importance in the treatment. Special oral rehydration solutions, e.g. sodium chloride and glucose powder (see Table 1.16), are available for use in severe episodes of diarrhoea in infants. These compounds were initially developed for use in cholera but are valuable in all severe diarrhoeas. Antidiarrhoeal drugs are thought to impair the clearance of any pathogen from the bowel but may be necessary for short-term relief, e.g. codeine phosphate 30 mg four times daily or loperamide 2 mg three times daily; antibiotics are sometimes given (see p. 31).

### Chronic diarrhoea

This always needs investigation. All patients should have a sigmoidoscopy and rectal biopsy. The flow diagram (Fig. 4.35) is illustrative; whether the large or the small bowel is investigated first will depend on the clinical story of, for example, bloody diarrhoea or steatorrhoea. The investigations and treatment are described in detail under the individual diseases.

### Some other causes of diarrhoea

PURGATIVE ABUSE. This is usually seen in females who surreptitiously take high-dose purgatives and are often

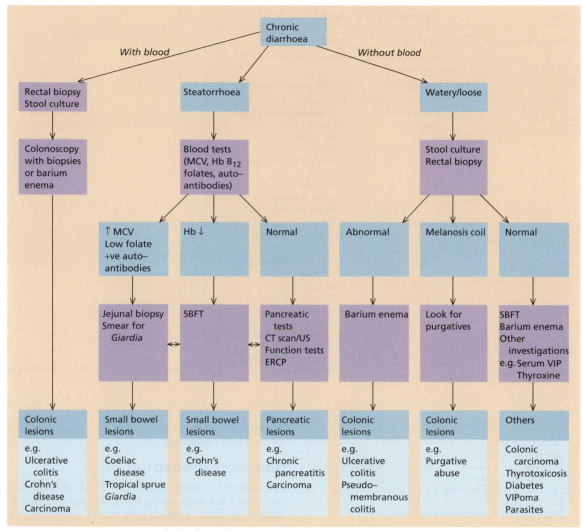

**Fig. 4.35** Flow diagram for the investigation of chronic diarrhoea. **ERCP**, endoscopic retrograde cholangiopancreatography; **MCV**, mean corpuscular volume; **SBFT**, small bowel follow-through; **US**, ultrasound; **VIP**, vasoactive intestinal polypeptide.

extensively investigated for chronic diarrhoea. The diarrhoea is usually of high volume (>1 litre daily). Sigmoidoscopy may show a pigmented mucosa, a condition known as *melanosis coli*. Histologically the rectal biopsy shows pigment-laden macrophages in patients taking an anthraquinone purgative (e.g. Senokot). Melanosis coli is also seen in people taking regular purgatives in normal doses.

Phenolphthalein laxatives can be detected by pouring an alkali, e.g. sodium hydroxide, on the stools, which then turn pink; a magnesium-containing purgative will give a high faecal magnesium content. Anthraquinones can be measured in the urine. A barium enema shows loss of haustral pattern and there may be mild abnormalities of absorption tests and a low serum potassium. Management is difficult as the patient usually denies purgative

ingestion. If the diagnosis is suspected, a locker or bed search (while the patient is out of the ward) is occasionally necessary.

The patient needs psychiatric help.

Pseudomembranous colitis (antibiotic-associated diarrhoea) (see p. 26). This colitis develops following the use of any antibiotic. Diarrhoea occurs in the first few days after taking the antibiotic or even up to 6 weeks after stopping the antibiotics. The causative agent is *Clostridium difficile*.

### Diarrhoea in patients with HIV infection

Chronic diarrhoea is a common symptom in HIV infection but its own role in the pathogenesis of diarrhoea is unclear. *Cryptosporidium* (see p. 74) and microsporidia

| Site | Symptoms | Problems |
|------|----------|----------|
| Mouth/oesophagus | Dysphagia | Candidiasis |
| | Retrosternal discomfort | Herpes simplex virus (HSV) |
| | Oral ulceration | Cytomegalovirus (CMV) |
| Small bowel ± colon | Chronic diarrhoea<br>Steatorrhoea<br>Weight loss | Parasites<br>  *Cryptosporidium parvum*<br>  *Isospora belli*<br>  Microsporidia<br>Viruses<br>  **CMV/HSV**, Adenovirus<br>Bacteria<br>  *Salmonella*<br>  *Campylobacter*<br>  *Mycobacterium avium intracellulare*<br>Non-infective enteropathy—cause unknown |
| Rectum/colon | Bloody diarrhoea | Bacterial infection e.g. Shigella |
| Any | Weight loss<br>Diarrhoea | Neoplasia<br>  Kaposi's sarcoma<br>  Lymphoma<br>  Squamous carcinoma<br>Infection—disseminated e.g. disseminated *Mycobacterium avium intracellulare* |

**Table 4.17** Gastrointestinal problems in patients with **HIV** infection.

Nausea alone
Vomiting alone
Bad breath (halitosis)
Belching
Abdominal bloating
Chronic right hypochondrial pain
Left iliac fossa pain
Frequent bowel actions in the morning

**Table 4.18** Chronic gastrointestinal symptoms suggestive of psychosomatic disorders.

are the commonest pathogens isolated. *Isospora belli* has also been found. An enteropathy has been described. The cause of the diarrhoea is often not found and treatment is symptomatic. Table 4.17 shows the conditions affecting the gastrointestinal tract in AIDS.

# Functional bowel disease

This is the general term used to embrace two syndromes:
1 Non-ulcer dyspepsia
2 The irritable bowel syndrome
These conditions are extremely common worldwide, making up to 60–80% of patients seen in a gastroenterology clinic. The two conditions overlap, with some symptoms being common to both. Table 4.18 gives some gastrointestinal symptoms that are suggestive of psychosomatic disorders.

## Non-ulcer dyspepsia

This consists of a heterogeneous group of patients whose symptoms are mainly stress-related. Patients complain of indigestion, wind, nausea, early satiety, heartburn, i.e. dyspepsia, when no ulcer is found. It can be difficult on the history to differentiate it from the symptoms of peptic ulceration, but typically patients with ulcers have nocturnal pain and also respond to antacids (Information box 4.5). Barium studies or endoscopy are often performed to exclude ulceration, but are best avoided in patients under 35 years, as no abnormality is found in the majority (80%). Chronic active gastritis due to *H. pylori* is found more frequently than in asymptomatic controls, but the relationship of this finding with symptoms is unclear.

Treatment is by reassurance. Antacids and $H_2$-receptor antagonists are probably of little benefit apart from the placebo effect. Cisapride 10 mg three times daily and metoclopramide 10 mg three times daily sometimes help particularly in the patients with fullness and early satiety, some of whom have been shown to have slow gastric emptying.

## The irritable bowel syndrome
### CLINICAL FEATURES
The pain is classically situated in the left iliac fossa and is usually relieved by defecation or the passage of wind.

| | Functional dyspepsia | Peptic ulceration |
|---|---|---|
| Site of pain | Diffuse 'all over' Fits no recognized pattern | Epigastric—points with one finger |
| Frequency of pain | Daily for long periods | Episodic |
| Food/meals | Pain unaffected Lasts all day | Exacerbate or help pain |
| Antacids | No help | Help pain |
| Nocturnal pain waking patient | Rare | Common |
| Vomiting | No effect | Reduces pain |

**Information box 4.5**  Clinical clues.

The patient may complain of constipation or diarrhoea with the passage of frequent small-volume stools and a feeling of incomplete emptying of the rectum. Stools may be ribbon-like or rabbity in appearance. True watery diarrhoea suggests organic disease. The pain, however, can be very variable and occur in any part of the abdomen and the bowel habit may be normal.

Abdominal distension and bloating are extremely common and if present strongly suggest the diagnosis of the irritable bowel. Women are more frequently affected than men, and often the symptoms occur at the time of the period. The length of history is usually long with frequent recurrent episodes and long symptom-free intervals. The patient may give a history of recurrent episodes of abdominal pain as a child and there is an increase of childhood or sexual abuse in some series. Mild episodes of pain occur frequently (approximately 40%) in the normal population and are often disregarded. The reason why some patients attend doctors is unclear, but it is sometimes related to other social factors. The patient with the irritable bowel syndrome looks well despite frequent episodes of pain, some of which can be very acute and require hospital admission to rule out an acute abdominal condition.

## PATHOPHYSIOLOGY

Motility abnormalities have been found in the irritable bowel syndrome, but these abnormal findings have not been consistent and do not always correlate with episodes of pain.

Psychological factors are important and most patients find the symptoms are exacerbated by stress. Some patients are depressed, and this fact may be missed unless carefully looked for.

## EXAMINATION

Examination reveals no abnormality. Rectal examination and sigmoidoscopy should be performed. Although sigmoidoscopy shows a normal mucosa, air insufflation may reproduce the pain. If diarrhoea is a feature, a rectal biopsy should be performed, even if the mucosa looks normal, to help rule out inflammatory bowel disease.

## INVESTIGATION

The amount of investigation varies in individual patients. A young girl with pain in the left iliac fossa exacerbated by stress will require no investigation. Conversely, an elderly person who has developed pain or diarrhoea for the first time must be investigated, with a full radiological assessment, before the diagnosis of functional bowel disease is made.

## MANAGEMENT

In many patients symptoms are not severe and are clearly stress-related. These patients often require nothing but a discussion of their life-style and reassurance. Over-investigation (Information box 4.6) and drug therapy should be avoided.

- Patients must be reassured of the benign nature of the condition. Cancer phobia must be dispelled. Patients are encouraged to learn to cope with their symptoms, as they tend to be recurrent.
- A high-fibre diet or even a change in diet help some patients.

*Beware of false correlations*. Diverticular disease is common in the elderly and because diverticular disease is seen on the barium enema it must not be assumed to be the cause of the pain. Hiatus hernias are also common findings and are also often asymptomatic.

*Gynaecological problems* must be excluded; on the other hand, it must not be assumed that all lower abdominal pain in women is due to some gynaecological problem. Many unnecessary operations are carried out as a consequence.

*Recurrent pain in the right iliac fossa* is not due to chronic appendicitis, but to the irritable bowel syndrome.

*Recurrent pain in the right hypochondrium* is usually not due to gallbladder disease, but to the irritable bowel syndrome.

*Abdominal bruits* are common and abdominal pain should not be ascribed to ischaemic bowel on this basis alone.

**Information box 4.6**  Traps for the unwary.

- Antispasmodics, e.g. mebeverine, are given.
- A small group of patients who are often hospital attenders have severe symptoms and treatment here is difficult. Many are depressed and improve with antidepressant therapy. Other therapies, i.e. biofeedback and hypnotherapy, have been tried.

# The acute abdomen

This section deals with acute abdominal conditions that cause the patient to be hospitalized within a few hours of the onset of their pain. It is important to make the diagnosis as quickly as possible to reduce morbidity and mortality. Although a specific diagnosis should be attempted, the immediate problem in management is to decide whether an 'acute abdomen' exists and whether surgery is required.

## History

This should include previous operations, any gynaecological problems and whether any concurrent medical condition is present.

### Pain

The onset, site, type and subsequent course of the pain should be determined as accurately as possible.

'Visceral' pain due to distension of a viscus or stretching of a capsule is poorly localized. However, in general, upper abdominal pain is produced by upper gastrointestinal tract lesions and lower abdominal pain by lesions of the lower gastrointestinal tract. Localized pain in the right iliac fossa suggests acute appendicitis.

Sudden pain suggests:
- A perforation, e.g. of a duodenal ulcer
- A rupture, e.g. of an aneurysm
- Torsion, e.g. of an ovarian cyst
- Acute pancreatitis
  Back pain suggests:
- Pancreatitis
- Rupture of an aortic aneurysm
- Renal tract disease

Inflammatory conditions, e.g. appendicitis, produce a more gradual onset of pain while in intestinal obstruction the pain is typically colic in nature. With peritonitis the pain is continuous and may be made worse by movement.

### Vomiting

Vomiting may accompany any acute abdominal pain, but if persistent it suggests an obstructive lesion of the gut. The character of the vomit should be asked—does it contain blood, bile or small bowel contents?

### Other symptoms

Any change in bowel habit or of urinary frequency should be documented and, in females, a gynaecological history taken.

## Physical examination

The general condition of the patient should be noted. Does he or she look ill? Is the patient shocked? Large volumes of fluid may be lost from the vascular compartment into the peritoneal cavity or into the lumen of the bowel giving rise to hypovolaemia, a pale cold skin, a weak rapid pulse and hypotension.

### Abdomen

INSPECTION. Look for the presence of scars, distension or masses.

PALPATION. The abdomen should be examined gently for sites of tenderness and the presence or absence of guarding. Guarding is involuntary spasm of the abdominal wall and it indicates peritonitis. This can be localized to one area or it may be generalized, involving the whole abdomen.

BOWEL SOUNDS. Increased high-pitch tinkling bowel sounds indicate obstruction; this occurs because of fluid movement within the large dilated bowel lumen. Absent bowel sounds suggest peritoneal involvement. In an obstructed patient, absent bowel sounds suggest strangulation or ischaemia.

It is essential that the hernial orifices are examined if intestinal obstruction is suspected.

### Pelvic and rectal examination

These can be very helpful, particularly in diagnosing gynaecological causes of an acute abdomen, e.g. a ruptured ectopic pregnancy. Rectal examination may detect localized tenderness or blood in the stools, which is suggestive of a vascular lesion.

### Other observations

1 Mouth—the tongue is furred in most acute abdominal disease and a fetor is present.
2 Temperature—fever is more common in acute inflammatory processes.
3 Urine—examine for:
   (a) Blood—suggests urinary tract infection or renal colic.
   (b) Glucose and ketones—ketoacidosis can present with acute pain.
   (c) Protein and white cells (to exclude acute pyelonephritis).
4 Think of other conditions, e.g.
   (a) Diabetes mellitus (ketoacidosis).
   (b) Pneumonia (referred pain).
   (c) Myocardial infarction (referred pain).
   (d) Lead poisoning.
   (e) The irritable bowel syndrome (this can produce acute severe pain).
   (f) Renal colic.
   (g) Porphyria is a rare cause of abdominal pain.

## Investigation

BLOOD COUNT A raised white cell count occurs with inflammatory conditions.

SERUM AMYLASE High levels of greater than five times normal indicate acute pancreatitis. Raised levels below this can occur in any acute abdomen and should not be considered diagnostic of pancreatitis.

SERUM ELECTROLYTES are not particularly helpful for diagnosis, but useful for general evaluation of the patient.

X-RAY OF THE ABDOMEN. Chest and supine X-rays of the abdomen are useful to detect air under the diaphragm (perforation) or dilated loops of bowel or fluid levels suggestive of obstruction.

ULTRASOUND—is useful in the diagnosis of acute cholangitis and in good hands is reliable in the diagnosis of acute appendicitis. Gynaecological and other pelvic causes of pain can also be detected.

LAPAROSCOPY—is being increasingly used in the diagnosis of the acute abdomen when, in addition, therapeutic manoeuvres, such as appendicectomy, can be performed.

## SPECIFIC CONDITIONS

## Acute appendicitis

This is the commonest surgical emergency. It affects all age groups, but is rare in the very young and the very old. Appendicitis should always be considered in the differential diagnosis if the appendix has not been removed.

Acute appendicitis mostly occurs when the lumen of the appendix becomes obstructed with a faecolith; however, in some cases there is only generalized acute inflammation. If the appendix is not removed at this stage, gangrene occurs with perforation, leading to a localized abscess or to generalized peritonitis.

### CLINICAL FEATURES AND MANAGEMENT

Most patients present with abdominal pain; in many it starts vaguely in the centre of the abdomen, becoming localized to the right iliac fossa in the first few hours. There is nausea, some vomiting and occasional diarrhoea. Because of the variable position of the appendix, symptoms and signs differ.

Examination of the abdomen reveals tenderness in the right iliac fossa, with guarding due to the localized peritonitis. Rectal examination may reveal tenderness to the right. There may be a tender mass in the right iliac fossa.

Laboratory tests are unhelpful, except that the white cell count may be raised. An ultrasound is accurate for the detection of an inflamed appendix and will also indicate an appendix mass or other localized lesion.

In the *differential diagnosis* all abdominal conditions must be considered, including:

- Non-specific mesenteric lymphadenitis may mimic appendicitis.
- Acute terminal ileitis (see p. 216)—due to Crohn's disease; *Yersinia* infection also gives similar symptoms and signs.
- Acute salpingitis—should be considered in women. There is usually a vaginal discharge and on vaginal examination adnexal tenderness is found.

- Inflamed Meckel's diverticulum.
- Functional bowel disease.

### TREATMENT

The appendix is removed by open surgery or laparoscopically.

If an appendix mass is present, the patient is treated conservatively with antibiotics. The pain subsides over a few days and the mass usually disappears over a few weeks. Appendicectomy is recommended at a later date to prevent further acute episodes.

## Acute peritonitis

### Localized peritonitis

There is virtually always some degree of localized peritonitis with all acute inflammatory conditions of the gastrointestinal tract, e.g. acute appendicitis, acute cholecystitis. Pain and tenderness are largely features of this localized peritonitis. The treatment is for the underlying disease.

### Generalized peritonitis

This is a serious condition resulting from irritation of the peritoneum due to infection, e.g. perforated appendix, or from chemical irritation due to leakage of intestinal contents, e.g. perforated ulcer. In the latter case, superadded infection gradually occurs; *E. coli* and *Bacteroides* are the commonest organisms.

The peritoneal cavity becomes acutely inflamed with production of an inflammatory exudate that spreads throughout the peritoneum leading to intestinal dilatation and paralytic ileus.

### CLINICAL FEATURES AND MANAGEMENT

In perforation the onset is sudden with acute severe abdominal pain, followed by general collapse and shock. The patient may improve temporarily, only to become worse later as generalized toxaemia occurs.

When the peritonitis is secondary to inflammatory disease, the onset is less rapid with the initial features being those of the underlying disease.

Investigations should always include an abdominal X-ray to detect free air under the diaphragm and a serum amylase to diagnose acute pancreatitis, which is treated conservatively.

Peritonitis is always treated surgically after initial treatment of the patient's general condition, including insertion of a nasogastric tube, intravenous fluids and antibiotics. Surgery has a two-fold objective:

1 Drainage of the abdominal cavity
2 Specific treatment of the underlying condition

### COMPLICATIONS

Any delay in treatment of peritonitis produces more profound toxaemia and septicaemia. In addition, local abscess formation occurs and should be suspected if the patient continues to remain unwell postoperatively with a swinging fever, high white cell count and continuing pain. Abscesses are commonly pelvic or subphrenic. Both are now localized chiefly by ultrasound examination; treatment is with antibiotics and drainage is often required.

## Intestinal obstruction

Most intestinal obstruction is due to a mechanical block. Sometimes the bowel does not function, leading to a paralytic ileus. This occurs temporarily after most abdominal operations and with peritonitis. Some causes of intestinal obstruction are shown in Table 4.19.

Obstruction of the bowel leads to bowel distension above the block, with increased secretion of fluid into the distended bowel. Bacterial contamination occurs in the distended stagnant bowel. In strangulation the blood supply is impeded, leading to gangrene, perforation and peritonitis unless urgent treatment of the condition is undertaken.

### CLINICAL FEATURES

The patient complains of colicky abdominal pain, vomiting and constipation without passage of wind. In upper gut obstruction the vomiting is profuse but in lower gut obstruction it may be absent.

Examination of the abdomen reveals distension with increased bowel sounds. Marked tenderness suggests strangulation and urgent surgery is necessary. Examination of the hernial orifices and rectum must be performed. X-ray of the abdomen reveals distended loops of bowel proximal to the obstruction. Fluid levels are seen in small bowel obstruction on an erect film. In large bowel obstruction, the caecum and ascending colon are distended. A water-soluble barium enema may help to demonstrate the site of the obstruction.

### MANAGEMENT

Initial management is by nasogastric intubation to decompress the bowel and replacement of fluid loss by intravenous fluids (mainly isotonic saline).

Laparotomy with removal of the obstruction is necessary in most cases of small bowel obstruction and if the bowel is gangrenous owing to strangulation gut resection will be required. A few patients, e.g. those with Crohn's disease, may have recurrent episodes of subacute intestinal obstruction that can be managed conservatively. Large bowel obstruction can often be managed conservatively with a defunctioning colostomy being performed, if necessary. Volvulus of the sigmoid colon can be managed by the passage of a rectal tube to unkink the bowel, but recurrent volvulus may require sigmoid resection.

Rarely the clinical features of obstruction are produced by a condition in which the nerve plexuses of the bowel are damaged—*intestinal pseudo-obstruction*. This condition is managed conservatively.

## Acute intestinal ischaemia

Mesenteric artery occlusion, either from an embolus or from thrombosis in an arteriosclerotic artery, leads to gut ischaemia and, if not dealt with promptly, necrosis of the intestine.

The patient presents with severe abdominal pain and vomiting. Bloody diarrhoea is a helpful indicator of the diagnosis but does not occur for some time. The abdomen is usually tender and bowel sounds are absent. The diagnosis must be considered in any elderly patient with arteriosclerotic disease or in patients with atrial fibrillation. Early surgery may prevent gut necrosis but sometimes massive resection of the dead gut is required to save the patient's life.

Mesenteric venous thrombosis occurs mainly in patients who have circulatory failure and can lead to gut necrosis. Often the patient is extremely ill from the underlying condition but surgery may be necessary if the patient is fit enough.

# The peritoneum

The peritoneal cavity is a closed sac lined by mesothelium. It normally contains a little fluid that allows the intra-abdominal organs to move freely. Some conditions that can affect the peritoneum are shown in Table 4.20.

*Peritonitis* can be acute or chronic, as seen in TB. Most cases of infective peritonitis are secondary to gastrointestinal diseases but it occasionally occurs without intra-abdominal sepsis in ascites due to liver disease. Very rarely, fungal and parasitic infections can also cause primary peritonitis, e.g. amoebiasis, candidiasis. Peritonitis is discussed further on p. 233.

The peritoneum can be involved by *secondary malignant deposits* and the commonest cause of ascites in a

| | |
|---|---|
| Small bowel obstruction | Adhesions |
| | Herniae |
| | Crohn's disease |
| Large bowel obstruction | Carcinoma of the colon |
| | Volvulus |
| | Diverticular disease |

**Table 4.19**  Some causes of intestinal obstruction.

*Infective (bacterial) peritonitis*
Secondary to gut disease, e.g.
   Appendicitis
   Perforation of any organ
Chronic peritoneal dialysis
Spontaneous, usually in ascites with liver disease
Tuberculosis

*Neoplasia*
Secondary deposits, e.g. from ovary, stomach
Primary mesothelioma

*Vasculitis*
Connective tissue disease

**Table 4.20**  Diseases of the peritoneum.

young to middle-aged woman is an ovarian carcinoma.

A *subphrenic abscess* is usually secondary to infection in the abdomen and is characterized by fever, malaise, pain in the right or left hypochondrium and shoulder-tip pain. A plain abdominal X-ray shows gas under the diaphragm, impaired movement of the diaphragm on screening and a pleural effusion. Ultrasound is usually diagnostic.

*Ascites* is associated with all diseases of the peritoneum. The fluid that collects is an exudate with a high protein content. It is also seen in liver disease. The mechanism, causes and investigation of ascites are discussed on p. 266.

## Tuberculous peritonitis (see p. 212)

This is due to reactivation of a tuberculous focus in the abdomen, often a lymph node. It is common in developing countries and is seen in the UK in debilitated patients, alcohol-dependent patients and in certain racial groups, e.g. Asians. Usually the onset is insidious, with fever, anorexia and weight loss. Abdominal pain is common, accompanied by ascites (75%) or an abdominal mass caused by an inflamed mesentery.

Diagnosis is made by examination of the peritoneal fluid, if present, which shows an increase in lymphocyte count; occasionally tubercle bacilli are seen on staining. Culture of the fluid should be performed. Ultrasound shows mesenteric thickening and enlargement of lymph nodes. At laparoscopy the peritoneum is seen to be studded with tubercles that can be biopsied and sent for culture and histology. Treatment is with conventional chemotherapy (see p. 686) for 18 months to 2 years.

## Retroperitoneal fibrosis

This is a rare condition in which there is a marked fibrosis over the posterior abdominal wall and retroperitoneum. The aetiology is usually unknown but it has been associated with the drug methysergide and occasionally with the carcinoid syndrome. The disease usually presents in middle age with malaise, fever and loss of weight. There is often anaemia and a raised ESR—a CT scan is diagnostic. The major complication is urinary tract obstruction from ureteric involvement, which may require surgery.

# *Further reading*

*Baillière's Clinical Gastroenterology*—quarterly reviews of gastroenterology. London: Baillière Tindall.

Field M *et al.* (1989) Intestinal electrolyte transport and diarrhoeal disease. *New England Journal of Medicine*, **321**, 879.

*Gastroenterology Clinics of North America* (1993), **22**. Review articles on *H. pylori* infection.

Lynch HT *et al.* (1993) Genetics, natural history, tumour spectrum and pathology of hereditary nonpolyposis colorectal cancer: an updated review. *Gastroenterology* **104**, 1535.

Sleisenger MH & Fordtran JS (1993) *Gastrointestinal Disease: Pathophysiology, Diagnosis, Management*, 5th edn. Philadelphia: WB Saunders.

## Introduction

In the Western World alcohol is the major cause of liver disease, whilst elsewhere the hepatitis B virus is still a significant factor. The longer term clinical consequences of hepatitis C are now being increasingly recognized. Health education and the improvement of social conditions should help stop the spread of viral infections.

Imaging techniques now enable the liver and biliary tree to be visualized with precision resulting in earlier diagnosis and the advent of laparoscopic surgery avoids the necessity of open surgery for biliary tract disease.

Results of liver transplantation continue to improve and transplantation can be of value in the treatment of both acute and chronic liver failure.

# THE LIVER AND BILIARY TRACT

## Structure

### Liver

The liver, the largest internal organ in the body, is situated in the right hypochondrium. Its upper border lies between the fifth and sixth ribs and its lower border can sometimes be palpated below the right costal margin on inspiration. The liver is divided into two main lobes—right and left. The right is larger and also contains the quadrate and caudate lobes. Riedel's lobe is an extension of the lateral portion of the right lobe and it can occasionally be palpated in a normal abdomen.

The blood supply to the liver, constituting 25% of the resting cardiac output, is via two main vessels:
1 The hepatic artery, which is a branch of the coeliac axis, supplies 25% of the total blood flow and 50% of the oxygen.
2 The portal vein drains most of the gastrointestinal tract and the spleen. It supplies 75% of the blood flow but only 50% of the total oxygen supply.

Both vessels enter the liver at the porta hepatis and the blood is distributed via the portal tracts into the sinusoids throughout the liver.

The functional component of the liver is the acinus. This consists of parenchyma supplied by the smallest portal tracts containing portal vein radicles, hepatic arterioles and bile ductules (Fig. 5.1). The hepatocytes near this triad (zone 1) are well supplied with oxygenated blood and are more resistant to damage than the cells nearer the central veins (zone 3). Blood passes from the portal tract via the sinusoids to the terminal hepatic vein (central vein). These sinusoids are lined by specialized endothelial cells, Kupffer's cells (phagocytic cells) and fat-storage cells (Ito cells) and are separated by plates of liver cells (hepatocytes). The potential space that lies between the sinusoids and hepatocytes is the space of Disse.

### Biliary system

Bile canaliculi form a network between the hepatocytes. These join to form thin bile ductules near the portal tract, which in turn enter the bile ducts in the portal tracts. These then combine to form the right and left hepatic ducts that leave each liver lobe. The hepatic ducts join at the porta hepatis to form the common hepatic duct. The

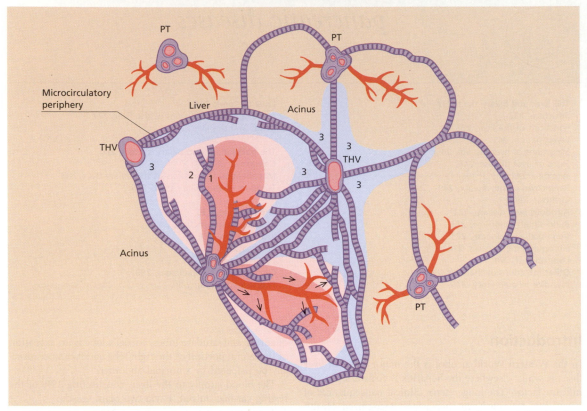

**Fig. 5.1**  Diagram of a functional acinus. Zones 1, 2 and 3 represent areas supplied by blood with zone 1 being best oxygenated. Zone 3 is supplied by blood remote from afferent vessels and is in the microcirculatory periphery of the acinus. The perivascular area (star shaped) is formed by the most peripheral parts of zone 3 of several adjacent acini and is the least well oxygenated. THV, terminal hepatic venule; PT, portal triad. From Sherlock S and Dooley J (1993) *Diseases of the Liver and Biliary System*, 9th edn. With permission from Blackwell Scientific Publications.

cystic duct connects the gallbladder to the lower end of the common hepatic duct. The gallbladder lies under the right lobe of the liver and stores and concentrates hepatic bile; it has a capacity of approximately 50 ml. The common bile duct is formed by the combination of the cystic and hepatic ducts and is approximately 8 mm in diameter, narrowing at its distal end to pass into the duodenum. The common bile duct and pancreatic duct open into the second part of the duodenum through a common channel at the ampulla of Vater. The lower end of the common bile duct contains the muscular sphincter of Oddi, which contracts rhythmically and prevents bile entering the duodenum in the fasting state.

# Functions of the liver

## Protein metabolism (see p. 155)

### Synthesis
The liver is the principal site of synthesis of all circulating proteins apart from $\gamma$-globulins, which are produced in the reticuloendothelial system. It receives amino acids from the intestine and muscles and, by controlling the rate of gluconeogenesis and transamination, regulates levels in the plasma. Plasma contains 60–80 g litre$^{-1}$ of protein, mainly in the form of albumin, globulin and fibrinogen.

Albumin has a half-life of 16–24 days and 10–12 g are synthesized daily. Its main functions are first to maintain the intravascular oncotic (colloid osmotic) pressure, and second to transport water-insoluble substances, e.g. bilirubin, hormones, fatty acids and drugs. Reduced synthesis of albumin over prolonged periods produces hypoalbuminaemia and is seen in chronic liver disease and malnutrition. Hypoalbuminaemia is also found in hypercatabolic states, e.g. trauma with sepsis, and in diseases where there is an excessive loss, e.g. nephrotic syndrome, protein-losing enteropathy.

Transport or carrier proteins such as transferrin and caeruloplasmin, and other proteins, e.g. $\alpha_1$-antitrypsin and $\alpha$-fetoprotein, are also produced in the liver.

The liver also synthesizes all coagulation factors (apart from factor VIII) i.e. fibrinogen, prothrombin, factors V, VII, IX, X, XIII, and components of the complement system (see Chapter 6).

## Degradation (nitrogen excretion)

Amino acids are degraded by transamination and oxidative deamination to produce ammonia, which is then converted to urea and excreted by the kidneys. This is a major pathway for the elimination of nitrogenous waste. Failure of this process occurs in severe liver disease.

# Carbohydrate metabolism

Glucose homeostasis and the maintenance of the blood sugar is an important function of the liver. It stores approximately 80 g of glycogen. In the immediate fasting state, blood glucose is maintained either by glucose released from the breakdown of glycogen (glycogenolysis) or by newly synthesized glucose (gluconeogenesis). Sources for gluconeogenesis are lactate, pyruvate, amino acids from muscles (mainly alanine and glutamine) and glycerol from lipolysis of fat stores. In prolonged starvation, ketone bodies and fatty acids are used as alternative sources of fuel and the body tissues adapt to a lower glucose requirement (see Chapter 3).

# Lipid metabolism

Fats are insoluble in water and are transported in the plasma as protein/lipid complexes (lipoproteins). These are discussed in detail on p. 854.

The liver plays a major role in the metabolism of lipoproteins. It synthesizes very low-density lipoproteins (VLDLs) and high-density lipoproteins (HDLs). HDLs are the substrate for lecithin–cholesterol acyltransferase (LCAT), which catalyses the conversion of free cholesterol to cholesterol ester (see below). Hepatic lipase removes triglyceride from intermediate-density lipoproteins (IDLs) to produce low-density lipoproteins (LDLs) which are degraded by the liver after uptake by specific cell-surface receptors (see Fig. 17.15).

Triglycerides may be of dietary origin but are also formed in the liver from circulating free fatty acids (FFA) and glycerol and incorporated into VLDLs. Oxidation or *de novo* synthesis of FFA also occurs in the liver, depending on the availability of dietary fat. Cholesterol may also be of dietary origin but most is synthesized from acetyl-CoA mainly in the liver, intestine, adrenal cortex and skin. It occurs either as free cholesterol or esterified with fatty acids, this reaction being catalysed by LCAT. This enzyme is reduced in severe liver disease, increasing the ratio of free cholesterol to ester, which alters membrane structures. One result of this is the red cell abnormalities, e.g. target cells, seen in chronic liver disease. Phospholipids, e.g. lecithin, are also synthesized in the liver.

The complex interrelationships between protein, carbohydrate and fat metabolism are shown in Fig. 5.2.

# Formation of bile

## Bile secretion

Bile consists of water, electrolytes, bile acids, cholesterol, phospholipids and bilirubin. Two processes are involved in bile secretion across the canalicular membrane of the hepatocyte:

1 In the *bile salt-dependent process* there is active secretion of bile salts; water and electrolytes follow down an osmotic and electrical gradient.
2 In the *bile salt-independent process*, bile flow is linked to sodium transport, which is dependent on Na+, K+ ATPase activity.

One-third of the bile flow emanates from the epithelial cells of the bile ductules. Secretion, particularly of bicarbonate, is stimulated mainly by secretin.

The average total bile flow is approximately 1 litre per day. In the fasted state half of the bile flows directly into the duodenum, half being diverted into the gallbladder. The mucosa of the gallbladder absorbs 80–90% of the water and electrolytes, but is impermeable to bile acids and cholesterol. Following a meal, cholecystokinin is secreted by the duodenal mucosa and stimulates contraction of the gallbladder and relaxation of the sphincter of Oddi, so that bile enters the duodenum. An adequate bile flow is dependent on bile salts being returned to the liver by the enterohepatic circulation.

## Bile acid metabolism

Bile acids are synthesized in hepatocytes from cholesterol. The rate-limiting step in their production is that catalysed by cholesterol-7$\alpha$-hydroxylase. They are excreted into the bile and then pass into the duodenum. The two primary bile acids—cholic acid and chenodeoxycholic acid (Fig. 5.3)—are conjugated with glycine or taurine (in a ratio of 3 : 1 in humans) and this process increases their solubility. Intestinal bacteria convert these acids into secondary bile acids—deoxycholic acid and lithocholic acid. Figure 5.4 shows the enterohepatic circulation of bile acids.

Bile acids act as detergents; their main function is lipid solubilization. Bile acid molecules contain both a hydrophilic and a hydrophobic end. In aqueous solutions they aggregate to form micelles, with their hydrophobic (lipid-soluble) ends in the centre. Micelles are expanded by cholesterol and phospholipids (mainly lecithin), forming mixed micelles.

## Bilirubin metabolism

Bilirubin is produced mainly from the breakdown of mature red cells in the Kupffer cells of the liver and in the reticuloendothelial system; 15% of bilirubin comes from the catabolism of other haem-containing proteins, such as myoglobin, cytochromes and catalases.

Normally, 250–300 mg of bilirubin are produced daily. The iron and globin are removed from the haem and are reutilized. Biliverdin is formed from the haem and this is reduced to form bilirubin. The bilirubin produced is unconjugated and water insoluble, and is transported to the liver attached to albumin. Bilirubin dissociates from albumin and is taken up by the hepatic cell membrane and transported to the endoplasmic reticulum by cytoplasmic proteins, where it is conjugated with glucuronic acid and excreted into bile. The microsomal enzyme uridine diphosphoglucuronyl transferase catalyses the formation of bilirubin monoglucuronide and then diglucuron-

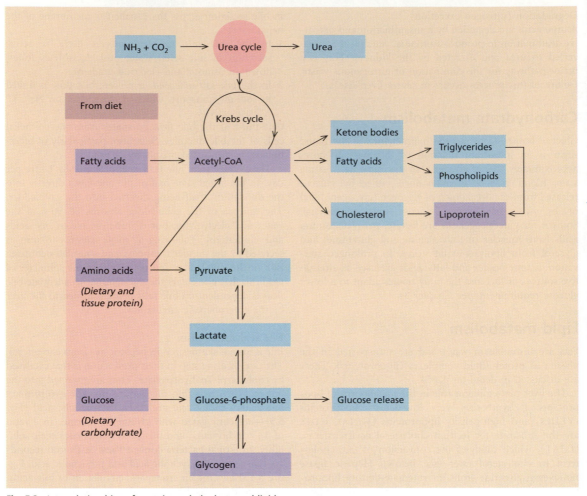

**Fig. 5.2** Interrelationships of protein, carbohydrate and lipid metabolism in the liver.

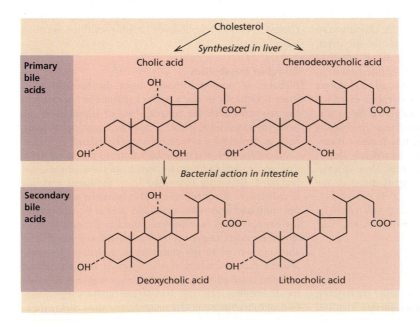

**Fig. 5.3** Primary and secondary bile acids. All bile acids are normally conjugated with glycine or taurine.

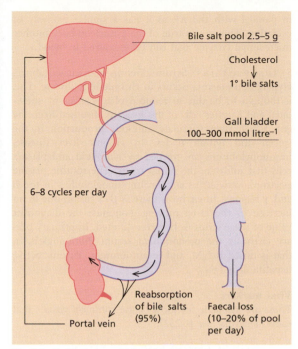

Bile salt pool 2.5–5 g

Cholesterol

↓

1° bile salts

Gall bladder
100–300 mmol litre⁻¹

6–8 cycles per day

Reabsorption
of bile salts
(95%)

Faecal loss
(10–20% of pool
per day)

Portal vein

**Fig. 5.4** Recirculation of bile acids. The bile salt pool is relatively small and the entire pool recycles six to eight times via the enterohepatic circulation. Up to 40 g are excreted daily into the bile and the synthesis of new bile acids only compensates for loss.

ide. This conjugated bilirubin is water soluble and is actively secreted into the bile canaliculi and excreted into the intestine with the bile. It is not absorbed from the small intestine because of its large molecular size. In the terminal ileum, bacterial enzymes hydrolyse the molecule, releasing free bilirubin, which is then reduced to urobilinogen. Some of this is excreted in the stools as stercobilinogen. The remainder is absorbed by the terminal ileum, passes to the liver via the enterohepatic circulation, and is re-excreted into the bile. Urobilinogen bound to albumin enters the circulation and is excreted in the urine via the kidneys. When hepatic excretion of conjugated bilirubin is impaired, a small amount of conjugated bilirubin is found strongly bound to serum albumin. It is not excreted by the kidney and accounts for the continuing hyperbilirubinaemia for a short time after cholestasis has resolved.

## Hormone and drug inactivation

The liver catabolizes hormones such as insulin, glucagon, oestrogens, growth hormone, glucocorticoids and parathyroid hormone. It is also the prime target organ for many hormones, e.g. insulin. It is the most important site for the metabolism of drugs (see p. 277) and alcohol (see p. 172). Fat-soluble drugs are converted to water-soluble substances that facilitate their excretion in the bile or urine.

## Immunological function

The reticuloendothelial system of the liver contains many immunologically active cells. The liver acts as a 'sieve' for the bacterial and other antigens carried to it via the portal tract from the gastrointestinal tract. These antigens are phagocytosed and degraded by Kupffer cells, which are macrophages attached to the endothelium. Kupffer cells have specific membrane receptors for ligands and are activated by several factors, e.g. infection. They secrete interleukins, tumour necrosis factor (TNF), collagenase and lysosomal hydrolases. Antigens are degraded without the production of antibody as there is very little lymphoid tissue. They are thus prevented from reaching other antibody-producing sites in the body and thereby prevent generalized adverse immunological reactions. The reticuloendothelial system is also thought to play a role in tissue repair, T and B lymphocyte interaction, and cytotoxic activity in disease processes. Thus in patients with liver disease immune response to infection is impaired. Furthermore immune-mediated damage can occur possibly initiated by antigens expressed on the hepatocyte surface itself.

# Investigation

Investigative tests can be divided into:
1 *Blood tests*
    (a) Liver 'function' tests
        (i)   Serum albumin
        (ii)  Prothrombin time
    (b) Liver biochemistry
        (i)   Reflecting hepatocellular damage—serum aspartate and alanine aminotransferases
        (ii)  Reflecting cholestasis—serum alkaline phosphatase, γ-glutamyl transpeptidase
    (c) Viral markers
    (d) Additional blood investigations, e.g. autoantibodies
2 *Imaging techniques*—to define gross anatomy
3 *Liver biopsy*—for histology

Most routine 'liver function tests' sent to the laboratory will be processed by an automated multichannel analyser to produce serum levels of bilirubin, aminotransferases, alkaline phosphatase, γ-glutamyl transpeptidase (γGT) and serum proteins. These routine tests are markers of liver damage but not actual tests of 'function' *per se*. Subsequent investigations are often based on these tests.

## Blood tests

### Liver function tests

SERUM ALBUMIN. This is a marker of synthetic function and is a valuable guide to the severity of chronic liver disease. A falling serum albumin in liver disease is a bad prognostic sign. In acute liver disease initial albumin levels may be normal.

PROTHROMBIN TIME (PT). This is also a marker of synthetic function. Because of its short half-life it is a sensitive indicator of both acute and chronic liver disease. Vitamin K deficiency should be excluded as the cause of a prolonged PT by giving an intravenous bolus (10 mg) of vitamin K. Vitamin K deficiency commonly occurs in biliary obstruction, as the low intestinal concentration of bile salts results in poor absorption of vitamin K.

### Liver biochemistry
BILIRUBIN. In the serum, bilirubin is normally almost all unconjugated. In liver disease increased serum bilirubin is usually accompanied by other abnormalities in liver biochemistry. Determination of whether the bilirubin is conjugated or unconjugated is only necessary in congenital disorders of bilirubin metabolism (see below) or to exclude haemolysis.

AMINOTRANSFERASES. These enzymes (often referred to as transaminases) are present in hepatocytes and leak into the blood with liver cell damage. The two enzymes measured are:
1 *Aspartate aminotransferase* (AST), which was previously known as serum glutamic oxaloacetic transaminase (SGOT). This is a mitochondrial enzyme and is also present in heart, muscle, kidney and brain. High levels are seen in hepatic necrosis, myocardial infarction, muscle injury and congestive cardiac failure.
2 *Alanine aminotransferase* (ALT), which was previously known as serum glutamic pyruvic transaminase (SGPT). This is a cytosol enzyme and is more specific to the liver than AST.

ALKALINE PHOSPHATASE (AP). This is present in the canalicular and sinusoidal membranes of the liver, but is also present in many other tissues, e.g. bone, intestine and placenta. If necessary, its origin can be determined by electrophoretic separation of isoenzymes or, alternatively, if there is also an abnormality of, for example, the γGT, the AP can be presumed to come from the liver.
  Serum AP is raised in cholestasis from any cause, whether intrahepatic or extrahepatic disease. The synthesis of AP is increased and this is released into the blood. In cholestatic jaundice, levels may be up to four to six times the normal limit. Raised levels may also occur in conditions with infiltration of the liver, e.g. metastases, and in cirrhosis, frequently in the absence of jaundice. The highest serum levels due to liver disease ($>1000$ IU litre$^{-1}$) are seen with hepatic metastases and primary biliary cirrhosis.

γ-GLUTAMYL TRANSPEPTIDASE. This is a microsomal enzyme that is present in many tissues as well as the liver. Its activity can be induced by such drugs as phenytoin and by alcohol. If the AP is normal, a raised serum γGT is a good guide to alcohol intake and can be used as a screening test (see p. 983). Mild elevation of the γGT is common even with a small alcohol consumption and does not necessarily indicate liver disease if the other liver biochemical tests are normal. In cholestasis the γGT rises in parallel with the AP as it has a similar pathway of excretion. This is also true of the 5-nucleotidase, another microsomal enzyme that can be measured in blood.

SERUM PROTEINS. Serum albumin is discussed above. Hyperglobulinaemia occurs in chronic liver disease. This is thought to be due to reduced phagocytosis by sinusoidal and Kupffer cells of the antigens absorbed from the gut, which then stimulate antibody production in the spleen and lymph nodes. In chronic liver disease, immunoglobulins are formed by lymphoid and plasma cells that infiltrate the portal tracts. The routine plasma electrophoretic strips contain immunoglobulins in the β and γ regions. In cirrhosis there is β–γ fusion due to an increase in the faster-moving globulins; the diagnostic value of these strips is, however, limited. In primary biliary cirrhosis the predominant serum immunoglobulin that is raised is IgM, and in autoimmune chronic active hepatitis it is IgG.

### Viral markers
These are available for most of the common viruses that cause hepatitis (see p. 252).

## ADDITIONAL BLOOD INVESTIGATIONS
### Haematological
A full blood count is always performed. Anaemia may be present. The red cells are often macrocytic and can have abnormal shapes—target cells and spur cells—owing to membrane abnormalities. Vitamin B$_{12}$ levels are normal or high, and folate levels are often low owing to poor dietary intake. Other changes are caused by the following:
● Bleeding produces a hypochromic, microcytic picture
● Alcohol causes macrocytosis, sometimes with leucopenia and thrombocytopenia
● Hypersplenism results in pancytopenia
● Cholestasis can often produce abnormal-shaped cells and also deficiency of vitamin K
● Haemolysis accompanies acute liver failure and jaundice
● Aplastic anaemia is present in up to 2% of patients with acute viral hepatitis
● Serum ferritin and transferrin saturation

### Biochemical

α$_1$-ANTITRYPSIN. A deficiency of this enzyme can produce cirrhosis.

α-FETOPROTEIN. This is normally produced by the fetal liver. Its reappearance in increasing and high concentrations in the adult indicates hepatocellular carcinoma. Increased concentrations in pregnancy in the blood and amniotic fluid suggest neural-tube defects of the fetus. Blood levels are also slightly raised in patients with hepatitis, chronic liver disease and also in teratomas.

### Immunological tests
There are no specific antibodies to the liver itself that are routinely measured. Autoantibodies found are:
ANTIMITOCHONDRIAL ANTIBODY (AMA) is found in

the serum in over 95% of patients with primary biliary cirrhosis (see p. 268). Many different AMA subtypes have been described, depending on their antigen specificity. AMA is demonstrated by an immunofluorescent technique and is neither organ nor species specific. Some subtypes are occasionally found in autoimmune chronic active hepatitis and other autoimmune diseases.

NUCLEIC, SMOOTH MUSCLE (ACTIN), LIVER/KIDNEY MICROSOMAL ANTIBODIES can be found in the serum in high titre in patients with autoimmune chronic active hepatitis. These antibodies can be found in the serum in other autoimmune conditions and other liver diseases.

### Bromsulphthalein (BSP) clearance test

This is now very rarely performed. The liver normally clears BSP from the blood. The level of BSP in the blood after an intravenous injection of BSP is a sensitive guide to hepatocellular damage. A second recirculation peak occurs in the congenital hyperbilirubinaemia of the Dubin–Johnson syndrome. Anaphylactic reactions may occur.

Useful blood tests for certain liver diseases are shown in Table 5.1.

## Imaging techniques

The main aim of these investigations is to delineate the anatomy and to look for any abnormality in the liver or biliary tree.

### Plain X-rays of the abdomen

These are rarely requested but may show:

GALLSTONES —10% contain enough calcium to be seen

AIR IN THE BILIARY TREE owing to its recent instrumentation, surgery or to a fistula between the intestine and the gallbladder

PANCREATIC CALCIFICATION

CALCIFICATION OF THE GALLBLADDER (porcelain gallbladder)—rare

### Ultrasound examination

This is a non-invasive, safe and relatively cheap technique. It involves the analysis of the reflected ultrasound beam detected by a probe moved across the abdomen. The normal liver appears as a relatively homogeneous structure. The gallbladder, common bile duct, pancreas, portal vein and other structures in the abdomen can be visualized.

It is useful in:

- A jaundiced patient (see p. 248)
- Hepatomegaly/splenomegaly
- The detection of gallstones (Fig. 5.5)
- Focal liver disease—lesions >1 cm
- General parenchymal liver disease
- Assessing portal and hepatic vein patency
- Lymph node enlargement

Other abdominal masses can be delineated and biopsies can be obtained under ultrasonic control. Doppler ultrasound can show the direction of blood flow in the portal and hepatic veins.

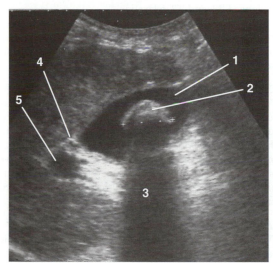

**Fig. 5.5** Ultrasound showing a large gallstone with acoustic shadowing. l, gallbladder; 2, gallstone; 3, acoustic shadow; 4, hepatic duct; 5, portal vein.

| Test | Disease |
|---|---|
| Antimitochondrial antibody | Primary biliary cirrhosis |
| Antinuclear, smooth muscle (actin), liver/kidney microsomal antibody | Autoimmune chronic active hepatitis |
| Serum immunoglobulins: | |
|   IgG | Autoimmune chronic active hepatitis |
|   IgM | Primary biliary cirrhosis |
| Viral markers (IgG and IgM) | Hepatitis A, B, C and others |
| $\alpha$-Fetoprotein | Primary hepatocellular carcinoma |
| Serum iron, transferrin saturation, serum ferritin | Haemochromatosis |
| Serum and urinary copper, serum caeruloplasmin | Wilson's disease |
| $\alpha_1$-Antitrypsin | Cirrhosis (± emphysema) |

**Table 5.1** Useful blood tests for certain liver diseases.

### Computed tomography (CT) examination

This is useful in all hepatobiliary problems and is complementary to ultrasound. Pancreatic disease, enlargement of regional lymph nodes, and lesions in the porta hepatis can be visualized. Abnormalities of size, shape and density as well as focal lesions of the liver can be detected. CT can detect calcification not seen on plain X-rays. It is not as useful as ultrasound for biliary tract disease but has advantages in obese subjects. As with ultrasound, biopsies can be taken under CT control.

### Magnetic resonance imaging (MRI)

In this technique, the amplitude of an MR signal depends on proton density, T1, T2 and flow. The higher the proton density of the tissue being imaged, the greater the signal obtained and thus the tissue will appear brighter on the image. T1 and T2 are relaxation time constants for the magnetism to return to equilibrium and these properties are intrinsic to different tissues, e.g. fat or muscle. The normal T1 and T2 can be altered by disease, for example, a focal hepatic mass such as a cyst will have a prolonged T1 and T2 relaxation.

MRI is useful in the detection and characterization of focal hepatic lesions (Fig. 5.6), diffuse parenchymal disease and hepatic and venous blood flow alteration. Its usefulness compared to CT scanning is still being evaluated.

### Cholecystogram

This has now been replaced in most centres by ultrasound. Oral iopanoic acid is absorbed from the gut, conjugated in the liver, secreted in bile and concentrated in the gallbladder, which opacifies homogeneously. A fatty meal is given to make the gall bladder contract. The dye is excreted by the liver via the same mechanism as bilirubin, so that non-visualization will occur in the jaundiced patient and in the patient with liver disease.

### Intravenous cholangiography

This has been replaced by ultrasound and endoscopic retrograde cholangiopancreatography.

### Radionuclide imaging—*scintiscanning*

TECHNETIUM-99M ($^{99m}$TC) COLLOID SCAN. This colloid, when injected intravenously, is taken up by the reticuloendothelial cells of the liver and spleen. It can show space-occupying lesions and a generalized decrease in uptake is found in parenchymal disease of the liver.

Since the introduction of ultrasound this technique is used less frequently. Currently its main uses are in:

ADVANCED CIRRHOSIS in which there is poor uptake in the liver and most of the colloid is taken up in the spleen and bone marrow

ALCOHOLIC HEPATITIS in which there is virtually no uptake in the liver owing to Kupffer cell damage by alcohol

$^{99m}$TC-HIDA SCAN. $^{99m}$Tc-HIDA (an imino-diacetic acid derivative) is taken up by the hepatocytes and excreted rapidly into the biliary system. Its main uses are in the diagnosis of:
- Acute cholecystitis
- Hepatitis due to biliary atresia in the neonatal period

### Endoscopy

This is used for the diagnosis and treatment of varices and for the detection of portal hypertensive gastropathy.

### Endoscopic retrograde cholangiopancreatography (ERCP)

This technique is used to outline the biliary and pancreatic ducts. It involves the passage of an endoscope into the second part of the duodenum and cannulation of the ampulla. Contrast is injected into both systems and the patient is screened radiologically. Contrast medium with a low iodine content of 1.5 mg ml$^{-1}$ is used for the common bile duct so that gallstones are not obscured; a higher iodine content of 2.8 mg ml$^{-1}$ is used for the pancreatic duct. In addition, other diagnostic and therapeutic procedures can be carried out:

REMOVAL OF COMMON BILE DUCT STONES after a diathermy cut to the sphincter has been performed to facilitate their withdrawal

DRAINING THE BILIARY SYSTEM by passing a tube (stent) through an obstruction

Complications include cholangitis, and broad-spectrum prophylactic antibiotics, e.g. i.v. cefotaxime 1 g 8-hourly, should be given to all patients with suspected biliary obstruction. A raised serum amylase is often seen and pancreatitis can occur. The presence of a pancreatic pseudocyst is a relative contraindication.

### Percutaneous transhepatic cholangiography (PTC)

Under a local anaesthetic a fine, flexible needle is passed into the liver. Contrast is injected slowly until a biliary radicle is identified and then further contrast is injected to outline the whole of the biliary tree. The main use of PTC is in jaundiced patients who have been shown to have dilated intrahepatic ducts demonstrated on ultrasound. The choice of ERCP or PTC often depends on local expertise. Sometimes the two techniques are performed together, PTC showing the biliary anatomy leading to an obstruction, while ERCP shows the more distal anatomy. If an obstruction in the bile ducts is seen, a bypass stent can sometimes be inserted either draining

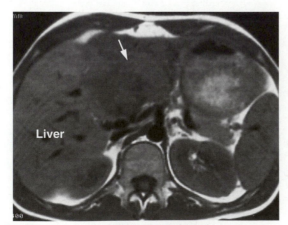

**Fig. 5.6**   MRI of a focal hepatic lesion (arrow).

externally or, for long-term use, internally. Contraindications are as for liver biopsy (see below). The main complications are bleeding and cholangitis with septicaemia, and prophylactic antibiotics should be given as for ERCP.

## Angiography

This can be performed by selective catheterization of the coeliac axis and hepatic artery, and is useful for detecting the abnormal vasculature of hepatic tumours. The portal vein can be demonstrated with increased definition using subtraction techniques, and splenoportography (by direct splenic puncture) is now rarely performed. In digital vascular imaging (DVI), contrast given intravenously or intra-arterially can be detected in the portal system using computerized subtraction analysis. Attempted visualization of the hepatic veins by venography is particularly important in the diagnosis of the Budd–Chiari syndrome. Hepatic venous cannulation also allows an indirect measurement of portal pressure to be made, although this has seldom been shown to be of any diagnostic or therapeutic value.

## Liver biopsy (Practical box 5.1)

Histological examination of the liver is valuable in the differential diagnosis of diffuse or localized parenchymal disease. Liver biopsy can be performed either on a day-case or overnight-stay basis. The indications and contraindications are shown in Table 5.2. The mortality rate is less than 0.02% when performed by experienced operators.

Liver biopsy is now often performed under ultrasound or CT control particularly when specific lesions need to be biopsied.

Laparoscopy with guided liver biopsy is performed through a small incision in the abdominal wall under local anaesthesia. General anaesthesia is preferred in some centres.

A transjugular approach is used when liver histology is essential for management but coagulation studies prevent the percutaneous approach.

### COMPLICATIONS

Most complications occur within 24 hours usually in the first 2 hours. They are usually minor and include abdomi-

---

*Indications*
Liver disease
  Unexplained hepatomegaly
  Some cases of jaundice (see p. 250)
  Persistently abnormal liver biochemistry
  Occasionally in acute hepatitis (p. 252)
  Cirrhosis
  Drug-related liver disease
  Infiltrations
  Tumours—primary or secondary
  Systemic disease
Screening relatives of patients with certain diseases,
  e.g. haemochromatosis
Pyrexia of unknown origin

*Usual contraindications to needle biopsy*
Uncooperative patient
Prolonged prothrombin time (by more than 3 s)
Platelets $\leqslant 80 \times 10^9$/litre
Ascites
Extrahepatic cholestasis

Table 5.2  Indications and contraindications for liver biopsy.

---

nal or shoulder pain which settles with analgesics. Minor intraperitoneal bleeding is common but this settles spontaneously. Rare complications include major intraperitoneal bleeding, pleurisy and perihepatitis, biliary peritonitis, haemobilia and transient septicaemia. Haemobilia produces biliary colic, jaundice and melaena within 3 days of the biopsy.

# Symptoms of liver disease

## Acute liver disease

Acute liver disease may be asymptomatic and anicteric. For example, an abnormality such as raised aminotransferases may be found during a routine biochemical screen.

Symptomatic acute liver disease, which is often viral, produces generalized symptoms of malaise, anorexia and fever. Jaundice may appear as the illness progresses.

---

This should only be performed by experienced doctors and with sterile precautions.

The patient's coagulation status (prothrombin time, platelets) is checked (see contraindications)
The patient's blood group is checked and serum saved for crossmatching
The patient lies on his back at the edge of the bed
The liver margins are delineated using percussion
Local anaesthetic is injected at the point of maximum dullness in the mid-axillary line through the intercostal space during
  expiration. Anaesthetic (1% lignocaine, approximately 5 ml) should be injected down to the liver capsule
A tiny cut is made in the skin with a scalpel blade
A special needle (Menghini, Trucut or Surecut) is used to obtain the liver biopsy whilst the patient holds his breath in
  expiration
The biopsy is laid on filter paper and placed in 10% formalin. If a culture of the biopsy is required it should be placed in a
  sterile pot
The patient should be observed, with pulse and blood pressure measurements taken regularly for 6 hours

**Practical box 5.1**  Needle biopsy of the liver.

## Chronic liver disease

Patients may be asymptomatic or complain of non-specific symptoms. Specific symptoms include:

- Abdominal distension due to ascites, ankle swelling and fluid retention
- Haematemesis and melaena from gastrointestinal haemorrhage
- Pruritus due to cholestasis; this is often an early symptom of primary biliary cirrhosis
- Breast swelling, loss of libido and amenorrhoea due to endocrine dysfunction
- Confusion and drowsiness due to neuropsychiatric complications

# Signs of liver disease

## Acute liver disease

There may be few signs apart from jaundice and an enlarged liver. Jaundice is a yellow coloration of the skin and mucous membranes and is best seen in the conjunctivae. In the cholestatic phase of the illness, pale stools and dark urine are seen. Spider naevi and liver palms usually indicate chronic disease but they can occur in severe acute disease.

## Chronic liver disease

The possible physical signs are shown in Fig. 5.7. However, it is possible for the physical examination to be normal in patients with advanced chronic liver disease.

### Common signs

THE SKIN. The chest and upper body may show spider naevi. These are telangiectases that consist of a central arteriole with radiating small vessels. They are found in the distribution of the superior vena cava, i.e. above the nipple line. They are also found in pregnancy. In haemochromatosis the skin may have a slate-grey appearance.

The hands may show palmar erythema, which is a nonspecific change indicative of a hyperdynamic circulation; it may also be seen in pregnancy, thyrotoxicosis or rheumatoid arthritis. Clubbing occasionally occurs, and a Dupuytren's contracture is often seen in alcoholic cirrhosis.

Xanthomas (cholesterol deposits) may be seen in the palmar creases or above the eyes in primary biliary cirrhosis.

THE ABDOMEN. Initial hepatomegaly will be followed by a small liver in well-established cirrhosis.

Splenomegaly is usually taken as an indication of portal hypertension.

THE ENDOCRINE SYSTEM. Gynaecomastia (occasionally unilateral) and testicular atrophy may be found in males.

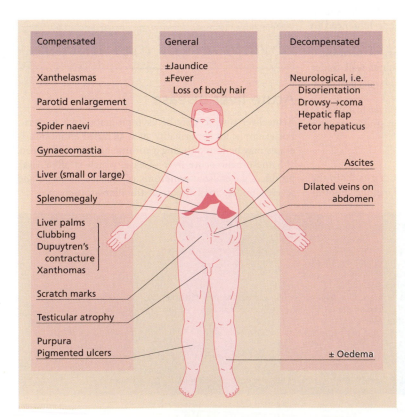

| Compensated | General | Decompensated |
|---|---|---|
| Xanthelasmas | ±Jaundice<br>±Fever<br>Loss of body hair | Neurological, i.e.<br>Disorientation<br>Drowsy→coma<br>Hepatic flap<br>Fetor hepaticus |
| Parotid enlargement | | |
| Spider naevi | | |
| Gynaecomastia | | |
| Liver (small or large) | | Ascites |
| Splenomegaly | | Dilated veins on abdomen |
| Liver palms<br>Clubbing<br>Dupuytren's contracture<br>Xanthomas | | |
| Scratch marks | | |
| Testicular atrophy | | |
| Purpura<br>Pigmented ulcers | | ± Oedema |

**Fig. 5.7** Physical signs in chronic liver disease.

The cause of gynaecomastia is complex, but it is probably related to altered oestrogen metabolism or to treatment with spironolactone.

IN DECOMPENSATED CIRRHOSIS, additional signs that can be seen are:
- Jaundice
- Ascites with or without peripheral oedema
- Evidence of portosystemic encephalopathy (PSE) (see p. 267) including drowsiness, stupor, fetor hepaticus and a flapping tremor of the outstretched hands
- Collateral veins and veins around the umbilicus (caput medusae) (rare)

# Jaundice

Jaundice (icterus) is detectable when the serum bilirubin is greater than 30–60 $\mu$mol litre$^{-1}$ (3 mg dl$^{-1}$). The usual division of jaundice into prehepatic, hepatocellular and obstructive (cholestatic) is an oversimplification as in hepatocellular jaundice there is invariably cholestasis and the clinical problem is whether the cholestasis is intrahepatic or extrahepatic. Jaundice will therefore be considered under the following headings:

HAEMOLYTIC JAUNDICE—increased bilirubin load for the liver cells

CONGENITAL HYPERBILIRUBINAEMIAS—defects in conjugation

CHOLESTATIC JAUNDICE, including hepatocellular (parenchymal) liver disease and large duct obstruction

## Haemolytic jaundice

The increased breakdown of red cells (see p. 310) leads to an increase in production of bilirubin. The resulting jaundice is usually mild (serum bilirubin of 68–102 $\mu$mol litre$^{-1}$ [4–6 mg dl$^{-1}$]) as normal liver function can easily handle the increased bilirubin derived from excess haemolysis. Unconjugated bilirubin is not water soluble and therefore will not pass into the urine, hence the term 'acholuric jaundice'. Urinary urobilinogen is increased.

The causes of haemolytic jaundice are those of haemolytic anaemia (see p. 310). The clinical features depend on the cause; anaemia, jaundice, splenomegaly, gallstones and leg ulcers may be seen.

Investigations show features of haemolysis (see p. 311). The level of unconjugated bilirubin is raised but the serum AP, transferases and albumin are normal. Serum haptoglobulins are low.

The differential diagnosis is from other forms of jaundice (see p. 248).

## Congenital hyperbilirubinaemias (non-haemolytic)

### Unconjugated
GILBERT'S SYNDROME. This is the commonest familial hyperbilirubinaemia and affects 2–5% of the population.

It is asymptomatic and is usually detected as an incidental finding of a slightly raised bilirubin (3–5 mg dl$^{-1}$; 51–85 $\mu$mol litre$^{-1}$) on a routine check. No signs of liver disease are seen. There is a family history of jaundice in 5–15% of patients. The aetiology of the syndrome is multifactorial and many abnormalities of bilirubin handling have been demonstrated. It is possible that this condition merely represents one end of the normal distribution curve.

The major importance of establishing this diagnosis is to inform the patient that this is not a serious disease and to prevent unnecessary investigation in the future. Investigations show only a raised unconjugated bilirubin, which rises on fasting and during a mild illness. The reticulocyte count is normal. No treatment is necessary.

CRIGLER–NAJJAR SYNDROME. This is very rare. Only type II (autosomal dominant) with a decrease rather than absence (Type I—autosomal recessive) of glucuronyl transferase can survive into adult life. Liver histology is normal. Transplantation is the only effective treatment.

### Conjugated
In the *Dubin–Johnson* (autosomal recessive) and *Rotor* (possibly autosomal dominant) syndromes, there are defects in bilirubin handling in the liver. The prognosis is good in both. In the former the liver is black due to melanin deposition.

## Cholestatic jaundice

This can be divided into:

INTRAHEPATIC CHOLESTASIS, due to the swelling of hepatocytes and oedema in parenchymal liver damage (hepatocellular) or to an excretory dysfunction of the bile canaliculi at a cellular level

EXTRAHEPATIC CHOLESTASIS, due to large duct obstruction of bile flow at any point in the biliary tract distal to the bile canaliculi

The causes are shown in Table 5.3.

*Extrahepatic*
Common duct stones
Carcinoma
   Head of pancreas
   Ampulla
   Bile duct
Biliary stricture
Pancreatitis ± pseudocyst
Sclerosing cholangitis

*Intrahepatic*
Viral hepatitis
Drugs
Alcoholic hepatitis
Cirrhosis—any type
Pregnancy
Recurrent idiopathic cholestasis
Some congenital disorders

**Table 5.3** Causes of cholestatic jaundice.

Clinically there is jaundice with pale stools and dark urine in both types and the serum bilirubin is conjugated.

Intrahepatic and extrahepatic cholestatic jaundice must be differentiated, as their clinical management is entirely different.

## The differential diagnosis of jaundice

### HISTORY

A careful history may give a clue to the diagnosis. Patients should be asked a series of questions, keeping in mind that certain causes of jaundice are more likely in particular categories of people. A young person is more likely to have hepatitis and therefore questions about drug and alcohol abuse and homosexuality should be asked. An elderly person with gross weight loss is more likely to have a carcinoma.

All patients may complain of malaise. Abdominal pain occurs in patients with biliary obstruction due to gallstones and, sometimes with an enlarged liver, there is pain due to distension of the capsule.

Questions should be appropriate to the particular situation and the following aspects of the history should be covered.

COUNTRY OF ORIGIN—the incidence of hepatitis B virus (HBV) infection is increased in Africa and the Far East
DURATION OF ILLNESS—a history of jaundice with prolonged weight loss in an older patient suggests malignancy; a short history, particularly with a prodromal illness of malaise, suggests a hepatitis
RECENT OUTBREAK of jaundice in the community— suggests hepatitis A virus (HAV)
RECENT CONSUMPTION of shellfish—suggests HAV
INTRAVENOUS DRUG ABUSE, RECENT INJECTIONS OR TATTOOS—all increase chance of HBV and hepatitis C virus (HCV) infection
MALE HOMOSEXUALITY—increases chance of HBV infection
FEMALE PROSTITUTION—increased HBV infection
BLOOD TRANSFUSIONS or infusion of pooled blood products—in developed countries all are screened for HBV and HCV
ALCOHOL CONSUMPTION—a careful history of drinking habits is taken, although many patients often lie about the actual amount they drink
DRUGS TAKEN, particularly in the previous 2–3 months—many drugs cause jaundice (see p. 279)
TRAVEL to areas with increased risk of HAV infection
RECENT ANAESTHETICS, e.g. halothane may cause jaundice
FAMILY HISTORY—patients with, for example, Gilbert's disease may have family members who get recurrent jaundice
RECENT SURGERY on the biliary tract or for carcinoma
PEOPLE ENGAGED IN RECREATIONAL ACTIVITIES in rural areas as well as farm and sewage workers are at risk for leptospirosis

FEVERS OR RIGORS—suggestive of cholangitis or possibly a liver abscess

### CLINICAL EXAMINATION

The signs of acute and chronic liver disease should be looked for (see p. 246). Certain additional signs may be useful:

HEPATOMEGALY—a smooth tender liver is seen in hepatitis and with extrahepatic obstruction, but a knobbly irregular liver suggests metastases. Causes of hepatomegaly are shown in Table 5.4.
SPLENOMEGALY indicates portal hypertension in patients when signs of chronic liver disease are present. The spleen can also be 'tipped' occasionally in viral hepatitis.
ASCITES is found in cirrhosis but can also be due to carcinoma (particularly ovarian) and many other causes (see Table 5.12).
A PALPABLE GALLBLADDER can suggest a carcinoma of the pancreas obstructing the bile duct.
GENERALIZED LYMPHADENOPATHY suggests a lymphoma.

### INVESTIGATION

Jaundice is not a diagnosis and the cause should always be sought. The two most useful tests are the viral markers and an ultrasound examination. The liver biochemistry confirms the jaundice and may help in the diagnosis. Investigations include:

1 Viral markers for HAV and HBV (antibodies to HCV develop late).

---

Apparent
  Low-lying diaphragm
  Reidel's lobe

Cirrhosis—early

Inflammation
  Hepatitis
  Schistosomiasis
  Abscesses—pyogenic or amoebic

Cysts
  Hydatid
  Polycystic

Metabolic
  Fatty liver
  Amyloid
  Glycogen storage disease

Haematological
  Leukaemias
  Lymphoma
  Myeloproliferative disorders

Tumours—primary and secondary carcinoma

Venous congestion
  Heart failure
  Hepatic vein occlusion

Biliary obstruction—particularly extrahepatic

Table 5.4  Causes of hepatomegaly.

2 An ultrasound should always be performed to exclude an extrahepatic obstruction unless the patient is young and the diagnosis of viral hepatitis is suspected.

An ultrasound will demonstrate:

SIZE OF THE BILE DUCTS which are dilated in extrahepatic obstruction (Fig. 5.8)

LEVEL OF THE OBSTRUCTION

CAUSE OF THE OBSTRUCTION in virtually all tumours and in 75% of patients with gallstones

The diagnosis of any mass lesion can be made by fine-needle aspiration cytology (sensitivity approximately 60%) or by needle biopsy using a spring-loaded device (sensitivity approximately 90%).

A flow diagram for the general investigation of the jaundiced patient is shown in Fig. 5.9.

### Liver biochemistry

In hepatitis the serum AST tends to be high early in the disease with only a small rise in the serum AP. Conversely, in extrahepatic obstruction the AP is high with a smaller rise in AST. These findings cannot, however, be relied on alone to make a diagnosis in an individual case. The PT is often prolonged in long-standing liver disease, and the serum albumin is also low.

### Haematological tests

These are helpful in a case of haemolytic jaundice (see p. 311). A raised white count may indicate infection, e.g. cholangitis. A leucopenia often occurs in viral hepatitis, while abnormal mononuclear cells suggest infectious mononucleosis and a Monospot test should be performed.

### Other blood tests

These include tests to exclude unusual causes of liver disease, e.g. cytomegalovirus antibodies, autoimmune antibodies, e.g. AMA for the diagnosis of primary biliary cirrhosis, and α-fetoprotein for a hepatocellular carcinoma.

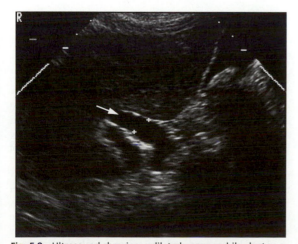

**Fig. 5.8** Ultrasound showing a dilated common bile duct (arrow), in front of the portal vein, at the porta hepatis.

# Parenchymal liver disease

The most common cause worldwide is viral hepatitis. Parenchymal liver disease can be divided into acute and chronic forms.

# Acute

Acute parenchymal liver damage can be caused by many agents (Fig. 5.10). If there is widespread damage of hepatocytes, the normal liver architecture may collapse. The extent of hepatocellular damage may be extremely variable.

### PATHOLOGY

Although some histological features are suggestive of the aetiological factor, most of the changes are essentially similar whatever the cause. Hepatocytes show degenerative changes (swelling, cytoplasmic granularity, vacuolation), undergo necrosis (becoming shrunken, eosinophilic Councilman bodies) and are rapidly removed. The distribution of these changes varies somewhat with the aetiological agent, but necrosis is usually maximal in zone 3. The extent of the damage is very variable between individuals affected by the same agent: at one end of the spectrum, single and small groups of hepatocytes die (spotty or focal necrosis), while at the other end multiple acini are destroyed (massive hepatic necrosis) resulting in fulminant hepatic failure. Between these extremes there is limited confluent necrosis of hepatocytes with collapse of the reticulin framework resulting in linking (bridging) between the central veins, the central veins and portal tracts, and between the portal tracts.

Centriacinar cholestasis is common, but fatty change is usually absent apart from certain types of hepatitis due to toxins such as alcohol or that seen in pregnancy. The extent of the inflammatory infiltrate is also variable, but portal tracts and lobules are infiltrated mainly by lymphocytes.

### MANAGEMENT

This will be discussed under the individual aetiological factors.

## VIRAL HEPATITIS

The differing features of the common forms of viral hepatitis are summarized in Table 5.5.

In HAV the damage is due to the virus itself, but in HBV infection it is due to an immunological reaction to the virus.

## Hepatitis A

### EPIDEMIOLOGY

This is the commonest type of viral hepatitis and causes 20–40% of clinically apparent hepatitis. It occurs world-

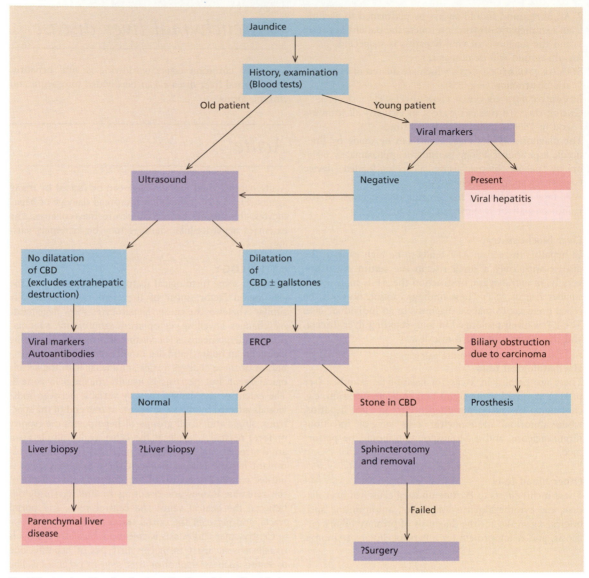

**Fig. 5.9**  An algorithm for the investigation of jaundice. Viral causes are rarer in the elderly, CBD, common bile duct; ERCP, endoscopic retrograde cholangiopancreatography.

wide, often in epidemics. The disease is commonly seen in the autumn and affects children and young adults. Spread of infection is mainly by the faecal–oral route and arises from the ingestion of contaminated food (e.g. shellfish, clams) or water. Overcrowding and poor sanitation facilitate spread. There is no carrier state.

### Hepatitis A virus

HAV is a picornavirus; its structure is shown in Fig. 5.11. It has a single serotype as only one epitope is immunodominant. It is excreted in the faeces of infected persons for about 2 weeks before the onset of the illness and for up to 7 days after. The disease is maximally infectious just before the onset of jaundice. HAV particles can be demonstrated in the faeces by electron microscopy.

### CLINICAL FEATURES

The preicteric or prodromal phase lasts up to 2 weeks. The viraemia causes the patient to feel unwell with nausea, vomiting, diarrhoea, anorexia, headaches, malaise and a distaste for cigarettes. Fever is usually mild and there may be upper abdominal discomfort. There are few physical signs at this stage; the liver is tender but not enlarged initially.

After 1 or 2 weeks the patient becomes icteric (although some may never do so) and symptoms often improve. The appetite returns and the patient feels better. As the jaundice deepens the urine becomes dark and the stools pale owing to intrahepatic cholestasis. The liver is moderately enlarged and the spleen is palpable in about 10% of patients. Occasionally, tender lymphadenopathy

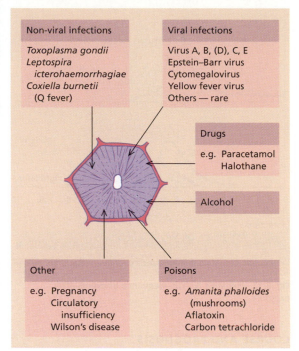

| Non-viral infections | Viral infections |
|---|---|
| *Toxoplasma gondii*<br>*Leptospira*<br>  *icterohaemorrhagiae*<br>*Coxiella burnetii*<br>  (Q fever) | Virus A, B, (D), C, E<br>Epstein–Barr virus<br>Cytomegalovirus<br>Yellow fever virus<br>Others — rare |

**Drugs**

e.g. Paracetamol
    Halothane

**Alcohol**

| Other | Poisons |
|---|---|
| e.g. Pregnancy<br>  Circulatory<br>    insufficiency<br>  Wilson's disease | e.g. *Amanita phalloides*<br>    (mushrooms)<br>  Aflatoxin<br>  Carbon tetrachloride |

**Fig. 5.10** Some causes of acute parenchymal damage.

is seen, with a transient rash in some cases. Thereafter the jaundice lessens and in the majority of cases the illness is over within 3–6 weeks. Extrahepatic complications are rare but include arthritis, vasculitis, myocarditis and renal failure. Relapses occasionally occur, with the return of jaundice. Rarely the disease may be very severe with fulminant hepatitis, liver coma and death. The sequence of events after HAV exposure is shown in Fig. 5.12.

## INVESTIGATIONS
### Liver biochemistry
In the prodromal stage the serum bilirubin is usually normal. However, there is bilirubinuria and increased urinary urobilinogen. A raised serum AST, which can sometimes be very high, precedes the jaundice.

In the icteric stage the serum bilirubin reflects the level of jaundice. Serum AST reaches a maximum 1–2 days after the appearance of jaundice, and may rise above 500 IU litre$^{-1}$. Serum AP is usually less than 300 IU litre$^{-1}$.

After the jaundice has subsided, the AST may remain elevated for some weeks and occasionally up to 6 months.

### Haematological tests
There is leucopenia with a relative lymphocytosis. Very rarely there is a Coombs'-positive haemolytic anaemia or

| | A | B | D | C | E |
|---|---|---|---|---|---|
| *Virus* | RNA<br>27 nm | DNA<br>42 nm | RNA<br>37 nm<br>(with HBsAg<br>coat) | RNA<br>30–60 nm | RNA<br>27 nm |
| | Picornavirus | Hepadnavirus | Unclassified<br>virus | Flavivirus | Calcivirus |
| *Spread* | | | | | |
| Faecal | Yes | No | No | No | Yes |
| Blood | Rare | Yes | Yes | Yes | No |
| Vertical | No | Yes | Rare | Yes | No |
| Saliva | Yes | Yes | Yes | ? | ? |
| Sexual | Rare | Yes | Yes (rare) | Occasionally | No |
| *Incubation* | Short<br>  (2–3 weeks) | Long<br>  (1–5 months) | Long | Intermediate | Short |
| *Age* | Young | Any | Any | Any | Any |
| *Carrier state* | No | Yes | ? | ? | No |
| *Chronic liver disease* | No | Yes | Yes | Yes | No |
| *Liver cancer* | No | Yes | Rare | Yes | No |
| *Mortality* (acute) | <0.5% | <1% | | <1% | 1–2% (pregnant<br>women 10–<br>20%) |
| *Immunization:* | | | | | |
| Passive | Normal<br>immunoglobulin<br>i.m.<br>(0.04–0.06 ml kg$^{-1}$) | Hepatitis B<br>immunoglobulin<br>(HBIG) | — | — | — |
| Active | Vaccine | Vaccine | HBV vaccine | — | — |

**Table 5.5** Some features of hepatitis viruses.

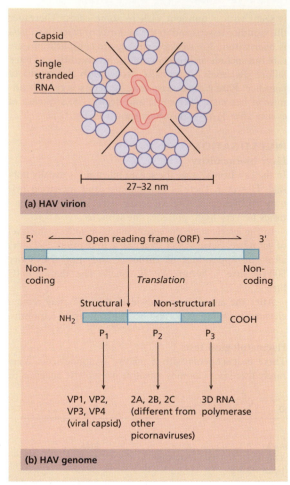

**Fig. 5.11** (a) The hepatitis A (HAV) virion consists probably of four polypeptides (VP1–VP4) which form a tight protein shell, or capsid, containing the RNA. The major antigenic component is associated with VP1. (b) Arrangement of HAV genome.

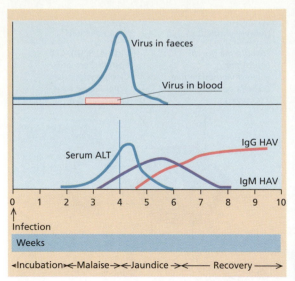

**Fig. 5.12** Hepatitis A virus—sequence of events after exposure.

## COURSE AND PROGNOSIS

The prognosis is excellent, with most patients making a complete recovery. The mortality in young adults is 0.1% but it increases with age. Death is due to fulminant hepatic necrosis. During convalescence 5–15% of patients may have relapse of the hepatitis but this settles spontaneously. Occasionally a more severe jaundice with cholestasis will run a prolonged course of 7–20 weeks and is called cholestatic viral hepatitis.

There is no reason to stop alcohol consumption other than for the few weeks when the patient is ill. Patients may complain of debility for several months following resolution of the symptoms and biochemical parameters. This is known as the posthepatitis syndrome; it is a functional illness. Treatment is by reassurance. HAV never progresses to chronic liver disease.

## TREATMENT

There is no specific treatment; rest and dietary measures are unhelpful. Corticosteroids have no benefit. Admission to hospital is not usually necessary. The condition is notifiable in the UK.

## PREVENTION AND PROPHYLAXIS

Control of hepatitis depends on good hygiene. The virus is resistant to chlorination but is killed by boiling water for 10 min. Ideally all individuals should have anti-HAV antibody tests to assess their requirement for prophylaxis.

ACTIVE IMMUNIZATION using a formaldehyde inactivated vaccine is commercially available. This is now preferable to repeated immunoglobulin injections for people frequently travelling to endemic areas.

PASSIVE IMMUNIZATION. Normal immunoglobulin (0.04–0.06 ml kg$^{-1}$ i.m.) gives protection for 2–3 months and is useful for persons at risk.

---

an associated aplastic anaemia. The PT is prolonged in severe cases. The erythrocyte sedimentation rate (ESR) is raised.

### Viral markers
ANTIBODIES TO HAV. IgG antibodies are common in the general population over the age of 50 years but an anti-HAV IgM means an acute infection.

### Other tests
ULTRASOUND. This should be performed if bile duct obstruction is suspected and always in an older patient.
LIVER BIOPSY. This is only indicated when there is doubt about the diagnosis.

## DIFFERENTIAL DIAGNOSIS

This is from all other causes of jaundice but, in particular, from other types of viral and drug-induced hepatitis.

## Hepatitis B

### EPIDEMIOLOGY

The virus (HBV) is present worldwide and has infected more than 2000 million people. There are an estimated 350 million carriers. The UK and the USA have a low prevalence but it rises to 10–15% in parts of Africa, the Middle and the Far East.

Spread of this virus is by the intravenous route, e.g. transfusion of infective blood or blood products, by contaminated needles used by drug addicts, tattooists or acupuncturists, or by close personal contact, e.g. sexual intercourse, particularly in male homosexuals. The virus can be found in semen and saliva. Vertical transmission from mother to child during parturition or soon after birth is the most important means of transmission worldwide. The role of insect vectors is controversial; there is no evidence that HBV replicates in these insects but the virus has been detected in mosquitoes and bed bugs.

#### Hepatitis B virus

Under electron microscopy a number of particles are seen (Fig. 5.13). The whole virus is the Dane particle, which consists of an inner core formed by the liver cell nucleus and an outer surface coat (HBsAg) produced by multiplication in the cytoplasm. The inner core contains double-stranded DNA, DNA polymerase, the core antigen (HBcAg) and the e antigen (HBeAg). Small spheres and tubules (100 nm long) of excess surface antigen protein are also produced.

The virus only replicates in the liver. The core antigen enters and replicates in the nucleus and eventually becomes integrated with the host nuclear DNA. The host DNA polymerase then transcribes for the virus. This may be an important link in the development of hepatocellular carcinoma. HBsAg particles have further antigenic determinants on their surface known as a, d, y, w and r. Combinations of these subdeterminants, e.g. adw, adr, ayw and ayr, are useful in epidemiology for studying geographical patterns of infection.

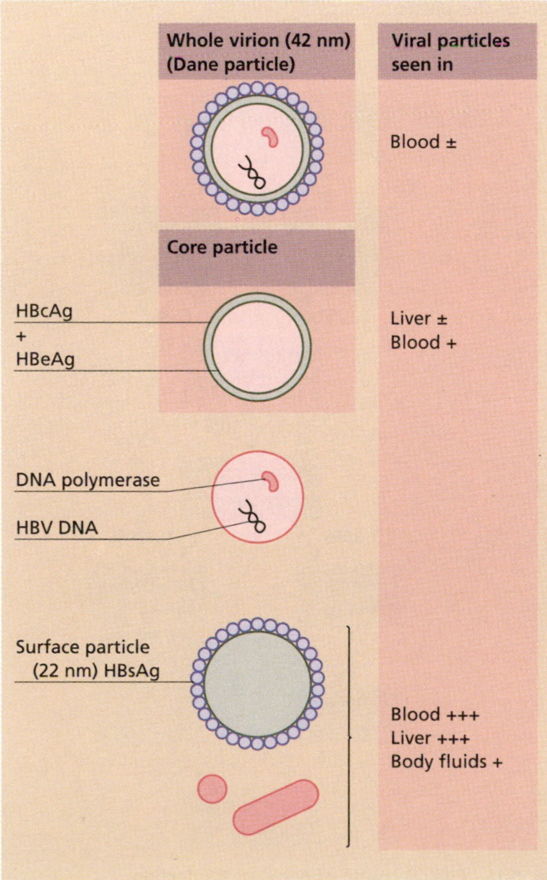
Whole virion (42 nm)
(Dane particle)
Viral particles
seen in
Blood ±
Core particle
HBcAg
+
HBeAg
Liver ±
Blood +
DNA polymerase
HBV DNA
Surface particle
(22 nm) HBsAg
Blood +++
Liver +++
Body fluids +

**Fig. 5.13** Hepatitis B virus—the antigenic components.

#### Hepatitis B mutants

Mutations are being increasingly described in the various reading frames of the HBV genome (Fig. 5.14). These mutants can emerge in chronic HBV carriers or can be acquired by infection. These variants of the HBV genome have also been found in patients with fulminant and fatal hepatitis who have HBsAg and anti-HBe rather than the e antigen itself. The amino acid sequence of the e antigen protein is almost identical to that of the core antigen which is involved in viral replication. Separate messenger RNAs have not been described for the two antigens but HBeAg is initiated several nucleotides upstream of HBcAg. A guanosine (G) to adenosine (A) mutation in the precore region of the genome creates a stop codon (TAG) that prevents the production of HBeAg but the synthesis of HBcAg is unaffected. Mutants have also been seen following interferon therapy. Their existence means that serological markers such as the HBeAg are less useful in detecting infectivity and HBV DNA must be measured.

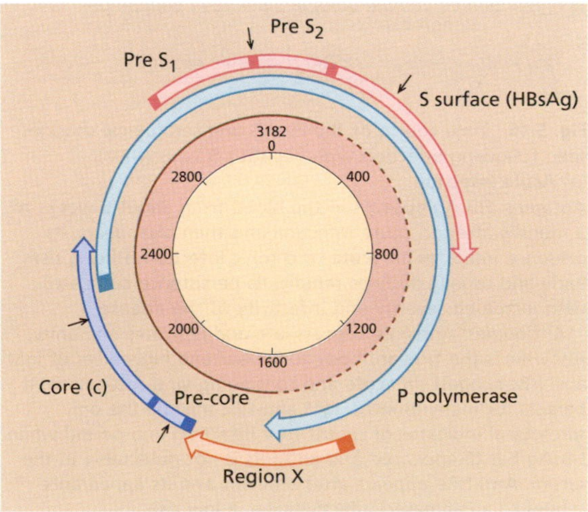
Pre $S_2$
Pre $S_1$
S surface (HBsAg)
3182
0
400
800
1200
1600
2000
2400
2800
Core (c)
Pre-core
P polymerase
Region X

**Fig. 5.14** Hepatitis B virus (HBV) genome. There are four open reading frames (S, P, C and X): S codes for the surface (HBsAg) polypeptide, P for the DNA polymerase, C for the core antigen (HBcAg), X for a protein with a transcriptional transactivating function. Pre $S_1$ domain is involved in the recognition of the virus by the hepatocyte receptors. Arrows mark sites of mutation.

## CLINICAL FEATURES

The sequence of events following acute HBV infection are shown in Fig. 5.15. Clinical features are the same as those found in HAV infection. In addition, a serum sickness-like immunological syndrome may be seen. This consists of rashes, e.g. urticaria or a maculopapular rash and polyarthritis affecting small joints occurring in up to 25% of cases in the prodromal period. Fever is usual. The illness may be more severe than hepatitis A. Extrahepatic immune complex-mediated conditions such as an arteritis or glomerulonephritis are occasionally seen.

## INVESTIGATION

This is generally the same as for hepatitis A.

### Specific tests

The markers for HBV are shown in Fig. 5.13. HBsAg is looked for initially; if it is found, a full viral profile is then performed. In acute infection HBsAg may be cleared rapidly and in such cases IgM anti-core antibodies are helpful. HBV DNA is the most sensitive index of viral replication; it is tested by the Southern blot technique or by the polymerase chain reaction (PCR).

## COURSE

The majority of patients recover completely, fulminant hepatitis occurring in up to 1%. Some patients go on to develop chronic hepatitis and hepatocellular carcinoma (see p. 277) or become asymptomatic carriers (Fig. 5.16. The outcome depends upon several factors, including the virulence of the virus and the immunocompetence and age of the patient.

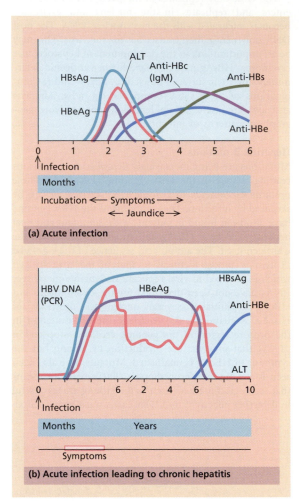

**Fig. 5.15** Time course of the events and serological changes seen following infection with hepatitis B virus (HBV).
(a) **Acute infection**
*Antigens*: HBsAg appears in the blood from about 6 weeks to 3 months after an acute infection and then disappears. Its presence indicates an acute or chronic infection. HBeAg rises early and usually declines rapidly. Its persistence correlates with increased severity and infectivity of the disease.
   *Antibodies*: Anti-HBs appears late and indicates immunity. Anti-HBc is the first antibody to appear and high titres of IgM anti-HBc suggest an acute and continuing viral replication. It persists for many months. IgM anti-HBc may be the only serological indicator of recent HBV infection in a period when HBsAg has disappeared and anti-HBs is not detectable in the serum. Anti-HBe appears after anti-HBc and its appearance relates to a decreased infectivity, i.e. a low risk.
(b) **Acute infection leading to chronic hepatitis B**
HbsAg persists and indicates a chronic infection (or carrier state). HBeAg persists and correlates with development of chronic liver disease when anti-HBe develops (seroconversion) the HBeAg disappears and there is usually a rise in alanine aminotransferase (ALT). HBV DNA suggests continual viral replication.

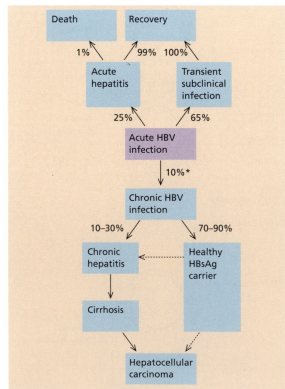

**Fig. 5.16** Clinical course of hepatitis B infection.
*, percentage variable worldwide.

## TREATMENT

There is no specific treatment apart from symptomatic therapy.

## PREVENTION AND PROPHYLAXIS

Prevention depends on avoiding risk factors, e.g. shared needles, multiple male homosexual partners and prostitutes. Infectivity is highest in those with the e antigen and HBV DNA in their blood. These patients should be counselled about their infection. In developing countries, blood and blood products are still a hazard. Standard safety precautions in laboratories and hospitals must be strictly enforced to avoid accidental needle punctures and contact with infected body fluids.

### Passive and active immunization

Vaccination should be given to:

- All health-care personnel in the UK
- Members of emergency and rescue teams
- Morticians and embalmers
- Long-term travellers, e.g. airline travellers
- Homosexual and bisexual men and prostitutes
- Children in high-risk areas
- Intravenous drug abusers
- Patients and staff of some psychiatric units

*Combined prophylaxis*, i.e. vaccination and immunoglobulin, should be given to:

- Staff with accidental needlestick injury
- All newborn babies of HBsAg-positive mothers
- Regular sexual partners of HBsAg-positive patients, who have been found to be HBV negative

Give 500 IU to adults (200 IU to newborn) of specific hepatitis B immunoglobulin (HBIG) and the vaccine i.m. at another site.

### Active immunization

This is with a recombinant yeast vaccine produced by insertion of a plasmid containing the gene of HBsAg into a yeast.

DOSAGE REGIMEN. Three (0, 1, 6 months) injections are given into the deltoid muscle and this gives short-term protection in over 90% of patients. Persons over 50 years or clinically ill and/or immunocompromised (including those with HIV infection or AIDS) have a poor antibody response; more frequent and larger doses are required. Antibody levels should be measured at 7–9 months after the initial dose in all at-risk groups. Antibody levels fall steadily after vaccination and booster doses may be required after approximately 3–5 years. It is not cost-effective to check antibody levels prior to active immunization. There are few side effects from the vaccine — soreness at the site of injection and very occasionally a fever, rash or a 'flu-like' illness.

## CHRONIC ASYMPTOMATIC CARRIERS

Following an acute HBV infection which may be subclinical, approximately 5–10% of patients will not clear the virus and will become carriers of HbsAg. Children are more likely to remain carriers than adults. There is a vast geographical variation in the incidence of carriers. In the UK, carriers are usually discovered incidentally on blood tests, e.g. when they are screened for donating blood for transfusion or when attending genital medicine clinics. Carriers with HBeAg or viral DNA in the serum (and thus having active viral replication) are highly infectious.

The progression of the disease in carriers is uncertain but most remain HBsAg positive. Some may seroconvert, i.e. develop HBe antibodies, and therefore are a lower infective risk to others. However, mutant strains occur (see p. 253). Some patients may carry the virus for many years without developing chronic liver disease, whereas others, particularly those with the e antigen, may go on to develop chronic hepatitis and cirrhosis and there is an increased risk of hepatocellular carcinoma.

### Treatment of chronic HBV carriers

Patients who are HBeAg positive or have HBV DNA in their serum should be treated with interferon-$\alpha$ (see p. 259). The aim of the treatment is to seroconvert and clear HBeAg and HBV DNA from the serum.

### HEPATITIS D

This is caused by the hepatitis D virus (HDV or delta virus). It is an incomplete RNA particle enclosed in a shell of HBsAg. It is unable to replicate on its own but is activated by the presence of HBV. It is particularly seen in intravenous drug abusers but can affect all risk groups for HBV infection. Active HBV synthesis is reduced by delta infection and patients are usually HBeAg and HBV DNA negative.

HDV infection can occur either as a coinfection with HBV or as a superinfection in an HBsAg-positive patient. Coinfection of HDV and HBV is clinically indistinguishable from an acute icteric HBV infection but a biphasic rise of serum AST may be seen. Diagnosis is confirmed by finding serum IgM anti-$\delta$ in the presence of IgM anti-HBc. IgM anti-$\delta$ appears at 1 week and disappears by 5–6 weeks (occasionally 12 weeks) when serum IgG anti-$\delta$ is seen. The infection may be transient but the clinical course is variable.

Superinfection results in an acute flare-up of previously quiescent chronic HBV infection. A rise in serum AST may be the only indication of infection. Diagnosis is by finding serum IgM anti-$\delta$ at the same time as IgG HBc; patients are usually negative for IgM anti-HBc. Fulminant hepatitis can follow both types of infection but is more common after coinfection.

HDV RNA in the serum and liver can be measured and is found in acute and chronic HDV infection. Chronic HDV is a severe form of liver disease. Spontaneous resolution is rare and 60–70% of patients will develop cirrhosis in the long term. In 15% the disease is rapidly progressive with the development of cirrhosis in a few years. $\alpha$ Interferon produces remission but relapse is common.

# Hepatitis C

## EPIDEMIOLOGY

HCV was identified in 1988 and was responsible for 70–90% of post-transfusion hepatitis in all countries where blood was tested for HBV markers. Since the screening of HCV in donor blood was introduced, this incidence has fallen to 4%. In the UK, 1 : 1800 samples of donated blood are positive for HCV antibodies; the prevalence may well be higher than this figure. HCV is much more common in southern Europe and Japan than in the UK, and in Egyptian blood donors the prevalence is as high as 19%. It is transmitted by blood and blood products and it is postulated that 76% of haemophiliacs in the UK may have been infected. The incidence in intravenous drug abusers is very high. A high prevalence amongst homosexual men (2.2% vs. 0.4% in heterosexuals) suggests sexual transmission and it may be transmitted from mother to child. Other routes of community-acquired infection, e.g. close contact, are unlikely. In many cases the exact mode of transmission is unknown.

### Hepatitis C virus

HCV is a single-stranded RNA virus arranged into structural and non-structural regions (Fig. 5.17). There are six subtypes based on differences in the non-structural region. Only types I, II and III are seen in Europe and type IV occurs in the Far East. Immunogenic peptides have been derived from these regions for use in HCV assays and are becoming increasingly sensitive. The concentration of viral antigens in the blood is very low.

### CLINICAL FEATURES

Symptoms are few in the acute phase with a mild flu-like illness and a rise in serum transferases. Less than 20% of patients develop jaundice and this is mild and self-limit-ing. Most patients will not be diagnosed until they present, years later, with complications of chronic liver disease. Extrahepatic manifestations are seen, including arthritis, agranulocytosis and aplastic anaemia, as well as diffuse neurological problems. Rarely, fulminant hepatic failure occurs. At least 50% of patients go on to develop chronic liver disease (see p. 259). Histologically, a chronic hepatitis leading to a cirrhotic picture is seen (see p. 258). Cirrhosis develops in about 10–20% within 5–30 years and of these patients about 15% will develop hepatocellular carcinoma.

### DIAGNOSIS

Antibodies to HCV are found in the serum. The first generation tests using the c100 antigen were relatively insensitive. Second generation tests (enzyme-linked immunosorbent assay (ELISA) and recombinant immunoblot assay (RIBA)) include c22 and c33 antigens and are more sensitive and specific. Anti-HCV-positive patients should have the presence of viral RNA confirmed by a PCR test. This is expensive and not generally available. Patients with a positive PCR should have a liver biopsy to detect chronic hepatitis and cirrhosis.

### TREATMENT

As most patients are not diagnosed in the acute stage, there are no clear guidelines for treatment. However, interferon has been used in some acute cases.

## HEPATITIS E

Hepatitis E virus (HEV) is an RNA virus which causes enteral (epidemic or water-borne) hepatitis. Epidemics have been seen in many developing countries. It has a mortality from fulminant hepatic failure of 1–2% which rises to 20% in pregnant women. There is no carrier state and it does not progress to chronic liver disease. Serological tests for HEV are being developed although HEV RNA can be detected in the serum or stools by PCR. Prevention and control depend on good sanitation and hygiene.

## Other viral hepatitides

Most of the non-A, non-B hepatitides (NANB) have now been identified. The letter F has been occasionally applied to fulminant hepatic failure (although several viruses are implicated) and G to granulomatous hepatitis.

## FULMINANT HEPATIC FAILURE (FHF)

This is defined as severe hepatic failure with encephalopathy developing in less than 8 weeks in a patient with a previously normal liver. Cases that evolve at a slower pace are called subacute or subfulminant hepatic failure. FHF is a rare but often life-threatening syndrome due to acute hepatitis from any cause (Table 5.6). The causes vary throughout the world; the majority are due to viral hepa-

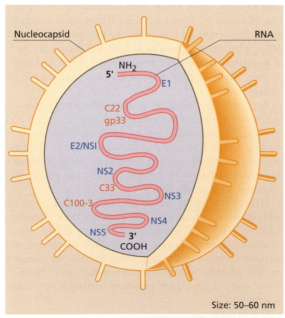

**Fig. 5.17** Hepatitis C virus. A schematic diagram showing single-stranded RNA genome with coding regions. C, nucleocapsid protein coding region; E, envelope protein coding region; GP, glycosylated protein; NS, non-structural region.

| Viral hepatitis | Toxins |
|---|---|
| A, B, (D), C, E | *Amanita* poisoning |
| | Halohydrocarbons |
| *Drugs, e.g.* | *Miscellaneous* |
| | Wilson's disease |
| Analgesics, e.g. paracetamol | Pregnancy |
| MAOIs, e.g. imipramine | Reye's syndrome |
| Anaesthetics, e.g. halothane | |
| Antituberculous, e.g. isoniazid | |
| Antiepileptic, e.g. valproate | |
| | |
| MAOIs, monoamine oxidase inhibitors. | |

**Table 5.6**  Fulminant hepatic failure—causes.

titis but paracetamol overdose is common in the UK.

Histologically there is massive necrosis of the whole liver lobule. Severe fatty degeneration in FHF is seen in pregnancy, Reye's syndrome, lymphoma or following i.v. tetracycline administration.

## CLINICAL FEATURES

Examination shows a jaundiced patient with the signs of hepatic encephalopathy developing usually within 2 weeks. The condition is called subfulminant if the encephalopathy develops between 2 and 8 weeks. The mental state varies from slight drowsiness, confusion and disorientation (grades I and II) to unresponsive coma (grade IV) with convulsions. Fetor hepaticus is common but signs of chronic liver disease, e.g. ascites and splenomegaly, are rare. The liver size is usually small. Fever, vomiting, hypertension and hypoglycaemia occur. Neurological examination shows spasticity and extension of the arms and legs; plantar responses remain flexor until late. Cerebral oedema is found in 80% of patients who die. Other complications include bacterial infections, vasodilatory hypotension, gastrointestinal bleeding, respiratory arrest, renal failure (hepatorenal syndrome and acute tubular necrosis) and pancreatitis.

## INVESTIGATION

This is as for acute liver disease. The PT is the most useful index of severity and when very high indicates a poor prognosis. The AST is high initially but is not a useful indicator of the course of the disease since it falls with progressive liver damage. The serum albumin falls and an EEG is sometimes helpful in grading the encephalopathy. An isotope scan may show no uptake in the liver.

## TREATMENT

There is no specific treatment but patients should be managed in an intensive care unit. Supportive therapy as for hepatic encephalopathy (see p. 267) is necessary. Cerebral oedema (which is measured directly) is the major cause of death and when signs of raised intracranial pressure are present 20% mannitol (1 g kg$^{-1}$ body weight) should be infused intravenously; this dose may need to be repeated. Dexamethasone is of no value.

Hypoglycaemia, hypokalaemia and hypocalcaemia should be anticipated and corrected with 10% dextrose infusion (checked by 2-hourly Dextrostix testing), potassium and calcium. Coagulopathy is managed with i.v. vitamin K, platelets, blood or fresh frozen plasma. Haemorrhage may be a problem and patients are given H$_2$-receptor antagonists to prevent gastrointestinal bleeding. Infection should be treated with suitable antibiotics, and renal and respiratory failure treated as appropriate. Flumazenil, a benzodiazepine receptor antagonist, may give a transient improvement in encephalopathy.

Liver transplantation has been a major advance for patients with FHF. It is difficult to judge the timing or the necessity for transplantation but various transplant centres have developed guidelines depending on prognosis (see below).

## COURSE AND PROGNOSIS

In mild cases (grades I and II), two-thirds of the patients will survive. The outcome of severe cases (grades III and IV) is related to the aetiology. In special units 70% of patients with paracetamol overdosage and grade IV coma survive, as do 30–40% of patients with HAV or HBV hepatitis. The survival is extremely poor in patients with HCV hepatitis. In patients with drug reactions and viral hepatitis, poor prognostic variables include aetiology (HCV or drugs), age (<10 years and >40 years), time interval from onset of jaundice to encephalopathy (more than 7 days—subfulminant), a serum bilirubin >300 $\mu$mol litre$^{-1}$ and a PT over 50 s. In addition, for paracetamol overdose an arterial pH <7.3, a serum creatinine >3 mg dl$^{-1}$, a PT >100 s with grade III–IV encephalopathy indicates a very poor prognosis and need for transplantation.

# ACUTE HEPATITIS DUE TO OTHER VIRUSES

INFECTIOUS MONONUCLEOSIS (see p. 49). This is due to the Epstein–Barr virus. Mild jaundice associated with minor abnormalities of liver biochemistry is extremely common but 'clinical' hepatitis is rare. Hepatic histological changes occur within 5 days of onset; the sinusoids and portal tracts are infiltrated with large mononuclear cells but the liver architecture is preserved. A Paul–Bunnell or Monospot test is usually positive and atypical lymphocytes are present in the peripheral blood. Treatment is symptomatic.

CYTOMEGALOVIRUS (see p. 48). This can cause acute hepatitis, particularly in patients with poor immune responses. The virus may be isolated from the urine. The liver biopsy shows intranuclear inclusions and giant cells.

YELLOW FEVER (see p. 54). This viral infection is carried by the mosquito *Aedes aegypti* and causes acute hepatic necrosis. There is no specific treatment.

HERPES SIMPLEX (see p. 47). Very occasionally the herpes simplex virus causes a generalized acute infection, particularly in the immunosuppressed patient. Liver biopsy shows extensive necrosis. Acyclovir is used for treatment.

OTHER INFECTIOUS AGENTS. Abnormal liver biochemistry is frequently found in a number of acute infections. The abnormalities are usually mild and have no clinical significance.

TOXOPLASMOSIS (see p. 67). Produces a similar clinical picture to infectious mononucleosis with abnormal liver biochemistry but the Paul–Bunnell test is negative.

Viral
    Hepatitis B ± δ virus
    Other viruses
Autoimmune

Drugs, e.g. methyldopa, oxyphenisatin (withdrawn in UK), isoniazid, ketoconazole, nitrofurantoin

Hereditary
    $\alpha_1$-Antitrypsin deficiency
    Wilson's disease

Others
    Inflammatory bowel disease—ulcerative colitis
    Alcohol—rarely

**Table 5.7**    Causes of chronic active hepatitis.

# Chronic hepatitis

Clinically this is defined as any hepatitis lasting 6 months or longer. The classification is usually based on histological grounds. There are three forms:
1  Chronic persistent hepatitis (CPH)
2  Chronic lobular hepatitis (CLH)
3  Chronic active hepatitis (CAH)
This simple histological classification has limitations as more becomes known about the aetiological factors. Morphological changes can be inaccurate due to sampling errors and also may show similar features at different clinical stages of the disease.
CHRONIC PERSISTENT HEPATITIS. There is marked expansion of the portal tracts with infiltration by mononuclear cells. The liver architecture is undisturbed and the limiting plate between hepatocytes is intact. This is often seen in HCV virus.
CHRONIC LOBULAR HEPATITIS. This histologically resembles acute viral hepatitis with predominant intra-acinar inflammation and necrosis. It is uncommon and presents with a hepatitic picture. The course is prolonged (greater than 3 months) with remissions and excerbations. It can follow HBV and HCV hepatitis often with coexistent CPH. Alternatively serum autoantibodies may be present and this often responds to steroids. It usually does not progress to cirrhosis.
CHRONIC ACTIVE HEPATITIS (Table 5.7). The hallmark of CAH is piecemeal necrosis. There is the destruction of liver cells at an interface between parenchyma and connective tissue leading to the erosion of the limiting plates of hepatocytes around portal tracts (zone 1). An inflammatory infiltrate, predominantly of lymphocytes and plasma cells, expands the portal area and infiltrates into the liver. The zone 1 hepatocytes with inflammatory infiltrates form rosettes with severe CAH; bridging necrosis (where fibrous septa extend between portal–central or portal–portal areas) is also

seen. Milder forms may only show slight erosion of the limiting plate and some piecemeal necrosis.

## CLINICAL FEATURES AND PRESENTATION
Patients may present in a variety of ways. Clinically, symptoms may range from none to mild fatigue or patients may present with the complications of cirrhosis. There may be no signs, but jaundice or signs of chronic liver disease (see p. 246) may be present. Alternatively a patient may have been identified by abnormal liver biochemical tests, e.g. a raised serum bilirubin, transaminase or AP. Always check the medication that a patient may be taking as many drugs, e.g. isoniazid, antithyroid drugs, nitrofurantoin, dantrolene, can cause abnormal liver biochemistry. The ethnic origin of the patient, homosexuality, intravenous drug abuse or blood transfusions may suggest HBV or HCV infection.

## INVESTIGATION
Test for viral markers—HBsAg and anti-HCV. If these are negative, check the autoantibodies and exclude Wilson's disease, iron overload and $\alpha_1$-antitrypsin deficiency.
    Liver biopsy should be carried out to assess activity and the presence or absence of cirrhosis.

## Chronic hepatitis B infection

This group makes up approximately 50% of all cases of CAH in some countries, e.g. Greece. It is much less common in the UK where only 3% of patients who have an acute HBV infection progress to CAH. Patients with a poor cell-mediated response to the virus develop chronic hepatitis: if the response is very poor, they become healthy carriers; if the response is slightly better there is continuing hepatocellular damage. Cytotoxic T cells recognize the viral antigen via HLA class I molecules on the infected hepatocyte; this mechanism may be defective in these patients. HBV infection goes through a replicative and an integrated phase. In the former there is active viral replication with hepatic inflammation and the patient is highly infectious with HBeAg and HBV DNA positivity. At some stage the viral genome becomes integrated into the host DNA and the viral genes are transcribed along with those of the host. This can cause malignant transformation to hepatocellular carcinoma. There is no association with autoimmune disease or any particular genetic markers.

Chronic hepatitis occurs mainly in men and it is often not preceded by an acute attack. The condition may be asymptomatic or may present as a mild, slowly progressive hepatitis; 50% present with established chronic liver disease.

Investigations show a moderately raised serum bilirubin and AST and a slightly raised AP. HBsAg is positive and HBeAg is usually present.

Histologically there may be a full spectrum of changes from near normal to CAH and cirrhosis. HBsAg may be seen as a 'ground-glass' appearance in the cytoplasm on haematoxylin and eosin staining and this can be confirmed on orcein staining or more specifically with immunohistochemical staining. HBcAg can also be demonstrated in hepatocytes by appropriate immunohistochemical staining.

### TREATMENT

Untreated patients seroconvert, i.e. converting from HBeAg to anti-HBe, at a rate of 15% per year; this varies with the age and ethnic origin of the patient. The aim of the treatment is to inhibit HBV replication. It is, however, difficult to achieve the eradication of HBsAg once it has been integrated into the host genome and most patients will have a biochemical and histological remission once HBeAg antigen, viral DNA and DNA polymerase have disappeared from the sera with seroconversion to anti-HBe.

Ideally, patients with CAH and asymptomatic carriers who have HBeAg and HBV DNA in the serum should be treated with antiviral agents. All patients with progressive liver disease should also be treated but decompensated cirrhosis is a contraindication.

#### Antiviral agents

Many antiviral agents have been tried but currently interferon seems to be the most successful. The dosage regimen is 5–9 MU three times per week. The response rate varies between 14 and 75% depending on the age of onset of infection, sexual preference and type of liver disease. HBsAg usually persists. During therapy patients often have a clinical relapse of their liver disease, suggesting an immunomodulatory effect of interferon. Side-effects of interferon treatment include a 'flu'-like illness with headaches, myalgia and non-specific malaise, diarrhoea, nausea, reversible hair loss and depression. The patient's blood and platelet counts should be monitored at frequent intervals. Drug trials are still being performed.

### PROGNOSIS

The progression is slow and remission may occur. Established cirrhosis is associated with a poor prognosis. Primary liver cell carcinoma is a frequent association and is one of the commonest carcinomas in HBV endemic areas such as the Far East.

## Chronic hepatitis C infection

Most patients are asymptomatic. Even with cirrhosis, the stigmata of chronic liver disease are few. The course is slow with persistently raised (mild-to-moderate) serum aminotransferases which fluctuate markedly over years. Serum albumin, bilirubin and PT are usually normal. Liver histology shows features of CPH with only minimal piecemeal necrosis although it can progress to cirrhosis.

Interferon-$\alpha$ therapy (3 MU three times weekly i.m. for 3–12 months) shows a 50–60% response rate but over 50% relapse. Indications for therapy are still being discussed but patients who have anti-HCV or HCV RNA, abnormal liver biochemistry and abnormal liver histology without cirrhosis should probably be given treatment. Side effects are few on this low dose. Preliminary studies suggest that type I responds poorly to treatment.

## Chronic autoimmune hepatitis

This condition occurs more frequently in young (10–20 years) and middle-aged women. There is an association with other autoimmune diseases, e.g. pernicious anaemia, thyroiditis and Coombs'-positive haemolytic anaemia, and 60% are associated with HLA-B8, DR3, Dw3.

The cause is unknown, but many immunological abnormalities are seen. There is a defect of suppressor (regulatory) T cells, which may be primary or secondary, resulting in the production of autoantibodies against hepatocyte surface antigens. Humoral disturbances are associated with a hypergammaglobulinaemia (mainly IgG) and nuclear, smooth muscle (actin), liver/kidney microsomal (LKM1) antibodies are found in the serum. The association with other diseases suggests immune complex formation and deposition. The condition was called 'lupoid hepatitis' as a positive lupus erythematosus (LE) cell test was found in 15%. CAH produced by some drugs (see below) may also be associated with the production of autoantibodies. HCV and HBV markers are negative in this condition.

The onset may be insidious but 25% present as acute hepatitis. Alternatively, patients can be asymptomatic for years and the signs of chronic liver disease are discovered on a routine examination. Amenorrhoea is common. Examination shows the signs of chronic liver disease, hepatosplenomegaly, cutaneous striae, acne, hirsuties and bruises. Jaundice may be present. In advanced cases the complications of cirrhosis occur. An ill patient can also have features of an autoimmune disease with a fever, migratory polyarthritis, glomerulonephritis, pleurisy, pulmonary infiltration or fibrosing alveolitis. The 'sicca' syndrome can occur (see p. 389).

### INVESTIGATION

The hallmark of this condition is positive antibodies against nuclei, smooth muscle (actin) and occasionally mitochondria. LKM1 antibodies are found in some patients who tend to be younger and have more aggressive disease. Additional antibodies to a soluble liver antigen and the measles virus are seen, possibly due to hyperfunction of the immune system. Serum bilirubin, globulins and aminotransferases are very high. A mild normochromic normocytic anaemia with thrombocytopenia and leucopenia is present even before portal hypertension and splenomegaly. Histology of the liver biopsy shows the changes of CAH with piecemeal necrosis.

## TREATMENT
Prednisolone 30 mg is given daily for 2 weeks followed by a maintenance dose of 10–15 mg daily along with azathioprine 1–2 mg kg$^{-1}$ daily.

## COURSE AND PROGNOSIS
Remissions and exacerbations occur, and 50% of patients will die of liver failure within 5 years if no treatment is given. The prognosis can be considerably improved with steroid and azathioprine therapy (90% 5-year survival), underlining the importance of establishing this diagnosis by liver histology and immune markers. Most patients, nevertheless, develop cirrhosis.

In a severe case with failure of medical treatment, orthotopic liver transplantation should be considered.

## Drug-induced chronic hepatitis

Many drugs (see Table 5.7) can cause a CAH which clinically bears many similarities to autoimmune hepatitis. Patients are often female, present with jaundice and hepatomegaly, have raised serum transaminases and globulin levels and LE cells and anti-LKM1 antibodies may be detected. Improvement follows drug withdrawal but exacerbations can occur with drug reintroduction.

## *Cirrhosis*

Cirrhosis results from the necrosis of liver cells followed by fibrosis and nodule formation. The liver architecture is diffusely abnormal and this interferes with liver blood flow and function. This derangement produces the clinical features of portal hypertension and impaired liver cell function.

## AETIOLOGY
The causes of cirrhosis are shown in Table 5.8. Alcohol is now the commonest cause in the Western World but HBV infection is the commonest cause worldwide and HCV is increasingly being diagnosed. With the identification of new hepatic viruses, idiopathic or cryptogenic cirrhosis is less commonly diagnosed. Young patients with cirrhosis must be carefully investigated as the cause may be treatable, e.g. Wilson's disease.

## PATHOLOGY
Two types have been described which give clues to the underlying cause:

1 *Micronodular cirrhosis*, in which regenerating nodules

*Common*
Alcohol
Hepatitis B
Hepatitis C
? Other non-A, non-B viruses

*Others*
Biliary cirrhosis
  Primary
  Secondary
Autoimmune chronic active hepatitis
Haemochromatosis
Hepatic venous congestion
Budd–Chiari syndrome
Wilson's disease
Drugs, e.g. methotrexate
$\alpha_1$-Antitrypsin deficiency
Cystic fibrosis
Intestinal bypass operations for obesity
Galactosaemia
Glycogen storage disease
Veno-occlusive disease
Idiopathic (cryptogenic)

**Table 5.8**  Causes of cirrhosis.

are usually less than 3 mm in size and are surrounded by fibrous septa and the condition uniformly involves the liver. This type is often caused by ongoing alcohol damage or biliary tract disease.

2 *Macronodular cirrhosis*, in which the nodules are of variable size and normal acini may be seen within the larger nodules. This type is often seen following previous hepatic illness, e.g. HBV infection.

A mixed picture with small and large nodules is sometimes seen and an aetiological cause cannot necessarily be inferred from the pathological picture.

Symptoms and signs are described on p. 246.

## INVESTIGATIONS
These are performed to assess the severity and type of liver disease.

### Severity
LIVER BIOCHEMISTRY. This can be normal depending on the severity of cirrhosis. In most cases there is at least a slight elevation in the serum AP and serum aminotransferases. In decompensated cirrhosis all biochemistry is deranged. The serum albumin is the best indicator of liver function.

SERUM ELECTROLYTES. A low sodium indicates severe liver disease because of dilution secondary to free water clearance or to excess diuretic therapy.

HAEMATOLOGY (see p. 242). The PT is prolonged commensurate to the severity of the liver disease.

SERUM $\alpha$-FETOPROTEIN is a useful screening test for a hepatocellular carcinoma.

### Type
This can be determined by the following:
VIRAL MARKERS.
SERUM AUTOANTIBODIES.

Serum immunoglobulins.

Miscellaneous: serum copper (see p. 270) and serum $\alpha_1$-antitrypsin (see p. 271) should always be measured in young cirrhotics. Serum iron, total iron binding capacity (TIBC) and ferritin should be measured to exclude haemochromatosis.

## Imaging

Ultrasound examination. This can demonstrate changes in size and shape of the liver. Fatty change and fibrosis produce a diffuse increased echogenicity. The patency of the portal and hepatic veins can be evaluated. It is useful to detect hepatocellular carcinoma.

CT is rarely necessary but can detect a fatty liver as well as excess iron deposition.

Barium swallow can detect varices.

Scintiscanning is only helpful in advanced cirrhosis (see p. 244) when clotting abnormalities preclude a biopsy.

Endoscopy is performed for the detection and treatment of varices.

## Liver biopsy

This is also necessary to confirm the severity and type of liver disease. The core of liver often fragments and sampling errors occur in macronodular cirrhosis. Special stains may be required for iron and copper.

## MANAGEMENT

Management is that of the complications seen in decompensated cirrhosis and patients should be followed up in order to detect complications as early as possible.

There is no treatment that will arrest or reverse the cirrhotic changes. Progression may be halted by correcting the underlying cause (see below). Patients with compensated cirrhosis should lead a normal life and no particular diet is helpful. Alcohol should be avoided, although if the cirrhosis is not due to alcohol, small amounts are not harmful.

## COURSE AND PROGNOSIS

This is extremely variable, depending on many factors, including the aetiology and the presence of complications. Poor prognostic indicators are given in Table 5.9. Development of any complication usually worsens the prognosis. In general, the 5-year survival rate is approximately 50% but this also varies depending on the aetiology and the stage at which the diagnosis is made. There are a number of prognostic classifications based on modifications of Child's grading (A, B and C). This is based on the presence of jaundice, ascites, encephalopathy and the level of serum albumin. Patients with good liver function—Child's Grade A—do better than patients with poor liver function (albumin $<30$ g litre$^{-1}$, bilirubin $>50$ $\mu$mol litre$^{-1}$ and ascites)—Child's Grade C.

Surgical procedures carry an operative mortality of 30% in non-bleeding cirrhotics (10% in Child's Grade A to 76% in Grade C patients).

---

*Blood tests*
Low albumin ($<25$ g litre$^{-1}$)
Low serum sodium ($<120$ mmol litre$^{-1}$)
Prolonged prothrombin time/INR

*Clinical*
Persistent jaundice
Failure of response to therapy
Ascites
Haemorrhage from varices, particularly with poor liver function
Neuropsychiatric complications developing with progressive liver failure
Small liver
Persistent hypotension
Aetiology, e.g. alcoholic cirrhosis (if the patient continues drinking)

---

INR, International Normalized Ratio.

**Table 5.9** Poor prognostic indicators in cirrhosis.

# LIVER TRANSPLANTATION

This is now an established treatment for a number of liver diseases and is becoming more widely available.

Indications include:

Acute liver disease—patients with fulminant hepatic failure of any cause including acute viral hepatitis.

Chronic liver disease, the indications for transplantation vary and the timing of the transplant is often difficult. All patients with end-stage (Child's Grade C) cirrhosis should be considered.

Primary biliary cirrhosis—patients with this disease should be transplanted when their serum bilirubin rises above 100 $\mu$mol litre$^{-1}$.

Chronic hepatitis B—recurrence of the hepatitis occurs in some transplanted cases and thus longer term survival is reduced.

Chronic hepatitis C—in end-stage disease the prognosis of the graft is good despite HCV RNA being found in the grafted liver, indicating re-infection.

Alcoholic liver disease—well-motivated patients who have stopped drinking can be offered a transplant.

Primary metabolic disorders, e.g. Wilson's disease.

Other conditions, e.g. sclerosing cholangitis.

## CONTRAINDICATIONS

Absolute contraindications include active sepsis outside the hepatobiliary tree, metastatic malignancy, AIDS infection and if the patient is not psychologically committed.

Relative contraindications are mainly anatomical considerations that would make surgery more difficult, e.g. portal vein thrombosis, previous portocaval shunts or complex surgery. With exceptions patients over 65 years are usually not transplanted. In hepatocellular carcinoma the recurrence rate is high and transplantation is not recommended.

## SURGICAL PROCEDURE

Pretransplant workup includes the confirmation of the diagnosis, ultrasound and CT scanning, radiological demonstration of the hepatic arterial and biliary tree. Because of the ethical and financial implications of this operation psychiatric counselling and regular psychosocial support are vital.

The donor should be ABO, but not necessarily HLA, compatible, be preferably less than 50 years of age and have no evidence of sepsis, malignancy, HIV or HBV infection.

The recipient operation takes approximately 8 hours and requires a large blood transfusion. Various immunosuppressive agents are used and include cyclosporin, methylprednisolone, azathioprine and FK506, a macrolide antibiotic which is more powerful than cyclosporin in inhibiting interleukin-2.

The operative mortality is low. Most postoperative deaths occur in the first 3 months. Sepsis, haemorrhage, metabolic acidosis and hyperkalaemia occur. Opportunistic infections (see p. 142) are still a problem due to immunosuppression.

## REJECTION

Rejection can be early (reversible) or late (irreversible). Acute or cellular rejection is usually seen 5–10 days post transplant; the patient feels ill with a pyrexia and tender hepatomegaly. Histologically there is portal inflammation, bile duct damage and endothelialitis of the liver. This type of rejection responds to immunosuppressive therapy. Irreversible chronic ductopenic rejection is seen 6 weeks to 9 months post-transplant with disappearing bile ducts (vanishing bile duct syndrome, VBDS) and an arteriopathy with narrowing and occlusion of the arteries. Ductopenic rejection is not reversed by immunosuppression and requires retransplantation. Graft-versus-host disease is extremely rare.

## PROGNOSIS

Elective liver transplantation in low-risk patients now has a 90% 1-year survival; 5-year survivals are as high as 70–85% largely due to the introduction of cyclosporin and FK 506. Patients require lifelong immunosuppression.

# Complications and effects of cirrhosis

These are shown in Table 5.10.

## PORTAL HYPERTENSION

The portal vein is formed by the union of the superior mesenteric and splenic veins. The pressure within it is normally 5–8 mmHg with only a small gradient across the liver to the hepatic vein in which blood is returned to the heart via the inferior vena cava. Portal hyperten-

| |
|---|
| Portal hypertension and gastrointestinal haemorrhage |
| Ascites |
| Portosystemic encephalopathy |
| Renal failure |
| Hepatocellular carcinoma |

**Table 5.10**   Complications and effects of cirrhosis.

sion can be classified according to the site of obstruction:

PREHEPATIC due to blockage of the portal vein before the liver

INTRAHEPATIC due to distortion of the liver architecture, which can be presinusoidal, e.g. in schistosomiasis, or postsinusoidal, e.g. in cirrhosis

POSTHEPATIC due to venous blockage outside the liver (rare)

As portal pressure rises above 10–12 mmHg the compliant venous system dilates and collaterals with the systemic venous system occur.

The main sites of the collaterals are at the gastro-oesophageal junction, the rectum, the left renal vein, the diaphragm, the retroperitoneum and the anterior abdominal wall via the umbilical vein.

The collaterals at the gastro-oesophageal junction (varices) are superficial in position and tend to rupture. Portosystemic anastomoses at other sites seldom give rise to symptoms. Rectal varices are frequently found (30%) if carefully looked for and can be differentiated from haemorrhoids, which are lower in the anal canal.

## PATHOPHYSIOLOGY

Portal vascular resistance is increased due to the deposition of collagen in the space of Disse and possibly hepatocyte enlargement. This increased resistance leads to portal hypertension and opening of portosystemic anastomoses in both precirrhotic and cirrhotic livers. Patients with cirrhosis have a hyperdynamic circulation. This is now thought to be due to the release of the mediators nitric oxide and glucagon (due to endotoxaemia) which leads to peripheral and splanchnic vasodilatation. This effect is followed by plasma volume expansion due to sodium retention (see ascites) and this has a significant effect in maintaining portal hypertension. The relevant roles of an impaired autonomic nervous system or of humoral factors, e.g. prostaglandins or serotonin, remain unclear.

## CAUSES (see Table 5.11)

The commonest cause is cirrhosis. Other causes include the following.

### Prehepatic causes

Extrahepatic blockage is due to portal vein thrombosis. The cause is often unidentifiable but some are due to portal vein occlusion secondary to congenital portal venous abnormalities or neonatal sepsis of the umbilical vein. Patients usually present with bleeding, often at a young age. They have normal liver function and, because

| |
|---|
| *Prehepatic*<br>Portal vein thrombosis<br><br>*Intrahepatic*<br>Cirrhosis<br>Hepatitis (alcoholic)<br>Idiopathic non-cirrhotic portal hypertension (subtle liver disease)<br>Schistosomiasis<br>Partial nodular transformation<br>Congenital hepatic fibrosis<br>Myelosclerosis (extramedullary haemopoiesis)<br>Granulomata<br><br>*Posthepatic*<br>Budd–Chiari syndrome<br>Veno-occlusive disease<br>Right heart failure—rare<br>Constrictive pericarditis |

**Table 5.11**  Causes of portal hypertension.

of this, their prognosis following bleeding is excellent. The portal vein blockage can be identified by ultrasound or Doppler imaging. A splenectomy should never be performed, as it may be possible to perform a splenorenal shunt in adult life. Treatment is usually with repeated sclerotherapy.

### Intrahepatic causes
Although cirrhosis is the commonest intrahepatic cause of portal hypertension, other causes include:

NON-CIRRHOTIC PORTAL HYPERTENSION or subtle change liver disease. Patients present with portal hypertension and variceal bleeding but without cirrhosis. Histologically, the liver shows mild portal tract fibrosis. The aetiology is unknown, but arsenic, vinyl chloride and other toxic agents have been implicated in some cases. A similar disease is found frequently in India. The liver lesion does not progress and the prognosis is therefore good.

SCHISTOSOMIASIS with extensive pipe-stem fibrosis is a common cause worldwide.

OTHER CAUSES include nodular regenerative hyperplasia, congenital hepatic fibrosis and partial nodular transformation. This latter condition is very rare and there is dispute about its existence.

### Posthepatic causes
Prolonged severe heart failure with tricuspid incompetence and constrictive pericarditis can both lead to portal hypertension. The Budd–Chiari syndrome is described on p. 273.

### CLINICAL FEATURES
Patients with portal hypertension are often asymptomatic and the only clinical evidence of portal hypertension is splenomegaly.

Presenting features are:
● Haematemesis or melaena from rupture of gastro-oesophageal varices
● Ascites and/or
● Encephalopathy

## Variceal haemorrhage

Approximately 70% of patients with cirrhosis will develop gastro-oesophageal varices but only one-third of these will bleed from them. Bleeding is likely to occur with large varices, high pressure and in severe liver disease.

### MANAGEMENT
The management can be divided into the active bleeding episode, the prevention of rebleeding and prophylactic measures to prevent the first haemorrhage. Despite all the therapeutic techniques available, the prognosis depends on the severity of the underlying liver disease.

#### Initial management of acute variceal bleeding (Fig. 5.18)
See also general management of gastrointestinal haemorrhage on p. 198.

RESUSCITATION
1 Assess the general condition of the patient—pulse and blood pressure.
2 Insert an intravenous line and obtain blood for grouping and crossmatching, haemoglobin, PT, urea, electrolytes and liver biochemistry.
3 Restore blood volume with plasma expanders or blood transfusion if possible. These measures are discussed in more detail in the treatment of shock (see p. 720). Prompt correction of hypovolaemia is necessary in patients with cirrhosis as their baroreceptor reflexes are diminished.

URGENT ENDOSCOPY should be performed to confirm

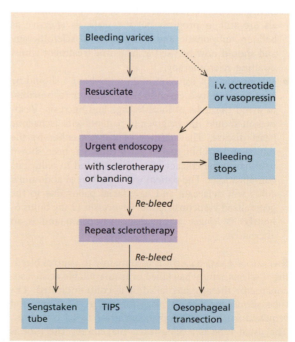

**Fig. 5.18**  Management of gastrointestinal haemorrhage due to oesophageal varices. TIPS, transjugular intrahepatic portocaval shunt.

the diagnosis of varices and to exclude bleeding from other sites (e.g. gastric ulceration), which are sometimes the source of haemorrhage in these patients. *Portal hypertensive (or congestive) gastropathy* is the term used for chronic gastric congestion, punctate erythema and gastric erosions and is a source of bleeding. Varices may or may not be present. Propranolol (see below) is the best treatment for this.

INJECTION SCLEROTHERAPY OR VARICEAL BANDING. The varices should be injected with a sclerosing agent that may arrest bleeding by producing vessel thrombosis. A needle is passed down the biopsy channel of the endoscope and a sclerosing agent is injected into the varices. Alternatively, the varices can be banded by mounting a band on the tip of the endoscope, sucking the varix just into the end of the scope and dislodging the band over the varix using a tripwire mechanism.

Acute variceal sclerotherapy and banding are the treatment of choice; this arrests bleeding in 80% of cases and reduces early rebleeding; 15–20% of bleeding comes from gastric varices and here results of sclerotherapy are poor.

### Other measures available

VASOCONSTRICTOR THERAPY. The main use of this is for emergency control of bleeding either whilst waiting for endoscopy and sclerotherapy or if the latter has failed to control the bleeding. The aim of vasoconstrictor agents is to restrict portal inflow by splanchnic arterial constriction.

- *Octreotide* (a *somatostatin* analogue—50 $\mu$g bolus followed by an infusion of 50 $\mu$g hour$^{-1}$ for 48 hours) will produce splanchnic vasoconstriction without significant systemic vascular effect or complications. Trials are still in progress but it is safe, as effective as balloon tamponade and comparable to sclerotherapy and should now be used as first-time treatment whilst awaiting sclerotherapy.
- *Vasopressin*. An infusion of 25 units hour$^{-1}$ should be administered by a central venous catheter (if possible) to avoid the risks of local leakage and necrosis. Vasopressin should not be given to patients with ischaemic heart disease. The addition of nitrates either by the intravenous, sublingual or patch route has been shown to enhance the efficacy of vasopressin and to reduce its complications. The patient will complain of abdominal colic, will defaecate and have facial pallor due to the generalized vasoconstriction. Glypressin (2 mg bolus 6-hourly) is longer acting than vasopressin and is an alternative.

BALLOON TAMPONADE is used mainly to control bleeding if sclerotherapy has failed or is unavailable or if vasoconstrictor therapy has failed or is contraindicated. The tube should be left in place for up to 12 hours and removed in the endoscopy room prior to sclerotherapy. The usual tube is a Sengstaken–Blakemore. The tube is passed into the stomach and the gastric balloon is inflated with air and pulled back. It should be positioned in close apposition to the gastro-oesophageal junction to prevent the cephalad variceal blood flow to the bleeding point. The oesophageal balloon should only be inflated if bleeding is not controlled by the gastric balloon alone. This technique is successful in up to 90% of patients and is very useful in the first few hours of haemorrhaging. However it has serious complications such as aspiration pneumonia, oesophageal rupture and mucosal ulceration, which produce a 5% mortality. The procedure is very unpleasant for the patient.

### Additional management of acute episode

REPEAT SCLEROTHERAPY once to control recurrent bleeding. Further sclerotherpy is not advisable if bleeding continues and other measures (see below) should be pursued.

MEASURES TO PREVENT ENCEPHALOPATHY. Portosystemic encephalopathy (PSE) can be precipitated by a large bleed (since blood contains protein). The management is described below.

NURSING. Patients require high-dependency/intensive-care nursing. They should have nil by mouth until bleeding has stopped.

SUCRALFATE 1 g four times daily is given to reduce oesophageal ulceration following sclerotherapy.

### Management of an acute rebleed

The source of bleeding should be re-established by endoscopy. It is sometimes due to an ulcer produced by previous sclerotherapy and this is difficult to manage.

REPEAT SCLEROTHERAPY for varices.

OCTREOTIDE INFUSION for 3–5 days.

TRANSJUGULAR INTRAHEPATIC PORTOCAVAL SHUNT (TIPS). This method can be used to reduce the portal venous pressure and is performed with a local anaesthetic. A guide wire is passed from the jugular vein into the liver and an expandable metal shunt is forced into the liver substance to form a channel between the systemic and portal venous systems. This method is used in cases where the bleeding cannot be stopped.

EMERGENCY SURGERY is used when sclerotherapy fails or if TIPS is not available, particularly if the bleeding is from gastric fundal varices. Oesophageal transection and ligation of the feeding vessels to the bleeding varices is the most common surgical technique. Acute portosystemic shunt surgery (see below) is infrequently performed in the UK.

### Prevention of recurrent variceal bleeding

Following an episode of variceal bleeding, the risk of recurrence is 60–80% over a 2-year period with an approximate mortality of 20% per episode; these facts justify the use of measures to prevent such rebleeding.

LONG-TERM INJECTION SCLEROTHERAPY OR BANDING. The use of repeated courses of injection sclerotherapy or banding at weekly intervals leads to the obliteration of the varices by fibrous tissue. This is now the method of choice. Follow-up endoscopy with treatment should be performed at intervals to keep varices ablated.

Results show a reduction in bleeding episodes but the effect on survival is controversial and probably small. Complications include oesophageal ulceration and mediastinitis and strictures occur in about 10% with repeated sclerotherapy. Banding has fewer complications, particularly in stricture formation.

$\beta$-Adrenoreceptor blockade. Oral propranolol in a dose sufficient to reduce resting pulse rate by 25% has been shown to decrease portal pressure. Portal inflow is reduced by two mechanisms: a decrease in cardiac output ($\beta_1$) and also by the blockade of $\beta_2$ vasodilator fibres on the splanchnic arteries, leaving an unopposed vasoconstrictor effect. This has been shown to decrease the frequency of rebleeding in patients with well-compensated liver disease and some studies show it to be as effective as sclerotherapy.

Surgical procedures. Portosystemic shunting is associated with an extremely low risk of rebleeding but the diversion of portal blood away from the liver produces significant *encephalopathy*. Operative mortality is low in patients with Child's Grade A (0–5%) but encephalopathy still occurs. Child's Grade C has a very poor prognosis. The 'shunts' performed today are usually an end-to-side portocaval anastomosis or a selective distal splenorenal shunt (Warren shunt), which maintains hepatic blood flow via the superior mesenteric vein. Oesophageal transection does not produce encephalopathy but rebleeding eventually occurs. Liver transplantation (see p. 261) should always be considered.

### Prophylactic measures

Patients with cirrhosis and varices should be prescribed non- selective $\beta$-blockers; this reduces variceal haemorrhage and may increase survival.

# ASCITES

Ascites is the presence of fluid within the peritoneal cavity and is a common complication of cirrhosis of the liver. The pathogenesis of the development of ascites is controversial but is probably secondary to renal sodium and water retention. Several factors are involved:

Sodium and water retention occur as a result of peripheral arterial vasodilatation and consequent reduction in the effective blood volume. Nitric oxide has been postulated as the putative vasodilator although other substances, e.g. atrial natriuretic peptide and prostaglandins, may be involved. The reduction in arterial blood volume activates various neurohumoral pressor systems such as the sympathetic nervous system and the renin–angiotensin system, thus promoting salt and water retention.

Portal hypertension exerts a local hydrostatic pressure and leads to increased hepatic and splanchnic production of lymph and transudation of fluid into the peritoneal cavity.

Low serum albumin (a consequence of poor synthetic liver function) may further contribute by a reduction in plasma oncotic pressure.

In patients with ascites, urine sodium excretion rarely exceeds 5 mmol in 24 hours. Loss of sodium from extra-renal sites accounts for approximately 30 mmol in 24 hours. The normal daily dietary sodium intake may vary between 120 and 200 mmol resulting in a positive sodium balance of approximately 90–170 mmol in 24 hours (equivalent to 600–1300 ml of fluid retained.

## CLINICAL FEATURES

The abdominal swelling associated with ascites may accumulate over many weeks or as rapidly as a few days. The presence of fluid is confirmed by the demonstration of shifting dullness. Mild generalized abdominal pain and discomfort are common but, if more severe, should raise the suspicion of spontaneous bacterial peritonitis (see below). Respiratory distress may accompany tense ascites. Many patients will also have peripheral oedema. A pleural effusion (usually on the right side) may infrequently be found and is believed to arise from the passage of ascites through congenital defects in the diaphragm.

## INVESTIGATION

A diagnostic aspiration of 10–20 ml of fluid should be obtained and the following performed:

Cell count: a neutrophil count >250 cells/mm$^3$ is indicative of an underlying (usually spontaneous) bacterial peritonitis.

Gram stain and culture for bacteria and acid-fast bacilli.

Protein: the ascitic protein level enables a division into transudative and exudative ascites. For this division the serum albumin must be used as a reference point. An ascitic protein of 11 g litre$^{-1}$ or more below the serum albumin level suggests a transudate. The level of ascitic protein provides an indirect estimate of opsonization capacity and thereby the risk of developing spontaneous bacterial peritonitis. Patients at most risk are those with ascitic protein levels <10 g litre$^{-1}$.

Cytology for malignant cells.

Amylase: to exclude pancreatic ascites.

The differential diagnosis of ascites is listed in Table 5.12.

## MANAGEMENT

The aim is to both reduce sodium intake and increase renal excretion and by doing so produce a net reabsorption of fluid from the ascites back into the circulating volume. The maximum rate at which ascites can be mobilized is 500–700 ml in 24 hours (see below).

The management is as follows:

Check serum electrolytes and creatinine at start and every other day, weigh daily, measure urinary output.

Bed rest—this alone will lead to a diuresis in a small proportion of people by improving renal perfusion but in practice is not helpful.

Dietary sodium restriction. It is possible to reduce sodium intake to 22 mmol in 24 hours and still

*Straw-coloured*
Malignancy—commonest cause
Cirrhosis
Infective
    Tuberculosis
    Following intra-abdominal perforation—any bacteria
        may be found, e.g. *E. coli*
    Spontaneous in cirrhotics
Hepatic vein obstruction (Budd–Chiari syndrome)—
        protein level high in fluid
Chronic pancreatitis
Constrictive pericarditis
Meig's syndrome (ovarian tumour)
Hypoproteinaemia, e.g. nephrotic syndrome

*Chylous*
Obstruction of main lymphatic duct, e.g. by
        carcinoma—chylomicrons are present

*Haemorrhagic*
Malignancy
Ruptured ectopic pregnancy
Abdominal trauma
Acute pancreatitis

**Table 5.12**  Causes of ascites divided according to the type of ascitic fluid.

maintain an adequate protein and calorie intake. Many patients find this difficult and a 40 mmol diet is frequently an adequate compromise.

FLUID RESTRICTION is probably not necessary unless the serum sodium is less than 120 mmol litre$^{-1}$.

DIURETICS. The diuretics of first choice are those acting on the distal nephron, namely spironolactone 200 mg daily, triamterene or amiloride 10 mg daily. These agents have only mild diuretic potency and are therefore without major risks of overdiuresis and renal impairment. The potassium-sparing action of these agents may give rise to hyperkalaemia.

The aim of diuretic therapy should be to produce a net loss of fluid approaching 700 ml in 24 hours (0.700 kg weight loss or 1.5 kg if peripheral oedema is present).

With this regimen diuresis is often poor. Spironolactone should be increased to 400 mg daily and a loop diuretic, such as frusemide 80 mg or bumetamide 1 mg daily, added. These diuretics have several potential disadvantages with hypokalaemia and volume depletion.

Diuretics should be temporarily discontinued if a rise in creatinine level (to approximately 160 $\mu$mol litre$^{-1}$) occurs, representing overdiuresis and hypovolaemia. Hyponatraemia occurring during therapy almost always represents haemodilution secondary to a failure to clear free water (usually a marker of reduced renal perfusion) and should be treated by stopping the diuretics if the sodium level falls below approximately 128 mmol litre$^{-1}$ as well as continued water restriction. Diuretics should also be stopped if there is hypokalaemia or precoma.

PARACENTESIS. This is used to relieve symptomatic tense ascites. It has also been reintroduced in some countries as a means of rapid therapy in patients with ascites and peripheral oedema, thus avoiding prolonged hospital stay. The main danger of this approach is the production of hypovolaemia as the ascites reaccumulates at the expense of the circulating volume. In patients with normal renal function and in the absence of hyponatraemia, this has largely been overcome by the administration of albumin (6 g per litre ascitic fluid removed) or a plasma expander, e.g. dextran-70 (8 g per litre ascitic fluid removed) or gelatin infusion (125 ml of a 3.5–4% solution per litre removed), to maintain the plasma volume. In practice, up to 20 litres can be removed over 4–6 hours. This should always be followed by the plasma expander given over half an hour, 3 hours after the paracentesis. This procedure should not be performed in end-stage cirrhosis or if the patient has renal failure.

PERITONEO-VENOUS SHUNT. The introduction of a catheter from the peritoneal cavity (subcutaneously) to the internal jugular vein, incorporating a one-way valve, allows passage of the ascites directly into the circulation. This is rarely used for patients with resistant ascites as it often blocks.

TRANS-JUGULAR INTRAHEPATIC PORTOCAVAL SHUNT (MPS) is useful for resistant ascites.

## SPONTANEOUS BACTERIAL PERITONITIS

This condition represents one of the more serious complications of ascites and occurs in approximately 8% of cirrhotics with ascites. The infecting organisms are believed to gain access to the peritoneum by haematogenous spread. The most frequently incriminated bacteria are *Escherichia coli*, *Klebsiella* and enterococci. The condition should be suspected in any patient with ascites with evidence of clinical deterioration. Features such as pain and pyrexia are frequently absent. Diagnostic aspiration should always be performed (see above). The raised neutrophil count in the ascites is alone sufficient evidence to start treatment immediately. A third-generation cephalosporin, such as cefotaxime or ceftazidime, is used and may be modified on the basis of culture results. The prognosis is grave and depends on the severity of the liver disease. It has a 50% mortality and recurs in 70% of patients within a year.

# PORTOSYSTEMIC ENCEPHALOPATHY

The term portosystemic encephalopathy refers to a chronic neuropsychiatric syndrome secondary to chronic liver disease. This condition occurs with cirrhosis, but a similar acute encephalopathy can occur in acute FHF (see p. 256). PSE is seen in patients with portal hypertension due to spontaneous 'shunting' or in patients following a portocaval shunt operation. Encephalopathy is potentially reversible. The mechanism is unknown but several factors are thought to play a part. In cirrhosis, the blood bypasses the liver via the collaterals and the 'toxic' metabolites pass directly to the brain to produce the encephalopathy. Many 'toxic' substances have been suggested as the causative factor, including ammonia, free fatty acids, mercaptans and accumulation of false neurotransmitters (octopamine) or activation of the $\gamma$-aminobutyric acid (GABA) inhibitory neurotransmitter system. Increased blood levels of aromatic amino acids (tyrosine and phenylalanine) and reduced branched-chain amino acids (valine, leucine and isoleucine) also occur. Nevertheless, ammonia seems to play a major role. Ammonia is produced by the breakdown of protein by intestinal bacteria and a high blood ammonia is seen in most patients. It may alter the blood–brain barrier and allow 'toxins' to interfere with cerebral metabolism. The factors that can precipitate PSE are shown in Table 5.13.

## CLINICAL FEATURES

An acute onset often has a precipitating factor (Table 5.13). The patient becomes increasingly drowsy and comatose.

Chronically, there is a disorder of personality, mood and intellect, with a reversal of normal sleep rhythm. These changes may be fluctuating and a history from a relative must be obtained. The patient is irritable, confused, disorientated and has slow slurred speech. General features include nausea, vomiting and weakness. Convulsions and coma occur as the encephalopathy becomes more marked. Hyperventilation and pyrexia are seen.

Signs include fetor hepaticus (a sweet smell to the breath) and a coarse flapping tremor seen when the hands are outstretched and the wrists hyperextended (asterixis). There is a constructional apraxia and the patient cannot write or draw, for example a five-pointed star. Mental function can be assessed by using the serial-sevens test (see p. 960). A trail-making test (the ability to join numbers and letters with a pen within a certain time—a standard psychological test for brain dysfunction) is prolonged and is a useful bedside test to assess encephalopathy.

Diagnosis is clinical and routine liver biochemistry merely confirms the presence of liver disease, not the presence of encephalopathy.

Additional investigations include:

ELECTROENCEPHALOGRAM (EEG). This shows a decrease in the frequency of the normal $\alpha$ waves (8–13 Hz) to $\delta$ waves (1.5–3 Hz). These changes occur before coma supervenes.

VISUAL EVOKED RESPONSES (see p. 877) also detect subclinical encephalopathy.

ARTERIAL BLOOD AMMONIA. This is occasionally useful in the differential diagnosis of the cause of the coma and to follow the course of the PSE, but is not readily available.

## MANAGEMENT

Management consists of restricting protein intake and sterilizing the bowel.

### Immediate

IDENTIFY AND REMOVE THE POSSIBLE PRECIPITATING CAUSE, e.g. drugs with cerebral depressant properties.

GIVE PURGATION AND ENEMAS to empty the bowels of nitrogenous substances. Lactulose (10–30 ml three times daily) is an osmotic purgative that reduces the colonic pH and limits ammonia absorption. Lactilol ($\beta$-galactoside sorbitol 30 g daily) is metabolized by colonic bacteria and is comparable in efficacy to lactulose. Hypernatraemia can result from water loss.

INSTITUTE A PROTEIN-FREE DIET, with adequate calories, given if necessary via a fine-bore nasogastric tube.

ANTIBIOTICS. Oral neomycin 1 g 6-hourly can be used if lactulose fails. Neomycin can also be used in retention enemas. It is mainly unabsorbed, but in the long term it can produce deafness. Metronidazole (200 mg four times daily) is also effective in the acute situation.

STOP OR REDUCE DIURETIC THERAPY.

CORRECT ANY ELECTROLYTE IMBALANCE.

GIVE INTRAVENOUS FLUIDS as necessary (beware of too much sodium).

TREAT ANY INFECTION.

FLUMAZENIL, a benzodiazepine receptor antagonist, can induce a transient improvement; controlled trials are in progress.

### Long term

INCREASE PROTEIN IN THE DIET to the limit of tolerance (20–50 g) as the encephalopathy improves.

AVOID CONSTIPATION.

GIVE LACTULOSE 10–30 ml three times daily.

AVOID PRECIPITATING FACTORS, e.g. narcotic drugs, which depress cerebral function, overdiuresis producing electrolyte imbalance.

### COURSE AND PROGNOSIS

Acute encephalopathy, often seen after FHF, has a very poor prognosis as the disease itself has a high mortality. In cirrhosis, chronic PSE is very variable and the prognosis is that of the underlying liver disease.

High dietary protein
Gastrointestinal haemorrhage
Constipation
Infection
Fluid and electrolyte disturbance due to:
  Diuretic therapy
  Paracentesis
Drugs, e.g. narcotics
Portosystemic shunt operations
Any surgical procedure

**Table 5.13** Factors precipitating portosystemic encephalopathy.

# Renal failure (hepatorenal syndrome)

The hepatorenal syndrome occurs typically in a patient with advanced cirrhosis with jaundice and ascites. The urine output is low with a low urinary sodium concentration, a residual capacity to concentrate urine (i.e. tubular function is intact) and an almost normal renal histology. The renal failure here is described as 'functional'. This is often precipitated by overvigorous diuretic therapy, diarrhoea or paracentesis, but often no precipitating factor is found. Advanced cases may progress beyond the 'functional' stage to produce an acute tubular necrosis.

The mechanism is similar to that producing ascites. The initiating factor is thought to be extreme peripheral vasodilation possibly due to nitric oxide, leading to an extreme decrease in the arterial blood volume and hypotension. This activates the homeostatic mechanisms causing a rise in plasma renin, aldosterone, noradrenaline and vasopressin leading to vasoconstriction of the renal vasculature. There is an increased preglomerular vascular resistance causing the blood flow to be directed away from the renal cortex. This leads to a reduced glomerular filtration rate and plasma renin remains high. Salt and water retention occur with reabsorption of sodium from the renal tubules. A number of other mediators have been incriminated in the pathogenesis of the hepatorenal syndrome, in particular the eicosanoids. This has been supported by the precipitation of the syndrome by inhibitors of prostaglandin synthetase such as non-steroidal anti-inflammatory agents.

The patient should be treated for prerenal failure and diuretic therapy should be stopped. The prognosis is poor.

# Primary hepatocellular carcinoma

This is discussed on p. 277.

# Types of cirrhosis

## Alcoholic

This is discussed in the section on alcoholic liver disease (see p. 271).

## Primary biliary cirrhosis (PBC)

This is a chronic disorder in which there is a progressive destruction of bile ducts, eventually leading to cirrhosis. It predominantly affects women aged 40–50 years (female to male ratio 6 : 1). It used to be considered rare but is now being diagnosed more frequently in its milder forms. PBC has been called 'chronic non-suppurative destructive cholangitis'; this term is more descriptive of the early lesion and emphasizes that true cirrhosis only occurs in the later stages of the disease.

### AETIOLOGY

The aetiology is unknown, but immunological mechanisms may play a part. Antibodies to mitochondria (AMA) are almost invariable and of the many mitochondrial proteins, the antigen M2 is specific to PBC. There are four M2 antigen polypeptides, all components of the pyruvate dehydrogenase complex of mitochondrial enzymes. Of these E2, a 74 kDa complex of lipoamide acyltransferase, and protein X, a 52 kDa peptide, appear to be specific to PBC and an ELISA test based against these antigens has been shown to be 98% sensitive for PBC in research laboratories. However, the presence of AMA in high titre is unrelated to the clinical or histological picture and may play no part in its pathogenesis.

Although damage to bile ducts is a feature, antibodies to bile ductules are not specific to PBC. Biliary epithelium from patients with PBC expresses aberrant class II HLAs but it is not known whether this expression is the cause or result of the inflammatory response. Cell-mediated immunity is impaired (demonstrated both *in vitro* and by skin testing) and this suggests that sensitized T lymphocytes might be involved in producing damage. There may be a defect in immunoregulation as a decrease in T suppressor cells may allow cytotoxic T cells to produce damage to the bile ducts; there is also evidence to suggest that lymphokine secretion and cell activation is impaired in T lymphocytes at the site of tissue destruction. There is an increased synthesis of IgM thought to be due to a failure of the switch from IgM to IgG antibody synthesis.

### CLINICAL FEATURES

Asymptomatic patients are discovered on routine examination or screening to have hepatomegaly, a raised serum alkaline phosphatase or autoantibodies.

The earliest symptom is pruritus, often preceding jaundice by a few years. When jaundice appears, hepatomegaly is usually found.

In the later stages patients are jaundiced with severe pruritus. Pigmented xanthelasma on eyelids or other deposits of cholesterol in the creases of the hands may be seen; hepatosplenomegaly is present.

### ASSOCIATIONS

Autoimmune disorders, e.g. Sjögren's syndrome, scleroderma, rheumatoid arthritis, occur with increased frequency. Keratoconjunctivitis sicca (dry eyes and mouth) is seen in 70% of cases. Renal tubular acidosis and membranous glomerulonephritis may occur.

### INVESTIGATION

MITOCHONDRIAL ANTIBODIES—measured routinely by indirect immunofluorescence on rat kidney substrate (in titres >1 : 160)—are present in over 95% of patients. M2 antibody is specific. Other non-specific antibodies, e.g. antinuclear factor and smooth muscle, may also be present.

High serum alkaline phosphatase is often the only abnormality in the liver biochemistry.

Serum cholesterol is raised.

Serum IgM may be very high.

Ultrasound shows diffuse alteration in liver architecture and is not always necessary (see below).

Liver biopsy shows characteristic histological features of a portal tract infiltrate mainly of lymphocytes and plasma cells, sometimes with granulomas. Most of the early changes are in zone 1. There is damage to and loss of small bile ducts, leading to portal tract fibrosis and, eventually, cirrhosis. Cholestasis occurs late.

*Hepatic granulomas* are also seen in sarcoidosis, tuberculosis, schistosomiasis, drug reactions (e.g. phenylbutazone), brucellosis, parasitic infestation (e.g. strongyloidiasis) and other conditions.

### DIFFERENTIAL DIAGNOSIS

The classical picture presents little difficulty with diagnosis (high serum alkaline phosphatase and the presence of AMA); this can be confirmed by the characteristic features on liver biopsy. There is a group of patients with the histological changes of PBC, but the serology of CAH (i.e. positive antinuclear and actin antibodies but negative AMA). This has been given the name of autoimmune cholangiopathy and responds to steroids.

In the jaundiced patient, extrahepatic biliary obstruction should be excluded by ultrasound and, if there is doubt about the diagnosis, ERCP should be performed to make sure that the bile ducts are normal.

### TREATMENT

Ursodeoxycholate (10–15 mg kg$^{-1}$) is of benefit in some patients with improvement in serum liver enzymes and pruritus. Azathioprine, corticosteroids and D-penicillamine have all been tried without beneficial effect, and corticosteroids are contraindicated because of bone thinning. Colchicine (0.6 mg twice daily) has been shown to improve liver function. Cyclosporin has been used in some trials with improvement in symptoms and reduced histological progression.

Malabsorption of fat-soluble vitamins (A, D and K) occurs and supplementation is required when deficiency is detected and in the jaundiced patient prophylactically. Calcium is required for osteoporosis. Hyperlipidaemia should be treated (see p. 858).

Pruritus is difficult to control but cholestyramine, one 4 g sachet three times daily, can be helpful, although it is unpalatable. Rifampicin and naloxone hydrochloride (an opioid antagonist) have been shown to be of benefit in trials.

The lack of effective medical therapy has made PBC a major indication for orthotopic liver transplantation (see p. 261).

### COMPLICATIONS

The complications are those of cirrhosis. In addition, osteoporosis, osteomalacia and a polyneuropathy can also occur.

### COURSE AND PROGNOSIS

This is very variable. Asymptomatic patients and those presenting with pruritus will survive for more than 20 years. Symptomatic patients with jaundice have a more rapidly progressive course and die of liver failure or bleeding varices in approximately 5 years. Liver transplantation should therefore be offered when the serum bilirubin reaches 100 $\mu$mol litre$^{-1}$. Transplantation has a 5 year survival of at least 70%.

## Secondary biliary cirrhosis

Cirrhosis can result from prolonged (for months) large duct biliary obstruction. Causes include bile duct strictures, gallstones and sclerosing cholangitis. An ultrasound examination, followed by ERCP or PTC is performed to outline the ducts and any remedial cause is dealt with.

## Haemochromatosis

Idiopathic haemochromatosis (IHC) is an inherited disease characterized by excess iron deposition in various organs leading to eventual fibrosis and functional organ failure.

### AETIOLOGY

The underlying metabolic defect is unknown, but abnormal enterocyte function resulting in inappropriate levels of iron absorption has been suggested. IHC is inherited as an autosomal recessive with only homozygotes manifesting the clinical features of the disease. It is associated with HLA-A3 (72% vs. 28% of general population); in addition HLA-B14 is increased in France and HLA-B7 in Australia. Dietary intakes of iron and chelating agents (ascorbic acid) are probably also important. Iron overload may be present in alcoholics, but alcohol excess *per se* does not cause IHC. There is a history of excess alcohol intake in 25% of patients. The iron accumulation is gradual and occurs throughout life.

### PREVALENCE

Prevalence of homozygotes (affected) varies between 0.3 and 0.5%, with a heterozygote (carrier) frequency of 9–14%.

### PATHOLOGY

In symptomatic patients the total body iron content is 20–40 g compared to 3–4 g in a normal person.

The iron content is particularly increased in the liver and pancreas (50–100 times normal) but is also increased in all other organs, e.g. the endocrine glands, heart and skin. Gonadal function is impaired despite a low testicular iron content.

Histologically the liver shows extensive pigmentation and fibrosis with iron deposition in dense, fibrous septae forming a network surrounding groups of acini. Early in the disease, iron is deposited in the periportal hepatocytes (in pericanalicular lysosomes). Later it is distributed widely throughout all acinian zones, biliary duct epithelium, Kupffer cells and connective tissue. Cirrhosis is a late feature.

## CLINICAL FEATURES

The course of the disease depends on a number of features including sex, dietary iron intake, presence of associated hepatotoxins (especially alcohol) and genotype. Overt clinical manifestations occur more frequently in men; the reduced incidence in women is probably explained by physiological blood loss and a smaller dietary intake of iron. Most affected individuals present in the fifth decade. The classic triad of bronze skin pigmentation (due to melanin deposition), hepatomegaly and diabetes mellitus is only present in cases of gross iron overload. Other more common features include gonadal atrophy and loss of libido.

Hypogonadism secondary to pituitary dysfunction is the commonest endocrine feature. Deficiency of other pituitary hormones is also found, but symptomatic endocrine deficiencies, e.g. loss of libido, are very rare. Cardiac manifestations, particularly heart failure and arrhythmias, are common, especially in younger patients. Calcium pyrophosphate is deposited asymmetrically in both large and small joints (chondrocalcinosis) leading to an arthropathy. The exact relationship of chondrocalcinosis to iron deposition is uncertain.

## COMPLICATIONS

Thirty per cent of patients with cirrhosis will develop primary hepatocellular carcinoma (HCC). HCC has only rarely been described in non-cirrhotic patients in whom the excess iron stores have been removed. This has important implications for early diagnosis.

## INVESTIGATION

**Homozygotes**

SERUM IRON is elevated ($>30\ \mu$mol litre$^{-1}$), with a reduction in the TIBC and complete or almost complete transferrin saturation ($>60\%$).

SERUM FERRITIN is elevated (usually $>500\ \mu$g litre$^{-1}$ or 240 nmol litre $^{-1}$).

LIVER BIOCHEMISTRY is often normal, even with established cirrhosis.

**Heterozygotes**

Heterozygotes may have normal biochemical tests or modest increases in serum iron transferrin saturation ($>50\%$) or serum ferritin (usually $>400\ \mu$g litre$^{-1}$).

**Liver biopsy**

This can define the extent of tissue damage, assess tissue iron, and the hepatic iron concentration can be measured ($>180\ \mu$mol g$^{-1}$ dry weight of liver indicates haemochromatosis).

Mild degrees of parenchymal iron deposition in patients with alcoholic cirrhosis can often cause confusion with true homozygous IHC. It is highly likely that many of this former group are heterozygotes for the haemochromatosis gene.

**Magnetic resonance imaging**

This shows a decreased T2 relaxation time but is not, as yet, accurate enough for diagnosis.

Causes of secondary iron overload such as multiple transfusions must be excluded.

## TREATMENT AND MANAGEMENT

**Venesection**

Venesection prolongs life and may reverse tissue damage; the risk of malignancy still remains if cirrhosis is present. All patients should have excess iron removed as rapidly as possible. This is achieved using venesection of 500 ml performed twice weekly for up to 2 years, i.e. 160 units $\times$ 250 mg of iron per unit, which equals 40 g removed. During venesection, serum iron and ferritin and the mean corpuscular volume (MCV) should be monitored. These fall only when available iron is depleted. Three or four venesections per year are required to prevent reaccumulation of iron. Serum ferritin should remain within the normal range. Liver biopsy is useful to ensure removal of iron and to assess progress of hepatic disease.

Manifestations of the disease usually improve or disappear, except for diabetes, testicular atrophy and chondrocalcinosis. The requirements for insulin often diminish in diabetic patients. Testosterone replacement is often helpful.

**Chelation therapy**

In rare patients who cannot tolerate venesection (because of severe cardiac disease or anaemia), chelation therapy with desferrioxamine either intermittently or continuously by infusion has been successful in removing iron.

**Screening of relatives**

In all cases of IHC all first-degree family members must be screened to detect early and asymptomatic disease. Serum ferritin is an excellent test with only occasional false-positives in hepatocellular necrosis and rare false-negatives in some family studies.

# Wilson's disease (hepatolenticular degeneration)

This is a very rare inborn error of copper metabolism that results in copper deposition in various organs to produce cirrhosis and degeneration of the basal ganglia of the brain. It is potentially treatable and all young patients with cirrhosis must be screened for this condition.

COPPER METABOLISM. Dietary copper is absorbed from the stomach and upper small intestine. It is transported to the liver loosely bound to albumin. Here it is incorporated into caeruloplasmin, a glycoprotein synthesized in the liver, and secreted into the blood. Copper is normally excreted in the bile.

## AETIOLOGY

It is inherited as an autosomal recessive gene located on chromosome 13. It occurs worldwide, particularly in countries where consanguinity is common. The basic problem is a failure to excrete copper but, although there is a low serum caeruloplasmin, the precise defect remains unknown.

## PATHOLOGY

The histology is not diagnostic and varies from that of CAH to macronodular cirrhosis. Stains for copper show a periportal distribution but this can be unreliable (see below). The basal ganglia are damaged and show cavitation, the kidneys show tubular degeneration, and erosions are seen in bones.

## CLINICAL FEATURES

Children usually present with hepatic problems, whereas young adults have more neurological problems, such as tremor, dysarthria, involuntary movements and eventually dementia (see p. 920).

Signs are of chronic liver disease with neurological signs of basal ganglia involvement. A specific sign is the Kayser–Fleischer ring, which is due to copper deposition in Descemet's membrane in the cornea. It appears as a greenish brown pigment at the corneoscleral junction just within the cornea. Identification of this ring frequently requires slit-lamp examination. It may be absent in young children.

## INVESTIGATION

The serum copper and caeruloplasmin are usually reduced but can be normal. The urinary copper is usually increased (100–1000 $\mu$g in 24 hours; normal levels <40 $\mu$g in 24 hours). The diagnosis depends on the measurement of the amount of copper in the liver, although high levels of copper are also found in the liver in chronic cholestasis. Measurement of $^{64}$Cu incorporation into the liver may be helpful. Haemolysis and anaemia may be present.

## TREATMENT

Long-term penicillamine, approximately 1 g daily, is effective in chelating copper and leads to clinical and biochemical improvement. Serious side-effects of the drug occur in 10% and include skin rashes, leucopenia and renal damage. Urine copper levels should be monitored. All siblings and children of patients should be screened. Homozygotes may have the above physical signs, Kayser–Fleischer rings and a low serum caeruloplasmin. Symptomless homozygous relatives should be treated.

## PROGNOSIS

Early diagnosis and effective treatment have improved the outlook. Neurological damage is, however, permanent. Death is from liver failure, bleeding varices or intercurrent infection.

## $\alpha_1$-Antitrypsin deficiency (see also p. 659)

A deficiency of $\alpha_1$-antitrypsin ($\alpha_1$AT) is sometimes associated with liver disease and pulmonary emphysema (particularly in smokers). $\alpha_1$AT is a glycoprotein and part of a family of protease inhibitors (Pi) that control various inflammatory cascades, e.g. complement (C1 inhibitor), coagulation (antithrombin). It is synthesized in the liver and comprises 90% of the serum $\alpha_1$-globulin seen on electrophoresis. The gene is located on chromosome 14. The genetic variants of $\alpha_1$AT are characterized by their electrophoretic mobilities as medium (M), slow (S) or very slow (Z). The normal genotype is PiMM, the homozygote for Z is PiZZ and the heterozygotes are PiMZ and PiSZ. S and Z variants are due to a single amino acid replacement of glutamic acid at positions 264 and 342 of the polypeptide, respectively, and this results in decreased synthesis and secretion of the normal protease inhibitor. S thus forms about 60% of that produced normally by M, whilst the Z variant forms only 15%.

$\alpha_1$AT is inherited as an autosomal dominant and 1 : 10 of northern Europeans carry a deficiency gene.

## CLINICAL FEATURES

The majority of patients with clinical disease have the PiZZ phenotype. Approximately 10–15% of these patients will develop cirrhosis usually over the age of 50 years and 75% will have respiratory problems. Approximately 5% of patients die of their liver disease.

## INVESTIGATION

The serum $\alpha_1$AT is low.

Liver biopsy. Periodic acid–Schiff (PAS)-positive, diastase-resistant globules are seen in periportal hepatocytes. These can be shown to be $\alpha_1$AT using immunodiagnostic techniques.

Phenotypes. PiM is associated with serum levels of $\alpha_1$AT of 2–4 g litre$^{-1}$. Homozygotes for the protease inhibitor Z (i.e. PiZZ) have low $\alpha_1$AT levels and are seriously affected with liver disease. Heterozygotes (e.g. PiSZ, PiMZ) exist and may develop signs of deficiency.

## TREATMENT

There is no treatment apart from dealing with the complications of liver disease. Patients with hepatic decompensation should be considered for liver transplantation. Patients should be advised to stop smoking (see p. 22).

## Alcoholic liver disease

This section gives the pathology and clinical features of liver disease. The amounts needed to produce liver damage, alcohol metabolism, and other clinical effects of alcohol are described on p. 173.

Ethanol is metabolized in the liver by two pathways (see p. 172) resulting in an increase in the NADH/NAD ratio. The altered redox potential results in increased hepatic fatty acid synthesis with decreased fatty acid oxidation, both events leading to accumulation of fatty acid that is then esterified to glycerides.

The changes in oxidation–reduction also impair carbohydrate and protein metabolism and are also the cause of the centrilobular necrosis of the hepatic acinus typical of alcohol damage.

Acetaldehyde is formed by the oxidation of ethanol and its effect on hepatic proteins may well be an important factor in producing liver cell damage. The exact mechanism of alcoholic hepatitis and cirrhosis is unknown, but since only 10–20% of people who drink excessively will suffer from cirrhosis, a genetic predisposition is proposed. Immunological mechanisms have also been proposed.

Alcohol can enhance the effects of toxic metabolites of drugs, e.g. paracetamol, on the liver, as it induces microsomal metabolism via the microsomal ethanol oxidizing system (MEOS).

## PATHOLOGY
Alcohol can produce a wide spectrum of liver disease from fatty change to hepatitis and cirrhosis.

### Fatty change
The metabolism of alcohol invariably produces fat in the liver, mainly in zone 3. This is minimal with small amounts of alcohol, but with larger amounts the cells become swollen with fat (steatosis) giving, eventually, a Swiss-cheese effect on haematoxylin and eosin stain. Steatosis can also be seen in obesity, diabetes, starvation and occasionally in chronic illness. There is no liver cell damage and therefore in general this is not precirrhotic. The fat disappears on stopping alcohol.

In some cases collagen is laid down around the central hepatic veins (perivenular fibrosis) and this can sometimes progress to cirrhosis without a preceding hepatitis.

### Alcoholic hepatitis
Here there is necrosis of liver cells and infiltration with polymorphonuclear leucocytes mainly in zone 3. A dense cytoplasmic material called a Mallory body is sometimes seen in hepatocytes. Steatosis is also frequently present and an established cirrhosis is often seen. Mallory bodies are suggestive of but not specific for alcoholic damage as they can also be found in other liver diseases, such as Wilson's disease and PBC. Alcoholic hepatitis usually goes on to become cirrhosis if alcohol consumption continues.

### Alcoholic cirrhosis
Destruction and fibrosis with regenerating nodules produces classically a micronodular cirrhosis; in later stages a macronodular pattern may be seen. There is bridging fibrosis between portal tracts and terminal hepatic veins. Fat may be present with the additional features of alcoholic hepatitis.

## CLINICAL FEATURES
### Fatty liver
There are often no symptoms or signs. Vague abdominal symptoms of nausea, vomiting and diarrhoea are due to the more general effects of alcohol on the gastrointestinal tract. Hepatomegaly, sometimes huge, can occur together with other features of chronic liver disease.

### Alcoholic hepatitis
The clinical features vary in degree:

THE PATIENT MAY BE WELL, with few symptoms, the hepatitis only being apparent on the liver biopsy in addition to fatty change.

MILD TO MODERATE SYMPTOMS OF ILL-HEALTH, occasionally with mild jaundice, may occur. Signs include all the features of chronic liver disease. Liver biochemistry is deranged and the diagnosis is made on liver histology.

IN THE SEVERE CASE, usually superimposed on patients with alcoholic cirrhosis, the patient is ill, with jaundice and ascites. Abdominal pain is frequently present, with a high fever associated with the liver necrosis. On examination there is deep jaundice, hepatomegaly, sometimes splenomegaly, and ascites with ankle oedema. The signs of chronic liver disease are also present.

### Alcoholic cirrhosis
This represents the final stage of liver disease from alcohol abuse. Nevertheless, patients can be very well with few symptoms. On examination, there are usually signs of chronic liver disease. The diagnosis is confirmed by liver biopsy.

Usually the patient presents with one of the complications of cirrhosis. In many cases there are features of alcohol dependency (see p. 983) as well as evidence of involvement of other symptoms, e.g. polyneuropathy.

## INVESTIGATION
### Fatty liver
An elevated MCV often indicates heavy drinking. Liver biochemistry shows mild abnormalities with elevation of both serum aminotransferase enzymes. The $\gamma$-GT level is a sensitive test for determining whether the patient is taking alcohol. With severe fatty infiltration, marked changes in all liver biochemical parameters can occur. Ultrasound or CT will demonstrate fatty infiltration as will liver histology.

### Alcoholic hepatitis
Investigations show a leucocytosis with markedly deranged liver biochemistry with elevated:
- Serum bilirubin
- Serum AST and ALT
- Serum alkaline phosphatase
- Prothrombin time

A low serum albumin may also be found. Rarely, hyperlipidaemia with haemolysis (Zieve's syndrome) may occur.

The prolonged PT makes liver biopsy impossible in the severe form. In these severe cases the mortality is at least 50%, and with a PT twice the normal, progressive encephalopathy and renal failure, the mortality approaches 90%.

### Alcoholic cirrhosis
Investigations are as for cirrhosis in general.

## MANAGEMENT AND PROGNOSIS

### General management

Patients should be advised to stop drinking. Delirium tremens (withdrawal symptoms) should be treated with diazepam or chlormethiazole. Bed rest with a diet high in protein and vitamin supplements is given. Dietary protein may have to be limited because of encephalopathy. Follow-up of patients with alcoholic liver disease show that apart from highly motivated groups, most patients continue to abuse alcohol.

### Fatty liver

In all but the mildest cases the patient is advised to stop drinking; the fat will disappear and the liver biochemistry usually returns to normal. Small amounts of alcohol can be drunk subsequently as long as patients are aware of the problems and can control their consumption.

### Alcoholic hepatitis

In severe cases the patient is confined to bed. Treatment for encephalopathy and ascites is commenced. Patients should be fed preferably via a fine-bore nasogastric tube or sometimes intravenously. Nitrogen solutions enriched with branched-chain amino acids, e.g. leucine, isoleucine and valine, may be helpful. Vitamins B and C should be given by injection. Corticosteroids are often given, but controlled trials have shown them to be of little benefit.

Patients are advised to stop drinking for life, as this is undoubtedly a precirrhotic condition. The prognosis is variable and, despite abstinence, the liver disease is progressive in many patients. Conversely, a few patients continue to drink heavily without developing cirrhosis.

### Alcoholic cirrhosis

The management of cirrhosis is described on p. 261.

Again, all patients are advised to stop drinking for life. Abstinence from alcohol results in an improvement in prognosis, with a 5-year survival of 90%, but with continued drinking this falls to 60%. With advanced disease (i.e. jaundice, ascites and haematemesis) the 5-year survival rate falls to 35%, with most of the deaths occurring in the first year. Liver transplantation is being widely used in some countries with good survival figures. Patients must demonstrate their ability to abstain from alcohol.

HCC is a complication in men in approximately 10–15% of cases.

# Budd–Chiari syndrome

In this condition there is obstruction to the venous outflow of the liver owing to occlusion of the hepatic vein. In one-third of patients the cause is unknown, but specific causes include hypercoagulability states, such as polycythaemia vera, taking the contraceptive pill, or leukaemia. Other causes include occlusion of the hepatic vein owing to posterior abdominal wall sarcomas, renal or adrenal tumours, HCC, hepatic infections (e.g. hydatid cyst), congenital venous webs, radiotherapy, or trauma to the liver.

The acute form presents with abdominal pain, nausea, vomiting, tender hepatomegaly and ascites. The liver histology shows centrilobular congestion with hepatocyte atrophy. In the chronic form there is enlargement of the liver (particularly the caudate lobe), mild jaundice, ascites, a negative hepatojugular reflex, and splenomegaly with portal hypertension.

## INVESTIGATION

Investigations show a high protein content in the ascitic fluid and characteristic liver histology. Ultrasound, CT or MRI will demonstrate hepatic vein occlusion and an enlarged caudate lobe which has a different venous drainage; there may be compression of the inferior vena cava. Venography may demonstrate the thrombosed vein. Pulsed Doppler sonography or a colour Doppler are useful as they show abnormalities in the direction of flow in the hepatic vein.

## TREATMENT

Ascites should be treated as well as any underlying cause, e.g. polycythaemia. Congenital webs should be resected surgically. A side-to-side portocaval or splenorenal anastomosis may decompress the congested liver, with considerable improvement in the clinical state of the patient. A peritoneal–jugular LeVeen shunt for resistant ascites is occasionally useful. Liver transplantation is becoming the treatment of choice.

## DIFFERENTIAL DIAGNOSIS

A similar clinical picture can be produced by inferior vena caval obstruction, right-sided cardiac failure or constrictive pericarditis, and appropriate investigations should be performed.

## PROGNOSIS

The prognosis depends on the aetiology, but some patients can survive for several years.

# Veno-occlusive disease

This is due to injury of the hepatic veins and presents clinically like the Budd–Chiari syndrome. It was originally described in Jamaica, where the ingestion of the toxic pyrrolizidine alkaloids in bush tea (made from plants of the genera *Senecio, Heliotropium* and *Crotolaria*) caused damage to the hepatic veins. It can be seen in other parts of the world. It is also seen as a complication of chemotherapy and total body irradiation before allogeneic bone transplantation. The development of veno-occlusive disease after transplantation carries a high mortality. Treatment is supportive with control of ascites and hepatocellular failure.

# Fibropolycystic diseases

These diseases are usually inherited and lead to the presence of cysts or fibrosis in the liver, kidney and occasionally the pancreas, and other organs.

## Polycystic disease of the liver

### Adult

This usually presents in middle age with abdominal swelling or right hypochondrial discomfort. It can also be detected by ultrasound scanning or may only be discovered at autopsy. There may or may not be hepatomegaly and bilateral irregular palpable kidneys. It is inherited as an autosomal dominant. The cysts are of variable size and consist of thin-walled cavities containing clear fluid or altered blood. Liver function is normal and complications such as oesophageal varices are very rare. The prognosis is excellent and is often dependent on whether the kidneys are involved.

### Child

Childhood polycystic disease is inherited in a different way from the adult type. It is an autosomal recessive condition presenting in the first few months of life. Renal involvement is common, with cystic changes in the renal tubules.

## Congenital hepatic fibrosis

In this rare condition the liver architecture is normal but there are broad collagenous fibrous bands extending from the portal tracts. It is often inherited as an autosomal recessive condition but can also occur sporadically. It usually presents in childhood with hepatosplenomegaly, and portal hypertension is common. It may present later in life and can be misdiagnosed as cirrhosis. A wedge biopsy of the liver may be required to confirm the diagnosis. The outlook is good and the condition should be distinguished from cirrhosis. Patients who bleed do well after variceal sclerotherapy or a portocaval anastomosis because of their good liver function.

## Congenital intrahepatic biliary dilatation (Caroli's disease)

In this rare, non-familial disease there are saccular dilatations of the intrahepatic or extrahepatic ducts. It can present at any age (although usually in childhood) with fever, abdominal pain and recurrent attacks of cholangitis with Gram-negative septicaemia. Jaundice and portal hypertension are absent. Diagnosis is by ultrasound, PTC or ERCP.

## Solitary non-parasitic cysts

These are rare and probably a variant of polycystic disease.

# Liver abscess

## Pyogenic abscess

These abscesses are uncommon, but may be single or multiple. The commonest cause used to be a portal pyaemia from intra-abdominal sepsis, e.g. appendicitis or perforations, but now in many cases the aetiology is not known. Biliary sepsis, particularly in the elderly, is a common cause. Other causes include trauma, bacteraemia and direct extension from, for example, a perinephric abscess.

The commonest organism found is *E. coli*. Other organisms include *Streptococcus faecalis, Proteus vulgaris* and *Staphylococcus aureus. Streptococcus milleri* and anaerobic organisms such as *Bacteroides* are now more frequently seen. Often the infection is mixed. Failure to culture an organism may be due to previous antibiotic therapy or inadequate anaerobic culture.

### CLINICAL FEATURES

Some patients are not acutely ill and present with malaise lasting several days or even months. Others can present with fever, rigors, anorexia, vomiting, weight loss and abdominal pain. In these patients a Gram-negative septicaemia with shock can occur. On examination there may be little to find. Alternatively, the patient may be toxic, febrile and jaundiced. In such patients, the liver is tender and enlarged and there may be signs of a pleural effusion or a pleural rub in the right lower chest.

### INVESTIGATION

Patients are often investigated as a 'pyrexia of unknown origin' (PUO) and in the mild chronic case most investigations will be normal. Often the only clue to the diagnosis is a raised serum alkaline phosphatase.

The serum bilirubin is raised in 25%. There is a normochromic normocytic anaemia, usually accompanied by a polymorphonuclear leucocytosis. The serum AP and ESR are often raised. The serum $B_{12}$ is very high, as vitamin $B_{12}$ is stored in and subsequently released from the liver.

Blood cultures are positive in only 30% of cases.

### Imaging

Ultrasound is useful for detecting fluid-filled lesions. A CT scan is of value for further localization. A chest X-ray will show elevation of the right hemidiaphragm with a pleural effusion in the severe cases.

### MANAGEMENT

Aspiration of the abscess should be attempted under ultrasound control. Antibiotics should initially cover Gram-positive, Gram-negative and anaerobic organisms until the causative organism is identified.

Further drainage via a large-bore needle under ultrasound control or surgically should almost always be performed if a localized abscess is found. The underlying cause must also be treated.

## PROGNOSIS

The overall mortality depends on the nature of the underlying pathology and has been reduced to approximately 16% with needle aspiration and antibiotics. A unilocular abscess in the right lobe has a better prognosis. Scattered multiple abscesses have a very high mortality, with only one in five patients surviving.

## Amoebic abscess (see p. 72)

This condition occurs worldwide and must be considered in patients travelling from endemic areas. *Entamoeba histolytica* (see p. 73) can be carried from the bowel to the liver in the portal venous system. Portal inflammation results, with the development of multiple microabscesses and eventually single or multiple large abscesses.

Clinically the onset is usually gradual but may be sudden. There is fever, anorexia, weight loss and malaise. There is often no history of dysentery. On examination the patient looks ill and has tender hepatomegaly and signs of an effusion or consolidation in the base of the right side of the chest. Jaundice is unusual.

## INVESTIGATION

This is as for pyogenic abscess, plus:

SEROLOGICAL TESTS FOR AMOEBA, e.g. haemagglutination inhibition, amoebic complement-fixation test, ELISA. These are always positive, particularly if there are bowel symptoms, and remain positive after a clinical cure and therefore do not indicate current disease. A repeat negative test, however, is good evidence against an amoebic abscess.

DIAGNOSTIC ASPIRATION OF FLUID looking like anchovy sauce.

## TREATMENT

Metronidazole 800 mg three times daily is given for 10 days. Some physicians recommend repeated aspirations in addition. Surgical drainage is used in patients failing to respond, in multiple and large abscesses, and in those with abscesses in the left lobe of the liver.

## COMPLICATIONS

Complications include rupture, secondary infection and septicaemia.

## *Other infections of the liver*

## Schistosomiasis (see p. 82)

*Schistosoma mansoni* and *S. japonicum* affect the liver, but *S. haematobium* rarely does so. During their life-cycle the ova reach the liver via the venous system and obstruct the portal branches, producing granulomas, fibrosis and inflammation but not cirrhosis. Clinically there is hepatosplenomegaly and presinusoidal portal hypertension, which is particularly severe with *S. mansoni*.

Investigations show a raised alkaline phosphatase, and ova can be found in the stools (centrifuged deposits) and in rectal and liver biopsies. Skin tests and other immunological tests often have false results and may also be positive because of past infection.

Treatment is with praziquantel, but fibrosis still remains with a potential of portal hypertension.

## Hydatid disease (see p. 86)

Cysts caused by *Echinococcus granulosus* are single or multiple. They usually occur in the lower part of the right lower lobe. The cyst has three layers: an outside layer derived from the host, an intermediate laminated layer, and an inner germinal layer that buds off brood capsules to form daughter cysts.

Clinically there may be no symptoms or a dull ache and swelling in the right hypochondrium. Investigations show a peripheral eosinophilia and usually a positive hydatid complement-fixation test or haemagglutination. The Casoni skin test is no longer used because of its lack of specificity. Plain abdominal X-ray may show calcification of the outer coat of the cyst. Ultrasound and CT scan demonstrate a space-occupying lesion and may show diagnostic daughter cysts.

Fine-needle aspiration under ultrasound control with chemotherapeutic cover is now used therapeutically. Surgery can be performed with removal of the cyst intact if possible after first sterilizing the cyst with formalin or alcohol. Medical treatment, e.g. with albendazole, which penetrates into large cysts, can result in reduction of cyst size. Chronic calcified cysts can be left.

Complications include rupture, secondary infection and involvement of other organs.

The prognosis without any complications is good, although there is always the risk of rupture. Preventative measures are important, including deworming of pet dogs and prevention of pets from eating infected carcasses where possible.

## Acquired immunodeficiency syndrome (see p. 96)

The liver is often involved but rarely causes significant morbidity or mortality. HIV itself is probably not the cause of the liver abnormalities. The following are seen:

PRE-EXISTING/COINCIDENTAL VIRAL HEPATITIS (HBV, HCV, HDV)

NEOPLASIA—Kaposi's sarcoma and non-Hodgkin's lymphoma

OPPORTUNISTIC INFECTION, e.g. *Mycobacterium tuberculosis*, *Mycobacterium avium intracellulare*, *Cryptococcus*, *Candida albicans*

DRUG HEPATOTOXICITY

SCLEROSING CHOLANGITIS (see p. 284)

Clinical hepatomegaly is common in 60% of patients.

# Jaundice in pregnancy

Liver function is not impaired in pregnancy. Any liver disease from whatever cause can occur incidentally and coincide with pregnancy. For example, viral hepatitis accounts for 40% of all cases of jaundice during pregnancy. Pregnancy does not necessarily exacerbate established liver disease, but it is uncommon for women with advanced liver disease to conceive.

The following changes take place:
1 Plasma and blood volumes increase during pregnancy but the hepatic blood flow remains constant.
2 The proportion of cardiac output delivered to the liver therefore falls from 35% to 29% in late pregnancy; drug metabolism can thus be affected.
3 The size of the liver remains constant.
4 Liver biochemistry remains unchanged apart from a rise in serum alkaline phosphatase from the placenta (up to three to four times) and a decrease in total protein and $\gamma$-globulins.
5 Triglycerides and cholesterol levels rise, and caeruloplasmin, transferrin, $\alpha_1$-AT and fibrinogen levels are elevated due to increased hepatic synthesis.

There are a number of liver diseases that complicate pregnancy.

## Hyperemesis gravidarum

Pathological vomiting during pregnancy can be associated with liver dysfunction and jaundice. This is never severe and resolves when vomiting subsides. Liver histology (biopsy seldom indicated) shows cholestasis.

## Pre-eclampsia and eclampsia

Pre-eclampsia complicates 10% of pregnancies of which 10% have deranged liver biochemistry (usually minor). In more severe cases disseminated intravascular coagulation (DIC) occurs. The HELLP syndrome refers to a combination of haemolysis, elevated liver enzymes and a low platelet count and can occur in association with pre-eclampsia.

If eclampsia supervenes, there is epigastric pain, nausea and vomiting with severe hepatic damage; fetal and maternal death can occur. Liver histology shows fibrin deposition, ischaemic necrosis and periportal haemorrhage thought to result from vasospasm. Hepatic haemorrhage and rupture are very rare. Urgent delivery of the fetus is required along with laparotomy to repair damage.

## Intrahepatic cholestasis of pregnancy

This condition of unknown aetiology presents usually with pruritus in the third trimester. It has a familial tendency and there is a higher prevalence in Scandinavia, Chile and Bolivia. Jaundice is not a prerequisite for diagnosis and the AST may be normal or rise three to four

times. Liver biopsy is not indicated but would show centrilobular cholestasis. Treatment is symptomatic with cholestyramine in high doses (up to 24 g daily). Prognosis is excellent and the condition resolves after delivery. Recurrent cholestasis may occur during subsequent pregnancies or with the ingestion of oestrogen containing oral contraceptive pills.

## Acute fatty liver of pregnancy

This is a rare, serious condition of unknown aetiology. It presents in the last trimester with symptoms of fulminant hepatitis, i.e. jaundice, vomiting, abdominal pain, possibly haematemesis and coma. Laboratory investigations show hepatocellular damage, hyperuricaemia and possible DIC. Liver biopsy is contraindicated but histology shows fine droplets of fat (microvesicles) in the liver cells with little necrosis. CT scanning is non-invasive and shows a low density of the liver due to the high fat content. Immediate delivery of the child may save both baby and mother. Early diagnosis and treatment has reduced the mortality to less than 20%. Treatment is as for acute liver failure.

# Liver tumours

The commonest liver tumour is a secondary (metastatic) tumour (Fig. 5.19), particularly from the gastrointestinal tract, breast or bronchus. Clinical features are variable but usually include hepatomegaly. MRI is comparable to CT at detecting metastases. However, ultrasound is cheaper and more readily available. Primary liver tumours may be benign or malignant. The commonest are malignant.

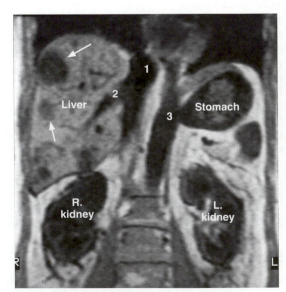

**Fig. 5.19**  MRI scan showing liver metastases (arrows). 1, inferior vena cava; 2, hepatic vein; 3, aorta.

# MALIGNANT TUMOURS

## Hepatocellular carcinoma (HCC)

This is one of the commonest cancers worldwide, although it is uncommon in the Western Hemisphere.

### AETIOLOGY

Carriers of HBV and HCV have an extremely high risk of developing HCC. In areas where HBV is prevalent, 90% of patients with this cancer are hepatitis B positive. Cirrhosis is present in over 80% of these patients. The development of HCC is related to the integration of viral DNA into the genome of the host hepatocyte. Primary liver cancer is also associated with other forms of cirrhosis, e.g. alcoholic cirrhosis and haemochromatosis. Males are affected more than females; this may account for the high incidence seen in haemochromatosis and low incidence in PBC. Other suggested aetiological factors are aflatoxin (a metabolite of a fungus found in groundnuts) and androgenic steroids, and there is an association with the contraceptive pill.

### PATHOLOGY

The tumour is either single or occurs as multiple nodules throughout the liver. Histologically it consists of cells resembling hepatocytes. It can metastasize via the hepatic or portal veins to the lymph nodes, bones and lungs.

### CLINICAL FEATURES

HCC usually presents below the age of 50 years. The clinical features include weight loss, anorexia, fever, an ache in the right hypochondrium and ascites. The rapid development of these features in a cirrhotic patient is suggestive of HCC. On examination, an enlarged, irregular, tender liver may be felt.

### INVESTIGATION

Serum $\alpha$-fetoprotein is raised. Ultrasound or radioisotope scans show large filling defects in 90% of cases. A liver biopsy, particularly under ultrasonic guidance, is performed for diagnosis.

### TREATMENT

Surgical resection is occasionally possible. Chemotherapy and radiotherapy are unhelpful.

### PROGNOSIS

Survival is seldom more than 6 months.

## Cholangiocarcinoma

Cholangiocarcinomas can be extrahepatic (see p. 285) or intrahepatic. Intrahepatic adenocarcinomas arising from the bile ducts account for approximately 10% of primary tumours. They are not associated with cirrhosis or hepatitis B. In the Far East they may be associated with infestation with *Clonorchis sinensis*. The clinical features are similar to primary HCC except that jaundice is frequent with hilar tumours. Treatment is unsuccessful and patients usually die within 6 months.

# BENIGN TUMOURS

The commonest benign tumour is a haemangioma. This is usually found incidentally on ultrasound or CT and requires no treatment. Hepatic adenomas are associated with oral contraceptives. They can present with abdominal pain or intraperitoneal bleeding. Resection is only required for symptomatic patients.

# Miscellaneous conditions of the liver

## Reye's syndrome

This syndrome is of unknown aetiology but has been associated with aspirin consumption in childhood. It consists of an acute encephalopathy with cerebral oedema and diffuse microvesicular fatty infiltration of the liver. It occurs mainly in children and the mortality rate is 50%.

## Benign recurrent intrahepatic cholestasis

This condition often presents in children and consists of bouts of cholestatic jaundice with pruritus. Jaundice may last for weeks or months. There is no treatment; cholestyramine 12 g daily may help relieve the itching.

## Indian childhood cirrhosis

This condition of children is seen in the Indian subcontinent. The cause is unknown. Eventually there is development of a micronodular cirrhosis with excess copper in the liver.

## Hepatic porphyrias

These are dealt with on p. 866.

## Cystic fibrosis (see p. 665)

This disease mainly affects the lung and pancreas, but patients can develop fatty liver, cholestasis and cirrhosis. The aetiology of the liver involvement is unclear.

# Drugs and the liver

## Drug metabolism

The liver is the major site of drug metabolism. Drugs are converted from fat-soluble to water-soluble substances that can be excreted in the urine or bile. This metabolism of drugs is mediated by a group of mixed-function enzymes, including cytochrome P450, located on the smooth endoplasmic reticulum of the liver cell. It takes place in two stages:

PHASE I METABOLISM involves oxidation, reduction or demethylation of the drug.

PHASE II METABOLISM involves the conjugation of the derivatives produced in Phase I with glucuronide, sulphate and glutathione. These conjugates are excreted in the urine and bile as they cannot be reabsorbed by renal tubular or bile ductular cells.

### Factors affecting drug metabolism

THE MICROSOMAL ENZYME SYSTEM. The *speed* of metabolism of drugs is dependent on the microsomal enzyme system. Certain drugs, e.g. phenytoin, barbiturates and alcohol, can themselves increase the activity of these enzymes such as cytochrome P450, i.e. cause 'enzyme induction', and are known as 'inducing agents'. Therapy with any of these drugs will produce increased metabolism of the drug and consequently a reduction in its effectiveness. Equally, if two drugs are metabolized by the same microsomal enzymes, metabolism of both drugs will be reduced, prolonging their actions.

ROUTE OF ADMINISTRATION. Many drugs are partially inactivated on passage through the liver (first-pass effect). If this is pronounced, drugs taken orally are inactive.

LIVER BLOOD FLOW. The rate of removal of the drug from the liver is influenced by the liver blood flow.

COMPETITIVE INHIBITION. Some drugs compete with bilirubin at various stages:
- Uptake by the liver, e.g. rifampicin
- Conjugation, e.g. novobiocin
- Excretion into the bile canaliculus, e.g. oral contraceptives

## Drug hepatotoxicity

Many drugs impair liver function and drugs should always be considered as a cause when mildly abnormal liver tests are found. Damage to the liver by drugs is usually classified as being either predictable (or dose related) or non-predictable (not dose related) (see p. 737). This classification should not be used rigidly, as there is considerable overlap and many mechanisms may be involved in the production of damage.

### Biochemical pathways

When a small amount of hepatotoxic drug whose effect is dose dependent, e.g. paracetamol, is ingested, a large proportion of it undergoes conjugation with glucuronide and sulphate, whilst the remainder is metabolized by microsomal enzymes to produce toxic derivatives that are immediately detoxified by conjugation with glutathione. If larger doses are ingested, the former pathway becomes saturated and the toxic derivative is produced at a faster rate. Once the hepatic glutathione is depleted large amounts of the toxic metabolite accumulate and produce damage.

The 'predictability' of drugs to produce damage can, however, be affected by metabolic events preceding their ingestion. For example, chronic alcohol abusers may become more susceptible to liver damage because of the enzyme-inducing effects of alcohol, or ill or starving patients may become susceptible because of the depletion of hepatic glutathione produced by starvation. Many other factors such as environmental or genetic effects may be involved in determining the 'susceptibility' of certain patients to certain drugs.

### Immunological mechanisms

These can be involved in the production of hepatic cell damage by certain drugs. The toxic metabolite produced by the microsomal enzymes may bind to the liver cell protein, thereby altering its antigenicity. The production of antibody against this will lead to immunologically mediated damage. An example of this mechanism is halothane-induced hepatic necrosis, which requires prior sensitization of the patient to halothane, although direct toxicity may also play a part.

Other pointers for the involvement of immunological mechanisms are the development of skin rashes, fever and arthralgia (serum-sickness syndrome) following ingestion of certain drugs. Eosinophilia and circulating immune complexes and antibodies may occasionally be detected.

## Hepatic damage

The type of damage produced by various drugs is shown in Table 5.14. The diagnosis of these conditions is usually by exclusion of other causes. Most reactions occur within 3 months of starting the drug. Monitoring liver biochemistry in patients on long-term treatment, e.g. antituberculosis therapy, is advisable. If a drug is suspected of causing hepatic damage, it should be stopped immediately. Liver biopsy is of limited help in confirming the diagnosis but occasionally hepatic eosinophilia or granulomas may be seen. Sometimes diagnostic challenge with subtherapeutic doses of the drug is required after the liver biochemistry has returned to normal to prove the diagnosis.

## Individual drugs

### Paracetamol

In high doses paracetamol produces liver cell necrosis (see above). The toxic metabolite binds irreversibly to liver cell membranes. Overdosage is discussed on p. 752.

### Halothane

This commonly used anaesthetic agent rarely produces a hepatitis in patients having repeated exposures. The mechanism is thought to be a hypersensitivity reaction. An unexplained fever occurs approximately 10 days after the second or subsequent halothane anaesthetic and is

| Types of liver damage | Drugs | |
|---|---|---|
| Zone 3 necrosis | Carbon tetrachloride<br>Paracetamol<br>Salicylates | Piroxicam<br>Cocaine |
| Zone 1 necrosis | Ferrous sulphate | |
| Microvesicular fat | Sodium valproate<br>Tetracyclines | |
| 'Alcoholic' hepatitis<br>(phospholipidosis) | Nifedipine<br>Amiodarone<br>Synthetic oestrogens | |
| Fibrosis | Methotrexate<br>Other cytotoxic agents<br>Arsenic | Vitamin A<br>Retinoids |
| Vascular<br>Sinusoidal dilatation | Contraceptive drugs<br>Anabolic steroids<br>Azathioprine | |
| Pelioses hepatis | Oral contraceptives<br>Anabolic steroids<br>Danazol | Azathioprine |
| Veno-occlusive | Pyrrolizidine alkaloids (*Senecio* in bush tea)<br>Cytotoxics—cyclophosphamide,<br>azathioprine | |
| Acute hepatitis | Isoniazid     Methyldopa<br>Rifampicin    Atenolol<br>            Enalapril<br>            Verapamil | Halothane<br>Ketoconazole<br>Cytotoxic drugs<br>Disulfiram<br>Niacin |
| Chronic active hepatitis | Methyldopa<br>Nitrofurantoin<br>Fenofibrate<br>Isoniazid | |
| General hypersensitivity | Sulphonamides e.g. Sulphasalazine<br>                    Co-trimoxazole<br>                    Fansidar<br><br>Penicillins e.g. Flucloxacillin, ampicillin, amoxycillin, co-amoxiclar<br><br>NSAIDs e.g. Salicylates<br>           Diclofenac<br><br>Allopurinol<br><br>Antithyroid e.g. Propylthiouracil<br>                Carbimazole<br><br>Quinine<br>Diltiazem<br><br>Anticonvulsants e.g. Phenytoin | |
| Canalicular cholestasis | Sex hormones | Cyclosporin |
| Hepato-canalicular<br>cholestasis | Chlorpromazine<br>Erythromycin<br>Nitrofurantoin<br>Azathioprine | Haloperidol<br>Cimetidine/ranitidine<br>Imipramine<br>Oral hypoglycaemics<br>Dextropropoxyphene |
| Biliary sludge | Ceftriaxone | |
| Sclerosing cholangitis | Hepatic arterial infusion of 5-fluorouracil<br>Thiabendazole into hydatid cysts | |
| Hepatic tumours | Pills with high hormone content<br>(adenomas) | |
| Hepatocellular carcinoma | Contraceptive pill<br>Danazol | |

NSAIDs, non-steroidal anti-inflammatory drugs.

**Table 5.14** Some drugs causing types of liver damage.

followed by jaundice, typically with a hepatic picture. Most patients recover spontaneously but there is a high mortality in severe cases. There are no chronic sequelae.

### Steroids

Cholestasis is caused by natural and synthetic oestrogens as well as methyltestosterone. These agents interfere with canalicular biliary flow and cause a pure cholestasis. Cholestasis is rare with the contraceptive pill because of the low dosage used. However, the contraceptive pill is associated with an increased incidence of gallstones, hepatic adenomas (rarely HCCs), the Budd–Chiari syndrome and peliosis hepatis. The latter condition, which also occurs with anabolic steroids, consists of dilatation of the hepatic sinusoids to form blood-filled lakes.

### Phenothiazines

Phenothiazines, e.g. chlorpromazine, can produce a cholestatic picture owing to a hypersensitivity reaction. It occurs in 1% of patients, usually within 4 weeks of starting the drug. Typically it is associated with a fever and eosinophilia. Recovery occurs on stopping the drug.

### Antituberculous chemotherapy

Isoniazid produces elevated aminotransferases in 10–20% of patients. Hepatic necrosis with jaundice occurs in a smaller percentage. The hepatotoxicity of isoniazid appears to be related to acetylator status, as the damage is due to the metabolites.

Rifampicin produces a hepatitis, usually within 3 weeks of starting the drug, particularly in patients on high doses.

Pyrazinamide produces abnormal liver biochemical tests and, rarely, liver cell necrosis.

## Drug prescribing in patients with liver disease

The metabolism of drugs is impaired in severe liver disease (with jaundice and ascites) as the removal of many drugs depends on liver blood flow and the integrity of the hepatocyte. In general, therefore, the effect of drugs is prolonged by liver disease and also by cholestasis. This is further accentuated by portosystemic shunting, which diminishes the first-pass extraction of drugs. With hypoproteinaemia there is decreased protein binding of some drugs and bilirubin competes with many drugs for the binding sites on serum albumin. In patients with portosystemic encephalopathy, care must be taken in prescribing drugs with a central depressant action.

# THE GALLBLADDER AND BILIARY SYSTEM

The main cause of disease of the gallbladder and biliary tract is gallstones. The structure, formation and function of bile is discussed on pp. 237 and 239.

# Gallstones

## Prevalence of gallstones

Gallstones are present in 10–20% of the population in the Western Hemisphere, but the exact prevalence is unknown. There is a geographical variation. Gallstones are rare in the Far East and Africa and very common in native North Americans and in Chile and Sweden. They occur twice as frequently in young women than in men but this difference decreases with increasing age.

## Types of gallstones

Gallstones can be divided into those composed of cholesterol and those composed of bile pigment. Cholesterol stones, which account for 80% of all gallstones in the Western Hemisphere, contain more than 70% cholesterol, often with some bile pigment and calcium (mixed stones). Pure cholesterol stones are often solitary.

### Cholesterol gallstones

Cholesterol is partly derived from dietary sources. In addition, it is synthesized, chiefly in the liver, but also in the small intestine, skin and adrenals. The rate-limiting step in cholesterol synthesis is $\beta$-hydroxy-$\beta$- methyl-glutaryl-CoA (HMG-CoA) reductase, which catalyses the first step, i.e. the conversion of acetate to mevalonate. The cholesterol formed is cosecreted with phospholipids into the biliary caniliculus as unilamellar vesicles.

Cholesterol stones only develop in bile that has an excess of cholesterol relative to bile salts and phospholipids (supersaturated bile). This could occur because of excess of cholesterol or because of a decrease in bile salts. There is a reduced bile salt pool in some patients with cholesterol gallstones and the pool circulates more frequently. This may account for the reduction in the rate-limiting cholesterol-7$\alpha$-hydroxylase found in some patients (feedback inhibition).

Diminished bile salt synthesis is not the only cause of supersaturated bile; there appears to be an increase in HMG-CoA reductase with an increase in cholesterol secretion into bile in some patients.

In supersaturated bile the bile acids solubilize phospholipids from the unilamellar vesicles more than cholesterol. This results in unstable vesicles which are more prone to aggregate, fuse and form multilamellar vesicles. It is from these vesicles that cholesterol crystals nucleate. Factors other than cholesterol saturation are required to form gallstones, as supersaturated bile is found in normal subjects during an overnight fast. The rate of cholesterol crystallization and gallbladder function also play a role. Glycoproteins in bile promote nucleation of cholesterol crystals, leading to stone formation, but why this occurs only in bile from patients with gallstones is unclear. It may depend on the presence or absence of solubilizing factors. The role of infection is unknown. Definite risk factors for gallstones are shown in Table 5.15.

Age
Sex (F > M)
Multiparity
Obesity
Diet, e.g. high in animal fat
Drugs, e.g. contraceptive pill
Ileal disease or resection
Diabetes
Acromegaly treated with octreotide

**Table 5.15**  Risk factors for cholesterol gallstones.

### Bile pigment stones

Black pigment stones contain calcium salts of bilirubin, phosphate and carbonate in addition to bilirubin polymers and mucin glycoproteins. The biliary lipids are normal. These stones form in the gallbladder and are seen in patients with chronic haemolysis, e.g. hereditary spherocytosis and sickle cell disease, where there is an increase in bilirubin, and also in cirrhosis. In other situations the pathogenesis is unclear.

Brown pigment stones have layers of cholesterol, calcium salts of fatty acids (mainly palmitate) and calcium bilirubinate. They tend to form in the common bile duct after cholecystectomy and are due to precipitation of bilirubin with calcium. They are also found with strictures, sclerosing cholangitis and Caroli's syndrome. In the Far East these stones are associated with parasitic infestation of the biliary tract.

## Clinical presentation of gallstones
(Fig. 5.20)

The majority of gallstones (approximately 80%) remain in the gall bladder and are asymptomatic.

A gallstone may impact in the neck of the gallbladder or in the cystic duct, giving biliary pain or acute cholecystitis.

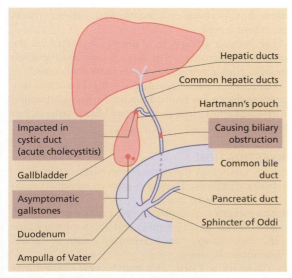

Hepatic ducts

Common hepatic ducts

Hartmann's pouch

Impacted in cystic duct (acute cholecystitis)

Causing biliary obstruction

Gallbladder

Common bile duct

Asymptomatic gallstones

Pancreatic duct

Duodenum

Sphincter of Oddi

Ampulla of Vater

**Fig. 5.20**  Clinical presentation of gallstones.

Finally, gallstones may pass into the common bile duct, giving rise to biliary obstruction that produces severe biliary pain and sometimes cholestatic jaundice. Bacterial infection can occur and produce cholangitis.

Clinically the type of pain is similar in the above situation. It occurs in the epigastrium and right hypochondrium and is not colicky. Biliary 'colic' therefore is a misnomer.

Rarely a gallstone may perforate through the wall of an inflamed gallbladder into the intestine, producing a fistula.

Gallstones do not give rise to any other symptom complex, and the idea that they produce indigestion, chronic right hypochondrial pain or intolerance to fatty food is based on a false correlation. Gallstones and upper abdominal symptoms are both common, so great care must be taken to establish that the two are truly related. Fair, fat, fertile females of 40 years of age have the same chance of having gallstones as the rest of the general population (10–20%). Thus, if they are investigated regardless of symptoms, gallstones will obviously be seen frequently by chance alone.

## Asymptomatic (silent) gallstones

Gallstones may be discovered accidentally when a patient is being investigated for some other reason. They require no treatment since the natural history is for them to remain asymptomatic, with only approximately 18% of patients having symptoms over a 15-year period.

## Acute cholecystitis

### PATHOPHYSIOLOGY

In over 90% of cases the gallbladder contains gallstones. Initially there is obstruction to the neck of the gallbladder or the cystic duct by an impacted stone, leading to distension and inflammation. The inflammation is usually sterile, but within 24 hours gut organisms can be cultured from the gallbladder. Occasionally the inflammation may be mild and quickly subsides, sometimes leaving a gallbladder distended by mucus (mucocele). In this situation the patient may only have slight abdominal pain with a palpable gallbladder.

More commonly, however, the inflammation is more severe, involving the whole wall and giving rise to localized peritonitis and acute pain. Occasionally the gallbladder can become distended by pus (an empyema) and rarely an acute gangrenous cholecystitis occurs with perforation and a more generalized peritonitis.

### CLINICAL FEATURES

The disease can occur at any age. The main symptoms are severe pain in the epigastrium and right hypochondrium. The pain is continuous, increasing in intensity over 24 hours. It can radiate to the back and shoulder. It may be accompanied by nausea and vomiting. Mild jaundice occurs in 20% of cases owing to accompanying common duct stones or to surrounding oedema occluding the common hepatic duct.

## EXAMINATION

The patient is usually ill with a fever and shallow respirations. Right hypochondrial tenderness is present, being worse on inspiration (Murphy's sign). There is guarding and rebound tenderness.

## INVESTIGATION

1 *Blood count.* A moderate leucocytosis is found.
2 *Biochemistry.* The serum bilirubin, alkaline phosphatase and AST may be slightly raised.
3 *Ultrasound examination* (Fig. 5.21). The detection of gallstones alone is insufficient for a diagnosis of acute cholecystitis. Additional criteria are:
   (a) Sonographic Murphy's sign (focal tenderness directly over the visualized gallbladder)
   (b) Gallbladder wall thickening—not specific for acute disease
   (c) Distension of gallbladder
   (d) The presence of biliary sludge
4 *HIDA scintiscan.* This is valuable and shows blockage of the cystic duct with the bile duct, but not the gallbladder, being visualized.
Ultrasound and HIDA scintiscans have a similar accuracy and the technique performed will depend on local facilities.
5 *X-ray.* A plain abdominal X-ray shows gallstones in 10% of cases; this is not useful diagnostically.

## DIFFERENTIAL DIAGNOSIS

The differential diagnosis includes other abdominal emergencies, such as a perforated peptic ulcer, retrocaecal appendicitis and acute pancreatitis. Right basal pneumonia and myocardial infarction must also be considered.

## MANAGEMENT

The majority of patients improve with conservative management consisting of bed rest, nil by mouth and intravenous fluids, with the addition of an antibiotic, usually amoxycillin or a cephalosporin. In all but the mild cases,

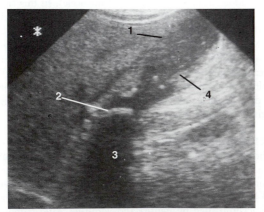

**Fig. 5.21** Ultrasound showing acute cholecystitis with impacted stone. Note distension of gallbladder with thickened wall and sludge. 1, thick wall; 2, stone; 3, acoustic shadow; 4, echogenic debris.

pain relief with an opiate is required.

In the absence of vomiting, the patient can soon tolerate oral fluids and nasogastric aspiration is not often required. Signs of complications such as generalized peritonitis or gangrene of the gallbladder (which causes increasing pain and fever) are an indication for urgent surgery, particularly in the elderly.

Cholecystectomy (see below) within days of the acute attack has been advocated for all patients who are not an anaesthetic risk. A firm diagnosis can usually be made using an HIDA scan or ultrasound. Alternatively, cholecystectomy can be performed 2–3 months later. However early surgery means only one hospital visit and no possibility of a recurrent attack while waiting for surgery to be performed. It does not increase operative morbidity or mortality and is, therefore, the recommended treatment.

## Chronic cholecystitis

There are no symptoms or signs that can conclusively be shown to be due to chronic cholecystitis. Symptoms attributed to this condition are vague with abdominal discomfort or distension. There is no doubt that gallbladders studied histologically can show signs of chronic inflammation and occasionally a small, shrunken gallbladder is found either radiologically or on ultrasound examination. However these findings can be seen in asymptomatic people and therefore this clinical diagnosis should not be made. Most patients with chronic right hypochondrial pain suffer from functional bowel disease.

## Common bile duct stones

These may be asymptomatic or they may present with any one or all of the triad of abdominal pain, jaundice and fever. The pain is usually severe and situated in the epigastrium and right hypochondrium.

The pain may be accompanied by vomiting. The pain usually lasts for a few hours and then clears up, only to return days, weeks or even months later. Between attacks the patient is well.

The jaundice is variable in degree, depending on the amount of obstruction. The urine is dark and the stools are pale. High fevers and rigors indicate cholangitis.

The liver is moderately enlarged if the obstruction lasts for more than a few hours. Prolonged biliary obstruction or repeated attacks lead to secondary biliary cirrhosis, but this is now rare.

## INVESTIGATION

BLOOD COUNT. A leucocytosis is present.
BLOOD CULTURES. These may grow an intestinal organism (*E. coli, Strep. faecalis*).
BIOCHEMISTRY. A cholestatic picture (see p. 249) with a raised conjugated bilirubin and alkaline phosphatase in the serum and relatively normal serum aminotransferases.
PROTHROMBIN TIME. This may become elevated over a few weeks owing to poor vitamin K absorption.

ULTRASOUND EXAMINATION. This reveals a dilated common bile duct (see Fig. 5.8) sometimes with a visible stone. Stones in the common bile duct can be missed and endoscopic ultrasound is a more accurate method of detecting a stone. Stones in the gallbladder suggest, but do not prove, that gallstones are the cause of the dilatation.

X-RAY. A plain abdominal X-ray may reveal gallstones.

ERCP. This is performed to confirm the diagnosis (Fig. 5.22) and to remove the stones (see below).

### DIFFERENTIAL DIAGNOSIS

The differential diagnosis includes all causes of jaundice.

### MANAGEMENT

The acute episode is usually allowed to settle and the serum bilirubin usually falls to normal levels. During this stage the patient normally only requires pain relief but occasionally antibiotics are necessary.

The serum AP falls more slowly than the serum bilirubin, and if the patient is seen some time after an acute attack elevation of this enzyme may be the only evidence of biliary tract disease.

Further management of common duct stones is discussed below.

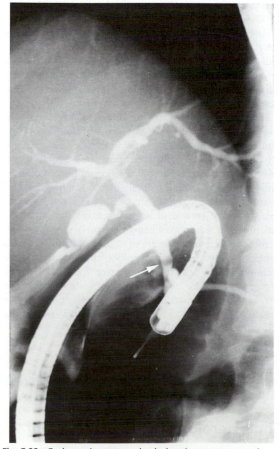

**Fig. 5.22** Endoscopic retrograde cholangiopancreatography showing gallstones in common bile duct (arrow).

## Acute cholangitis

Acute cholangitis is due to bacterial infection of the bile ducts and is always secondary to bile duct abnormalities. The common causes are common duct stones, biliary strictures, neoplasms, or following ERCP in the presence of large duct obstruction.

The symptoms are fever, often with a rigor, upper abdominal pain and jaundice. All three symptoms are present in 70% of cases. Older patients can present with collapse and Gram-negative septicaemia.

Specific signs may be minimal but tenderness over the liver occurs.

When all three symptoms are present the diagnosis is not difficult, but the patient can present with only a fever and an accompanying leucocytosis. Blood cultures are often positive (usually for *E. coli*) and a severe Gram-negative septicaemia can occur.

Treatment is with intravenous amoxycillin 1 g 6-hourly with intravenous gentamicin 2–5 mg kg$^{-1}$ daily in divided doses for severe cases. Ceftazidime is also used.

Suppurative cholangitis can occur as a complication. The fever continues and shock develops despite adequate antibiotics. Urgent decompression of the duct should be performed, usually endoscopically with placement of a nasobiliary drain. The subsequent treatment of the obstruction is either endoscopic or surgical (see below).

## MANAGEMENT OF GALLSTONES

### Stones in the gallbladder

#### Cholecystectomy

This is the treatment of choice for virtually all patients with gallbladder stones and symptoms.

LAPAROSCOPIC CHOLECYSTECTOMY is now the operation of choice. The abdominal cavity is insufflated with carbon dioxide under a general anaesthetic and the laparoscope and operating channels are inserted through the umbilicus and three other small incisions. The gallbladder is dissected from its bed on the liver and removed whole after the cystic duct and vessels have been clipped and haemostasis achieved with electrocautery or laser. The mortality is less than 0.1% and the patients can leave hospital in 24–48 hours. Complications are low and include wound sepsis, bile duct injury and retained gallstones in the common bile duct. Patients can return to full activity in approximately 7 days, compared to 3 weeks for the open operation.

OPEN CHOLECYSTECTOMY. This is also a safe procedure with a mortality of less than 0.1% in experienced hands. An increased mortality occurs in obese and elderly patients.

Only patients who refuse surgery should be considered for alternative therapy (see below).

POSTCHOLECYSTECTOMY SYNDROME. Some patients continue to complain of right hypochondrial pain, flatulence, indigestion and intolerance to fatty foods after cho-lecystectomy, despite a normal radiological appearance of the biliary tree. In the vast majority of these patients the original diagnosis was incorrect and the patient was suffering from functional bowel disease, the gallstones being an incidental finding. The occurrence of severe pain with jaundice suggests a retained stone in the common duct.

### Gallstone dissolution or disruption

*Cholesterol gallstones* can be dissolved by the bile acids chenodeoxycholic acid and ursodeoxycholic acid, which increase cholesterol solubility in bile. They only dissolve radiolucent stones in a functioning gallbladder and not calcified stones. Only about 10% of patients are suitable for this therapy.

Gallstone dissolution takes anything from 6 months to 2 years and when the treatment is stopped 50% of the gallstones recur. Chenodeoxycholate also produces diarrhoea.

Shock-wave treatment of gallstones can be carried out using ultrasound-guided lithotripters that do not require a general anaesthetic or water bath.

Laparoscopic cholecystectomy has made the above techniques redundant except in a very few cases where an anaesthetic is contraindicated.

## Stones in the common bile duct

Endoscopic sphincterotomy with removal of the common bile duct stone, if possible, is performed initially. The sphincter of Oddi is cut with a diathermy wire. Stones can then pass from the common bile duct following this sphincterotomy either naturally through the enlarged opening or they can be removed endoscopically using a Dormia basket. The duct is 'swept' with a balloon to ensure that all stones have been removed; a cholangiogram is performed.

Large stones (>15 cm in diameter) that cannot be removed whole, can be crushed with a mechanical lithotripter or fragmented later by extracorporeal shock-wave lithotripsy. Alternatively a double pig-tail endoprosthesis can be inserted to allow biliary drainage.

In a patient with an intact gallbladder containing stones, the endoscopic removal of a stone is usually followed by a laparoscopic cholecystectomy. Whether this is necessary in all cases is debatable as further problems are only encountered in 20% of patients.

Some surgeons can remove common bile duct stones at the time of laparoscopic cholecystectomy, but most prefer the stones to be removed endoscopically.

If an open operation is performed, the duct should always be explored.

*Retained stones* after surgery can be treated by:

1  Removal via the T-tube: this is possible if the T-tube is large (14 French gauge) using a steerable catheter under fluoroscopic control
2  Chemical dissolution by infusion of monooctanoin down the T-tube
3  Endoscopic removal
4  Further surgery if the above fail.

# COMPLICATIONS OF GALLSTONES

PANCREATITIS (p. 287)

GALLSTONE ILEUS AND BILIARY ENTERIC FISTULA. Gallstones can occasionally erode through the wall of the gallbladder into the intestine. They can cause obstruction, mainly in the terminal ileum but occasionally in the duodenum.

CARCINOMA OF THE GALLBLADDER may be causally related.

# Miscellaneous conditions of the biliary tract

## Primary sclerosing cholangitis

Primary sclerosing cholangitis results from inflammation and fibrosis of the bile ducts leading to multiple areas of narrowing throughout the biliary system. The cause is unknown but immunological mechanisms have been implicated. HLA associations have been reported with HLA-B8, DR3; HLA-DR52a and HLA-DW2. DR4 marks for rapid disease progression.

Fifty per cent or more of patients have inflammatory bowel disease, but this may be asymptomatic. Patients with AIDS have been found to have sclerosing cholangitis. The cause here is unclear but infection particularly with *Cryptosporidium parvum* is a probable aetiological factor.

There may be no symptoms and the diagnosis is suggested by a raised serum AP but a negative mitochondrial antibody. Symptoms that may fluctuate are pruritus, jaundice and occasionally abdominal pain. Portal hypertension can develop. Liver biopsy shows a fibrous obliterating cholangitis with eventual loss of interlobular and adjacent septal bile ducts. An ERCP will show the multiple strictures. Treatment is unsatisfactory. In half of the patients the disease runs a benign course over many years. Steroids and azathioprine are of unproven value but seem to help some patients. The results with methotrexate are encouraging. In associated ulcerative colitis, colectomy does not affect the progress of the condition. Obvious extrahepatic biliary strictures can sometimes be dilated or stented at endoscopy. Liver transplantation is now being performed for this condition.

## Non-calculous cholecystitis

Occasionally cholecystitis occurs in patients with diabetes mellitus, polyarteritis nodosa and systemic infections.

## Cholesterolosis of the gallbladder

In this condition, deposits of cholesterol are seen in the mucosal wall, producing a fine yellow pattern on a red background (strawberry gallbladder). Cholesterol stones may or may not be present. The relationship to symptoms is unclear.

## Adenomyomatosis of the gallbladder

This may be found as an incidental finding on a cholecystogram and consists of thickening of the mucosal and muscle layers with the presence of Rokitansky–Aschoff sinuses, often associated with small gallstones. It does not usually produce symptoms.

## Choledochal cyst

This is a congenital cystic dilatation of the extrahepatic ducts producing jaundice and abdominal pain. Fifty per cent of the patients do not present until early adult life. Treatment is surgical.

## Haemobilia

Haemobilia can occur due to hepatic trauma, sometimes from a tumour, and rarely after liver biopsy. Blood enters the biliary tree and produces either obstructive jaundice or gastrointestinal bleeding.

# Tumours of the biliary tract

## Primary carcinoma of the gallbladder

This adenocarcinoma represents <1% of all cancers. It occurs chiefly in those over 70 years of age and is commoner in females. Gallstones are usually present but a definite relationship is uncertain. The presenting features are of jaundice and occasionally right hypochondrial pain. A mass may be palpable in the right hypochondrium. The diagnosis is often made at operation and cholecystectomy is performed if possible. Few patients survive 1 year.

## Cholangiocarcinoma (see p. 277)

This sometimes affects the extrahepatic biliary tree, giving rise to jaundice. Surgery, if possible, is the only effective treatment. Alternatively, a stent or tube can be passed through the obstruction during PTC or ERCP. The prognosis is poor.

## Malignant tumours of the ampulla

These present with a cholestatic jaundice which may occasionally be intermittent. They may ulcerate and prod-

uce gastrointestinal haemorrhage. The diagnosis is usually made at ERCP. Carcinoma of the ampulla can sometimes be resected with a 40% 5-year survival rate (compare with pancreatic carcinoma, p. 290).

# THE PANCREAS

# Structure and function

The pancreas extends retroperitoneally across the posterior abdominal wall from the second part of the duodenum to the spleen. The head is encircled by the duodenum; the body, which forms the main bulk of the organ, ends in a tail that lies in contact with the spleen. The main pancreatic duct usually joins the common bile duct to enter the duodenum as a single duct at the ampulla of Vater. The main pancreatic duct has many tributary ductules and gradually tapers towards the tail of the pancreas. Pancreas divisum is an anatomical variant in which a small proportion of the pancreas drains through an accessory duct into the duodenum.

Exocrine cells form 98% of the human pancreas. The pancreatic acinar cells form a ductal system that eventually joins into the main pancreatic duct.

Pancreatic acini synthesize digestive enzymes which are stored in secretory glands and released by exocytosis in response to stimulation by several hormones (Fig. 5.23).

These receptors have been divided into two categories: vasoactive intestinal polypeptide (VIP) and secretin that act via cyclic AMP, and another group that stimulate cellular metabolism of membrane phosphoinositides and calcium.

The main regulators of pancreatic exocrine secretion are the hormones secretin and cholecystokinin (CCK). Secretin is released when acid enters the duodenum; it stimulates pancreatic juice containing water and electrolytes, chiefly bicarbonate. CCK is released, via cholinergic pathways, when fatty acids and amino acids enter the duodenum, stimulating pancreatic enzyme secretion. Enzymes produced are amylase, lipase, colipase, phospholipase and proteases (trypsinogen and chymotrypsinogen). The proteases are secreted in the inactive form but are then activated in the duodenum by enterokinase.

The endocrine pancreas consists of hormone-producing cells arranged in nests or islets—the islets of Langerhans. They do not connect directly to the duct system. There are four main types of islet cell and these have different secretory granules in their cytoplasm:

1 $\beta$-Cells, which are the commonest cells, produce insulin.
2 $\alpha$-Cells produce glucagon.
3 D cells produce somatostatin.

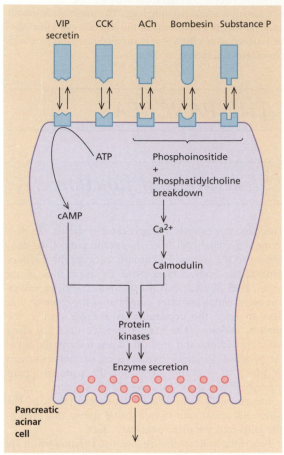

**Fig. 5.23** Diagram showing stimulus–secretion coupling of pancreatic acinar cell protein secretion. VIP, vasoactive intestinal polypeptide; CCK, cholecystokinin; ACh, acetylcholine.

4  PP cells produce pancreatic polypeptide (PP).
5  A number of other hormones, e.g. bombesin, neuropeptide Y and galanin, are present in pancreatic neurones and probably act as neurotransmitters.

## Investigation (Table 5.16)

### Exocrine function

The choice of individual tests is made on the clinical situation.

SERUM AMYLASE MEASUREMENT is useful in acute disease but is of no value in chronic disease.

SERUM LIPASE is raised in acute pancreatitis.

MEASUREMENT OF DUODENAL ENZYMES, either after hormone stimulation or after food, is only sometimes helpful in the diagnosis of chronic pancreatitis because of

---

*Exocrine*
Serum amylase
Duodenal enzymes after:
   Hormone stimulation with CCK and secretin
   Food stimulation (Lundh meal)
PABA test
Fat excretion
   Faecal fat (see p. 202)
   Breath tests

*Endocrine*
Serum levels of:
   Insulin
   Glucagon
   Pancreatic polypeptide
Glucose tolerance test measuring glucose and insulin

*Visualization of the pancreas*
Abdominal X-ray—to detect calcification
Barium meal—to show an abnormal duodenal loop
ᵃUltrasound  ⎱  to demonstrate size, presence of
CT scan     ⎰  calcification, tumours or pseudocyst
MRI         ⎰  (NB percutaneous biopsies can be taken)
ERCP—to examine the ductular system
Angiography—to detect tumours

———

ᵃUltrasound can also be performed endoscopically.
CCK, cholecystokinin; ERCP, endoscopic retrograde cholangiopancreatography; PABA, p-aminobenzoic acid.

**Table 5.16** Investigations available for the assessment of pancreatic disease.

---

the large reserve in enzyme capacity. A tube is passed into the duodenum and pancreatic secretions are collected after stimulation. *Stimulation with secretin or CCK causes a rise in bicarbonate and enzyme*, e.g. trypsin levels, which are low with chronic disease. The differential diagnosis between pancreatic tumour and pancreatitis is difficult. These tests have been largely superseded by imaging techniques. *The Lundh test* is performed in a similar fashion, the stimulation being produced by a meal. Measurement of trypsin and lipase is undertaken. These are low in chronic pancreatitis. The Lundh meal test is particularly useful in the investigation of steatorrhoea.

PABA TEST. *N*-benzoyl-L-tyrosyl *p*-aminobenzoic acid is a synthetic peptide hydrolysed by pancreatic chymotrypsin to release free PABA, which is absorbed, metabolized and excreted in the urine. Reduction in absorption of free PABA occurs (after an oral load of the peptide) in pancreatic insufficiency and the test is highly specific in expert hands, although not widely utilized.

FAECAL FAT ESTIMATION is performed to demonstrate steatorrhoea. A breath test can also be used; here the amount of $^{14}CO_2$ in expired air is measured following oral ingestion of a labelled fatty acid compared with that after a labelled triglyceride (e.g. [$^{14}C$]oleic acid compared with [$^{14}C$]triolein). Impaired triglyceride absorption with normal fatty acid absorption indicates that pancreatic disease is the cause of the steatorrhoea.

### Endocrine function

Assessment of endocrine function is only useful if a hormone-secreting tumour is suspected and the serum measurements are often diagnostic. Plasma PP is raised with all endocrine tumours. The glucose tolerance test is seldom performed as it is affected by so many parameters.

### Visualization of the pancreas

This now largely depends on ultrasound examination and CT scan to detect pancreatic size and shape, and the presence of cysts or tumours. An ERCP can be used to outline the pancreatic ducts. MRI with or without dynamic enhancement with contrast is slightly more sensitive than CT. Endoscopic ultrasound is particularly useful in the diagnosis of small endocrine tumours. Arteriography with selective catheterization of the splenic artery shows irregularity and encasement in carcinoma.

A combination of two or three tests is often necessary and none of the investigations is diagnostic. Fine-needle aspiration of any abnormality discovered can be performed under ultrasound or CT scan control. The presence of malignant cells in the aspirate indicates tumour but, of course, a negative sample does not exclude malignancy.

*Acute*
Gallstones
Alcohol
Infections, e.g. mumps, Coxsackie B
Pancreatic tumours
Drugs, e.g. azathioprine, oestrogens, corticosteroids
Iatrogenic, e.g. postsurgical, ERCP
Hyperlipidaemias
Miscellaneous
  Trauma
  Scorpion bite
  Cardiac surgery
Idiopathic

*Chronic*
Alcohol (>85%)
Idiopathic
Tropical (nutritional)
Hereditary
Trauma
Hypercalcaemia

———

ERCP, endoscopic retrograde cholangiopancreatography.

**Table 5.17** Causes of pancreatitis.

# Pancreatitis

### Classification

The classification of pancreatitis is difficult due to the inability to clearly separate acute and chronic pancreatitis. The original 1983 Marseilles classification was reviewed in 1984 and 1988 and simplified into acute and chronic forms. It was agreed that alcohol, which previously was classified as only causing chronic pancreatitis, can now cause the first episode acutely.

By definition, acute pancreatitis may occur as isolated or as recurrent attacks. It is distinguished from chronic pancreatitis by the absence of continuing inflammation, irreversible structural changes and permanent loss of exocrine and endocrine pancreatic function. The causes of pancreatitis are shown in Table 5.17.

## Acute pancreatitis

This is an acute condition presenting with abdominal pain and raised pancreatic enzymes in the blood or urine, due to inflammatory disease of the pancreas.

### PATHOGENESIS

The exact mechanism by which pancreatic necrosis occurs is unclear. Associated gallstones are mainly found in the gallbladder and only occasionally in the common bile duct. Reflux of bile up the pancreatic duct associated with occlusion of the ampulla may play a role in the pathogenesis. Autodigestion of the pancreas by proteolytic enzymes (particularly trypsin and phospholipase A) released in the pancreas rather than in the intestinal lumen may also be involved in the pathogenesis. Active enzymes could digest cell membranes, leading to proteolysis, oedema, vascular damage and necrosis. The mildest form of pancreatitis is characterized by intestinal oedema with an inflammatory exudate (oedematous pancreatitis), while in the severe form there is pancreatic necrosis and haemorrhage (haemorrhagic pancreatitis).

### CLINICAL FEATURES

These vary depending on the severity of the attack. In all patients the principal symptom is abdominal pain that is usually localized to the epigastrium or upper abdomen. It may radiate to the back between the scapulae. The pain will vary from mild discomfort to excruciating pain in severe cases. Rarely, acute pancreatitis can occur in the absence of pain.

Nausea and vomiting accompany the pain in most cases.

In severe cases there may be multisystem failure and/or development of a complication, e.g. pseudocyst.

Physical examination may reveal tenderness, guarding and rigidity of the abdomen, with varying degrees of shock depending on the severity of the attack. Rarely, body wall ecchymoses occur, e.g. umbilical (Cullen's sign) or in the flanks (Grey Turner's sign). The remaining clinical features depend on the local and systemic complications that occur (Table 5.18).

Local pancreatic complications can occur with mild attacks of pancreatitis but systemic complications only occur with severe attacks.

### INVESTIGATION AND DIAGNOSIS

The clinical manifestations are so varied that pancreatitis must be considered in the differential diagnosis of all causes of upper abdominal pain. Most present as an acute

Pancreatic
  Phlegmon
  Pseudocyst
  Abscess
  Ascites

Intestinal
  Paralytic ileus
  Gastrointestinal haemorrhage

Hepatobiliary
  Jaundice
  Obstruction of common bile duct
  Portal vein thrombosis

Systemic
  Metabolic
    Malnutrition
    Hypocalcaemia
    Hyperglycaemia
  Haematological
    Disseminated intravascular coagulation
    Portal vein thrombosis
  Renal
    Acute renal failure
  Cardiovascular
    Circulatory failure (shock)
  Respiratory
    Hypoxic acute respiratory failure

Fat necrosis

**Table 5.18** Complications of acute pancreatitis.

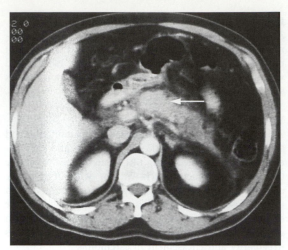

**Fig. 5.24** CT showing severe acute pancreatitis (arrow) with a small effusion around the pancreas.

| Age | >55 years |
|---|---|
| WBC | $>15 \times 10^9$/litre |
| Blood glucose | >10 mmol litre$^{-1}$ |
| Blood urea | >16 mmol litre$^{-1}$ |
| Serum albumin | <30 g litre$^{-1}$ |
| Serum aminotransferase | >200 U litre$^{-1}$ |
| Serum calcium | <2 mmol litre$^{-1}$ |
| Serum LDH | >600 U litre$^{-1}$ |
| $P_aO_2$ | <8.0 kPa (60 mmHg) |

LDH, lactate dehydrogenase; WBC, white blood cell count.

**Table 5.19** Factors during the first 48 hours that indicate severe pancreatitis and a poor prognosis.

abdomen and differentiation from an acute perforated ulcer is the most difficult, as both may give rise to abdominal rigidity.

The diagnosis of acute pancreatitis depends on the serum amylase. A raised serum amylase level can be seen in other acute abdominal emergencies such as acute cholecystitis and perforated peptic ulcer, but if the serum amylase level is five times greater than normal, acute pancreatitis is very likely. However, the serum amylase cannot be entirely relied upon and must be evaluated in conjunction with the history and physical signs. A plain abdominal X-ray may show ileus initially limited to the loop of bowel (sentinel loop) or calcification in acute or chronic pancreatitis. If there is doubt about the diagnosis, exploratory laparotomy must be performed to exclude a potentially fatal but treatable non-pancreatic lesion.

Peritoneal aspiration and lavage, with estimation of amylase in the peritoneal fluid obtained, is particularly useful in difficult cases. Ultrasound or contrast enhanced CT scan (Fig. 5.24) may reveal a swollen pancreas, sometimes with peripancreatic fluid collections and gallstones, all of which help with the diagnosis.

The differential diagnosis includes all acute abdominal conditions. Factors indicating the severity, which is assessed chiefly on blood investigations, are given in Table 5.19. APACHE II score (see p. 735) is also used to grade severity.

### TREATMENT

Nasogastric suction is necessary to reduce vomiting and abdominal distension even in mild cases. All feeding is stopped and in severe cases nothing is given by mouth for weeks and intravenous nutrition is required (see p. 170). Water and electrolyte replacement and analgesia with an opiate (other than morphine) are necessary. No form of drug therapy has been shown to help; results of trials of somatostatin infusion have been disappointing. The efficacy of peritoneal lavage, which is sometimes used for severe cases, is in doubt. In some countries, surgery is used mainly to remove devitalized pancreatic tissue.

Management of shock plus respiratory failure (see p. 720) is required.

### LOCAL COMPLICATIONS

PHLEGMON. This is a solid inflammatory mass of pancreatic tissue that usually resolves spontaneously.

PSEUDOCYSTS (see also p. 290). Small pseudocysts are seen on ultrasound or CT in up to 50% of cases of severe pancreatitis, but do not usually require treatment *per se*. Large collections persisting for weeks can be aspirated under ultrasonic control or removed surgically.

PANCREATIC ABSCESSES. Secondary infection of a peripancreatic collection of fluid may occur, usually after about 2 weeks. The clinical features are persistent fever, leucocytosis and abdominal distension, with a possible palpable mass. Patients are usually very ill with the accompanying respiratory, cardiac and renal problems.

Drainage (either surgically or percutaneously under ultrasound or CT guidance) is performed with vigorous antibiotic therapy. General support of the patient is required, as the disease has a long clinical course of several months.

PANCREATIC ASCITES. This is usually associated with chronic pancreatitis and has a high amylase content.

## PROGNOSIS

The mortality rate varies from 1% in mild cases to 50% in severe cases. With multiple complications and the presence of all the bad prognostic signs, the mortality is nearer 100%. The patients who recover may have recurrent attacks, depending on the aetiology and whether accompanying gallstones are dealt with.

# Chronic pancreatitis

This is defined as a continuing inflammatory disease of the pancreas characterized by irreversible morphological change and typically causing pain and/or permanent impairment of function.

## PATHOGENESIS

The majority of cases occur as a result of high alcohol consumption and it is in these cases that the pathology has been most studied. The earliest change appears to be deposition of protein plugs within pancreatic ducts. These then lead to ductular dilatation followed by acinar atrophy. There is some accompanying infiltration but this is variable. Extensive fibrous tissue is deposited near the pancreatic ducts. Eventually only a few acinar and islet cells remain, with widely dilated pancreatic ducts. Intraluminal calcification of the protein plugs occurs, leading to stone formation. There is controversy as to whether this results from repeated bouts of acute inflammation and necrosis or whether it is due to an insidious chronic process.

Chronic pancreatitis is not reversible, but it is possible that the disease will arrest if the patient stops drinking. However, because patients often continue to take small amounts of alcohol, the disease is most often progressive.

The causes of chronic pancreatitis are shown in Table 5.17. Other suggested risk factors include excess smoking in males and an added risk factor of a low-protein and high-fat diet in alcohol abusers.

## CLINICAL FEATURES

The major symptom is abdominal pain situated mainly in the epigastrium and upper abdomen and radiating to the back. The pain can be severe; in some cases it is comparable to that occurring in acute pancreatitis.

Continuing episodes of pain may occur; sometimes these are mild and of brief duration. In other cases there may be chronic pain interspersed with acute episodes (relapsing pancreatitis). The relationship to alcohol is variable; nevertheless, some acute episodes seem to be precipitated by heavy alcohol consumption. The abdominal pain is accompanied by severe weight loss due to anorexia.

Steatorrhoea occurs when the secretion of pancreatic lipase is reduced by 90%. It occurs in about half the patients. The development of diabetes is more common. The steatorrhoea is often severe and the patient may notice drops of oil in the lavatory pan. Both diabetes and steatorrhoea occur more commonly with calcified pancreatitis.

Less common presentations include biliary obstruction with jaundice and occasionally cholangitis. Obstruction of the splenic vein can lead to portal hypertension.

## INVESTIGATION

This includes assessment of some of the endocrine and exocrine functions as outlined earlier, as well as visualization of the pancreas. The serum amylase is of little value in chronic pancreatitis but may be raised during an acute episode of pain.

PATIENTS WITH PAIN are investigated using ultrasound or CT scan, which show abnormalities in size and duct dilatation or the presence of calcification (Fig. 5.25) not seen on a plain X-ray. An ERCP is also useful in these patients to confirm the diagnosis. A dilated pancreatic duct, sometimes associated with stones or stenotic areas, can be identified. Early cases are difficult to diagnose and a combination of all tests with a strong clinical suspicion is necessary. Endoscopic ultrasound can visualize the pancreas and is being assessed.

PATIENTS PRESENTING WITH STEATORRHOEA require a Lundh test to estimate exocrine function (see p. 286).

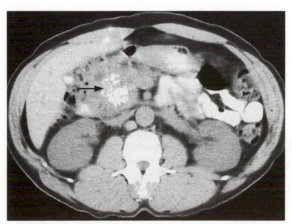

**Fig. 5.25**   CT showing chronic calcific pancreatitis (arrow).

## DIFFERENTIAL DIAGNOSIS

Carcinoma of the pancreas must be suspected, particularly when the history is short; occasionally laparotomy may be necessary to distinguish between these two conditions.

## TREATMENT

In alcoholic pancreatitis the patient should stop drinking alcohol. The pain needs to be controlled, often with narcotics, with the problem of addiction. Surgery is used for the treatment of intractable pain, pancreatic resection combined with drainage of an obstructed pancreatic duct into the small bowel being required. The use of surgery is controversial; good results are only obtained in a small number of cases, usually those who stop drinking.

Steatorrhoea is treated with a low-fat diet, pancreatic supplements, e.g. pancreatin 2–4 g with each meal, with occasionally cimetidine 400 mg twice daily. Diabetes mellitus is treated with diet, oral hypoglycaemic agents and/or insulin as appropriate. The insulin requirement is greater than in idiopathic diabetes, and patients may experience frequent or severe hypoglycaemia. This may be because pancreatic glucagon is lacking.

## COMPLICATIONS

The commonest complication is a pancreatic pseudocyst. These are found very frequently if careful ultrasound examinations are performed. Small cysts require no treatment. Large cysts can give rise to increased pain, nausea and vomiting 3–4 weeks after the onset of the most recent attack of pain. A smooth, tender mass may be palpable and the cyst can be easily identified using ultrasound. Surgical treatment has been used for most large pseudocysts but a more conservative approach, with aspiration and close follow-up using ultrasound examination, is preferable.

Pancreatic ascites occurs, usually in alcoholic pancreatitis, when there is a communication between the pancreatic duct and the peritoneal cavity. The amylase content of the ascitic fluid is high.

A good prognosis depends on complete abstention from alcohol.

## Cystic fibrosis (see p. 665)

This is the commonest cause of pancreatic disease in childhood. It is inherited as an autosomal recessive condition and a specific gene deletion has been identified in 70% of cases. It has been suggested that the resultant protein defect produces an abnormality in the regulation of a β-adrenergic-gated chloride channel in the cell membrane. This cystic fibrosis gene product has been named cystic fibrosis transmembrane conductance regulator (CFTR)(see Fig. 2.9). This basic defect in all exocrine glands produces thick viscoid secretions causing cystic dilatation of the ducts. Increased numbers of patients are now surviving into adult life because of improved therapy.

## CLINICAL FEATURES

See p. 665.

## DIAGNOSIS

SWEAT TESTING (see p. 665) of symptomatic people and siblings of patients with cystic fibrosis identifies 77% by 2 years of age and 95% by the age of 12 years.

IN INFANTS, immunoreactive trypsin assay in dried blood.

PANCREATIC FUNCTION TESTS (see p. 286).

## TREATMENT

Treatment is required for pancreatic insufficiency and respiratory problems (see p. 666). Steatorrhoea is treated with pancreatic supplements. High-dose pancreatin-containing trypsin and lipase can be given in microsphere-containing capsules which deliver high doses of enzyme to the duodenum for fat digestion. Recently, colonic strictures have been reported in a few patients and patients should be carefully monitored. $H_2$ antagonists are not usually required with these new preparations and the fat content of the diet can be kept normal. Optimal nutrition has been recognized as improving prognosis and a high calorie intake (150% of recommended daily allowance) with vitamin supplements should be given.

## Carcinoma of the pancreas

The incidence of pancreatic carcinoma is steadily increasing in Western countries. This tumour is now the fourth commonest cause of cancer death in the UK and USA. The incidence increases with age and most patients are over 60 years of age. Males are affected more than females.

There are no known aetiological factors, but the increasing incidence has been attributed to an increase in both smoking and the consumption of alcohol. Excessive coffee and dietary fats have also been implicated.

Most carcinomas of the pancreas are adenocarcinomas arising from duct epithelium. In 60% of cases the tumour is in the head of the pancreas. The tumour spreads locally to involve lymph nodes and the liver.

## CLINICAL FEATURES

CARCINOMA OF THE HEAD OF THE PANCREAS OR THE AMPULLA OF VATER presents with painless jaundice due to obstruction of the common duct. However, most patients will have pain at some time in the course of their disease. Weight loss also occurs.

CARCINOMA OF THE BODY OR TAIL OF THE PANCREAS presents with abdominal pain, anorexia and weight loss. The pain is often a dull, boring pain that radiates through to the back. It may be relieved by sitting forward. Jaundice is rare. Diabetes may occur due to insulin resistance. This is now thought to be caused by islet amyloid polypeptide, a hormonal factor secreted from pancreatic β cells. There is an increased incidence of thrombophlebitis.

In carcinoma of the head of the pancreas, examination will reveal jaundice with the dilated gallbladder sometimes being palpable (Courvoisier's sign). A dilated gallbladder is not found with gallstone disease because of the accompanying chronic inflammation of the gallbladder.

A palpable mass can be felt in 20% of patients, with hepatomegaly being present in most cases eventually.

### INVESTIGATION
Haematological or biochemical tests (including blood glucose) are not helpful.

Diagnosis is usually made using ultrasound (Fig. 5.26) or CT scan and confirmed by fine-needle or Trucut biopsy (see p. 243). However, in almost all cases, by the time the tumour is detected resection is impossible. Duodenoscopy with ERCP may detect tumours of the head of the pancreas or of the ampulla. MRI or endoscopic ultrasound may become useful aids to imaging.

### DIFFERENTIAL DIAGNOSIS
The differential diagnosis includes all causes of painless jaundice and persistent upper abdominal pain in the elderly.

### MANAGEMENT
The 5-year survival rate is miserably low at 2%. Resection of the tumour with total pancreatectomy is not usually possible, and, as this operation carries a very high mortality (20%) and morbidity, it is seldom attempted. Jaundice from carcinoma of the head of the pancreas is usually relieved by a bypass procedure. This is now performed endoscopically with the placement of a stent through the narrowed area of the common bile duct to allow drainage. An expandable metal stent is now being used which

remains patent longer. Surgical bypass where the common bile duct is anastomosed to the jejunum is now reserved for cases where the tumour has obstructed the duodenum. Chemotherapy and radiotherapy have had little success in decreasing mortality. Ampullary tumours have a better prognosis than pancreatic carcinomas and every attempt should be made to diagnose these rare lesions, as a resection in these cases can be performed. Pain and symptoms of anxiety and depression are an important part of management and analgesia with long-acting oral morphines should be used liberally (see p. 376). Addiction is not a problem in these terminally ill patients. Palliative care teams play an important role in this distressing condition.

# Endocrine tumours

These tumours arise in the pancreas from APUD (*a*mine *p*recursor *u*ptake and *d*ecarboxylation) cells and are sometimes called apudomas.

Pancreatic endocrine tumours can occur in association with other endocrine tumours, particularly parathyroid adenoma and pituitary adenoma, as part of multiple endocrine neoplasias (see p. 824). Endocrine tumours predominantly secrete one hormone that produces its clinical effect, but other hormones are often synthesized and can be detected either in the blood or in the resected tumour.

## Gastrinoma (Zollinger–Ellison syndrome)

These tumours mainly arise from G cells in the pancreas and secrete large amounts of gastrin. This stimulates maximal gastric acid secretion, so that the main clinical problem is peptic ulceration. Peptic ulcers occur in the usual areas of the stomach and duodenum and also in the jejunum. The ulcers are often large and deep and sometimes multiple. Haemorrhage and perforation can occur.

Diarrhoea due to the low pH in the upper intestine is also a common feature. Jejunal mucosal abnormalities are also seen. A high serum gastrin confirms the diagnosis. Acid studies show high acid output. Treatment is with omeprazole (which inhibits the $H^+$–$K^+$ proton pump necessary for acid secretion). Octreotide is also used. Surgery is reserved for removal of the primary tumour only. The tumour may be demonstrated by scans or local venous sampling for gastrin. These tumours are malignant and although they grow slowly the patients now die of malignancy rather than gastrointestinal problems if the primary cannot be removed.

## Other endocrine tumours

ISLET CELL TUMOURS. These are described on p. 852.

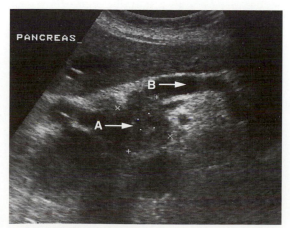

**Fig. 5.26** Ultrasound showing carcinoma of head of pancreas (A) with dilated pancreatic duct (B).

VIPOMAS. These rare pancreatic tumours produce severe intestinal secretion and watery diarrhoea leading to dehydration. VIP is a neurotransmitter that stimulates adenyl cyclase to produce intestinal secretion. Plasma concentrations of VIP are very high and are diagnostic. Levels of PP hormone are also raised. The role of peptide histidine isoleucine (PHI), levels of which are also raised in this condition, is uncertain but this hormone may be involved in secretion.

Corticosteroids help reduce the stool volume but octreotide is the most effective agent. An attempt should be made to localize the tumour and, if possible, it should be resected.

GLUCAGONOMAS. These are $\alpha$-cell tumours of the pancreas that produce pancreatic glucagon. The patients have diabetes mellitus and a unique characteristic necrolytic migratory erythematous rash. The diagnosis is made by measuring pancreatic glucagon in the serum.

A tumour originating in the right kidney has been described that produces marked hypertrophy of the villi in the jejunum and produces enteroglucagon (enteroglucagonoma).

SOMATOSTATINOMAS. These have also been described; they produce diabetes, steatorrhoea and weight loss.

# Further reading

Go VL, Dimagno EP, Gardner J, Lebenthal E, Reber HA & Scheele GA (1993) *The Pancreas, Biology, Pathology and Disease*, 2nd edn. New York: Raven Press.

Millward-Sadler GH, Wright R & Arthur MJP (1993) *Wright's Liver and Biliary Disease*, 3rd edn, Volumes I and II. London: WB Saunders.

Sherlock S & Dooley J (1993) *Diseases of the Liver and Biliary System*, 9th edn. Oxford: Blackwell Scientific Publications.

Sleisenger MH & Fordtran JS (1993) *Gastrointestinal Disease*, 5th edn. Philadelphia: WB Saunders.

*New England Journal of Medicine* progress reports and current concepts, e.g. Runyon BA (1993) Current concepts. Care of patients with ascites. *New England Journal of Medicine* **330** (5), 337–342.

*Baillières Clinical Gastroenterology* series, e.g. Sackmann M (ed) (1992) Diagnosis and Management of Biliary Stones. London: Baillière Tindall.

*Current Opinions in Gastroenterology*—useful updates with extensive references.

Major journals such as *Gastroenterology*, *Gut* and *Hepatology*—monthly reviews and progress reports of current topics.

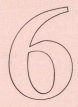

# Diseases of the blood

## Introduction

Blood consists of:

- Red cells
- White cells
- Platelets
- Plasma, in which the above elements are suspended

Plasma is the liquid component of blood, which contains soluble fibrinogen. Serum is what remains after the formation of the fibrin clot.

### The formation of blood cells (haemopoiesis)

Around the third week of development of the embryo, blood islands are formed in the yolk sac and produce primitive blood cells which migrate to the liver and spleen. These organs are the chief sites of haemopoiesis from 6 weeks to 6–7 months of fetal life. The bone marrow becomes the main source of blood cells for the remainder of fetal life and is the only source of blood cells during normal childhood and adult life.

At birth, haemopoiesis occurs in the marrow of nearly every bone. As the child grows the marrow cavity starts to be replaced by fat so that haemopoiesis in the adult becomes confined to the central skeleton and the proximal ends of the long bones. Only if the demand for blood cells increases and persists do the areas of red marrow extend once again. Pathological processes interfering with normal haemopoiesis may result in resumption of haemopoietic activity in the liver and spleen, which is referred to as *extramedullary haemopoiesis*.

All peripheral blood cells are derived from pluripotential stem cells by a number of *differentiation* steps (Fig. 6.1). Stem cells probably resemble small lymphocytes, although their exact appearance remains unknown. However, their presence can be shown by bone marrow culture techniques, involving the detection of *colony-forming units* (CFUs) in agar culture medium. The earliest detectable CFU is CFU-S (spleen); this gives rise to CFU-GEMM, which produces CFU 'committed' to the production of:

- Granulocytes
- Erythroid cells
- Monocytes
- Megakaryocytes

Stem cells also produce lymphoid cells.

Stem cells have the capability for *self-renewal*, as well as differentiation, and maintain a constant cellularity in a normal healthy marrow.

### Haemopoietic growth factors

Haemopoietic growth factors are glycoproteins which regulate the differentiation and proliferation of haemopoietic progenitor cells and the function of mature blood cells. They act on receptors expressed on haemopoietic cells at various stages of development to maintain the haemopoietic progenitor cells and to stimulate increased production of one or more cell lines in response to stresses such as blood loss and infection. More than one growth factor is often needed to stimulate a particular cell to differentiate or proliferate (Fig. 6.1).

Haemopoietic growth factors include erythropoietin, colony-stimulating factors (CSFs, the prefix indicating the cell type, see Fig. 6.1) and interleukins (IL). T lymphocytes, monocytes and bone marrow stromal cells such as fibroblasts, endothelial cells and macrophages are the major sources except for erythropoietin, which is mainly produced in the kidney. Many growth factors have been produced by recombinant DNA techniques and are being used clinically. Examples include G-CSF which is used to accelerate haemopoietic recovery after chemotherapy and bone marrow transplantation, and erythropoietin which is used to treat anaemia in patients with chronic renal failure.

### Peripheral blood—normal values (Table 6.1)

Automated cell counters are used to measure the level of haemoglobin (Hb) and the number and size of red cells, white cells and platelets. Other indices can be derived from these values. The mean corpuscular volume (MCV) of red cells is the most useful of the indices and is used to classify anaemia (p. 298).

The white cell count (WCC) gives the total number of circulating leucocytes and many automated cell counters produce differential counts as well.

Normally less than 2% of the red cells are *reticulocytes* (p. 295). The reticulocyte count gives a guide to the erythroid activity in the bone marrow. An increased count is seen with haemorrhage or haemolysis, or after the response to treatment with a specific haematinic. A low count in the presence of anaemia indicates an inappropriate response by the bone marrow and may be seen

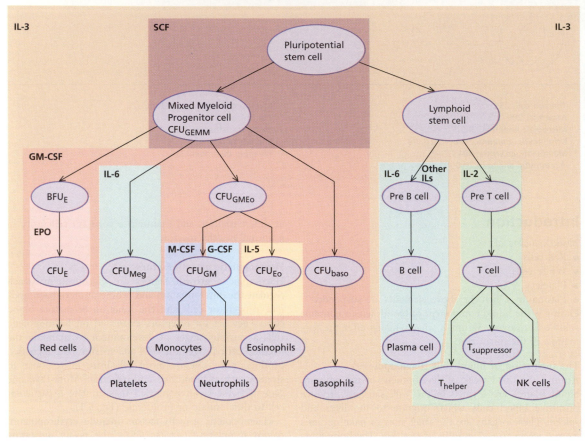

**Fig. 6.1** A diagram of the role of growth factors in normal haemopoiesis. Multiple growth factors act on stem cells and early progenitor cells. BFU, burst-forming unit; CFU, colony forming unit; CSF, colony-stimulating factor; E, erythroid; Eo, eosinophil; EPO, erythropoietin; G, granulocyte; GEMM, mixed granulocyte, erythroid, monocyte, megakaryocyte; GM, granulocyte, monocyte; IL, interleukin; M, monocyte; Meg, megakaryocyte; SCF, stem cell factor.

| | Male | Female |
|---|---|---|
| Hb (g dl$^{-1}$) | 13–18 | 11.5–15.5 |
| PCV (haematocrit) (litre litre$^{-1}$) | 0.42–0.53 | 0.36–0.45 |
| RCC (10$^{12}$/litre) | 4.5–6.0 | 3.9–5.1 |
| MCV (fl) | 80–96 | |
| MCH (pg) | 27–33 | |
| MCHC (g dl$^{-1}$) | 32–35 | |
| WCC (10$^9$/litre) | 4.0–11.0 | |
| Platelets (10$^9$/litre) | 150–400 | |
| ESR (mm hour$^{-1}$) | < 20 | |
| Reticulocytes (%) | 0.5–2.5 | |

———

ESR, erythrocyte sedimentation rate; Hb, haemoglobin; MCH, mean corpuscular haemoglobin; MCHC, mean corpuscular haemoglobin concentration; MCV, mean corpuscular volume of red cells; PCV, packed cell volume; RCC, red cell count; WCC, white cell count.

**Table 6.1** Normal values for peripheral blood.

in bone marrow failure (from whatever cause) or where there is a deficiency of a haematinic.

A carefully evaluated *blood film* is still an essential adjunct to the above, as definitive abnormalities of cells can be seen.

ERYTHROCYTE SEDIMENTATION RATE (ESR). This is the rate of fall of red cells in a column of blood and is a measure of the acute phase response. The pathological process may be immunological, infective, ischaemic, malignant or traumatic. A raised ESR reflects an increase in the plasma concentration of large proteins, such as fibrinogen and immunoglobulins. The proteins cause rouleaux formation, when cells clump together like a stack of coins, and therefore fall more rapidly. The ESR increases with age, and is higher in females than males. It is low in polycythaemia vera due to the high red cell concentration and increased in patients with severe anaemia.

PLASMA VISCOSITY measurement is being used instead of the ESR in many laboratories. As with the ESR, the level is dependent on the concentration of large molecules such as fibrinogen and immunoglobulins. There is no difference between levels found in males and females and viscosity only increases slightly in the elderly. It is not affected by the level of Hb and the result may be obtained within 15 min.

C-REACTIVE PROTEIN is one of the proteins produced in the acute phase response. It is synthesized exclusively in the liver and rises within 6 hours of an acute event. It rises with temperature (possibly triggered by IL-1) and in inflammatory conditions and after trauma. It follows the clinical state of the patient much more rapidly than the ESR and is unaffected by the level of Hb. Its measurement is easy and quick to perform using an immunoassay that can be automated. It is being increasingly used instead of the ESR, although more sophisticated equipment is required and it is more expensive, particularly when assayed in small numbers.

# The Red Cell

## Erythropoiesis

Red cell precursors pass through several stages in the bone marrow. The earliest morphologically recognizable cells are *pronormoblasts*. Smaller *normoblasts* result from cell divisions and precursors at each stage progressively contain less RNA and more Hb in the cytoplasm. The nucleus becomes more condensed and is eventually lost from the late normoblast in the bone marrow, when the cell becomes a *reticulocyte*.

Reticulocytes contain residual ribosomal RNA and are still able to synthesize Hb. They remain in the marrow for about 1–2 days and are released into the circulation, where they lose their RNA and become mature red cells (or erythrocytes) after another 1–2 days. Mature red cells are non-nucleated biconcave discs. Nucleated red cells (normoblasts) are not normally present in peripheral blood, but are present if there is extramedullary haemopoiesis and in some marrow disorders (see leucoerythroblastic anaemia, p. 335).

About 10% of erythroblasts die in the bone marrow even during normal erythropoiesis. Such *ineffective erythropoiesis* is substantially increased in some anaemias such as thalassaemia major and megaloblastic anaemia.

Erythropoiesis is controlled by the hormone *erythropoietin*. The gene for erythropoietin on chromosome 7 codes for a heavily glycosylated polypeptide of 165 amino acids. Erythropoietin has a molecular weight of 30 400 and is produced in the peritubular cells in the kidneys (90%) and in the liver (10%). Its production is mainly regulated by tissue oxygen tension. Production is increased if there is hypoxia from whatever cause, for example anaemia or cardiac or pulmonary disease. Erythropoietin stimulates an increase in the proportion of bone marrow precursor cells committed to erythropoiesis and CFU-E are stimulated to proliferate and differentiate. Increased 'inappro-priate' production of erythropoietin is also seen in patients with renal disease and neoplasms in other sites resulting in polycythaemia (see Table 6.15).

OTHER REQUIREMENTS FOR NORMAL ERYTHROPOIESIS
- Iron for Hb synthesis
- Vitamin $B_{12}$ and folate for normal DNA synthesis
- Other vitamins—$B_6$ (pyridoxine), thiamine, riboflavin, and vitamins C and E
- Trace metals such as cobalt
- Hormones—androgens and thyroxine

### Haemoglobin synthesis

Hb performs the main functions of red cells of carrying $O_2$ to the tissues and returning $CO_2$ from the tissues to the lungs.

Each normal adult Hb molecule, Hb A, has a molecular weight of 68 000 and consists of two $\alpha$ and two $\beta$ polypeptide chains ($\alpha_2\beta_2$) which have 141 and 146 amino acids respectively. Hb A comprises about 97% of the Hb in adults. Two other Hbs, Hb $A_2$ ($\alpha_2\delta_2$) and Hb F ($\alpha_2\gamma_2$), are found in adults in small amounts (1.5–3.2% and <1%, respectively).

Hb synthesis occurs in the mitochondria of the developing red cell (Fig. 6.2). The major rate-limiting step is the conversion of glycine and succinic acid to $\delta$-aminolaevulinic acid (ALA) by ALA synthetase producing porphobilinogen (see Fig. 17.18).

Vitamin $B_6$ is a coenzyme for this reaction which is inhibited by haem and stimulated by erythropoietin. Pyrrole rings are formed and then grouped in fours to produce protoporphyrins. Finally, iron is inserted to form haem. Haem is then inserted into the globin chains to form Hb. The structure of Hb is shown in Fig. 6.3.

### Haemoglobin function

The biconcave shape of red cells provides a large surface area for the uptake and release of $O_2$ and $CO_2$. Hb becomes saturated with $O_2$ in the pulmonary capillaries where the partial pressure of $O_2$ is high and Hb has a high affinity for $O_2$. $O_2$ is released in the tissues where the partial pressure of $O_2$ is low and Hb has a low affinity for $O_2$.

The four haem units in Hb molecules successively unload $O_2$ in the tissues and as they do the $\beta$ chains are pulled apart allowing the entry of 2,3-diphosphoglycerate (2,3-DPG). This causes the affinity of Hb for $O_2$ to decrease and improves delivery of $O_2$ to the tissues (Fig. 6.4). Most molecules carry no $O_2$ or are fully oxygenated. This is responsible for the sigmoid shape of the *oxygen dissociation curve* (see Fig. 13.5). Hb is efficient for oxygen transport largely because the steepest part of the curve occurs at the partial pressures of $O_2$ which occur in the tissues.

The *oxygen affinity* of Hb is expressed as the $P_{50}$, which is the partial pressure of $O_2$ at which 50% saturation occurs. When oxygen affinity increases, the oxygen dissociation curve shifts to the left and the $P_{50}$ falls and vice versa.

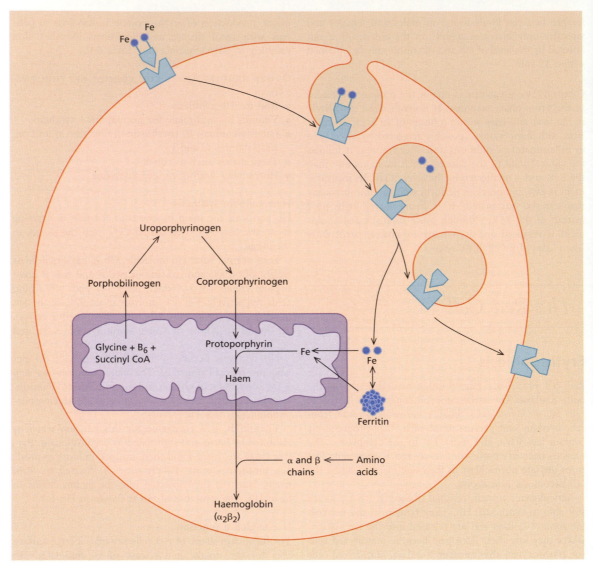

**Fig. 6.2** Haemoglobin synthesis. Transferrin attaches to a surface receptor on developing red cells. Iron is released and transported to the mitochondrion, where it combines with protoporphyrin to form haem. Haem combines with $\alpha$ and $\beta$ chains (formed on ribosomes) to make haemoglobin.

The oxygen dissociation curve is influenced by 2,3-DPG, which is an intermediate in red cell glycolysis, the pH, the concentration of $CO_2$ in the red cell and the structure of Hb. High concentrations of 2,3-DPG or $CO_2$, a low pH and certain Hbs such as sickle Hb (Hb S) shift the curve to the right, thus decreasing oxygen affinity. A shift in the curve to the left occurs with Hb F which is unable to bind 2,3-DPG and some rare abnormal Hbs where erythrocytosis may result from the increased oxygen affinity and decreased release of $O_2$ to the tissues.

A summary of normal red cell production and destruction is given in Fig. 6.5.

# Anaemia

Anaemia is present when there is a decrease in the level of Hb in the blood below the reference level for the age and sex of the individual (Table 6.1). Alterations in the level of Hb may occur as a result of changes in the plasma volume, as shown in Fig. 6.6. A reduction in the plasma volume will lead to a spuriously high Hb—this is seen with dehydration and in the clinical condition of *stress polycythaemia*. A high plasma volume, such as in preg-

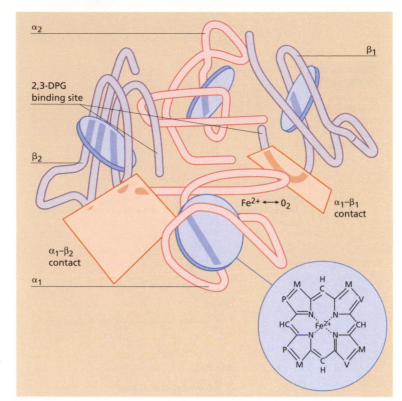

**Fig. 6.3** Model of the haemoglobin molecule showing $\alpha$ (pink) and $\beta$ (blue) chains. 2,3-DPG binds in the centre of the molecule and stabilizes the deoxygenated form by cross-linking the $\beta$ chains (also see Fig. 6.4). M, Methyl; P, propionic acid; V, vinyl. (From Schrier, S. L. (1988) *Scientific American* **10**. With permission.)

nancy, may produce a spurious anaemia.

After a major bleed, anaemia may not be apparent for several days until the plasma volume returns to normal.

## CLINICAL FEATURES

Patients with anaemia may be asymptomatic. A very slowly falling level of Hb allows for haemodynamic compensation and enhancement of the oxygen-carrying capacity of the blood. A rise in 2,3-DPG causes a shift of the oxygen dissociation curve to the right, so that oxygen is more readily given up to the tissues. Where blood loss is more rapid or severe, particularly in elderly people, symptoms may occur.

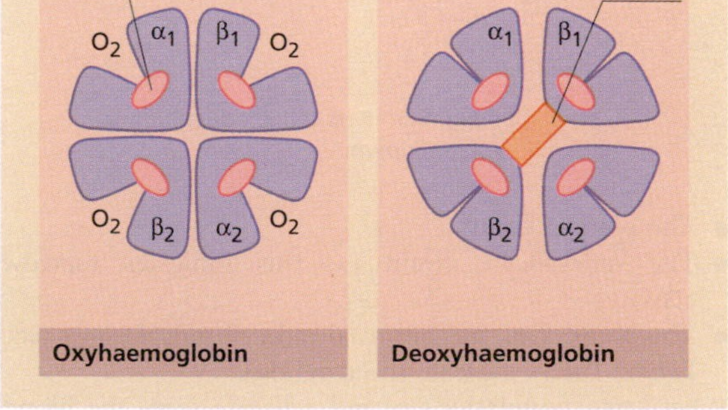

**Symptoms (all non-specific)**
- Fatigue
- Headaches $\left.\right\}$ NB Very common in the normal
- Faintness $\qquad$ population.
- Breathlessness
- Angina of effort
- Intermittent claudication
- Palpitations

**Signs**
- Pallor
- Tachycardia
- Systolic flow murmur
- Cardiac failure
- Rarely papilloedema and retinal haemorrhages after an acute bleed (can be accompanied by blindness)

Specific signs of the different types of anaemia will be discussed in the appropriate section. Examples include:
- Koilonychia—spoon-shaped nails seen in iron deficiency anaemia
- Jaundice—found in haemolytic anaemia
- Bone deformities—found in thalassaemia major
- Leg ulcers—occur in association with sickle cell disease

**Fig. 6.4** The oxygenated and deoxygenated haemoglobin molecule. The haemoglobin molecule is predominantly stabilized by $\alpha$—$\beta$ chain bonds rather than $\alpha$—$\alpha$ and $\beta$—$\beta$ chain bonds. The structure of the molecule changes during $O_2$ uptake and release. When $O_2$ is released, the $\beta$ chains rotate on the $\alpha_1\beta_2$ and $\alpha_2\beta_1$ contacts allowing the entry of 2,3-DPG which causes a lower affinity of haemoglobin for $O_2$ and improved delivery of $O_2$ to the tissues. (From Hoffbrand AV & Pettit JE (1993) *Essential Haematology*, 3rd edn. Oxford: Blackwell Scientific Publications. With permission.)

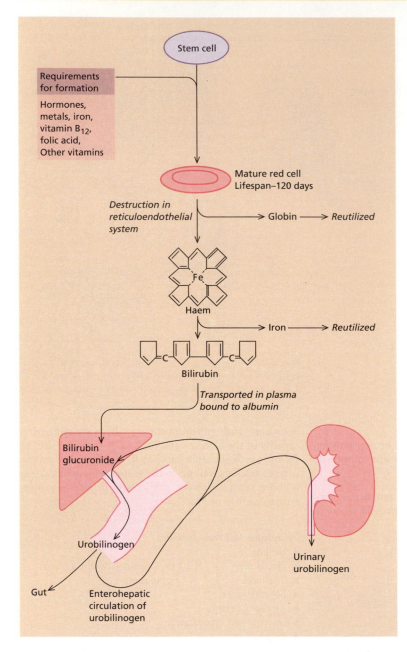

**Fig. 6.5** Red cell production and breakdown.

It must be emphasized that anaemia is not a diagnosis, and a cause must be found.

## CLASSIFICATION
The various types of anaemia, classified in terms of the red cell indices, particularly the MCV, are shown in Fig. 6.7. There are three major types of anaemia:
- Hypochromic microcytic with a low MCV
- Normochromic normocytic with a normal MCV
- Macrocytic with a high MCV

## INVESTIGATIONS
### Peripheral blood
A low Hb should always be considered in relation to:
- The white cell count (WCC)
- The platelet count
- The reticulocyte count (as this indicates marrow activity)
- The blood film, as abnormal red cell morphology (see Fig. 6.8) may indicate the diagnosis

Where two populations of red cells are seen, the blood film is said to be *dimorphic*. This may, for example, be seen in patients with 'double deficiencies', i.e. combined iron and folate deficiency in coeliac disease, or following treatment of anaemic patients with the appropriate haematinic.

### Bone marrow
Examination of the bone marrow is performed to investigate abnormalities found in the peripheral blood

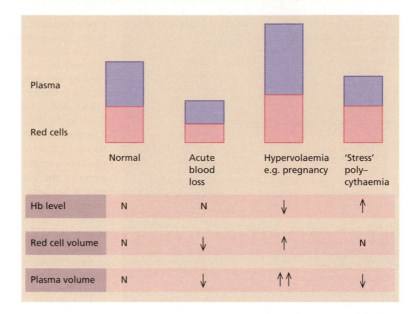

**Fig. 6.6** Alterations of haemoglobin in relation to plasma.

| | Normal | Acute blood loss | Hypervolaemia e.g. pregnancy | 'Stress' poly–cythaemia |
|---|---|---|---|---|
| Hb level | N | N | ↓ | ↑ |
| Red cell volume | N | ↓ | ↑ | N |
| Plasma volume | N | ↓ | ↑↑ | ↓ |

(Practical box 6.1). Aspiration provides a film which can be examined by microscopy for the morphology of the developing haemopoietic cells. The trephine provides a core of bone which is processed as a histological specimen and allows an overall view of the bone marrow architecture, cellularity and presence/absence of abnormal infiltrates. The following are assessed:

- Cellularity of the marrow
- Type of erythropoiesis, e.g. normoblastic or megaloblastic
- Cellularity of the various cell lines
- Infiltration of the marrow
- Assessment of iron stores
- Special tests may be performed: cytogenetic, immunological, cytochemical markers, biochemical analyses (e.g. deoxyuridine suppression test), microbiological culture

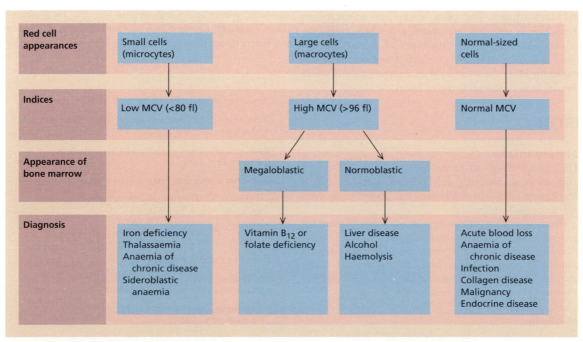

**Fig. 6.7** Classification of anaemia.

**Aspiration**
Site—usually iliac crest
Give local anaesthetic injection
Use special bone marrow needle (e.g. Salah)
Aspirate marrow
Make smear on a glass slide
Stain with:
(a) Romanowsky technique
(b) Perls' reaction (acid ferrocyanide) for iron

**Trephine**
Indications include:
  'Dry tap' obtained with aspiration
  Better assessment of cellularity, e.g. aplastic anaemia
  Better assessment of presence of infiltration or fibrosis

*Technique*
Site—usually posterior iliac crest
Give local anaesthetic injection
Use special needle (e.g. Jamshidi—longer and wider than
  for aspiration)
Obtain core of bone
Fix in formalin; decalcify—this takes a few days
Stain with:
(a) Haematoxylin and eosin
(b) Reticulin stain

**Practical box 6.1**  Techniques for obtaining bone marrow.

# Microcytic anaemia

Iron deficiency is the commonest cause of anaemia in the world. This is because of the body's limited ability to absorb iron and the frequent increased loss of iron due to haemorrhage. The other causes of a microcytic hypochromic anaemia are anaemia of chronic disease, sideroblastic anaemia and thalassaemia. In thalassaemia (described on p. 313), there is a defect in globin synthesis unlike the other three causes of microcytic anaemia where the defect is in the synthesis of haem.

## IRON

### Dietary intake
The average daily diet in the UK contains 15–20 mg of iron, although normally only 10% of this is absorbed. Absorption may be increased to 20–30% in iron deficiency and pregnancy.

Haem iron forms the main part of dietary iron and is derived from Hb and myoglobin in red or organ meats. Non-haem iron is mainly derived from cereals which are commonly fortified with iron. Haem iron is better absorbed than non-haem iron whose availability is more affected by other dietary constituents.

### Absorption
This takes place in the duodenum and jejunum. The absorption of iron is a complex process; some of the fac-

tors influencing it are shown in Table 6.2. Haem iron is partly broken down to non-haem iron but some haem iron is absorbed intact into mucosal cells. Absorption is favoured by factors such as the acidity of the stomach keeping the iron soluble and in the ferrous rather than the ferric form.

The iron content of the body is kept within narrow limits and its loss and intake are normally finely balanced. The precise mechanisms by which iron is absorbed and transported across the epithelial cell are uncertain but its absorption appears to be closely related to the total iron stores of the body. The body is unable to excrete iron once it has been absorbed. Iron overload may occur due to excessive absorption of iron (haemochromatosis, see p. 269) or due to the breakdown of transfused blood (transfusion haemosiderosis, see p. 316).

Iron absorption seems to be controlled by mucosal cells in the small intestine, possibly at both the stages of uptake of iron into the cells and transfer of iron into the portal blood. Excess iron in mucosal cells is joined to apoferritin to form ferritin. Ferritin is lost into the gut lumen when the mucosal cells are shed. In iron deficiency, more iron enters the cells and a greater proportion of the intracellular iron is transported to the portal vein. In iron overload, less iron enters the cells and a greater proportion is shed into the gut lumen.

### Transport in the blood
The normal serum iron level is about 11–30 $\mu$mol litre$^{-1}$; there is a diurnal rhythm with higher levels in the morning. Iron is transported in the plasma bound to transferrin, a $\beta$-globulin that is synthesized in the liver. Each transferrin molecule binds two atoms of ferric iron and is normally one-third saturated. Most of the iron bound to transferrin comes from macrophages in the reticuloendothelial system and not from iron absorbed by the intestine. Transferrin-bound iron becomes attached by specific receptors to erythroblasts and reticulocytes in the marrow

---

Ferrous iron is absorbed better than ferric.

Gastric acidity helps to keep iron in the ferrous state and soluble in the upper gut.

Reducing agents, e.g. ascorbic acid, increase iron absorption.

Haem iron is absorbed better than non-haem iron.

Iron absorption is increased with low iron stores and decreased in iron overload.

Increased erythropoietic activity, e.g. bleeding, haemolysis, high altitude, increases absorption.

Alcohol increases absorption.

Formation of insoluble complexes with phytate or phosphate decreases iron absorption.

There is increased absorption in idiopathic haemochromatosis.

**Table 6.2**  Factors influencing iron absorption.

and the iron is removed (Fig. 6.2).

In an average adult male, 20 mg of iron, chiefly obtained from red cell breakdown in the macrophages of the reticuloendothelial system, is incorporated into Hb every day.

### Iron stores

About two-thirds of the total body iron is in the circulation as Hb (2.5–3 g in a normal adult man). Iron is stored in reticuloendothelial cells, hepatocytes and skeletal muscle cells as ferritin and haemosiderin (500–1500 mg); about two-thirds as ferritin and one-third as haemosiderin in normal individuals. Small amounts of iron are also found in plasma, with some in myoglobin and enzymes.

*Ferritin* is a water-soluble complex of iron and protein. It is more easily mobilized than haemosiderin for Hb formation. It is present in small amounts in plasma.

*Haemosiderin* is an insoluble iron–protein complex found in macrophages in the bone marrow, liver and spleen. Unlike ferritin, it is visible by light microscopy in tissue sections and bone marrow films after staining by Perls' reaction.

### Requirements

Each day 0.5–1 mg of iron is lost in the faeces, urine and sweat. Menstruating women lose 40 ml of blood per month, an average of about 0.7 mg of iron per day. Blood loss through menstruation in excess of 100 ml will usually result in iron deficiency as increased iron absorption from the gut cannot compensate for such losses of iron. The demand for iron also increases during growth (about 0.6 mg per day) and pregnancy (1–2 mg per day).

In the normal adult the iron content of the body remains relatively fixed. Increases in the body iron content (haemochromatosis) are classified into primary and secondary forms. Primary (idiopathic) haemochromatosis is discussed on p. 269. Secondary haemochromatosis (transfusion siderosis) is due to iron overload in conditions where repeated transfusion is the only therapy.

# IRON DEFICIENCY

Iron deficiency anaemia develops when there is inadequate iron for Hb synthesis. A normal level of Hb is maintained for as long as possible after the iron stores are depleted; *latent iron deficiency* is said to be present during this period.

## CAUSES OF IRON DEFICIENCY
- Blood loss
- Increased demands such as growth and pregnancy
- Decreased absorption, e.g. postgastrectomy
- Poor intake

Most iron deficiency occurs from *blood loss*, usually from the uterus or gastrointestinal tract. Premenopausal women are always in a state of precarious iron balance owing to menstruation. Isolated nutritional iron deficiency is rare in developed countries. The commonest cause of iron deficiency worldwide is blood loss from the gastrointestinal tract due to hookworm infestation. The poor quality of the diet, predominantly containing vegetables, also contributes to the high prevalence of iron deficiency in developing countries.

## CLINICAL FEATURES

The symptoms of anaemia are described on p. 297. Other clinical features occur as a result of tissue iron deficiency. These are mainly epithelial changes induced by the effect of inadequate iron in the cells:
- Brittle nails
- Spoon-shaped nails (koilonychia)
- Atrophy of the papillae of the tongue
- Angular stomatitis
- Brittle hair
- A syndrome of dysphagia and glossitis (Plummer–Vinson or Paterson–Brown Kelly syndrome)

The diagnosis of iron deficiency anaemia relies on a good clinical history with questions about dietary intake, regular self-medication with aspirin (which may give rise to gastrointestinal bleeding) and the presence of blood in the faeces (which may be a sign of haemorrhoids or carcinoma of the lower bowel). No examination of an iron-deficient patient is complete without a rectal examination. In women, a careful inquiry about the duration of periods, the occurrence of clots and the number of sanitary towels or tampons used should be made.

## INVESTIGATION

### Blood count and film

A characteristic blood film is shown in Fig. 6.8. The red cells are microcytic (MCV $<80$ fl) and hypochromic (MCH $<27$ pg). There is *poikilocytosis* (variation in shape) and *anisocytosis* (variation in size). Target cells are seen.

### Serum iron and iron-binding capacity

The values for serum iron and iron-binding capacity in iron deficiency are included in Fig. 6.9; the serum iron falls and the total iron-binding capacity (TIBC) rises compared with normal. Iron deficiency is regularly present when the transferrin saturation (i.e. serum iron divided by TIBC) falls below 19%.

### Serum ferritin

The level of serum ferritin reflects the amount of stored iron, probably more accurately than the saturation of the serum iron-binding capacity. The normal values for serum ferritin are 30–300 $\mu$g litre$^{-1}$ (11.6–144 nmol litre$^{-1}$) in males and 15–200 $\mu$g litre$^{-1}$ (5.8–96 nmol litre$^{-1}$) in females.

### Bone marrow

Erythroid hyperplasia with ragged normoblasts are seen in the marrow in iron deficiency. Staining using Perls' reaction (acid ferrocyanide) does not show the characteristic Prussian-blue granules of stainable iron in the bone marrow fragments or in the erythroblasts.

Examination of the bone marrow is not essential for

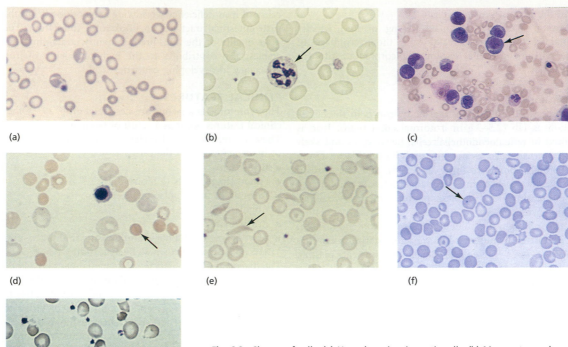

(a)    (b)    (c)

(d)    (e)    (f)

(g)

**Fig. 6.8**  Shapes of cells. (a) Hypochromic microcytic cells. (b) Macrocytes and a hypersegmented neutrophil (arrowed). (c) Megaloblasts (arrowed) in the bone marrow. (d) Spherocytes (arrowed), reticulocytes (polychromasia) and a nucleated erythroblast. (e) Sickle cells (arrowed) and target cells. (f) Postsplenectomy film with Howell–Jolly bodies (arrowed), target cells and irregularly contracted cells. (g) 'Blister' cells (arrowed) in G6PD deficiency.

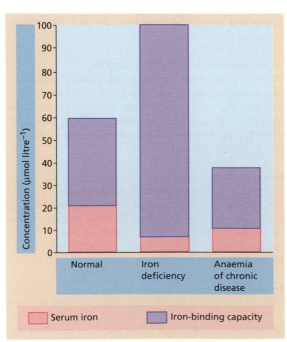

**Fig. 6.9**  Serum iron and total iron-binding capacity in normal subjects and in iron deficiency anaemia and anaemia of chronic disease.

the diagnosis of iron deficiency but it may be helpful in the investigation of complicated cases of anaemia.

### Other investigations
These will be indicated by the clinical history and examination; investigations of the gastrointestinal tract are often required (see p. 199).

### DIFFERENTIAL DIAGNOSIS
The presence of anaemia with microcytosis and hypochromia does not necessarily indicate iron deficiency. The commonest other causes are thalassaemia, sideroblastic anaemia and anaemia of chronic disease. In all of these disorders the iron stores are normal or increased. The differential diagnosis of microcytic anaemia is shown in Table 6.3.

### TREATMENT
The correct management of iron deficiency is to find and treat the underlying cause, and to give iron to correct the anaemia and replace iron stores. The response to iron therapy can be monitored using the reticulocyte count and Hb level with an expected rise in haemoglobin of 1 g per week.

Oral iron is all that is required in most cases. The best preparation is ferrous sulphate (600 mg daily, 120 mg ferrous iron) which is absorbed best when the patient is fasting. If the patient has side-effects such as nausea, diarrhoea or constipation, taking the tablets with food or reducing the dose using a preparation with less iron such as ferrous gluconate (600 mg daily, 70 mg ferrous iron) is all that is usually required to reduce the symptoms. The use of expensive iron compounds, particularly the slow-release ones which release iron beyond its main sites of absorption, is unnecessary.

Oral iron should be given for long enough to correct the Hb and to replenish the iron stores which usually takes six months. Failure of response to oral iron may be due to:

- Lack of compliance
- Continuing haemorrhage
- Severe malabsorption
- Another cause for the anaemia

These possibilities should be considered before parenteral iron is used. However, parenteral iron is required by occasional patients, including those who have general intolerance of oral preparations even at low dose, those with severe malabsorption and those who have chronic gastrointestinal diseases such as ulcerative colitis or Crohn's disease. Iron stores are replaced much faster with parenteral iron than with oral iron but the haematological response is no quicker. Parenteral iron can be given as repeated injections of iron dextran or iron-sorbitol or as a total dose infusion over about 6 hours using iron dextran.

## ANAEMIA OF CHRONIC DISEASE

One of the commonest types of anaemia, particularly in hospital patients, is the anaemia of chronic disease, occurring in patients with chronic infections such as infective endocarditis and tuberculosis and osteomyelitis in developing countries, chronic inflammatory diseases such as rheumatoid arthritis, systemic lupus erythematosus (SLE) and polymyalgia rheumatica and in patients with malignant disease. There is decreased release of iron from the bone marrow to developing erythroblasts, an inadequate erythropoietin response to the anaemia and decreased red cell survival. The exact mechanisms responsible for these effects are not clear but they seem to be mediated by inflammatory cytokines such as IL-1,

tumour necrosis factor and interferons.

The serum iron is low and the TIBC is also low (Fig. 6.9). Serum ferritin is normal or raised. There is stainable iron present in the bone marrow and, therefore, patients do not respond to iron therapy. However, iron is not seen in the developing erythroblasts. Treatment is, in general, that of the underlying disorder, although trials are being carried out with recombinant erythropoietin in some patients, for example those with rheumatoid arthritis.

## SIDEROBLASTIC ANAEMIA

Sideroblastic anaemias are inherited or acquired disorders characterized by a refractory anaemia, a variable number of hypochromic cells in the peripheral blood, and excess iron and ring sideroblasts in the bone marrow. The presence of *ring sideroblasts* is the diagnostic feature of sideroblastic anaemia; there is disordered accumulation of iron in the mitochondria of erythroblasts due to disordered haem synthesis. A ring of iron granules is formed round the nucleus that can be seen with Perls' reaction. The blood film is often dimorphic; ineffective haem synthesis is responsible for the microcytic hypochromic cells. Sideroblastic anaemias can be classified as shown in Table 6.4. Primary acquired sideroblastic anaemia is one of the myelodysplastic syndromes (see p. 327).

### TREATMENT

Some patients respond when drugs or alcohol are withdrawn if these are the causative agents. In some cases, particularly the inherited type, there is a response to pyridoxine. Treatment with folic acid may be required to treat accompanying folate deficiency.

## LEAD POISONING

The causes, clinical features and treatment are discussed on p. 756. The characteristic haematological features include:

SIDEROBLASTIC ANAEMIA, due to inhibition by lead of

| | Iron deficiency | Anaemia of chronic disease | Thalassaemia trait (α or β) | Sideroblastic anaemia |
|---|---|---|---|---|
| MCV | Reduced | Low normal or normal | Very low for degree of anaemia | Low in inherited type but often raised in acquired type |
| Serum iron | Reduced | Reduced | Normal | Raised |
| Serum TIBC | Raised | Reduced | Normal | Normal |
| Serum ferritin | Reduced | Normal or raised | Normal | Raised |
| Iron in marrow | Absent | Present | Present | Present |
| Iron in erythroblasts | Absent | Absent or reduced | Present | Ring forms |

TIBC, Total iron binding capacity.

**Table 6.3**  Differential diagnosis of microcytic anaemia.

*Inherited*
X-linked disease—transmitted by females

*Acquired*
Primary (one of the myelodysplastic syndromes, see
    p. 327)

Secondary:
Other types of myelodysplasia
Myeloproliferative disorders
Myeloid leukaemia
Drugs, e.g. isoniazid
Alcohol
Lead
Other disorders, e.g. rheumatoid arthritis, carcinoma,
    megaloblastic and haemolytic anaemias

**Table 6.4**   Classification of sideroblastic anaemia.

several enzymes involved in haem synthesis including
δ-aminolaevulinic acid synthetase

HAEMOLYSIS, which is usually mild, due to damage to
the red cell membrane

PUNCTATE BASOPHILIA (the blood film shows red cells
with small, round, blue particles), due to aggregates of
RNA in red cells due to inhibition by lead of pyrim-
idine-5-nucleotidase, which normally disperses residual
RNA to produce a diffuse blue staining seen in
reticulocytes on blood films (*polychromasia*)

## Normocytic anaemia

Normocytic, normochromic anaemia is seen in anaemia
of chronic disease, in some endocrine disorders (e.g.
hypopituitarism, hypothyroidism and hypoadrenalism)
and in some haematological disorders (e.g. aplastic anaemia and some haemolytic anaemias) (Fig. 6.7). In
addition, this type of anaemia is seen acutely following
blood loss before iron stores are depleted.

## Macrocytic anaemia

This can be divided into megaloblastic and non-mega-
loblastic types, depending on bone marrow findings.

## Megaloblastic anaemia

Megaloblastic anaemia is characterized by the presence in
the bone marrow of erythroblasts with delayed nuclear
maturation because of defective DNA synthesis (*megaloblasts*). Megaloblasts are large and have large immature

nuclei. The nuclear chromatin is more finely dispersed
than normal and has an open stippled appearance
(Fig. 6.8). A characteristic abnormality of white cells,
*giant metamyelocytes*, is frequently seen in megaloblastic
anaemia. These cells are about twice the size of normal
cells and often have twisted nuclei. Megaloblastic changes
occur in:

- Vitamin $B_{12}$ deficiency or abnormal vitamin $B_{12}$ metabolism
- Folic acid deficiency or abnormal folate metabolism
- Other defects of DNA synthesis, e.g. congenital enzyme
  deficiencies in DNA synthesis such as orotic aciduria,
  therapy with drugs interfering with DNA synthesis
  and myelodysplasia

**Haematological values**
Anaemia may be present. The MCV is characteristically
>96 fl unless there is a coexisting cause of microcytosis.
The peripheral blood film shows macrocytes with *hypersegmented polymorphs* with six or more lobes in the
nucleus (Fig. 6.8). If severe, there may be leucopenia
and thrombocytopenia.

**Biochemical basis of megaloblastic anaemia**
The key biochemical problem common to both vitamin
$B_{12}$ and folate deficiency is a block in DNA synthesis due
to an inability to methylate deoxyuridine monophosphate
to deoxythymidine monophosphate, which is then used
to build DNA (Fig. 6.10). The methyl group is supplied
by the folate coenzyme, methylene tetrahydrofolate poly-
glutamate. Deficiency of folate reduces the supply of this
coenzyme; deficiency of vitamin $B_{12}$ also reduces its supply by slowing the demethylation of methyl tetrahydrofolate and preventing cells receiving tetrahydrofolate for synthesis of methylene tetrahydrofolate.

Other congenital and acquired forms of megaloblastic
anaemia are due to interference with purine or pyrimidine synthesis causing an inhibition in DNA synthesis.

**Deoxyuridine suppression test**
Tritiated thymidine is added to the patient's bone marrow *in vitro*. In a normoblastic marrow, the thymidine
requirement is supplied by the methylation of deoxyuridine and this 'suppresses' the requirement for preformed
tritiated thymidine to less than 5%. In a megaloblastic
marrow, however, much more tritiated thymidine is used
(5–50%). If the addition of $B_{12}$ corrects the abnormality,
it suggests that $B_{12}$ is the cause of the deficiency. The
addition of folate corrects the abnormality in both vitamin $B_{12}$ and folate deficiency.

This is a useful method for rapidly determining the
nature and severity of the vitamin deficiency in severe or
complex cases of megaloblastic anaemia.

## VITAMIN $B_{12}$

Vitamin $B_{12}$ is synthesized by certain microorganisms,
and humans are ultimately dependent on animal sources.
It is found in meat, fish, eggs and milk, but not in plants.

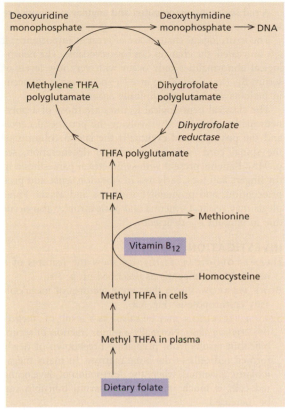

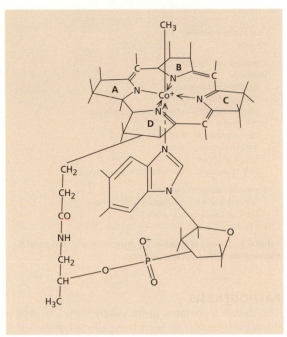

**Fig. 6.10** Biochemical basis of megaloblastic anaemia. The metabolic relationship between vitamin $B_{12}$ and folate and their role in DNA synthesis. THFA, tetra hydrofolic acid.

**Fig. 6.11** The structure of methylcobalamin, the main form of vitamin $B_{12}$ in the plasma.

Vitamin $B_{12}$ is not usually destroyed by cooking. The average daily diet contains 5–30 $\mu g$ of vitamin $B_{12}$, of which 2–3 $\mu g$ are absorbed. The average adult stores some 2–3 mg, mainly in the liver, and it may take 2 years or more after absorptive failure before $B_{12}$ deficiency develops, as the daily losses are small (1–2 $\mu g$).

### Structure
Cobalamins consist of a planar group with a central cobalt atom (corrin ring) and a nucleotide set at right angles (Fig. 6.11). Vitamin $B_{12}$ was first crystallized as cyanocobalamin but the main natural cobalamins have deoxyadenosyl, methyl and hydroxycobalamin groups attached to the cobalt atom.

### Function
Methylcobalamin is a coenzyme for the methylation of homocysteine to methionine by methyltetrahydrofolate, as described above (Fig. 6.10).

Deoxyadenosylcobalamin is a coenzyme for the conversion of methylmalonyl CoA to succinyl CoA. Measurement of methylmalonic acid in urine was used as a test for vitamin $B_{12}$ deficiency but it is no longer routinely carried out.

### Absorption and transport
Vitamin $B_{12}$ is liberated from protein complexes in food by gastric enzymes and then binds to two vitamin $B_{12}$-binding proteins, intrinsic factor and 'R'-binder. Vitamin $B_{12}$ bound to 'R' binder is released by pancreatic enzymes and also becomes bound to intrinsic factor.

*Intrinsic factor* is a glycoprotein with a molecular weight of over 44 000 that is secreted by gastric parietal cells with $H^+$ ions. It combines with vitamin $B_{12}$ and carries it to specific receptors on the surface of the mucosa of the ileum.   Vitamin $B_{12}$ enters the ileal cells and intrinsic factor remains in the lumen. Vitamin $B_{12}$ is transported from the enterocytes to the bone marrow and other tissues by the glycoprotein *transcobalamin II* (TC II). Although TC II is the essential carrier protein for vitamin $B_{12}$, the amount of $B_{12}$ on TC II is low. Vitamin $B_{12}$ in plasma is mainly bound to *transcobalamin I* (TC I) (70–90%) and *transcobalamin III* (TC III) (<10%) but neither protein plays a role in delivering $B_{12}$ to the bone marrow.

## VITAMIN $B_{12}$ DEFICIENCY

There are a number of causes of $B_{12}$ deficiency and abnormal $B_{12}$ metabolism (Table 6.5). The commonest cause of vitamin $B_{12}$ deficiency in adults is *pernicious anaemia*. Malabsorption of vitamin $B_{12}$ due to pancreatitis, coeliac disease or treatment with metformin is mild and does not usually result in significant vitamin $B_{12}$ deficiency.

## Pernicious anaemia (PA)

PA is a condition in which there is atrophy of the gastric mucosa with consequent failure of intrinsic factor production and vitamin $B_{12}$ malabsorption.

*Low dietary intake*
Vegans

*Impaired absorption*
Stomach
    Pernicious anaemia
    Gastrectomy
    Congenital deficiency of intrinsic factor
Small bowel
    Ileal disease or resection
    Bacterial overgrowth
    Tropical sprue
    Fish tapeworm (*Diphyllobothrium latum*)

*Abnormal metabolism*
    Congenital transcobalamin II deficiency
    Nitrous oxide (inactivates $B_{12}$)

**Table 6.5**  Causes of vitamin $B_{12}$ deficiency and abnormal $B_{12}$ metabolism. Other causes—see text.

## PATHOGENESIS

This disease is common in the elderly, with 1 in 8000 of the population over 60 years being affected in the UK. It can be seen in all races, but is particularly common in fair-haired and blue-eyed people. It is commoner in females than males.

There is an association with other autoimmune diseases, particularly thyroid disease, Addison's disease and vitiligo. Approximately one-half of all patients with PA have thyroid antibodies. There is a higher incidence of gastric carcinoma in males with PA than in the general population; females have a normal life expectancy with replacement therapy.

Parietal cell antibodies are present in the serum in 90% of patients with PA—and also in many older patients with gastric atrophy. Conversely, intrinsic factor antibodies, although found in only 50% of patients with PA, are specific for this diagnosis. Two types of intrinsic factor antibodies are found: a *blocking* antibody, which inhibits binding of intrinsic factor to $B_{12}$ and a *precipitating* antibody, which inhibits the binding of the $B_{12}$–intrinsic factor complex to its receptor site in the ileum. Their role in pathogenesis is unknown.

$B_{12}$ deficiency may rarely occur in children due to a congenital deficiency or abnormality of intrinsic factor, or due to early onset of the adult autoimmune type.

## PATHOLOGY

Atrophic gastritis (see p. 190) is present with plasma cell and lymphoid infiltration. There is achlorhydria and absent secretion of intrinsic factor. The histological abnormality can be improved by corticosteroid therapy, which supports an autoimmune basis for the disease.

## CLINICAL FEATURES

The onset of PA is insidious with progressively increasing symptoms of anaemia. Patients are sometimes said to have a lemon yellow colour due to a combination of pallor and jaundice caused by excess breakdown of Hb due to ineffective erythropoiesis in the bone marrow.

A red sore tongue (glossitis) and angular stomatitis are sometimes present.

The neurological changes are of greatest importance; if left untreated, the changes can be irreversible. The neurological abnormalities only occur with very low levels of serum $B_{12}$ (less than 60 ng litre$^{-1}$) and occasionally occur in patients who are not clinically anaemic.

The classical neurological features are those of a polyneuropathy progressively involving the peripheral nerves and the posterior and eventually the lateral columns of the spinal cord (subacute combined degeneration, see p. 948). Patients present with symmetrical paraesthesia in the fingers and toes, early loss of vibration sense and proprioception, and progressive weakness and ataxia. Paraplegia may result. Dementia and optic atrophy also occur due to vitamin $B_{12}$ deficiency.

## INVESTIGATION

Haematological findings show the features of a megaloblastic anaemia as described on p. 304.

Bone marrow shows the typical features of megaloblastic erythropoiesis (Fig. 6.8).

Serum bilirubin may be raised as a result of *ineffective erythropoiesis*. Normally a minor fraction of serum bilirubin results from premature breakdown of newly formed red cells in the bone marrow. In many megaloblastic anaemias, where the destruction of developing red cells is much increased, the serum bilirubin can be increased.

Serum vitamin $B_{12}$ is usually well below the normal level of 160 ng litre$^{-1}$. Serum vitamin $B_{12}$ can be assayed using microbiological or radioisotope dilution assays.

Serum folate level is normal or high, and the red cell folate is normal or reduced due to inhibition of normal folate synthesis.

### Absorption tests

The absorption of $B_{12}$ can be measured using the Schilling test (Practical box 6.2). This test may give a falsely low

---

**Part I**
Give 1 $\mu$g $^{58}$Co-$B_{12}$ orally to fasting patient
Give 1000 $\mu$g $B_{12}$ (non-radioactive) by intramuscular injection to saturate $B_{12}$-binding proteins and to flush out $^{58}$Co-$B_{12}$
Collect urine for 24 hours
Normal subjects excrete more than 10% of the radioactive dose

*If abnormal:*

**Part II**
Repeat part I with oral intrinsic factor capsules

*Result*
If excretion now normal, diagnosis is pernicious anaemia or gastrectomy
If excretion still abnormal, lesion is in the terminal ileum or there is bacterial overgrowth. Vitamin $B_{12}$ malabsorption due to bacterial overgrowth may be corrected by antibiotic therapy

**Practical box 6.2**  Schilling test.

*Nutritional* (major cause)
Poor intake:
   Old age
   Poor social conditions
   Starvation
   Alcohol excess (also causes impaired utilization)
Poor intake due to anorexia
   Gastrointestinal disease, e.g. partial gastrectomy,
     coeliac disease, Crohn's disease
   Cancer

*Excess utilization*
Physiological
   Pregnancy
   Lactation
   Prematurity
Pathological:
   Haematological disease with excess red cell production,
     e.g. haemolysis
   Malignant disease with increased cell turnover
   Inflammatory disease
   Metabolic disease, e.g. homocystinuria
   Haemodialysis or peritoneal dialysis

*Malabsorption*
Occurs in small bowel disease, but the effect is minor
   compared with that of anorexia

*Antifolate drugs*
Anticonvulsants
   Phenytoin
   Primidone
Methotrexate
Pyrimethamine
Trimethoprim

**Table 6.6**  Causes of folate deficiency.

result if there is an incomplete 24-hour collection of urine or if renal function is impaired. An alternative to the Schilling test is whole-body counting where a radioactive dose of $B_{12}$ is given orally and the total body activity is measured. The level of radioactivity is counted no less than 7 days later to measure how much vitamin $B_{12}$ has been retained. A normal result is retention of 50% or more of the 1 $\mu$g dose of radioactive $B_{12}$.

### Gastrointestinal investigations

In PA there is marked gastric atrophy with achlorhydria and intubation studies can be performed to confirm this but are rarely carried out in routine practice. Endoscopy or barium meal examination of the stomach are performed only if gastric symptoms are present.

## DIFFERENTIAL DIAGNOSIS

Vitamin $B_{12}$ deficiency must be differentiated from other causes of megaloblastic anaemia, principally folate deficiency, but usually this is quite clear from the blood level of these two vitamins.

PA must be distinguished from other causes of vitamin $B_{12}$ deficiency, which are briefly indicated below:

GASTROINTESTINAL DISEASE. Any disease involving the terminal ileum or bacterial overgrowth in the small bowel can produce vitamin $B_{12}$ deficiency (see p. 203).

VEGANS. These are patients who are strict vegetarians and eat no meat or animal products. A careful dietary history should be obtained.

## FOLIC ACID

Folic acid is formed from three building blocks: a pteridine (similar to xanthopterin), *p*-aminobenzoic acid and glutamic acid (Fig. 6.12). It is not present in nature but is the parent compound of folates, which are polyglutamates (extra glutamic acid residues).

Folates are present in food in the reduced dihydrofolate or tetrahydrofolate forms (Fig. 6.12) with methyl ($CH_3$), formyl (CHO) or methylene ($CH_2$) groups attached to the pteridine part of the molecule. Polyglutamates are broken down to monoglutamates in the upper gastrointestinal tract and during the absorptive process these are converted to methyltetrahydrofolate, monoglutamate which is the main form in the serum. Vitamin $B_{12}$ converts methyltetrahydrofolate to tetrahydrofolate, which is the substrate for the synthesis of folate polyglutamates in cells. These intracellular folates are the active forms of folate and act as coenzymes in the transfer of single carbon units in amino acid metabolism and DNA synthesis (Fig. 6.10).

### Dietary intake

Folate is found in green vegetables such as spinach and broccoli, and offal, such as liver and kidney. Cooking causes a loss of 60–90% of the folate. The minimal daily requirement is about 100 $\mu$g.

## FOLATE DEFICIENCY

The causes of folate deficiency are shown in Table 6.6. The main cause is poor intake which may occur alone or in combination with excessive utilization or malabsorption. Unlike vitamin $B_{12}$, the body's reserves of folate are low. On a deficient diet, folate deficiency develops over

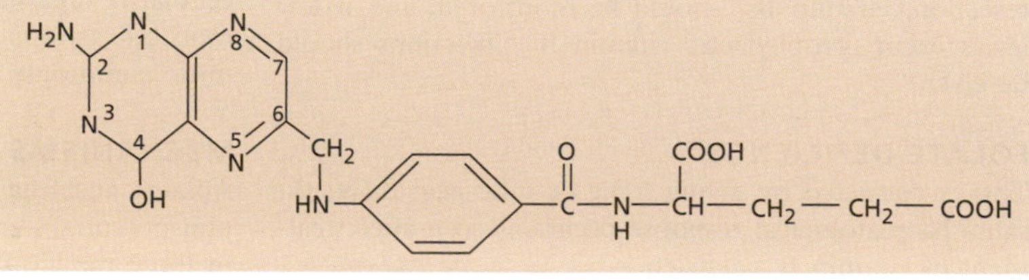

**Fig. 6.12**  The structure of folic acid. Tetrahydrofolate has additional hydrogen atoms at positions 5, 6, 7 and 8.

the course of about 4 months, but folate deficiency may develop rapidly in patients who have both a poor intake and excess utilization of folate, for example patients in intensive care units.

## CLINICAL FEATURES
Patients with folate deficiency may be asymptomatic. The clinical manifestations are megaloblastic anaemia and glossitis.

## INVESTIGATION
The haematological findings are those of a megaloblastic anaemia as discussed on p. 304.

### Blood measurements
Serum folate can be assayed by radioisotope dilution assays or microbiologically using the *Lactobacillus casei* method; antibiotic therapy may lead to falsely low results. Normal levels of serum folate are 4–18 $\mu$g litre$^{-1}$. The amount of folate in the red cells is a better measure of tissue folate; the normal range is 160–640 $\mu$g ml$^{-1}$.

### Further investigations
In many cases of folate deficiency the cause is not obvious from the clinical picture or dietary history. Occult gastro-intestinal disease should then be suspected and appropriate investigations, such as jejunal biopsy, should be performed (p. 205).

## TREATMENT AND PREVENTION OF MEGALOBLASTIC ANAEMIA

Treatment depends on the type of deficiency. Blood transfusion is not indicated in chronic anaemia; indeed, it is dangerous to transfuse elderly patients, as heart failure may be precipitated. Folic acid may produce a haematological response in vitamin B$_{12}$ deficiency but may aggravate the neuropathy. Large doses of folic acid alone should not be used to treat megaloblastic anaemia unless the serum vitamin B$_{12}$ level is known to be normal.

### VITAMIN B$_{12}$ DEFICIENCY
This is treated with hydroxycobalamin 1000 $\mu$g intramuscularly to a total of 5000–6000 $\mu$g over the course of 3 weeks; 1000 $\mu$g is then necessary every 3 months for the rest of the patient's life. Clinical improvement may occur within 48 hours and a reticulocytosis can be seen some 2–3 days after starting therapy, peaking at 5–7 days. Improvement of the peripheral neuropathy may occur over 6–12 months, but long-standing spinal cord damage is irreversible.

In patients who have had a total gastrectomy or an ileal resection, vitamin B$_{12}$ should be monitored, and if low levels occur, prophylactic vitamin B$_{12}$ injections should be given.

### FOLATE DEFICIENCY
This is corrected by giving 5 mg of folic acid daily; the same haematological response occurs as seen after treatment of vitamin B$_{12}$ deficiency.

Prophylactic folate is recommended for all women planning a pregnancy, and particularly in those who have had a child with a neural tube defect. Many authorities also recommend prophylactic administration of folate throughout pregnancy but this is not essential for those women with good diets. Prophylactic folate is also given in chronic haematological disorders where there is rapid cell turnover.

# Macrocytosis without megaloblastic changes

A raised MCV with macrocytosis on the peripheral blood film can occur with a normoblastic rather than a megaloblastic bone marrow. Common causes of macrocytosis include the following.

**Physiological**
- Pregnancy
- Newborn

**Pathological**
- Alcohol excess
- Liver disease
- Reticulocytosis
- Hypothyroidism
- Some haematological disorders, e.g. aplastic anaemia, sideroblastic anaemia

In all these conditions, normal levels of vitamin B$_{12}$ and folate will be found. The exact mechanisms in each case are uncertain, but in some there is increased lipid deposition in the red cell membrane. An increased number of reticulocytes leads to a raised MCV because they are large cells. Alcohol is a frequent cause of a raised MCV in an otherwise normal individual. Megaloblastic anaemia may occur in people who abuse alcohol; this is due to a toxic effect of alcohol on erythropoiesis or to dietary folate deficiency.

# Anaemia due to marrow failure (aplastic anaemia)

Aplastic anaemia is defined as pancytopenia with hypocellularity (aplasia) of the bone marrow. It is an uncommon but serious condition that may be inherited but is more commonly acquired.

## MECHANISMS
Aplastic anaemia is due to a reduction in the number of pluripotential stem cells (see Fig. 6.1) together with a fault in those remaining or an immune reaction against them

| |
|---|
| *Primary* |
| Congenital, e.g. Fanconi's anaemia |
| Idiopathic acquired (50% of cases) |
| |
| *Secondary* |
| Chemicals, e.g. benzene |
| Drugs |
| Insecticides |
| Ionizing radiation |
| Infections, e.g. viral hepatitis, measles |
| Miscellaneous infections, e.g. tuberculosis |
| Thymoma |
| Pregnancy |

**Table 6.7**  Causes of aplastic anaemia.

so that they are unable to repopulate the bone marrow. Failure of one cell line may occur resulting in isolated deficiencies such as the absence of red cell precursors in pure red cell aplasia.

## CAUSES

A list of causes of aplasia is given in Table 6.7. An immune mechanism is probably responsible for most cases of idiopathic acquired aplastic anaemia; immune suppression of stem cells by T suppressor cells has been implicated in many of these cases.

In contrast, secondary aplastic anaemia is due to direct damage to the bone marrow caused by drugs, chemicals, radiation or infection. Many drugs may cause marrow aplasia, including cytotoxic drugs such as busulphan and doxorubicin, which are expected to cause transient aplasia. However, some individuals develop aplasia after exposure to non-cytotoxic drugs such as chloramphenicol, gold, carbimazole, chlorpromazine, phenytoin, tolbutamide and many others which have been reported to cause occasional cases of aplasia.

Congenital aplastic anaemias are rare. Fanconi's anaemia is inherited as an autosomal recessive and is associated with skeletal, renal and central nervous system abnormalities. It usually presents between the ages of 5 and 10 years.

## CLINICAL FEATURES

The clinical manifestations of marrow failure are anaemia, bleeding and infection. Physical findings include ecchymoses, bleeding gums and epistaxis. Mouth infec-

tions are common. Lymphadenopathy and hepatosplenomegaly are rare in aplastic anaemia.

## INVESTIGATION

The laboratory diagnosis is made on the basis of:
- Pancytopenia
- The virtual absence of reticulocytes
- A hypocellular or aplastic bone marrow with increased fat spaces (Fig. 6.13)

## DIFFERENTIAL DIAGNOSIS

This is from other causes of pancytopenia (Table 6.8). A bone marrow trephine is essential for assessment of the bone marrow cellularity.

## TREATMENT AND PROGNOSIS

The cause of aplastic anaemia must be eliminated if possible. Supportive care including transfusions of red cells and platelets and antibiotic therapy should be given as necessary.

The course of aplastic anaemia can be variable, ranging from a rapid spontaneous remission to a persistent increasingly severe pancytopenia, which may lead to death through haemorrhage or infection. The most reliable determinants for the prognosis are the number of neutrophils, reticulocytes, platelets, and the cellularity of the bone marrow.

**Bad prognostic features**
- A neutrophil count $<0.5 \times 10^9$/litre
- A platelet count of $<20 \times 10^9$/litre

| |
|---|
| Aplastic anaemia (Table 6.7) |
| Megaloblastic anaemia |
| Bone marrow infiltration or replacement |
|    Hodgkin's and non-Hodgkin's lymphoma |
|    Acute leukaemia |
|    Myeloma |
|    Secondary carcinoma |
|    Myelofibrosis |
| Hypersplenism |
| Systemic lupus erythematosus |
| Disseminated tuberculosis |
| Paroxysmal nocturnal haemoglobinuria |
| Overwhelming sepsis |

**Table 6.8**  Causes of pancytopenia.

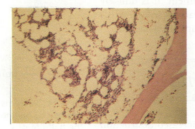

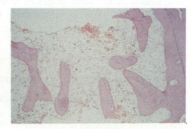

**Fig. 6.13**  Low power views of bone marrow trephine biopsies: (a) normal cellularity, and (b) hypocellularity in aplastic anaemia.

(a)                    (b)

- A reticulocyte count of $10 \times 10^9$/litre (0.1%)
- Severe hypocellularity of the bone marrow

In *severe aplastic anaemia* (with three of the four bad prognostic features) there is less than 50% chance of survival beyond 6 months. Bone marrow transplantation (see p. 371) is the treatment of choice for patients under 20 years of age who have an HLA-identical sibling donor. Older patients up to the age of 45 years with *very severe aplastic anaemia* (i.e. all the above criteria and a neutrophil count $<0.2 \times 10^9$/litre) should also be treated by transplantation if an HLA-identical sibling is available. A successful graft occurs in 70–80% of patients. Patients between 20 and 45 years with severe aplastic anaemia might also be considered for bone marrow transplantation if an HLA-identical sibling is available, but, if not, treatment with immunosuppressive therapy is used (see below).

About 70% of patients with aplastic anaemia eligible for bone marrow transplantation do not have an HLA-identical sibling. The results of bone marrow transplantation using unrelated donors or mismatched family donors is still too unsatisfactory to warrant its widespread use. Such treatment is currently restricted to very young patients ($<6$ years) with severe aplastic anaemia and adults with very severe aplastic anaemia; both groups have a poor chance of survival if treated with immunosuppressive therapy. Patients failing to respond to immunosuppressive therapy may also be considered for this treatment.

Immunosuppressive therapy is used for those patients outlined above and for patients with severe aplastic anaemia over the age of 45 years; antilymphocyte globulin (ALG), steroids and cyclosporin are used alone or in combination. Patients over the age of 45 are not eligible for bone marrow transplantation whether an HLA-identical donor is available or not, because the high risk of graft-versus-host disease is a complication of bone marrow transplantation. ALG alone produces a haematological recovery in 50–60% of cases and this is increased to 80% in patients receiving ALG, steroids and cyclosporin.

Steroids are used to treat children with congenital pure red cell aplasia (Diamond–Blackfan syndrome). Adult pure red cell aplasia is associated with a thymoma in 30% of cases and thymectomy may induce a remission. It may also be associated with autoimmune disease or may be idiopathic. Steroids and cyclosporin are effective treatment in some cases.

Recombinant haemopoietic growth factors (see Fig. 6.1) are being used in aplastic anaemia to prevent infective deaths in the early stages of treatment. It is unlikely that the use of haemopoietic growth factors will be effective as primary treatment for severe aplastic anaemia.

## Haemolytic anaemia

Haemolytic anaemias are caused by increased destruction of red cells. The red cell normally survives about 120 days

but in haemolytic anaemias the red cell survival times are considerably shortened (Fig. 6.14).

There is no definite explanation why red cells are removed from the circulation at the end of their life-span. Breakdown of normal red cells occurs in the macrophages of the bone marrow, liver and spleen (see Fig. 6.5).

## Consequences of haemolysis

Shortening of red cell survival does not always cause anaemia as there is a compensatory increase in red cell production by the bone marrow. If the red cell loss can be contained within the marrow's capacity for increased output, then a haemolytic state can exist without anaemia (*compensated haemolytic disease*). The bone marrow can increase its output by six to eight times by increasing the proportion of cells committed to erythropoiesis (*erythroid hyperplasia*) and by expanding the volume of active marrow. In addition, immature red cells (*reticulocytes*) are released prematurely. These cells are larger than mature cells and stain light blue on a peripheral blood film (the description of the appearance of the blood film is *polychromasia*). They may be counted accurately as a percentage of all red cells on a blood film using a supravital stain for residual RNA e.g. new methylene blue.

## Sites of haemolysis

### Extravascular haemolysis

In most haemolytic conditions red cell destruction is extravascular. The red cells are removed from the circulation by macrophages in the reticuloendothelial system, particularly the spleen.

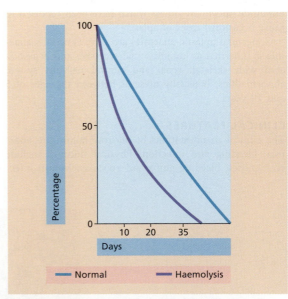

**Fig. 6.14** Patterns of survival of normal red cells and cells affected by haemolysis, using labelling of red cells with $^{51}$Cr. The half-life of normal cells is about 30 days and is reduced to less than 15 days in patients with haemolytic anaemia.

**Intravascular haemolysis**

When red cells are rapidly destroyed within the circulation, Hb is liberated (Fig. 6.15). This is initially bound to *plasma haptoglobins* but these may soon become saturated.

Excess free plasma Hb is filtered by the renal glomerulus and enters the urine, although small amounts are reabsorbed by the renal tubules. In the renal tubular cell, Hb is broken down and becomes deposited in the cells as *haemosiderin*. This can be detected in the spun sediment of urine using Perls' reaction. Some of the free plasma Hb is oxidized to *methaemoglobin*, which dissociates into *ferrihaem* and globin. *Plasma haemopexin* binds ferrihaem but if its binding capacity is exceeded, ferrihaem becomes attached to albumin, forming *methaemalbumin*. On spectrophotometry of the plasma, methaemalbumin forms a characteristic band; this is the basis of *Schumm's test*.

The *liver* plays an important role in removing Hb bound to haptoglobin and haemopexin and any remaining free Hb.

## Evidence for haemolysis

Increased red cell breakdown leads to:
- Elevated serum bilirubin (unconjugated)
- Excess urinary urobilinogen (resulting from bilirubin breakdown in the intestine, Fig. 6.5)
- Reduced plasma haptoglobin
- Raised serum lactic dehydrogenase (LDH)

Increased red cell production leads to:
- Reticulocytosis
- Erythroid hyperplasia of the bone marrow

There may be evidence of abnormal red cells in some haemolytic anaemias:
- Spherocytes (see Fig. 6.8)
- Sickle cells (see Fig. 6.8)
- Red cell fragments

Demonstration of shortened red cell life-span: Red cell survival studies using $^{51}$Cr-labelled red cells are useful in complicated cases and also for quantitation of the severity of haemolysis. The dominant site of red cell destruction can be shown with external body counting over the liver and spleen.

INTRAVASCULAR HAEMOLYSIS. This is suggested by raised levels of plasma Hb, haemosiderinuria, very low or absent haptoglobins and the presence of methaemalbumin (positive Schumm's test).

Various laboratory studies will be necessary to determine the exact type of haemolytic anaemia present. The causes of haemolytic anaemias are shown in Table 6.9.

# Inherited haemolytic anaemias

## RED CELL MEMBRANE DEFECTS

The normal red cell membrane consists of a lipid bilayer crossed by integral proteins with an underlying lattice of proteins (or cytoskeleton), including spectrin, actin, ankyrin and protein 4.1, attached to the integral proteins (Fig. 6.16).

## Hereditary spherocytosis (HS)

HS is the commonest inherited haemolytic anaemia in northern Europeans, affecting 1 in 5000. It is inherited in an autosomal dominant manner but in 25% of patients neither parent is affected and it is presumed that HS has occurred by spontaneous mutation. HS is due to a defect in the red cell membrane, resulting in the cells losing part of the cell membrane as they pass through the spleen, possibly because the lipid bilayer is inadequately supported by the cytoskeleton. The surface-to-volume ratio decreases, and the cells become spherocytic. Spherocytes

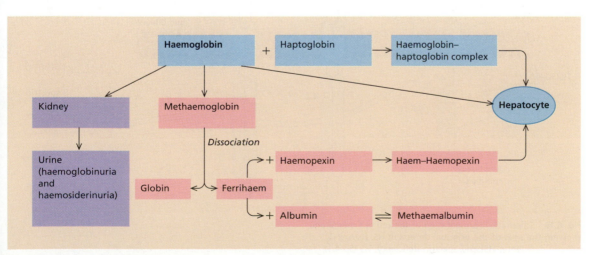

**Fig. 6.15** The fate of haemoglobin in the plasma.

**Inherited**
*Red cell membrane defect*
Hereditary spherocytosis
Hereditary elliptocytosis

*Haemoglobin abnormalities*
Thalassaemia
Sickle cell disease

*Metabolic defects*
Glucose-6-phosphate dehydrogenase deficiency
Pyruvate kinase deficiency

**Acquired**
*Immune*
Autoimmune:
  Warm
  Cold
Alloimmune:
  Haemolytic transfusion reactions
  Haemolytic disease of the newborn
  After allogeneic bone marrow or organ transplantation
Drug-induced

*Non-immune*
Acquired membrane defects
  Paroxysmal nocturnal haemoglobinuria
Mechanical
  Microangiopathic haemolytic anaemia
  Valve prosthesis
  March haemoglobinuria
Secondary to systemic disease:
  Renal and liver failure

*Miscellaneous*
Infections, e.g. malaria, *Clostridium welchii*
Drugs and chemicals causing damage to the red cell
  membrane or oxidative haemolysis
Hypersplenism
Burns

**Table 6.9**  Causes of haemolytic anaemia.

are more rigid and less deformable than normal red cells. They are unable to pass through the splenic microcirculation and they die. Several defects in the cell membrane have been identified in HS (Fig. 6.16). The best characterized is a deficiency in the structural protein spectrin, but quantitative defects in other membrane proteins have been identified such as a deficiency of ankyrin. There may also be functional abnormalities of membrane proteins such as defective binding of spectrin to protein 4.1. The abnormal red cell membrane in HS is associated functionally with an increased permeability to sodium, and this requires an increased rate of active transport of sodium out of the cells which is dependent on ATP produced by glycolysis.

## CLINICAL FEATURES

The condition may present with jaundice at birth. However, the onset of jaundice can sometimes be delayed for many years and some patients may go through life with no symptoms and are only detected during family studies. The patient may eventually develop anaemia, splenomegaly and ulcers on the leg. As in many haemolytic anaemias, the course of the disease may be interrupted by aplastic, haemolytic and megaloblastic crises. Aplastic anaemia usually occurs after infections, particularly with parvovirus, whereas megaloblastic anaemia is the result of folate depletion due to the hyperactivity of the bone marrow. Chronic haemolysis leads to the formation of pigment gallstones (see p. 281).

## INVESTIGATION

ANAEMIA is usually mild, but occasionally can be severe.
BLOOD FILM shows spherocytes and reticulocytes.
HAEMOLYSIS is evident, e.g. the serum bilirubin and urinary urobilinogen will be raised.
OSMOTIC FRAGILITY: when red cells are placed in solutions of increasing hypotonicity, they take in water, swell, and eventually lyse. Spherocytes tolerate hypo-

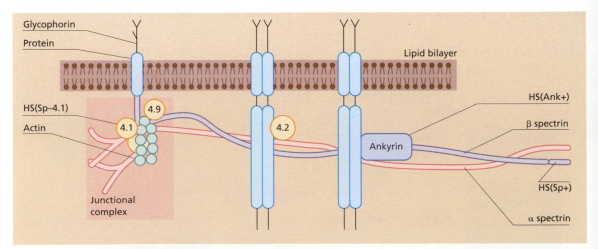

**Fig. 6.16**  Schematic representation of the red cell membrane showing the sites of the principal defects in HS. Hs(Ank+), ankyrin deficiency; HS(Sp+), spectrin deficiency; HS (Sp-4.1), abnormal spectrin/protein 4.1 binding.

tonic solutions less well than normal biconcave red cells. Osmotic fragility tests are infrequently carried out in routine practice, but may be useful to confirm a suspicion of spherocytosis on a blood film.

DIRECT ANTIGLOBULIN (COOMBS') TEST (p. 323) is negative in spherocytosis, virtually ruling out autoimmune haemolytic anaemia where spherocytes are also commonly present.

### TREATMENT

The spleen, which is the site of cell destruction, should be removed in all but the mildest cases. The decision about splenectomy in symptomless patients is difficult, but a raised bilirubin and especially the presence of gallstones should encourage splenectomy.

It is best to postpone splenectomy until after childhood, as sudden overwhelming fatal infections, usually due to encapsulated organisms such as pneumococci, may occur (see p. 330).

Following splenectomy, the spherocytosis is reduced and Hb usually returns to normal as the red cells are no longer destroyed. Folate deficiency often occurs in chronic haemolysis with rapid cell turnover. Folate levels should be monitored, or folic acid can be given prophylactically.

## Hereditary elliptocytosis

This disorder of the red cell membrane is inherited in an autosomal dominant manner. The red cells are elliptical. It is a similar condition to HS but milder clinically. Only a minority of patients have anaemia and only occasional patients require splenectomy.

## Hereditary stomatocytosis

*Stomatocytes* are red cells in which the pale central area appears slit-like. Their presence in large numbers may occur in a hereditary haemolytic anaemia associated with a membrane defect but excess alcohol intake is a common cause.

## HAEMOGLOBIN ABNORMALITIES

### Normal haemoglobin

Normal adult Hb (Hb A) has two polypeptide globin chains, the $\alpha$ and $\beta$ chains (Table 6.10), which have 141 and 146 amino acids, respectively. These are folded so that haem molecules can be held within the fold and are yet able to combine reversibly with oxygen.

In early embryonic life, haemoglobins Gower 1, Gower 2 and Portland predominate (Fig. 6.17). Later, fetal haemoglobin (Hb F), which has two $\alpha$ and two $\gamma$ chains, is produced. There is increasing synthesis of $\beta$ chains from 13 weeks of gestation and at term there is 80% Hb F and 20% Hb A. The switch from Hb F to Hb A occurs 3–6 months after birth when the genes for $\gamma$ chain production are further suppressed and there is rapid increase in the synthesis of $\beta$ chains. The exact mechanism responsible

for the switch remains unknown. There is little Hb F produced (normally less than 1%) from 6 months after birth. The $\delta$ chain is synthesized just before birth and Hb $A_2$ ($\alpha_2\delta_2$) remains at a level of about 2% throughout adult life.

Globin chains are synthesized in the same way as any protein (see Chapter 2). Four globin chain genes are required to control $\alpha$-chain production (Fig. 6.17). Two are present on each haploid genome (genes derived from one parent). These are situated close together on chromosome 16. The genes controlling the production of $\epsilon$, $\gamma$, $\delta$ and $\beta$ chains are close together on chromosome 11. The globin genes are arranged on chromosomes 16 and 11 in the order in which they are expressed.

### Abnormal haemoglobins

Abnormalities occur in:

- Globin chain production, e.g. thalassaemia
- Structure of the globin chain, e.g. sickle cell disease
- Combined defects of globin chain production and structure, e.g. sickle cell $\beta$-thalassaemia

Genetic defects in haemoglobin are the commonest of all genetic disorders.

## Thalassaemia

The thalassaemias (Greek *thalassa* = sea) are anaemias originally found in people living on the shores of the Mediterranean but are now known to affect people throughout the world (Fig. 6.18).

Normally there is balanced (1 : 1) production of $\alpha$ and $\beta$ chains. The defective synthesis of globin genes in thalassaemia leads to 'imbalanced' globin chain production, leading to precipitation of globin chains within the red cell precursors and resulting in ineffective erythropoiesis. Precipitation of globin chains in mature red cells leads to haemolysis.

## β-Thalassaemia

In homozygous $\beta$-thalassaemia either no normal $\beta$ chains are produced ($\beta^0$) or $\beta$-chain production is very reduced ($\beta^+$). There is an excess of $\alpha$ chains which precipitate in erythroblasts and red cells causing ineffective erythropoiesis and haemolysis. The excess $\alpha$ chains combine with whatever $\beta$, $\delta$ and $\gamma$ chains are produced, resulting in increased quantities of Hb $A_2$ and Hb F and, at best, small amounts of Hb A. In heterozygous $\beta$-thalassaemia there is usually symptomless microcytosis with or without mild anaemia. Table 6.11 shows the findings in the homozygote and heterozygote for the common types of $\beta$-thalassaemia.

### MOLECULAR GENETICS

The molecular errors accounting for over 100 genetic defects leading to $\beta$-thalassaemia genes have been characterized. Unlike $\alpha$-thalassaemia, the defects are mainly point mutations rather than gene deletions. The mutations result in defects in transcription, RNA splicing

| | Haemoglobin | Structure | Comment |
|---|---|---|---|
| Normal | A | $\alpha_2\beta_2$ | Comprises 92% of adult haemoglobin |
| | $A_{1c}$ | $\alpha_2\beta_2$ ($\beta$-NH glucose) | Comprises 5% of adult haemoglobin. This glycosylated haemoglobin is increased in patients with uncontrolled diabetes |
| | $A_2$ | $\alpha_2\delta_2$ | Comprises 2% of adult haemoglobin. Elevated in $\beta$-thalassaemia |
| | F | $\alpha_2\gamma_2$ | Normal haemoglobin in fetus from 3rd to 9th month. Increased in $\beta$-thalassaemia Comprises <1% of haemoglobin in adult |
| Abnormal chain production | H | $\beta_4$ | Found in $\alpha$-thalassaemia. Biologically useless |
| | Barts | $\gamma_4$ | Comprises 100% of haemoglobin in homozygous $\alpha$-thalassaemia. Biologically useless |
| Abnormal chain structure | S | $\alpha_2\beta_2$ | Substitution of valine for glutamic acid in position 6 of $\beta$ chain |
| | C | $\alpha_2\beta_2$ | Substitution of lysine for glutamic acid in position 6 of $\beta$ chain |

**Table 6.10**  Some types of haemoglobin.

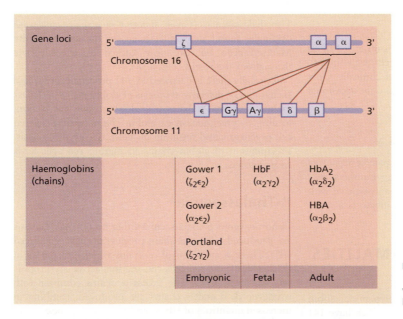

**Fig. 6.17**  Loci of genes on chromosomes 16 and 11 and the combination of various chains to produce different haemoglobins.

and modification, translation via frame shifts and nonsense codons producing highly unstable $\beta$-globin which cannot be utilized.

## CLINICAL SYNDROMES
Clinically, $\beta$-thalassaemia can be divided into the following:
- Thalassaemia major with severe anaemia requiring regular transfusions
- Thalassaemia intermedia, with moderate anaemia, rarely requiring transfusions
- Thalassaemia minor (or trait), the symptomless heterozygous carrier state

### $\beta$-Thalassaemia trait
This common carrier state is asymptomatic. Anaemia is mild or absent. The red cells are hypochromic and microcytic with a low MCV and MCH and it may be confused with iron deficiency. However, the two are easily distinguished as in thalassaemia trait the serum iron, the serum ferritin and the iron stores are normal (see Table 6.3). Hb electrophoresis usually shows a raised Hb $A_2$ and

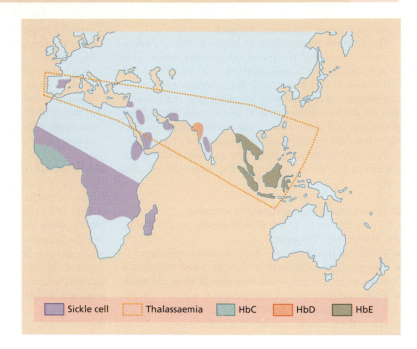

**Fig. 6.18** Geographical distribution of the major haemoglobin abnormalities.

Sickle cell    Thalassaemia    HbC    HbD    HbE

often a raised Hb F (Fig. 6.19). Iron should not be given to these patients unless they develop coincidental iron deficiency.

### Thalassaemia intermedia

Thalassaemia intermedia includes patients who are symptomatic with moderate anaemia (Hb 7–10 g dl⁻¹) and who do not require regular transfusions, i.e. more severe than in β-thalassaemia trait but milder than in trans-

| Type of thalassaemia | Findings in homozygote | Findings in heterozygote |
|---|---|---|
| $\beta^+$ | Thalassaemia major Hb A + F + A$_2$ | Thalassaemia minor Hb A$_2$ raised |
| $\beta^0$ | Thalassaemia major Hb F + A$_2$ | Thalassaemia minor Hb A$_2$ raised |
| $\delta\beta$ | Thalassaemia intermedia Hb F only | Thalassaemia minor Hb F 5–15% Hb A$_2$ normal |
| $\delta\beta$ (Lepore) | Thalassaemia major or intermedia Hb F and Lepore | Thalassaemia minor Hb Lepore 5–15% Hb A$_2$ normal |
| $\gamma\delta\beta$ | Not viable | Neonatal haemolysis Thalassaemia minor in adults with normal Hb F and A$_2$ |

Adapted from Weatherall DJ (1988) Disorders of the synthesis or function of haemoglobin. In: Weatherall DJ, Ledingham JGG & Warrell DA (eds) *Oxford Textbook of Medicine* pp. 19.108–19.130. Oxford: Oxford University Press. With permission.

**Table 6.11** Findings in $\beta$-, $\delta\beta$- and $\gamma\delta\beta$-thalassaemias.

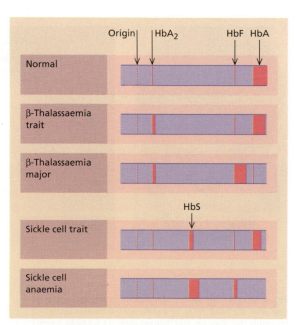

**Fig. 6.19** Patterns of haemoglobin electrophoresis.

fusion-dependent thalassaemia major.

Thalassaemia intermedia may be due to a combination of homozygous mild $\beta^+$- and $\alpha$-thalassaemia, where there is reduced $\alpha$ chain precipitation and less ineffective erythropoiesis and haemolysis. The inheritance of hereditary persistence of Hb F with homozygous $\beta$-thalassaemia also results in a milder clinical picture than unmodified $\beta$-thalassaemia major because the excess $\alpha$ chains are partially removed by the increased production of $\gamma$ chains.

Patients may have splenomegaly and bone deformities. Recurrent leg ulcers, gallstones and infections are also seen.

### β-Thalassaemia major (Cooley's anaemia)

Children affected by severe $\beta$-thalassaemia present during the first year of life with:

- Failure to thrive and recurrent bacterial infections
- Severe anaemia from 3–6 months when the switch from $\gamma$- to $\beta$-chain production should normally occur
- Extramedullary haemopoiesis that soon leads to hepatosplenomegaly and bone expansion, giving rise to the classical thalassaemic facies (Fig. 6.20a)

Skull X-rays in these children show the characteristic 'hair on end' appearance of bony trabeculation as a result of expansion of the bone marrow into cortical bone (Fig. 6.20b).

### INVESTIGATION

BLOOD COUNT shows a moderate to severe anaemia with reduced MCV and MCH. The reticulocyte count is raised and nucleated red cells are present in the peripheral blood. The WCC and the number of platelets are normal unless hypersplenism is present.

BLOOD FILM shows a hypochromic and predominantly microcytic picture. Postsplenectomy features will be present after splenectomy has been carried out (see Fig. 6.8).

SATURATED IRON-BINDING CAPACITY AND HIGH SERUM FERRITIN LEVELS are caused by multiple blood transfusions.

HB ELECTROPHORESIS shows an increase in Hb F, markedly reduced or absent Hb A, and Hb $A_2$ is normal or slightly increased (Fig. 6.19).

### MANAGEMENT

The aims of treatment are to suppress ineffective erythropoiesis, prevent bony deformities and allow normal activity and development. Regular transfusions should be given to keep the Hb above 10 g dl$^{-1}$. Blood transfusions may be required every 4–6 weeks. Febrile transfusion reactions can be prevented by the use of leucocyte-depleted blood (p. 333). If transfusion requirements increase, splenectomy should be considered although this is usually delayed until after the age of 6 years because of the risk of infection. Prophylaxis against infection is required for patients undergoing splenectomy (see p. 330).

Iron overload caused by repeated transfusions (*transfusion haemosiderosis*) may lead to damage to the endocrine glands, liver, pancreas and the myocardium by the time patients reach adolescence. The iron-chelating agent of choice remains desferrioxamine although it has to be administered parenterally. It is given as an overnight subcutaneous infusion on five to seven nights each week. Ascorbic acid 200 mg daily is given, as it increases the urinary excretion of iron in response to desferrioxamine.

With current therapy, normal growth and sexual development occur but compliance may be a problem

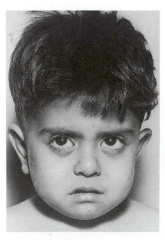
(a)

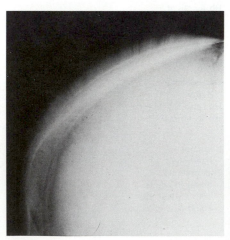
(b)

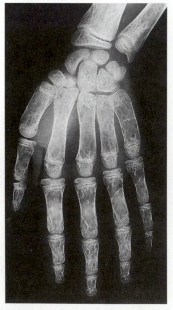
(c)

**Fig. 6.20**(a) A child with thalassaemia, showing the typical features. (b) Skull X-ray of a child with $\beta$-thalassaemia, showing the 'hair on end' appearance. (c) X-ray of hand, showing expansion of the marrow and a thinned cortex.

especially in teenagers. Intensive treatment with desferrioxamine has been reported to reverse damage to the heart in patients with severe iron overload but excessive doses of desferrioxamine may cause cataracts, retinal damage and nerve deafness. Infection with *Yersinia enterocolitica* occurs in iron-loaded patients treated with desferrioxamine. There are some promising reports of the use of oral iron-chelating agents and clinical trials are in progress. Iron overload should be periodically assessed by measuring the serum ferritin and assessing damage to organs, particularly the heart, liver and endocrine glands.

Bone marrow transplantation has been used in young patients with HLA-matched siblings. It has been successful in about 80% of cases but there is a mortality of 5–10% due to graft-versus-host disease or other transplant-related complications.

Prenatal diagnosis and gene therapy are discussed on p. 124.

### δβ-Thalassaemias, Hb Lepore and hereditary persistence of fetal haemoglobin (HPFH) (see Table 6.11)

These variants are due to deletions of the α- and β-globin genes and produce a milder form of thalassaemia than homozygous $\beta^0$ thalassaemia because the reduced β-chain production is partially compensated by increased γ-chain synthesis.

## α-Thalassaemia

### MOLECULAR GENETICS

In contrast to β-thalassaemia, α-thalassaemia is caused by gene deletions. The gene for α chains is duplicated on both chromosomes 16, i.e. there are four genes. Deletion of one α-chain gene ($\alpha^+$) or both α-chain genes ($\alpha^0$) on each chromosome 16 may occur (Table 6.12).

If all four genes are absent (deletion of both genes on both chromosomes) there is no α-chain synthesis and only Hb Barts ($\gamma_4$) is present. Hb Barts cannot carry oxygen and is incompatible with life (Tables 6.10 and 6.12). Infants are either stillborn at 28–40 weeks or die very shortly after birth. They are pale, oedematous and have enormous livers and spleens—a condition called *hydrops fetalis.*

If three genes are deleted, there is moderate anaemia (Hb 7–10 g dl$^{-1}$) and splenomegaly (*Hb H disease*). The patients are not usually transfusion dependent. Hb A, Hb Barts and Hb H ($\beta_4$) are present.

If one or two genes are deleted (*α-thalassaemia traits*) there is microcytosis with or without mild anaemia. Hb H bodies may be seen on staining a blood film with brilliant cresyl blue. Globin chain synthesis studies for the detection of a reduced ratio of α- to β chains may be necessary for the definitive diagnosis of α-thalassaemia trait.

Less commonly, α-thalassaemia may result from genetic defects other than deletions, for example mutations in the stop codon producing an α chain with many extra amino acids (Hb Constant Spring) (Table 6.12).

| Type of thalassaemia | Findings in homozygote | Findings in heterozygote |
|---|---|---|
| $\alpha^+$ | Thalassaemia minor 5–10% Hb Barts at birth Normal Hb A$_2$ | Thalassaemia minor 1–2% Hb Barts |
| $\alpha^0$ | Hydrops 80% Hb Barts at birth Fatal | Thalassaemia minor 5–10% Hb Barts at birth Normal Hb A$_2$ |
| Hb Constant Spring | Thalassaemia minor 5–6% Hb Constant Spring Moderate anaemia | $\cong$ 1% Hb Constant Spring No clinical abnormality |

From Weatherall DJ (1988) Disorders of the synthesis or function of haemoglobin. In: Weatherall DJ, Ledingham JGG & Warrell DA (eds) *Oxford Textbook of Medicine*, pp. 19.108–19.130. Oxford: Oxford University Press. With permission.

**Table 6.12**   The α-thalassaemias.

## Sickle syndromes

The most important structural abnormality of the Hb chain is sickle cell haemoglobin (Hb S). Hb S results from a single-base mutation of adenine to thymine which produces a substitution of valine for glutamine at the sixth codon of the β-globin chain. In the homozygous state (*sickle cell anaemia*) both genes are abnormal (Hb SS), whereas in the heterozygous state (*sickle cell trait*, Hb AS) only one chromosome carries the gene. As the synthesis of Hb F is normal, the disease usually does not manifest itself until the Hb F decreases to adult levels at about 6 months of age.

The disease occurs mainly in Africans (25% carry the gene) but is also found in India, the Middle East, and southern Europe (see Fig. 6.18).

### PATHOGENESIS

Deoxygenated Hb S molecules are insoluble and polymerize. The flexibility of the cells is decreased and they become rigid and take up their characteristic sickle appearance (see Fig. 6.8). This process is initially reversible but, with repeated sickling, the cells eventually lose their membrane flexibility and remain in the sickle form. Sickling can produce:

1 A shortened red cell survival
2 Impaired passage of cells through the microcirculation leading to obstruction of small vessels and tissue infarction

Sickling is *precipitated* by infection, dehydration, cold, acidosis or hypoxia. In many cases the cause is unknown. Hb S releases its oxygen to the tissues more easily than normal Hb (see Fig. 13.5) and patients therefore feel well despite being anaemic except during crises or complications.

# SICKLE CELL ANAEMIA

Symptoms vary from a mild asymptomatic disorder to a severe haemolytic anaemia and recurrent severe painful crises. The condition may present in childhood with anaemia and mild jaundice. The hand-and-foot syndrome due to infarcts of small bones is quite common in children and may result in digits of varying lengths.

In the older patient, vaso-occlusive problems occur owing to sickling in the small vessels of any organ, mimicking many medical and surgical emergencies.

Typical infarctive sickle crises include:
- Bone pain (commonest)
- Chest—pleuritic pain
- Cerebral—hemiparesis, fits
- Kidney—papillary necrosis causing haematuria, renal tubular defect resulting in lack of concentration of the urine
- Spleen—painful infarcts
- Penis—priapism
- Liver—pain with abnormal biochemistry

Attacks of pain with low-grade fever last from a few hours to a few days. In a given patient the degree of anaemia is usually stable and during a crisis Hb does not fall unless there is one or more of the following:

APLASIA: due to decreased erythropoiesis, associated with viral infections particularly parvovirus.

ACUTE SEQUESTRATION: the liver and spleen become engorged with sickle cells.

HAEMOLYSIS: due to drugs, acute infection or associated G6PD deficiency.

### Long-term problems

SUSCEPTIBILITY TO INFECTIONS: particularly to *Streptococcus pneumoniae*, which can cause a fatal meningitis or pneumonia. Osteomyelitis can occur in necrotic bone, often due to *Salmonella*

CHRONIC LEG ULCERS: due to ischaemia

GALLSTONES: pigment stones from persistent haemolysis

ASEPTIC NECROSIS OF BONE: particularly of the femoral heads

BLINDNESS: due to retinal detachment and proliferative retinopathy

CHRONIC RENAL DISEASE

## INVESTIGATION

BLOOD COUNT: the level of Hb may be 6–8 g dl$^{-1}$ with a high reticulocyte count (10–20%).

BLOOD FILMS can show features of hyposplenism (see Fig. 6.8).

SICKLING of red cells on a blood film can be induced in the presence of sodium metabisulphite.

SICKLE SOLUBILITY TEST: a mixture of Hb S in a reducing solution such as sodium dithionite gives a turbid appearance due to precipitation of Hb S whereas normal Hb gives a clear solution.

HB ELECTROPHORESIS (see Fig. 6.19) confirms the diagnosis. There is no Hb A, 80–95% Hb SS and 2–20% Hb F.

THE PARENTS of the affected child will show features of sickle cell trait.

## MANAGEMENT

The 'steady state' anaemia requires no treatment. Precipitating factors (see above) should be avoided or treated quickly. Acute attacks require supportive therapy with intravenous fluids, oxygen, antibiotics and adequate analgesia. Prophylaxis is given to prevent pneumococcal infection (see p. 330). Folic acid is given to pregnant women and those with severe haemolysis.

Regular transfusions are given only if there is severe anaemia or if patients are having frequent crises in order to suppress the production of Hb S. Before elective operations and during pregnancy repeated transfusions may be used to reduce the proportion of circulating Hb S to less than 20% to prevent sickling. Exchange transfusions may be necessary in patients with severe or recurrent crises, or before emergency surgery. Transfusion and splenectomy may be life-saving for young children with splenic sequestration.

Research is being carried out to find a way to increase production of Hb F to reduce the number of sickle cells and sickle cell crises; hydroxyurea in combination with recombinant human erythropoietin and butyrate are currently being investigated.

## PROGNOSIS

Some patients with Hb SS die in the first few years of life from either infection or episodes of sequestration. However, there is marked individual variation in the severity of the disease and some patients have a relatively normal life-span with few complications.

# SICKLE CELL TRAIT

These individuals have no symptoms unless extreme circumstances cause anoxia, such as flying in non-pressurized aircraft or problems with anaesthesia. Anaesthesia should always be carried out with care to avoid hypoxia. Sickle cell trait protects against *Plasmodium falciparum* malaria (see p. 71). Typically there is 60% Hb A and 40% Hb S. The blood count and film are normal. The diagnosis is made by a positive sickle test or by Hb electrophoresis (see Fig. 6.19).

# Other structural globin chain defects

There are many Hb variants (e.g. Hb C, D), many of which are not associated with clinical manifestations.

Hb C disease may be associated with Hb S (Hb SC disease). The clinical course is similar to Hb SS but there is an increased likelihood of thrombosis, and in particular this may lead to life-threatening episodes of thrombosis in pregnancy and retinopathy.

# Combined defects of globin chain production and structure

Abnormalities of Hb structure, e.g. Hb S, C can occur in combination with thalassaemia. The combination of β-thalassaemia trait and sickle cell trait (sickle cell β-thalassaemia) resembles sickle cell anaemia (Hb SS) clinically. Hb E is the commonest Hb variant in South East Asia. Homozygous Hb E causes a mild microcytic anaemia but the combination of Hb E and β-thalassaemia produces the clinical and haematological features of β-thalassaemia major.

# Prenatal diagnosis of severe haemoglobin abnormalities

Of the offspring of parents who both have either β-thalassaemia or sickle cell trait, 25% will have β-thalassaemia major or sickle cell anaemia, respectively. Recognition of these heterozygous states in parents and family counselling provides a basis for antenatal diagnosis.

If a pregnant woman is found to have a Hb defect, her partner should be tested. Antenatal diagnosis is offered if both are affected and there is a risk of a severe fetal Hb defect, particularly β-thalassaemia major. Fetal blood samples can be taken from the umbilical cord in the second trimester and tested for the rate of β-globin chain synthesis. Abortion is offered if the fetus is found to be affected. Alternatively, fetal DNA analysis of amniotic fluid or chorionic villus samples can be used. Chorionic villus biopsy can be carried out in the first trimester and thus second trimester abortions can be avoided.

# Gene therapy

The ultimate corrective therapy for severe Hb abnormalities would be gene therapy. This might involve inserting normal Hb genes into the patient's haemopoietic cells *in vitro* and then transplanting these cells back into the patient after ablative treatment had been given to remove the abnormal bone marrow. However, numerous problems remain to be overcome before gene therapy for Hb defects becomes a practical option.

# METABOLIC DISORDERS OF THE RED CELL

### Red cell metabolism

The mature red cell has no nucleus, mitochondria or ribosomes and is therefore unable to synthesize proteins. Red cells have only limited enzyme systems but they are of major importance in maintaining the viability and function of the cells. In particular, energy is required in the form of ATP for the maintenance of the flexibility of the membrane and the biconcave shape of the cells to allow passage through small vessels, and for regulation of the sodium and potassium pumps to ensure osmotic equilibrium. In addition, it is essential that Hb is maintained in the reduced state. The enzyme systems (Fig. 6.21) responsible for producing energy and reducing power are:

GLYCOLYTIC (EMBDEN–MEYERHOF) PATHWAY, in which glucose is metabolized to pyruvate and lactic acid with production of ATP

HEXOSE MONOPHOSPHATE (PENTOSEPHOSPHATE) PATHWAY, which provides reducing power for the red cell in the form of NADPH

About 90% of glucose is metabolized by the former and 10% by the latter. The importance of the hexose monophosphate shunt is that it maintains glutathione (GSH) in a reduced state. Glutathione is important in combating oxidative stress to the red cell, and failure of this mechanism may result in:

1 Rigidity due to cross-linking of spectrin, which decreases membrane flexibility (see Fig. 6.16) and causes 'leakiness' of the red cell membrane
2 Oxidation of the Hb molecule, producing methaemoglobin and precipitation of globin chains as Heinz bodies localized on the inside of the membrane; these bodies are removed from circulating red cells by the spleen

2,3-DPG is formed from a side-arm of the glycolytic pathway. It binds to the central part of the Hb tetramer, fixing it in the low affinity state. A decreased affinity with a shift in the oxygen dissociation curve to the right enables more oxygen to be delivered to the tissues (see Fig. 13.5).

# Glucose-6-phosphate dehydrogenase (G6PD) deficiency

The enzyme G6PD holds a vital position in the hexose monophosphate shunt. G6PD deficiency is a common condition that presents with a haemolytic anaemia and affects millions of people throughout the world, particularly in Africa, around the Mediterranean, the Middle East and South East Asia.

The gene for G6PD is sex-linked, being carried on the X chromosome. The deficiency therefore affects males. It is carried by females, who show half the normal levels of the enzyme and who have some protection against *Plasmodium falciparum*.

There are over 400 structural types of G6PD. The commonest with normal activity are type B, which is present in almost all Caucasians and about 70% of Blacks, and type A, which is present in about 20% of Blacks. There are many variants with reduced activity but only two are common. In the African, or A type, the degree of deficiency is mild (enzyme activity about 10% of normal). Haemolysis is self-limiting as the young red cells newly produced by the bone marrow have nearly normal enzyme activity. However, in the Mediterranean type, both young and old red cells have very low enzyme activity. After an oxidant shock the Hb level may fall precipitously; death may follow unless the condition is recognized and the patient is transfused urgently.

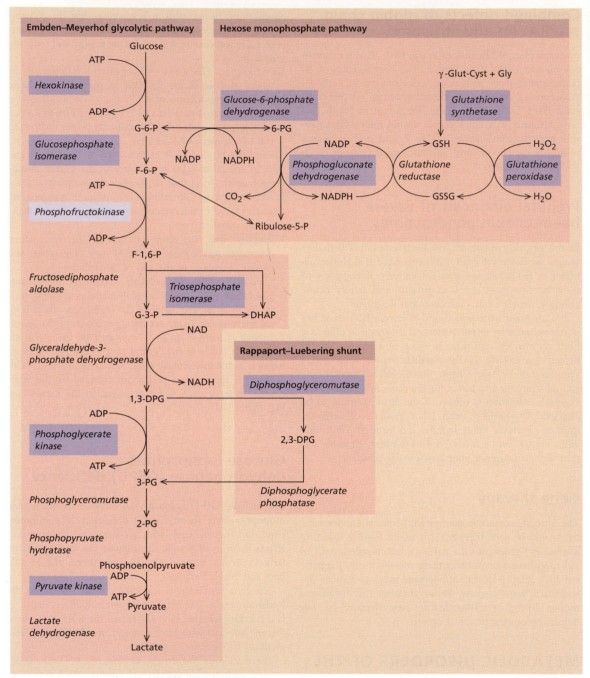

**Fig. 6.21**  Metabolic pathways (simplified) in the red cell. Enzymes in purple boxes indicate documented hereditary deficiency diseases. DHAP, dihydroxyacetone phosphate; DPG, diphosphoglycerate; F, fructose; G, glucose; GSH, reduced glutathione; GSSG, oxidized glutathione; P, phosphate; PG, phosphoglycerate.

## CLINICAL SYNDROMES
- Acute drug-induced haemolysis (Table 6.13)
- Favism (ingestion of fava beans)
- Chronic haemolytic anaemia
- Neonatal jaundice
- Infections and acute illnesses will also precipitate haemolysis in patients with G6PD deficiency

The clinical features are due to rapid intravascular hae-molysis with symptoms of anaemia, jaundice and haemo-globinuria.

## INVESTIGATION
BLOOD COUNT is normal between attacks.

DURING AN ATTACK the blood film may show irregu-larly contracted cells, bite cells (cells with an inden-tation of the membrane), blister cells (cells in which

*Analgesics*, e.g.
Aspirin
Phenacetin (withdrawn in the UK)
Acetanilide

*Antimalarials*, e.g.
Primaquine
Pyrimethamine
Quinine
Chloroquine
Pamaquine

*Antibacterials*, e.g.
Most sulphonamides
Dapsone
Nitrofurantoin
Nitrofurazone
Furazolidone
Chloramphenicol

*Miscellaneous drugs*, e.g.
Vitamin K
Probenecid
Nalidixic acid
Quinidine
Dimercaprol
Phenylhydrazine
p-Aminosalicylic acid

**Table 6.13** Drugs causing haemolysis in glucose-6-phosphate dehydrogenase deficiency.

the Hb appears to have become partially detached from the cell membrane) (see Fig. 6.8), Heinz bodies (best seen on films stained with methyl violet) and reticulocytosis.

HAEMOLYSIS is evident (see p. 311).

G6PD DEFICIENCY can be detected using several screening tests, such as demonstration of the decreased ability of G6PD-deficient cells to reduce dyes. The level of the enzyme may also be directly assayed.

**TREATMENT**

- Any offending drugs should be stopped
- Underlying infection should be treated
- Blood transfusion may be life-saving
- Splenectomy is not usually helpful

## Pyruvate kinase deficiency

This is the most common defect of red cell metabolism after G6PD deficiency, affecting thousands rather than millions of people. The site of the defect is shown in Fig. 6.21. There is reduced production of ATP causing rigid red cells. Homozygotes have haemolytic anaemia and splenomegaly. It is inherited as an autosomal recessive.

**INVESTIGATION**

ANAEMIA of variable severity is present (Hb 5–10 g dl$^{-1}$). The oxygen dissociation curve is shifted to the right as a result of the rise in intracellular 2,3-DPG (Fig. 6.21), and this reduces the severity of symptoms due to anaemia.

BLOOD FILM shows distorted ('prickle') cells and a reticulocytosis.

PYRUVATE KINASE activity is low (affected homozygotes have levels of 5–20%).

**TREATMENT**

Blood transfusions may be necessary during infections and pregnancy. Splenectomy may improve the clinical condition and is usually advised for patients requiring frequent transfusions.

In addition to G6PD and pyruvate kinase deficiencies, there are a number of rare enzyme deficiencies that need specialist investigation.

# Acquired haemolytic anaemia

These anaemias may be divided into those due to immune, non-immune, or other causes (see Table 6.9).

1 *Immune destruction* of red cells by:
   (a) autoantibodies,
   (b) drug-induced antibodies,
   (c) alloantibodies.
2 *Non-immune destruction* of red cells may be due to:
   (a) acquired membrane defects, e.g. paroxysmal nocturnal haemoglobinuria (see p. 326),
   (b) mechanical factors, e.g. prosthetic heart valves, or microangiopathic haemolytic anaemia (see p. 326),
   (c) secondary to systemic disease, e.g. renal and liver disease.
3 *Miscellaneous*: Various toxic substances can disrupt the red cell membrane and cause haemolysis, e.g. arsenic, products of *Clostridium welchii*. Anaemia is frequent in *malaria* and this is due to a combination of a reduction in red cell survival and reduced production of red cells. *Hypersplenism* (p. 330) results in a reduced red cell survival, which may also contribute to the anaemia seen in malaria. Extensive *burns* result in denaturation of red cell membrane proteins and reduced red cell survival. Some drugs, e.g. dapsone, sulphasalazine, cause oxidative haemolysis with Heinz bodies in normal subjects; some chemicals, e.g. weed killers such as sodium chlorate may cause severe oxidative haemolysis causing acute renal failure.

## AUTOIMMUNE HAEMOLYTIC ANAEMIA

Autoimmune haemolytic anaemias (AIHA) are acquired disorders resulting from increased red cell destruction due to red cell autoantibodies. These anaemias are characterized by the presence of a positive direct antiglobulin (Coombs') test, which detects the autoantibody on the surface of the patient's red cells (Fig. 6.22).

AIHA is divided into 'warm' and 'cold' types, depending on whether the antibody attaches better to the red cells at body temperature (37°C) or at lower temperatures. The major features and the causes of these two forms of AIHA are shown in Table 6.14. In warm AIHA, IgG antibodies predominate and the direct antiglobulin test is positive with IgG alone, IgG and complement or complement only. In cold AIHA, the antibodies are usually IgM. They easily elute off red cells leaving complement which is detected as C3d.

### Immune destruction of red cells

IgM or IgG red cell antibodies which fully activate the complement cascade cause lysis of red cells in the circulation (*intravascular haemolysis*).

IgG antibodies frequently do not activate complement and the coated red cells undergo *extravascular haemolysis* (Fig. 6.23). They are either completely phagocytosed in the spleen through an interaction with Fc receptors on macrophages, or they lose part of the cell membrane due to partial phagocytosis and circulate as spherocytes until they too become sequestered in the spleen. Some IgG antibodies partially activate complement leading to deposition of C3b on the red cell surface and this may enhance phagocytosis as macrophages also have receptors for C3b.

Non-complement-binding IgM antibodies are rare and have little or no effect on red cell survival. IgM antibodies which partially rather than fully activate complement cause adherence of red cells to C3b receptors on macrophages, particularly in the liver, although this is an ineffective mechanism of haemolysis. Most of the red cells are released from the macrophages when C3b is cleaved to C3d and then circulate with C3d on their surface.

## 'Warm' autoimmune haemolytic anaemias

### CLINICAL FEATURES

These anaemias may occur at all ages and in both sexes. They can present as a short episode of anaemia and jaundice but they often remit and relapse and may progress to an intermittent chronic pattern. The spleen is often palpable. Infections or folate deficiency may provoke a profound fall in the Hb level.

In more than 30% of cases, the cause remains unknown. These anaemias may be associated with lymphoid malignancies or diseases such as rheumatoid arthritis and SLE or drugs (Table 6.14).

### INVESTIGATION

HAEMOLYTIC ANAEMIA is evident (see p. 311).

SPHEROCYTOSIS is present as a result of red cell damage.

DIRECT ANTIGLOBULIN TEST is positive, with either IgG alone (67%), IgG and complement (20%) or complement alone (13%) being found on the surface of the red cells.

AUTOANTIBODIES may have specificity for the Rh blood group system, e.g. for the e antigen.

AUTOIMMUNE THROMBOCYTOPENIA AND/OR NEUTROPENIA may be associated with the condition (Evans' syndrome).

### TREATMENT AND PROGNOSIS

Corticosteroids (e.g. prednisolone in doses of 40–60 mg daily for adults) are effective in inducing a remission in about 80% of patients. Steroids reduce both production of the red cell autoantibody and destruction of antibody-coated cells. Splenectomy may be necessary if there is no response to steroids or if the remission is not maintained when the dose of prednisolone is reduced. Other immunosuppressive drugs, such as azathioprine and cyclophos-

|  | Warm | Cold |
|---|---|---|
| Temperature at which antibody attaches best to red cells: | 37°C | Lower than 37°C |
| Type of antibody: | IgG | IgM |
| Direct Coombs' test: | Strongly positive | Positive |
| Causes of primary condition: | Idiopathic | Idiopathic |
| Causes of secondary condition: | Autoimmune disorders, e.g. systemic lupus erythematosus<br>Lymphomas<br>Chronic lymphatic leukaemias<br>Hodgkin's disease<br>Carcinomas<br>Drugs, e.g. methyldopa | Infections, e.g. infectious mononucleosis,<br>*Mycoplasma pneumoniae*<br>Other viral infections (rare)<br>Lymphomas<br>Paroxysmal cold haemoglobinuria (IgG) |

**Table 6.14** Causes and major features of autoimmune haemolytic anaemias.

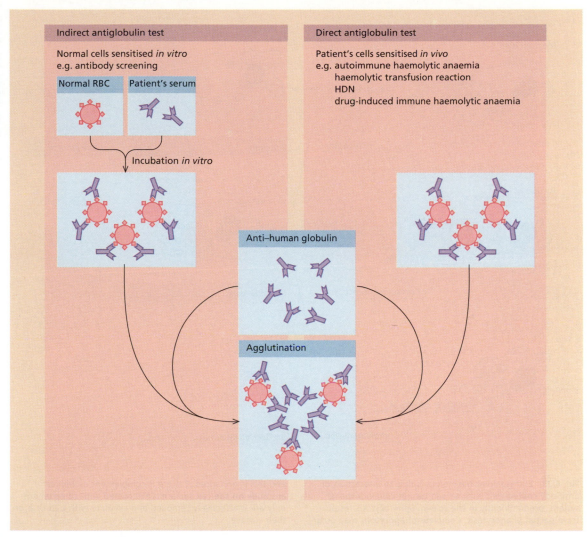

**Fig. 6.22**  Antiglobulin (Coombs') tests. The human antiglobulin forms bridges between the sensitized cells causing visible agglutination. The direct test detects patients' cells sensitized *in vivo* and the indirect test detects normal cells sensitized *in vitro*. HDN, haemolytic disease of newborn.

phamide, may be effective in patients failing to respond to steroids and splenectomy.

# 'Cold' autoimmune haemolytic anaemias

These disorders are due to antibodies, usually of the IgM type, that attach to red cells at low temperatures and cause agglutination of red cells in the cold peripheries of the body. Activation of complement may cause intravascular haemolysis when the cells return to the higher temperatures in the core of the body.

Low titres of IgM cold agglutinins reacting at 4°C are normally present in serum and are harmless. After certain infections (such as *Mycoplasma*, cytomegalovirus (CMV), Epstein–Barr virus (EBV)) there is increased synthesis of

*polyclonal* cold agglutinins with a higher thermal range and they may produce transient mild to moderate haemolysis if the thermal range reaches peripheral body temperatures (30–32°C).

## CHRONIC COLD HAEMAGGLUTININ DISEASE (CHAD)

This usually occurs in the elderly with a gradual onset of haemolytic anaemia due to the production of *monoclonal* IgM cold agglutinins. After exposure to cold the patient develops an acrocyanosis similar to Raynaud's (see p. 108) due to red cell autoagglutination.

### Investigation

RED CELLS agglutinate in the cold or at room temperature. Agglutination is sometimes seen in the sample

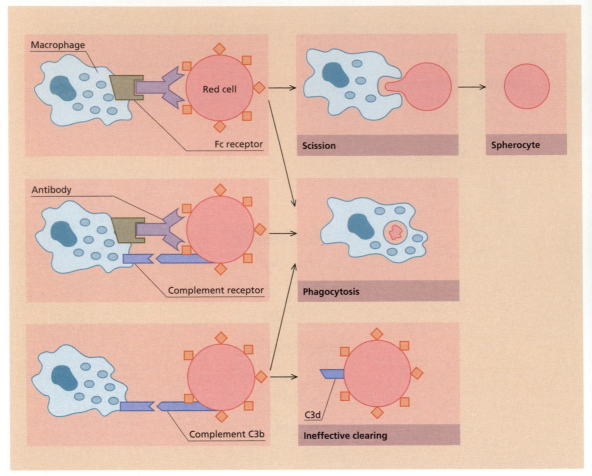

**Fig. 6.23** Extravascular haemolysis is due to interaction of antibody-coated cells with cells in the reticuloendothelial system, predominantly in the spleen. Spherocytosis results from partial phagocytosis. Complete phagocytosis may occur and this is enhanced if there is complement as well as antibody on the cell surface. Cells coated with complement only are ineffectively removed and circulate with C3d or b on their surface.

tube after cooling but is more easily seen on the peripheral blood film made at room temperature. The agglutination is reversible after warming the sample.

DIRECT ANTIGLOBULIN TEST is positive with complement alone.

AUTOANTIBODIES often have specificity for the Ii blood group system, usually for the I antigen.

### Treatment

The underlying cause should be treated, if possible. Patients should avoid exposure to cold. Treatment with steroids, alkylating agents and splenectomy is usually ineffective.

### PAROXYSMAL COLD HAEMOGLOBINURIA (PCH)

This is a rare condition associated with common childhood infections, such as measles, mumps and chickenpox, but was originally described in association with syphilis. Intravascular haemolysis is associated with polyclonal IgG complement-fixing antibodies. These antibodies are *biphasic*, reacting with red cells in the cold in the peripheral circulation with lysis occurring due to complement activation when the cells return to the central circulation. The antibodies have specificity for the P red cell antigen. The lytic reaction is demonstrated *in vitro* by incubating the patient's red cells and serum at 4°C and then warming the mixture to 37°C (*Donath–Landsteiner test*). Haemolysis is self-limiting but supportive transfusions may be necessary.

## DRUG-INDUCED HAEMOLYTIC ANAEMIA

Drugs have been classically thought to cause immune haemolytic anaemia by the following mechanisms:

IMMUNE COMPLEX. The formation of drug–antibody immune complexes that become attached to red cells, activating complement and resulting in cell destruction. Example: quinine.

MEMBRANE ADSORPTION. An antigenic drug–red cell

complex is formed. Production of IgG antibodies results in cell destruction. Example: penicillin.

AUTOANTIBODY. The drug induces the production of a red cell autoantibody. Example: methyldopa.

New data suggest that the mechanisms involved in drug-induced haemolytic anaemia may be simpler than indicated above. The interaction between a drug and red cell membrane is now thought to cause a composite antigenic structure (or *neoantigen*), which provokes two types of antibodies:

1 Drug-dependent antibodies, which bind to both the drug and the cell membrane but not to either separately. Clinically there is usually severe complement-mediated intravascular haemolysis, which resolves quickly after withdrawal of the drug.

2 Drug-independent antibodies, which are induced by a subtle alteration of the red cell membrane. Such antibodies react with red cells *in vitro* in the absence of the drug and are indistinguishable from 'true' autoantibodies. There is extravascular haemolysis and the clinical course tends to be more protracted.

This new concept for drug-induced immune haemolytic anaemia probably also applies to drug-induced thrombocytopenia and neutropenia.

# ALLOIMMUNE HAEMOLYTIC ANAEMIA

Antibodies produced in one individual react with the red cells of another. This situation occurs in haemolytic disease of the newborn, haemolytic transfusion reactions (see p. 331) and after allogeneic bone marrow, renal, liver or cardiac transplantation when donor lymphocytes transferred in the allograft may produce red cell antibodies against the recipient and cause haemolytic anaemia.

## Haemolytic disease of the newborn (HDN)

HDN is due to fetomaternal incompatibility for red cell antigens; maternal alloantibodies against fetal red cell antigens pass from the maternal circulation via the placenta into the fetus, where they destroy the fetal red cells. Only IgG antibodies are capable of transplacental passage from mother to fetus.

The commonest type of HDN is that due to ABO incompatibility, where the mother is usually group O and the fetus group A.

HDN due to ABO incompatibility is usually mild and exchange transfusion is rarely needed.   HDN due to RhD incompatibility has become much less common following the introduction of anti-D prophylaxis (see below). HDN may be caused by antibodies against antigens in many blood group systems, e.g. other Rh antigens such as c and E, and Kell, Duffy and Kidd (see p. 330).

Sensitization occurs due to passage of fetal red cells into the maternal circulation which most readily occurs at the time of delivery, so that first pregnancies are rarely affected. However, sensitization may occur at other times, for example after a miscarriage, ectopic pregnancy or blood transfusion, or due to episodes during pregnancy which cause transplacental bleeding such as amniocentesis, chorionic villus sampling and threatened miscarriage.

## CLINICAL FEATURES

These vary from a mild haemolytic anaemia of the newborn to intrauterine death from 18 weeks' gestation with the characteristic appearance of *hydrops fetalis* (hepatosplenomegaly, oedema and cardiac failure).

*Kernicterus* occurs due to severe jaundice in the neonatal period, where the unconjugated (lipid-soluble) bilirubin exceeds 250 $\mu$mol litre$^{-1}$ and bile pigment deposition occurs in the basal ganglia. This results in mental deficiency, deafness, epilepsy and spasticity.

## INVESTIGATION
### Routine antenatal serology
All mothers should have their ABO and RhD groups determined and their serum tested for atypical antibodies after attending the antenatal booking clinic. The serum should be tested again for antibodies at 26 and 34 weeks of gestation.

If an antibody is detected, its blood group specificity should be determined and the mother's serum should be tested more frequently. A rising antibody titre is an indication for amniocentesis to assess the level of bilirubin in the amniotic fluid which gives an indication of the severity of HDN.

### At the birth of an affected infant
A sample of cord blood is obtained. This shows:
- Anaemia with a high reticulocyte count
- A positive direct antiglobulin test
- A raised serum bilirubin

## TREATMENT
### Management of the baby
In mild cases phototherapy may be used to convert bilirubin to water-soluble biliverdin. Biliverdin can be excreted by the kidneys and this therefore reduces the chance of kernicterus.

In more severely affected cases, exchange transfusion may be necessary to replace the infant's red cells and to remove bilirubin. Indications for exchange transfusion include:
- A cord Hb of <14 g dl$^{-1}$
- A cord bilirubin of >60 $\mu$mol litre$^{-1}$
- A later bilirubin of >300 $\mu$mol litre$^{-1}$
- A rapidly rising bilirubin level

Further exchange transfusions may be necessary to remove the unconjugated bilirubin.

The blood used for exchange transfusions should be ABO compatible with the mother and infant, lack the antigen against which the maternal antibody is directed, be as fresh as possible and seronegative for cytomegalovirus.

A fetus severely affected before 33 weeks of gestation

may need intrauterine blood transfusions carried out in a special unit.

### Prevention of RhD immunization in the mother

Anti-D should be given after delivery when all of the following are present:

- The mother is RhD negative
- The fetus is RhD positive
- There is no maternal anti-D detectable in the mother's serum, i.e. mother not already immunized

The dose is 500 i.u. of IgG anti-D intramuscularly within 48 hours of delivery. The *Kleihauer test* is used to assess the number of fetal cells in the maternal circulation. A blood film prepared from maternal blood is treated with acid, which elutes Hb A. Hb F is resistant to this treatment and can be seen when the film is stained with eosin. If large numbers of fetal red cells are present in the maternal circulation, a higher dose of anti-D is necessary.

It may be necessary to give prophylaxis to RhD-negative women at other times when sensitization may occur, for example after an ectopic pregnancy, threatened miscarriage or amniocentesis. The dose of anti-D is 500 i.u. after 20 weeks of gestation and 250 i.u. before 20 weeks.

Of previously non-immunized RhD-negative women carrying RhD-positive fetuses, 1–2% are immunized by the time of delivery. *Antenatal prophylaxis* with administration of anti-D to RhD-negative women at 28 and 34 weeks of gestation has been shown to reduce the incidence of immunization in some studies. Antenatal prophylaxis is already used in some centres but further evidence is required before a recommendation for its routine use can be given.

## NON-IMMUNE HAEMOLYTIC ANAEMIA

## Paroxysmal nocturnal haemoglobinuria (PNH)

This is a rare acquired red cell defect in which a clone of red cells is particularly sensitive to destruction by activated complement. These cells are continually haemolysed intravascularly. Platelets and granulocytes are also affected and there may be thrombocytopenia and neutropenia.

The underlying defect is an inability of PNH cells to make glycosyl-phosphatidylinositol (GPI) which anchors proteins such as delay accelerating factor (DAF) and membrane inhibitor of reactive lysis (MIRL) to cell membranes. These and other proteins are involved in complement degradation and in their absence the haemolytic action of complement is not regulated.

### CLINICAL FEATURES

Patients present with haemolysis which may be precipitated by infection, iron therapy or surgery. Characteristically only the urine voided at night and in the morning on waking is dark in colour although the reason for this phenomenon is not clear. In severe cases all urine samples are dark. Urinary iron loss may be sufficient to cause iron deficiency.

The condition may be complicated by thrombotic episodes, giving acute abdominal pain, myocardial infarction or stroke. The Budd–Chiari syndrome (hepatic vein occlusion) can occur.

### INVESTIGATION

INTRAVASCULAR HAEMOLYSIS is evident (see p. 311).
HAM'S TEST. Cells from a patient with PNH lyse more readily in acidified serum than do normal cells.
BONE MARROW is sometimes hypoplastic despite haemolysis.

### TREATMENT AND PROGNOSIS

There is no specific treatment for PNH. It is a chronic disorder requiring supportive measures such as blood transfusions, which are necessary for patients with severe anaemia. Leucocyte-depleted blood should be used in order to prevent transfusion reactions resulting in complement activation and acceleration of the haemolysis.

Long-term anticoagulation may be necessary for patients with recurrent thrombotic episodes. Bone marrow transplantation has been successfully carried out in a small number of patients.

The course of PNH is variable. It may remain stable for many years and the PNH clone may even disappear. The median survival is 10 years.

PNH may transform into aplastic anaemia or acute leukaemia.

## MECHANICAL HAEMOLYTIC ANAEMIA

Red cells may be injured by physical trauma in the circulation. Direct injury may cause immediate cell lysis or may be followed by resealing of the cell membrane with the formation of distorted red cells or 'fragments'. These cells may circulate for a short period before being destroyed prematurely in the reticuloendothelial system.

The causes of mechanical haemolytic anaemia include *damaged artificial heart valves*, *March haemoglobinuria*, where there is damage to red cells in the feet associated with prolonged marching or running, and *microangiopathic haemolytic anaemia* (MAHA) where fragmentation of red cells occurs in an abnormal microcirculation caused by malignant hypertension, eclampsia, haemolytic uraemic syndrome, thrombotic thrombocytopenic purpura, vasculitis or disseminated intravascular coagulation.

## *Myeloproliferative disorders*

In these disorders there is uncontrolled clonal proliferation of one or more of the cell lines in the bone marrow, namely erythroid, myeloid, megakaryocyte lines. Myeloproliferative disorders include *polycythaemia vera* (PV), *essential thrombocythaemia* (ET), *myelofibrosis* and *chronic myeloid leukaemia*. These disorders are grouped together as there can be transition from one disease to another, for example PV can lead to myelofibrosis. They may also transform to acute myeloblastic leukaemia. The *non-leukaemic myeloproliferative disorders* (PV, ET and myelo-fibrosis) will be discussed in this section. Chronic myeloid leukaemia is described on p. 365.

Myelodysplasia describes a group of acquired bone marrow disorders, also resulting from defects in stem cells, characterized by quantitative and qualitative abnor-malities of myeloid cells. They occur mainly in the elderly and present with increasing bone marrow failure. Trans-formation into acute myeloblastic leukaemia may occur.

# Polycythaemia

Polycythaemia (or erythrocytosis) is defined as an in-crease in Hb, PCV and red cell count. PCV is a more reliable indicator of polycythaemia than Hb, which may be disproportionately low in iron deficiency. Polycythae-mia can be divided into *absolute erythrocytosis* where there is a true increase in red cell volume or *relative erythro-cytosis* where the red cell volume is normal but there is a decrease in the plasma volume (see Fig. 6.6).

Absolute erythrocytosis may be due to primary polycy-thaemia (PV) or secondary polycythaemia. Secondary polycythaemia may be due to an *appropriate* increase in red cells in response to anoxia, or may be due to an *inap-propriate* increase associated with tumours, such as a renal carcinoma. The causes of polycythaemia are given in Table 6.15.

## PRIMARY POLYCYTHAEMIA— POLYCYTHAEMIA VERA

PV is a clonal stem cell disorder in which there is an alteration in the pluripotent progenitor cell leading to excessive proliferation of erythroid, myeloid and megaka-ryocytic progenitor cells.

The main clinical problems are due to the increased volume and viscosity of the blood and the bone mar-row overactivity.

### CLINICAL FEATURES

The onset is insidious. It usually presents in patients over 60 years with tiredness, depression, vertigo, tinnitus and visual disturbance. It should be noted that these symp-toms are also common in the normal population over the age of 60 and consequently PV is easily missed. These features, together with hypertension, angina, intermittent claudication and a tendency to bleed are suggestive evi-dence for PV.

Severe itching after a hot bath or when the patient is warm is common. Gout due to increased cell turnover may be a feature and peptic ulceration occurs in a min-ority of patients. Thrombosis and haemorrhage are the major complications of PV.

**Primary**
Polycythaemia vera

**Secondary**
*Due to an appropriate increase in erythropoietin*
High altitude
Lung disease
Cardiovascular disease (right-to-left shunt)
Heavy smoking
Increased affinity of haemoglobin, e.g. familial
    polycythaemia

*Due to an inappropriate increase in erythropoietin*
Renal disease, renal cell carcinoma, Wilms' tumour
Hepatocellular carcinoma
Adrenal tumours
Cerebellar haemangioblastoma
Massive uterine fibroma

**Relative**
Stress or spurious polycythaemia
Dehydration
Burns

**Table 6.15**  Causes of polycythaemia.

## Physical signs
The patient is usually plethoric and has a deep dusky cyanosis. Injection of the conjunctivae is commonly seen. The spleen is palpable in 70% and is useful in dis-tinguishing PV from secondary causes. The liver is enlarged in 50% of patients.

### INVESTIGATION
Hb and PCV are increased. The WCC is raised in about 70% of cases of PV and the platelet count is elevated in about 50%.

The bone marrow shows erythroid hyperplasia and increased numbers of megakaryocytes.

Red cell volume measured using $^{51}$Cr-labelled red cells is increased ($>36$ ml kg$^{-1}$ in males and 32 ml kg$^{-1}$ in females). Measurement of plasma vol-ume shows normal or increased values (normal range is $45 \pm 5$ ml kg$^{-1}$).

Serum uric acid levels may be raised.

Leucocyte alkaline phosphatase (LAP) score is usually high.

Serum vitamin B$_{12}$ and vitamin B$_{12}$-binding protein (TC I) levels may be high, although these are not rou-tinely measured.

### DIFFERENTIAL DIAGNOSIS
An increase in the red cell volume should be established. Raised WCC and platelet counts with splenomegaly makes a diagnosis of PV very likely. The principal sec-ondary causes can often be excluded by the history and examination but a renal ultrasound, an arterial $Po_2$ and carboxyhaemoglobin levels are usually performed. The serum erythropoietin level is not diagnostic but may be helpful in distinguishing PV from secondary polycythae-mia: in PV the level is low or normal; in secondary poly-cythaemia the level may be raised, as expected, but may be normal.

## COURSE AND MANAGEMENT

Treatment is designed to maintain a normal blood count and to prevent the complications of the disease, particularly thromboses and haemorrhage. Treatment is aimed at keeping the PCV below 0.45 litre litre$^{-1}$ and the platelet count below $400 \times 10^9$/litre. There are three types of treatment:

VENESECTION. This will successfully relieve many of the symptoms of PV. Iron deficiency limits erythropoiesis. Venesection is often used as the sole treatment and other therapy is reserved to control the thrombocytosis.

CHEMOTHERAPY. Continuous or intermittent treatment with agents such as busulphan or hydroxyurea is used particularly for controlling the thrombocytosis. Hydroxyurea is now being used frequently because of the ease of controlling thrombocytosis and general safety in comparison to the alkylating agents such as busulphan which carry an increased risk of acute leukaemia.

RADIOACTIVE $^{32}$P. One dose may give control for up to 18 months but the administration of $^{32}$P carries an increased risk of transformation to acute leukaemia. $^{32}$P is usually confined to the over 70 years age group.

Allopurinol is given to block uric acid production. The pruritus is lessened by avoiding very hot baths. $H_1$-receptor antagonists have largely proved unsuccessful in relieving distressing pruritus but $H_2$-receptor antagonists such as cimetidine are occasionally effective.

It should be noted that patients with uncontrolled PV have a high operative risk; 75% of patients have severe haemorrhage following surgery and 30% of these patients die. Polycythaemia should be controlled before surgery. In an emergency, reduction of the haematocrit by venesection and appropriate fluid replacement must be carried out.

## PROGNOSIS

PV develops into myelofibrosis in 30% of cases and into acute myeloblastic leukaemia in 5% as part of the natural history of the disease.

## SECONDARY POLYCYTHAEMIAS

The causes of these are shown in Table 6.15. The treatment is that of the precipitating factor; for example, renal or posterior fossa tumours need to be resected. Heavy smoking can produce as much as 10% carboxyhaemoglobin and this can produce polycythaemia because of a reduction in the oxygen-carrying capacity of the blood. Complications are similar to those seen in PV, including thrombosis, haemorrhage and cardiac failure, but the complications due to myeloproliferative disease such as progression to myelofibrosis or acute leukaemia do not develop. Venesection may be symptomatically helpful in the hypoxic patient, particularly if the PCV is above 0.55 litre litre$^{-1}$.

### 'Relative' or 'stress' polycythaemia (Gaisböck's syndrome)

This condition was originally thought to be stress-induced. The red cell volume is normal but, as the result of a decreased plasma volume, there is a *relative* polycythaemia. 'Stress' polycythaemia is commoner than PV and occurs in middle-aged men, particularly in smokers who are obese and hypertensive. The condition may present with cardiovascular problems such as myocardial or cerebral ischaemia. For this reason, it may be justifiable to venesect the patient. Smoking should be stopped.

### Essential thrombocythaemia (ET)

ET is a rare condition that is closely related to PV. The patient has $>1000 \times 10^9$/litre platelets. It presents with bruising, bleeding and cerebrovascular symptoms. Initially splenic hypertrophy may be seen but, as the condition progresses, recurrent thromboses due to the increased number of platelets reduce the size of the spleen and it may atrophy.

ET has to be distinguished from *secondary thrombocytosis* that is seen in haemorrhage, connective tissue disorders, malignancy, after splenectomy and in other myeloproliferative disorders.

Treatment is with hydroxyurea or busulphan to control the platelet count at less than $400 \times 10^9$/litre. Alpha-interferon is also effective but it is expensive and is administered by subcutaneous injection. ET may eventually transform into PV, myelofibrosis or acute leukaemia but the disease may not progress for many years.

# Myelofibrosis (myelosclerosis)

The terms myelosclerosis and myelofibrosis are interchangeable. There is clonal proliferation of stem cells and extramedullary haemopoiesis in the liver and spleen. There is increased fibrosis in the bone marrow caused by hyperplasia of abnormal megakaryocytes which release fibroblast-stimulating factors such as platelet-derived growth factor. In about 25% of cases there is a preceding history of PV.

## CLINICAL FEATURES

The disease presents insidiously with lethargy, weakness and weight loss. Patients often complain of a 'fullness' in the upper abdomen due to splenomegaly. Severe pain related to respiration may indicate perisplenitis secondary to splenic infarction, and bone pain and attacks of gout can complicate the illness. Bruising and bleeding may occur due to thrombocytopenia or abnormal platelet function.

### Physical signs

- Anaemia
- Fever
- Massive splenomegaly (for other causes, see p. 329)

## INVESTIGATION

ANAEMIA with leucoerythroblastic features is present (p. 335). Poikilocytes and red cells with characteristic tear-drop forms are seen. The WCC may be over $100 \times 10^9$/litre, and the differential WCC may be very similar to that seen in chronic myeloid leukaemia; later leucopenia may develop.

THE PLATELET COUNT may be very high but, in later stages, thrombocytopenia occurs.

BONE MARROW ASPIRATION is often unsuccessful and this gives a clue to the presence of the condition. A bone marrow trephine is necessary to show the markedly increased fibrosis. Increased numbers of megakaryocytes may be seen.

THE PHILADELPHIA CHROMOSOME is absent; this helps to distinguish myelofibrosis from most cases of chronic myeloid leukaemia.

THE LAP SCORE is normal or high.

A HIGH SERUM URATE is present.

LOW SERUM FOLATE levels may occur owing to the increased haemopoietic activity.

## DIFFERENTIAL DIAGNOSIS

The major diagnostic difficulty is the differentiation of myelofibrosis from chronic myeloid leukaemia as in both conditions there may be marked splenomegaly and a raised WCC with many granulocyte precursors seen in the peripheral blood. The main distinguishing features are the appearance of the bone marrow and the absence of the Philadelphia chromosome in myelofibrosis.

Fibrosis of the marrow, often with a leucoerythroblastic anaemia, can occur secondarily to leukaemia or lymphoma, tuberculosis or malignant infiltration with metastatic carcinoma, or to irradiation.

## TREATMENT

This consists of general supportive measures such as blood transfusion, folic acid, analgesics and allopurinol. Drugs such as busulphan, chlorambucil and hydroxyurea are used to reduce metabolic activity and high WCC and platelet levels; hydroxyurea is the commonest drug used. Chemotherapy and radiotherapy are used to reduce splenic size. If the spleen becomes very large and painful, and transfusion requirements are high, it may be advisable to perform splenectomy. Splenectomy may also result in relief of severe thrombocytopenia.

## PROGNOSIS

Patients may survive for 10 years or more; median survival is 3 years. Death may occur from transformation to acute myeloblastic leukaemia in 10–20%. The most common causes of death are cardiovascular disease, infection and gastrointestinal bleeding.

# The spleen

The spleen is the largest lymphoid organ in the body and is situated in the left hypochondrium. There are two anatomical components:

1 The red pulp, consisting of sinuses lined by endothelial macrophages and cords (spaces)
2 The white pulp, which has a structure similar to lymphoid follicles

Blood enters via the splenic artery and is delivered to the red and white pulp. During the flow the blood is 'skimmed', with leucocytes and plasma preferentially passing to white pulp. Some red cells pass rapidly through into the venous system while others are held up in the red pulp.

### Functions

SEQUESTRATION AND PHAGOCYTOSIS. Normal red cells, which are flexible, pass through the red pulp into the venous system without difficulty. Old or abnormal cells are damaged by the hypoxia, low glucose and low pH found in the sinuses of the red pulp and are therefore removed by phagocytosis along with other circulating foreign matter. Howell–Jolly and Heinz bodies and sideroblastic granules have their particles removed by 'pitting' and are then returned to the circulation. IgG-coated red cells are removed through their Fc receptors by macrophages.

EXTRAMEDULLARY HAEMOPOIESIS. Pluripotential stem cells are present in the spleen and proliferate during severe haematological stress, e.g. haemolytic anaemia, thalassaemia major.

IMMUNOLOGICAL FUNCTION. About 25% of the body's T lymphocytes and 15% of B lymphocytes are present in the spleen. The spleen shares the function of production of antibodies with other lymphoid tissues.

BLOOD POOLING. Up to one-third of the platelets are sequestrated in the spleen and can be rapidly mobilized. Enlarged spleens pool a significant percentage (up to 40%) of the red cell mass.

# Splenomegaly

A clinically palpable spleen has many causes including:
1 Infection
   (a) acute—septicaemia, infective endocarditis, typhoid, infectious mononucleosis
   (b) chronic—tuberculosis and brucellosis
   (c) parasitic—malaria, kala-azar and schistosomiasis
2 Inflammation: rheumatoid arthritis, sarcoidosis, SLE
3 Haematological: haemolytic anaemia, haemoglobinopathies and the leukaemias, lymphomas and myeloproliferative disorders
4 Portal hypertension: liver disease
5 Miscellaneous: storage diseases, amyloid, primary and secondary neoplasias, tropical splenomegaly

*Massive splenomegaly* is seen in myelofibrosis, chronic myeloid leukaemia, chronic malaria, kala-azar or, rarely, Gaucher's disease.

*Investigation* is that of the primary disorder. The spleen can be visualized by ultrasound or CT scanning. Splenic function can be assessed with isotope scanning.

## HYPERSPLENISM

This can result from splenomegaly due to any cause. It is commonly seen with splenomegaly due to haematological disorders, portal hypertension, rheumatoid arthritis (Felty's syndrome) and lymphoma. Hypersplenism produces:

- Pancytopenia
- Haemolysis due to sequestration and destruction of red cells in the spleen
- Increased plasma volume

Treatment is often dependent on the underlying cause but splenectomy is sometimes required for severe anaemia or thrombocytopenia.

## SPLENECTOMY

Splenectomy is performed mainly for:

- Trauma
- Autoimmune thrombocytopenic purpura (p. 341)
- Haemolytic anaemias (p. 310)
- Hodgkin's disease—staging (p. 368), although this is less frequently performed as occult abdominal disease can be detected by CT and MRI scanning
- Hypersplenism

### Postsplenectomy problems

IMMEDIATE: increased platelet count (usually 600–$1000 \times 10^9$/litre) for 2–3 weeks, thromboembolic phenomena may occur.

LONG-TERM: increased risk of overwhelming infections, particularly pneumococcal infections.

### Prophylaxis against infection after splenectomy or splenic dysfunction

All patients should receive a single dose of polyvalent antipneumococcal vaccine, which should be given 2–3 weeks before splenectomy. It is effective if the types of pneumonia are reflected in the polysaccharides contained in the serum. The vaccine may need to be repeated in 5–10 years. Long-term prophylactic penicillin is given.

### Postsplenectomy haematological features

THROMBOCYTOSIS persists in about 30%

THE WCC is usually normal but there may be a mild lymphocytosis and monocytosis

ABNORMALITIES IN RED CELL MORPHOLOGY are the most prominent changes and include Howell–Jolly bodies, Pappenheimer bodies, target cells and irregular contracted red cells (see Fig. 6.8). Pitted red cells can be counted.

## SPLENIC ATROPHY

This is seen in sickle cell disease due to infarction. It is also seen in coeliac disease, dermatitis herpetiformis and occasionally in ulcerative colitis and essential thrombocythaemia. Postsplenectomy haematological features are seen.

# Blood transfusion

The cells and proteins in the blood express antigens which are controlled by polymorphic genes, i.e. a specific antigen may be present in some individuals but not others. A blood transfusion may immunize the recipient against donor antigens that the recipient lacks (*alloimmunization*); repeated transfusions increase the risk of the occurrence of alloimmunization. Similarly, the transplacental passage of fetal blood cells during pregnancy may alloimmunize the mother against fetal antigens inherited from the father. Antibodies stimulated by blood transfusion or pregnancy are termed *immune* antibodies, in contrast to *naturally occurring* antibodies, such as ABO antibodies, which are made in response to environmental antigens present in food and bacteria.

## BLOOD GROUPS

The blood groups are determined by antigens on the surface of red cells; more than 400 blood groups have been found. The ABO and Rh systems are the two most important blood groups but incompatibilities involving many other blood groups (such as Kell, Duffy, Kidd) may cause haemolytic transfusion reactions and/or HDN.

### ABO system

This is the most important blood group system because naturally occurring IgM anti-A and anti-B antibodies are capable of producing rapid and severe intravascular haemolysis of incompatible red cells.

The ABO system is under the control of a pair of allelic genes, *H* and *h*, and also three allelic genes, *A*, *B* and *O*, producing the genotypes and phenotypes shown in Table 6.16. The A, B and H antigens are very similar in structure; differences in the terminal sugars determine their specificity. The *H* gene codes for enzyme H, which attaches fructose to the basic glycoprotein backbone to form H substance, which is the precursor for A and B antigens.

The *A* and *B* genes control specific enzymes responsible for the addition to H substance of *N*-acetylgalactosamine for Group A and D-galactose for Group B. The *O* gene is amorphic and does not transform H substance and therefore O is not antigenic. The A, B and H antigens are present on most body cells. These antigens are also found in soluble form in tissue fluids such as saliva and gastric juice in the 80% of the population who possess secretor genes.

### Rh system

This is the second most clinically important blood group system because of the high frequency of development of

| Phenotype | Genotype | Antigens | Antibodies | Frequency, UK (%) |
|-----------|----------|----------|------------|-------------------|
| O | OO | None | Anti-A and anti-B | 44 |
| A | AA or AO | A | Anti-B | 45 |
| B | BB or BO | B | Anti-A | 8 |
| AB | AB | A and B | None | 3 |

**Table 6.16**  Antigens and antibodies in the ABO system.

IgG RhD antibodies in RhD-negative individuals after exposure to RhD-positive red cells following blood transfusions or during pregnancy. The antibodies formed are of major importance in causing HDN and haemolytic transfusion reactions.

This system is coded by allelic genes, *C* and *c*, *E* and *e*, *D* and no *D*, which is signified as *d*; they are inherited as triplets on each chromosome, one from each pair of genes, i.e. *CDE/cde*. The presence of the d antigen has not been demonstrated and the presence or absence of the D antigen determines whether an individual is characterized as RhD positive or negative.

## PROCEDURE FOR BLOOD TRANSFUSION

The safety of blood transfusion depends on meticulous attention to detail at each stage leading to and during the transfusion. Prevention of simple errors involving patient and blood sample identification would avoid most serious haemolytic transfusion reactions, almost all of which involve the ABO system. About 50% of fatalities associated with blood transfusion are due to immediate haemolytic transfusion reactions; the remainder are mainly due to post-transfusion hepatitis.

**Pretransfusion compatibility testing**

1 Blood grouping. The ABO and RhD groups of the patient are determined.
2 Antibody screening. The patient's serum is screened for atypical antibodies that may cause a significant reduction in the survival of the transfused red cells. The patient's serum is tested against red cells from at least two Group O donors, expressing a wide range of red cell antigens, for detection of IgM red cell alloantibodies (using a direct agglutination test of cells suspended in saline) and IgG antibodies (using an indirect antiglobulin test, see p. 323). If there is a positive result, the blood group specificity of the antibody should be determined using a comprehensive panel of typed red cells.
3 Donor blood of the same ABO and RhD group as the patient is selected.
4 Crossmatching
   (a) *Patients without atypical red cell antibodies.* The full crossmatch involves testing the patient's serum against the donor red cells suspended in saline in a direct agglutination test and also using an indirect antiglobulin test. In some hospitals this has been shortened to an *immediate spin crossmatch* where the patient's serum is briefly incubated with the donor red cells, followed by centrifugation and examination for agglutination; this rapid crossmatch is an acceptable method of excluding ABO incompatibility in patients known to have a negative antibody screen.
   (b) *Patients with atypical red cell antibodies.* Donor blood lacking the relevant red cell antigen(s), as well as being the same ABO and RhD group as the patient should be selected. A full crossmatch should always be carried out.

Many hospitals have guidelines for blood ordering for elective surgery (*maximum surgical blood ordering schedules*), aiming to reduce unnecessary crossmatching and the amount of blood that eventually becomes outdated. Many operations in which blood is only occasionally required for unexpectedly high blood loss can be classified as 'group and save serum'; this means that, where the antibody screen is negative, blood is not reserved in advance but can be made available quickly if necessary. If a patient has atypical antibodies, compatible blood should always be reserved in advance.

## The complications of blood transfusion (Table 6.17)

### IMMUNOLOGICAL

ALLOIMMUNIZATION. All transfusions carry a risk of immunization to the many antigens present on red cells, leucocytes, platelets and plasma proteins. Alloimmunization does not usually cause clinical problems with the first transfusion but these may occur with subsequent transfusions. There may also be important delayed consequences of alloimmunization such as HDN and rejection of tissue transplants.

INCOMPATIBILITY. This may result in poor survival of transfused cells, such as red cells and platelets, and also in the harmful effects of antigen–antibody reaction.

**Haemolytic transfusion reactions**

IMMEDIATE. This is the most serious complication of blood transfusion and is usually due to ABO incompatibility. There is complement activation by the antigen–antibody reaction, usually due to IgM antibodies, leading to rigors, lumbar pain, dyspnoea, hypotension, haemo-

**Immunological**
*Alloimmunization*

*Incompatibility*
Red cells
  Immediate haemolytic transfusion reactions
  Delayed haemolytic transfusion reactions
Leucocyte and platelets
  Non-haemolytic (febrile) transfusion reactions
  Post-transfusion purpura
  Poor survival of transfused platelets and granulocytes
  Graft-versus-host disease
Plasma proteins
  Urticarial and anaphylactic reactions

**Non-immunological**

Transmission of infection
  Hepatitis
  HIV
  Other viruses—CMV, EBV, HTLV-1
  Parasites—malaria, trypanosomiasis, toxoplasmosis
  Syphilis
  Transfusion of blood contaminated with bacteria
Circulatory failure due to volume overload
Iron overload due to multiple transfusions (see. p. 316)
Massive transfusion of stored blood may cause bleeding
    and electrolyte changes (see p. 346)
Thrombophlebitis
Air embolism

**Table 6.17**  Complications of blood transfusion.

globinuria and renal failure. Activation of coagulation may also occur; bleeding due to disseminated intravascular coagulation (DIC) is a bad prognostic sign. Emergency treatment may be needed to maintain the blood pressure and renal function.

The diagnosis is confirmed by finding evidence of haemolysis, such as haemoglobinuria, and incompatibility between donor and recipient. All documentation should be checked to detect errors such as:
- Failure to confirm the identity of the patient when taking the sample for compatibility testing, i.e. sample taken from the wrong patient
- Mislabelling the blood sample with the wrong patient's name
- Simple labelling or handling errors in the laboratory
- Failure to perform proper identity checks before the blood is transfused, i.e. blood transfused to the wrong patient

The blood grouping of the patient's sample (used for the original compatibility testing), a new sample taken from the patient after the reaction and the donor units should all be checked to confirm where the error occurred. The serious consequences of such failures emphasize the need for meticulous checks at all stages in the procedure of blood transfusion.

At the first suspicion of any transfusion reaction the transfusion should always be stopped and the donor units returned to the blood transfusion laboratory with a new blood sample from the patient to exclude a haemolytic transfusion reaction.

DELAYED. This may occur in patients alloimmunized by previous transfusions or pregnancies. The antibody level is too low to be detected by pretransfusion compatibility testing but a secondary immune response occurs after transfusion, resulting in destruction of the transfused cells, usually by IgG antibodies.

Haemolysis is usually extravascular and the patient may develop anaemia and jaundice about a week after the transfusion, although most are clinically silent. The blood film shows spherocytosis and reticulocytosis. The direct antiglobulin test is positive and detection of the antibody is usually straightforward.

### Non-haemolytic (febrile) transfusion reactions

Febrile reactions are a common complication of blood transfusion in patients who have previously been transfused or pregnant. The usual cause is the presence of leucocyte antibodies in the recipient acting against transfused leucocytes, leading to release of pyrogens. Typical signs are flushing and tachycardia, fever (>38°C), chills and rigors. Aspirin may be used to reduce the fever, although it should not be used in patients with thrombocytopenia. Febrile reactions may be prevented after further transfusions by the use of leucocyte-depleted blood.

Potent leucocyte antibodies in the plasma of donors, who are usually multiparous women, may cause severe pulmonary reactions (called *transfusion-related acute lung injury* or TRALI) characterized by dyspnoea, fever, cough, and shadowing in the perihilar and lower lung fields on the chest X-ray.

### Urticaria and anaphylaxis

Urticarial reactions are often attributed to plasma protein incompatibility but, in most cases, they are unexplained. They are common but rarely severe; stopping or slowing the transfusion and administration of chlorpheniramine 10 mg i.v. are usually sufficient treatment.

Anaphylactic reactions (see p. 147) occasionally occur; severe reactions are seen in patients lacking IgA who produce anti-IgA that reacts with IgA in the transfused blood. The transfusion should be stopped and adrenaline 0.5 mg i.m. and chlorpheniramine 10 mg i.v. should be given immediately; endotracheal intubation may be required.    Patients who have had severe urticarial or anaphylactic reactions should receive either washed red cells, autologous blood or blood from IgA-deficient donors for patients with IgA deficiency.

### NON-IMMUNOLOGICAL
### Transmission of infection

The incidence of post-transfusion hepatitis was estimated to be about 1% in the UK before testing for antibodies against hepatitis C virus (HCV) was introduced in 1991. As most cases were due to non-A, non-B hepatitis due to HCV, the incidence of post-transfusion hepatitis is expected to decrease. Each donation has been tested for HBsAg for many years and the incidence of post-transfusion hepatitis due to hepatitis B is very low. Other viruses which may cause post-transfusion hepatitis include CMV, EBV and other as yet unidentified viruses.

In the UK the incidence of transmission of HIV by blood transfusion is extremely low, probably in the order of one in one million units. Prevention is based on self-exclusion of donors in 'high-risk' groups and testing each donation for anti-HIV. There is an increased risk of transmission of hepatitis viruses and HIV from coagulation factor concentrates prepared from large pools of plasma. However, these are now subjected to measures for inactivating viruses such as treatment with heat, solvents and detergents. The problem of viral transmission is still a major problem in the developing world.

Transfusion-transmitted syphilis is now very rare in the UK. Spirochaetes do not survive for more than 72 hours in blood stored at 4°C and each donation is tested using the *Treponema pallidum* haemagglutination assay (TPHA).

### Autologous transfusion

An alternative to the use of blood from volunteer donors for the replacement of blood lost during surgery is the patient's own blood. Interest in autologous transfusion was mainly stimulated by concern about transmission of infection, especially HIV, by blood transfusion. There are three types:

1 Pre-deposit. The patient donates 2–5 units of blood at approximately weekly intervals before elective surgery.
2 Preoperative haemodilution. One or two units of blood are removed from the patient immediately before surgery and retransfused to replace operative losses.
3 Blood salvage. Blood lost during or after surgery may be collected and retransfused. Several techniques of varying levels of sophistication are available. The operative site must be free of bacteria, bowel contents and tumour cells.

There has been little demand for autologous transfusion in the UK as blood is generally perceived as being 'safe'. In addition, there would be considerable costs in setting up a predeposit autologous transfusion service, which would only benefit a minority of patients. In developing countries, however, autologous blood and blood from relatives is increasingly being used.

# Blood, blood components and blood products

Most blood collected from donors is processed into:

1 Blood components, such as red cell and platelet concentrates, fresh frozen plasma (FFP) and cryoprecipitate, are prepared from a single donation of blood by simple separation methods such as centrifugation and transfused without further processing.
2 Blood products, such as coagulation factor concentrates and albumin and immunoglobulin solutions, are prepared by complex processes using the plasma from many donors as the starting material.

In most circumstances it is preferable to transfuse only the blood component or product required by the patient rather than using whole blood (*component therapy*). This is the most effective way of using donor blood, which is a scarce resource, and reduces the risk of complications from transfusion of unnecessary components of the blood.

WHOLE BLOOD. The average volume of blood withdrawn is 450 ml, taken into 63 ml of anticoagulant. Blood stored at 4°C has a 'shelf-life' of 5 weeks when at least 70% of the transfused red cells should survive normally. Whole blood should be reserved for acute blood loss; packed cells or red cell concentrates plus crystalloid or colloid solutions are acceptable alternatives.

PACKED RED CELLS. 200–250 ml of plasma are removed from whole blood to be frozen as FFP or to be further processed.

RED CELL CONCENTRATES. Virtually all the plasma is removed and it is replaced by about 100 ml of an *optimal additive solution*, such as SAG-M which contains sodium chloride, adenine, glucose and mannitol. The PCV is about 0.65 litre litre$^{-1}$ but the viscosity is low as there are no plasma proteins in the additive solution, and this allows fast administration if necessary.

LEUCOCYTE-DEPLETED RED CELL CONCENTRATES are usually prepared by filtration. They are used in patients who have had recurrent febrile transfusion reactions and to prevent alloimmunization to leucocyte antigens in patients likely to receive repeated transfusions such as patients with thalassaemia major.

WASHED RED CELL CONCENTRATES are preparations of red cells suspended in saline, produced by cell separators to remove all but traces of plasma proteins. They are used in patients who have had severe recurrent urticarial or anaphylactic reactions.

PLATELET CONCENTRATES are prepared either from whole blood by centrifugation or by plateletpheresis of single donors using cell separators. They may be stored for up to 5 days at 22°C. They are used to treat bleeding in patients with severe thrombocytopenia and prophylactically to prevent bleeding in patients with bone marrow failure.

GRANULOCYTE CONCENTRATES are prepared from single donors using cell separators. They are used for patients with severe neutropenia with definite evidence of bacterial infection where antibiotic therapy has failed. They are rarely used now.

FRESH FROZEN PLASMA is prepared by freezing the plasma from 1 unit of blood at 0°C within 6 hours of donation. The volume is approximately 200 ml. FFP contains all the coagulation factors present in fresh plasma and is mostly used for replacement of coagulation factors in acquired coagulation factor deficiencies.

CRYOPRECIPITATE is obtained by allowing the frozen plasma from a single donation to thaw at 4–8°C and removing the supernatant. The volume is about 20 ml and it is stored at 0°C. It contains factor VIII:C, factor VIII:vWF and fibrinogen. It is no longer used for the treatment of haemophilia A and von Willebrand's disease because of the greater risk of virus transmission compared to virus-inactivated coagulation factor concentrates.

FACTOR VIII AND IX CONCENTRATES are freeze-dried preparations of specific coagulation factors prepared from large pools of plasma. They are used for treating patients with haemophilia and von Willebrand's disease.

*High purity* products are prepared using purification procedures involving chromatography columns and either monoclonal antibodies or ion exchanges. *Intermediate purity* products are prepared by conventional fractionation methods. Solvents, detergents and heat treatment are used for viral inactivation. High purity products should be used in preference to the intermediate purity products because of their greater safety and because they cause less immunosuppression in HIV-seropositive patients with haemophilia.

ALBUMIN. There are two preparations: *Human albumin solution (4.5%)*, previously called plasma protein fraction (PPF), contains 45 g litre$^{-1}$ albumin and 160 mmol litre$^{-1}$ sodium. It is produced in 50, 100, 250 and 500 ml bottles.

*Human albumin solution 20%*, previously called 'salt-poor' albumin contains approximately 200 g litre$^{-1}$ albumin and 130 mmol litre$^{-1}$ sodium and is produced in 50 and 100 ml bottles.

Human albumin solutions are generally considered to be inappropriate fluids for acute volume replacement or the treatment of shock because they are no more effective in these situations than synthetic colloid solutions such as polygelatins (*Gelofusine*) or hydroxyethyl starch (*Haemaccel*). However, albumin solutions are indicated for treatment of acute severe hypoalbuminaemia and as the replacement fluid for plasma exchange. The 20% albumin solution is particularly useful for patients with nephrotic syndrome or liver disease who are fluid overloaded and resistant to diuretics. Albumin solutions should not be used to treat patients with malnutrition or chronic renal or liver disease.

NORMAL IMMUNOGLOBULIN is prepared from normal plasma. It is used in patients with hypogammaglobulinaemia to prevent infections and in patients with immune thrombocytopenia.

SPECIFIC IMMUNOGLOBULINS are obtained from donors with high titres of antibodies. Many preparations are available, such as anti-D, anti-hepatitis B, anti-varicella-zoster.

# *The white cell* (see also Chapter 2)

The five types of leucocytes found in peripheral blood are neutrophils, eosinophils and basophils (which are all called granulocytes) and lymphocytes and monocytes. The development of these cells is shown in Fig. 6.1.

## NEUTROPHILS

The earliest morphologically identifiable precursors of neutrophils in the bone marrow are *myeloblasts*, which are large cells constituting up to 3.5% of the nucleated cells in the marrow. The nucleus is large and contains two to five nucleoli. The cytoplasm is scanty and contains no granules. *Promyelocytes* are similar to myeloblasts but have some primary cytoplasmic granules containing enzymes such as myeloperoxidase. *Myelocytes* are smaller cells without nucleoli but with more abundant cytoplasm and both primary and secondary granules. Indentation of the nucleus marks the change from myelocyte to *metamyelocyte*. The mature *neutrophil* is a smaller cell with a nucleus with two to five lobes with predominantly secondary granules in the cytoplasm which contain lysozyme, collagenase and lactoferrin.

Peripheral blood neutrophils are equally distributed into a circulating pool and a marginating pool lying along the endothelium of blood vessels. In contrast to the prolonged maturation time of about 10 days for neutrophils in the bone marrow, their half-life in the peripheral blood is extremely short, only 6–8 hours. In response to stimuli (e.g. infection, corticosteroid therapy) neutrophils are released into the circulating pool from both the marginating pool and the marrow. Immature white cells are released from the marrow when a rapid response (within hours) occurs in acute infection (described as a 'shift to the left' on a blood film).

### Function

The prime function of neutrophils is to ingest and kill bacteria, fungi and damaged cells. Neutrophils are attracted to sites of infection or inflammation by chemotaxins. Recognition of foreign or dead material is aided by coating of particles with immunoglobulin and complement (*opsonization*) as neutrophils have Fc and C3b receptors (see p. 130). The material is ingested into vacuoles where it is subjected to enzymic destruction, which is either oxygen-dependent with the generation of hydrogen peroxide (myeloperoxidase) or oxygen-independent (lysosomal enzymes and lactoferrin).

## Neutrophil leucocytosis

A rise in the number of circulating neutrophils to $>10 \times 10^9$/litre occurs in bacterial infections or as a result of tissue damage. This may also be seen in pregnancy, during exercise and after corticosteroid administration

Bacterial infection
Tissue necrosis, e.g. myocardial infarction
Inflammation
Corticosteroid therapy
Myeloproliferative disease
Leukaemoid reaction
Leucoerythroblastic anaemia
Acute haemorrhage or haemolysis
Physiological e.g. pregnancy, exercise

**Table 6.18**  Causes of neutrophil leucocytosis.

(Table 6.18). With any tissue necrosis there is a release of various soluble factors, causing a leucocytosis. Interleukin-1 is also released in tissue necrosis and causes a pyrexia. The pyrexia and leucocytosis accompanying a myocardial infarction are a good example of this and may be wrongly attributed to infection.

A *leukaemoid reaction* (an overproduction of white cells, with many immature cells) may occur in severe infections, tuberculosis, malignant infiltration of the bone marrow and occasionally after haemorrhage or haemolysis.

In *leucoerythroblastic anaemia*, nucleated red cells and white cell precursors are found in the peripheral blood; causes include marrow infiltration with metastatic carcinoma, myelofibrosis, osteopetrosis, myeloma, lymphoma and occasionally severe haemolytic or megaloblastic anaemia.

## Neutropenia and agranulocytosis

Neutropenia is defined as a circulatory neutrophil count below $1.5 \times 10^9$/litre. A virtual absence of neutrophils is called agranulocytosis. The causes are given in Table 6.19.

### CLINICAL FEATURES
Infections may be frequent, often serious, and are more likely as the neutrophil count falls. A characteristic glazed mucositis occurs in the mouth and ulceration is common.

### INVESTIGATION
The blood film shows marked neutropenia. The appearance of the bone marrow will indicate whether the neutropenia is due to depressed production or increased destruction of neutrophils. Neutrophil antibody studies may be performed if an immune mechanism is suspected.

Congenital (Kostmann's syndrome)
Racial (neutropenia is common in black races)
Viral infection
Severe bacterial infection, e.g. typhoid
Felty's syndrome
Autoimmune neutropenia
Pancytopenia from any cause (see Table 6.8), including
    drug-induced marrow aplasia
Cyclic (genetic defect with neutropenia every 2–3 weeks)

**Table 6.19**  Causes of neutropenia.

### TREATMENT
Antibiotic therapy should be given to patients with acute severe neutropenia as necessary (see p. 358).

If the neutropenia seems likely to have been caused by a drug, all current drug therapy should be stopped. Recovery of the neutrophil count usually occurs after about 10 days. G-CSF (see p. 360) is used after chemotherapy.

Steroids and high-dose intravenous immunoglobulin are used to treat patients with severe autoimmune neutropenia and recurrent infections.

## EOSINOPHILS

Eosinophils are slightly larger than neutrophils and are characterized by a nucleus with usually two lobes and large cytoplasmic granules that stain deeply red. The eosinophil seems to play some part in allergic responses and in the defence against infections with helminths and protozoa.

Eosinophilia is said to occur when the number of eosinophils is $>0.4 \times 10^9$/litre in the peripheral blood. It is associated with a wide variety of disorders. The causes of eosinophilia are listed in Table 6.20.

## BASOPHILS

The nucleus of basophils is similar to neutrophils but the cytoplasm is filled with large black granules. The granules contain histamine, heparin and enzymes such as myeloperoxidase. The physiological role of the basophil is not known. Binding of IgE causes the cells to degranulate and

*Parasitic infestations*, e.g.
*Ascaris*
*Strongyloides*

*Allergic disorders*, e.g.
Hayfever (allergic rhinitis)
Other hypersensitivity reactions, including drug reactions

*Skin disorders*, e.g.
Urticaria
Pemphigus
Eczema

*Pulmonary disorders*, e.g.
Bronchial asthma
Tropical pulmonary eosinophilia
Allergic bronchopulmonary aspergillosis
Polyarteritis nodosa (Churg–Strauss syndrome)

*Malignant disorders*, e.g.
Hodgkin's disease
Carcinoma
Eosinophilic leukaemia

*Miscellaneous*, e.g.
Hypereosinophilic syndrome
Sarcoidosis
Hypoadrenalism
Eosinophilic gastroenteritis

**Table 6.20**  Causes of eosinophilia.

release histamine and other contents involved in acute hypersensitivity reactions.

Basophils are usually few in number ($<1 \times 10^9$/litre) but are significantly increased in myeloproliferative disorders.

## MONOCYTES

Monocytes are slightly larger than neutrophils. The nucleus has a variable shape and may be round, indented or lobulated. The cytoplasm contains less granules than neutrophils. Monocytes are precursors of tissue macrophages and spend only a few hours in the blood but can continue to proliferate in the tissues for many years.

A monocytosis ($>0.8 \times 10^9$/litre) may be seen in chronic bacterial infections such as tuberculosis or infective endocarditis, chronic neutropenia and patients with myelodysplasia particularly chronic myelomonocytic leukaemia.

## LYMPHOCYTES

Lymphocytes form nearly half the circulating white cells. They descend from pluripotential stem cells. Circulating lymphocytes are small cells, a little larger than red cells, with a dark-staining central nucleus. There are two main types: the thymus-dependent or T lymphocytes, which are concerned with cellular immunity and form about 80% of the circulating lymphocytes, and the 'bursa dependent' or B lymphocytes, which are concerned with humoral immunity (see p. 133).

Lymphocytosis (lymphocyte count $>5 \times 10^9$/litre) occurs in response to viral infections, particularly EBV, CMV and HIV and chronic infections such as tuberculosis and toxoplasmosis. It also occurs in chronic lymphocytic leukaemia and in some lymphomas.

## *Bleeding disorders*

Blood is normally separated from the activators of haemostasis by the endothelial cell. Injury to the vessel wall exposes collagen and sets in motion a series of events leading to haemostasis.

## Haemostasis

Haemostasis is a complex process depending on interactions between the vessel wall, platelets and coagulation factors (Fig. 6.24).

### Vessel wall

An immediate reflex vasoconstriction of the injured vessel and adjacent vessels results in a transient reduction of blood flow to the affected area. Damage to the endothelium of the vessel results in activation of platelets and coagulation; release of serotonin and thromboxane $A_2$ ($TXA_2$) from activated platelets contributes to the vasoconstriction.

### Platelets

*Platelet adhesion* to collagen is dependent on platelet membrane receptors, glycoprotein Ia (GPIa), which binds directly to collagen, and glycoprotein Ib (GPIb), which binds to von Willebrand factor (VIII:vWF) in the plasma and VIII:vWF in turn adheres to collagen. Following adhesion, platelets undergo a shape change from a disc to a sphere, spread along the subendothelium and *release* the contents of their cytoplasmic granules, i.e. the dense bodies (containing ADP and serotonin) and the $\alpha$-granules (containing platelet-derived growth factor, platelet factor 4, $\beta$-thromboglobulin, fibrinogen, VIII:vWF and other factors).

The release of ADP leads to exposure of a fibrinogen receptor, the glycoprotein IIb–IIIa complex (GPIIb–IIIa), on surfaces of adherent platelets; fibrinogen binds platelets into activated aggregates (*platelet aggregation*) and further platelet release occurs. A self-perpetuating cycle of events is set up leading to formation of a platelet plug at the site of the injury.

Further platelet membrane receptors are exposed during aggregation, providing a surface for the interaction of coagulation factors; this platelet activity is referred to as platelet factor 3 (PF-3). The presence of thrombin encourages *fusion of platelets*, and fibrin formation reinforces the stability of the platelet plug.

Central to normal platelet function is platelet prostaglandin synthesis, which is induced by platelet activation and leads to the formation of $TXA_2$ in platelets (Fig. 6.25). $TXA_2$ is a powerful vasoconstrictor and also lowers cyclic AMP levels and initiates the platelet release reaction.

Prostacyclin ($PGI_2$) is synthesized in vascular endothelial cells and opposes the actions of $TXA_2$. It produces vasodilatation and increases the level of cyclic AMP, preventing platelet aggregation on the normal vessel wall as well as limiting the extent of the initial platelet plug after injury.

### Coagulation and fibrinolysis

Coagulation involves a series of enzymatic reactions leading to the conversion of soluble plasma fibrinogen to fibrin clot (Fig. 6.26). The coagulation factors are either enzyme precursors (factors XII, XI, X, IX and thrombin) or cofactors (V and VIII), except for fibrinogen, which is the subunit of fibrin. The enzymes apart from factor XIII are serine proteases and hydrolyse peptide bonds.

EXTRINSIC PATHWAY. Coagulation is initiated by tissue factor, which is expressed on the surface of perivascular tissue cells, coming into contact with plasma after an injury. The complex of activated factor VII and tissue factor activates factor X but its main role *in vivo* is to activate factor IX in the intrinsic pathway.

INTRINSIC PATHWAY. Factor XII was thought to be activated by 'contact' with the injured surface and then

**Fig. 6.24** Formation of the haemostatic plug. Sequential interactions of the vessel wall, platelets and coagulation factors. (a) Contact of platelets with collagen, either via the platelet receptor GPIb and factor VIII:vWF in plasma or directly via GPIa, activates platelet prostaglandin synthesis which stimulates release of ADP from the dense bodies. Vasoconstriction of the vessel occurs as a reflex and by release of serotonin and TXA₂ from platelets. (b) Release of ADP from platelets induces platelet aggregation and formation of the platelet plug. The coagulation pathway is stimulated leading to formation of fibrin. (c) Fibrin strands are cross-linked by factor XIII and stabilize the haemostatic plug by binding platelets and red cells.

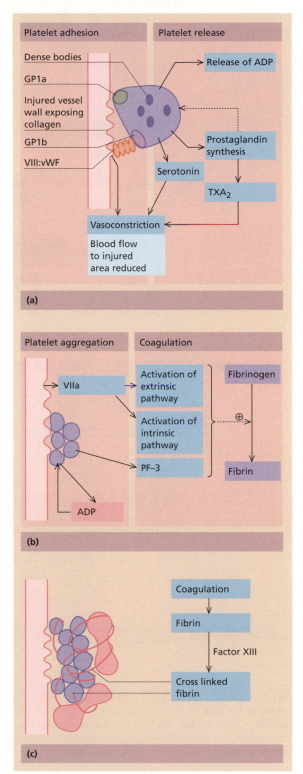

to initiate a series of reactions beginning with activation of factor XI and leading to activation of factor X. The upper part of the intrinsic pathway includes kallikrein and high molecular weight kininogen (HMWK) but recent evidence suggests that this part of the intrinsic pathway is not important for *in vivo* haemostasis. It is now thought that factor IX is activated by a complex of tissue factor and factor VII. Activated factor IX together with factor VIII and calcium ions activate factor X. Factor XI is activated *in vivo* by thrombin and only makes an important contribution after major trauma.

Factor VIII is a complex protein consisting of a small molecule with coagulant activity (VIII:C) and a larger part, von Willebrand factor (VIII:vWF), which is associated with platelet adhesion. VIII:C is a single chain protein with a molecular weight of about 350 000. VIII:vWF is a glycoprotein with a molecular weight of about 200 000. It readily forms multimers in the circulation with molecular weights of up to $20 \times 10^6$. The high molecular weight multimeric forms of VIII:vWF are the most effective in producing platelet adhesion.

COMMON PATHWAY. Activated factor X eventually leads to the conversion of prothrombin to thrombin. Thrombin hydrolyses the peptide bonds of fibrinogen, releasing fibrinopeptides A and B, and allowing polymerization between fibrinogen molecules to form fibrin. At the same time thrombin, in the presence of calcium ions, activates factor XIII, which stabilizes the fibrin clot by cross-linking adjacent fibrin molecules. The presence of thrombin helps in the activation of factors XI, V, VIII and XIII.

LIMITATION OF COAGULATION. Coagulation is limited to the site of injury by removal of activated coagulation factors by rapid blood flow at the periphery of the damaged area, by plasma inhibitors of activated coagulation factors and by fibrinolysis.

Antithrombin III (AT-III) is the most potent inhibitor of coagulation; it inactivates the serine proteases by forming stable complexes with them and its action is greatly potentiated by heparin. Active protein C is generated from its vitamin K-dependent precursor by the action of thrombin; thrombin activation of protein C is enhanced when thrombin is bound to thrombomodulin, which is an endothelial cell receptor (Fig. 6.27). Active protein C destroys factor V and factor VIII reducing further throm-

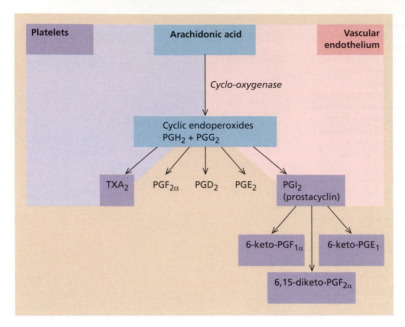

**Fig. 6.25** Prostaglandin synthesis (simplified).

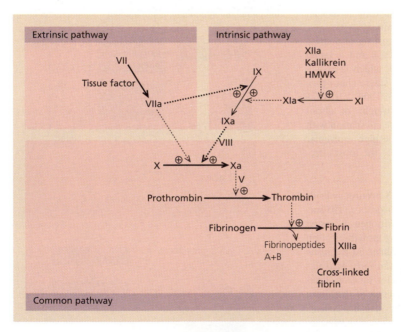

**Fig. 6.26** Coagulation sequence. The intrinsic pathway *in vivo* begins with activation of factor IX by factor VIIa. The factor XII and kallikrein reactions are probably only relevant *in vitro*. Factor XI is activated by thrombin *in vivo*. HMWK, high molecular weight kininogen.

bin generation. Protein S is a cofactor for protein C by allowing binding of activated protein C to the platelet surface. Other natural inhibitors of coagulation are $\alpha_2$-macroglobulin, $\alpha_1$-antitrypsin, $\alpha_1$-antiplasmin and heparin cofactor II.

FIBRINOLYSIS, which helps to restore vessel patency, also occurs in response to vascular damage. In this system (Fig. 6.28), an inactive plasma protein, plasminogen, is converted to plasmin by plasminogen activators derived from the plasma or blood cells (intrinsic activation) or the tissues (extrinsic activation).

Plasmin is a serine protease which breaks down fibrinogen and fibrin into fragments X, Y, D and E, collectively known as fibrin (and fibrinogen) degradation products (FDPs). Degradation of cross-linked fibrin also yields D-dimer and D-dimer-E fragments. Plasmin is also capable of breaking down coagulation factors such as factors V and VIII.

The fibrinolytic system is activated by the presence of fibrin. Plasminogen is specifically adsorbed to fibrin and fibrinogen by lysine-binding sites. However, little plasminogen activation occurs in the absence of fibrin, as fibrin also has a specific binding site for plasminogen

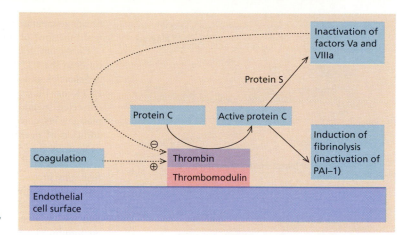

**Fig. 6.27** Activation of protein C. PAI-1, plasminogen activator inhibitor 1.

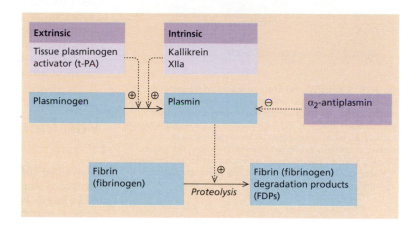

**Fig. 6.28** Fibrinolytic system.

activators, whereas fibrinogen does not (Fig. 6.29).

The most important plasminogen activator is tissue-type plasminogen activator (t-PA); vascular endothelium is the major source of t-PA in plasma. Its release is stimulated by thrombin. Another plasminogen activator is urokinase, synthesized in the kidney and released into the urogenital tract. Intrinsic plasminogen activators such as factor XII and kallikrein are of minor physiological importance.

t-PA is inactivated by plasminogen activator inhibitor-1 (PAI-1). Activated protein C inactivates PAI-1 and therefore induces fibrinolysis (Fig. 6.27). Inactivators of plasmin (such as $\alpha_2$-antiplasmin) are also present in the plasma and contribute to the regulation of fibrinolysis (Fig. 6.29).

## Investigation of bleeding disorders

Although the precise diagnosis of a bleeding disorder may depend on laboratory tests, much information may be obtained from the history and physical examination, which should aim to determine the following:

1 Is there a generalized haemostatic defect? Supportive evidence for this includes bleeding from multiple sites, spontaneous bleeding and bleeding into the skin.

2 Is the defect inherited or acquired? A family history of a bleeding disorder should be sought. Severe inherited defects usually become apparent in infancy, while mild inherited defects may only come to attention later in life, for example with excessive bleeding after surgery, childbirth, dental extractions or trauma.

3 Is the bleeding suggestive of a vascular/platelet defect or a coagulation defect?

VASCULAR/PLATELET BLEEDING is characterized by easy bruising and spontaneous bleeding from small vessels. The bleeding is mainly into the skin (the term purpura includes both petechiae, which are small skin haemorrhages varying from pinpoint size to a few millimetres in diameter and which do not blanch on pressure, and ecchymoses, which are small bruises) and from mucous membranes, often from the nose and mouth.

COAGULATION DISORDERS are typically associated with haemarthroses and muscle haematomas.

### LABORATORY INVESTIGATION

BLOOD COUNT AND FILM show the number and morphology of platelets and any blood disorder such as leukaemia.

BLEEDING TIME measures platelet plug formation *in vivo*. It is determined by applying a sphygmoman-

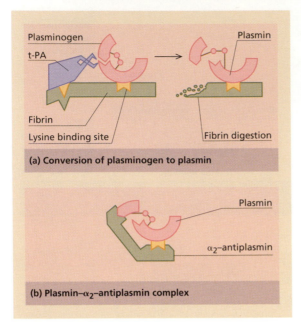

**(a) Conversion of plasminogen to plasmin**

Plasminogen
t-PA
Fibrin
Lysine binding site
Plasmin
Fibrin digestion

**(b) Plasmin–α₂–antiplasmin complex**

Plasmin
α₂–antiplasmin

**Fig. 6.29** Fibrinolysis. (a) The conversion of plasminogen to plasmin by plasminogen activator (t-PA) occurs most efficiently on the surface of fibrin which has binding sites for both plasminogen and t-PA. (b) Free plasmin in the blood is rapidly inactivated by $\alpha_2$-antiplasmin. Plasmin generated on the fibrin surface is partially protected from inactivation. The lysine-binding sites on plasminogen are important for the interaction between plasmin(ogen) and fibrin and between plasmin and $\alpha_2$-antiplasmin.

ometer cuff to the arm and inflating it to 40 mmHg. Two 1 mm deep, 1 cm long incisions are made in the forearm with a template. Each wound is blotted every 30 s and the time taken for bleeding to stop is recorded, normally between 3 and 10 min. Prolonged bleeding times are found in patients with platelet function defects and there is a progressive prolongation with platelet counts less than $80 \times 10^9$/litre. The Hess or capillary resistance test parallels the bleeding time but is unreliable and not routinely used.

COAGULATION TESTS are performed using blood collected into citrate, which neutralizes calcium ions and prevents clotting.

The *prothrombin time* (PT) (see p. 349) is measured by adding tissue thromboplastin in the form of animal brain extract and calcium to patient's plasma. The normal PT is 16–18 s and it is prolonged with abnormalities of either the extrinsic or common pathways (see Fig. 6.26).

The *partial thromboplastin time with kaolin* (PTTK) is also known as the APTT (activated PTT). It is performed by adding a surface activator, kaolin, phospholipid (as platelet substitute) and calcium to patients' plasma. The normal PTTK is 30–50 s depending on the exact methodology, and it is prolonged with abnormalities of either the intrinsic or common pathways (see Fig. 6.26).

The *thrombin time* (TT) is performed by adding thrombin to patients' plasma. The normal TT is about 12 s, and it is prolonged with fibrinogen deficiency, dys-

fibrinogenaemia (normal level of fibrinogen but abnormal function) or inhibitors such as heparin or FDPs.

*Correction tests* are used to differentiate prolonged times in the PT, PTTK and TT due to coagulation factor deficiencies and inhibitors of coagulation. Prolonged PT, PTTK or TT due to coagulation factor deficiencies are corrected by addition of normal plasma to the patient's plasma; no correction of an abnormal result after the addition of normal plasma is suggestive of the presence of an inhibitor of coagulation.

*Special tests of coagulation* will often be required to confirm the precise haemostatic defect. Such tests include estimation of fibrinogen and FDPs, assays of coagulation factors, platelet function tests such as platelet aggregation and tests of the fibrinolytic pathway which include the euglobulin clot lysis time (ELT) and assays of plasminogen, t-PA and PAI-1. The ELT involves precipitation by acidification of the euglobulin fraction of plasma which contains fibrinogen, plasminogen and plasminogen activators. The euglobulin is clotted with thrombin and the time taken for lysis of the fibrin clot is a measure of fibrinolytic activity; the normal range is 60–270 min.

# Vascular disorders

The vascular disorders (Table 6.21), sometimes previously classified as non-thrombocytopenic purpuras, are characterized by easy bruising and bleeding into the skin. Bleeding from mucous membranes sometimes occurs but the bleeding is rarely severe. Laboratory investigations includ-

*Congenital*
Hereditary haemorrhagic telangiectasia (Osler–Weber–Rendu disease)
Connective tissue disorders (Ehlers–Danlos syndrome, osteogenesis imperfecta, pseudoxanthoma elasticum, Marfan's syndrome)

*Acquired*
Severe infections:
    Septicaemia
    Meningococcal infections
    Measles
    Typhoid

*Allergic*
Henoch–Schönlein purpura
Connective tissue disorders (SLE, rheumatoid arthritis)

*Drugs*
Steroids
Sulphonamides

*Others*
Senile purpura
Easy bruising syndrome
Scurvy
Factitial purpura

**Table 6.21** Vascular disorders.

ing the bleeding time are normal. The vascular disorders include the following.

HEREDITARY HAEMORRHAGIC TELANGIECTASIA. This is a rare disorder with autosomal dominant inheritance. Dilatation of capillaries and small arterioles produces characteristic small red spots that blanch on pressure in the skin and mucous membranes, particularly the nose and gastrointestinal tract. Recurrent epistaxis and chronic gastrointestinal bleeding are the major problems and may cause chronic iron deficiency anaemia.

EASY BRUISING SYNDROME. This is a benign disorder occurring in otherwise healthy women. It is characterized by bruises on the arms, legs and trunk with minor trauma, possibly due to skin vessel fragility. It may give rise to the suspicion of a serious bleeding disorder.

SENILE PURPURA AND PURPURA DUE TO STEROIDS. These are both due to atrophy of the vascular supporting tissue.

PURPURA DUE TO INFECTIONS. This is mainly due to damage to the vascular endothelium.

HENOCH–SCHÖNLEIN PURPURA. This usually occurs in children. It is a type III hypersensitivity reaction that is often preceded by an acute upper respiratory tract infection. Purpura is mainly seen on the legs and buttocks. Abdominal pain, arthritis, haematuria and nephritis also occur. Recovery is usually spontaneous but some patients develop renal failure.

FACTITIAL PURPURA. Episodes of inexplicable bleeding or bruising may represent abuse, either self-inflicted or caused by others. These various forms of artificial or factitious purpuras are often expressions of severe emotional or psychiatric disturbances.

# Platelet disorders

Bleeding due to thrombocytopenia or abnormal platelet function is characterized by purpura and bleeding from mucous membranes. Bleeding is uncommon with platelet counts above $50 \times 10^9$/litre, and severe spontaneous bleeding is unusual with platelet counts above $20 \times 10^9$/litre.

## THROMBOCYTOPENIA

This is caused by reduced platelet production in the bone marrow or excessive peripheral destruction of platelets (Table 6.22). A bone marrow aspirate to assess whether the numbers of megakaryocytes are reduced or normal/increased is an essential part of the investigation.

*Impaired production*
Generalized bone marrow failure
   Leukaemia
   Aplastic anaemia
   Megaloblastic anaemia
   Myeloma
   Myelofibrosis
   Marrow infiltration by solid tumours
Selective reduction in megakaryocytes
   Drugs, e.g. co-trimoxazole
   Chemicals
   Viral infections

*Excessive destruction*
Immune
   Autoimmune thrombocytopenic purpura
   Secondary immune thrombocytopenia (SLE, chronic
      lymphatic leukaemia, viral infections, drugs)
   Alloimmune neonatal thrombocytopenia
   Post-transfusion purpura
Coagulation
   Disseminated intravascular coagulation
   Thrombotic thrombocytopenic purpura
   Haemolytic uraemic syndrome (see p. 452)

*Sequestration*
Hypersplenism

*Dilutional loss*
Massive transfusion of stored blood

**Table 6.22**   Causes of thrombocytopenia.

## Autoimmune thrombocytopenic purpura (AITP)

Thrombocytopenia is due to immune destruction of platelets. The sensitized platelets are removed by the reticuloendothelial system. There are two distinct clinical syndromes.

Acute AITP is usually seen in children, often following a viral infection. It has been suggested that the thrombocytopenia is due to the deposition of immune complexes on platelets, but the acute development of platelet autoantibodies is probably responsible for the shortened platelet survival.

Chronic AITP is characteristically seen in adult women. It is usually idiopathic but may occur in association with other autoimmune disorders such as SLE, thyroid disease and autoimmune haemolytic anaemia (Evans' syndrome), in patients with chronic lymphocytic leukaemia and solid tumours and after viral infections with viruses such as HIV. Platelet autoantibodies are detected in about 60–70% of patients, and are presumed to be present, although not detectable, in the remaining patients.

### CLINICAL FEATURES
Major haemorrhage is rare and is only seen in patients with severe thrombocytopenia. Easy bruising, purpura, epistaxis and menorrhagia are common.

Physical examination is normal except for evidence of bleeding. Splenomegaly is rare.

**INVESTIGATION**

The only blood count abnormality is thrombocytopenia. Normal or increased numbers of megakaryocytes are found in the bone marrow, which is otherwise normal. The detection of platelet autoantibodies is not essential for confirmation of the diagnosis, which often depends on exclusion of other causes of excessive destruction of platelets.

**TREATMENT**

Acute AITP in children usually remits spontaneously. It is still not clear whether treatment in the acute phase with steroids or high-dose intravenous immunoglobulin is effective in minimizing the period of thrombocytopenia or in reducing the incidence of chronic AITP, which develops in 5–10% of children.

Spontaneous remissions are rare in chronic AITP. The main aims of treatment are to reduce the production of platelet autoantibodies and the removal of antibody-coated platelets. Initial treatment is with prednisolone, 40–60 mg daily in adults with cautious reduction of the dose after remission has occurred.

Twenty per cent of patients have a complete response and require no further treatment; 60% have a partial response, and half of these have little bleeding associated with mild or moderate thrombocytopenia (platelet count 30–100 × 10⁹/litre) and may require small doses of steroids, such as prednisolone 5–15 mg daily, or no further treatment. The other half of the partial responders eventually relapse and require splenectomy, as do the 20% of patients who failed to respond to steroids at all.

Splenectomy should be avoided in young children because of the subsequent risk of severe pneumococcal infection (see p. 330). There is a 90% response rate to splenectomy, although about 30% of responders eventually relapse. Some of these refractory patients may respond to immunosuppressive drugs such as azathioprine, cyclophosphamide or vincristine or to danazol, which is a non-virilizing androgen.

Intravenous infusion of high-dose immunoglobulin produces a rapid rise in the platelet count due to blockade of Fc receptors in the spleen. The increase in platelet count is usually transient but may be useful in patients with acute haemorrhage and in preparing patients with chronic AITP for surgery.

Transfused platelets survive no longer than the patient's own platelets but may sometimes be beneficial in patients with life-threatening bleeding.

## Other immune thrombocytopenias

DRUGS cause immune thrombocytopenia by the same mechanisms as described for drug-induced immune haemolytic anaemia (p. 324). The same drugs may be responsible for immune haemolytic anaemia, thrombocytopenia or neutropenia in different patients; it is not known what determines the target cell in each case.

FETOMATERNAL ALLOIMMUNE THROMBOCYTO-PENIA is due to fetomaternal incompatibility for platelet-specific antigens, usually for HPA-1a (human platelet alloantigen, previously called Pl^{A1}), and is the platelet equivalent of HDN. The mother is HPA-1a-negative and produces antibodies which destroy the HPA-1a-positive fetal platelets.

Thrombocytopenia is self-limiting after delivery, but platelet transfusions may be required to prevent or treat bleeding associated with severe thrombocytopenia; platelets may be prepared from HPA-1a-negative volunteers or the mother herself. Recently, it has been recognized that severe bleeding such as intracranial haemorrhage may occur *in utero*. Antenatal treatment of the mother with steroids and/or high-dose intravenous immunoglobulin or platelet transfusions given directly to the fetus by ultrasound-guided needling of the umbilical vessels have been effective in preventing haemorrhage in severely affected cases.

POST-TRANSFUSION PURPURA (PTP) is rare, occurring 2–12 days after a blood transfusion. PTP is associated with a platelet-specific alloantibody, usually anti-HPA-1a in a HPA-1a-negative individual. PTP almost invariably occurs in females who have been previously immunized by pregnancy or blood transfusion. The cause of the platelet destruction is uncertain. PTP is self-limiting but high-dose intravenous immunoglobulin may limit the period of thrombocytopenia.

## PLATELET FUNCTION DISORDERS

These are usually associated with excessive bruising and bleeding and, in some of the acquired forms, with thrombosis. The platelet count is normal or increased and the bleeding time is prolonged. The rare inherited defects of platelet function require more detailed investigations such as platelet aggregation studies and factor VIII:C and VIII:vWF assays, if von Willebrand's disease is suspected.

Acquired forms of platelet dysfunction include:

- Myeloproliferative disorders
- Uraemia and liver disease
- Paraproteinaemias
- Drugs, e.g. aspirin and dipyridamole

If there is serious bleeding or if the patient is about to undergo surgery, drugs with antiplatelet activity should be withdrawn and any underlying condition should be corrected if possible. In patients with renal failure, the haematocrit should be increased to greater than 0.30 litre litre⁻¹ and the use of desmopressin (DDAVP) may be helpful. Platelet transfusions may be required if these measures are unsuccessful.

---

# Coagulation disorders

---

Coagulation disorders may be inherited or acquired. The inherited disorders are uncommon and usually involve deficiency of one factor only. The acquired disorders occur more frequently and almost always involve several coagulation factors.

# INHERITED COAGULATION DISORDERS

Deficiencies of all factors have been described. They are rare apart from haemophilia A (factor VIII deficiency), haemophilia B (factor IX deficiency) and von Willebrand's disease.

## Haemophilia A

In haemophilia A, the level of factor VIII:C is reduced but the level of factor VIII:vWF is normal (Fig. 6.30). It is inherited as an X-linked recessive. The incidence of haemophilia A varies from 1 in 5000 to 1 in 10 000 of the male population.

The human factor VIII gene was cloned in 1984. The gene is enormous, constituting about 0.1% of the X chromosome, encompassing 186 kilobases of DNA. Various genetic defects have been found, including deletions, point mutations and insertions. There is a high mutation rate with one-third of cases being apparently sporadic with no family history of haemophilia.

### CLINICAL FEATURES

The clinical features depend on the level of factor VIII:C. Levels of less than 1% are associated with frequent spontaneous bleeding from early life. Haemarthroses are common and may lead to joint deformity and crippling if adequate treatment is not given. Bleeds into muscles are also common.

Levels of less than 5% are associated with severe bleeding, following injury and occasional spontaneous epi-

sodes, and levels above 5% with milder disease usually with post-traumatic bleeding only.

The most frequent cause of death in patients with severe haemophilia is AIDS. HIV was transmitted to many patients by coagulation factor concentrates in the 1980s.

### LABORATORY FEATURES

The main laboratory features of haemophilia A are shown in Table 6.23. The abnormal findings are a prolonged PTTK and a reduced level of factor VIII:C; the PT, bleeding time and factor VIII:vWF level are normal.

### TREATMENT

Bleeding is treated by administration of factor VIII concentrate by intravenous injection. For minor bleeding the factor VIII level should be raised to 20–30% of normal, and for severe bleeding episodes it should be raised to at least 50%. For major surgery the level should be raised to 100% preoperatively and maintained above 50% until healing has occurred.

| | Haemophilia A | von Willebrand's disease | Vitamin K deficiency |
|---|---|---|---|
| Bleeding time | Normal | ↑ | Normal |
| PT | Normal | Normal | ↑ |
| PTTK | ↑⁺ | ↑± | ↑ |
| VIII:C | ↓⁺⁺ | ↓ | Normal |
| VIII:vWF | Normal | ↓ | Normal |

**Table 6.23**  Blood changes in haemophilia A, von Willebrand's disease and vitamin K deficiency.

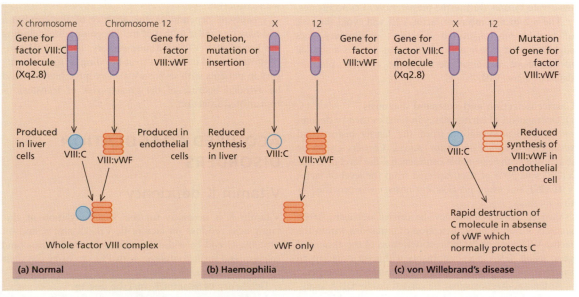

(a) Normal

(b) Haemophilia

(c) von Willebrand's disease

**Fig. 6.30**  Normal factor VIII synthesis (a) and defective synthesis in haemophilia A (b) and von Willebrand's disease (c).

Factor VIII has a half-life of 12 hours and therefore must be administered twice daily to maintain the required therapeutic level. Factor VIII concentrate may be stored in domestic refrigerators and so may be administered by the patient immediately after bleeding has started, reducing the likelihood of chronic damage to joints and the need for inpatient care. High purity factor VIII concentrates are now preferred to intermediate purity concentrates (see p. 334). Factor VIII:C produced by recombinant DNA technology is undergoing clinical trials.

DDAVP (i.v.) produces a rise in factor VIII proportional to the initial level of factor VIII. It avoids the complications associated with blood products and is useful for treating bleeding episodes in mild haemophiliacs and as prophylaxis before minor surgery.

All haemophiliacs should be registered at haemophilia centres, who take responsibility for their full medical care, including social and psychological support. Each haemophiliac carries a special medical card giving details of the defect and treatment.

### COMPLICATIONS

About 10% of severe haemophiliacs develop antibodies to factor VIII:C. Inhibitors develop almost exclusively in patients with no detectable VIII:C. Management of such patients may be very difficult, and extremely high doses of factor VIII may be needed to produce a rise in the plasma level of factor VIII:C. Alternative treatment includes recombinant factor VIIa, purified porcine factor VIII which may not cross-react with the patient's antibody, and some factor IX concentrates containing activated factor X, which may 'bypass' the inhibitor and stop the bleeding. Following numerous transfusions there is a high risk of acquiring transfusion-transmitted infections, particularly hepatitis and HIV. The risk has been reduced by excluding high risk blood donors, testing all donations for HBsAg and HIV antibody, and by including steps to inactivate viruses during the preparation of concentrates.

The use of recombinant factor VIII will avoid the risk of transfusion-transmitted infection; preliminary data suggest that it is safe and effective but there is a similar incidence of inhibitor development as with plasma-derived factor VIII.

#### Carrier detection and antenatal diagnosis

Determination of carrier status in females used to depend on detailed information from the family history and results of coagulation factor assays. Carriers could be diagnosed with reasonable confidence if the level of factor VIII:C was 50% of that expected from the level of factor VIII:vWF but often no clear-cut answer was provided by this method.

Carrier detection can now be carried out using DNA analysis either by direct detection of mutations within the factor VIII gene or by indirect detection of the abnormal gene using DNA polymorphisms within or adjacent to the factor VIII gene as markers of the abnormal gene.

Antenatal diagnosis may be carried out by DNA analysis of fetal tissue obtained by chorionic villus biopsy at 9–11 weeks' gestation or by using ultrasound-guided fetal blood sampling to detect low plasma levels in a fetus at 18–20 weeks of gestation.

## Haemophilia B (Christmas disease)

Haemophilia B is caused by a deficiency of factor IX. The inheritance and clinical features are identical to haemophilia A, but the incidence is only about 1:30 000 males. It is treated with factor IX concentrates.

## von Willebrand's disease (vWD)

In vWD, there is defective platelet function as well as factor VIII:C deficiency and both are due to a deficiency or abnormality of factor VIII:vWF (Fig. 6.30). Factor VIII:vWF plays a role in platelet adhesion to damaged subendothelium as well as stabilizing factor VIII:C in plasma (see p. 337).

The VIII:vWF gene is on chromosome 12 and numerous mutations of the gene have been identified. vWD has been classified into three types:

TYPE I is characterized by a mild reduction in factor VIII:vWF and is inherited as an autosomal dominant.

TYPE II is due to a decrease in the proportion of high molecular weight multimers and is also inherited as an autosomal dominant.

TYPE III is recessively inherited and patients have barely detectable levels of factor VIII:vWF (and therefore factor VIII:C).

The clinical features of vWD are variable. Type I and type II patients usually have mild clinical features. Bleeding follows minor trauma or surgery and epistaxis and menorrhagia often occur. Haemarthroses are rare. Type III patients have clinical features resembling haemophilia A.

Characteristic laboratory findings are shown in Table 6.23. These also include defective platelet aggregation with ristocetin.

Treatment depends on the severity of the condition and may be similar to that of mild haemophilia, including the use of DDAVP for minor surgery. Factor VIII concentrates should be used to treat bleeding or to cover surgery in patients with severe vWD. Cryoprecipitate should be avoided because of the greater risk of transfusion-transmitted infection.

## ACQUIRED COAGULATION DISORDERS

### Vitamin K deficiency

Vitamin K is necessary for the γ-carboxylation of glutamic acid residues on factors II, VII, IX and X and on proteins C and S; without it, these factors cannot bind calcium and form complexes with PF-3 to carry out their normal functions.

Deficiency of vitamin K may be due to:

- Inadequate stores, as in haemorrhagic disease of the newborn and protein-energy malnutrition (see p. 158)

- Malabsorption of vitamin K, which particularly occurs in cholestatic jaundice as it is a fat-soluble vitamin
- Oral anticoagulant drugs, which are vitamin K antagonists

The PT and PTTK are prolonged (Table 6.23) and there may be bruising, haematuria and gastrointestinal or cerebral bleeding. Minor bleeding is treated with phytomenadione (vitamin $K_1$) 10 mg intravenously. Some correction of the PT is usual within 6 hours but it may not return to normal for 2 days.

Newborn babies have low levels of vitamin K, and this may cause minor bleeding in the first week of life (*classical haemorrhagic disease of the newborn*). Vitamin K deficiency may also cause *late haemorrhagic disease of the newborn* which occurs between 2 and 26 weeks after birth and may result in severe bleeding such as intracranial haemorrhage. Most infants with these syndromes have been exclusively breastfed and both may be prevented by administering 1 mg intramuscular vitamin K to all neonates. There has been recent concern that the administration of intramuscular vitamin K is associated with the development of cancer in childhood but the evidence for the association is not conclusive and further studies will be needed to resolve the uncertainty.

## Liver disease

Liver disease may result in a number of defects in haemostasis:

VITAMIN K DEFICIENCY due to intra- or extra-hepatic cholestasis.

REDUCED SYNTHESIS of coagulation factors due to severe hepatocellular damage. The use of vitamin K does not improve the results of abnormal coagulation tests, but it is generally given because of the accompanying malabsorption.

THROMBOCYTOPENIA may result from hypersplenism due to splenomegaly associated with portal hypertension.

FUNCTIONAL ABNORMALITIES of platelets and fibrinogen are found in many patients with liver failure.

DISSEMINATED INTRAVASCULAR COAGULATION may occur in acute liver failure.

## Disseminated intravascular coagulation

There is widespread generation of fibrin within blood vessels, due to activation of the extrinsic pathway by release of coagulant material, activation of the intrinsic pathway by diffuse endothelial damage or generalized platelet aggregation.

There is consumption of platelets and coagulation factors and secondary activation of fibrinolysis leading to production of FDPs, which may contribute to the coagulation defect by inhibiting fibrin polymerization (Fig. 6.31).

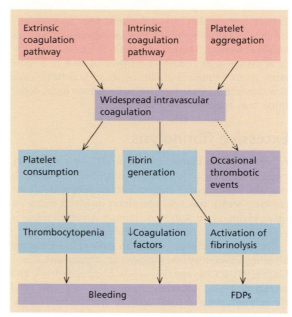

**Fig. 6.31** Disseminated intravascular coagulation. FDP, fibrin degradation products.

### CAUSES
These are numerous and include Gram-negative and meningococcal septicaemia, disseminated malignant disease, haemolytic transfusion reactions, obstetric conditions such as abruptio placentae and amniotic fluid embolism, widespread tissue damage after trauma, burns or surgery, falciparum malaria and snake bites.

### CLINICAL FEATURES
The underlying disorder is usually obvious. The patient is often acutely ill and shocked. The clinical presentation of DIC varies from no bleeding at all to complete haemostatic failure with widespread haemorrhage. Bleeding may occur from the mouth, nose and venepuncture sites and there may be widespread ecchymoses.

Thrombotic events may occur as a result of vessel occlusion by fibrin and platelets; any organ may be involved but the skin and kidneys are most often affected.

### INVESTIGATIONS
The diagnosis is often suggested by the underlying condition of the patient. In severe cases with haemorrhage, the PT, PTTK and TT are usually very prolonged and the fibrinogen level markedly reduced. High levels of FDPs are found due to the intense fibrinolytic activity stimulated by the presence of fibrin in the circulation. There is severe thrombocytopenia and the blood film may show fragmented red blood cells. In mild cases without bleeding, increased synthesis of coagulation factors and platelets may result in normal PT, PTTK, TT and platelet counts, although the FDPs will be raised.

### TREATMENT
Treatment of the underlying condition is most important and may be all that is necessary in non-bleeding patients.

Transfusions of platelet concentrates, FFP, cryoprecipitate and red cell concentrates may be indicated in patients who are bleeding. The use of heparin to prevent intravascular coagulation remains controversial and it is now rarely given. Inhibitors of fibrinolysis such as tranexamic acid should not be used in DIC as dangerous fibrin deposition may result.

## Excessive fibrinolysis

Activation of fibrinolysis occurs in DIC as a secondary event in response to intravascular deposition of fibrin. It may also occur during surgery involving tumours of the prostate, breast, pancreas and uterus owing to release of tissue plasminogen activators. *Primary hyperfibrinolysis* is very rare.

The clinical picture is similar to DIC with widespread bleeding. Laboratory investigations are similar with a prolonged PT, PTTK and TT, a low fibrinogen level, and increased FDPs, although fragmented red cells and thrombocytopenia are not seen as disseminated coagulation is not present.

If the diagnosis is certain, fibrinolytic inhibitors such as ε-aminocaproic acid (EACA) or tranexamic acid should be considered. If DIC cannot be excluded, it is safer to treat as for DIC.

## Massive transfusion

Stored blood contains few platelets and has reduced levels of factors V and VIII, although there are adequate amounts of the other coagulation factors. During *massive transfusion* (defined as transfusion of a volume of blood equal to the patient's own blood volume within 24 hours, e.g. approximately 10 units in an adult), the platelet count and PT and PTTK should be checked at intervals. Transfusion of platelet concentrates and FFP should be considered if thrombocytopenia or defective coagulation are thought to be contributing to continued blood loss.

Citrate binds ionized calcium and potentially lowers plasma calcium levels. This is rarely a problem as citrate is rapidly metabolized but neonates and hypothermic patients may have a reduced capacity for removal of citrate. Where there is clinical and ECG evidence of hypocalcaemia, 5 ml of 10% calcium gluconate should be given at 5 min intervals until the ECG is normal. The plasma potassium content of blood increases during storage but hyperkalaemia is rarely a problem unless very large volumes of blood are transfused rapidly.

Lactic acid is produced by red cell glycolysis in the blood pack and might contribute to the acidosis of hypoxic shocked patients. However, acidosis is usually improved by transfusion because of reversal of hypoxia and improved tissue perfusion.

Hypothermia may result from rapid transfusion of stored blood. Blood warmers should be used if the rate of infusion exceeds 1 unit in 10 min in adults and proportionately less in children.

Although it might be expected that massive transfusion of stored blood with high oxygen affinity due to low levels of 2,3-DPG would impair tissue oxygenation, there is little evidence that this occurs. Regeneration of 2,3-DPG is complete within a few hours following transfusion.

The combination of *hyperkalaemia, hypocalcaemia, hypothermia* and *acidosis* might impair cardiac performance and even cause cardiac arrest. Careful monitoring of the patient's temperature, plasma potassium and ECG for evidence of hypocalcaemia are essential in patients receiving rapid transfusions of large volumes of stored blood.

## Inhibitors of coagulation

In addition to the factor VIII:C *alloantibodies* that arise in up to 10% of severe haemophiliacs, factor VIII:C *autoantibodies* occasionally arise in patients with autoimmune disorders such as SLE, in elderly patients and sometimes after childbirth. There may be severe bleeding. The antibodies may disappear spontaneously but treatment such as plasma exchange and immunosuppressive drugs may be required.

Lupus anticoagulants are IgG autoantibodies directed against phospholipids. They are found in about 10% of patients with SLE and may also occur in otherwise healthy individuals. They lead to prolongation of phospholipid-dependent coagulation tests, particularly the PTTK, but do not inhibit coagulation factor activity. Bleeding does not occur unless there is coexistent severe immune thrombocytopenia. The main clinical problems are thrombosis, perhaps due to platelet activation due to inhibition of $PGI_2$, and recurrent abortions.

# *Thrombosis*

A thrombus is defined as a solid mass formed in the circulation from the constituents of the blood during life. Fragments of thrombi (emboli) may break off and block vessels downstream. Thromboembolic disease is much more common than abnormal bleeding; nearly half of adult deaths in England and Wales are due to coronary artery thrombosis, cerebral artery thrombosis or pulmonary embolism.

A thrombus results from a complex series of events involving coagulation factors, platelets, red blood cells and the vessel wall.

## Arterial thrombosis

This usually occurs in association with atheroma, which tends to form at areas of turbulent blood flow such as the bifurcation of arteries. Platelets adhere to the damaged vascular endothelium and aggregate in response to ADP and $TXA_2$ to form a 'white thrombus'. The growth of the platelet thrombus is limited at its margins by $PGI_2$. Eventually blood coagulation may be activated at the site of the thrombus, resulting either in complete occlusion of the vessel or embolization that produces distal obstruction. The risk factors for arterial thrombosis are related to the development of atherosclerosis (p. 578).

Arterial thrombi may form in the heart, as mural thrombi in the left ventricle after myocardial infarction, in the left atrium in mitral valve disease or on the surfaces of prosthetic valves.

## Venous thrombosis

Unlike arterial thrombosis, venous thrombosis often occurs in normal vessels. Important causes are stasis and hypercoagulability. The majority of venous thrombi occur in the deep veins of the leg, originating around the valves as 'red thrombi' consisting mainly of red cells and fibrin. The propagating thrombus is formed of fibrin and platelets and is particularly liable to embolize. Chronic venous obstruction in the deep veins of the leg results in a permanently swollen limb and may lead to ulceration (post-phlebitic syndrome).

Risk factors for venous thrombosis are shown in Table 6.24. Both arterial and venous thrombosis may occur with changes in blood cells such as polycythaemia, thrombocythaemia and sickle cell anaemia.

The clinical features and diagnosis of venous thrombosis are discussed on p. 629.

## Thrombophilia

Thrombophilia is a term describing inherited or acquired defects of haemostasis leading to a predisposition to venous or arterial thrombosis. It should be considered in patients with:
- Recurrent venous thrombosis
- Venous thrombosis for the first time under 40
- A family history of venous thrombosis
- An unusual venous thrombosis such as mesenteric vein thrombosis
- Neonatal thrombosis
- Recurrent abortions

- Arterial thrombosis in the absence of arterial disease

Laboratory investigation of such patients includes:
- Full blood count including platelet count
- Coagulation screen including a fibrinogen level
- Screen for a coagulation factor inhibitor including a lupus anticoagulant
- Assays for naturally occurring anticoagulants such as AT-III, protein C and protein S
- Tests of the fibrinolytic pathway (see p. 340)

## Prevention and treatment of arterial thrombosis

Attempts to prevent or reduce arterial thrombosis are mainly directed at minimizing factors predisposing to atherosclerosis. Treatment of established arterial thrombosis includes the use of antiplatelet drugs and thrombolytic therapy.

### Antiplatelet drugs

Platelet activation at the site of vascular damage is crucial to the development of arterial thrombosis, and this can be altered by the following drugs (Table 6.25):

ASPIRIN inhibits the enzyme cyclo-oxygenase (see Fig. 6.25) and this results in reduced platelet production of $TXA_2$.

DIPYRIDAMOLE, which inhibits platelet phosphodiesterase causing an increase in cyclic AMP with potentiation of the action of $PGI_2$, has been widely used as an antithrombotic agent but there is little evidence that it is effective.

The indications for and results of antiplatelet therapy are discussed in the appropriate sections.

### Thrombolytic therapy

STREPTOKINASE is a purified fraction of the filtrate obtained from cultures of haemolytic streptococci. It forms a 1:1 complex with plasminogen, resulting in a conformational change in plasminogen, revealing an active site which activates other plasminogen molecules to form plasmin. Streptokinase is given as an infusion of

| Patient factors | Disease or surgical procedure |
|---|---|
| Age | Trauma or surgery, especially of pelvis, hip or lower limb |
| Obesity | |
| Varicose veins | |
| Immobility (bed rest >4 days) | Malignancy |
| | Cardiac failure |
| Pregnancy and puerperium | Recent myocardial infarction |
| | Infection |
| High doses of oestrogens | Inflammatory bowel disease |
| Previous deep vein thrombosis or pulmonary embolism | Nephrotic syndrome |
| | Polycythaemia, thrombocythaemia |
| Thrombophilia, e.g. AT-III deficiency | Paroxysmal nocturnal haemoglobinuria |
| | Sickle cell anaemia |
| | Homocystinuria |

**Table 6.24** Risk factors for venous thromboembolism.

*Antiplatelet drugs*
Aspirin
Dipyridamole

*Thrombolytic therapy*
Streptokinase
Anisoylated plasminogen streptokinase activator complex (APSAC or antistreplase)
Urokinase
Single-chain urokinase-type plasminogen activator (scu-PA)
Tissue-type plasminogen activator (t-PA or alteplase)

*Anticoagulant drugs*
Heparin
Warfarin

**Table 6.25** Drugs used in the treatment of thrombotic disorders.

1 500 000 units over 1 hour in acute myocardial infarction. Laboratory monitoring of such short-term thrombolytic therapy is not necessary.

The main problem with streptokinase is its indiscriminate activation of plasminogen so that both fibrin in clots and free fibrinogen are lysed, leading to low fibrinogen levels and the risk of haemorrhage.

ANISOYLATED PLASMINOGEN STREPTOKINASE ACTIVATOR COMPLEX (APSAC) is a complex of plasminogen and an anisoylated form of streptokinase. The complex binds to any fibrin within intravascular clots where the anisoyl group is hydrolysed and the streptokinase–plasminogen complex produces fibrinolysis. The advantage of APSAC over streptokinase is its more sustained duration of action and it is given as a single bolus dose.

UROKINASE is produced naturally by the kidney. It cleaves plasminogen directly to produce plasmin.

TISSUE-TYPE PLASMINOGEN ACTIVATOR (t-PA) and single-chain urokinase-type plasminogen activator (scu-PA) are produced using recombinant gene technology. They were claimed to be relatively 'clot-specific', i.e. to have a greater affinity for fibrin-bound plasminogen than circulating plasminogen, and therefore to cause less systemic fibrinolysis and bleeding than streptokinase. However, the use of these newer thrombolytic agents has not yet been shown to produce fewer bleeding episodes than streptokinase. An accelerated dosage schedule of t-PA seems to produce a more rapid restoration of coronary flow.

THROMBOLYTIC THERAPY. The indications for and results of the use of thrombolytic therapy in myocardial infarction are discussed on p. 586. The combination of aspirin with thrombolytic therapy produces better results than thrombolytic therapy alone.

The main risk of thrombolytic therapy is bleeding and treatment should not be given to patients who have had recent bleeding, uncontrolled hypertension or a stroke, or surgery or other invasive procedures within the previous 10 days.

## Prevention and treatment of venous thromboembolism

Venous thromboembolism is a common problem after surgery, particularly in high-risk patients such as elderly patients, those with malignant disease and those with a history of previous thrombosis (Table 6.26). The incidence is also high in patients confined to bed following trauma, myocardial infarction or other illnesses.

Prevention and treatment of venous thrombosis includes the use of anticoagulants.

### Anticoagulants

HEPARIN is not a single substance but a mixture of polysaccharides. Commercially available unfractionated heparin consists of components with molecular weights varying from 5000 to 35 000 and an average of about 13 000. It was extracted initially from liver, hence its name, but it is now prepared from porcine gastric mucosa.

Heparin has an immediate effect on coagulation by potentiation of the formation of irreversible complexes between AT-III and activated serine protease coagulation factors (thrombin, XIIa, XIa, Xa, IXa and VIIa).

LOW MOLECULAR WEIGHT HEPARINS are produced by enzymatic or chemical degradation of standard heparin producing fractions with molecular weights in the range of 2000–8000. Potentiation of thrombin inhibition (anti-IIa activity) requires a minimum length of the heparin molecule with an approximate molecular weight of 5400, whereas the inhibition of factor Xa only requires a smaller heparin molecule with a molecular weight of about 1700. Low molecular weight heparins have the following properties:

1 They have greater activity against factor Xa than against factor IIa, suggesting that they may produce an equivalent anticoagulant effect as standard heparin but have a lower risk of bleeding, although this still awaits confirmation in clinical studies. In addition, low molecular weight heparins cause less inhibition of platelet function.

2 They have a longer half-life than standard heparin and so can be given as a once daily subcutaneous injection instead of every 8–12 hours.

3 They produce little effect on tests of overall coagulation, such as the PTTK at doses recommended for prophylaxis.

4 They are being increasingly used for antithrombotic prophylaxis of high-risk surgical patients. Fixed-dose low molecular weight heparin regimens are being studied for the treatment of established thrombosis.

The main *complication* of treatment with heparin is bleeding. This is managed by stopping heparin. Very occasionally it is necessary to neutralize heparin with protamine. Other complications include osteoporosis with prolonged therapy and thrombocytopenia.

ORAL ANTICOAGULANTS act by interfering with vitamin K metabolism. There are two types of oral anticoagulants, the coumarins and indanediones. The coumarin warfarin is most commonly used because it has a low incidence of side-effects other than bleeding.

The dosage is controlled by PT tests. Thromboplastin reagents for PT testing are derived from a variety of sources and give different PT results for the same plasma. It is now standard practice to compare each thromboplastin with an international reference preparation so that they can be assigned an international sensitivity index (ISI). The international normalized ratio (INR) is the ratio of the patient's PT to a normal control when using the international reference preparation (Information box 6.1).

Each laboratory develops a chart adapted to the ISI of their thromboplastin to convert the patient's PT to the INR and reports both values. The use of this system

| | Deep vein thrombosis | Proximal vein thrombosis | Fatal pulmonary embolism |
|---|---|---|---|
| Low-risk groups | <10% | <1% | 0.01% |
| Moderate-risk groups | 10–40% | 1–10% | 0.1–1% |
| High-risk groups | 40–80% | 10–30% | 1–10% |

| | |
|---|---|
| Low-risk groups: | Minor surgery (<30 min); no risk factors other than age<br>Major surgery (>30 min); age <40 years; no other risk factors<br>Minor trauma or medical illness |
| Moderate-risk groups: | Major surgery; age > 40 years or other risk factor<br>Major medical illness, e.g. cancer, severe cardiac or pulmonary disease<br>Major trauma or burns<br>Minor surgery, trauma or illness in patients with previous deep vein thrombosis, pulmonary embolism or thrombophilia |
| High-risk groups: | Fracture or major orthopaedic surgery of pelvis, hip or lower limb<br>Major pelvic or abdominal surgery for cancer<br>Major surgery, trauma or illness in patients with previous deep vein thrombosis, pulmonary embolism or thrombophilia |

Modified from Salzman EW & Hirsch J (1982) Prevention of venous thromboembolism. In: Colman RW, Hirsch J, Marder V & Salzman EW (eds) *Haemostasis and Thrombosis: Basic Principles and Clinical Practice*, p. 986. New York: Lippincott.

**Table 6.26** Incidence of venous thromboembolism in hospital patients according to risk group.

| INR | Clinical state |
|---|---|
| 2.0–2.5 | Prophylaxis of deep venous thrombosis including high-risk surgery<br>INR 2.0–3.0 for hip surgery and operations of fractured femur |
| 2.0–3.0 | Treatment for deep venous thrombosis, pulmonary embolism and systemic embolism; transient ischaemic attacks; atrial fibrillation; mitral stenosis with embolism; prophylaxis of venous thromboembolism in myocardial infarction |
| 3.0–4.5 | Recurrent deep venous thrombosis and pulmonary embolism; arterial disease including myocardial infarction; arterial grafts; cardiac prosthetic valves and grafts |

**Information box 6.1** Therapeutic ranges for oral anticoagulation proposed by the British Society for Haematology (1990).

means that PT tests on a given plasma sample using different thromboplastins result in the same INR and that anticoagulant control is comparable in different hospitals across the world.

Contraindications to the use of oral anticoagulants are seldom absolute and include:
- Severe hypertension
- Non-thrombo-embolic strokes
- Peptic ulceration
- Severe liver and renal disease
- Pre-existing haemostatic defects
- Pregnancy. Oral anticoagulants should be avoided in pregnancy because they are teratogenic in the first trimester and may be associated with fetal haemorrhage later in pregnancy. When anticoagulation is considered essential in pregnancy, self-administered subcutaneous heparin should be used as an alternative, although this may not be as effective for women with prosthetic cardiac valves. Specialist advice should be sought about anticoagulation in pregnancy.

Many drugs interact with warfarin (see Chapter 14). More frequent PT testing should accompany changes in medication, which should occur with the full knowledge of the anticoagulant clinic.

An *increased anticoagulant effect due to warfarin* (Emergency box 6.1) is usually produced by:
- Drugs causing a reduction in the metabolism of warfarin include tricyclic antidepressants, cimetidine, sulphonamides, phenothiazines and amiodarone.
- Drugs such as clofibrate and quinidine increase the sensitivity of hepatic receptors to warfarin.
- Drugs interfering with vitamin K absorption (such as broad-spectrum antibiotics and cholestyramine) may also potentiate the action of warfarin.
- The displacement of warfarin from its binding site on serum albumin by drugs such as sulphonamides is not usually responsible for clinically important interactions.
- Drugs that inhibit platelet function (such as aspirin) increase the risk of bleeding.
- Alcohol excess, cardiac failure, liver or renal disease, thyrotoxicosis and febrile illnesses may result in potentiation of the effect of warfarin.

A *decreased anticoagulant effect due to warfarin* is usually

*Life-threatening haemorrhage*
Immediately give vitamin K 5 mg by slow intravenous infusion and either a concentrate of factor II, IX, X with frozen VII concentrate (if these are available) or fresh frozen plasma

*Less severe haemorrhage, e.g. haematuria* or *epistaxis*
Withhold warfarin for one or more days and consider giving vitamin K 0.5–2 mg intravenously

*INR of >4.5 without haemorrhage*
Withdraw warfarin for 1 or 2 days and then review

*Unexpected bleeding at therapeutic levels*
Investigate possibility of underlying cause such as unsuspected renal or alimentary tract disease

**Emergency box 6.1**    Management of over-anticoagulation with warfarin. Recommendations of British Society of Haematology (1990).

produced by drugs that increase the clearance of warfarin by induction of hepatic enzymes that metabolize warfarin, such as rifampicin and barbiturates.

Side-effects of warfarin other than bleeding are rare.

**Prophylaxis to prevent venous thromboembolism**

Prophylactic measures to prevent venous thrombosis during surgery are aimed at procedures for preventing stasis, such as early mobilization, elevation of the legs, compression stockings, and possibly calf-muscle stimulation and passive calf-muscle exercises during surgery, and methods for preventing hypercoagulability, usually using heparin.

*Low-risk patients* (Table 6.26) require no specific measures other than early mobilization. *Moderate-risk patients* should receive specific prophylaxis such as low-dose heparin at a dose of 5000 units subcutaneously every 8 or

12 hours until the patient is ambulatory; no laboratory monitoring is required.

Low molecular weight heparin once daily has been shown to be more effective than standard low-dose heparin in preventing thrombosis in *high-risk patients*. However, in general surgical practice there is no clear evidence that low molecular weight heparin is superior to low-dose heparin and it is much more expensive. Before the introduction of low molecular weight heparin, other approaches were used in high-risk surgical patients such as low-dose warfarin and higher doses of subcutaneous heparin to keep the PTTK between 1.25 and 1.5 times the control value.

**Treatment of established venous thromboembolism** (Information box 6.2)

The aim of anticoagulant treatment is to prevent further thrombosis and pulmonary embolization while resolution of venous thrombi occurs by natural fibrinolytic activity.

Anticoagulation is started with heparin as it produces an immediate anticoagulant effect. There is no evidence that it is necessary to use heparin for any longer than it takes for simultaneously administered warfarin to produce an anticoagulant effect, usually about 3–4 days. Anticoagulation for 6 weeks is sufficient for patients after their first thrombosis as long as there are no persisting risk factors. Long-term treatment should be considered in patients with repeated episodes or continuing risk factors.

Outpatient anticoagulation is best supervised in anticoagulant clinics. Patients are issued with national booklets for recording INR results and anticoagulant doses.

The role of *thrombolytic therapy* in the treatment of venous thrombosis is not established. It is sometimes used in patients with massive pulmonary embolism and in patients with extensive deep venous thrombi.

For these conditions it is necessary to give a bolus dose of streptokinase, 250 000 units over 30 min to inactivate

Obtain objective evidence of thrombosis using venography, ultrasound imaging or pulmonary ventilation/perfusion scanning as soon as possible (see p. 629).

Perform a coagulation screen and platelet count before starting treatment to exclude a pre-existing haemostatic effect.

Give an intravenous loading dose of 5000 units of standard heparin (except in severe pulmonary embolism when 10 000 units should be given).

Heparinization should be continued with either:
(a) an intravenous infusion of 1000–2000 units hour$^{-1}$ or
(b) subcutaneous injections of 15 000 units every 12 hours.

The dose of intravenous or subcutaneous heparin is adjusted by laboratory monitoring 4–6 hours after the dose of heparin to prolong the PTTK to between 1.5 and 2.5 times the control value. Monitoring should be carried out at least once each day.

Administer warfarin 5–10 mg depending on the size and age of the patient at the same time the heparin is started. Give the same dose the next day and check the INR on the third day.

Heparin is stopped when the INR reaches the therapeutic range, usually 2.0 and the dose of warfarin is adjusted to maintain the INR in the therapeutic range.

The maintenance dose of warfarin is usually 3–9 mg daily. The INR is measured frequently until stability is achieved. The maximum interval between tests for patients on long-term anticoagulation is 6 weeks.

**Information box 6.2**    Treatment of established venous thromboembolism.

antibodies formed by previous streptococcal infection followed by a continuous infusion, approximately 100 000 units every hour, for 24–72 hours. The dose of streptokinase is adjusted to maintain the TT between two and four times the control value.

Thrombolytic therapy should be followed by anticoagulation with heparin for a few days and then by oral anticoagulants for a few months to prevent rethrombosis.

New agents are being evaluated as antithrombotic agents including direct inhibitors of thrombin such as hirudin. Hirudin can inactivate thrombin bound to fibrin more efficiently than AT-III potentiated by heparin. Clinical studies are required to establish the antithrombotic effect in relation to the risk of bleeding.

# Further reading

Bloom AL, Forbes CD, Thomas DP and Tuddenham EGD (1994) *Haemostasis and Thrombosis*, 2nd edn. Edinburgh: Churchill Livingstone.

Chanarin I (1979) *The Megablastic Anaemias*, 3rd edn. Oxford: Blackwell Scientific Publications.

Dacie JV (1985 (volume 1), 1988 (volume 2), 1992 (volume 3)) *The Haemolytic Anaemias*, 3rd edn. Edinburgh: Churchill Livingstone.

Firkin F, Chesterman C, Pennington D & Rush B (eds) (1989) *de Gruchy's Clinical Haematology in Medical Practice*, 5th edn. Oxford: Blackwell Scientific.

Furie B & Furie BC (1992) Molecular and cellular biology of blood coagulation. *New England Journal of Medicine* **326**, 800–806.

Groopman JE, Molina JM & Scadden DT (1989) Haemopoietic growth factors: Biology and clinical applications. *New England Journal of Medicine* **321**, 1449–1459.

Hows JM (1991) Severe aplastic anaemia: The patient without a HLA-identical sibling. *British Journal of Haematology* **77**, 1–4.

Mollison PL, Engelfriet CP & Contreras M (1993) *Blood Transfusion in Clinical Medicine*, 9th edn. Oxford: Blackwell Scientific Publications.

Pippard MJ, Hughes RT & Cotes PM (1992) Erythropoietin. In: *Recent Advances in Haematology* 6 (ed. Hoffbrand AV & Brenner MK). Edinburgh: Churchill Livingstone.

Thein SL & Weatherall DJ (1988) The thalassaemias. In: *Recent Advances in Haematology* 5 (ed. Hoffbrand AV). Edinburgh: Churchill Livingstone.

Williams WJ, Beutler E, Erslev AJ & Lichtman MA (1990) *Hematology*, 4th edn. New York: McGraw-Hill.

# Medical oncology

## Introduction

The term cancer encompasses a wide range of diseases including common illnesses such as lung cancer and colon cancer, as well as more esoteric ones, such as the acute leukaemias. Malignant disease is widely prevalent and, in the Western world, is second only to cardiovascular disease as the cause of death.

Cancer is thus not one illness and the treatment therefore involves multidisciplinary teams including surgeons, radiotherapists, medical oncologists, specialist nurses and palliative care teams. Treatment is given with either curative or palliative intent.

Many advances have been made in the last 30 years, both in treatment and in understanding the biology of the disease. Molecular biology techniques have opened up new possibilities of determining the aetiology of cancer, at least at the molecular level. However, for most cancers, the consequences of the molecular changes have not been determined.

### AETIOLOGY

Although in most patients the cause of the illness remains unknown, various factors have been identified as being associated with the development of malignant disease (Table 7.1). Usually the cause is multifactorial, although the association of smoking with lung cancer is so strong that it almost certainly represents a single cause-and-effect relationship.

# Epidemiology

### Geographical distribution

The incidence of various cancers varies with geographical location. England, Scotland and Wales in fact have the highest death rate from malignant disease in the world, mainly as a result of the very high incidence of lung cancer. Breast, colon and prostatic cancer all have a low incidence in Asian countries compared to Europe and North America. In contrast, liver cancer is very common worldwide but is rare in Europe and North America.

Many of these geographical differences are due to

Geographic
Age
Environmental
  Tobacco
  Alcohol
  Diet
  Ultraviolet light
  Ionizing radiation (see p. 765)
Occupational (see Table 7.3)
Drugs
Infective agents
Genetic

**Table 7.1** Possible factors associated in the causation of cancer.

environmental factors; for example, people who move from countries with a low incidence of breast and colon cancer to countries where the incidence is high eventually acquire the cancer incidence of the country to which they have moved. Japanese people moving to North America acquire the incidence of colon cancer typical of North America within one generation but take two generations to show an increase in the incidence of breast cancer. These changes in incidence can be due to infective agents (see below).

### Age distribution

Age has a strong influence upon the incidence of most common cancers. For lung, breast and colon cancer the frequency rises with increasing age; for Hodgkin's disease, a bimodal age distribution is seen, with peaks occurring in early adult life and in old age.

### Environmental factors

Some causative factors that have been associated with an increased risk of cancer are shown in Table 7.2. It could therefore be concluded that most common cancers in the Western world are potentially avoidable.

TOBACCO. Smoking is associated with lung cancer but also with cancer of the pharynx, oesophagus, bladder, pancreas and cervix. There is also evidence that the risk of lung cancer is influenced by an interaction between tobacco and exposure to other agents including asbestos, radon (in uranium miners) and nickel.

| Smoking | Mouth, pharynx, oesophagus, larynx, lung, bladder, lip |
|---|---|
| Alcohol | Mouth, pharynx, larynx, oesophagus, colorectal |
| Drugs (alkylating agents) | Bladder, bone marrow |
| Asbestos | Lung, mesothelium |
| Oestrogens | Endometrium, vagina |
| Vinyl chloride | Liver (angiosarcoma) |
| Polycyclic hydrocarbons | Skin, lung |
| Aromatic amines | Bladder |
| Aflatoxin | Liver |
| Hepatitis B virus | Liver |
| Ultraviolet light | Skin, lip |

**Table 7.2**  Some causative factors associated with the development of cancer at different sites.

ALCOHOL. Alcohol is associated with cancers of the upper respiratory and gastrointestinal tracts but also interacts with tobacco in the aetiology of these cancers. Alcohol may also increase the risk of breast cancer.

DIET. There are large international differences in dietary fat intake which correlate with the incidence of cancer of the breast, colon, ovary, prostate, endometrium and pancreas. However, these correlations may be due to other differences in life-style. Gastrointestinal cancers in particular have been associated with dietary factors. Conversely increased dietary fibre may protect against colon cancer. Food contamination may also play a role, e.g. aflatoxins found in mouldy peanuts and grains.

ULTRAVIOLET (UV) LIGHT is known to increase the risk of skin cancer of all types (basal cell, squamous cell and melanoma). The incidence of melanoma is particularly high in areas of Australia, New Zealand and South Africa.

### Occupational factors
Percival Pott, in 1775, first described the association between carcinogenic hydrocarbons in soot and the development of scrotal epitheliomas in chimney sweeps.

Subsequently, other chemicals used in industry have been found to cause cancer, e.g. asbestos increases the risk of mesothelioma and lung cancer and vinyl chloride (used in the manufacture of PVC) causes angiosarcoma of the liver. Some of the agents known or suspected of causing cancer are listed in Table 7.3.

### Infective agents
Clustering of certain malignancies has been shown to be related to infective agents. A specific type of T-cell leukaemia, seen predominantly in the Southern Island of Japan and in the West Indies, is associated with the retrovirus human T-cell leukaemia virus: (HTLV-1) (see below) which is endemic in these areas; a high incidence of liver cancer is related to hepatitis B virus infection and *Helicobacter pylori* infection is becoming increasingly recognized as a causative agent in stomach cancer and lymphoma. The Epstein–Barr virus (EBV) has been implicated in Burkitt's lymphoma and patients with AIDS due to HIV infection have an increased incidence of lymphoma and Kaposi's sarcoma. The risk of cervical cancer is increased by early onset of sexual activities and by the number of sexual partners, suggesting that an infectious agent may be involved and there is evidence that papillomavirus is associated with cervical cancer.

### Drugs
Oestrogens have been implicated in both vaginal and endometrial carcinoma. Cytotoxic drugs given, for example, for lymphoma, are associated with a subsequent increased incidence of secondary acute myelogenous leukaemia.

# Cancer genetics

The development of cancer is associated with a fundamental genetic change within the cell and there is overwhelming evidence that mutations can cause cancer (a mutation being defined as a change in the genome).

### Mutations
Evidence for the genetic origin of cancer is based on the following:
- Most known carcinogens induce mutations.
- Genetically determined traits associated with a

| Occupation | Agent | Site of disease |
|---|---|---|
| Dye manufacturers, rubber workers | Aromatic amines | Bladder |
| Asbestos mining and handling | Asbestos | Lung, mesothelium |
| Cadmium workers | Cadmium | Prostate |
| Uranium miners | Ionizing radiation | Lung |
| Coal gas manufacturers, asphalters and others | Polycyclic hydrocarbons | Skin, lung |
| Farmers, sailors | Ultraviolet light | Skin, lip |
| Hardwood furniture manufacturers | Unknown | Nasal sinuses |

**Table 7.3**  Some occupational exposures that influence cancer risk.

deficiency in the enzymes required for DNA repair are associated with an increased risk of cancer.

- Many types of cancer are associated with chromosome instability.
- Some cancers are inherited.
- Malignant tumours are clonal.
- Some tumours contain mutated oncogenes (see p. 122).
- Susceptibility to some carcinogens depends on the ability of cellular enzymes to convert them to a mutagenic form.

Mutations may occur in the germ line and therefore can be in every cell in the body, or they may occur in only a single somatic cell and therefore be found in the tumour following clonal proliferation.

### Chromosome abnormalities

Genetic changes in cells are often manifest as a chromosome change that can be picked up by examination of mitotic cells. Most of these observations have been made in leukaemic cells because they can be obtained easily. Chromosome changes are usually reciprocal translocations. A non-reciprocal exchange results in either deletion or addition of a chromosome region, or an increase in the amount of DNA from a specific region of a chromosome.

Examples of chromosome changes that are associated with malignancy are:

CHRONIC MYELOID LEUKAEMIA (see p. 365).

ACUTE PROMYELOCYTIC LEUKAEMIA (APML) (also see p. 363). Almost all patients with APML have the t(15;17) reciprocal translocation, which occurs at the q25 band on chromosome 15 and the q22 band on chromosome 17. It is of especial interest because the translocation breakpoint on chromosome 17 occurs in the gene encoding the retinoic acid receptor. This is, in turn, of great interest in view of the responsiveness of patients with APML to all-*trans*-retinoic acid (see p. 364).

BURKITT'S LYMPHOMA. This was the first tumour where a chromosome change was shown to involve the translocation of a specific gene. The translocations involving chromosome 8 and chromosomes 2, 14 or 22 result in the relocation of the *MYC* oncogene near to the genes that encode for immunoglobulin molecules.

The most frequent change in Burkitt's lymphoma is a reciprocal translocation between chromosomes 8 and 14 in which the *MYC* oncogene moves from chromosome 8 to a position near the constant region of the immunoglobulin heavy chain gene on chromosome 14. The variable region of the immunoglobulin gene is transferred from chromosome 14 to chromosome 8. Similar rearrangements involving the light chain loci are seen in the translocations between chromosome 8 and either chromosome 2 ($\kappa$ chain) or 22 ($\lambda$ chain).

### DNA REPAIR

There are four autosomal recessive diseases that predispose to the development of cancer:
1 Xeroderma pigmentosum (XP)
2 Ataxia telangiectasia (AT)
3 Bloom's syndrome (BS)
4 Fanconi's anaemia (FA)

Patients with XP have a defect in their ability to repair DNA damage caused by UV light and by some chemicals. This leads to a high incidence of skin cancer. The AT mutation results in an increased sensitivity to ionizing radiation and increased susceptibility to lymphoid tumours. People with BS and FA also have an increased susceptibility to lymphoid malignancy. It is not known why these chromosome-break syndromes predispose to tumours of lymphatic tissue.

### INHERITED CANCERS

The following are examples of inherited cancers that exhibit dominant inheritence:
- Retinoblastoma
- Familial adenomatous polyposis (FAP) (see p. 225)
- Wilms' tumour
- Basal-cell naevus syndrome
- Neurofibromatosis
- Multiple-endocrine-adenomatosis syndromes
- Neuroblastoma
- 'Family' cancer syndrome

Retinoblastoma is an eye tumour found in young children. It occurs in both hereditary (40%) and non-hereditary (60%) forms. The 40% of patients with the hereditary form have a germ-line mutation on the long arm of chromosome 13 that predisposes to retinoblastoma. In addition to the latter, people inheriting this mutation at the so-called *RBL* locus are at risk for developing other tumours particularly osteosarcoma.

# The diagnosis of malignancy

The diagnosis of cancer may be suspected by both doctor and patient but obviously needs to be confirmed. Patients with cancer and their families are likely to be frightened; the very word cancer, often avoided by doctors and patients alike, is, often incorrectly, assumed to imply certain death. Reassurance and advice on therapy can only be given on the basis of a tissue diagnosis obtained via a needle biopsy or at surgery. Alternatively a fine needle aspiration can be obtained for cytological diagnosis. This has the advantage of being simple and quick to perform but an experienced cytologist is necessary.

Malignant lesions can be distinguished by the pleomorphism of the cells, increased numbers of mitoses, nuclear aberration and evidence of invasion into surrounding tissues. The degree of differentiation or anaplasia of the tumour is a factor in deciding the treatment and determining the prognosis.

Immunohistochemistry using monoclonal antibodies against tumour antigens is being used to differentiate cell types.

### Staging

Before a decision about treatment can be made, it is important to establish not only the type of tumour but also its extent, i.e. which other organs are involved. Various staging investigations will therefore be performed before a treatment decision is made.

Staging systems vary according to the type of tumour. One widely used system is the TNM classification (T, tumour; N, node; M, metastasis) which can be applied to most cancers. T describes the size of the tumour (where in T0 there is no evidence of tumour and T1–3 indicates a progressive increase in size); N describes the increasing involvement of nodes (N1–N3) and M describes the absence (M0) or presence (M1) of metastases. Specific tumours, e.g. Hodgkin's disease, are classified according to more specific classifications (see p. 367).

In addition to anatomical staging, the person's general state of health obviously needs to be taken into account when planning treatment. This has been ascribed a 'performance scale' which is also of important prognostic significance (Table 7.4).

### Tumour markers

These can be useful in diagnosis and in following the response to treatment. Relatively specific markers include $\alpha$-fetoprotein (see p. 242), $\beta$-human chorionic gonadotrophin ($\beta$-HCG) and prostate-specific antigen (PSA). Other less disease-specific antigens can be useful particularly in following up treatment, e.g. carcinoembryonic antigen (CEA) in gastrointestinal adenocarcinomas and Ca 125 in ovarian or other epithelial cancers.

## Measuring response to treatment

Response to treatment can be subjective or objective. A subjective response is one perceived by the patient in terms of, for example, relief of pain, dyspnoea or improvement in appetite, weight gain or energy. Quantitative measurements of these subjective symptoms form an increasingly important part of the assessment of response to chemotherapy especially in those situations where cure is not possible and where the aim of treatment is to provide good-quality prolongation of life. In these circumstances, measures of quality of life enable an estimate of the balance of benefit and side-effects to be made.

Objective response to treatment is measured either as a partial response, which is defined as more than a 50% reduction in the size of the tumour, or complete response, which is a complete disappearance of all detectable disease clinically and radiologically. The terms used to evaluate the responses of tumours are given in Table 7.5. Partial remission is often associated with a reduction in symptoms and improvement in quality of life. The rate of regrowth of the tumour is dependent on the underlying doubling time of that particular tumour. For more rapidly growing tumours a partial response may not be associated with very much prolongation of life, whereas with more slow growing tumours responses may continue for a long time. Complete remission is a necessary prerequisite for cure but unfortunately many patients who achieve complete remission will subsequently relapse because of the presence of residual microscopic disease. Many strategies have been developed to try and increase the proportion of patients with complete remission who go on to long-term remission or cure.

## Principles of chemotherapy

The ability to give anticancer treatment via the bloodstream was a major advance as it enabled therapy to potentially reach metastatic disease in any part of the

| | |
|---|---|
| 100 | Normal; no complaints |
| 90 | Able to carry on normal activity. Minor symptoms of disease |
| 80 | Normal activity with effort. Some symptoms of disease |
| 70 | Cares for self. Unable to carry on normal activity or to work |
| 60 | Requires occasional assistance but is able to care for most of own needs |
| 50 | Requires considerable assistance and frequent medical care |
| 40 | Disabled. Requires special care and assistance |
| 30 | Severely disabled. Hospitalization indicated although death not imminent |
| 20 | Very sick. Hospitalization necessary, active supportive treatment necessary |
| 10 | Moribund. Fatal processes progressing rapidly |

Table 7.4  Karnowsky performance status.

| | |
|---|---|
| *Complete response* | Complete disappearance of all detectable disease |
| *Partial response* | More than 50% reduction in the size of the tumour |
| *No response* | No change or less than 50% reduction |
| *Progressive disease* | Increase in size of tumour at any site |

Table 7.5  Definitions of response.

body. The toxicity of chemotherapy determined that drugs could only be given intermittently and that time had to be allowed for normal tissues to recover between each administration of new cytotoxic drugs. Furthermore, it quickly became apparent in the early development of cytotoxic chemotherapy that tumours rapidly developed resistance to single agents given on their own. For this reason the principle of intermittent combination chemotherapy was developed. Several drugs were combined together, chosen on the basis of differing mechanisms of action and non-overlapping toxicities. These drugs were given over a period of a few days followed by a rest of a few weeks, during which time the normal tissues had the opportunity to recuperate. Although the tumour cells also had the same opportunity for regrowth, it became apparent that normal tissues repaired more rapidly than cancer cells and it was therefore possible to continually deplete the tumour while allowing the restoration of normal tissues between chemotherapy cycles (Fig. 7.1). In many experimental tumours it has been shown that there is a log linear relationship between drug dose and number of cancer cells killed. With a chemosensitive tumour a relatively small increase in dose may have a large effect on tumour cell kill. It is therefore apparent that where cure is a realistic option the dose administered may be critical and may need to be maintained despite toxicity. In situations where cure is not a realistic possibility and palliation is the aim, dose is less critical particularly as quality of life becomes paramount.

## Classification of cytotoxic drugs (Table 7.6)

### ALKYLATING AGENTS

The alkylating agents were first developed for use in chemical warfare. They act by covalently bonding alkyl groups and their major effect is to cross-link DNA strands, interfering with DNA synthesis. Despite being among the earliest cytotoxic drugs developed they maintain a central position in the treatment of cancer in the 1990s. Common alkylating agents include cyclophosphamide, chlorambucil, melphalan and busulphan.

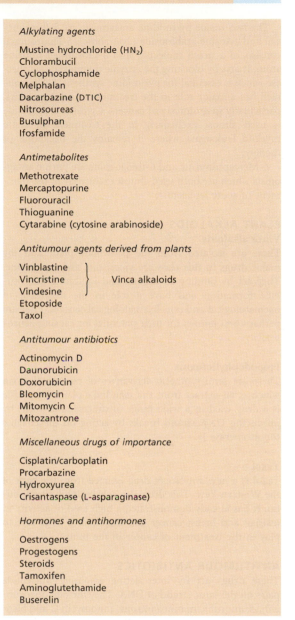

*Alkylating agents*

Mustine hydrochloride (HN₂)
Chlorambucil
Cyclophosphamide
Melphalan
Dacarbazine (DTIC)
Nitrosoureas
Busulphan
Ifosfamide

*Antimetabolites*

Methotrexate
Mercaptopurine
Fluorouracil
Thioguanine
Cytarabine (cytosine arabinoside)

*Antitumour agents derived from plants*

Vinblastine
Vincristine ⎫
Vindesine ⎬ Vinca alkaloids
Etoposide
Taxol

*Antitumour antibiotics*

Actinomycin D
Daunorubicin
Doxorubicin
Bleomycin
Mitomycin C
Mitozantrone

*Miscellaneous drugs of importance*

Cisplatin/carboplatin
Procarbazine
Hydroxyurea
Crisantaspase (L-asparaginase)

*Hormones and antihormones*

Oestrogens
Progestogens
Steroids
Tamoxifen
Aminoglutethamide
Buserelin

**Table 7.6** Antitumour agents.

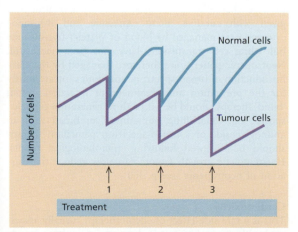

**Fig. 7.1** Effects of multiple courses of cytotoxic chemotherapy.

### ANTIMETABOLITES

Antimetabolites are usually structural analogues of naturally occurring metabolites and interfere with normal synthesis of nucleic acids by falsely substituting purines and pyrimidines in metabolic pathways. Antimetabolites can be divided into folic acid antagonists, pyrimidine antagonists and purine antagonists. The classic folic acid antagonist methotrexate is structurally very similar to folic acid and binds preferentially to dihydrofolate reductase, the enzyme responsible for the conversion of folic acid to folinic acid. It is widely used in the treatment of solid tumours and haematological malignancies and also has a role in non-malignant conditions such as rheumatoid arthritis.

The two major pyrimidine antagonists are 5-fluorouracil and cytosine arabinoside (cytarabine). 5-Fluorouracil consists of a uracil molecule with a substituted fluorine atom. It acts by blocking the enzyme thymidylate synthetase which is essential for pyrimidine synthesis. 5-Fluorouracil has a major role in the treatment of solid tumours, particularly gastrointestinal cancers. Cytosine arabinoside is used almost exclusively in the treatment of acute myeloid leukaemia where it remains the backbone of therapy.

6-Mercaptopurine and 6-thioguanine are purine antagonists which are both used almost exclusively in the treatment of acute leukaemia.

## PLANT ALKALOIDS
### Vinca alkaloids
These are isolated from the periwinkle plant and the major drugs in this class are vincristine and vinblastine. They act by binding to tubulin and inhibiting microtubule formation and have a role in the treatment of haematological and non-haematological cancers. They are perhaps best known for their potential for causing neurotoxicity.

### Epipodophyllotoxins
These are semi-synthetic derivatives of podophyllotoxin which is an extract from the mandrake plant. Etoposide is a drug used in a wide range of cancers and works by producing DNA strand breaks by acting on the enzyme topoisomerase II.

### Taxol
Taxol is a new anticancer drug isolated from the bark of the Western Yew. This drug also acts by inhibiting tubulin. It has already demonstrated a high level of activity in ovarian and breast cancer and may have a large role to play in the treatment of cancer in the future.

## ANTITUMOUR ANTIBIOTICS
These drugs act by intercalating adjoining nucleotide pairs on the same strand of DNA. They include doxorubicin, daunorubicin, mitozantrone, mitomycin C and bleomycin. These drugs have a wide spectrum of activity in haematological and solid tumours. Doxorubicin is one of the most widely used of all cytotoxic drugs.

## PLATINUM ANALOGUES
Cisplatin and carboplatin cause interstrand cross-links of DNA and are often regarded as non-classical alkylating agents. They have transformed the treatment of testicular cancer and have a major role to play in many other tumours including ovarian cancer and head and neck cancer.

# Side-effects of chemotherapeutic drugs

The side-effects of anticancer drugs are legendary and have created fear in both the medical profession and the general public. The situation in the 1990s has improved vastly from the early days of cytotoxic chemotherapy where persistent and prolonged nausea and vomiting were the rule, and life-threatening complications from myelosuppression were not uncommon. Modern cytotoxic chemotherapy has improved out of all recognition to those early days and newer cytotoxic drugs, often analogues of the original drugs, are frequently associated with significantly lesser side-effects. Modern antiemetics such as the 5 hydroxy tryptamine (5HT$_3$) antagonists can prevent or reduce vomiting to a minimum in a majority of patients. In those intensive chemotherapy regimens where myelosuppression is a major feature, the use of growth factors can now reduce this to a certain extent. Despite these advances, chemotherapy still carries many potentially serious side-effects and should only be used by practitioners with considerable skill and experience.

## MAJOR SIDE-EFFECTS
### Nausea and vomiting
This common side-effect can be eliminated or reduced by choice of drugs and by using modern antiemetics. Nausea and vomiting are particular problems with platinum analogues and with doxorubicin. Antiemetics such as metoclopramide and domperidone are used initially but the 5HT$_3$ serotonin antagonists (ondansetron and granisetron) have revolutionized management of vomiting and many patients are now given platinum drugs as an outpatient.

### Hair loss
Many but not all cytotoxic drugs are capable of causing hair loss. Scalp cooling can sometimes be used to reduce hair loss with doxorubicin but in general this side-effect can only be prevented by selection of drugs where this is possible. Hair always regrows on completion of chemotherapy.

### Bone marrow suppression
Suppression of the production of haemoglobin, white cell series and platelets may occur with many cytotoxic drugs and is a dose-related phenomenon. Severely myelosuppressive chemotherapy is only used when treatment is given with curative intent. Anaemia and thrombocytopenia are managed by blood or platelet transfusions but white cell transfusions have not been successful. Neutropenic patients are therefore managed by the early introduction of broad-spectrum antibiotics intravenously for the prevention and treatment of infection. Initial 'blind' therapy should be with a third generation cephalosporin, e.g. ceftazidime, sometimes combined with an aminoglycoside or a broad-spectrum penicillin; therapy should be reviewed following microbiological results. Haemopoietic growth factors can now reduce the duration of neutropenia (see p. 360).

### Cardiotoxicity
This is a rare side-effect of chemotherapy, usually associated with doxorubicin. It is dose related and can largely

be prevented by keeping the total dose within the safe range.

### Neurotoxicity
This occurs predominantly with the plant alkaloids and platinum analogues. It is dose related and chemotherapy is usually stopped before the development of a significant polyneuropathy. This is only partially reversible.

### Nephrotoxicity
A number of cytotoxic drugs, particularly platinum analogues, can potentially cause renal damage but this can usually be prevented by maintaining an adequate diuresis during treatment.

### Sterility
Some anticancer drugs, particularly alkylating agents, may cause sterility which can be irreversible. In males the storage of sperm is an important consideration when chemotherapy is given with curative intent.

### Secondary malignancies
Anticancer drugs have mutagenic potential and the development of secondary malignancies, particularly acute leukaemia, is an uncommon but particularly unwelcome long-term side-effect in patients otherwise cured of their malignancies. The alkylating agents are particularly implicated in this very severe complication.

## Drug resistance

Drug resistance is one of the major obstacles to curing cancer with chemotherapy. Some tumours have an inherently low level of resistance to currently available treatment and are often cured. These include testicular teratomas, Hodgkin's disease and childhood acute leukaemia. Solid tumours such as small-cell lung cancer initially appear to be chemosensitive with the majority of patients responding but most patients eventually relapse with resistant disease. In other tumours such as melanoma the disease is largely chemoresistant from the start. It is now thought that most resistance occurs as a result of genetic mutation and becomes more likely as the number of tumour cells increases. It has also been shown that anticancer drugs can themselves increase the rate of mutation to resistance. Unfortunately resistance to cytotoxic drugs is often multiple and is known as multidrug resistance (MDR). An example of this is resistance to anthracyclines (e.g. doxorubicin) which is often associated with resistance to vinca alkaloids and epipodophyllotoxins. It is thought that this resistance is mediated via increased expression of P-glycoprotein, which mediates an efflux of cytotoxic drugs. A second important mechanism for MDR concerns altered drug binding to topoisomerase II, an enzyme which is important in bringing about DNA strand breaks in association with cytotoxic drugs. Treating patients as early as possible in the disease, using maximal doses of drugs and combination chemotherapy may help to reduce the likelihood of MDR. Many innovative approaches are currently being examined experimentally.

## Adjuvant therapy

When a patient first presents with a tumour, it is possible that small amounts of tumour tissue have already spread to the lungs, liver, bone marrow and other sites. This micrometastatic disease consists of relatively few cells with a good blood supply, and might be particularly amenable to the action of anticancer drugs. Therefore, if the primary tumour is removed and the tumour has a great likelihood of relapse, chemotherapy can be given to destroy the residual micrometastatic disease, and the chance of long-term survival and cure might be improved. This was dramatically demonstrated in the childhood renal sarcoma, Wilms' tumour, when the use of actinomycin D given after nephrectomy resulted in a doubling of the number of children who survived. Chemotherapy used in this way is known as adjuvant therapy, and has been employed in a number of other childhood tumours. In adults adjuvant chemotherapy has been shown to be of value in breast cancer and colon cancer.

## Treatment of malignancy in sanctuary sites

A 'sanctuary site' is the term used to indicate that metastatic disease has involved a site that is not accessible to conventional drug therapy. An example of this is leukaemic infiltration of the meninges in children with acute lymphoblastic leukaemia. Because of the blood–brain barrier, agents such as vincristine and prednisolone do not enter the subarachnoid space in sufficient quantity to eliminate all the leukaemic cells, and are therefore ineffective in preventing the development of meningeal infiltration. In order to treat these cells, intrathecal chemotherapy and/or cranial irradiation are required.

## Principles of endocrine therapy

It has long been known that oestrogen is capable of stimulating the growth of breast cancer and androgens the growth of prostate cancer. Manipulation of the hormonal environment may result in regression of a number of tumours particularly breast cancer, endometrial cancer and prostate cancer. Hormonal therapy is in general not curative. It may, however, provide control of a tumour for a period of time often with few side-effects. The presence of cell surface receptors for the hormone in question is a prerequisite for the therapy to be effective. The binding of hormone to receptor and translocation of the hormone–receptor complex into the nucleus, where it reacts

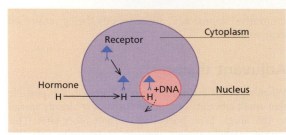

**Fig. 7.2** Mechanism of the cell receptor system. A hormone H combines with a receptor and the complex is transported to the nucleus, where it reacts with DNA.

with the DNA, is shown diagrammatically in Fig. 7.2. Patients with breast cancer frequently have receptors for oestrogens and progesterones. Hormonal manipulation includes the use of the anti-oestrogen tamoxifen, the reduction of endogenous oestrogen by oophorectomy or 'medical oophorectomy' via pituitary down-regulation using a luteinizing hormone releasing hormone (LHRH) analogue. Progestogens and aromatase inhibitors also have antitumour activity.

Endometrial tumours also have receptors for both oestrogens and progesterones. These tumours frequently respond to the administration of progesterone and also to the anti-oestrogen tamoxifen.

In prostate cancer the commonest hormonal manipulation used to be the administration of oestrogen. By a negative feedback on the pituitary this resulted in anorchid levels of testosterone and was associated with a response of the tumour in the majority of patients. Unfortunately the severe side-effects with oestrogens, including increased mortality from cardiovascular and cerebrovascular disease, significantly reduced the overall benefit. Another alternative was to carry out an orchidectomy, which reduced circulating testosterone but without the oestrogenic side-effects. More recently the use of an LHRH analogue to create a 'medical' orchidectomy and the availability of antiandrogenic drugs have revolutionized the medical treatment of prostate cancer, achieving a response in most patients with few side-effects.

# Principles of biological therapy

The term 'biological therapy' encompasses a wide range of treatments and adjuncts to the treatment of cancer. Most are still being evaluated—a few examples are discussed below.

## Interferons (IFNs) (see p. 139)

Interferons are naturally occurring lymphokines that are normally produced in response to viral infection. Their mechanism of action in malignant disease is uncertain; they have specific antiproliferative activity but can also induce natural killer cells and other immunological changes that might have an antitumour effect.

IFN-$\alpha$ is now commercially available and is being used in several haematological malignancies, e.g. hairy cell leukaemia and chronic myeloid leukaemia. In the latter, it results in a reduction in the proportion of Philadelphia (Ph) chromosome positive cells in at least 50% of patients, with total elimination in 10%. It remains to be established whether these effects will translate into prolongation of survival. IFNs are also being tested in an 'adjuvant' setting in follicular lymphoma and myeloma.

The treatment has side-effects, mainly flu-like symptoms which tend to diminish with time. The main disadvantage is that IFN has to be given as a subcutaneous injection.

## Colony stimulating factors (growth factors) (see p. 294)

Granulocyte and granulocyte/macrophage colony stimulating factors (G-CSF and GM-CSF) are being evaluated in patients with cancer:
- To reduce the duration of neutropenia following chemotherapy
- In conjunction with chemotherapy, to stimulate the proliferation of haemopoietic progenitor cells in the marrow so that they enter the circulation and can be collected from the peripheral blood to support very intensive therapy
- In acute myelogenous leukaemia, to induce leukaemic blast cells into cycle in the hope of increasing cell kill by cell-cycle specific drugs such as cytosine arabinoside

## Monoclonal antibodies

Monoclonal antibodies directed against tumour cell surface antigens are being investigated in three experimental settings:

1 *In vitro*, in conjunction with complement, to deplete autologous bone marrow of tumour cells in patients with leukaemia and lymphoma receiving very intensive therapy with autologous bone marrow transplantation
2 *In vitro*, in conjunction with complement to deplete allogeneic bone marrow of mature T cells which cause graft-versus-host disease (see p. 371)
3 *In vitro*, conjugated to a toxin, e.g. ricin, or *in vivo* to a radioactive element, e.g. iodine/yttrium, to deliver the cell killing substance directly to the tumour cell

# Haematological malignancy

### Introduction

Leukaemia, lymphoma and myeloma constitute only a small proportion of all malignant diseases. They share common origins in the myeloproliferative and lympho-proliferative systems but are a heterogeneous group, with a natural history resulting in survival ranging from a few months to several years. Their importance lies in their responsiveness to both chemotherapy and radiotherapy, so that many patients with acute leukaemia, Hodgkin's disease, and high grade non-Hodgkin's lymphoma, can now be cured. However, the majority of patients with haematological malignancy still die as a consequence of the illness, it is therefore essential to explain the disease, its treatment and the chance of success to the patient and to the family.

## LEUKAEMIA

Leukaemia is rare, with an annual overall incidence of 5 per 100 000. Both subtypes of acute leukaemia can occur in all age groups but acute lymphoblastic leukaemia (ALL) is predominantly a disease of childhood, whereas acute myelogenous leukaemia (AML) is most frequently seen in older adults.

### AETIOLOGY

In the majority of cases, the aetiology is unknown. Feline leukaemia virus has been shown to cause the disease in cats; there is, however, no evidence for a viral aetiology in humans apart from the association of a specific subtype of T-cell leukaemia, found predominantly in the Sou-thern Island of Japan and the Caribbean, with the retro-virus HTLV-1. However, many people in the endemic areas have antibodies to the virus, implying past infection, but may never develop leukaemia.

### Genetic factors

Many patients with acute leukaemia have a chromosomal abnormality. When complete remission (CR) is achieved, the chromosomal translocation/deletion often becomes undetectable, but returns at recurrence. Such a cyto-genetic change usually implies a worse prognosis but not always: 99% of patients with acute promyelocytic leu-kaemia (APML) have the t(15;17) translocation; the latter and the t(8;21) translocation in AML in fact confer a better long-term prognosis once CR has been achieved (see p. 363).

The first non-random chromosomal abnormality to be described was the Ph chromosome (see p. 365) which is associated in 95% of cases with chronic myeloid leu-kaemia (CML). The Ph chromosome is also found in some patients with ALL, the incidence in the latter increasing with age. The translocation is shown sche-matically in Fig. 7.3. The Ph chromosome is an abnormal chromosome 22, resulting from a reciprocal translocation between part of the long arm of chromosome 22 and chromosome 9. The resulting karyotype is described as t(9;22)(q34;q11). The molecular consequences of the translocation have been defined as follows: the oncogene (C-ABL) normally present on chromosome 9 is translo-cated to chromosome 22, where it comes into juxtapo-sition with a region of chromosome 22 named the 'break-point cluster region' (BCR). The translocation thus

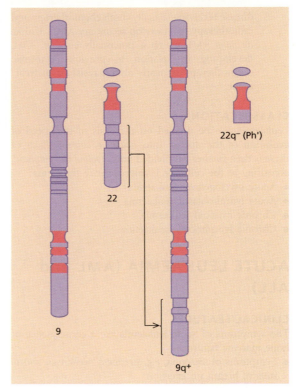

**Fig. 7.3** The Philadelphia chromosome (Ph'). The long arm (q) of chromosome 22 has been shortened by the reciprocal translo-cation with chromosome 9.

creates a hybrid transcription unit consisting of the 5′ end of the BCR gene and the C-ABL proto-oncogene. The new gene is capable of being expressed as a chimeric mRNA which has been identified in cells from patients with CML. When translated, this produces a fusion pro-tein that has tyrosine kinase activity and enhanced phos-phorylating activity compared to the normal C-ABL pro-tein. The contribution of these molecular events to the disease process is at present unclear. The precise break-point differs in CML and Ph-positive ALL, leading to the production of two different tyrosine kinase proteins.

### Environmental factors

1 Chemicals, e.g. benzene compounds used in industry.
2 Drugs, e.g. cytotoxic agents such as chlorambucil and procarbazine.
3 Radiation—the evidence for radiation causing leu-kaemia comes from three sources:
  (a) The atomic bombs exploded in Hiroshima and Nagasaki resulted in an increased incidence of both AML and, in particular, CML in people living in surrounding areas. There is therefore concern about the population living round Chernobyl.
  (b) In the past, patients with ankylosing spondylitis (see p. 394) were treated with radiotherapy, lead-ing to an increased incidence of secondary AML.
  (c) A small proportion of patients with Hodgkin's

disease receiving (usually) both chemotherapy and radiotherapy will develop secondary AML. Unlike *de novo* AML which is potentially curable, AML developing in relation to previous cytotoxic chemotherapy is nearly always resistant to treatment.

## CLASSIFICATION

Leukaemia can be divided on the basis of the speed of evolution of the disease into *acute* or *chronic*. Each of these is then further subdivided into *myeloid* or *lymphoid*, according to the cell type involved, hence the terms:
- Acute myelogenous leukaemia
- Acute lymphoblastic leukaemia
- Chronic myeloid leukaemia
- Chronic lymphocytic leukaemia

# ACUTE LEUKAEMIA (AML and ALL)

## CLINICAL FEATURES

The symptoms of acute leukaemia are a consequence of bone marrow failure:
- Symptoms of anaemia, e.g. tiredness, weakness, shortness of breath on exertion
- Repeated infections, e.g. sore throat, pneumonia
- Bruising and/or bleeding
- Occasionally, lymph node enlargement and/or symptoms relating to enlargement of the liver and spleen

There may be few or no signs; commonly patients have:
- Signs of anaemia
- Bruises, petechial haemorrhages, purpura, fundal haemorrhages
- Signs of infection
- Sometimes peripheral lymphadenopathy and/or hepatosplenomegaly

## INVESTIGATIONS

The definitive diagnosis is made on the peripheral blood film and a bone marrow aspirate. Additional investigations such as cytogenetic analysis and immunophenotyping of the leukaemic blast cells are not mandatory but can be helpful. If the patient has a fever, blood cultures and a chest X-ray are essential.

BLOOD COUNT:
A low haemoglobin (Hb).
White cell count (WCC) usually raised, but can be decreased or normal.
Platelets usually reduced.

PERIPHERAL BLOOD FILM shows characteristic leukaemic blast cells.

BONE MARROW ASPIRATE usually shows increased cellularity with a high percentage of abnormal lymphoid or myeloid blast cells.

## MANAGEMENT—GENERAL

The decision to treat a patient with curative intent will depend on the person's age, their general state of health, the point in the course of the illness (presentation or recurrence), and the person's wishes. The use of intensive combination chemotherapy may, for example, be entirely inappropriate at the time of recurrence in an older person. The diagnosis, its implications, the treatment options and the likely outcome of such treatment, together with its side-effects, need to be explained to the patient and to the family. People often find it difficult to assimilate all of this information on one occasion; it is therefore essential to give them the opportunity to ask questions, particularly as circumstances change.

Before starting treatment, the following need to be considered:

CORRECTION OF ANAEMIA AND THROMBOCYTOPENIA by administration of blood and platelets.

TREATMENT OF INFECTION with intravenous antibiotics.

LEUKAEMIC BLAST CELLS can infiltrate the brain and the lungs resulting in coma and respiratory failure respectively. If the blast cell count in the peripheral blood is very high ($>100 \times 10^9$/litre) the patient may need leucophoresis (i.e. blood is collected from a vein and centrifuged so as to remove some of the leukaemic cells; the red cells and plasma are then returned to the patient via another vein). Leucophoresis can be life saving; an alternative is to use high doses of the drug hydroxyurea.

ADMINISTRATION OF ALLOPURINOL, a xanthine oxidase inhibitor to treat and prevent hyperuricaemia.

In certain types of leukaemia where the rate of cell division is very fast, e.g. B-ALL, T-ALL, patients may develop the 'tumour lysis' syndrome when chemotherapy is given. The latter is characterized by hypercalcaemia and high serum levels of phosphate and potassium resulting from a high rate of cellular breakdown. This is a potentially life-threatening situation and difficult to treat once it has happened. It can usually be prevented by making sure that chemotherapy is not given whilst the uric acid level is high, by giving intravenous fluids before starting chemotherapy and monitoring the relevant biochemical parameters at regular intervals. Patients may require haemodialysis to correct the metabolic imbalance.

Specific treatment programmes for the different subtypes of leukaemia will be mentioned only briefly since treatment regimens are evolving. Good 'supportive care' in terms of antibiotics and blood products is as important as the specific combination of drugs used; patients with acute leukaemia should therefore be treated in specialist centres where the medical and nursing staff are familiar with the management of neutropenia and thrombocytopenia. Patients need to be informed of what is going on as the situation changes.

## Acute myelogenous leukaemia

AML is a potentially curable disease. The aim of treatment is to restore the bone marrow to normal and the patient to a normal state of health, i.e. complete remission (CR). AML is classified on the basis of the morphological appearance of the bone marrow into seven subtypes, FAB M1-M7, which differ depending on the predominant cell type involved (Table 7.7).

## TREATMENT

Treatment has traditionally been regarded in two parts: remission/induction and postremission/consolidation therapy. The rationale for going on with treatment beyond the point of CR is based on data from an experimental mouse model (L1210 leukaemia) and from children with ALL in whom it has been calculated that, at the time of presentation, the number of leukaemic blast cells is of the order of $10^{12}$ or $10^{13}$. At the point of CR, i.e. when there is no morphologically detectable leukaemia, there are still $10^8$ or $10^9$ leukaemic blast cells present. It is therefore not surprising that if no postremission therapy is given, the majority of patients develop recurrent leukaemia.

Remission/induction therapy usually includes an anthracycline drug such as daunorubicin or doxorubicin, given in conjunction with cytosine arabinoside. The first cycle of treatment is given in hospital; the patient needs to stay for about 4 weeks due to the risk of infection and bleeding consequent upon neutropenia and thrombocytopenia. Subsequent cycles of treatment are given as much as possible on an outpatient basis.

There is much debate as to the best postremission therapy. Alternatives include:

- Further cycles of chemotherapy which is the same as that given to induce remission
- Chemotherapy different from that given to induce remission
- Myeloablative therapy with allogeneic/autologous bone marrow transplantation (BMT) (see below)

With modern combination chemotherapy, approximately 70% of younger people (aged <60 years) would be expected to return to normal health. However, within 1–3 years, the disease will recur in at least 60% of the latter, the remainder almost certainly having been cured. In general, treatment has become more intensive over the last 20 years with a concomitant improvement in overall survival. Survival curves for patients treated at St Bartholomew's Hospital during three consecutive time periods are shown in Fig. 7.4.

Following recurrence, it is possible to give further treatment in an attempt to induce secondary remission but such remissions are rarely durable, hence the use of very intensive treatment involving BMT (see p. 371).

## TREATMENT AT RECURRENCE

Second remissions are more difficult to achieve and are virtually never durable. The decision to treat a person at the time of recurrence will therefore (even more than at presentation) depend on the patient's overall situation and his/her wishes. In younger patients, provided a second remission can be achieved, cure is still a possibility for a proportion, with the use of myeloablative therapy with allogeneic/autologous BMT (see p. 371).

In older patients, the options lie between further intensive combination chemotherapy and keeping the person as well as possible for as long as possible, with supportive measures such as blood transfusions for anaemia, antibiotics for infection and the judicious use of palliative oral drugs that help to lower the circulating blast cell count.

# Acute promyelocytic leukaemia (FAB-M3)

APML has a specific association with disseminated intravascular coagulation (DIC) (see p. 345). Patients may present with severe bleeding and this tends to increase when treatment is started as the leukaemic blast cells break down, leading to further consumption of clotting factors and platelets. Treatment consists of regular, twice daily, platelet transfusions and maintenance of the fibrinogen level with fresh frozen plasma. Provided remission can be achieved, patients with APML (which is associated with the chromosome translocation t(15;17)) have a somewhat better prognosis overall than patients with other subtypes of AML. Ensuring that they survive this early period of DIC is therefore critical.

It has recently been demonstrated that the use of a

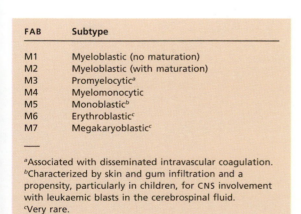

| FAB | Subtype |
|-----|---------|
| M1 | Myeloblastic (no maturation) |
| M2 | Myeloblastic (with maturation) |
| M3 | Promyelocytic[a] |
| M4 | Myelomonocytic |
| M5 | Monoblastic[b] |
| M6 | Erythroblastic[c] |
| M7 | Megakaryoblastic[c] |

[a]Associated with disseminated intravascular coagulation.
[b]Characterized by skin and gum infiltration and a propensity, particularly in children, for CNS involvement with leukaemic blasts in the cerebrospinal fluid.
[c]Very rare.

**Table 7.7** FAB classification of acute myelogenous leukaemia.

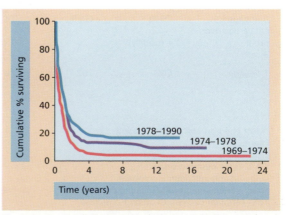

**Fig. 7.4** Acute myelogenous leukaemia—overall survival over three time periods.

| FAB | Cell type |
|-----|-----------|
| L1 | Homogeneous population of small cells (childhood ALL) |
| L2 | More heterogeneous population of cells (more often seen in adults) |
| L3 | Rare — cells like those in Burkitt's lymphoma |

**Table 7.8**   FAB classification of acute lymphoblastic leukaemia.

differentiating agent, all-*trans*-retinoic acid (ATRA), given orally can lead to the achievement of CR in some patients with APML. ATRA has a differentiating effect on leukaemic promyelocytes, both *in vitro* and *in vivo*. It does not appear to be effective in other subtypes of AML. Unfortunately such remissions do not last and need to be consolidated with conventional chemotherapy. The advantage is that patients receiving ATRA do not usually develop DIC, with a decrease in the risk of fatal haemorrhage.

## Acute lymphoblastic leukaemia

Predominantly a disease of children, ALL is also potentially curable. Overall, 90% of children respond to treatment and 50–60% are cured. The results in adults are not as good, with only approximately 30% being cured. ALL is classified on the basis of the morphology of the leukaemic blast cells into subtypes L1–L3 (Table 7.8).

There is also an 'immunological' classification which is continually evolving as more sophisticated techniques are developed for detecting the B- or T-cell origin of lymphoid cells (Table 7.9).

### TREATMENT

The principles of treatment are the same as for AML, the aim being to return the bone marrow to normal and the person to a normal state of health. The sequence of treatment is, however, somewhat different because ALL has a propensity for involvement of the central nervous system (CNS); thus treatment also includes prophylactic intrathecal drugs (methotrexate or cytosine arabinoside) with or without prophylactic cranial radiotherapy to the meninges. Most patients also receive oral maintenance therapy for 2–3 years. The sequence of treatment is shown in Fig. 7.5.

Cyclical combination chemotherapy comprising vincristine, prednisolone and an anthracycline such as doxorubicin forms the basis of most treatment regimens. Other drugs such as L-asparaginase, cyclophosphamide and/or cytosine arabinoside (also known as cytarabine) are also increasingly being used in patients (both adults and children) considered to be at high risk of recurrence.

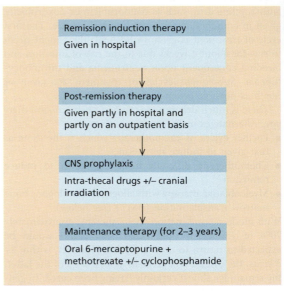

**Fig. 7.5**   Treatment regimen for acute lymphoblastic leukaemia.

| Phenotypic markers | | | | | | |
|---|---|---|---|---|---|---|
| *B lineage* | CD10 | CD19 | TdT | Ia | CyIg | SmIg |
| cALLa positive[a] | + | + | + | + | − | − |
| pre-B | + (usually) | + | + | + | + | − |
| B-cell[b] | ± | + | − | + | ± | + |
| *T lineage* | CD7 | CD2 | TdT | | | |
| pre-T | + | − | + | | | |
| T-cell | + | + | + | | | |

——

[a]Most children and >50% of adults.
[b]Rare.
cALLa, Common ALL antigen.
CD, Cluster designation.
CyIg, Cytoplasmic immunoglobulin.
SmIg, Surface membrane immunoglobulin.
TdT, Terminal deoxynucleotidyl transferase.

**Table 7.9**   Immunological categories of acute lymphoblastic leukaemia.

Although a proportion of adult patients are cured with the initial therapy, in the rest the disease recurs and ultimately proves fatal unless secondary remission can be achieved and further treatment involving BMT given, when a further 20–30% of patients will survive long term.

## TREATMENT AT RECURRENCE

Recurrence of ALL occurs most frequently in the bone marrow and is associated with a worse prognosis if it occurs during maintenance therapy. CNS recurrence, detected by the presence of leukaemic blast cells in the cerebrospinal fluid, is now less frequent since the regular use of CNS prophylaxis. Treatment comprises intrathecal drugs plus radiotherapy to the meninges surrounding the brain and spinal cord, followed by reinduction chemotherapy if the recurrence is limited to the CNS. Unfortunately, it often occurs in association with bone marrow recurrence, when induction of a second CR followed by myeloablative therapy with allogeneic or autologous BMT is the only potentially curative option.

Testicular recurrence is usually manifest by painless enlargement of one or both testicles. It can occur in isolation, shortly before, or concurrent with bone marrow recurrence. Treatment involves radiotherapy to the testes, followed by reinduction chemotherapy (for isolated testicular recurrence) or, if the marrow is also involved, the latter followed by myeloablative therapy with allogeneic or autologous BMT, provided a second remission can be achieved.

# Chronic myeloid leukaemia

The majority of patients die within 5 years of diagnosis. The illness has a progressive clinical course which starts with a chronic phase of 3–4 years' duration. This evolves into an accelerated phase which may be manifest by fever, weight loss, increasing splenomegaly, anaemia, thrombocythaemia and refractory leukocytosis with increasing numbers of blast cells. The duration of the accelerated phase is variable though blastic transformation usually supervenes within a few months. Unlike *de novo* acute leukaemia, the blastic phase of CML is characterized by the development of acute leukaemia which may be myeloid (60%), lymphoid (30%) or erythroid (10%) in origin. The blastic phase is generally refractory to treatment, the median survival being less than 6 months. Less frequently, CML transforms into myelofibrosis, death ensuing from bone marrow failure.

## CLINICAL FEATURES
### Symptoms
These are usually of insidious onset:
● Anaemia
● Sweating at night, fever, weight loss
● Abdominal discomfort due to splenic enlargement

### Signs
● Anaemia
● Splenomegaly

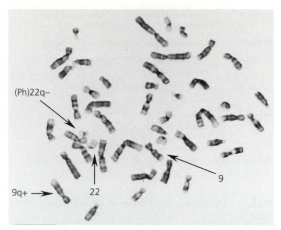

**Fig. 7.6** Philadelphia chromosome. This is formed by a reciprocal translocation of part of the long arm (q) of chromosome 22 to chromosome 9. It is seen in 90–95% of patients with chronic granulocytic leukaemia. The karyotype is expressed as 46XX, t(9;22)(q34;q11).

## INVESTIGATION

BLOOD COUNT:
  Hb low or normal.
  WCC raised with characteristically the whole spectrum of myeloid precursors, including a few blast cells.
  Platelet count low, normal or raised.
BONE MARROW ASPIRATE shows a hypercellular marrow with an increase in myeloid precursors. On cytogenetic analysis, the Ph chromosome t(9;22) is present in most patients (Fig. 7.6).

## TREATMENT

CONVENTIONAL TREATMENT — the aim is to relieve symptoms, keep the WCC under control and reduce the size of the spleen. Most patients are currently treated with hydroxyurea (or busulphan) given orally with allopurinol to prevent hyperuricaemia.

MYELOABLATIVE THERAPY SUPPORTED BY ALLOGENEIC BMT can be curative but the approach is limited by donor availability, the age of the patient, and the morbidity and mortality of the transplant procedure (see below).

EXPERIMENTAL TREATMENT — trials involving IFN are currently in progress to determine whether this drug is any 'better' than the conventional treatment (see p. 360).

# Chronic lymphocytic leukaemia

CLL is an incurable disease of older people, characterized by an uncontrolled proliferation and accumulation of mature B lymphocytes (although T-cell CLL does occur). The symptoms are a consequence of bone marrow failure, i.e. anaemia, infection and bleeding. A proportion of patients remain asymptomatic and never need any treatment, dying of an unrelated cause; in the remainder, the disease can usually be kept under control for 9–10 years, infection being the predominant cause of death.

| Stage 0 | Lymphocytosis only (in blood and bone marrow) |
| Stage I | Lymphocytosis with lymphadenopathy |
| Stage II | Lymphocytosis with hepatic and/or splenic enlargement |
| Stage III | Lymphocytosis with anaemia (Hb <11 g dl⁻¹) |
| Stage IV | Lymphocytosis with thrombocytopenia (platelets <100 × 10⁹/litre) |

---

Lymphocytosis: white cell count >15 × 10⁹/litre of which >40% are lymphocytes.

**Table 7.10**  RAI staging classification of chronic lymphoblastic leukaemia.

## CLINICAL FEATURES

As mentioned above, some patients may be asymptomatic, the diagnosis being a chance finding on the basis of a blood count done for a quite different reason.

**Symptoms**
- Symptoms of anaemia may develop rapidly in the context of haemolysis, which is usually precipitated by infection.
- Recurrent infections are due to neutropenia with or without reduced immunoglobulin levels.
- Painless lymph node enlargement.

**Signs**
Any combination of:
- Signs of anaemia
- Lymph node enlargement
- Enlarged liver and/or spleen

## INVESTIGATIONS

BLOOD COUNT:
    Hb low or normal
    WCC >15 × 10⁹/litre of which at least 40% are lymphocytes
    Platelets low or normal
SERUM IMMUNOGLOBULINS low or normal
COOMBS' TEST positive if haemolysis is occurring
Two different staging classifications are in use (Tables 7.10 and 7.11). They are useful because they correlate closely with prognosis. The median survival of patients with stage 0 (or stage A) CLL is 8 years as compared with 2 years for patients presenting with stages III or IV (or stage C) disease.

## TREATMENT

The disease may remain stable for several years. There is no advantage to starting treatment before there is a clinical indication, e.g. anaemia, recurrent infections, bleeding, 'bulky' lymphadenopathy or increasing splenomegaly. Chlorambucil is most often used. The purine analogues, fludarabine and 2-chloroadenosine acetate, are being evaluated, interest lying in the fact that CR can be achieved although such remissions are rarely durable.

# Hairy cell leukaemia (HCL)

A rare disease of late middle age, HCL represents again a clonal proliferation of abnormal B (or very rarely, T) cells which, as in CLL, accumulate in the bone marrow and spleen. The bizarre name relates to the appearance of the cells on a blood film where they have an irregular outline due to the presence of filament-like cytoplasmic projections.

## CLINICAL FEATURES
**Symptoms**
- Symptoms of anaemia
- Recurrent infections
- Abdominal discomfort due to splenic enlargement

**Signs**
- Signs of anaemia
- Palpable spleen

## INVESTIGATIONS
BLOOD COUNT:
    Hb usually low
    WCC usually low (or raised with circulating 'hairy cells')
    Platelets usually low
BONE MARROW shows increased cellularity with characteristic infiltration by 'hairy' cells

## TREATMENT
The use of IFN (see p. 360) has revolutionized the management of patients with this illness. Although CR is rarely achieved, in the majority of cases the blood count

| Stage A | < Three involved lymphoid areasᵃ | Hb > 10 g dl⁻¹ |
| Stage B | > Three involved lymphoid areas | Platelets <100 × 10⁹/litre |
| Stage C | Any number of involved lymphoid areas | Hb <10 g dl⁻¹ |
| | | Platelets <100 × 10⁹/litre |

---

ᵃThe cervical, axillary and inguinal lymph node groups (whether unilateral or bilateral), the spleen and the liver each count as one area; therefore, the number of involved areas can be any value between 0 and 5.

**Table 7.11**  Binet staging classification of chronic lymphoblastic leukaemia.

reverts to normal obviating the need for regular blood transfusions and admissions to hospital with life-threatening infections. Such remissions are temporary but treatment can be given repeatedly. Two new drugs, deoxycoformycin and 2-chloroadenosine acetate (2-CDA), are of interest because CR is achieved much more frequently than with IFN.

## Prolymphocytic leukaemia

Another rare B-cell disorder, often mistaken for CLL, prolymphocytic leukaemia, is characterized by bone marrow failure (anaemia, neutropenia and thrombocytopenia) and, as in HCL, splenomegaly. Treatment is generally with chlorambucil as for CLL, though splenectomy may be indicated and, again, fludarabine is being evaluated.

# The lymphomas

Lymphomas represent abnormal proliferations of different parts of the lymphoid system and are currently classified on the basis of histological appearance into:

- Hodgkin's disease
- Various subtypes of non-Hodgkin's lymphoma

## Hodgkin's disease (HD)

With modern treatment (radiotherapy, chemotherapy or both), HD is now a potentially curable illness. The choice of treatment is determined largely by the distribution and extent of disease (i.e. the 'stage') (Table 7.12).

| | |
|---|---|
| I | Involvement of a single LN region (I) or a single extralymphatic organ or site (I$_E$) |
| II | Involvement of two or more LN regions on the same side of the diaphragm (II) or one or more LN regions plus an extralymphatic site (II$_E$) |
| III | Involvement of LN regions on both sides of the diaphragm (III) (the spleen is included in stage III, e.g. splenic involvement plus cervical LN enlargement = stage III) |
| IV | Involvement of one or more extralymphatic organs, e.g. lung, liver, bone, bone marrow, with or without LN involvement |

LN, lymph node.
'Bulky' disease, a LN mass >10 cm in diameter, or if involving the mediastinum a mass greater than one-third of the intrathoracic diameter at the level of T10 is denoted by the suffix X.

**Table 7.12** Staging classification of Hodgkin's disease (modified Ann Arbor classification). All stages subclassified as A (asymptomatic) or B (fever, night sweats and loss of >10% of body weight).

## CLINICAL FEATURES

### Symptoms

- Painless lymph node enlargement (most often the cervical nodes). The majority of patients present with lymph node enlargement; the latter however in itself does not imply the diagnosis of lymphoma. The differential diagnosis of cervical lymph node enlargement is shown in Table 7.13.
  - 'B' symptoms: fever, drenching night sweats, weight loss of >10% body weight (see Table 7.12).
- Other constitutional symptoms, e.g. pruritus, fatigue, anorexia and alcohol-induced pain at the site of enlarged lymph nodes.
- Symptoms due to involvement of other organs, e.g. lung, bone, liver.

### Signs

- Peripheral lymph node enlargement
- Enlargement of the spleen/liver depending on stage

## INVESTIGATIONS

BLOOD COUNT: normal or a normochromic, normocytic anaemia

---

*Infections*
Acute
  Pyogenic infections
  Infective mononucleosis
  Toxoplasmosis
  Cytomegalovirus infection
  Infected eczema
  Cat scratch fever
  Acute childhood exanthema

Chronic
  Tuberculosis
  Syphilis
  Sarcoidosis
  HIV infection

*Connective tissue disorders*
Rheumatoid arthritis

*Drug reactions*
Phenytoin

*Primary lymph node malignancies*
Hodgkin's disease
Non-Hodgkin's lymphoma
Chronic lymphocytic leukaemia
Acute lymphoblastic leukaemia

*Secondary malignancies*
Nasopharyngeal
Thyroid
Laryngeal
Lung
Breast
Stomach

*Miscellaneous*
Sinus histiocytosis
Kawasaki's syndrome

**Table 7.13** Differential diagnosis of cervical lymph node enlargement.

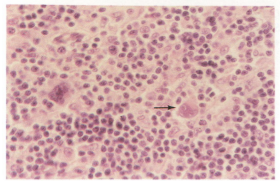

**Fig. 7.7** Histological appearance of Hodgkin's disease showing a background rich in small lymphocytes and histocytes together with scattered mononuclear Hodgkin's cells and a classical binucleate Sternberg–Reed cell (arrow) to the right of centre. Courtesy of Dr A.J. Norton.

ERYTHROCYTE SEDIMENTATION RATE (ESR) usually raised

LIVER BIOCHEMISTRY — abnormal if liver involved

URIC ACID — normal or raised

CHEST X-RAY — may show mediastinal (with or without lung involvement)

CT SCANS — may show involvement of intrathoracic, abdominal or pelvic lymph nodes

BONE MARROW ASPIRATE AND TREPHINE BIOPSY — may show involvement in patients with advanced disease

LYMPH NODE BIOPSY — required for a definitive diagnosis. Classically, Sternberg–Reed cells (Fig. 7.7) are present together with a characteristic admixture of lymphocytes and histiocytes

A typical chest X-ray and CT scan of the same patient are shown in Fig. 7.8.

## 'STAGING'

The 'stage' of disease, i.e. its extent and distribution, will influence the choice of treatment. There is currently debate as to the need for a 'staging laparotomy'. The aim of the latter is to biopsy any intra-abdominal lymph nodes which appear enlarged and to perform a splenectomy, the spleen being notoriously difficult to demonstrate as being involved with lymphoma by any radiological technique.

The original Ann Arbor staging classification has been modified (see Table 7.12) to take into account the volume of lymph node masses and the use of modern imaging techniques such as CT scanning.

The long-term outcome is closely related to stage (Fig. 7.9).

## TREATMENT

Treatment is virtually always given with curative intent and consists of radiotherapy, cyclical combination chemotherapy or both. The choice of treatment will depend predominantly on:

- Stage
- Involved sites
- 'Bulk' of lymph node masses
- Presence or absence of B symptoms (see Table 7.12)

### Stages IA and IIA

The majority of patients are treated with radiotherapy, provided that all the involved sites can be encompassed within a radiation field. Patients with a large 'bulky' mediastinal mass are usually given chemotherapy initially, since otherwise too much lung tissue would be irradiated with potential long-term lung damage. Such patients receive radiotherapy subsequently (see below).

### Stages IIB, IIIA/B, IVA/B

Most patients are treated with chemotherapy in the first instance, with subsequent radiotherapy to sites of 'bulky' disease to prevent local recurrence. (In practice, the latter applies mainly to patients with a large mediastinal mass at presentation as above.)

The first effective chemotherapy for HD, a regimen comprising mustine, vincristine (oncovin), procarbazine and prednisolone (MOPP) was used until recently, when the combination ABVD (doxorubicin (previously known as Adriamycin), bleomycin, vinblastine and dacarbazine) was developed and added to MOPP, as alternating cycles.

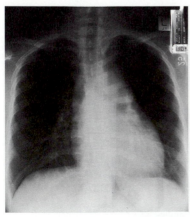

(a)

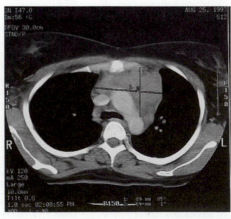

(b)

**Fig. 7.8** (a) A chest X-ray and (b) a CT scan of a large mediastinal mass (indicated by cross lines) due to Hodgkin's disease.

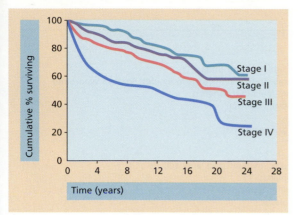

**Fig. 7.9** Survival in Hodgkin's disease related to stage at presentation.

Apart from the immediate side-effects of nausea, vomiting and hair loss, potential long-term side-effects, namely infertility and second malignancy, have caused concern. Current 'MOPP-EVA' so-called 'HYBRID' treatment programmes have therefore been designed to minimize these long-term effects, by reducing the amount of alkylating agent and adding drugs such as doxorubicin. The emphasis has been on using alternating, non-cross-resistant drug combinations, given as cycles of treatment, e.g. every 4 weeks for about 6 months. Treatment can usually be given on an outpatient basis and most people are able to lead a normal life. The prognosis correlates closely with stage (Fig. 7.9). However, survival of patients in whom recurrence occurs is inferior to that of those who remain in continuous remission (Fig. 7.10).

### RESISTANT DISEASE AND RECURRENCE
Failure to achieve an initial complete or almost complete response and early recurrence (within 1 year of remission being achieved) are both associated with a very poor prognosis. Similarly, patients who develop recurrent HD

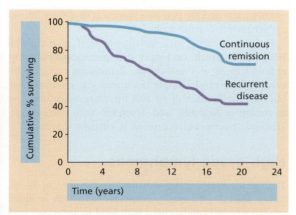

**Fig. 7.10** Survival courses of patients with Hodgkin's disease. (After Oza A.M. *et al*. (1993) Patterns of survival in patients with Hodgkin's disease: long follow up in a single centre. *Annals of Oncology* **4**, 385–392. Reprinted by permission of Kluwer Academic Publishers.)

more than once will almost certainly die of HD eventually. Hence, the use of myeloablative therapy with autologous bone marrow or peripheral blood progenitor cell support in these situations (see p. 371). In contrast, patients who develop recurrent HD, e.g. within the abdomen, a few years after receiving radiotherapy for localized, supradiaphragmatic disease can be given combination chemotherapy, still with curative intent.

## Non-Hodgkin's lymphoma (NHL)

The term non-Hodgkin's lymphoma encompasses many different histological subtypes. The basic subdivision into high and low grade (Kiel classification) reflects the rate at which the cells are dividing. Ironically, high-grade lymphomas (those in which the cells are dividing quickly) are potentially curable, whereas low-grade lymphomas are generally considered to be incurable with conventional therapy, although patients may live for a number of years and respond to treatment several times. A further subdivision is made on the basis of B- or T-cell origin. Most NHLs are of B-cell phenotype although T-cell tumours are increasingly being recognized. Several different histological groupings have been suggested; the two most widely used at present are the Kiel classification (Table 7.14) and the 'Working Formulation' (Table 7.15). The latter (which looks much simpler) is not really a histological classification but an attempt to group together diseases which behave in a relatively similar way, to allow comparison between treatment results.

### CLINICAL FEATURES
Most patients present with peripheral lymph node enlargement, with or without systemic symptoms. Patients with low-grade lymphoma often have bone marrow infiltration and may have symptoms of anaemia, recurrent infections or bleeding. In addition to peripheral lymphadenopathy, NHLs frequently also involve mediastinal, intra-abdominal and pelvic lymph nodes with resulting symptoms. In contrast, they may involve only an extranodal site, e.g. part of the gastrointestinal tract.

### INVESTIGATIONS
FULL BLOOD COUNT AND ESR — anaemia; an elevated WCC or thrombocytopenia would be suggestive of bone marrow infiltration.

UREA AND ELECTROLYTES — patients may, for example, have renal impairment as a consequence of ureteric obstruction, secondary to intra-abdominal or pelvic lymph node enlargement.

LIVER BIOCHEMISTRY may be abnormal if there is hepatic involvement.

CHEST X-RAY.

CT SCANS of chest, abdomen and pelvis.

BONE MARROW ASPIRATE AND TREPHINE BIOPSY.

LYMPH NODE BIOPSY (or Trucut needle biopsy in the case of surgically inaccessible nodes).

### TREATMENT
Treatment will depend on the extent and distribution of disease as well as on histological subtype. Patients with

| B cell | T cell |
|--------|--------|
| *Low grade* | |
| Lymphocytic (CLL and others)[a] | Lymphocytic (CLL and others)[a] |
| Lymphoplasmacytoid | Small cerebriform cell (mycosis fungoides, Sézary's syndrome) |
| Plasmacytic | Lymphoepithelioid (Lennert's) |
| Centroblastic/centrocytic (follicular or diffuse) | Angioimmunoblastic |
| Centrocytic | T zone |
| | Pleomorphic, small cell |
| *High grade* | |
| Centroblastic | Pleomorphic, medium and large cell |
| Immunoblastic | Immunoblastic |
| Large cell anaplastic (Ki-1+)[b] | Large cell anaplastic (Ki-1+)[b] |
| Burkitt's lymphoma | Lymphoblastic |
| Lymphoblastic | |

[a]CLL, chronic lymphocytic leukaemia.
[b]Ki-1 is an activation marker; + indicates expression of this marker.
From Stansfeld AG (1988) *Lancet* **i**, 292–293.

**Table 7.14**  Updated Kiel classification of non-Hodgkin's lymphomas.

| *Low grade* | |
|---|---|
| A | Small lymphocytic |
| B | Follicular small-cleaved |
| C | Follicular mixed histiocytic |
| *Intermediate grade* | |
| D | Follicular large-cell |
| E | Diffuse small-cleaved |
| F | Diffuse mixed histiocytic |
| G | Diffuse large-cell |
| *High grade* | |
| H | Immunoblastic |
| I | Lymphoblastic |
| J | Small non-cleaved |

**Table 7.15**  Working Formulation for non-Hodgkin's lymphoma.

stage I disease can be cured with radiotherapy alone (or radiotherapy plus chemotherapy); those with more extensive involvement require systemic therapy.

## Low-grade lymphomas (Tables 7.14 and 7.15)

Three subtypes will be discussed.

### Follicular lymphoma

Repeated remissions can usually be achieved with relatively simple treatment, e.g. the alkylating agent chlorambucil. More intensive treatment has thus far not been shown to improve survival. The response rate at presentation, first and second recurrence is approximately 75%, with a median survival of 9 years. With such conventional therapy, the disease remains incurable, and new approaches such as IFN and the use of myeloablative therapy with allogeneic or autologous BMT are therefore being investigated.

### Low-grade B-cell diffuse lymphomas (generally either lymphoplasmacytoid or centrocytic)

The majority of patients present with advanced disease, the bone marrow frequently being involved. In the small proportion of patients who present with localized disease, the site may be extranodal, most frequently the gastrointestinal tract. The prognosis for patients with low-grade B-cell diffuse lymphoma is worse than that of patients with equivalent stage follicular lymphoma, with a median survival of 3.5 years, fewer than 20% surviving more than 5 years.

### Low-grade T-cell lymphoma

These tumours are less common than their B-cell counterparts and are part of a spectrum of disease known as 'peripheral T-cell lymphomas'.

Patients present with enlargement of a peripheral lymph node which, on biopsy and immunophenotyping, is found to be of T-cell origin. Remissions can be achieved with relatively simple treatment, e.g. chlorambucil, but are usually short-lived and therefore more intensive treatment is generally used. However, with current conventional treatment, recurrence is virtually inevitable.

## High-grade lymphomas

High-grade lymphomas are more commonly of B-cell, rather than T-cell, origin. Some patients with localized (stage I disease) can be cured with local radiotherapy with or without chemotherapy, or chemotherapy alone. However, the majority present with more advanced disease, chemotherapy being usually given with curative intent. Achievement of a CR is a prerequisite for cure.

## TREATMENT

Treatment usually comprises an anthracycline, e.g. doxorubicin given with cyclophosphamide, vincristine (oncovin) and prednisolone (CHOP). Variations on a theme of CHOP have since been tried but thus far none has been shown to be definitively superior in terms of survival. Three factors correlate with survival: advanced disease (stage III and IV), a high serum lactate dehydrogenase (LDH) and poor performance status (an estimate of the person's general state of health) are all associated with a poor prognosis.

With modern combination chemotherapy, 60–70% of patients respond to treatment and about one-third overall are cured. The treatment is inevitably myelosuppressive and therefore, particularly in older patients, the main problem is potentially fatal infection as a consequence of neutropenia. Recurrent high-grade lymphoma has a grave prognosis. However, a proportion of patients who respond to further chemotherapy at recurrence can still be cured with myeloablative therapy supported by autologous BMT or peripheral blood progenitor cells.

## Burkitt's lymphoma

Burkitt's lymphoma was first described by Dennis Burkitt in children in West Africa who presented with a specific syndrome comprising a lesion in the jaw (Fig. 7.11), extranodal abdominal involvement and ovarian tumours. This specific type of lymphoma is found in areas of Africa where there is a high incidence of the Epstein Barr virus (EBV) and in areas where malaria is common. Most patients have EBV antibodies in the serum. The tumour can be treated with both radiation and chemotherapy and is associated with a chromosome change, most commonly t(18;14) (see p. 122).

## *Myeloablative therapy with bone marrow transplantation*

High doses of chemotherapy, such as cyclophosphamide, and radiation both kill cells indiscriminately; myelo-

suppression is therefore the main dose-limiting toxicity. Thus, without a 'transplant' the person would die of bone marrow failure.

The indications for this type of treatment are shown in Table 7.16.

## Allogeneic BMT

The donor is usually an HLA-identical brother or sister. The patient (recipient) receives the myeloablative therapy (drugs or drugs plus total body irradiation [TBI]), over a period of several days. The donor supplies approximately 1 litre of bone marrow, aspirated from the posterior iliac crests, which is then given intravenously to the recipient, together with immunosuppressive drugs (e.g. steroids, cyclosporin) to prevent rejection and graft-versus-host disease (GVHD). The patient's blood count usually recovers within 3–4 weeks.

Allogeneic BMT has a mortality of 25–40%, depending mainly on the person's age; the main causes of death are infection (bacterial, fungal or viral, cytomegalovirus pneumonitis being the greatest problem) and GVHD. The latter is a syndrome that can occur to varying degrees, in which mature T lymphocytes in the donor marrow infiltrate the skin, gut and liver. Acute GVHD occurs in the first 3 months but may also run a chronic course. Patients who develop GVHD have a lower incidence of recurrent leukaemia than those who do not, e.g. the recipients of syngeneic (twin) transplants. Thus, not only does the 'marrow ablative' chemoradiotherapy have an antileukaemic effect, but T cells within the donor

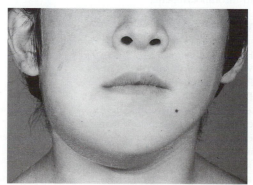

**Fig. 7.11** A child with Burkitt's lymphoma.

> **Allogeneic BMT**
> Genetic disorders, e.g. thalassaemia
> Aplastic anaemia
> AML in first CR (patients aged <20 years)
> AML and ALL in second CR
> CML in chronic phase
>
> **Myeloablative therapy with autologous BMT/PBPC**
> This is still an experimental treatment in many situations, e.g.
> AML in first CR
> Adult ALL in first CR
> AML and ALL in second CR
> Low-grade NHL and HD once recurrence has occurred (with regard to HD, either very early recurrence or more than one)
> High-grade NHL in first remission in patients at high risk of recurrence
> High-grade NHL in second remission
>
> ——
>
> ALL, acute lymphoblastic leukaemia; AML, acute myelogenous leukaemia; BMT, bone marrow transplantation; CML, chronic myeloid leukaemia; CR, complete remission; HD, Hodgkin's disease; NHL, non-Hodgkin lymphoma; PBPC, peripheral blood progenitor cells.

**Table 7.16** Possible indications for the use of myeloablative therapy.

marrow appear to have an immunological role, the 'graft vs. leukaemia' effect, which itself correlates with the development of GVHD.

The use of allogeneic transplantation is primarily limited by donor availability; using a 'matched unrelated donor' increases the likelihood of GVHD, which, as mentioned above, is the major cause of mortality and long-term morbidity (chronic GVHD). T-cell depletion of the donor marrow has been attempted but this also removes the putative 'graft vs. leukaemia' effect, resulting in an increased risk of recurrence.

## Autologous BMT

Using the patient's own bone marrow is limited by the potential risk of reinfusing malignant cells.

A remission is first induced; 1 litre of marrow is then aspirated from the patient's iliac crests under general anaesthetic and (usually) cryopreserved. The myeloablative therapy is given and the thawed marrow reinfused intravenously, as with an allogeneic transplant. The time to blood count recovery after an autograft is usually somewhat longer than after an allograft. Methods to remove malignant cells, as well as methods to induce a 'graft vs. leukaemia' effect, are currently being investigated.

The mortality is considerably lower than with allogeneic BMT (5–10%), GVHD not being a problem. Bacterial and fungal infection are the greatest risk; viral and fungal infections can continue to be a problem for up to 1 year afterwards due to a reversal of the normal T helper : suppressor cell ratio.

## The use of peripheral blood progenitor cells (PBPC) instead of autologous bone marrow to support myeloablative therapy

It is possible, by using chemotherapy for ablation followed by the growth factor G-CSF (see p. 360), to stimulate haemopoietic progenitor cells in the marrow to proliferate, so that they can be collected from the peripheral blood. PBPC are increasingly being used instead of autologous bone marrow since, because they are more differentiated cells, the time to recovery of the blood count is only 2–3 weeks, with obvious advantages in both human and economic terms. PBPC have predominantly been used in patients with HD and NHL in an experimental setting.

## The paraproteinaemias

## Multiple myeloma

Myeloma is part of a spectrum of diseases characterized by the presence of a paraprotein in the serum that can be demonstrated as a monoclonal, dark-staining band on protein electrophoresis. The paraprotein is produced by abnormal, proliferating plasma cells that produce, most often, IgG or IgA and rarely IgD. The paraproteinaemia may be associated with excretion of light chains in the urine, which are either κ or λ; the excess light chains have for many years been known as Bence-Jones protein.

### CLINICAL FEATURES

Myeloma is a disease of the elderly, the median age at presentation being 60 years. It is a complex illness which represents the interrelationship between:

BONE DESTRUCTION causing fractures, vertebral collapse (which can cause spinal cord compression) and hypercalcaemia.

BONE MARROW INFILTRATION resulting in anaemia, neutropenia and thrombocytopenia, together with production of an abnormal protein which may (rarely) result in symptoms of hyperviscosity.

RENAL IMPAIRMENT due to a complex combination of factors, i.e. deposition of light chains, hypercalcaemia, hyperuricaemia and, usually in patients who have had the disease for some time, deposition of amyloid.

All of this is further complicated by a reduction in the normal immunoglobulin levels contributing to the tendency for patients with myeloma to have recurrent infections.

### PROGNOSIS

Severe anaemia and renal failure at presentation used to be the two main factors associated with a very poor prognosis, with 50% of patients dying within 9 months. The availability of renal dialysis has reduced the impact of renal failure. In patients without these features at presentation, the median survival with treatment is of the order of 2 years.

### SYMPTOMS

- Bone pain, most commonly backache due to vertebral involvement
- Symptoms of anaemia
- Recurrent infections
- Symptoms of renal failure
- Symptoms of hypercalcaemia
- Rarely, symptoms of hyperviscosity and bleeding due to thrombocytopenia

### INVESTIGATIONS

FULL BLOOD COUNT:
  Hb normal or low
  WCC normal or low
  Platelets normal or low
  ESR almost always high

BLOOD FILM — there may be rouleaux formation as a consequence of the paraprotein

UREA AND ELECTROLYTES — there may be evidence of renal failure (see above)

SERUM CALCIUM — normal or raised

SERUM ALKALINE PHOSPHATASE — usually normal

TOTAL PROTEIN — normal or raised

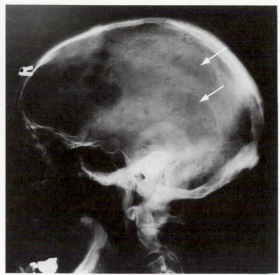

**Fig. 7.12** Myeloma affecting the skull. Note the rounded lytic translucencies produced by infiltration of the skull with myeloma cells.

SERUM ALBUMIN — normal or low
PROTEIN ELECTROPHORESIS — characteristically shows a monoclonal band
URIC ACID — normal or raised
SKELETAL SURVEY — characteristic lytic lesions, most easily seen in the skull (Fig 7.12)
URINE — for assessment of light chain excretion
BONE MARROW ASPIRATE — shows characteristic infiltration by plasma cells (Fig 7.13)

## TREATMENT
### General
Bone pain can be helped by radiotherapy. Pathological fractures may be prevented by prompt orthopaedic surgery with pinning of lytic bone lesions seen on the skeletal survey. Renal impairment requires urgent attention and patients may need to be considered for long-term peritoneal dialysis or haemodialysis. Renal impairment is

often a consequence of hypercalcaemia which requires correction with bisphosphonates (disodium etidronate: i.v. infusion 7.5 mg kg$^{-1}$ for 3 days) (see p. 432) or hydration and systemic steroids if bisphosphonates are not available. Anaemia should be corrected and infection treated. Patients with spinal cord compression known to be due to myeloma are treated with dexamethasone, followed by radiotherapy to the lesion delineated by a myelogram. Hyperviscosity is treated by plasmapheresis, together with systemic therapy.

### Specific
The use of alkylating agents, e.g. melphalan or cyclophosphamide, given in conjunction with prednisolone has increased the survival from 7 months to 2.5 years. Recently, more intensive doxorubicin-containing regimens have been used, and in selected patients high-dose melphalan with allogeneic or autologous BMT or PBPC rescue have been tried. Adjuvant IFN therapy following both standard chemotherapy and very intensive treatment involving allogeneic or autologous BMT is being evaluated.

# Waldenström's macroglobulinaemia

An illness most often seen in elderly men, the clinical features may be more like those of lymphoma, i.e. peripheral lymph node enlargement and symptoms due to bone marrow infiltration, or symptoms of hyperviscosity may predominate.

## CLINICAL FEATURES
- General malaise and weight loss
- Lymph node enlargement
- Symptoms of hyperviscosity (headaches, visual disturbance)
- Symptoms of anaemia
- A bleeding tendency

## INVESTIGATION
BLOOD COUNT:
  Hb normal or low
  WBC normal or low
  Platelets normal or low
  ESR usually raised
BLOOD FILM usually shows rouleaux formation
BONE MARROW ASPIRATE usually shows infiltration with lymphoplasmacytoid cells
PROTEIN ELECTROPHORESIS shows an IgM paraprotein

## TREATMENT
Alkylating agents and, in younger patients, more intensive doxorubicin-containing regimens produce meaningful responses but recurrence is inevitable. In patients in whom hyperviscosity is the main problem, regular plasmapheresis can be helpful. Death results from progressive bone marrow infiltration and infection.

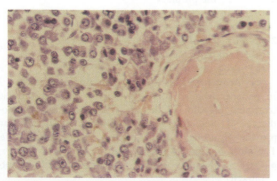

**Fig. 7.13** Multiple myeloma showing replacement of the medullary cavity by abnormal plasma cells with some binucleate forms. A residual bony trabeculum is present to the right of the figure. Courtesy of Dr A.J. Norton.

## Monoclonal gammopathy of undetermined significance (MGUS)

This is characteristically seen in older people; a paraprotein is found in the blood but the level is low ($<2$g litre$^{-1}$). Patients may be quite asymptomatic and the paraprotein detected as a result of investigations for some quite different reason. The blood count is usually normal and there is no renal impairment or bone destruction. In such patients, no specific treatment is required but they should be followed up regularly in case they later develop lymphoma or myeloma.

# Solid tumours

The treatment of solid tumours involves the combined use of surgery, radiotherapy and chemotherapy. In the earlier stages surgery alone may be curative in many solid tumours, but may fail because of inadequate local excision with residual microscopic disease or because of disseminated micrometastases present at the time of diagnosis. Radiotherapy, similarly, is a local treatment which can often be used after surgery to reduce the chance of local recurrence. Good examples of this are breast cancer, where the use of surgery plus radiotherapy makes it possible to carry out breast-conserving surgery, and in rectal cancer, where local relapse in the pelvis can be reduced by the addition of radiotherapy. In some solid tumours, like early laryngeal cancer, radiotherapy can be used on its own with curative intent. It also has an important role in palliative treatment.

Chemotherapy is systemic treatment which can reach any part of the body with an adequate blood supply and is therefore normally used to treat disseminated cancer. Only a minority of metastatic solid cancers can routinely be cured with chemotherapy. These include testicular cancer, choriocarcinoma and childhood solid tumours. In other advanced solid tumours, chemotherapy may cure a small minority but it is usually given with the intention of prolonging life and relieving symptoms. In this situation it may be used to reduce the volume of the tumour without any realistic hope of eradicating disease. When chemotherapy is used without prospect of cure it is essential that care is taken choosing drugs with the least side-effects. The development of new less toxic chemotherapeutic drugs and more effective antiemetics have done much to reduce the side-effects of chemotherapy.

Chemotherapy is increasingly being used in patients who have had surgical clearance of their primary tumour but are at high risk of relapse from metastatic disease at distant sites. When used in this situation as adjuvant chemotherapy, there is a much greater chance of eradicating the tumour than when chemotherapy is given at the time of clinical relapse.

## Breast cancer

Breast cancer is the commonest cancer in women. Although surgical removal of the primary tumour is usu-

ally possible, most women will eventually relapse with metastatic disease.

### Adjuvant therapy

Adjuvant therapy immediately following surgery has reduced the number of women dying from breast cancer by about 25%. A meta-analysis of all randomized trials of adjuvant therapy in breast cancer has shown conclusively that *adjuvant chemotherapy*, most commonly cyclophosphamide, methotrexate and 5-fluorouracil, for 6 months reduces the death rate by about 25% in premenopausal node-positive women. *Adjuvant tamoxifen* given for 2–5 years reduces death from breast cancer by a similar amount in postmenopausal patients.

Trials to improve these results further are in progress.

### Advanced disease

Patients with established metastatic disease are treated with hormonal therapy or chemotherapy. Women who have high levels of oestrogen receptors in their tumour have a greater chance of responding to hormonal treatments. In addition certain clinical features can predict the likelihood of responding to hormonal manipulations.

1 *More likely to respond to hormonal treatment*
   (a) Receptor positive
   (b) Long interval from initial surgery to time of relapse
   (c) Metastatic disease in bone and soft tissue
2 *Less likely to respond to hormonal treatments*
   (a) Receptor negative
   (b) Short interval from initial surgery to relapse
   (c) Liver metastases or lymphangitis carcinomatosa

Endocrine therapy is usually tried first in those patients who have characteristics suggesting they are likely to respond. Useful remissions can be obtained for years and many elderly patients may live a normal life expectancy despite still having residual breast cancer. A range of hormonal manipulations are available:

1 *Premenopausal*
   (a) Cessation of ovarian function
       (i) Oophorectomy
       (ii) Radiation-induced ovarian ablation
       (iii) LHRH analogue with down-regulation of the pituitary
   (b) Anti-oestrogen—tamoxifen
   (c) Progesterone
2 *Postmenopausal*
   (a) Tamoxifen
   (b) Progesterone
   (c) Aromatase inhibitors, e.g. aminoglutethamide

In patients who are unlikely to respond to hormonal treatment or who fail therapy with hormones, chemotherapy is used. If chosen carefully chemotherapy can provide good quality palliation and prolongation of life. The most common regimens used include:

- CMF (cyclophosphamide, methotrexate, 5-fluorouracil)
- MMM (mitozantrone, methotrexate and mitomycin C)
- Doxorubicin and cyclophosphamide

The first two regimens are often very well tolerated and

cause little in the way of nausea and vomiting and do not usually cause hair loss. Single agent mitozantrone is often used in elderly unfit patients and is usually well tolerated.

## Lung cancer

This is the commonest cancer in males, and second commonest cancer in females after breast cancer. It is also the most preventable cancer as over 90% is directly related to cigarette smoking. For practical purposes lung cancer can be divided into small-cell lung cancer, comprising about 20%, and non-small-cell lung cancer, comprising 80%. In non-small-cell lung cancer surgery should be considered in all cases although only one-quarter of patients will be operable and only one-quarter of them will be cured. Radiotherapy may provide useful palliation in inoperable patients and very good symptom relief in metastatic disease. Chemotherapy is still experimental in non-small-cell lung cancer and its role is not yet established.

In small-cell lung cancer the disease has almost always disseminated by the time of diagnosis and surgery is thus inappropriate. As opposed to non-small-cell lung cancer, this tumour is very chemosensitive and radiosensitive and the majority of patients will respond to combination chemotherapy (e.g. mitomycin, ifosfamide and cisplatin) with good relief of symptoms and modest prolongation of life. A small proportion of limited small-cell lung cancer patients will be cured. In patients with extensive disease, who are incurable, single agent etoposide orally or intravenously is a possible alternative to combination chemotherapy. As in non-small-cell lung cancer, radiotherapy can provide very useful palliative relief.

## Gastrointestinal cancer

Surgery is the primary treatment for gastrointestinal cancer with radiotherapy sometimes being used after surgery to prevent local relapse. Chemotherapy is playing an increasingly important role.

### OESOPHAGEAL CANCER

In early-stage squamous cell carcinoma of the oesophagus surgery is the treatment of choice. In patients who are inoperable radiotherapy is given as primary treatment. More recently it has been shown that chemotherapy, comprising 5-fluorouracil and cisplatin, given concurrently with radiotherapy improves the cure rate and is now part of standard therapy.

### GASTRIC CANCER AND COLONIC CANCER

#### Adjuvant therapy

Adjuvant therapy has not yet been shown to be useful in gastric cancer. In contrast, in Dukes' B and C colon cancer, the use of adjuvant chemotherapy following surgery has reduced the number of people relapsing and dying with metastatic disease by about one-third.

#### Advanced disease

In advanced metastatic gastric and colonic cancer relatively mild chemotherapy can provide good quality palliation and improvement in quality and quantity of life in some patients. Chemotherapy is based on 5-fluorouracil and cisplatinum in gastric cancer and 5-fluorouracil and folinic acid in colonic cancer. With the appropriate support these regimens are usually very well tolerated.

## Ovarian cancer

Surgery plays a major role in the treatment of ovarian cancer in all stages. In patients where the disease is confined to the ovary, the surgery can be curative, sometimes without the need for further therapy. In patients with more advanced disease, with spread throughout the pelvis and abdomen, surgery still has a role in improving response and survival from chemotherapy. It has been shown that the response to chemotherapy is much enhanced if the tumour is debulked to leave only small amounts of metastatic disease. The most important drugs used to treat ovarian cancer are cisplatinum and its analogue carboplatin, which is associated with less side-effects. More recently taxol, from the bark of the Western Yew, has been shown to have substantial activity in carcinoma of the ovary.

## Testicular cancer

This is the commonest cancer in young men 15–35 but comprises only 1–2% of all cancers. There are two histological types, seminomas and teratomas.

### Seminomas

Seminomas are the least common of these tumours and are very radiosensitive. These can almost always be cured with surgery and radiotherapy to the para-aortic lymph nodes. When there is more widespread disease chemotherapy cures the majority of patients.

### Teratomas

This disease often presents with para-aortic and pulmonary metastases. It is very rapidly growing and most patients have a raised $\alpha$-fetoprotein or $\beta$ human chorionic gonadotrophin ($\beta$-HCG) in the peripheral blood which can be used as tumour markers to follow the response of the disease to treatment. Chemotherapy is the treatment of choice once the disease has spread and radiotherapy has very little role. The great majority of patients can be cured with chemotherapy. The major drugs used include cisplatinum, etoposide, bleomycin and ifosfamide.

## Management of patients with cancer of an unknown primary site

Approximately 5% of all cancers present with no obvious primary site. The aim of investigation and searching for a primary is to identify tumours that are likely to respond to treatment, and to be able to provide the most appropriate palliative care. It is also important to avoid expensive and unnecessary diagnostic procedures. The most important initial distinction is between well-differentiated and poorly differentiated carcinomas because a subset of poorly differentiated carcinomas may be extremely responsive to chemotherapy and may occasionally be cured.

### Well-differentiated adenocarcinoma

The most important primaries to exclude are those that respond well to the treatment. In females breast cancer should always be considered especially if they have axillary lymphadenopathy. Even in the absence of a clinically palpable mass in the breast mammography will sometimes detect an unsuspected primary.

Ovarian cancer and thyroid cancer may also respond well to therapy and should be excluded. In men prostatic carcinoma and thyroid cancer similarly should always be considered.

With improvements in the palliative chemotherapy of advanced gastric and colonic carcinoma, younger fitter patients should also be considered for investigations of the upper and lower gastrointestinal tract to exclude these tumours.

### Poorly differentiated carcinomas

In addition to the above investigations, in patients with poorly differentiated carcinomas detailed immunoperoxidase tumour staining is very important as a subgroup of these patients will turn out to have lymphoma, germ cell tumours or neuroendocrine tumours which may all be very responsive to chemotherapy.

Patients under the age of 50, particularly those with peripheral lymphadenopathy or lymph nodes in the mediastinum and retroperitoneum, may have highly responsive tumours that respond well to teratoma-type cisplatin-based chemotherapy. There are a high proportion of complete responders and a minority will achieve long-term remission.

# Palliative medicine and symptom control

Palliative medicine may be defined as the active, total care of patients whose disease is no longer responsive to curative treatment. The goal of this care is to achieve the best quality of life for patients and their families by controlling physical symptoms and psychological, social and spiritual problems.

Many symptoms suffered by such patients have a complex aetiology in which the physical component may be overlaid by psychosocial issues which require considerable input from a multidisciplinary team of professionals to resolve. Palliative care for the family unit accepts that death is a normal process which will neither be hastened nor postponed, and provides a support system for the family in bereavement. The first step in providing care is often to deal with physical symptoms.

## Pain

Pain is the most feared symptom, although only two-thirds of cancer patients suffer significant pain throughout the course of their disease. The principles of pain relief are careful assessment and diagnosis of the cause of the pain, use of analgesics according to the analgesic ladder and regular review of the effectiveness of the prescription.

The analgesic ladder, adopted by the Cancer Pain Relief Programme from the World Health Organization, groups drugs into three main classes:
1 Non-opioids, e.g. non-steroidal anti-inflammatory drugs including aspirin and paracetamol
2 Weak opioids, e.g. codeine and dextropropoxyphene or combinations of codeine with paracetamol
3 Strong opioids, e.g. morphine and diamorphine
The ladder states that should optimum use of a drug, e.g. paracetamol 1 g 6-hourly, not result in satisfactory pain relief, the prescription should be increased to a weak opioid. If codeine 60 mg 4-hourly is not sufficient to control pain, the patient will require a strong opioid.

### Strong opioid drugs

Morphine is the drug of choice and it should be given regularly by mouth. The dose can be tailored to the individual patient's needs by the addition of 'as required' doses; morphine has no ceiling of analgesic effect. A suitable starting dose of morphine is 10 mg 4-hourly, with a reduction to 5 mg if the patient is elderly or frail. Patients with renal failure may receive morphine in single doses, but should be carefully observed for the return of pain in order to determine the rate of excretion of morphine metabolites. If the 10 mg dose does not last for 4 hours, a 50% increase in the dose should be made, i.e., 10, 15, 20, 30, 45, 60, 90, 120, 180 mg, until satisfactory pain control is achieved.

Once the patient's 24 hour morphine requirement has been established, the prescription may be converted to a controlled-release preparation, e.g. MST.

20 mg morphine elixir 4-hourly = 120 mg in 24 hours = 60 mg MST twice daily

If the patient is unable to take oral medication because of nausea or vomiting, gastrointestinal obstruction or altering levels of consciousness, the opiate should be given rectally or parenterally. In cancer patients in whom longer term treatment is required, continuous subcutaneous infusion is preferred. Diamorphine is used in this situation, because of its greater solubility. By subcutaneous or intramuscular injection diamorphine is about twice as potent as morphine.

The conversion from oral morphine may be calculated:

30 mg morphine 4-hourly = 180 mg over 24 hours = 90 mg diamorphine over 24 hours

SIDE-EFFECTS. Constipation caused by opioid drugs is almost universal. The prescription of a stimulant laxative such as co-danthrusate 1–3 capsules at night should be mandatory at the same time as morphine is started.

Nausea or vomiting can occur in up to 60% of patients started on morphine. However, for those who have worked up the analgesic ladder and who have no other cause for vomiting, the prescription of an 'as required' antiemetic is usually sufficient.

Confusion, nightmares and hallucinations occur in a small percentage of patients. Tolerance to these symptoms does not develop and a change of treatment is usually required.

### Other drugs

Not all pains are clinically opioid responsive and in these situations the addition of co-analgesic drugs will result in improved analgesia.

Non-steroidal anti-inflammatory drugs are used for bone pain in addition to an analgesic drug. Published studies have most frequently used naproxen (500 mg twice daily) but there is no clear evidence of any one drug being superior in effect.

Neuropathic pains are generally only marginally improved by opiates. Several classes of drug have been found to be helpful. In cases of constant burning dysaesthesiae, the tricyclic antidepressants, usually amitriptyline, are helpful. Amitriptyline 25 mg at night increasing incrementally to 75–100 mg is usually sufficient (unlike the doses required for mood elevation) and a response, if achieved, can be expected in about 1 week. Anticonvulsant drugs are useful in the management of lancinating, neuropathic pains. Carbamazepine starting at a dose of 100 mg twice daily is most commonly used, but recent interest has turned to sodium valproate 300 mg twice daily which may cause fewer adverse side-effects.

In addition to drugs many other techniques, such as radiotherapy, anaesthesia and neurosurgery, are employed for the treatment of specific pains.

## Other physical symptoms

Anorexia, malaise and weakness are among the most frequently troublesome symptoms. Current research suggests that endogenously produced cytokines, e.g. tumour necrosis factor, are mediators of the anorexia/cachexia syndrome. The approach to therapy at present depends simply on the adequate treatment of associated symptoms such as pain, nausea and psychological factors as well as attention to nutrition and the judicious use of steroids.

Nausea and vomiting occur in up to two-thirds of cancer patients in the last 2 months of life. The approach to treatment should be similar to that required for pain. It may, however, be more difficult to reach a diagnosis on the cause of the symptom and a somewhat empirical approach to treatment is used. In order to ensure adequate absorption of an antiemetic, parenteral administration for the first 24 hours can be helpful.

Antiemetics are classified according to their pharmacological effects on neurotransmitters. A gastrokinetic dopamine antagonist such as metoclopramide 10 mg 6–8 hourly would be helpful in vomiting related to upper gastrointestinal tract stasis or to liver metastases. As it increases peristalsis in the upper bowel, metoclopramide should be avoided in cases of intestinal obstruction. Centrally acting antiemetics such as the anticholinergic phenothiazine cyclizine 50 mg 8-hourly or the dopamine-antagonist butyrophenone haloperidol 1.5 mg 8-hourly would be the drug of choice in vomiting due to metabolic disturbance or drugs.

## Bowel obstruction

Active medical management of malignant bowel obstruction includes the relief of intestinal colic using antispasmodics such as hyoscine butylbromide 60–80 mg daily; treating continuous pain with diamorphine; and vomiting, especially if nausea is a problem, with a centrally acting emetic, e.g. cyclizine 150 mg daily or haloperidol 5–10 mg daily.

Patients are allowed to drink and eat low-residue diets which are mostly absorbed in the proximal gastrointestinal tract. It is usually possible, with adequate mouth care, to prevent a sensation of thirst and parenteral fluids are not required. A few patients with intractable vomiting due to a high intestinal block may benefit from nasogastric aspiration.

## Respiratory symptoms

Respiratory symptoms cause great distress to patients. Management is based on an accurate diagnosis of the cause and active treatment of all potentially reversible situations. Pleural and pericardial effusions should be drained, infections treated and symptomatic anaemic patients transfused. Sensations of breathlessness and a cycle of respiratory panic may be partially relieved by the prescription of diazepam 2 mg at night. Regular doses of short-acting morphine 5–20 mg 4-hourly are also helpful, as there may be morphine receptors within the lung. Nebulization of a morphine solution will reduce the sensation of breathlessness in a proportion of patients.

Persistent unproductive cough is a very troublesome symptom. Opiates, codeine, methadone or morphine elixir are helpful as antitussive agents. Nebulized local anaesthetic can be helpful.

## Psychological symptoms

Communication with all patients and their families is a basic tenet of care, but is particularly important in the stressful situations which surround fatal disease. Basic skills include allowing time for the patient to talk, using language which is appropriate to the circumstances, being prepared to repeat information and being aware that both patients and their families often receive bad news by blocking or denying it. It is important to remember that it is not always necessary to have an answer or a solution to every problem that is presented, but that considerable support may be given by sympathetic listening.

Care of cancer patients should be designed to allow them to spend as much time as possible at home. Effective liaison between the hospital and the primary health care team is essential to ensure total care. It is especially important to avoid misinterpretation of information regarding treatment and prognosis that may be given.

Approximately 60% of cancer patients will die in general hospital wards under the care of the physician or surgeon who first diagnosed their tumour. Anxiety or depression will be present in up to half of these patients. Caring for this group of patients requires detailed attention to alleviating physical symptoms and establishing a secure environment for the patient and their family to obtain information and support.

The practice of palliative medicine has traditionally been confined to patients with cancer although some services now cover HIV and AIDS and some of the rapidly fatal neurological diseases. These are all conditions in which the clinical situation is changing rapidly and where difficult symptoms exist. There are undoubtedly patients with non-malignant disease who would benefit from a similar multidisciplinary approach to their care. The patient-orientated principles of palliative medicine can however be usefully applied throughout medical practice.

# Further reading

Armitage J (1993) Treatment of non-Hodgkin's lymphoma. *New England Journal of Medicine* **328**, 1023.

Doyle D, Hanks G & MacDonald N (1993) *Oxford Textbook of Palliative Medicine.* Oxford: Oxford University Press.

Rohatiner AZS & Lister TA (1990) The treatment of acute myelogenous leukaemia. In: Henderson ES & Lister TA (eds) *Leukaemia.* Philadelphia: WB Saunders.

Rohatiner AZS & Lister TA (1993) The challenge of acute myelogenous leukaemia. *British Journal of Haematology* **85**, 641–645.

Urba WJ & Longo DL (1992) Hodgkin's disease. *New England Journal of Medicine* **326**, 678.

Yarbro JW (ed) *Seminars in Oncology.* Orlando: Grune & Stratton.

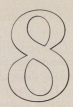

# Rheumatology and bone disease

# RHEUMATOLOGY

## Introduction

Rheumatology is concerned with medical disorders of the locomotor system, which can be divided into three categories: arthritis, back pain and soft-tissue rheumatism. Most of these diseases are seen worldwide, although the prevalence of individual conditions varies. Rheumatic diseases constitute about 20% of the work-load of a primary-care physician.

## The normal joint

The structure of a typical synovial joint is shown in Fig. 8.1. The joint itself is made up of two articulating bone surfaces, each covered with articular cartilage, and a fibrous capsule lined by synovium. The space within the joint is filled with synovial fluid, which acts as a lubricant. Inflammation of the above structures is described as arthritis. The term arthropathy is sometimes used to describe joint disease of any type. The joint is surrounded by so-called 'soft tissues', including tendons, ligaments and bursae. The specialized junction of tendon and bone is called an enthesis; this can also become inflamed.

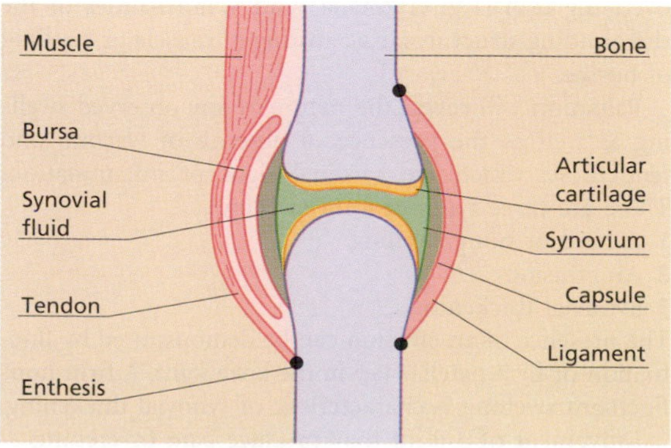

**Rheumatological terminology**
The main terms used in rheumatology are outlined in Information box 8.1.

# Clinical features

### HISTORY
The main features are listed in Table 8.1 and some of these points are discussed below.

### Background information
This may be helpful in assessing the type of arthritis. For example:

**Fig. 8.1** A typical synovial joint.

Muscle
Bone
Bursa
Synovial fluid
Articular cartilage
Synovium
Tendon
Capsule
Ligament
Enthesis

| Term | Meaning |
| --- | --- |
| Monoarticular | One joint involved |
| Polyarticular | Many joints involved |
| Oligoarticular or pauciarticular | Two, three or four joints involved |
| Migratory | Arthritis moving from joint to joint |
| Arthralgia | Joint pain without swelling |
| Small joints | Joints of hands and feet |
| Large joints | Any other joint |
| Seropositive | Rheumatoid factor positive |
| Seronegative | Rheumatoid factor negative |

**Information box 8.1** Rheumatological terms.

379

> Background information—age, sex
> Main complaint
> Pain, e.g. site, duration, radiation
> Other symptoms, e.g. morning stiffness
> Resultant problems
> Pattern of joint involvement
> Time relationships, e.g. duration, frequency of attacks
> Associated symptoms
> Past medical history
> Family history
> Social history
> Previous treatment

**Table 8.1** Main features in the history of a patient with arthritis.

AGE. Osteoarthritis commonly presents at 50 years of age.

SEX. Rheumatoid arthritis is commoner in women, whilst Reiter's syndrome is commoner in men.

RACE. Some arthropathies are particularly associated with diseases occurring in particular races, e.g. in sickle cell disease.

OCCUPATION. This can be an important factor in soft-tissue rheumatism or osteoarthritis.

### Joint pain

The type of pain is of little help as all joint pains feel much the same to the patient. The following points are of some value:

1 *Duration.* For example, a long history is suggestive of rheumatoid arthritis, whilst a short history may suggest gout.
2 *Onset.* Some conditions like gout start suddenly.
3 *Precipitating factors.* For example, injury may lead to osteoarthritis, diuretic therapy can precipitate gout, and a sore throat precedes rheumatic fever.

### Characteristics

(a) Site of the pain—this usually indicates the site of the pathology although hip disease may present with knee pain and pain in the arm or leg may arise from the neck or back.
(b) Radiation—a lesion of the cervical or lumbar spine will give pain in the distribution of the affected roots.
(c) Severity—excruciating pain is characteristic of acute gout.
(d) Aggravating and relieving factors—inflammatory joint pains are usually better with activity; patients are stiff and painful after rest. Mechanical problems are made worse by activity and relieved by rest.
(e) Diurnal variation—pain due to inflammation is characteristically worst in the mornings and improves during the day.
(f) Episodic arthritis—the frequency, regularity and duration of attacks should be noted.

### Other joint symptoms

Enquire about:

MORNING STIFFNESS. This is characteristic of inflam-

matory arthropathies. The duration of stiffness gives some guide to the activity of the inflammatory process.

JOINT SWELLING. This always indicates local disease.

PATTERN OF JOINT INVOLVEMENT. For example, recurrent attacks in the big toe are suggestive of gout.

CLICKING AND CREAKING OF THE JOINT. These are not important and can be felt in normal joints.

DISABILITY. This is a very individual problem, depending on joints affected and the demands made upon them. It is however important in determining the right approach to treatment.

### Associated non-articular symptoms

Nodules or a pleural effusion may be a clue to the diagnosis of rheumatoid arthritis. The cause of a particular arthritis may also lie in disease of other systems such as psoriasis or ulcerative colitis.

### Past medical history

A history of trauma or of some other disease like psoriasis may be helpful.

### Family history

Some conditions run in families, e.g. osteoarthritis, ankylosing spondylitis and gout. Patients with psoriatic arthritis do not necessarily have psoriatic skin lesions but may give a family history of psoriasis.

### Social history

The occupation of the patient may have a bearing on the arthritis. In addition, the development of a chronic arthritis has a major influence on the life-style of both patient and family.

### Treatment record

A record of the previous treatments tried and their success is important for the future management.

## EXAMINATION OF JOINTS

There are three stages in the examination of an individual joint:

1 Look at it
2 Feel it
3 Move it

Inspection will reveal swelling, deformities, changes in the overlying skin (e.g. erythema) and abnormalities of the surrounding structures, e.g. wasting of muscle or swelling of bursae.

Palpation will reveal the nature of any observed swelling as well as the presence or absence of warmth and tenderness, which are cardinal signs of inflammation. There are three types of joint swelling:

1 A hard or bony swelling
2 An effusion
3 Synovial thickening

The presence of an effusion can be demonstrated by fluctuation or by a patellar tap in the knee joint. A firm non-fluctuant swelling is characteristic of synovial thickening.

Movement of a joint may produce pain or crepitus—a sensation of grating that is characteristic of osteoarthritis. The range of movement should be noted. Excessive abnormal movement is called instability. Posture and gait should also be assessed.

Movement of joints is described in terms of flexion, extension, abduction, adduction and rotation. Deformities are described as valgus (like knock knees) or varus (like bow legs).

A system of examination should be followed so that no joint is missed.

# Investigation (Table 8.2)

Investigations are often unnecessary in patients with rheumatic complaints. In patients with tennis elbow, osteoarthritis and many other conditions, the diagnosis can be made on the basis of history and examination findings. There are no diagnostic tests in osteoarthritis and tests are only requested to exclude some other condition.

## ERYTHROCYTE SEDIMENTATION RATE (ESR) AND C-REACTIVE PROTEIN (CRP)

These provide a guide to the activity of inflammation and are characteristically raised in inflammatory conditions such as rheumatoid arthritis but are normal in osteoarthritis.

## TESTS FOR RHEUMATOID FACTOR

Rheumatoid factors are autoantibodies found in the serum, usually of the IgM class, which are directed against human IgG. They are detected by agglutination of either latex particles (the latex test) or sheep red cells (the Rose–Waaler test) (Fig. 8.2). The major value of rheumatoid factor tests is in the diagnosis of rheumatoid arthritis (Table 8.3). The latex test is quicker and easier to perform; it is more sensitive, and therefore more often positive, but is less specific than the sheep red cell test.

## ANTINUCLEAR ANTIBODIES (Fig. 8.3 and Table 8.4)

Antinuclear antibodies in the serum are detected using immunofluorescent staining of the nuclei of a tissue such as rat liver or human cells in tissue culture. A low titre of less than 1 : 40 is weakly positive and of little significance.

### Antibodies to other nuclear antigens

A variety of antinuclear antibodies have been described with particular disease associations that are summarized in Table 8.5. It seems likely that the pattern of disease is determined by the nature of the autoantibodies produced.

---

**Useful tests**

ESR/CRP
Rheumatoid factor
Antinuclear antibodies
Serum uric acid
Synovial fluid examination
X-rays

**Occasionally useful tests**

White blood cell count
HLA-B27
Serum alkaline phosphatase
ASO titre—in rheumatic fever
Protein electrophoresis, immunoglobulin, urinalysis for
   Bence-Jones protein, bone marrow—for myeloma
Serum ferritin
Complement
ANCA
Anticardiolipin antibodies
Arthroscopy ± synovial biopsy
Arthrogram
Bone scan
MRI scan

---

ANCA, antineutrophil cytoplasmic antibodies; ASO, antistreptolysin-O; CRP, C-reactive protein; ESR, erythrocyte sedimentation rate; MRI, magnetic resonance imaging.

**Table 8.2** Investigations in rheumatic diseases.

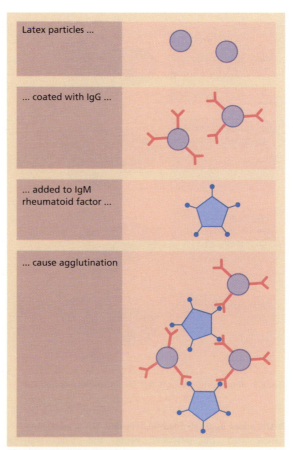

Latex particles ...

... coated with IgG ...

... added to IgM rheumatoid factor ...

... cause agglutination

**Fig. 8.2** The rheumatoid factor test using latex particles. The coated latex particles are added to the patient's serum and if this contains IgM rheumatoid factor, agglutination is seen.

*Diseases involving joints*

Sjögren's syndrome (90%)
Rheumatoid arthritis (80%)
Systemic lupus erythematosus (50%)
Systemic sclerosis (30%)
Polymyositis/dermatomyositis (50%)
Mixed connective tissue disease

*Chronic infections* (low titres), e.g.

Tuberculosis
Leprosy
Infective endocarditis
Kala-azar

*'Normal' population*

Elderly
Relatives of patients with rheumatoid arthritis

*Miscellaneous*

Autoimmune chronic active hepatitis
Fibrosing alveolitis
Sarcoidosis
Waldenström's macroglobulinaemia

**Table 8.3** Conditions in which rheumatoid factor is found in the serum.

Systemic lupus erythematosus (95%)
Systemic sclerosis (80%)
Sjögren's syndrome (60%)
Polymyositis and dermatomyositis (30%)
Still's disease (30%)

*Occasionally seen in*:
Autoimmune chronic active hepatitis
Primary biliary cirrhosis
Infections, e.g. infective endocarditis
Normal elderly people

**Table 8.4** Conditions in which antinuclear antibodies are found in the serum.

| Antibody to | Clinical association |
|---|---|
| dsDNA | SLE |
| ENA; ribonucleoprotein (RNP) | Mixed connective tissue disease and SLE |
| Ro (SSA)[a] | SLE and primary Sjögren's syndrome |
| La[a] | Primary Sjögren's syndrome |
| Sm[a] | SLE |
| Centromere | CREST syndrome |
| Nucleolus | Systemic sclerosis |
| Scl-70[a] | Systemic sclerosis |
| Jo-1[a] | Polymyositis |
| Cardiolipin | SLE and cardiolipin syndrome |

———

[a]Fractions of nuclear material.
CREST, calcinosis (C), Raynaud's phenomenon (R), oesophageal involvement (E), sclerodactyly (S), telangiectasia (T); dsDNA, double-stranded DNA; ENA, extractable nuclear antigen; SLE, systemic lupus erythematosus.

**Table 8.5** Serum antinuclear antibodies and their clinical associations.

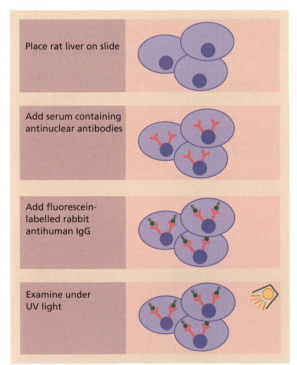

| | |
|---|---|
| Place rat liver on slide | |
| Add serum containing antinuclear antibodies | |
| Add fluorescein-labelled rabbit antihuman IgG | |
| Examine under UV light | |

**Fig. 8.3**  Immunofluorescent test for antinuclear antibodies.

## Antibodies against double-stranded DNA (dsDNA)

These can be detected using the Farr test, a radioimmunoassay measuring the percentage antibody binding of added labelled dsDNA. Antibodies are found in about 50% of cases of systemic lupus erythematosus

(SLE) but seldom in any other condition. They are therefore a much more specific test than antinuclear antibodies. They are also associated with more severe disease and renal involvement.

**Antibodies against extractable nuclear antigen (ENA)**
IgG class antibodies against soluble nuclear antigens are characteristic of mixed connective-tissue disease, the overlap syndrome described on p. 405, but are also found in patients with SLE.

## OTHER ANTIBODIES
### Anticardiolipin antibodies
These are found in the antiphospholipid syndrome, which is described on p. 403.

## Antineutrophil cytoplasmic antibodies (ANCA)

These are detected by immunofluorescence and by enzyme-linked immunosorbent assay (ELISA) in the serum, and are of two types:

1 cANCA (cytoplasmic staining) is directed against serine proteinase C.

2 pANCA (perinuclear staining) is mainly directed against myeloperoxidase.

*cANCA* is seen in Wegener's granulomatosis with a specificity of about 90%. It is found in 50% of early cases and almost 100% of cases with full-blown systemic disease. It disappears with treatment and rising titres may predict relapse, making it a very useful marker of progress. It is very occasionally found in other types of vasculitis such as microscopic polyarteritis (see p. 451).

*pANCA* is much less specific and is found in:

- Various types of vasculitis including microscopic poly-arteritis, Churg–Strauss syndrome and sometimes polyarteritis nodosa
- Glomerulonephritis
- Rheumatoid arthritis
- Connective tissue disorders such as SLE and Sjögren's syndrome, not necessarily associated with vasculitis
- Chronic inflammatory bowel disease, in primary sclerosing cholangitis and in autoimmune hepatitis
- Drug treatment, e.g. hydralazine.

## SERUM URIC ACID

A raised serum uric acid is a good confirmatory test for gout, but is not diagnostic. A low level of uric acid excludes gout. In known cases of gout, the uric acid level is helpful in deciding treatment (see p. 410).

## JOINT PUNCTURE

See Procedure box 8.1.

## SYNOVIAL FLUID EXAMINATION

The characteristics of synovial fluid in normal and diseased joints are shown in Table 8.6.

Polarized light microscopy reveals the presence of negatively birefringent crystals in gout. In pyrophosphate arthropathy, crystals of calcium pyrophosphate, which are weakly positively birefringent, are seen. Crystals of hydroxyapatite are too small to be seen in polarized light microscopy and need to be identified using electron microscopy. Gram stain may identify organisms in septic arthritis but the fluid should also be cultured.

## X-RAYS

X-rays show characteristic abnormalities in many rheumatic conditions; these are described in the appropriate sections. Degenerative changes are present in almost everyone by the age of 65 years and often before; their presence on an X-ray does not necessarily therefore mean osteoarthritis.

X-rays are of little value in acute conditions such as septic arthritis.

## OCCASIONALLY USEFUL TESTS (see Table 8.2)

WHITE BLOOD CELL COUNT is useful in infections and leukaemia presenting with arthritis.

---

*Indications*

Diagnosis—particularly septic arthritis and crystal deposition disease
Drainage—in septic arthritis and to relieve pain from tense effusions
Drugs—intra-articular steroids for rheumatoid and other inflammatory arthropathies

*Risks*

Infection—1 in 10 000 punctures with luck and care!
Destruction—deterioration of cartilage reported in weight-bearing joints of patients given frequent steroid injections who increased their activities
Inflammation—some preparations of steroids contain crystals that may cause a transient inflammatory reaction

*Precautions*

Asepsis—no-touch technique
Advice to patients:
    Report at once if symptoms worsen
    Avoid weight-bearing for 2 days—care for 2 weeks after injection
Administer only three steroid injections in one joint in one lifetime

*Procedure*

Wash hands thoroughly
Examine joint and identify correct site for puncture
Clean the skin and do not touch it again
Draw up steroid if required
Infiltrate with local anaesthetic if necessary, for nervous patients or difficult joints
Insert untouched sterile needle into joint
Aspirate and inject through same needle

*Synovial fluid handling*

Inspect for volume, colour and viscosity
Divide into three portions for
    (a) WBC and differential (Sequestrene tube)
    (b) Polarized light microscopy for crystals (slide or plain tube)
    (c) Gram stain and culture (sterile bottle)

**Procedure box 8.1** Joint puncture.

---

RAISED SERUM ALKALINE PHOSPHATASE is characteristic of Paget's disease (see p. 428) but is also sometimes seen in active rheumatoid arthritis and polymyalgia rheumatica.

A MONOCLONAL PROTEIN BAND on serum electrophoresis is found in myeloma (see p. 372).

RAISED ANTISTREPTOLYSIN-O (ASO) titre indicates recent streptococcal infection. Very high levels are characteristic of rheumatic fever.

HIGH SERUM TRANSFERRIN SATURATION OR FERRITIN LEVEL occurs in haemochromatosis, which may present with arthritis.

LOW SERUM COMPLEMENT may be found in the active phase of SLE.

ARTHROSCOPY is useful for the demonstration of mech-

| | Appearance | White blood cells (×10⁶/litre) | Crystals | Culture |
|---|---|---|---|---|
| Normal | Clear viscous fluid | <200 Mononuclear | None | Sterile |
| Osteoarthritis | Increased volume; viscosity retained | 3000 Mononuclear | 5% have pyrophosphate | Sterile |
| Rheumatoid arthritis | Sometimes turbid, yellow or green in colour; viscosity lost | 30 000 Neutrophils | None | Sterile |
| Septic arthritis | Turbid; low viscosity | 50 000–100 000 Neutrophils | None | Positive |
| Gout | Clear; low viscosity | 10 000 Neutrophils | Needle-shaped negatively birefringent | Sterile |
| Pyrophosphate arthropathy | Clear; low viscosity | 10 000 Neutrophils | Brick-shaped, positively birefringent | Sterile |

**Table 8.6**   Typical synovial fluid changes in some rheumatic diseases.

anical lesions in the knee joint such as a torn meniscus and if necessary a synovial biopsy can be obtained during the procedure. This investigation is particularly useful in persistent monoarticular arthritis, e.g. in tuberculosis.

AN ARTHROGRAM can also be used to visualize the meniscus or to demonstrate knee-joint rupture.

RADIOISOTOPE BONE SCAN is useful in demonstrating malignant deposits. Increased uptake also occurs around osteoarthritic joints and also in inflammatory arthropathies, but these abnormalities can usually be distinguished from malignant disease.

HISTOCOMPATIBILITY ANTIGEN HLA-B27 is found in 96% of patients with ankylosing spondylitis and only 5% of normal people in the UK. There are marked differences between the incidence of the antigen in different populations that roughly parallel the frequency of ankylosing spondylitis. In addition, about 60% of patients with Reiter's disease are B27 positive.

MRI SCANNING is useful for the detection of mechanical problems in joints, for example a torn meniscus or ruptured cruciate ligament in the knee or a rotator cuff tear in the shoulder. It is also useful to detect avascular necrosis for example in the hip joint, and is replacing myelography for the detection of spinal disease.

## Arthritis

The causes of arthritis are given in Table 8.7.

## Osteoarthritis

Osteoarthritis (OA) is the commonest type of arthritis, occurring in about 20% of the population as a whole and

| Osteoarthritis |
| Rheumatoid arthritis |
| Spondylarthropathies, e.g. |
|   Ankylosing spondylitis |
|   Reactive arthritis and Reiter's disease |
| Connective tissue disorders |
|   Systemic lupus erythematosus |
|   Polymyositis/dermatomyositis |
|   Systemic sclerosis |
| Polymyalgia rheumatica and other types of vasculitis |
| Crystal deposition diseases |
|   Gout |
|   Pyrophosphate arthropathy |
|   Acute calcific periarthritis |
| Infective arthritis |
| Juvenile arthritis, e.g. Still's disease |
| Arthritis associated with other diseases, e.g. psoriasis |
| Rare rheumatic disease |

**Table 8.7**   Main causes of arthritis.

in 50% of those aged over 60 years. It is a disease of cartilage, which becomes eroded and progressively thinned as the disease proceeds.

The pattern of development of joint disease in osteoarthritis is additive. The disease moves slowly from joint to joint and also progresses very slowly (in most cases) within individual joints. Its greatest impact is on weight-bearing joints such as the hips and knees, and involvement of these joints is the commonest cause of disability in an elderly population.

### EPIDEMIOLOGY

OA occurs throughout the world and has occurred throughout the history of humanity. It is twice as common in women as in men. It is particularly common in British populations but this has nothing to do with climate, latitude or longitude and is therefore presumably genetic. OA is uncommon in black populations; when it does occur it usually affects the knees and hand involvement is rare.

## PATHOGENESIS

OA is a disease of cartilage. Normal cartilage is composed of a matrix of collagen fibres stuffed with proteoglycan molecules that attract water and thereby maintain a positive pressure within the structure. There are just a few chondrocytes scattered within normal cartilage. It is likely that different stimuli can initiate the degenerative process but the two most obvious are:

1 Mechanical insults
2 Biochemical abnormalities of cartilage

The chondrocyte is believed to start the deterioration, releasing enzymes that degrade collagen and proteoglycans. Breaks in the collagen fibres allow the uptake of water; cartilage swells and splits. Crystals are released into the joint and are one of the mechanisms of the synovial inflammation that follows and which may perpetuate the destruction of cartilage. Attempts at repair include remodelling of bone, which produces the characteristic osteophytes.

Identifiable aetiological factors in primary OA include:

AGE. The disease tends to start at the age of 50 years.

GENETICS. There is a strong familial tendency. Specific abnormalities of collagen caused by a single aminoacid defect have recently been identified in a few families with an OA-like disease.

OBESITY AND OTHER SYSTEMIC FACTORS. Obesity is associated with OA of the knees. Chondrocytes may be influenced by sex hormones, growth hormone and other systemic factors.

It is probably a mistake to think of primary OA as a single disease. It is probably a common response to a variety of insults and has identifiable pathophysiological features which vary according to the joint site as well as the cause. Current concepts of the aetiology of primary OA are summarized in Fig. 8.4. The relative importance of different factors varies at different sites. With OA of the small joints of the hand, genetic factors are particularly important, while in the hip abnormal biomechanics may be more relevant.

Most OA is primary but in a small proportion of patients there is an obvious cause. The causes of secondary OA are listed in Table 8.8.

## PATHOLOGY

There is fibrillation of the superficial layer of cartilage with fissures (splits) developing and extending into the

*Congenital abnormalities of joints*
Hypermobility
Congenital dysplasias

*Structural disorders in children*
Slipped femoral epiphysis
Perthes' disease

*Trauma and mechanical problems*
Intra-articular fractures
Meniscectomy
Obesity
Recurrent dislocation
Occupational hazards, e.g. repetitive actions

*Crystal deposition disease and metabolic abnormalities of cartilage*
Pyrophosphate arthropathy
Ochronosis
Haemochromatosis

*Avascular necrosis*, e.g.
Sickle cell disease
Corticosteroid therapy
Caisson disease

*Other conditions in which cartilage is destroyed*, e.g.
Septic arthritis
Recurrent haemarthrosis
Inflammatory arthropathy such as rheumatoid arthritis

**Table 8.8** Causes of secondary osteoarthritis.

deeper layers. The bases of these fissures contain clusters of chondrocytes, which are increased in number. As the disease advances there is progressive cartilage loss until hard eburnated bone is all that remains. The synovial membrane is heavily infiltrated with mononuclear cells. There is thickening of subchondral bone with cyst formation.

## CLINICAL FEATURES

### Symptoms

PAIN, typically in the knees, hips or hands, worst in the evenings and aggravated by use and relieved by rest. Sometimes intermittent at first but later chronic with inflammatory exacerbations in particular joints.

MORNING STIFFNESS, usually lasting up to half an hour and stiffness after sitting.

DISABILITY depends upon the joints affected.

### Signs

SWELLING: characteristically hard and bony, sometimes with associated effusion.

CREPITUS on movement.

SIGNS OF INFLAMMATION: warmth in the knees and erythema in the small joints of the hands, particularly in the early stages and during exacerbations.

LIMITATION OF MOVEMENT follows with wasting of muscles around the affected joint.

JOINT DEFORMITIES are particularly important in the knee. Valgus, varus or flexion deformities are seen with instability in the later stages of the disease.

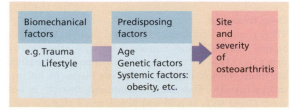

**Fig. 8.4** Current view of osteoarthritis.

## Pattern of disease
Occasionally monoarticular; usually one, two, three or four sites including knees (commonest), hands, hips, feet, ankles and lumbar spine; bilateral and symmetrical.

HANDS. Bony swellings occur at the distal interphalangeal joints of the fingers (Heberden's nodes) and also at the proximal interphalangeal joints (Bouchard's nodes). At first the joints are often red, warm, swollen and very tender ('hot Heberden's nodes'). Later the inflammation disappears, leaving knobbly but often painless swellings. The pattern of hand involvement is shown in Fig. 8.5; the distal interphalangeal and first carpometacarpal joints are most often affected.

FEET. The metatarsophalangeal joint of the big toe is often affected, sometimes called 'poor man's gout'. Problems may arise from valgus deformity (hallux valgus) or progressive restriction of movement (hallux rigidus).

OA is characterized by inflammation of joints but, unlike rheumatoid arthritis, there is no systemic involvement. Thus there are no non-articular features and there is no systemic illness.

## DIFFERENTIAL DIAGNOSIS
The pattern of hand involvement should be contrasted with that of rheumatoid arthritis (see later), in which metacarpophalangeal and proximal interphalangeal joint involvement is usual and the distal interphalangeal joints are characteristically spared. The pattern of involvement of other joints in OA is contrasted with that in rheumatoid arthritis in Fig. 8.6. The number of joints affected in OA is much less than in rheumatoid arthritis.

Apophyseal joints in the cervical and lumbar spine are not uncommonly involved but it is difficult to distinguish OA at this site from chronic disc disease.

## INVESTIGATION
### X-ray changes
The X-ray changes in OA are shown in Fig. 8.7. Narrowing of the joint space is due to loss of cartilage and

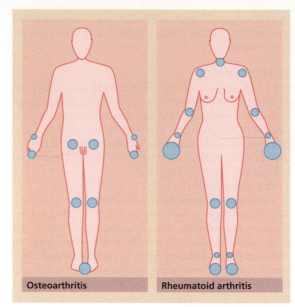

Osteoarthritis    Rheumatoid arthritis

**Fig. 8.6** The pattern of joint involvement in osteoarthritis compared with rheumatoid arthritis. Both conditions are usually bilateral and symmetrical in distribution.

is the most important change. It is accompanied by the formation of osteophytes at the margins of the joint, sclerosis of the underlying bone and cyst formation. There is often calcification, which takes one of two forms:
1 Linear calcification, which is characteristic of pyrophosphate deposition
2 Spotty calcification, which is characteristic of hydroxyapatite deposition

### Blood tests
There are no diagnostic markers for OA. The ESR is normal and there are no biochemical abnormalities. Rheumatoid factor and antinuclear antibodies are negative but remember that positive low titre tests can occur in the elderly.

### Synovial fluid (see Table 8.6)

## MANAGEMENT
The nature of the condition, treatment and prognosis should be discussed with the patient.

There are three main types of treatment: drugs, physical measures and surgery. Obese patients should be encouraged to lose weight but, apart from this, it is seldom possible to alter the aetiological factors of the disease.

### Drug treatment
There is no specific therapy to control the disease process. Simple analgesics and non-steroidal anti-inflammatory drugs (NSAIDs) are used to control symptoms. The latter are more effective because of the part played by inflammation in OA. Systemic corticosteroid therapy is not used. Drugs such as gold and pencillamine that are used for rheumatoid arthritis are not effective in OA.

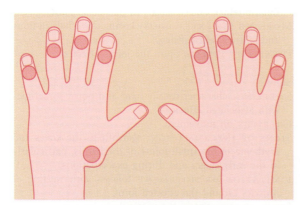

**Fig. 8.5** The pattern of hand involvement in osteoarthritis. Bony swelling of the first carpometacarpal joints gives rise to the appearance of 'square hands'.

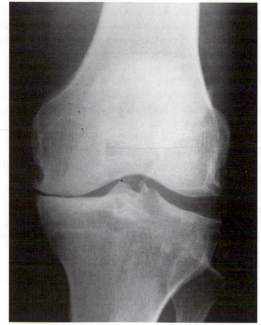

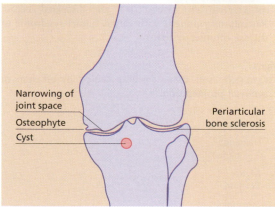

Narrowing of
joint space

Osteophyte

Cyst

Periarticular
bone sclerosis

**Fig. 8.7**  X-ray changes of osteoarthritis of the knee.

Intra-articular corticosteroids can be used for inflammatory exacerbations. Injection should be preceded by aspiration of any fluid in the joint.

### Physical therapy
The application of heat to an osteoarthritic joint may provide pain relief. Exercises are useful to maintain muscle power and are especially required for the quadriceps muscle in patients with knee involvement. Hydrotherapy is particularly useful for the hip joint, sometimes enabling a stiff joint to be mobilized and providing symptomatic relief. A walking stick may be useful for a patient with involvement of one hip or knee and should be held in the opposite hand.

### Surgery
The greatest advance in the management of OA has been joint replacement. Many joints can be successfully replaced. For example, a total hip replacement offers a 99% chance of almost complete pain relief and increased mobility. Knee replacements are now as successful. For disease of the first carpometacarpal joint, the trapezium can be removed or replaced with a plastic prosthesis. The first metatarsophalangeal joint can also be replaced.

Replacements of knees and hips have a limited lifespan. Hip replacements fail at the rate of 1% per year, the cement fixation becoming loose and the joint becoming painful. X-rays often fail to show this loosening but a bone scan becomes 'hot' and is a useful way of confirming the diagnosis. Treatment is surgical revision but the success rate falls with each procedure. A much less common but much more serious problem with replacements is infection. Antibiotics seldom solve the problem of infection around a metal prosthesis, which acts as a foreign body; it is often necessary to remove the prosthesis, drain the site and replace the prosthesis at a later date using cement containing antibiotics. An uncemented hip prosthesis is sometimes used in young people needing total hip replacement when it is anticipated that revision will be required. It is easy to remove such a prosthesis and replace it with the cemented variety.

# Rheumatoid arthritis

Rheumatoid arthritis (RA) is a common, chronic, systemic disease producing:
- A symmetrical inflammatory polyarthritis
- Extra-articular involvement, e.g. in the lungs and many other organs
- Progressive joint damage causing severe disability in young people, demanding considerable resources in terms of doctors, drugs and surgery

### EPIDEMIOLOGY
RA affects about 2% of the population worldwide and is just as common in tropical countries as in cold, damp Britain. It is about three times as common in women as in men. It can begin at any age from 10 to 70 years but it most often starts between the ages of 30 and 40 years. There is an increased incidence in those with a family history of RA (5–10%) and an association with HLA-DR4 (70%) in most ethnic groups. HLA-DR1 is found in the majority of HLA-DR4-negative patients, particularly in Indians and Israelis.

### PATHOGENESIS
The cause of RA is unknown. Toxic substances produced by the inflammatory reaction in the synovium are thought to lead to the destruction of cartilage, the characteristic feature of progressing RA.

Many immunological disturbances are seen and RA is considered to be an autoimmune disease for the following reasons.

AUTOANTIBODIES are seen. Rheumatoid factor is also

found in other diseases and therefore may play little part in the pathogenesis of RA.

IMMUNE COMPLEXES are common in the synovial fluid and the circulation.

LOCALLY SYNTHESIZED IMMUNOGLOBULINS AND LYMPHOKINES are found in the synovial fluid.

CELL-MEDIATED IMMUNITY is defective.

ASSOCIATION OF OTHER ORGAN-SPECIFIC AUTO-IMMUNE DISEASES such as primary hypothyroidism and pernicious anaemia.

A likely hypothesis for the chronicity of the inflammatory process is a persistent foreign antigen, perhaps a bacterium or virus, that is taken up by macrophages but not destroyed or removed. This leads to a systemic inflammatory reaction, not unlike adjuvant arthritis in rats, mediated by the immune system and characterized by an inflammation of many joints, vasculitis and granuloma formation (nodules). Figure 8.8 shows possible pathogenic mechanisms leading to joint damage and destruction.

## PATHOLOGY

RA is a disease of the synovium. There are two main pathological characteristics—inflammation and proliferation. The synovium shows signs of a chronic inflammatory reaction, with infiltration of lymphocytes, plasma cells and macrophages. It then proliferates and grows out over the surface of the cartilage, producing a tumour-like mass called 'pannus'.

The subcutaneous nodules seen in RA, usually called rheumatoid nodules, have a central area of necrosis surrounded by a palisade of macrophages and fibrous tissue. Similar lesions occur in the pleura, pericardium and lung. The lymph nodes are often hyperplastic.

## CLINICAL FEATURES

RA usually presents with the insidious onset of pain and stiffness in the small joints of the hands and feet, which eventually goes on to the characteristic chronic bilateral symmetrical peripheral polyarthritis. In 25% of cases it presents as arthritis of a single joint, such as the knee.

An acute onset of the disease is characteristic in the elderly and is sometimes called 'explosive RA'.

### Symptoms

JOINT PAIN. The pain is worst on waking in the morning and may improve with activity. There is often pain at night and disturbed sleep.

MORNING STIFFNESS, often lasting for several hours.

GENERAL SYMPTOMS. Fatigue and general malaise are common.

DISABILITY depends upon the changes in individual joints.

NON-ARTICULAR SYMPTOMS are discussed below. Patients may present with carpal tunnel syndrome or disease of other systems.

### Signs

SWELLING: soft tissue swelling caused by effusion or synovial proliferation.

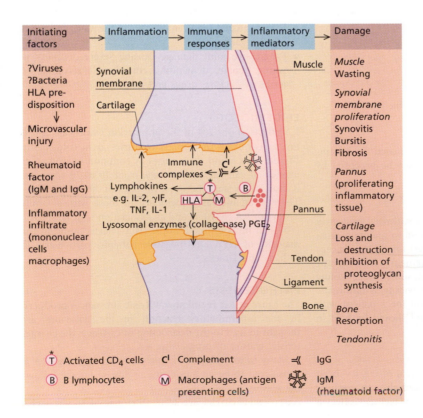

**Fig. 8.8** Pathogenesis of rheumatoid arthritis. The earliest changes are microvascular injury, oedema and a proliferation of mononuclear cells and lymphocytes. Activation of T cells by antigen-presenting cells releases lymphokines, lysosomal enzymes and prostaglandins, which leads to the degradation of cartilage and bone erosions. Rheumatoid factor is produced locally in the synovium and immune complexes are formed with the activation of complement. Proliferating inflammatory tissue (pannus) leads to further intra-articular damage and eventually the joint is destroyed.

WARMTH.

TENDERNESS on pressure or movement.

LIMITATION OF MOVEMENT with muscle wasting around affected joints.

DEFORMITIES occurring in the later stages of the disease.

NODULES and other extra-articular features.

### Pattern of joint involvement

The characteristic pattern of joint involvement is shown in Fig. 8.6. Most patients eventually have many joints involved, including the hands, wrists, elbows, shoulders, cervical spine, knees, ankles and feet. The dorsal and lumbar spines are not involved.

THE HIPS. The hip joint is involved in about 50% of patients. This seldom occurs at the onset of the disease but usually develops within the first few years.

THE HANDS AND WRISTS. The pattern of joint involvement is shown in Fig. 8.9. In contrast to OA the distal interphalangeal joints are only involved in 30% of cases. Early in the disease there is spindling of the fingers due to swelling of the proximal but not distal interphalangeal joints; the metacarpophalangeal and wrist joints are also swollen. As the disease progresses, there is weakening of joint capsules causing laxity and deformity. The characteristic deformities of the rheumatoid hand are shown in Fig. 8.10.

THE FEET. Deformities in the feet are similar to those seen in the hands and wrists. There is lateral deviation of the toes and subluxation of the metatarsophalangeal joints so that the heads of the metatarsals become palpable in the soles of the feet. Patients often describe a sensation of walking on marbles.

THE KNEES. Synovial effusions and quadriceps wasting are early features. Later flexion, valgus or varus deformities appear with joint instability. The pressure of fluid within the knee leads to the formation of a Baker's cyst in the popliteal fossa. With the increased pressure, the knee joint may rupture, releasing irritant synovial fluid

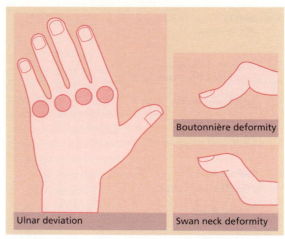

**Fig. 8.10** Characteristic hand deformities in rheumatoid arthritis.

into the muscles of the calf. The sudden onset of pain with swelling of the ankle and a positive Homan's sign may be mistaken for deep vein thrombosis but the correct diagnosis can be confirmed by ultrasound or arthrogram.

### Progression and prognosis of joint involvement

The activity and rate of progression of joint changes in RA are very variable. New joints are involved in an additive pattern in most cases. The pattern of joint involvement is usually established within months of its onset. Partial remissions and relapses follow. In some, the disease is mild with little or no progression. In others, the characteristic deformities and complications occur. About 10% of patients become seriously disabled and 40% develop significant disability.

PALINDROMIC RHEUMATISM. Episodes of arthritis may precede the development of chronic RA. Palindromic rheumatism is described on p. 413.

### Non-articular features (Fig. 8.11)

SOFT TISSUES SURROUNDING JOINTS.

1  *Rheumatoid* nodules are found in about 20% of cases. They are most often felt on the ulnar surface of the forearm just below the elbow but they can appear almost anywhere. Patients with nodules are usually seropositive.

2  *Bursitis.* The olecranon and other bursae may be swollen.

3  *Tenosynovitis*, particularly affecting the flexor tendons in the palm of the hand, can cause trigger finger as well as pain and swelling and may contribute to flexion deformities. Swelling of the extensor tendon sheath over the dorsum of the wrist is common.

4  *Muscle wasting.* There is wasting of muscles around affected joints, particularly in the hands.

THE EYES.

1  The commonest eye problem in RA is *secondary Sjögren's syndrome*, occurring in about 15% of cases. It

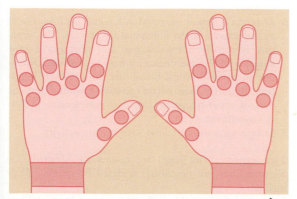

**Fig. 8.9** The pattern of hand involvement in rheumatoid arthritis.

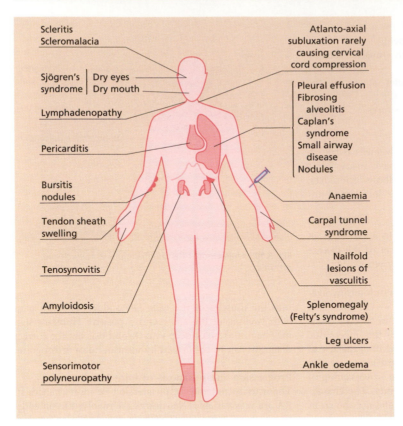

Scleritis
Scleromalacia

Sjögren's | Dry eyes
syndrome | Dry mouth

Lymphadenopathy

Pericarditis

Bursitis
nodules

Tendon sheath
swelling

Tenosynovitis

Amyloidosis

Sensorimotor
polyneuropathy

Atlanto-axial
subluxation rarely
causing cervical
cord compression

Pleural effusion
Fibrosing
  alveolitis
Caplan's
  syndrome
Small airway
  disease
Nodules

Anaemia

Carpal tunnel
syndrome

Nailfold
lesions of
vasculitis

Splenomegaly
(Felty's syndrome)

Leg ulcers

Ankle oedema

**Fig. 8.11**  The non-articular manifestations of rheumatoid arthritis.

comprises dry eyes (keratoconjunctivitis sicca), a dry mouth (xerostomia) and RA. This syndrome is also seen in other connective tissue disorders, e.g. SLE. The lacrimal and salivary glands are infiltrated with lymphocytes and plasma cells, suggesting that this syndrome is part of the immunological process of rheumatoid disease. The development of dry eyes is particularly important because tear production protects the cornea. Artificial tears such as hypromellose 0.3% eyedrops should be prescribed. Primary Sjögren's syndrome is described on p. 405.
2  *Scleritis* may occur, causing a painful red eye. Scleromalacia presents as a bluish discoloration of the sclera around the iris; perforation rarely occurs.

THE NERVOUS SYSTEM.
1  *Carpal tunnel syndrome* is the commonest neurological abnormality (see p. 945).
2  Atlanto-axial subluxation can cause serious neurological abnormality. In this condition rheumatoid involvement of an adjacent bursa leads to weakening of the transverse ligament of the atlas. This in turn allows the odontoid process to separate from the anterior arch of the atlas and to move posteriorly on flexion of the cervical spine with potential infringement on the cervical cord. Atlanto-axial subluxation is a common X-ray finding, but cervical cord compression is fortunately rare.
3  *Polyneuropathy* occurs rarely causing glove and stock-

ing sensory loss and sometimes motor weakness. It is usually symmetrical and often involves the legs.
Multiple mononeuropathy (mononeuritis multiplex) can also occur as a result of vasculitis.

THE SPLEEN, LYMPH NODES AND BLOOD.
1  *Palpable lymph nodes* are common, usually in the distribution of affected joints.
2  The spleen may be enlarged. RA with splenomegaly and neutropenia is known as *Felty's syndrome*. Recurrent infections may occur. HLA-DRW4 is found in 95% of such patients compared with 70% of patients with RA and 30% of controls. Skin pigmentation also occurs.
3  Anaemia is almost universal in RA and is proportional to the activity of the inflammatory process. The anaemia is usually normochromic and normocytic—the anaemia of chronic disease; it may be iron-deficient—due to gastrointestinal blood loss from NSAID ingestion, or rarely, haemolytic (positive Coombs' test) or part of a pancytopenia due to hypersplenism in Felty's syndrome.
3  Thrombocytosis correlates with disease activity.

THE LUNGS.  The lungs are commonly affected; the abnormalities are described in detail on p. 690. They include:
1  *Pleural effusion*—this is the commonest lung problem and occurs particularly in middle-aged men but seldom

in women. It may precede the development of arthritis. The fluid has a high protein and low sugar content.

2 *Diffuse fibrosing alveolitis* is rare.

3 *Rheumatoid nodules* in the lungs can be up to 3 cm in diameter and mistaken for carcinoma.

4 *Caplan's syndrome* is the occurrence of nodular pulmonary fibrosis in patients with RA exposed to various industrial dusts.

5 *Small airway disease* is commoner in patients with RA who smoke than in normal people who smoke.

THE HEART. A pericardial rub is often heard in patients with RA (up to 30%). Pericarditis is seldom a clinical problem but occasionally a large pericardial effusion causes tamponade. Constrictive pericarditis is rare.

THE KIDNEYS. RA is a common cause of amyloidosis affecting the kidneys. It usually presents as proteinuria and may go on to renal failure or to the nephrotic syndrome. Analgesic nephropathy is nowadays very rare (see p. 461).

THE SKIN. The skin is not directly involved in RA but leg ulcers may occur, particularly in patients with Felty's syndrome and in those with a vasculitis. Vasculitis most often appears as nail fold lesions in the hands and, very occasionally, it produces gangrene of the fingers or toes. Ankle oedema is often seen in active RA and is due to increased vascular permeability.

## DIAGNOSIS

This relies on clinical features. Useful pointers are the presence of morning stiffness, symmetrical arthritis at multiple joints including the hands lasting 6 or more weeks and the presence of rheumatoid nodules. A positive rheumatoid factor and X-ray changes are also helpful. These American Rheumatism Association criteria are useful for disease classification.

## INVESTIGATION

### X-ray changes

The X-ray changes of RA are shown in Fig. 8.12. The characteristic lesion is an erosion that has the appearance of a mouse-bite on the surface of the affected bone. Erosions are best seen in X-rays of the hands and feet. Other changes include loss of joint space, which indicates thinning of the cartilage, porosis of the periarticular bone and cysts. In advanced disease, destruction of bone ends occurs.

### Full blood count

A full blood count in RA shows anaemia (see above) and ESR and CRP are raised in proportion to the activity of the inflammatory process.

### Other tests

Tests for rheumatoid factor are positive in about 80% of cases and for antinuclear antibodies in about 30%.

Aspirated synovial fluid will show the changes outlined in Table 8.6. Fluid from a suddenly painful rheumatoid

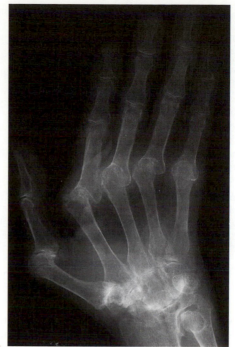

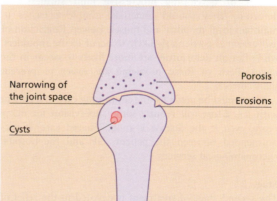

**Fig. 8.12** X-ray changes in rheumatoid arthritis. Erosions are best seen in the small joints of the hands and feet.

joint should always be aspirated and cultured, as septic arthritis can occur in patients with RA.

## MANAGEMENT (see Table 8.9)

### Stage 1

The diagnosis of RA inevitably causes concern and patients require a lot of information, explanation and reassurance. Assessment is part of the diagnostic process and includes the activity of the inflammatory process, the severity of anatomical changes, the rate of progression and particular problems which have arisen, all factors which will determine the right approach to treatment. All aspects of a patient's life-style should be reviewed including home, work and leisure activities with the emphasis on preserving as many activities as possible. RA is entirely consistent with a full, normal and busy life.

*Stage 1*
Making the diagnosis, telling the patient
Joint protection and maintenance
Management planning

*Stage 2*
Symptomatic treatment with NSAIDs and other
    measures

*Stage 3*
The control of the disease with long-term suppressive
    drugs

*Stage 4*
Regular supervision and the management of
    complications

*Stage 5*
Rehabilitation of the disabled patient

———

NSAIDs, non-steroidal anti-inflammatory drugs.

**Table 8.9**  Stages in the management of rheumatoid arthritis.

Physical activity does not increase the rate of deterioration of joints in RA and since patients are particularly at risk of developing progressive joint stiffness and deformity they should undertake simple exercises to maintain joint mobility and muscle power. Restriction of movement is particularly likely to occur in the shoulders, while flexion deformities are more likely to occur in the knees. Both of these problems are easier to prevent than correct.

Plans must be made for the continuing care of a patient with RA. Most will require some supervision for many years, even if the disease is mild. 'Shared care' is recommended between the patient, GP and the hospital rheumatological services.

### Stage 2

The second stage of treatment is devoted to the relief of symptoms. NSAIDs are the mainstay of such treatment and are more effective than simple analgesics.

INDIVIDUAL RESPONSE TO NSAIDS varies greatly. It is therefore desirable to try several different drugs for a particular patient in order to find the best. Each compound should be given for 1 week. Drugs with a low incidence of side-effects, a good safety record and a convenient dosage schedule should be tried first. Piroxicam 20 mg daily is a reasonable first choice, but many NSAIDs of equal efficacy are available. The major side-effects of NSAIDs are gastrointestinal with haemorrhage being a major problem in the elderly. Other side-effects include fluid retention, tubulo-interstitial nephritis and problems with drug interactions.

The relief of night pain and morning stiffness is particularly important in RA and slow-release indomethacin (75 mg) taken on retiring usually works well and can be given in addition to regular daytime therapy if necessary. If patients require additional relief, a simple analgesic can be taken as required. Paracetamol can be used but many patients prefer a combination such as dextropropoxyphene and paracetamol.

CORTICOSTEROIDS are effective but are seldom used because of their side-effects. In explosive RA in the elderly, small doses of prednisolone (10 mg daily) are usually dramatically effective;the dose can be reduced over the years. In the younger patient, however, much larger doses of prednisolone, often for long periods, are necessary to control symptoms and because of side-effects such treatment is best avoided.

REST IN HOSPITAL is often useful, either to produce a remission of the disease or to encourage a dispirited disabled patient. Localized rest for individual joints can be provided with splints, which are particularly useful for the wrist.

INTRA-ARTICULAR CORTICOSTEROID INJECTIONS are of value for particularly troublesome joints to avoid the risk of systemic steroids.

### Stage 3

The third stage consists of long-term suppressive drug therapy with drugs such as penicillamine (Table 8.10). The indications for this type of treatment are:
● Progressive disease
● Troublesome extra-articular problems
● Failure of NSAIDs to control symptoms
● Excessive corticosteroid requirements

The current trend is to use these drugs very early in the treatment of RA with the aim of controlling the disease before structural damage appears in the joints.

The characteristics of long-term suppressive therapy are:

A SLOW ACTION: these drugs start to work after 4–6 weeks and take 6 months to produce their full effect. For this reason, NSAIDs should be continued for a few months at least.

IMPROVEMENT IN JOINT SYMPTOMS is accompanied by a fall in ESR and the titre of rheumatoid factor.

COMPLETE REMISSION or very effective suppression of disease can be achieved, delaying or preventing joint destruction.

The mode of action of these drugs is unknown and it is impossible to predict which patient will respond to a particular compound. It is often necessary to try several, as with NSAIDs.

The most effective drugs are penicillamine, azathioprine and methotrexate. Hydroxychloroquine, sulphasalazine and auranofin are a little less effective but safer. Intramuscular gold is as effective as penicillamine but because of the inconvenience of injections and the frequency of side-effects, which produces a low ultimate success rate, it is less used. Penicillamine is often the first choice of drug for younger patients, but because of failures due to lack of effect or side-effects one must be prepared to use all these drugs. Combinations are increasingly used for the difficult case. All of these drugs have side-effects and require careful monitoring with blood tests at appropriate intervals. Patients should be informed of the potential for side-effects and told to report new symptoms immediately. The antimalarial drug hydroxychloroquine may

| Drug | Usual dose | Possible side-effects |
|------|-----------|----------------------|
| Penicillamine | 250 mg daily | Rash<br>Loss of taste<br>Thrombocytopenia<br>Proteinuria |
| Gold (sodium aurothiomalate) | 50 mg weekly i.m. | Rash<br>Thrombocytopenia |
| Oral gold (auranofin) | 3 mg twice daily | Diarrhoea<br>Rash |
| Azathioprine | 50 mg twice daily | Neutropenia<br>Nausea and vomiting<br>Infections |
| Methotrexate | 7.5–15 mg weekly | As for azathioprine |
| Hydroxychloroquine | 400 mg daily | Retinopathy |
| Sulphasalazine | 1 g twice daily | Nausea<br>Mild depression<br>Male infertility |

Table 8.10    Drugs used in long-term suppressive therapy for rheumatoid arthritis.

affect the eyes and vision must be checked before therapy and immediately if any disturbance of vision is noted.

### Stage 4
Regular supervision is required to assess the course of the disease and to treat complications (Table 8.11).

ARTICULAR COMPLICATIONS. Joints may become stiff and painful and require intra-articular injections of corticosteroids and exercises to mobilize the joint and improve muscle power. Deformities can also sometimes be corrected by steroid injections and exercises.

Rupture of the knee joint is treated with aspiration, injection of corticosteroid and rest. A Baker's cyst behind the knee does not itself require treatment since it merely reflects inflammatory changes in the knee joint. Steps should be taken to control the activity of the disease in the affected knee.

Painful feet may be treated with insoles; metatarsal bar insoles are particularly useful for subluxed metatarsal heads. More complex foot deformities may require special shoes such as space shoes.

At this stage in the disease replacement surgery plays an increasingly important role in the management of a patient with a wrecked joint. Not only can hips be replaced, but also knees, shoulders, elbows and the small joints of the hands.

Excision arthroplasty is of value in two situations. First, the painful subluxed metatarsal heads in the feet can be excised (Fowler's operation) and the lateral deviation of the toes corrected at the same time. Second, the head of the ulna can be excised at the wrist, often relieving pain and allowing better movement. Osteotomy is occasionally used at the knee joint to relieve pain and correct deformity.

NON-ARTICULAR COMPLICATIONS. Many different symptoms require treatment. For example, the patient who develops carpal tunnel syndrome will require an injection of corticosteroid or surgical decompression of the median nerve.

SOCIAL AND DOMESTIC COMPLICATIONS. RA strains relationships and makes life difficult. Crises arise in these matters and patients often turn to a sympathetic physician for advice and help.

### Stage 5
Despite all treatments, the disease may continue to progress and become disabling. Priorities in treatment then change. It is no longer relevant to control the disease and the aims of treatment become relief of symptoms and maintenance of a reasonable life-style. It may be useful to visit a patient's home with a view to making life easier. A wheelchair may be required and many other aids and appliances can be used to reduce disability. Steps should be taken to preserve as much as possible of all aspects of the patient's life. Successful management can make an enormous difference to the quality of life of rheumatoid patients.

Ruptured tendons ✓
Joint infection
Ruptured joints, e.g. Baker's cysts
Side-effects of therapy
  Anaemia
  Marrow hypoplasia ✓
  Renal impairment ✓
  Gastrointestinal bleeding/dyspepsia ✓
Spinal cord compression
Amyloidosis

Table 8.11    Complications of rheumatoid arthritis.

Inflammatory back pain
Synovitis—lower limbs and asymmetrical
Sacroiliitis on X-ray
Overlap of features (see Fig. 8.13)
Familial aggregation
HLA-B27 positivity
Absence of rheumatoid factor and nodules
   ('seronegativity')
Anterior uveitis

**Table 8.12**   Clinical and laboratory features of spondylarthropathies.

# The spondylarthropathies

This term describes a family of diseases with common features which are summarized in Table 8.12. The major members of the family are shown in Fig. 8.13 which emphasizes the overlap of features between the different syndromes. There is a common genetic basis to these conditions: HLA-B27 is found in all of them but more frequently in classical ankylosing spondylitis with sacroiliitis and a bamboo spine on X-ray than in other syndromes. The same patient may have several different syndromes from the group either simultaneously or at different times: thus a patient with enteropathic synovitis may also have anterior uveitis. Similarly, the same conditions may occur within families, e.g. patients with reactive arthritis may have uncles and aunts with psoriasis or nephews and nieces with juvenile arthritis. In some cases it is impossible to describe the condition of a particular patient except as an 'undifferentiated spondylarthropathy'.

## PATHOGENESIS

The tendency to develop these conditions is inherited but there is increasing interest in the role of gut inflammation in precipitating the development of the various clinical features. It is well known that gut or venereal infections precipitate reactive arthritis, but recent studies show that gut inflammation is often present in ankylosing spondylitis and other spondylarthropathies. It is thought that microbial antigens are disseminated from the gut to, for example, joints where, as in the gut, they cause lymphocyte activation, cytokine production and inflammation.

## Ankylosing spondylitis

Ankylosing spondylitis is the most important cause of inflammatory back pain. It affects young adults, with men more severely afflicted than women. It presents with back pain and morning stiffness, and is typically associated with sacroiliitis on X-ray. Other important associations include peripheral arthritis and non-articular features such as iritis.

It is a genetically determined disease, susceptibility to which is related to the presence of HLA-B27. This antigen is found in about 5% of European people and 95% of patients with ankylosing spondylitis. Studies of large populations of B27-positive subjects such as blood donors suggest that about 20% of B27-positive individuals have

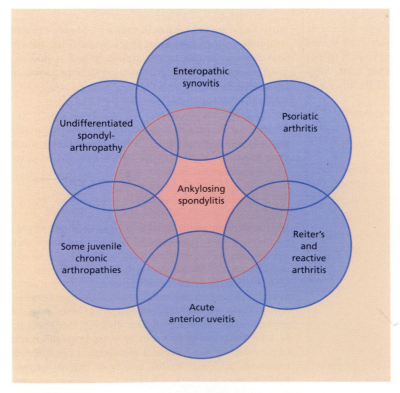

**Fig. 8.13**   The spondylarthropathy family.

ankylosing spondylitis or a related disease. The prevalence of ankylosing spondylitis in the population can thus be calculated as 1%. Since HLA-B27 is found equally in men and women, the incidence of the disease should also be equal. Population surveys using radiological sacroiliitis as the main criterion for diagnosis have shown both a much lower incidence than 1% and a male preponderance. It is now clear that there are many mild cases, especially in women, that present as pain and stiffness but with no other features. The disease is probably almost as common in women as in men and the presence of X-ray changes are not essential to the diagnosis.

The frequency of ankylosing spondylitis in different populations is roughly paralleled by the incidence of HLA-B27: Africans and Japanese have a low incidence of both HLA-B27 and ankylosing spondylitis. Some native American tribes have a correspondingly higher incidence of both.

## CLINICAL FEATURES

The typical case presents with an insidious onset of low back pain in the late teens or early twenties. The pain is typically inflammatory in type (Table 8.13). The first symptoms may arise from sacroiliitis, with pain in the buttocks radiating down the back of both legs. Peripheral polyarthritis may also occur; the joints of the lower limbs are particularly affected. Plantar fasciitis may cause heel pain. Iritis occurs at some time in 30% of cases.

Inspection of the spine in a patient with ankylosing spondylitis reveals two characteristic abnormalities:

1  Loss of lumbar lordosis and increased kyphosis
2  Variable limitation of spinal flexion and a reduction in chest expansion

In addition, tenderness is commonly found around the pelvis and chest wall.

## INVESTIGATION

THE ESR AND CRP are often raised.

X-RAYS OF THE LUMBAR SPINE AND PELVIS are often but not always abnormal. In the early stages, the sacro-iliac joints are eroded, with irregular margins, and there is sclerosis of adjacent bone. As the disease advances, the sacroiliac joints may fuse. In the spinal column, the characteristic abnormality is a syndesmo-phyte that grows between the margins of the vertebrae. There is calcification and ossification of the inter-spinous ligaments so that with the syndesmophytes, the PA X-ray shows three continuous lines, the so-called tramline appearance. Vertebrae appear square as a

result of the erosion of their corners. These changes are particularly seen at the dorsolumbar junction, but may occur throughout the spine (Fig. 8.14).

HLA-B27 (measured in blood lymphocytes) is useful supporting evidence in the difficult case but one must remember that many normal people carry the gene.

## COURSE AND PROGNOSIS

In all but the mild case there is progressive limitation of spinal movement over the course of a few years. In severe cases the spine becomes completely fused. There is a tendency for patients to develop a kyphosis, but this can usually be prevented. Despite the limitation of spinal movement, most patients are able to lead a normal active life and remain at work. In women, the disease is usually mild, with little restriction and no deformity. In contrast to RA, the disease does not remit in pregnancy but nor does it cause problems with childbirth. It tends to improve with age but seldom resolves completely.

Most cases of ankylosing spondylitis do well. Death is seldom related to the disease except in rare complications like amyloidosis and neck fractures. The disease tends to be more severe when it starts earlier: hip disease is more likely when the disease starts in teenagers; when it starts after the age of 22 years, hip replacement is almost never required. Neck problems are also more likely with a younger onset. While men are more likely to have aggressive spinal disease, women are more likely to have peripheral joint disease.

## MANAGEMENT

NSAIDS ARE VERY EFFECTIVE; slow-release indo-methacin is often the best choice (75 mg at night). It is

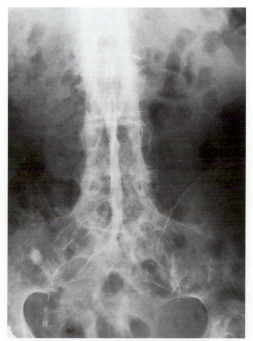

**Fig. 8.14**  X-ray of ankylosing spondylitis with sacroiliitis.

|  | Inflammatory | Mechanical |
|---|---|---|
| Onset | Gradual | Sudden |
| Worse pain | In the morning | In the evening |
| Morning stiffness | Present | Absent |
| Effect on exercise | Relieves pain | Aggravates pain |

**Table 8.13**  Points of distinction between inflammatory and mechanical back pain.

particularly useful in relieving night pain and morning stiffness. Useful alternatives include piroxicam or flurbiprofen.

AN EXERCISE PROGRAMME is essential to maintain movement, relieve symptoms and prevent deformity, particularly kyphosis. Exercises should be carried out at least twice daily. In addition, patients should be encouraged to take part in whatever sports they like.

SULPHASALAZINE is useful as a long-term suppressive drug in the difficult case but penicillamine and gold are not effective. Azathioprine may be useful for peripheral arthritis but not for spondylitis.

Radiotherapy has been used but should seldom be necessary and carries a small risk of leukaemia.

Surgery plays little part, but hip replacement is occasionally required.

## Reiter's syndrome

This syndrome consists of the triad of a seronegative reactive arthritis, non-specific urethritis and conjunctivitis. Two types are recognized:

1 Following a gastrointestinal infection with *Shigella, Salmonella, Yersinia* or *Campylobacter* (enteric)

2 Following non-specific urethritis (venereal) (p. 90)

The male-to-female ratio is 20 : 1 and most cases occur in young adults. HLA-B27 is present about 60% of cases.

### CLINICAL FEATURES (Fig. 8.15)

ARTHRITIS begins within 2 weeks of the enteric or venereal infection, which may have been mild and asymptomatic. The joints of the lower limbs are particularly affected in an asymmetrical pattern; the knees, ankles and feet are the commonest sites. The wrists and other joints of the upper limbs are occasionally involved, and there may be localized pain and tenderness in the spine due to sacroiliitis. The arthritis is often very acute at presentation but resolves over the course of a few months. It is occasionally associated with non-articular inflammatory lesions, including plantar fasciitis and Achilles tendinitis.

URETHRITIS is associated with a sterile urethral discharge and mild dysuria. Prostatism can occur. Circinate balanitis, a superficial penile lesion characterized by a circle of erythema with a pale centre, is rare.

CONJUNCTIVITIS is usually mild and bilateral, resolving spontaneously. It occurs in only one-third of patients. Acute anterior uveitis develops later in the disease, in approximately 10% of patients.

KERATODERMA BLENNORRHAGICA is seen in 10% of patients with postvenereal Reiter's syndrome. It is characterized by intense scaling of the skin of the soles of the feet, resembling pustular psoriasis. Nail dystrophy with subungual keratosis may lead to shedding of the nails.

Patients with Reiter's syndrome may have a low-grade fever. Very rarely cardiac (e.g. pericarditis, aortitis), respiratory (mainly pleurisy) or neurological (peripheral neuropathy) complications occur.

### DIAGNOSIS

The diagnosis in these conditions is entirely clinical; there are no diagnostic blood tests. The ESR is raised in the acute stage. Tests for rheumatoid factor and other autoantibodies are negative; 60% of patients are HLA-B27 positive. X-rays are of no value in the acute stage of the disease, though signs of sacroiliitis may appear with the development of ankylosing spondylitis. Aspirated synovial fluid is inflammatory in nature, with a high polymorphonuclear leucocyte count; the fluid is sterile.

### TREATMENT

Treatment is with NSAIDs such as indomethacin. It is often useful to aspirate acutely inflamed joints and to inject them with a corticosteroid preparation.

If the acute arthritis fails to resolve quickly, and in rare chronic cases, sulphasalazine or azathioprine can be used.

### PROGNOSIS

Although the acute arthritis resolves within a few months, there is a very high incidence of long-term problems. About 50% of patients with Reiter's syndrome will go on to develop recurrences of arthritis, iritis or ankylosing spondylitis. Recurrent synovitis is the commonest problem and typically presents with effusions in the knee. Recurrences are not necessarily preceded by further enteric or venereal infection and are not associated with progressive deterioration of joints.

## Reactive arthritis

This has all the characteristics of the arthritis described above but without the other associations of Reiter's syndrome and is called reactive arthritis. The full triad of Reiter's syndrome is rare, but reactive arthritis following enteric or venereal infection is common. It is the commonest cause of arthritis in young men.

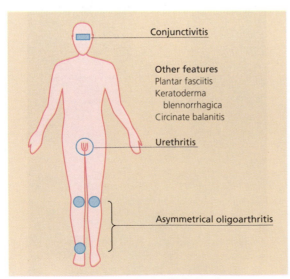

**Fig. 8.15**  The clinical features of Reiter's syndrome.

Conjunctivitis

Other features
Plantar fasciitis
Keratoderma
   blennorrhagica
Circinate balanitis

Urethritis

Asymmetrical oligoarthritis

# Psoriatic arthritis

This is a seronegative arthritis occurring in 10% of patients with psoriasis. The aetiology is unknown, but there is an increased incidence of HLA-B27 and of a history of psoriasis in the family.

The skin lesions, which are described on p. 999, may be minimal or absent. The nail changes of psoriasis are usually present (85%). Differing patterns of arthritis are seen.

The commonest pattern of psoriatic arthropathy is a polyarthritis affecting the small joints of the hands, including the distal interphalangeal joints, in an asymmetrical pattern. This is a mild but chronic condition, and in most cases is benign. It can usually be controlled with analgesics but NSAIDs are sometimes necessary.

Less often the pattern of the arthritis is similar to that in RA, i.e. a bilateral, symmetrical polyarthritis.

Rarely the disease is rapidly progressive, producing destruction of the ends of the small bones of the hands and feet (arthritis mutilans), a condition that can also occur in RA. Because of the shortening of the bones of the fingers there is an excess of soft tissue and the fingers can be pulled in and out like an opera glass, after which the condition is sometimes named.

Finally, patients with psoriasis have an increased incidence of ankylosing spondylitis.

Blood tests are unhelpful in the diagnosis. The ESR is often normal and tests for rheumatoid factor are negative. X-rays may show characteristic changes in the terminal interphalangeal joints, with erosions and periarticular osteoporosis.

Treatment is with analgesic and anti-inflammatory drugs. In progressive cases, immunosuppressive drugs such as azathioprine are particularly effective. Gold is sometimes effective in psoriatic arthropathy, but penicillamine is not.

## Juvenile chronic arthritis (see p. 407)

Juvenile ankylosing spondylitis, which accounts for 50% of cases of juvenile chronic arthritis, can be classified as a spondylarthropathy and is discussed on p. 394.

## Enteropathic synovitis

Enteropathic synovitis occurs in 11% of patients with ulcerative colitis and 14% of patients with Crohn's disease. This type of arthritis is always related to the activity of the underlying disease, although in a small proportion of cases it is the first manifestation of underlying bowel problems. The aetiology is unknown but deposition of immune complexes in the joint may play a part. Enteropathic synovitis usually affects the knees and ankles as a monoarthritis or asymmetrical oligoarthritis. It presents with painful swollen joints and large effusions. Attacks last for a few months only and resolve without joint damage. Enteropathic synovitis should be distinguished from ankylosing spondylitis. The latter occurs in about 5% of patients with inflammatory bowel disease but is an associ-

ated lesion rather than a complication of the bowel disease and is not therefore related to disease activity. Other non-articular features of inflammatory bowel disease, e.g. iritis, may be present.

X-rays of affected joints are normal and investigations are otherwise unhelpful. The first priority for treatment is to control the underlying inflammatory bowel disease. Aspiration and injection of affected joints and oral anti-inflammatory drugs may help the symptoms while the underlying disease is being brought under control.

# Infective arthritis

Infection of joints is fortunately uncommon but is important because of the damage it produces. The possibility of infection as a cause of arthritis must always be kept in mind. If its presence is suspected, synovial fluid must be obtained for culture. Infection with pyogenic organisms (septic arthritis) can be caused by a number of bacteria, including mycobacteria (see below). Arthritis also occurs with viral infections and less commonly from infection with spirochaetes or fungi.

Apart from direct infection, arthritis can also occur as a result of an immunological reaction to infection elsewhere (see p. 399).

## Septic arthritis

Septic arthritis results from infection of joints with pyogenic organisms, of which *Staphylococcus aureus* is the commonest. It can also occur with other types of staphylococci, streptococci, *Neisseria* or Gram-negative bacilli.

Organisms reach the joint in septic arthritis via the bloodstream, sometimes from an identifiable site of infection such as otitis media or a boil. Less commonly, infection spreads from osteomyelitis adjacent to the joint or the organism is introduced directly as a result of trauma, surgery or intra-articular injection.

Septic arthritis particularly occurs at the extremes of life and in immunologically compromised individuals, e.g. patients receiving immunosuppressive drugs or with RA.

### CLINICAL FEATURES

The clinical features of septic arthritis are similar for all the different causative organisms. The presentation is usually dramatic. The patient typically presents with a single painful joint, often the knee. The joint is red, warm and swollen, with a demonstrable effusion. Fever is usual and there may be evidence of infection elsewhere.

In RA, the presentation may be misleading; patients are often afebrile and do not necessarily have a systemic reaction or a leucocytosis. Any suddenly painful joint in a patient with RA should be aspirated to exclude infection.

Systemic and local reactions can also be absent in patients receiving corticosteroids.

## INVESTIGATION

ASPIRATION OF THE JOINT is the only important diagnostic manoeuvre (see Table 8.6). The synovial fluid is often purulent and typically contains over $50\,000 \times 10^6$/litre white blood cells, predominantly neutrophils. A Gram stain may show the presence of organisms. Culture of the fluid, including special techniques for detecting anaerobes and gonococci, usually gives a definite answer.

BLOOD LEUCOCYTOSIS may be present.

BLOOD CULTURE may be positive.

X-RAYS are of no value in the diagnosis of septic arthritis; they become abnormal only when joint destruction is advanced.

## TREATMENT

This should be started immediately the diagnosis is made, as cartilage destruction can occur within a few days of the onset of the joint infection and the situation can be life-threatening. The joint should be immobilized.

### Antibiotic therapy

The choice of antibiotic will depend upon the organism concerned. If the identification of this is delayed, 'blind' therapy should be started immediately with a slow i.v. infusion of flucloxacillin 500 mg 6-hourly together with clindamycin 300 mg i.v. 6-hourly or fusidic acid 500 mg 8-hourly by mouth. Antibiotics given by the intramuscular or intravenous route will pass into joints, especially when they are inflamed; antibiotics should not be injected intra-articularly. Antibiotic levels in the synovial fluid should be checked during the acute illness. Antibiotics should be continued for 6 weeks.

### Drainage

Drainage of infected joints is best achieved by needle aspiration, which should be performed daily until no further fluid is obtainable. For inaccessible joints such as the hip, surgical drainage may be required. If infection is allowed to continue, debris that cannot be removed with a needle collects within the joint and this delays recovery. In these circumstances, the effusion will fail to resolve and surgical debridement will be required.

## PROGNOSIS

The resolution of septic arthritis with complete recovery usually occurs within a few days or weeks.

# SPECIFIC TYPES OF BACTERIAL ARTHRITIS

## Tuberculous arthritis

Of patients with tuberculosis, 1% have skeletal involvement. Tuberculous arthritis affecting children usually occurs in the primary stage of the disease. In adults, it is invariably secondary to pulmonary or renal disease and is due to haematogenous spread to the subchondral bone or the spinal intervertebral discs. Predisposing factors for tuberculous arthritis are those for developing tuberculosis anywhere in the body, e.g. alcohol dependence, diabetes mellitus or any other chronic debilitating disease.

### PATHOLOGY

The synovial membrane and periarticular tissues become inflamed and oedematous; histologically, caseating granulomas are seen. Later there is destruction of cartilage and this may lead to fibrous ankylosis. When the spine is involved, the infection may track along the fascial planes to produce a psoas abscess.

### CLINICAL FEATURES

There is usually a monoarticular arthritis affecting the hip or knee (30%) or the sacroiliac or other joints (20%); in 50% of patients there is spinal involvement. There is an insidious onset of pain and dysfunction of the joint, with swelling and synovial proliferation very like that seen in RA, and restriction of movement associated with general symptoms of malaise, anorexia and night sweats.

### DIAGNOSIS

The mycobacterium may be cultured from the synovial fluid; however, negative results do not exclude the diagnosis and if suspicion remains, synovial biopsy is required. X-rays are at first normal but later there is narrowing of the joint space and bony erosions.

### TREATMENT

Drug treatment is as for tuberculosis elsewhere (see p. 686). The joint should be immobilized in the acute phase. If infection is allowed to continue, the effusion cannot be aspirated via a needle because of debris and surgical debridement is necessary.

## Meningococcal arthritis

Meningococcal arthritis usually occurs as part of a generalized meningococcal septicaemia. It is a migratory polyarthritis and organisms cannot usually be recovered from the synovial fluid. Joint destruction does not occur. This type of arthritis is due to circulating immune complexes containing meningococcal antigens. Occasionally the effusion is purulent and contains meningococcal organisms. Treatment is with penicillin.

## Gonococcal arthritis

Gonococcal arthritis is similar to meningococcal arthritis. It particularly affects young adult females and also homosexual men. It presents with a mildly inflammatory polyarthritis. It is usually asymmetrical and occasionally migratory. A useful clue to the diagnosis is the presence of small pustular skin lesions, often near the affected joints. The organism can be recovered from the bloodstream and in 25% of cases from the joints. In the remainder the arthritis is a reaction to the infection, and is probably immunologically mediated.

If neglected, gonococcal septicaemia may go on to

produce a typical septic arthritis. Treatment is with penicillin 1 g orally, daily for 2 weeks.

## *Salmonella* arthritis

*Salmonella* infection differs from septic arthritis in being polyarticular. It is also less dramatic than septic arthritis and is therefore easily missed. It occurs with types of *Salmonella* that invade the bloodstream rather than staying within the gastrointestinal tract. Gastrointestinal features may therefore be minor or absent, deflecting attention away from the correct diagnosis.

Treatment with systemic antibiotics, e.g. i.v. amoxycillin 500 mg 6-hourly, is curative.

## Lyme disease (see p. 43)

Arthritis is seen in patients with Lyme disease, first described in the USA but now known to occur throughout the world. It is caused by a spirochaete, *Borrelia burgdorferi* (which has recently been detected in synovial fluid by PCR) and is transmitted from deer by a tick. It occurs mainly in children and is easily mistaken for Still's disease. The arthritis is characteristically episodic with attacks of arthritis affecting about three large joints and lasting 1 week but may eventually become chronic. There are associated skin lesions, erythema chronicum migrans and a variety of other manifestations, particularly neurological, have been described (see p. 43).

## Infective endocarditis

Infective endocarditis (see p. 602) may present with arthritis, which occurs particularly in the early stages of the disease. Like other clinical features, the arthritis may be due to circulating immune complexes; direct infection of the joints is much less common. Asymmetrical arthritis of a few large joints is characteristic, but other patterns may occur. Localized back pain associated with fever is another manifestation.

## VIRAL ARTHRITIS

A number of different viral infections cause arthritis. The commonest and most important is *rubella*, where the virus can occasionally be isolated from the joint. Arthritis is particularly a complication of the disease in young adult females, occurring in 15% of cases. Arthritis may follow either rubella or the rubella vaccine. It begins a few days after development of the rash, or 2 weeks after vaccination. It may be associated with other complications such as lymphadenopathy. It presents as a bilateral, symmetrical polyarthritis, closely resembling RA, for which it is often mistaken. However, it resolves within a few weeks in most cases. Occasionally there is persistent or recurrent arthralgia that may continue for years. Treatment is symptomatic.

Arthritis may also complicate *mumps*. A few large joints are typically affected and, as in rubella, the condition is self-limiting.

Arthralgia and sometimes arthritis may be features of the prodromal stage of *hepatitis B* infection, but resolve when the jaundice appears. As in meningococcal arthritis, this prodromal syndrome is associated with circulating immune complexes.

Patients with Reiter's syndrome or psoriatic arthropathy may develop a severe exacerbation following HIV infection (see p. 49).

Human *parvovirus B19* (see p. 49) causes an acute asymmetrical short-lived polyarthritis in adults, particularly women. It often occurs without the rash. A specific anti-B19 IgM antibody is found in the serum.

Transient polyarthritis is also seen in *infectious mononucleosis, chickenpox* and other viral infections.

## FUNGAL AND OTHER INFECTIONS

Fungal infections of joints occur rarely. Actinomycosis can affect the mandible or vertebrae. Bone abscesses may be seen. Destructive joint lesions can also occur with blastomycosis. A benign polyarthritis accompanied by erythema nodosum occasionally occurs in coccidioidomycosis and histoplasmosis. Culture of purulent synovial fluid and skin tests for fungi may help the diagnosis.

---

# *Arthritis following infection*

Much more common than direct infection of joints is a condition in which arthritis is associated with an immunological reaction to infection. There are two different types, which are summarized in Table 8.14. Rheumatic fever and Henoch–Schönlein purpura follow streptococcal infections and predisposition to these disorders is not related to the presence of the antigen HLA-B27. By contrast, HLA-B27-positive individuals are particularly likely to develop reactive arthritis following enteric or venereal infection (see p. 396).

## Rheumatic fever (see p. 590)

This poststreptococcal condition is associated with a migratory polyarthritis. A joint such as the wrist or elbow becomes acutely painful and swollen for about 2 days. As resolution occurs, another joint becomes involved. The arthritis lasts for a few weeks or months but eventually resolves completely without any long-term problems. Its importance is the association of carditis in 40% of cases.

## Henoch–Schönlein purpura (see p. 449)

This childhood condition also follows a streptococcal infection. It presents as a generalized purpuric rash associated with abdominal pain or a symmetrical poly-

|  | HLA-B27 associated | Not associated with HLA-B27 |
|---|---|---|
| *Type of infection* | Enteric or venereal | Streptococcal |
| *Resulting arthropathies* | Reactive arthritis<br>Reiter's syndrome | Rheumatic fever<br>Henoch–Schönlein purpura |

**Table 8.14** Classification of arthropathies following infections.

arthritis, and lasts for a few weeks. Its importance is the association of glomerulonephritis in 40% of cases.

# Connective tissue diseases

The term connective tissue disease is used for three diseases—systemic lupus erythematosus (SLE), systemic sclerosis, and polymyositis and dermatomyositis, whose relationship is illustrated in Fig. 8.16. The collective term 'connective tissue disease' means little but, since the aetiology of these conditions is unknown, it is difficult to suggest a better alternative. The diseases have a number of features in common, including the occurrence of arthritis or arthralgia, multisystem involvement, vasculitis and immunological abnormalities such as circulating autoantibodies and immune complex deposition. Features of all three diseases appear in mixed connective tissue disease.

## Systemic lupus erythematosus

SLE is the commonest of the connective tissue disorders and is characterized by the presence in the serum of antibodies against nuclear components. It is a multisystem disease, with arthralgia and rashes as the commonest clinical features, and cerebral and renal disease as the most serious problems.

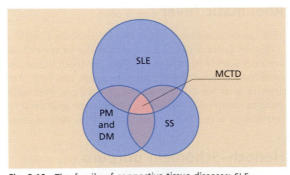

**Fig. 8.16** The family of connective-tissue diseases: SLE, systemic lupus erythematosus; PM, polymyositis; DM, dermatomyositis; SS, systemic sclerosis; MCTD, mixed connective tissue disease.

## EPIDEMIOLOGY

The disease probably affects about 0.1% of the population and is thus about 20 times less common than RA. It is much commoner in black women in the USA, with a prevalence of up to 1 in 250. It is about nine times as common in women as men, with a peak age of onset between 20 and 40 years.

## PATHOGENESIS

The cause of SLE is unknown but is probably multifactorial, including a variable genetic predisposition and environmental factors that trigger the disease. In some cases, genetic predisposition is so strong that minor additional triggers are sufficient. Known predisposing factors include:

HEREDITY: the identical twin of a patient with SLE has a 30% chance of developing the disease; first-degree relatives have a 5% chance. Certain races are especially prone, including Sioux Indians, Africans and Polynesians.

COMPLEMENT DEFICIENCIES of all types.

SEX HORMONE STATUS: women are much more often affected than men.

Known environmental triggers include:

DRUGS such as hydralazine.

ULTRAVIOLET LIGHT.

INFECTION: a virus infection is a popular theory for the cause of lupus and it is easy to see how a DNA virus could lead to the production of antibodies to nuclear material.

The immunological mechanisms of the disease include:

POLYCLONAL B-CELL ACTIVATION. Increased numbers of B cells lead to hyperglobulinaemia.

ANTINUCLEAR ANTIBODIES AND OTHER AUTOANTIBODIES are produced.

IMPAIRED T-CELL REGULATION of the immune response.

FAILURE TO REMOVE IMMUNE COMPLEXES FROM THE CIRCULATION. Circulating immune complexes cause arthralgia; deposition of immune complexes in tissues causes vasculitis and many other features of the disease, including glomerulonephritis.

Many immunological abnormalities are seen, including antibodies to human IgG, nuclear protein, smooth muscle, cytoplasm, organ-specific antibodies, e.g. thyroid, leucocytes, platelets, red cells, clotting factors and cryoglobulins with varying clinical effects. Their role in the pathogenesis, if any, is unknown.

## PATHOLOGY

SLE is characterized by a widespread vasculitis affecting capillaries, arterioles and venules. Fibrinoid (an eosinophilic amorphous material) is found along blood vessels and tissue fibres. The synovium of joints may be oedematous and may contain fibrinoid deposits. Haematoxylin bodies (rounded blue homogeneous haematoxylin-stained deposits) are seen in inflammatory infiltrates and are thought to result from the interaction of antinuclear antibodies and cell nuclei.

Lesions of other organs are described in the appropriate chapters.

## CLINICAL FEATURES (Fig. 8.17)

SLE is extremely variable in its manifestation and most of the clinical features are due to the consequences of vasculitis. Mild cases may present only with arthralgia, whilst in severe cases there may be multisystem involvement.

GENERAL FEATURES. Fever is common in exacerbations, occurring in up to 80% of cases. Patients complain of malaise and tiredness.

THE JOINTS. Joint involvement is the commonest clinical feature (>90%). Patients often present with symptoms that sound like RA. Joints are painful but characteristically appear clinically normal, although sometimes there is slight soft-tissue swelling surrounding the joint. Aseptic necrosis affecting the hip or knee is a rare complication of the disease.

THE SKIN. This is affected in 80% of cases (see p. 1020). Erythema in a butterfly distribution on the cheeks of the face and across the bridge of the nose is characteristic. Vasculitic lesions on the fingertips and around the nail folds, purpura and urticaria occur. In one-third of cases there is photosensitivity and prolonged exposure to sunlight can lead to exacerbations of the disease. Livedo reticularis, palmar and plantar rashes, pigmentation and alopecia may be seen. Raynaud's phenomenon is common and may precede the development of arthralgia and other clinical problems by years. Immunofluorescence of 'normal' skin will show immunoglobulin and complement deposition at the dermo-epidermal junction, which is known as the positive band test.

DISCOID LUPUS. See p. 1020.

THE LUNGS. Up to two-thirds of patients will have lung involvement sometime during the course of the disease (see p. 691). Recurrent pleurisy and pleural effusions (exudates) are the commonest manifestations. Pneumonitis and atelectasis may be seen; eventually a restrictive lung defect develops. Rarely, pulmonary fibrosis occurs.

THE HEART. This is involved in over 40% of cases. Pericarditis, with small pericardial effusions detected by echo-

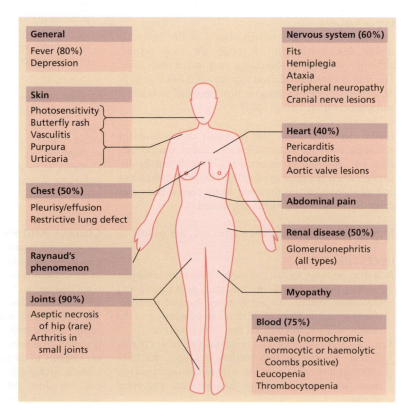

**General**

Fever (80%)
Depression

**Skin**

Photosensitivity
Butterfly rash
Vasculitis
Purpura
Urticaria

**Chest (50%)**

Pleurisy/effusion
Restrictive lung defect

**Raynaud's phenomenon**

**Joints (90%)**

Aseptic necrosis
  of hip (rare)
Arthritis in
  small joints

**Nervous system (60%)**

Fits
Hemiplegia
Ataxia
Peripheral neuropathy
Cranial nerve lesions

**Heart (40%)**

Pericarditis
Endocarditis
Aortic valve lesions

**Abdominal pain**

**Renal disease (50%)**

Glomerulonephritis
  (all types)

**Myopathy**

**Blood (75%)**

Anaemia (normochromic
  normocytic or haemolytic
  Coombs positive)
Leucopenia
Thrombocytopenia

**Fig. 8.17** Clinical features of systemic lupus erythematosus.

cardiography, is common. A mild myocarditis also occurs. Aortic valve lesions and a cardiomyopathy can rarely be present. Endocarditis involving the mitral valve (Libman–Sacks syndrome) is very rare.

THE KIDNEYS. These are affected in 30–50% of cases. Proteinuria (>1 g per 24 hours) is common. The renal histological lesions consist of minimal change, proliferative changes (either focal, diffuse or crescentic) or a membranous glomerulonephritis (see p. 448). Most patients with or without renal disease have immune complex deposits in their kidneys.

Hypertension may occur owing to progression to either the nephrotic syndrome or renal failure.

THE NERVOUS SYSTEM. Involvement of the nervous system occurs in 60% of cases. There may be a mild depression but occasionally more severe psychiatric disturbances occur. Epilepsy, cerebellar ataxia, aseptic meningitis, cranial nerve lesions, cerebrovascular accidents or peripheral neuropathy may be seen. These lesions may be due to vasculitis or immune-complex deposition.

THE EYES. Retinal lesions include cytoid bodies, which appear as hard exudates, and haemorrhages. Blindness is uncommon. Secondary Sjögren's syndrome may be seen.

THE GASTROINTESTINAL SYSTEM. SLE often causes gastrointestinal symptoms, although these are usually not a major presenting feature. Symptoms include nausea, vomiting, anorexia and diarrhoea.

### Lupus variants

DISCOID LUPUS. is a benign variant of the disease in which skin involvement is often the only feature, although systemic abnormalities may occur with time. The rash is characteristic and appears on the face as well-defined erythematous plaques that progress to scarring and pigmentation (see p. 1020).

DRUG-INDUCED SLE. This is usually characterized by arthralgia and mild systemic features, rashes and pericarditis, but seldom renal or cerebral disease. It usually disappears when the drug causing it is stopped. Hydralazine and procainamide are the most likely causes, but other drugs have occasionally been implicated.

MIXED CONNECTIVE TISSUE DISEASE. See p. 405.

### INVESTIGATION

A FULL BLOOD COUNT usually shows an anaemia (usually normochromic normocytic), neutropenia and thrombocytopenia. An autoimmune haemolytic anaemia may occur. The ESR is raised in proportion to the disease activity. In contrast, the CRP is normal.

SERUM ANTINUCLEAR ANTIBODIES ARE POSITIVE in almost all cases. dsDNA binding is specific for SLE, although it is only present in 50% of cases, particularly those with severe systemic involvement, e.g. renal disease.

SERUM RHEUMATOID FACTOR is positive in half of the patients.

SERUM COMPLEMENT LEVELS are reduced during active disease. Immunoglobulins are raised (usually IgG and IgM).

CHARACTERISTIC HISTOLOGICAL ABNORMALITIES are seen in biopsies from, for example, the kidney.

## MANAGEMENT
### Drug therapy

Systemic corticosteroid therapy is the mainstay of treatment in SLE, although patients with mild disease and arthralgia can be managed with NSAIDs. In cases where steroids are required, they should be used in small doses for short periods just sufficient to suppress the disease in order to minimize complications. Active SLE, with fever and pleurisy, should be treated with prednisolone 30 mg daily, the dose being reduced over the course of a few weeks to a maintenance level of around 5–10 mg daily. It may be possible to stop treatment in such a patient within a few months.

Two other types of drug are used in the management of SLE:

1 The antimalarial drug hydroxychloroquine (400 mg daily) is useful for suppressing the disease activity in patients with minor manifestations such as arthralgia that cannot be controlled with NSAIDs or troublesome skin lesions. Ocular toxicity may occur (see p. 393).

2 Immunosuppressive drugs are used for patients with more serious disease manifestations such as renal disease, usually in combination with steroids. Azathioprine (2 mg kg$^{-1}$ daily) is most often used; chlorambucil is an alternative and cyclophosphamide is reserved for patients with life-threatening disease. Immunosuppressive drugs also have a useful steroid-sparing effect.

### General management

Patients should be told about their disease and its management. Patients with photosensitivity problems should avoid excessive exposure to sunlight.

There is no major contraindication to pregnancy. However, there is an increased rate of fetal loss and complications may arise during the pregnancy; specialist care should therefore be available.

### COURSE AND PROGNOSIS

An episodic course is characteristic, with exacerbations and complete remissions that may last for long periods of time. These remissions may occur even in patients with renal disease. A chronic course is occasionally seen. Earlier estimates of the mortality in SLE were exaggerated; 5-year survival rate is about 95%. In most cases the pattern of the disease becomes established in the first few years; if serious problems have not developed in this time, they are unlikely to do so. The arthritis is usually intermittent. Chronic progressive destruction of joints as seen in RA and OA does not occur, but a few patients develop deformities such as ulnar deviation.

# Antiphospholipid syndrome

This condition was first described in a small proportion of patients with SLE but over the years it has become clear that it is much commoner than SLE and that most patients do not have SLE. The syndrome is characterized by the presence of antiphospholipid antibodies, which are thought to play a role in thrombosis by an effect on platelet membranes, endothelial cells and on clotting compounds such as prothrombin, protein C and protein S.

## CLINICAL FEATURES

The major features are:

THROMBOCYTOPENIA.

ARTERIAL AND VENOUS THROMBOSES—17% of strokes occurring under the age of 45 years are thought to be due to the antiphospholipid syndrome. Thromboses of different types occur and cause other features of the disease including the Budd–Chiari syndrome and Addison's disease.

ABORTIONS—27% of women who have had more than two abortions have the antiphospholipid syndrome.

CHOREA, MIGRAINE AND EPILEPSY.

VALVULAR HEART DISEASE.

ATHEROMA. The syndrome may also be important in the development of accelerated atheroma.

CUTANEOUS MANIFESTATIONS—see p. 1028.

## INVESTIGATIONS

Anti-cardiolipin antibodies are diagnostic. The ESR is usually normal and antinuclear antibodies are usually negative.

## TREATMENT

Anticoagulants: small doses of aspirin in mild cases; warfarin in severe cases; heparin in early pregnancy because warfarin is toxic to the fetus.

# Systemic sclerosis

Systemic sclerosis is a multisystem disease that predominantly affects the skin and presents with Raynaud's phenomenon in over three-quarters of cases. It is less common than SLE. The major features distinguishing systemic sclerosis from polymyositis and SLE are shown in Fig. 8.18. It is commoner in women than men (3 : 1) and can appear at any age under 50 years.

## AETIOLOGY

The aetiology of systemic sclerosis is unknown. Abnormalities in both humoral and cellular immunity have been documented. A positive speckled or nucleolar antinuclear antibody is found in up to 60% of patients. Familial cases have been documented and HLA-B8, DR3 has been reported to occur with greater frequency in systemic sclerosis. A similar syndrome can be produced by certain chemicals, including polyvinyl chloride and in poisoning with adulterated oil (toxic epidermal syndrome).

## PATHOLOGY

In the early phase the skin is oedematous, with perivascular lymphocyte infiltration and degeneration of collagen fibres. Later there is an increase in collagen. Small blood vessels show intimal proliferation and obliteration. Progressive fibrosis is the major feature of visceral involvement.

## CLINICAL FEATURES

The involvement of various organs is shown in Table 8.15.

### The skin

The cutaneous changes that occur are described on p. 1021. Sclerosis of the skin can lead to beaking of the

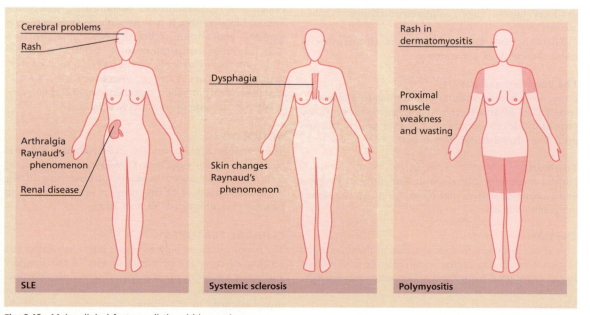

**Fig. 8.18** Major clinical features distinguishing various connective-tissue diseases.

| Organ | Involved in |
|---|---|
| Skin | 90% |
| Vascular system— | |
|    Raynaud's phenomenon | 80% |
| Oesophagus | 80% |
| Lungs | 45% |
| Heart | 40% |
| Kidneys | 35% |
| Joints | 25% |
| Muscle | 20% |

**Table 8.15**  Involvement of various organs in systemic sclerosis.

nose and difficulty in opening the mouth. Other changes seen in the skin include telangiectasis, pigmentation or depigmentation, ulceration and calcinosis. Raynaud's phenomenon often occurs; it is described on p. 628.

**The gastrointestinal system** (see p. 184)
Oesophageal involvement is almost invariable, although only half of these patients will have symptoms of heartburn or dysphagia. A barium swallow may show delayed peristalsis, dilatation or stricture formation, but oesophageal manometry is the most sensitive test. This shows lack of distal oesophageal peristalsis and a reduced oesophageal sphincter pressure.

The small bowel can be involved, producing malabsorption from bacterial overgrowth due to dilatation and atony. Dilatation and atony may also affect the colon.

**The joints and muscles**
The fibrotic process can affect tendons, causing flexion deformities of the fingers. The small joints of the hands are affected in 25% of patients, particularly in the early stages of the disease. Soft-tissue swelling of the fingers produces 'sausage fingers'. Progressive changes in joints are not seen.

Myopathy and myositis occur and electromyogram EMG abnormalities are common.

**The lungs** (see also p. 691)
Lower-lobe fibrosis leads to cyst formation and honeycombing in advanced cases. Gas transfer and restrictive ventilatory defects are seen. Aspiration pneumonia and pulmonary hypertension may occur.

**The heart**
Diffuse myocardial fibrosis with arrhythmias (in 25%) and conduction defects may occur. Effusions accompany pericardial disease.

**The kidneys**
This is the most serious manifestation of the disease and is caused by an obliterative endarteritis of renal vessels. It can cause renal failure and malignant hypertension.

**The eyes**
Sjögren's syndrome with keratoconjunctivitis sicca may be seen.

## VARIANTS OF SYSTEMIC SCLEROSIS
MORPHOEA—see p. 1021.
CREST SYNDROME consists of calcinosis (C), Raynaud's phenomenon (R), oesophageal involvement (E), sclerodactyly (S) and telangiectasia (T). Antinuclear antibodies to the centromere are found in the blood.
MIXED CONNECTIVE TISSUE DISEASE—see p. 405.

### INVESTIGATION
SERUM ANTINUCLEAR ANTIBODIES are often positive. Antinucleolar and anticentromere antibodies are specifically elevated. A positive rheumatoid factor is found in 30% of cases.

A NORMOCHROMIC NORMOCYTIC ANAEMIA can be seen. An acquired haemolytic anaemia with 'cold' agglutinins may occur. The ESR may be raised.

X-RAYS OF THE HANDS may show deposits of calcium around the fingers. In severe cases there is erosion and resorption of the tufts of the distal phalanges.

BARIUM SWALLOW to detect oesophageal involvement is often a useful confirmatory test.

### TREATMENT
No treatment has been shown to influence the progress of this condition. Management is therefore symptomatic.

### PROGNOSIS
In some patients the disease is mild, whilst in others it is severe and complicated by systemic features such as renal disease. The mean 5-year survival rate is 50%.

## Polymyositis and dermatomyositis

Polymyositis is a disorder of muscle in which the pathological features are necrosis of muscle fibres together with evidence of regeneration and inflammation, particularly around blood vessels. It presents with proximal muscular weakness and wasting. When this is accompanied by a rash, it is called dermatomyositis. Its incidence is comparable with that of systemic sclerosis, i.e. it is less common than SLE. It occurs at any age, even in children, but with a peak incidence in adults aged between 30 and 60 years. It is twice as common in women as in men.

### AETIOLOGY
The aetiology is unknown, but immunological and viral factors have been suggested. Dermatomyositis is associated with an increased incidence of carcinoma of the bronchus in men or of the ovary in women, mainly in patients presenting after 50 years of age.

### CLINICAL FEATURES
The major feature of polymyositis is muscle weakness and wasting affecting the proximal muscles of the shoulder and pelvic girdles. It may be very acute in onset, particularly in children, and is sometimes accompanied by myoglobinuria. In the chronic form there is gradually progressive muscular weakness. Muscle pain and tenderness are found in about one-half of the cases, but weak-

ness is the chief complaint. The rash of dermatomyositis is characteristic (see p. 1022). As in other connective tissue diseases, systemic features are often found:

ARTHRALGIA OR ARTHRITIS occur in about half of all patients and may be the presenting feature, occurring before the onset of the muscular symptoms. The small joints of the hands are particularly affected but the arthritis may extend in a distribution resembling that of RA. Joints are often swollen but the arthritis is intermittent and not progressive.

DYSPHAGIA is found in 50% of cases and is due to oesophageal muscle involvement.

RAYNAUD'S PHENOMENON is common.

SJÖGREN'S SYNDROME AND RESPIRATORY PROBLEMS may occur.

## INVESTIGATION

The diagnosis of polymyositis is made on the basis of three tests, two of which at least should be positive:

1 *Muscle enzymes.* Serum creatine phosphokinase and aldolase are raised and can be used to follow the progress of the disease during treatment.
2 *EMG.* Short polyphasic motor potentials, sometimes spontaneous fibrillation and high-frequency repetitive discharges (see p. 951) are almost pathognomonic of polymyositis.
3 *Muscle biopsy.* This shows necrosis of muscle fibres with swelling and disruption of muscle cells. Vacuolation, fragmentation and fibrosis of the fibres are seen, with thickening of the blood vessels. There are also inflammatory changes.

### Other tests

THE ESR IS USUALLY RAISED. A normochromic normocytic anaemia and a polymorphonuclear leucocytosis are seen in acute cases.

SERUM ANTINUCLEAR ANTIBODIES AND TESTS FOR RHEUMATOID FACTOR may be positive.

## MANAGEMENT

Systemic corticosteroids, starting with 60 mg of prednisolone daily and reducing to a maintenance dose of about 15 mg daily are used. In most cases this produces a gradual remission of the disease. Physiotherapy may be required to restore muscle power. Treatment is required for a variable period, usually months but sometimes years. Some patients fail to respond to steroids, and immunosuppressive drugs such as methotrexate or azathioprine may be required.

## PROGNOSIS

Fifty per cent of affected children die within 2 years. In adults the prognosis is better, except in association with malignancy.

## Mixed connective tissue disease

The existence of this rare disorder emphasizes the overlap between the connective tissue diseases, although it may not itself be a distinct entity. It is a useful term for cases with features of more than one of the connective tissue diseases together with high titres of antibody to an extractable nuclear antigen such as RNP. Like the other conditions, it affects women more often than men and presents in young adults.

Clinical features include arthralgia, Raynaud's phenomenon, proximal muscle weakness and wasting, and a puffy swelling of the skin of the hands that somewhat resembles the changes occurring in scleroderma. Other features of SLE, polymyositis or scleroderma may appear, but serious problems such as renal disease are unusual.

The condition tends to be benign and often responds well to small doses of prednisolone.

## Primary Sjögren's syndrome

The syndrome of dry eyes (keratoconjunctivitis sicca), in the absence of RA, is known as primary Sjögren's syndrome. There is an association with HLA-B8, DR3. Dryness of the mouth, skin or vagina may also be a problem. Salivary and parotid gland enlargement is seen.

Systemic associations include:

- Arthralgia and occasionally non-progressive polyarthritis like that seen in SLE
- Raynaud's phenomenon
- Dysphagia and abnormal oesophageal motility as seen in systemic sclerosis
- Other organ-specific autoimmune diseases, including thyroid disease, myasthenia gravis, primary biliary cirrhosis and chronic active hepatitis
- Renal tubular defects causing nephrogenic diabetes insipidus and renal tubular acidosis
- Pulmonary diffusion defects and fibrosis
- Polyneuropathy, fits and depression
- Vasculitis
- Increased incidence of lymphoma

### PATHOLOGY

Biopsies of the salivary gland or of the lip show a focal infiltration of lymphocytes and plasma cells.

### DIAGNOSIS

THE SCHIRMER TEAR TEST, in which a standard strip of filter paper is placed on the inside of the lower eyelid; wetting of less than 10 mm in 5 min indicates defective tear production

ROSE BENGAL STAINING of the eyes showing punctate or filamentary keratitis

LABORATORY ABNORMALITIES include raised immunoglobulin levels, circulating immune complexes and many autoantibodies. Rheumatoid factor is usually positive, antinuclear antibodies are found in 60–70% and antimitochondrial antibodies in 10% of cases. Anti-Ro (SSA) antibodies are found in 70% of cases compared with 10% of cases of RA and secondary Sjögren's syndrome. This antibody is of particular interest because it can cross the placenta and cause congenital heart block.

# Vasculitis (see also p. 1027)

The 'vasculitides' encompass a wide range of diseases with considerable overlap between them. Many different classifications have been suggested and only better understanding of these conditions will clarify the situation. In the meantime, they are usually classified according to the predominant type of vessel involvement (Table 8.16).

## Polyarteritis nodosa (PAN) group

There is much overlap within this group. The classic PAN is a rare condition and, unlike other connective tissue disorders, it usually presents in middle-aged men. It is accompanied by severe systemic manifestations and its association with hepatitis B antigenaemia suggests a vasculitis secondary to the deposition of immune complexes. Pathologically, there is fibrinoid necrosis of vessel walls with microaneurysm formation, thrombosis and infarction. Classic PAN does not involve the lung.

The Churg–Strauss syndrome is associated with allergic angiitis and granuloma formation accompanied by an intense eosinophilic infiltration that affects the pulmonary arteries and causes asthma and pneumonia (see p. 693) .

Microscopic polyarteritis is an inflammation of capillaries involving many organs, e.g. kidneys (see p. 452) and the lungs resulting in pulmonary haemorrhage.

ANCA is particularly associated with microscopic polyarteritis and is usually negative in classic PAN. It may play a role in the pathogenesis of this condition.

### CLINICAL FEATURES
In classic PAN the initial features are non-specific, being fever, malaise, severe weight loss, myalgia and arthralgia. Later the most characteristic features are renal impairment, hypertension, polyneuropathy, lung disease and cardiac problems, including arrhythmia, heart failure and myocardial infarction. The polyneuropathy in vasculitic disorders characteristically takes the form of a mononeuritis multiplex (see p. 945). A migratory arthralgia or arthritis with fever are seen, and abdominal pain, due to liver and gastrointestinal tract involvement, is common. Death is usually from renal disease.

### INVESTIGATION
The ESR is raised but the diagnosis depends upon either histological examination of biopsy material from an affected organ or angiographic demonstration of microaneurysms in hepatic, intestinal or renal vessels.

### TREATMENT
Treatment is with corticosteroids, usually in combination with immunosuppressive drugs such as azathioprine.

## Essential mixed cryoglobulinaemia

In this disorder a cutaneous vasculitis is associated with cryoglobulinaemia. It is exacerbated by exercise and the cold, and there is an association with hepatitis B infection. Multisystem involvement occurs as in other connective tissue disorders.

## Vasculitis associated with granulomas

Two forms of vasculitis associated with granulomas are Wegener's granulomatosis and the Churg–Strauss syndrome (see p. 693). *Wegener's granulomatosis* classically consists of the triad of upper respiratory tract granuloma, fleeting pulmonary shadows, and glomerulonephritis; it is discussed on pp. 690 and 451.

## Polymyalgia rheumatica and giant-cell arteritis

Polymyalgia rheumatica and giant-cell arteritis (also known as temporal or cranial arteritis) can be regarded as two conditions at the ends of a spectrum, with giant-cell arteritis as the basic pathological lesion. The cause is unknown. Occasionally the syndrome of polymyalgia is

---

**Infective**

Bacterial, spirochaetal (Lyme disease and syphilis), fungal, mycobacterial, viral, rickettsial, protozoal

**Non-infective**
*Involving large, medium sized and small blood vessels*

Takayasu's arteritis
Giant cell arteritis (temporal arteritis and polymyalgia rheumatica)

*Involving predominantly medium sized and small vessels*

Buerger's disease
Polyarteritis nodosa
Microscopic polyarteritis
Wegener's granulomatosis
Churg–Strauss syndrome
Sarcoidosis
Vasculitis of connective tissue disorder, e.g. SLE
Vasculitis associated with rheumatoid arthritis

*Involving predominantly small vessels (hypersensitivity or leucocytoclastic vasculitis)*

Serum sickness
Henoch–Schönlein purpura
Drug-induced vasculitis
Essential mixed cryoglobulinaemia
Hypocomplementaemia
Vasculitis associated with malignancy, inflammatory bowel disease and primary biliary cirrhosis
Goodpasture syndrome

---

SLE, systemic lupus erythematosus.

**Table 8.16**  Classification of vasculitis.

due to some underlying condition, e.g. a severe infection or a malignancy.

## CLINICAL FEATURES

Polymyalgia rheumatica is characterized by pains and morning stiffness in the proximal muscles of the shoulder and pelvic girdle, and a high ESR.

The onset is sudden. It is rare before the age of 50 years and usually occurs in those aged 60–70 years. Women are three times more commonly affected than men. Severe pains and stiffness occur in the girdle muscles and also in the muscles of the cervical and lumbar spines. The hands and feet are never affected. Early morning stiffness often causes difficulty in getting out of bed. Systemic symptoms include malaise, anorexia, weight loss and a low-grade fever. Painful restriction of movement of the shoulders and hips is characteristic. The distribution of joint involvement is bilateral and symmetrical. Occasionally knees and wrists are involved. There may be no physical signs if the patient is examined in the afternoon when the stiffness has worn off.

Headache, particularly if localized and accompanied by temporal tenderness and loss of pulsation, suggests a temporal arteritis (see p. 936), which rarely occurs with polymyalgia.

## INVESTIGATION

ESR is usually raised to a very high level (around 100 mm hour$^{-1}$) but returns to normal with treatment.
MILD NORMOCHROMIC NORMOCYTIC ANAEMIA is present.
RHEUMATOID FACTOR TESTS are negative, though false-positive results are found particularly in older people.
SERUM ALKALINE PHOSPHATASE LEVELS are sometimes raised but return to normal with treatment.
There is no specific test. It is not usual to carry out a temporal artery biopsy in polymyalgia, although a giant-cell arteritis can be demonstrated in 20% of cases. Temporal artery biopsy is often performed in temporal arteritis, but is not necessary in classic cases.

## MANAGEMENT

Corticosteroids are the treatment of choice in polymyalgia rheumatica, starting with 15 mg of prednisolone daily. NSAIDs are less effective and, as they do not control the arteritis, should not be used. Treatment should be started immediately the diagnosis is made and before waiting for the results of tests, in order to prevent irreversible blindness, although this is rare in the absence of temporal arteritis. With steroid therapy, patients feel better within days, though mobilization of stiff shoulders may take a month or two. The dose of prednisolone is slowly reduced over the course of the next 2 years in amounts not exceeding 1 mg and at intervals not less than 1 month. Relapses are common. In most patients it is possible to stop treatment after 2–4 years.

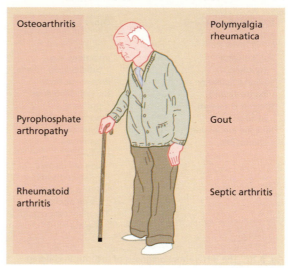

**Fig. 8.19**  The differential diagnosis of arthritis in the elderly.

# Differential diagnosis of arthritis in the elderly

Common conditions are summarized in Fig. 8.19. OA is common from the age of 50 years onwards but is easily distinguished from polymyalgia rheumatica by its less dramatic onset, peripheral distribution and normal ESR; if there is any doubt, a 1 week trial of prednisolone should be given.

RA can begin in elderly patients. It is often sudden in onset, with very dramatic joint inflammation ('explosive' RA). Unlike the disease in young patients, it often responds very well to small doses of steroids (prednisolone 10–15 mg daily) and has a good prognosis.

Pyrophosphate deposition is common in elderly patients, typically presenting as a painful swollen knee.

Gout and septic arthritis are other causes of acute problems in the elderly.

# Arthritis in children (Fig. 8.20)

Joint pain is a common problem in childhood but arthritis is fortunately rare. Benign limb pain in childhood is sometimes called 'growing pain' and, though meaningless, this is probably a convenient term that parents readily accept.

## JUVENILE CHRONIC ARTHRITIS

Juvenile chronic arthritis is a general term used to cover a group of diseases in which an exact diagnosis is not

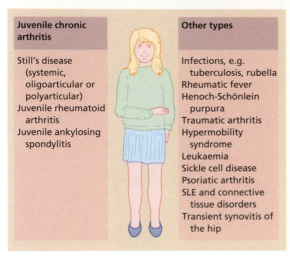

| Juvenile chronic arthritis | Other types |
|---|---|
| Still's disease (systemic, oligoarticular or polyarticular) | Infections, e.g. tuberculosis, rubella |
| Juvenile rheumatoid arthritis | Rheumatic fever |
| | Henoch-Schönlein purpura |
| Juvenile ankylosing spondylitis | Traumatic arthritis |
| | Hypermobility syndrome |
| | Leukaemia |
| | Sickle cell disease |
| | Psoriatic arthritis |
| | SLE and connective tissue disorders |
| | Transient synovitis of the hip |

**Fig. 8.20**   The differential diagnosis of arthritis in children.

always possible. There are three main types: Still's disease, juvenile RA and juvenile ankylosing spondylitis.

## Still's disease

This is the commonest type of juvenile chronic arthritis, accounting for about 70% of cases. It is entirely distinct from RA, being distinguished by a number of clinical features and negative tests for rheumatoid factor. There are two peaks in the age of onset: the first and largest is between the ages of 2 and 5 years, and the second between the ages of 10 and 15 years. Still's disease occasionally begins after the age of 16 years, and rarely in the twenties. The disease is often episodic, with bouts of fever and arthritis. It can be divided into three subtypes:

1  *The systemic type* is usually seen in children under the age of 5 years. They present with a high fever, a characteristic rash and various other features, including lymphadenopathy, splenomegaly and pericarditis. The rash is characterized by patches of erythema on the trunk or limbs, often appearing in the evening and brought out by warmth. Arthritis or arthralgia are minor features of the illness and may be absent. Arthritis may, however, develop later in the course of the disease.

2  *The pauciarticular or oligoarticular type* of Still's disease affects up to four of the large joints such as the hips, knees or ankles. These patients are particularly liable to chronic iritis, which may lead to blindness without any preceding symptoms. Antinuclear antibodies are often positive and provide a useful warning that iritis may develop. Slit-lamp examination should be performed at regular intervals in these patients.

3  *Polyarticular Still's disease* presents with a bilateral symmetrical polyarthritis not unlike that of RA, but with less prominent and less frequent involvement of the small joints of the hands and feet.

The characteristic systemic features described above may be associated with arthritis, whether polyarticular or pauciarticular.

## DIAGNOSIS

The non-articular features of Still's disease are often helpful in making a diagnosis. A high swinging fever is also characteristic. This can be misleading to the unwary, as it suggests the possibility of infection.

The joints themselves are swollen, but pain and tenderness are much less prominent than in adult RA. The ESR is usually raised and there is frequently an anaemia.

### TREATMENT

Treatment is with NSAIDs as in RA. Gold and penicillamine are effective but probably in a smaller proportion of cases than in RA. Corticosteroids should be avoided because of their effect on growth. It is important to protect the joints and prevent deformity during relapses, particularly as spontaneous remissions occur in 85% of patients before the age of 20 years. Long periods of rest and splinting of joints may be necessary. The patient's education and normal life-style should be continued if possible.

## Juvenile rheumatoid arthritis

RA may begin before 16 years of age. The clinical features are identical to those of adults and tests for rheumatoid factor are usually positive. However, the prognosis is much worse than in adults. Juvenile RA accounts for about 15% of cases of juvenile chronic arthritis.

## Juvenile ankylosing spondylitis

This accounts for the remaining 15% of cases of juvenile chronic arthritis. It is the most benign of the subtypes and usually presents between the ages of 10 and 15 years. A peripheral arthritis occurs, with the lower limb joints being particularly affected. Joints are swollen and painful in the acute stage, but often respond well to anti-inflammatory drugs and usually settle within a few years. These patients may develop iritis and there may be other features of HLA-B27-associated diseases (see p. 394). Back pain is not a prominent feature at this age. A family history of ankylosing spondylitis or related diseases is sometimes helpful in the diagnosis. Tests for rheumatoid factor are negative. Although the arthritis usually resolves, 50% of these patients go on to develop ankylosing spondylitis in adult life.

## OTHER CONDITIONS

Other types of arthritis that are seen in childhood are summarized in Fig. 8.20.

Some soft tissue syndromes particularly affect children including Osgood–Schlatter disease, which is characterized by localized pain over the tibial tubercle and is usually seen in athletic teenagers.

A mysterious condition called transient synovitis of the hip, which causes hip pain, may give rise to concern because of the possibility of tuberculosis or other serious conditions. It presents as painful limitation of movement of one hip, and usually resolves within a few weeks or months.

# Crystal deposition diseases

Three types of crystal are deposited in joints; each is associated with a characteristic clinical syndrome (Fig. 8.21):

1 *Monosodium urate deposition* is associated with acute gout, typically affecting the big toe.
2 *Calcium pyrophosphate deposition* causes many different syndromes including pseudogout, which most often affects the knee.
3 *Hydroxyapatite deposition* causes acute calcific periarthritis and most often affects the shoulder.

In addition, calcium pyrophosphate and hydroxyapatite crystals are found in the joints of patients with OA and may contribute to the inflammation.

## Gout

Gout is an abnormality of uric acid metabolism that results in the deposition of sodium urate crystals in:
JOINTS—causing acute gouty arthritis
SOFT TISSUE—causing tophi and tenosynovitis
URINARY TRACT—causing urate stones

### EPIDEMIOLOGY

The prevalence varies from approximately 0.2% in Europe and the USA to 10% in the adult male Maori of New Zealand. Filipinos have high prevalences in the USA but not in the Philippines, suggesting an environmental factor. Gout is commoner in the upper social classes and one-third of patients give a family history. At least 50% are regular alcohol drinkers.

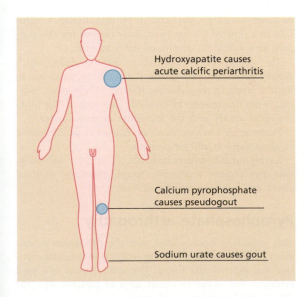

**Fig. 8.21** The typical patterns of joint involvement seen in crystal deposition disease.

### PATHOGENESIS

The biochemical abnormality is hyperuricaemia resulting from overproduction or under-excretion of uric acid. A high dietary intake of purines can be an additional factor, but does not in itself produce hyperuricaemia.

### Uric acid production

Uric acid is the last step in the breakdown pathway of nucleoprotein and purines. The last two steps—the conversion of hypoxanthine to xanthine and of xanthine to uric acid—are catalysed by the enzyme xanthine oxidase.

### Uric acid excretion

Uric acid is completely filtered by the glomerulus; 100% is then reabsorbed in the proximal tubule and 75% is secreted by the distal tubule. Some postsecretory reabsorption also takes place.

### Causes of hyperuricaemia

In most patients with idiopathic (primary) gout the major cause of the hyperuricaemia is increased urate production, but there is also impaired renal excretion. Conditions in which hyperuricaemia occur are shown in Table 8.17.

### CLINICAL FEATURES

Gout is predominantly a disease of men. Hippocrates was the first to note that it does not occur in men before puberty or in women until after the menopause. It is a disease that mostly begins in middle life. Asymptomatic hyperuricaemia is 10 times more common than gout.

There are two stages in the natural history of the dis-

---

*Impaired excretion of uric acid*
Idiopathic (primary) gout
Chronic renal disease (clinical gout unusual)
Drug therapy, e.g. thiazide diuretics, low-dose aspirin
Hypertension
Lead toxicity
Primary hyperparathyroidism
Hypothyroidism
Increased lactic acid production from alcohol, exercise, starvation
Glucose-6-phosphatase deficiency (interferes with renal excretion)

*Increased production of uric acid*
Idiopathic (primary) gout
Increased purine synthesis de novo due to:
  Hypoxanthine-guanine-phosphoribosyl transferase (HGPRT) reduction (an X-linked inborn error causing the Lesch–Nyhan syndrome)
  Phosphoribosyl-pyrophosphate synthetase overactivity
  Glucose-6-phosphatase deficiency with glycogen storage disease type 1 (patients who survive develop hyperuricaemia due to increased production as well as decreased excretion)
Increased turnover of purines due to:
  Myeloproliferative disorders, e.g. polycythaemia vera
  Lymphoproliferative disorders, e.g. leukaemia
  Others, e.g. carcinoma, severe psoriasis

**Table 8.17** Causes of hyperuricaemia.

ease. First, recurrent acute attacks of arthritis occur. Secondly, the attacks fail to resolve completely and there are persistent symptoms associated with the permanent deposition of urate in and around joints; this stage is known as chronic tophaceous gout.

The typical acute attack begins suddenly in the early hours of the morning with excruciating pain in the big toe. Attacks may be precipitated by events such as:
• A surgical operation (hence postoperative arthritis is usually due to gout)
• Dietary or alcoholic excess
• Starvation
• Drugs, e.g. diuretics, particularly thiazides
In 25% of attacks, a joint other than the big toe is the site of the disease. Joints of the lower limb are most often affected, including the toes, ankles and knees. Occasionally attacks occur in the upper limb, particularly in the distal interphalangeal joints of the fingers. One joint only is affected in 90% of attacks.

### Signs

The typical gouty joint is red, warm, swollen and exquisitely tender. The presence of tophi in the ear lobes or around joints may provide a clue to the correct diagnosis, but they usually occur in the later stages of the disease, by which time the nature of the problem is obvious.

### Associated features

Patients with gout have a higher than expected incidence of vascular disease, hypertension and renal disease. Renal disease may be due to uric acid stones or very rarely to deposition of uric acid in the kidney itself, a condition known as chronic hyperuricaemic nephropathy (see p. 462). However, most often the renal disease is due to hypertension and vascular disease, which are genetic associations of gout rather than complications of hyperuricaemia.

### INVESTIGATION

SYNOVIAL FLUID EXAMINATION. The affected joint is aspirated and the synovial fluid is examined under polarized light microscopy. In acute gout, the presence of long, needle-shaped, negatively birefringent crystals is diagnostic. The test takes just a few minutes and is the best way to make the diagnosis if this is in doubt.

SERUM URIC ACID has a number of limitations as a diagnostic test. It takes time, and a high incidence of false-positive and false-negative results makes interpretation difficult. Acute gout never occurs with a serum uric acid in the lower half of the normal range. However, in the first few attacks, which are the most difficult to diagnose, the serum uric acid is often below the upper limit of normal. The level also falls after an acute attack. Thus, a normal serum uric acid does not exclude the diagnosis of gout. Similarly, a high level alone is not diagnostic. However, the serum uric acid is useful in monitoring treatment.

## MANAGEMENT
### Acute attacks

Acute gout is treated with anti-inflammatory drugs:

INDOMETHACIN, 50 mg three to four times daily, should produce substantial relief within 24–48 hours, when the dose should be reduced to 25 mg three to four times daily. The attack should resolve completely within a few weeks. Azapropazone, 600 mg twice daily, is an alternative.

COLCHICINE works slowly and produces diarrhoea; it is rarely used.

INTRAMUSCULAR ADRENOCORTICOTROPHIN (ACTH) is very effective in difficult cases.

EFFUSIONS IN LARGE JOINTS should be aspirated and a corticosteroid injected to reduce inflammation.

### Long-term therapy

Long-term therapy should be considered when the acute attack has settled. Simple measures to reduce uric acid levels include:
• Weight reduction
• Reduction in alcohol intake
• Avoidance of foods and drinks containing high levels of purine, e.g. game and lager
• Good fluid intake
• Withdrawal of drugs such as salicylates and thiazides

DRUGS. Allopurinol (a xanthine oxidase inhibitor) is the drug of choice. Indications include:
• Frequent acute attacks
• Tophi or chronic gouty arthritis
• Renal stones
• Very high serum uric acid levels (0.55 mmol litre$^{-1}$ or >9 mg dl$^{-1}$)
• Prophylaxis when treating malignant disease
Allopurinol should not be started until 4 weeks after the last acute attack. It may precipitate acute gout and should be given with a prophylactic to prevent attacks. Colchicine in a dose of 0.5 mg twice daily is ideal for this purpose and should be continued for 6 months.

The dosage of allopurinol is 300 mg daily, which should be sufficient to bring the serum urate down to normal levels. In renal disease 100 mg daily is given. Side-effects are uncommon but include skin rashes. The tophi disappear slowly with the reduction in serum urate.

Probenecid, a uricosuric drug, is used as an alternative to allopurinol in allergic patients.

Asymptomatic hyperuricaemia, found on screening, does not require treatment. Simple measures outlined above are, however, usually advised.

## Pyrophosphate arthropathy

This condition is associated with the deposition of calcium pyrophosphate dihydrate (CPPD) in articular cartilage and periarticular tissue. The acute attacks of crystal synovitis that occur in about 25% of patients with the disease are known as pseudogout.

The aetiology of CPPD arthropathy is unknown but there is an association with primary hyperparathyroidism, haemochromatosis, hypothyroidism, hypophosphatasia and true gout. CPPD crystal deposition often complicates OA, particularly in the knees and hips.

Pyrophosphate arthropathy is a disease of older people, with the typical age of onset being 60 years. It is equally common in men and women.

### CLINICAL FEATURES

Pyrophosphate arthropathy is not dissimilar to primary OA but tends to be polyarticular, sometimes with involvement of unusual joints such as the wrist. The course of OA associated with pyrophosphate deposition may be punctuated by attacks of pseudogout.

Acute attacks most commonly affect the knee but they can affect other joints, usually large ones and mainly one at a time. The attacks begin suddenly with pain and swelling. The affected joint is warm and swollen with a large effusion. The attack resolves within weeks or months but recurs at irregular intervals. Patients may have other changes associated with OA, such as Heberden's nodes.

Occasionally, pyrophosphate deposition is entirely asymptomatic. Rarely, it causes a polyarthritis resembling RA, a severe destructive arthritis of weight-bearing joints (resembling a Charcot joint), an acute spinal syndrome or polymyalgia rheumatica.

### INVESTIGATION

SERUM CALCIUM is normal.

ESR may be raised during an attack.

ASPIRATION OF SYNOVIAL FLUID and identification of crystals by polarized light microscopy is diagnostic. Calcium pyrophosphate crystals are smaller than urate crystals. They are brick-shaped and postively birefringent, and are therefore easily distinguished from urate crystals.

X-RAYS OF THE KNEE and occasionally the wrist may show linear calcification lying between and parallel to the articular surfaces (chondrocalcinosis articularis). X-rays may also show changes of OA, with joint space narrowing and osteophyte formation.

### MANAGEMENT

Pyrophosphate arthropathy is not as easy to treat and control as gout. Rest and aspiration of as much fluid as possible from an affected joint and an injection of corticosteroid are helpful. NSAIDs are less dramatic in their effects than in gout but are, nevertheless, useful.

## Acute calcific periarthritis

This syndrome is associated with deposition of hydroxyapatite in the soft tissues around joints. It is the least common of the crystal deposition diseases, but is by no means rare. It typically occurs in adults aged about 40 years and is equally common in men and women.

The shoulder joint is the commonest site, but it can affect the small joints of the hands and feet, the wrists, the knees and other joints. When the big toe is affected, the condition is often confused with gout. There is a sudden onset of pain, which is often very severe. The affected joint is red, warm and swollen, and there is sometimes a small effusion. The attack resolves within days or weeks, but attacks recur at irregular intervals.

X-rays are diagnostic: there is a rounded well-defined radiopaque deposit in the soft tissue adjacent to the joint.

Treatment is with NSAIDs such as indomethacin. Potent analgesics such as opiates are sometimes required in the acute stage. It is often useful to inject the affected joint or soft tissues with a combination of local anaesthetic and corticosteroid. It is seldom, if ever, necessary to remove the calcific deposit.

# Arthritis associated with other diseases

## Gastrointestinal and liver disease

### Enteropathic synovitis

This is associated with HLA B27 and is described on p. 395.

### Autoimmune chronic active hepatitis (see p. 259)

This may be accompanied by an arthralgia that is like that seen in SLE. Joint pain occurs in a bilateral, symmetrical distribution, with the small joints of the hands being prominently affected. Joints usually look normal but sometimes there is a slight soft-tissue swelling. These patients often have positive tests for antinuclear antibodies.

### Primary biliary cirrhosis

Patients occasionally have a similar symmetrical arthropathy to the above.

### Haemochromatosis

This is associated with osteoarthritis in 50% of cases; it is often the first sign of the disease and chondrocalcinosis is common. The metacarpophalangeal joints of the hands are particularly affected and the disease tends to be polyarticular, severe and progressive. Iron depletion does not solve the problem of the arthritis.

### Whipple's disease (see p. 211)

This is accompanied by fever and arthralgia.

## Malignant dissease

### Hypertrophic pulmonary osteoarthropathy

Hypertrophic osteoarthropathy is most often associated with carcinoma of the bronchus. It is a non-metastatic complication and may be the presenting feature of the disease. It occurs only rarely with other conditions that cause clubbing. It is seen most often in middle-aged men, who present with pain and swelling of the wrists and ankles. Other joints are occasionally involved.

The diagnosis is made on the presence of clubbing of

the fingers, which is usually gross, and periosteal new bone formation along the shafts of the distal ends of the radius, ulna, tibia and fibula seen on X-ray. A chest X-ray usually shows the malignancy.

Treatment should be directed at the underlying carcinoma; if this can be removed, the arthropathy disappears. NSAIDs may help to relieve the symptoms.

### Other disorders

Secondary gout occurs in conditions such as chronic myeloid leukaemia. Pain in the shoulder or back may be referred from malignant disease of the chest or abdomen. Secondaries around the joints may present with pain, but primary joint tumours are very rare. A synovioma presents as a painless soft-tissue swelling adjacent to joints. It is highly malignant but extremely rare.

## Skin disease

### Psoriatic arthritis

This is a seronegative arthritis occurring in patients with psoriasis (see p. 999).

### Erythema nodosum

Erythema nodosum (see p. 1005) can be due to several conditions, e.g. sarcoidosis, and is accompanied by arthritis in over 50% of cases. The knees and ankles are particularly affected and are swollen, red and tender. The arthritis subsides, along with the skin lesions, within a few months. Treatment is with NSAIDs or occasionally steroids.

## Neurological disease

Neuropathic joints (Charcot's joints) are joints damaged by trauma as a result of the loss of the protective pain sensation. They were first described by Charcot in relation to tabes dorsalis. They are also seen in syringomyelia, diabetes mellitus and leprosy. The site of the neuropathic joint depends upon the localization of the pain loss:

- In tabes dorsalis, the knees and ankles are most often affected.
- In diabetes mellitus, the joints of the tarsus are involved.
- In syringomyelia, the shoulder is involved.

Neuropathic joints are not painful, although there may be painful episodes associated with crystal deposition. Presentation is usually with swelling and instability and eventually grotesque deformities appear.

The characteristic finding is a swollen joint with abnormal but painless movement. This is associated with neurological findings that depend upon the underlying disease, e.g. dissociated sensory loss in syringomyelia or peripheral neuropathy in diabetes. X-ray changes are characteristic, with gross joint disorganization and bony distortion.

Treatment is symptomatic; surgery may be required in advanced cases.

## Blood disease

Arthritis due to haemarthrosis is a common presenting feature of *haemophilia*. Attacks begin in early childhood in most cases and are recurrent. The knee is the commonest affected joint but the elbows and ankles are sometimes involved. The arthritis can lead to bone destruction and disorganization of joints. Apart from replacement of factor VIII, affected joints require initial immobilization followed by physiotherapy to restore movement and measures to prevent and correct deformities.

*Sickle cell crises* are often accompanied by joint pain that particularly affects the hands and feet in a bilateral, symmetrical distribution. Affected joints usually look normal but are occasionally swollen. This condition may also be complicated by avascular necrosis (see below) and by *Salmonella* osteoarthritis.

Arthritis can also occur in *acute leukaemia*; it may be the presenting feature in childhood. The knee is particularly affected and is very painful, warm and swollen. Treatment is directed at the underlying leukaemia. Arthritis may also occur in chronic leukaemia, with leukaemic deposits in and around the joints.

## Endocrine and metabolic disorders

Hypothyroid patients may complain of pain and stiffness of proximal muscles, resembling polymyalgia rheumatica. They may also have carpal tunnel syndrome. Less often, there is an arthritis accompanied by joint effusions, particularly in the knees, wrist and small joints of the hands and feet. These problems respond rapidly to thyroxine.

In acromegaly an arthritis occurs in about 50% of patients. It resembles OA and particularly affects the small joints of the hands and knees. It may be associated with the carpal tunnel syndrome.

Diabetes mellitus-related joint disorders are described on p. 850.

Familial hypercholesterolaemia is associated with oligoarthritis or polyarthritis usually with tendon xanthomata. Arthritis also occurs in combined hyperlipidaemia.

# *Less-common arthropathies*

## Amyloidosis (see p. 866)

Primary amyloidosis causes a polyarthritis that resembles RA in distribution and it is also often associated with carpal tunnel syndrome and subcutaneous nodules.

## Ankylosing vertebral hyperostosis (Forrestier's disease)

This is a condition of elderly people in which exuberant osteophytes are found in the spine, particularly the dorsal region. It is often asymptomatic, but it may be confused with ankylosing spondylitis. Sometimes there is stiffness and occasionally some discomfort. It may be accompanied by peripheral soft-tissue problems associated with calcification, ossification and spur formation, when it is called diffuse idiopathic skeletal hyperostosis (DISH).

## Avascular necrosis

In this condition, bone infarction disrupts the surface of the joint and often leads to changes resembling OA. The hip is particularly affected, for example following fractures of the neck of the femur, perhaps because of its precarious blood supply. It also occurs in various systemic conditions, including sickle cell disease, prolonged steroid therapy, SLE, alcohol abuse and Gaucher's disease. It occurs in deep-sea divers (caisson disease). It may occur for no obvious reason, particularly in middle-aged men.

Avascular necrosis presents with a single painful joint. X-rays are usually diagnostic in the latter phases, showing rarefaction and dense bone in the subcortical areas with distortion of the epiphysis. In the early stages, a bone scan will show increased uptake and an MRI scan will confirm the diagnosis.

## Behçet's syndrome

This is a rare condition characterized by oral and genital ulceration, iritis, and a polyarthritis of variable distribution that may be either chronic or episodic. There are many less-common features of the disease, including erythema nodosum, pustular skin lesions, and neurological and gastrointestinal manifestations. Treatment is with oral steroids but response is variable.

## Drugs

Drugs may cause arthritis. SLE may be induced by procainamide, hydralazine and other drugs. Certain drugs may also precipitate or aggravate gout.

## Familial Mediterranean fever

This condition occurs in certain ethnic groups, particularly Jews and Arabs. The aetiology is unknown. It is characterized by recurrent attacks of fever, arthritis and abdominal or chest pain due to pleurisy. The arthritis is usually monoarticular and attacks last up to 1 week. The condition may be mistaken for palindromic rheumatism, but such attacks are not usually accompanied by fever. In familial Mediterranean fever, attacks can usually be prevented by regular treatment with colchicine 1.0–1.5 mg daily. In general the disorder is benign but in some cases amyloidosis develops.

## Hypermobility syndrome

Hypermobility syndrome occurs in children or young adults with lax joints. The musculoskeletal manifestations of this syndrome include recurrent attacks of joint pain and effusion, dislocation, ligamentous injuries, low back pain and premature OA. Hypermobility is also associated with some rare congenital disorders such as the Ehlers–Danlos syndrome. Joints become stiffer with increasing age. Treatment should be directed at improving muscle power.

## Osteochondritis dissecans

This is a rare condition of adolescent sportsmen in which there is separation of an avascular osteochondral fragment in the knee joint. It results in disruption of the joint surface and the formation of loose bodies within the joint. OA may develop.

## Osteochondromatosis

In this condition, foci of cartilage form within the synovial membrane. These foci become calcified and then ossified (osteochondromas). They may give rise to loose bodies within the joint. The condition occurs in a single joint of a young adult and X-rays are usually diagnostic. Treatment involves removal of loose bodies and synovectomy.

## Palindromic rheumatism

This condition is a variant of RA, characterized by recurrent attacks of arthritis. They occur at irregular intervals, sometimes with long periods of freedom between them, begin suddenly, reach a peak after a few hours and fade over the course of the next 2 days. A single joint is affected in each attack and during the attack it is red, warm, swollen and very painful. Between attacks the joints are normal. Tests for rheumatoid factor are positive in 50% and one-third of cases go on to develop chronic RA.

## Pigmented villonodular synovitis

This is characterized by exuberant synovial proliferation that occurs either in joints or in tendon sheaths. The main manifestation in joints is recurrent haemarthrosis. Treatment is synovectomy. In tendons, the condition gives rise to a nodular mass that requires excision.

## Relapsing polychondritis

Relapsing polychondritis is a rare condition of cartilage. It gives rise to a polyarthritis accompanied by chest disease due to tracheal or bronchial involvement. The diagnosis is often made on the basis of recurrent attacks of pain and swelling of the nose or external ear.

## Temporomandibular pain/dysfunction syndrome

This is a functional disorder of the temporomandibular joint associated with abnormalities of bite. It particularly occurs in anxious people who grind their teeth at night. It gives rise to pain and clicking in one or both temporomandibular joints. Treatment is dental—correction of the bite.

## Sarcoidosis

The commonest type of arthritis is that associated with erythema nodosum, which occurs in 20% of cases of sarcoidosis at or soon after the onset of the disease. The most useful diagnostic test is a chest X-ray, which shows hilar lymphadenopathy in 80% of cases.

Other patterns of arthritis including a transient rheumatoid-like polyarthritis and an acute monoarthritis that can be mistaken for gout occur later in the course of the disease. If NSAIDs fail to control the symptoms, corticosteroids are usually very effective.

# Back pain

Back pain is extremely common. It can be mild and transient, or chronic and disabling. In many cases, the exact cause is not established. In Britain 375 000 people lose some time from work each year because of back pain, an annual loss of 11.5 million working days, and back pain accounts for 6% of general-practice consultations. Back pain is not usually serious and mostly resolves; in one survey 44% of cases resolved within a week and 12% within 2 months.

Most back pain can be readily diagnosed from a simple clinical history and physical examination. A diagnostic approach to back pain is shown in Table 8.18.

In many patients (30%) no cause will be found. It is foolish to label such patients as having 'spondylosis' or arthritis of the spine, terms that merely cause anxiety. It is better to use a term such as non-specific low back pain and explain to the patient what this means.

The back is a common site of psychogenic pain. If possible a positive diagnosis of psychogenic back pain, rather than a diagnosis by exclusion, should be made. Supportive treatment can then be given.

### HISTORY
The following factors should be considered.

### Site
LUMBAR PAIN. This is usually due to degenerative disease, disc prolapse and OA, which are almost never seen in the thoracic spine.

THORACIC PAIN. This is a characteristic site of osteoporotic crush fractures.

### Radiation
Sciatic radiation of pain suggests root compression; however, sacroiliac pain can also radiate down the back of the thigh to the knee.

### Onset
- Sudden, e.g. disc prolapse or mechanical injury
- Gradual, e.g. ankylosing spondylitis

### Aggravating factors
Pain in the back and leg on walking and relieved by stopping, suggestive of intermittent claudication, can be due to spinal stenosis.

| | Question | Possible causes |
|---|---|---|
| 1 | Is it serious? | Infection<br>Septic discitis<br>Tuberculosis<br>Malignancy<br>Metastases<br>Myeloma<br>Spinal tumour<br>Referred pain |
| 2 | Is it inflammatory? | Ankylosing spondylitis |
| 3 | Is it disc disease?<br>or osteoarthritis? | Acute disc prolapse<br>Chronic disc disease/osteoarthritis (spondylosis) |
| 4 | Is it bone disease? | Osteoporosis<br>Osteomalacia<br>Paget's disease<br>Hyperparathyroidism<br>Renal osteodystrophy |
| 5 | Is it a mechanical problem—perhaps amenable to surgery? | Spondylolisthesis<br>Spinal stenosis<br>Posture<br>Pregnancy<br>Obesity<br>Congenital abnormalities |
| 6 | Is it a soft-tissue problem? | Fibromyalgia, sprains and strains |
| 7 | Is it psychogenic? | |
| | If not, it is non-specific back pain | |

Table 8.18  A diagnostic approach to back pain.

*The back*
Appearance—deformity
Movement
Palpation for tenderness

*The nerve roots*
Straight leg raising; femoral stretch test
Sensation; weakness
Reflexes; plantar responses

*Complete physical examination ESSENTIAL*
Look for abdominal masses, lymph nodes, iritis

**Table 8.19**  Examination of patients with back pain.

## Time pattern

- Disc disease is recurrent.
- Ankylosing spondylosis is chronic.

## Inflammatory vs. mechanical

The differences in the history given in inflammatory and in mechanical back pain are shown in Table 8.13.

## EXAMINATION

Examination of the patient is summarized in Table 8.19.

## INVESTIGATION (Table 8.20)

In back pain, investigations are less important than the history and examination. They can also be misleading; for example, degenerative changes on X-ray are virtually always present in older people and may not be the cause of the pain.

X-rays are particularly useful for excluding serious bone disease. Normal X-rays usually exclude metastases but not invariably. They are of little value in acute disc disease, although a narrowed disc space may suggest a prolapse.

Bone scans are useful to detect metastases; a slightly increased uptake in areas of degenerative disease is usually easily distinguished.

MRI scans are now the investigation of choice in disc disease. Abnormal discs are distinguished on MRI scans because of changes in their water content. Impingement of disc material on the nerve roots is usually well seen and it is seldom neccesary to undertake the old-fashioned and invasive radiculogram.

## Blood tests

ESR OR CRP is a particularly useful investigation. A

Plain X-rays
Blood count and ESR
Serum calcium, phosphate and alkaline phosphatase
Serum acid phosphatase and prostate-specific antigen
protein electrophoresis; immunoglobulins
HLA-B27
Bone scan
MRI

**Table 8.20**  Investigations to consider in a patient with back pain.

normal ESR or CRP makes serious disease unlikely. A very high ESR suggests myeloma.

CALCIUM, PHOSPHATE AND ALKALINE PHOSPHATASE LEVELS are measured to look for metabolic bone disease such as osteomalacia.

ACID PHOSPHATASE AND PROSTATE-SPECIFIC ANTIGEN are measured to look for metastases from prostatic carcinoma.

PROTEIN ELECTROPHORESIS, IMMUNOGLOBULINS (AND BONE MARROW ASPIRATION) are performed to look for myeloma.

# Back pain due to serious disease

Back pain is seldom serious but, nevertheless, is important because conditions such as infection are readily treatable. Some features that suggest serious back pain are shown in Table 8.21.

## Spinal infections

Spinal infections include osteomyelitis, discitis and epidural abscess. Infections tend to affect the disc, while malignant processes affect the vertebra itself.

Discitis can be due to pyogenic organisms such as *Staph. aureus*, *Mycobacterium tuberculosis* or rare organisms such as *Brucella*.

### INVESTIGATION

X-RAYS AND BONE SCAN to confirm the diagnosis
BLOOD COUNT—leucocytosis, high ESR
BLOOD CULTURE
NEEDLE ASPIRATION of disc for culture

### TREATMENT

Immobilization in the acute stage and prolonged appropriate antibiotic therapy are required.

## Malignant disease

Bone metastases are classically from primaries in the bronchus, breast, kidney, thyroid or prostate. These are discussed on p. 432. Multiple myeloma produces osteolytic lesions of the spine (see p. 372). Primary tumours of the spinal cord rarely cause back pain (see p. 938).

Recent onset
Weight loss
Symptoms elsewhere, e.g. cough
Localized pain in the dorsal spine
Fever
Raised ESR

**Table 8.21**  Features that suggest that back pain is serious.

## Referred pain

Sources of referred pain are shown in Table 8.22.

# Inflammatory back pain

Ankylosing spondylitis is described on p. 394 and is the most important cause of inflammatory back pain.

# Disc disease

The term 'disc disease' is used to describe two common clinical problems which are due to degenerative change in the intervertebral disc, a process in cartilage which is not unlike OA. There is an acute syndrome in which disc prolapse causes conditions that are known to the public as either lumbago or sciatica, depending upon the presence or absence of radiation of the pain to the areas supplied by the sciatic nerve. It is also used to describe a chronic syndrome in which back pain is associated with 'degenerative changes' on X-ray. This chronic syndrome is sometimes called spondylosis. Chronic disc disease is often associated with OA of the apophyseal joints of the spine and it is difficult or impossible to separate the role of these two pathologies in the pathogenesis of symptoms. There is a very poor correlation between the presence of radiological changes and symptoms. Severe X-ray changes can be seen in patients without any appropriate symptoms and chronic back pain may also occur in patients with little radiological change.

## Acute disc disease

Acute disc disease causes acute back pain (lumbago) with or without sciatic radiation (sciatica). The severity of this syndrome is enormously variable, from a brief and trivial

episode to a long and difficult illness that occasionally requires surgical intervention. It is predominantly a disease of younger people with a peak incidence between the ages of 20 and 40 years, since the disc degenerates with age and is no longer capable of prolapse in the elderly. In older patients, sciatica is more likely to be due to compression of the nerve root by osteophytes in the lateral recess of the spinal canal.

### CLINICAL FEATURES

The back pain is sudden, often severe and often continuous at first. Its onset may be associated with a feeling that something has 'gone' in the back. This may occur after some strenuous activity, typically with the back in forward flexion. The pain is often clearly related to position and at first the back may be fixed in forward flexion. The pain is aggravated by movement and by certain activities. The radiation of the pain and various examination findings are dependent upon the disc affected; these features are summarized in Table 8.23. The three lowest discs account for most cases of disc disease; in order of frequency, they are the L5/S1, L4/L5 and L3/L4 discs.

In a mild case there may be no signs at all, but characteristic findings include loss of lumbar lordosis, sometimes a compensatory scoliosis (Fig. 8.22) and limitation of movement in all directions. Severe neurological problems such as foot-drop or bladder or bowel dysfunction are fortunately rare.

### INVESTIGATION

Investigations are of very limited value in acute disc disease. X-rays do not visualize the disc itself, although there may be narrowing at the level of the lesion. MRI scanning is usually reserved for patients in whom surgery is being considered and is unnecessary in most cases.

### MANAGEMENT

Treatment probably has little effect on the duration of the disease and is therefore aimed at the relief of symptoms and the maintenance of a reasonable way of life for the duration of the illness.

In the *acute* stage:

REST for a few days on a firm bed. Longer periods of rest are unnecessary except in the most severe cases.

CORSETS may be used in the acute stage.

DRUGS: analgesics to relieve pain; anti-inflammatory drugs if required, for example for pain at night or morning stiffness; diazepam for short periods as a muscle relaxant.

EPIDURAL CORTICOSTEROID INJECTION reduces pain and speeds recovery but is unpleasant and requires hospitalization. It is worth considering for acute sciatica that is not responding to simpler measures.

SURGERY is required in the acute stage only for severe or increasing neurological impairment, e.g. foot-drop or bladder symptoms.

In the *recovery* stage, which usually begins within a few days of the acute episode:

PHYSIOTHERAPY to relieve pain, correct posture and restore movement. A particularly useful technique is

| Kidney | Stomach and duodenum |
|---|---|
| Stones | Peptic ulcer |
| Tumours | Carcinoma |
| Infection | |
| Hydronephrosis | *Pancreas* |
| | Pancreatitis |
| *Uterus* | Carcinoma |
| Dysmenorrhoea | |
| Pelvic infection | *Aorta* |
| Tumours | Aneurysm |
| | Peri-aortitis |
| *Ovary* | |
| Tumour | *Bowel* |
| Cysts | Diverticulitis |
| | Abscess |
| *Oesophagus* | Tumour |
| Oesophagitis | |
| Carcinoma | *Gallbladder* |
| Hiatus hernia | Cholecystitis |

**Table 8.22**   Sources of referred pain in the back.

| Root lesion | Pain | Sensory loss | Motor weakness | Reflex lost | Other signs |
|---|---|---|---|---|---|
| S1 | From buttock down back of thigh and leg to ankle and foot | Sole of foot and posterior calf | Plantar flexion of ankle and toes | Ankle jerk | Diminished straight-leg raising |
| L5 | From buttock to lateral aspect of leg and dorsum of foot | Dorsum of foot and anterolateral aspect of lower leg | Dorsiflexion of foot and toes | None | Diminished straight-leg raising |
| L4 | Lateral aspect of thigh to medial side of calf | Medial aspect of calf and shin | Dorsiflexion and inversion of ankle; extension of knee | Knee jerk | Femoral stretch test (hyperextension of hip with patient lying prone) |

**Table 8.23**  Symptoms and signs of common root compression syndromes produced by lumbar disc prolapse.

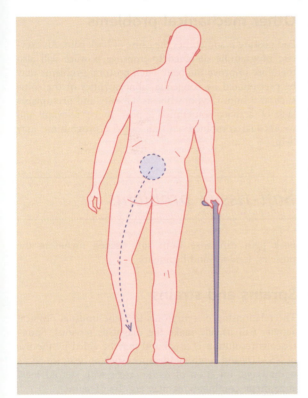

**Fig. 8.22**  Acute lumbar disc prolapse and sciatica, showing the area of the pain and the compensatory scoliosis.

Maitland mobilization, which begins with careful assessment by the therapist to determine levels involved and restriction of movement. Applied movements with local pressure are then used to mobilize individual segments of the lumbar spine. An exercise programme is often useful at this stage. The MacKenzie approach to back care is a self-help system of exercises that emphasize extension, and includes advice about everyday activities that is useful both in treatment and in the prevention of recurrence.

SURGERY will be required for a small proportion of patients (<1%) who fail to recover after an adequate period of conservative therapy.

## COURSE AND PROGNOSIS

Most cases of acute lumbar disc prolapse recover completely, though the process may take as long as 1 year. A small proportion of patients fail to recover and may require surgery. An MRI scan is required to pin-point the lesion as closely as possible, thus improving the prospects of surgery. The simplest operation is removal of the prolapsed disc (microdiscectomy).

# Chronic disc disease and osteoarthritis

This very common syndrome is characterized by the presence of chronic low back pain associated with 'degenerative' changes in the lower lumbar discs and apophyseal joints. Pain in these cases is of the mechanical type and is typically aggravated by exercise, although there may be an inflammatory component, reflected in a brief period of morning stiffness. Sciatic radiation of the pain may occur and there may be a past history of acute disc prolapse. In many cases, the pain is long-standing and the prospects for cure are very limited. Nevertheless, there are measures that will alleviate a difficult situation:

DRUGS. Analgesic or anti-inflammatory drugs to relieve pain.

PHYSIOTHERAPY. The same techniques are used as in acute disc prolapse, described above, and with the same aims. Maitland mobilization is useful when there is restriction of movement. An exercise programme, such as the MacKenzie approach, is usually required and it may be necessary to try different types of programme to achieve the desired result.

BACK CARE. Advice about way of life, lifting, firm beds and other aspects of daily living is essential to identify and remove aetiological factors as well as preventing recurrence. Many physiotherapy departments have 'back' schools for this purpose.

CORSETS should be avoided. They may be useful for patients with mechanical abnormalities, such as instability, or a spondylolisthesis, but are grossly overprescribed. Fortunately, many patients have the good sense not to wear them!

SURGERY should be considered especially for a patient with severe pain of mechanical origin, arising from a single identifiable level, that has failed to respond to conservative measures. Fusion at this level would be appropriate together with decompression of affected nerve roots. The results of surgery for chronic disc disease are not particularly good—about 50% of patients recovering completely—and a failed operation is a demoralizing event in the course of a chronic illness.

WEIGHT REDUCTION may help obese patients.

PAIN RELIEF can be achieved in many other ways including acupuncture, transcutaneous nerve stimulation, massage, hypnosis and faith healing.

# Mechanical problems

There are two mechanical problems in the spine that are of particular importance because they are amenable to surgical treatment: spondylolisthesis and spinal stenosis.

## Spondylolisthesis

This condition arises because of a defect in the pars interarticularis of the vertebra, which may be either congenital or acquired. It gives rise to a slipping forward of one vertebra on another, most commonly at L4/L5. The acquired variety is usually the result of a fairly major traumatic episode that the patient will remember. A small spondylolisthesis is sometimes found in patients with degenerative disease of the lumbar spine and may contribute to the symptoms. The patients have mechanical pain that is not present on waking in the morning but develops as the day goes on and is aggravated by activities such as standing or walking. The pain may radiate to one or other leg and there may be signs of root irritation. More often there are no physical signs, though there may be some limitation of back movement. The diagnosis is confirmed by X-ray.

Small spondylolistheses are common, especially in patients with degenerative disease of the lumbar spine, and may be managed conservatively. It is appropriate to use simple analgesics to relieve the pain and there is no particular need for anti-inflammatory agents. A corset may provide support; this is one of the few indications for its use. A large spondylolisthesis causing severe pain, especially in a younger patient without associated degenerative changes, requires spinal fusion. This is usually a very successful procedure.

## Spinal stenosis

This is sometimes called spinal claudication because of the resemblance of the symptoms to those of intermittent claudication due to vascular occlusion. The anatomical change in spinal stenosis is narrowing of the central canal, compressing the cauda equina. This can result from a variety of causes:

- Disc prolapse
- Degenerative osteophyte formation
- Tumour—rare
- Congenital narrowing of the spinal canal

The patient typically presents with pain in one or sometimes both legs. The absence of back pain makes the diagnosis difficult. The pain comes after a period of walking and tends to diminish with the passage of time. The symptoms are relieved by rest and occasionally by leaning forward. Signs of root compression such as limitation of straight-leg raising or absent reflexes may be precipitated by exertion.

If spinal stenosis is suspected, CT or MRI scans will be required to confirm the diagnosis. Treatment is by surgical decompression.

## Other mechanical problems

Bad posture is sometimes the cause of back pain. An exercise programme designed to improve posture will also therefore improve the pain. Such postural problems may be precipitated by congenital abnormalities of the spine such as a minor kyphoscoliosis. Obesity and presumably lack of activity sometimes appear to be relevant and weight-loss combined with an exercise programme may help.

# Soft-tissue problems

Back pain can arise from soft tissues, including the muscles, tendons and ligaments.

## Sprains and strains

The relationship of symptoms to some unusual physical activity will usually make the diagnosis obvious. Spontaneous resolution is usual and may be aided by the use of NSAIDs and soothing measures such as heat, ice packs or massage. Injection of tender areas with steroid–local anaesthetic combinations may also be of value.

### Sacroiliac strain

This usually results from some physical activity and is particularly common in people whose occupation requires lifting, such as nurses. The pain radiates from the sacroiliac joint to the buttock and sometimes down the back of the thigh. It is a sudden acute problem that usually resolves within a few weeks with rest, avoidance of lifting and NSAIDs. Unfortunately, it has a great tendency to recur.

## Coccydynia

This is a soft-tissue problem in which pain arises from the region of the coccyx, often in anxious women (see Fig. 8.23). Reassurance and protection with a soft ring cushion are usually sufficient treatment since the condition is self-limiting.

## Fibromyalgia

This is described on p. 421.

## Psychogenic back pain

Diagnostic points include:
- Young adult females predominantly affected
- Continuous unvarying pain, often described in vivid terms; no relief from rest, which usually helps even the most severe organic conditions
- Long history of treatment failures, including with analgesics
- Associated symptoms, e.g. headaches; history of fruitless investigation of symptoms from other systems
- Sometimes depression but more often difficult life situations
- No signs—normal tests

### MANAGEMENT
- Reassure and explain
- Explore causes
- Treat depression if appropriate
- Avoid inappropriate diagnoses, e.g. 'arthritis of the spine' and repeated referrals
- Avoid confrontation
- Avoid prescribing drugs or predicting cures—the drugs will not work and the cures will not happen

## Non-specific low back pain

This is an appropriate term for those cases that defy diagnosis with current knowledge and techniques. Patients will vary from those with acute pain that will quickly resolve to those with long-standing symptoms and little prospect of recovery. Without the possibility of definitive treatment, one must rely on simple symptomatic measures such as analgesic drugs.

## Neck pain

Pain in the neck may be caused by RA, ankylosing spondylitis, soft-tissue rheumatism or fibromyalgia. In addition, disc disease, both acute and chronic, the latter in association with OA, may occur in the neck as well as in the lumbar spine. The three lowest cervical discs are most often affected and there is pain and stiffness of the neck with or without root pain radiating to the arm (see p. 949). Chronic cervical disc disease is known as cervical spondylosis.

Painful stiff necks are common clinical problems, often attributed, without much evidence, to disc disease. The essence of treatment is to mobilize the neck with physiotherapy techniques such as traction or Maitland mobilization. Pain may be relieved with simple analgesics. While cervical collars may be required in the acute stage of cervical disc prolapse and occasionally in patients with cervical spondylosis, they can also perpetuate the problem of a painful stiff neck when the right treatment is mobilization.

## Soft-tissue rheumatism

Soft-tissue rheumatism is a convenient term for a number of conditions with similar features (Table 8.24). They cause musculoskeletal or joint pain that arises, not from the joint itself, but from surrounding structures such as the tendon sheaths and bursae. These conditions are benign and in most cases self-limiting. They are often regarded as trivial except by those who have them. Many are best treated by local corticosteroid injection rather than by anti-inflammatory drugs. It is also important to remove aetiological factors whenever possible; mechanical factors such as overuse and repetitive strain are probably particularly important.

Common soft-tissue rheumatic syndromes are shown in Fig. 8.23.

### Bursitis

There are numerous bursae around the body and any of these can become inflamed; olecranon bursitis (student's elbow) and prepatellar bursitis (housemaid's knee) are two examples. Bursitis may appear for no obvious reason or it can be secondary to trauma, repetitive injury or an arthritis such as RA or gout. Occasionally, bursitis is due to infection, when aspiration will be necessary. In many cases no treatment is required other than protection of the inflamed site. Injection of corticosteroid may be useful and, very occasionally, large and troublesome bursae may require excision. Ischial bursitis causes pain over the ischial tuberosity and makes sitting difficult. A ring cushion is usually helpful.

---

Bursitis
Tenosynovitis or peritendonitis
Enthesitis
Nerve compression
Periarthritis or capsulitis
Muscle tension and dysfunction

**Table 8.24** Mechanisms of soft-tissue rheumatism.

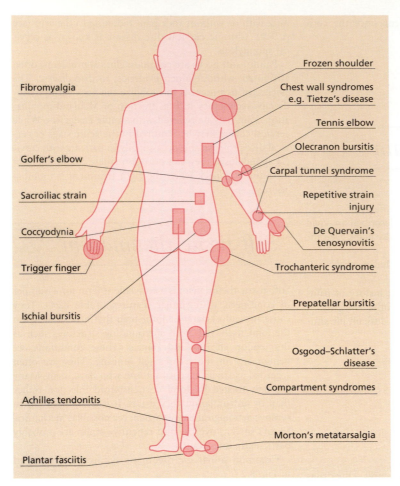

Fibromyalgia

Golfer's elbow

Sacroiliac strain

Coccyodynia

Trigger finger

Ischial bursitis

Achilles tendonitis

Plantar fasciitis

Frozen shoulder

Chest wall syndromes e.g. Tietze's disease

Tennis elbow

Olecranon bursitis

Carpal tunnel syndrome

Repetitive strain injury

De Quervain's tenosynovitis

Trochanteric syndrome

Prepatellar bursitis

Osgood–Schlatter's disease

Compartment syndromes

Morton's metatarsalgia

**Fig. 8.23** Common soft-tissue rheumatic syndromes.

## Tenosynovitis

Tenosynovitis can occur in any tendon sheath. The flexor tendons of the fingers are often affected and cause the condition known as trigger finger. Patients characteristically wake with one finger fixed in flexion. Some force is needed to extend the finger and this produces pain. There is a palpable nodule in the flexor tendon. Injection of this nodule with a corticosteroid preparation usually provides relief.

De Quervain's tenosynovitis gives rise to pain in the anatomical snuff box and may be mistaken for OA of the first carpometacarpal joint. The point of maximum tenderness should be injected with a combination of corticosteroid and local anaesthetic.

## Enthesitis

The enthesis is the specialized area at the junction of tendons or ligaments and bone.

Inflammation of the junction of the common extensor origin of the muscles of the forearm and the lateral humeral epicondyle results in 'tennis elbow'. This condition is seldom due to tennis, more often it is caused by housework or some repetitive manual occupation. Often

there is no obvious cause. There is pain in the elbow, but it is not clearly localized. However, on examination, the joint is normal and there is an area of exquisite tenderness over the lateral epicondyle. It is usually treated by injecting this tender area with a combination of corticosteroid and local anaesthetic. Since the condition resolves within a year or two whatever is done, in mild cases it may be best ignored.

Golfer's elbow is a similar problem at the junction of the origin of the flexor muscles of the forearm and the medial humeral epicondyle. Another common site is the greater trochanter of the femur (trochanteric syndrome).

In plantar fasciitis, the inflammation arises on the undersurface of the heel at the origin of the plantar fascia. This common condition is best treated with an injection of corticosteroid and a protective heel pad; it normally resolves within a year or two.

## Nerve compression syndromes

Carpal tunnel syndrome is described on p. 945. A similar condition in the foot, tarsal tunnel syndrome, gives rise to burning pain with pins and needles in the sole of the foot and toes. As in carpal tunnel syndrome, the pain is often worse at night and may wake the patient from sleep. In cases of diagnostic difficulty, nerve conduction studies will show a block at the appropriate level.

In Morton's metatarsalgia, pain arises from a digital nerve in the foot, usually between the third and fourth metatarsal heads. It is due either to a neuroma or to compression by a bursa. There is pain in the forefoot that radiates into the toes. It is usually aggravated by wearing shoes and relieved by removing them. Manual compression of the forefoot reproduces the symptoms. The condition sometimes responds to local injection and to the use of a metatarsal pad. If not, surgical exploration and excision of the bursa or digital nerve is required.

## Frozen shoulder

This is a convenient term for a group of soft-tissue syndromes that produce the same clinical picture—a painful stiff shoulder. Some people reserve the term for the later stage of the disease when the glenohumeral joint is completely immobile. Many other terms, such as periarthritis or capsulitis, are used to describe this condition, but without much pathological justification. In some cases, local tenderness points to a lesion such as supraspinatus tendinitis, bicipital tendinitis or subacromial bursitis. In most cases, however, it is not possible to identify a specific cause and differentiation makes little difference to the outcome or treatment.

Frozen shoulder is a common condition occurring in adults at any age. It is usually but not always unilateral. There is pain in the shoulder that may radiate to the arm and is usually most troublesome at night. In most cases the condition appears without obvious cause but it may occasionally be related to overuse or injury. A similar clinical picture is produced by acute calcific periarthritis (see p. 411). Examination shows restriction of glenohumeral movement. Analgesics and exercises to prevent stiffness are sufficient treatment in mild cases. If there is restriction of movement, intra-articular injection of corticosteroid is required, followed by exercises to mobilize the joint. The response is variable but the condition usually resolves eventually.

### Shoulder–hand syndrome

Shoulder–hand syndrome is a rare condition in which a frozen shoulder is followed by sympathetic nervous system-mediated abnormalities in the corresponding hand, diffuse swelling, warmth and erythema. It may be idiopathic but also occurs after strokes and head injuries. Untreated, hand involvement may progress to atrophy and contractures. ACTH is usually very effective, combined with an exercise programme to restore function.

## Fibromyalgia

This term is used to describe a functional condition of voluntary muscle that gives rise to widespread pains arising from muscles and their insertions. In some cases there is a large psychogenic component and in this respect the condition has a lot in common with irritable bowel syndrome, with which it is often associated. It begins in early adult life, with females being particularly affected. Widespread aches and pains are characteristic, moving from place to place, varying in severity and often aggravated by cold and stress. Patients have a characteristic sleep disturbance, lacking non-rapid eye movement (REM, $\delta$) sleep, waking unrefreshed and feeling tired. Interruption of sleep in normal volunteers will reproduce the syndrome.

The characteristic physical sign in fibromyalgia is multiple areas of localized soft-tissue tenderness known as trigger points. They are particularly found around the dorsal spine in the interscapular region, around the base of the neck, over both sacroiliac joints, over the lateral epicondyles of the elbows (resembling tennis elbows), and over the medial sides of the knees. In some patients, crops of nodules appear in the muscles, but these have no consistent pathological basis and are believed to be part of the functional abnormality. Blood tests and X-rays are normal.

The condition is chronic or recurrent but entirely benign. Treatment measures include:

AN EXERCISE PROGRAMME. The rationale for this is the observation that it is difficult to induce fibromyalgia experimentally in trained athletes.

MEASURES TO IMPROVE SLEEP. Amitriptyline at night is particularly useful.

HEAT, MASSAGE AND LOCAL OINTMENTS to relieve pain. Analgesic and anti-inflammatory drugs are seldom helpful.

LOCAL INJECTION of trigger points.

REASSURANCE AND EXPLANATION.

## Chest pain

Musculoskeletal conditions are sometimes a cause of chest pain. An example is Tietze's disease. In this condition, pain arises from the costosternal junctions. It is usually unilateral and affects one, two or three joints. There is local tenderness, which helps to make the diagnosis. The condition is benign and self-limiting. It often responds well to anti-inflammatory drugs, or may be treated with local injections of corticosteroid and local anaesthetic.

## Compartment syndromes

The muscles of the lower leg are enclosed in a compartment of fascia, with little room for expansion to occur. Compartment syndromes may be acute (anterior tibial syndrome), e.g. following exercise, or chronic. The former sometimes requires immediate surgical decompression to prevent muscle necrosis. Chronic compartment syndromes produce pain in the lower leg that is aggravated by exercise and may therefore be mistaken for a vascular or neurological disorder.

## Repetitive strain syndrome

This term describes a muscular condition which arises as a result of excessive repetitive activity, usually involving the hands in occupations such as keyboard workers and those who work on assembly lines. Although overuse is the fundamental cause, the condition is more likely to arise in stressful circumstances and when other workers are affected. It presents with pain in the hands and forearms together with various other symptoms such as weakness, cramps, sensory disturbances and a feeling of swelling. There are usually no objective abnormalities. It is important to distinguish this condition from others like tennis elbow, tenosynovitis and carpal tunnel syndrome which can also arise from repetitive manual work. Treatment involves remaining at work but stopping or reducing the activity which caused the problem, exercise and physiotherapy. The condition recovers with time but in severe cases this takes years. Prevention is therefore most important and involves ensuring a good ergonomic position at work, taking regular breaks and recognizing problems quickly if they occur.

# BONE DISEASE

## INTRODUCTION

Bone forms 25% of the weight of a normal adult; its major mineral constituents are calcium, phosphate and, to a much lesser extent, magnesium. While obviously there is major growth in childhood, bone is not a static framework in the adult. There is a continuous process of bone remodelling with bone formation by osteoblasts and resorption by osteoclasts. While exchange of calcium between bone and plasma is only 10–15 mmol daily, over 1 year 20% of total bone calcium is exchanged; minor imbalances of control of the remodelling processes can therefore lead to substantial changes in bone mass or mineralization over the years.

# Physiology, structure and formation of bone

Bone is subdivided into cortical and cancellous bone. In an adult long bone, cortical bone forms the diaphyseal shaft within which is the medullary cavity containing bone marrow. Cancellous bone consists of a network of interconnecting trabecular plates and rods, and is found within the medullary cavity at the epiphyses.

Bone remodelling takes place at four bone surfaces: the periosteum, the Haversian systems, at the endosteum of cortical bone and the cancellous bone surface, which is continuous with the endosteal surface.

In normal adult bones, 80% of surfaces are quiescent. The rest are remodelled by a coupling process, resorption by osteoclasts being followed in sequence by bone matrix

synthesis and mineralization by osteoblasts. This process takes 4 months with no net change in bone mass.

Bone metabolism and mineralization is thus dependent on:

- Collagen synthesis
- Absorption and availability of calcium, affected by vitamin D
- Bone resorption and deposition, largely under hormonal control with local factors affecting bone resorption and remodelling

## CALCIUM HOMEOSTASIS

## Calcium absorption and distribution

Normal Western adult calcium consumption is approximately (20–25 mmol $Ca^{2+}$) (800–1000 mg) daily, though it is much lower in some less affluent countries. Calcium deficiency does not appear to be a significant cause of bone disease, probably because calcium absorption increases in states of dietary calcium deficiency. Absorption is, however, sometimes reduced by generalized malabsorption.

Calcium fluxes between gut, plasma, bone and kidney are shown in Fig. 8.24. The circulating pool of calcium (about 12 mmol in total) is tiny compared with the bony reservoir and small compared with the daily fluxes.

## Regulation

### Vitamin D metabolism

The metabolism and actions of vitamin D are shown in Fig. 8.25. Vitamin D is produced in the skin as cholecalciferol (vitamin $D_3$) by photoactivation of 7-dehydrocholesterol. This, rather than dietary vitamin D, is the chief source of vitamin D metabolites in humans and poor nutrition is of only small importance in producing vitamin D deficiency. These metabolites are transported in the circulation bound to vitamin D-binding protein. In the *liver* cholecalciferol is hydroxylated to 25-hydroxycholecalciferol $(25(OH)D_3)$ and the measurement of this in the blood is a good indicator of vitamin D bioavailability.

The next step in the metabolism occurs in the *kidney* where, in the tubules, the enzyme $1\alpha$-hydroxylase is concentrated and the highly biologically active 1,25-dihydroxycholecalciferol $(1,25(OH)_2D_3)$ is produced. The kidney also produces a second metabolite, $24,25(OH)_2D_3$, as well as $1,25(OH)_2D_3$ if vitamin D supplies are adequate. The production of $1,25(OH)_2D_3$ is strictly regulated by parathyroid hormone (PTH), phosphate and by a feedback inhibition by $1,25(OH_2)D_3$ itself. Hypocalcaemia also stimulates $1,25(OH_2)D_3$ production probably via PTH.

*Extra-renal* sources of $1,25(OH)_2D_3$ production are small under normal conditions but it can be produced in lymphomatous and sarcoid tissue.

The *mode of action* is similar to that of other steroid hormones, i.e. interaction with a specific receptor in the target cell (Fig. 8.26): $1,25(OH)_2D_3$ attaches non-coval-

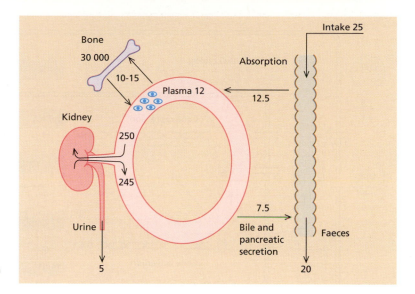

**Fig. 8.24** Calcium exchange in the normal human. The fluxes are shown in mmols per day.

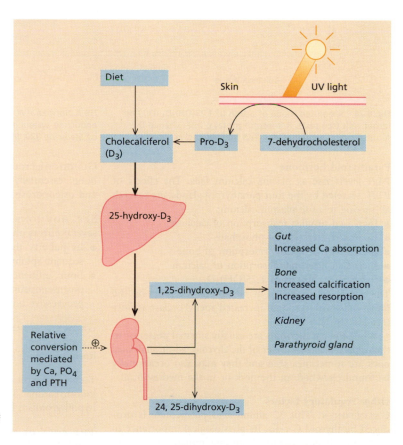

**Fig. 8.25** The metabolism and actions of vitamin D. PTH, parathyroid hormone.

ently to an intracellular receptor protein; this complex is transported through the nuclear membrane into the nucleus, where it interacts with DNA to initiate or suppress the synthesis of RNA-encoding proteins. The control of this is regulated by several factors; for example, interleukin, interferons and C-*MYC* down-regulate, and prolactin and fibronectin up-regulate. The biological potencies of the $D_3$ metabolites influence their ligand affinities for the receptor proteins. Bone, gut, kidney and the parathyroid gland are the prime target organs, but many other tissues respond to $1,25(OH)_2D_3$, e.g. the skin, activated lymphocytes and cancer cells. This suggests a much wider role, e.g. immunoregulation and cellular differentiation, for vitamin D.

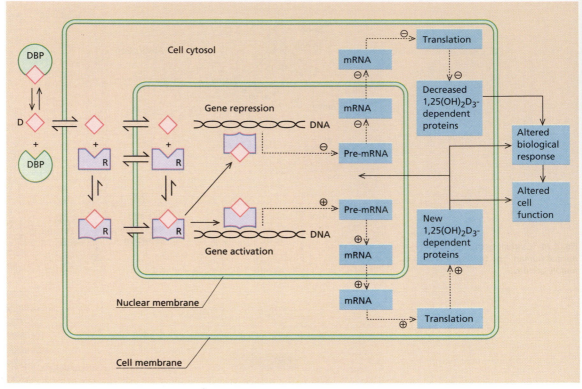

**Fig. 8.26** Suggested mode of action of 1,25(OH)$_2$D$_3$ (D◇) on target cells (see text). R, receptor protein; DBP, vitamin D serum-binding protein. (Modified from Reichel H, Kaeffler HP & Norman AW (1989) The role of vitamin D in the endocrine system in health and disease. *New England Journal of Medicine* **320**, 984. With permission.)

## Parathyroid hormone

PTH levels rise as plasma calcium falls. The effects of PTH, secreted by the four parathyroid glands, are several, all serving to raise plasma calcium:

- Increased tubular reabsorption of calcium
- Increased excretion of phosphate
- Increased osteoclastic resorption of bone
- Increased intestinal absorption of calcium
- Increased synthesis of 1,25(OH)$_2$D$_3$

The effects are mediated at membrane receptors on the target cells, with resultant increased adenyl cyclase activity (see Fig. 16.1).

While the parathyroids are usually situated posterior to the upper and lower lobes of the thyroid, additional local ones are sometimes seen and they may also occasionally be found elsewhere in the neck or in the mediastinum.

## Other regulatory factors

CALCITONIN. This 32 amino acid polypeptide is produced by thyroid C-cells. Its physiological importance in man as a hypocalcaemic hormone remains uncertain. Plasma levels rise with increasing plasma calcium, and it is known to inhibit osteoclastic bone resorption and increased renal excretion of calcium and phosphate. However, total thyroidectomy (absent calcitonin) and medullary carcinoma (excess calcitonin, see p. 826) have few skeletal or other noticeable clinical effects. It is, however, used in the treatment of Paget's disease (see p. 428) and, rarely, in hypercalcaemia.

GLUCOCORTICOIDS. Steroids have complex actions on bone, essentially leading to excessive bone resorption and osteoporosis.

SEX HORMONES. Androgens and/or oestrogens have several effects on the skeleton:

- In puberty they induce the growth spurt and subsequent epiphyseal closure
- Both influence skeletal calcium content, especially postmenopausal oestrogen deficiency, which leads to progressive bone loss

GROWTH HORMONE. Acting via IGF-1 (insulin-like growth factor-1 or somatomedin C, see p. 797) growth hormone stimulates growth of cartilage.

THYROID HORMONES. Excess thyroxine (T$_4$) and tri-iodothyronine (T$_3$) cause increased bone turnover, while hypothyroidism leads to growth delay.

THE ROLE OF MAGNESIUM. Total body magnesium is about 25 g. Plasma magnesium ranges between 0.7 and 1.1 mmol litre$^{-1}$, and generally follows plasma calcium. Magnesium deficiency prevents the release of PTH; the level should be measured when there are signs and symptoms of hypocalcaemia unresponsive to calcium administration.

THE ROLE OF PHOSPHATE. Phosphate forms an essential part of most biochemical systems from nucleic acids downwards. About 80% of all body phosphorus is within bone, plasma phosphate normally ranging from 0.80 to 1.40 mmol litre$^{-1}$. Phosphate reabsorption from the kidney is decreased by PTH, thus hyperparathyroidism is associated with low plasma levels of phosphate. High levels are found in hypoparathyroidism and in renal failure when normal excretion does not occur.

## Measurement of plasma calcium, phosphate and PTH

Total plasma calcium is normally 2.2–2.6 mmol litre$^{-1}$ (8.5–10.5 mg dl$^{-1}$). Usually only 40% of total plasma calcium is ionized and physiologically relevant; the remainder is protein bound or complexed and thus unavailable to the tissues. Ionized calcium is difficult to measure, but is very dependent upon protein, in particular albumin, concentration. An approximate correction for plasma calcium is to add or subtract 0.02 mmol litre$^{-1}$ for every gram per litre by which the simultaneous albumin lies below or above a standard figure (normally 40 or 47 g litre$^{-1}$). Thus, a total calcium of 2.22 mmol litre$^{-1}$ with an albumin of 35 g litre$^{-1}$ will become 2.32 mmol litre$^{-1}$ (corrected to 40 g litre$^{-1}$).

For critical measurements, samples should be taken in the fasting state without use of a cuff, as this affects protein concentration.

Improved two-site immunoradiometric assays for PTH are now available that only measure the intact molecule and not fragments; interpretation requires simultaneous plasma calcium and phosphate measurements.

# *Metabolic bone disease*

## Osteomalacia

### Pathophysiology
This results from inadequate mineralization of the osteoid framework, leading to soft bones. It is thus usually caused by a defect in vitamin D availability or metabolism. The effect on bone is shown in Fig. 8.27.

### CAUSES
DEFICIENCY OF VITAMIN D
- Dietary plus inadequate sunlight exposure often seen in Asian immigrant females in Western countries. Increased melanin in skin decreases vitamin D$_3$ formation and as many Asians are vegans they do not benefit from the small amounts of dietary vitamin D.
- Elderly people who are immobile and not exposed to sunlight.
- Malabsorption: patients after gastric surgery, those with coeliac disease and those with deficient bile salt production.
- Renal disease leading to inadequate conversion of 25(OH)D$_3$ to 1,25(OH)$_2$D$_3$ (see p. 439).

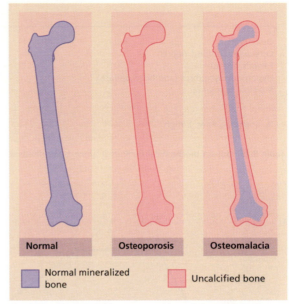

**Fig. 8.27** Diagrammatic representation of the effects of osteoporosis and osteomalacia on the density and calcification of bone.

Less common causes are hepatic failure (reduced 25(OH)D$_3$ causes) and phenytoin or barbiturate therapy (which induce the mixed function oxidase system and affect vitamin D metabolism). Vitamin D-resistant rickets (familial hypophosphataemia) is an X-linked disorder with hypophosphataemia, phosphaturia and rickets.

### CLINICAL FEATURES
Childhood rickets usually presents with bony deformity or failure of adequate growth. In the adult, osteomalacia may produce bone and muscle pain and tenderness, often due to subclinical fractures. There is often a marked proximal myopathy, with a characteristic 'waddling' gait, but a high degree of clinical suspicion is needed.

### DIAGNOSIS
Certain diagnosis can only be made by bone biopsy with demonstration of increased unmineralized bone; undecalcified bone must be used. The procedure is uncomfortable and clinically rarely necessary.

The biochemical (Table 8.25) and radiological findings are characteristic:
- low serum phosphate
- increased serum alkaline phosphatase
- low or low-normal plasma calcium, corrected for albumin (see above)
- a low phosphate–calcium product is a useful screening test, but use the local laboratory normal ranges
- X-rays show defective mineralization, especially in the pelvis, long bones and ribs, often with Looser's zone (linear areas of low density)

### TREATMENT
The simplest treatments are exposure to sunlight and oral vitamin D$_2$ supplements (calciferol); 250 $\mu$g daily will

|  | Calcium | Phosphate | Alkaline phosphatase |
|---|---|---|---|
| Osteoporosis | N | N | N |
| Osteomalacia (and rickets) | N or ↓ | N or ↓ | ↑ |
| Paget's disease | N | N | ↑↑ |
| Hyperparathyroidism (and bone disease) | ↑ | ↓ | ↑ |
| Multiple myeloma | N or ↑ | ↓, N or ↑ | N |

N, normal; ↓, low; ↑, high.

**Table 8.25**   Serum biochemical findings in some bone diseases.

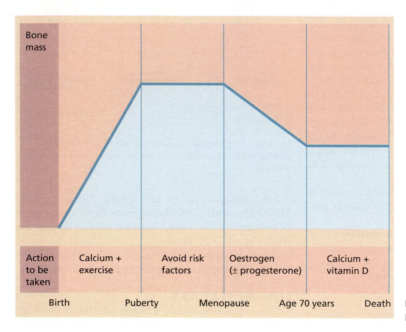

**Fig. 8.28**   A whole-life strategy to prevent osteoporosis.

cure rickets and osteomalacia and should be given until the serum alkaline phosphatase returns to normal. An adequate calcium intake is necessary. Vitamin D 1 mg (40 000 units) daily should be given as a supplement to patients with chronic fat malabsorption. 1α-Hydroxy-cholecalciferol (alfacalcidol) (1 μg daily) is the usual treatment for vitamin D deficiency in renal disease and other conditions. 1,25(OH)$_2$D$_3$ (calcitriol) is also available for anephric patients.

All patients receiving pharmacological doses of vitamin D should have their serum calcium measured regularly. Hypervitaminosis D presents with nausea and vomiting and other features of hypercalcaemia.

PREVENTION. Education to ensure a balanced diet, exposure to sunlight and the taking of vitamin D supplements when necessary will prevent both rickets and osteomalacia.

## Osteoporosis

### EPIDEMIOLOGY
Osteoporosis means thin bone and the term implies a reduction in bone mass including all components of bone

and not just calcium. It is already a major problem; it is said that 40% of Caucasian women and 20% of men will suffer fractures as a result of osteoporosis. The risk in women will triple as a result of increasing life expectancy. One-third of women will have had a fracture by the age of 90 years.

### PATHOPHYSIOLOGY
Changes in bone mass with age are shown in Fig. 8.28. Bone mass increases up to the age of puberty and remains stable until the menopause. After the menopause, there is a progressive reduction as a result of oestrogen deficiency. The rate of reduction in bone mass is much less in men. When bone mass falls below the fracture threshold, there is a risk of fracture, which is increased in the elderly by other factors such as failing eyesight, incoordination and falls.

### RISK FACTORS AND CAUSES
Osteoporosis is not a disease but a condition which exists to a variable extent as a result of a number of different factors, shown in Table 8.26. The most important risk factors are age and sex: osteoporosis has its biggest impact in postmenopausal women.

*Risk factors*
Age and sex
Early menopause
Hysterectomy
White skin
Slender habitus
Smoking
Lack of exercise
Family history
Excess alcohol

*Diseases*
Endocrine
   Cushing's disease
   Diabetes mellitus
   Thyrotoxicosis
   Hypogonadism
   Acromegaly
Rheumatoid arthritis
Chronic renal failure

*Drugs*
Corticosteroids

**Table 8.26**  Risk factors and diseases associated with osteoporosis.

## TYPES OF OSTEOPOROSIS

There are two types of osteoporosis: type 1 the typical postmenopausal osteoporosis and type 2 the more recently recognised senile osteoporosis which occurs in the over-seventies. Their features are summarized in Table 8.27. Four factors are thought to be important in the pathogenesis of type 2 osteoporosis:
1 Less sunshine
2 Lower calcium intake
3 Less vitamin D-containing foods
4 Less vitamin D synthesis in the skin
Increased parathyroid activity is the result, leading to cortical bone resorption.

## CLINICAL FEATURES

Osteoporosis is not itself painful. The pain results from fractures and is usually therefore self-limiting although long-standing pain can result from structural problems, for example as a result of vertebral crush fractures. The typical history in osteoporosis of the spine is thus an episode of very severe pain in the dorsal spine which resolves slowly over the course of about 6 weeks. Fractures can also occur in the lumbar spine. The typical sites of fractures in osteoporosis are vertebrae, the distal radius (Colles fracture) and the neck of the femur.

Other symptoms which result from vertebral osteoporosis are loss of height, increasing kyphosis and abdominal protruberance.

Similar symptoms can occur in such conditions as multiple myeloma and metastatic deposits.

## INVESTIGATION

X-RAYS will demonstrate most fractures. Bone scans are sometimes useful to demonstrate a recent fracture and to distinguish an osteoporotic crush fracture from a metastatic lesion. These often appear identical on X-ray but metastatic lesions are likely to be associated with multiple lesions elsewhere. X-rays are however of limited value in diagnosing osteoporosis itself because the whiteness of the bone depends on the penetration of the film.

SERUM CALCIUM, PHOSPHATES AND ALKALINE PHOSPHATASE are usually normal. Osteoporosis is not a disorder of calcium metabolism (see Table 8.25).

HISTOLOGICAL EXAMINATION of a bone biopsy may occasionally be required to confirm the diagnosis.

BONE DENSITOMETRY (DEXA SCANNING) is of increasing importance in screening people at risk and in monitoring the effects of treatment.

APPROPRIATE INVESTIGATIONS to exclude diseases that are associated with osteoporosis are shown in Table 8.26.

## MANAGEMENT

Treatment of the established disease is unsatisfactory because bone mass has already been lost. Prophylaxis for high-risk individuals is, therefore, preferable. Elderly patients should be educated about the risks of falling.

FRACTURES should be treated by conventional orthopaedic means. Fresh fractures of the spine require short-term bed rest with adequate analgesia and, if necessary, muscle relaxants.

## PREVENTION

Prevention of osteoporosis is important, particularly in postmenopausal women and in the elderly. The following measures are used:

OESTROGEN THERAPY is of proven value and is being increasingly used as evidence accumulates that the

|  | Type 1 | Type 2 |
|---|---|---|
| Age (years) | 51–75 | 70+ |
| Mechanism | Oestrogen deficiency | Senile secondary hyperparathyroidism |
| Pathology | Thinning, perforation and disappearance of trabeculae | Reduction in cortical thickness |
| Outcome | Vertebral fractures | Hip fractures |
| Management | Oestrogen ± progesterone | Calcium and vitamin D |

**Table 8.27**  The two types of osteoporosis.

potential side-effects (thrombosis, endometrial carcinoma, hypertension) are less than the benefits. Those with premature menopause or ovariectomy, those with high-risk factors, e.g. nullipara, the hypogonadal, those with family history of osteoporosis, should certainly be treated and many believe hormone replacement therapy (HRT) should be given to most postmenopausal women (see p. 786).

It is now clear that androgens should be given to hypogonadal men, though prostatic hypertrophy is a problem.

DIETARY CALCIUM should be increased to above 1.5 g daily (40 mmol $Ca^{2+}$), especially for postmenopausal women, with or without vitamin D supplements. This gives a small benefit. Vitamin D is necessary for housebound elderly people.

COURSES OF DIPHOSPHONATES which inhibit bone resorption (see p. 427) may be used and seem to be safe.

MODERATE EXERCISES AGAINST GRAVITY, e.g. walking, running and competitive sports, also retard bone loss and should be encouraged.

FLUORIDE increases bone density but is difficult to use and is not recommended.

CALCITONIN AND PTH remain under investigation and the field is changing rapidly.

## Paget's disease

### DEFINITION AND CAUSATION

Strictly this is a disorder of bone remodelling rather than a metabolic bone disease, although the metabolic changes are considerable. Recent evidence involving apparent viral inclusion bodies suggests a possible 'slow viral' aetiology, for which canine distemper virus is a prime candidate. The condition causes uncontrolled bone turnover with local excessive osteoclastic resorption followed by disorded osteoblastic activity leading to abundant new bone formation which is structurally abnormal and weak.

### EPIDEMIOLOGY

It is a common disorder, most often seen in Europe and particularly northern England, affecting up to 10% of adults by the age of 90 years, though rarely before the age of 40 years. It is relatively rare in North America, Africa and Asia. Probably less than 2% of those affected show any symptoms.

### SITES OF INVOLVEMENT AND CLINICAL FEATURES

The commonest sites are the femur, pelvis, tibia, skull and lumbosacral spine, although any bone can be involved. Most cases are entirely asymptomatic, but features include (Fig 8.29):

● Bone pain, usually spine or pelvis
● Apparent joint pain, when involved bone is close to a joint
● Deformities, particularly bowed tibia and skull changes
● Complications, e.g. deafness due to nerve compression, a high-output cardiac state from shunting, fracture

through abnormal bone and, rarely, osteogenic sarcoma.

### RADIOLOGY AND SCANNING

Characteristic changes are seen most often in the pelvis, skull or spine involving resorption fronts, osteolytic lesions, sclerosis and thickening of bone trabeculae, long bones and vertebrae.

Bone scans will show the extent of skeletal involvement, often including unsuspected areas, but may be difficult to distinguish from metastatic carcinoma, sometimes a major clinical differential diagnosis.

### BIOCHEMISTRY

The hallmark of Paget's disease is an increased serum alkaline phosphatase with normal serum calcium and phosphate, reflecting the increased bone turnover (see Table 8.25). The serum alkaline phosphatase levels may exceed 1000 mU litre$^{-1}$. The levels are normal only when bone involvement is limited. Mild hypercalcaemia only follows immobilization. Bone turnover can also be monitored by 24 hour urinary hydroxyproline excretion, which is frequently increased.

### TREATMENT

When asymptomatic, Paget's disease requires no therapy. Pain is the usual indication for treatment:

SIMPLE ANALGESICS OR NSAIDs are sometimes adequate.

DIPHOSPHONATES, most often disodium etidronate 5 mg kg$^{-1}$ daily over 3–12 months, will reduce osteoclastic activity and frequently induce remissions of up to 2 years. Diphosphonates are pyrophosphate analogues which are resistant to enzymatic hydrolysis. Serum alkaline phosphatase activity frequently falls, reflecting the effect of the drug. Disodium etidronate must be given away from meals as absorption is erratic, and higher doses may lead to osteomalacia.

CALCITONIN (salmon or porcine) 50 IU three times weekly to 160 IU daily inhibits bone resorption and turnover, but is extremely expensive and the side-effects of flushing and nausea are frequent problems. Antibody formation is a further difficulty.

SEVERE CASES may benefit from courses of intravenous diphosphonates under specialist supervision.

MITHRAMYCIN is very occasionally used in severe cases. The dose is 10–15 $\mu$g kg$^{-1}$ i.v. and requires monitoring of platelets and liver biochemistry.

# Calcium disorders

## Hypocalcaemia and hypoparathyroidism

### PATHOPHYSIOLOGY

Hypocalcaemia may be due to deficiencies of calcium homeostatic mechanisms, secondary to high phosphate

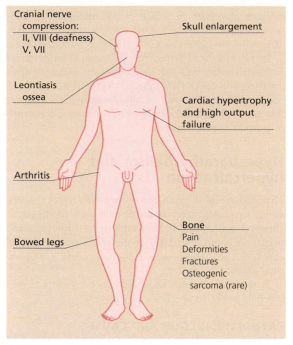

Cranial nerve
compression:
II, VIII (deafness)
V, VII

Skull enlargement

Leontiasis
ossea

Cardiac hypertrophy
and high output
failure

Arthritis

Bone
Pain
Deformities
Fractures
Osteogenic
    sarcoma (rare)

Bowed legs

(a)

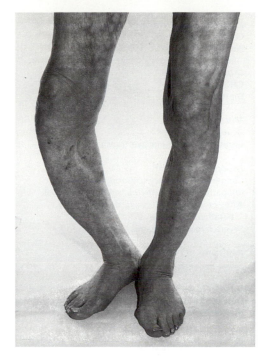

(b)

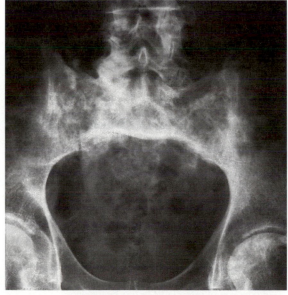

(c)

**Fig. 8.29** Paget's disease.
(a) Clinical features.
(b) Paget's disease of the tibia showing bowing due to increased bone growth.
(c) X-ray appearance of Paget's disease of the pelvis.

levels or other causes of hypocalcaemia (Table 8.28). Hypoparathyroidism is uncommon.

## CAUSES

1 Renal failure is the commonest cause of hypocalcaemia.
2 Immediately following thyroidectomy and parathyroidectomy, hypocalcaemia is usually transient.
3 Idiopathic hypoparathyroidism is one of the rarer

autoimmune disorders. Vitiligo, cutaneous moniliasis and other autoimmune diseases are often seen.
4 The DiGeorge syndrome is a familial condition and associated with intellectual impairment, cataracts, calcified basal ganglia and occasionally with organ-specific autoimmune disease.
5 Pseudohypoparathyroidism is a syndrome of end-organ resistance to PTH. It is associated with short

*Increased phosphate levels*
Chronic renal failure
Phosphate therapy

*Drugs*
Calcitonin
Diphosphonates

*Miscellaneous*
Acute pancreatitis
Citrated blood in massive transfusion

*Hypoparathyroidism*
Congenital deficiency (DiGeorge's syndrome)
Idiopathic hypoparathyroidism (autoimmune)
After neck exploration e.g. thyroidectomy,
    parathyroidectomy
Severe hypomagnesaemia

*Resistance to PTH*
Pseudohypoparathyroidism

*Vitamin D*
Deficiency
Resistance to vitamin D

———

PTH, parathyroid hormone.

**Table 8.28**   Causes of hypocalcaemia.

stature, short metacarpals and intellectual impairment. Pseudopseudohypoparathyroidism describes the phenotypic defects without the calcium abnormalities.

### CLINICAL FEATURES

The symptoms are those of neuromuscular irritability and neuropsychiatric manifestations. Paraesthesiae, circumoral numbness, cramps, anxiety and tetany are followed by convulsions, laryngeal stridor, dystonia and psychosis.

Two important signs of hypocalcaemia are Chvostek's sign—gentle tapping over the facial nerve causes twitching of the facial muscles—and Trousseau's sign, where inflation of the sphygmomanometer cuff above diastolic blood pressure for 3 min induces tetanic spasm of the fingers and wrist. Severe hypocalcaemia may cause papilloedema and a prolonged Q–T interval on the ECG.

### INVESTIGATION

The clinical picture is usually diagnostic and is confirmed by a low serum calcium. Additional tests include:
- Serum urea and creatinine
- High phosphate levels
- Absent or low PTH levels
- Parathyroid antibodies (not widely available)
- Vitamin D metabolite levels
- X-rays of metacarpals showing short fourth metacarpals, which occur in pseudohypoparathyroidism

### TREATMENT

Urgency of treatment depends upon severity of symptoms and degree of hypocalcaemia. If severe, e.g. tetany, intravenous calcium (10 ml initially, then 10–40 ml of 10%

calcium gluconate in 1 litre of 150 mmol litre$^{-1}$ saline over 4–8 hours) is given. Oral calcium supplements (2–10 g daily, 40–200 mmol $Ca^{2+}$) are rarely sufficient alone.

$1\alpha$-Hydroxylated derivatives of vitamin D are preferred for their shorter half-life. Usual daily maintenance doses are 1 $\mu$g for $1\alpha(OH)D_3$ (alfacalcidol) and $1,25(OH)_2D_3$ (calcitriol) and 0.25 mg of dihydrotachysterol. During treatment, plasma calcium must be monitored frequently to prevent hypercalcaemia.

## Hyperparathyroidism and hypercalcaemia

Hypercalcaemia is much commoner than hypocalcaemia and is frequently detected incidentally with multichannel chemical analysers. Mild, asymptomatic hypercalcaemia occurs in about 1 in 1000 of the population, especially elderly females, and is usually due to primary hyperparathyroidism.

True hypercalcaemia should always be confirmed on a carefully collected specimen (see p. 425).

### PATHOPHYSIOLOGY AND CAUSES

Major causes of hypercalcaemia are listed in Table 8.29; primary hyperparathyroidism and malignant disease are the commonest.

Hyperparathyroidism may be primary, secondary or tertiary.

PRIMARY HYPERPARATHYROIDISM is caused by single (80%+) or multiple (5%) parathyroid adenomas or by

*Excess PTH*
Primary hyperparathyroidism
Tertiary hyperparathyroidism
Ectopic PTH secretion (very rare indeed)

*Excess action of vitamin D*
Iatrogenic or self-administered excess
Sarcoidosis

*Excess calcium intake*
'Milk alkali' syndrome

*Drugs*
Thiazides

*Malignant disease*
Secondary deposits
Production of osteoclastic factors by tumours
Myeloma

*Other endocrine disease*
Thyrotoxicosis
Addison's disease

*Miscellaneous*
Long-term immobility
Familial hypocalciuric hypercalcaemia

———

PTH, parathyroid hormone.

**Table 8.29**   Causes of hypercalcaemia.

hyperplasia (10%). Parathyroid carcinoma is rare (2%) though usually with severe hypercalcaemia.

SECONDARY HYPERPARATHYROIDISM is physiological compensatory hypertrophy of all four parathyroids due to hypocalcaemia (e.g. in renal failure or vitamin D deficiency). PTH levels are raised, but calcium levels are low or normal; PTH levels fall to normal after correction of the cause of hypocalcaemia.

TERTIARY HYPERPARATHYROIDISM is the development of apparently autonomous parathyroid hyperplasia after long-standing secondary hyperparathyroidism, most often in renal failure. Plasma calcium and PTH are both raised, the latter often grossly so. Parathyroidectomy is necessary at this stage.

## CLINICAL FEATURES

The symptoms and signs of hypercalcaemia are now more often mild and general rather than the severe renal and bone problems seen years ago:

GENERAL—malaise, depression.

RENAL—renal colic from stones, polyuria/nocturia, haematuria and hypertension. The polyuria results from the effect of hypercalcaemia on the renal tubules reducing concentrating ability, a form of nephrogenic diabetes insipidus.

BONES—bone pain.

ABDOMINAL—abdominal pain, sometimes due to peptic ulceration.

Particular points of note are:

MALIGNANT DISEASE is usually advanced by the time hypercalcaemia occurs as a result of bony metastases. The common primary tumours are bronchus, breast, myeloma, oesophagus, thyroid, prostate, lymphoma and renal cell carcinoma. 'Ectopic PTH secretion' is very rare. There is evidence of a PTH-related protein, a 141 amino acid polypeptide, the sequence of which shows an initial approximate homology with PTH. The biological action appears to lie in the first 34 amino acids. Local bone-resorbing cytokines and prostaglandins may be important locally where there are metastatic skeletal lesions leading to local mobilization of calcium by osteolysis with subsequent hypercalcaemia. They probably rarely cause hypercalcaemia by a generalized 'hormonal' action as previously thought.

SEVERE HYPERCALCAEMIA ($>3$ mmol litre$^{-1}$) is usually associated with malignant disease, hyperparathyroidism, renal dialysis or vitamin D therapy.

CORNEAL CALCIFICATION is a marker of long-standing hypercalcaemia.

IN PRIMARY HYPERPARATHYROIDISM, only 5–10% have definite bony lesions and 20–40% renal involvement.

## INVESTIGATION AND DIFFERENTIAL DIAGNOSIS

SEVERAL FASTING SERUM CALCIUM AND PHOSPHATE SAMPLES should be taken. Hypophosphataemia is common in primary hyperparathyroidism.

SERUM PTH LEVELS should be measured. Detectable levels during hypercalcaemia are inappropriate and imply hyperparathyroidism.

ABDOMINAL X-RAYS may show renal calculi or nephrocalcinosis. Renal function must be measured.

HIGH-DEFINITION HAND X-RAYS may show subperiosteal erosions in the middle or terminal phalanges.

HYDROCORTISONE SUPPRESSION TEST is often helpful; plasma calcium in hyperparathyroidism is resistant to suppression by steroids (10 days of hydrocortisone 40 mg three times daily); this also occurs with some malignancies. In sarcoidosis, vitamin D-mediated hypercalcaemia and some malignancies, suppression to normal or near-normal levels is seen.

PROTEIN ELECTROPHORESIS FOR MYELOMA.

SERUM TSH, T$_3$ FOR THYROTOXICOSIS.

BIOPSY TO EXCLUDE SARCOIDOSIS.

PLASMA CHLORIDE is elevated and the bicarbonate reduced in primary hyperparathyroidism due to PTH which reduces renal tubular reabsorption of bicarbonate.

If primary hyperparathyroidism is confirmed, the following may be helpful in localization, although adenomas are usually small:

ULTRASOUND, though insensitive to small tumours, is simple and safe.

CT SCAN, though very high resolution is needed. MRI may prove more sensitive.

RADIOISOTOPE 'SUBTRACTION' SCANS: a picture of the parathyroid tissue is derived from the difference in uptake between thallium-201 (taken up by thyroid and parathyroid) and technetium-99m (thyroid only). Reports on its efficacy are conflicting.

BARIUM SWALLOW may show indentation of the oesophagus by an adenoma.

VENOUS CATHETERIZATION of parathyroids to measure PTH. This is usually reserved for previous operative failures.

## TREATMENT OF PRIMARY HYPERPARATHYROIDISM

Indications for surgery in hyperparathyroidism remain controversial. All agree that with renal disease or bone involvement surgery is indicated, there being no long-term medical treatment. The situation in which the plasma calcium is mildly raised (2.65–3.0 mmol litre$^{-1}$) is disputed; most physicians feel that probable symptoms of hypercalcaemia, which may be mild and non-specific, should lead to parathyroidectomy. Those who are asymptomatic should receive careful follow-up; development of renal, bone or other symptoms then warrants surgery.

### Surgery

Parathyroid surgery should only be performed by experienced surgeons. Ninety per cent of these patients have adenomas rather than hyperplasia, but the minute glands may be very difficult to define. It is also very difficult to distinguish between an adenoma and normal parathyroid.

If initial exploration is unsuccessful, venous catheteriz-

This is an emergency, leading to nausea and vomiting, nocturia and polyuria, drowsiness and altered consciousness. The serum calcium is greater than 3 mmol litre$^{-1}$, sometimes as high as 5 mmol litre$^{-1}$.

While investigations of the cause (if unknown) is underway, immediate treatment is mandatory if the patient is seriously ill or plasma calcium is very high (>3.5 mmol litre$^{-1}$):

Adequate rehydration (3–4 litres daily of saline for 2–3 days) is essential in all cases

Intravenous diphosphonates (e.g. etidronate disodium, sodium clodronate and pamidronate disodium) are now probably the **treatment of choice** for hypercalcaemia of malignancy. The i.v. dose for etidronate is 7.5 mg kg$^{-1}$ per day for 3 successive days, and for pamidronate disodium 15–60 mg as an infusion in normal saline or 5% dextrose over 2–8 hours, or in smaller doses over 2–4 days

Prednisolone (30–60 mg daily) is effective in a few states, especially myeloma, sarcoidosis and vitamin D excess. In others it has little or no value

Mithramycin (plicamycin) (10–25 $\mu$g kg$^{-1}$ i.v. over 4–6 hours) is often effective for 48 hours in severe cases, but platelet counts and liver biochemistry must be monitored

Calcitonin (200 units 6-hourly i.v.) has an acute but very short-lived hypocalcaemic action; it is now little used

Oral phosphate (sodium cellulose phosphate 5 g three times daily) produces diarrhoea; i.v. phosphate rapidly lowers calcium levels but is dangerous

Once the calcium is reduced to levels where the patient is no longer acutely ill, routine investigation can proceed.

**Emergency box 8.1**   Treatment of acute hypercalcaemia.

ation for PTH levels may be helpful if CT or MRI is not; a few parathyroids lie in ectopic sites elsewhere in the neck and upper mediastinum.

**Postoperative care**

The main danger postoperatively is hypocalcaemia (see above):

CHVOSTEK AND TROUSSEAU SIGNS should be sought regularly.

DAILY PLASMA CALCIUM MEASUREMENTS are needed for 2–5 days.

MILD TRANSIENT HYPOPARATHYROIDISM often occurs for 1–2 weeks, possibly owing to suppression of other parathyroids. Depending on severity, oral or intravenous calcium should be given temporarily.

LONG-STANDING SURGICAL HYPOPARATHYROIDISM develops in a few patients.

**TREATMENT OF ACUTE HYPERCALCAEMIA**

See Emergency box 8.1

**TREATMENT OF SECONDARY HYPERPARATHYROIDISM**

Treatment depends upon the primary pathology, although steroids are often useful. Emergency treatment is discussed below.

# Infections of bone

## Osteomyelitis

*Staphylococcus* is the organism responsible for 90% of cases of acute osteomyelitis (see p. 19). Other organisms include *Haemophilus influenzae* and *Salmonella*; infection with the latter may occur as a complication of sickle cell anaemia.

Osteomyelitis can be due either to metastatic haematogenous spread (e.g. from a boil) or to local infection. Malnutrition, debilitating disease and decreased immunity may play a part in the pathogenesis.

Chronic osteomyelitis may follow an acute infection. Another variety of chronic osteomyelitis is due to infection being localized to form a chronic abscess within the bone (Brodie's abscess). Patients may be asymptomatic for months or years or may have intermittent local pain.

Treatment of osteomyelitis is with immobilization and antibiotic therapy with flucloxacillin and fusidic acid.

**Tuberculous osteomyelitis**

This is usually due to haematogenous spread from a primary focus in the lungs or gastrointestinal tract. The disease starts in intra-articular bone. The spine is commonly involved (Pott's disease), with damage to the bodies of two neighbouring vertebrae leading to vertebral collapse and later abscess formation ('cold abscess'). Pus can track along tissue planes and discharge at a point far from the affected vertebrae. Symptoms consist of local pain and later swelling if pus has collected. Systemic symptoms of malaise, fever and night sweats occur. Treatment is as for pulmonary tuberculosis (see p. 686) together with immobilization.

# Neoplastic bone disease

Malignant tumours of bone are shown in Table 8.30. The most common tumours are *metastases* from the bronchus, breast and prostate. Metastases from kidney and thyroid are less common. Symptoms are usually related to the anatomical position of the tumour, with local bone pain over the area. Systemic symptoms including malaise and pyrexia, and aches and pains occur and are some-

Metastases (osteolytic)
    Bronchus
    Breast
    Prostate (often osteosclerotic as well)
    Thyroid
    Kidney

Multiple myeloma

Primary bone tumours (rare; seen in the young), e.g.
    Osteosarcomas
    Fibrosarcomas
    Chondromas
    Ewing's tumour

**Table 8.30** Malignant neoplasms of bone.

times related to the hypercalcaemia (see p. 431). The diagnosis of metastases can often be made from the history and examination, particularly if the primary has already been diagnosed. Symptoms from bony metastases may, however, be the first presenting feature.

### INVESTIGATION

SKELETAL ISOTOPE SCANS can pick up bony metastases as 'hot' areas before radiological changes occur.

X-RAYS may show metastases as osteolytic areas with bony destruction. Osteosclerotic metastases are characteristic of prostatic metastases.

SERUM ALKALINE PHOSPHATASE (from the bone) is usually raised.

HYPERCALCAEMIA is seen in 10–20% of patients with malignancies. It is chiefly associated with metastases.

SERUM ACID PHOSPHATASE is raised in prostatic metastases.

PROSTATIC SPECIAL ANTIGEN (PSA) is also raised in prostatic metastases.

### TREATMENT

Treatment is usually symptomatic with analgesics and anti-inflammatory drugs like indomethacin. Local radiotherapy over bone metastases may be the best way of relieving pain. Depending on the tumour, cytotoxic chemotherapy is occasionally helpful. Some tumours are hormone-dependent and a remission can be obtained by hormonal therapy. Occasionally pathological fractures require internal fixation.

PRIMARY BONE TUMOURS are rare and usually seen in children and young adults.

## *Connective tissue*

All connective tissues have a large proportion of extracellular matrix as well as cells. This matrix consists of extracellular macromolecules containing collagens, elastins, non-collagenous glycoproteins and proteoglycans.

### Collagens

These consist of three polypeptide chains ($\alpha$ chains) wound around one another in a triple helical confirmation. These $\alpha$ chains contain repeating sequences of Gly-X-Y triplets where X and Y are often prolyl and hydroxyprolyl residues. There is much genetic heterogeneity in collagen fibres and the gene for different chains is located on several chromosomes.

Functionally the tissue depends on the type of collagen. Thirteen distinct collagen types have been described so far, although the exact function of many remains undefined. For example, type I collagen fibres are seen in structures with a high tensile strength, e.g. tendons, type II collagen molecules form the cartilaginous structures and type III collagen is seen in more distensible tissues such as blood vessels.

### Elastin

Elastic fibres in the extracellular matrix consist of elastin and microfibrils. Elastin is an insoluble protein polymer and its gene has been characterized. Its precursor, tropoelastin, is synthesized by vascular smooth muscle cells and skin fibroblasts. Elastin fibres are cross-linked with desmosine and isodesmosine which are specific to elastin.

### Glycoproteins

Fibronectin is the major non-collagenous glycoprotein in the extracellular matrix. Its molecule contains a series of functional domains, or cell recognition sites, that bind ligands and are involved in cell adhesion. A synthetic peptide sequence (Arg-Gly-Asp), which mimics some of the functions of fibronectin, is also found in other adhesion proteins, e.g. vitronectin, laminin and collagen type VI. Fibronectin plays a major role in tissue remodelling. It is stimulated by interferon-$\gamma$ and transforming growth factor-$\beta$ and inhibited by tumor necrosis factor and interleukin-1.

### Proteoglycans

These are of different shapes and sizes. Their function is that of a multipurpose glue in that they bind extra cellular matrix together, mediate cell binding and inhibit soluble molecules.

## Osteogenesis imperfecta (fragilitas ossium, brittle bone syndrome)

This rare group of inherited disorders is due to an abnormality of connective tissue. The major feature is very fragile and brittle bones; other collagen-containing tissues are also involved, such as tendons, the skin and the eyes. Osteogenesis imperfecta tarda is a mild, dominantly inherited condition with milder bony deformities, blue sclerae, defective dentine, early-onset deafness, hypermobility of joints, and heart valve disorders. More severe forms present with multiple fractures and gross deformities. Prognosis is variable, depending on the severity of the disease.

## Achondroplasia

This is one of a group of heterogeneous disorders that affect the normal development of bone and cartilage. Achondroplasia (dwarfism) is diagnosed in the first years of life. The disease is inherited in an autosomal dominant manner. The trunk is of normal length but the limbs are very short and broad. The vault of the skull is enlarged, the face is small and the nose bridge is flat. Intelligence is normal.

# Other hereditary diseases

## Osteopetrosis (marble bone disease)

This condition may be inherited in either an autosomal dominant or an autosomal recessive manner; the recessive type is severe and the dominant type is mild. In the severe form, bone density is increased throughout the skeleton but bones tend to fracture easily. Involvement of the bone marrow leads to a leucoerythroblastic anaemia. There is mental retardation and early death.

In the mild form there may only be X-ray changes, but fractures and infection can occur. The acid phosphatase level is raised.

## Hypophosphatasia

This rare autosomal recessive condition is due to a deficiency of alkaline phosphatase and pyrophosphatase. It is not known where the primary defect lies, but it may be in the osteoblasts. It varies in severity from unmineralized bones *in utero* resulting in death, to rickets in infancy or recurrent fractures in adults.

# Further reading

Huskisson EC & Hart FD (1987) *Joint Disease: All the Arthropathies*, 4th edn. Bristol: John Wright.

Kelley WN *et al* (eds) (1993) *Textbook of Rheumatology*, 4th edn. Philadelphia: WB Saunders.

Maddison PJ *et al* (eds) (1993) *Oxford Textbook of Rheumatology*. Oxford: Oxford University Press.

McCarty DJ & Koopman WJ (eds) (1993) *Arthritis and Allied Conditions: A Textbook of Rheumatology*, 12th edn. Philadelphia: Lea & Febiger.

Bilezikian JP (ed) (1994) *The Parathyroids: Basic and Clinical Concepts*. New York: Raven Press.

Nordin BC (1993) *Metabolic Bone and Stone Disease*, 3rd edn. Edinburgh: Churchill Livingstone.

Smith R (ed) (1990) *Osteoporosis 1990*. London: Royal College of Physicians.

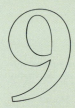
# Renal function and structure

The kidneys' principal role is the elimination of waste material and the regulation of the volume and composition of body fluid (Table 9.1). The kidneys have a unique system involving the free ultrafiltration of water and non-protein-bound low-molecular-weight compounds from the plasma and the selective reabsorption and/or excretion of these as the ultrafiltrate passes along the tubule.

The functioning unit is the *nephron*, of which there are approximately one million in each kidney. A conventional diagrammatic representation is shown in Fig. 9.1a and a physiological version in Fig. 9.1b.

An essential feature of renal function is that a large volume of blood—25% of cardiac output or approximately 1300 ml min$^{-1}$—passes through the two million glomeruli.

A hydrostatic pressure gradient of approximately 10 mmHg (a capillary pressure of 45 mmHg minus 10 mmHg of pressure within Bowman's space and 25 mmHg of plasma oncotic pressure) provides the driving force for ultrafiltration of virtually protein-free and fat-free fluid across the glomerular capillary wall into Bowman's space and so into the renal tubule (Fig. 9.2).

The ultrafiltration rate (glomerular filtration rate;

GFR) varies with age and sex but is approximately 120–130 ml min$^{-1}$ per 1.73 m$^2$ surface area in adults. This means that each day ultrafiltration of between 170 and 180 litres of water and unbound small-molecular-weight constituents of blood occurs. The 'need' for this high filtration rate relates to the elimination of compounds present in relatively low concentration in plasma (e.g. urea). If these large volumes of ultrafiltrate were excreted unchanged as urine, it would be necessary to ingest huge amounts of water and electrolytes to stay in balance. This is avoided by the selective reabsorption of water, essential electrolytes and other blood constituents, such as glucose and amino acids, from the filtrate in transit along the nephron. Thus, 60–80% of filtered water and sodium are reabsorbed in the proximal tubule along with virtually all the potassium, bicarbonate, glucose and amino acids (see Fig. 9.1b). Further water and sodium chloride are reabsorbed more distally, and fine tuning of salt and water balance is achieved in the distal and collecting tubules under the influence of aldosterone and antidiuretic hormone (ADH). The final urine volume is thus 1–2 litres daily. Calcium, phosphate, and magnesium are also selectively reabsorbed in proportion to need to maintain a normal electrolyte composition of body fluids.

The urinary excretion of some compounds is more complicated. For example, potassium is freely filtered at the glomerulus, almost completely absorbed in the proximal tubule, and excreted in the distal tubule and collecting ducts. An important clinical consequence of this is that the ability to eliminate unwanted potassium is less dependent on GFR than is the elimination of urea or creatinine. Other compounds filtered and reabsorbed or excreted to a variable extent include urate and many organic acids, including many drugs or their metabolic breakdown products. The more tubular secretion of a compound occurs, the less dependent is elimination on the GFR; penicillin and cephradine are examples of compounds secreted by the tubules.

Tubular function is also critical to the control of acid–base balance. Thus, filtered bicarbonate is largely reabsorbed and hydrogen ion is excreted mainly buffered by phosphate (see p. 515).

---

*Excretory*—excretion of waste products, drugs

*Regulatory*—control of body fluid volume and composition

*Endocrine*—production of erythropoietin, renin, prostaglandins

*Metabolic*—metabolism of vitamin D, small molecular weight proteins

**Table 9.1** Functions of the kidney.

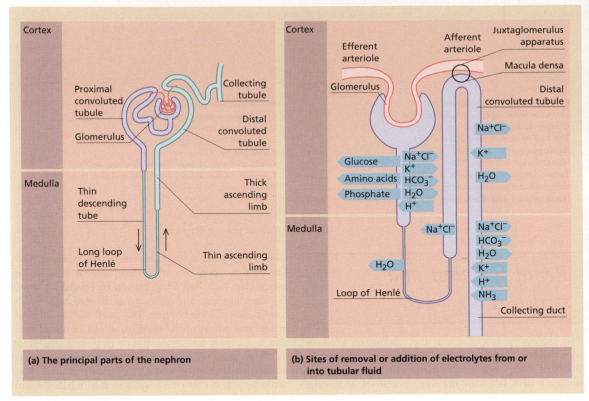

| Cortex | | Cortex | |
|---|---|---|---|

(a) The principal parts of the nephron

(b) Sites of removal or addition of electrolytes from or into tubular fluid

**Fig. 9.1** (a) The principal parts of the nephron. (b) Sites of removal or addition of electrolytes from or into tubular fluid.

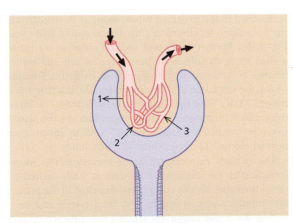

**Fig. 9.2** Pressures controlling glomerular filtration. 1, capillary hydrostatic pressure (45 mmHg); 2, hydrostatic pressure in Bowman's space (10 mmHg); 3, plasma protein oncotic pressure (25 mmHg). Arrows indicate direction of pressure gradient.

# Glomerular filtration rate

In health the GFR remains remarkably constant owing to intrarenal regulatory mechanisms. In disease, with a reduction in intrarenal blood flow, damage to or loss of glomeruli, or obstruction to the free flow of ultrafiltrate along the tubule, the GFR will fall and the ability to eliminate waste material and to regulate the volume and composition of body fluid will decline. This will be manifest as a rise in the blood level of urea or the plasma level of creatinine and in a reduction in *measured* GFR.

## Uraemia

The concentration of urea or creatinine in blood or plasma, respectively, represents the dynamic equilibrium between production and elimination. In healthy subjects there is an enormous reserve of renal excretory function and serum urea and creatinine do not rise above the normal range until there is a reduction of 50–60% in the GFR. Thereafter, the level of urea depends both on the GFR and the production rate (Table 9.2). The latter is heavily influenced by protein intake and tissue catabolism. The level of creatinine is much less dependent on diet but is more related to age, sex and muscle mass. Once it is elevated, serum creatinine is a better guide to GFR than urea and, in general, measurement of serum creatinine is a good way to monitor further deterioration in the GFR.

It must be re-emphasized that a normal serum urea or creatinine is *not* synonymous with a normal GFR.

### Measurement of the glomerular filtration rate
Measurement of the GFR is necessary to define the exact level of renal function. It is essential when the blood urea or serum creatinine are within the normal range.

Inulin clearance—the gold standard of physiologists—

| Production | Elimination |
|---|---|
| *Increased by* | *Increased by* |
| High-protein diet | Elevated GFR, e.g. |
| Increased catabolism | pregnancy |
| Surgery | |
| Infection | *Decreased by* |
| Trauma | Glomerular disease |
| Corticosteroid therapy | Reduced renal blood flow |
| Tetracyclines | Hypotension |
| Gastrointestinal bleeding | Dehydration |
| Cancer | Urinary obstruction |
| | Tubulo-interstitial nephritis |
| *Decreased by* | |
| Low-protein diet | |
| Reduced catabolism, e.g. | |
| old age | |
| Liver failure | |

GFR, glomerular filtration rate.

**Table 9.2** Factors influencing serum urea levels.

is not practical or necessary in clinical practice. The most widely used measurement is the creatinine clearance (Fig. 9.3).

The use of creatinine clearance is dependent on the fact that daily production of creatinine (principally from muscle cells) is remarkably constant and little affected by protein intake. Serum creatinine and urinary output thus vary very little throughout the day. This permits the use

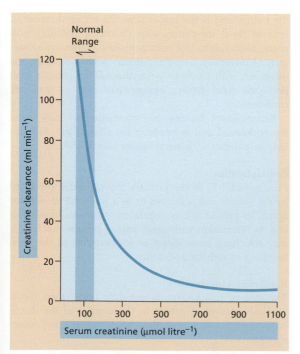

**Fig. 9.3** Creatinine clearance versus serum creatinine. Note that the serum creatinine does not rise above the normal range until there is a reduction of 50–60% in the glomerular filtration rate (creatinine clearance).

of 24-hour urine collections, which reduce collection errors, and the measurement of a single serum creatinine value during the 24 hours (Practical box 9.1).

Creatinine excretion is, however, by both glomerular filtration and tubular secretion, although at normal serum levels the latter is relatively small. As most laboratory methods for measurement of serum creatinine give slight overestimates, the calculation of clearance fortuitously gives a value close to that of inulin.

With progressive renal failure, creatinine clearance may overestimate GFR but, in clinical practice, this is seldom important. Certain drugs—for example cimetidine, trimethoprim, spironolactone and amiloride—reduce tubular secretion of creatinine, leading to a rise in serum creatinine and a fall in measured clearance.

Given these observations, creatinine clearance, nevertheless, is a reasonably accurate measure of GFR in those situations in which it is most required—normal or near normal renal function.

Where urine collections are difficult (e.g. with ileal conduits) or deemed inaccurate, the GFR may be measured by the single injection of compounds such as [51Cr]EDTA (ethylenediamine tetra-acetic acid), [99mTc]DTPA (diethylenetriaminepenta-acetic acid) or [125I]iothalamate, their excretion being primarily by glomerular filtration. Following intravenous injection of the compound, three blood samples are obtained at 2, 3 and 4 hours (or rather longer intervals if the patient is oedematous or if renal failure is suspected). The GFR may then be calculated from the slope of the exponential fall in blood level of the compound.

Urea clearance is not an accurate measure of GFR, particularly when urine flow rate is low, and should not be used as a measure of GFR.

Empty bladder at beginning of collection period. Discard the urine. Note time
*All* urine passed (including overnight) during subsequent 24 hours to be collected
Exactly 24 hours after commencement of collection, empty bladder. Urine thus voided to be included in collection

**Measurement of creatinine clearance**

Urine is collected over 24 hours for measurement of urinary creatinine; a 24-hour collection diminishes collection errors
A plasma level of creatinine is measured sometime during the 24-hour period
Given the rate of urine flow (*V*), the urine (*U*) and plasma (*P*) concentrations of creatinine, clearance is obtained from the formula:

$$\frac{U \times V}{P} \times 100$$

where *U* and *P* are measured in mmol litre⁻¹, and *V* is measured in ml min⁻¹
Normal range: men 90–140 ml min⁻¹
women 80–125 ml min⁻¹

**Practical box 9.1** To obtain a timed 24-hour urine collection and to measure creatinine clearance.

# TUBULAR FUNCTION

The major function of the tubule is the selective reabsorption or excretion of water and various cations and anions to keep the volume and electrolyte composition of body fluid normal (see Chapter 10).

The active reabsorption from the glomerular filtrate of compounds such as glucose and amino acids also takes place. Within the normal range of blood concentrations these substances are completely reabsorbed by the proximal tubule. However, if blood levels are elevated above the normal range, the amount filtered (filtered load = GFR × plasma concentration) may exceed the maximal absorptive capacity of the tubule and the compound 'spills over' into the urine. Examples of this occur with hyperglycaemia in diabetes mellitus or elevated plasma phenylalanine in phenylketonuria.

Conversely, inherited or acquired defects in tubular function may lead to incomplete absorption of a *normal* filtered load, with loss of the compound in the urine (a lowered 'renal threshold'). This is seen in renal glycosuria, in which there is a genetically determined defect in tubular reabsorption of glucose. It is diagnosed by demonstrating glycosuria in the presence of normal blood glucose levels. Inherited or acquired defects in the tubular reabsorption of amino acids, phosphate, sodium, potassium and calcium also occur, either singly or in combination. Examples include cystinuria and the Fanconi syndrome (see p. 863). Tubular defects in the reabsorption of water (nephrogenic diabetes insipidus) or bicarbonate (proximal renal tubular acidosis) and defective acidification of the urine (distal renal tubular acidosis) are dealt with on p. 517.

## Investigation of tubular function in clinical practice

### Proximal tubular function

Five tests of proximal tubular function are employed in clinical practice: measurement of serum potassium and serum phosphorus concentrations, and detection of glycosuria, generalized aminoaciduria and 'tubular' proteinuria.

Hypokalaemia in the face of a normal or increased urinary potassium excretion (>40 mmol in 24 hours) is indicative of proximal tubular failure of potassium reabsorption. Unless other explanations exist such as treatment with thiazide diuretics or hyperaldosteronism, the defect can be assumed to lie in the proximal tubule. Similarly, hypophosphataemia may be attributed to a proximal tubular abnormality, provided alternative explanations, such as the use of gut phosphorus binders and primary hyperparathyroidism, can be ruled out. Glycosuria in the absence of hyperglycaemia and generalized aminoaciduria are also indicative of failure of proximal tubular reabsorption of glucose and amino acids, respectively. Proteins derived from tubular cells, such as $\beta_2$-microglobulin, are reabsorbed in the proximal nephron. If proteinuria is present, and urine electrophoresis shows the characteristic 'tubular' as distinct from 'glomerular'

pattern (i.e. albumin) a proximal tubular defect is demonstrated.

### Distal tubular function

Two tests of distal tubular function are commonly applied in clinical practice: measurement of urinary concentrating capacity in response to water deprivation, and measurement of urinary acidification. These tests are dealt with on pp. 518 and 1050.

# ENDOCRINE FUNCTION

### Renin–angiotensin system

The juxtaglomerular apparatus is made up of specialized arteriolar smooth muscle cells that are sited on the afferent glomerular arteriole as it enters the glomerulus (see Fig. 9.1b). These cells secrete renin, which converts angiotensinogen in blood to angiotensin I. Renin release is controlled by:

- Pressure changes in the afferent arteriole
- Sympathetic tone
- Chloride and osmotic concentration in the distal tubule via the macula densa (see Fig. 9.1b)
- Local prostaglandin release

Angiotensin II is generated from angiotensin I by angiotensin-converting enzyme (ACE). Angiotensin II is both a vasoconstrictor and the most important stimulus for the release of aldosterone by the adrenal cortex. It also modifies intrarenal blood flow.

### Erythropoietin (see p. 295)

Erythropoietin is a glycoprotein produced principally by the kidney and is the major stimulus for erythropoiesis. Loss of renal substance, with decreased erythropoietin production, results in a normochromic, normocytic anaemia. Conversely, erythropoietin secretion may be increased, with resultant polycythaemia, in patients with polycystic renal disease, benign renal cysts or renal cell carcinoma.

Recombinant human erythropoietin has now been biosynthesized and is available for clinical use, particularly in patients with renal failure (see p. 484).

### Prostaglandins

Prostaglandin $E_2$ is the primary prostaglandin produced by the kidney and is known to be a powerful vasodilator agent. Its precise role in regulating intrarenal blood flow and its interaction with renin release remains unclear. It may also have some direct or indirect role in the renal handling of sodium and water.

### Kallikrein–kinin system

The role of this system is not fully understood but it probably also plays a part in the control of the distribution of renal blood flow and in salt and water excretion.

### Natriuretic hormones (see p. 823)

There is considerable evidence that atrial tissue contains a group of peptides that contribute to the regulation of sodium balance—atrial natriuretic peptides (ANP). Intravenous infusion of one of these is followed by a marked natriuresis with a rise in GFR and a fall in blood pressure. These peptides appear to oppose the renin–angiotensin system in four ways: reduced renin secretion, reduced aldosterone secretion, opposition to the action of angiotensin II and to the sodium-retaining action of aldosterone on the renal tubule. Their role in the long-term regulation of sodium balance and blood pressure in humans remains to be clarified.

Endopeptidase inhibitors are becoming available and show therapeutic promise as potent new diuretic agents.

### Vitamin D metabolism (see p. 422)

Naturally occurring vitamin D requires hydroxylation in the liver and again by a $1\alpha$-hydroxylase enzyme in the kidney to produce the powerfully metabolically active 1,25-dihydroxycholecalciferol (1,25-$(OH)_2D_3$). Reduced $1\alpha$-hydroxylase activity in diseased kidneys results in relative deficiency of 1,25-$(OH)_2D_3$. As a result, gastrointestinal calcium absorption is reduced and bone mineralization impaired. Receptors for 1,25-$(OH)_2D_3$ exist in the parathyroid glands and reduced occupancy of the receptors by the vitamin alters the set-point for release of parathyroid hormone (PTH) in response to a given decrement in plasma calcium concentration. Gut calcium malabsorption, which induces a tendency to hypocalcaemia, and relative lack of 1,25-$(OH)_2D_3$ contribute therefore to the hyperparathyroidism seen regularly in patients with renal impairment, even of modest degree.

### Protein and polypeptide metabolism

It is clear that the kidney is a major site for the catabolism of many small molecular-weight proteins and polypeptides, including many hormones such as insulin, PTH and calcitonin. In renal failure the metabolic clearance of these substances is reduced and their half-life is prolonged. This accounts, for example, for the reduced insulin requirements of diabetic patients as their renal function declines.

## Tests for renal disease or malfunction

Renal disease is suspected if there are:
- Symptoms referable to the urinary tract
- Hypertension
- An elevated blood urea or creatinine concentration
- Abnormalities on urinalysis

## THE URINE

### Appearance

This is of little value in the differential diagnosis of renal disease except in the diagnosis of haematuria. Overt 'bloody' urine is usually unmistakable but should be checked using dipsticks (Stix testing). Very concentrated urine may also appear dark or smoky. Other causes of discoloration of urine include cholestatic jaundice, haemoglobinuria, drugs such as rifampicin, use of fluorescein or methylene blue, and ingestion of beetroot. Discoloration of urine after standing for some time occurs in porphyria, alkaptonuria and in patients ingesting the drug L-dopa. In patients with frequency or dysuria the passage of crystal clear urine usually indicates that significant bacteriuria is absent.

### Volume

In health, the volume of urine passed is primarily determined by diet and fluid intake. In temperate climates it lies within the range 800–2500 ml per 24 hours. The minimum amount passed to stay in fluid balance is determined by the amount of solute—mainly urea and electrolytes—being excreted and the maximum concentrating power of the kidneys. On a normal diet, some 800 mosmol of solute are passed daily. Since the maximum urine concentration is approximately 1200 mosmol litre$^{-1}$, the minimum volume of urine obligated by excretion of 800 mosmol of solute would thus be approximately 650 ml (Table 9.3). Fluid intake is generally greater than this, so that larger volumes of more dilute urine are passed. A diet rich in carbohydrate and fat and low in protein and salt results in a lower solute excretion and as little as 300 ml of urine per day may be required. Conversely, a high-salt, high-protein intake obligates a larger urine flow and, via the thirst mechanism, a higher fluid intake. The appropriateness of a given daily urine output must therefore be related to factors such as diet, body size and fluid intake.

In disease, impairment of concentrating ability requires increased volumes of urine to be passed, given the same

| Diet | Approximate solute output (mosmol/24 hours) | Minimum urine volume required to excrete solute load (ml/24 hours) | |
|---|---|---|---|
| | | With normal urine concentration (maximum 1200 mosmol kg$^{-1}$) | In disease (impaired urine concentration—maximum 300 mosmol kg$^{-1}$) |
| Normal | 800 | 667 | 2667 |
| High-protein/salt | 1200 | 1000 | 4000 |
| Low-protein/salt | 360 | 300 | 1200 |

**Table 9.3** Relationship between diet, kidney function and urine volume.

daily solute output (Table 9.3). An increased solute output, e.g. in glycosuria or increased protein catabolism following surgery or associated with sepsis, also demands increased urine volumes.

The maximum urine output depends on the ability to produce a dilute urine. Intakes of 10 or even 20 litres daily can be tolerated by normal humans but, given a daily solute output of 800 mosmol, require the ability to dilute to 80 and 40 mosmol litre$^{-1}$, respectively. Where diluting ability is impaired, the ability to excrete large volumes of ingested water is also impaired.

### Oliguria

Oliguria, usually defined as the excretion of less than 300 ml of urine per day, may be 'physiological', e.g. in patients with hypotension and hypovolaemia, where urine is maximally concentrated in an attempt to conserve water. More often, it is due to intrinsic renal disease or obstructive nephropathy (see p. 471).

Anuria (no urine) suggests urinary tract obstruction until proved otherwise; bladder outflow obstruction must always be considered first.

### Polyuria

Polyuria is a persistent, large increase in urine output, usually associated with nocturia. It must be distinguished from frequency of micturition with the passage of small volumes of urine. Documentation of fluid intake and output may be necessary. Polyuria is the result of an excessive (hysterical) intake of water, an increased excretion of solute (as in hyperglycaemia and glycosuria), or a defective renal concentrating ability or failure of production of ADH.

## Specific gravity and osmolality

Urine specific gravity is a measure of the weight of dissolved particles in urine, whereas urine osmolality reflects the number of such particles. Usually the relationship between the two is close. An exception exists when a relatively small number of relatively large particles are present in urine, as occurs in multiple myeloma. Measurement of urine specific gravity or osmolality is only required under limited circumstances, such as the differential diagnosis of oliguric renal failure or the investigation of polyuria or inappropriate ADH secretion.

## pH

Measurement of urinary pH is unnecessary except in the investigation and treatment of renal tubular acidosis (see p. 517).

## Chemical (Stix) testing

Routine Stix testing of urine for blood, protein and sugar is obligatory in all patients suspected of having renal disease.

### Blood

Haematuria may be overt, with bloody urine, or microscopic and found only on chemical testing. A positive Stix test must always be followed by microscopy of fresh urine to confirm the presence of red cells and so exclude the relatively rare conditions of haemoglobinuria or myoglobinuria. Bleeding may come from any site within the urinary tract (Fig. 9.4):

OVERT BLEEDING FROM THE URETHRA is suggested when blood is seen at the start of voiding and then the urine becomes clear.

BLOOD DIFFUSELY PRESENT THROUGHOUT THE URINE comes from the bladder or above.

BLOOD ONLY AT THE END OF MICTURITION suggests bleeding from the prostate or bladder base.

Careful urine microscopy is mandatory as the presence of red-cell casts is diagnostic of bleeding from the kidney, most often due to glomerulonephritis. In the absence of red-cell casts, further investigations, such as urine cytology, intravenous urography and cystoscopy, are required to define the site of bleeding. Renal biopsy may be required (see p. 444).

### Protein

Proteinuria is one of the most common signs of renal disease. Detection is now primarily by Stix testing. Most reagent strips can detect a concentration of 150 mg litre$^{-1}$ or more in urine. They react primarily with albumin and are relatively insensitive to globulin and Bence–Jones proteins.

If proteinuria is confirmed on repeated Stix testing, protein excretion in 24-hour urine collections should be measured. Normal values for urinary protein excretion are dependent on the laboratory methods used and in

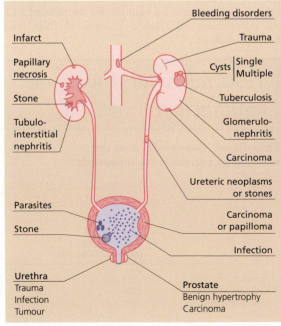

**Fig. 9.4** Sites and causes of bleeding from the urinary tract.

particular whether or not the method measures Tamm–Horsfall glycoprotein, which is a normal constituent of urine. Results must therefore take account of the laboratory's normal reference range. Given this caveat, healthy adults excrete approximately 60–100 mg of protein daily but up to 150–200 mg daily is within the acceptable range. Slightly higher values—up to 300 mg daily—may be excreted by adolescents. Pyrexia, exercise and adoption of the upright posture all increase urinary protein output. Proteinuria, while occasionally benign, always requires further investigation.

POSTURAL PROTEINURIA. This term is used to refer to proteinuria present on dipstick testing which becomes undetectable after a period of hours lying flat. Typically, a negative dipstick result is obtained on the first urine passed on rising in the morning, whereas subsequent specimens give a positive result. This is regarded by many—including some insurance companies—as a benign condition. Renal biopsy sometimes discloses glomerular abnormalities but progressive renal failure is rare.

### Glucose

Renal glycosuria is uncommon, so that a positive test for glucose always requires exclusion of diabetes mellitus.

### Bacteriuria

Dipsticks are available for testing for bacteriuria based on detection of nitrite produced from the reduction of urinary nitrate by bacteria. Unfortunately, there is an unacceptable false-negative detection rate and urine culture is still required.

### Microalbuminuria

The term microalbuminuria is an unfortunate one since the albumin referred to is of normal molecular size and weight. Normal urine contains albumin in a concentration of less than 20 mg litre$^{-1}$. Dipsticks, however, only detect albumin in a concentration around 150 mg litre$^{-1}$. An increase in albumin between these two levels—so-called microalbuminuria—is now known to be an early indicator of diabetic glomerular disease. It is now widely used as a predictor of the development of nephropathy in diabetics and may be extended to other conditions.

Measurement is done by radioimmunoassay. Timed 24-hour urinary excretion may be measured. Microalbuminuria is then defined as an excretion rate between 30 and 150 $\mu g$ min$^{-1}$. Equally reliable results may be more conveniently obtained using random samples in which albumin concentration is related to urinary creatinine concentration (normal range <0.2–2.8 mg of albumin per mmol litre$^{-1}$ creatinine).

## Microscopy

An unspun sample of urine may be examined by placing a drop on a slide using a pipettte, covering with a coverslip and examining by low-power and higher power microscopy. Phase-contrast microscopy is a helpful additional tool. Frequently, a spun-urine sample is examined. Urine is centrifuged, the supernatant is discarded and an aliquot of the residuum placed on a glass slide employing a Pasteur pipette.

Urine microscopy should be carried out in all patients suspected of having renal disease. Care must be taken to obtain a 'clean' sample of mid-stream urine (Practical box 9.2). The presence of numerous skin squames suggests a contaminated, poorly collected sample that cannot be properly interpreted.

If a clean sample of urine cannot be obtained, suprapubic aspiration is required in suspected urinary-tract infections.

Most urines are examined by microscopy in hospital practice by microbiology laboratory technicians who must process large numbers of such urines each day. Best results are obtained in nephrological practice if microscopy is carried out by the physician caring for the patient.

### White cells

The presence of 10 or more white blood cells (WBC) per cubic millimetre in fresh unspun mid-stream urine samples is abnormal and indicates an inflammatory reaction within the urinary tract. Most commonly it is due to urinary tract infection (UTI) but it may also be found in sterile urine in patients during antibiotic treatment of urinary infection or within 14 days of treatment. Sterile pyuria also occurs in patients with stones, tubulo-interstitial nephritis, papillary necrosis, tuberculosis, and interstitial cystitis.

### Red cells

The presence of one or more red cells per cubic millimetre in unspun urine samples results in a positive Stix test for blood and is abnormal. It is claimed that red

**Female**

The patient's bladder should be full ('desperate to go')
The patient removes underpants and *stands* over the toilet pan
The labia are separated using the left hand
The vulva is cleansed front to back with sterile swabs
The patient voids downward into the toilet and continues until 'half-done'
*Without stopping the urine flow*, the sterile container is plunged into the stream of urine with the right hand. Only a small volume is required
The patient then completes voiding into the toilet

**Male**

The patient's bladder should be full
The foreskin, if present, is retracted
The glans penis is cleaned with a sterile swab
The patient voids into the toilet until 'half-done'
*Without stopping the urine flow*, the sterile container is plunged into the stream of urine
The patient then completes voiding into the toilet

**Practical box 9.2**  Collection of mid-stream specimens of urine.

cells of glomerular origin can be identified by their dysmorphic appearance, especially on phase-contrast microscopy, but this is not yet generally available or accepted.

### Casts (Fig. 9.5)

These cylindrical bodies, which are moulded ('cast') in the shape of the distal tubular lumen, may be hyaline, granular or cellular. Hyaline casts and fine granular casts represent precipitated protein and may be seen in normal urine, particularly after exercise. More coarsely granular casts occur with pathological proteinuria in glomerular and tubular disease. Red-cell casts—even one—always indicate renal disease. If red cells degenerate, a rusty-coloured 'haemoglobin' granular cast is seen. White cell casts may be seen in acute pyelonephritis. They may be confused with the tubular cell casts that occur in patients with acute tubular necrosis.

### Bacteria

The demonstration of bacteria on Gram staining of the centrifuged deposit of a clean-catch mid-stream urine sample is highly suggestive of urinary infection and can be of value in the *immediate* differential diagnosis of UTI. If accompanied by pyuria it may be accepted as evidence of UTI in the ill and febrile patient and treatment should be initiated.

Urine for quantitative culture (see p. 459) must always be obtained prior to starting antibiotic treatment in order to confirm the diagnosis and to allow definition of bacterial antibiotic sensitivities.

Stix testing for blood or protein is of no value in the diagnosis of UTI, as both are absent from the urine of many patients with bacteriuria.

## QUANTITATIVE TESTS OF RENAL FUNCTION

The use of blood urea, serum creatinine and GFR as measures of renal function is discussed on p. 436. Quanti-

fication of proteinuria, including the investigation of selective proteinuria, is discussed on p. 455. Other quantitative tests of disturbed renal function such as measurements of urine output of calcium, sodium or potassium or urine acidification are described under the relevant disorders.

## IMAGING TECHNIQUES

### Plain X-ray

A plain radiograph of the abdomen is always taken prior to urography. Its main value is to identify renal calcification or radiodense calculi in the kidney pelvis, line of the ureters or bladder (Fig. 9.6). Care must be taken in viewing the X-ray in order not to miss calculi obscured by bowel shadows or bone. Renal size and outline are best assessed during excretion urography or by ultrasound.

### Excretion urography

This is also known as intravenous urography (IVU) or intravenous pyelography (IVP). If carefully executed and properly interpreted, the urogram is one of the most valuable diagnostic tools for the investigation of renal disease. Carefully timed serial X-rays are taken of the kidneys and the full length of abdomen following a slow intravenous injection of an organic iodine-containing contrast medium. Films taken at the end of the injection show opacification of the parenchyma, allowing definition of size and renal outline. The kidneys are normally

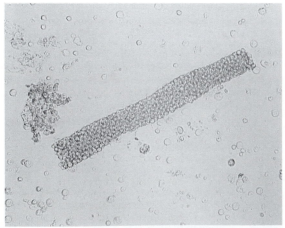

**Fig. 9.5**  Red-cell cast. Note aggregation of red cells as a 'cast' of the tubule.

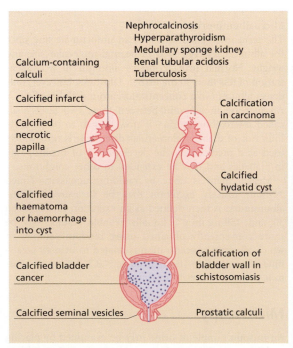

**Fig. 9.6**  Calcification in the renal tract. Calculi can occur at any site.

smooth in outline. In adults they measure 11–14 cm in length, differing by less than 2 cm. An irregular outline due to cortical scarring is abnormal. Reduction in size indicates chronic disease either primarily of the renal parenchyma or of the renal vasculature.

The application of a compression band to the abdomen, designed to partially obstruct ureteral emptying, helps distension of the upper tracts. Special attention is paid to the size, shape and disposition of the calyces and pelvis for evidence of anatomical abnormality such as calyceal clubbing, abnormal dilatation, cavitation or filling defects. The significance of these are described under the particular diseases.

After 10–20 min, the compression bands are removed and full-length films are obtained before and after voiding to study emptying of the upper tract, ureters and bladder.

Reactions to the contrast media include anaphylactic reactions and, rarely, convulsions. Non-ionic contrast media have reduced these complications. Patients with a history of allergy to iodine, those who have had a previous contrast reaction, those with multiple allergies, and asthmatics should receive prednisolone 40 mg 24 hours before and on the day of the examination. Contrast media may also be nephrotoxic (see p. 453).

## Ultrasonography

Ultrasonography of the kidneys, bladder and prostate is well established. Unfortunately, it is often used indiscriminately. An ultrasound scan cannot provide the detailed visualization of the calyces and pelvis required to demonstrate pelvicalyceal abnormalities such as reflux nephropathy or papillary necrosis. It does not visualize the greater part of the ureter and gives no functional information on the upper tract. It requires considerable operator skill in performance. For the general investigation of suspected renal disease, IVU remains the imaging technique of first choice.

The particular value of ultrasound is in defining:

RENAL MASSES OR CYSTIC DISEASE

PRESENCE OR ABSENCE OF OBSTRUCTION in patients with renal failure when urography is unlikely to provide calyceal detail and the administration of contrast medium may be less safe

RENAL SIZE in a patient with renal failure

BLADDER EMPTYING combined with urodynamic studies

THE PROSTATE by means of a rectal transducer

## Computed tomography (CT)

CT has a valuable role in the diagnosis of renal tumours when this is not possible by ultrasound or excretion urography, and in the diagnosis of retroperitoneal masses. It is also valuable in defining the presence and spread of bladder or prostatic tumours and in visualizing uric acid stones which are radiolucent on conventional X-ray.

## Antegrade urography (Fig. 9.7)

Antegrade urography involves percutaneous puncture of a renal calyx, with the insertion of a fine catheter and the injection of contrast medium in an antegrade fashion. It is the procedure of choice in patients with upper urinary tract obstruction demonstrated by ultrasound. Not only does it allow definition of the site of obstruction but also the catheter may be left *in situ* to allow urine drainage in oliguric patients.

## Retrograde urography

Following cystoscopy, preferably under screening control, a catheter is either impacted in the ureteral orifice or passed a short distance up the ureter, and contrast medium is injected; this is followed by X-ray filming.

This investigation is less often used as it is invasive, commonly requires a general anaesthetic and may result in the introduction of infection. It is mainly used to investigate lesions of the ureter and to define the lower level of ureteral obstruction shown on excretion urography or ultrasound plus antegrade studies.

## Micturating cystourography (MCU)

This involves catheterization and the instillation of contrast medium into the bladder. The patient is then screened and filmed during voiding to demonstrate or exclude vesicoureteric reflux and to study bladder emptying. It is primarily used in children with recurrent infection (see p. 459) and in adults with disturbed bladder function,

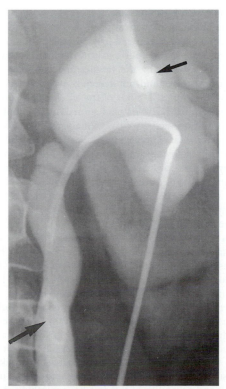

**Fig. 9.7** Antegrade pyelography via percutaneous catheter (small arrow) of obstructed system. Percutaneous drainage catheter (large arrow) has been inserted.

when it may be combined with urodynamic studies of bladder pressure and urethral flow. MCU is not an appropriate part of the investigation of the adult female with recurrent bacterial cystitis in whom IVU, including an after-micturition bladder film, is normal.

The presence or absence of vesicoureteric reflux may also be investigated by scintigraphy.

## Aortography or renal arteriography

Conventional or digital subtraction angiography (DSA) are used. The latter allows the use of smaller doses of contrast medium which can be injected via a central venous catheter (venous DSA) or via a fine transfemoral arterial catheter (arterial DSA). Angiography is mainly used for extrarenal or intrarenal arterial disease and the presence and extent of renal tumours.

## Renal scintigraphy

Renal scintigraphy using a gamma camera is divided into:
1 Dynamic studies in which the function of the kidney is examined serially over a period of time, most often using a radiopharmaceutical excreted by glomerular filtration
2 Static studies involving imaging of tracer that is taken up and *retained* by the renal tubule

### Dynamic scintigraphy
The radiopharmaceutical most often used is [$^{99m}$Tc]DTPA. It is excreted by glomerular filtration. $^{123}$I-labelled *ortho*-iodohippuric acid (Hippuran) is both filtered and secreted by the tubules and is also used but is more expensive and not generally available. Following venous injection of a bolus of tracer, emissions from the kidney can be recorded and stored on computer for analysis of time–activity curves. Analogue images can also be generated at intervals as the study proceeds. This information allows examination of blood perfusion of the kidney, uptake of tracer as a result of glomerular filtration, transit of tracer through the kidney and the outflow of tracer-containing urine from the collecting system.

Dynamic studies are used for:
RENAL BLOOD FLOW. To investigate patients in whom renal artery stenosis is suspected as a cause for hypertension and in patients with severe oliguria (post-traumatic, post-aortic surgery, or after a kidney transplant) to establish whether and to what extent there is renal perfusion. In patients with unilateral renal artery stenosis there is, typically, a slowed and reduced uptake of tracer with delay in reaching a peak. Studies carried out before and after administration of an ACE inhibitor may demonstrate a fall in uptake that is suggestive of functional arterial stenosis. The usefulness and reliability of this test has recently been questioned. In patients with total renal artery occlusion, no kidney uptake of tracers is observed.

INVESTIGATION OF OBSTRUCTION. Renography can demonstrate the severity of obstruction. The results obtained from overall uptake and outflow curves must be treated with caution because of the large 'dead space' commonly contributed by dilated calyces and pelves. Dynamic scintigraphy combined with the injection of frusemide can commonly distinguish functional obstruction from a dilated non-obstructed system.

BLADDER EMPTYING. At the end of dynamic studies, bladder emptying may be investigated and any post-micturition residual measured. Vesicoureteric reflux may be observed, although the sensitivity for detection of this is low. Increased sensitivity can be obtained by direct isotope cystography when a dilute isotope solution is instilled into the bladder by catheter.

GLOMERULAR FILTRATION RATE (see p. 437).

### Static renal scintigraphy
This is usually performed using [$^{99m}$Tc]DMSA (dimercaptosuccinic acid), which is taken up by tubular cells. Uptake is proportional to renal function. Static studies are used for:

RELATIVE RENAL FUNCTION. Function is normally evenly divided between the kidneys with a range of 45–55%. Static studies are particularly useful in unilateral renal disease, where the relative uptake of the two kidneys can be calculated.

KIDNEY VISUALIZATION. Normal kidneys show a uniform uptake with a smooth renal outline. Scars can be identified as photon-deficient 'bites'. Static scintigraphy is of considerable value in identifying ectopic kidneys or 'pseudotumours' of the kidneys, i.e. normally functioning renal tissue abnormally placed within the kidney.

LOCALIZATION OF INFECTION. The use of citrate labelled with gallium-67 or isotopically labelled leucocytes that are taken up by inflammatory tissue may be of value in defining localized infection, such as renal abscesses or infection within a renal cyst.

## TRANSCUTANEOUS RENAL BIOPSY (Practical box 9.3)

Indications and contraindications for renal biopsy are shown in Table 9.4.

The biopsies are carried out under ultrasound control using a spring loaded biopsy needle. Tissue must be examined by conventional histochemical staining, by electron microscopy and by immunofluorescence.

The complications of transcutaneous renal biopsy are shown in Table 9.5.

## *Glomerulonephritis*

Glomerulonephritis is a general term for a **group** of disorders in which:

**Table 9.4**   Renal biopsy.

**Practical box 9.3**   Transcutaneous renal biopsy.

**Table 9.5**   Complications of transcutaneous renal biopsy.

- There is immunologically mediated injury to glomeruli.
- The kidneys are involved symmetrically.
- Secondary mechanisms of glomerular injury come into play following an initial immune insult (see below).
- The renal lesion may be part of a generalized disease, e.g. systemic lupus erythematosus (SLE).

## PATHOGENESIS

Two chief pathogenetic mechanisms are recognized:

1 Deposition or *in situ* formation of immune complexes (most human glomerulonephritides)
2 Deposition of antiglomerular basement membrane antibody (less than 5% of glomerulonephritides)

Both of these pathogenetic mechanisms activate secondary mechanisms that produce glomerular damage.

### Immune complex nephritis

Circulating antigen–antibody complexes (see p. 149) are deposited in the kidney or complexes are formed locally when circulating free antigen has become trapped in the glomerulus. The nature of the antigen involved in the complex formation is important in many instances.

The antigen may be:

EXOGENOUS (e.g. bacterial). For example, a nephrito-genic Lancefield group A $\beta$-haemolytic *Streptococcus* can cause glomerulonephritis in previously healthy individuals.

ENDOGENOUS. For example, patients with SLE may form antibodies to host DNA, leading to a glomerulonephritis.

Harmful immune complexes can also occur when there is impaired host ability to produce appropriate antibody. Certain strains of black mice regularly develop glomerulonephritis as a result of an impaired ability to produce antibody of appropriate quality or quantity, and it is likely that there are human counterparts of this phenomenon. There is an association between HLA markers and certain nephritides.

Impaired ability on the part of the host to clear immune complexes from the circulation and deficiencies in the complement system are each associated with an increased incidence of glomerulonephritis.

### Antiglomerular basement membrane (anti-GBM) antibody

Anti-GBM antibody reacts with an antigen in the glomerular basement membrane, producing a rare form of glomerular damage. It is of the IgG type. The antibody can also react with alveolar capillary basement membrane (owing to shared antigens) and can cause both lung haemorrhage and glomerulonephritis (Goodpasture's syndrome).

### Secondary mechanisms of glomerular injury

Several events can be triggered by the above immunological insults:

- Complement activation
- Fibrin deposition
- Platelet aggregation

- Inflammation with neutrophil-dependent mechanisms
- Activation of kinin systems

Immune complex or anti-GBM antibody deposition trigger these mechanisms to varying degrees, resulting in an increase in capillary permeability and glomerular damage.

In experimentally induced glomerulonephritis in animals, prior anticoagulation, prevention of complement activation, and depletion of polymorphonuclear leucocytes have all been shown to reduce the severity of the induced glomerular injury. However, in humans presenting with most forms of glomerulonephritis these measures do not help.

T-cell dysfunction may play a part in the production of lesions when immune complexes are not seen.

## CAUSES

In the majority of patients with immune complex-mediated glomerulonephritis, the cause is unknown, i.e. the nature of the antigen involved is not determined. Antigen derived from viruses, bacteria, parasites, drugs and from the host may be involved (Table 9.6). The reasons for the development of anti-GBM antibody are not known; viral or solvent damage to alveolar capillary basement membrane, rendering it antigenic, has been suggested as a possible cause.

## PATHOLOGY

### Macroscopic appearances

In acute glomerulonephritis, the kidneys are normal in size or enlarged and oedematous, and the surface of the kidney may show punctate haemorrhages.

In long-standing progressive chronic glomerulo-

nephritis the kidneys may be normal in size or small with finely granular cortical scarring.

### Microscopic appearances

Different immunological insults may induce similar or identical histological changes. For example, the immune complex-mediated glomerulonephritis in mumps is not distinguishable from that following β-haemolytic streptococcal infection. Conversely, different histological responses may occur in the same disease process in different individuals, e.g. in SLE (see below).

The histological response to immune complex deposition probably depends on the size of the complexes, their rate of deposition and the efficiency of host clearance mechanisms.

Renal tissue, obtained at transcutaneous renal biopsy, is examined by:

LIGHT MICROSCOPY to assess the extent and histological type of disease.

ELECTRON MICROSCOPY to define the type of disease and to correlate with immunofluorescence, e.g. to see the exact sites of deposits.

IMMUNOFLUORESCENCE to assess the type of immunological injury. Immunoperoxidase methods may also be applied.

All three methods of examination are necessary for proper histopathological assessment.

Immune complex deposition results in a diffuse granular pattern of staining, with IgG, IgM, IgA, components of the complement system and, in addition, fibrin and fibrinogen all present (Fig. 9.8).

The presence of anti-GBM antibody produces a smooth linear pattern of staining for IgG on immunofluorescence (Fig. 9.9).

### Histopathological types

There is not a complete correlation between the histopathological types and the clinical features of the disease; Table 9.7 shows the commonest associations.

PROLIFERATIVE GLOMERULONEPHRITIS. Proliferative changes occur in many immune complex-mediated

---

Viruses
    Mumps
    Measles
    Hepatitis B
    Epstein–Barr
    Coxsackie
    Varicella

Bacteria
    Lancefield group A β-haemolytic streptococci
    *Streptococcus viridans* (infective endocarditis)
    Staphylococci
    *Treponema pallidum*
    Gonococci, *Salmonella*

Parasites
    *Plasmodium malariae*
    *Schistosoma*
    Filiariasis

Host antigens
    DNA (systemic lupus erythematosus)
    Cryoglobulin
    Malignant tumours

Drugs
    Penicillamine

**Table 9.6**  Some causes of immune complex-mediated glomerulonephritis.

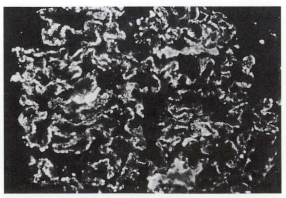

**Fig. 9.8**  Immunofluorescence showing immune complex deposition in a diffuse granular pattern.

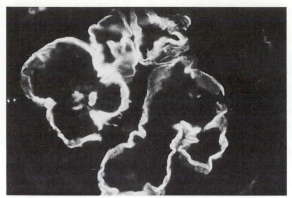

**Fig. 9.9** Immunofluorescence showing antiglomerular basement membrane antibody (anti-GBM) deposition in a linear pattern typical of Goodpasture's syndrome.

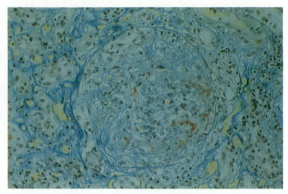

**Fig. 9.10** A glomerulus showing proliferative glomerulonephritis.

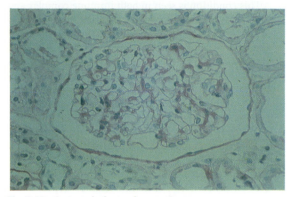

**Fig. 9.11** A normal glomerulus.

| Histological type | Most common clinical presentation |
|---|---|
| *Proliferative glomerulonephritis* | |
| Diffuse | Acute nephritic syndrome |
| Focal segmental | Haematuria, proteinuria |
| With crescent formation (rapidly progressive glomerulonephritis) | Progressive renal failure |
| Mesangiocapillary (membranoproliferative) | Haematuria, proteinuria, acute nephritic or nephrotic syndrome |
| *Membranous glomerulonephritis* | Nephrotic syndrome in adults |
| *Minimal-change nephropathy* | Nephrotic syndrome especially in children |
| *IgA nephropathy* | Asymptomatic haematuria |
| *Focal glomerulosclerosis* | Proteinuria or nephrotic syndrome |

**Table 9.7** Correlation between the histological type of glomerulonephritis and the clinical picture.

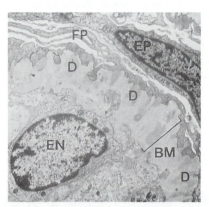

**Fig. 9.12** An electron micrograph showing immune complex-mediated glomerulonephritis. BM, basement membrane; D, electron-dense deposits (antigen–antibody complexes); EN, endothelial cell; EP, epithelial podocyte; FP, foot process.

nephritides and also in anti-GBM nephritis. It has the following subtypes:

1 *Diffuse proliferative glomerulonephritis.* All the glomeruli are similarly affected; Fig. 9.10 shows the typical histological appearances. There is proliferation of endothelial and mesangial cells and several polymorphonuclear leucocytes are present. The glomerulus is swollen, packed with cells and bulges into the opening of the proximal tubule. A normal glomerulus is shown in Fig. 9.11 for comparison. Electron microscopy of the lesions shows subepithelial humps present on the glomerular basement membrane (Fig. 9.12) and immunofluorescence shows granular deposits of immunoglobulin and C3.

This type of glomerulonephritis, presenting as an acute nephritis, is commonly seen after a streptococcal infection (see below).

2 *Focal segmental glomerulonephritis.* Only some of the glomeruli here show proliferative changes whilst others are normal, hence the term focal. The affected glomeruli show segmental involvement of the tufts, i.e. changes are present in one or more parts of the glomerulus.

This condition may occur as a primary renal disease, but it is also seen in SLE, subacute infective endocarditis, with infected atrioventricular shunts (shunt nephritis), and in disorders with IgA deposits, e.g.

Henoch–Schönlein purpura and IgA nephropathy. A severe focal necrotizing form is seen in polyarteritis nodosa and Wegener's granulomatosis. Special sub-types (IgA nephropathy and focal glomerulosclerosis) are discussed below.

3 *Proliferative glomerulonephritis with crescent formation (rapidly progressive glomerulonephritis; RPGN) or crescentic glomerulonephritis* (Fig. 9.13). The term 'crescent' is applied to an aggregate of macrophages and epithelial cells in Bowman's space. Crescents are associated with severe damage to the glomerular tuft and are seen in occasional glomeruli in several types of glomerulonephritis. However, if most glomeruli show crescents the glomerulonephritis is usually placed in this subtype, as clinical progression to renal failure is rapid.

This condition is seen in both immune complex and anti-GBM antibody-mediated nephritis. It particularly occurs in polyarteritis nodosa, Wegener's granulomatosis and Goodpasture's syndrome.

4 *Mesangiocapillary (membranoproliferative) glomerulonephritis (MCGN).* In *type 1* there is mesangial cell proliferation, with mainly subendothelial immune complex deposition and apparent splitting of the capillary basement membrane, giving a 'tram-line' effect. It may be idiopathic or may occur with shunt nephritis. It can be associated with persistently reduced levels of C3 and normal levels of C4.

In *type 2* there is mesangial cell proliferation with electron-dense, linear intramembranous deposits that usually stain for C3 only. This type may be idiopathic or may occur after measles. Partial lipodystrophy (loss of subcutaneous fat in various parts of the body) may be seen. MCGN affects young adults. Patients present with haematuria, proteinuria, the nephrotic syndrome or renal failure. Most patients eventually go on to develop renal failure over several years.

MEMBRANOUS GLOMERULONEPHRITIS (Fig. 9.14). Thickening of the capillary basement membrane due to immune complex deposition is the main feature of this disease. In the majority of patients the antigenic component of the complex is unknown. Associations include

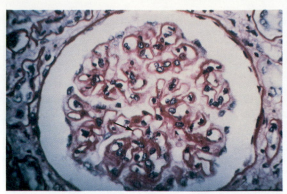

**Fig. 9.14** Membranous glomerulonephritis showing thickened basement membrane (arrow).

SLE (where the antigen is host DNA), malignancy of the bowel and bronchus (tumour-derived antigen) and penicillamine therapy. *Plasmodium malariae* is a common cause in the tropics. A strong association with HLA-DR3 has been found.

This condition occurs mainly in adults, predominantly in males. Patients present with proteinuria or frank nephrotic syndrome. Approximately one-third of patients develop end-stage renal failure within 10–20 years of diagnosis. Younger patients, females and those with asymptomatic proteinuria of modest degree at the time of presentation do best. Spontaneous remission occurs in about one-third of patients, particularly females.

Controversy exists as to the value or otherwise of corticosteroid and immunosuppressive treatment with, for example, chlorambucil, azathioprine and cyclophosphamide, which is not surprising in view of the fact that a significant proportion of patients are destined to do well without specific treatment. It may well be that a subgroup of patients who develop progressive renal impairment benefit from such treatment.

MINIMAL CHANGE GLOMERULAR LESION (MINIMAL CHANGE NEPHROPATHY). This is not a true glomerulonephritis and is included here for convenience. In this condition the glomeruli appear normal on light microscopy. The only abnormality seen on electron microscopy is fusion of the foot processes of epithelial cells (podocytes). This is a non-specific finding and is seen in many conditions associated with proteinuria.

Neither immune complexes nor anti-GBM antibody can be demonstrated by immunofluorescence. However, the immunological pathogenesis of this condition is suggested by three factors:

1 Its response to steroids and immunosuppressive drugs
2 Its occurrence in Hodgkin's disease, with remission following successful treatment
3 Patients with the condition and family members having a higher incidence of asthma and eczema—remission following desensitization or antigen avoidance has been described

A suggested explanation for the proteinuria is the pro-

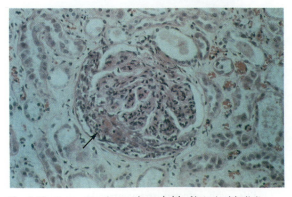

**Fig. 9.13** Crescentic glomerulonephritis. Note 'epithelial' crescent at the periphery of the glomerulus (arrow).

duction by lymphocytes of a factor that increases glomerular permeability to protein.

Minimal change nephropathy is commonest in children, particularly males, accounting for the large majority of cases of nephrotic syndrome in childhood. The condition accounts for 20–25% of cases of adult nephrotic syndrome. It does not lead to chronic renal failure.

Specific treatment is with corticosteroids, cyclophosphamide and cyclosporin (see p. 455).

IgA nephropathy. This disease consists of focal proliferative glomerulonephritis and mesangial deposits of IgA. In some cases IgG, IgM or C3 and properdin may also be seen in the glomerular mesangium.

Glomerulonephritis in Henoch–Schönlein purpura has a similar pathological picture and is sometimes regarded as the same condition (see below).

IgA nephropathy tends to occur in children and young males. They present with asymptomatic microscopic haematuria or recurrent macroscopic haematuria, which is sometimes related to upper respiratory infection. Proteinuria occurs and 5% can be nephrotic. The prognosis is usually good especially in those with normal blood pressure, normal renal function and absence of proteinuria at presentation. Surprisingly, recurrent macroscopic haematuria is a good prognostic sign. There is no specific treatment. Up to 20% of patients eventually develop renal failure.

Henoch–Schönlein syndrome. This clinical syndrome comprises a characteristic skin rash, abdominal colic, joint pain and glomerulonephritis. The rash is of purpuric type and the synonym Henoch–Schönlein purpura is often used. It occurs at all ages and in both sexes, but is mainly a disease of early childhood. Males are twice as often affected as females. A recent history of infection, often respiratory, is common. The disease is rare in adults. Serum concentrations of IgA are increased in about half the patients during the first 3 months of the disease and IgA-containing immune complexes have been detected in serum in a high proportion of cases. The renal lesion is a focal segmental proliferative glomerulonephritis, sometimes with mesangial hypercellularity. Epithelial crescents may be present. Immunoglobulin deposition, mainly of IgA, is seen in the glomerular mesangium and to a lesser extent in the capillary walls on immunofluorescence. IgG, IgM and components of the complement system may also be detectable. Electron-dense deposits, presumably immune complexes, are seen in the mesangium and subendothelial position on electron microscopy. No treatment is of proven benefit.

Focal segmental glomerulosclerosis (FSGS). This is a disease of unknown pathogenesis. It is particularly prone to recur in kidneys transplanted into affected individuals, sometimes within days of transplantation. A circulating factor may be involved. It presents as proteinuria or nephrotic syndrome and is usually resistant to steroid therapy. All age groups are affected.

On light microscopy, segmental glomerulosclerosis is seen, which later progresses to global sclerosis. The deep glomeruli at the corticomedullary junction are affected first. These may be missed on transcutaneous biopsy, leading to a mistaken diagnosis of minimal change glomerular lesion. Immunofluorescence may show deposits of C3 and IgM in affected portions of the glomerulus, but non-specific fixation to damaged tissue, rather than immune complex deposition, may well be the explanation for this.

About 50% of patients progress to end-stage renal failure within 10 years of diagnosis.

## CLINICAL FEATURES

Glomerulonephritis presents in one of four ways:

1 Asymptomatic proteinuria and/or microscopic haematuria
2 Acute nephritic syndrome (see below)
3 Nephrotic syndrome (see p. 453)
4 Chronic renal failure (see p. 478)

Asymptomatic proteinuria and/or microscopic haematuria is discovered incidentally, e.g. at a routine medical examination. Some causes of haematuria are shown in Fig. 9.4. Overt haematuria may occur after exercise.

## INVESTIGATION

Since false-positives are often obtained using Stix methods, the presence of significant proteinuria must be demonstrated by measuring the 24-hour urinary output of protein on two consecutive occasions (see p. 440).

Urine microscopy is performed to look for haematuria. A positive Stix test for blood may result from haematuria or haemoglobinuria. These can be differentiated on microscopy since red cells are only seen in patients with haematuria. Red cell morphology may provide a guide to diagnosis (see p. 441).

Further investigations will include:

Urine microscopy for red-cell casts

Assessment of renal function by estimation of blood urea, serum creatinine and endogenous creatinine clearance

Renal imaging, usually by excretion urography

# Acute nephritic syndrome

This comprises:

- Haematuria (macroscopic or microscopic)—red cell casts are typically seen on urine microscopy
- Proteinuria
- Hypertension } owing to salt and
- Oedema (periorbital, } water retention
  leg or sacral) }
- Oliguria
- Uraemia

## CLINICAL FEATURES

In classical poststreptococcal glomerulonephritis the patient, usually a child, will have suffered a streptococcal infection 1–3 weeks before the onset of the acute nephritic syndrome. Streptococcal tonsillitis or pharyngitis, otitis media or cellulitis may be responsible.

The infecting organism is a Lancefield group A β-haemolytic *Streptococcus* of a nephritogenic type. The latent interval between the infection and development of symptoms and signs of renal involvement reflects the time taken for immune complex formation and deposition and glomerular injury to occur.

### INVESTIGATION

A list of investigations is given in Table 9.8.

If the clinical diagnosis of a nephritic illness is clearcut, e.g. in poststreptococcal glomerulonephritis, renal imaging and renal biopsy are usually unnecessary. A biopsy is required if the diagnosis is uncertain, if the clinical features are unusual, or if renal failure is rapidly progressive, suggesting the presence of crescentic glomerulonephritis (RPGN).

### MANAGEMENT

In the majority of patients with glomerulonephritis, neither corticosteroid nor immunosuppressive therapy is of benefit. The same applies to treatment with agents that alter coagulation and platelet function. Important exceptions to this general rule include glomerulonephritis complicating SLE, systemic vasculitides such as polyarteritis nodosa and Wegener's granulomatosis, Goodpasture's syndrome and some forms of rapidly progressive crescentic glomerulonephritis (see later) and probably idiopathic membranous nephropathy with progressive renal impairment.

As spontaneous remissions usually occur in acute glomerulonephritis, the aim of management is to prevent patients dying from pulmonary oedema, uraemia or hypertensive encephalopathy while awaiting improvement in renal function.

Hospital admission is advisable for all children with oliguria and marked hypertension; levels of blood press-

ure that are of no risk to adults may be associated with hypertensive fits in the young.

Otherwise, hospital admission is not mandatory, providing the general practitioner is able to visit daily to examine the patient and check the blood pressure. Blood for measurement of urea or serum creatinine concentrations should be taken every few days.

### Management in hospital

Most patients require:
- Daily recording of fluid intake and output
- Daily weighing (as a check on change in body fluid status)
- Regular measurement of blood pressure

Strict bed rest is unnecessary unless the patient feels ill, is severely hypertensive or has pulmonary oedema.

Dietary protein restriction is required only if severe uraemia occurs, but salt restriction is always necessary. In oliguric patients, fluid restriction is necessary to maintain body weight at a level at which severe hypertension, pulmonary congestion and gross oedema are prevented.

Mild to moderate hypertension and oedema may respond to salt restriction and diuretic therapy, e.g. frusemide given orally or parenterally. Other hypotensive agents may be required. β-Adrenergic receptor blocking therapy should be used with caution for hypertension as it may precipitate pulmonary oedema in those on the brink of heart failure.

The prognosis in immune complex-mediated glomerulonephritis is improved if the antigen responsible can be eradicated. In patients with poststreptococcal glomerulonephritis, a course of penicillin should be given.

### Management of life-threatening complications

HYPERTENSIVE ENCEPHALOPATHY. In this condition the priorities are to maintain the airway and to reduce the blood pressure using a parenteral agent such as hydralazine 5–20 mg by slow intravenous infusion over 20 min. Fits should be controlled with parenteral diazepam (10 mg i.v.), but this may induce respiratory depression and facilities for resuscitation must be available.

PULMONARY OEDEMA. This should be treated in the usual way (see p. 576). Because of the renal failure, high doses of potent diuretics such as frusemide given parenterally may be required. If this fails to produce a diuresis, salt and water may be removed osmotically by peritoneal dialysis, or by haemofiltration, or by ultrafiltration during haemodialysis (see p. 486).

SEVERE URAEMIA. Peritoneal dialysis, haemodialysis or haemofiltration will be required pending recovery of the renal function.

OUTBREAK OF POSTSTREPTOCOCCAL GLOMERULONEPHRITIS IN A CLOSED COMMUNITY. Prophylactic penicillin (phenoxymethylpenicillin 500 mg daily) should be given to all individuals at risk, providing that they are

| Investigations | Positive findings |
|---|---|
| Urine microscopy | Red cells, red-cell casts |
| Blood urea | May be elevated |
| Serum creatinine | May be elevated |
| Culture (throat swab, discharge from ear, swab from inflamed skin) | Nephritogenic organism—not always |
| Antistreptolysin-O titre | Elevated in poststreptococcal nephritis |
| C3 level | May be reduced |
| Antinuclear antibody | Present in significant titre in systemic lupus erythematosus |
| Creatinine clearance | Reduced |
| Urinary protein output | Increased |
| Chest X-ray | Cardiomegaly ⎫ Not<br>Pulmonary oedema ⎬ always |
| Renal imaging | Usually normal |
| Renal biopsy | Glomerulonephritis |

**Table 9.8**  Investigation of acute nephritic syndrome.

not allergic to penicillin. If one member of a family living in overcrowded conditions develops the disorder, other members should be treated prophylactically. Evidence in support of long-term penicillin prophylaxis after the development of glomerulonephritis is lacking.

## PROGNOSIS
### Poststreptococcal glomerulonephritis
The prognosis in children is excellent. A small number of adults develop hypertension and/or renal impairment later in life. Therefore in older patients, an annual blood pressure check, and less frequently an estimation of serum creatinine, is a reasonable precaution, even after apparent complete recovery.

### Acute glomerulonephritis of unknown cause
The prognosis is less good and the need for follow-up is correspondingly greater.

### Systemic vasculitides and progressive crescentic glomerulonephritis occurring in isolation
The prognosis is often poor and severe renal failure with oliguria and hypertension often occurs within a few weeks or months of the onset of the illness. This group of conditions constitute a nephrological emergency since specific treatment is beneficial (see p. 452).

## Goodpasture's syndrome (see p. 693)

This rare condition is mediated by anti-GBM antibody. It presents with recurrent haemoptysis and a severe progressive proliferative, often crescentic, glomerulonephritis. There is a strong association with HLA-DR2. Lung haemorrhage, which occurs more commonly in cigarette smokers, responds to repeated plasma exchange (which removes the anti-GBM antibody) combined with immunosuppressive therapy. The effect of this treatment upon the glomerulonephritis is less clear-cut; when oliguria occurs or serum creatinine rises above 0.6–0.7 mmol litre$^{-1}$, renal failure is almost always irreversible.

## The kidney in systemic disease

## GLOMERULONEPHRITIS AS A PART OF SYSTEMIC VASCULITIS

### Systemic lupus erythematosus
(see p. 400)

Renal disease in SLE is 10 times as common in women as in men. All varieties of histological abnormality are seen, ranging from a minimal-change lesion to crescentic glomerulonephritis. Serial renal biopsies show that in approximately 25% of patients, histological appearances alter from one histological classification to another during the interbiopsy interval. The prognosis is better in patients with the minimal-change and membranous lesions than in those with proliferative glomerulonephritis.

Pregnancy is associated with significant risk to the lupus patient, not only owing to hypertension and premature delivery, but also to more rapid progression of the glomerular lesion following delivery.

Whilst corticosteroid therapy improves the extrarenal manifestations of SLE, evidence is lacking that this treatment alters the renal prognosis. Both azathioprine and cyclophosphamide improve renal function, but long-term studies suggest that cyclophosphamide is better. Intermittent intravenous 'pulse' cyclophosphamide treatment may be safer and is likely to be as effective as continuous oral therapy.

The indications for treatment vary. Those whose urine sediment contains many red cells and red-cell casts and those in whom renal function is impaired or is observed to deteriorate are strong candidates for treatment. A histological diagnosis should be obtained before commencing such potentially hazardous treatment.

## Systemic vasculitides (see p. 406)

In this group of disorders there is considerable overlap between individual varieties. The common feature is an immunologically mediated inflammation of vessels of varying size. A major advance in understanding has followed the discovery of autoantibodies directed against constituents of the cytoplasm of normal human granulocytes and monocytes in patients with systemic vasculitis. Antineutrophil cytoplasmic antibodies (ANCA) are now established as a marker for vasculitides involving the kidney with or without signs of systemic disease. Two forms of ANCA can be demonstrated by immunofluorescence, one with cytoplasmic staining, named c-ANCA, and one with perinuclear staining, named p-ANCA. In most instances, c-ANCA is directed to a serine protease called proteinase C, whereas p-ANCA is, at least in renal disease, mainly directed at myeloperoxidase. Whether ANCA is only a marker of disease or whether it takes part in the pathogenic process is currently undetermined. ANCA levels can be measured by enzyme-linked immunosorbent assay (ELISA) and variations in the ANCA titre have been used in the assessment of disease activity.

### Polyarteritis nodosa (PAN) (see p.406)
Classical PAN is a multisystem disorder. Aneurysmal dilatation of medium-sized arteries may be seen on renal arteriography. The condition is commoner in men and in the elderly and, typically, the patient is ANCA negative. Hypertension and haematuria occur and eventually renal failure which is the usual cause of death.

### Microscopic polyarteritis
In this condition necrotizing crescentic glomerulonephritis without immune complex deposition occurs

with p-ANCA positivity. The lungs may be involved but granuloma are not seen.

**Wegener's granulomatosis** (see p. 690)
In this condition, glomerulonephritis occurs together with necrotizing granulomatous lesions affecting the nasopharynx, lungs and kidneys. The necrotizing glomerular lesions do not appear to be due to immune complex deposition. c-ANCA positivity is the rule.

## Treatment of systemic vasculitis

The sooner treatment is instituted the more chance there is of recovery of renal function. Corticosteroids and cyclophosphamide are of benefit: pulsed high dose methylprednisolone and plasmapheresis may reverse advanced disease. Once remission has been achieved, azathioprine may be substituted for cyclophosphamide.

## RENAL INVOLVEMENT IN OTHER DISEASES

## Diabetes mellitus

Renal disease is a major complication of diabetes; it is discussed on p. 847.

## Systemic sclerosis (see p. 403)

Interlobular renal arteries are affected with intimal thickening and fibrinoid changes occur in afferent glomerular arterioles. Glomerular changes are non-specific. The pathogenesis is unknown and neither steroid nor immunosuppressive therapy is of value. ANCA are not present.

## Amyloidosis

The kidney is often affected in amyloidosis (see p. 866). Presentation is with asymptomatic proteinuria, nephrotic syndrome or renal failure.

### PATHOLOGY
On light microscopy eosinophilic deposits are seen in the mesangium, capillary loops and arteriolar walls. Staining with Congo red renders these deposits pink and they show green birefringence under polarized light. Immunofluorescence is unhelpful but on electron microscopy the characteristic fibrils of amyloid can be seen. Amyloid consisting of immunoglobulin light chains (AL amyloid) can be distinguished by immunological techniques from the protein found in secondary amyloid (amyloid protein A, AA amyloid). AL amyloid is found in disorders associated with lymphoproliferative diseases such as myeloma, Waldenström's macroglobulinaemia or non-Hodgkin's lymphoma. It is also present in cases of so-called primary amyloidosis where an abnormal clone of cells is presumed to be responsible, although at present not identifiable. AA amyloid is found following long-standing inflammatory

conditions such as suppurative infections or rheumatoid arthritis and familial Mediterranean fever.

### DIAGNOSIS
The diagnosis can often be made clinically when features of amyloidosis are present elsewhere. On imaging, the kidneys are often large. Renal biopsy is necessary in doubtful cases.

### TREATMENT
Treatment of the underlying cause should be undertaken. In primary amyloid, treatment also used in myeloma such as corticosteroids and melphalan are of benefit. The success of dialysis and kidney transplantation is dependent upon the extent of amyloid deposition in extrarenal sites, especially the heart.

## Haemolytic uraemic syndrome (HUS)

HUS is a disorder of infancy and childhood that is characterized by intravascular haemolysis with red-cell fragmentation (microangiopathic haemolysis), thrombocytopenia and acute renal failure. The syndrome often follows a febrile illness, particularly gastroenteritis or upper respiratory tract infection. A few particular strains of pathogenic *Escherichia coli* have been isolated in many cases. Clustering of cases and the occurrence of 'epidemics' of HUS provide further support for an infective aetiology. It has been suggested that infection triggers endothelial damage and that derangements of the haemostatic coagulation system then occur in susceptible individuals. Recurrent episodes of HUS have been described in the same individual. Fibrin deposition is seen in the vascular endothelium, particularly in the renal arterioles and glomerular capillaries. Most children recover spontaneously.

Treatment with heparin, inhibitors of platelet aggregation, synthetic prostacyclins, infusion of fresh frozen plasma and plasma exchange have been employed, but controlled trials of treatment are lacking.

## Thrombotic thrombocytopenic purpura (TTP)

TTP is characterized by the presence of widespread hyaline thrombi in small vessels. Young adults are most commonly affected. Microangiopathic haemolysis, renal failure and evidence of neurological disturbance are characteristically found. The pathogenesis is unknown. Some patients with TTP have underlying SLE or polyarteritis nodosa and there is clearly considerable overlap between HUS, TTP and the connective tissue disorders. Corticosteroid therapy and measures employed in HUS may be of benefit.

## Multiple myeloma

Acute renal failure is relatively common in myeloma, occurring in 2–8% of affected individuals. Histological appearances may be simply those of acute tubular necrosis; tubular blockage by Tamm–Horsfall glycoprotein, light chains and immunoglobulin may be apparent. Dehydration and the administration of intravenous or intra-arterial contrast medium to the volume-depleted patient with myeloma predispose to the development of actue renal failure.

In myeloma, free $\kappa$ and $\lambda$ light chains are excreted. Blockage of tubules by casts composed in part at least of light chains, and perhaps their toxic effects upon tubular cells, account for the proteinuria and chronic renal impairment associated with 'myeloma kidney'. Renal amyloid deposition often complicates myeloma, accounting both for proteinuria—sometimes of nephrotic proportions—and chronic renal failure.

Hypercalcaemia, renal sepsis and—rarely—urinary tract obstruction due to bulky myeloma deposits are further causes of renal impairment in myelomatosis.

## Contrast nephropathy

Iodinated radiological contrast media are nephrotoxic, possibly by causing renal vasoconstriction. The effect is dose dependent and therefore more commonly seen in procedures which require large amounts of contrast media such as angiography with or without angioplasty. In many patients the effect is mild, transient, fully reversible and of no clinical significance. The risk and severity of contrast nephropathy is amplified by the presence of coexisting conditions which also cause renal hypoperfusion:

- Pre-existing renal impairment
- Hypovolaemia
- Low cardiac output
- Diabetes mellitus
- Hyperviscosity (myeloma)

As many as possible of these risk factors should be corrected prior to the use of contrast media. The dose should be minimized. The newer non-ionic and low osmolality media carry less risk of allergic contrast reactions but do *not* decrease the risk of contrast nephropathy. The use of calcium antagonists to prevent contrast nephropathy is under investigation. Mannitol and dopamine may also protect against nephrotoxicity in non-diabetics but not in diabetics.

# Nephrotic syndrome

The nephrotic syndrome consists of heavy urinary protein loss, hypoalbuminaemia and oedema. Hypercholesterolaemia is almost always present.

## PATHOPHYSIOLOGY

Urinary protein loss of the order of 3–5 g daily or more in an adult is required to cause hypoalbuminaemia. In children, proportionately less proteinuria results in hypoalbuminaemia.

The normal dietary protein intake in the UK is of the order 70 g daily and the normal liver can synthesize albumin at a rate of 10–12 g daily. How then does a urinary protein loss of the order of 3–5 g daily result in hypoalbuminaemia? The explanation appears to be that in normal individuals there is some catabolism within the kidney of albumin filtered at the glomeruli. In nephrotic patients with heavy proteinuria, catabolism is substantially increased, limiting the amount of protein appearing in the urine and concealing the extent of protein loss through the glomerulus.

The mechanism of the proteinuria is complex. It occurs partly because structural damage to the glomerular basement membrane leads to an increase in the size and numbers of pores, allowing passage of more and larger molecules. Electrical charge is also involved in glomerular permeability. Fixed negatively charged components are present in the glomerular capillary wall, which repel negatively charged protein molecules. Reduction of this fixed charge occurs in glomerular disease and appears to be an important factor in the genesis of heavy proteinuria.

### Pathogenesis of oedema in hypoalbuminaemia

The pathogenesis of the oedema is incompletely understood. The conventional explanation is that a reduction in the concentration of osmotically active albumin molecules in the blood results in a reduction in the oncotic force that retains fluid within blood vessels, and salt and water escapes into the extravascular compartment, i.e. oedema occurs. Such loss of salt and water results in a fall in blood volume and a reduction in pressure within afferent glomerular arterioles. This activates the renin–angiotensin–aldosterone system (see p. 822). The consequent hyperaldosteronism promotes sodium and water reabsorption in the distal nephron, increasing the tendency to oedema. However, measurements of these various parameters do not always support this concept. The plasma renin activity in nephrotic patients is often normal and measured blood volume may be normal or high in nephrotic patients, even those without renal failure.

### CAUSES (Table 9.9)

All types of glomerulonephritis can produce the nephrotic syndrome.

Although proliferative glomerulonephritis is commoner than membranous disease, the latter is the commonest cause of nephrotic syndrome in adults in the UK.

Minimal change glomerular disease accounts for most cases of the nephrotic syndrome in childhood compared

All glomerulonephritides and minimal-change
glomerular lesions
Systemic vasculitides, mainly systemic lupus
erythematosus
Diabetic glomerulosclerosis
Amyloidosis
Drugs
Allergies

**Table 9.9** Causes of the nephrotic syndrome.

with approximately 20% of adult cases. In tropical areas minimal change is present in fewer than 10% of nephrotic children owing to the high incidence of nephrotic syndrome due to infections such as malaria. Minimal-change disease does not progress to chronic renal failure (see p. 448).

Diabetic glomerular disease can also cause the nephrotic syndrome. The histological lesion seen on light microscopy in diabetes may comprise amorphous nodular deposits, which are not immune complexes, in the glomeruli or a diffuse glomerulosclerosis. There is associated glomerular basement membrane thickening.

Diabetes is also a cause of renal papillary necrosis, but patients with this lesion alone do not have sufficiently heavy proteinuria to become nephrotic.

### Drugs
Many drugs can cause sufficiently heavy proteinuria to result in the nephrotic syndrome. Penicillamine, which in all probability combines with a plasma protein to form an antigen hapten, induces an immune complex-mediated membranous glomerulonephritis, as may high dose captopril. Various metals, whether used therapeutically (e.g. gold) or in industry (e.g. mercury and cadmium), can induce proteinuria severe enough to cause the nephrotic syndrome.

### Allergic reactions
Reactions to many allergens such as poison ivy, pollens, bee stings and cows' milk may be associated with the nephrotic syndrome, but evidence of a causal relationship is lacking in most cases.

Most lists of causes of the nephrotic syndrome include renal vein thrombosis, but this is probably a complication rather than a cause of the syndrome. It is particularly likely to complicate membranous glomerulonephritis. In nephrotic patients the blood is more coagulable than normal and the circulation may be sluggish owing to hypovolaemia, both of which are likely to induce thrombosis. Estimates of the incidence of this complication range from 5% to approximately 50% in nephrotic syndrome due to membranous glomerulonephritis.

### Renal disorders not associated with the nephrotic syndrome
Proteinuria severe enough to cause the nephrotic syndrome is not a feature of reflux nephropathy (chronic atrophic pyelonephritis), chronic tubulo-interstitial nephritis, renal tuberculosis, polycystic disease or many other renal disorders.

### HISTORY
The history may provide clues to the aetiology, e.g. exposure to a drug or allergen. Patients with minimal-change lesion may give a history or family history of atopy. There may be a family history of renal disease.

Patients with heavy proteinuria may have noted that their urine has been frothy; the onset of the renal lesion can be timed from this observation.

### EXAMINATION
Examination will reveal oedema; ascites may also be present, particularly in children. Genital oedema is sometimes seen. The oedema may involve the face (periorbital oedema) and arms. Neither elevation of the jugular venous pressure nor pulmonary oedema are features of the nephrotic syndrome, though either or both may be present if renal and/or cardiac failure are present in the nephrotic patient.

Features of the underlying disorder may be evident, such as the butterfly facial rash of SLE or the neuropathy and retinopathy associated with diabetes mellitus.

Exclude:

PRIMARY CARDIAC FAILURE: here, the venous pressure is high, oedema is not usually present in the face, and the proteinuria is less severe.

LIVER DISEASE, and other causes of hypoalbuminaemia (Table 9.10), with oedema and ascites.

### INVESTIGATION
The presence of the nephrotic syndrome is established by measuring:

24-HOUR URINARY PROTEIN—usually more than 3–5 g daily in adults

SERUM ALBUMIN CONCENTRATION—usually less than 30 g litre$^{-1}$

Increased hepatic albumin synthesis is accompanied by increased cholesterol synthesis and there is an approximate reciprocal relationship between the serum albumin and the serum cholesterol concentration. Low-density lipoprotein (LDL) cholesterol concentrations are elevated but high-density lipoprotein (HDL) cholesterol is usually normal. Hypertriglyceridaemia is present in about 50% of patients.

Renal function is assessed by measuring:
- Serum urea and creatinine
- Creatinine clearance, to determine the GFR

Further investigations are required to elucidate the cause:

MICROSCOPY OF THE URINE may show red cells and red-cell casts; the latter are virtually diagnostic of glomerulonephritis. Minimal-change lesions do not usually result in red cells or red-cell casts in the urine.

SERUM C3 COMPLEMENT CONCENTRATIONS may be decreased in immune complex-mediated glomerulonephritis.

THROAT SWAB AND SERUM ASO titre may show evidence of streptococcal infection.

PRESENCE OF ANTINUCLEAR FACTOR may suggest SLE and of ANCA (see p. 451) a systemic vasculitis.

SERUM ELECTROPHORESIS. In the nephrotic syndrome

| Inadequate protein intake—protein–energy malnutrition |
| Failure of protein production—liver disease |
| Excessive protein loss—nephrotic syndrome, protein-losing enteropathy, extensive burns |
| Pregnancy |

**Table 9.10**  Causes of hypoalbuminaemia.

there is always a reduced serum albumin, commonly with an increase in the α- and β-globulin fractions (Fig. 9.15) on serum electrophoresis. In myeloma, abnormal protein bands may be found, including Bence–Jones protein in the urine. Ten per cent of patients with myeloma have amyloid and can develop the nephrotic syndrome.

RAISED BLOOD GLUCOSE indicates diabetes mellitus.

SELECTIVE PROTEIN CLEARANCE may be measured. Blood and urine samples are taken at the same time; a timed urine collection is not required. The clearance of large-molecular-weight protein such as IgG is compared with that of a smaller molecule such as albumin or transferrin. A low ratio (selective protein leak) is found in minimal-change glomerulopathy, early diabetes and renal amyloidosis. Severe glomerulonephritides, e.g. diffuse proliferative glomerulonephritis with crescent formation, are more typically associated with an unselective protein leak. Overlap between the groups exists. Measurement of selective protein clearance is unnecessary if renal biopsy is to be carried out. Its main use is in children in whom a minimal-change lesion is suspected. An unselective protein leak in such a child would bring this diagnosis into question and might prompt renal biopsy (see below).

### Renal biopsy (see p. 444)

Transcutaneous biopsy is performed to make a histological diagnosis when management will be affected, particularly when the major question is whether a steroid-sensitive minimal-change lesion is present or not. It is *not* indicated in three groups of patients:

1 In young children (particularly males) who have a highly selective protein leak, no hypertension and no red cells or red-cell casts in the urine. The diagnosis is almost certain to be a minimal-change lesion, so that a trial of steroids should be instituted first.

2 In long-standing, insulin-dependent diabetes with associated retinopathy or neuropathy, since the diagnosis is in little doubt.

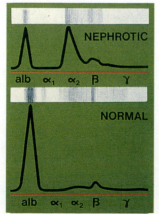

**Fig. 9.15** Serum electrophoresis in a normal person and a patient with nephrotic syndrome. Note the reduced albumin and increased α- and β-globulin in the nephrotic patient.

3 In patients on drugs such as penicillamine, which should be stopped first.

## MANAGEMENT
### General measures

Initial treatment should be with dietary sodium restriction and a thiazide diuretic, e.g. bendrofluazide 5 mg daily. Unresponsive patients require frusemide 40–120 mg daily with the addition of amiloride (5 mg daily), but the serum potassium concentration should be monitored carefully. Patients are often hypovolaemic, and moderate oedema may have to be accepted in order to avoid postural hypotension.

A high-protein diet (approximately 80–90 g protein daily) confers no benefit and normal protein intake is advisable.

Infusion of albumin produces only a transient effect and is normally employed only in diuretic-resistant patients. Such infusion is combined with diuretic therapy. Diuresis, when once initiated in this way, often continues with diuretic treatment alone.

### Specific measures

The aim is to reverse the abnormal urinary protein leak.

MINIMAL-CHANGE GLOMERULAR LESION. High-dose corticosteroid therapy with prednisolone 60 mg daily (dose corrected to a normal body surface area of 1.73 m$^2$) for 8 weeks corrects the urinary protein leak in more than 95% of children. Response rates in adults are significantly lower and response may occur only after many months of steroid therapy. Spontaneous remission also occurs and steroid therapy should, in general, be withheld if urinary protein loss is insufficient to cause hypoalbuminaemia or oedema.

In both children and adults, if remission lasts for 4 years after steroid therapy, further relapse is very rare. In children, approximately one-third do not subsequently relapse, but in the remainder further courses of corticosteroids are indicated. One-third of these patients relapse regularly on steroid withdrawal and in these patients remission is induced with steroid therapy once more and a course of cyclophosphamide 3 mg kg$^{-1}$ daily is given for 6–8 weeks. This increases the likelihood of long-term remission. Steroid-unresponsive patients may also respond to cyclophosphamide. No more than two courses of cyclophosphamide should be prescribed in children because of the risk of side-effects, which include azoospermia.

An alternative to cyclophosphamide is cyclosporin, which is effective but must be continued long term to prevent relapse on stopping treatment. Excretory function must be monitored carefully as cyclosporin is potentially nephrotoxic.

MEMBRANOUS GLOMERULONEPHRITIS (see p. 448)

OTHER CAUSES. Remission occurs if the underlying disease can be treated. In patients with SLE, treatment with steroids and cyclophosphamide or azathioprine usually induces long-term remission.

When the glomerular lesion causing the nephrotic syndrome progresses and the GFR declines, the degree of proteinuria often diminishes so that the hypoalbuminaemia and oedema improve.

### Prevention and management of complications

VENOUS THROMBOSIS. Hypovolaemia and a hypercoagulable state predispose to venous thrombosis. Prolonged bed rest should therefore be avoided.

Once renal vein thrombosis has occurred, prolonged anticoagulation is required. Thromboembolism is exceptionally common in nephrotic syndrome due to membranous glomerulonephritis and prophylactic anticoagulation may be warranted.

SEPSIS. Sepsis is an important cause of death in nephrotic patients. The increased susceptibility to infection is partly due to loss of immunoglobulin in the urine. Pneumococcal infections are particularly common.

Early detection and aggressive treatment of infections, rather than long-term antibiotic prophylaxis, is the best approach.

OLIGURIC RENAL FAILURE. A low blood volume and hypotension may lead to underperfused kidneys. Acute tubular necrosis may therefore readily develop when renal ischaemia occurs from other complications such as blood loss or septicaemia. In some patients, uraemia appears to result from derangements in renal perfusion in the absence of hypotension.

Albumin infusion combined with mannitol or another diuretic may initiate a diuresis in oliguric renal failure.

LIPID ABNORMALITIES. It is suggested that these are responsible for an increase in the risk of myocardial infarction or peripheral vascular disease. There is no consensus on whether lipid-lowering agents should be prescribed routinely.

## Urinary tract infection

Urinary tract infection (UTI) is common in women, uncommon in men and of special importance in children. Recurrent infection causes considerable morbidity; if complicated, it can cause severe renal disease including end-stage renal failure. It is also a common source of life-threatening Gram-negative septicaemia.

### PATHOGENESIS

Infection is most often due to bacteria from the patient's own bowel flora (Table 9.11). Transfer to the urinary tract may be via the bloodstream, the lymphatics or by direct extension (e.g. from a vesicocolic fistula), but is most often via the ascending transurethral route (Fig.

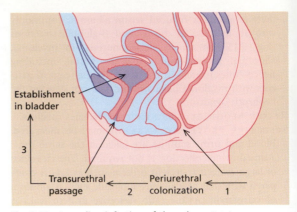

**Fig. 9.16**  Ascending infection of the urinary tract.

9.16). For the latter route, three important steps are involved:

1 The periurethral area is heavily colonized with bacteria. This may be facilitated by the adhesion of bacteria to uroepithelial surfaces by pili or fimbriae present on their surface. Previous UTIs may also predispose to further colonization, initiating a vicious circle. Other factors involved are unclear, although gross lack of personal hygiene, the wearing of nappies or sanitary towels, local infection (e.g. vaginitis) and the use of bubble baths or chemicals in bath water have all been incriminated.

2 Bacteria are transferred along the urethra to the bladder. This step is facilitated by catheterization or sexual intercourse. Spontaneous transfer along the short female urethra is easy, while the longer male urethra protects against transfer of bacteria to the bladder; in addition, prostatic fluid has defensive bactericidal properties.

3 The most important step is the *establishment* and *multiplication* of bacteria within the bladder. Bladder urine is normally sterile, owing to bladder defence mechanisms that are the main protection against UTI. These include hydrokinetic and bladder mucosal factors. A low flow rate and infrequent and poor bladder emptying predispose to infection.

Mucosal defence mechanisms are poorly understood. The establishment of infection may be facilitated by fimbriated bacteria adhering to the bladder uroepithelium or previous damage to this epithelium. Neither humoral nor cell-mediated immune mechan-

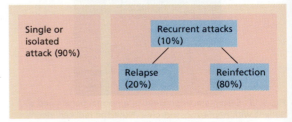

**Fig. 9.17**  The natural history of urinary tract infection.

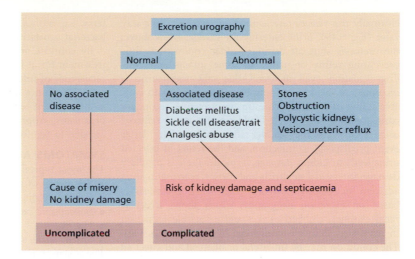

**Fig. 9.18** Complicated versus uncomplicated urinary tract infection.

isms have been shown to play any part in maintaining the sterility of bladder urine.

The first phase in the development of UTI is the entry and establishment of bacteria within the bladder. Extension of infection up the ureters to the kidneys is relatively easy and is facilitated by vesicoureteric reflux and dilated hypotonic ureters. Once infection is established it can pass up or down the system quite readily.

### NATURAL HISTORY

UTI is commonly an isolated, never (or rarely) repeated event (Fig. 9.17). At least 50% of women will experience an episode of 'cystitis' at some time in their lives. Although often unpleasant, such single episodes of UTI rarely result in significant kidney damage. Recurrent or persistent infections are much more important.

### Complicated versus uncomplicated infection (Fig. 9.18)

It is important to distinguish between UTI occurring in patients with:

Functionally normal urinary tracts (with normal excretion urography). Here, persistent or recurrent infection rarely results in serious kidney damage (*uncomplicated* UTI).

Abnormal urinary tracts (e.g. with stones) or associated diseases (e.g. diabetes mellitus) which themselves cause kidney damage may be made worse with infection (*complicated* UTI). UTI, particularly with *Proteus*, may predispose to stone formation. The combination of infection and obstruction results in severe, sometimes rapid, kidney damage (obstructive pyonephrosis) and is an important cause of Gram-negative septicaemia.

### Chronic pyelonephritis

Chronic pyelonephritis (also called atrophic pyelonephritis or reflux nephropathy) is now known to result from a combination of:

- Vesicoureteric reflux, and
- Infection acquired in infancy or early childhood

| Organism | Approximate frequency (%) |
|---|---|
| *Escherichia coli* and other 'coliforms' | 68+ |
| *Proteus mirabilis* | 12 |
| *Klebsiella aerogenes*[a] | 4 |
| *Enterococcus faecalis*[a] | 6 |
| *Staphylococcus saprophyticus* or *epidermidis*[b] | 10 |

[a]More common in hospital practice.
[b]More common in young women (20–30%).

**Table 9.11** Organisms causing urinary tract infection in domiciliary practice.

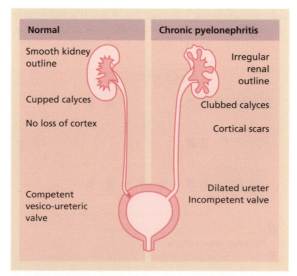

**Fig. 9.19** Chronic pyelonephritis with vesicoureteric reflux compared with the normal state.

Normally the vesicoureteric junction acts as a one-way valve (Fig. 9.19), urine entering the bladder from above; the ureter is shut off during bladder contraction, thus preventing reflux of urine. In some infants and children—possibly even *in utero*—this valve mechanism is incompetent, bladder voiding being associated with variable reflux of a jet of urine up the ureter. A secondary consequence is incomplete bladder emptying, as refluxed urine returns to the bladder after voiding. This latter event predisposes to infection, and the reflux of infected urine leads to kidney damage. Typically there is papillary damage, interstitial nephritis and cortical scarring in areas adjacent to 'clubbed calyces' (Fig. 9.19). Diagnosis is based on excretion urography, which shows irregular renal outlines, clubbed calyces and a variable reduction in renal size. Reflux is confirmed by MCU (see p. 443). The condition may be unilateral or bilateral and affect all or part of the kidney.

Reflux usually ceases around puberty with growth of the bladder base. Damage already done persists and progressive renal fibrosis and further loss of function occurs in severe cases even though there is no further infection. This condition does not develop in the absence of reflux and does not begin in adult life. It is therefore important to reassure adult females with bacteriuria and a normal urogram that kidney damage due to reflux nephropathy will not develop. Chronic pyelonephritis acquired in infancy predisposes to hypertension in later life and, if severe, is a relatively common cause of end-stage renal failure in childhood or adult life. Early detection and treatment of infection, with or without ureteral reimplantation to create a competent valve, can prevent further scarring and allow normal growth of the kidneys.

### Reinfection versus relapsing infection

When UTI is recurrent it is important to distinguish between relapse and reinfection.

Relapse is diagnosed by recurrence of bacteriuria with the *same* organism within 7 days of treatment and implies failure to eradicate infection (Fig. 9.20). It usually occurs in conditions in which it is difficult to eradicate the bacteria, e.g. stones, scarred kidneys, polycystic disease or bacterial prostatitis.

By contrast, in reinfection bacteriuria is absent after treatment for at least 14 days, usually longer, followed by recurrence of infection with the same or different organisms. This is not due to failure to eradicate infection, but is the result of reinvasion of a susceptible tract with new organisms. Approximately 80% of recurrent infections are due to reinfection.

### SYMPTOMS AND SIGNS

The most typical symptoms of UTI are:

- Frequency of micturition by day and night
- Painful voiding (dysuria)
- Suprapubic pain and tenderness
- Haematuria
- Smelly urine

These symptoms relate to bladder and urethral inflammation, commonly called 'cystitis', and suggest lower urinary tract infection. Loin pain and tenderness, with fever and systemic upset, suggest extension of the infection to the pelvis and kidney, known as pyelitis or pyelonephritis. However, localization of the site of infection on the basis of symptoms alone is unreliable.

UTI may also be present with minimal or no symptoms or may be associated with atypical symptoms such as abdominal pain, fever or haematuria in the absence of frequency or dysuria.

In small children, who cannot complain of dysuria, symptoms are often 'atypical'. The possibility of UTI must always be considered in the fretful, febrile sick child who fails to thrive.

### Abacteriuric frequency or dysuria ('urethral syndrome')

Symptoms of frequency and/or dysuria are *not* synonymous with UTI and 50% of symptomatic young women may have no demonstrable bacteriuria. Alternative causes include postcoital bladder trauma, vaginitis, atrophic vaginitis or urethritis in the elderly, and interstitial cystitis (Hunner's ulcer).

Interstitial cystitis is an uncommon but distressing complaint, most often affecting women over the age of 40 years. It presents with frequency, dysuria and often severe suprapubic pain. Urine cultures are sterile. Cystoscopy shows typical inflammatory changes with ulceration of the bladder base. The cause is unclear but it is commonly thought to be an autoimmune disorder. Various treatments are advocated with variable success. These include oral prednisolone therapy, bladder instillation of sodium cromoglycate and bladder stretching under anaesthesia.

Careful history-taking will identify a group with predominant frequency and passage of small volumes of urine who have 'irritable bladders', possibly consequent on previous UTI or conditioned by psychosexual factors. Such patients must be distinguished from those with frequency due to polyuria. Repeated courses of antibiotics in patients with abacteriuric frequency or dysuria are quite inappropriate and detract from identifying the true nature of the problem.

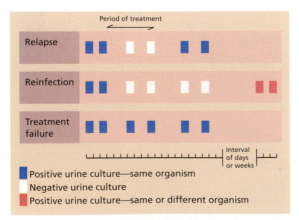

**Fig. 9.20**  A comparison of reinfection, relapse and treatment failure in urinary tract infection.

## DIAGNOSIS

The diagnosis is based on *quantitative* culture of a clean-catch mid-stream specimen of urine. Details on the collection of urine samples are given on p. 441. Once collected, samples must be sent to the laboratory immediately or refrigerated pending despatch in order to prevent further multiplication of bacteria. More than 100 000 of the same organism per millilitre of urine indicates bladder infection ('significant bacteriuria'). Lower counts may be accepted as evidence of infection in patients passing large volumes of urine. If in doubt, urine must be obtained by suprapubic bladder aspiration, when any growth of a uropathogenic organism is evidence of infection. Pyuria is not a constant feature of UTI and its absence does not exclude the diagnosis. Dipstick tests for nitrite have a high false-negative detection rate (see p. 441).

## SPECIAL INVESTIGATIONS

### Excretion urography

Excretion urography is not indicated in women with one or two isolated episodes of UTI if post-treatment urinalysis, including microscopy and urine culture, are normal. If there are further attacks or if post-treatment urinalysis is abnormal, excretion urography should be performed to identify or exclude anatomical or functional abnormalities predisposing to or complicating infection, e.g. impaired bladder emptying.

Excretion urography should be carried out in all males and children following a first proven episode of bacteriuria to identify complicating factors.

### Micturating cystourography

MCU is indicated in children with abnormal excretion urograms and may be required to evaluate abnormal bladder emptying at any age. Otherwise it is of no value in the management of UTI.

### Cystoscopy

Cystoscopy in patients with known UTI has a very limited role. It is indicated only to investigate abnormal bladder or ureteral emptying, or haematuria in bacteriuric women over the age of 40 years, since bladder cancer becomes more common with age. It is more appropriately performed in abacteriuric frequency or dysuria to exclude bladder lesions such as carcinoma or interstitial cystitis (Hunner's ulcer).

## TREATMENT

### Single isolated attack

Pretreatment urine cultures are desirable.

IF SYMPTOMS ARE MILD, symptomatic treatment with potassium citrate mixture (10 ml three times daily) can be given pending the result of urine culture.

IF SYMPTOMS ARE SEVERE, treatment with 3–5 days of amoxycillin (250 mg three times daily), nitrofurantoin (50 mg three times daily) or trimethoprim (200 mg twice daily) should be started immediately without waiting for the result of urine culture. A high (2 litres daily) fluid intake should be encouraged during treatment and for some subsequent weeks.

Urinalysis, microscopy and culture should be repeated 5 days after treatment. 'Single-shot' treatment with 3 g of amoxycillin or 1.92 g of co-trimoxazole can be used for patients with bladder symptoms of less than 36 hours duration who have no previous history of UTI.

IF THE PATIENT IS ACUTELY ILL with high fever, loin pain and tenderness (acute pyelonephritis), intravenous ampicillin or amoxycillin (1 g 6-hourly) or intravenous gentamicin (2–5 mg kg$^{-1}$ daily in divided doses) should be given switching to a further 7 days' treatment with oral therapy as symptoms improve. Intravenous fluids may be required to achieve a good urine output.

In patients presenting for the first time with high fever, loin pain and tenderness, urgent renal ultrasound examination is required to exclude an obstructed pyonephrosis. If this is present it should be drained by percutaneous nephrostomy.

### Recurrent infection

Pretreatment and post-treatment urine cultures are mandatory to confirm the diagnosis and identify whether recurrent infection is due to relapse or reinfection.

IN RELAPSE, a search should be made for a cause, e.g. stones or scarred kidneys, and this should be eradicated if possible, for example by the removal of stones. Intense or prolonged treatment—intravenous or intramuscular aminoglycoside for 7 days or oral antibiotics for 4–6 weeks—is required. If this fails, long-term antibiotics are required.

REINFECTION implies that the patient has poor defence systems; such patients must undertake prophylactic measures:

- A 2-litre daily fluid intake
- Voiding at 2–3 hour intervals with double micturition if reflux is present
- Voiding before bedtime and after intercourse
- Avoidance of bubble baths and other chemicals in bath water
- Avoidance of constipation, which may impair bladder emptying

Evidence of impaired bladder emptying on excretion urography requires urological assessment. If UTI continues to recur, treatment for 6–12 months with low-dose prophylaxis (trimethoprim 100 mg, co-trimoxazole 480 mg, or cephradine 250–500 mg) is required; it should be taken last thing at night when urine flow is low. Intravaginal oestrogen therapy has been shown to produce a reduction in the number of episodes of UTI in elderly women.

# Urinary infections in the presence of an indwelling catheter

Colonization of the bladder by a urinary pathogen is common after a urinary catheter has been present for more than a few days. Because antibiotic treatment while the catheter is in place is thought to encourage the development of resistant organisms, antibiotic treatment is only recommended if the patient has symptoms or evidence of systemic infection. There may be a place for antibiotic treatment prior to catheter removal, as catheter-introduced infections are often slow to clear spontaneously. Bladder stones may form in patients with long-term indwelling catheters, further complicating the situation.

Infection by *Candida* sp. is a frequent complication of prolonged bladder catheterization. Treatment should be reserved for patients with evidence of invasive infection or those who are immunosuppressed, and should consist of removal or replacement of the catheter and possibly intravesical antifungals.

## Bacteriuria in pregnancy

The urine of pregnant women must always be cultured as 2–6% have asymptomatic bacteriuria. Failure to treat this may result in severe symptomatic pyelonephritis later in pregnancy, with the possibility of premature labour. Asymptomatic bacteriuria, particularly in the presence of previous renal disease, may predispose to pre-eclamptic toxaemia, anaemia of pregnancy, and small or premature babies. Therefore bacteriuria must always be treated and be shown to be eradicated. Reinfection may require prophylactic therapy. Tetracycline drugs must be avoided in pregnancy, as should trimethoprim in the first trimester and sulphonamides in the third.

## Bacterial prostatitis

Bacterial prostatitis is a relapsing infection which is difficult to treat. It presents as perineal pain, recurrent epididymo-orchitis and prostatic tenderness, with pus in expressed prostatic secretion. Treatment is with drugs that penetrate the prostate—trimethoprim, tetracylines or ciprofloxacin—for 4–6 weeks. Long-term low-dose treatment may be required.

## Renal carbuncle

Renal carbuncle is an abscess in the renal cortex caused by a blood-borne *Staphylococcus*, usually from a boil or carbuncle of the skin. It presents with high swinging fevers, loin pain and tenderness, and fullness in the loin. The urine shows no abnormality as the abscess does not communicate with the renal pelvis, more often extending into the perirenal tissue. Staphylococcal septicaemia is common. Diagnosis is by ultrasound or CT scanning. Treatment involves antibacterial therapy with flucloxacillin and surgical drainage.

## Tuberculosis of the urinary tract

Tuberculosis of the urinary tract should still be kept in mind in patients presenting with frequency, dysuria or haematuria, particularly in the Asian immigrant population of the UK. Cortical lesions result from haematogenous spread in the primary phase of infection. Most heal, but in some, infection persists and spreads to the papillae, with the formation of cavitating lesions and the discharge of mycobacteria into the urine. Infection of the ureters and bladder commonly follows, with the potential for the development of ureteral stricture and a contracted bladder. Rarely, cold abscessses may form in the loin. In males the disease may present with testicular or epididymal discomfort and thickening.

Diagnosis depends on constant awareness, especially in patients with sterile pyuria. Excretion urography may show cavitating lesions in the renal papillary areas, commonly with calcification. There may also be evidence of ureteral obstruction with hydronephrosis. Diagnosis of active infection depends on culture of mycobacteria from early-morning urine samples. The urogram may be normal in diffuse interstitial renal tuberculosis when diagnosis is made by renal biopsy. Some patients present with small unobstructed kidneys when the diagnosis is easy to miss.

The treatment is as for pulmonary tuberculosis (see p. 686). Renal ultrasonography or excretion urography should be carried out 2–3 months after initiation of treatment as ureteric strictures may first develop in the healing phase.

## Xanthogranulomatous pyelonephritis

This is an uncommon chronic interstitial infection of the kidney, most often due to *Proteus* spp., in which there is fever, weight loss, loin pain and a palpable enlarged kidney. It is usually unilateral and associated with staghorn calculi. CT scanning shows up intrarenal abscesses as lucent areas within the kidney. Nephrectomy is the treatment of choice; antibacterial treatment rarely, if ever, eradicates the infection.

## Malakoplakia

This is a rare condition in which plaques of abnormal inflammatory tissue grow within the urinary tract in the presence of urinary infection. The histological appearances are characteristic. It is thought that the condition is caused by an acquired inability of macrophages to kill phagocytosed bacteria. Cholinergic agonists and ascorbic acid may improve macrophage function; ciprofloxacin penetrates the macrophage well and is the antibiotic of choice. Prolonged treatment may be needed.

## Viral renal infections

Viruses are commonly present in the urine in a wide range of common viral infections, but very few viruses cause significant renal disease. Secondary immune complex glomerulonephritis may result from chronic viral infections; for instance, membranous nephropathy complicating hepatitis B and cryoglobulinaemic mesangiocap-illary glomerulonephritis complicating hepatitis C infection. The role of cytomegalovirus in renal disease is unclear. Haemorrhagic fever with renal syndrome is the name given to a spectrum of diseases caused by Hanta viruses; renal failure may be severe, and is caused by an acute haemorrhagic interstitial nephritis. Human immunodeficiency virus infection is associated both with focal glomerulosclerosis and with haemolytic uraemic syndrome, but the pathogenesis of these complications remains uncertain.

## Tubulo-interstitial nephritis

Interstitial inflammation with tubular damage is a regular feature of bacterial pyelonephritis but, contrary to former belief, it rarely, if ever, leads to chronic renal damage in the absence of reflux, obstruction or other complicating factors. However, there is growing concern that tubulo-interstitial disease due to other causes is more common than was previously diagnosed. The major stimulus for this interest came from recognition that it could be due to analgesic abuse. Subsequently, tubulo-interstitial disease due to a variety of drugs has been recognized and this condition should be considered in all patients presenting with otherwise unexplained renal failure. Presentation may be with acute, often oliguric renal failure or more commonly as chronic slowly progressive renal disease.

## ACUTE TUBULO-INTERSTITIAL NEPHRITIS

Acute tubulo-interstitial nephritis is most often due to a hypersensitivity reaction to drugs (Table 9.12), most commonly drugs of the penicillin family and non-steroidal anti-inflammatory drugs (NSAIDs). Patients present with fever, arthralgia, skin rashes and acute oliguric or non-oliguric renal failure. Many have eosinophilia and eosinophiluria. Renal biopsy shows an intense interstitial cellular infiltrate, often including eosinophils, with variable tubular necrosis.

Treatment involves withdrawal of offending drugs. High-dose steroid therapy (prednisolone 60 mg daily) is commonly given but its efficacy has not been proved. Patients may require dialysis for management of the acute renal failure. Most patients have good recovery of kidney function, but some may be left with significant interstitial fibrosis.

## CHRONIC TUBULO-INTERSTITIAL NEPHRITIS

The major causes of chronic tubulo-interstitial nephritis are set out in Table 9.13. In many cases no cause is found. The patient usually either presents with polyuria and nocturia, or is found to have proteinuria or uraemia. Proteinuria is usually slight (less than 1 g daily). Papillary necrosis with ischaemic damage to the papillae occurs in a number of interstitial nephritides, e.g. in analgesic abuse, diabetes mellitus, sickle cell disease or trait. The papillae can separate and be passed in the urine. Chronic tubulo-interstitial nephritis may be associated with microscopic or overt haematuria or sterile pyuria, and occasionally a sloughed papilla may cause ureteral colic or produce acute ureteral obstruction. The radiological appearances must be distinguished from those of chronic pyelonephritis (Fig. 9.21).

Tubular damage to the medullary area of the kidney leads to defects in urine concentration and sodium conservation with polyuria and salt wasting. Fibrosis progressing into the cortex leads to loss of excretory function and uraemia.

### Analgesic nephropathy

The chronic consumption of *large* amounts of analgesics (especially those containing phenacetin) leads to chronic tubulo-interstitial nephritis and papillary necrosis. This also seems to be true of NSAIDs. In Australia, the incidence of end-stage renal failure due to analgesic nephropathy has declined as 'over-the-counter' purchase of nephrotoxic analgesics has been reduced by legislation.

#### CLINICAL FEATURES

Analgesic nephropathy is twice as common in women as in men and presents typically in middle-age. Patients are

Penicillins
Sulphonamides
Non-steroidal anti-inflammatory drugs
Phenindione
Allopurinol
Cephalosporins
Rifampicin
Diuretics—frusemide, thiazides
Cimetidine
Phenytoin

**Table 9.12**  Common causes of acute tubulo-interstitial nephritis.

*Common*
Chronic pyelonephritis
Non-steroidal anti-inflammatory drugs
Diabetes
Sickle cell disease or trait
Cadmium or lead intoxication

*Uncommon*
Alport's syndrome
Balkan nephropathy
Irradiation
Sjögren's syndrome
Hyperuricaemic nephropathy

**Table 9.13**  Causes of chronic tubulo-interstitial nephritis.

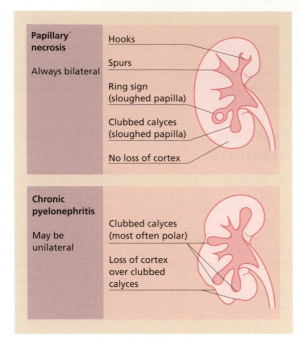

**Fig. 9.21**  A comparison of radiological appearances of papillary necrosis and chronic pyelonephritis.

often depressed or neurotic. Presentation may be with anaemia, chronic renal failure, symptoms of urinary infection (which may be difficult to eradicate), haematuria, or urinary tract obstruction (due to sloughing of a renal papilla). Salt and water-wasting renal disease may occur.

Chronic analgesic abuse also predisposes to the development of uroepithelial tumours.

**MANAGEMENT**
The consumption of analgesics should be discouraged. If necessary, dihydrocodeine or paracetamol are reasonable alternative choices. This may result in the arrest of the disease and even in improvement in function.

UTI, hypertension (if present) and saline depletion will require appropriate management.

The development of flank pain or an unexpectedly rapid deterioration in renal function should prompt ultrasonography or urography to screen for urinary tract obstruction due to a sloughed papilla.

## Balkan nephropathy

This is a chronic tubulo-interstitial nephritis endemic in the central Danube basin in the former Yugoslavia, Bulgaria and Rumania. Primarily restricted to rural areas, its cause is unknown. The disease is insidious in onset, with mild proteinuria progressing to renal failure in 3 months to 10 years. Patients exhibit a high incidence of uroepithelial tumours. There is no treatment.

Other forms of chronic tubulo-interstitial nephritis are rare (see Table 9.13). Diagnosis of all forms depends on

a careful history being taken, with special attention to drug-taking and industrial exposure to nephrotoxins. In patients with unexplained renal impairment with normal-sized kidneys, renal biopsy must always be undertaken to exclude a treatable interstitial nephritis.

# Hyperuricaemic nephropathy (gouty nephropathy)

Three patterns of renal disease have been described in patients with hyperuricaemia or hyperuricosuria:
1 Gouty or chronic hyperuricaemic nephropathy
2 Acute hyperuricaemic nephropathy
3 Uric acid stone formation (see p. 466)

## Chronic hyperuricaemic nephropathy

Considerable controversy surrounds the possible role of chronic hyperuricaemia as a cause of tubulo-interstitial disease and progressive renal damage. While uric acid 'tophi' may be found in the kidneys of patients with gout, there is no convincing evidence that chronic hyperuricaemia *per se* causes progressive renal failure, nor that allopurinol treatment improves renal function. There is one important exception: a rare form of familial hyperuricaemia and gout occurring in adolescence is associated with renal impairment and allopurinol therapy both improves and protects kidney function.

## Acute hyperuricaemic nephropathy

This is a well-recognized cause of acute renal failure in patients with marked hyperuricaemia due to lympho-proliferative or myeloproliferative disorders. This may occur prior to treatment but most often occurs on commencement of treatment, when there is rapid lysis of malignant cells, release of large amounts of nucleoprotein and increased uric acid production. Renal failure is due to intrarenal and extrarenal obstruction caused by deposition of uric acid crystals in the collecting ducts, pelvis and ureters. The condition is manifest in oliguria or anuria with increasing uraemia. There may be flank pain or colic. Plasma urate levels are above 0.75 mmol litre$^{-1}$ and may be as high as 4.5 mmol litre$^{-1}$. Diagnosis is based on the hyperuricaemia and the clinical setting. Ultrasound demonstrates extrarenal obstruction due to stones but a negative scan does not exclude this where there is coexistent intrarenal obstruction.

**PREVENTION**
It is now regular practice to prescribe allopurinol 100–200 mg three times daily for 5 days prior to and continu-

ing throughout treatment with radiotherapy or cytotoxic drugs. A high rate of urine flow must be maintained by oral or parenteral fluid and the urine kept alkaline by the administration of sodium bicarbonate 600 mg four times daily and acetazolamide 250 mg three times daily.

## TREATMENT

Allopurinol treatment should be commenced immediately and a forced alkaline diuresis attempted with intravenous 1.26% sodium bicarbonate plus acetazolamide (500 mg dose, then 250 mg three times daily). In severely oliguric or anuric patients, dialysis is required to lower the plasma urate, which allows urate to diffuse out of the obstructed collecting ducts into the peritubular capillaries. Percutaneous nephrostomy (see p. 473) may be required to relieve extrarenal obstruction due to stones in the pelvis or ureters. Such stones may subsequently be passed spontaneously or may require surgical removal (see p. 468).

# Hypertension and the kidney

Hypertension can be the cause or the result of renal disease. It is often difficult to differentiate between the two on clinical grounds. Routine tests as described on p. 621 should be performed on all patients, but IVU is usually unnecessary. A guide to which patients should be fully investigated is given on p. 822.

## ESSENTIAL HYPERTENSION

### PATHOPHYSIOLOGY

In *benign essential hypertension*, arteriosclerosis of major renal arteries and changes in the intrarenal vasculature (nephrosclerosis) occur as follows:

IN SMALL VESSELS AND ARTERIOLES, intimal thickening with reduplication of the internal elastic lamina occurs and the vessel wall becomes hyalinized.

IN LARGE VESSELS, concentric reduplication of the internal elastic lamina and endothelial proliferation produce an 'onion skin' appearance.

REDUCTION IN SIZE OF BOTH KIDNEYS may occur; this may be asymmetrical if one major renal artery is more affected by atheromatous change than the other.

THE PROPORTION OF SCLEROTIC GLOMERULI is increased compared with age-matched controls.

Deterioration in excretory function accompanies these changes, but severe renal failure is unusual in Whites. In Afro-Caribbeans, by contrast, such hypertension much more often results in the development of renal failure.

In *accelerated, or malignant phase hypertension*:

ARTERIOLAR FIBRINOID NECROSIS occurs, probably as a result of plasma entering the media of the vessel through splits in the intima.

FIBRINOID NECROSIS in afferent glomerular arterioles is a prominent feature.

FIBRIN DEPOSITION within small vessels is often associated with thrombocytopenia and red-cell fragmentation seen in the peripheral blood film (microangiopathic haemolytic anaemia).

Microscopic haematuria, proteinuria, usually of modest degree (1–3 g daily), and progressive uraemia occur. If untreated, fewer than 10% of patients survive 2 years.

### MANAGEMENT

Management of benign essential and malignant hypertension is described on p. 621.

If treatment is begun before renal impairment has occurred, the prognosis for renal function is good. Stabilization or improvement in renal function with healing of intrarenal arteriolar lesions and resolution of microangiopathic haemolysis occur with effective treatment of malignant phase hypertension. Lifelong follow-up of the patient is mandatory.

## RENAL HYPERTENSION

### Bilateral renal disease

Hypertension commonly complicates bilateral renal disease such as chronic glomerulonephritis, bilateral reflux nephropathy (chronic atrophic pyelonephritis of childhood), polycystic disease and analgesic nephropathy.

Two main mechanisms are responsible:

1 Activation of the renin–angiotensin–aldosterone system

2 Retention of salt and water with impairment in excretory function leading to an increase in blood volume and hence blood pressure.

The second of these assumes greater importance as renal function deteriorates.

Hypertension occurs earlier, is more common and tends to be more severe in patients with renal cortical disorders such as glomerulonephritis than in those with disorders affecting primarily the renal interstitium, such as reflux or analgesic nephropathy.

Management is described on p. 621. Good control of the blood pressure is necessary to prevent further deterioration of renal function secondary to vascular changes produced by the hypertension itself.

### Unilateral renal disease

A small proportion of cases of hypertension are due to unilateral renal disease. The main causes are:

UNILATERAL RENAL ARTERY STENOSIS due to fibromuscular hyperplasia (typically in young women) or atheroma in the elderly

UNILATERAL REFLUX NEPHROPATHY (atrophic pyelonephritis)

#### Mechanism of hypertension

Unilateral renal ischaemia results in a reduction in the pressure in afferent glomerular arterioles. This leads to an increase in the production and release of renin from the juxtaglomerular apparatus (see p. 823) with a consequent increase in angiotensin II.

**Physiological changes in renal artery stenosis**

In unilateral renal artery stenosis, renal perfusion pressure is reduced and nephron transit time is prolonged on the side of the stenosis; salt and water reabsorption is therefore increased. As a result, urine from the ischaemic kidney is more concentrated but has a lower sodium concentration than urine from the contralateral kidney. Inulin, creatinine and *p*-aminohippuric acid (PAH) clearances are decreased on the ischaemic side.

**Screening for unilateral renovascular disease**

RAPID SEQUENCE EXCRETION UROGRAPHY is still widely employed.

INTRAVENOUSLY INJECTED CONTRAST MEDIUM is filtered at the glomerulus more slowly and concentrated within the nephron to a greater extent on the side of the stenosis. Rapid sequence films taken after injection of contrast may show a small kidney and a delayed and denser pyelogram on the side of the stenosis.

RADIONUCLIDE STUDIES (see p. 444) using labelled DTPA can demonstrate decreased renal perfusion on the affected side. In recent years, the captopril renogram has been employed in this connection. In unilateral renal artery stenosis, a disproportionate fall in uptake of isotope on the affected side following administration of an ACE inhibitor such as captopril has been claimed to be a useful screening test for significant renal artery stenosis. The value of this investigation has recently been called into question.

DIVIDED RENAL FUNCTION STUDIES that involve ureteric catheterization are seldom used.

RENAL ARTERIOGRAPHY remains the gold standard for the diagnosis of renal artery stenosis.

**TREATMENT**

Surgical options in renal artery stenosis include transluminal angioplasty to dilate the stenotic region, reconstructive vascular surgery and nephrectomy. With good selection of patients, more than 50% are cured or improved by intervention. In recent years, increasing interest has focused upon the diagnosis and correction of unilateral and bilateral renal arterial disease with a view to improving renal perfusion and excretory function rather than to correcting hypertension alone. No test can predict the results of vascular surgery and many patients will do well on hypotensive therapy with or without surgery. ACE inhibitors must be avoided as they can lead to acute renal failure in the presence of renal artery stenoses.

UNILATERAL ATROPHIC PYELONEPHRITIS. In this condition prediction of the outcome after nephrectomy is currently not possible. The case for nephrectomy is strengthened if isotope renography demonstrates the abnormal kidney to be making an insignificant contribution to overall excretion function, particularly if the patient is young and medical treatment has proved unsatisfactory. About one-third of patients with unilateral atrophic pyelonephritis benefit from nephrectomy.

## Other vascular disorders of the kidney

## Renal artery occlusion

This occurs from thrombosis *in situ* usually in a severely damaged arteriosclerotic vessel or more commonly from embolization. Both result in renal infarction resulting in a wide spectrum of clinical manifestations depending on the size of the artery involved. Occlusion of a small branch artery may produce no effect but occlusion of larger vessels results in dull flank pain and varying degrees of renal failure.

Embolization may occur from the heart, e.g. in atrial fibrillation. It can also occur from the aorta and renal artery where showers of cholesterol-rich atheromatous material from ulcerated arteriosclerotic plaques lodge in the small renal vessels. This leads to renal insufficiency usually with hypertension. Occasionally acute renal failure occurs, sometimes complicating catheterization of the abdominal aorta.

Anticoagulants and thrombolytic agents may also precipitate cholesterol embolism.

## Renal vein thrombosis

This is usually of insidious onset occurring in the nephrotic syndrome, with a renal cell carcinoma and in conditions with increased thrombosis, e.g. antithrombin III deficiency or with anticardiolipin antibodies.

## Calculi and nephrocalcinosis

## Renal and vesical calculi

Approximately 2% of the population in the UK have a urinary tract stone at any given time. A much higher prevalence of stone disease has been recorded elsewhere, notably in the Middle East. In the Western World, most stones occur in the upper urinary tract.

The incidence of bladder stones has declined in the UK since the eighteenth and nineteenth centuries, whereas in some developing countries they are still common.

Most stones are composed of calcium oxalate and

| Type of renal stone | Approximate frequency (%) |
|---|---|
| Calcium oxalate | 65 |
| Calcium phosphate | 15 |
| Magnesium ammonium phosphate | 10–15 |
| Uric acid | 3–5 |
| Cystine | 1–2 |

**Table 9.14** Type and frequency of renal stones.

phosphate; these are commoner in men (Table 9.14). Mixed infective stones, which account for about 20% of all calculi, are twice as common in women as in men. The overall male/female ratio of stone disease is 2 : 1.

Stone disease is frequently a recurrent problem. More than 50% of patients with a calculus will have formed a further stone or stones within 10 years. The risk of recurrence increases if a metabolic or other abnormality predisposing to stone formation is present and is not modified by treatment.

## AETIOLOGY

It is in a sense surprising that stones are not universal, since some constituents of urine are at times present in concentrations that exceed their maximum solubility in water. The presence of inhibitors of crystal formation in normal urine appears to be of importance in preventing stones.

Many stone-formers have no detectable metabolic defect, although microscopy of warm, freshly passed urine reveals both more and larger calcium oxalate crystals than are found in normal subjects. Factors predisposing to stone formation in these so-called 'idiopathic stone-formers' are:

CHEMICAL COMPOSITION OF URINE that favours stone crystallization

PRODUCTION OF A CONCENTRATED URINE as a consequence of dehydration associated with life in a hot climate or work in a hot environment

IMPAIRMENT OF INHIBITORS that prevent crystallization in normal urine.

Recognized causes of stone formation are listed in Table 9.15.

| |
|---|
| Dehydration |
| Hypercalcaemia |
| Hypercalciuria |
| Hyperoxaluria |
| Hyperuricaemia and hyperuricosuria |
| Infection |
| Cystinuria |
| Renal tubular acidosis |
| Primary renal disease (polycystic kidneys, medullary sponge kidneys) |

**Table 9.15** Causes of urinary tract stone formation.

### Hypercalcaemia

If the GFR is normal, hypercalcaemia almost invariably leads to hypercalciuria. The common causes of hypercalcaemia leading to stone formation are:
- Primary hyperparathyroidism
- Vitamin D ingestion
- Sarcoidosis

Of these, primary hyperparathyroidism (see p. 430) is the commonest cause of stones.

### Hypercalciuria

This is by far the commonest metabolic abnormality detected in calcium stone-formers.

Approximately 8% of men excrete in excess of 7.5 mmol calcium per 24 hours. Calcium stone formation is commoner in this group, but as most patients do not form stones the definition of 'pathological' hypercalciuria is arbitrary. A reasonable definition of pathological hypercalciuria is excretion of more than 7.5 mmol calcium per 24 hours in male and more than 6.25 mmol calcium per 24 hours in female stone-formers.

Causes of hypercalciuria are:
- Hypercalcaemia
- An excessive dietary intake of calcium
- Excessive resorption of calcium from the skeleton, such as occurs with prolonged immobilization or weightlessness
- Idiopathic hypercalciuria

The majority of patients with idiopathic hypercalciuria can be shown to have increased absorption of calcium from the gut. Dietary calcium restriction in this group markedly reduces urinary calcium excretion. However, a proportion of these patients appear to have a renal tubular calcium leak with secondary compensatory hyperabsorption of calcium from the gut. Calcium restriction has less effect on urinary calcium excretion in this group.

### Hyperoxaluria

Two inborn errors of glyoxalate metabolism that cause increased endogenous oxalate biosynthesis are known. Both are inherited in an autosomal recessive manner. In type I (primary hyperoxaluria) there is increased glycolate excretion as well as hyperoxaluria. In type II L-glycerate excretion is increased. In both types, calcium oxalate stone formation occurs.

The prognosis is poor owing to widespread calcium oxalate crystal deposition in the kidneys. Renal failure typically develops in the late teens or early twenties.

Much commoner causes of mild hyperoxaluria are:

EXCESS INGESTION OF HIGH OXALATE-CONTAINING FOOD, such as spinach, rhubarb and tea.

DIETARY CALCIUM RESTRICTION, with compensatory increased absorption of oxalate.

GASTROINTESTINAL DISEASE, such as Crohn's disease, usually with an intestinal resection is associated with increased absorption of oxalate from the colon. Dehydration secondary to fluid loss from the gut also plays a part in stone formation.

### Hyperuricaemia and hyperuricosuria

Uric acid stones account for 3–5% of all stones in the UK, but in Israel the proportion is as high as 40%.

Uric acid is the end-point of purine metabolism. Hyperuricaemia (see p. 409) can occur as a primary defect in idiopathic gout, and as a secondary consequence of increased cell turnover, e.g. in myeloproliferative disorders. Increased uric acid excretion occurs in these conditions, and stones will develop in some patients. Some uric acid stone-formers have hyperuricosuria (>4 mmol/24 hours on a low purine diet) without hyperuricaemia.

Dehydration alone may also cause uric acid stones to form. Patients with ileostomies are at particular risk both from dehydration and from the fact that loss of bicarbonate from gastrointestinal secretions results in the production of an acid urine (uric acid is more soluble in an alkaline than an acid medium).

Some patients with calcium stones also have hyperuricaemia and/or hyperuricaciduria; it is believed the calcium salts precipitate upon an initial nidus of uric acid in such patients.

### Urinary tract infection

Mixed infective stones are composed of magnesium ammonium phosphate together with variable amounts of calcium. Such stones are often large, forming a cast of the collecting system (staghorn calculus). They are believed to form as a result of infection of the urinary tract with organisms such as *Proteus mirabilis* that hydrolyse urea, with formation of the strong base ammonium hydroxide.

$$\begin{array}{c} NH_2 \\ \diagdown \\ \phantom{xx}C = O + HOH \rightleftharpoons 2NH_3 + CO_2 \\ \diagup \\ NH_2 \end{array}$$

$$NH_3 + HOH \rightleftharpoons NH_4OH \rightleftharpoons NH_4^+ + OH^-$$

The availability of ammonium ions and the alkalinity of the urine favour stone formation. An increased amount of mucoprotein resulting from infection also creates an organic matrix on which stone formation can occur.

### Cystinuria (see p. 863)

Cystinuria results in the formation of cystine stones. About 1–2% of all stones are composed of cystine.

### Primary renal diseases

There is a moderate increase in prevalence of stone disease in patients with polycystic renal disease (see p. 492).

Medullary sponge kidney is another primary renal disorder associated with stones. In this congenital (though not inherited) condition there is dilatation of the collecting ducts with associated stasis and calcification (Fig. 9.22). Approximately 20% of these patients have hypercalciuria and a similar proportion have a renal tubular acidification defect.

The renal tubular acidoses, both inherited and acquired, are associated with nephrocalcinosis and stone

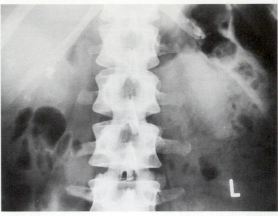

(a)

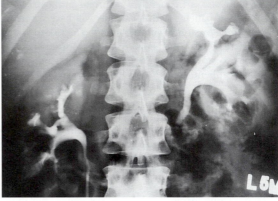

(b)

**Fig. 9.22**  Medullary sponge kidney. (a) Plain film showing 'spotty' calcification in the renal areas. (b) After injection of contrast, the calcification is shown to be small calculi in the papillary zones.

formation owing, in part at least, to the production of a persistently alkaline urine and reduced urinary citrate excretion.

### Aetiology of bladder stones

Bladder stones are endemic in some developing countries. The cause of this is unknown but dietary factors are probably important. Stones forming in the bladder do so as a result of:

BLADDER OUTFLOW OBSTRUCTION, e.g. urethral stricture, neuropathic bladder, prostatic obstruction

THE PRESENCE OF A FOREIGN BODY, e.g. catheters, non-absorbable sutures.

Significant bacteriuria is usually found in patients with bladder stones. Some stones found in the bladder have been passed down from the upper urinary tract.

### PATHOLOGY

Stones may be single or multiple and vary enormously in size from sand-like minute particles to staghorn calculi or large stone concretions in the bladder. They may be located within the renal parenchyma or within the col-

| |
|---|
| Asymptomatic |
| Pain—renal colic |
| Haematuria |
| Urinary tract infection |
| Urinary tract obstruction |
| Strangury |

**Table 9.16** Clinical features of urinary tract stones.

lecting system. Pressure necrosis from a large calculus may cause direct damage to the renal parenchyma and stones regularly cause obstruction, leading to hydronephrosis. They may ulcerate through the wall of the collecting system, including the ureter. A combination of obstruction and infection accelerates damage to the kidney.

## CLINICAL FEATURES (Table 9.16)

Most people with urinary tract calculi are asymptomatic. Pain is the commonest symptom and may be sharp or dull, constant, intermittent or colicky.

When urinary tract obstruction is present, measures that increase urine volume, such as copious fluid intake or diuretics, including alcohol, make the pain worse. Physical exertion may cause mobile calculi to move, precipitating pain and, occasionally, haematuria. Calyceal colic, i.e. pain resulting from movement of stones within the calyces, is a real entity, but whether small calyceal calculi are the cause of backache or not is often difficult to decide.

Ureteric colic occurs when a stone enters the ureter and either obstructs it or causes spasm during its passage down the ureter (Fig. 9.23). This is one of the most severe pains known. Radiation from the flank to the iliac fossa and testis or labium in the distribution of the first lumbar nerve root is common. Pallor, sweating and vomiting often occur and the patient is restless, tending to assume a variety of positions in an unsuccessful attempt to obtain relief from the pain. Haematuria often occurs. Untreated, the pain of ureteric colic typically subsides after a few hours.

When urinary tract obstruction and infection are present, the features of acute pyelonephritis or of a Gram-negative septicaemia may dominate the clinical picture.

Vesical calculi associated with bladder bacteriuria may present with frequency, dysuria and haematuria; severe introital or perineal pain may occur if trigonitis is present. A calculus at the bladder neck or an obstruction in the urethra may cause bladder outflow obstruction, resulting in anuria and painful bladder distension.

Physical examination should include a search for corneal or conjunctival calcification, gouty tophi and arthritis and features of sarcoidosis.

## DIAGNOSIS AND INVESTIGATION

A history of possible aetiological factors should be obtained, including:

- Occupation and residence in hot countries likely to be associated with dehydration
- A history of vitamin D consumption
- Gouty arthritis

Calcified papillae may mimic ordinary calculi, so that causes of papillary necrosis such as analgesic abuse should be considered.

Investigations should include a mid-stream specimen of urine for culture and measurement of the blood urea and electrolytes and serum creatinine and calcium levels.

Plain abdominal X-ray, renal tomography and excretion urography are the mainstay of diagnosis.

Pure uric acid stones are radiolucent. Mixed infective stones in which organic matrix predominates are barely radiopaque. Calcium-containing and cystine stones are radiopaque. Calculi overlying bone are easily missed (Fig. 9.24). Staghorn calculi may be missed on excretion urography (Fig. 9.25). Uric acid stones may present as a filling defect after injection of contrast medium (Fig. 9.26). Such stones are readily seen on CT scanning (Fig. 9.27).

Excretion urography is carried out during the episode of pain; a normal urogram excludes the diagnosis of pain due to calculous disease. The urographic appearances in a patient with acute left ureteric obstruction are shown in Fig. 9.23. The urine of the patient should be passed

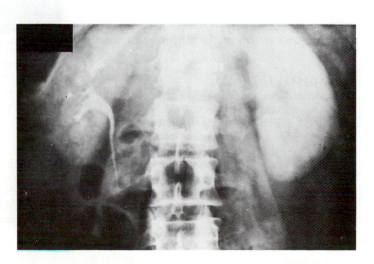

**Fig. 9.23** X-ray showing acute left ureteric obstruction. Note the increased density of the nephrogram and the absence of a pyelogram on the left side 15 min after contrast injection. (From Weatherall DJ, Ledingham JGG & Warrell DA (eds) (1987) *Oxford Textbook of Medicine*, 2nd edn. Oxford: Oxford University Press. With permission.)

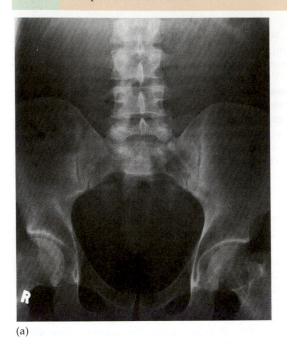

(a)

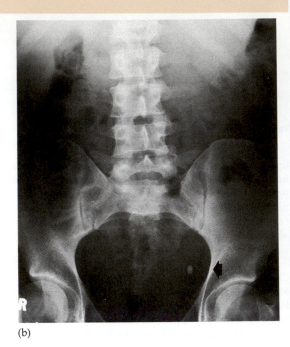

(b)

**Fig. 9.24**   X-rays showing calculus. (a) The calculus is overlying bone on the left (easily missed). (b) The same patient 1 week later. The calculus has descended and is easily seen in the pelvis of the left side (arrowed).

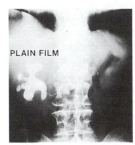
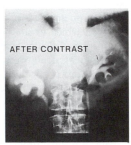

**Fig. 9.25**   Staghorn calculus. X-ray appearances before and after contrast on the right side are identical owing to a staghorn calculus in a non-functioning right kidney. A plain film may be confused with those taken after contrast injection.

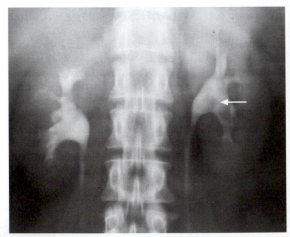

**Fig. 9.26**   An excretion urogram showing a lucent filling defect (uric acid stone) in the left renal pelvis. The differential diagnosis includes a sloughed papilla and a transitional cell tumour.

through a sieve to trap any calculi passed for chemical analysis.

### MANAGEMENT
Adequate analgesia should be given, e.g. morphine 15–30 mg i.m. repeated as necessary. Alternatively an NSAID can be tried. A high fluid intake and, if feasible, increased physical activity are recommended but the efficacy of these measures is doubtful.

Stones less than 0.5 cm in diameter usually pass spontaneously and can be left. Stones greater than 1 cm in diameter usually require intervention.

Persistent pain, frequent bouts of severe pain, or anuria, are indications for further therapy. Intervention is also required if a stone is not moving though causing only partial obstruction in the absence of infection. With the advent of percutaneous surgery and extracorporeal shock-wave lithotripsy (see below) there has developed a trend towards earlier intervention in such cases. Complete obstruction or the coexistence of UTI with partial obstruction should prompt even earlier intervention owing to the increased risk of permanent kidney damage in these circumstances.

Stones may be removed by a cutting operation:
NEPHROLITHOTOMY for renal calculi
PYELOLITHOTOMY for stones in the renal pelvis

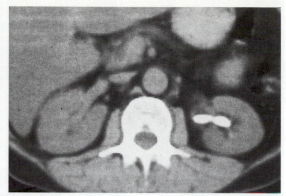

**Fig. 9.27** CT scan showing a uric acid stone, which appears as a bright lesion in the left kidney.

URETEROLITHOTOMY for ureteric stones

Cutting operations can now be avoided by using either percutaneous nephrolithotomy or extracorporeal shock-wave lithotripsy. In the former, stones in the calyces and renal pelvis are removed by creating a percutaneous track down to the collecting system followed by endoscopic removal along this track. In the latter, shock waves are focused upon the renal calculi, causing them to fragment. Most of the fragments then pass spontaneously via the urethra. Fragments that do not pass can be removed percutaneously.

Ureteric stones may be removed endoscopically or may be pushed up into the upper urinary tract, to allow percutaneous nephrolithotomy or extracorporeal shock-wave lithotripsy.

Large renal stones need to be reduced in bulk by percutaneous means before lithotripsy can be expected to be successful. Some staghorn calculi are best dealt with by open operation.

Bladder stones can be removed endoscopically. They may be dealt with by direct electrohydraulic disintegration at cystoscopy or may be gripped in a lithotrite and crushed, the stone fragments then being washed out. Open cystotomy is required for very large bladder stones.

## INVESTIGATING THE CAUSE OF STONE FORMATION

In an elderly patient who has had a single episode with one stone, only limited investigation is required. Younger patients and those with recurrent stone formation require detailed investigation.

AN EXCRETION UROGRAM is necessary to define the presence of a primary renal disease predisposing to stone formation.

SIGNIFICANT BACTERIURIA may indicate mixed infective stone formation but relapsing bacteriuria may be a consequence of stone formation rather than the original cause.

CHEMICAL ANALYSIS of any stone passed may be of great value and may be all that is required to make a diagnosis of cystinuria or uric acid stone formation.

SERUM CALCIUM CONCENTRATION should be estimated and corrected for serum albumin concentration (see p. 425). Hypercalcaemia, if present, should be investigated further (see p. 431).

SERUM URATE CONCENTRATION is often, but not invariably, elevated in uric acid stone-formers.

A SCREENING TEST FOR CYSTINURIA should be carried out by adding sodium nitroprusside to a random unacidified urine sample; a purple colour indicates that cystinuria may be present. Urine chromatography is required to define the diagnosis precisely.

URINARY CALCIUM, OXALATE AND URIC ACID OUTPUT should be measured in two consecutive carefully collected 24-hour urine samples. After withdrawing aliquots for estimation of uric acid, it is necessary to add acid to the urine in order to prevent crystallization of calcium salts upon the walls of the collection vessel, which would give falsely low results for urinary calcium and oxalate.

PLASMA BICARBONATE is low in renal tubular acidosis. The finding of a urine pH that does not fall below 5.5 in the face of metabolic acidosis is diagnostic of this condition (see p. 517).

## PROPHYLAXIS

The age of the patient and the severity of the problem affect both the need for and the type of prophylaxis.

### Idiopathic stone-formers

Where no metabolic abnormality is present, the mainstay of prevention is maintenance of a high intake of fluid throughout the day and night. The aim should be to ensure a daily urine volume of 2–2.5 litres, which requires a fluid intake in excess of this, substantially so in the case of those who live in hot countries or work in a hot environment. A large glass of water should be drunk before retiring for the night and on waking during the night if this occurs. Special dietary measures are not warranted, although avoidance of excessive consumption of calcium-rich dairy products seems sensible.

### Idiopathic hypercalciuria

Dietary calcium restriction is recommended, although the value of this has recently been questioned. Intake of milk, cheese, and white bread if this is fortified (as it is in the UK) with calcium and vitamin D is reduced. Vitamin D supplements should be avoided. Dietary calcium restriction results in hyperabsorption of oxalate and foods containing large amounts of oxalate should also be limited. The advice of a dietitian is helpful. A high fluid intake should be advised as for idiopathic stone-formers. Patients who live in a hard-water area may benefit from drinking softened water.

If hypercalciuria persists and stone formation continues, a thiazide, e.g. bendrofluazide 2.5 or 5 mg each morning is used. Thiazides reduce urinary calcium excretion by a direct effect on the renal tubule. They may occasionally cause hypercalciuria or gout and worsen hypercholesterolaemia. Sodium cellulose phosphate reduces calcium absorption from the gut but increases oxalate absorption, causes diarrhoea and has largely been abandoned. Avoidance of excessive sodium intake is also advisable as sodium and calcium excretion are linked.

### Mixed infective stones

Recurrent stones should be prevented by maintenance of a high fluid intake and meticulous control of bacteriuria. This will require long-term follow-up and may demand the use of long-term low-dose prophylactic antibacterial agents.

### Uric acid stones

Dietary measures are probably of little value and are difficult to implement. Effective prevention can be achieved by the long-term use of the xanthine oxidase inhibitor allopurinol to maintain the serum urate and urinary uric acid excretion in the normal range. A high fluid intake should also be maintained. Uric acid is more soluble at alkaline pH and long-term sodium bicarbonate supplementation to maintain an alkaline urine is an alternative approach in those few patients unable to take allopurinol. However, alkalinization of the urine facilitates precipitation of calcium oxalate and phosphate.

### Cystine stones

These can be prevented and indeed will dissolve slowly if there is obsessional attention to maintenance of a high fluid intake—5 litres of water must be drunk each 24 hours, and the patient must wake twice during the night to ingest 500 ml or more of water. Many patients cannot tolerate this regimen. An alternative, though potentially more troublesome, option is the long-term use of the chelating agent penicillamine; this causes cystine to be converted to the more soluble penicillamine–cysteine complex. Side-effects include drug rashes, blood dyscrasias and immune complex-mediated glomerulonephritis and are by no means uncommon. In addition, the drug is expensive. It is, however, especially effective in promoting dissolution of cystine stones already present.

### Mild hyperoxaluria with calcium oxalate stones

A high fluid intake and dietary oxalate restriction are required.

## Nephrocalcinosis

The term nephrocalcinosis means diffuse renal parenchymal calcification that is detectable radiologically (Fig. 9.28). The condition is typically painless. Hypertension and renal impairment commonly occur.

The main causes of nephrocalcinosis are listed in Table 9.17.

Dystrophic calcification occurs following renal cortical necrosis. In hypercalcaemia and hyperoxaluria, deposition of calcium oxalate results from the high concentration of calcium and oxalate within the kidney.

In renal tubular acidosis (see p. 517) failure of urinary acidification and a reduction in urinary citrate excretion both favour calcium phosphate and oxalate precipitation, since precipitation occurs more readily in an alkaline medium and the calcium-chelating action of urinary citrate is reduced.

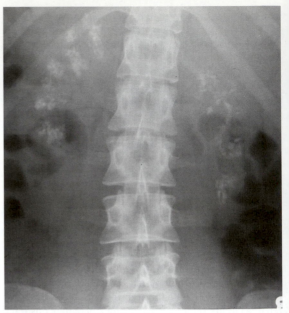

**Fig. 9.28**    An X-ray of nephrocalcinosis.

| |
|---|
| *Mainly cortical (rare)* |
| Renal cortical necrosis (tram-line calcification) |
| |
| *Mainly medullary* |
| Hypercalcaemia (primary hyperparathyroidism, hypervitaminosis D, sarcoidosis) |
| Renal tubular acidosis (inherited and acquired) |
| Primary hyperoxaluria |
| Medullary sponge kidney |
| Tuberculosis |

**Table 9.17**    Common causes of nephrocalcinosis.

Treatment and prevention of nephrocalcinosis consists of treatment of the cause.

## Urinary tract obstruction

The urinary tract may be obstructed at any point between the kidney and the urethral meatus. This results in dilatation of the tract above the obstruction. Dilatation of the renal pelvis is known as hydronephrosis.

### AETIOLOGY

Obstructing lesions may lie within the lumen, or in the wall of the urinary tract, or outside the wall, causing obstruction by external pressure. The major causes of obstruction are shown in Table 9.18. Overall the frequency is the same in men and women. However, in the elderly, urinary tract obstruction is more common in men owing to the frequency of bladder outflow obstruction.

*Within the lumen*
Calculus
Blood clot
Sloughed papilla (diabetes; analgesic abuse; sickle cell
    disease or trait)
Tumour of renal pelvis or ureter
Bladder tumour

*Within the wall*
Pelviureteric neuromuscular dysfunction (congenital, 10%
    bilateral)
Ureteric stricture (tuberculosis, especially after treatment;
    calculus; after surgery)
Ureterovesical stricture (congenital; ureterocele; calculus;
    schistosomiasis)
Congenital megaureter
Congenital bladder neck obstruction
Neuropathic bladder
Urethral stricture (calculus; gonococcal; after
    instrumentation)
Congenital urethral valve
Pin-hole meatus

*Pressure from outside*
Pelviureteric compression (bands; aberrant vessels)
Tumours (e.g. retroperitoneal tumour or glands,
    carcinoma of colon)
Diverticulitis
Aortic aneurysm
Retroperitoneal fibrosis
Accidental ligation of ureter
Retrocaval ureter (right-sided obstruction)
Prostatic obstruction
Tumours in pelvis (e.g. carcinoma of cervix)
Phimosis

**Table 9.18**  Causes of urinary tract obstruction.

## PATHOPHYSIOLOGY

Obstruction with continuing urine formation results in:
1 Progressive rise in intraluminal pressure
2 Dilatation proximal to the site of obstruction
3 Compression and thinning of the renal parenchyma,
    eventually reducing it to a thin rim and resulting in a
    decrease in the size of the kidney.

## CLINICAL FEATURES

### Symptoms

UPPER TRACT OBSTRUCTION. Loin pain occurs which
can be dull or sharp, constant or intermittent. It may be
provoked by measures that increase urine volume and
hence distension of the collecting system, such as a high
fluid intake or diuretics, including alcohol.

Complete anuria is strongly suggestive of complete
bilateral obstruction or complete obstruction of a single
kidney.

Conversely, polyuria may occur in partial obstruction
owing to impairment of renal tubular concentrating
capacity. Intermittent anuria and polyuria indicates intermittent complete obstruction.

Infection complicating the obstruction may give rise to
malaise, fever and septicaemia.

BLADDER OUTFLOW OBSTRUCTION. Symptoms may
be minimal. Hesitancy, narrowing and diminished force
of the urinary stream, terminal dribbling and a sense of
incomplete bladder emptying are typical features. The frequent passage of small volumes of urine occurs if a large
volume of residual urine remains in the bladder after urination. Incontinence of such small volumes of urine is
known as 'overflow incontinence' or 'retention with overflow'.

Infection commonly occurs, causing increased
frequency, urgency, urge incontinence, dysuria and the
passage of cloudy smelly urine. It may precipitate acute
retention.

### Signs

Loin tenderness may be present. An enlarged hyd-
ronephrotic kidney may be palpable.

In acute or chronic retention the enlarged bladder may
be felt or percussed.

Examination of the genitalia, rectum and vagina are
essential, since prostatic obstruction and pelvic malignancy are common causes of urinary tract obstruction.
However, the apparent size of the prostate on digital
examination is a poor guide to the presence of prostatic
obstruction.

## INVESTIGATION

Routine blood and biochemical investigations may be
abnormal, e.g. there may be a raised blood urea or serum
creatinine, hyperkalaemia, anaemia of chronic disease or
blood in the urine, but the diagnosis of obstruction cannot be made on these tests alone and further investigations must be performed.

### Ultrasonography (see p. 443)

This is a reliable means of ruling out upper urinary tract
dilatation. Ultrasound cannot distinguish a baggy, low-
pressure unobstructed system from a tense, high-pressure
obstructed one, so that false-positive scans are seen. However, a normal scan does rule out urinary tract obstruction.

### Radionuclide studies (see p. 444)

In obstructive nephropathy, the relative uptake may be
normal or reduced on the side of obstruction, peak
activity may be delayed and parenchymal (as distinct
from pelvic) transit time prolonged. If doubt exists as to
whether obstruction at the pelviureteric junction is present, frusemide may be administered; satisfactory 'washout' of a radionuclide rules out obstruction and vice
versa. In general, absence of uptake of radiopharmaceutical indicates renal damage sufficiently severe to render
correction of obstruction unprofitable.

### Excretion urography

This is the most widely used investigation. Urography can
usually exclude obstruction even in the presence of severe
renal failure, provided that a high dose of contrast
medium, renal tomography and, if necessary, delayed
films are employed.

A plain film is necessary to detect calcification. However, calculi overlying bone are easily missed.

In recent unilateral obstruction, the affected kidney is enlarged and smooth in outline. The nephrogram is delayed due to a reduction in the GFR. The calyces and pelvis fill with contrast medium later than on the normal side.

In time the nephrogram on the affected side becomes denser than normal, owing to the prolonged nephron transit time, which allows greater than normal concentration of contrast medium within the tubules. Later, the site of obstruction may be seen, with dilatation of the system proximal to the level of the block (Fig. 9.29).

A full-length film should be taken after an attempt at bladder emptying by the patient. Complete emptying indicates either that no obstruction to bladder outflow exists or that intravesicular pressure can be raised sufficiently to overcome it. Apparent bladder outflow impairment may be the result of nervousness or embarrassment on the part of the patient or failure to carry out the X-ray before the bladder has refilled with contrast medium from above, or may be due to an atonic but non-obstructed bladder. Vesicoureteric reflux can result in contrast medium returning to the bladder from above, giving the appearance of a partially full bladder.

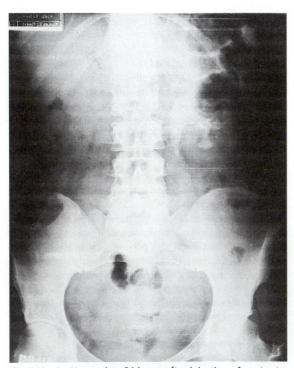

**Fig. 9.29** An X-ray taken 24 hours after injection of contrast, showing a delayed nephrogram and pyelogram on the left side and dilatation of the system to the level of the block. By this time contrast medium has disappeared from the normal right side. (From Weatherall DJ, Ledingham JGG & Warrell DA (eds) (1987) *Oxford Textbook of Medicine*, 2nd edn. Oxford: Oxford University Press. With permission).

**Antegrade pyelography and ureterography** (see p. 443)
This defines the site and cause of obstruction. It can be combined with drainage of the collecting system by percutaneous needle nephrostomy.

**Retrograde ureterography** (see p. 443)
This is indicated if antegrade examination cannot be carried out or if there is the possibility of dealing with ureteric obstruction from below at the time of examination. The technique carries the risk of introducing infection into an obstructed urinary tract.

In obstruction due to neuromuscular dysfunction at the pelviureteric junction or retroperitoneal fibrosis, the collecting system may fill normally from below.

**Cystoscopy, urethroscopy and urethrography**
Obstructing lesions within the bladder and urethra can be seen directly by endoscopic examination.

Urethrography involves introducing contrast medium into the bladder by catheterization or suprapubic bladder puncture, and taking X-ray films during voiding to show obstructing lesions in the urethra. It is of particular value in the diagnosis of urethral valves and strictures.

**Pressure–flow studies**
Pressure changes within the bladder during filling and emptying can be recorded. Demonstration that a high voiding pressure is required to maintain urine flow is indicative of bladder outflow obstruction. This may be combined with video cystography and urethrography to define the site of obstruction.

Normally, while the bladder is being filled there is only a small pressure rise before the voluntary initiation of urination. Uninhibited contractions of the detrusor muscle during filling may be seen in upper motor neurone bladder neuropathy, such as occurs in multiple sclerosis. Less commonly, a neuropathic bladder may be 'hypotonic', readily accepting large volumes of fluid before the initiation of weak contractions at a low intravesical pressure. A common cause of such lower motor neurone bladder neuropathy is diabetes mellitus.

Pressure–flow and video studies may enable a logical decision to be taken as to whether surgery to relieve bladder outflow impairment should be carried out.

### TREATMENT
#### Aims
Treatment involves:
- Relieving the obstruction
- Treating the underlying cause
- Preventing and treating infection

The ultimate aim of treatment is to relieve symptoms and to preserve renal function.

Temporary external drainage of urine by nephrostomy may be valuable, as this allows time for further investigation when the site and nature of the obstructing lesion is uncertain and doubt exists as to the viability of the obstructed kidney, or when immediate definitive surgery would be hazardous.

Recent, complete upper urinary tract obstruction

demands urgent relief to preserve kidney function, particularly if infection is present.

In contrast, with partial urinary tract obstruction, particularly if spontaneous relief is expected, e.g. by passage of a calculus, there is no immediate urgency.

In recent years, increasing use has been made of the insertion of stents to relieve obstruction, either temporarily or on a long-term basis.

**Surgical management**
This depends on the cause of the obstruction (see below). Dialysis may be required in the ill patient prior to surgery.

Nephrectomy or nephroureterectomy is justified when obstruction is due to malignant disease or when it is judged that no worthwhile amount of renal excretory function will be conserved by, or will return after, relief of obstruction.

Permanent urinary diversion is required when the obstruction cannot be relieved; in such cases malignant disease is usually present. Ureteric anastomosis to an ileal conduit opening on to the abdominal wall is often a satisfactory method of diversion. In some patients, obstruction is best relieved by the insertion of indwelling catheters or stents into the ureter. An obstruction high in the urinary tract may require a permanent nephrostomy.

In obstruction due to untreatable malignant disease it is wise to consider carefully whether urinary diversion or stent insertion is justified, since this may exchange a pain-free death from renal failure for a painful one with malignant invasion of bones or nerves.

Diuresis usually follows relief of obstruction at any site in the urinary tract. Massive diuresis may occur following relief of bilateral obstruction owing to previous sodium and water overload and the osmotic effect of retained solutes combined with a defective renal tubular reabsorptive capacity (as in the diuretic phase of recovering acute tubular necrosis). This diuresis is associated with increased blood volume and high levels of atrionatriuretic peptide (ANP). Defective renal tubular reabsorptive capacity cannot be the sole mechanism of severe diuresis since this phenomenon is not observed following relief of unilateral obstruction. The diuresis is usually self-limiting, but a minority of patients will develop severe sodium, water and potassium depletion requiring appropriate intravenous replacement. In milder cases oral salt and potassium supplements together with a high water intake are sufficient.

# Specific causes of obstruction

## Calculi
These are discussed on p. 464.

## Pelviureteric junction obstruction (Fig. 9.30)
This appears to result from a functional disturbance in peristalsis of the collecting system in the absence of mechanical obstruction. Surgical attempts at correction of the obstruction by open or percutaneous pyeloplasty should be limited to patients with recurrent loin pain and those in whom serial excretion urography, background-subtrac-

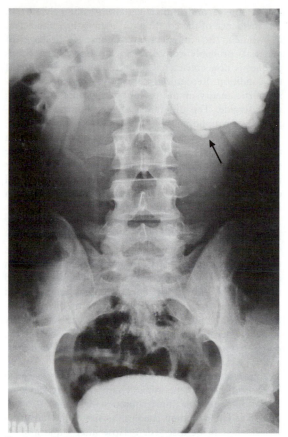

**Fig. 9.30** An X-ray showing left pelviureteric junction obstruction.

tion isotope renography or measurements of GFR indicate progressive kidney damage. Nephrectomy to remove the risk of developing pyonephrosis and septicaemia is indicated if long-standing obstruction has destroyed kidney function.

## Obstructive megaureter
This childhood condition may only become evident in adult life. It results from the presence of a region of defective peristalsis at the lower end of the ureter adjacent to the ureterovesical junction. The condition is commoner in males. It presents with UTI, flank pain or haematuria. The diagnosis is made on excretion urography or, if necessary, ascending ureterography. Excision of the abnormal portion of ureter with reimplantation into the bladder is always indicated in children, and is indicated in adults when the condition is associated with evidence of progressive deterioration in renal function, bacteriuria that cannot be controlled by medical means or recurrent stone formation.

## Retroperitoneal fibrosis (chronic periaortitis)
In this condition the ureters become embedded in dense retroperitoneal fibrous tissue with resultant unilateral or bilateral obstruction. The condition may extend from the

level of the second lumbar vertebra to the pelvic brim. The incidence of the condition in men is three times that in women. An autoallergic response to leakage of material, probably ceroid, derived from atheromatous plaques is now considered to be the underlying cause of the condition. Recognized associations are with abdominal aortic aneurysm and prolonged exposure to the drug methysergide. The differential diagnosis includes retroperitoneal lymphoma or cancer.

Malaise, back pain, normochromic anaemia, uraemia and a raised erythrocyte sedimentation rate (ESR) are typical features. Excretion urography shows bilateral or unilateral ureteric obstruction commencing at the level of the pelvic brim. A periaortic mass may be seen on a CT scan.

Obstruction is relieved surgically by ureterolysis. Biopsy should be performed at operation to determine whether there is an underlying lymphoma or carcinoma. Corticosteroids are of benefit, and in bilateral obstruction in frail patients it may be best to free only one ureter and to rely upon steroid therapy to induce regression of fibrous tissue on the contralateral side, since bilateral ureterolysis is a major operation. In some patients, surgery alone or steroid therapy alone may suffice, but in the majority both surgery and subsequent corticosteroid therapy appear to be necessary.

Response to treatment and disease activity are assessed by serial measurements of ESR and GFR supplemented by isotopic and imaging techniques including CT scanning. The latter method enables the size of the retroperitoneal mass to be assessed. Relapse after withdrawal of steroid therapy may occur and treatment may need to be continued for years. Long-term follow-up is mandatory.

### Benign prostatic hypertrophy

Benign prostatic hypertrophy is a common cause of urinary tract obstruction. It is described on p. 495.

## Prognosis of urinary tract obstruction

The prognosis depends upon the cause and the stage at which obstruction is relieved. In obstruction, four factors influence the rate at which kidney damage occurs, its extent and the degree and rapidity of recovery of renal function after relief of obstruction. These are:
1 Whether obstruction is partial or complete
2 The duration of obstruction
3 Whether or not infection occurs
4 The site of obstruction
Complete obstruction for several weeks will lead to irreversible or only partially reversible kidney damage. If the duration of complete obstruction is several months, total irreversible destruction of the affected kidney will result.

Partial obstruction carries a better prognosis, depending upon its severity.

Bacterial infection coincident with obstruction rapidly increases kidney damage.

Obstruction at or below the bladder neck may induce hypertrophy and trabeculation of the bladder without a rise in pressure within the upper urinary tract, in which case the kidneys are protected from the effects of back-pressure.

# Drugs and the kidney

## Drug-induced impairment of renal function

### Prerenal

Impaired perfusion of the kidneys can result from drugs that cause:
1 Hypovolaemia due to:
  (a) Potent loop diuretics such as frusemide, especially in elderly patients
  (b) Renal salt and water loss, e.g. from hypercalcaemia induced by vitamin D therapy (since hypercalcaemia adversely affects renal tubular salt and water conservation)
2 Decrease in cardiac output, which impairs renal perfusion, e.g. due to β-blockers
3 Decreased renal blood flow, e.g. ACE inhibitors

### Renal

Several mechanisms of drug-induced renal damage exist and may coexist. These include:

ACUTE TUBULAR NECROSIS PRODUCED BY DIRECT NEPHROTOXICITY. Examples include prolonged or excessive treatment with aminoglycosides (kanamycin, gentamicin, streptomycin), amphotericin B and cephaloridine, heavy metals or carbon tetrachloride. The combination of aminoglycosides or cephaloridine with frusemide is particularly nephrotoxic (see p. 744).

ACUTE TUBULO-INTERSTITIAL NEPHRITIS (SEE P. 461) WITH INTERSTITIAL OEDEMA AND INFLAMMATORY CELL INFILTRATION. This cell-mediated hypersensitivity nephritis occurs with many drugs, including penicillins, particularly methicillin, sulphonamides and some NSAIDS.

CHRONIC TUBULO-INTERSTITIAL NEPHRITIS due to drugs (see p. 461).

IMMUNE COMPLEX-MEDIATED GLOMERULO-NEPHRITIS—examples include penicillamine.

### Postrenal

Retroperitoneal fibrosis with urinary tract obstruction may result from the use of methysergide.

## Use of drugs in patients with impaired renal function

(Information box 9.1)

Many aspects of drug handling are altered in patients with renal impairment.

Safe prescribing in renal failure demands knowledge of the clinical pharmacology of the drug and its metabolites in normal individuals and in uraemia. The clinician should ask the following questions when prescribing:

1    Is treatment mandatory? Unless it is, it should be withheld.
2    Can the drug reach its site of action?
     For example, there is little point in prescribing the urinary antiseptic nitrofurantoin in renal failure since bacteriostatic concentrations will not be attained in the urine.
3    Is the drug's metabolism altered in uraemia?
4    Will accumulation of the drug or metabolites occur?
     Even if accumulation is a potential problem owing to the drug or its metabolites being excreted by the kidneys, it is not necessarily an indication to change the drug given. The size of the loading dose will depend upon the size of the patient and is unrelated to renal function. Avoidance of toxic levels of drug in blood and tissues subsequently requires the administration of normal doses of the drug at longer time intervals than usual or smaller doses at the usual time intervals.
5    Is the drug toxic?
6    Are the effective concentrations of the drug in biological tissues similar to the toxic concentrations?
7    Should blood levels of the drug be measured?
8    Will the drug worsen the uraemic state by means other than nephrotoxicity, e.g. steroids, tetracycline?
9    Is the drug a sodium or potassium salt? These are potentially hazardous in uraemia.

Not surprisingly, adverse drug reactions are more than twice as common in renal failure as in normal individuals. Elderly patients, in whom unsuspected renal impairment is common, are particularly at risk. Careful attention to the above and careful titration of the dose of drugs employed should reduce this problem.

The dose may be titrated by:

Observation of its clinical effect, e.g. hypotensive agents
Early detection of toxic effects
Measurement of drug levels in the blood, e.g. gentamicin levels

**Information box 9.1**   Safe prescribing in renal disease.

ABSORPTION. This may be unpredictable in uraemia as nausea and vomiting are frequently present.

METABOLISM. Oxidative metabolism of drugs by the liver may be altered in uraemia. This is rarely of clinical significance.

The rate of drug metabolism by the kidney may be reduced as a result of two factors:

1  Reduced drug catabolism. Insulin, for example, is in part catabolized by the normal kidney. In renal disease, insulin catabolism is reduced. The insulin requirements of diabetics decline as renal function deteriorates for this reason.
2  Reduced conversion of a precursor to a more active metabolite, e.g. the conversion of 25-hydroxycholecalciferol to the more active $1,25\text{-}(OH)_2D_3$. The $1\alpha$-hydroxylase enzyme responsible for this conversion is located in the kidney. In renal disease, production of the enzyme declines and deficiency of $1,25\text{-}(OH)_2D_3$ results.

PROTEIN BINDING. Reduced protein binding of a drug potentiates its activity and increases the potential for toxic side-effects. Measurement of the total plasma concentration of such a drug can give misleading results. For example, the serum concentration of phenytoin required to produce an antiepileptic effect is much higher in normal individuals than in those with renal failure, since in the latter proportionately more drug is present in the free form.

Some patients with renal disease are hypoproteinaemic and reduced drug-binding to protein results. This is not the sole mechanism of reduced drug-binding in such patients. For example, hydrogen ions, which are retained in renal failure, bind to receptors for acidic drugs such as sulphonamides, penicillin and salicylates, thus enhancing their potential for causing toxicity.

VOLUME OF DISTRIBUTION. Salt and water overload or depletion may occur in patients with renal disease. This affects the concentration of drug obtained from a given dose.

END-ORGAN SENSITIVITY. The renal response to drug treatment may be reduced in renal disease. For example, mild thiazide diuretics have little diuretic effect in patients with severe renal impairment.

RENAL ELIMINATION. By far the most important problem in the use of drugs in renal failure concerns the reduced elimination of many drugs normally excreted by the kidneys.

Water-soluble drugs such as gentamicin that are poorly absorbed from the gut, typically given by injection and are not metabolized by the liver give rise to far more problems than lipid-soluble drugs such as propranolol, which are well absorbed and principally metabolized by the liver. Metabolites of lipid-soluble drugs, however, may themselves be water-soluble and potentially toxic.

### Drugs causing uraemia by effects upon protein anabolism and catabolism

Tetracyclines, with the exception of doxycycline, have a catabolic effect and as a result the concentration of nitrogenous waste products is increased. They may also cause impairment of GFR by a direct effect. Corticosteroids have a catabolic effect and so also increase the production of nitrogenous wastes. A patient with moderate impairment of renal function may therefore become severely uraemic if given tetracyclines or corticosteroid therapy.

Drugs and toxic agents causing specific renal tubular syndromes include mercury, lead, cadmium and vitamin D.

### Problem patients

Particular problems are presented by patients in whom renal function is altering rapidly, such as those with recovering acute tubular necrosis and those on regular dialysis treatment. In addition, drugs may be removed by dialysis, which will affect the dosage required.

## Renal failure

The term 'renal failure' means failure of renal excretory function due to depression of GFR. This is accompanied to a variable extent by failure of erythropoietin production (see p. 438), vitamin D hydroxylation (see p. 422), regulation of acid–base balance (see p. 514), and regulation of salt and water balance and blood pressure (see p. 463).

'Acute renal failure' means a decrease in renal function lasting days or weeks, whereas 'chronic renal failure' means renal failure lasting months or years. Acute renal failure is more likely than chronic renal failure to be reversible, depending on the cause. Chronic renal failure is often progressive, whatever the cause. Acute renal failure may cause sudden, life-threatening biochemical disturbances and is a medical emergency. The distinction between acute and chronic renal failure is therefore important in the initial management of a patient presenting with uraemia.

Clinical features are often non-specific (see p. 478).

## ACUTE RENAL FAILURE

This may be (i) prerenal, (ii) renal or (iii) postrenal. This distinction is useful in generating a logical approach to a patient with renal disease, but it is important to remember that more than one category of cause may be present in an individual patient. Other causes of altered serum urea and creatinine concentrations are shown in Table 9.19.

### Prerenal

Failure of perfusion with blood of the kidneys is present in pre-renal failure. This results either from hypovolaemia and hypotension or from impaired cardiac pump

| | Decreased concentration | Increased concentration |
|---|---|---|
| Urea | Low protein intake<br>Liver failure<br>Sodium valproate treatment | Corticosteroid treatment<br>Tetracycline treatment<br>Gastrointestinal bleeding |
| Creatinine | Low muscle mass | High muscle mass<br>Red meat ingestion<br>Muscle damage (rhabdomyolysis)<br>Decreased tubular secretion (cimetidine, trimethoprim) therapy |

**Table 9.19** Causes of altered serum urea and creatinine concentrations other than altered renal function.

efficiency or both. Normally the kidney is able to maintain glomerular filtration close to normal despite wide variations in renal perfusion pressure and volume status—so-called 'autoregulation'. Maintenance of a normal GFR in the face of decreased systemic pressure depends on the intrarenal production of prostaglandins and angiotensin II. Increased sodium and water reabsorption in response to sympathetic stimulation, aldosterone and vasopressin lead to decreased urine flow which results in decreased urea clearance, even when GFR is preserved. This leads to an elevated blood urea and urea : creatinine ratio. Further depression of renal perfusion leads to a drop in glomerular filtration, termed prerenal failure.

Drugs which impair renal autoregulation, such as ACE inhibitors and NSAIDs, increase the risk of prerenal failure in hypovolaemia.

By definition, renal function in prerenal failure returns to normal completely once normal renal perfusion has been restored.

A number of criteria have been proposed to differentiate between prerenal and intrinsic renal causes of renal failure (Table 9.20); laboratory tests however are no substitute for careful clinical assessment. If hypovolaemia or hypotension are present, these should be corrected whether the renal failure is prerenal or intrinsic in origin; failure to do so may prolong the course of intrinsic renal disease. The criteria suggested rely on the fact that renal tubular function is intact in prerenal states; in particular, sodium and water reabsorption, both of which should be maximal in hypovolaemia.

| | Prerenal | Intrinsic |
|---|---|---|
| Urine specific gravity | >1.020 | <1.010 |
| Urine osmolality (mosmol litre$^{-1}$) | >500 | <350 |
| Urine sodium (mmol litre$^{-1}$) | <20 | >40 |
| FE$_{Na}$ (U$_{Na}$·P$_{Cr}$/P$_{Na}$·U$_{Cr}$) × 100% | <1% | >1% |

FE, fractional excretion; P, plasma; U, urine.

**Table 9.20** Criteria for distinction between prerenal and intrinsic causes of renal dysfunction.

URINE SPECIFIC GRAVITY AND URINE OSMOLALITY are easily obtained parameters of concentrating ability but are unreliable in the presence of glycosuria or other osmotically active substances in the urine. Interpretation of these measurements also depends critically on the clinical context. Dilute urine may be a perfectly normal response to water overload, for instance.

URINE SODIUM is low if there is avid tubular reabsorption, but may be increased by diuretics or dopamine.

FRACTIONAL EXCRETION OF SODIUM (FE$_{Na}$), the ratio of sodium clearance to creatinine clearance, increases the reliability of this index but may remain low in some 'intrinsic' renal diseases, including contrast nephropathy and myoglobinuria.

## Renal

Given that normal renal function requires arterial and venous blood supply, normal glomeruli and normal tubules, it is not surprising that a large range of diseases may cause acute renal failure (Table 9.21).

### Acute tubular necrosis

This is a common and important cause of acute renal failure, particularly in hospital practice, and can be caused by a number of different insults to the renal circulation (Table 9.22). The renal medulla is normally relatively hypoxic, despite the high fraction of the cardiac output which is delivered to the kidneys, due to countercurrent exchange of oxygen; this increases its susceptibility to ischaemic damage. In early hypoperfusion, blood flow is

*Systemic hypotension*
Haemorrhage
Severe hypovolaemia
  Burns
  Diarrhoea
  Pancreatitis
  Hypoalbuminaemia
  Diuretics
Decreased cardiac output
  Myocardial infarction
  Massive pulmonary embolism
  Congestive cardiac failure
Endotoxic shock
Iatrogenic—antihypertensives
Snake bite

*Renal vasoconstriction*
Sepsis
Hepatorenal syndrome
Radiological contrast agents
Non-steroidal anti-inflammatory drugs

*Systemic vasodilatation*
Liver disease
Sepsis
Drugs

*Complications of pregnancy*
Abruptio placentae
Pre-eclampsia and eclampsia

*Intrinsic renal disease*

**Table 9.22**   Some causes of acute tubular necrosis.

diverted from the cortex to medulla, resulting in a moderate decrease in GFR but protecting the hypoxic medulla from ischaemic injury. More severe hypoperfusion overcomes this protective mechanism and tubular damage results. Ischaemic tubular damage results in a further fall in glomerular filtration by a number of interrelated mechanisms:

GLOMERULAR CONTRACTION, reducing surface area available for filtration

REFLEX AFFERENT ARTERIOLAR SPASM

'BACKLEAK' OF FILTRATE in the proximal tubule due to loss of function of the tubular cells

OBSTRUCTION OF THE TUBULE by debris shed from ischaemic tubular cells

The clinical course of acute renal failure due to acute tubular necrosis is variable depending on how severe or prolonged the insult is. Oliguria is common in the early stages; non-oliguric renal failure is usually a result of a less severe renal insult. In the recovery phase of acute tubular necrosis GFR may remain low while urine output increases, sometimes to many litres a day, due to defective tubular reabsorption of filtrate. Even after a relatively short-lived insult acute tubular necrosis may last for up to 6 weeks. Eventually, renal function usually returns towards normal. The outcome is critically dependent on the severity and reversibility of the underlying cause and on age.

*Renal perfusion*
Arterial hypotension
Decreased systemic vascular resistance (e.g. sepsis)
Defective renal autoregulation (ACE inhibitors, NSAIDs)
Hepatorenal syndrome (p. 261)

*Renal vasculature*
Renal artery stenosis
Renal embolism
Renal arterioles
  Polyarteritis nodosa
  Accelerated hypertension
Glomerular capillaries
  Goodpasture's syndrome (p. 693)
  Wegener's disease and microscopic polyarteritis
  Accelerated hypertension (p. 620)
  Pre-eclampsia (p. 620)
  Haemolytic uraemic syndrome
  Cholesterol embolism
Renal vein thrombosis (p. 464)

*Glomeruli*
Glomerulonephritis

*Tubules*
Interstitial nephritis
Drug-induced nephrotoxicity
Contrast nephropathy
Urate nephropathy
Acute tubular necrosis

**Table 9.21**   Causes of acute renal failure.

### Acute cortical necrosis

Renal hypoperfusion results in diversion of blood flow from the cortex to the medulla, with a drop in GFR. Medullary ischaemic damage is largely reversible due to the capacity of the tubular cells for regeneration. In contrast, glomerular ischaemic injury heals not with regeneration but with scarring—glomerulosclerosis. Prolonged cortical ischaemia therefore leads to irreversible loss of renal function, termed cortical necrosis. Any cause of acute tubular necrosis, if sufficiently severe or prolonged, may also lead to cortical necrosis. This outcome is particularly common in pregnancy, for reasons that are not well understood.

## Postrenal

The causes and presentation of urinary tract obstruction are dealt with on p. 470. Although patients may present as acute uraemic emergencies, renal failure due to obstruction is often relatively chronic. The longer obstruction has been present, the worse the prognosis for recovery of renal function after relief of obstruction.

## CHRONIC RENAL FAILURE

A list of causes of chronic renal failure, together with their relative frequencies in European patients starting dialysis, is given in Table 9.23. In the early stages, a specific diagnosis is often possible but with near end-stage renal failure with small kidneys a specific diagnosis is often impossible even with a renal biopsy. Hypertension is frequently found, but whether this is the cause or the result of the renal disease is often impossible to determine (see p. 463).

| | |
|---|---|
| Uncertain | 14.4 |
| Glomerulonephritis | 24.1 |
| Pyelonephritis, e.g. | 16.6 |
|     Reflux nephropathy | |
|     Stones/obstruction | |
|     Congenital obstruction | |
| Diabetes IDDM and NIDDM | 13.1 |
| Renal vascular disease | 9.8 |
| Polycystic kidney disease | 8.2 |
| Multisystem diseases (e.g. SLE) | 4.8 |
| Analgesic nephropathy | 2.6 |
| Nephrotoxic agents (e.g. cisplatinum) | 0.2 |
| Alport's syndrome | 0.5 |
| Other hereditary diseases | 0.6 |
| Hypoplastic kidneys | 1.0 |
| Renal vasculitis | 0.7 |
| Amyloidosis | 1.6 |
| Miscellaneous | 3.2 |

SLE, systemic lupus erythematosus.

**Table 9.23** Causes of end-stage renal failure (%) in patients starting dialysis in Europe in 1987 (n = 22 489). Figures from the European Dialysis and Transplant Registry. Diabetes and renal vascular disease are underrepresented owing to selection bias against diabetics and the elderly.

## CLINICAL APPROACH TO THE PATIENT WITH RENAL FAILURE

At first presentation it is often impossible to determine whether a uraemic patient has acute or chronic renal disease.

### HISTORY

Particular attention should be paid to:

DURATION OF SYMPTOMS

DRUG INGESTION, including non-prescription medications or dietary supplements

PREVIOUS MEDICAL AND SURGICAL HISTORY, e.g. previous chemotherapy, multisystem diseases such as SLE

PREVIOUS OCCASIONS on which urinalysis or measurement of urea and creatinine might have been performed, e.g. pre-employment or insurance medical examinations, new patient checks

FAMILY HISTORY of renal disease

### SYMPTOMS

The early stages of renal failure are often completely asymptomatic, despite the accumulation of thousands of metabolites. Symptoms are common when the blood urea concentration is over 40 mmol litre$^{-1}$, but many patients develop uraemic symptoms at lower levels of blood urea. It is not the accumulation of urea itself which causes symptoms, but a combination of many different metabolic abnormalities. Symptoms include:

- Malaise, loss of energy
- Loss of appetite
- Insomnia
- Nocturia and polyuria due to impaired concentrating ability
- Bed-wetting in children may be due to nocturia rather than to emotional disturbance
- Itching
- Nausea and vomiting
- Paraesthesiae due to polyneuropathy
- Restless legs syndrome
- Bone pain due to metabolic bone disease
- Paraesthesiae and tetany due to hypocalcaemia
- Symptoms due to salt and water retention—peripheral or pulmonary oedema
- Symptoms due to anaemia (see p. 297)
- Amenorrhoea in women; erectile impotence in men

In more advanced uraemia (blood urea >50–60 mmol litre$^{-1}$), these symptoms become more severe, and CNS symptoms are common:

- Mental slowing, clouding of consciousness, and seizures
- Myoclonic twitching

Severe depression of glomerular filtration can result in oliguria. This can occur with either acute renal failure or the terminal stages of chronic renal failure.

However, even if the GFR is profoundly depressed, failure of tubular reabsorption may lead to very high urine volumes. For instance, a GFR of 5 ml min$^{-1}$ without any tubular reabsorption would produce a urine output of 300 ml hour$^{-1}$ or over 7 litres a day! Because tubular dysfunction always accompanies glomerular disease to some extent, the urine output is therefore not a useful guide to renal function.

## EXAMINATION

There are few specific physical signs of uraemia *per se*. Findings may include:

SHORT STATURE—in patients who have had chronic renal failure in childhood

PALLOR—due to anaemia

INCREASED PHOTOSENSITIVE PIGMENTATION— which may make the patient look misleadingly healthy

BROWN DISCOLORATION of the nails

SCRATCH MARKS due to uraemic pruritis

SIGNS OF FLUID OVERLOAD

PERICARDIAL FRICTION RUB

FLOW MURMURS—mitral regurgitation due to mitral annular calcification; aortic and pulmonary regurgitant murmurs due to volume overload

GLOVE AND STOCKING PERIPHERAL SENSORY LOSS (rare)

The kidneys themselves are usually impalpable unless grossly enlarged due to polycystic disease, obstruction or tumour. Rectal and vaginal examination may disclose evidence of an underlying cause of renal failure, particularly urinary obstruction and should always be performed.

In addition to these findings, there may be physical signs of any underlying disease which may have caused the renal failure, for instance:

● Cutaneous vasculitic lesions in systemic vasculitides
● Retinopathy in diabetes
● Evidence of peripheral vascular disease
● Evidence of spina bifida or other causes of neurogenic bladder

An assessment of the central venous pressure, skin turgor, blood pressure both lying and standing, and peripheral circulation should also be made. The major symptoms and signs of chronic renal failure are shown in Fig. 9.31.

## INVESTIGATION

### Urinalysis

HAEMATURIA may indicate glomerulonephritis but other sources must be considered. Haematuria should not be assumed to be due to the presence of an indwelling catheter.

PROTEINURIA is strongly suggestive of glomerular disease, but may occur with tubular disease. Urinary infection may also cause proteinuria.

GLYCOSURIA with normal blood glucose indicates tubular disease (failure of tubular reabsorption of glucose).

### Urine microscopy (see p. 441)

WHITE CELLS in the urine usually indicate active bacterial urinary infection, but this is an uncommon cause of acute renal failure; sterile pyuria suggests papillary necrosis (see p. 461) or renal tuberculosis.

EOSINOPHILURIA is strongly suggestive of allergic tubulo-interstitial nephritis.

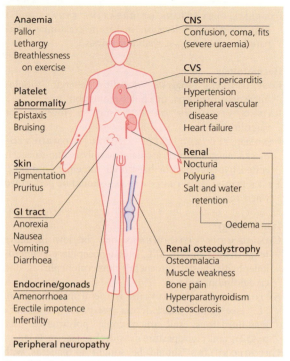

**Fig. 9.31** Symptoms and signs of chronic renal failure. Oedema may be due to a combination of primary renal salt and water retention and heart failure.

GRANULAR CASTS are formed from abnormal cells within the tubular lumen, and indicate active renal disease.

RED CELL CASTS are highly suggestive of glomerulonephritis.

RED CELLS in the urine may be from anywhere between the glomerulus and the urethral meatus.

### Urine biochemistry

24-HOUR CREATININE CLEARANCE is useful in assessing the severity of renal failure.

MEASUREMENTS OF URINARY ELECTROLYTES are unhelpful in chronic renal failure. The use of urinary sodium in the distinction between prerenal and intrinsic renal disease is discussed on p. 476.

URINE OSMOLALITY is a measure of concentrating ability. A low urine osmolality is normal in the presence of a high fluid intake but indicates renal disease when the kidney should be concentrating urine, e.g. in hypovolaemia or hypotension.

URINE ELECTROPHORESIS is necessary for the detection of light chains, which can be present without a detectable serum paraprotein.

### Plasma biochemistry

UREA AND CREATININE.

SERUM ELECTROPHORESIS should be performed for myeloma.

SERUM LDH—acute elevation occurs in renal infarction due to embolism.

EXTREME ELEVATIONS OF CREATINE KINASE and a disproportionate elevation in serum creatinine compared to urea suggest rhabdomyolysis.

### Haematology

EOSINOPHILIA suggests vasculitis, allergic tubulo-interstitial nephritis, or cholesterol embolism.

RAISED VISCOSITY OR ESR suggests myeloma or vasculitis.

FRAGMENTED RED CELLS AND/OR THOMBOCYTOPENIA suggests intravascular haemolysis due to accelerated hypertension or haemolytic uraemic syndrome.

TESTS FOR SICKLE CELL DISEASE should be performed when relevant.

### Immunology

COMPLEMENT COMPONENTS may be low in active renal disease due to SLE, mesangiocapillary glomerulonephritis, poststreptococcal glomerulonephritis, and cryoglobulinaemia.

AUTOANTIBODY SCREENING is useful in detection of SLE (see p. 400), scleroderma (see p. 403), Wegener's granulomatosis and microscopic polyarteritis (see p. 452), and Goodpasture's syndrome (see p. 451).

CRYOGLOBULINS should be sought in patients with unexplained glomerular disease, particularly mesangiocapillary glomerulonephritis.

### Microbiology

URINE CULTURE should always be performed.

EARLY-MORNING URINE SAMPLES should be cultured if tuberculosis is possible.

ANTIBODIES TO STREPTOCOCCAL ANTIGENS (ASOT, antiDNAase B) should be sought if post streptococcal glomerulonephritis is possible.

ANTIBODIES TO HEPATITIS B AND C may point to polyarteritis nodosa or membranous nephropathy (hepatitis B) or to cryoglobulinaemic renal disease (hepatitis C).

ANTIBODIES TO HIV raise the possibility of HIV-associated glomerulonephritis.

MALARIA is an important cause of glomerular disease in the tropics.

### Radiological investigation

ULTRASOUND. Every patient should undergo ultrasonography (for renal size and to exclude hydronephrosis), and plain abdominal radiography and renal tomography to exclude low-density renal stones or nephrocalcinosis, which may be missed on ultrasound.

INTRAVENOUS UROGRAPHY is seldom diagnostic in advanced renal disease.

CT is useful for the diagnosis of retroperitoneal fibrosis and some other causes of urinary obstruction, and may also demonstrate cortical scarring.

### Renal biopsy (see p. 444)

This should be considered in every patient with unexplained renal failure and normal-sized kidneys, unless there are strong contraindications. If rapidly progressive glomerulonephritis is possible, this investigation must be performed within 24 hours of presentation if at all possible, to guide immunosuppressive treatment.

## ACUTE OR CHRONIC RENAL FAILURE?

Distinction between acute and chronic renal failure depends on the history, duration of symptoms and previous urinalyses or measurements of renal function.

The rapid rate of change of urea and creatinine with time suggests an acute process. A normochromic normocytic anaemia suggests chronic disease, but anaemia may complicate many of the diseases which cause acute renal failure, due to a combination of haemolysis, bleeding, and deficient erythropoietin production.

The ultrasound estimation of renal echogenicity and size is helpful. Small kidneys of increased echogenicity are diagnostic of a chronic process, although the reverse is not always true: the kidneys may remain normal in size in diabetes and amyloidosis, for instance.

Renal osteodystrophy suggests chronic disease.

The measurement of carbamylated haemoglobin (product of non-enzymatic reaction between urea and haemoglobin, cf. glycosylated haemoglobin) is not yet widely available.

## COMPLICATIONS OF CHRONIC RENAL FAILURE

### Anaemia

Anaemia is present in the great majority of patients with chronic renal failure. Several factors have been implicated:

ERYTHROPOIETIN DEFICIENCY is the most important

BONE MARROW TOXINS such as polyamines, aluminium, arsenic, copper, lead

BONE MARROW FIBROSIS secondary to hyperparathyroidism

HAEMATINIC DEFICIENCY—iron, vitamin $B_{12}$, folate

INCREASED RED CELL DESTRUCTION due to mechanical, oxidant and thermal damage during haemodialysis

ABNORMAL RED CELL MEMBRANES causing increased osmotic fragility

INCREASED BLOOD LOSS—occult gastrointestinal bleeding, blood sampling, blood loss during haemodialysis or due to platelet dysfunction

ACE inhibitors may cause anaemia in chronic renal failure, probably by interfering with the control of endogenous erythropoietin release.

### Bone disease

RENAL OSTEODYSTROPHY. The term renal osteodystrophy embraces the various forms of bone disease that develop in chronic renal failure, i.e. osteomalacia and osteoporosis, secondary and tertiary hyperparathyroidism and osteosclerosis (Fig. 9.32). Covert renal osteodystrophy is present in most patients with severe renal failure. Phosphate retention results in hyperphosphataemia, which lowers the concentration of ionized serum calcium.

Other effects include decreased renal production of $1,25(OH)_2D_3$, which leads to decreased calcium absorption and a fall in serum calcium. This in turn stimulates the release of PTH, which may already be increased due to the loss of the normal inhibitory effect of $1,25(OH)_2D_3$.

OSTEOMALACIA AND OSTEOPOROSIS (see p. 425).

HYPERPARATHYROIDISM. Poor absorption of dietary calcium and phosphate retention lowers the serum calcium. PTH is released in response to hypocalcaemia and promotes resorption of calcium from bone and increased proximal tubular reabsorption of calcium in the kidney in an attempt to correct the low serum calcium. Over months or years, this 'secondary' hyperparathyroidism can lead to severe decalcification of the skeleton associated with the classical radiological appearances listed in Fig. 9.32.

A common, but not inevitable, sequel to long-standing secondary hyperparathyroidism is hyperplasia of the glands, leading to autonomous or 'tertiary' hyperparathyroidism. In this condition PTH is released inappropriately, resulting in hypercalcaemia and severe bone disease. Hyperparathyroidism causes bone and joint pains and a high serum alkaline phosphatase. Histologically there is increased osteoclastic activity, cyst formation and bone marrow fibrosis (osteitis fibrosa cystica or von Recklinghausen's disease of bone).

OSTEOSCLEROSIS. This literally means 'hardening of bone' and may be a direct result of excess PTH. Alternate bands of sclerotic and porotic bone in the vertebrae produce the characteristic 'rugger-jersey spine' X-ray appearance.

### Skin disease

Itching is a common and frequently intractable problem in dialysis patients. The cause is multifactorial and includes:

- Elevated calcium × phosphate product—the most important remediable cause
- Hypermagnesaemia
- Hyperparathyroidism (even if calcium and phosphate levels are well controlled)
- Iron deficiency
- Inadequate dialysis
- Dry skin—simple aqueous creams are helpful

Chronic renal failure may also cause pseudoporphyria, a blistering photosensitive skin rash. The pseudoporphyria is due to suppression of hepatic uroporphyrin decarboxylase combined with a decreased clearance of porphyrins in the urine or by dialysis.

### Gastrointestinal complications

These include:

DECREASED GASTRIC EMPTYING and increased risk of reflux oesophagitis.

INCREASED RISK OF PEPTIC ULCERATION.

INCREASED RISK OF ACUTE PANCREATITIS—particularly in continuous ambulatory peritoneal dialysis (CAPD) (see p. 488). However, elevations of serum amylase of up to three times normal may be found in chronic renal failure without any evidence of pancreatic disease, due to retention of high-molecular-weight forms of amylase normally excreted in the urine. In patients on CAPD, presence of amylase in the peritoneal effluent is diagnostic of pancreatitis.

CONSTIPATION—particularly in patients on CAPD.

### Metabolic abnormalities

GOUT. Urate retention is a common feature of chronic renal failure, particularly in renal vascular disease. Treatment of asymptomatic hyperuricaemia does not (as once thought) protect against further deterioration in renal function. Treatment of clinical gout is complicated by the nephrotoxic potential of NSAIDs. Colchicine is useful in treatment of the acute attack, and allopurinol should be introduced later under colchicine cover to prevent further attacks. The dose of allopurinol should be reduced in renal impairment.

INSULIN RESISTANCE is a feature of advanced renal impairment, and may contribute to hypertension and

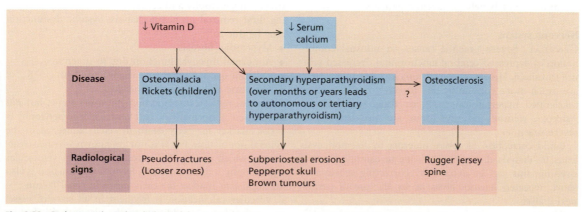

**Fig. 9.32** Pathogenesis and radiological features of renal osteodystrophy.

lipid abnormalities, but rarely causes clinically significant hyperglycaemia.

LIPID METABOLISM ABNORMALITIES are common in renal failure and include:
- Impaired clearance of triglyceride-rich particles
- Hypercholesterolaemia (particularly in advanced renal failure)

The situation is further complicated in end-stage renal disease, when regular heparinization (in haemodialysis), excessive glucose absorption (in CAPD) and immunosuppressive drugs (in transplantation) may all contribute to lipid abnormalities.

## Endocrine abnormalities

These include:

HYPERPROLACTINAEMIA, which may present with galactorrhoea in men as well as women.

INCREASED LUTEINIZING HORMONE (LH) LEVELS in both sexes, and abnormal pulsatility of LH release.

DECREASED SERUM TESTOSTERONE LEVELS (only rarely below the normal levels). Impotence and decreased spermatogenesis are common.

ABSENCE OF NORMAL CYCLICAL CHANGES IN FEMALE SEX HORMONES, resulting in oligomenorrhoea or amenorrhoea.

COMPLEX ABNORMALITIES OF GROWTH HORMONE SECRETION AND ACTION, resulting in impaired growth in uraemic children. Pharmacological treatment with recombinant growth hormone and insulin-like growth factor is being studied.

ABNORMAL THYROID HORMONE LEVELS, partly due to altered protein binding. Sensitive assays for thyroid-stimulating hormone are the best way to assess thyroid function. True hypothyroidism occurs with increased frequency in renal failure. Function of the posterior pituitary is normal in renal failure.

## Muscle dysfunction

Uraemia appears to interfere with muscle energy metabolism, but the mechanism for this interference is uncertain. Decreased physical fitness (cardiovascular deconditioning) also contributes; exercise training programmes are of benefit in uraemic patients.

## Nervous system

CENTRAL. Severe uraemia causes an unusual combination of depressed cerebral function and decreased seizure threshold. However, convulsions in a uraemic patient are much more commonly due to other causes such as accelerated hypertension, TTP, or drug accumulation. Asterixis, tremor and myoclonus are also features of severe uraemia.

Rapid correction of severe uraemia by haemodialysis leads to 'dialysis disequilibrium' due to osmotic cerebral swelling; this can be avoided by correcting uraemia by short, repeated haemodialysis or by the use of peritoneal dialysis.

'Dialysis dementia' is a syndrome of progressive intellectual deterioration, speech disturbances, myoclonus and fits which is now known to be due to aluminium intoxication; it may be accompanied by aluminium bone disease and by microcytic anaemia. Low-grade aluminium exposure may also cause more subtle, subclinical deterioration in intellectual function.

AUTONOMIC. Reversible autonomic dysfunction is common in renal impairment. Findings include:
- Increased circulating catecholamine levels associated with down-regulation of $\alpha$-receptors
- Impaired baroreceptor sensitivity
- Impaired efferent vagal function

All of these abnormalities improve to some extent after institution of regular dialysis and resolve completely after successful renal transplantation.

PERIPHERAL. Median nerve compression in the carpal tunnel is common, and usually due to $\beta_2$-microglobulin-related amyloidosis.

Restless legs syndrome is common in uraemia. Patients complain of an irresistible need to move their legs, often interfering with sleep. The syndrome is difficult to treat. Iron deficiency should be treated if present. Attention should be paid to adequacy of dialysis. Symptoms may improve with the correction of anaemia by erythropoietin. Clonazepam and codeine phosphate are sometimes useful. Renal transplantation cures the problem.

A polyneuropathy occurs in patients who are inadequately dialysed.

## Cardiovascular disease

Life expectancy remains severely reduced compared to the normal population due to a greatly increased incidence of cardiovascular disease, particularly myocardial infarction, cardiac failure, sudden cardiac death and stroke.

Hypertension is a frequent complication of renal failure.

Cardiac hypertrophy is common, even in patients without hypertension. Causative factors include anaemia, causing increased cardiac work, hyperparathyroidism, hypertension, sympathetic overactivity, recurrent volume overload and possibly uraemia *per se*.

Systolic and diastolic dysfunction are also common. Diastolic dysfunction is largely attributable to left ventricular hypertrophy and contributes to hypotension during fluid removal on haemodialysis. Systolic dysfunction may be due to:
- Myocardial fibrosis
- Abnormal myocyte function due to uraemia
- Calcium overload and hyperparathyroidism
- Carnitine and selenium deficiency

Successful renal transplantation improves some, but not all, of these abnormalities. Left ventricular hypertrophy is a risk marker for early death in renal failure, as in the general population, but it is not yet known whether treatments which result in regression of left ventricular hypertrophy reduce mortality. Systolic dysfunction is also an important marker for early death in renal failure.

Vascular calcification is frequent in all sizes of vessel in renal failure. In addition to the classical risk factors for atherosclerosis, a raised calcium × phosphate product causes medial calcification. Hyperparathyroidism may also contribute independently to the pathogenesis by increasing intracellular calcium. Diffuse calcification of the myocardium is also common; the causes are similar.

There is no good evidence that dialysis *per se* results in accelerated atherosclerosis; the excess risk of cardiovascular death is highest in the predialysis phase of chronic renal failure.

Pericarditis is common and occurs in two clinical settings:

URAEMIC PERICARDITIS is a feature of severe, pre-terminal uraemia or of underdialysis. Haemorrhagic pericardial effusion and atrial arrhythmias are often associated. There is a danger of pericardial tamponade and anticoagulants should be used with caution. Pericarditis usually resolves with intensive dialysis.

DIALYSIS PERICARDITIS occurs as a result of an intercurrent illness or surgery in a patient receiving apparently adequate dialysis.

## MANAGEMENT OF RENAL FAILURE

### Acute renal failure

The principles of management are outlined in Information box 9.2 and Practical box 9.4. Obviously, treatment should be directed at the underlying disease. However, many causes of acute renal failure result in the 'final common path' of acute tubular necrosis.

No treatment has been shown to affect the natural history of acute tubular necrosis. Clearly as many of the factors leading to hypoperfusion should be controlled as quickly as possible. Often this requires fluid replacement, guided by measurements of central venous pressure or pulmonary capillary wedge pressure. The polyuric phase of acute tubular necrosis requires extremely careful clinical care in order to avoid further renal injury from hypo-

---

Correction of hyperkalaemia

Aggressive correction of hypovolaemia and/or hypotension

Treatment of underlying cause

Avoidance of further insults to renal circulation e.g.
  Hypotension
  Hypovolaemia
  Sepsis

Avoidance of potentially nephrotoxic agents where possible
  Aminoglycosides
  NSAIDs
  Contrast media

Adequate nutrition—enteral or parenteral

Good nursing care, e.g. prevention of pressure sores

Correction of uraemia by dialysis

Full explanation and reassurance

**Information box 9.2** General management of acute renal failure.

---

1   *Weigh* daily to ensure stable fluid balance
    Check:
    (a) Jugular venous pressure and presence or absence of peripheral oedema
    (b) Lying and standing blood pressure
    (c) Daily serum electrolytes
    Careful measurement of fluid input and output

2   Intravenous access
    Central venous pressure line where necessary

3   Fluid balance—patients may be hypervolaemic, normovolaemic or hypovolaemic
    *Normovolaemic*
    If possible give fluids by mouth or by nasogastric tube, otherwise i.v.
    Maintain balance by daily intake of 300–500 ml plus amount equal to total fluid output on previous day (i.e. urine, stools, vomit, fistula drainage)

    *Hypervolaemic*
    Indicated by an increase in weight, rise in jugular venous pressure or development of peripheral oedema
    Give no fluid with only minimal fluid for parenteral drugs (usually 5% glucose)
    Trial of frusemide 180 mg i.v. or 500–1000 mg orally
    If no diuresis and clinical evidence of pulmonary congestion use ultrafiltration or dialysis

    *Hypovolaemic*
    Indicated by an excessive fall in weight or postural hypotension
    Replace fluid quickly with normal saline or appropriate fluid (see Table 10.5)

**Practical box 9.4** Practical management of acute renal failure.

volaemia. Inotropic support is rational treatment in patients with cardiac disease (see p. 723) and poor renal perfusion; low-dose dopamine (see p. 724) selectively improves renal perfusion.

The role of loop diuretics and mannitol remain controversial. Theoretically these agents may help to flush out tubular debris, prevent reflex vasoconstriction in response to tubular injury, and decrease renal work and oxygen consumption. Controlled trials have shown that loop diuretics in very high doses may increase urine volumes in acute tubular necrosis without much effect on GFR or the subsequent need for dialysis. This marginal benefit must be weighed against the risk of exacerbating hypovolaemia if they are used without adequate monitoring, the risk of auditory toxicity, and (with mannitol) the risk of causing volume expansion and pulmonary oedema if an adequate diuresis is not achieved.

Acute renal failure can be treated by dialysis. Particular care should be used to avoid haemodynamic disturbance and because of this continuous haemofiltration, haemodialysis or peritoneal dialysis are often preferred to intermittent haemodialysis, particularly in patients with persistent cardiovascular instability.

### Chronic renal failure

The underlying cause of renal disease should be treated aggressively wherever possible, e.g. tight metabolic control in diabetes.

## Blood pressure control

Antihypertensive treatment is thought to decrease the rate of deterioration of renal function in chronic progressive renal disease, whatever the initiating cause. Blood pressure should probably be reduced to around 140/80 mmHg. Captopril (an ACE inhibitor) has been proven to slow the rate of deterioration in GFR in diabetic nephropathy to a greater extent than with other hypotensive agents inducing the same degree of blood pressure reduction. ACE inhibitors are under investigation for other renal disease but are now the drugs of choice for hypotensive therapy. ACE inhibitors must be used with caution in the presence of coexistent renal vascular disease. Adequate blood pressure control may require a combination of drugs together with large doses of diuretics to correct sodium and water retention. In patients receiving regular dialysis blood pressure can often be controlled by removal of sodium and water during dialysis.

## Hyperkalaemia

Hyperkalaemia often responds to dietary restriction of potassium intake. Drugs which cause potassium retention (see p. 511) should be stopped. Occasionally it may be necessary to presribe ion-exchange resins to remove potassium in the gastrointestinal tract.

## Acidosis

Correction of acidosis helps to correct hyperkalaemia in chronic renal failure, and may also decrease muscle catabolism. Sodium bicarbonate supplements are often effective, but may cause oedema and hypertension due to extracellular fluid expansion. Calcium carbonate, also used as a calcium supplement and phosphate binder, also has a beneficial effect on acidosis.

## Calcium and phosphate

Hypocalcaemia and hyperphosphataemia should be aggressively treated, preferably with regular (e.g. 3-monthly) measurements of serum PTH to assess how effectively hyperparathyroidism is being suppressed. Dietary restriction of phosphorus is seldom effective alone, because so many important foods contain it. Oral calcium carbonate acts as a calcium supplement and also reduces bioavailability of dietary phosphorus. $1\alpha$-Cholecalciferol and $1,25\text{-}(OH)_2D_3$ increase calcium absorption and also directly suppress parathyroid activity, but must be used with great caution to avoid hypercalcaemia. They have the disadvantage that they also increase phosphorus absorption and may therefore exacerbate hyperphosphataemia. $H_2$ antagonists decrease the effectiveness of phosphate binders.

## Dietary restrictions

In advanced renal disease, reduction of protein intake lessens the amount of nitrogenous waste products generated, and this may delay the onset of symptomatic uraemia. There is some evidence to suggest that dietary protein restriction may slow the rate of progression towards end-stage disease but this remains controversial.

## Fluid and salt intake

A high fluid intake is probably beneficial in chronic renal failure, allowing excretion of metabolites despite poor concentrating ability, and suppressing vasopressin (which may contribute to progressive renal disease). Fluid restriction is sometimes necessary in patients with oedema, but is less important than sodium restriction.

## Hyperlipidaemia

The treatment of lipid abnormalities in chronic renal failure is controversial. Reducing excessive dietary fat intake is sensible. Many lipid-lowering drugs are unsafe in renal failure.

## Anaemia

The anaemia of erythropoietin deficiency can be treated with synthetic (recombinant) human erythropoietin, starting at a dose of $25–50\ U\ kg^{-1}$ three times a week; subcutaneous administration is more effective than intravenous. Blood pressure, haemoglobin concentration and reticulocyte count are measured every 2 weeks and the dose adjusted to maintain a target haemoglobin of $10–12\ g\ dl^{-1}$. Failure to respond to $300\ U\ kg^{-1}$ weekly, or a fall in haemoglobin after a satisfactory response, may be due to iron deficiency, bleeding, malignancy or infection. Partial correction of anaemia with erythropoietin has been clearly shown to improve quality of life, exercise tolerance, sexual function and cognitive function in dialysis patients, and to result in regression of left ventricular hypertrophy. Avoidance of blood transfusion also lessens the chance of sensitization to HLA antigens, which may otherwise be a barrier to successful renal transplantation.

The disadvantages of erythropoietin therapy are that it is expensive and causes a rise in blood pressure in up to 30% of patients, particularly in the first 6 months. Peripheral resistance rises in all patients, due to loss of hypoxic vasodilatation and to increased blood viscosity. A rare complication is encephalopathy with fits, transient cortical blindness and hypertension. Other causes of anaemia should be looked for and treated appropriately (see p. 298).

# Patient education

Involvement at an early stage in various aspects of treatment helps prepare the way for the complicated training that may lie ahead. Dietary and drug therapy should be explained. As dialysis and/or transplantation may be required in the future, forward planning may be necessary. The patient's home may need to be assessed and converted to take dialysis equipment. Job prospects and economic resources need to be considered.

# RENAL REPLACEMENT THERAPY

Approximately 100 individuals per million population reach end-stage renal failure per annum. The aim of all renal replacement techniques is to mimic the excretory functions of the normal kidney, including excretion of

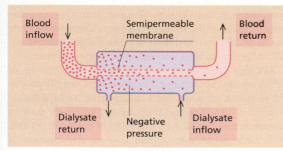

**Fig. 9.33** Changes across a semi-permeable dialysis membrane.

nitrogenous wastes, e.g. urea, maintenance of normal electrolyte concentrations, and maintenance of a normal extracellular volume.

## Haemodialysis

### Basic principles

In haemodialysis blood from the patient is pumped through an array of semi-permeable membranes (the dialyser, often called an 'artificial kidney') which bring the blood into close contact with dialysate, flowing countercurrent to the blood. The plasma biochemistry changes towards that of the dialysate due to diffusion of molecules down their concentration gradients (Fig. 9.33).

THE DIALYSIS MACHINE comprises a series of blood pumps, with pressure monitors and bubble detectors and a proportionating unit, also with pressure monitors and blood leak detectors. Blood flow during dialysis is usually 200–300 ml min$^{-1}$ and dialysate flow usually 500 ml min$^{-1}$. The efficiency of dialysis in achieving biochemical change depends on blood and dialysate flow and the surface area of the dialysis membrane.

*Dialysate* is prepared by a proportionating unit which mixes specially purified water with concentrate, resulting in fluid with the composition described in Table 9.24. A large number of semi-permeable membranes are now available. Cellulose-based membranes are the most widely used and cheapest. The total surface area of the dialyser is about 1 m$^2$ while the thickness is about 10 $\mu$m. Numerous configurations have been invented; the one in most common use is the hollow fibre dialyser, in which blood from the patient is distributed to thousands of hollow

fibres made from a semi-permeable material, with the dialysate flowing around the outside of the fibres (Fig. 9.34). Newer highly permeable synthetic membranes allow more rapid haemodialysis than with cellulose-based membranes (high-flux haemodialysis).

### Access for haemodialysis

Adequate dialysis requires a blood flow of at least 200 ml min$^{-1}$. The most reliable long-term way of achieving this is surgical construction of an *arteriovenous fistula*, using the radial or brachial artery and the cephalic vein. This results in distension of the vein and thickening ('arterialization') of its wall, so that after 6–8 weeks large-bore needles may be inserted to take blood to and from the dialysis machine.

Arteriovenous *shunts* are large-bore plastic cannulae surgically tied into a superficial artery and adjacent vein. These allow direct flow of arterial blood into the dialysis machine, which is returned directly into a vein. Between dialysis sessions flow between artery and vein is restored by a plastic connector between the two cannulae, which lie outside the body, usually on the forearm. Disadvantages include a high rate of infection, thrombosis and the potential for disconnection which could result in exsanguination.

If dialysis is needed immediately, a large-bore double-lumen cannula may be inserted into a central vein — usually the subclavian, jugular or femoral. Semi-permanent dual-lumen venous catheters may also be inserted with a skin tunnel to lessen the risk of infection.

### Dialysis prescription

Dialysis must be tailored to an individual patient to obtain optimal results.

DRY WEIGHT is the weight at which a patient is neither fluid overloaded nor depleted. Patients are weighed at the start of each dialysis session and the transmembrane pressure adjusted to achieve fluid removal equal to the amount by which they exceed their dry weight.

| | |
|---|---|
| Sodium | 130–145 |
| Potassium | 0.0–4.0 |
| Calcium | 1.0–1.6 |
| Magnesium | 0.25–0.85 |
| Chloride | 99–108 |
| Bicarbonate | 35–40 |
| or | |
| Acetate | 35–40 |
| Glucose | 0–10 |

**Table 9.24** Range of concentrations (mmol litre$^{-1}$) in routinely available final dialysates used for haemodialysis.

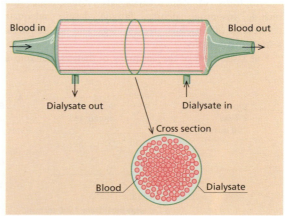

**Fig. 9.34** A hollow fibre dialyser.

THE DIALYSATE BUFFER is usually acetate or bicarbonate. The sodium and calcium concentration of the dialysate buffer are carefully monitored. A high dialysate sodium causes thirst and hypertension. A high dialysate calcium causes hypercalcaemia, whilst a low calcium dialysate combined with poor compliance of medication with oral calcium carbonate and vitamin D may result in hyperparathyroidism.

FREQUENCY AND DURATION of dialysis is adjusted to achieve adequate removal of uraemic metabolites and to avoid excessive fluid overload between dialysis sessions. An adult of average size usually requires 4–5 hours' treatment three times a week if standard Cuprophane dialysers are used. Twice weekly dialysis is only adequate if the patient has considerable residual renal function. All patients are anticoagulated (usually with heparin) during treatment as contact with foreign surfaces activates the clotting cascade. In the UK, many patients have self-supervised home haemodialysis.

### Complications of haemodialysis

Hypotension during dialysis is the major complication. Contributing factors include: an excessive removal of extracellular fluid, inadequate 'refilling' of the blood compartment from the interstitial compartment during fluid removal, abnormalities of venous tone, autonomic neuropathy, acetate intolerance (acetate acts as a vasodilator) and left ventricular hypertrophy.

Very rarely patients may develop anaphylactic reactions to ethylene oxide, which is used to sterilize most dialysers. Patients receiving ACE inhibitors are at risk of anaphylaxis if polyacrylonitrile dialysers are used.

Other potential, rare, complications include the hard water syndrome (caused by failure to soften water resulting in a high calcium concentration prior to mixing with dialysate concentrate), haemolytic reactions and air embolism.

### Adequacy of dialysis

Morbidity and mortality in dialysis patients are influenced by the adequacy of dialysis and nutrition of the patient.

Symptoms of underdialysis are non-specific and include insomnia, itching, fatigue despite adequate correction of anaemia, restless legs and a peripheral sensory neuropathy.

Full assessment of the adequacy of dialysis demands a computerized calculation of urea kinetics, requiring measurement of the residual renal urea clearance, the rate of rise of urea concentration between dialysis sessions and the reduction in urea concentration during dialysis.

Machine haemodialysis is the most efficient way of achieving rapid biochemical improvement, for instance in the treatment of acute renal failure or severe hyperkalaemia. This advantage is offset by disadvantages such as haemodynamic instability, especially in acutely ill patients with multi-organ disease, and over-rapid correction of uraemia can lead to 'dialysis disequilibrium'. This is characterized by nausea and vomiting, restlessness, headache, hypertension, myoclonic jerking, and in severe instances seizures and coma due to rapid changes in plasma osmolality leading to cerebral oedema.

These problems have led to the increasing adoption of gentler continuous methods for the treatment of acute renal failure (see below).

## Haemofiltration

This removes plasma water and its dissolved constituents, e.g. $K^+$, $Na^+$, urea, phosphate, by convective flow across a high-flux semi-permeable membrane, and replacing it with a solution of the desired biochemical composition (Fig. 9.35). Lactate is used as buffer in the replacement solution because rapid infusion of acetate causes vasodilatation and bicarbonate may cause precipitation of calcium carbonate. Haemofiltration can be used for both acute and chronic renal failure. High volumes need to be exchanged in order to achieve adequate small molecule removal; typically a 22-litre exchange three times a week for maintenance treatment and 1000 ml hour$^{-1}$ in acute renal failure.

## Haemodiafiltration

This is a combination of high-flux haemodialysis, using dialysate made from highly purified water for countercurrent dialysis, plus haemofiltration combined with infusion of replacement fluid. Advantages include a better small molecule clearance than with haemofiltration alone, a good clearance of middle molecules and an excellent haemodynamic stability. However, it is expensive.

## Continuous treatments

Continuous treatments are used in acute renal failure and have the advantage of slow continuous correction of

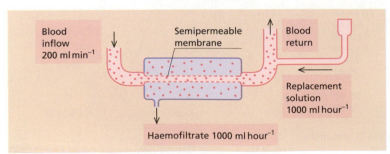

**Fig. 9.35** Principles of haemofiltration.

metabolic and fluid balance. They are particularly suitable for patients with haemodynamic instability. Blood flow may be achieved either by using the patient's own blood pressure to generate flow through a dialyser (*continuous arteriovenous* treatment, CAVH) or by the use of a blood pump to draw blood from the 'arterial' lumen of a dual-lumen catheter placed in the jugular, subclavian or femoral vein, through the dialyser, and back to the 'venous' lumen (*continuous venovenous* treatment, CVVH).

Continuous haemofiltration (CAVH, CVVH) refers to the continuous removal of ultrafiltrate from the patient, usually at rates of up to 1000 ml hour$^{-1}$, combined with simultaneous infusion of replacement solution. For instance, in a fluid-overloaded patient one might remove filtrate at 1000 ml hour$^{-1}$ and replace at a rate of 900 ml hour$^{-1}$, achieving a net fluid removal of 100 ml hour$^{-1}$. Haemofiltration may have an advantage over continuous haemodialysis of removing cardio-depressant substances which appear to accumulate in acute renal failure and septic shock.

Continuous haemodialysis (CAVHD, CVVHD) involves the continuous passage of dialysate countercurrent to the flow of blood. Dialysate is pumped (using an intravenous fluid pump) through the dialysate compartment of a synthetic membrane hollow fibre dialyser at a rate of around 1000 ml hour$^{-1}$.

Continuous haemodiafiltration (CAVHDF, CVVHDF) is a combination of haemofiltration and haemodialysis, involving both the net removal of ultrafiltrate from the blood and its replacement with a replacement solution, together with the countercurrent passage of dialysate (which may be identical to the replacement solution). Both the ultrafiltrate and the spent dialysate appear as 'waste'.

Slow continuous ultrafiltration (SCUF) is the removal of ultrafiltrate from the patient by convection across the dialyser without infusion of replacement fluid or dialysate flow. Fluid is normally removed at a rate of 100–200 ml hour$^{-1}$. This results in a gradual reduction in plasma volume and is useful for the treatment of severe volume overload, for instance in severe cardiac failure prior to definitive treatment. No biochemical improvement occurs, and this is not really a renal replacement technique, but is mentioned here for completeness.

## Peritoneal dialysis

Peritoneal dialysis utilizes the peritoneal membrane as a semi-permeable membrane, avoiding the need for extracorporeal circulation of blood. This is a very simple, low technology treatment compared to haemodialysis. The principles are simple (Fig. 9.36):

1 A tube is placed into the peritoneal cavity through the anterior abdominal wall.
2 Dialysate is run into the peritoneal cavity, usually under gravity.
3 Urea, creatinine, phosphate, and other uraemic toxins pass into the dialysate down their concentration gradients.
4 Water (with solutes) is attracted into the peritoneal cavity by osmosis, depending on the osmolarity of the dialysate. This is determined by the dextrose content of the dialysate (Table 9.25).
5 The fluid is changed regularly to repeat the process.

For acute peritoneal dialysis a stiff catheter is inserted under local anaesthetic in the midline, one-third of the way down between the umbilicus and the symphysis pubis.

Chronic peritoneal dialysis requires insertion of a soft catheter, with its tip in the pelvis, exiting the peritoneal cavity in the midline and lying in a skin tunnel with an

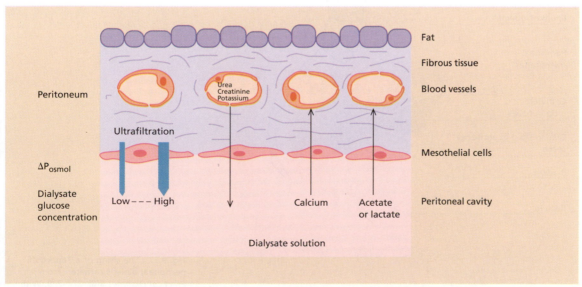

**Fig. 9.36** The principles of peritoneal dialysis.

| Sodium | 130–134 |
|---|---|
| Potassium | 0 |
| Calcium | 1.0–1.75 |
| Magnesium | 0.25–0.75 |
| Chloride | 95–104 |
| Lactate | 35–40 |
| Glucose | 77–236 |
| Total osmolarity | 356–511 |

**Table 9.25**  Range of concentrations (mmol litre$^{-1}$) in routinely available CAPD dialysate. Glucose content is often expressed as gram per decilitre of anhydrous glucose, e.g. 1.36% = 77 mmol litre$^{-1}$. An even more hypertonic dialysate (6.36%) is available for acute (intermittent) peritoneal dialysis.

exit site in the lateral abdominal wall (Fig. 9.37).

This form of dialysis can be adapted in several ways.

CONTINUOUS AMBULATORY PERITONEAL DIALYSIS.
Dialysate is present within the peritoneal cavity continuously, apart from when dialysate is being exchanged. Dialysate exchanges are performed three to five times a day, using a sterile no-touch technique to connect 1.5–3 litre bags of dialysate to the peritoneal catheter; each exchange takes 20–40 min. This is the technique most often used for maintenance dialysis in patients with end-stage renal failure.

INTERMITTENT PERITONEAL DIALYSIS (IPD).
Dialysate is exchanged every 60–120 min, requiring the patient to remain in bed during the treatment. This form of treatment is often used for acute renal failure and as maintenance treatment for end-stage renal failure when 20–40 hours' treatment per week is given as two or more overnight sessions.

NIGHTLY INTERMITTENT PERITONEAL DIALYSIS (NIPD). An automated device is used to perform exchanges each night while the patient is asleep. Sometimes dialysate is left in the peritoneal cavity during the day in addition, to increase the time for which biochemical exchange is occurring.

TIDAL DIALYSIS. A residual volume is left within the peritoneal cavity with continuous cycling of smaller volumes in and out.

FLUID BALANCE CONTROL. Ultrafiltration, i.e. removal of excess plasma water and solutes, is achieved using hypertonic dialysate, which exerts an osmotic 'drag'. Depending on the patient's fluid intake and residual urine output, it may be necessary to use one or more hypertonic dialysate bags daily to achieve fluid balance in CAPD. Fluid overload is a relatively common problem in CAPD, and is due to failure of transport across the peritoneal membrane.

### Complications of peritoneal dialysis

PERITONITIS. Bacterial peritonitis is the commonest serious complication of CAPD and other forms of peritoneal dialysis. Clinical presentations include abdominal pain of varying severity (guarding and rebound tenderness are unusual), and a cloudy peritoneal effluent—without which the diagnosis cannot be made. Microscopy reveals a neutrophil count of >100 cells/ml. Nausea, vomiting, fever and paralytic ileus may be seen if peritonitis is severe.

CAPD peritonitis must be investigated with culture of peritoneal effluent. Empirical antibiotic treatment must be started immediately, with a spectrum which covers both Gram-negative and Gram-positive organisms, e.g.

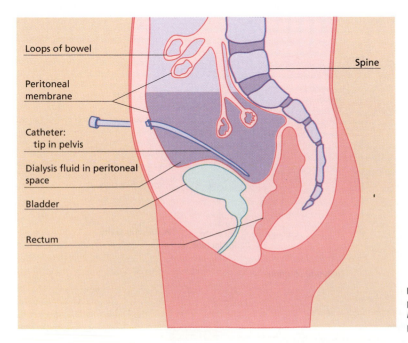

Loops of bowel

Peritoneal membrane

Catheter: tip in pelvis

Dialysis fluid in peritoneal space

Bladder

Rectum

Spine

**Fig. 9.37**  The siting of a Tenckhoff peritoneal dialysis catheter. From *Practical Diabetes* **9(6)**: 224–229. With permission.

third generation cephalosporin intravenously. Antibiotics may be given by the oral, intravenous or intraperitoneal route; most centres rely on intraperitoneal antibiotics. Common causative organisms are listed in Table 9.26.

*Staph. aureus* peritonitis should lead to a search for nasal carriage of this organism and *Staph. epidermidis* peritonitis usually indicates contamination from the patient's (or helper's) skin. Relapsing *Staph. epidermidis* peritonitis with an organism with the same antibiotic sensitivity pattern on each occasion may indicate that the Tenckhoff catheter has become colonized: often this is difficult to eradicate without replacement of the tube under antibiotic cover.

Gram-negative peritonitis may complicate septicaemia from urinary or bowel infection. A mixed growth of Gram-negative and anaerobic organisms strongly suggests bowel perforation, and is an indication for formal laparotomy.

Fungal peritonitis often follows antibacterial treatment but may occur *de novo*. Clinical presentation is very variable. It is rare to be able to cure fungal peritonitis without catheter removal as well as antifungal treatment. Intraperitoneal amphotericin has been associated with the formation of peritoneal adhesions.

INFECTION AROUND THE SITE where the catheter exits through the skin is relatively common. It should be treated aggressively (with systemic and/or local antibiotics) to prevent spread of the infection into the subcutaneous tunnel and the peritoneum; the commonest causative organisms are staphylococci.

## Other complications

CAPD is often associated with constipation, which in turn may impair flow of dialysate in and out of the pelvis. Occasionally dialysate may leak through a diaphragmatic defect into the thoracic cavity, causing a massive pleural 'effusion'. The glucose content of the effusion is usually diagnostic or the diagnosis may be made by instillation of methylene blue with dialysate and the demonstration of a blue colour on pleural tap. Dialysate may also leak into the scrotum down a patent processus vaginalis.

Failure of peritoneal membrane function is a predictable complication of long-term CAPD, resulting in worsening biochemical exchange and decreased ultrafiltration with hypertonic dialysate. It is thought that this problem may be accelerated by excessive reliance on hypertonic dialysate to remove fluid.

Sclerosing peritonitis is a rare but potentially fatal complication of CAPD. The causes are often unknown, but recurrent peritonitis, contamination of the peritoneal cavity with chlorhexidine, and some drugs have been implicated. Progressive thickening of the peritoneal membrane occurs in association with adhesions and strictures, turning the small bowel into a mass of matted loops and causing repeated episodes of small bowel obstruction. There is no known way of reversing the process. CAPD should be abandoned.

## Contraindications to peritoneal dialysis

There are few absolute contraindications apart from unwillingness or inability on the patient's part to learn the technique.

Previous peritonitis causing peritoneal adhesions may make peritoneal dialysis impossible: but the extent of adhesions is difficult to predict, and it may be worth an attempted surgical placement of a dialysis catheter.

The presence of a stoma (colostomy, ileostomy, ileal urinary conduit) makes successful placement of a dialysis catheter extremely unlikely.

Active intra-abdominal sepsis, for instance due to diverticular abscesses, is an absolute contraindication to peritoneal dialysis although diverticular disease *per se* is not.

Abdominal hernias may often expand during CAPD as a result of increased intra-abdominal pressure, and should ideally be repaired before or at the time of CAPD catheter insertion.

Visual impairment may make it difficult for a patient to perform dialysate exchanges, but completely blind patients can be trained in the technique if adequately motivated.

Severe arthritis makes it difficult to perform the exchanges, but a large number of mechanical aids are available. Sterilization of connections by heat or ultraviolet light reduces the risk of peritonitis.

## Adequacy of peritoneal dialysis

No consensus yet exists on how the adequacy of peritoneal dialysis should be measured. Symptoms of underdialysis (see p. 486) should be noted. A protein intake of at least 1.1 g kg$^{-1}$ ideal body weight together with dialysis adequate to keep peak or average blood urea concentration below 25 mmol litre$^{-1}$ probably indicates adequate dialysis.

Renal function declines less rapidly in CAPD patients than in those receiving intermittent haemodialysis, but with total renal failure it is often difficult to maintain adequacy of dialysis with CAPD alone, necessitating conversion to haemodialysis. CAPD is an excellent treatment for those patients likely to receive a renal transplant or for elderly patients with limited life expectancy, but is probably not the treatment of choice in the small minority in whom long-term dialysis is contemplated.

| | Approximate percentage of cases |
|---|---|
| *Staphylococcus epidermidis* | 40–50 |
| *Escherichia coli, Pseudomonas* and other Gram-negative organisms | 25 |
| Staphylococcus aureus | 15 |
| *Mycobacterium tuberculosis* | 2 |
| *Candida* and other fungal species | 2 |

**Table 9.26** Some causes of CAPD peritonitis. In approximately 20%, no bacteria are found.

## Complications of long-term dialysis

Cardiovascular disease (see p. 482) and sepsis are the leading causes of death in long-term dialysis patients.

Causes of fatal sepsis include peritonitis complicating peritoneal dialysis and *Staph. aureus* infection (including endocarditis) complicating the use of indwelling access devices for haemodialysis.

DIALYSIS AMYLOIDOSIS is caused by the accumulation of amyloid protein as a result of failure of clearance of $\beta_2$-microglobulin, a molecule of 11.8 kDa. This protein is the light chain of the class I HLA antigens and is normally freely filtered at the glomerulus but is not removed by cellulose-based haemodialysis membranes. Complement activation resulting from the use of cellulose-based membranes may increase the generation rate of the protein. The protein polymerizes to form amyloid deposits, which may cause median nerve compression in the carpal tunnel or a dialysis arthropathy—a clinical syndrome of pain and disabling stiffness in the shoulders, hips, hands, wrists and knees. $\beta_2$-Microglobulin-related amyloid may be demonstrated in the synovium. There is little inflammation and the pathogenesis is ill understood. Rapid improvement after renal transplantation is probably due to steroid therapy. Low-dose prednisolone alone can also cause an improvement. A change to a biocompatible synthetic membrane has also been reported to be of benefit: again, the mechanism for this improvement is not clear. Amyloid deposits can also cause pathological bone cysts and fractures, pseudotumours and gastrointestinal bleeding caused by amyloid deposition around submucosal blood vessels.

The extent of amyloid deposition is best assessed by nuclear imaging, either using [$^{99m}$Tc]DMSA, or, more specifically, by the use of radiolabelled serum amyloid P component.

## Transplantation

Successful renal transplantation offers the potential for complete rehabilitation in end-stage renal failure. It allows freedom from dietary and fluid restriction, anaemia and infertility are corrected and the need for parathyroidectomy is reduced.

The technique involves the anastomosis of an explanted human kidney, either from a cadaveric donor or, less frequently, from a living close relative, on to the iliac vessels of the recipient (Fig. 9.38). The donor ureter is placed into the recipient's bladder. Unless the donor is genetically identical (i.e. an identical twin), immunosuppressive treatment is needed, for as long as the transplant remains in place, to prevent rejection. Eighty per cent of grafts now survive for 5–10 years in the best centres, and 60% for 10–30 years.

Success of transplantation is affected by numerous factors:

ABO (BLOOD GROUP) COMPATIBILITY.

MATCHING DONOR AND RECIPIENT FOR HLA TYPE.

DR matching appears to have the most impact on sur-

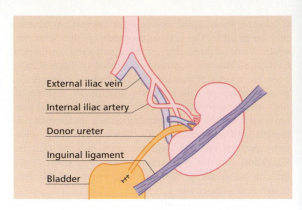

**Fig. 9.38** The anatomy of a renal transplant operation.

vival, followed by the B and, least importantly, the A loci. Complete compatibility at A, B and DR offers the best chance of success, and this has led to nationwide matching schemes for kidneys retrieved from cadaver donors.

ADEQUATE IMMUNOSUPPRESSIVE TREATMENT (see below).

PREOPERATIVE BLOOD TRANSFUSION appears to exert a non-specific immunosuppressive effect, decreasing the incidence of rejection; however this effect is modest compared to the immunosuppressive effects of cyclosporin, and blood transfusion carries a risk of HLA sensitization.

THE 'CENTRE EFFECT': graft survival is higher in those centres with extensive experience of medical management of transplant recipients.

### Donor kidney

CADAVERIC DONATION. Most countries allow the removal of kidneys and other organs from patients who have suffered irretrievable brain damage ('brain stem death') while their hearts are still beating (see p. 734).

LIVING RELATED DONATION. Occasionally a close relative may volunteer as a potential donor. A sibling donor may be HLA identical or share one or no haplotypes with the potential recipient. Most transplant centres accept one haplotype matches as well as HLA-identical donors. Most avoid using child-to-parent donation unless the circumstances are exceptional.

Potential living related donors are subjected to an intensive preoperative evaluation, including clinical examination and measurement of renal function, tests for carriage of hepatitis B, C, HIV and cytomegalovirus, and detailed imaging of renal anatomy with IVU and then arteriography, to be sure that transplantation will be technically feasible.

### Immunosuppression for transplantation

Long-term drug treatment for the prevention of rejection is employed in all cases apart from living related donation from an identical twin. Some degree of immunological tolerance does develop, and the risk of rejection is highest in the first 3 months after transplantation. A combination of immunosuppressive drugs is usually used.

CORTICOSTEROIDS have a non-specific immunosuppressive action. High-dose methylprednisolone is used as the primary treatment for acute rejection.

AZATHIOPRINE prevents cell-mediated rejection by interfering with nucleic acid synthesis and preventing replication of lymphocytes. Adverse effects include suppression of red cell and platelet production and an increased incidence of infections (particularly viral).

CYCLOSPORIN prevents the activation of T lymphocytes in response to new antigens and is highly effective in preventing rejection, while leaving the function of the rest of the immune system largely intact. Its introduction has revolutionized organ transplantation. Disadvantages include variable bioavailability, high cost and nephrotoxicity. Even with careful adjustment of the dose in response to trough blood levels, renal function may be adversely affected due to renal vasoconstriction which may result in irreversible interstitial fibrosis.

NEW IMMUNOSUPPRESSIVE AGENTS such as FK506 and rapamycin are becoming available and are undergoing clinical trials.

ANTIBODIES AGAINST T CELLS are potent and relatively specific immunosuppressive agents whose role is increasing. Antibodies may be polyclonal or monoclonal, derived from mouse, rabbit, horse, or 'humanized', and directed against any of a number of lymphocyte surface marker proteins, enabling neutralization or killing of lymphocytes with certain functions, e.g. T cells, activated T cells, cells expressing adhesion molecules, cells expressing the interleukin-2 receptor. These antibodies may be used both in the prevention and the treatment of rejection, but are highly immunosuppressive; some may increase the risk of virus-associated malignancy, e.g. lymphomas.

IN FUTURE attention will turn increasingly to the induction of immunological tolerance to grafted organs and to the use of organs from genetically modified animals.

### Complications of renal transplantation
These include:

TECHNICAL FAILURES.

OPPORTUNISTIC INFECTIONS, e.g. *Pneumocystis*, cytomegalovirus.

LIPID ABNORMALITIES and a high risk of cardiovascular events.

HYPERTENSION—often attributable to cyclosporin.

RECURRENCE OF THE DISEASE WHICH CAUSED RENAL FAILURE—this is uncommon but may occur in specific diseases, e.g. primary oxalosis, mesangiocapillary glomerulonephritis, focal segmental glomerulosclerosis, Goodpasture's syndrome.

DE NOVO GLOMERULONEPHRITIS in the grafted kidney.

MALIGNANCY, particularly lymphomas and skin cancers—these are often attributable to viral induction of malignancy.

ASEPTIC NECROSIS OF BONE resulting from high-dose corticosteroid treatment.

## Choice of renal replacement therapy

For the majority of patients with end-stage renal failure a renal transplant is the treatment of choice, but because of the limited availability of donor organs many patients remain on dialysis for years while waiting for a transplant. Sensitization to HLA antigens, for instance by pregnancy, blood transfusion or a previous failed transplant, makes finding a compatible organ more difficult. In addition, there are a number of patients who are thought unsuitable for transplantation, e.g.

- Previous malignancy
- Severe non-renal disease likely to limit survival and the degree of rehabilitation after transplantation
- Elderly patients

The choice between CAPD and haemodialysis is influenced by medical, social, psychological and financial factors. Nearly all renal units offer a choice of modalities.

## PREVENTION OF CHRONIC RENAL FAILURE (Information box 9.3)

Detection and treatment of ascending urinary infections in children—preventing reflux nephropathy

Tight metabolic control in diabetes decreases the risk of diabetic nephropathy

Early detection and treatment of urinary obstruction (e.g. due to prostatic enlargement)

Avoidance of unnecessary nephrotoxins

Care with the use of ACE inhibitors and NSAIDs in patients with any degree of pre-existing renal impairment

Amelioration of the progression of chronic renal failure:
  Antihypertensive therapy (? specific protective effect of ACE inhibitors)
  Protein restriction
  ? Avoidance of hyperlipidaemia
  ? Avoidance of phosphate retention

Attention to vascular risk factors

Colchicine in familial Mediterranean fever

Early detection and treatment of systemic vasculitis

Prevention or adequate treatment of hypertension

Greater understanding of the pathogenesis of many renal diseases is required before a rational approach to prevention can be devised.

**Information box 9.3** Prevention of chronic renal failure.

# Cystic, congenital and familial disease

## Cystic renal disease

Solitary or multiple renal cysts are common, especially with advancing age: 50% of those aged 50 years or more have one or more such cysts. They have no special significance except in the differential diagnosis of renal tumours (see p. 495). Such cysts are often asymptomatic and are found on excretion urography or ultrasound examination performed for some other reason. Occasionally they may cause pain and/or haematuria due to their large size or bleeding may occur into the cyst.

## Adult polycystic renal disease

Adult polycystic renal disease (APCD) is an important cystic disease of the kidney that is relatively common. In the large majority of cases, inheritance is in an autosomal dominant manner as a single gene defect linked to the α-haemoglobin gene locus on the short arm of chromosome 16. It is manifested in infancy as tiny cystic lesions distributed throughout both kidneys and should be distinguished from juvenile nephronophthisis (see below). The precise mechanism for cyst formation is disputed. With advancing age the cysts enlarge at a variable rate, often at the same rate within family groups but at different rates between different families. There is progressive asymmetric renal enlargement, with compression of intervening renal tissue and progressive loss of excretory function.

Clinical presentation may be at any age from the second decade. Presenting symptoms include:

- Acute loin pain and/or haematuria due to haemorrhage into a cyst
- Vague loin or abdominal discomfort due to the increasing size of the kidneys
- Development of hypertension or symptoms of uraemia

The natural history of the disease is one of progressive renal impairment, sometimes punctuated by acute episodes of loin pain and haematuria and commonly associated with the development of hypertension. It is popularly believed that there is an increased incidence of UTI in patients with APCD. There is little evidence to support this, but if such patients do develop infection it may be more difficult to eradicate. As mentioned earlier, the rate of progression to renal failure is variable but tends to follow the same pattern in families. Some may reach end-stage renal failure at 40 years but others survive to 70 years or more.

Approximately 30% of patients with APCD have hepatic cysts; these rarely cause liver dysfunction. Cysts may more rarely develop in the pancreas, spleen, ovary and other organs. Berry aneurysms of the cerebral vessels (10–30%) are not infrequent and may result in subarachnoid or cerebral haemorrhage. Renal neoplasms may develop

in polycystic kidneys and are difficult to diagnose.

Polycythaemia and mitral valve prolapse are not uncommon associations.

### DIAGNOSIS

Physical examination commonly reveals large, irregular kidneys and possibly hepatomegaly. Definitive diagnosis was previously based on excretion urography, but is now more easily established by ultrasound examination (Fig. 9.39). However, such renal imaging techniques may be equivocal, especially in subjects under the age of 20 years.

### TREATMENT

The disease is always progressive. The most important aspect of management is regular blood pressure recording in affected patients, with control of hypertension as it develops. Uncontrolled hypertension accelerates the loss of kidney function. Some patients may develop salt and water wasting as the disease advances (see p. 505), when salt replacement with Slow Sodium can improve excretory function. Many patients will require renal replacement by dialysis and/or transplantation.

### SCREENING

The children and siblings of patients with established APCD should be routinely offered screening. We believe that this should be offered to identify patients with this disorder, who must then have regular blood pressure checks and should be offered genetic counselling in respect of family planning. Screening should not be carried out before the age of 20 years, as excluding the condition may be difficult and hypertension is unusual before this age. Even at this age, renal ultrasonography may give a false-negative result. Gene linkage analysis can be utilized in many families.

## Medullary cystic disease ('juvenile nephronophthisis')

Developing early in childhood, juvenile nephronophthisis is commonly inherited in an autosomal recessive manner. A similar condition developing later in childhood (medullary cystic disease) is inherited as an autosomal dominant trait, but sporadic cases occur in both conditions. Despite its name, the dominant histological finding is interstitial inflammation and tubular atrophy, with later development of medullary cysts. Progressive glom-

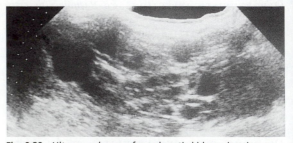

**Fig. 9.39** Ultrasound scan of a polycystic kidney showing an enlarged kidney with many cysts of varying size.

erular failure is a secondary consequence.

The dominant features are polyuria, polydipsia and growth retardation. Diagnosis is based on the family history and renal biopsy, the cysts rarely being visualized by imaging techniques.

## Medullary sponge kidney

Medullary sponge kidney is an uncommon but not rare condition that usually presents with renal colic or haematuria. Although it is most often sporadic, a few affected families have been reported. The condition is characterized by dilatation of the collecting ducts in the papillae, sometimes with cystic change. In severe cases the medullary area has a sponge-like appearance. The condition may affect one or both kidneys or only part of one kidney. Cyst formation is commonly associated with the development of small calculi within the cyst. In about 20% of patients there is associated hypercalciuria or renal tubular acidosis (see p. 517). Hemihypertrophy of the skeleton has been described in this condition.

The diagnosis is made by excretion urography, which shows small calculi in the papillary zones with an increase in radiodensity *around* these following injection of contrast medium as the dilated or cystic collecting ducts are filled with contrast (see Fig. 9.22).

The natural history is one of intermittent colic with passage of small stones or haematuria. Renal function is usually well maintained and renal failure is unusual, except where obstructive nephropathy develops owing to the growth of stones in the pelvis or ureters.

## CONGENITAL ABNORMALITIES

### Agenesis

Agenesis may be bilateral or unilateral. Unilateral agenesis ('solitary kidney') occurs in 1 in 1000 of the population. It is usually associated with compensatory hypertrophy of the single kidney and normal renal function. Save for the potential hazard of trauma to this solitary kidney, it has no clinical significance.

### Hypoplasia

Renal hypoplasia (failed development) of one kidney is uncommon, and hypoplasia of both kidneys is rare. It may be difficult to distinguish unilateral renal hypoplasia from a small kidney due to renal artery stenosis, obstruction or reflux nephropathy in early life. Clinical interest in the condition most often arises in patients with hypertension, where the small kidney may be considered the cause. If the small kidney is shown by radioisotope studies to contribute no useful renal function and if the hypertension has developed in a young subject or is difficult to control by medical treatment, nephrectomy should be undertaken.

### Ectopic kidneys

Defects in embryological renal development may lead to ectopic or maldeveloped renal systems. At the risk of oversimplification, the kidneys may be thought of as developing in the embryo as one structure in the 'pelvic' area, migrating upwards and separating with growth. Failure in normal development may result in failure of the kidneys to migrate normally and indeed they may fail to separate. This results in a 'pelvic kidney' when one or both remain in the pelvis, a 'crossed ectopic kidney' when both have moved to the same side of the spine, a horseshoe or discoid kidney when there is partial (usually fusion of the lower poles) or total failure of separation.

In clinical practice the main problem associated with ectopic kidneys usually relates to impaired urinary drainage with secondary obstruction or stone formation. This may be compounded if infection supervenes, the poor drainage making eradication of infection difficult and predisposing to stone formation. Pelvic kidneys may interfere with parturition.

## OTHER FAMILIAL RENAL DISEASE

Familial renal disease is in general rare, but there are a number of familial conditions that, among other things, can affect the kidneys.

### Alport's syndrome

Alport's syndrome is a rare condition characterized by hereditary nephritis with haematuria, progressive renal failure and high-frequency nerve deafness. It is principally expressed in males and both X-linked and dominant modes of inheritance have been postulated. Some 15% of cases may have ocular abnormalities such as cataract, conical cornea and dislocated small lens. The disease is progressive and accounts for some 5% of cases of end-stage renal failure in childhood or adolescence. Anti-GBM antibody does not adhere normally to the glomerular basement membrane of affected individuals.

### Congenital nephrotic syndrome

This syndrome is rare.

### Renal tubular transport defects

Renal tubular transport defects include cystinuria, X-linked hypophosphataemia, Hartnup's disease, adult Fanconi syndrome, galactosaemia and fructosaemia. They are discussed in more detail on p. 863.

### Renal glycosuria

Renal glycosuria, in which there is glucose in the urine in subjects demonstrated to have normal blood glucose levels, who are not starved and who have no other urinary abnormality, is uncommon. Such patients have either a defect in the tubular threshold for reabsorption of glucose in the proximal tubule (a 'splayed' reabsorption curve) or a defect in the maximal tubular reabsorption of glucose. Both autosomal dominant and recessive inheritance have been postulated. It has no clinical significance except in the differential diagnosis of patients with diabetes mellitus or other tubular disorders such as the Fanconi syndrome.

# Tumours of the kidney and genitourinary tract

## MALIGNANT RENAL TUMOURS

These comprise 1–2% of all malignant tumours, and the male/female ratio is 2 : 1.

## Renal cell carcinoma

Renal cell carcinomas (previously called hypernephromas or Grawitz tumours) arise from proximal tubular epithelium. They are the commonest renal tumour in adults. They rarely present before the age of 40 years, the average age of presentation being 55 years.

### PATHOLOGY
The tumours may be solitary, multiple or occasionally bilateral. The tumour lies within the kidney but it may eventually penetrate the capsule. Macroscopically, its cut surface appears as a yellow mass, sometimes containing areas of haemorrhage and cystic degeneration. Local invasion of renal veins and spread to the opposite kidney may occur, as may metastasis to lymph nodes, liver, bone and lung (often as an apparently solitary metastasis). Renal cell carcinomas are highly vascular tumours. Microscopically the tumour is composed of large cells containing clear cytoplasm.

### CLINICAL FEATURES
Patients present with haematuria, loin pain and a mass in the flank. Malaise, anorexia and weight loss may occur, and occasionally patients present with polycythaemia (see p. 327). Pyrexia is present in about one-fifth of patients and approximately one-quarter present with metastases. Rarely, a left-sided varicocele may be associated with left-sided tumours that have invaded the renal vein and caused obstruction to drainage of the left testicular vein.

### DIAGNOSIS
Excretion urography will reveal a space-occupying lesion in the kidney; 10% of these show calcification.

Ultrasonography is used to demonstrate the solid lesion and to examine the patency of the renal vein and inferior vena cava. CT scanning can also be used to identify the renal lesion and involvement of the renal vein or inferior vena cava. MRI is proving to be better than CT for tumour staging. Renal arteriography will reveal the

tumour's circulation (Fig. 9.40). Urine cytology for malignant cells is of no value. The ESR is usually raised.

### TREATMENT
Treatment is by nephrectomy unless bilateral tumours are present or the contralateral kidney functions poorly, in which case conservative surgery such as partial nephrectomy may be indicated. If metastases are present, nephrectomy may still be warranted since regression of metastases has been reported after removal of the main tumour mass. Severe flank pain may also demand nephrectomy despite the presence of metastases. Radiotherapy has no proven value. Medroxyprogesterone acetate is of some value in controlling metastatic disease. Treatment with interferon-α produces up to a 20% response rate in the short term.

### PROGNOSIS
The prognosis depends upon the degree of differentiation of the tumour and whether or not metastases are present. The 5-year survival rate is 60–70% with tumours confined to the renal parenchyma, 15–35%, with lymph node involvement, and only approximately 5% in those who have distant metastases.

## Nephroblastoma (Wilms' tumour)

This tumour is seen mainly within the first 3 years of life and may be bilateral. It presents as an abdominal mass,

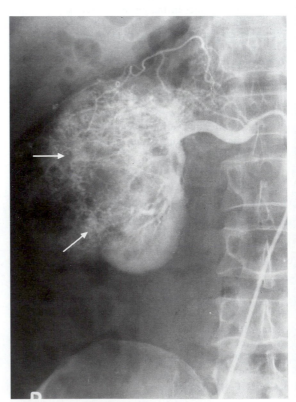

**Fig. 9.40**   Renal arteriogram in a patient with renal carcinoma. Note the abnormal tumour circulation.

rarely with haematuria. Diagnosis is established by excretion urography followed by arteriography. A combination of nephrectomy, radiotherapy and chemotherapy has much improved survival rates, and the majority of children, even those with metastatic disease, are cured.

# BENIGN RENAL TUMOURS

## Renal adenoma

Benign adenomas are usually an incidental finding, presenting as a space-occupying lesion on excretion urography. They seldom cause symptoms. On urography they may be difficult to distinguish from a renal cell carcinoma.

## Simple cysts

Simple cysts are common. They are discussed in more detail on p. 492.

### Differentiation of benign renal cyst from malignant tumour

If a space-occupying lesion is a chance finding on excretion urography in a patient with no relevant symptoms and no haematuria, ultrasonography should be carried out. If the lesion is transonic with no features suggesting a tumour, no further investigation is required. If haematuria has been present, a needle should be inserted into the transonic lesion and cyst fluid aspirated and examined for malignant cells. Contrast medium may be injected to delineate the walls of the cyst. Lesions shown to be solid or non-homogeneous on ultrasonography require further investigation by CT or arteriography.

# UROTHELIAL TUMOURS

The calyces, renal pelvis, ureter, bladder and urethra are lined by transitional cell epithelium. Transitional cell tumours account for about 3% of deaths from all forms of malignancy. Such tumours are uncommon below the age of 40 years, and the male/female ratio is 4 : 1. Bladder tumours are about 50 times as common as those of the ureter or renal pelvis.

## PREDISPOSING FACTORS

These include:
CIGARETTE SMOKING.
EXPOSURE TO INDUSTRIAL CARCINOGENS such as β-naphthylamine and benzidine. Workers in the chemical, cable and rubber industries are at particular risk.
EXPOSURE TO DRUGS, e.g. phenacetin, cyclophosphamide.
CHRONIC INFLAMMATION, e.g. schistosomiasis (usually associated with squamous carcinoma).

## PRESENTATION

Painless haematuria is the commonest presenting symptom of bladder malignancy, although pain may occur owing to clot retention. Symptoms suggestive of UTI may develop in the absence of significant bacteriuria. In patients with bladder cancer, pain may also result from local nerve involvement.

Presenting symptoms may result from local metastases.

Transitional cell carcinomas in the kidney and ureter may present with haematuria. They may also give rise to flank pain, particularly if urinary tract obstruction is present.

## INVESTIGATION

Investigation includes:
CYTOLOGICAL EXAMINATION of urine for malignant cells
EXCRETION UROGRAPHY
CYSTOSCOPY if no evidence of upper urinary tract pathology has been found

Cystoscopy may be omitted in men under 20 and women under 30 years if significant bacteriuria accompanies the haematuria and both cease following control of the infection, and if urine cytology and excretion urography are normal. With these exceptions, it is essential that haematuria is always investigated.

In cases where the tumour is not clearly outlined on excretion urography, abdominal CT scanning and/or retrograde ureterography may be helpful.

## TREATMENT

### Pelvic and ureteric tumours

These are treated by nephroureterectomy. Radiotherapy and chemotherapy appear to be of little or no value.

Subsequently cystoscopy should be regularly carried out, since about half the patients will develop bladder tumours.

### Bladder tumours

Treatment depends upon the stage of the tumour (in particular whether it has penetrated the bladder muscle) and its degree of differentiation. Treatment options include local cystodiathermy and/or resection with follow-up check cystoscopies, cytological examination of urine/cystoscopy, cystectomy, radiotherapy, or local and systemic chemotherapy.

## PROGNOSIS

The prognosis ranges from a 5-year survival rate of 80% for lesions not involving bladder muscle to 5% for those presenting with metastases.

# DISEASES OF THE PROSTATE GLAND

## Benign enlargement of the prostate gland

Benign prostatic enlargement occurs most often in men over the age of 60 years. Such enlargement is much less common in African and Asian individuals. It is unknown in eunuchs. The aetiology of the condition is unknown.

Microscopically, hyperplasia affects the glandular and connective tissue elements of the prostate. Enlargement of the gland stretches and distorts the urethra, obstructing bladder outflow. The bladder musculature hypertrophies so that a higher than usual pressure is generated within the bladder in order to overcome the obstruction and allow voiding of urine. Bands of muscle fibre are seen at cystoscopy (trabeculation). Eventually the bladder becomes dilated and the muscle hypotonic. The sphincter mechanism at the vesicoureteric junction may be impaired and reflux of urine from the bladder into the ureters and upper urinary tract may occur.

### CLINICAL FEATURES
Frequency of urination, usually first noted as nocturia, is a common early symptom. Difficulty or delay in initiating urination, with variability and reduced forcefulness of the urinary stream and post-void dribbling are often present. Suprapubic pain occurs if bladder bacteriuria is present, if a bladder calculus has formed as a result of stagnation of urine within the bladder, or in acute retention of urine. Flank pain may accompany dilatation of the upper tracts. Acute retention of urine (see below) or retention with overflow incontinence may occur. Occasionally, severe haematuria results from rupture of prostatic veins or as a consequence of bacteriuria or stone disease. Some patients present with severe renal failure.

Abdominal examination for bladder enlargement together with examination of the rectum are essential. A benign prostate feels smooth. An accurate impression of prostatic size cannot be obtained on rectal examination.

### INVESTIGATION
This should include urine culture, assessment of renal function by measuring the serum urea and creatinine concentrations, measurement of prostate-specific antigen (markedly raised in prostatic cancer), a plain abdominal X-ray, and renal ultrasonography to define whether upper tract dilatation is present. Excretion urography is not usually necessary. The completeness of bladder emptying after an act of voiding can be assessed by ultrasonography or by inspection of the after-voiding radiograph carried out during excretion urography. Cystourethroscopy is essential.

### MANAGEMENT AND PROGNOSIS
Patients with moderate prostatic symptoms can be treated medically. A number of drugs have been tried including α-blockers. Finasteride is a competitive inhibitor of 5α-reductase, which is the enzyme involved in the conversion of testosterone to dihydrotestosterone. This is the androgen primarily responsible for prostatic growth and enlargement. Finasteride decreases prostatic volume with an increase in urine flow. This new treatment must be compared with transurethral resection which is quick and safe.

Deterioration in renal function or the development of upper tract dilatation requires surgery. Transurethral resection is usually successful unless the gland is very large. It carries a lower morbidity and mortality with a shorter stay in hospital than open prostatectomy. Microwave hyperthermia, balloon dilatation and prostatic stents are all being tried, but long-term results are unavailable as yet. Very large glands require open transvesical prostatectomy.

*In acute retention* or retention with overflow, the first priorities are to relieve pain and to establish urethral catheter drainage. The bladder should be decompressed slowly to prevent bleeding from the mucosa. If urethral catheterization is impossible, suprapubic catheter drainage should be carried out. The choice of further management is then between immediate prostatectomy, a period of catheter drainage followed by prostatectomy, or the acceptance of a permanent indwelling suprapubic or urethral catheter.

# Prostatic carcinoma

Prostatic carcinoma accounts for 7% of all cancers in men and is the fourth commonest cause of death from malignant disease in men in England and Wales. Malignant change within the prostate becomes increasingly common with advancing age. By the age of 80 years, 80% of men have malignant foci within the gland, but most of these appear to lie dormant. Histologically, the tumour is an adenocarcinoma. Hormonal factors are thought to play a role in the aetiology.

### CLINICAL FEATURES
Presentation is usually with symptoms of lower urinary tract obstruction or of metastatic spread, particularly to bone. The diagnosis may be made by the incidental finding of a hard irregular gland on rectal examination or as an unexpected histological result after prostatectomy for what was believed to be benign prostatic hypertrophy.

### INVESTIGATION
Investigation is as for benign enlargement of the prostate gland, with in addition measurement of prostate-specific antigen level, supplemented by transrectal ultrasound of the prostate and prostatic biopsy.

A histological diagnosis is essential before treatment is considered. This may be obtained by:
CYTOLOGICAL STAINING of biopsy material from the prostate
HISTOLOGICAL EXAMINATION of biopsy material or material obtained at transurethral or open prostatectomy

If metastases are present, serum acid phosphatase and serum prostate-specific antigen are usually elevated; it is a myth that elevated levels occur as a result of rectal examination.

Ultrasonography and transrectal ultrasonography are of value in defining the size of the gland and staging any tumour present. The upper renal tracts can be examined by ultrasonography for evidence of dilatation. Bone metastases may appear as osteosclerotic lesions on X-ray or may be detected by isotopic bone scans.

## TREATMENT

Microscopic, not clinically palpable tumour can be managed by watchful waiting. Treatment for disease confined to the gland is radical prostatectomy or radiotherapy, both resulting in an 80–90% 5-year survival. There have, however, been no controlled trials of this therapy and survival may be good without therapy. Locally extensive disease is managed with radiotherapy. Metastatic disease can be treated with orchidectomy, but many men refuse. Luteinizing hormone-releasing hormone (LHRH) analogues such as buserelin or goserelin are equally effective and preferred by many. The addition of an antiandrogen, e.g. cyproterone or flutamide, seems to increase median survival. Non-hormonal chemotherapy is unhelpful.

## PROGNOSIS

The duration of survival depends on the age of the patient and the degree of differentiation and extent of the tumour.

## SCREENING

A yearly rectal examination for men over 40 years of age remains a reasonable screening technique. Transrectal ultrasonography and measurement of serum prostate-specific antigen are being evaluated.

## TESTICULAR TUMOURS

Testicular tumours, though uncommon, are the commonest malignant disease in men between the ages of 29 and 34 years. All such tumours should nowadays be regarded as curable. Patient survival depends upon early diagnosis, accurate staging of the tumour and appropriate treatment and follow-up. The expertise of a specialist centre is invaluable.

More than 96% of testicular tumours arise from germ cells. Two main types of tumour exist:
1 Seminomas (about one-third)
2 Teratomas (about two-thirds)

## AETIOLOGY

The aetiology is unknown. The risk of malignant change is much greater in undescended testes and there is a history of orchidopexy in about 10% of patients.

## CLINICAL FEATURES

Common presenting symptoms are:
- Testicular swelling, which may be painless or painful
- Symptoms from metastases

## DIFFERENTIAL DIAGNOSIS

The differential diagnosis includes:
- Epididymo-orchitis
- Torsion
- Chronic infection, e.g. tuberculosis, syphilitic gumma

## INVESTIGATION

Diagnosis may only be possible after surgical exploration of the testis through the groin. Scrotal exploration and scrotal testicular biopsy should be avoided owing to the high incidence of tumour implantation.

Staging of the tumour will require:
- Chest X-ray to look for metastases
- Estimation of $\alpha$-fetoprotein and $\beta$-human chorionic gonadotrophin concentrations (tumour markers)
- Abdominal CT scanning

## TREATMENT

Seminomas are radiosensitive, so tumours confined to the testis or with metastases below the diaphragm only are treated by radiotherapy. More widespread tumours require chemotherapy.

Teratomas are treated by orchidectomy if the growth is confined to the testis. Chemotherapy is required for more widespread disease (see p. 375).

## Renal disease in the elderly

Renal disease and renal failure are common in the elderly. Acceptance of patients aged 65 years and over for renal replacement therapy approximately doubles the number of such patients in whom renal replacement is initiated.

Renal failure in the elderly more often results from renal vascular disease or urinary tract obstruction than in younger age groups. In males, obstruction is most often due to benign or malignant prostatic enlargement, while in females it results from pelvic cancer.

Progressive sclerosis of glomeruli occurs with ageing and this, together with the development of atheromatous renal vascular disease, accounts for the progressive reduction in GFR seen with advancing years. A GFR of 50–60 ml min$^{-1}$ (about half the normal value for a young adult) may be regarded as 'normal' in patients in their eighties. The reduction in muscle mass often seen with ageing may mask this deterioration in renal function in that the serum creatinine concentration may be less than 0.12 mmol litre$^{-1}$ in an elderly patient whose GFR is 50 ml min$^{-1}$ or lower. The use of serum creatinine as a measure of renal function in the elderly must take this into account. This is especially important in the elderly when prescribing drugs whose excretion is in whole or in part by the kidney.

URINARY TRACT INFECTIONS are more common in the elderly, in whom impaired bladder emptying due to prostatic disease in males and neuropathic bladder—especially common in females—is frequently found. Symptoms may be atypical, the major complaints being incontinence, nocturia, smelly urine or vague change in well-being with little in the way of dysuria. Demonstration of significant bacteriuria in the presence of such symptoms requires treatment.

URINARY INCONTINENCE is one of the major disabilities of the elderly. Correctable factors, such as chronic constipation, infections and treatable bladder outflow impairment need to be excluded. An expert and committed incontinence advisory and treatment service combining nursing and medical skills is invaluable in elderly patients with this distressing problem. Home visits to ensure the availability of commodes and toilets is essential. For established incontinence, catheterization may be necessary.

## Further reading

Cameron JS, Davison AM, Grunfeld JP, Kerr DNS & Ritz E (eds) (1991) *Oxford Textbook of Clinical Nephrology.* Oxford: Oxford University Press.

Coe FL, Parks JH & Asplin JR (1992) Medical progress: The pathogenesis and treatment of kidney stones. *New England Journal of Medicine* **327**, 1141–1152.

Feehally J (1988) Immune mechanisms in glomerular IgA deposition. *Nephrology Dialysis Transplantation* **3**, 361–378.

Jacobson HS (1991) Chronic renal failure: pathophysiology. *Lancet* **338**, 419–423.

Klahr S (1991) Chronic renal failure: management. *Lancet* **338**, 423–427.

Lee DBN, Goodman WG & Coburn JW (1988) Renal osteodystrophy: some new questions on an old disorder. *American Journal of Kidney Diseases* **XI**, 365–376.

Lewis EJ, Hunsicker LG, Bain RP & Rohde RD (1993) The effect  of angiotensin-converting enzyme inhibition on diabetic nephropathy. *New England Journal of Medicine* **329**: 1456–1462.

Nolph KD, Lindblad AS & Novak JW (1988) Current concepts: Continuous ambulatory peritoneal dialysis. *New England Journal of Medicine* **318**, 1595–1600.

Robinson AJ (1994) Antineutrophil cytoplasmic antibodies (ANCA) and the systemic vasculitides. *Nephrology, Dialysis, Transplantation* **9**, 119–126.

Weatherall DJ, Ledingham JGG & Warrell JDA (eds) (1994) *Oxford Textbook of Medicine*, 3rd edn, section on nephrology. Oxford: Oxford University Press.

*Current Opinions in Nephrology and Hypertension*, ed Brenner BM. Current Science. Monthly journal with review articles: each issue devoted to one or two topics.

*Nephrology, Dialysis, Transplantation.* Oxford University Press. This is the major European journal devoted to the subject, with review articles, editorial comments and original papers.

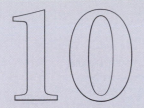

# 10 Water and electrolytes and acid–base homeostasis

## Introduction

In health, the volume and biochemical composition of both extracellular and intracellular fluid compartments in the body remains remarkably constant. Many different disease states result in changes of control either of extracellular fluid volume, leading to clinical abnormalities such as oedema and hypotension or hypertension, or of the electrolyte composition of extracellular fluid. A sensible approach to these abnormalities is therefore essential in a wide range of clinical settings.

## Body fluid compartments

Water accounts for 50–60% of total body weight. This percentage varies with age, sex and body build, being less in women and the obese, as fat has a lower water content. Changes in total body water from one day to the next is, in an individual, reflected by changes in body weight.

In a healthy, 70-kg male, total body water is approximately 42 litres, distributed between several compartments. Two-thirds (28 litres) is intracellular fluid (ICF); the remainder is extracellular fluid (ECF), comprising the interstitial fluid (10.5 litres) and the vascular compartment (3.5 litres).

There is no barrier to the passage of water between the extracellular and intracellular compartments as the distribution of water is governed by osmotic forces and all compartments have the same osmolality (280–290 mosmol kg$^{-1}$). The major intracellular solute is potassium, balanced largely by phosphate and ionic protein, whilst the major extracellular solute is sodium chloride.

Osmolality is determined by the concentration of osmotically active particles. Fully ionized (dissociated) molecules (e.g. NaCl) have twice the osmolality of undissociated particles (urea, glucose). The major determinant of plasma osmolality is sodium concentration: plasma osmolality can be approximated as

$$(2 \times [Na^+]) + [urea] + [glucose],$$

unless there is an unmeasured osmotically active substance present. For instance, plasma alcohol or ethylene glycol concentration can be estimated by subtracting calculated from measured osmolality.

The distribution of extracellular water between the vascular and extravascular (interstitial space) is determined by the equilibrium between hydrostatic and oncotic pressures (Fig. 10.1). The composition of intracellular

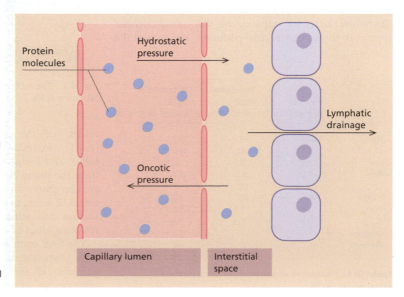

**Fig. 10.1** Distribution of water between the vascular and extravascular (interstitial) spaces is determined by the equilibrium between hydrostatic pressure, which tends to force fluid out of the capillaries, and oncotic pressure, which acts to retain fluid within the vessel. The net flow of fluid outwards is balanced by 'suction' of fluid into the lymphatics, which returns it to the bloodstream. Similar principles govern the volume of the peritoneal and pleural spaces.

and extracellular fluids is shown in Table 10.1.

Figure 10.2 shows the relative effect of the addition of identical volumes of water, saline and colloid solutions on the different compartments. Thus, 1 litre of water given intravenously as 5% dextrose is distributed equally into all compartments, whilst 1 litre of 0.9% saline remains in the extracellular compartment. The latter is thus the correct treatment for extracellular water depletion—sodium keeping the water in this compartment. The addition of 1 litre of colloid with its high oncotic pressure stays in the vascular compartment and is the treatment for hypovolaemia.

### Regulation of extracellular volume (Fig. 10.3)

The extracellular volume is controlled by the total body content of sodium. Sodium is 'diluted' by water to keep it at the right concentration.

It is essential to distinguish between the *concentration* of sodium in the ECF (in practice the plasma sodium) and the *amount* of sodium. Concentration only implies the relative amounts of sodium to water and does not suggest the absolute amounts or volumes of either.

Control of the body's sodium is exerted by tight control over renal excretion. This is achieved by activation of receptors which respond to extracellular volume rather than the change in sodium concentration. These 'volume' receptors can be divided into extrarenal and intrarenal baroreceptors.

EXTRARENAL. These are located in the vascular tree in the left atrium and major thoracic veins and also in the sinus body and aortic arch. These volume receptors respond to a slight reduction in effective circulating volume and result in increased sympathetic nerve activity and a rise in catecholamines. In addition volume receptors in the cardiac atria control the release of a powerful natriuretic hormone—atrial natriuretic peptide (ANP)—from granules located in the atrial walls.

INTRARENAL. Receptors in the walls of the afferent glomerular arterioles respond, via the juxtaglomerular apparatus, to changes in renal perfusion, and control the

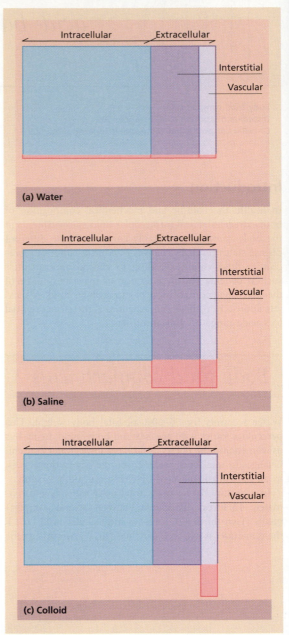

(a) Water

(b) Saline

(c) Colloid

**Fig. 10.2** The relative effects of addition of 1 litre of water (a), saline 0.9% (b), and a colloid solution (c).

activity of the renin–angiotensin–aldosterone system (p. 822). In addition sodium concentration in the distal tubule and sympathetic nerve activity alter renin release from the juxtaglomerular cells. Prostaglandins $I_2$ and $E_2$ are also generated within the kidney in response to angiotensin II, acting to maintain glomerular filtration rate and sodium and water excretion, modulating the sodium-retaining effect of this hormone.

The final common pathway for all the regulatory systems discussed is to increase or decrease the renal excretion of sodium in the event of an increase or decrease in effective circulating blood volume. An

| | Plasma (mmol litre⁻¹) | Interstitial fluid (mmol litre⁻¹) | Intracellular fluid (mmol litre⁻¹) |
|---|---|---|---|
| Na⁺ | 142 | 144 | 10 |
| K⁺ | 4 | 4 | 160 |
| Ca²⁺ | 2.5 | 2.5 | 1.5 |
| Mg²⁺ | 1.0 | 0.5 | 13 |
| Cl⁻ | 102 | 114 | 2 |
| HCO₃⁻ | 26 | 30 | 8 |
| PO₄²⁻ | 1.0 | 1.0 | 57 |
| SO₄²⁻ | 0.5 | 0.5 | 10 |
| Organic acid | 3 | 4 | 3 |
| Protein | 16 | 0 | 55 |

**Table 10.1** Electrolyte composition of intracellular and extracellular fluids.

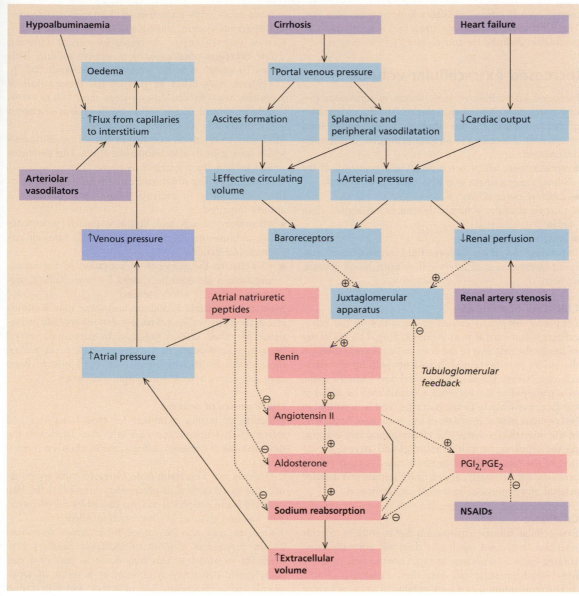

**Fig. 10.3** Regulation of extracellular volume in health and disease.

increase in the reabsorption of salt, with concomitant retention of water (due to a change in osmolality) expands the vascular and interstitial compartments while increased sodium excretion has the opposite effect.

## Regulation of body water content

Body water homeostasis is effected by thirst and the urine concentrating and diluting functions of the kidney. These in turn are controlled by intracellular osmoreceptors, principally in the hypothalamus, to some extent by volume receptors in capacitance vessels close to the heart, and via the renin–angiotensin system. Of these, the major and best-understood control is via osmoreceptors.

An increase in intracellular osmolality—for example

after water deprivation—stimulates both thirst and release of anti-diuretic hormone (ADH) from the posterior pituitary. Thirst stimulates increased water intake while ADH increases the reabsorption of water from the tubular fluid by its action on the distal tubules of the kidney. This causes a reduction in the urine output. The increased intake of water and reduced urinary excretion results in a net gain of water that returns body fluid osmolality to normal. A decrease in intracellular osmolality in the osmoreceptors has the reverse effect. By this method the amount of water in body fluid is adjusted to ensure normal osmolality in the face of varying increase or loss of water or solute.

In addition non-osmotic stimuli may cause ADH

release even if serum osmolality is normal or even low. These include hypovolaemia, stress (e.g. surgery, trauma), psychiatric disturbance and nausea.

# Increased extracellular volume

Increased extracellular volume occurs in numerous disease states. The physical signs depend on the distribution of excess volume and on whether the increase is local or systemic. According to Starling principles, distribution depends on

- venous tone, which determines the capacitance of the blood compartment and thus hydrostatic pressure
- capillary permeability
- oncotic pressure—mainly dependent on serum albumin
- lymphatic drainage

Depending on these factors, fluid accumulation may result in expansion of interstitial volume, blood volume, or both.

## CLINICAL FEATURES

Peripheral oedema is caused by expansion of the extracellular volume by at least 2 litres (15%). The ankles are normally the first part of the body to be affected, although the ankles may be spared in patients with lipodermatosclerosis (where the skin is tethered and cannot expand to accommodate the oedema). Oedema may be noted in the face, particularly in the morning, and in a patient in bed oedema may accumulate in the sacral area. Expansion of the interstitial volume also causes pulmonary oedema, pleural effusion, pericardial effusion and ascites. Expansion of the blood volume causes a raised jugular venous pressure, cardiomegaly, added heart sounds and a raised arterial blood pressure in certain circumstances.

## CAUSES

Extracellular volume expansion is due to sodium chloride retention. Increased salt intake does not normally cause volume expansion because of rapid homeostatic mechanisms which increase salt excretion. However, a rapid intravenous solution of a large volume of saline will cause volume expansion. Thus most causes of extracellular volume expansion are associated with *renal* sodium chloride retention:

HEART FAILURE: due to increased venous pressure causing oedema formation, activation of the renin-angiotensin-aldosterone system, and increased activity of the renal sympathetic nerves.

HYPOALBUMINAEMIA (see Table 9.10, p. 454): the major mechanism is loss of plasma oncotic pressure leading to loss of water from the vascular space to the interstitial space. This activates the renin-angiotensin-aldosterone system. However, other factors may be involved as in the nephrotic syndrome measured plasma volume may be normal, decreased, or increased. There is some evidence that the nephrotic syndrome itself alters renal sodium handling.

HEPATIC CIRRHOSIS: the mechanism is again complex, but involves peripheral vasodilatation, possibly due to

nitric oxide with activation of the renin-angiotensin-aldosterone system causing sodium retention.

RENAL IMPAIRMENT: decreased glomerular filtration rate decreases renal capacity to excrete sodium. This may be acute, as in the acute nephritic syndrome (p. 449), or may occur as part of the presentation of chronic renal failure. In end-stage renal failure extracellular volume is controlled by the balance between salt intake and its removal by dialysis.

Mild sodium retention can also be caused by oestrogens which have a weak aldosterone-like effect. This produces weight gain in the premenstrual phase.

Numerous other *drugs* may cause renal sodium retention, particularly in patients whose renal function is already impaired:

- Mineralocorticoids and liquorice (which potentiates the sodium-retaining action of cortisol) have aldosterone-like actions
- NSAIDs, in the presence of activation of the renin-angiotensin-aldosterone system by heart failure, cirrhosis and renal artery stenosis

Substantial amounts of sodium and water may accumulate in the body without clinically obvious oedema or evidence of raised venous pressure. In particular, several litres may accumulate in the pleural space or as ascites; these spaces are then referred to as 'third spaces'. Bone may also act as a 'sink' for sodium and water.

### Other causes of oedema

Initiation of insulin treatment for type 1 diabetes and refeeding after malnutrition are both associated with the development of transient oedema; the mechanism is complex.

Oedema may also result from increased capillary pressure due to relaxation of precapillary arterioles; the best example is the peripheral oedema caused by dihydropyridine calcium channel blockers such as nifedipine.

Oedema may also be caused by *increased interstitial oncotic pressure* as a result of increased capillary permeability to proteins. This may occur as part of a rare complement-deficiency syndrome; as a result of septicaemia; with therapeutic use of interleukin-2 in cancer chemotherapy; or in ovarian hyperstimulation syndrome.

IDIOPATHIC OEDEMA OF WOMEN, by definition, occurs in women without heart failure, hypoalbuminaemia, renal or endocrine disease. Oedema is intermittent and often worse in the premenstrual phase. The condition remits after the menopause. Patients complain of swelling of the face, hands, breasts and thighs and a feeling of being bloated. Sodium retention during the day and increased sodium excretion during recumbency are characteristic; an abnormal fall in plasma volume on standing caused by increased capillary permeability to proteins may be the cause of this. The oedema may respond to diuretics, but returns when they are stopped. A similar syndrome of diuretic-dependent sodium retention can be caused by abuse of diuretics, for instance as part of an attempt to lose weight, but not all women with idiopathic oedema admit to having taken diuretics, and the syndrome was described before diuretics were introduced for clinical use.

Local increase in oedema does not reflect disturbances of extracellular volume control *per se*, but can cause clinical confusion, e.g. ankle oedema due to venous damage following thrombosis or surgery, ankle or leg oedema due to immobility, oedema of the arm due to subclavian thrombosis, facial oedema due to superior vena caval obstruction. Local loss of oncotic pressure may result from increased capillary permeability to proteins, caused by inflammatory mediators including histamine and interleukins, e.g. bee stings. Lastly, local loss of lymphatic drainage causes lymphoedema (see p. 1026).

## TREATMENT

The underlying cause should be treated where possible. For instance, treat heart failure, or withdraw offending drugs, e.g. NSAIDs.

Sodium restriction has a limited role, but is useful in patients who are resistant to diuretics. Sodium intake can easily be reduced to approximately 100 mmol daily; reductions below this are often difficult to achieve without affecting the palatability of food.

Manoeuvres which increase venous return stimulate salt and water excretion by effects on cardiac output and ANP release. This is the rationale for strict bed rest in congestive cardiac failure. Water immersion also causes redistribution of blood towards the central veins, but is seldom of practical use. Venous compression stockings or bandages may help to mobilize oedema in heart failure.

The mainstay of treatment is the use of diuretic agents, which increase sodium, chloride and water excretion in the kidney (Table 10.2). These agents act by interfering with membrane ion pumps which are present on numerous cell types, but most achieve specificity for the kidney by being secreted into the proximal tubule, resulting in much higher concentrations in the tubular fluid than in other parts of the body.

### Clinical use of diuretics

Loop diuretics are widely used, potent diuretics which are useful in the treatment of any cause of systemic extracellular volume overload. They stimulate excretion of both sodium chloride and water, and are useful in stimulating water excretion in states of relative water overload. They also act by causing increased venous capacitance, resulting in rapid clinical improvement in patients with left ventricular failure, preceding the diuresis. Unwanted effects include:

- Urate retention causing gout
- Hypokalaemia
- Hypomagnesaemia
- Decreased glucose tolerance
- Allergic tubulo-interstitial nephritis and other allergic reactions
- Myalgia (especially with bumetanide)
- Ototoxicity (due to an action on sodium pump activity in the inner ear)—particularly frusemide
- Interference with excretion of lithium, resulting in toxicity

In most situations there is little to choose between the drugs in this class. Ethacrynic acid is now very seldom used because of ototoxicity. Bumetanide has a better oral

| Class | Major action | Examples | Clinical uses | Potency |
|---|---|---|---|---|
| Carbonic anhydrase inhibitors | ↓ Na$^+$ HCO$_3^-$ reabsorption in the proximal tubule<br>↓ Aqueous humour formation | Acetazolamide | Metabolic alkalosis<br>Glaucoma | + |
| Loop diuretics | ↓ Na$^+$ Cl$^-$ K$^+$ cotransport in thick ascending limb | Frusemide<br>Bumetanide<br>Piretanide | Volume overload (CCF, nephrotic syndrome, CRF)<br>Sodium-dependent hypertension<br>Hypercalcaemia<br>?Acute renal failure<br>SIADH | +++ |
| Thiazide diuretics | ↓ Na$^+$ Cl$^-$ cotransport early distal tubule | Bendrofluazide<br>Hydrochlorothiazide<br>Metolazone | Hypertension<br>Volume overload (CCF)<br>Hypercalciuria | ++ |
| Potassium sparing | ↓ Na$^+$ reabsorption (in exchange for K$^+$) collecting duct | Aldosterone antagonist e.g. spironolactone<br>Others:<br>Amiloride<br>Triamterene | Hyperaldosteronism (primary and secondary)<br>Bartter's syndrome<br>Prevention of K$^+$ deficiency in combination with loop or thiazide<br>Cirrhosis with fluid overload | + |

CCF, congestive cardiac failure.
CRF, chronic renal failure.

**Table 10.2** Types and clinical uses of diuretics.

bioavailability, particularly in patients with severe peripheral oedema, and may have more beneficial effects on venous capacitance in left ventricular failure than frusemide. It may cause severe muscle cramps when used in high doses.

THIAZIDE DIURETICS are weaker diuretics than loop diuretics. They cause relatively more urate retention, glucose intolerance and hypokalaemia. They interfere with water excretion and may cause hyponatraemia, particularly if combined with amiloride or triamterene. This effect is clinically useful in diabetes insipidus. Thiazides reduce peripheral vascular resistance by mechanisms which are not completely understood but which do not appear to depend on their diuretic action, and are widely used in the treatment of essential hypertension. They are also used extensively in mild to moderate cardiac failure. Thiazides reduce calcium excretion. This effect is useful in patients with idiopathic hypercalciuria, but may cause hypercalcaemia. Numerous agents are available, with varying half-lives but little else to choose between them. Metolazone is not dependent for its action on glomerular filtration, and therefore retains its potency in renal impairment.

POTASSIUM-SPARING DIURETICS are relatively weak and are most often used in combination with thiazides or loop diuretics to prevent potassium depletion. These are of two types. Spironolactone, an aldosterone antagonist, competes with aldosterone in the collecting ducts reducing sodium absorption. Amiloride and triamterene inhibit sodium uptake in collecting duct epithelial cells and reduce renal potassium excretion.

CARBONIC ANHYDRASE INHIBITORS are relatively weak diuretics and are seldom used except in the treatment of glaucoma. They may cause metabolic acidosis and hypokalaemia.

RESISTANCE TO DIURETICS may occur as a result of:
- Poor bioavailability
- Reduced GFR, which may be due to decreased circulating volume despite oedema (e.g. nephrotic syndrome, local causes of oedema) or intrinsic renal disease
- Activation of sodium-retaining mechanisms, particularly aldosterone

Intravenous administration may establish a diuresis. High doses of loop diuretics may be required to achieve adequate concentrations in the tubule if GFR is depressed: the daily dose of frusemide must be limited to a maximum of 2 g for an adult, because of ototoxicity. Intravenous albumin solutions restore plasma oncotic pressure temporarily in the nephrotic syndrome and may allow mobilization of oedema. Combinations of different classes of diuretics are extremely helpful in patients with resistant oedema. A loop diuretic plus a thiazide inhibits two major sites of sodium reabsorption; this effect may be further potentiated by addition of a potassium-sparing agent. Metolazone in combination with a loop diuretic is particularly useful in refractory congestive cardiac failure,

because its action is less dependent on glomerular filtration. However, this potent combination can cause severe electrolyte imbalance.

Both aminophylline and dopamine increase renal blood flow and may be useful in refractory cardiogenic sodium retention.

EFFECTS ON RENAL FUNCTION. All diuretics may increase blood urea concentrations by increasing urea reabsorption in the medulla. Thiazides may also promote protein breakdown. In certain situations diuretics may also decrease GFR:
- Excessive diuresis may cause volume depletion and prerenal failure.
- Diuretics may cause allergic tubulo-interstitial nephritis.
- Thiazides may directly cause a drop in GFR; the mechanism is complex.

# Decreased extracellular volume

Deficiency of sodium and water causes shrinkage both of the interstitial space and of the blood volume and may have profound effects on organ function.

## CLINICAL FEATURES

SYMPTOMS are variable. Thirst, muscle cramps, nausea and vomiting, and postural dizziness may occur. Severe depletion of circulating volume causes hypotension and impairs cerebral perfusion, causing confusion and eventual coma.

SIGNS can be divided into those due to loss of interstitial fluid and those due to loss of circulating volume.

Loss of interstitial fluid leads to loss of skin elasticity ('turgor')—the rapidity with which the skin recoils to normal after being pinched. Skin turgor decreases with age, particularly at the peripheries. The turgor over the anterior triangle of the neck or on the forehead is a very useful sign in all ages.

Loss of circulating volume leads to decreased pressure in the venous and (if severe) arterial compartments. Loss of up to 1 litre of extracellular fluid in an adult may be compensated for by venoconstriction and may cause no physical signs. Loss of more than this causes:

POSTURAL HYPOTENSION. Normally the blood pressure rises if a subject stands up, as a result of increased venous return due to venoconstriction (this maintains cerebral perfusion). Loss of extracellular fluid prevents this and causes a fall in blood pressure. This is one of the earliest and most reliable signs of volume depletion, as long as the other causes of postural hypotension are excluded (Table 10.3).

LOW JUGULAR VENOUS PRESSURE. In hypovolaemic patients, the jugular venous pulsation can only be seen with the patient lying completely flat, or even head down, because the left atrial pressure is lower than $5 \text{ cmH}_2\text{O}$.

PERIPHERAL VENOCONSTRICTION causes cold skin

Decreased circulating volume (hypovolaemia)

Autonomic failure
  Diabetes
  Systemic amyloidosis
  Shy–Drager syndrome

Interference with autonomic function by drugs
  Ganglion blockers
  Tricyclic antidepressants

Interference with peripheral vasoconstriction by drugs
  Nitrates
  Calcium channel blockers
  Alpha-adrenergic receptor antagonists

Prolonged bed-rest (cardiovascular deconditioning)

**Table 10.3**  Some causes of a fall in blood pressure from lying to standing (postural hypotension).

*Haemorrhage*
External
Concealed, e.g. leaking aortic aneurysm

*Burns*

*Gastrointestinal losses*
Vomiting
Diarrhoea
Ileostomy losses

*Renal losses*
Diuretic use
Impaired tubular sodium conservation
  Reflux nephropathy
  Papillary necrosis
    Analgesic nephropathy
    Diabetes
    Sickle cell disease

**Table 10.4**  Causes of extracellular volume depletion.

with empty peripheral veins, which are difficult to cannulate, just when the patient needs intravenous therapy the most! This sign is absent in sepsis, where peripheral vasodilatation contributes to effective hypovolaemia.

TACHYCARDIA (not always reliable). Beta-blockers and other antiarrhythmics may prevent this and hypovolaemia may activate vagal mechanisms and actually cause bradycardia.

ARTERIAL HYPOTENSION. A late sign.

## CAUSES

Salt and water may be lost either from the kidneys, from the gastrointestinal tract, or from the skin. Examples are given in Table 10.4.

In addition to these causes, there are a number of situations where signs of volume depletion occur despite a normal or increased body content of sodium and water:

1 Septicaemia causes vasodilatation both of arterioles and veins, resulting in greatly increased capacitance of the vascular space. In addition, increased capillary permeability to plasma proteins leads to loss of fluid from the vascular space to the interstitium.
2 Diuretic treatment of heart failure or nephrotic syndrome may lead to rapid reduction in plasma volume; mobilization of oedema may take much longer.
3 Inappropriate diuretic treatment of oedema e.g. when the cause is local rather than systemic.

| | Na$^+$ (mmol litre$^{-1}$) | K$^+$ (mmol litre$^{-1}$) | HCO$_3^-$ or equivalent (mmol litre$^{-1}$) | Cl$^-$ (mmol litre$^{-1}$) | Ca$^{2+}$ (mmol litre$^{-1}$) | Indication (see footnotes) |
|---|---|---|---|---|---|---|
| Normal plasma values | 142 | 4.5 | 26 | 103 | 2.5 | |
| Sodium chloride 0.9% ('normal saline') | 150 | — | — | 150 | — | 1 |
| Sodium chloride 0.18% + glucose 4% ('1/5 normal saline') | 30 | — | — | 30 | — | 2 |
| Glucose 5% | — | — | — | — | — | 3 |
| Sodium bicarbonate 1.26% | 150 | — | 150 | — | — | 4 |
| Compound sodium lactate (Hartmann's) | 131 | 5 | 29 | 111 | 2 | 5 |

1. Volume expansion in hypovolaemic patients. Rarely to maintain fluid balance when there are large doses of sodium. The sodium (150 mmol litre$^{-1}$) is greater than plasma and hypernatraemia can result. It is often necessary to add KCl 20–40 mmol litre$^{-1}$.
2. Maintenance of fluid balance in normovolaemic, normonatraemic patients.
3. To replace *water*. May be alternated with normal saline as an alternative to (2).
4. For volume expansion in hypovolaemic, *acidotic* patients alternating with (1). Occasionally for maintenance of fluid balance combined with (2) in salt-wasting, acidotic patients. To induce forced alkaline diuresis, e.g. in severe salicylate poisoning.
5. Used for maintenance of fluid balance after surgery. The potassium content may be dangerous in renal failure but occasionally useful in the diuretic phase of acute tubular necrosis where hypokalaemia occurs.

**Table 10.5**  Intravenous fluids in general use for fluid and electrolyte disturbances.

## INVESTIGATION

Blood tests are in general not helpful in assessment of extracellular volume. Blood urea may be raised due to increased urea reabsorption and, later, to prerenal failure (when the creatinine rises as well) but is very non-specific. Urinary sodium is low if the kidneys are functioning normally, but is misleading if the cause of the volume depletion involves the kidneys (e.g. diuretics, intrinsic renal disease). Urine osmolality is high in volume depletion (due to increased water reabsorption) but may also often mislead.

## TREATMENT

The overriding principle is: aim to replace what is missing.

HAEMORRHAGE involves the loss of whole blood. The rational treatment of acute haemorrhage is therefore whole blood, or a combination of red cells and a plasma substitute. (Chronic anaemia causes salt and water retention rather than volume depletion; correction therefore involves replacement of red cells with the minimum of salt, water and albumin, combined with diuretics.)

LOSS OF PLASMA, as in burns or severe peritonitis, should be treated with human plasma or a plasma substitute (see p. 721).

LOSS OF WATER AND ELECTROLYTES, as in vomiting, diarrhoea, or excessive renal losses, should be treated by replacement of water and electrolytes. If possible, this should be done with oral water and sodium salts. These are available as slow sodium 600 mg (approximately 10 mmol NaCl per tablet). The usual dose is 6–12 tablets per day with 2–3 litres of water. It is used in mild or chronic salt and water depletion, e.g. associated with renal salt wasting.

Sodium bicarbonate 500 mg (6 mmol $NaHCO_3$ per tablet) is used in doses of 6–12 tablets per day with 2–3 litres of water. This is used in milder chronic sodium depletion with acidosis, e.g. chronic renal failure, post-obstructive renal failure, renal tubular acidosis. Sodium bicarbonate is less effective in causing positive sodium balance than sodium chloride.

Oral rehydration solutions are described in Table 1.16 (see p. 30). Intravenous fluids may sometimes be required (Table 10.5). Rapid infusion (e.g. 1000 ml hour$^{-1}$ or even faster) is necessary if there is hypotension and evidence of impaired organ perfusion (e.g. oliguria, confusion); in these situations plasma expanders (colloids) are often used in the first instance to restore an adequate circulating volume (see p. 721). Repeated clinical assessments are vital in this situation, usually complemented by frequent measurements of central venous pressure (see Management of Shock, p. 720). Severe hypovolaemia induces venoconstriction, which maintains venous return; over-rapid correction does not give time for this to reverse, resulting in signs of circulatory overload (e.g. pulmonary oedema) even if a total body ECF deficit remains. In less severe ECF depletion, (e.g. a patient with postural hypo-

tension complicating acute tubular necrosis) the fluid should be replaced at a rate of 1000 ml every 4–6 hours, again with repeated clinical assessment. If all that is required is avoidance of fluid depletion during surgery, 1–2 litres may be given over 24 hours, remembering that surgery is a stimulus to sodium and water retention and that over-replacement may be as dangerous as under-replacement.

LOSS OF WATER ALONE only causes extracellular volume depletion in severe cases, because the loss is spread evenly between all the compartments of body water. In the rare situations where there is a true deficiency of water alone, as in diabetes insipidus in a patient who is unable to drink (after surgery, for instance), the correct treatment is to give water. If intravenous treatment is required, water is given as 5% dextrose, because pure water would lead to osmotic lysis of blood cells.

# Disorders of sodium concentration

These are best thought of as disorders of body water content. As discussed above, sodium content is regulated by volume receptors; water content is adjusted to maintain, in health, a normal osmolality and (in the absence of abnormal osmotically active solutes) a normal sodium concentration. Disturbances of *sodium concentration* are caused by disturbances of *water* balance.

## HYPONATRAEMIA

Hyponatraemia is one of the commonest abnormalities detected in biochemistry laboratories. It may be associated with normal (Table 10.6), decreased (Table 10.7), or increased (Table 10.8) extracellular volume and total body sodium content. The differential diagnosis of hyponatraemia depends on an assessment of extracellular volume. Rarely hyponatraemia may be pseudohyponatraemia, where in hyperlipidaemia or hyperproteinaemia there is a spuriously low measured sodium concentration, the sodium being confined to the aqueous phase but having its concentration expressed in terms of the total volume of plasma. In this situation plasma osmolality is normal and therefore treatment of 'hyponatraemia' is unnecessary. It is also important to exclude artefactual 'hyponatraemia' caused by taking blood from the limb into which fluid of low sodium concentration is being infused.

### Salt-deficient hyponatraemia

This is due to salt loss in excess of water; the causes are listed in Table 10.7. In this situation ADH secretion is initially suppressed (via the hypothalamic

Abnormal ADH release
  Vagal neuropathy (failure of inhibition of ADH
    release)
  Deficiency of ACTH or glucocorticoids (Addison's
    disease)
  Hypothyroidism
  Severe potassium depletion

Syndrome of inappropriate antidiuretic hormone (see
    Table 16.38)

Stress
  Surgery
  Nausea

Major psychiatric illness
  'Psychogenic polydipsia'
  Non-osmotic ADH release?

Increased sensitivity to ADH
  Chlorpropamide
  Tolbutamide

ADH-like substances
  Oxytocin
  DDAVP

Unmeasured osmotically active substances stimulating
    osmotic ADH release
  Glucose
  Alcohol
  Mannitol
  Sick cell syndrome (leakage of intracellular ions)

**Table 10.6**  Causes of hyponatraemia with normal
extracellular volume.

Gut
  Vomiting
  Diarrhoea
  Haemorrhage

Kidney
  Osmotic diuresis (e.g. hyperglycaemia, severe uraemia)
  Excessive use of diuretics
  Adrenocortical insufficency
  Tubulo-interstitial renal disease
  Unilateral renal artery stenosis
  Recovery phase of acute tubular necrosis

**Table 10.7**  Causes of hyponatraemia with decreased
extracellular volume.

Heart failure
Liver failure
Oliguric renal failure
Hypoalbuminaemia

**Table 10.8**  Causes of hyponatraemia with increased
extracellular volume.

osmoreceptors), but as fluid volume is lost, volume receptors override the osmoreceptors and stimulate both thirst and the release of ADH. This is an attempt by the body to defend circulating volume at the expense of osmolality.

With extrarenal losses and normal kidneys, the urinary excretion of sodium falls in response to the volume depletion, as does water excretion, leading to concentrated urine containing less than 10 mmol litre$^{-1}$ of sodium. However, in salt wasting kidney disease, renal compensation cannot occur and the only physiological protection is increased water intake in response to thirst.

### CLINICAL FEATURES
With sodium depletion the clinical picture is usually dominated by features of volume depletion (p. 504).

The diagnosis is usually obvious where there is a history of gut losses, diabetes mellitus or diuretic abuse. Table 10.9 shows the potential daily losses of water and electrolytes from the gut. Losses due to renal or adrenocortical disease may be less easily identified and are suggested by a urinary sodium concentration of more than 20 mmol litre$^{-1}$ in the presence of clinically evident volume depletion.

### TREATMENT
This is directed at the primary cause whenever possible. Increased salt intake as Slow Sodium 60–80 mmol daily is all that is required in the relatively healthy patient who can take this by mouth. In the face of vomiting or severe volume depletion, intravenous infusion of normal saline is given. Potassium supplements and correction of acid–base abnormalities may also be required.

## Hyponatraemia due to water excess

This results from an intake of water in excess of the kidney's ability to excrete it. It is uncommon with normal

| | Na$^+$ (mmol litre$^{-1}$) | K$^+$ (mmol litre$^{-1}$) | Cl$^-$ (mmol litre$^{-1}$) | Volume (ml 24 hours) |
|---|---|---|---|---|
| Stomach | 50 | 10 | 110 | 2500 |
| Small intestine | | | | |
|   Recent ileostomy | 120 | 5 | 110 | 1500 |
|   Adapted ileostomy | 50 | 4 | 25 | 500 |
|   Bile | 140 | 5 | 105 | 500 |
|   Pancreatic juice | 140 | 5 | 60 | 2000 |
| Diarrhoea | 130 | 10–15 | 95 | 1000–2000+ |

**Table 10.9**  Average concentrations and potential daily losses of water and electrolytes from the gut.

kidney function, requiring an intake of approximately 1 litre hour$^{-1}$. Overgenerous infusion of 5% glucose into postoperative patients is one of the commonest causes, in which situation it is exacerbated by increased ADH secretion in response to stress. Some degree of hyponatraemia is usual in acute oliguric renal failure, while in chronic renal failure it is most often due to ill-given advice to 'push' fluids.

The commonest presentation of hyponatraemia due to water excess is in patients with severe cardiac failure, hepatic cirrhosis or the nephrotic syndrome in which there is evidence of volume overload. In all these conditions there is usually an element of reduced glomerular filtration rate with avid reabsorption of sodium and chloride in the proximal tubule. This leads to reduced delivery of chloride to the 'diluting' ascending limb of Henle's loop and a reduced ability to generate 'free water', with a consequent inability to excrete dilute urine. This is commonly compounded by the administration of diuretics that block chloride reabsorption and interfere with the dilution of filtrate either in Henle's loop (loop diuretics) or distally (thiazides).

### CLINICAL FEATURES

Symptoms are common with dilutional hyponatraemia when this develops acutely. They are principally neurological and are due to the movement of water into brain cells in response to the fall in extracellular osmolality. Symptoms rarely occur until the serum sodium is less than 120 mmol litre$^{-1}$ and are more usually associated with values around 110 mmol litre$^{-1}$ or lower. Symptoms and signs of hyponatraemia are non-specific and include headache, confusion, and restlessness leading to drowsiness, myoclonic jerks, generalized convulsions and eventually coma. Other features depend on the cause, e.g. signs of congestive cardiac failure or liver disease.

### INVESTIGATION

No further investigation of hyponatraemia is usually necessary if it is associated with clinically detectable extracellular volume excess. The cause of hyponatraemia with apparently normal extracellular volume is usually less obvious, and this category requires careful investigation to:
- exclude Addison's disease
- exclude hypothyroidism
- consider 'syndrome of inappropriate ADH secretion' (SIADH) (p. 821) and drug-induced water retention
- remember potassium and magnesium depletion potentiate ADH release and are an important cause of diuretic-associated hyponatraemia

The syndrome of inappropriate ADH secretion is often over-diagnosed. Some causes are associated with a lower set point for ADH release, rather than completely autonomous ADH release; an example is chronic alcohol abuse.

### TREATMENT

The underlying cause should be corrected where possible. Most cases are simply managed by restriction of water intake (to 1000 or even 500 ml per day) with review of diuretic therapy. Magnesium and potassium deficiency must be corrected. The use of hypertonic saline is restricted to patients with acute water retention in which there are severe neurological signs, e.g. fits and coma. It must be given slowly (not more than 70 mmol per hour) the aim being to increase the serum sodium to more than 125 mmol litre$^{-1}$. If hyponatraemia has developed slowly, as in the majority of patients, the brain will have adapted by decreasing intracellular osmolality; a rapid rise in extracellular osmolality, particularly if there is an 'overshoot' to high serum sodium and osmolality will then result in severe shrinking of brain cells, and the syndrome of 'central pontine myelinolysis', which may be fatal. Hypertonic saline must not be given to patients who are already fluid overloaded because of the risk of acute heart failure; in this situation 100 ml of 20% mannitol may be infused in an attempt to increase renal water excretion.

## Syndrome of inappropriate ADH secretion

This is described in Chapter 16.

## HYPERNATRAEMIA

This is much rarer than hyponatraemia and nearly always indicates a water deficit. This may be due to (Table 10.10):
- Pituitary diabetes insipidus (see p. 820) (failure of ADH secretion)
- Nephrogenic diabetes insipidus (failure of response to ADH)
- Osmotic diuresis
- Excessive loss of water through the skin or lungs

Excessive administration of hypertonic sodium may also contribute, for example:
- Excessive reliance on 0.9% (150 mmol litre$^{-1}$) saline for volume replacement
- Administration of drugs with a high sodium content, e.g. piperacillin
- Use of 8.4% sodium bicarbonate after cardiac arrest

ADH deficiency
  Diabetes insipidus (p. 820)

Iatrogenic
  Administration of hypertonic sodium solutions

Insensitivity to ADH (nephrogenic diabetes insipidus)
  Lithium
  Tetracyclines
  Amphotericin B
  Acute tubular necrosis

Osmotic diuresis
  Total parenteral nutrition
  Hyperosmolar diabetic coma

*Plus*
Deficient water intake

**Table 10.10**  Causes of hypernatraemia.

Hypernatraemia is always associated with increased plasma osmolality, which is a potent stimulus to thirst. None of the above causes hypernatraemia unless thirst sensation is abnormal or access to water limited. For instance, a patient with diabetes insipidus will maintain a normal serum sodium concentration by maintaining a high water intake until an intercurrent illness prevents this. Thirst is frequently deficient in elderly people, making them more prone to water depletion. Hypernatraemia may occur in the presence of normal, reduced or expanded extracellular volume, and does not necessarily imply that total body sodium is increased.

## CLINICAL FEATURES

SYMPTOMS of hypernatraemia are non-specific. Nausea, vomiting, fever and confusion may occur. A history of long-standing polyuria, polydipsia and thirst suggests diabetes insipidus. There may be clues to a pituitary cause. A drug history may reveal ingestion of nephrotoxic drugs.

SIGNS. Assessment of extracellular volume status is important in guiding resuscitation. Mental state should be assessed. Convulsions occur in severe hypernatraemia.

## INVESTIGATION

Simultaneous urine and plasma osmolality and sodium should be measured. Serum osmolality is high in hypernatraemia. Passage of urine with an osmolality lower than that of plasma in this situation is clearly abnormal and indicates diabetes insipidus. In pituitary diabetes insipidus, urine osmolality will increase after administration of desmopressin; the drug (a vasopressin analogue) has no effect in nephrogenic diabetes insipidus. If urine osmolality is high this suggests either an osmotic diuresis due to an unmeasured solute (e.g. in parenteral feeding) or excessive extra-renal loss of water (e.g. heat stroke).

## TREATMENT

Treatment is that of the underlying cause: replacement of ADH in the form of desmopressin, a stable non-pressor analogue of ADH, in ADH deficiency; withdrawal of nephrogenic drugs where possible; and replacement of water, either orally, if possible, or intravenously. In severe ($>170$ mmol litre$^{-1}$) hypernatraemia 0.9% (150 mmol litre$^{-1}$) saline should be used initially, to avoid too rapid a drop in serum sodium concentration; the aim is correction over 48 hours, as over-rapid correction may lead to cerebral oedema. In less severe (e.g. $>150$ mmol litre$^{-1}$) hypernatraemia the treatment is 5% dextrose or 0.45% saline; the latter is obviously preferable in hyperosmolar diabetic coma. Very large volumes—5 litres a day or more—may need to be given in diabetes insipidus.

If there is clinical evidence of volume depletion (see p. 504), this implies that there is a sodium deficit as well as a water deficit. Treatment of this is discussed on p. 506.

# Disorders of potassium content and concentration

## Regulation of serum potassium concentration

The usual dietary intake varies between 80 and 150 mmol daily depending upon fruit and vegetable intake. Most of the body's potassium (3500 mmol in an adult man) is intracellular. Serum potassium levels are controlled by:

- Uptake of K$^+$ into cells
- Renal excretion
- Extra-renal losses (e.g. gastrointestinal)

Uptake of potassium into cells is governed by the activity of the Na$^+$, K$^+$ ATPase in the cell membrane and by H$^+$ concentration. Uptake is stimulated by:

- Insulin
- Beta-adrenergic stimulation
- Theophyllines

and decreased by:

- Alpha-adrenergic stimulation
- Acidosis—K$^+$ exchanged for H$^+$ across cell membrane
- Cell damage or cell death—resulting in massive K$^+$ release.

Excretion of potassium is increased by aldosterone, which stimulates K$^+$ and H$^+$ secretion in exchange for Na$^+$ in the collecting duct. Because H$^+$ and K$^+$ are interchangeable in the exchange mechanism, acidosis decreases and alkalosis increases the secretion of K$^+$. Aldosterone secretion is stimulated by hyperkalaemia and increased angiotensin II levels, as well as by some drugs, and acts to protect the body against hyperkalaemia and against extracellular volume depletion. The body adapts to dietary deficiency of potassium by reducing aldosterone secretion. However, because aldosterone is also influenced by volume status, conservation of potassium is relatively inefficient, and significant potassium depletion may therefore result from prolonged dietary deficiency.

A number of drugs affect K$^+$ homeostasis by affecting aldosterone release (e.g. heparin, NSAIDs) or by directly affecting renal potassium handling.

Normally only about 10% of daily potassium intake is excreted in the gastrointestinal tract. Vomit contains around 5–10 mmol litre$^{-1}$ K$^+$, but prolonged vomiting may cause hypokalaemia by inducing sodium depletion, stimulating aldosterone, which increases renal potassium excretion. Potassium may be secreted by the colon, and diarrhoea contains 10–50 mmol litre$^{-1}$ K$^+$; profuse diarrhoea can therefore induce marked hypokalaemia. Villous adenomas may rarely produce profuse diarrhoea and K$^+$ loss.

## HYPOKALAEMIA

### CAUSES

The commonest causes of chronic hypokalaemia are diuretic treatment (particularly thiazides) and hyperaldosteronism. Acute hypokalaemia is more often caused by redistribution into cells. The common causes are shown in Table 10.11.

### Rare causes

BARTTER'S SYNDROME consists of hypokalaemia, alkalosis, normal blood pressure, and elevated plasma renin and aldosterone. Numerous causes of this syndrome probably exist. Diagnostic pointers include high urinary potassium and chloride despite low serum values, increased plasma renin, hyperplasia of the juxtaglomerular apparatus on renal biopsy, and careful exclusion of diuretic abuse. Excess production of renal prostaglandins is often found. Magnesium wasting may also occur.

LIDDLE'S SYNDROME is also characterized by potassium wasting, hypokalaemia, and alkalosis, but is associated with low aldosterone production and high blood pressure.

HYPOKALAEMIC PERIODIC PARALYSIS may be precipitated by carbohydrate intake, suggesting that insulin-mediated potassium influx into cells may be responsible. This syndrome also occurs in association with hyperthyroidism in Chinese patients.

### CLINICAL FEATURES

Hypokalaemia is usually asymptomatic, but severe hypokalaemia may cause muscle weakness. Potassium depletion may also cause symptomatic hyponatraemia (see p. 506).

Hypokalaemia is associated with an increased frequency of atrial and ventricular ectopic beats. This association may not always be causal, because adrenergic activation (for instance after myocardial infarction) causes both hypokalaemia and increased cardiac irritability. Hypokalaemia in patients without cardiac disease is unlikely to lead to serious arrhythmias.

Hypokalaemia seriously increases the risk of digoxin toxicity by increasing binding of digoxin to cardiac cells, potentiating its action, and decreasing its clearance. The same may be true of some other drugs which cause arrhythmias.

Chronic hypokalaemia is associated with interstitial renal disease, but the pathogenesis is not completely understood.

### TREATMENT

The underlying cause should be identified and treated where possible; for examples see Table 10.12.

Acute hypokalaemia may correct spontaneously. In most cases, withdrawal of oral diuretics or purgation, accompanied by the oral administration of potassium supplements in the form of slow-releasing potassium or effervescent potassium, is all that is required. Intravenous potassium replacement is only required in conditions such as cardiac arrhythmias, muscle weakness or severe diabetic ketoacidosis when the potassium is <2.5 mmol litre$^{-1}$. When used, intravenous therapy must take account of renal function and replacement at rates >20 mmol hour$^{-1}$ should only be used with hourly

---

*Increased renal excretion*
Diuretics
  Thiazides
  Loop diuretics
Increased aldosterone secretion
  Liver failure
  Heart failure
  Nephrotic syndrome
  Conn's syndrome
  ACTH-producing tumours
Exogenous mineralocorticoid
  Corticosteroids
  Carbenoxolone
  Liquorice (potentiates renal actions of cortisol)
Renal tubular acidosis type 1 and 2
Renal tubular damage
  Acute leukaemia
  Cytotoxic treatment
  Nephrotoxicity
    Amphotericin
    Aminoglycosides
Bartter's syndrome
Liddle's syndrome

*Severe dietary deficiency*

*Redistribution into cells*
Beta-adrenergic stimulation
  Acute myocardial infarction
  Beta-agonists
    Fenoterol, salbutamol
Insulin treatment, e.g.
  treatment of diabetic ketoacidosis
Correction of megaloblastic anaemia
Alkalosis
Hypokalaemic periodic paralysis

*Gastrointestinal losses*
Vomiting
Severe diarrhoea
Purgative abuse
Villous adenoma
Ileostomy or uterosigmoidostomy
Fistulae

**Table 10.11**  Causes of hypokalaemia.

---

| Cause | Treatment |
|---|---|
| Dietary deficiency | Increase intake of fresh fruit/vegetables or oral potassium supplements (20–40 mmol daily). (Potassium supplements can cause gastrointestinal irritation) |
| Hyperaldosteronism | Spironolactone or, in heart failure, ACE inhibitors |
| Thiazides | Co-prescription of a potassium-sparing diuretic with a similar onset and duration of action. |
| Bartter's syndrome | Amiloride with or without indomethacin. |

**Table 10.12**  Treatment of hypokalaemia, as a function of its cause.

monitoring of serum potassium and ECG changes.

The treatment of adrenal disorders is described on p. 814.

Failure to correct hypokalaemia may be due to concurrent hypomagnesaemia; serum magnesium should be measured and deficiency corrected.

# HYPERKALAEMIA

## CAUSES

Acute self-limiting hyperkalaemia occurs normally after vigorous exercise and is of no pathological significance. Hyperkalaemia in all other situations is due either to increased release from cells or to failure of excretion (Table 10.13). The commonest causes are renal impairment and drug interference with potassium excretion. The combination of ACE inhibitors with potassium-sparing diuretics or NSAIDs is particularly dangerous.

### Rare causes

HYPORENINAEMIC HYPOALDOSTERONISM is also known as type 4 renal tubular acidosis (see p. 517).

PSEUDOHYPOALDOSTERONISM is a disease of infancy apparently due to resistance to the action of aldosterone, characterized by hyperkalaemia and evidence of sodium wasting (hyponatraemia, extracellular volume depletion).

HYPERKALAEMIC PERIODIC PARALYSIS is precipitated by exercise, and is caused by a genetically determined abnormality of the sodium pump.

GORDON'S SYNDROME appears to be a mirror image of Bartter's syndrome, in which primary renal retention of sodium causes hypertension, volume expansion, low renin/aldosterone, hyperkalaemia and acidosis. The disorder may be due to deficiency of ANP.

SUXAMETHONIUM AND OTHER DEPOLARIZING MUSCLE RELAXANTS cause release of potassium from cells. Induction of muscle paralysis during general anaesthesia may result in a rise of plasma potassium of up to 1 mmol litre$^{-1}$. This is not usually a problem unless there is pre-existing hyperkalaemia.

## CLINICAL FEATURES

Serum potassium of greater than 7.0 mmol litre$^{-1}$l is a medical emergency and is associated with ECG changes (Fig. 10.4). Severe hyperkalaemia may be asymptomatic and may predispose to sudden death from asystolic cardiac arrest. Muscle weakness is often the only symptom, unless (as is commonly the case) the hyperkalaemia is associated with metabolic acidosis, causing Kussmaul respiration. Hyperkalaemia causes hyperpolarization of cell membranes leading to decreased cardiac excitability, hypotension, bradycardia, and eventual asystole.

---

*Decreased excretion*
Renal failure
Drug: direct effect on potassium handling
  Amiloride
  Triamterene
  Spironolactone
Aldosterone deficiency
Hyporeninaemic hypoaldosteronism
Addison's disease
ACE inhibitors
NSAIDs
Cyclosporin treatment
Heparin treatment
Acidosis
Gordon's syndrome

*Increased release from cells (decreased Na$^+$, K$^+$ ATPase activity)*
Acidosis
Diabetic ketoacidosis
Rhabdomyolysis
Tumour lysis
Succinylcholine (amplified by muscle denervation)
Digoxin poisoning
Vigorous exercise (alpha-adrenergic: transient)

*Increased extraneous load*
Potassium chloride
  Iatrogenic
  Salt substitutes
Potassium citrate
Transfusion of stored blood
Transfusion of irradiated blood

*Spurious*
Increased *in vitro* release from abnormal cells
  Leukaemia
  Infectious mononucleosis
  Thrombocytosis
  Familial pseudohyperkalaemia
Increased release from muscles
  Vigorous fist clenching during phlebotomy

**Table 10.13**  Causes of hyperkalaemia.

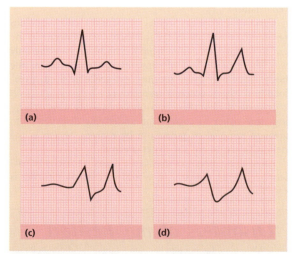

**Fig. 10.4**  Progressive ECG changes with increasing hyperkalaemia. (a) Normal. (b) Tented T wave. (c) Reduced P wave with increased QRS complex. (d) 'Sine wave' pattern (pre-cardiac arrest).

*Protect myocardium*

10 ml 10% calcium gluconate given in the presence of ECG change; effect is temporary but dose can be repeated.

*Drive K⁺ into cells*

Insulin 10 units + 50 ml 50% dextrose followed by regular checks of blood glucose and plasma K⁺

Repeat as necessary

and/or correction of severe acidosis—$NaHCO_3$ (1.26%)

and/or salbutamol 0.5 mg in 100 ml 5% dextrose over 15 min (rarely used)

*Deplete body K⁺*

Calcium or sodium resonium
    15 g orally up to three times daily with laxatives
    30 g rectally followed 3–6 hours later by an enema

Haemodialysis or peritoneal dialysis

**Practical Box 10.1**   Correction of hyperkalaemia.

## TREATMENT

Treatments for hyperkalaemia are summarized in Practical Box 10.1 and should also include treatment of the cause.

Calcium ions protect the cell membranes from the effects of hyperkalaemia but do not alter the potassium concentration. Insulin drives potassium into the cell, but must be accompanied by glucose to avoid hypoglycaemia. Regular measurements of blood glucose *must* be used for at least 6 hours after use of insulin in this situation, and extra glucose must be available for immediate use.

Intravenous salbutamol has not yet found widespread acceptance and may cause disturbing muscle tremor at the doses required. Correction of acidosis with hypertonic (8.4%) sodium bicarbonate causes volume expansion and should be used with extreme caution, particularly in renal failure.

Cation exchange resins (sodium and calcium resonium) make use of the ion fluxes which occur in the gut to remove potassium from the body, and are the only way short of dialysis of removing potassium from the body. They may cause sodium (extracellular fluid) overload and hypercalcaemia respectively.

In general all of these measures are simply ways of buying time either to correct the underlying disorder or to arrange removal of potassium by dialysis, which is the definitive treatment for hyperkalaemia.

All of these measures may cause digoxin toxicity in patients receiving digoxin, in whom cardiac monitoring is essential.

# Disorders of magnesium concentration

Plasma magnesium levels are normally maintained within the range 0.7–1.1 mmol litre⁻¹. Like potassium, mag-

nesium is principally an intracellular cation (Table 10.1). Regulation of magnesium balance is mainly via the kidney. Primary disturbance of magnesium balance is uncommon, hypo- or hypermagnesaemia usually developing on a background of more obvious fluid and electrolyte disturbances. Disturbance in magnesium balance should always be suspected in association with other fluid and electrolyte disturbances when the patient develops unexpected neurological signs or symptoms.

## HYPOMAGNESAEMIA

This most often develops as a result of deficient intake, defective gut absorption, or excessive gut or urinary loss (see Table 10.14). It can also occur with acute pancreatitis, possibly due to the formation of magnesium soaps in the areas of fat necrosis. Calcium deficiency usually develops with hypomagnesaemia.

### CLINICAL FEATURES

Symptoms and signs include irritability, tremor, ataxia, carpopedal spasm, hyperreflexia, confusional and hallucinatory states and epileptiform convulsions. The serum magnesium is usually <0.7 mmol litre⁻¹. An ECG may show a prolonged QT interval, broad flattened T waves and occasional shortening of the ST segment.

### TREATMENT

This involves the withdrawal of precipitating agents such as diuretics or purgatives and the parenteral infusion of 50 mmol of magnesium chloride in 1 litre of 5% dextrose

*Decreased magnesium absorption*
Malabsorption
Malnutrition
Alcohol excess

*Increased renal excretion*
Drugs
    Loop diuretics
    Thiazide diuretics
    Digoxin
Diabetic ketoacidosis
Bartter's syndrome
Hyperaldosteronism
SIADH
Alcohol excess
Hypercalciuria
1,25-(OH)-vitamin D deficiency
Drug toxicity
    Amphotericin
    Aminoglycosides
    Cisplatinum
    Cyclosporin

*Gut losses*
Prolonged nasogastric suction
Excessive purgation
Gastrointestinal/biliary fistulae
Severe diarrhoea

*Miscellaneous*
Acute pancreatitis

**Table 10.14**   Causes of hypomagnesaemia.

| |
|---|
| Impaired renal excretion |
|     Chronic renal failure |
|     Acute renal failure |
| |
| Increased magnesium intake |
|     Purgatives, e.g. magnesium sulphate |
|     Antacids, e.g. magnesium trisilicate |
| |
| Haemodialysis with high dialysate [Mg] |

**Table 10.15**   Causes of hypermagnesaemia.

| |
|---|
| Hyperparathyroidism |
| Vitamin D deficiency or resistance |
| Carbohydrate administration after fasting |
|     Total parenteral nutrition |
|     Anorexia nervosa |
| Hypomagnesaemia |
| Rise in pH—treatment of acidosis or development of alkalosis |
| Alcohol withdrawal |
| Diabetic ketoacidosis |
| Gut phosphate binders, e.g. aluminium hydroxide |
| Paracetamol poisoning (phosphaturia) |
| Acute liver failure |

**Table 10.16**   Causes of hypophosphataemia.

or other isotonic fluid over 12–24 hours. This should be repeated daily until the plasma magnesium level is normal.

## HYPERMAGNESAEMIA

This primarily occurs in patients with acute or chronic failure given magnesium-containing laxatives or antacids. It can also be induced by magnesium-containing enemas. Mild hypermagnesaemia may occur in patients with adrenal insufficiency. Causes are given in Table 10.15.

### CLINICAL FEATURES

Symptoms and signs relate to neurological and cardiovascular depression, and include weakness with hyporeflexia proceeding to narcosis, respiratory paralysis and cardiac conduction defects. Symptoms usually develop when the plasma magnesium level exceeds 2 mmol litre$^{-1}$.

### TREATMENT

Treatment requires withdrawal of any magnesium therapy. An intravenous injection of 10 ml of calcium gluconate 10% (2.25 mmol calcium), is given to antagonize the effects of hypermagnesaemia and dextrose and insulin (as for hyperkalaemia) to lower the plasma magnesium level. Dialysis may be required in patients with severe renal failure. Respiratory failure requires artificial ventilation until the plasma magnesium level returns to normal level.

## Disorders of phosphate concentration

## HYPOPHOSPHATAEMIA

Significant hypophosphataemia may occur in a number of clinical situations, either due to redistribution into cells, to renal losses, or to decreased intake (Table 10.16), and may cause:

- Muscle weakness—diaphragmatic weakness, decreased cardiac contractility, skeletal muscle rhabdomyolysis
- Left-shifted oxyhaemoglobin dissociation (reduced 2,3-diphosphoglycerate (2,3-DPG)).
- Confusion, hallucinations and convulsions

Mild hypophosphataemia often resolves without specific treatment. However, diaphragmatic weakness may be severe in acute hypophosphataemia, and may impede weaning a patient from a ventilator. Interestingly, chronic hypophosphataemia (in X-linked hypophosphataemia) is associated with normal muscle power.

Treatment of acute hypophosphataemia, if warranted, is with intravenous phosphate at a maximum rate of 9 mmol every 12 hours, with repeated measurements of calcium and phosphate, as over-rapid administration of phosphate may lead to severe hypocalcaemia, particularly in the presence of alkalosis. Chronic hypophosphataemia can be corrected, if warranted, with oral effervescent sodium phosphate.

## HYPERPHOSPHATAEMIA

Hyperphosphataemia is common in patients with chronic renal failure (see p. 484) (Table 10.17). Hyperphosphataemia is usually asymptomatic but may result in precipitation of calcium phosphate, particularly in the presence of a normal or raised calcium or of alkalosis. Uraemic itching may be caused by a raised calcium × phosphate product. Prolonged hyperphosphataemia causes hyperparathyroidism, and periarticular and vascular calcification.

No treatment is usually required for acute hyperphosphataemia, as the causes are self-limiting. Treatment of chronic hyperphosphataemia is with gut phosphate binders and dialysis (see p. 484).

| |
|---|
| Chronic renal failure |
| Phosphate-containing enemas |
| Tumour lysis |
| Myeloma—abnormal phosphate-binding protein |

**Table 10.17**   Causes of hyperphosphataemia.

# Disorders of acid–base balance

The concentration of hydrogen ions in both extracellular and intracellular compartments is extremely tightly controlled; very small changes may lead to major cell dysfunction. Hydrogen ion concentration has traditionally been expressed as pH, the negative logarithm of $[H^+]$, but this may contribute to complacency about the real magnitude of changes in $[H^+]$ (Table 10.18).

## Basic principles

CARBOHYDRATE AND FAT METABOLISM. Complete combustion of carbohydrate and fat in the liver and muscle produces $CO_2$, which forms carbonic acid. If respiratory function is normal, the partial pressure of $CO_2$ remains constant.

- Respiratory acidosis is due to decreased removal of $CO_2$.
- Respiratory alkalosis is due to increased removal of $CO_2$.

Incomplete combustion of these metabolic fuels results in the formation of organic acids such as lactic acid, hydroxybutyric acid, acetoacetic acid and free fatty acids. These may cause significant acidosis if their production exceeds the capacity of the liver to metabolize them completely, as in lactic acidosis and diabetic ketoacidosis.

AMINO ACID METABOLISM. Amino acids, by definition, contain $-COOH$ and $-NH_2$ groups; metabolism of amino acids produces $HCO_3^-$ and $NH_4^+$ ions. These may be combined to form urea:

$$2NH_4^+ + 2HCO_3^- \rightarrow NH_2 - CO - NH_2 + CO_2 + 3H_2O$$

resulting in no net acid or base production (assuming $CO_2$ is removed by respiration).

Alternatively, if $NH_4^+$ is excreted in the urine, this leaves $HCO_3^-$ within the body, resulting in alkali retention, which is equivalent to $H^+$ excretion.

Both the liver and the kidney appear to have important regulatory roles in acid–base balance. The liver regulates the degree to which $NH_4^+$ and $HCO_3^-$ are metabolized to urea in response to acid–base balance; ureagenesis is increased by alkalosis (thus consuming bicarbonate) and decreased by acidosis (thus sparing bicarbonate). $NH_4^+$ not utilized for ureagenesis is incorporated into glutamine, which is transported to the kidney: hydrolysis of glutamine in the kidney also appears to be regulated by acid–base balance and is an important mechanism by which $NH_4^+$ is excreted in the urine. $NH_4^+$ excretion in urine increases in response to acidosis, and defective $NH_4^+$ excretion in tubular diseases (distal renal tubular acidosis) causes systemic acidosis.

Some amino acids also contain sulphur and chlorine groups, metabolism of which yields sulphuric acid and hydrochloric acid. Metabolism of phosphorus-containing compounds yields phosphoric acid. These are all known as 'fixed acids' because they cannot be metabolized further to $CO_2$ and removed by respiration; removal requires renal excretion both of sulphate, phosphate, or chloride and of $H^+$.

EXOGENOUS ACIDS. Absorption of ingested acids and alkalis results in acidosis and alkalosis respectively. The commonest example is ingestion of salicylic acid.

RENAL $H^+$ HANDLING. Secretion of $H^+$ into the distal nephron is dependent on an aldosterone-sensitive pump which exchanges $Na^+$ for $H^+$ or $K^+$.

Excretion of hydrogen ions is therefore dependent on delivery of sodium to the distal tubule:

- Increased sodium delivery (for instance caused by diuretics) and hyperaldosteronism cause increased excretion of $H^+$ and $K^+$, leading to hypokalaemia and alkalosis.
- Decreased sodium delivery (e.g. hypovolaemia) or aldosterone deficiency cause hyperkalaemia and acidosis.

By the same mechanism, increased $K^+$ delivery leads to acidosis and alkaline urine. In this respect, the requirement for control of acid–base balance is overridden by the requirement to maintain extracellular volume.

RENAL $HCO_3^-$ HANDLING. Bicarbonate filtered at the glomerulus must be reabsorbed, otherwise there would be massive losses of bicarbonate causing severe acidosis.

Sodium bicarbonate reabsorption in the proximal tubule is complicated by the fact that $CO_2$ diffuses freely across the membrane of the tubular cell, whereas $HCO_3^-$ and $H^+$ cannot diffuse freely (Fig. 10.5).

The capacity for bicarbonate reabsorption is limited, so that bicarbonate is lost into the urine if the plasma concentration exceeds the threshold of around 28 mmol litre$^{-1}$. This threshold is lowered by parathyroid hormone and raised by intracellular acidosis (allowing bicarbonate retention to balance $CO_2$ retention in respiratory acidosis).

BUFFERING SYSTEMS. Buffers are weak acids, present in blood and urine, which prevent large fluctuations of hydrogen ion concentration.

| pH | $[H^+]$ (nmol litre$^{-1}$) |
|----|-----|
| 6.9 | 126 |
| 7.0 | 100 |
| 7.1 | 79 |
| 7.2 | 63 |
| 7.3 | 50 |
| 7.4 | 40 |
| 7.5 | 32 |
| 7.6 | 25 |

**Table 10.18** Relationship between $[H^+]$ and pH.

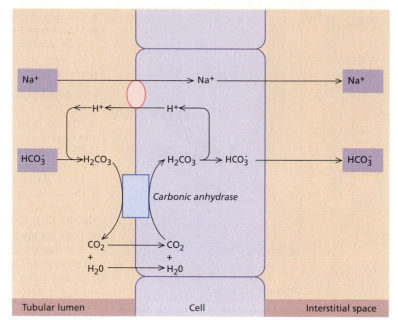

**Fig. 10.5** Reabsorption of sodium bicarbonate in the renal (mainly proximal) tubule. Bicarbonate is reclaimed by the secretion of H⁺ into the tubule in exchange for Na⁺. This results in the formation of $H_2CO_3$ which is then broken down to $CO_2$. This is reabsorbed and converted back to $H_2CO_3$ which now dissociates into H⁺ and $HCO_3^-$. The net result is reabsorption of Na⁺ and $HCO_3^-$. This process is dependent on carbonic anhydrase within the cells and on the luminal surface of the tubular cell.

In blood hydrogen ions are buffered partly by phosphate and haemoglobin but mainly by the bicarbonate/carbonic acid system:

$$H^+A^- + Na^+HCO_3^- = H_2CO_3 + Na^+A^-$$

where A is any fixed acid.

Equilibrium between bicarbonate and carbonic acid is related to hydrogen ion concentration by the Henderson–Hasselbach relationship:

$$[H^+] = k\frac{[H_2CO_3]}{[HCO_3^-]}$$

where $k$ is the dissociation coefficient of carbonic acid. If [H⁺] is expressed in nmoles per litre, $[H_2CO_3]$ as $P_{CO_2}$ in kPa, and $[HCO_3^-]$ in mmoles litre$^{-1}$,

$$[H^+] = \frac{181 \times P_{CO_2}}{[HCO_3^-]}.$$

Alternatively the relationship may be expressed as

$$pH = pK + \log\frac{[HCO_3^-]}{[H_2CO_3]},$$

where $pK = 6.1$.

Control of the concentration of $CO_2$ by the respiratory system and of $HCO_3^-$ by the liver and kidneys results in tight control of [H⁺].

In urine, hydrogen ions are buffered mainly by the phosphate buffer system:

$$H^+A^- + HPO_4^{2-} = A^- + H_2PO_4^-.$$

Some textbooks refer to $NH_3$ and $NH_4^+$ as a buffer system. This is not strictly accurate, although, as discussed above, $NH_4^+$ excretion in the urine results in $HCO_3^-$ retention.

## CAUSES AND DIAGNOSIS

Acid–base disturbances may be caused by:

- Abnormal $CO_2$ removal in the lungs ('respiratory' acidosis and alkalosis), or by
- Abnormalities in the regulation of bicarbonate and other buffers in the blood ('metabolic' acidosis and alkalosis).

Both may, and usually do, coexist. For instance, metabolic acidosis causes hyperventilation (via medullary chemoreceptors, see p. 635), leading to increased removal of $CO_2$ in the lungs and partial compensation for the acidosis. Conversely, respiratory acidosis is accompanied by renal bicarbonate retention, which could be mistaken for primary metabolic alkalosis. The situation is even more complex if a patient has both respiratory disease and a metabolic disturbance.

Clinical history and examination usually point to the correct diagnosis. In complicated patients, the acid–base nomogram (Fig. 10.6) is invaluable. The H⁺ and $P_aCO_2$ are measured in arterial blood (for precautions see p. 727) as well as the bicarbonate. If the values from a patient lie in one of the bands in the diagram, it is likely that only one abnormality is present. If the [H⁺] is high (pH low) but the $P_{CO_2}$ is normal, the intercept lies between two bands: the patient has respiratory dysfunction, leading to failure of $CO_2$ elimination, but this is partly compensated for by metabolic acidosis, stimulating respiration and $CO_2$

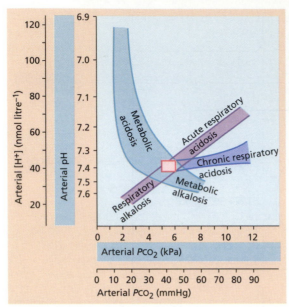

**Fig. 10.6**  The Flenley acid–base nomogram. This was derived from a large number of observations in patients with 'pure' respiratory or metabolic disturbances. The bands show the 95% confidence limits representing the individual varieties of acid–base disturbance. The pink area shows the approximate limits of arterial pH and $P\text{co}_2$ in normal individuals.

removal (this is the commonest 'combined' abnormality in practice).

## Respiratory acidosis

This is caused by retention of $CO_2$. The $P_a\text{co}_2$ and $[H^+]$ rise. Renal retention of bicarbonate may partly compensate, returning the $[H^+]$ towards normal (see p. 727).

## Respiratory alkalosis

Increased removal of $CO_2$ is caused by hyperventilation so there is a fall in $P_a\text{co}_2$ and $[H^+]$ (see p. 727).

## Metabolic acidosis

This is due to the accumulation of any acid other than carbonic acid (see above). The most common cause is lactic acid production during shock or following cardiac arrest.

### Differential diagnosis of metabolic acidosis: the anion gap

The first step is to identify whether the acidosis is due to retention of $H^+Cl^-$ or to another acid. This is achieved by calculation of the anion gap. The principles underlying this calculation are straightforward:

- The normal cations present in plasma are $Na^+$, $K^+$, $Ca^{2+}$, $Mg^{2+}$.
- The normal anions present in plasma are $Cl^-$, $HCO_3^-$, negative charges present on albumin, phosphate, sulphate, lactate, and other organic acids.

- The sum of the positive and negative charges are equal.
- Measurement of $Na^+$, $K^+$, $Cl^-$ and $HCO_3^-$ are usually easily available. The sum

$$\{[Na^+] + [K^+]\} - \{[Cl^-] + [HCO_3^-]\}$$

$$= [\text{unmeasured anions}] - [\text{unmeasured cations}]\}$$

is referred to as the *anion gap*. Because there are more unmeasured anions than cations, the normal anion gap is 10–18 mmol litre$^{-1}$.

- *Beware*: some textbooks leave $[K^+]$ out of the calculation, giving a lower 'normal range'.

If the anion gap is normal in the presence of acidosis, one may conclude that $H^+Cl^-$ is being retained or $Na^+HCO_3^-$ is being lost. Causes of a normal anion gap acidosis are given in Table 10.19.

If the anion gap is increased, one may conclude that an unmeasured anion is present in increased quantities. This may either be one of the acids normally present in small, but unmeasured quantities, such as lactate, or an exogenous acid. Causes of a high anion gap acidosis are given in Table 10.20.

The anion gap involves a number of assumptions and uncertainties, such as the negative charge attributable to albumin. An albumin concentration of 40 g litre$^{-1}$ gives a negative charge of around 10 mmol; a fall in albumin concentration to 20 g litre$^{-1}$ would lower the normal anion gap by 5 mmol litre$^{-1}$. Both types of acidosis may co-exist. For instance, cholera would be expected to cause a normal anion gap acidosis due to massive gastrointestinal losses of bicarbonate, but the anion gap is often increased due to renal failure and lactic acidosis as a result of hypovolaemia.

### Lactic acidosis

Increased lactic acid production occurs when cellular respiration is abnormal, either due to lack of oxygen in the tissues ('type A') or to a metabolic abnormality, e.g. drug-induced ('type B') (Table 10.20). The commonest cause

---

Increased gastrointestinal bicarbonate loss
  Diarrhoea
  Ileostomy
  Ureterosigmoidostomy

Increased renal bicarbonate loss
  Acetazolamide
  Proximal (type 2) renal tubular acidosis
  Hyperparathyroidism
  Tubular damage, e.g. drugs, heavy metals, paraproteins

Decreased renal hydrogen ion excretion
  Distal (type 1) renal tubular acidosis
  Type 4 renal tubular acidosis (aldosterone deficiency)

Increased HCl production
  Ammonium chloride ingestion
  Increased catabolism of lysine, arginine

**Table 10.19**  Causes of metabolic acidosis with a normal anion gap.

Renal failure (sulphate, phosphate)

Accumulation of organic acids

Lactic acidosis
  L-lactic
    Type A—anaerobic metabolism in tissues
      Hypotension/cardiac arrest
      Sepsis
      Poisoning—ethylene glycol, methanol, others
    Type B—decreased hepatic lactate metabolism
      Insulin deficiency (decreased pyruvate
      dehydrogenase activity)
      Metformin accumulation (chronic renal failure)
      Haematological malignancies
      Other drugs
      Rare inherited enzyme defects
  D-lactic (fermentation of glucose in bowel by
  abnormal bowel flora, complicating abnormal small
  bowel anatomy, e.g. blind loops)

Ketoacidosis
  Insulin deficiency
  Alcohol excess
  Starvation

Exogenous acids
  Salicylate

**Table 10.20** Causes of metabolic acidosis with an increased anion gap.

in clinical practice is type A lactic acidosis, occurring in septicaemic or cardiogenic shock. Significant acidosis can occur despite a normal blood pressure and $P_aO_2$, due to splanchnic and peripheral vasoconstriction. Acidosis worsens cardiac function and vasoconstriction further, contributing to a downward spiral and fulminant production of lactic acid.

### Diabetic ketoacidosis (see p. 841)
This is a high anion gap acidosis due to the accumulation of organic acids, acetoacetic acid and hydroxybutyric acid due to increased production and some reduced peripheral utilization.

### Renal tubular acidosis
This term refers to systemic acidosis caused by impairment of the ability of the renal tubules to maintain acid–base balance. This group of disorders is uncommon and only rarely a cause of significant clinical disease. Renal tubular acidosis may be secondary to immunological, drug-induced or structural damage to the tubular cells, an inherited abnormality, or an isolated ('primary') abnormality. As with most disorders which are not well understood, the nomenclature is confusing.

TYPE 4 RENAL TUBULAR ACIDOSIS, also called hyporeninaemic hypoaldosteronism, is probably the commonest of these disorders. The cardinal features are hyperkalaemia and acidosis occurring in a patient with mild chronic renal insufficiency, usually caused by tubulo-interstitial disease (e.g. reflux nephropathy) or diabetes. Plasma renin and aldosterone are found to be low even

after measures which would normally stimulate their secretion (Table 10.21). An identical syndrome may be caused by NSAIDs, which impair renin and aldosterone secretion. In the presence of acidosis, urine pH may be low. Treatment is with fludrocortisone, sodium bicarbonate, diuretics, or ion exchange resins to remove potassium, or some combination of these. Dietary potassium restriction alone is ineffective.

TYPE 3 RENAL TUBULAR ACIDOSIS is vanishingly rare, and represents a combination of type 1 and type 2.

TYPE 2 ('PROXIMAL') RENAL TUBULAR ACIDOSIS is very rare in adult practice. It is caused by failure of sodium bicarbonate reabsorption in the proximal tubule. The cardinal features are acidosis, hypokalaemia, an inability to lower the urine pH below 5.5 despite systemic acidosis, and the appearance of bicarbonate in the urine despite a subnormal plasma bicarbonate. This disorder normally occurs as part of a generalized tubular defect, together with other features such as glycosuria and amino aciduria. Treatment is with sodium bicarbonate: massive doses may be required to overcome the renal 'leak'.

TYPE 1 ('DISTAL') RENAL TUBULAR ACIDOSIS is due to a failure of $H^+$ excretion in the distal tubule and consists of:
- Acidosis
- Hypokalaemia
- Inability to lower the urine pH below 5.5 despite systemic acidosis
- Low urinary ammonium production

These features may only be present in the face of increased acid production; hence the need for an acid load test in diagnosis (see Practical Box 10.2). Other features include:
- Low urinary citrate
- Hypercalciuria

These abnormalities result in osteomalacia, renal stone formation and recurrent urinary infections.

Osteomalacia is caused by buffering of $H^+$ by $Ca^{2+}$ in bone resulting in depletion of calcium from bone.

Renal stone formation is caused by hypercalciuria, hypocitraturia (citrate inhibits calcium phosphate

Hyperkalaemia (in the absence of drugs known to cause hyperkalaemia) (low plasma bicarbonate)

Normal ACTH stimulation test

Low basal 24 hour urinary aldosterone

Subnormal response of plasma renin and plasma aldosterone to stimulation: samples taken after 2 hours supine and again after 40 mg frusemide (80 mg if creatinine >120 $\mu$mol litre$^{-1}$) and 4 hours upright posture

Correction of hyperkalaemia by fludrocortisone 0.1 mg daily

**Table 10.21** Diagnosis of hyporeninaemic hypoaldosteronism (type 4 renal tubular acidosis).

Plasma $HCO_3^-$ <21 mmol litre$^{-1}$, urine pH >5.3: renal tubular acidosis

To differentiate between proximal (very rare) and distal (rare) requires bicarbonate infusion test

Plasma $HCO_3^-$ >21 mmol litre$^{-1}$ but suspicion of partial renal tubular acidosis (e.g. nephrocalcinosis, associated diseases): Acid load test required

Give 100 mg kg$^{-1}$ ammonium chloride by mouth. Check urine pH hourly and plasma bicarbonate at 3 hours. Plasma $HCO_3^-$ should drop below 21 mmol litre$^{-1}$ unless the patient vomits (in which case the test should be repeated with an antiemetic). If urine pH remains >5.3 despite a plasma $HCO_3^-$ of 21 mmol litre$^{-1}$, the diagnosis is confirmed

**Practical box 10.2**   Diagnosis of renal tubular acidosis.

precipitation), and alkaline urine (which favours precipitation of calcium phosphate).

Recurrent urinary infections are caused by renal stones. This disorder is associated with numerous diseases including any cause of nephrocalcinosis (causing structural tubular damage), immunological damage (for instance, in association with Sjögren's syndrome), and a number of drugs. Treatment is with sodium bicarbonate, potassium supplements and citrate.

Thiazide diuretics are useful by causing volume contraction and increased proximal sodium bicarbonate reabsorption.

### Uraemic acidosis

Kidney disease may cause acidosis in several ways. Reduction in the number of functioning nephrons decreases the capacity to excrete $NH_4^+$ and $H^+$ in the urine. In addition, tubular disease may cause bicarbonate wasting. Acidosis is a particular feature of those types of chronic renal failure in which the tubules are particularly affected, such as reflux nephropathy and chronic obstructive uropathy.

Chronic acidosis is most often caused by chronic renal failure, where there is a failure to excrete fixed acid. Up to 40 mmol of hydrogen ions may accumulate daily. These are buffered by *bone*, in exchange for calcium. Chronic acidosis is therefore a major risk factor for renal osteodystrophy and hypercalciuria.

Chronic acidosis has also been shown recently to be a risk factor for muscle wasting in renal failure, and may also contribute to the inexorable progression of some types of renal disease.

Uraemic acidosis should be corrected because of the effects of chronic acidosis on growth, muscle turnover and bones. Sodium bicarbonate 2–3 mmol kg$^{-1}$ daily is usually enough to maintain serum bicarbonate above 20 mmol litre$^{-1}$, but may contribute to sodium overload. Calcium carbonate improves acidosis and also acts as a phosphate binder and calcium supplement, and is increasingly used. Acidosis in end-stage renal failure is usually fully corrected by adequate dialysis.

### Clinical features of acidosis

Clinically the most obvious effect is stimulation of respiration, leading to the clinical sign of 'air hunger', or Kussmaul's sign. Interestingly, patients with profound hyperventilation may not complain of breathlessness, although in others it may be a presenting complaint.

Acidosis increases delivery of oxygen to the tissues by shifting the oxyhaemoglobin dissociation curve to the right, but also leads to inhibition of 2,3-DPG production, which returns the curve towards normal (see Chapter 13).

Cardiovascular dysfunction is common in acidotic patients, although it is often difficult to dissociate the numerous possible causes of this. There is no doubt that acidosis is negatively inotropic. Severe acidosis causes venoconstriction, resulting in redistribution of blood from the peripheries to the central circulation, and increased systemic venous pressure, which may worsen pulmonary oedema caused by myocardial depression. Arteriolar vasodilatation also occurs, further contributing to hypotension.

Cerebral dysfunction is variable. Severe acidosis is often associated with confusion and fits, but numerous other possible causes are usually present.

As mentioned earlier, acidosis stimulates potassium loss from cells, which may lead to potassium deficiency if renal function is normal or to hyperkalaemia if renal potassium excretion is impaired.

### Treatment of acidosis

In lactic acidosis caused by poor tissue perfusion ('type A'), treatment should be aimed at maximizing oxygen delivery to the tissues and usually requires inotropic agents, mechanical ventilation and invasive monitoring. In 'type B' lactic acidosis treatment is that of the underlying disorder, e.g.

- Insulin in diabetic ketoacidosis
- Treatment of methanol and ethylene glycol poisoning with ethanol
- Removal of salicylate by dialysis

The question of whether severe acidosis should be treated with bicarbonate is extremely controversial. Severe acidosis ([$H^+$] >100 nmol litre$^{-1}$, pH <7.0) is associated with a very high mortality, which makes many doctors keen to correct it. Since acidosis is known to impair cardiac contractility it would seem sensible to correct acidosis with bicarbonate in a sick patient. However:

- Rapid correction of acidosis may result in tetany and fits due to a rapid decrease in ionized calcium.
- Administration of sodium bicarbonate may lead to extracellular volume expansion, exacerbating pulmonary oedema.
- Bicarbonate therapy increases $CO_2$ production and will therefore only correct acidosis if ventilation can be increased to remove the added $CO_2$ load.
- The increased amounts of $CO_2$ generated may diffuse more readily into cells than bicarbonate, worsening intracellular acidosis.

Administration of sodium bicarbonate (50 mmol, as 50 ml of 8.4% sodium bicarbonate intravenously) is sometimes given during cardiac arrest and is often necessary before arrhythmias can be corrected. Correction of hyperkalaemia associated with acidosis is also of undoubted benefit. In other situations there is no clinical evidence to show that correction of acidosis improves outcome, but it remains standard practice to administer sodium bicarbonate when [H$^+$] is >126 nmol litre$^{-1}$ (pH <6.9) using intravenous 1.26% (150 mmol litre$^{-1}$) bicarbonate.

## Metabolic alkalosis

Renal excretion of excess bicarbonate is normally very efficient, and for this reason metabolic alkalosis is much rarer than acidosis. A number of factors stimulate bicarbonate reabsorption and hydrogen ion excretion despite the presence of alkalosis:

- Extracellular volume depletion
- Potassium deficiency
- Excess mineralocorticoids
- Thiazide and loop diuretics

All of these may be thought of as increasing secretion of H$^+$ in exchange for Na$^+$ in the distal tubule.

Vomiting causes alkalosis both by causing volume depletion and by causing loss of gastric acid.

Exogenous alkalis, such as those found in effervescent preparations of analgesics or in proprietary antacids, may also contribute to metabolic alkalosis, particularly if combined with another contributory factor.

### Effects of alkalosis

Cerebral dysfunction is an early feature of alkalosis. The oxyhaemoglobin dissociation curve is shifted to the left. Respiration may be depressed.

### Treatment of alkalosis

Replacement of sodium, potassium and chloride allows renal excretion of bicarbonate. Clearly sodium chloride administration should be avoided in patients on diuretics as appropriate treatment for heart failure. Acetazolamide may be useful in patients without sodium depletion.

# Further reading

Arieff AI (1993) Management of hyponatraemia. *British Medical Journal* **307**, 305–308.

Atkinson DE & Bourke E (1987) Metabolic aspects of the regulation of systemic pH. *American Journal of Physiology* **252**, F947–F956.

Cameron *et al.* (eds) (1993) Water, electrolyte or acid–base disorders. In: *Oxford Textbook of Clinical Nephrology*, pp. 867–917. Oxford: Oxford University Press.

Editorial (1988) What causes oedema? *Lancet* **i**, 1028–1030.

Field MJ & Giebisch GJ (1985) Hormonal control of renal potassium excretion. *Kidney International* **27**, 379–387.

Jamieson MJ (1985) Clinical algorithms: Hyponatraemia. *British Medical Journal* **290**, 1723–1728.

# 11 Cardiovascular disease

## Introduction

In the Western Hemisphere approximately 50% of deaths are related to cardiovascular disease. This is due mainly to ischaemic heart disease that could, perhaps, be significantly reduced if smoking were prohibited, life-style moderated (e.g. weight reduction) and the intake of cholesterol and saturated fats reduced. Whilst the incidence of rheumatic heart disease is decreasing in the West, it is still an important problem worldwide, predominantly in countries with poor sanitation, overcrowding and malnutrition. Up to one-third of all cardiac cases admitted to hospital in, for example, India, Jamaica, Egypt or the Philippines are due to rheumatic heart disease. Hypertension is another major cause of mortality, being responsible for 10% of deaths worldwide. The incidence of hypertension usually increases with age and is higher in Western countries. There is also a wide geographical variation in other cardiac diseases: endomyocardial fibrosis is seen in the tropics; cardiac problems associated with protein–energy malnutrition are seen in countries where famine and malnutrition occur; cardiomyopathy is seen with beriberi and myocarditis is seen with other diseases associated with the tropics, e.g. Chagas' disease, typhoid fever and diphtheria.

Congenital heart disease is important in the young and is responsible for approximately 1% of deaths in patients below 15 years of age.

Lastly, pulmonary heart disease is common in countries with a high incidence of smoking.

## Essential anatomy, physiology and embryology of the heart

### The cellular basis of myocardial contraction

Myocardial cells contain bundles of parallel myofibrils. Each myofibril is made up of a series of sarcomeres (Fig. 11.1). A sarcomere is bound by two transverse Z lines, to each of which is attached a perpendicular filament of the protein actin. The actin filaments from each of the two Z bands overlap with thicker parallel protein filaments known as myosin. Actin and myosin filaments are attached to each other by cross-bridges that contain ATPase.

During cardiac contraction the length of the actin and myosin monofilaments does not change. Rather, the actin filaments slide between the myosin filaments when a high-energy bond of ATP is split by ATPase. Magnesium ions are required to facilitate this reaction. To supply the

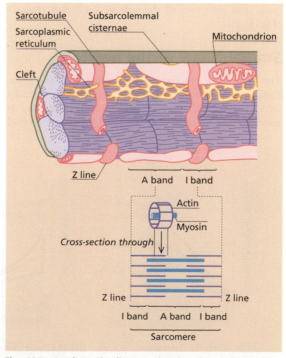

**Fig. 11.1** A schematic diagram showing the structure of a myofibril. The myofibrils are made up of a series of sarcomeres joined at the Z line.

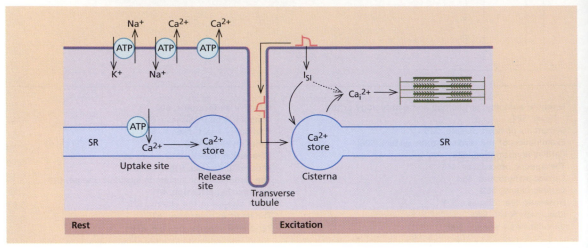

**Fig. 11.2** The calcium cycle. *Right*: Ca²⁺ ions stored in the cisternae of the sarcoplasmic reticulum (SR) are released when the depolarization spike travels into the cell along the T-tubule. A second inward current ($I_{SI}$) causes release of extra calcium. *Left*: Calcium levels are restored by sarcolemmal Na⁺–Ca²⁺ pump and SR pump. From Levick *et al. Introduction to Cardiovascular Physiology*.

ATP, the myocyte (which cannot stop for a rest) has an extraordinarily high mitochondrial density (35% of the cell volume). Calcium ions initiate contraction by inactivating another protein called troponin C, which ordinarily inhibits the actin–myosin interaction. Calcium is made available during the plateau phase (phase 2) of the action potential (see Fig. 11.33) by calcium ions entering the cell and by being mobilized in mass from the sarcoplasmic reticulum. The force of cardiac muscle contraction ('inotropic state') is thus regulated by the influx of calcium ions into the cell through slow calcium channels (Fig. 11.2).

## Starling's law of the heart

The contractile function of an isolated strip of cardiac tissue can be described by the relationship between the velocity of muscle contraction, the load that may be moved by the contracting muscle, and the extent to which the muscle is stretched before contracting. As with all other types of muscle, the velocity of contraction of myocardial tissue is reduced by increasing the load against which the tissue must contract. However, in the non-failing heart, prestretching of cardiac muscle improves the relationship between the force and velocity of contraction (Fig. 11.3).

This phenomenon was described in the intact heart as an increase of stroke volume (ventricular performance) with an enlargement of the diastolic volume (pre-load), and is known as 'Starling's law of the heart' or the 'Frank–Starling relationship'. It has been transcribed into more clinically relevant indices. Thus, stroke work (aortic pressure × stroke volume) is increased as ventricular end-diastolic volume is raised. Alternatively, within certain limits, cardiac output rises as pulmonary capillary wedge pressure increases. This clinical relationship is described by the ventricular function curve (Fig. 11.3, which also shows the effect of sympathetic stimulation).

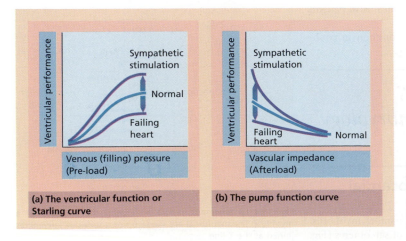

**Fig. 11.3** The Frank–Starling mechanism, showing the effect on ventricular contraction of alteration in filling pressures and outflow impedance in the normal, failing and sympathetically stimulated ventricle.

# The law of Laplace

This is also relevant to the contractile function of the heart. Laplace stated that the pressure within a sphere is proportional to wall stress (in the heart this is equivalent to after-load) and inversely proportional to its radius. Thus, as the heart enlarges beyond the point at which Starling's law conferred an advantage, the wall stress increases and cardiac output falls.

# The conduction system of the heart

Each natural heart beat begins in the heart's pacemaker—the sinoatrial (SA) node. This is a crescent-shaped structure that is located around the medial and anterior aspect of the junction between the superior vena cava and the right atrium (Fig. 11.4). Progressive loss of the diastolic resting membrane potential is followed, when the threshold potential has been reached, by a more rapid depolarization of the sinus node tissue. This depolarization triggers depolarization of the atrial myocardium. The atrial tissue is activated like a 'forest fire', but the activation peters out when the insulating layer between the atrium and the ventricle—the annulus fibrosus—is reached.

The depolarization continues to conduct slowly through the atrioventricular (AV) node. This is a small, bean-shaped structure that lies beneath the right atrial endocardium within the lower interatrial septum. The AV node continues as the His bundle, which penetrates the annulus fibrosus and conducts the cardiac impulse rapidly towards the ventricle. The His bundle reaches the crest of the interventricular septum and divides into the right bundle branch and the main left bundle branch.

The right bundle branch continues down the right side of the interventricular septum to the apex, from where it radiates and divides to form the Purkinje network, which spreads throughout the subendocardial surface of the right ventricle.

The main left bundle branch is a short structure which fans out into many strands on the left side of the inter-ventricular septum. These strands can be grouped into an anterior superior division (the anterior hemibundle) and a posterior inferior division (the posterior hemibundle). The anterior hemibundle supplies the subendocardial

Purkinje network of the anterior and superior surfaces of the left ventricle, and the inferior hemibundle supplies the inferior and posterior surfaces. Impulse conduction through the AV node is slow and depends on action potentials largely produced by slow transmembrane calcium flux. In the atria, ventricles and His–Purkinje system conduction is rapid and is due to action potentials generated by rapid transmembrane sodium diffusion.

# Nerve supply of the cardiovascular system

Adrenergic nerves supply atrial and ventricular muscle fibres as well as the conduction system. $\beta_1$ Receptors predominate in the heart with both adrenaline and nor-adrenaline having positive inotropic and chronotropic effects. $\beta_2$ Receptors predominate in the vascular smooth muscle.

Cholinergic nerves from the vagus supply mainly the SA and AV nodes via M2 muscarinic receptors. The ventricular myocardium is sparsely innervated by the vagus.

Under basal conditions vagal inhibitory effects predominate over the sympathetic excitatory effects resulting in a slow heart rate.

# The coronary circulation

The coronary arterial system (Fig. 11.5) consists of the right and left coronary arteries. The right coronary artery arises from the right coronary sinus and courses through the right side of the atrioventricular groove, giving off vessels that supply the right atrium and the right ventricle. The vessel usually continues as the posterior descending coronary artery, which runs in the posterior interventricular groove and supplies the posterior part of the interventricular septum and the posterior left ventricular wall.

The left coronary artery arises from the left coronary sinus. The first part is known as the left main coronary artery, and is usually not more than 2.5 cm long. It then divides into the left anterior descending and the left circumflex arteries. The left anterior descending artery runs in the anterior interventricular groove and supplies the anterior septum and the anterior left ventricular wall. The left circumflex artery travels along the left atrioventricular groove and gives off branches to the left atrium and the left ventricle (marginal branches).

The sinus node and the AV node are supplied by the right coronary artery in 60% and 90% of people, respectively. Therefore, disease in this artery may cause sinus bradycardia and AV nodal block. The majority of the left ventricle is supplied by the left coronary artery, so that stenosis in the left main artery is extremely dangerous; total obstruction of this vessel is rarely compatible with life.

# Functions of the vascular endothelium

The vascular endothelium is a cardiovascular endocrine organ which occupies a strategic interface between blood

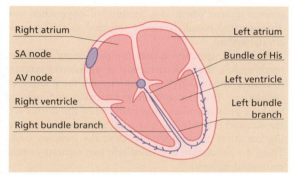

Right atrium

Left atrium

SA node

AV node

Bundle of His

Left ventricle

Right ventricle

Left bundle branch

Right bundle branch

**Fig. 11.4** The normal cardiac conduction system. AV, atrioventricular; SA, sinoatrial.

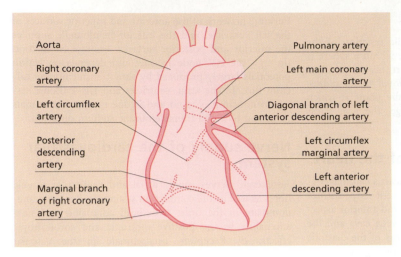

Aorta

Right coronary artery

Left circumflex artery

Posterior descending artery

Marginal branch of right coronary artery

Pulmonary artery

Left main coronary artery

Diagonal branch of left anterior descending artery

Left circumflex marginal artery

Left anterior descending artery

**Fig. 11.5** Diagram of the normal coronary arterial anatomy.

and body and has many regulatory roles:

- modulation of immunoresponses
- regulation of vascular cell growth
- vasomotor control
- pro- and antithrombotic mechanism
- metabolic and immunological functions.

Enzymes located on the endothelial surface control the level of circulating compounds, such as bradykinin, serotonin, angiotensin and adenine nucleotides. In addition, the endothelium releases substances which affect vascular tone and platelet function. Many endothelium-derived substances have now been characterized and play an important role in the physiological control of the coronary circulation through the production of endothelium-derived relaxing and contracting factors.

One of the most powerful substances, endothelium-derived relaxing factor (EDRF), has now been identified as nitric oxide (NO). The release of NO can be triggered by sheer stress (flow) and by a number of autocoids including bradykinin, histamine, noradrenaline, substance P, platelet-derived products, serotonin and thrombin. NO evokes relaxation of vascular smooth muscle and inhibits platelet function through activation of soluble guanylate cyclase, which leads to an increase in the intracellular levels of cyclic 3,5-guanosine monophosphate. The potent vasomotor and anti-platelet properties of NO suggest a functional role of the endothelium in the maintenance of an adequate organ blood flow. Dysfunction of endothelial cells in controlling the underlying smooth muscle is an early sign of vascular disease, such as atherosclerosis, hypertension and cerebral or coronary vasospasm.

The normal endothelium is a non-thrombogenic surface, which under physiological circumstances does not react with platelets or blood constituents. NO inhibits platelet aggregation, adhesion and secretion. Several other factors contribute to the antiaggregatory activity of the endothelium. Endothelial cells offer a negatively charged surface which repels the negatively charged platelets. The endothelial lining of blood vessels forms prostacyclin which inhibits platelet aggregation and formation of platelet derived growth factors.

In addition to their inhibitory effects on platelet function, prostacyclin and NO act together to antagonize procoagulant factors such as thrombin and thromboxane A2.

Other endothelium-derived compounds are also specific antagonists of the procoagulant activity of thrombin. Endothelial cells generate specific thrombin inhibitors that remove thrombin from the circulation and convert its procoagulant activity into anticoagulant activity. Examples of these are thrombomodulin, a surface receptor and heparin sulphate, a glycosaminoglycan, which activates antithrombin III. The endothelium also modulates fibrinolysis by generation of fibrinolytic components.

## The fetal circulation

*In utero*, the pulmonary circulation is largely unnecessary because fetal blood is oxygenated by placental blood flow, a parallel and integral element in the systemic circulation. In the fetus, systemic venous blood returning to the right atrium is partly deflected through the foramen ovale to the left atrium. Blood that passes through the right ventricle is diverted away from the pulmonary arteries to the aorta through the ductus arteriosus. Thus, the systemic venous return, which is a mixture of oxygenated and deoxygenated blood, is mostly returned to the systemic arterial system.

*At birth,* inspiration dilates the pulmonary arterioles, resulting in a dramatic reduction of pulmonary vascular resistance. Blood therefore flows through the pulmonary circulation. The increased oxygen tension and reduced levels of prostaglandins trigger closure of the ductus arteriosus, and the reduced right atrial pressure and increasing left atrial pressure tend to close the foramen ovale. Thus, the circulation is divided into two separate circuits connected in series.

In the fetus the left and right heart both propel blood from the systemic veins to the systemic arteries; thus, severe abnormalities of the heart may not compromise fetal blood flow.

## The cardiac cycle (Fig. 11.6)

The first event in the cardiac cycle is atrial depolarization (a P wave on the surface ECG) followed by right atrial and then left atrial contraction. Ventricular activation (the QRS complex on the ECG) follows after a short interval (the PR interval). Left ventricular contraction starts and shortly thereafter right ventricular contraction begins. The increased ventricular pressures exceed the atrial pressures, and close first the mitral and then the tricuspid valves. Until the aortic and pulmonary valves open, the ventricles contract with no change of volume (isovolumetric contraction). When ventricular pressures rise above the aortic and pulmonary artery pressures, the pulmonary valve and then the aortic valve open and ventricular ejection occurs. As the ventricles begin to relax, their pressures fall below the aortic and pulmonary arterial pressures, and aortic valve closure is followed by pulmonary valve closure. Isovolumetric relaxation then occurs. After the ventricular pressures have fallen below the right atrial and left atrial pressures, the tricuspid and mitral valves open.

The cardiac cycle can be graphically depicted as the relationship between the pressure and volume of the ventricle. This is illustrated in Fig. 11.7 which illustrates the changing pressure–volume relationships in response to increased contractility and to exercise.

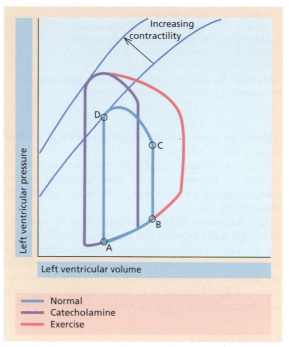

**Fig. 11.7** Pressure–volume loop. AB, diastole—ventricular filling; BC, systole—isovolumetric ventricular contraction; CD, systole—ventricular emptying; DA, diastole—isovolumetric ventricular relaxation.

## Symptoms of heart disease

Patients even with severe heart disease may be asymptomatic. However, symptoms include the following.

## Dyspnoea

Dyspnoea is an awareness of breathlessness. It can be due to cardiac or respiratory causes. It is also a symptom during exercise in healthy people.

Breathlessness may occur only on exercise or may be present at rest. The New York Heart Association has

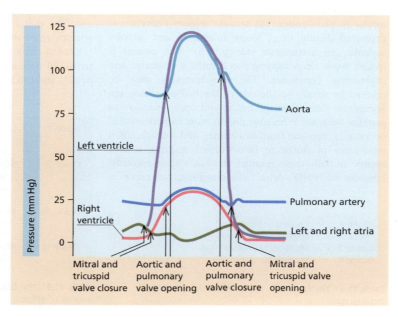

**Fig. 11.6** The cardiac cycle.

| Grade 1 | No breathlessness |
| Grade 2 | Breathlessness on severe exertion |
| Grade 3 | Breathlessness on mild exertion |
| Grade 4 | Breathlessness at rest |

**Table 11.1**  The New York Heart Association functional and therapeutic classification applied to dyspnoea.

replaced by a very similar grading known as 'cardiac status' (Table 11.2).

It is also clinically valuable to grade dyspnoea by the amount of physical exertion possible before breathlessness occurs, e.g. climbing 14 stairs or walking 200 yards on the flat.

Left ventricular failure causes dyspnoea because of a rise in left atrial pressure and pulmonary capillary pressure leading to interstitial and alveolar oedema. This makes the lung stiff (less compliant) and this increases the amount of respiratory effort necessary to breathe. Usually a fast breathing rate (tachypnoea) is also present due to stimulation of the pulmonary stretch receptors.

## Orthopnoea

This is a form of breathlessness that occurs when the patient lies flat. Orthopnoea occurs because lying flat results in the redistribution of blood, leading to an increased central and pulmonary blood volume. Recumbency also causes the abdominal contents to press up against the diaphragm. Both factors increase the difficulty of breathing. Patients usually cope with orthopnoea by propping themselves up with pillows.

## Paroxysmal nocturnal dyspnoea (PND)

This occurs when there is an accumulation of fluid in the lungs (pulmonary oedema) at night. The mechanism is similar to orthopnoea, but because sensory awareness is depressed during sleep, severe interstitial and alveolar oedema can accumulate (see p. 576). The patient is woken from sleep fighting for breath, a dramatic and frightening experience. The breathlessness may be relieved by sitting on the side of the bed or getting up. Sometimes the patient will get up and open a window to gasp for fresh air. Wheezing, due to bronchial endothelial oedema, is common (cardiac asthma), and a cough, often productive of frothy or blood-tinged sputum, usually occurs. Initially these episodes terminate spontaneously. Episodes of 'PND', often with coughing, can occur in

| Grade 1 | Uncompromised |
| Grade 2 | Slightly compromised |
| Grade 3 | Moderately compromised |
| Grade 4 | Severely compromised |

**Table 11.2**  The New York Heart Association grading of 'cardiac status'.

asthma, but conventionally the term is reserved for cardiac problems.

## Cheyne–Stokes respiration (see also p. 902)

In very severe heart failure, alternate hyperventilation and apnoea known as Cheyne–Stokes respiration may occur. This may also develop in the elderly without obvious heart failure. It is related to depression of the respiratory centre, which is partly due to prolonged circulation time and cerebrovascular disease. This type of respiration is also seen after morphine administration.

## Chest pain

Pain in the chest is the most common symptom associated with ischaemic heart disease.

### Angina pectoris

Angina pectoris literally means a strangling sensation (angina) in the chest (pectoris). It is a gripping or crushing central chest pain (or discomfort) that may be felt around the whole chest or deep within the chest. The pain may radiate into the neck or jaw and, rarely, into the teeth, back or abdomen. It is associated with heaviness, paraesthesia or pain in one (usually the left) or both arms. It is typically provoked by exercise and is promptly relieved by rest. A pain of similar distribution and type also occurs at rest in myocardial infarction (see p. 583). The mechanism of the pain is myocardial hypoxia secondary to inadequate coronary blood flow. Sharp pains over the heart are not usually angina. Angina should be classified according to the Canadian Cardiovascular Society grading of angina of effort (Table 11.3), although most physicians find that a verbal description is adequate.

### Other causes of chest pain

The pain of pericarditis is felt in the centre of the chest and, like that of pleurisy, is aggravated by movement, posture, respiration and coughing. It is sharp and severe.

Central chest pain that radiates to the back is characteristic of a dissecting or enlarging aortic aneurysm (see p. 627) and can mimic the pain of myocardial infarction.

| Grade I | Ordinary physical activity does not cause angina (strenuous physical activity provokes angina) |
| Grade II | Slight limitations of ordinary physical activity (climbing more than one flight of stairs or walking uphill provokes angina) |
| Grade III | Marked limitation of ordinary physical activity (walking on the level or climbing one flight of stairs provokes angina) |
| Grade IV | Inability to carry on any physical activity (angina may be present at rest) |

**Table 11.3**  The Canadian Cardiovascular Society grading of angina of effort.

It is important to consider and exclude a dissection since the administration of a thrombolytic agent in this circumstance would be catastrophic.

Left, submammary stabbing pain, known as 'precordial catch' is usually associated with anxiety and is sometimes known as effort (Da Costa's) syndrome. Occasionally, cardiac conditions such as mitral valve prolapse cause similar pain. Central chest pain similar to angina can occur with oesophageal disease and can be difficult to differentiate (see p. 186).

Other causes of chest pain are pulmonary embolism, pulmonary hypertension, costochondritis, pleurisy, pneumothorax and mediastinitis.

## Palpitations

A palpitation is an increased awareness of the normal heart beat or the sensation of slow or rapid heart rate or an irregular heart rhythm. The normal heart beat is sensed when the patient is anxious, excited, exercising, or lying on the left side. The most common arrhythmias to be felt as palpitations are premature ectopic beats and paroxysmal tachycardias.

### Premature beats
These are usually felt as 'missed beats' because the premature beat is followed by a pause before the next normal beat, which is rather forceful because of the longer diastolic filling period. Premature beats often occur in clusters and may cause the patient much anxiety.

### Paroxysmal tachycardias
These start abruptly and may terminate equally suddenly. Often, however, the tachycardia slows before terminating and therefore seems to fade away. Paroxysmal atrial fibrillation is noticeably irregular, whereas other forms of paroxysmal supraventricular or ventricular tachycardia are regular. Paroxysms of rapid tachycardia, especially when prolonged, may be associated with syncope, presyncope, dyspnoea or chest pain. Palpitations can be graded in a similar way to the grading of dyspnoea or angina. Supraventricular tachycardias, such as atrial fibrillation or junctional tachycardias, may produce polyuria.

### Bradycardias
An unduly slow heart rate may be appreciated as slow, regular, 'heavy' or forceful beats. Most often bradycardias are not felt as palpitations.

## Syncope

Syncope can be due to many causes (see p. 916), the most common of which is situational or vasovagal syncope. These attacks may be provoked by fright, anxiety, phobias or other situations such as micturition or coughing. The basic mechanism is vasodilatation leading to venous pooling followed by emptying of the heart. Vigorous contraction of the near-empty heart stimulates mechanoreceptors in the infero-posterior wall of the left ventricle.

Consequent reflexes via the central nervous system leads to further vasodilatation and sometimes profound bradycardia. This is known as 'neurocardiogenic' syncope. The episodes are usually associated with a prodome that consists of dizziness, nausea, sweating, ringing in the ears, a sinking feeling and yawning. Recovery occurs within a few seconds.

Cardiovascular syncope is usually sudden and brief. The classical variety is known as a Stokes–Adams attack and is due to a disturbance of cardiac rhythm, e.g. a profound bradycardia related to complete heart block. Without warning the patient falls to the ground, pale and deeply unconscious. The pulse is usually very slow or absent. After a few seconds the patient flushes brightly and recovers consciousness as the pulse quickens. If the period of unconsciousness is prolonged the patient may suffer a generalized convulsion but this is not usual. Often there are no sequelae but patients may injure themselves during falls.

Other causes of syncope due to heart disease can be grouped as cardiac arrhythmias or valvular or vascular obstruction (Table 11.4).

## Fatigue

This symptom, which consists of tiredness and lethargy, is associated with heart failure, persistent cardiac arrhythmias and cyanotic heart disease. It is due to poor cerebral and peripheral perfusion and poor oxygenation. When severe cardiac disorders are not present, an active infection such as infective endocarditis may be responsible. However, disorders of most systems may produce this non-specific symptom. Drugs prescribed for angina or hypertension, particularly $\beta$-blockers, may cause fatigue.

## Oedema

Heart failure results in salt and water retention. Retained fluid accumulates in the feet and ankles of ambulant patients and over the sacrum of bed-bound patients. The oedema associated with heart failure becomes progress-

*Arrhythmias*
Ventricular tachycardia
Rapid supraventricular tachycardia
Sinus arrest
Atrioventricular block
Artificial pacemaker failure

*Obstruction*
Aortic/pulmonary stenosis
Hypertrophic obstructive cardiomyopathy
Fallot's tetralogy
Pulmonary hypertension/embolism
Atrial myxoma
Atrial thrombus
Defective prosthetic valve

*Situational*
Neurocardiogenic (vasovagal)

**Table 11.4** Cardiac causes of syncope.

ively worse during the day and is often absent on initial rising as the fluid is reabsorbed on lying down. When severe, the calf and thigh may become oedematous and ascites or a pleural effusion may develop.

# Examination of the cardiovascular system

## GENERAL EXAMINATION

General features of the patient's well-being should be noted as well as the presence of anaemia, obesity, jaundice and cachexia.

## Clubbing (see also p. 641)

The most common cardiac causes of severe clubbing are subacute infective endocarditis and congenital cyanotic heart disease, particularly Fallot's tetralogy. Clubbing takes many months to develop and is therefore not seen in acute endocarditis or in neonates or infants with cyanotic heart disease. Clubbing seen in cor pulmonale is due to the underlying pulmonary disease (e.g. bronchiectasis or fibrosing alveolitis).

## Splinter haemorrhages

These small, subungual linear haemorrhages are most frequently due to trauma but are also caused by infective endocarditis when they may be florid.

## Cyanosis

This is a dusky blue discoloration of the skin (particularly at the extremities) or of the mucous membranes. It is due to the presence of unoxygenated haemoglobin (traditionally at least $5 \text{ g dl}^{-1}$ of blood) and occasionally of other reduction products of haemoglobin such as sulphaemoglobin or methaemoglobin. Cyanosis is more readily provoked in the presence of polycythaemia and is uncommon when anaemia is present.

### Central cyanosis
This is present when the tongue is cyanosed. It is caused by cardiac failure or respiratory disorders. The central cyanosis of pulmonary or cardiac failure is improved by breathing oxygen if the degree of shunting is small.

### Peripheral cyanosis
This is due to vasoconstriction and stasis of blood in the extremities, and increased oxygen extraction by peripheral tissues. Peripheral cyanosis occurs in congestive heart failure, shock, exposure to cold temperatures and with abnormalities of the peripheral circulation.

## THE ARTERIAL PULSE

A pulse is felt by compressing an artery against a bone. The first pulse to be examined is the right radial pulse. The timings of the left radial and femoral pulses are then compared with that of the right radial pulse. Delayed pulsation occurs because of a proximal stenosis, particularly of the aorta (coarctation).

## Rate

The pulse rate should be between 60 and 80 beats per minute (b.p.m.) when an adult patient is lying quietly in bed. Young children may have higher pulse rates and athletes and elderly adults may have slower rates. The exact rate is unimportant but changes (seen on a pulse chart) are helpful. When the pulse is irregular, not all beats may be transmitted to the wrist and it is therefore best to count the pulse whilst at the same time listening to the heart beat with a stethoscope. An apex–radial (pulse) deficit is common in atrial fibrillation.

## Rhythm

In normal subjects the pulse is regular except for a slight quickening in early inspiration and a slowing in expiration (sinus arrhythmia). Irregularities of the pulse rhythm are usually due to premature beats, intermittent heart block or atrial fibrillation.

Premature beats occur as occasional or repeated irregularities superimposed on a regular pulse rhythm. Similarly, intermittent heart block is revealed by occasional beats dropped from an otherwise regular rhythm. A more irregular pattern (irregularly irregular) of heart beats occurs in atrial fibrillation. This irregular pattern persists when the pulse quickens in response to exercise in contrast to pulse irregularity due to ectopic beats, which usually disappears on exercise. However, this is not a reliable way to distinguish ectopic beats from other causes of pulse irregularity.

## Carotid pulse

The amplitude and shape of the carotid pulse is examined. Usually carotid pulsation is not visible, but a very large-volume pulse may be apparent as pulsation of the neck (Corrigan's sign). A large-volume pulse occurs in high output states and in aortic regurgitation. The carotid pulse is also visible when the carotid artery is aneurysmal or kinked. The right carotid is palpated lightly in order to detect a thrill.

A large-volume pulse with a brisk rise and fall is known as a collapsing or waterhammer pulse (Fig. 11.8). It is found in the elderly when the aorta is rigid, or when the cardiac output is high, e.g. in thyrotoxicosis, anaemia or fever. Aortic valvular regurgitation or a persistent ductus arteriosus also cause a collapsing pulse. A large-volume pulse that is not collapsing in nature is associated with the large stroke volume that is necessary if bradycardia is present.

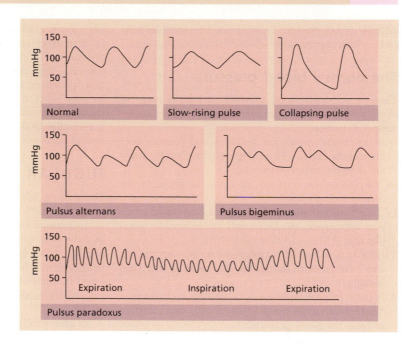

**Fig. 11.8**   Various arterial waveforms.

A small-volume pulse is seen in cardiac failure, shock and obstructive vascular or valvular disease. It is also present when tachycardia occurs. The pulse of aortic stenosis is not only small in volume but is slow in rising to a peak (plateau pulse) and is often associated with a notch on the upstroke (anacrotic pulse) or a systolic shudder or thrill.

## Other changes in arterial pulse

### Paradoxical pulse (pulsus paradoxus) (Fig. 11.8)
Paradoxical pulse is a misnomer as it is actually an exaggeration of the normal pattern. In normal subjects, the systolic pressure and the pulse pressure (the difference between the systolic and diastolic blood pressures) fall during inspiration. The normal fall of systolic pressure is less than 10 mmHg and this can be measured using a sphygmomanometer. The reason for this fall in pressure is that the right heart responds directly to changes in intrathoracic pressure while the filling of the left depends on the pulmonary intravascular volume. Thus as the return of blood to the left ventricle falls there is a drop in systolic pressure. At high respiratory rates this is exaggerated with the volumes of the right and left ventricles being unequal. In severe airflow limitation (especially severe asthma) there is an increased and sudden negative intrathoracic pressure on inspiration and this will enhance the normal fall in blood pressure. In patients with cardiac tamponade the fluid in the pericardium increases the intrapericardial pressure thereby reducing the heart's filling capacity. The inspiratory increase in the right ventricle occurs very much at the expense of the left ventricle as both ventricles are confined within a relatively 'fixed' pericardium. Through a similar mechanism, paradox can occur in constrictive pericarditis but is less common.

### Alternating pulse (pulsus alternans)
This is characterized by alternate beats that are weak and strong but with a regular rhythm. It is a feature of severe myocardial failure and is due to the prolonged recovery time of damaged myocardium; it indicates a very poor prognosis. It is easily noticed when taking the blood pressure because the systolic blood pressure may vary from beat to beat by as much as 50 mmHg. Pulsus alternans may also occur when there is rapid, abnormal tachycardia. In this case it acts as a compensatory mechanism and does not indicate a poor prognosis. Pulsus alternans should be distinguished from a bigeminal pulse (see below).

### Bigeminal pulse (pulsus bigeminus)
This is due to premature ectopic beats following every sinus beat. The rhythm is not regular (see Fig. 11.8) because every weak pulse is premature.

### Pulsus bisferiens
This is a pulse that is found in hypertrophic obstructive cardiomyopathy and in aortic regurgitation combined with aortic stenosis. The first systolic wave is the 'percussion' wave produced by the transmission of the left ventricular pressure in early systole. The second peak is the 'tidal' wave caused by recoil of the vascular bed. This normally happens in diastole (the dicrotic wave), but when the left ventricle empties slowly or is obstructed from emptying completely, the tidal wave occurs in late systole. The result is a palpable double pulse.

## BLOOD PRESSURE (Practical box 11.1)

The peak systemic arterial blood pressure is produced by transmission of left ventricular systolic pressure. The diastolic blood pressure is maintained by vascular tone and an intact aortic valve.

## The normal blood pressure

There is no single blood pressure or limited range of blood pressures that is normal in all subjects and circumstances. However:

In a resting adult the systolic blood pressure does not usually exceed 150 mmHg and the diastolic pressure does not exceed 90 mmHg.

In children or young adults the pressures are correspondingly less.

In the elderly the rigidity of the arterial vessels produces an increase, predominantly in the systolic blood pressure.

There is a diurnal variation of blood pressure, the pressure during the day being greater than at night.

Anxiety (for example when consulting a physician— 'white coat' hypertension, see p. 619) and exertion increase the blood pressure.

Note that a cuff that is too small leads to overestimation of the pressure. For example, if a standard arm cuff size (12 cm) is used in an obese patient, the pressure measured will be too high. Similarly, if an arm cuff is used on the thigh (with the diaphragm of the stethoscope applied over the popliteal artery), the femoral pressure will be overestimated. The usual thigh cuff is 15 cm wide. Smaller cuff sizes are available for children and thin adults.

## Variations in blood pressure

The systolic blood pressure varies by up to 10 mmHg between the right and left brachial arteries. Standing usu-ally causes a slight reduction of the systolic pressure (<20 mmHg) and an increase in the diastolic blood pressure (<10 mmHg). In postural (orthostatic) hypotension, a large postural fall of both the systolic and diastolic pressures is associated with dizziness. When an irregular heart rhythm such as atrial fibrillation is present, the blood pressure is variable. Because the blood pressure is normally liable to variation it must be estimated on several occasions before it can be declared elevated.

## JUGULAR VENOUS PULSE (JVP)

There are no valves between the internal jugular vein and the right atrium and observation of the column of blood in the internal jugular system is therefore a good measure of right atrial pressure (Practical box 11.2). The external jugular cannot be relied upon because of its valves and because it may be obstructed by the fascial and muscular layers through which it passes; it can only be used if typical venous pulsation is seen, indicating no obstruction to flow.

An abnormally low jugular venous pressure cannot be measured clinically. Causes include haemorrhage and other forms of hypovolaemia.

Elevation of the jugular venous pressure occurs in heart failure (see p. 571). It is also produced by:

● Constrictive pericarditis
● Cardiac tamponade
● Renal disease with salt and water retention
● Overtransfusion or excessive infusion of fluids
● Superior vena caval obstruction (but in this case pulsation is absent)

In constrictive pericarditis or cardiac tamponade, ventricular filling is reduced during inspiration because the ventricles are squeezed by the pericardial fluid or non-

---

The blood pressure is taken in the (right) arm with the patient relaxed and comfortable

The sphygmomanometer cuff is wrapped around the upper arm with the inflation bag placed over the brachial artery

The cuff is inflated until the pressure exceeds the arterial pressure and the radial pulse is no longer palpable

The diaphragm of the stethoscope is positioned over the brachial artery just below the cuff

The cuff pressure is slowly reduced until sounds (Korotkoff sounds) can be heard (phase 1). This is the systolic pressure

The pressure is allowed to fall further until the Korotkoff sounds become suddenly muffled (phase 4)

The pressure is allowed to fall still further until they disappear (phase 5)

The diastolic pressure is usually taken as phase 5 because this phase is more reproducible and nearer to the intravascular diastolic pressure. The Korotkoff sounds may disappear (phase 2) and reappear (phase 3) between the systolic and diastolic pressures. It is important not to mistake phase 2 for the diastolic pressure or phase 3 for the systolic pressure.

**Practical box 11.1** Taking the blood pressure.

---

The patient is positioned at about 45° to the horizontal (between 30° and 60°, wherever the top of the venous pulsation can be seen in a good light)

The head is supported by a pillow and the neck is slightly flexed to allow the skin and muscle overlying the vein to relax

The jugular venous pressure is measured as the vertical distance between the manubriosternal angle and the top of the venous column

The normal jugular venous pressure is usually less than 3 cmH$_2$O, which is equivalent to a right atrial pressure of 8 cmH$_2$O when measured with reference to a point midway between the anterior and posterior surfaces of the chest. The venous pulsations are not usually palpable (except for the forceful venous distension associated with tricuspid regurgitation)

Pulsations should be looked for before touching the neck

Gentle pressure at the root of the neck may abolish visible venous pulsation and may make a vein visible by causing distension above the occlusion.

Hepatojugular reflex. Abdominal compression causes a temporary increase in central and hence jugular venous pressure. It is a simple way of confirming the venous nature of a pulsation in the neck

**Practical box 11.2** Measurement of the jugular pressure.

compliant pericardium, which tightens as the diaphragm descends. Thus, the level of venous pressure increases during inspiration (Kussmaul's sign). Other causes of an increased jugular pressure also distort the shape of the pressure wave and are considered below.

## The jugular venous pressure wave

This consists of three peaks and two troughs (Fig. 11.9). The peaks are described as *a*, *c* and *v* waves and the troughs are known as *x* and *y* descents:
1 The *a wave* is produced by atrial systole.
2 The *x descent* occurs when the atrial contraction finishes.
3 As the pressure falls there is a small transient increase that produces a positive deflection called the *c wave*. This is caused by transmission of the rapidly increasing right ventricular pressure before the tricuspid valve closes.
4 The *v wave* develops as the venous return fills the right atrium during continued ventricular systole.
5 The *y descent* follows the *v* wave when the tricuspid valve opens.
The *a* wave can be distinguished from the *v* wave by observing the venous pulse while palpating the carotid artery. The *a* wave occurs immediately before carotid pulsation and the *v* wave occurs simultaneously with carotid pulsation.

The main abnormalities of the shape of the jugular venous pressure wave are elevations of the *a* and *v* waves and steepness of the *y* descent (Fig. 11.9).

### Large *a* waves

These are caused by increased resistance to ventricular filling, as seen with right ventricular hypertrophy due to pulmonary hypertension or pulmonary stenosis. They may also be caused by tricuspid stenosis, but this is unusual because patients with tricuspid stenosis are usually in atrial fibrillation and therefore do not have *a* waves.

A very large *a* wave occurs when the atrium contracts against a closed tricuspid valve. This is known as a 'cannon wave'. Cannon waves occur irregularly in complete heart block and in ventricular tachycardia. In both these situations there is atrioventricular dissociation, and by random chance there is occasional simultaneous atrial and ventricular contraction. In junctional rhythms the atria and ventricles usually contract simultaneously and rapid, regular cannon waves are produced.

### Large *v* waves

Tricuspid regurgitation results in giant *v* waves (systolic waves) because the right ventricular pressure is transmitted directly to the right atrium and the great veins.

### Steep *y* descent

Diastolic collapse of elevated venous pressure can occur in right ventricular failure but is more dramatic in constrictive pericarditis and tricuspid regurgitation. At the end of ventricular systole the elevated atrial pressure suddenly falls when the tricuspid valve opens. However, the ventricles are stiff and cannot be distended. The venous pressure therefore rapidly rises again. This rapid fall and rise of the jugular venous pulse is known as Friedreich's sign.

## EXAMINATION OF THE PRECORDIUM

### Inspection

Deformities should be looked for as they can mimic cardiac abnormalities. For example, pectus excavatum (funnel chest) or kyphoscoliosis may cause an ejection systolic murmur. The position of the apex beat and other cardiac pulsations should be noted; a left ventricular aneurysm may produce an eccentric and abnormal pulsation.

### Palpation

The apex beat is defined as the most inferior and most lateral point of cardiac pulsation. It is usually felt just inside the mid-clavicular line at the level of the fourth or fifth left intercostal space. Cardiac enlargement, particularly left ventricular dilatation, displaces the apex beat to the left. The apex beat may also be displaced by a pneumothorax, pulmonary collapse or skeletal abnormalities such as scoliosis. The apex beat is normally just palpable and confined to a point that can be covered by one finger. There are several abnormal forms:
TAPPING—a sudden but brief cardiac impulse felt in mitral stenosis.
THRUSTING—vigorous but non-sustained pulsation

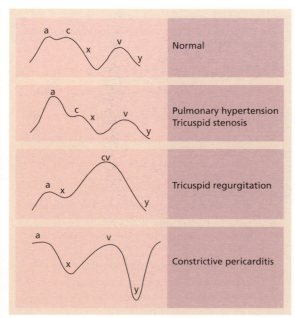

**Fig. 11.9**  Various jugular venous waveforms.

typical of 'volume overload' due to mitral or aortic regurgitation.

HEAVING—vigorous and sustained pulsation due to 'pressure overload' as in aortic stenosis and systemic hypertension.

IMPALPABLE—occurs in emphysema, pleural effusion, obesity and pericardial effusion.

DOUBLE—two apical pulsations with each heart beat may be felt in hypertrophic cardiomyopathy. This may be due to a palpable atrial impulse. A double apex can also be due to accentuated outward movement in late systole in ventricular aneurysm.

A parasternal heave is elicited by pressing the outstretched hand flat against the sternum or against the costal cartilages just to the left of the sternum. It occurs because of right ventricular hypertrophy. An enlarged left atrium may also cause a parasternal heave. Left atrial pulsation can be distinguished from pulsation due to right ventricular hypertrophy because it occurs before the apex beat or carotid pulsation.

Vigorous pulmonary artery pulsation may be appreciated by palpation in the second left interspace. This is usually due to pulmonary hypertension.

Thrills are palpable murmurs that are most easily appreciated with the flat or ulnar border of the hand rather than with the fingers. A thrill implies a definite abnormality. Systolic thrills in the aortic area are usually due to aortic stenosis, whereas at the apex a systolic thrill is due to mitral regurgitation. A diastolic thrill is usually caused by mitral stenosis; a diastolic thrill due to aortic regurgitation is uncommon.

Heart sounds that are very loud may also be palpated. In systemic hypertension the aortic second sound may be felt, and in pulmonary hypertension the pulmonary component of the second sound may be felt. Occasionally a third or fourth heart sound may be palpated.

## Percussion

Percussion is not usually undertaken, but it may allow the approximate position and size of the heart to be determined.

## Auscultation

The sounds best heard with the bell or the diaphragm of the stethoscope are shown in Table 11.5.

| Bell (for low-frequency sounds) | Diaphragm (for high-frequency sounds) |
|---|---|
| Mid-diastolic rumbles of mitral stenosis and tricuspid stenosis | Early diastolic murmurs of aortic and pulmonary regurgitation |
| Third and fourth heart sounds | Second heart sound Systolic clicks and opening snaps |

Table 11.5   Use of the stethoscope.

There are four areas where the heart sounds and valvular murmurs are best heard:

1 The *aortic area* is in the second intercostal space immediately to the right of the sternum. The aorta arches upwards and forwards from the aortic valve and the murmur of aortic stenosis is transmitted best to this area.

2 The *pulmonary area* is in the second interspace just to the left of the sternum. This is the closest point to the pulmonary valve, where the murmur of pulmonary stenosis and the pulmonary component of the second heart sound are loudest.

3 The *tricuspid area* is in the fourth interspace to the left of the sternum (left sternal edge). Not only is this close to the tricuspid valve but is also over the ventricles. Therefore, as well as the murmurs and sounds from the tricuspid valve, the murmurs of pulmonary and aortic regurgitation and third and fourth right ventricular sounds are heard well here.

4 The *mitral area or apex* is the point at which the apex beat is felt. The first heart sound and mitral murmurs are loudest here, and aortic regurgitation and third and fourth left ventricular sounds are often heard best at this point.

The sequence of cardiac auscultation is summarized in Table 11.6.

### Heart sounds

THE FIRST HEART SOUND. This is caused by the closure of the mitral and tricuspid valves and is best heard at the cardiac apex. The sound is usually single but may be slightly split. If split, this 'double' sound at the beginning of systole must be distinguished from the combination of the first heart sound with a fourth heart sound or with an ejection click.

The first heart sound is loud when the patient is thin

The mitral, tricuspid, pulmonary and aortic areas should be auscultated in turn

1    *Supine*
First heart sound—mitral area
Second heart sound—pulmonary and aortic areas, during respiration
Third and fourth heart sounds—mitral and tricuspid areas
Clicks, snaps, plops, knocks—mitral and tricuspid areas
Systolic murmurs—all four auscultation areas, also the neck, axilla and back

2    *Sitting forward*
Aortic diastolic murmur—tricuspid and mitral areas

3    *Lying on the left side*
Mitral diastolic murmur—mitral area (exactly over the apex beat)

4    *During inspiration and expiration*—see Table 11.8

5    *Exercise, squatting, Valsalva manoeuvres*
Can be used to accentuate murmurs

Table 11.6   Summary of the auscultation procedure.

and when the circulation is hyperdynamic, e.g. due to anaemia or thyrotoxicosis. The sound is also loud if the valve is still open when ventricular systole begins, e.g. in mitral stenosis.

A soft first heart sound occurs in patients with obesity, emphysema or pericardial effusion. It is also present when the valve leaflets are immobile, e.g. in severe calcific mitral stenosis, or when the leaflets are partly closed when systole begins, which occurs when the PR interval is long. A soft first heart sound also occurs when the valve does not close properly, as in mitral regurgitation. Heart failure and cardiogenic shock are also associated with a soft first heart sound.

The intensity of the first heart sound is variable when the relationship between atrial and ventricular systole is not constant, e.g. during ventricular tachycardia or complete heart block: when the PR interval is short the sound is loud, and when the PR interval is long the sound is soft.

THE SECOND HEART SOUND. This is caused by the closure of the aortic and pulmonary valves. Unless excessively loud, the pulmonary component of the second sound is only heard in the pulmonary area. Left heart emptying is usually finished just before right heart emptying; therefore the pulmonary component of the second sound closely follows the aortic component. Inspiration results in increased venous return to the right heart, which further delays right heart emptying. The pulmonary sound is therefore delayed further on inspiration and the second heart sound becomes audibly split (Fig. 11.10). Splitting of the second heart sound on inspiration is known as normal or physiological splitting and is most commonly heard in children or young adults.

Reversed splitting of the second heart sound (when the aortic component follows the pulmonary component) occurs on expiration. It is due to a fixed delay in left heart emptying caused by aortic stenosis, left bundle branch block or left ventricular failure. Thus, when right heart emptying is delayed during inspiration, the two sounds move together, and when the right heart empties more quickly during expiration, the sounds move apart.

The fixed delay in the emptying of the right ventricle produced, for example, by right bundle branch block or pulmonary stenosis will result in wide splitting of the second heart sound. With an atrial septal defect there is usually some degree of right bundle branch block, and because of shunting of blood from the left to the right atrium the right-sided cardiac output is high and ventricular emptying is further delayed. The second heart sound is therefore widely split. Because communication at atrial level prevents differential changes of the venous return during inspiration and expiration, the wide splitting of the second heart sound is not varied by respiration. This is called fixed splitting.

The aortic second sound is louder in systemic hypertension and when a hyperdynamic circulation is present. It is soft in aortic stenosis because the valve is relatively immobile, and it is soft in cardiac failure because of low blood flow. Similarly, the pulmonary component of the second heart sound is loud in pulmonary hypertension and soft in pulmonary stenosis.

ADDITIONAL HEART SOUNDS (Fig. 11.11). Third and fourth heart sounds are diastolic in timing, representing ventricular filling, and are heard as soft 'thudding' noises immediately before the first sound (fourth sound) or after the second sound (third sound). The presence of a third or fourth sound produces a triple rhythm that, when associated with sinus tachycardia, sounds like a galloping horse—a gallop rhythm. The cadence of a gallop rhythm due to a third heart sound has been likened to 'Kentucky', whilst that due to a fourth heart sound resembles 'Tennessee'. When both third and fourth heart sounds occur there is usually a marked sinus tachycardia, which results in a short diastolic period so that third and fourth sounds occur simultaneously. This is known as a summation gallop.

THE THIRD SOUND is due to rapid ventricular filling as soon as the mitral and tricuspid valves open. It is a normal finding in children and young adults when it is heard at the apex, especially in the left lateral position. In those over 40 years it represents heart failure or volume overload, e.g. due to mitral regurgitation. It is therefore sometimes referred to as a sound of 'distress'. A right ventricular third sound is heard best at the left sternal edge, and a left ventricular third sound is heard at the apex.

THE FOURTH SOUND is caused by the surge of ventricular filling that accompanies atrial systole. It therefore occurs in late diastole. It may be a normal finding in an elderly subject, but in younger patients it usually indicates increased ventricular stiffness associated with

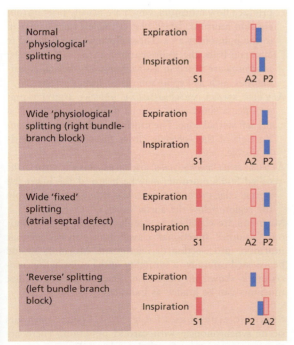

**Fig. 11.10** Variations of the second heart sound. A$_2$, aortic component; P$_2$, pulmonary component.

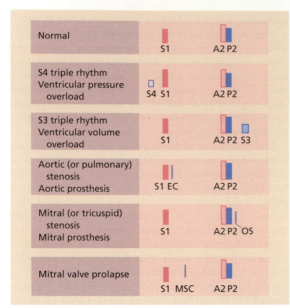

| | | |
|---|---|---|
| Normal | S1 | A2 P2 |
| S4 triple rhythm Ventricular pressure overload | S4 S1 | A2 P2 |
| S3 triple rhythm Ventricular volume overload | S1 | A2 P2 S3 |
| Aortic (or pulmonary) stenosis Aortic prosthesis | S1 EC | A2 P2 |
| Mitral (or tricuspid) stenosis Mitral prosthesis | S1 | A2 P2 OS |
| Mitral valve prolapse | S1 MSC | A2 P2 |

**Fig. 11.11** Normal and additional heart sounds and the conditions in which they are found. A2, aortic component of the second sound; EC, ejection click; MSC, mid-systolic click; OS, opening snap; P2, pulmonary component of the second sound; S1, first heart sound; S3, third heart sound; S4, fourth heart sound.

hypertension, aortic stenosis or acute myocardial infarction. It is called the sound of cardiac 'stress', and can sometimes be felt.

ABNORMAL HEART VALVES may cause an audible signal when opening. An *ejection click* sound occurs immediately following the first heart sound. It is produced by the sudden opening of a deformed but mobile aortic or pulmonary valve. It is most commonly heard in association with a bicuspid aortic valve when it is easily heard throughout the respiratory cycle. A stenotic pulmonary valve also produces an ejection click, but this is best heard on expiration. A dilated aorta or pulmonary artery may also give rise to an ejection click.

A STENOTIC MITRAL OR TRICUSPID VALVE may produce a high-frequency opening snap that occurs just after the second heart sound. It can be distinguished from a split second sound or a third sound by the site at which it is best heard, its higher frequency and its lack of respiratory variation.

A MID-SYSTOLIC CLICK (OR CLICKS) is due to sudden prolapse of the mitral valve into the left atrium during ventricular systole. It occurs when the mitral valve is congenitally deformed or has undergone myxomatous degeneration, as in the mitral valve prolapse syndrome. These auscultatory features are inconsistent and wax and wane with time.

TUMOUR PLOPS are low-frequency sounds produced by the sudden checking of the travel of an atrial tumour when it reaches the valve. Such sounds occur after an opening snap, but before a third sound would be expected. The pericardial knock is another sound that

occurs in this position in the cardiac cycle. Like a third heart sound, it is low frequency. It is heard in constrictive pericarditis and is due to rather early, sudden and marked halting of ventricular filling due to constriction.

**Prosthetic sounds**

Mechanical replacement heart valves produce loud clicks due to the opening and closing of the valve. These prosthetic sounds may be muffled or absent if valve movement is impeded by thrombus or vegetations.

**Heart murmurs**

Turbulent blood flow causes heart murmurs. Turbulence may be produced when there is high blood flow through a normal valve, or when there is normal blood flow through an abnormal valve or into a dilated chamber. Turbulence is also caused by the regurgitation of blood through a leaking valve. Murmurs produced by high-velocity blood flow (e.g. the systolic murmur of mitral regurgitation) are high frequency and are often described as 'blowing' in quality. The intensity of murmurs is determined not only by the blood velocity but also by the volume of blood producing the murmur and the distance of the source of the murmur from the stethoscope. Right-sided murmurs tend to become louder on inspiration because inspiration increases the venous return to the right heart.

Heart murmurs may occur with a normal or near-normal heart (innocent murmurs). They are usually soft and short, and occur early in systole. Murmurs also occur in the following situations:

ANAEMIA, THYROTOXICOSIS, PREGNANCY AND OTHER CAUSES OF A HIGH CARDIAC OUTPUT produce flow murmurs, which are usually brief systolic ejection murmurs heard best at the left sternal edge or in the pulmonary area. These murmurs are believed to emanate from the pulmonary or aortic valve. Similar murmurs are heard in association with skeletal abnormalities such as kyphoscoliosis or funnel chest.

A VERY SMALL VENTRICULAR SEPTAL DEFECT may produce a short early systolic murmur, heard well at the left sternal edge. The murmur is short because contraction of the ventricle closes the small defect early in systole.

A BUZZING, TWANGING OR VIBRATORY MURMUR, called Still's murmur, may be heard at the lower left sternal edge or cardiac apex. It is thought to arise from the region below the aortic valve.

Murmurs are classified as systolic, diastolic or continuous. Another functional classification divides systolic murmurs into ejection or regurgitant. Murmurs should be assessed carefully; a summary of the auscultation procedure is shown in Table 11.6. The intensity of cardiac murmurs can be graded as indicated in Table 11.7.

SYSTOLIC MURMURS (Table 11.8) Systolic murmurs occur synchronously with carotid pulsation. There are three main varieties of pathological systolic murmur:

**1** *Ejection mid-systolic murmurs* are heard separately from

| Grade | Systolic murmurs | Diastolic murmurs |
|---|---|---|
| 1 | Very soft (heard only in good circumstances) | Very soft (heard only in good circumstances) |
| 2 | Soft | Soft |
| 3 | Moderate | Moderate |
| 4 | Loud | Loud or associated with palpable thrill |
| 5 | Very loud | — |
| 6 | Very loud (no stethoscope needed) or associated with palpable thrill | — |

**Table 11.7**  The grading of murmur intensity.

the first and second heart sounds. Their intensity rises then falls, being greatest in mid-systole.

2 *Pan-systolic murmurs* extend from the first to the second heart sound and tend to be of constant intensity throughout the whole of systole.

3 *Late systolic murmurs* are separated from the first sound but extend up to the second sound.

DIASTOLIC MURMURS (Table 11.8). Diastolic murmurs are always associated with cardiac disease. They are of two types:

1 *Mid-diastolic murmurs* usually arise from the mitral and tricuspid valves. In aortic regurgitation the flow of blood back into the left ventricle may partially close and obstruct the mitral valve, producing a mitral mid-diastolic murmur (Austin Flint murmur).

2 *Early diastolic murmurs* usually result from aortic regurgitation and rarely from pulmonary regurgitation. These murmurs begin with the second heart sound and are blowing (high-pitched) in quality. Pulmonary hypertension secondary to mitral stenosis may lead to pulmonary valve regurgitation (Graham Steell murmur).

CONTINUOUS MURMURS. A continuous murmur may occur because of a combination of systolic and diastolic murmurs, due to connections between the aorta and pulmonary artery (e.g. patent ductus arteriosus) or due to arteriovenous anastomoses and collateral circulations such as those associated with coarctation of the aorta. High venous flow, especially in young children, can produce a continuous venous hum in the neck. This is reduced by occluding the vein or by lying the child flat. Similarly, high mammary blood flow in pregnant or lactating women can produce a continuous murmur known as a mammary souffle.

**Extra cardiac sounds**
Bruits, usually due to arterial stenoses, are murmurs arising from a peripheral artery, including the distal aorta.

| Murmur | Position where murmur is best heard |
|---|---|
| **Systolic** | |
| *Ejection (mid-)systolic* | |
| Aortic stenosis | Aortic area and clavicles |
| Pulmonary stenosis ⎱ Atrial septal defect ⎰ | Left sternal edge on inspiration |
| Left (e.g. hypertrophic cardiomyopathy, HOCM) and right (e.g. Fallot's tetralogy) outflow tract obstruction may also cause mid-systolic murmurs | |
| **Pan-systolic** | |
| Mitral regurgitation (blowing) | Apex to axilla |
| Tricuspid regurgitation (low-pitched) | Left sternal edge |
| Ventricular septal defect (loud and rough) | Left sternal edge |
| **Late systolic** | |
| Dynamic outflow tract obstruction (HOCM) | Accentuated on standing |
| Mitral valve prolapse | Apex |
| Coarctation of the aorta | Left sternal edge |
| **Diastolic** | |
| *Mid-diastolic* | |
| Mitral stenosis (low-frequency rumbling) | Apex, patient on left side, accentuated on exertion |
| Tricuspid stenosis | Left sternal edge, accentuated on inspiration |
| Austin Flint murmur | Apex |
| **Early diastolic** | |
| Aortic regurgitation (blowing, high-pitched) | Left sternal edge and apex, patient sitting forward and in expiration |
| Pulmonary regurgitation (blowing, variable pitch) | Right of sternum, louder on inspiration |
| Graham Steell in pulmonary hypertension (due to mitral stenosis) | Left sternal edge |
| **Combined systolic and diastolic** | |
| Patent ductus arteriosus Aortic stenosis and regurgitation | Left sternal edge |

**Table 11.8**  Some common structural causes of murmurs.

A pericardial friction rub is a scratching or crunching noise produced by the movement of inflamed pericardium. Since it is relatively high frequency, it is best heard with the diaphragm. It is most obvious in systole but may also be heard in early diastole or synchronously with atrial contraction. It should be listened for during both held inspiration and expiration.

# Cardiac investigation

## Chest X-ray

This is taken in the postero-anterior (PA) direction at maximum inspiration with the heart close to the X-ray film to minimize magnification with respect to the thorax. A lateral may give additional information if the PA is abnormal. The cardiac structures and great vessels that can be seen on these X-rays are indicated in Fig. 11.12.

### Heart size

Heart size can be reliably assessed only from the PA chest film; the maximum transverse diameter of the heart is compared with the maximum transverse diameter of the chest (see Fig. 11.12) measured from the inside of the ribs.

The cardiothoracic ratio (CTR) is usually less than 50%, except in neonates, infants, athletes and patients with skeletal abnormalities such as scoliosis and funnel chest in general. A transverse cardiac diameter of more than 15.5 cm is abnormal. Pericardial effusion or cardiac dilatation causes an increase in the ratio.

A pericardial effusion produces a globular, sharp-edged shadow. This enlargement may occur quite suddenly and, unlike heart failure, there is no associated change in the pulmonary vasculature. The echocardiogram is more specific than the chest X-ray for the diagnosis of pericardial effusion, particularly because at least 250 ml of fluid must accumulate before X-ray changes are apparent.

Certain patterns of specific chamber enlargement may be seen on the chest X-ray:

LEFT ATRIAL DILATATION results in prominence of the left atrial appendage on the left heart border, a double atrial shadow to the right of the sternum, and splaying of the carina because a large left atrium elevates the left main bronchus (Fig. 11.13). On a lateral chest X-ray an enlarged left atrium bulges backwards, displacing the left main stem branches.

LEFT VENTRICULAR ENLARGEMENT results in an increase in the CTR and a smooth elongation and increased convexity of the left heart border. A left ventricular aneurysm may produce a distinct bulge or distortion of the left heart border.

RIGHT ATRIAL ENLARGEMENT results in the right border of the heart projecting into the right lower lung field.

RIGHT VENTRICULAR ENLARGEMENT, due to congenital heart disease, results in an increase of the CTR and an upward displacement of the apex of the heart because the enlarging right ventricle pushes the left ventricle leftwards, upwards and eventually backwards. Differentiation of left from right ventricular enlargement may be difficult from the shape of the left heart border alone, but the lateral view shows enlargement anteriorly for the right ventricle and posteriorly for the left ventricle.

ASCENDING AORTIC DILATATION OR ENLARGEMENT is seen as a prominence of the aortic shadow to the right of the mediastinum between the right atrium and superior vena cava.

DISSECTION OF THE ASCENDING AORTA is seen as a

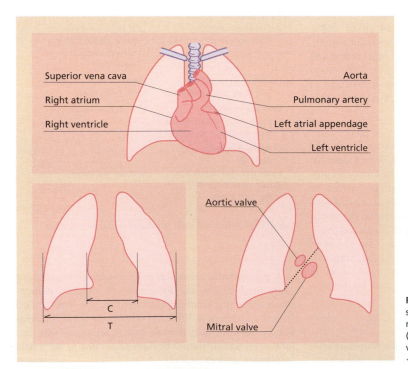

**Fig. 11.12** Diagrams to show the heart silhouette on the chest X-ray, measurements of the cardiothoracic ratio (CTR) and the location of the cardiac valves. CTR = (C/T) × 100%; normal CTR <50%.

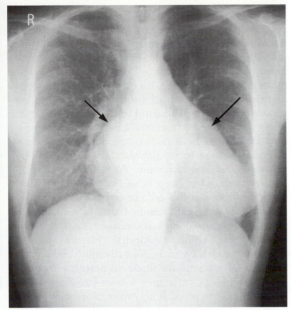

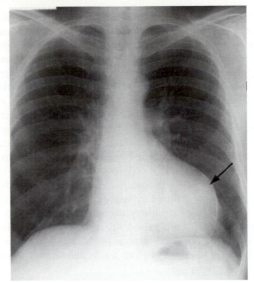

**Fig. 11.14**   Plain PA chest X-ray demonstrating a cardiac silhouette with a 'bulge' on the left lateral border. This bulge is due to aneurysm formation of many years following a myocardial infarction. A thin line of calcification can be seen along the edge of this bulge.

**Fig. 11.13**   This plain PA chest X-ray is taken from a patient with mixed mitral valve disease. The left atrium is markedly enlarged. Note the large bulge on the left heart border (left atrium) and the 'double shadow' on the right side of the heart (border of the right and left atria). There is cardiac (left ventricular) enlargement due to mitral regurgitation.

widening of the mediastinum, although this is often difficult to assess on an AP chest X-ray. A left-sided pleural effusion may be evident if the aneurysm is leaking or there may be blood around the apex of the lung ('capping').

Enlargement of the pulmonary artery in pulmonary hypertension, pulmonary artery stenosis and left-to-right shunts produces a prominent bulge on the left-hand border of the mediastinum below the aortic knuckle.

## Calcification

Calcification in the cardiovascular system occurs because of tissue degeneration. Calcification is visible on a lateral or a penetrated PA film, but is best studied by fluoroscopy or CT scanning. Various types of calcification can occur:

Pericardial calcification may be seen as plaque-like opacities over the surface of the heart, but particularly concentrated in the atrioventricular groove. Such calcification often results from tuberculous pericarditis and may be associated with pericardial constriction.

Valvular calcification may result from long-standing rheumatic or bicuspid aortic valve disease. The aortic and mitral valves are most commonly affected. On the lateral film, a calcified aortic valve is seen on or above a line joining the carina to the sterno-phrenic angle. Mitral valvular calcification is seen below and behind this line (see Fig. 11.12).

Myocardial calcification may occur after myocardial infarction, especially in association with a left ventricular aneurysm (Fig. 11.14).

Calcification of the aorta is a common, normal finding in patients over the age of 40 years and appears as a curvilinear opacity around the circumference of the aortic knuckle. Calcification in the ascending aorta usually denotes syphilitic aortitis, whereas in the descending aorta it is due to atheroma or, in the younger patient, to non-specific aortitis.

Coronary arterial calcification, especially of the proximal left coronary artery, is associated with coronary atheroma but does not necessarily correspond to the site of maximal stenosis.

## Lung fields

Pulmonary plethora results from left-to-right shunts, e.g. atrial or ventricular septal defects. It is seen as a general increase in the vascularity of the lung fields and as an increase in the size of hilar vessels, e.g. in the right lower lobe artery, which normally should not exceed 16 mm in diameter.

Pulmonary oligaemia is a paucity of vascular markings and a reduction in the width of the arteries. It occurs in situations where there is reduced pulmonary blood flow, such as pulmonary embolism, severe pulmonary stenosis and Fallot's tetralogy.

Pulmonary arterial hypertension may result from pulmonary embolism, chronic lung disease or chronic left heart disease such as shunts due to a ventricular septal defect or mitral valve stenosis. In addition to X-ray features of these conditions, the pulmonary arteries are prominent close to the hili but are very reduced in size (pruned) in the peripheral lung fields. This pattern is usually symmetrical.

Pulmonary venous hypertension occurs in left ventricular failure or mitral valve disease. Normal pulmonary venous pressure is 5–14 mmHg at rest. Mild pulmonary venous hypertension (15–20 mmHg) produces isolated dilatation of the upper zone vessels. Interstitial oedema occurs when the pressure is between 21 and 30 mmHg. This manifests as fluid collections in the interlobar fissures, interlobular septa (Kerley B lines) and pleural spaces. This gives rise to indistinctness of the hilar regions and haziness of the lung fields. Alveolar oedema occurs when the pressure exceeds 30 mmHg, appearing as areas of consolidation and mottling of the lung fields (Fig. 11.15) and pleural effusions. Patients with long-standing elevation of the pulmonary venous pressure have reactive thickening of the pulmonary arteriolar intima, which protects the alveoli from pulmonary oedema. Thus, in these patients the pulmonary venous pressure may increase to well above 30 mmHg before frank pulmonary oedema develops.

### Fluoroscopy

Fluoroscopy has been largely superseded by echocardiography. However, it is still essential for the insertion of cardiac catheters and pacemaker electrodes.

## Electrocardiography

The electrocardiogram (ECG) is a recording of the electrical activity of the heart. It is the vector sum of the depolarization and repolarization potentials of all myocardial cells (see Fig. 11.33). At the body surface these generate potential differences of about 1 mV and the fluctuations of these potentials create the familiar P–QRS–T pattern. At rest the intracellular voltage of the myocardium is polarized at −90 mV compared with that of the extracellular space. This diastolic voltage difference occurs because of the high intracellular potassium concentration, which is maintained by the sodium–potassium pump despite the free membrane permeability to potassium. Depolarization of cardiac cells occurs when there is a sudden increase in the permeability of the membrane to sodium. Sodium rushes into the cell and the negative resting voltage is lost (stage 0; see Fig. 11.33). The depolarization of a myocardial cell causes the depolarization of adjacent cells and, in the healthy heart, the entire myocardium is depolarized in a coordinated fashion. During repolarization, cellular electrolyte balance is slowly restored (stages 1, 2 and 3). Slow diastolic depolarization (stage 4) follows until the threshold potential is reached. Another action potential then follows (see Fig. 11.33).

The ECG is recorded from two or more simultaneous points of skin contact (electrodes). When cardiac activation proceeds towards the positive contact, an upward deflection is produced on the ECG. Correct representation of a three-dimensional spatial vector requires recordings from three mutually perpendicular (orthogonal) axes. The shape of the human torso does not make this easy, so the practical ECG records 12 projections of the vector, called 'leads' (Fig. 11.16 and Practical box 11.3). Six of these are obtained by recording voltages from the

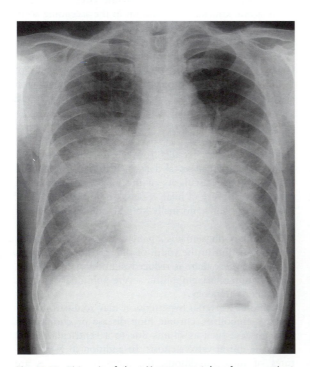 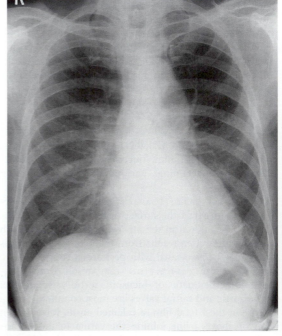

**Fig. 11.15**  This pair of chest X-rays were taken from a patient before (left) and after (right) treatment of acute pulmonary oedema. The chest X-ray taken when the oedema was present demonstrates hilar haziness, Kerley B lines, upper lobe venous engorgement and fluid in the right horizontal interlobar fissure. These abnormalities are resolved on the film taken after successful treatment.

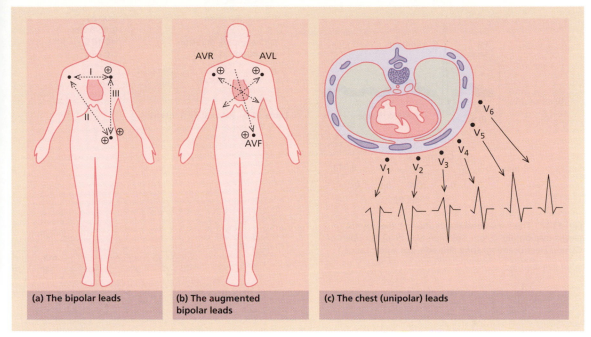

**Fig. 11.16** The connections or directions that comprise the 12-lead electrocardiogram. (a) The bipolar leads. (b) The unipolar leads. (c) The chest leads.

**Standard leads** (bipolar) are derived:
Lead 1 Right arm (−ve) to left arm (+ve)
Lead 2 Right arm (−ve) to left leg (+ve)
Lead 3 Left arm (−ve) to left leg (+ve)

**Augmented leads** (augmented bipolar) are derived:
AVR    Right arm (+ve) to left arm and left leg (−ve)
AVL    Left arm (+ve) to left leg and right arm (−ve)
AVF    Left leg (+ve) to left arm and right arm (−ve)

**Chest leads** (unipolar) are derived by connecting the V lead against the three extremity leads—the exploring electrodes are placed as follows:

V1    4th intercostal space just to the right of the sternum
V2    4th intercostal space just to the left of the sternum
V3    Halfway between V2 and V4
V4    5th intercostal space in the left mid-clavicular line
V5    On same horizontal as V4 in anterior axillary line
V6    On same horizontal as V4 in mid-axillary line

**Practical box 11.3**  ECG leads.

limbs (I, II, III, AVR, AVL and AVF). The other six leads record potentials between points on the chest surface and an average of the three limbs: RA, LA and LL. These are designated $V_1$–$V_6$ and aim to select activity from the right ventricle ($V_1$–$V_2$), interventricular septum ($V_3$–$V_4$) and left ventricle ($V_5$–$V_6$). Note that leads AVR and $V_1$ are oriented towards the cavity of the heart, leads II, III and AVF face the inferior surface and leads I, AVL and $V_6$ face the lateral wall of the left ventricle.

The ECG potentials are picked up by electrodes attached to the patient. Disposable, self-adhesive electrodes are more convenient and hygienic than the nickel plates and cup electrodes which are still used with some older machines. The electrodes are connected to the ECG recorder by a multicolour or coded cable.

Although some single-channel ECG machines still exist, most are simultaneous three-channel recorders with output either as a continuous strip or with automatic channel switching. Many modern ECG machines present the ECG (all 12 standard leads and a rhythm strip) in a convenient page-sized format. Many ECG machines also analyse the recordings and print the analysis on the record. Usually the machine interpretation is correct, but many arrhythmias still defy automatic analysis.

### ECG waveform

The shape of the normal ECG waveform (Fig. 11.17) has important similarities, whatever the orientation. The first deflection is caused by atrial depolarization, and it is a low-amplitude slow deflection called a P wave. The QRS complex results from ventricular depolarization and is sharper and larger in amplitude than the P wave. The T wave is another slow and low-amplitude deflection that results from ventricular repolarization.

The atrial repolarization wave is not seen in a conventional ECG because it is low in voltage and is hidden by the QRS complex.

The *PR interval* is the length of time from the start of the P wave to the start of the QRS complex. It is the time taken for activation to pass from the sinus node, through the atrium, AV node and the His–Purkinje system to the ventricle.

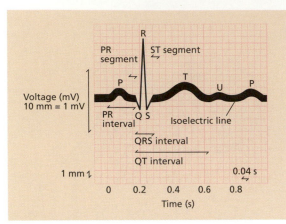

**Fig. 11.17** The waves and elaboration of the normal electrocardiogram. (From Goldman MJ (1976) *Principles of Clinical Electrocardiography*, 9th edn. Los Altos: Lange.)

| | |
|---|---|
| P wave duration | ≤0.12 s |
| PR interval | 0.12–0.22 s |
| QRS complex duration | ≤0.10 s |
| Corrected QT (QT$_c$) | ≤0.44 s |

$$QT_c = \frac{QT}{\sqrt{RR\ interval}}$$

**Table 11.9**  Normal ECG intervals.

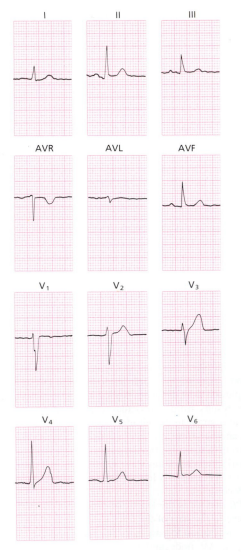

**Fig. 11.18**  A normal 12-lead electrocardiogram.

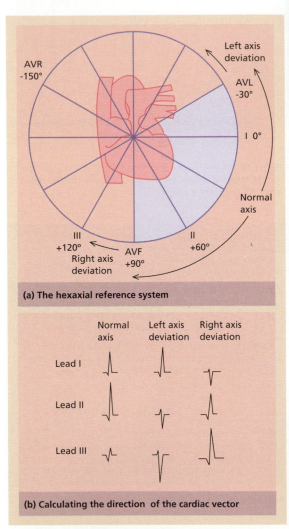

**(a) The hexaxial reference system**

**(b) Calculating the direction of the cardiac vector**

**Fig. 11.19**  (a) The hexaxial reference system illustrating the six leads in the frontal plane, e.g. lead I is 0°, lead II is +60°, lead III is +120°. (b) Calculating the direction of the cardiac vector. In the first column the QRS complex with zero net amplitude (i.e. when the positive and negative deflections are equal) is seen in lead III. The mean QRS vector is therefore perpendicular to lead III and is either −150° or +30°. Lead I is positive, so the axis must be +30°, which is normal. In left axis deviation (second column) the main deflection is positive (R wave) in lead I and negative (S wave) in lead III. In right axis deviation (third column) the main deflection is negative (S wave) in lead I and positive (R wave) in lead III.

The *QT interval* extends from the start of the QRS complex to the end of the T wave. This interval represents the time taken to depolarize and repolarize the ventricular myocardium.

The *ST segment* is the period between the end of the QRS complex and the start of the T wave. In the normal heart, all cells are depolarized by this phase of the ECG.

The normal values for the electrocardiographic intervals are indicated in Table 11.9. A normal ECG is shown in Fig. 11.18. Leads that face the lateral wall of the left ventricle have predominantly positive deflections, and leads looking into the ventricular cavity are usually negative. Detailed patterns depend on the size, shape and rhythm of the heart and the characteristics of the torso.

### Cardiac vectors (Fig. 11.19)

At any point in time during depolarization and repolarization, electrical potentials are being propagated in different directions. Most of these cancel each other out and only the net force is recorded. This net force in the frontal plane is known as the cardiac vector.

The mean QRS vector can be calculated from the six standard leads (Fig. 11.19); it normally lies between $-30°$ and $+90°$. Left axis deviation lies between $-30°$ and $-90°$ and right axis deviation between $+90°$ and $+150°$. Calculation of this vector is useful in the diagnosis of cardiac disorders.

### Exercise electrocardiography

This is a technique used to assess the cardiac response to exercise. The ECG is recorded whilst the patient walks or runs on a motorized treadmill or cycles on a stationary cycle ergometer. Recording the ECG after the exercise is not an adequate form of stress test. Normally there is little change in the T wave or ST segment.

Myocardial ischaemia provoked by exertion results in ST segment depression ($>1$ mm) in leads facing the affected area. Although most abnormalities are detected in leads $V_5$ (anterior and lateral ischaemia) or AVF (inferior ischaemia), it is best to record a full 12-lead ECG. The form of ST segment depression provoked by ischaemia is characteristic: it is either planar or shows down-sloping depression (Fig. 11.20). Up-sloping depression is a non-specific finding. During an exercise test the exercise tolerance, blood pressure and rhythm responses to exercise are also assessed. Exercise causes an increase in heart rate and blood pressure. A sustained fall in blood pressure indicates severe coronary artery disease.

The usual indications and contraindications for the test are shown in Table 11.10. Its use in angina is described on p. 580.

### 24-Hour ambulatory taped electrocardiography

This is a technique for recording transient changes such as a brief paroxysm of tachycardia, an occasional pause

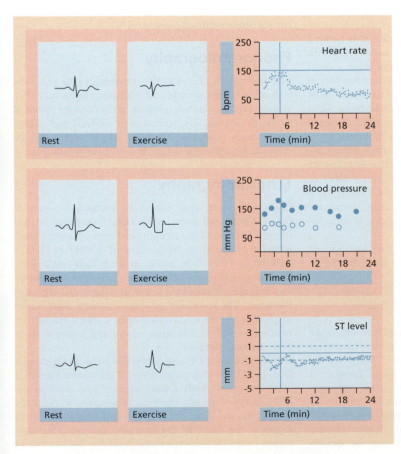

**Fig. 11.20** Electrocardiographic, heart rate and blood pressure changes on exercise. The middle (planar) and lower (downsloping) depression are characteristic in response to 4 min of exercise in a patient with myocardial ischaemia. The top exercise ECG shows upsloping depression which is non-specific. The end of the exercise period is indicated by the vertical dotted line in the graphs.

NB   Provided that adequate precautions are observed (doctor and resuscitation facilities available, continuous ECG and blood pressure monitoring), the mortality from exercise testing is less than 0.01%. Myocardial infarction occurs in less than 0.05%.

**Table 11.10**   Indications and contraindications for exercise electrocardiography.

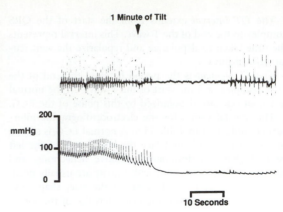

**Fig. 11.21**   ECG (top trace) and arterial blood pressure recorded during a tilt test. After 1 min of tilt, hypotension, bradycardia and syncope occur.

in the rhythm, or intermittent ST segment shifts. A conventional 12-lead ECG is recorded in less than a minute and usually samples less than 20 complexes. In a 24-hour period over 100 000 complexes are recorded. Such a large amount of data must be analysed by automatic or semi-automatic methods. This technique is called 'Holter' electrocardiography after its inventor.

Event recording is another technique that may be used to record rare arrhythmias. The patient is provided with a pocket-sized device that can record and store a short segment of the ECG. The device may be kept for several days or weeks until the arrhythmia is recorded. Most units of this kind will also allow transtelephonic ECG transmission so that the physician can determine the need for treatment or the continued need for monitoring.

Heart rate variability (HRV) can be assessed from a 24-hour ECG. HRV is decreased in some patients following myocardial infarction and represents an abnormality of autonomic tone or cardiac responsiveness. Low HRV is a major risk factor for sudden death and ventricular arrhythmias in patients discharged following myocardial infarction.

Ambulatory ECG recordings may also be used to monitor the level of the ST segment and to record transient ST segment depression.

## Tilt testing

Patients with suspected neurocardiogenic syncope (see p. 527) should be investigated by upright tilt. The patient is secured to a table which is tilted to +60° to the vertical for 45 min or more. The ECG and blood pressure is monitored throughout. If neither symptoms nor signs develop, isoprenaline may be slowly infused and the tilt repeated. A positive test results in hypotension, sometimes bradycardia (Fig. 11.21) and presyncope/syncope. If symptoms and signs appear, they can be quickly

reversed by placing the patient flat. The effect of treatment can be evaluated by repeating the tilt test.

## Carotid sinus massage

Carotid sinus massage (see p. 563) may lead to asystole (≥ 3 s) and/or fall of blood pressure (> 50 mmHg). This hypersensitive response occurs in many of the normal (especially elderly) population, but may also be responsible for loss of consciousness in some patients with carotid sinus syndrome (see p. 916).

## Phonocardiography

The application of a sensitive microphone to the chest wall allows heart sounds and murmurs to be recorded. Usually cardiac, carotid or jugular pulsations are recorded at the same time. The technique is difficult and, except for research purposes, has been largely superseded by echocardiography and other non-invasive techniques.

## Echocardiography

Echocardiography uses echoes of ultrasound waves to map the heart and study its function. To provide detailed images, ultrasound wavelengths of 1 mm or less are used, which correspond to frequencies of 2 MHz (1 MHz = 1 000 000 cycles s$^{-1}$) or more. At such high frequencies, the ultrasound waves behave more like light and can be focused into a 'beam' and aimed at a particular region of the heart. The waves are generated in very short bursts or pulses a few microseconds long by a crystal transducer, which also detects returning echoes and converts them into electrical signals.

When the crystal transducer is placed on the body surface, the ultrasound pulses emitted encounter interfaces between various body tissues as they pass through the body. In crossing each interface, some of the wave energy is reflected, and if the beam path is approximately at right angles to the plane of the interface, the reflected waves return to the transducer as an echo. Since the velocity of sound in body tissues is almost constant ($1550$ m s$^{-1}$), the time delay for the echo to return measures the distance of the reflecting interface. Thus, if a single ultrasound pulse is transmitted, a series of echoes return, the first from the closest interface, and so on, until the distance becomes too great for further echoes to be detected.

To document in detail the motion patterns of individual structures, a technique called M-mode is used. The echo signals from a particular beam direction are recorded as a column of dots on a roll of photosensitive paper which is pulled past the cathode-ray tube display at constant speed. Stationary structures thus generate straight lines, the distances of which from the top of the paper indicate their depths, and movements, such as those of heart valves, are indicated by zig-zag lines (Fig. 11.22c).

Calibration markers indicate depth at 1 cm intervals and lines along the edges of the paper show time intervals of 0.04 s. It is customary to add an ECG trace as an aid to identifying the phases of the heart cycle.

Alternatively a series of views from different positions can be obtained in the form of a two-dimensional image (cross-sectional 2-D echocardiography) (Fig. 11.22a,b,d). This method is useful for delineating anatomical structures.

### Transoesophageal echocardiography

This technique is being increasingly used. The ultrasound probe in the oesophagus which is nearer the heart. It is particularly useful for detecting dissecting aneurysm.

### Doppler echocardiography

Echocardiography imaging utilizes echoes from tissue interfaces. Using high amplification, it is also possible to detect weak echoes scattered by small targets, including those from red blood cells. If the blood is moving relative to the direction of the ultrasound beam, the frequency of the returning echoes will be changed according to the Doppler phenomenon. The Doppler shift frequency is directly proportional to the blood velocity.

Blood velocity data can be acquired and displayed in several ways. Continuous-wave (CW) Doppler collects all the velocity data from the path of the beam and analyses it to generate a spectral display. The outline of the envelope of the spectral display shows the value of peak velocity throughout the cardiac cycle. Normal velocities are of the order of $1$ m s$^{-1}$, but if there is an obstructive lesion, such as a stenotic valve, velocities of $5$ m s$^{-1}$ or more can occur. These velocities are generated by the pressure gradient that exists across the lesion. According to the Bernoulli equation:

$$\text{Pressure gradient} = 4 \times (\text{velocity})^2.$$

This equation has been validated in a wide variety of clinical situations, including valve stenoses, and ventricular septal defects, and makes it unnecessary to resort to invasive methods to measure intracardiac pressure gradients in many cases.

CW Doppler does not provide any depth information. Pulsed-wave (PW) Doppler extracts velocity data from

the pulse echoes used to form a two-dimensional image and gives useful qualitative information. It can be thought of as a small intracardiac 'stethoscope' the location of which can be determined precisely. Doppler colour flow imaging uses one colour for blood flowing towards the transducer and another colour for blood flowing away. This technique allows the direction, velocity and timing of the flow to be measured with a simultaneous view of cardiac structure and function.

### The echocardiographic examination

Echocardiography is a 'non-invasive' procedure that causes the patient no discomfort and is harmless. Studies are performed by a physician or technician and a comprehensive examination takes 15–30 min.

The major problem of echocardiography is that access to the heart is restricted by the lungs and rib cage, both of which form impenetrable barriers to ultrasound in the adult subject. Small 'windows' can usually be found in the third and fourth left intercostal spaces (termed left parasternal); just below the xiphoid process of the sternum (subcostal); and, with the subject turned to the left and exhaling, from the point where the apical beat is palpated (apical). By positioning the transducer successively over these sites and angling and rotating it to align the scan plane, a series of standard sectional views is obtained. In children, and some adults, the aortic arch can be visualized from a suprasternal position.

The standard nomenclature for two-dimensional echocardiographic images is shown in Fig. 11.22(a). The left parasternal position gives access to the long-axis and short-axis planes. The apical approach gives a second view of the long-axis plane, but with the apex in the foreground, and also shows the four-chamber plane (Fig. 11.22(e)). Note that the convention of showing the trans-

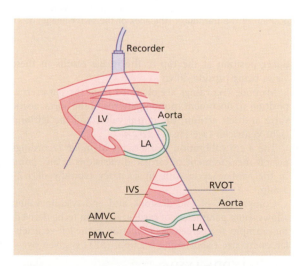

**Fig. 11.22(a)** The diagram shows the anatomy of the area scanned and a diagrammatic representation of the echocardiogram. LV, left ventricle; LA, left atrium; RVOT, right ventricular outflow tract; IVS, interventricular septum; PMVC, posterior mitral valve cusp; AMVC, anterior mitral valve cusp.

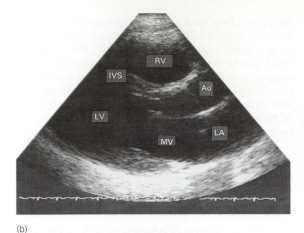

(b)

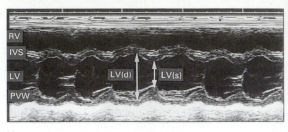

(c)

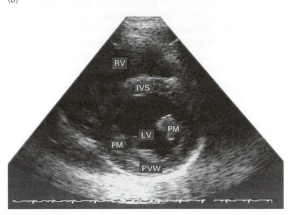

(d)

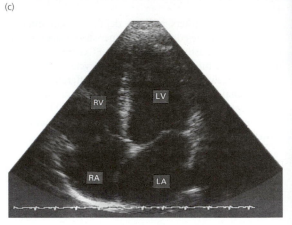

(e)

**Fig. 11.22(b)–(e)** Echocardiograms from a normal subject: (b) two-dimensional long-axis view; (c) M-mode recording with the ultrasound beam directed across the left ventricle, just below the mitral valve; (d) two-dimensional short-axis view at the level of the tips of the papillary muscles; (e) apical four-chamber view. Note that the convention that shows the position of the transducer (the apex of the sector image) at the top of the paper causes the heart to appear 'upside down' in these views: RA = right atrium; RV, right ventricle; IVS, interventricular septum; LV, left ventricle; LV(d), LV(s), left ventricular end-diastolic and end-systolic dimensions; PVW, posterior ventricular wall; PM, papillary muscle; MV, mitral valve; LA, left atrium; Ao, aorta.

ducer position at the top of the image results in these views being 'upside-down'.

M-mode recordings are obtained from the parasternal position to document motion patterns of the aorta, aortic valve and left atrium, the mitral valve, and the left and right ventricles (see Fig. 11.22(c)).

The 1 cm calibration markers on M-mode recordings permit measurement of cardiac dimensions at any point in the cardiac cycle with an accuracy typically of ± 2–3 mm.

Comparison of end-diastolic and end-systolic values allows some parameters of cardiac function to be derived: for example, the percentage reduction in the left ventricular cavity size ('shortening fraction' (SF)) is given by:

$$SF = \frac{LVDD - LVSD}{LVDD} \times 100 \; (\%)$$

(normal range 30–45%)

where LVDD is left ventricular diastolic diameter and

LVSD is left ventricular systolic diameter.

The echocardiographic findings in particular conditions are discussed in relevant sections, but a brief overview is given below.

VALVE STENOSIS. Congenitally abnormal aortic or pulmonary valves show a characteristic 'dome' shape in systole because the cusps cannot separate fully and a bicuspid configuration may be demonstrated. The presence of calcium in a valve gives rise to intense echoes that generate multiple, parallel lines on M-mode recordings. CW Doppler directed from the apex measures velocity of the jet crossing the diseased valve, from which the pressure gradient can be calculated (Fig. 11.23).

In mitral stenosis, the M-mode shows restriction and reversal of direction of the posterior leaflet motion (Fig. 11.24(c)). A short-axis view shows the shape of the mitral orifice in diastole and its area can be measured directly from the image (Fig. 11.24). Peak, mean and end-

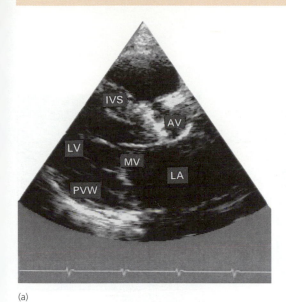

(a)

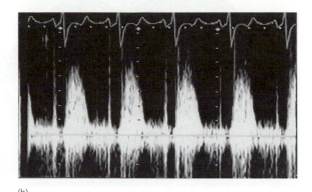

(b)

**Fig. 11.23** (a) Two-dimensional echocardiogram (long-axis view) in a patient with calcific aortic stenosis. The calcium in the valve generates abnormally intense echoes. There is some evidence of the associated left ventricular hypertrophy. (b) Continuous-wave (CW) Doppler signals obtained from the right upper parasternal edge, where the high velocity jet from the stenotic valve is coming towards the transducer. The peak jet velocity is 5 m s$^{-1}$, corresponding to a pressure gradient of 100 mmHg. AV, aortic valve; LA, left atrium; MV, mitral valve; LV, left ventricle; IVS, interventricular septum; PVW, posterior ventricular wall.

diastolic pressure gradients can be obtained from CW Doppler (Fig. 11.24d). Additional imaging views indicate the size of the left atrium, and may show the presence of left atrial thrombus.

VALVE REGURGITATION. Doppler is extremely sensitive for detecting valve regurgitation and, indeed, demonstrates mild physiological regurgitation through the tricuspid and pulmonary valves in the majority of normal subjects. It is hard to quantify the amount of regurgitation with echo Doppler techniques but echocardiography is an excellent way to determine the underlying cause of valve regurgitation, e.g. rheumatic disease or mitral valve prolapse.

AORTIC ANEURYSMS AND DISSECTIONS. Dilatation of the aortic root can be measured accurately and the presence of a reflecting structure within the lumen of the aorta is strongly suggestive of an intimal flap associated with dissection.

PROSTHETIC HEART VALVES. Each type of heart valve prosthesis has characteristic echocardiographic features. Irregularity or restriction of movement can be shown on M-mode recordings. The presence of stenosis or regurgitation may be documented by Doppler.

INFECTIVE ENDOCARDITIS. Vegetations >2 mm can be detected (see Fig. 11.74).

CARDIAC FAILURE. Left ventricular function and response to treatment is readily assessed and should be performed in all patients with heart failure.

CARDIOMYOPATHIES. Dilated cardiomyopathy is characterized by an enlarged, globular-shaped, thin-walled left ventricle with poor function and low stroke output shown by reduced movements of the valves (see Fig. 11.87).

In hypertrophic cardiomyopathy (see Fig. 11.88), the left ventricle is small, with a grossly thickened, immobile interventricular septum (asymmetric septal hypertrophy (ASH)). There is a characteristic, though poorly understood, displacement of the mitral valve apparatus towards the septum in systole (systolic anterior motion (SAM)).

PERICARDIAL EFFUSION. Fluid in the pericardial cavity shows as an echo-free region between the myocardium and the intense echo of the parietal pericardium (Fig. 11.25).

MASSES WITHIN THE HEART. Echocardiography is a sensitive method for detecting masses within the heart (see Fig. 11.86).

ISCHAEMIC DISEASE. Coronary arteries cannot be imaged adequately using echo techniques but images may be useful for the diagnosis of complications related to myocardial infarction, such as mitral papillary muscle rupture, tamponade or ventricular septal rupture.

In the postinfarction period, echocardiography and

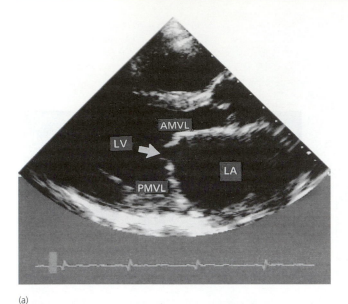

(a)

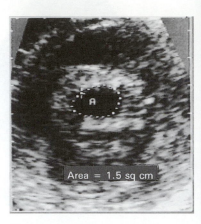

(b)

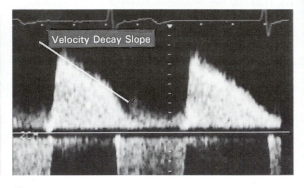

(c)

(d)

**Fig. 11.24** Echocardiograms in rheumatic mitral valve disease. (a) Two-dimensional long-axis view showing enlarged left atrium and 'hooked' appearance of the mitral valve leaflets resulting from commisural fusion. (b) Magnified short axis view showing the mitral valve orifice as seen from the direction of the arrow in (a). The orifice area can be planimetered to assess the severity; in this case it is 1.5 cm², indicating moderately severe disease. (c) M-mode recording of the mitral valve showing restricted motion of the thickened leaflets; (d) continuous-wave (CW) Doppler recording showing slow rate of decay of flow velocity from the left atrium to the left ventricle during diastole. It is also possible to derive the valve orifice area from the velocity decay rate. LA, left atrium; LV, left ventricle, AMVL, PMVL, anterior and posterior mitral valve leaflets; MVA, mitral valve orifice area.

Doppler are used to diagnose left ventricular aneurysm, left ventricular thrombus, mitral regurgitation and pericardial effusion as well as to assess left ventricular function (ejection fraction).

CONGENITAL HEART DISEASE. Echocardiography has largely replaced cardiac catheterization and angiography. The aim of the examination is first to establish the sequence of blood flow through the heart, and to define anatomical abnormalities.

## Nuclear imaging

Nuclear imaging techniques are primarily used in ischaemic heart disease. Myocardial structure and function can be assessed by radionuclide-imaging techniques.

### Thallium-201 imaging

This is used to detect myocardial ischaemia and infarction. Thallium, which behaves like potassium, is taken up by healthy myocardium. Ischaemia or infarction produces a nuclear image with a 'cold' spot (Fig. 11.26). The isotope is usually administered during exercise and an image is taken soon after the exercise. Three or four hours later the heart is scanned again to obtain a redistribution image. The disappearance of the cold spot on the redistribution image implies ischaemia provoked by exertion and reversed by rest, whereas a persistent cold spot indicates infarction.

### Pyrophosphate scan

Pyrophosphate labelled with technetium-99m concentrates in bone and acutely infarcted myocardium. The iso-

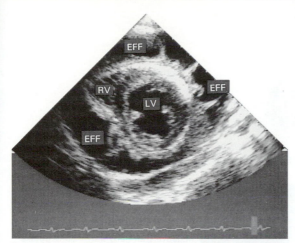

**Fig. 11.25** Two-dimensional echocardiogram (short-axis view) from a patient with a large pericardial effusion associated with pulmonary tuberculosis. The exudate is seen between the visceral and parietal layers of the pericardium and would give a false impression of cardiomegaly on a chest X-ray. Note the multiple fibrous strands within the effusion, showing that it is consolidating and will probably lead to constriction of cardiac function. LV, left ventricle; RV, right ventricle; EFF, effusion.

tope should be injected intravenously between 1 and 5 days (best on the second or third day) following a myocardial infarction. Imaging a few hours later detects a 'hot spot' (Fig. 11.27a) in the region of the infarction. Scans are difficult to interpret because calcified costal cartilage and breast tissue may both concentrate the isotope. On the other hand, infarction may not result in the expected hot spot because the isotope is prevented from reaching the infarct owing to complete occlusion of coronary vessels to the infarcted myocardium. False-positive scans may occur in unstable angina.

### Radionuclide ventriculography

Two methods are used to obtain blood pool images:

1 A *MUGA* (multigated acquisition) or equilibrium image is obtained by intravenous injection of technetium-99m which attaches to the patient's own red cells *in vivo* and which is therefore retained in the vascular space. Over 200 heart beats are imaged. Comparison of the study with the ECG allows systolic and diastolic points of the cycle to be identified.

2 A *first-pass study* images the heart as a bolus of isotope makes a single pass through the circulation.

These techniques are complementary, but both outline the cardiac chambers, particularly the left ventricle, by imaging the isotope within the central circulation during systole and diastole. The percentage of the left ventricular volume ejected with each systole (the ejection fraction) can be accurately measured, and any section of the left ventricular wall that contracts abnormally (a wall motion defect) can be visualized (Fig. 11.27b). Radionuclide studies may be performed at rest and during exercise to assess changes in cardiac function. A deterioration on exercise suggests coronary disease or myocardial abnormality.

## Cardiac catheterization

Cardiac catheterization is the introduction of a thin radiopaque tube (catheter) into the circulation.

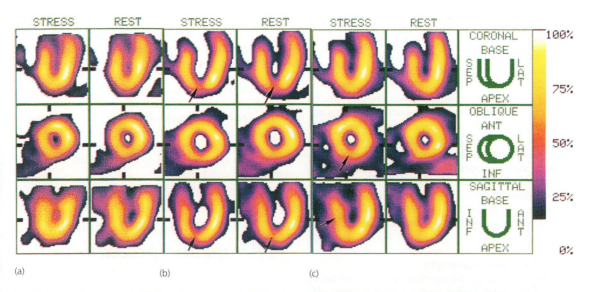

**Fig. 11.26** Thallium or sestamibi myocardial scintigram during stress and afterwards at rest in three patients. (a) Normal perfusion at rest and during stress. (b) Similar (fixed) defect at rest and during stress. This is due to a previous myocardial infarction. (c) Poor reperfusion in the inferior wall during stress which is largely resolved at rest due to 'reversible ischaemia'.

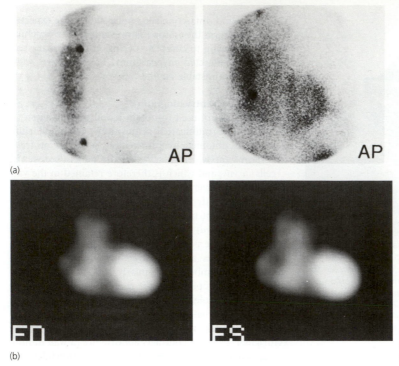

Fig. 11.27 (a) Infarct-avid scans using technetium-labelled pyrophosphate. A negative scan (left) shows bone uptake in the ribs and sternum; the darker circles are position markers. A positive scan (right) shows myocardial uptake with a density greater than the ribs but slightly less than the sternum. AP, anterior–posterior.
(b) This MUGA scan shows a large, dilated left ventricle with virtually no difference between end systolic (ES) and end diastolic (ED) frames.

The right heart is catheterized by introducing the catheter into a peripheral vein and advancing it through the right atrium and ventricle into the pulmonary artery. The left heart is reached by way of a peripheral artery. The catheter is manipulated through the aortic valve into the left ventricle.

The pressures in the right heart chambers, left ventricle, aorta and pulmonary artery can be measured directly. An indirect measure of left atrial pressure can be obtained by 'wedging' a catheter into the distal pulmonary artery (see also p. 720). In this position the pressure from the right ventricle is obstructed by the catheter and only the pulmonary venous and left atrial pressures are recorded. Pressure measurements are used to quantify stenoses or measure contractile function.

During cardiac catheterization, blood samples may be withdrawn to measure the concentration of ischaemic metabolites, e.g. lactate, and the oxygen content. These estimations are used to gauge ischaemia, quantify intracardiac shunts, and measure cardiac output.

Contrast cine-angiograms are also taken during catheterization. Radio-opaque contrast material is injected into the cardiac chambers (Fig. 11.28), arterial trunks or coronary arteries. Figure 11.29 shows a normal angiogram compared with angiograms showing an aneurysm and cardiomyopathy.

**Digital subtraction angiography**
This technique permits the injection of small volumes of radiocontrast agents during cardiac catheterization with the production of computer-analysed high-quality angiograms.

Unfortunately, peripheral injection of contrast does not give adequate visualization of the coronary arteries, but aortic lesions can be visualized.

## CT scanning

CT scanning is particularly useful for showing the size and shape of the cardiac chambers as well as the thoracic aorta and mediastinum.

## Magnetic resonance imaging (MRI)

MRI is a non-invasive imaging technique which does not involve harmful radiation. A powerful magnetic field is used to line up the protons in the hydrogen atoms of the body, each of which can be thought of as a tiny magnet. A radiofrequency emission distorts this line-up, but when the radio waves are turned off, the atoms return to their previous position and give off energy. This energy can be reconstituted as an image. MRI of the heart is complicated because the heart is a moving structure, but the technique is already finding clinical application for imaging vascular structures.

Synchronization with the ECG allows cardiac images in systole and diastole to be obtained (Fig. 11.30).

# Therapeutic procedures

## Cardiac resuscitation

No matter where cardiac arrest occurs it is essential that someone close to the victim institutes basic life support.

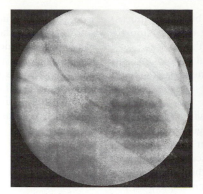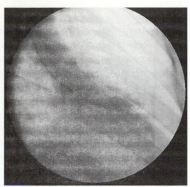

**Fig. 11.28** Diastolic (left) and systolic (right) frames recorded after X-ray contrast was injected into the left ventricle (contrast left ventriculogram). Normal left ventricular function is demonstrated.

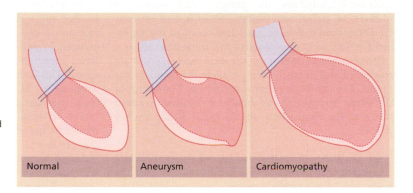

**Fig. 11.29** Diagrams of left ventricular angiograms. A normal picture is compared with those showing an aneurysm and cardiomyopathy. The solid line represents the end-diastolic perimeter and the dotted line the end-systolic perimeter of the left ventricle. The double line marks the plane of the aortic valve.

Normal    Aneurysm    Cardiomyopathy

The longer the period of respiratory and circulatory arrest, the less the possibility of restoring healthy life. After 3 min there will be permanent cerebral dysfunction. Because sudden unexpected cardiac arrest is relatively common in the hospital, medical students and all doctors must know what to do. A cardiac arrest usually causes a great deal of excitement and some panic. Therefore, it is very important that the basic procedure is well known. A standard procedure must be used in order that a variety of personnel may work easily together.

**Basic life support**

The first step is to establish whether the victim is unconscious (shake and shout at the patient) and whether there is a pulse. It is best to feel the carotid pulse by pressing backwards just to the side of the thyroid cartilage. If there is no pulse, immediately call for help. Quickly place the victim in an accessible position with firm underlying support (e.g. on his/her back on the floor), and begin basic life support. This can be remembered as A (airway) and B (breathing) and C (circulation).

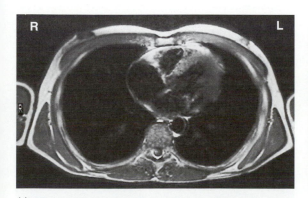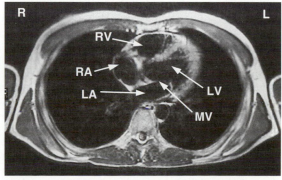

(a)                                          (b)

**Fig. 11.30** Magnetic resonance image (MRI) showing a pair of axial images taken through the mid-thorax at the level of the mitral valve. Image (a) is a view of end-systole, image (b) is taken at end-diastole. Note the clear differentiation between the atria and ventricles. This is a normal study. LA, left atrium; LV, left ventricle; MV, mitral valve; RA, right atrium; RV, right ventricle.

AIRWAY. Any loose obstruction (e.g. blood and mucus) in the mouth and pharynx should be quickly removed. Unless already detached, leave false teeth in place because they give form and support to the oral cavity. Open the airway by flexing the neck and extending the head ('sniffing the morning air' position).

BREATHING. Look for the rise and fall of the chest and abdomen. If there is no respiration, begin expired air respiration. With the head of the victim tilted backwards and the chin pulled forward the rescuer takes a deep breath and seals his/her lips around the mouth or nose of the victim. Four quick puffs are given. Expired air respiration is the only method of artificial respiration that successfully ventilates the patient. The mechanical methods of Holger and Neilson, Shaeffer and Sylvester are completely useless because they result in the movement of less air than is required to fill the dead space.

If the airway is obstructed, the head, neck and jaw are readjusted and another check is made for debris in the mouth. If obstruction persists, any foreign body stuck in the larynx or upper airway should be removed by a firm thrust to the epigastrium (the *Heimlich manoeuvre*, see p. 656).

CIRCULATION. Circulation is achieved by external chest compression. The heel of one hand is placed over the lower half of the victim's sternum and the heel of the second hand is placed over the first with the fingers interlocked. The arms are kept straight and the sternum is rhythmically depressed by 1–2 inches. Chest compression does not massage the heart. The thorax acts as a pump and the heart provides a system of one-way valves to ensure forward circulation.

Respiration and compression is now continued as follows:

SINGLE RESCUER—compression at a rate of 80 b.p.m. with two respirations after 15 compressions.

TWO RESCUERS—continuous compressions at a rate of 60 b.p.m. and one respiration given after every 5 compressions.

If possible, it is better to give compressions without interruption. This maintains adequate cerebral and coronary perfusion pressures. Ventilation can easily be achieved despite continued chest compression.

### Advanced cardiac life support

By the time effective life support has been established, more help should have arrived and advanced cardiac life support can begin. This consists of ECG monitoring, endotracheal intubation and setting up an intravenous infusion in a large peripheral vein or a central vein. Immediate therapy includes defibrillation, oxygen and cardioactive drugs. It is not possible to recommend an exact sequence of management because it will depend on the arrival of skilled personnel and equipment and the nature of the cardiac arrest. However, as soon as possible the ECG should be connected. At first this is easily achieved by monitoring the ECG through the paddles of a defibrillator. Later, electrodes, leads and specific ECG

scopes can be set up. If the ECG shows ventricular fibrillation, no time should be lost before defibrillating the patient. If initial defibrillation attempts are unsuccessful, time can then be spent intubating the patient and setting up an intravenous infusion whilst the circulation is supported by external chest compression. If there is any difficulty in intubating the patient, ventilation should be continued by means of an airway, a ventilating bag and oxygen.

There are three main mechanisms of sudden unexpected cardiac arrest (Information box 11.1):

1 Ventricular fibrillation
2 Asystole
3 Electromechanical dissociation

Three-quarters of arrests are due to ventricular fibrillation. Only a very small proportion are due to electromechanical dissociation, and the remainder are due to asystole. In patients dying of other causes, such as terminal pneumonia, the heart rhythm is described as being agonal. This is characterized by an inexorable slowing and widening of the QRS complexes associated with falling blood pressure and cardiac output. This type of arrhythmia is very difficult to reverse and usually no attempt should be made because it is the result rather than the cause of death.

Arrests are treated in the following ways:

VENTRICULAR FIBRILLATION is readily treated with defibrillation, antiarrhythmic drugs and cardiac stimulants.

ASYSTOLE is more difficult to treat but the heart may respond to atropine or adrenaline. If there is any sign of electrocardiographic activity, emergency pacing should be used.

ELECTROMECHANICAL DISSOCIATION is often due to a severe mechanical problem such as pericardial tamponade or massive pulmonary embolism. These conditions should be treated urgently. Toxic levels of cardiodepressant drugs, such as β-blockers, may also cause electromechanical dissociation. If there is an antidote, such as adrenaline, it should be administered. Figure 11.31 shows the treatments recommended by

---

Each year in the UK there are approximately 100 000 unexpected deaths occurring within 24 hours of the development of cardiac symptoms. About half of these deaths are almost instantaneous. There are several causes:

Cardiac arrhythmias (e.g. ventricular fibrillation)
Sudden pump failure (e.g. acute myocardial infarction)
Acute circulatory obstruction (e.g. pulmonary embolism)
Cardiovascular rupture (e.g. dissecting aneurysm of the aorta, myocardial rupture)
Vasomotor collapse (e.g. pulmonary hypertension)

Most deaths are due to ventricular fibrillation, and a small proportion are due to severe bradyarrhythmias. Although coronary disease is frequent in these victims, acute coronary occlusion and myocardial infarction is relatively uncommon (~40%).

**Information box 11.1**    Sudden death.

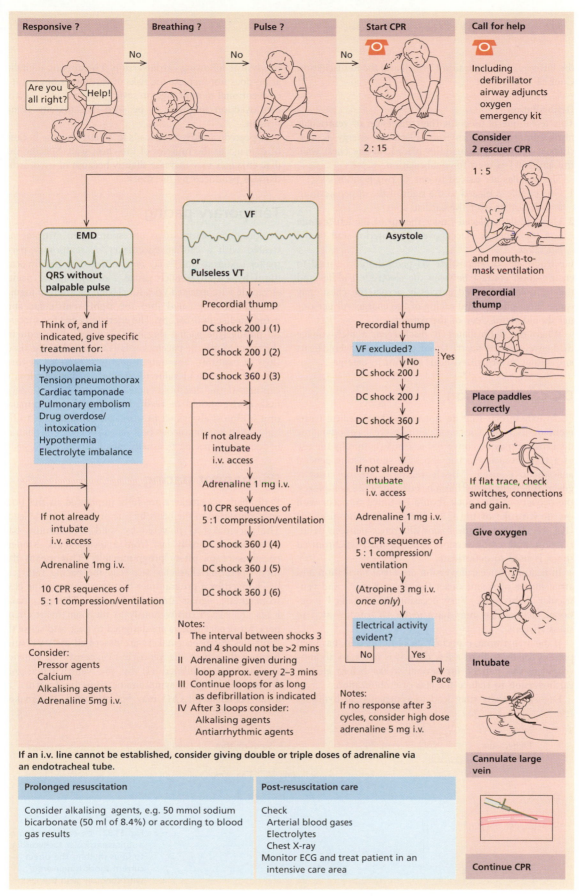

**Responsive ?**

Are you all right? Help!

No →

**Breathing ?**

No →

**Pulse ?**

No →

**Start CPR**

2 : 15

**Call for help**

Including defibrillator airway adjuncts oxygen emergency kit

**Consider 2 rescuer CPR**

1 : 5

and mouth-to-mask ventilation

**Precordial thump**

**Place paddles correctly**

If flat trace, check switches, connections and gain.

**Give oxygen**

**Intubate**

**Cannulate large vein**

**Continue CPR**

---

**EMD**

**QRS without palpable pulse**

Think of, and if indicated, give specific treatment for:

Hypovolaemia
Tension pneumothorax
Cardiac tamponade
Pulmonary embolism
Drug overdose/ intoxication
Hypothermia
Electrolyte imbalance

If not already intubate i.v. access

Adrenaline 1mg i.v.

10 CPR sequences of 5 : 1 compression/ventilation

Consider:
Pressor agents
Calcium
Alkalising agents
Adrenaline 5mg i.v.

---

**VF**

**or Pulseless VT**

Precordial thump

DC shock 200 J (1)

DC shock 200 J (2)

DC shock 360 J (3)

If not already intubate i.v. access

Adrenaline 1 mg i.v.

10 CPR sequences of 5 :1 compression/ventilation

DC shock 360 J (4)

DC shock 360 J (5)

DC shock 360 J (6)

Notes:
I   The interval between shocks 3 and 4 should not be >2 mins
II  Adrenaline given during loop approx. every 2–3 mins
III Continue loops for as long as defibrillation is indicated
IV  After 3 loops consider:
    Alkalising agents
    Antiarrhythmic agents

---

**Asystole**

Precordial thump

VF excluded? — Yes

↓ No

DC shock 200 J

DC shock 200 J

DC shock 360 J

If not already intubate i.v. access

Adrenaline 1 mg i.v.

10 CPR sequences of 5 : 1 compression/ ventilation

(Atropine 3 mg i.v. *once only*)

Electrical activity evident?

No        Yes

         Pace

Notes:
If no response after 3 cycles, consider high dose adrenaline 5 mg i.v.

---

**If an i.v. line cannot be established, consider giving double or triple doses of adrenaline via an endotracheal tube.**

| Prolonged resuscitation | Post-resuscitation care |
|---|---|
| Consider alkalising agents, e.g. 50 mmol sodium bicarbonate (50 ml of 8.4%) or according to blood gas results | Check<br>  Arterial blood gases<br>  Electrolytes<br>  Chest X-ray<br>Monitor ECG and treat patient in an<br>  intensive care area |

**Fig. 11.31** Advanced cardiac life support. (Recommended by the European Resuscitation Council and Resuscitation Council UK.) EMD, electromechanical dissociation.

the European Resuscitation Council and the Resuscitation Council UK.

### Defibrillation

This technique is used for the conversion of ventricular fibrillation to sinus rhythm. Electrical energy is discharged through two paddles placed on the chest wall. Initially 200 J is used for defibrillation.

The paddles are placed in one of two positions:

1 One paddle is placed to the right of the upper sternum and the other over the cardiac apex.
2 One paddle is placed under the tip of the left scapula and the other is placed over the anterior wall of the left chest.

Electrode jelly or electrolyte gel pads should be used to ensure good contact between the electrode paddles and the skin. Jelly smeared carelessly across the chest may cause short-circuits and arcing of the charge. All personnel should stand clear of the patient.

When the defibrillator is discharged, a high-voltage field envelopes the heart. This depolarizes the whole heart and allows an organized heart rhythm to emerge.

## DC-cardioversion

Tachyarrhythmias that do not respond to medical treatment or that are associated with severe haemodynamic disturbance may be converted to sinus rhythm by the use of a transthoracic electric shock. A short-acting general anaesthetic is used. Muscle relaxants are not usually given. When the arrhythmia has definite QRS complexes, the delivery of the shock should be timed to occur with the downstroke of the QRS complex (synchronization) (Fig. 11.32). This is the major difference between defibrillation and cardioversion, since a non-synchronized shock is used to defibrillate.

Indications for cardioversion are atrial fibrillation and atrial flutter of recent onset (less than 1 year), and ventricular tachycardia. Very occasionally, sustained junctional tachycardias may have to be DC-cardioverted to sinus rhythm.

If the arrhythmia, especially atrial fibrillation, has been present for more than a few days, it is necessary to anticoagulate the patient for several weeks before elective cardioversion to reduce the risk of embolization.

Digoxin toxicity may lead to ventricular arrhythmias or asystole following cardioversion. Therapeutic digitalization does not increase the risks of cardioversion, but it is conventional to omit digoxin several days prior to elective cardioversion in order to be sure that toxicity is not present.

Repeated cardioversion leads to an enzyme rise because of damage to the muscles of the chest wall. Specific cardiac enzymes may increase slightly because of myocardial damage produced by the shock.

## Temporary pacing

Symptomatic bradycardias unresponsive to atropine are treated with a cardiac pacemaker. A temporary pacemaker (external unit) may be connected to the myocardium by a thin (French gauge 5 or 6), bipolar pacing electrode wire inserted via a subclavian or internal jugular vein and manipulated into the right ventricular apex using cardiac fluoroscopy. The energy needed for successful pacing (the pacing threshold) is assessed by reducing the energy until the pacemaker fails to stimulate the tissue (loss of capture). The output energy is then set at three times the threshold value to prevent inadvertent loss of capture. If the threshold increases above 5 V, the pacemaker wire should be re-sited. A temporary pacemaker unit is almost always set to work 'on demand', i.e. to fire only when a spontaneous beat has not occurred. The rate of temporary pacing is usually 60–80 b.p.m.

## Permanent pacing

Permanent pacemakers are fully implanted in the body and connected to the heart by one or two electrode leads. The pacemaker is powered by solid-state lithium batteries, which usually last from 5 to 10 years. Modern pacemakers are often 'programmable'. This means that their operating characteristics (e.g. the pacing rate) can be changed by a programmer that transmits specific electromagnetic signals through the skin. The pacemaker leads are passed transvenously to the right heart chambers. Most pacemakers are designed to pace and sense the ventricles. Such pacemakers are described as 'VVI' units because they pace the ventricle (V), sense the ventricle (V) and are inhibited (I) by the ventricular signal. Occasionally, e.g. in symptomatic sinus bradycardia, an atrial pacemaker (AAI) may be implanted. Pacemakers

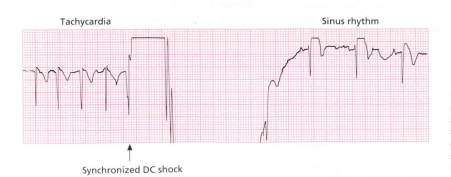

Tachycardia

Sinus rhythm

Synchronized DC shock

**Fig. 11.32** DC-cardioversion of a supraventricular tachycardia to sinus rhythm. The direct current shock is delivered synchronously with the QRS complex.

that are connected to both the right atrium and ventricle ('dual chamber' pacemaker) are increasingly being used in order to simulate the natural pacemaker and activation sequence of the heart. This form of pacemaker is called DDD because it paces the two (Dual) chambers, senses both (D) and reacts in two (D) ways—pacing in the same chamber is inhibited by spontaneous atrial and ventricular signals, and ventricular pacing is triggered by spontaneous atrial events. Another form of 'physiological' pacemaker is the 'rate-responsive' system, which, by measuring activity, respiration, biochemical or electrical indicators, changes its rate of pacing so that it is appropriate to the level of exertion. The choice of pacemaker mostly depends on the underlying condition (e.g. sick sinus syndrome must be treated with a dual chamber device) and the general condition of the patient (old and infirm patients do not usually benefit from the most sophisticated units).

Permanent pacemakers are inserted under local anaesthetic using fluoroscopy to guide the insertion of the electrode leads. The pacemaker is usually positioned subcutaneously in front of the pectoral muscle. Following surgery, which usually takes 30 min to 1 hour, the patient rests in bed for 6–24 hours before being discharged. Patients may not drive until the pacemaker has been shown to be working correctly at least 1 month after implantation, and must inform the licensing authorities and their motor insurers. Antibiotics may be prescribed prophylactically.

Complications are few but include:

INFECTION. When a pacemaker system is infected, antibiotic treatment is not sufficient and the pacemaker must usually be removed before antibiotics will subdue the infection. Another pacemaker is fitted later.

EROSION. The pacemaker may erode through the skin. This is usually due to a low-grade infection. Mechanical factors may also be responsible.

LEAD DISPLACEMENT. In most cases the pacing lead is securely wedged into the trabeculae of the right ventricle. It rarely displaces but when it does it may lead to sudden loss of pacing and a recurrence of pre-pacing symptoms.

PACEMAKER MALFUNCTION. This is now a very uncommon complication but requires the replacement of the pacemaker.

Electromagnetic interference of the function of a modern pacemaker is not common, except in the hospital or industrial environment. High tension cables, high energy radars and some medical equipment, such as MRI machines and lithotripters, may transiently inhibit the output of a pacemaker or convert it to interference mode (continuous pacing despite an adequate underlying rhythm).

## Pericardiocentesis

A pericardial effusion is an accumulation of fluid between the parietal and visceral layers of pericardium. Fluid is removed to relieve symptoms due to haemodynamic embarrassment or for diagnostic purposes. Pericardial aspiration or pericardiocentesis is performed by inserting a needle into the pericardial space, usually via a subxiphisternal route. If a large volume of fluid is to be removed, a wide-bore needle and cannula are inserted. The needle may be removed and the cannula left *in situ* to drain the fluid. Fluid that is removed is sent for chemical analysis, microscopy, including cytology, and culture. If a re-accumulation of pericardial fluid is anticipated, the cannula may be left in place for several days or an operation can be performed to cut a window in the parietal pericardium (fenestration) or to remove a large section of the pericardium.

## Right heart bedside catheterization

Bedside catheterization of the pulmonary artery with a Swan–Ganz catheter may be performed in patients with:
- Cardiac failure
- Cardiogenic shock
- Doubtful fluid status

The catheter is used to measure cardiac output, pulmonary artery pressure, right atrial pressure and the pulmonary artery wedge pressure (an indirect measurement of left atrial pressure). The measurement of these pressures and the cardiac output allows appropriate therapy to be prescribed and the effects of that therapy to be monitored. The catheter also provides a route for the delivery of drugs to the central circulation (see Fig. 13.14).

## Intra-aortic balloon pumping

This is a technique used to assist temporarily the failing left ventricle. A catheter with a long sausage-shaped balloon at its tip is introduced percutaneously into the femoral artery and manipulated under X-ray control so that the balloon lies in the descending aorta just below the aortic arch. The balloon is rhythmically deflated and inflated with carbon dioxide gas. Using the ECG or intra-aortic pressure changes, the inflation is timed to occur during ventricular diastole to increase diastolic aortic pressure and consequently to improve coronary and cerebral blood flow. During systole the balloon is deflated, resulting in a reduction in the resistance to left ventricular emptying.

Balloon pumping is used:

TO IMPROVE CARDIAC OUTPUT when there is a transient or reversible depression of left ventricular function, e.g. in a patient with severe mitral valve regurgitation who is awaiting surgical replacement of the mitral valve or in a patient with a ventricular septal defect due to septal infarction.

TO TREAT UNSTABLE ANGINA PECTORIS by improving coronary flow and decreasing myocardial oxygen consumption by reducing the 'after-load'. This technique may be successful, even when medical therapy has failed. It is followed by early arteriography and appropriate definitive therapy such as surgery or coronary angioplasty.

Balloon pumping should not be used when there is no remediable cause of cardiac dysfunction. It is also unsuitable in patients with aortic valve regurgitation or dissection of the aorta.

Complications of balloon pumping occur in about 20% of patients and include aortic dissection, leg ischaemia, emboli from the balloon, and balloon rupture. Embolic complications are reduced by anticoagulation with heparin.

# Cardiac arrhythmias

An abnormality of the cardiac rhythm is called a cardiac arrhythmia. Such a disturbance of rhythm may cause sudden death, syncope, dizziness, palpitations or no symptoms at all. There are two main types of arrhythmia:

1 *Bradycardia*, where the heart rate is slow (<60 b.p.m.). The slower the heart rate the more likely the arrhythmia will be symptomatic.
2 *Tachycardia*, where the heart rate is fast (>100 b.p.m.). Tachycardias are more symptomatic when the arrhythmia is fast and sustained. Tachycardias are subdivided into *supraventricular tachycardias*, which arise from the atrium or the atrioventricular junction, and *ventricular tachycardias*, which arise from the ventricles.

Ventricular tachyarrhythmias tend to be more symptomatic than supraventricular tachycardias. Some arrhythmias occur in patients with apparently normal hearts, and in others arrhythmias reflect underlying cardiac abnormalities. When myocardial function is poor, arrhythmias tend to be more symptomatic and are potentially life-threatening.

## Mechanisms of arrhythmia production

There are four main mechanisms of tachycardia production:

TWO ARE ABNORMALITIES OF AUTOMATICITY, which might theoretically arise from a single disordered cell.

TWO ARE ABNORMALITIES OF CONDUCTION, which require abnormal interaction between cells.

Figure 11.33 shows the mechanisms of arrhythmias.

### Accelerated automaticity

The normal mechanism of cardiac rhythmicity is slow depolarization of the transmembrane voltage during diastole until the threshold potential is reached and the pacemaker fires. This mechanism may be accelerated by increasing the rate of diastolic depolarization or changing the threshold potential. Such changes are thought to produce sinus tachycardia, escape rhythms and accelerated AV nodal rhythms.

### Triggered activity

Myocardial damage can result in oscillations of the end of the action potential. These oscillations may reach threshold potential and produce an arrhythmia. The abnormal oscillations can be exaggerated by pacing and by catecholamines and these stimuli can be used to trigger this abnormal form of automaticity. Some of the arrhythmias produced by digoxin toxicity are due to triggered activity.

### Reflection

If adjacent cells repolarize at different rates, the cells that repolarize more quickly may be restimulated by those cells that have not yet repolarized. The ventricular tachyarrhythmias associated with the long-QT syndrome may result from this mechanism.

### Re-entry (or circus movement)

A wave of depolarization may be forced to travel in one direction around a ring of cardiac tissue. If the time to conduct around the ring is longer than the recovery of any tissue within the ring, circus movement will result, producing a tachycardia. The majority of regular paroxysmal tachycardias are thought to be produced by this mechanism.

## SINUS RHYTHMS

The normal cardiac pacemaker is the sinus node and, like most cardiac tissue, it depolarizes spontaneously (see p. 538). Its rate of discharge is controlled by the autonomic nervous system. Normally the parasympathetic system predominates, resulting in slowing of the spontaneous discharge rate from approximately 100 to 70 b.p.m. A reduction of parasympathetic tone or an increase in sympathetic stimulation leads to tachycardia; conversely, increased parasympathetic tone and decreased sympathetic stimulation produces bradycardia. The sinus rate in women is slightly faster than in men. Normal sinus rhythm is characterized by P waves that are upright in leads I and II of the ECG (see Fig. 11.18), but are inverted in the cavity leads AVR and $V_1$ (Fig. 11.34).

## Sinus arrhythmia

Fluctuations of autonomic tone result in phasic changes of the sinus discharge rate. Thus, during inspiration, parasympathetic tone falls and the heart rate quickens, and on expiration the heart rate falls. This variation is normal, particularly in children and young adults.

## Sinus bradycardia

A sinus rate of less than 60 b.p.m. during the day or less than 50 b.p.m. at night is known as sinus bradycardia. It is usually asymptomatic unless the rate is very slow. It is normal in athletes and in elderly patients. Causes include:

- Hypothermia, hypothyroidism, cholestatic jaundice and raised intracranial pressure
- Drug therapy with $\beta$-blockers, digitalis and other antiarrhythmic drugs
- Acute ischaemia and infarction of the sinus node

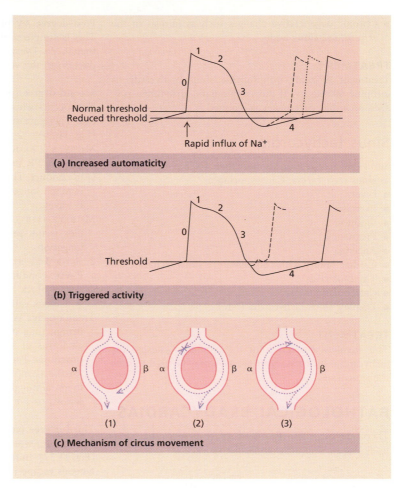

**Fig. 11.33** Mechanisms of arrhythmogenesis.
(a) and (b) Action potentials (i.e. the potential difference between intracellular and extracellular fluid) of ventricular myocardium after stimulation.
(a) Increased automaticity due to a reduced threshold potential or an increased slope of phase 4 depolarization (see p. 538).
(b) Triggered activity due to 'after' depolarizations reaching threshold potential.
(c) Mechanism of circus movement or re-entry. In panel (1) the impulse passes down both limbs of the potential tachycardia circuit. In panel (2) the impulse is blocked in the α pathway but proceeds slowly down the β pathway and returns along the α pathway. In panel (3) the impulse travels so slowly along the β pathway that when it returns along the α pathway to its starting point it is able to travel again down the β pathway, producing a circus movement tachycardia.

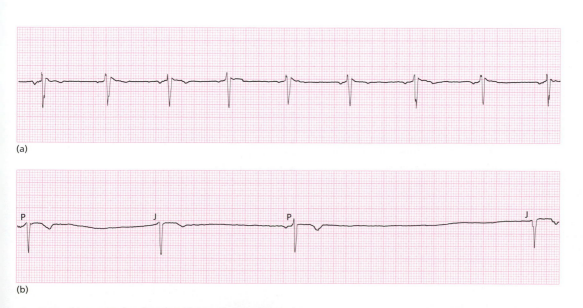

**Fig. 11.34** (a) An ECG showing normal sinus rhythm. (b) An ECG from a patient with sick sinus syndrome. This shows sinus arrest (only occasional sinus P waves) and junctional escape beats (J). P waves are inverted in these cavity leads.

- Chronic degenerative changes such as fibrosis of the atrium and sinus node

### TREATMENT

Treatment of acute symptomatic sinus bradycardia is atropine 600 $\mu$g i.v. If the symptomatic arrhythmia persists, a cardiac pacemaker is required.

## Sinus tachycardia

Sinus rate acceleration to more than 100 b.p.m. is known as sinus tachycardia. Causes include:

- Fever
- Exercise
- Emotion
- Pregnancy
- Anaemia
- Cardiac failure with compensatory sinus tachycardia
- Thyrotoxicosis
- Catecholamine excess
- Primary sinus tachycardia (rare)

### TREATMENT

This involves correction of the condition causing the tachycardia. If necessary, $\beta$-blockers may be used to slow the sinus rate.

## PATHOLOGICAL BRADYCARDIAS

There are two main forms of severe bradycardia: sinus node disease and atrioventricular block.

## Sinus node disease (sick sinus syndrome)

Sinus node disease is caused by ischaemia, infarction or degenerative disease of the sinus node. It is characterized by long intervals between consecutive P waves (>2 s) on the ECG (Fig. 11.34). These sinus pauses may be an exact multiple of the basic sinus interval (sinoatrial exit block) or not (sinus arrest). Both conditions have a similar prognosis.

Sinus pauses and sinus bradycardia may allow cardiac tachyarrhythmias to emerge. A combination of fast and slow supraventricular rhythms is known as the tachycardia–bradycardia (tachy–brady) syndrome.

### TREATMENT

Treatment of chronic symptomatic sick sinus syndrome requires permanent pacing, with additional antiarrhythmic drugs to manage any tachycardia element. Thromboembolism is common in sick sinus syndrome and patients should be anticoagulated unless there is a contraindication.

## Atrioventricular block

There are three forms: first-degree block, second-degree (partial) block and third-degree (complete) block.

### First-degree AV block

This is simple prolongation of the PR interval to more than 0.22 s. Every atrial depolarization is followed by conduction to the ventricles but with delay (Fig. 11.35).

### Second-degree (partial) AV block

This occurs when some P waves conduct and others do not. There are several forms of second-degree AV block (Fig. 11.36).

Mobitz I block (Wenckebach phenomenon) is progressive PR interval prolongation until a P wave fails to conduct. The PR interval before the blocked P wave is much longer than the PR interval after the blocked P wave.

Mobitz II block occurs when a dropped QRS complex is not preceded by progressive PR interval prolongation.

2:1 or 3:1 block occurs when every second or third P wave conducts to the ventricles. This form of second-degree block is neither Mobitz I nor II. A 4:1 block, 5:1 block can also occur.

Traditionally, Wenckebach block was said to be more benign than other forms of second-degree block, but all forms of second-degree AV block have a similar prognosis. Patients with this conduction problem are usually asymptomatic. A close watch should be kept on them, although no treatment is necessary unless more serious or symptomatic heart block develops.

### Third-degree (complete) AV block

This occurs when no P waves conduct to the ventricles (Fig. 11.37). In this situation life is maintained by a spontaneous escape rhythm that has either broad (≥0.1 s) or narrow (<0.1 s) QRS complexes.

Narrow complex (Fig. 11.37a). This is due to disease in the AV node or the proximal His bundle. The escape rhythm occurs with an adequate rate (50–60 b.p.m.) and is relatively reliable. It occurs in association with:

- Congenital heart disease (such as transposition of the great arteries)
- An isolated congenital problem (congenital heart block)
- Inferior wall myocardial infarction
- Diphtheria
- Rheumatic fever

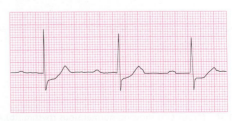

**Fig. 11.35**   An ECG showing first-degree atrioventricular block with a prolonged PR interval. In this trace coincidental ST depression is also present.

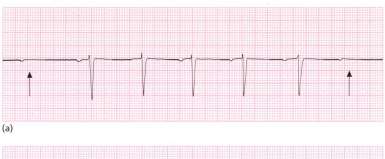

(a)

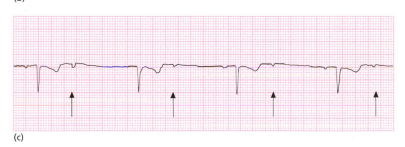

(b)

**Fig. 11.36** Three varieties of second-degree atrioventricular (AV) block. (a) Wenckebach (Mobitz type I) AV block. The PR interval gradually prolongs until the P wave does not conduct to the ventricles (arrows). (b) Mobitz type II AV block. The P waves that do not conduct to the ventricles (arrows) are not preceded by gradual PR interval prolongation. (c) Two P waves to each QRS complex. The PR interval prior to the dropped P wave is always the same. It is not possible to define this type of AV block as type I or type II Mobitz block and it is, therefore, a third variety of second-degree AV block.

(c)

- Toxic concentrations of drugs such as digitalis, verapamil or β-blockers

Treatment is often unnecessary except for the eradication of toxic causes. Recent-onset narrow-complex AV block due to acute myocardial infarction may respond to intravenous atropine but a temporary pacemaker may be necessary. Chronic narrow-complex AV block requires permanent pacing if it is symptomatic or associated with heart disease.

Occasionally, permanent pacing is advocated for asymptomatic, isolated, congenital AV block.

BROAD COMPLEX (Fig. 11.37b). This occurs because of disease in the Purkinje system. The escape pacemaker arises from the distal Purkinje network or the ventricular myocardium. The resulting rhythm is slow (15–40 b.p.m.) and relatively unreliable. Dizziness and blackouts (Stokes–Adams attacks) often occur. In the elderly, it is usually caused by degenerative fibrosis and calcification of the distal conduction system (Lenegre's disease) or the more proximal conduction system (Lev's disease). In younger patients, broad-complex AV block may be caused by ischaemic heart disease.

A permanent pacemaker should always be inserted, as the mortality from the condition, even when asymptomatic, is considerably reduced by pacing.

# Intraventricular conduction disturbances

The intraventricular conduction system consists of the His bundle, the right and left bundle branches and the antero-superior and postero-inferior divisions of the left bundle branch. Various conduction disturbances can occur:

HIS BUNDLE DELAY may produce a long PR interval but it is often too small a delay to be noticed on the surface ECG.

BLOCKED HIS BUNDLE CONDUCTION produces AV block.

BUNDLE BRANCH CONDUCTION DELAY produces trivial widening of the QRS complex (up to 0.11 s). This is known as incomplete bundle branch block.

COMPLETE BLOCK OF A BUNDLE BRANCH is associated with a wider QRS complex (0.12 s or more). The shape of the QRS depends on whether the right or the left bundle is blocked. *Right bundle branch block* (an example is shown in Fig. 11.63) produces late activation of the right ventricle. This is seen as deep S waves in leads I and $V_6$ and as a tall late R wave in lead $V_1$ (see Fig. 11.82) (late activation moving towards right and away from left-sided leads). *Left bundle branch block* (Fig. 11.38) produces the opposite, i.e. a deep S wave in lead $V_1$ and a tall late R wave in leads

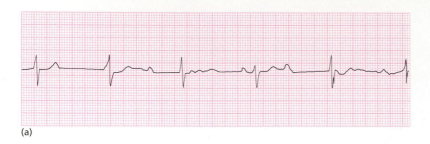

(a)

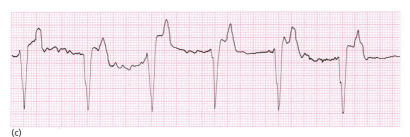

(b)

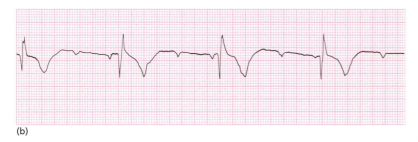

(c)

**Fig. 11.37** Three examples of complete heart block.
(a) Congenital complete heart block. The QRS complex is narrow (0.08 s) and the QRS rate is relatively rapid (52 b.p.m.).
(b) Acquired complete heart block. The QRS complex is broad (0.13 s) and the QRS rate is relatively slow (38 b.p.m.).
(c) Drug-induced complete heart block in a patient with atrial fibrillation rather than sinus rhythm (note the undulating baseline but the regular and slow ventricular rate).

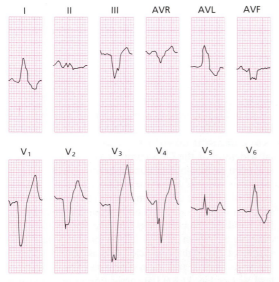

**Fig. 11.38** A 12-lead ECG showing left bundle branch block. The QRS duration is greater than 0.12 s. Note the broad notched R waves with ST depression in leads I, AVL, and V₆, and the broad QS waves in V₁–V₃.

I and $V_6$. Because left bundle branch conduction is normally responsible for the initial ventricular activation, left bundle branch block also produces abnormal Q waves.

Delay or block in the divisions of the left bundle branch produces a swing in the direction of depolarization (electrical axis) of the heart. When the antero-superior division is blocked, the left ventricle is activated from inferior to superior. This produces a superior (leftwards) movement of the axis. Delay or block in the postero-inferior division swings the QRS axis inferiorly.

BISFASCICULAR BLOCK (see Fig. 11.63) is a combination of a block of any two of the following: the right bundle branch, the left antero-superior division and the left postero-inferior division. Block of the remaining fascicle will result in complete AV block.

## CLINICAL FEATURES

Intraventricular conduction disturbances other than complete block of the His bundle are usually asymptomatic. Sometimes left bundle branch block actually seems to provoke chest pain.

Right bundle branch block causes wide but physiological splitting of the second heart sound. Left bundle branch block may cause reverse splitting of the second

*Congenital heart disease*
Atrial septal defect
Fallot's tetralogy
Pulmonary stenosis
Ventricular septal defect

*Pulmonary disease*
Cor pulmonale
Recurrent pulmonary embolism
Acute pulmonary embolism (transient)

*Myocardial disease*
Acute myocardial infarction
Cardiomyopathy
Conduction system fibrosis

*Drugs and electrolytes*
Hyperkalaemia
Class Ia drugs (see p. 568)

*Right ventriculotomy*

**Table 11.11**  Causes of right bundle branch block. It is also a normal finding in 1% of young adults and 5% of elderly adults.

sound. Patients with intraventricular conduction disturbances may complain of syncope. This is due to intermittent complete heart block or to ventricular tachyarrhythmias. ECG monitoring and electrophysiological study is needed to determine the cause of syncope in these patients.

## CAUSES

Right bundle branch block (Table 11.11) occurs as an isolated congenital anomaly or is associated with right ventricular overload. Left bundle branch block (Table 11.12) is almost always caused by disease of the left ventricle. All forms of intraventricular conduction disturbance may be caused by ischaemic heart disease and cardiomyopathy.

Conduction system fibrosis and calcification (Lenegre's disease and Lev's disease, see above) are progressive conditions that may present with bundle branch block or bifascicular block and eventually lead to complete heart block, when a pacemaker will be required.

## Bradycardic syndromes

Carotid sinus syndrome (which occurs predominantly in the old) and neurocardiogenic syndrome (which often

*Left ventricular outflow obstruction*
Aortic stenosis
Hypertension

*Coronary artery disease*
Acute myocardial infarction
Severe coronary disease (two- to three-vessel disease)

*Cardiomyopathy*

*Conduction system fibrosis*

**Table 11.12**  Causes of left bundle branch block.

occurs in the young), both present with recurrent syncope and presyncope. These two autonomic syndromes are characterized by bradycardia (AV block and/or sinus arrest) and hypotension. Carotid sinus syndrome is primarily bradycardic and the neurocardiogenic syndrome is primarily hypotensive. Fainting in the carotid sinus syndrome is due to stimulation of the carotid sinus by turning the neck, wearing stiff collars or coughing. In neurocardiogenic syndrome, syncope results from a variety of situations that stimulate the sympathetic nervous system. Carotid sinus syndrome often requires treatment with a dual chamber pacemaker. Only rarely is neurocardiogenic syncope helped by pacemaker treatment. Compression of the lower legs with hose and drugs such as β-blockers, α-agonists or myocardial negative inotropes (such as disopyramide) may be helpful.

# PATHOLOGICAL TACHYCARDIAS

## Atrial tachyarrhythmias

Ectopic beats, tachycardia, flutter and fibrillation may all arise from the atrial myocardium. They share common aetiologies, which are listed in Table 11.13.

### Atrial ectopic beats

These often cause no symptoms although they may be sensed as an irregularity or heaviness of the heart beat. On the ECG they appear as early and abnormal P waves, and are usually, but not always, followed by normal QRS complexes (see Fig. 11.40a).

Treatment is not normally required unless the ectopic beats provoke more significant arrhythmias, when β-blockade may be effective.

### Atrial tachycardia

This is an uncommon arrhythmia. (Previously, arrhythmias arising from the AV junction were wrongly called 'atrial tachycardias'.) There are three varieties of true atrial tachycardia:
1 Paroxysmal tachycardia
2 Chronic tachycardia
3 Atrial tachycardia with block
All are usually associated with heart disease, but chronic atrial tachycardia may occur in young children with no

Ischaemic heart disease
Rheumatic heart disease
Thyrotoxicosis
Cardiomyopathy
Lone atrial fibrillation (i.e. no cause discovered)
Wolff–Parkinson–White syndrome
Pneumonia
Atrial septal defect
Carcinoma of the bronchus
Pericarditis
Pulmonary embolus
Acute and chronic alcohol abuse

**Table 11.13**  Causes of atrial arrhythmias.

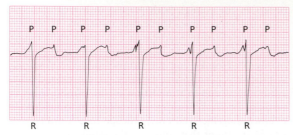

**Fig. 11.39**   Atrial tachycardia with second-degree atrioventricular block. Note the fast atrial (P wave) rate of 150 min⁻¹ and the slower ventricular (R wave) rate of 75 min⁻¹. This arrhythmia is most commonly due to digoxin toxicity.

obvious heart disease. Atrial tachycardia with block is often a result of digitalis poisoning.

Figure 11.39 demonstrates an atrial tachycardia at an atrial rate of 150 min⁻¹. The P waves are abnormally shaped and occur in front of the QRS complexes. Carotid sinus massage may increase AV block during tachycardia but does not usually terminate the arrhythmia. Treatment

with class Ia, Ic or III drugs (see p. 568) is usually successful, e.g. disopyramide 2 mg kg⁻¹ over 10 min.

### Atrial flutter

This is a rhythm disturbance that is usually associated with organic heart disease. The atrial rate varies between 280 and 350 min⁻¹ but is usually around 300 min⁻¹.

Symptoms are largely related to the degree of AV block. Most often, every second flutter beat conducts, giving a ventricular rate of 150 min⁻¹. Occasionally, every beat conducts, producing a heart rate of 300 min⁻¹. More often, especially when patients are receiving treatment, AV conduction block reduces the heart rate to approximately 75 min⁻¹.

The ECG shows regular sawtooth-like atrial flutter waves (F waves) between QRST complexes (Fig. 11.40b, c). If they are not clearly visible, AV conduction may be transiently impaired by carotid sinus massage or by the administration of AV nodal blocking drugs such as verapamil.

Treatment of an acute paroxysm is electrical cardioversion. Prophylaxis is achieved with class Ia, Ic or III drugs

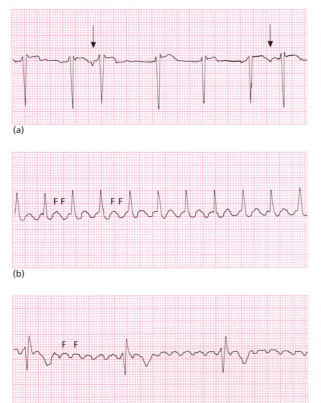

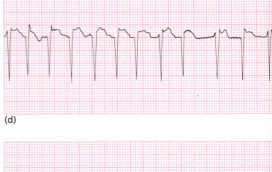

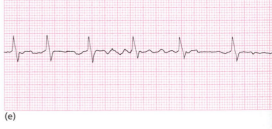

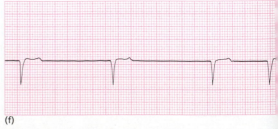

**Fig. 11.40**   ECGs of a variety of atrial arrhythmias. (a) Atrial premature beats (arrows). The premature P wave is different to the sinus P wave and conducts to the ventricle with a slightly prolonged PR interval. (b) Atrial flutter. The flutter waves are marked with an F. In this case the flutter frequency is 270 min⁻¹. Every second flutter wave is transmitted to the ventricles, and the ventricular rate is therefore 135 min⁻¹. (c) Atrial flutter at a frequency of 305 min⁻¹. The ventricular rate

is approximately 38 min⁻¹. Therefore, only one in eight flutter waves is transmitted to the ventricles. (d) Irregular ventricular response. This is typical of rapidly conducted atrial fibrillation. (e) Moderate conduction of atrial fibrillation. The underlying baseline undulations can now be appreciated. (f) So-called 'slow' atrial fibrillation. The ventricular response rate is slow and the underlying atrial fibrillation is seen as minor fluctuations of the baseline.

(see p. 568). If the arrhythmia is chronic, AV nodal blocking drugs (classes II or IV, or digitalis) are used.

### Atrial fibrillation

This is a common arrhythmia, occurring in between 5 and 10% of patients over 65 years of age. It also occurs, particularly in a paroxysmal form, in younger patients. It is caused by a raised atrial pressure, increased atrial muscle mass, atrial fibrosis, or inflammation and infiltration of the atrium.

Atrial fibrillation is continuous, rapid ($\geq 400$ min$^{-1}$) activation of the atria by multiple meandering wavelets. The atria respond electrically at this rate but there is practically no mechanical action and only a proportion of the impulses are conducted.

The aetiology (see Table 11.13) includes most cardiac disorders, but in some patients no cause can be found—'lone atrial fibrillation'. Thyrotoxicosis may provoke atrial fibrillation, sometimes as virtually the only feature of the disease (apathetic hyperthyroidism). Thyroid function tests are mandatory in any patient with unaccounted atrial fibrillation. When caused by rheumatic mitral stenosis, the onset of atrial fibrillation results in considerable worsening of cardiac failure.

Clinically the patient has a very irregular pulse, as opposed to a basically regular pulse with an occasional irregularity (e.g. extrasystoles) or recurring irregular patterns (e.g. Wenckebach block). The irregular nature of the pulse in atrial fibrillation is maintained during exercise.

The ECG shows fine oscillations of the baseline (so-called fibrillation or f waves) and no clear P waves. The QRS rhythm is rapid and irregular. Untreated, the ventricular rate is usually 120–180 min$^{-1}$, but it slows with treatment (Fig. 11.40d, e, f).

When atrial fibrillation is due to an acute precipitating event such as alcohol toxicity, chest infection or thyrotoxicosis, the provoking cause should be treated before attempting to convert the arrhythmia. Conversion to sinus rhythm can then be achieved by electrical DC-cardioversion (see p. 552) in about 80% of patients.

Intravenous infusion of some antiarrhythmic drugs, e.g. classes Ia, Ic and III drugs, is often used to restore sinus rhythm. This is known as medical cardioversion, but electrical cardioversion is often also necessary. Recurrent paroxysms may be prevented by oral medication with class Ia, Ic or III drugs.

If the arrhythmia is chronic and cannot be converted to sinus rhythm, AV nodal blocking drugs should be used to control the ventricular response rate. The most usual drug for this purpose is digoxin.

Anticoagulation is essential when atrial fibrillation is associated with valvular heart disease, left ventricular dysfunction or hypertension. Anticoagulation is also advised if there has been a previous thromboembolus. In most other patients aspirin is prescribed. Young patients (< 60 years) with no heart disease (lone AF) may not require any treatment unless the cause is alcoholic heart disease (the patient no longer drinking), thyrotoxicosis or sick sinus syndrome.

## Junctional tachycardia

Almost all junctional tachycardia is paroxysmal in nature. There is usually no associated structural heart disease but there may be demonstrable electrophysiological or electrocardiographic abnormalities such as the Wolff–Parkinson–White syndrome (Fig. 11.41) (see p. 563) or the Lown–Ganong–Levine syndrome (in which there is an anomalous connection between the atrium and the bundle of His).

There are two main varieties of junctional tachycardia:
1 Intra-AV nodal re-entry tachycardia (AVNRT)
2 Atrioventricular tachycardia (AVRT)
Both tachycardias are re-entry in type. In the intra-AV nodal re-entry tachycardia the entire tachycardia circuit is confined to the AV node and its surrounding myocardium. In atrioventricular re-entry tachycardia there is a large circuit comprising the AV node, the His bundle, the ventricle, an abnormal connection and the atrium. The abnormal connection linking the ventricle to the atrium completes the circuit necessary to sustain the tachycardia.

Typically, the tachycardia strikes suddenly without obvious provocation, but exertion, coffee, tea and alcohol may aggravate or induce the arrhythmia. The rhythm is rapid (140–280 min$^{-1}$) and regular. An attack may stop spontaneously or may continue indefinitely until medical intervention. The predominant symptom is palpitations, but chest pain, dyspnoea and polyuria may develop. The polyuria occurs because tachycardia leads to an elevated atrial pressure and the release of atrial natriuretic peptide and other hormones.

The rhythm is recognized by normal QRS complexes at a rate of 140–280 min$^{-1}$. Sometimes the QRS com-

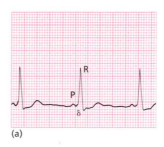

(a)

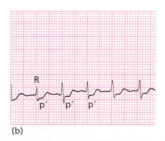

(b)

**Fig. 11.41** An ECG showing Wolff–Parkinson–White syndrome. (a) A trace is taken during sinus rhythm demonstrating a short PR interval (0.09 s) and broad QRS complex (0.12 s). (b) A trace demonstrating the paroxysmal junctional tachycardia associated with this syndrome. Notice the tachycardia p′ waves, which closely follow each QRS complex. δ, delta wave.

plexes will show typical bundle branch block (aberration). The P waves may occur simultaneously with the QRS complex (AV nodal tachycardia) or just after the QRS in the ST segment or the T wave (atrioventricular tachycardia).

## Treatment of acute supraventricular tachycardia

An acute paroxysm of tachycardia is easy to treat.

### Vagotonic manoeuvres
Most supraventricular arrhythmias require conduction through the AV node for their continuation or their expression at ventricular level. An intense efferent vagal discharge increases AV nodal conduction time and the AV nodal recovery time. Thus, atrial arrhythmias may be revealed by vagotonic stimulation, which blocks the transmission of these arrhythmias to the ventricles, and junctional tachycardias that involve continuous circulation (circus movement or re-entry) involving the AV node may be terminated by these manoeuvres.

Carotid sinus massage (Practical box 11.4), ocular pressure, immersion of the face in water (diving reflex) and the Valsalva manoeuvre may be used to stimulate the vagal efferent discharge. Of these techniques the Valsalva manoeuvre is the best and often easier for the patient to perform successfully. It should be undertaken when the patient is resting in the supine position (thus avoiding elevated background sympathetic tone). Several seconds after the release of strain, the resulting intense vagal effect may terminate a junctional re-entry tachycardia or may produce sufficient AV block to reveal an underlying atrial tachyarrhythmia.

### Drug treatment (Fig. 11.42)
If physical manoeuvres have not been successful, intravenous adenosine (up to 0.25 mg kg$^{-1}$) may be tried. This is a very short-acting (half-life < 10 s) naturally occurring purine nucleoside that causes complete heart block for a fraction of a second following intravenous administration (usual dose in adult 3 mg; maximum 12 mg). It is highly effective at terminating junctional tachycardias or revealing atrial tachycardias. It rarely affects ventricular

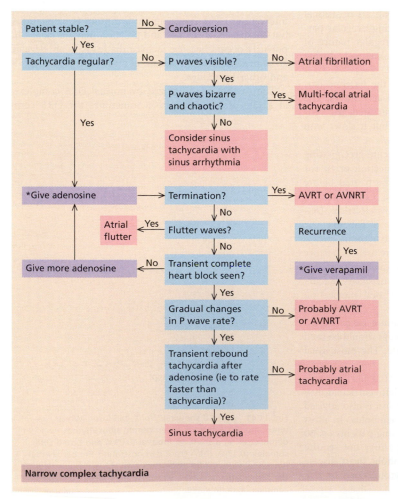

**Fig. 11.42**  Management of tachycardia. Narrow complex.

Carotid sinus message is performed for three reasons:
  To break supraventricular tachycardia by blocking AV
    nodal conduction
  To reveal on the ECG the P wave pattern of an atrial
    arrhythmia by reducing the frequency of AV nodal
    conduction during the tachycardia so that the QRS
    complexes do not mask the atrial activity
  To test for carotid sinus hypersensitivity, which is a severe
    fall in blood pressure or heart rate in response to
    carotid sinus stimulation

The carotid sinus is stimulated by firm rotary pressure of
    the carotid sinus against the transverse processes of the
    third cervical vertebrum. Provided that there is no
    carotid bruit, each carotid should be tried in turn. In
    general, right carotid pressure tends to slow the sinus
    rate and left carotid pressure tends to impair AV nodal
    conduction.

**Practical Box 11.4**   Carotid sinus massage.

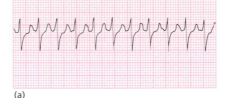

(a)

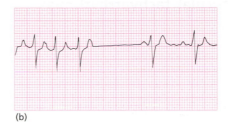

(b)

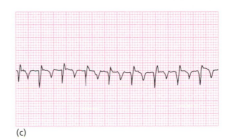

(c)

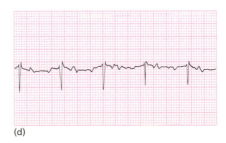

(d)

**Fig. 11.43** Two examples of the slowing of tachycardia following the administration of antiarrhythmic drugs. (a) A supraventricular tachycardia (rate 205 b.p.m.) before treatment with verapamil. (b) The result 60 s later. The tachycardia slows to 130 b.p.m. before terminating abruptly and revealing sinus rhythm. (c) Atrial tachycardia at a rate of 170 b.p.m. It is difficult to discern the atrial tachycardia waves. Verapamil is administered and the result is shown in (d). Now the atrial tachycardia is easily seen. The proportion of atrial tachycardia beats transmitted to the ventricles has been reduced following the administration of verapamil.

tachycardia. The side-effects of adenosine are very brief but include bronchospasm, chest pain and heaviness of the limbs. An alternative treatment is verapamil 10 mg i.v. over 5–10 min (Fig. 11.43). It is important not to give verapamil if β-blockers have been previously administered or if the tachycardia presents with broad (>0.14 s) QRS complexes.

### Other treatments

Rarely, medical therapy fails to terminate a tachycardia and rapid atrial pacing (directly or via the oesophagus) or DC-cardioversion may be considered.

### Prophylaxis

To prevent recurrences, drugs may be used to impair AV nodal conduction (classes II and IV and digoxin), impair abnormal connection conduction (classes Ia and III) or suppress the ectopic beats that initiate the arrhythmia (classes I, II and III) (see p. 568). In most cases, however, AV nodal modification, by a radiofrequency ablation technique, is used to destroy the tachycardia circuit and prevent recurrences.

## Wolff–Parkinson–White (WPW) syndrome

This is a congenital condition caused by an abnormal myocardial connection between atrium and ventricle (bundle of Kent). During sinus rhythm the electrical impulse can conduct quickly over this abnormal connection to depolarize the ventricles abnormally. This results in the typical ECG pattern of WPW syndrome—a short PR interval and a wide QRS complex that begins as a slurred part known as the δ wave (see Fig. 11.41). About half of those with WPW pattern on the ECG have tachycardias (see Fig. 11.41b). The tachycardias are of two sorts:

ATRIOVENTRICULAR RE-ENTRY. This is a circus movement tachycardia in which a depolarization wave travels from the atrium to the ventricle, usually through the AV node, and from the ventricle to the atrium through the abnormal pathway. Intravenous verapamil will terminate most of these tachycardias.

ATRIAL FIBRILLATION. During atrial fibrillation the ventricles may be depolarized by impulses travelling over both the abnormal and the normal pathways. The conduction ability of the abnormal pathway is depressed by drugs that affect the atrium (e.g. disopyramide and amiodarone) but not by verapamil and digoxin, which, paradoxically, may improve conduction over the abnormal pathway. Therefore, neither verapamil nor digoxin should be used to treat atrial fibrillation associated with the WPW syndrome.

Symptomatic patients should be treated by radiofrequency ablation of the abnormal pathway. Drugs, such as class Ia, Ic and III, may be used if ablation is (rarely) unsuccessful or not wanted.

## Ventricular tachyarrhythmias

There are four main types of ventricular tachyarrhythmia:

1 Ventricular premature beats
2 Ventricular tachycardia
3 Ventricular fibrillation
4 Torsades de pointes (twisting of points)

Except for torsades de pointes, most ventricular arrhythmias are caused by coronary heart disease, hypertension or cardiomyopathy. Torsades de pointes arises when ventricular repolarization is greatly prolonged (long QT interval). The causes of QT prolongation and torsades de pointes are listed in Table 11.14. Congenital QT prolongation may be associated with syncope, and torsades de pointes which may cause sudden death. Congenital QT prolongation may (Jervell–Lange–Nielsen syndrome) or may not (Romano–Ward syndrome) be associated with congenital deafness.

### Ventricular premature beats

These may be uncomfortable, especially when frequent. The patient may complain of extra beats, missed beats or heavy beats because it may be the premature beat, the post-ectopic pause or the next sinus beat that is noticed by the patient. The pulse is irregular owing to the premature beats. Some early beats may not be felt at the wrist.

When a premature beat occurs regularly after every normal beat, 'pulsus bigeminus' may occur.

On the ECG (Fig. 11.44) the premature beat has a broad (>0.12 s) and bizarre QRS complex because it arises from an abnormal (ectopic) site in the ventricular myocardium. Following the premature beat there is usually a complete compensatory pause because the timing of sinus rhythm is not influenced by the premature beat.

Ventricular premature beats have been graded in order of severity. The 'Lown Classification' (Table 11.15) is designed for premature beats occurring in the setting of

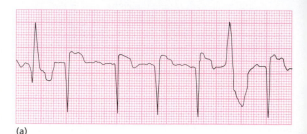

(a)

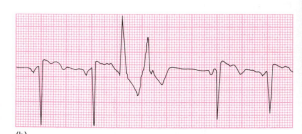

(b)

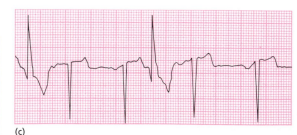

(c)

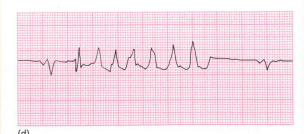

(d)

**Fig. 11.44**  Varieties of ventricular ectopic activity. (a) Two ventricular ectopic beats of different morphology (multimorphological). (b) Two ventricular premature beats (VPBs) occurring one after the other (a pair or couplet of VPBs). (c) Frequently repetitive ventricular ectopic activity of a single morphology. (d) A brief run of ventricular tachycardia (non-sustained ventricular tachycardia) that follows previous ectopic activity.

---

*Congenital syndromes*
Jervell–Lange–Nielsen (autosomal recessive)
Romano–Ward (autosomal dominant)

*Electrolyte abnormalities*
Hypokalaemia
Hypomagnesaemia
Hypocalcaemia

*Drugs*
Quinidine (and other class Ia antiarrhythmic drugs)
Amiodarone (and other class III antiarrhythmic drugs)
Amitriptyline (and other tricyclic antidepressants)
Chlorpromazine (and other phenothiazine drugs)
Terfenadine and astemizole
Terodiline
Erythromycin

*Poisons*
Organophosphate insecticides

*Miscellaneous*
Bradycardia
Mitral valve prolapse
Acute myocardial infarction
Prolonged fasting and liquid protein diets (long term)
Central nervous system diseases

**Table 11.14**  Causes of prolonged repolarization syndrome (long QT interval and torsades de pointes tachycardia).

| Grade | Description |
|---|---|
| 0 | No VPBs |
| 1 | Occasional VPBs (<30 hour$^{-1}$, not >1 min$^{-1}$) |
| 2 | Frequent VPBs (≥30 hour$^{-1}$) |
| 3 | Multiform VPBs |
| 4A | Couplets (two consecutive VPBs) |
| 4B | Repetitive VPBs (3 or more) |
| 5 | Early VPBs (R-on-T) |

**Table 11.15** Grading system for ventricular premature beats (VPBs) following acute myocardial infarction, as proposed by Lown.

VT is more likely than SVT with bundle branch block when there is:

| | |
|---|---|
| 1 | A very broad QRS (>0.14 s) |
| 2 | Atrioventricular dissociation |
| 3 | A bifid, upright QRS with a taller first peak in V$_1$ |
| 4 | A deep S wave in V$_6$ |
| 5 | A concordant (same polarity) QRS direction in all chest leads (V$_1$–V$_6$) |

**Table 11.16** ECG distinction between supraventricular tachycardia (SVT) with bundle branch block and ventricular tachycardia (VT).

acute myocardial infarction, but has been wrongly applied to other situations. This is particularly true of R-on-T ventricular premature beats (occurring simultaneously with the upstroke or peak of the T wave of the previous beat). Following myocardial infarction, such premature beats may induce ventricular fibrillation. This is extremely uncommon in other circumstances.

Treatment of ventricular ectopics may be advised because of symptoms or because they may provoke or threaten to provoke more serious arrhythmias. If structural heart disease is present and premature beats are frequent or run together (three or more beats at a time), treatment is offered. Drugs from classes I, II or III (see p. 568) are used. In the absence of heart disease, ventricular premature beats may safely be ignored.

### Ventricular tachycardia

This is defined as three or more ventricular beats occurring at a rate of 120 b.p.m. or more. Often the patient will be hypotensive and ill but some ventricular tachycardias are well tolerated.

Examination reveals a pulse rate of 120–220 b.p.m. Usually there are clinical signs of atrioventricular dissociation, i.e. intermittent cannon *a* waves and variable intensity of the first heart sound.

The ECG shows a rapid ventricular rhythm with broad (often 0.14 s or more), abnormal QRS complexes. Dissociated P wave activity may be seen (Fig. 11.45). Supraventricular tachycardia with bundle branch block (aberration) may resemble ventricular tachycardia on the ECG; the diagnostic features are indicated in Table 11.16. In all cases of doubt, a ventricular tachycardia should be diagnosed.

Treatment may be urgent depending on the haemodynamic situation (Fig. 11.46). If the cardiac output and the blood pressure are very depressed, emergency DC-cardioversion must be considered. On the other hand, if the blood pressure and cardiac output are well maintained, intravenous therapy with class I drugs is usually advised. First-line drug treatment consists of lignocaine (50–100 mg i.v. over 5 min) followed by a lignocaine infusion (2–4 mg min$^{-1}$ i.v.). DC-cardioversion may be necessary if medical therapy is unsuccessful. The administration of multiple antiarrhythmic drugs should be avoided.

Prophylaxis against relapse is extremely important. If possible, the likely success of therapy should be judged by Holter monitoring, exercise testing or other provocative techniques. Initial therapy is usually with a β-blocker if exercise induces the arrhythmia, or a class I drug if exercise is not responsible. If these drugs fail, a class III drug such as amiodarone or sotalol is tried. When severe left ventricular dysfunction is present, most antiarrhythmic drugs cannot be used because they cause further depression of myocardial function (negative inotropic effect). In such cases amiodarone or mexiletine may be the agent of choice.

### Ventricular fibrillation

This is very rapid and irregular ventricular activation with no mechanical effect. The patient is pulseless and becomes rapidly unconscious, and respiration ceases. The ECG shows shapeless, rapid oscillations and there is no hint of organized complexes (Fig. 11.47). It is usually provoked by a ventricular ectopic beat (especially in acute myocardial infarction), ventricular tachycardia or torsades de pointes. Ventricular fibrillation rarely reverses spontaneously. The only effective treatment is electrical defibrillation or, on rare occasions, intravenous bretylium 5–10 mg kg$^{-1}$ over 5 min. Basic and advanced cardiac life support is needed (see p. 551).

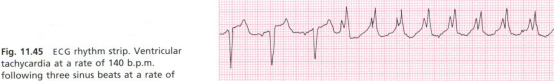

**Fig. 11.45** ECG rhythm strip. Ventricular tachycardia at a rate of 140 b.p.m. following three sinus beats at a rate of 92 b.p.m.

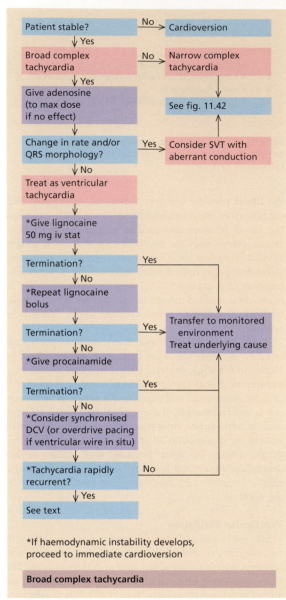

**Fig. 11.46**  Management of tachycardia. Broad complex.

If the attack of ventricular fibrillation occurs during the first day or two of an acute myocardial infarction, it is probable that prophylactic therapy will be unnecessary. If the ventricular fibrillation was not related to an acute infarction, prophylaxis with antiarrhythmic drugs, especially amiodarone or β-blockers, and possibly an implantable defibrillator (see p. 569) may be necessary.

**Torsades de pointes** (see Table 11.14)
This arrhythmia is usually short in duration and spontaneously reverts to sinus rhythm. It does, however, give rise to presyncope or syncope and occasionally converts to ventricular fibrillation, and sudden death may occur. It is characterized on the ECG by rapid, irregular, sharp complexes that continuously change from an upright to an inverted position (Fig. 11.48a). Between spells of tachycardia the ECG shows a prolonged QT interval: the corrected QT (see Table 11.9) is equal to or greater than 0.44 s. Figure 11.48b shows a further example of a prolonged QT interval. The arrhythmia is treated as follows:
1 Any electrolyte disturbance is corrected.
2 Causative drugs are stopped.
3 The heart rate is maintained with atrial or ventricular pacing.
4 Intravenous isoprenaline may be effective when QT prolongation is acquired.
5 β-Blockade or left stellectomy is advised if the QT prolongation is congenital. (Isoprenaline is contraindicated for congenital long-QT syndrome.)

# MANAGEMENTS AVAILABLE FOR ARRHYTHMIAS

Many cardiac arrhythmias are symptomatic, and some are life-threatening. Usually arrhythmias can only be suppressed, but occasionally, for example with surgical treatment, a complete cure can be effected.

Arrhythmias such as ventricular tachycardia must be terminated, but others, such as atrial fibrillation, may not easily convert to sinus rhythm. In this case, control of the ventricular rate response is the best treatment available.

Arrhythmias can be managed by a wide variety of means (Table 11.17), ranging from simple techniques that increase vagal tone to expensive and sophisticated treatments such as surgery or implantable electronic devices. Antiarrhythmic drugs remain the most important form of treatment.

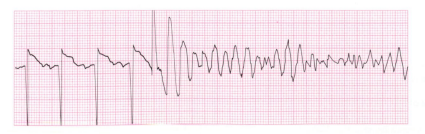

**Fig. 11.47**  A rhythm strip demonstrating four beats of sinus rhythm followed by a ventricular ectopic beat that initiates ventricular fibrillation. The ST segment during sinus rhythm is elevated owing to acute myocardial infarction.

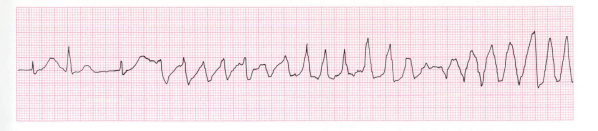

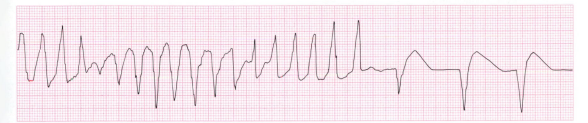

**Fig. 11.48(a)** An ECG demonstrating a supraventricular rhythm with a long QT interval giving way to atypical ventricular tachycardia (torsades de pointes). The tachycardia is short-lived and is followed by a brief period of idioventricular rhythm.

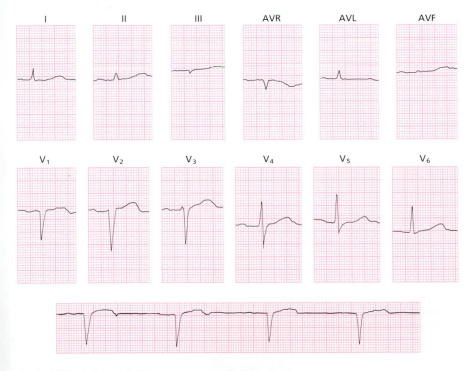

**Fig. 11.48(b)** A 12-lead ECG from an 11-year-old child with a history of syncope, demonstrating sinus bradycardia with a long QT interval (560 ms). The ECG is typical of the hereditary long-QT syndrome.

# Antiarrhythmic drugs

Drugs that modify the rhythm and conduction of the heart are used to prevent cardiac arrhythmias. All such drugs may aggravate or produce arrhythmias and they may also depress ventricular contractility and must therefore be used with caution. There are more than 30 antiarrhythmic drugs. They are classified according to their effect on the action potential (Vaughan Williams' classification; Table 11.18 and Fig. 11.49).

*Aims*
Cure
Prevention (suppression)
Termination
Reduction of ventricular rate

*Techniques available*
Vagotonic methods
DC cardioversion
Antiarrhythmic drugs
Pacemakers and other electronic devices
Surgery and other ablation methods

**Table 11.17**  Management of arrhythmias.

| Class I | |
|---|---|
| Ia | Quinidine, procainamide, disopyramide |
| Ib | Lignocaine, mexiletine, tocainide |
| Ic | Flecainide, propafenone |
| Class II | β-Adrenergic blocking drugs |
| Class III | Amiodarone, sotalol, bretylium |
| Class IV | Verapamil, diltiazem |
| (Other | Adenosine, digoxin) |

**Table 11.18**  Vaughan Williams' classification of antiarrhythmic drugs.

### Class I drugs

These are membrane-depressant drugs that reduce the rate of entry of sodium into the cell. They may slow conduction, delay recovery or reduce the spontaneous discharge rate of myocardial cells. Class Ia drugs (e.g. disopyramide) lengthen the action potential, Class Ib drugs (e.g. lignocaine) shorten the action potential, and Class Ic (flecainide, propafenone) do not affect the duration of the action potential.

In one postinfarction study in the USA (cardiac arrhythmia suppression trial—CAST), mortality in the patient group receiving flecainide was twice that of the control group. In view of this, flecainide should be reserved for life-threatening ventricular arrhythmias or supraventricular arrhythmias causing disabling symptoms in patients who do not have significant left ventricular dysfunction or a previous myocardial infarction.

### Class II drugs

These antisympathetic drugs prevent the effects of catecholamines on the action potential. Most are β-adrenergic antagonists. Cardioselective β-blockers ($\beta_1$) include metoprolol, atenolol and acebutalol.

### Class III drugs

These prolong the action potential and do not affect sodium transport through the membrane. There are two major drugs in this class: amiodarone and sotalol. Sotalol is also a β-blocker.

### Class IV drugs (see also Table 11.25)

The non-dihydropyridine calcium antagonists that reduce the plateau phase of the action potential are particularly effective at slowing conduction in nodal tissue. Verapamil and diltiazem are the most important drugs in this group.

Another clinical classification is based on the part of the heart that is affected by the antiarrhythmic drug (Fig. 11.50).

The features of the major antiarrhythmic drugs are given in Table 11.19.

## Other management techniques

Ventricular tachycardia can be eradicated by surgical removal of the focus of the arrhythmia, but this operation

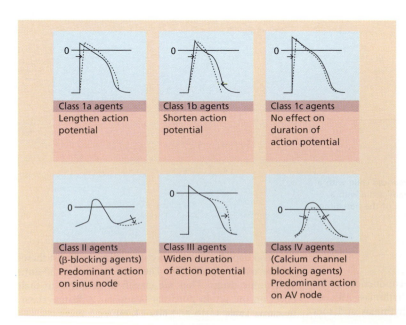

**Fig. 11.49**  Vaughan Williams' classification of antiarrhythmic drugs based on their effect on cardiac action potentials. 0, 0 mV. The dotted curves indicate the effects of the drugs.

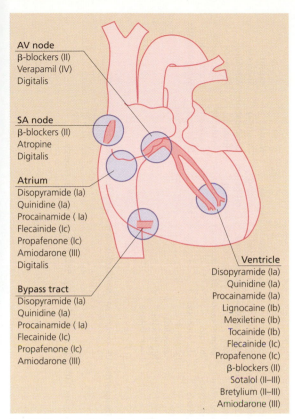

**AV node**
β-blockers (II)
Verapamil (IV)
Digitalis

**SA node**
β-blockers (II)
Atropine
Digitalis

**Atrium**
Disopyramide (Ia)
Quinidine (Ia)
Procainamide ( Ia)
Flecainide (Ic)
Propafenone (Ic)
Amiodarone (III)
Digitalis

**Bypass tract**
Disopyramide (Ia)
Quinidine (Ia)
Procainamide ( Ia)
Flecainide (Ic)
Propafenone (Ic)
Amiodarone (III)

**Ventricle**
Disopyramide (Ia)
Quinidine (Ia)
Procainamide (Ia)
Lignocaine (Ib)
Mexiletine (Ib)
Tocainide (Ib)
Flecainide (Ic)
Propafenone (Ic)
β-blockers (II)
Sotalol (II–III)
Bretylium (II–III)
Amiodarone (III)

**Fig. 11.50** Drugs that affect different parts of the heart. The Vaughan Williams class is given in parentheses.

carries considerable risk and is reserved for very serious problems.

The AV node or His bundle may be destroyed by electrical energy delivered through a catheter electrode placed close to the AV conduction system. This procedure effectively prevents the AV conduction of atrial arrhythmias. A ventricular pacemaker is then needed to prevent ventricular bradycardia. Pacemakers of another sort can also be used to interrupt repetitive paroxysms of tachycardia. Steerable electrode catheters can be used to deliver radiofrequency energy to any part of the heart responsible for the generation or continuation of tachycardias. Atrial tachycardia, AV nodal tachycardia and the abnormal pathways responsible for WPW syndrome can be successfully treated. The catheter ablation techndique is very successful and safe.

## Implantable automatic cardioverter–defibrillator

Serious ventricular arrhythmias (ventricular fibrillation or rapid ventricular tachycardia with hypotension) carry a mortality within 1 year of up to 40%. Antiarrhythmic drug therapy, particularly with amiodarone, may reduce the mortality. An important alternative therapy is the implantable cardioverter–defibrillator (ICD), which can recognize ventricular tachycardia or fibrillation and auto-

matically deliver a defibrillating shock to the heart. It is relatively small and is powered by lithium batteries sufficient to provide energy for about 100 shocks each of 25–30 J. The device is usually implanted behind the rectus abdominis muscle and is connected to the heart by several wires and electrodes. When an arrhythmia develops that requires treatment, the device takes about 15 s to recognize the arrhythmia and charge its capacitors. It then delivers the defibrillating discharge. The shock may be painful, particularly if the patient is still fully conscious.

The use of this device has cut the sudden death rate in patients with serious ventricular arrhythmias to between 1 and 2% in the first year. However, because of its expense it is not widely available.

# Cardiac failure

Cardiac failure occurs when, despite normal venous pressures, the heart is unable to maintain sufficient cardiac output to meet the demands of the body. The incidence of heart failure is estimated at 10 per 1000 over 65 years of age. Irrespective of the aetiology of heart failure, the prognosis is poor. Approximately 50% of patients with severe heart failure die within 2 years of diagnosis from either progression of heart failure or sudden death. The causes of heart failure include:

MYOCARDIAL DYSFUNCTION, e.g. ischaemic heart disease, cardiomyopathy, hypertension

VOLUME OVERLOAD, e.g. valvular regurgitation (aortic and mitral)

OBSTRUCTION TO OUTFLOW, e.g. aortic stenosis

OBLIGATORY HIGH OUTPUT, e.g. anaemia, thyrotoxicosis, Paget's disease, beri-beri, systemic to pulmonary shunts

COMPROMISED VENTRICULAR FILLING, e.g. constrictive pericarditis, pericardial tamponade, restrictive cardiomyopathy

ALTERED RHYTHM, e.g. atrial fibrillation

## Haemodynamic effects of myocardial failure

When the heart fails, considerable changes occur to the heart and peripheral vascular system in response to the haemodynamic changes associated with heart failure (Table 11.20). These physiological changes are compensatory and maintain cardiac output and peripheral perfusion. However, as heart failure progresses, these mechanisms are overwhelmed and become pathophysiological. The development of pathophysiological peripheral vasoconstriction and sodium retention in heart failure reflects loss of beneficial compensatory mechanisms and represents cardiac decompensation and are manifest by the onset of clinical heart failure. Factors involved are the venous return, the outflow resistance, the contractility of the myocardium, and salt and water retention.

| | Quinidine | Disopyramide | Lignocaine | Mexiletine | Flecainide | Propafenone | Amiodarone | Sotalol | Verapamil | Diltiazem | Digoxin |
|---|---|---|---|---|---|---|---|---|---|---|---|
| Class: | Ia | Ia | Ib | Ib | Ic | Ic | III | III | IV | IV | N/A |
| Daily dose: | 250–500 mg orally | 100–250 mg ×3 orally | 1–4 mg min$^{-1}$ (50–150 mg i.v. loading dose) | 400–800 mg orally loading, 150–300 mg maintenance | 100 mg ×2 orally | 150 mg ×3 300 mg ×2 or 300 mg ×3 | 200 mg ×1–2 orally | 80–160 mg ×2–3 orally | 0.1 mg kg$^{-1}$ i.v. 40–160 mg ×3–4 orally | 60–120 mg ×3–4 orally | 0.25 mg ×1 orally |
| Protein binding: | 75% | 40–90% | 50–80% | 70% | 50% | 85% | 98% | <10% | 90% | 80% | 25% |
| Half-life: | 6 hours | 5 hours | 1½ hours | 15 hours | 18 hours | 6 hours | 50 days + | 24 hours | 6 hours | 2–8 hours | 36 hours |
| Plasma therapeutic range: | 2–5 µg ml$^{-1}$ | 3–6 µg ml$^{-1}$ | 2–6 µg ml$^{-1}$ | 0.5–2.0 µg ml$^{-1}$ | 0.2–0.8 µg ml$^{-1}$ | 0.2–1.5 µg ml$^{-1}$ | 0.2–5.0 µg ml$^{-1}$ | 0.3–1.5 µg ml$^{-1}$ | 0.1–0.3 µg ml$^{-1}$ | 0.02–0.16 µg ml$^{-1}$ | 1.3–2.6 nmol litre$^{-1}$ |
| Indications: | AF PSVT VT VPBs WPW | AF PSVT VT VPBs WPW | VT/VF associated with myocardial infarction | VT, especially after myocardial infarction | VT PSVT WPW | VT/VF PSVT | VT/VF WPW PSVT AF | VT WPW PSVT | PSVT | PSVT | AF/AFL PSVT |
| Side-effects: | Nausea Diarrhoea Rash Fever Cinchonism Syncope Blood dyscrasia | Hypotension Anticholinergic effects Dry mouth Urinary hesitancy Blurred vision Heart failure AV block | Confusion Convulsions | Confusion Tremor Bradycardia Hypotension | Dizziness Visual disturbance Arrhythmogenesis | Light-headedness Unusual taste Headache Constipation Arrhythmogenesis | Corneal deposits Photosensitivity Skin pigmentation Thyroid disturbance Pulmonary alveolitis Nightmares Liver disease | Ventricular arrhythmias Bradycardia Heart failure Bronchospasm | Nausea Vomiting Constipation Flushing Headache Bradycardia Fluid retention | Nausea Vomiting Constipation Flushing Headache Bradycardia Fluid retention | Nausea Anorexia Vomiting Visual disturbance Bradycardia Gynaecomastia |

AF, atrial fibrillation; AFL, atrial flutter; N/A, not applicable; PSVT, paroxysmal supraventricular tachycardia; VF, ventricular fibrillation; VPBs, ventricular premature beats; VT, ventricular tachycardia; WPW, Wolff–Parkinson–White syndrome.

**Table 11.19**   Details of antiarrhythmic drugs. (For class II drugs (β-blockers) see Table 11.39.) Adenosine 0.05–0.25 mg kg$^{-1}$ (see p. 562) only given intravenously.

Ventricular dilatation
Ventricular hypertrophy
Increased inotropy
Neurohumoral activation
Peripheral vasoconstriction
Skeletal muscle and vascular deconditioning

**Table 11.20** Compensatory mechanisms in heart failure.

### Venous return (pre-load)

In the intact heart, myocardial failure leads to a reduction of the volume of blood ejected with each heart beat and an increase in the volume of blood remaining after systole. This increased diastolic volume stretches the myocardial fibres and, as Starling's law of the heart would suggest, myocardial contraction is restored. However, the failing myocardium results in depression of the ventricular function curve (cardiac output plotted against the ventricular diastolic volume) (see Fig. 11.3).

Slight myocardial depression is not associated with a reduction in cardiac output because it is maintained by an increase in venous pressure (and hence diastolic volume). However, the proportion of blood ejected with each heart beat (ejection fraction) is reduced early in heart failure. Sinus tachycardia also ensures that any reduction of stroke volume is compensated for by the increase in heart rate; cardiac output (stroke volume × heart rate) is therefore maintained.

When there is more severe myocardial dysfunction, cardiac output can only be maintained by a large increase in venous pressure and/or marked sinus tachycardia. This eventually results in further depression of the ventricular function curve and reduced contractility; the resultant increased venous pressure contributes to the development of dyspnoea, owing to the accumulation of interstitial and alveolar fluid, and to the occurrence of hepatic enlargement, ascites and dependent oedema, owing to increased systemic venous pressure. Despite symptoms due to increased venous pressure, the cardiac output at rest may not be much depressed, but myocardial and haemodynamic reserve is so compromised that a normal increase in cardiac output cannot be produced by exercise.

In very severe heart failure the cardiac output at rest is depressed, despite high venous pressures. The inadequate cardiac output is redistributed to maintain perfusion of vital organs, such as the heart, brain and kidneys, at the expense of the skin and muscle.

### Outflow resistance (after-load) (see Figs 13.2 and 13.4)

This is the load or resistance against which the ventricle contracts. It is formed by:
● Pulmonary and systemic resistance
● Physical characteristics of the vessel walls
● Volume of blood that is ejected

An increase in after-load decreases the cardiac output. This decrease in function with further increase of end-diastolic volume and dilatation of the ventricle itself further exacerbates the problem of after-load. This is expressed by Laplace's law: the tension of the myocar-

dium ($T$) is proportional to the intraventricular pressure ($P$) multiplied by the radius of the ventricular chamber ($R$), i.e. $T \propto PR$ (see p. 523).

### Myocardial contractility (inotropic state)

The state of the myocardium also influences performance. Increased contractility (positive inotropism) can result from increased sympathetic drive, and this is a normal part of the Frank–Starling relationship (see Fig. 11.3). Conversely, myocardial depressants (e.g. hypoxia) decrease myocardial contractility (negative inotropism).

### Salt and water retention

The increase in venous pressure that occurs when the ventricles fail leads to retention of salt and water and their accumulation in the interstitium, producing many of the physical signs of heart failure. Reduced cardiac output also leads to diminished renal perfusion, activating the renin–angiotensin system and enhancing fluid retention (see p. 501). This increased salt and water retention further increases venous pressure, which in the early stages of heart failure improves cardiac output by the Starling mechanism. In severe heart failure the ventricular function curve plateaus such that further increases in venous pressure do not provoke an increase in cardiac output. This retention of sodium is in part compensated by the action of circulating atrial natriuretic peptides. These are short-chain peptides secreted by the atria in response to distension. These atrial peptides are potent vasodilators with natriuretic properties and levels rise considerably in heart failure. The effect of their action may represent a beneficial, albeit inadequate, compensatory response tending to reduce cardiac load (pre-load and after-load) by vasodilatation and by enhancing sodium and water excretion.

The precise way in which haemodynamic and neurohumoral factors interact and contribute to the progression of heart failure remains unclear. Both increase ventricular wall stress which promote ventricular dilatation and further worsen contractile efficiency. In addition, prolonged activation of the sympathetic nervous and renin–angiotensin–aldosterone systems exerts direct toxic effects on myocardial cells. The realization over recent years that heart failure was not just a mechanical disorder but involved considerable pathophysiological changes has improved our understanding of many clinical aspects of the heart failure syndrome and also has provided a more rational basis for treatment.

## Clinical syndromes of heart failure

It is clinically useful to divide heart failure into the syndromes of right, left and biventricular (congestive) cardiac failure, but it is rare for any part of the heart to fail in isolation.

### Right heart failure

This syndrome occurs in association with:
● Chronic lung disease (cor pulmonale)

- Pulmonary embolism or pulmonary hypertension
- Tricuspid valve disease
- Pulmonary valve disease
- Left-to-right shunts, e.g. atrial or ventricular septal defects
- Isolated right ventricular cardiomyopathy
- Mitral valve disease with pulmonary hypertension

The most frequent cause of right heart failure is secondary to left heart failure.

SYMPTOMS include fatigue, breathlessness, anorexia and nausea and relate to distension and fluid accumulation in areas drained by the systemic veins.

PHYSICAL SIGNS are usually more prominent than the symptoms, with:
- Jugular venous distension ($\pm\ v$ waves of tricuspid regurgitation)
- Tender smooth hepatic enlargement
- Dependent pitting oedema
- Development of free abdominal fluid (ascites)
- Pleural transudates (commonly right-sided)

Dilatation of the right ventricle produces cardiomegaly and may give rise to functional tricuspid regurgitation. Tachycardia and a right ventricular third heart sound are usual.

### Left heart failure

Causes include:
- Ischaemic heart disease (commonest)
- Systemic hypertension (chronic or 'malignant')
- Mitral and aortic valve disease
- Cardiomyopathies

Mitral stenosis causes left atrial hypertension and signs of left heart failure but does not itself cause failure of the left ventricle.

SYMPTOMS are predominantly fatigue, exertional dyspnoea, orthopnoea and paroxysmal nocturnal dyspnoea.

PHYSICAL SIGNS are few and not prominent until a late stage or if the ventricular failure is acute. Cardiomegaly is demonstrable with a displaced and often sustained apical impulse. Auscultation reveals a left ventricular third or fourth heart sound that, with tachycardia, is described as a gallop rhythm. Dilatation of the mitral annulus results in functional mitral regurgitation. Crackles are heard at the lung bases. In severe left heart failure the patient has pulmonary oedema. In this circumstance a chest X-ray is the most useful investigation. Rarely the cause of left ventricular failure is apparent, e.g. ventricular aneurysm at the site of previous infarction.

### Biventricular failure (congestive)

This term is used variously but is best restricted to cases where right heart failure is a result of pre-existing left heart failure. The physical signs are thus a combination of the above syndromes.

### Acute heart failure

Acute failure of the heart most commonly occurs in the setting of acute myocardial infarction when there is extensive loss of ventricular muscle. The condition may also occur with rupture of the interventricular septum producing a ventricular septal defect, or due to acute valvular regurgitation. Common examples of valvular regurgitation are papillary or chordal rupture producing mitral regurgitation or sudden aortic valve regurgitation in infective endocarditis. Other causes of acute heart failure include obstruction of the circulation due to acute pulmonary embolus and cardiac tamponade. In each case severe cardiac failure can occur with a relatively normal heart size.

### High-output heart failure

The heart may not be able to meet the demands placed on it in conditions such as anaemia, thyrotoxicosis, beri-beri and Gram-negative septicaemia. This form of heart failure presents in much the same manner as low-output states but is associated with tachycardia and a gallop rhythm. Patients are often warm with distended superficial veins. Unlike low-output failure the oxygen content of systemic venous blood is high owing to the delivery of large amounts of arterial blood to non-metabolizing tissues.

## Factors aggravating or precipitating heart failure

Any factor that increases myocardial work may aggravate existing heart failure or initiate failure. These factors must be carefully considered in patients who present with heart failure. The most common are arrhythmias, anaemia, thyrotoxicosis, pregnancy, infective endocarditis, pulmonary infection or adjustment of heart failure therapy.

## Investigation

The diagnosis 'heart failure' is inadequate and a cause should be determined. In many cases the cause will be evident from the clinical history and examination. Investigations are determined by the suspected cause of heart failure and include the following.

### General/diagnostic

CHEST X-RAY/ECG for cardiac size and evidence of ischaemia or hypertension

ECHOCARDIOGRAPHY for valvular disease and assessment of left ventricular function

BLOOD TESTS: full blood count, liver biochemistry, urea and electrolytes

CARDIAC ENZYMES IN ACUTE heart failure to diagnose myocardial infarction

THYROID FUNCTION

CARDIAC CATHETERIZATION, see p. 547

### Functional/prognostic

EXERCISE TESTING and a 6 min exercise walk

Resting and stress radionuclide angiography (MUGA)—ejection fraction, regional wall motion abnormality
24–48-Hour ambulatory ECG monitoring—if arrhythmia suspected

# Treatment of heart failure

Treatment of chronic heart failure is aimed at relieving symptoms, retarding disease progression and improving survival. The management of heart failure requires that any factor aggravating the failure should be identified and treated. Similarly the cause of heart failure must be elucidated and where possible corrected. Nursing care of the mouth and pressure areas is necessary and patients should be nursed in a comfortable upright position.

## GENERAL TREATMENT
### Reduction of physical activity
Bed rest reduces the demands of the heart and is useful for a few days. Migration of fluid from the interstitium promotes a diuresis, reducing heart failure. Prolonged bed rest may, however, lead to development of deep vein thrombosis; this can be avoided by daily leg exercises, low-dose subcutaneous heparin and elastic support stockings.

### Dietary modifications
Large meals should be avoided and if necessary weight reduction instituted. Salt restriction is important and foods rich in salt or added salt in cooking and at the table should be avoided. A low-sodium diet is unpalatable and of questionable value. Alcohol has a negatively inotropic effect and patients should abstain.

## DRUG MANAGEMENT
The pharmacological management of heart failure relies on the following categories of drugs: diuretics, vasodilators, positive inotropic agents including digitalis glycosides, and antiarrhythmic agents.

### Diuretics (see Table 10.2)
These act by promoting the renal excretion of salt and water by blocking tubular reabsorption of sodium and chloride. The resulting loss of fluid reduces ventricular filling pressures (pre-load) and produce consistent haemodynamic and symptomatic benefits in patients with heart failure and rapidly relieve dyspnoea and peripheral oedema. The intravenous administration of loop diuretics such as frusemide relieves pulmonary oedema rapidly by means of arteriolar vasodilatation reducing after-load, an action that is independent of its diuretic effect.

Diuretics act in different ways.

Loop diuretics such as frusemide and bumetanide act by reducing sodium and chloride reabsorption in the ascending limb of the loop of Henle. They cause a brisk and generally short-lived diuresis as the concentrating power of the kidney is reduced. These agents also produce marked potassium loss and promote hyperuricaemia.

Thiazide diuretics such as bendrofluazide have a mild diuretic effect and act on the distal convoluted tubule, reducing sodium reabsorption. Potassium excretion is enhanced. Metolazone is a powerful thiazide producing profound diuresis acting synergistically with loop diuretics. This combination is useful in treating severe and resistant heart failure.

Potassium-sparing diuretics. Spironolactone is a specific competitive antagonist to aldosterone, producing a weak diuresis but with a potassium-sparing action. Amiloride and triamterene act at the distal tubule preventing potassium secretion in exchange for sodium. These drugs are weak diuretics but are useful in combination with more powerful loop diuretics. They should be avoided in the presence of renal failure.

Although heart failure symptoms are improved by diuretic treatment alone, they do not provide any survival benefit. In addition, their use may be complicated by over-diuresis, electrolyte depletion (potassium and magnesium) which may predispose to the development of lethal ventricular arrhythmias, hyperkalaemia (potassium-sparing diuretics) and other metabolic disturbances (hyperuricaemia and dyslipidaemia).

### Vasodilator therapy (Table 11.21)
Diuretics and sodium restriction serve to activate the renin–angiotensin system, promoting formation of angiotensin (a potent vasoconstrictor) and an increase in after-load. A variety of other neural and hormonal reactions also serve to increase pre-load and after-load. These compensatory mechanisms are initially beneficial in maintaining blood pressure and redistributing blood flow, but in the later stages of heart failure they are deleterious and reduce cardiac output. The high venous pressures found in heart failure are also related to the activation of the sympathetic nervous system and the presence of circulating vasoconstrictors, thus shifting the Starling curve to the right.

Several large controlled trials, e.g. CONSENSUS and

| | Reduction in | |
|---|---|---|
| | Pre-load | After-load |
| Nitroprusside | + | +++ |
| Glyceryl trinitrate | +++ | + |
| Isosorbide di/mono nitrate | +++ | + |
| Prazosin | + | ++ |
| ACE inhibitors | ++ | ++ |
| Hydralazine | 0 | +++ |
| Calcium antagonists | + | ++ |

ACE, angiotensin-converting enzyme.

**Table 11.21**  Effects of vasodilator drugs used in heart failure.

SOLVD, have established the benefit of vasodilator ther-apy in heart failure. The trials have shown that in addition to producing considerable symptomatic improvement in patients with symptomatic heart failure, vasodilators markedly improve prognosis and limit the development of progressive heart failure. Whether there are significant clinical differences between treatment with different angiotensin-converting enzyme (ACE) inhibi-tors (see Table 11.22) or between ACE inhibitors and combined nitrate/hydralazine treatment remains uncer-tain. The recent SAVE study has confirmed the benefit of ACE inhibitor therapy in patients with asymptomatic heart failure following myocardial infarction in whom the development of overt heart failure was reduced by this treatment.

ARTERIOLAR VASODILATORS (Fig. 11.51). Drugs such as $\alpha$-adrenergic blockers (e.g. prazosin) and direct smooth-muscle relaxants (e.g. hydralazine) are potent arteriolar vasodilators. Calcium antagonists (see Table 11.25), e.g. nifedipine, are also used and reduce after-load. The reduction in after-load causes an increase in cardiac output. Any tendency to hypotension is usually offset by the increased output.

VENODILATORS (Fig. 11.51). Short- and long-acting nitrates (e.g. glyceryl trinitrate and isosorbide mononitrate) act by reducing pre-load and lowering venous pressure with resulting reduction in pulmonary and dependent oedema. Reduction of filling pressure does not significantly enhance cardiac output because the heart is operating on the flat portion of the ventricular filling curve. With chronic use, tolerance develops with loss of efficacy and consequent worsening of heart failure.

ANGIOTENSIN-CONVERTING ENZYME INHIBITORS (Table 11.22 and Fig. 16.28). ACE inhibitors lower sys-temic vascular resistance, venous pressure and reduce lev-els of circulating catecholamines, thus improving myocar-dial performance. The beneficial haemodynamic effect of these drugs appears to be independent of their inhibition of ACE as they are equally effective when plasma renin activity is normal.

These drugs should be carefully introduced to patients with heart failure because of the risk of first-dose hypo-tension. This is a particular risk in patients who are receiving large doses of diuretics and in the presence of hyponatraemia (<130 mmol litre$^{-1}$). In such cases a test dose of ACE inhibitor should be commenced and the preceding diuretic doses omitted. Some of these agents are prodrugs (e.g. enalapril) and require conversion to the active metabolite (enalaprilat) by liver enzymes; these drugs have a delayed onset of action and first-dose hypo-tension may not occur for several hours. Prodrugs are best avoided if heart failure results in significantly altered hepatic function. Serious hypotension may result in acute renal failure. Concomitant potassium-sparing diuretics should be discontinued, as ACE inhibitors tend to pro-mote potassium retention.

**Inotropic agents** (Fig. 11.52)
Recently, several orally active positive inotropic drugs have become available, supplementing digoxin and those currently available for intravenous use. They can be classified as follows:
- Digitalis glycosides
- $\beta$-Adrenergic agonists
- Phosphodiesterase inhibitors
Efficacy of these agents is variable and must be judged both in terms of objective and symptomatic improvement on an individual patient basis.

DIGITALIS GLYCOSIDES. Digitalis glycosides are no longer extensively used in the management of heart fail-

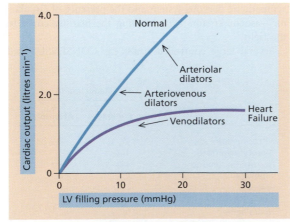

**Fig. 11.51** Effect of vasodilators on cardiac output and left ventricular filling pressure. Agents with arteriolar and arteriovenous dilating properties reduce the after-load and increase cardiac output. Venodilators reduce the left ventricular filling pressure (and pulmonary oedema) but do not increase cardiac output.

| Drug | First dose | Maintenance dose |
|------|-----------|------------------|
| Captopril | 6.25 mg | 25–50 mg twice daily |
| Enalapril | 5 mg | 10–20 mg daily |
| Lisinopril | 2.5 mg | 10–20 mg daily |
| Perindopril | 2 mg | 4–8 mg daily |
| Fosinopril | 10 mg | 20–40 mg |
| Quinapril | 5 mg | 20–40 mg |

Note: (a) All ACE inhibitors should be given with caution to patients who have received diuretics, when the first dose may cause marked hypotension. It is therefore recommended that the first dose is given at bedtime after withholding diuretics for a few days. In severe heart failure therapy should be initiated in hospital.
(b) Renal impairment may occur or be aggravated by treatment with ACE inhibitors, particularly when co-administered with non-steroidal anti-inflammatory drugs.
(c) Other side-effects of ACE inhibitors include: dry cough, loss of taste, rash, abdominal pain and angioedema.

**Table 11.22** Angiotensin-converting enzyme (ACE) inhibitors.

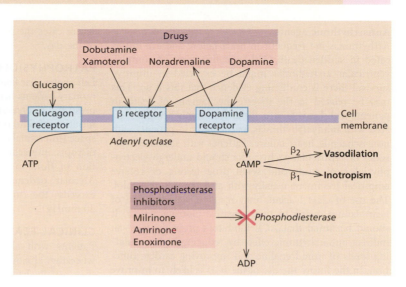

**Fig. 11.52** Diagrammatic representation of the action of inotropic drugs. Dopamine stimulates the myocardium by activating the $\beta_1$-adrenergic receptors; it also acts indirectly by releasing noradrenaline from sympathetic nerve terminals. Dopamine is unselective and also activates widespread dopaminergic receptors causing vasodilatation. Dobutamine and xamoterol act through the $\beta_1$-receptor to produce cAMP. Phosphodiesterase inhibitors, e.g. amrinone, prevent the breakdown of cAMP which accumulates and increases contractility and causes vasodilatation by acting on peripheral vascular $\beta_2$-receptors.

ure, although they remain effective positive inotropic agents. Digoxin usage is of particular benefit in congestive heart failure associated with atrial fibrillation when the rapid ventricular response is effectively controlled. Studies have suggested that digoxin may also be beneficial in patients with heart failure and sinus rhythm. The withdrawal of digoxin in these patients is associated with clinical deterioration and increased hospitalization. Further studies are currently underway to determine if digoxin provides useful adjunctive therapy in conjunction with ACE inhibitors. Digoxin is the most common glycoside in use with a half-life of approximately 36 hours. It is highly protein-bound, making it liable to drug interaction. Ninety per cent is excreted unchanged in the urine, causing accumulation in renal failure. Digoxin acts as a positive inotrope by competitive inhibition of $Na^+,K^+$ ATPase, producing high intracellular levels of sodium. The intracellular sodium is exchanged for extracellular calcium. High intracellular levels of calcium ions allow increased binding of the contractile proteins actin and myosin, enhancing the force of cardiac contractility (see Fig. 11.2). Digoxin is usually administered orally (1 mg loading and 0.125–0.25 mg daily). In elderly patients and in patients with impaired renal function digoxin may accumulate, resulting in serious toxicity. Careful titration of the dose is important with monitoring of trough serum levels (1.3–2.6 nmol litre$^{-1}$) and avoidance of hypokalaemia. Patients with hypothyroidism are particularly sensitive to digitalis glycosides. In patients with fluctuating renal function the administration of the liver-metabolized digitoxin may be preferable.

With improvement in formulation, digoxin toxicity has become less problematic but is prone to occur in the elderly and in patients with renal impairment. The most common features of *digoxin toxicity* are:

• Anorexia, nausea, altered vision
• Arrhythmia, e.g. ventricular premature beats especially bigeminy, ventricular tachycardia and AV block
• Digoxin levels >2.5 ng ml$^{-1}$.

Digoxin toxicity is treated by discontinuing the drug, res-

toration of serum potassium levels and management of arrhythmias. Digoxin antibodies (Fab fragments) are a specific antidote that are useful for life-threatening toxicity.

$\beta$-ADRENERGIC AGONISTS. Dopamine and dobutamine are adrenergic agonists but are only effective intravenously. Dobutamine is a selective agonist of the $\beta_1$-receptor, increasing intracellular cyclic AMP, which in turn increases calcium availability for the contractile process. Dopamine is a less potent inotrope than dobutamine but because of its unselective action on the adrenergic system it also improves renal perfusion. Xamoterol is a $\beta$-blocking drug with high intrinsic sympathomimetic activity (ISA) and is effective in improving cardiac performance. Xamoterol competes competitively with endogenous catecholamines at the $\beta_1$-receptor. At states of low sympathetic tone (rest) this produces a positive inotropic effect together with lowering of filling pressures. At states of high sympathetic tone (e.g. exercise), xamoterol produces a $\beta$-blocking effect, blunting the chronotropic response. In mild to moderate heart failure xamoterol (200 mg twice daily) is as effective as intravenous dobutamine in improving cardiac performance. Chronic high levels of circulating catecholamines in severe heart failure may lead to down-regulation of the $\beta$-receptors; the administration of xamoterol to these patients may precipitate acute heart failure.

PHOSPHODIESTERASE INHIBITORS. Amrinone, milrinone and enoximone are in a class of so-called 'inodilator' drugs that act by inhibiting phosphodiesterase, thus preventing breakdown of cyclic AMP. Accumulation of cAMP produces an increase in contractility and also peripheral vasodilatation. The Starling curve is shifted upwards. Although these agents are effective in improving myocardial performance acutely, there is evidence that they have a deleterious effect on myocardial cells when administered in the long term with an increased mortality. They are not often used.

### Antiarrhythmic agents

Arrhythmias are frequent in heart failure and are implicated in sudden death. Although treatment of complex ventricular arrhythmias might be expected to improve survival there is conflicting evidence that this is so. This may be related to the diverse mechanisms of death in patients with heart failure, death commonly being associated with bradyarrhythmias, particularly in patients with non-ischaemic heart failure. Patients with sustained episodes of ventricular tachycardia should undergo electrophysiological study and serial drug testing or receive empirical treatment usually with amiodarone or sotalol. The use of class I agents may result in deterioration of heart failure owing to their negative inotropic effect. It should be noted that ACE inhibitors probably exert an indirect antiarrhythmic effect by reducing high circulating levels of noradrenaline and improving cardiac function. In the future the use of the ICD is likely to improve the survival prospects of patients with serious ventricular arrhythmias. Several reports have suggested that chronic β-blocker therapy, most often metoprolol, may improve haemodynamic and clinical function in patients with heart failure despite its negative inotropic effect.

### Summary

It is now recommended that all patients with clinical heart failure should receive treatment with diuretics and an ACE inhibitor. Patients in atrial fibrillation should be digitalized but patients in sinus rhythm may also be improved by the addition of digoxin or a β-blocker. Patients with asymptomatic left ventricular dysfunction are at risk of progressive deterioration and should be treated with prophylactic ACE inhibitor therapy. Patients with ischaemic heart failure and ongoing ischaemia and patients intolerant of ACE inhibitors or in whom they are contraindicated (hypotension, renal insufficiency or hyperkalaemia) may benefit from nitrate/hydralazine therapy.

## CARDIAC TRANSPLANTATION

Since the advent of cyclosporin in the late 1970s and improved immunosuppression regimens, cardiac transplantation has become the treatment of choice for younger patients with severe intractable heart failure, whose life expectancy is less than 6 months. With careful recipient selection the expected 1-year survival for patients following transplantation is over 80%, and is 70% at 5 years; irrespective of survival, quality of life is dramatically improved for the majority of patients.

## Pulmonary oedema

This is a very frightening, life-threatening emergency characterized by extreme breathlessness. The dyspnoea may first occur at night in the form of paroxysmal dyspnoea due to pulmonary congestion. This occurs because of reabsorption of dependent oedema when lying flat and the relative insensitivity of the respiratory centre at night allows pulmonary congestion to develop. In more severe cases the patient is severely breathless at all times of the day.

### PATHOPHYSIOLOGY

Left ventricular failure and mitral valve disease cause pulmonary oedema because of increased pulmonary capillary pressure. A pressure above 20 mmHg causes increased filtration of fluid out of the capillaries into the interstitial space (interstitial oedema). Further accumulation of fluid disrupts intercellular membranes, leading to the collection of fluid in the alveolar spaces (alveolar oedema). Alveolar oedema occurs when the capillary pressure exceeds the total oncotic pressures (approximately 30 mmHg).

### CLINICAL FEATURES

Patients with alveolar oedema are acutely breathless, wheezing, anxious and perspiring profusely. In addition, they usually have a cough productive of frothy, blood-tinged (pink) sputum, which can be copious. The patient is tachypnoeic with peripheral circulatory shutdown. There is a tachycardia, a raised venous pressure and a gallop rhythm. Crackles and wheeze are heard throughout the chest. The arterial $P_O_2$ falls and initially the $P_aCO_2$ also falls owing to overbreathing. Later, however, the $P_aCO_2$ increases because of impaired gas exchange. The chest X-ray shows diffuse haziness due to alveolar fluid and the Kerley B lines of interstitial oedema (see Fig. 11.15). The abnormality can be unilateral, giving the appearance of a tumour that disappears on treatment (a pseudotumour).

### TREATMENT

1 The patient should be placed in the sitting position.
2 High-concentration oxygen (60% via a variable performance mask) is given unless it is suspected that there is a coexisting chronic hypercapnia due to long-standing respiratory failure. In severe cases it may be necessary to ventilate the patient (see p. 728).
3 Intravenous diuretic treatment with frusemide or bumetanide is given. These diuretics produce *immediate* vasodilatation in addition to the more delayed diuretic response.
4 Morphine (10–20 mg i.v. depending on the size of the patient) together with an antiemetic such as metoclopramide (10 mg i.v.) or cyclizine (50 mg i.v.) is given. Morphine sedates the patient and causes systemic vasodilatation; it must be avoided if the systemic arterial pressure is less than 90 mmHg. Respiratory depression occurs with large doses of morphine.
5 Venous vasodilators, such as glyceryl trinitrate, may produce prompt relief by reducing the pre-load. Cardiac output may be increased by using arterial vasodilatation, such as occurs with hydralazine (see Table 11.21).
6 Aminophylline (250–500 mg or 5 mg kg$^{-1}$ i.v.) is infused over 10 min. Aminophylline is a phosphodiesterase inhibitor that causes bronchodilatation, vasodilatation and increased cardiac contractility. It must be given slowly because of the risk of precipitating ventricular arrhythmias. It is now only used when bronchospasm is present.

7 Venesection and mechanical methods of reducing venous return (e.g. sphygmomanometer cuffs inflated to 10 mmHg below diastolic blood pressure and placed around the thighs) are inefficient and rarely used.

In a severe case, after the acute emergency is controlled, a pulmonary artery balloon catheter may be inserted to monitor progress and treatment. Any factor that precipitated the heart failure, such as cardiac arrhythmias or chest infection, should be corrected. The underlying cardiac problem should be diagnosed and treated.

## Cardiogenic shock

Shock is a severe failure of tissue perfusion, usually characterized by hypotension, a low cardiac output and signs of poor tissue perfusion such as oliguria, cold extremities and poor cerebral function. Cardiogenic shock (pump failure) is an extreme type of cardiac failure with a high mortality of approximately 90%. Its most common cause is myocardial infarction.

Cardiogenic shock must be differentiated from other forms of shock. Cardiogenic shock is diagnosed when the shock syndrome occurs despite an adequate or elevated pulmonary capillary wedge pressure and in the absence of mechanical circulatory obstruction. An essential element in this diagnosis is the measurement of the pulmonary capillary wedge pressure (see p. 720). In situations where the vascular capacity has expanded or the circulatory fluid volume has decreased, the wedge pressure will be low. In cardiogenic shock the wedge pressure is normal or elevated.

The mortality rate in cardiogenic shock is so high because of the vicious downward spiral that occurs: hypotension due to pump failure results in a reduction of coronary flow, which results in further impairment of pump function, and so on.

**TREATMENT** (see also p. 721)

1 Patients require intensive care (see Chapter 13).
2 General measures such as complete rest, continuous 60% oxygen administration and pain relief are essential.
3 The infusion of fluid is necessary if the pulmonary capillary wedge pressure is below 18 mmHg, which is probably the optimal 'filling pressure' with which to prime a failing heart.
4 Short-acting venous dilators such as glyceryl trinitrate or sodium nitroprusside should be administered intravenously if the wedge pressure is 25 mmHg or more.
5 Cardiac inotropes such as dobutamine and dopamine may be used to increase aortic diastolic pressure (coronary perfusion pressure). Dopamine also selectively increases renal perfusion.
6 Mechanical assist devices such as an intra-aortic balloon pump may be used (see p. 553). Although leading to a temporary improvement, long-term prognosis is not improved unless there is a surgically correctable cause, such as a ruptured interventricular septum or acute mitral regurgitation.

# Ischaemic heart disease

An imbalance between the supply of oxygen (and other essential myocardial nutrients) and the myocardial demand for these substances results in myocardial ischaemia. The causes are as follows:

1 The coronary blood flow to a region of the myocardium may be reduced by an obstruction due to:
   (a) Atheroma
   (b) Thrombosis
   (c) Spasm
   (d) Embolus
   (e) Coronary ostial stenosis (e.g. syphilis)
   (f) Coronary arteritis (e.g. polyarteritis)
2 There can be a decrease in the flow of oxygenated blood to the myocardium due to:
   (a) Anaemia
   (b) Carboxyhaemoglobinaemia
   (c) Hypotension causing decreased coronary perfusion pressure
3 An increased demand for oxygen may occur owing to an increase in cardiac output (e.g. during exercise or in thyrotoxicosis) or myocardial hypertrophy (e.g. from aortic stenosis or hypertension).

In types 2 and 3, ischaemia may occur despite normal coronary arteries. In a small number of cases, ischaemia develops despite normal coronary arteries and a normal demand for oxygen. This condition is known as syndrome X and is possibly caused by an abnormality of small coronary vessels, resulting in a reduction of coronary flow reserve.

The most common cause of ischaemic heart disease is coronary atheroma, which causes a fixed obstruction to coronary blood flow. Variations in the tone of smooth muscle in the wall of a coronary artery may add an important element of dynamic or variable obstruction. Sometimes an extreme increase in coronary tone may produce coronary spasm and severely reduced coronary blood flow in the absence of any underlying coronary atheroma.

## Atheroma

This condition, which affects medium-sized arteries, is characterized by the development of atherosclerotic plaques. Such a plaque consists of a necrotic core, rich in cholesterol and other lipids, surrounded by smooth muscle cells and fibrous tissue.

### PATHOGENESIS

The pathogenesis of atherosclerosis is complex. The two major hypotheses of the nineteenth century (the 'incrustation' and 'lipid' hypotheses) have been combined to form the 'response to injury' hypothesis. Experimentally, this divides the formation of atheroma into three stages (Fig. 11.53).

*Stage I* consists of functional alteration of endothelial

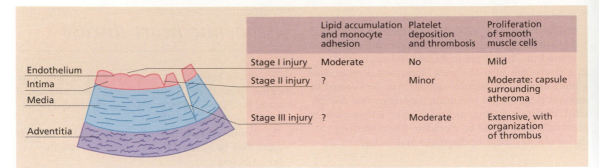

| | | Lipid accumulation and monocyte adhesion | Platelet deposition and thrombosis | Proliferation of smooth muscle cells |
|---|---|---|---|---|
| Endothelium<br>Intima<br>Media<br>Adventitia | Stage I injury | Moderate | No | Mild |
| | Stage II injury | ? | Minor | Moderate: capsule surrounding atheroma |
| | Stage III injury | ? | Moderate | Extensive, with organization of thrombus |

**Fig. 11.53**  Classification of vascular injury or damage and vascular response.

cells without substantial morphological changes. In *stage II* there is endothelial denudation and intimal damage with intact internal elastic lamina and in *stage III* there is endothelial damage to both intima and media.

Stage I injury may occur at branching points of vessels and can be caused by a high circulating cholesterol, vasoactive amines, immunocomplexes, infection and chemical irritants in tobacco smoke. This leads to an accumulation of lipids and macrophages at these sites of injury. Toxic products released by the latter lead to stage II damage with adhesion of platelets. There is a proliferation of smooth muscle cells, disruption of the endothelium and thrombus formation. This thrombus becomes organized and leads to the development of an atherosclerotic plaque. Cholesterol-rich material accumulates within the plaque and this becomes surrounded by a fibrotic cap which narrows the lumen of the vessel. The rate of development of these lesions is variable and depends on risk factors (see below). Fissuring and disruption of the plaque triggers the release of mediators, e.g. serotonin, ADP, and the formation of a thrombus leading to total occlusion of the vessel. These thrombotic occlusions can resolve spontaneously or can be treated with thrombolytic therapy.

### RISK FACTORS FOR CORONARY ARTERY DISEASE (Table 11.23)

A number of 'risk' factors are known to predispose to coronary artery disease. Some of these, such as age, sex and family history, cannot be modified, whereas other major risk factors, such as serum cholesterol, smoking habits and hypertension, can be changed.

### Age

Atherosclerosis develops progressively as age advances. It is rarely present in early childhood, except in familial hyperlipidaemia, but it is often detectable in post-mortem specimens of young men between 20 and 30 years. It is almost universal in the elderly in the Western World.

### Sex

Men are more affected than premenopausal women. However, after the menopause the incidence of atheroma in women becomes similar to that in men. The cause of this difference in incidence is not clearly understood.

*Fixed*
Age
Male sex
Positive family history
Deletion polymorphism in the ACE gene (DD)

*Potentially changeable with treatment*
Strong association
  Hyperlipidaemia
  Cigarette smoking
  Hypertension
  Diabetes mellitus

Weak association
  Personality
  Obesity
  Gout
  Soft water
  Lack of exercise
  Contraceptive pill
  Heavy alcohol consumption

———

ACE, angiotensin-converting enzyme.

**Table 11.23**  Risk factors for coronary disease.

### Family history

Coronary artery disease is often found in several members of the same family. Because the disease is so prevalent and because other risk factors are familial, it is uncertain whether family history is an independent risk factor.

### Hyperlipidaemia (see p. 855)

Atherosclerotic plaques contain cholesterol. A high serum cholesterol, especially when associated with low values of high-density lipoproteins (HDLs), is strongly associated with coronary atheroma. High triglyceride levels are less definitely linked with coronary atheroma.

Familial hypercholesterolaemia, familial combined hyperlipidaemia and remnant hyperlipidaemia are associated with an increased risk of coronary atherosclerosis.

Measurement of total cholesterol, HDL cholesterol with calculation of low-density lipoprotein (LDL) cholesterol and HDL ratio as well as triglycerides should be performed on all patients. Lowering the serum cholesterol has been shown to decrease the incidence of coronary artery disease and slow the progression of coronary atheroma. Management is described on p. 858.

## Smoking

In men, the risk of developing coronary artery disease is directly related to the number of cigarettes smoked. This relationship is less certain, but still important, in women, and in cigar and pipe smokers. The risk from smoking declines to almost normal after 10 years of abstention.

## Hypertension

Both systolic and diastolic hypertension are associated with an increased risk of coronary artery disease. The risk is the same for men and women. Reduction of blood pressure with hypotensive therapy reduces the risks of a cerebrovascular accident but does not affect the risk of cardiac events such as myocardial infarction.

## Other factors

Lack of exercise increases the risk of coronary artery disease, and regular exercise probably protects against its development. Diabetes mellitus, or even just an abnormal glucose tolerance test, is associated with vascular disease. Obesity is certainly associated with coronary artery disease, but it is not certain whether obesity itself is independently linked with the condition.

Recently it has been shown that possession of an ACE gene polymorphic marker (D) (deletion of a 287 base pair *Alu* repeat sequence) has been shown to be a risk factor for coronary artery disease. DD genotype, which is associated with higher concentrations of circulating ACE, is significantly more frequent in people who have had a myocardial infarction than in age-matched controls. This is seen particularly in young people assumed to be at low risk by standard criteria.

A certain kind of personality type known as 'type A', which is characterized by unsuccessful aggression, ambition, compulsion and competitiveness, is said to be associated twice as frequently with coronary artery disease than is 'type B' (the converse of type A). Gout, oral contraceptives, alcohol and soft water have also been suggested as risk factors for coronary atheroma.

It is clear that many factors influence the development of coronary atheroma. It is not certain that modification of any of these can substantially reverse the established atherosclerotic process.

## Angina (see p. 526)

Angina ranges from a mild ache to a most severe pain that provokes sweating and fear. It is generally described as 'heavy', 'crushing' or 'gripping', and the patient may indicate the type of pain by clenching the fist or gripping the hands together. Occasionally these symptoms may occur in the arms without any chest pain.

There are several types of angina; these are described below.

### Classical or exertional angina

Physical exertion, especially after a meal, in cold weather or walking against the wind, provokes this pain. It is also aggravated by anger or excitement. The pain usually fades quickly (in less than 3 min) when the patient ceases exertion. Sometimes the pain will disappear even though exertion continues ('walking through the pain'); the exertion threshold for the development of pain is very variable. Usually, pain is more easily provoked in the early morning than later in the day. This type of angina can be graded as in Table 11.3.

### Decubitus angina

This is angina that occurs when the patient lies down. It usually occurs in association with heart failure because of the increased central blood volume and consequent myocardial tensions that develop in the recumbent position. Patients with this symptom usually have severe coronary artery disease.

### Nocturnal angina

This is angina that wakes the patient from sleep. It may be provoked by vivid dreams. Patients with this symptom usually have critical coronary artery disease, or the angina may be associated with coronary spasm.

### Variant (Prinzmetal's) angina

A classical attack of variant angina, as described by Prinzmetal, has no obvious provocation. It occurs at rest, especially at night or in the early morning, and is rarely induced by exertion. It occurs more frequently in women and the pain is usually more severe and more prolonged than in classical angina. It produces a characteristic electrocardiographic feature of ST segment elevation developing during the pain. Arrhythmias—both heart block and ventricular tachycardia—are common in the ischaemic episode.

Prinzmetal's angina is caused by spasm of a coronary artery often in association with an eccentric coronary artery atheromatous lesion. More often, variant angina is not classical Prinzmetal's angina but is due to variation in coronary arterial tone rather than frank coronary arterial spasm. Such patients have a varying exercise threshold for the provocation of angina.

### Unstable angina

Unstable angina includes angina of very recent onset, worsening angina or angina at rest. A number of terms, such as crescendo angina, preinfarction angina and intermediate chest pain syndrome, have been used to describe angina that is provoked more easily and persists for a longer duration than ordinary angina or that fails to respond readily to therapy. Whilst the pain is present, myocardial infarction must be considered, but with angina the ECG changes (T wave inversion or ST segment depression) are only transient and cardiac enzyme levels are not elevated. Unless vigorously treated, a large proportion of patients with unstable angina will proceed to develop a myocardial infarction within weeks.

### EXAMINATION

There are usually no abnormal findings in angina, although a fourth heart sound may be heard. Any factor responsible for angina (e.g. thyrotoxicosis) or risk factors may lead to physical signs such as nicotine staining, hypertension or xanthelasma.

## DIAGNOSIS

The primary diagnosis rests on the description of the chest pain as investigations may be normal.

## INVESTIGATION

### Resting ECG

This is usually normal between attacks, although an old myocardial infarction, left ventricular hypertrophy or other unrelated heart disease may be present. During an attack, transient ST segment depression, symmetrical T wave inversion or tall, pointed, upright T waves may appear.

A normal ECG between attacks or even during an attack cannot definitely exclude angina pectoris. Typical ECG changes during an attack are strong pointers to the diagnosis of angina.

### Exercise ECG (see p. 541)

When angina is provoked by exertion, an exercise stress ECG should be performed. ST segment depression greater than or equal to 1 mm suggests myocardial ischaemia, especially if typical chest pain occurs at the same time. The severity of the electrocardiographic changes indicates the extent of the coronary artery disease. Approximately 75% of patients with severe coronary artery disease will give a positive test. Stress testing is less reliable in women and is confused by electrolyte abnormalities, therapy with digoxin, and intraventricular conduction disturbances. A normal stress test does not definitely exclude coronary disease.

### Cardiac scintigraphy

UPTAKE OF THALLIUM-201 (see p. 546). This is useful:
● When the exercise test is equivocal
● In deciding whether stenotic vessels on angiography are giving rise to ischaemic areas on exercise
A normal perfusion scan after exercise makes significant coronary artery disease unlikely.

RADIONUCLIDE VENTRICULOGRAPHY (see p. 547). This can be used to outline the left ventricle. When part of the left ventricular wall is ischaemic it does not contract normally, producing an abnormal image. This test can be performed at rest and during exertion. The ejection fraction is a good index of ventricular function and is useful in the assessment of patients for coronary artery bypass surgery.

### Echocardiography (see p. 542)

This can be used to assess ventricular wall involvement and ventricular function. An abnormal resting echocardiogram reflects previous ventricular damage. Exercise echocardiography, although technically difficult, may be useful in patients with an equivocal exercise ECG.

### Coronary angiography

This is occasionally useful in patients with chest pain when the cause is unclear. More often, the test is per-

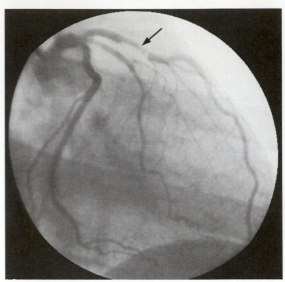

**Fig. 11.54** X-ray contrast material is injected into the ostium of the left main coronary artery in order to perform a left coronary angiogram. In this example, the left main artery divides into three vessels: left anterior descending (top) diagonal and circumflex (bottom) vessels. In the proximal part of the left anterior descending artery is a severe narrowing due to an atherosclerotic plaque.

formed to delineate the exact coronary anatomy (Fig. 11.54) prior to coronary grafting or coronary angioplasty. Coronary angiography should only be performed when the benefit in terms of diagnosis and potential treatment outweighs the small risk associated with the procedure (a mortality of less than 1 in 1000 cases) (Table 11.24).

A coronary angiogram may not reveal coronary spasm unless an intracoronary injection of dihydroergotamine has been given. This test is not often performed because the induction of coronary spasm may prove difficult to reverse and its clinical relevance is uncertain.

## TREATMENT

### Management of an acute attack

An acute attack is treated by stopping exercise (exertional angina) or by getting up (decubitus angina) and dissolving a fresh glyceryl trinitrate tablet (0.5 mg) under the tongue. After 2–3 min the angina usually recedes. When the pain is relieved the glyceryl trinitrate tablet is spat out or swallowed to inactivate it. This minimizes the main side-effect, which is a severe pounding headache. Some

---

Angina refractory to medical therapy
Severely abnormal exercise ECG
Unstable angina
Angina occurring after myocardial infarction
Subendocardial myocardial infarction (non-Q-wave infarction), especially if exercise test is abnormal
Angina or myocardial infarction in a young (<50 years) patient, especially if exercise test is abnormal

**Table 11.24** Indications for coronary angiography.

prefer to use an aerosol formulation of glyceryl trinitrate; this, unlike the tablets, is stable for a long period. If glyceryl trinitrate cannot be tolerated, a capsule of nifedipine may be chewed or sucked. However, this has similar side-effects to glyceryl trinitrate.

## General management

Patients should be reassured that their condition is not uniformly or rapidly fatal. Many have a good prognosis—30% survive for more than 10 years and spontaneous remission does occur. Any underlying problems such as obesity, thyrotoxicosis, anaemia or aortic stenosis should be treated. Risk factors should be evaluated and steps made to correct them. Smoking must be stopped. Patients must be encouraged not to do things that they know provoke their angina, but this must not lead to a severe restriction of life-style. Regular exercise sufficient to improve the fitness of the patient will tend to increase the threshold to angina. More severe exercise is not recommended unless the cardiovascular response to exertion (treadmill ECG test) has been documented. Emotional crises and overexcitement must be minimized.

## Medical treatment

Patients should be told to suck a tablet of glyceryl trinitrate before exertion rather than waiting for the pain to commence. They must be specifically encouraged to do this, because many prefer to believe that it is better to suffer the pain than to take more tablets. When angina occurs frequently, or with only modest exertion, regular prophylactic therapy should be advised. This consists of nitrates, β-adrenergic blocking drugs or calcium antagonists.

Nitrates such as glyceryl trinitrate are available in a variety of slow-release formulations, particularly infiltrated skin plasters and buccal pellets. Alternatively, tablets of long-acting nitrate preparations such as isosorbide dinitrate or isosorbide mononitrate may be used. Nitrates are successful in the treatment of angina pectoris because they reduce venous and hence intracardiac diastolic pressures, reduce the impedance to the emptying of the left ventricle, and relax the tone of the coronary arteries.

β-Adrenergic blocking drugs reduce heart rate (negative chronotropic effect) and the force of ventricular contraction (negative inotropic effect), both of which reduce myocardial oxygen demand, especially on exercise. Sufficient β-blocker to reduce the resting heart rate to about 60 b.p.m. is usually necessary to achieve relief from angina. Very high doses of β-blockers are no longer used because of side-effects and the possibility of infarction or arrhythmia on withdrawal, and because many alternative therapies are available. Propranolol 40–80 mg three times daily is the most conventional therapy.

Relatively cardioselective β-blockers (β₁-antagonists) such as atenolol (50–100 mg daily) or metoprolol (50 mg three times daily) are often preferred because they have fewer side-effects.

Calcium channel blockers (Table 11.25) such as nifedipine, nicardipine, amlodipine, verapamil and diltiazem block calcium flux into the cell and the utilization of calcium within the cell. They relax coronary arteries and other vascular systems and also reduce the force of left ventricular contraction, reducing the oxygen demand and improving angina. Nifedipine 20–30 mg daily is the calcium antagonist most commonly used in angina.

## Coronary angioplasty

This is a technique of dilating coronary atheromatous obstructions by inflating a balloon against the obstruction (Fig. 11.55). The balloon, which is mounted on the tip of a very thin catheter, is inserted through the obstruction using X-ray fluoroscopy, and it is then inflated with dilute contrast material. Multiple inflations of the balloon using a pressure of several atmospheres will squash and crack the atheroma and relieve the obstruction. This technique is widely applied for the treatment of angina due to isolated, proximal, non-calcified, atheromatous plaques, usually in patients with a relatively short history of

| Class | 1 (non-dihydropyridine) | 2 (dihydropyridine) |
|---|---|---|
| Example | Verapamil<br>Diltiazem | Nifedipine<br>Nicardipine |
| *Effects* | | |
| Sinus node suppression | +++ | + |
| AV node suppression | +++ | + |
| Myocardial depression | ++ | ++ |
| Arteriolar vasodilatation | + | +++ |
| *Side-effects* | | |
| Flushing, ankle oedema, palpitations | + | ++ |
| Bradycardia, impaired AV conduction | ++ | + |
| Aggravation of heart failure | ++ | + |
| Combination with β-blockers | No | Yes |

AV, atrioventricular.

Table 11.25 Calcium channel blockers.

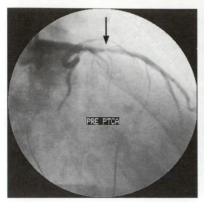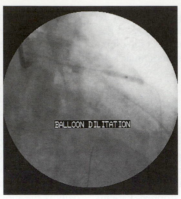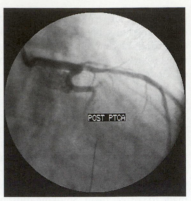

**Fig. 11.55**   This sequence of three films demonstrates percutaneous transluminal coronary angioplasty (PTCA) in a patient with a 90% stenosis in the proximal left anterior descending coronary artery (left film taken during coronary angiogram). The middle X-ray shows the inflated angioplasty balloon across the arterial lesion. The right film is taken from the post PTCA coronary angiogram. It shows virtually complete alleviation of the stenosis.

coronary ischaemia. Multiple lesions may be treated and repeat procedures can be undertaken. Two complications are acute coronary occlusion (2–4%) and chronic restenosis, which occurs in 30% in the first 6 months after angioplasty.

### Surgical management

When angina worsens or persists despite general measures and optimal medical treatment, the option of surgery should be considered. The patient should be assessed using exercise testing and angiography. Symptomatic patients with left main stem obstructions, two- or three-vessel involvement and good ventricular function are often treated surgically.

There are three operations currently used for the relief of myocardial ischaemia:

1  Coronary artery vein bypass grafting (CAVBG) (Fig. 11.56) involves taking a vein, usually from the leg (saphenous) and bypassing the coronary obstruction by suturing the vein (reversed because of the venous valves) between the aorta and the coronary artery distal to the obstruction.

2  An internal mammary artery may be mobilized and implanted into the left anterior descending coronary artery distal to an obstruction (Fig. 11.56).

3  Endarterectomy (removal of an atheromatous obstruction) can sometimes be successful when combined with bypass or internal mammary artery grafting. Surgery provides dramatic relief from angina in about 90% of those operated on. When surgery is performed for left main stem obstruction or for three-vessel disease involvement, an improved life-span and quality of life can be expected. Surgical mortality is well below 1% in patients with normal left ventricular function. Progressive slow occlusion of grafts with atheroma occurs in a significant number of cases (5–10% a year).

### Treatment of variant angina

The treatment of variant angina is slightly different. Nitrates and calcium antagonists are useful, but β-blockers may increase coronary tone and exacerbate the angina, so should not be used. It may be necessary to treat the arrhythmias provoked by the spasm. Surgical relief is rarely necessary or possible.

### Treatment of unstable angina

Unstable angina should be managed vigorously. If rest pain persists despite the use of agents such as sublingual glyceryl trinitrate, the patient should be treated with bed rest, mild sedation, intravenous heparin and/or oral aspirin as well as standard medical antianginal therapy. Oxygen may also be beneficial. Calcium antagonists are particularly valuable for the treatment of this condition but usually β-blockers, nitrates and calcium antagonists are all used in combination. Aspirin decreases both death and myocardial infarction. If medical therapy fails, urgent coronary arteriography is desirable with a view to coronary artery surgery or angioplasty. Fibrinolytic therapy may be of benefit if myocardial infarction is suspected. Alter-

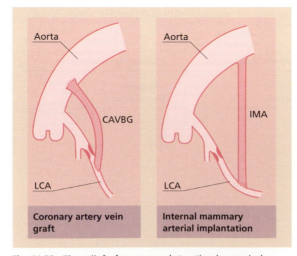

**Fig. 11.56**   The relief of coronary obstruction by surgical techniques: coronary artery vein bypass grafting (CAVBG) or internal mammary arterial implantation (IMA). In both of these examples, the graft bypasses a coronary obstruction in the left coronary artery (LCA).

natively, intra-aortic balloon pumping (see p. 553) may help to stabilize the patient.

Irrespective of the immediate success of treatment, early coronary angiography and, depending on the results, urgent referral for surgery are usually advised.

# Myocardial infarction

Myocardial infarction is now the most common cause of death in the UK and other developed countries, but was hardly known before 1910. It almost always occurs in patients with coronary atheroma because of sudden coronary thrombosis. This usually develops at the site of a fissure or rupture of the intimal surface of an atheromatous plaque. Haemorrhage may occur into a plaque and local coronary spasm may develop. Sometimes thrombosis results from stasis at a critical stenosis or in association with coronary spasm. About 6 hours after the onset of infarction the myocardium is pale and swollen, and at 24 hours the necrotic tissue appears deep red owing to haemorrhage. In the next weeks an inflammatory reaction develops, lymphocytes infiltrate and the infarcted tissue turns grey. Necrotic tissue is replaced by mononuclear cells, and gradually a thin fibrous scar develops.

## CLINICAL PRESENTATION

Myocardial infarction presents with chest pain, similar in character to exertional angina pectoris, but usually occurring at rest and lasting for some hours. The pain may be so severe that the patient may fear imminent death ('angor animi'), but it may be less severe and mistaken for indigestion. It is usually sudden in onset, but it may develop gradually. The pain of myocardial infarction is often associated with restlessness and the patient usually cannot remain still. Sweating, nausea and vomiting are often associated with myocardial infarction.

About 20% of patients with myocardial infarction have no pain. Diabetics, hypertensives and elderly patients often have 'silent' myocardial infarctions. In these cases the myocardial infarction may go unnoticed or may produce hypotension, breathlessness or arrhythmias.

### Physical signs

Often there are no specific physical signs unless complications develop, but the patient appears pale, sweaty and grey. Hypotension, which may first occur several hours after the onset of infarction and may increase over the following 3–4 days, abnormal precordial pulsation due to the systolic bulging of the infarcted myocardium, an additional heart sound (particularly a fourth heart sound), and sinus tachycardia may be noted in some patients. A raised venous pressure and basal crackles are common. As the infarction progresses, a modest fever (up to 38°C) due to muscle necrosis and lasting for up to 7 days occurs. A pericardial friction rub may develop.

## INVESTIGATION
### Non-specific tests

Non-specific abnormalities such as an increased erythrocyte sedimentation rate (ESR) (up to 70 mm in the first hour) and a polymorphonuclear leucocytosis (up to $20 \times 10^9$/litre) may occur in the first few days following myocardial infarction.

### Cardiac enzymes (Fig. 11.57)
Necrotic cardiac tissue releases cellular enzymes:

CREATINE KINASE (CK) is released by infarcted myocardium and peaks within 24 hours. It is usually back to normal before 48 hours. It is also produced by damaged skeletal muscle and brain. The myocardial-bound (MB) isoenzyme fraction of CK is specific for heart muscle damage. A several-fold increase in total CK, but not in CK-MB, can be produced by an intramuscular injection. Cardioversion can increase both the total CK and the MB isoenzyme fraction of CK. The size of the infarction determines the total enzyme release with larger infarcts producing higher serum levels.

ASPARTATE AMINOTRANSFERASE (AST), which was formerly called serum glutamic oxaloacetic transaminase (SGOT), peaks at 24–48 hours and may fall to normal by 72 hours. AST is also released by damaged red blood cells, kidney, liver and lungs.

LACTIC DEHYDROGENASE (LDH) peaks at 3–4 days and remains elevated for 10–14 days. LDH is not only present in cardiac muscle but is also released from damaged liver, skeletal muscle and red blood cells. There are five isoenzymes, and cardiac necrosis causes a predominant increase of LDH 1, which can also be measured as hydroxybutyrate dehydrogenase (HBD).

TROPONIN T AND MYOGLOBIN are also released early (2–4 hours) following myocardial infarction. Troponin T is a regulatory protein with a high specificity for cardiac injury and is not raised if skeletal muscle damage is present. Elevation of cardiac troponin persists for up to 7 days.

Enzymes are usually estimated for the first 3 days following a suspected myocardial infarction. The first assay is often normal and subsequent assays will show a threefold or more increase in the majority of cases. With reper-

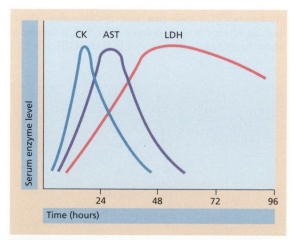

**Fig. 11.57** The enzyme profile in acute myocardial infarction. AST, aspartate aminotransferase; CK, creatine kinase; LDH, lactic dehydrogenase.

fusion after thrombolytic therapy the enzyme rise may be curtailed.

CK or CK-MB are the enzymes which should be requested within 24 hours of the suspected infarction. After this period, AST and LDH are more likely to be elevated.

### The ECG

A Q wave (Fig. 11.58) is a broad (>1 mm) and deep (>2 mm or more than 25% of the amplitude of the following R wave) negative deflection that starts the QRS complex. It may occur normally in leads AVR and $V_1$ (and sometimes in lead III), but in other leads it is abnormal. Abnormal Q waves are produced by several abnormalities such as left bundle branch block, ventricular tachycardia and the WPW syndrome. The gradual development of Q waves over minutes or hours suggests the occurrence of a full-thickness (as opposed to a subendocardial) myocardial infarction. They develop because the electrical silence of infarcted cardiac tissue results in a so-called 'window' through which the normal endocardial-to-epicardial activation of the opposite non-infarcted ventricular wall is 'seen' resulting in an unopposed depolarization front moving away from an electrode situated over the epicardial surface of the infarct (Fig. 11.58). Q waves are usually permanent electrocardiographic features following full-thickness myocardial infarction.

T wave and ST segment changes result from ischaemia and injury. They are therefore often transient, occurring only during the acute attack. The progressive changes or evolution of the ECG during the course of a full-thickness myocardial infarction are illustrated in Fig. 11.59.

With subendocardial infarction (Fig. 11.60) only the endocardial surface is infarcted and Q waves do not develop. ST segment and T wave changes are therefore the only ECG features of a subendocardial infarction. Because the injury is endocardial rather than predominantly epicardial, ST segment depression rather than elevation is usual.

Typically ECG changes (Table 11.26) are usually confined to the ECG leads that 'face' the infarction. Therefore, an inferior wall myocardial infarction is diagnosed when the ECG findings are seen in leads II, III and AVF

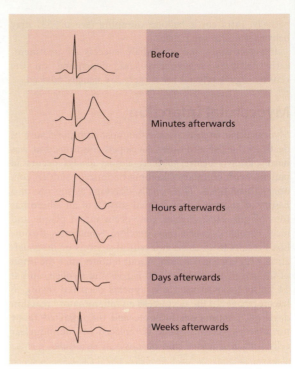

**Fig. 11.59**  Electrocardiographic evolution of myocardial infarction. After the first few minutes the T waves become tall, pointed and upright and there is ST segment elevation. After the first few hours the T waves invert, the R wave voltage is decreased and Q waves develop. After a few days the ST segment returns to normal. After weeks or months the T wave may return to upright but the Q wave remains.

| Infarct site | Leads showing main changes |
|---|---|
| Anterior | |
|   Small | $V_3$–$V_4$ |
|   Extensive | $V_2$–$V_5$ |
| Anteroseptal | $V_1$–$V_3$ |
| Anterolateral | $V_4$–$V_6$, I, AVL |
| Lateral | I, II, AVL |
| Inferior | II, III, AVF |
| Posterior | $V_1$, $V_2$ (reciprocal) |
| Subendocardial | Any lead |

**Table 11.26**  Typical ECG changes in myocardial infarction.

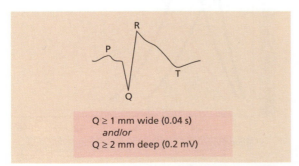

    Q ≥ 1 mm wide (0.04 s)
    *and/or*
    Q ≥ 2 mm deep (0.2 mV)

**Fig. 11.58**  The electrocardiographic features of myocardial infarction, showing a Q wave, ST elevation and T wave inversion.

(Fig. 11.61). Lateral infarction produces changes in leads I, II and AVL. In anterior infarction, leads $V_2$–$V_5$ may be affected. Changes seen in an anterolateral infarction are shown in Fig. 11.62. Because there are no posterior leads, a true posterior wall infarct is usually diagnosed by the appearance of mirror image or reciprocal changes in leads $V_1$ and $V_2$, i.e. the development of a tall initial R wave, ST segment depression and tall, upright T waves. These reciprocal changes can also be seen in association with other infarctions. For example, in an inferior wall myocardial infarction, anterior ST segment depression may be seen.

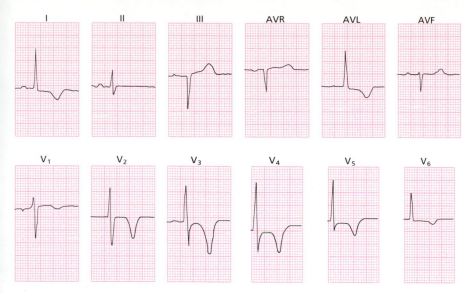

**Fig. 11.60**  A 12-lead ECG showing a widespread (anterolateral) subendocardial myocardial infarction. Note the deeply inverted, symmetrical T waves in addition to ST depression.

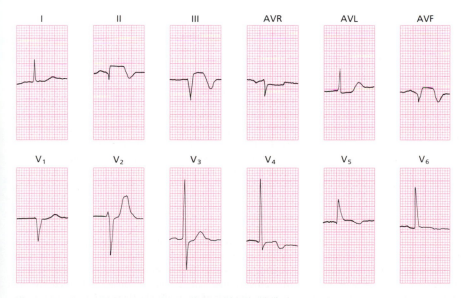

**Fig. 11.61**  A 12-lead ECG showing an acute inferior wall myocardial infarction. Notice the raised ST segment and Q waves in the inferior leads (II; III and AVF). The additional T wave inversion in V₄ and V₅ probably represents anterior wall ischaemia.

A normal ECG, especially early in the presentation, does not exclude myocardial infarction.

### Pyrophosphate scanning (see p. 547)

This test is particularly useful when the ECG is unhelpful because of pre-existing abnormalities such as left bundle branch block. Imaging is performed about 2 hours after the injection of the isotope to detect the infarcted area.

### MANAGEMENT

Fibrinolytic therapy (see below) should be given as soon as possible because it results in coronary vessel recanalization and a significant reduction in mortality. During an acute myocardial infarction, lethal arrhythmias may occur. Patients should therefore be admitted to the coronary care unit (CCU) as soon as possible. Here, the ECG should be monitored continuously for the first 48 hours

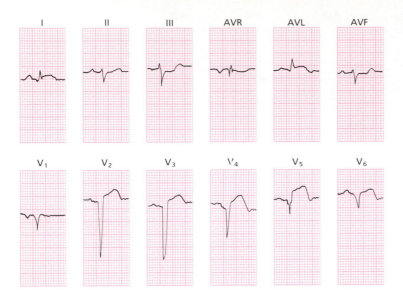

**Fig. 11.62** A 12-lead ECG showing an acute anterolateral myocardial infarction. Notice the ST segment elevation in leads I, AVL, and $V_2$–$V_6$. The T wave is inverted in leads I, AVL and $V_3$–$V_6$. Pathological Q waves are seen in leads $V_2$–$V_6$.

to allow the detection of arrhythmias such as 'R on T' ventricular ectopic beats, which may precipitate ventricular fibrillation. Ventricular fibrillation must be recognized promptly and resuscitation started immediately. Therefore, patients should not be kept in casualty departments waiting for ECGs and chest X-rays but should be admitted immediately to the CCU. If this is not possible then the accident and emergency department must have the staff and facilities to provide the treatment required in the first few hours.

AN INTRAVENOUS CANNULA is always inserted so that emergency intravenous medication can be administered, e.g. i.v. magnesium.

THE PAIN OF MYOCARDIAL INFARCTION should be treated promptly with powerful analgesics such as morphine (10–20 mg i.v. or s.c.) or diamorphine (5–10 mg i.v. or s.c.) combined with antiemetics such as cyclizine (50 mg i.v.) or metoclopramide (10 mg i.v.).

OXYGEN is usually given routinely because during an acute myocardial infarction the arterial $Po_2$ is reduced. Oxygen at 60% is administered by face mask or nasal cannulae for several hours following myocardial infarction.

FIBRINOLYTIC THERAPY should be considered as soon as the diagnosis is suspected regardless of age if there is no contraindication. These agents can achieve early reperfusion in 50–70% of patients (compared with a spontaneous reperfusion rate of less than 30%) and have been shown to reduce the extent of ventricular damage, and the early and 1-year mortality rates associated with myocardial infarction. A reduction in expected mortality of up to 30% is possible if these agents are given within the first 3–6 hours following infarction, but some benefit may be achieved even up to 24 hours. Although many physicians administer these drugs on the history alone, pro-

vided there are no contraindications it is desirable that typical electrocardiographic evidence of early infarction should also be available prior to their administration. Oral aspirin therapy (150 mg daily) should accompany the fibrinolytic therapy and be continued for at least 4 weeks after infarction.

Three fibrinolytic agents are currently licensed for use in acute myocardial infarction. Streptokinase is most commonly used. The recommended doses of these drugs are shown in Table 11.27. Recombinant tissue plasminogen activator (rt-PA) achieves higher reperfusion rates than the other two agents, and when it is administered early and in association with full heparinization leads to a definite (14%) reduction of 30 day mortality. It is, however, associated with a slight increase in stroke and is more expensive than non-selective fibrinolytics. Although the single-injection administration of anistreplase confers some advantage over the other two agents (both of which are given as an intravenous infusion of at least 1 hour), this is also considerably more expensive than streptokinase. Both streptokinase and anistreplase increase the patient's antistreptokinase antibody level, which falls to baseline levels after 3–6 months. These antibodies reduce the effectiveness of a repeat dose and theoretically increase the risk of an anaphylactic reaction. Repeat usage of these drugs within 3 months is therefore not rec-

| Agent | Intravenous dose regimen |
|---|---|
| Streptokinase | 1.5 million U over 1 hour |
| Anistreplase (APSAC) | 30 U over 4–5 min |
| Alteplase (rt-PA, recombinant tissue-type plasminogen activator) | 10 mg bolus, followed by 50 mg in the first hour, and 40 mg over the subsequent 2 hours |

**Table 11.27** Fibrinolytic therapy for acute myocardial infarction.

ommended. If repeat administration is deemed necessary, it should be preceded by intravenous methylprednisolone. The use of rt-PA, or even urokinase (neither of which provokes antibody formation), is preferable in these circumstances. Because of the small risk of bleeding following fibrinolytic therapy, all patients should have their blood group assessed in case of the need for transfusion. Because of the risk of reperfusion arrhythmias, patients should be monitored during and after fibrinolytic therapy. The ventricular arrhythmias that develop are usually short-lived and do not require treatment, but, rarely, ventricular fibrillation can occur.

An alternative approach is immediate coronary angioplasty, which is particularly useful when there are contraindications to thrombolysis. The results are perhaps better than thrombolytic therapy, but angioplasty is only available in large centres.

ANTICOAGULATION is given to myocardial infarction patients to prevent thromboembolic complications from prolonged immobilization. Usually subcutaneous heparin (5000 U, 8-hourly) is sufficient for this purpose. Patients who receive rt-PA must receive immediate and full doses of heparin (10 000 U bolus, plus 1000 U hourly).

ACE INHIBITORS. Patients who suffer from transient or chronic heart failure or who have a depressed ejection fraction on echocardiography following an acute myocardial infarction should receive an ACE inhibitor. This therapy reduces mortality and slows the progression of left ventricular function after infarction.

PERSISTENT PAIN can be treated with nitrates. If there is no hypotension, sublingual glyceryl trinitrate should be given. Alternatively, especially if the haemodynamic situation is not stable, continuous intravenous infusion of either isosorbide dinitrate or glyceryl trinitrate should be considered.

ANXIOUS PATIENTS should be reassured and mild sedation, in addition to analgesia, may be necessary. A quiet atmosphere should reduce anxiety.

BED REST is advised for the first 24–48 hours, after which the patient is progressively mobilized. Smoking is not allowed.

## Home versus hospital care of myocardial infarction victims

CCUs were developed to facilitate the detection and treatment of arrhythmias occurring in the immediate postinfarction period. However, it has been suggested that the coronary care ward is a frightening environment that may itself increase the incidence of these arrhythmias. There have been several studies comparing home care and coronary ward care of patients with myocardial infarction. The conclusions have been controversial, but home care can be considered if:

- The patient has suffered a myocardial infarction 24 hours or more previously

- There are no complications such as shock or arrhythmia
- The patient is aged 70 years or older
- The patient has concurrent terminal disease

However, most patients suffering from myocardial infarction should be cared for in the CCU of a hospital, where sudden and perhaps fatal complications can be promptly recognized and effectively treated.

## Mobile coronary care units

Because a large proportion of deaths from myocardial infarction are due to arrhythmias that occur in the first few minutes of the infarction, it is logical to train ambulance personnel in methods of advanced cardiac life support and to provide them with the equipment to perform these techniques (intravenous infusion, endotracheal intubation and ventilation and ECG monitoring and defibrillation). Ambulances manned and equipped in this way are called mobile CCUs, coronary rescue vehicles or cardiac resuscitation vehicles. This kind of ambulance is sent to those patients who have severe chest pain or who have collapsed unconscious. Together with the training in basic life support of a significant proportion (at least one-third) of the general public, mobile CCUs have reduced the incidence of sudden unexpected cardiac death, whether due to myocardial infarction or to arrhythmias unrelated to acute myocardial infarction. This service is now becoming generally available throughout the UK as part of the statutory ambulance service.

## COMPLICATIONS

In the acute phase, i.e. the first 2–3 days following a myocardial infarction, cardiac arrhythmias, cardiac failure and pericarditis are the most common complications. Later, recurrent infarction, angina, thromboembolism, mitral valve regurgitation, and ventricular septal or free wall rupture may occur. Late complications include the postmyocardial infarction syndrome (Dressler's syndrome), shoulder–hand syndrome, ventricular aneurysm and recurrent cardiac arrhythmias.

### Cardiac arrhythmias

These are described in detail on pp. 554–569.

VENTRICULAR EXTRASYSTOLES. These commonly occur after myocardial infarction. Their occurrence may precede the development of ventricular fibrillation. If they are frequent (more than 5 min$^{-1}$), multiform (different shapes) or R-on-T (falling on the upstroke or peak of the preceding T wave), they may be treated with lignocaine 50–100 mg i.v. over 5 min followed by 1–4 mg min$^{-1}$ by continuous infusion, which is slowly reduced and discontinued over 24 hours. Such treatment has not been shown to reduce the likelihood of subsequent ventricular tachycardia or fibrillation.

VENTRICULAR TACHYCARDIA. This may degenerate into ventricular fibrillation or may itself produce serious haemodynamic consequences. It is treated with intravenous lignocaine. If haemodynamic deterioration occurs, the tachycardia is immediately treated with synchronized cardioversion (initially 200 J).

VENTRICULAR FIBRILLATION. This may occur in the first few hours or days following a myocardial infarction in the absence of severe cardiac failure or cardiogenic shock. This is known as primary ventricular fibrillation. It is treated with prompt defibrillation (200–400 J). Intravenous lignocaine is usually prescribed in an attempt to prevent recurrences of ventricular fibrillation. The prognosis is usually very good because the electrical derangement is only transient.

When ventricular fibrillation occurs in the setting of heart failure, shock or aneurysm, it is called secondary ventricular fibrillation. It is treated in a similar way to primary ventricular fibrillation, but the prognosis is very poor unless the underlying haemodynamic or mechanical cause can be corrected.

ATRIAL FIBRILLATION. This occurs in about 10% of patients with myocardial infarction. It is due to atrial irritation caused by heart failure, pericarditis and atrial ischaemia or infarction. It may be managed with intravenous digoxin or intravenous amiodarone and by treatment of the underlying pathology. It is not usually a long-standing problem.

SINUS BRADYCARDIA. This is especially associated with acute inferior wall myocardial infarction. Symptoms emerge only when the bradycardia is severe. When symptomatic, treatment consists of elevating the foot of the bed and giving intravenous atropine 600 $\mu$g if necessary. When sinus bradycardia occurs, an escape rhythm such as idioventricular rhythm (wide QRS complexes with a regular rhythm at 50–100 b.p.m.) or idiojunctional rhythm (narrow QRS complexes) may occur. Usually no specific treatment is required.

It has been suggested that sinus bradycardia following myocardial infarction may predispose to the emergence of ventricular fibrillation. Severe sinus bradycardia associated with symptoms or the emergence of unstable rhythms may need treatment with temporary pacing.

SINUS TACHYCARDIA. This is produced by heart failure, fever and anxiety. Usually no specific treatment is needed.

CONDUCTION DISTURBANCES. These are common following myocardial infarction. AV nodal delay (first-degree AV block) or higher degrees of block may occur during acute myocardial infarction, especially of the inferior wall. First-degree block does not need treatment, but progressive or complete block may need treatment with atropine or an artificial temporary pacemaker. Such blocks may last for only a few minutes but frequently persist for days or several weeks; they are rarely permanent.

Acute anterior wall myocardial infarction may produce damage to the distal conduction system (the His bundle or the bundle branches). The development of complete heart block usually implies a large myocardial infarction and a poor prognosis. The ventricular escape rhythm is slow and unreliable and a temporary pacemaker is necessary. This form of block is often permanent.

The development of complete AV block (Table 11.28) can be expected in 20–30% of cases where progressive bundle branch block (right bundle branch block and then right bundle branch block with a QRS axis shift) has already occurred (Fig. 11.63).

## Cardiac failure and cardiogenic shock

Heart failure after acute myocardial infarction is graded according to a clinical classification (Table 11.29).

Mild left heart failure (a few basal crackles that persist after coughing, an extra heart sound and upper lobe blood division on the chest X-ray) occur in about 40% of patients with acute myocardial infarction. Treatment for a few days with a mild diuretic such as a thiazide is usually all that is needed for symptomatic relief but an ACE inhibitor should be given (see p. 587).

A large myocardial infarction may lead to severe heart failure and pulmonary oedema. In such cases more prolonged and powerful diuretics and vasodilator treatment is necessary.

In very severe cases a pulmonary artery balloon catheter is used to measure the pulmonary artery and 'left atrial' pressures and the cardiac output. Treatment is with loop diuretics, vasodilators (see p. 573) and, occasionally, digoxin.

Severe heart failure may also follow ventricular septal rupture or mitral valve papillary muscle rupture. Both of these conditions present with worsening heart failure, a systolic thrill and a loud pan-systolic murmur, widely heard over the precordium. Often, echocardiography and right heart catheterization with a balloon catheter is needed to differentiate between these two conditions. Both are associated with a poor prognosis, but vigorous treatment including early surgical correction may be successful.

| Type of fascicular block | Percentage progressing to complete heart block |
|---|---|
| LAH | 4 |
| LPH | 8 |
| Long PR interval | 10 |
| LBBB | 10 |
| RBBB | 20 |
| RBBB + LAH | 30 |
| RBBB + LPH | 40 |
| RBBB + (LPH or LAH) + Long PR interval | 40 |

LAH, left anterior hemiblock; LBBB, left bundle branch block; LPH, left posterior hemiblock; RBBB, right bundle branch block.

Table 11.28 Progression from different types of fascicular block to complete heart block in patients with acute myocardial infarction.

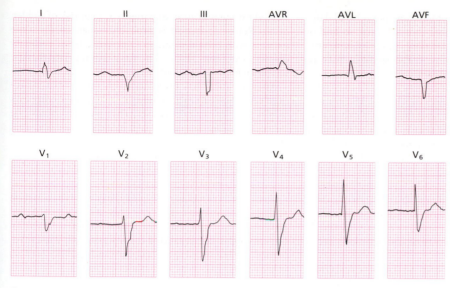

**Fig. 11.63** A 12-lead ECG demonstrating a prolonged PR interval (0.32 s), a broad QRS complex with a deep S wave in leads I and $V_6$ (right bundle branch block) and left axis deviation (−75°). This electrocardiographic picture is consistent with bifascicular block with delay in the AV node on the third fascicle.

| Class | Description | Incidence (%) | Mortality (%) |
|-------|-------------|---------------|---------------|
| I | No heart failure | 40 | 5 |
| II | Mild left ventricular failure | 40 | 20 |
| III | Pulmonary oedema | 10 | 40 |
| IV | Cardiogenic shock | 10 | 90 |

**Table 11.29** Killip (clinical) classification of heart failure in patients with acute myocardial infarction.

Ventricular asynergy and papillary muscle dysfunction (not rupture) may produce mild mitral regurgitation in association with heart failure. This causes a transient, soft, pan-systolic murmur in up to half of those with acute myocardial infarction. In these cases no specific treatment is necessary for the mitral regurgitation.

Cardiac rupture results in almost immediate cardiac tamponade and is usually fatal within a few minutes. Electromechanical dissociation, i.e. no pulse or cardiac output but a persistently normal rhythm on the ECG, is the classical presentation. Treatment is rarely successful.

Cardiogenic shock is an extreme form of cardiac failure or circulatory collapse. Its features and management are described on p. 577. The mortality from this condition is about 90%. The majority of those rescued have a complication that can be treated surgically (e.g. left ventricular aneurysm, torrential mitral regurgitation or ventricular septal perforation).

## Thromboembolism

Bed rest and cardiac failure contribute to the common occurrence of thrombosis and embolism associated with myocardial infarction. Only 10% of patients have clinical features of thromboembolism, but in almost 50% of patients who die there is evidence of emboli. Deep venous thrombosis (see p. 629) is the most common manifestation, and pulmonary embolism may result from this. A left ventricular mural thrombus may form on the endocardial surface of the infarcted region. Such a thrombus is dislodged, forming a systemic embolus, in 15% of cases. Prophylactic anticoagulation with subcutaneous heparin probably reduces the risk of this complication.

## Other complications

THE SHOULDER–HAND SYNDROME. This consists of pain and immobility of the left arm in the weeks and months following an acute myocardial infarction. Early mobilization reduces the incidence of this symptom and physiotherapy improves those symptoms that do occur.

PERICARDITIS. This is characterized by sharp chest pain and a pericardial rub. It frequently occurs in the first few days after an acute myocardial infarction, especially following anterior wall infarction. Anticoagulation should be avoided in these patients and anti-inflammatory medication is usually a successful treatment.

POSTMYOCARDIAL INFARCTION SYNDROME (DRESSLER'S SYNDROME). This occurs weeks to months after an acute myocardial infarction, and consists of a combination of pericarditis, fever and a pericardial effusion. It is caused by an autoimmune response to damaged cardiac tissue and is more common after second or subsequent myocardial infarction. Anti-inflammatory medication, including systemic corticosteroids, may be necessary. Anticoagulation should be avoided.

LEFT VENTRICULAR ANEURYSM. This is a late complication. Patients present with heart failure, arrhythmias or emboli. It is characterized by ventricular asynergy, often palpable as a double impulse, a fourth heart sound, persistent ST segment elevation on the ECG and sometimes a visible bulge on the chest X-ray. Diagnosis is confirmed by 2-D echocardiography (Fig. 11.64). Treatment includes suitable antiarrhythmic drugs, anticoagulants and medication for heart failure. Surgical removal of the aneurysm (aneurysmectomy) may be necessary if arrhythmias or embolic or haemodynamic complications occur.

## REHABILITATION AND RISK STRATIFICATION

If possible, full mobilization should be achieved within 1 week to 10 days to reduce the degree of physical and mental debility inflicted by this illness. Strong reassurance and constant encouragement are very important. Prior to discharge it is ideal to assess:

- Cardiovascular response to stress (limited or submaximal exercise test)
- Signal-averaged ECG
- Arrhythmia profile (24-hour taped ECG)
- Ventricular function (echocardiogram or nuclear angiogram)
- Autonomic status as evidenced by heart rate variability and baroreceptor sensitivity

Any abnormalities that are detected should stimulate further investigations such as coronary angiography and left ventriculography. Attempts to provoke ventricular tachycardia by right ventricular pacing must be considered for identification of patients at high risk of sudden death. Revascularization is probably beneficial for some patients with certain arteriographic patterns of coronary disease (see Table 11.24). The most appropriate therapy for other high-risk patients is under investigation.

After a patient has presented with myocardial infarction every opportunity should be taken to modify risk factors for coronary disease. The patient should be instructed to stop smoking. High blood pressure and lipid abnormalities should be corrected.

The families of young patients who present with myocardial infarction should be screened for lipid abnormalities and other risk factors.

Structured psychological and physical rehabilitation schemes are valuable but are only available in a few centres. The patient may return to work after 3 months. Car driving is not permitted for 6 weeks following myocardial infarction. Heavy goods (and public service) vehicle driving licences are withdrawn pending evaluation of the patient's status.

### Follow-up treatment

The patient should be discharged taking regular β-blockade (e.g. propranolol 80 mg twice daily or metoprolol 50 mg twice daily), which has been shown to reduce the incidence of sudden death in the 6 months following acute myocardial infarction. Timolol 10–20 mg daily and probably other β-blockers are similarly effective. Routine treatment with other antiarrhythmic drugs has not proved beneficial in reducing the incidence of sudden death following myocardial infarction. Long-term aspirin (150 mg daily) further reduces cardiac events following myocardial infarction and long term anticoagulation may be advised for patients with large antero-apical infarction. ACE inhibitors should be continued probably indefinitely.

### PROGNOSIS

Statistics concerning sudden death from acute myocardial infarction and from other cardiac causes are so often combined that it is difficult to accurately assess the mortality specifically from myocardial infarction. Assuming that all sudden unexpected cardiac death is due to myocardial infarction, then about 50% of those who die do so within the first 2–3 hours, and 75% of the deaths occur within 24 hours. Of those who leave hospital alive, about 15–25% die in the first year, and thereafter the annual mortality is 5–10%. Fifty per cent of myocardial infarction victims survive for 10 years. Factors suggesting an unfavourable prognosis include a large myocardial infarction, heart failure, a large heart on chest X-ray, ventricular arrhythmias, multiple infarction, recurrent angina, and an abnormal exercise test.

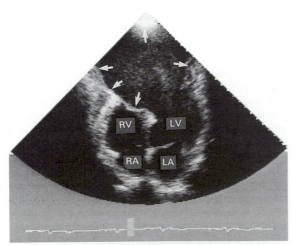

**Fig. 11.64** Two-dimensional echocardiogram (apical four-chamber view) showing a very large apical left ventricular aneurysm (arrowed). The relatively static blood in the aneurysm produces a swirling 'smoke' effect. This aneurysm was successfully resected surgically. LV, left ventricle; LA, left atrium; RV, right ventricle; RA, right atrium.

# Rheumatic fever

Rheumatic fever is an inflammatory disease that occurs in children and young adults (the first attack usually occurs between 5 and 15 years of age) as a result of infection with group A streptococci. It affects the heart, skin, joints and central nervous system. It is common in the Middle and Far East, eastern Europe and South America, but it is now rare in the UK, western Europe and North America. This decline in the incidence of rheumatic fever (from 10% of children in the 1920s to 0.01% today) parallels the reduction in all streptococcal infections and is largely due to improved sanitation and also to the use of antibiotics.

Pharyngeal infection with group A *Streptococcus* may be followed by the clinical syndrome of rheumatic fever. This is thought to develop because of an autoimmune reaction triggered by the infecting *Streptococcus*. The condition is not due to direct infection of the heart or to the production of a toxin.

## PATHOLOGY

All three layers of the heart may be affected. The characteristic lesion of rheumatic carditis is the Aschoff nodule, which is a granulomatous lesion with a central necrotic area occurring in the myocardium, particularly in the subendocardium of the left ventricle. Small, warty vegetations may develop on the endocardium, particularly on the heart valves. This leads to some degree of valvular regurgitation. A serofibrinous effusion characterizes the acute pericarditis that occurs.

The synovial membranes are acutely inflamed during rheumatic fever, and subcutaneous nodules (which are also granulomatous lesions) are seen in the acute stage of the disease.

## CLINICAL FEATURES

The disease presents suddenly, with fever, joint pains, malaise and loss of appetite. The clinical features depend on the organs that are involved. Diagnosis relies on the presence of two or more major clinical manifestations or one major manifestation plus two or more minor features. These are known as the Duckett Jones criteria (Table 11.30).

Carditis manifests as:
- New or changed heart murmurs
- Development of cardiac enlargement or cardiac failure
- Appearance of a pericardial effusion and ECG changes of pericarditis (raised ST segments) or myocarditis (inverted or flattened T waves), first-degree or greater AV block or other cardiac arrhythmias
- Transient diastolic mitral (Carey–Coombs) murmur due to mitral valvulitis

Non-cardiac features include the following.

A FEVER with an apparently excessive tachycardia is usually present.

THE ARTHRITIS ASSOCIATED WITH RHEUMATIC FEVER is classically a fleeting polyarthritis affecting large joints such as the knees, elbows, ankles and wrists. The joints are swollen, red and tender. As the inflammation in one joint recedes, another becomes affected. Once the acute inflammation disappears, the rheumatic process leaves the joints normal.

SYDENHAM'S CHOREA (or St Vitus' dance) (see p. 921)

| |
| --- |
| *Major criteria* |
| Carditis |
| Polyarthritis |
| Chorea |
| Erythema marginatum |
| Subcutaneous nodules |
| |
| *Minor criteria* |
| Fever |
| Arthralgia |
| Previous rheumatic fever |
| Raised ESR/C-reactive protein |
| Leucocytosis |
| Prolonged PR interval on ECG |
| |
| Plus evidence of antecedent streptococcal infection, e.g. positive throat cultures for group A streptococci, elevated antistreptolysin O titre (>250 U) or other streptococcal antibodies, or a history of recent scarlet fever |
| — |
| ESR, erythrocyte sedimentation rate. |

**Table 11.30** Revised Duckett Jones criteria for the diagnosis of rheumatic fever. The diagnosis is made on the basis of two or more major criteria, or one major plus two or more minor criteria.

is involvement of the central nervous system that develops late after a streptococcal infection. Sufferers are noticeably 'fidgety' and display spasmodic, unintentional movements. Speech is often affected.

SKIN MANIFESTATIONS include erythema marginatum, a transient pink rash with slightly raised edges, which occurs in 20% of cases. The erythematous areas found mostly on the trunk and limbs coalesce into crescent- or ring-shaped patches. Subcutaneous nodules, which are painless, pea-sized, hard nodules beneath the skin, may also occur, particularly over tendons, joints and bony prominences.

## INVESTIGATION

THROAT SWABS are cultured for the group A *Streptococcus*.

SEROLOGICAL CHANGES may indicate a recent streptococcal infection. The antistreptolysin O titre, and sometimes others such as the antistreptokinase titre, are performed.

NON-SPECIFIC INDICATORS OF INFLAMMATION such as the ESR and the C-reactive protein levels are usually elevated.

## TREATMENT

Patients with fever, active arthritis or active carditis should be completely rested in bed. When the clinical syndrome has subsided (e.g. no pyrexia, normal pulse rate, normal ESR, normal white count) the patient may be mobilized.

Residual streptococcal infections should be eradicated with a single intramuscular injection of 916 mg of benzathine penicillin or oral phenoxymethylpenicillin 500 mg four times daily for 1 week. This therapy should be administered even if nasal or pharyngeal swabs do not culture the streptococci.

High-dose salicylate (preferably acetyl salicylate, i.e. aspirin) therapy is given to the limit of tolerance determined by the development of tinnitus. If carditis is present, systemic corticosteroids may be given. Prednisolone 60–120 mg in four divided doses each day is administered until the clinical syndrome is improved and the ESR has fallen to normal. Steroids are then tapered off over 2–4 weeks. However, the efficacy of steroids is in doubt.

Recurrences are most common when persistent cardiac damage is present, and are prevented by the continued administration of oral phenoxymethylpenicillin 250 mg daily or by monthly injections of 916 mg of benzathine penicillin until the age of 20 years or for 5 years after the latest attack (see p. 10). A sulphonamide (e.g. sulphadimidine) may be used if the patient is allergic to penicillin. Any streptococcal infection that does develop should be very promptly treated.

## Chronic rheumatic heart disease

More than 50% of those who suffer acute rheumatic fever *with carditis* will later (after 10–20 years) develop chronic rheumatic valvular disease, predominantly affecting the mitral and aortic valves (Table 11.31).

# Valvular heart disease

## MITRAL STENOSIS

Almost all mitral stenosis is due to rheumatic heart disease:

- At least 50% of sufferers have a history of rheumatic fever or chorea.
- The single most common valve lesion due to rheumatic fever is pure mitral stenosis (50%).
- The mitral valve is affected in over 90% of those with rheumatic valvular heart disease.
- Rheumatic mitral stenosis is much more common in women.
- The pathological process results after some years in valve thickening, cusp fusion, calcium deposition, a narrowed (stenotic) valve orifice and progressive immobility of the valve cusps.

**Other causes**

- Lutembacher's syndrome is the combination of acquired mitral stenosis and an atrial septal defect.
- A rare form of congenital mitral stenosis can occur.
- In the elderly a syndrome similar to mitral stenosis can develop because of calcification and fibrosis of the valve, valve ring and subvalvular apparatus (chordae tendineae).

### PATHOPHYSIOLOGY

When the normal valve orifice area of $5 \text{ cm}^2$ is reduced to approximately $1 \text{ cm}^2$, severe mitral stenosis is present. In order that sufficient cardiac output will be maintained, the left atrial pressure increases and left atrial hypertrophy and dilatation occurs. Consequently, pulmonary venous, pulmonary arterial and right heart pressures also increase. The increase in pulmonary capillary pressure is followed by the development of pulmonary oedema. This is partially prevented by alveolar and capillary thickening and pulmonary arterial vasoconstriction (reactive pulmonary hypertension). Pulmonary hypertension leads to right ventricular hypertrophy, dilatation and failure. Right ventricular dilatation results in tricuspid regurgitation. The complications of mitral stenosis (Table 11.32) are frequent.

### SYMPTOMS

Usually there are no symptoms until the valve orifice is moderately stenosed, i.e. has an area of $2 \text{ cm}^2$. In Europe this does not usually occur until several decades after the first attack of rheumatic fever, but in the Middle or Far East, children of 10–20 years of age may have severe calcific mitral stenosis.

Because of pulmonary venous hypertension and recurrent bronchitis, progressively severe dyspnoea develops. A cough productive of blood-tinged, frothy sputum is quite common, and occasionally frank haemoptysis may occur. The development of pulmonary hypertension eventually leads to right heart failure and its symptoms of weakness, fatigue and abdominal or lower limb swelling.

The large left atrium favours atrial fibrillation, giving rise to symptoms such as palpitations. Atrial fibrillation may result in systemic and pulmonary emboli, which give rise to cerebral, mesenteric, renal and pulmonary infarcts.

### SIGNS (see Clinical memo in Fig. 11.65)

### Face

Severe mitral stenosis with pulmonary hypertension is associated with the so-called mitral facies or malar flush.

| Valves involved | Percentage of cases |
|---|---|
| Mitral valve alone | 50 |
| Mitral and aortic valves | 40 |
| Mitral, aortic and tricuspid | 5 |
| Aortic valve alone | 2 |
| All other combinations | 3 |

**Table 11.31** Rheumatic valvular lesions.

Atrial fibrillation
Systemic embolization
Pulmonary hypertension
Pulmonary infarction
Chest infections
Infective endocarditis (rare)
Tricuspid regurgitation
Right ventricular failure

**Table 11.32** Complications of mitral stenosis.

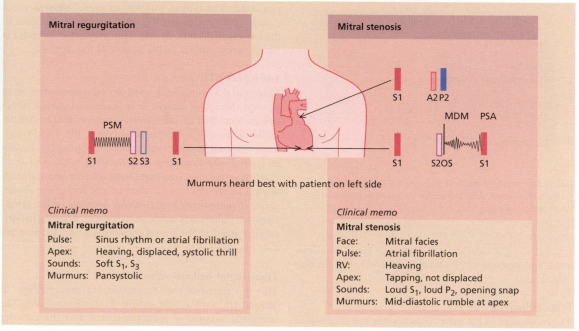

**Fig. 11.65** Auscultatory features associated with mitral regurgitation and mitral stenosis. $A_2$, aortic component of the second heart sound; MDM, mid-diastolic murmur; OS, opening snap; $P_2$, pulmonary component of the second heart sound; PSA, presystolic accentuation; PSM, pan-systolic murmur; $S_1$, first heart sound; $S_2$, second heart sound; $S_3$, third heart sound.

---

This is a bilateral, cyanotic or dusky pink discoloration over the upper cheeks that is due to arteriovenous anastomoses and vascular stasis.

### Pulse

At first the pulse is regular (sinus rhythm) but later the irregular pulse of atrial fibrillation usually develops. The onset of atrial fibrillation often causes a dramatic clinical deterioration.

### Jugular veins

If right heart failure develops there is obvious distension of the jugular veins. If pulmonary hypertension or tricuspid stenosis is present, the *a* wave will be prominent provided that atrial fibrillation has not supervened.

### Apex beat

The apex beat is 'tapping' in quality. This is the result of a palpable first heart sound combined with left ventricular backward displacement produced by an enlarging right ventricle. A parasternal heave due to right ventricular hypertrophy may also be felt.

### Auscultation

Auscultation (Fig. 11.65) reveals a loud first heart sound because the cusps are kept open until the beginning of ventricular systole. In early diastole a sound is produced when the mitral valve opens (opening snap). This is followed by a diastolic rumbling murmur due to turbulent blood flow through the narrowed valve. If the patient is in sinus rhythm the murmur becomes louder when atrial systole occurs. This is called presystolic accentuation.

The severity of mitral stenosis is judged by the time between the closure of the aortic valve and the opening of the mitral valve. Thus the shorter the $A_2$–OS time the more severe the stenosis. This is because it takes less time for the left ventricular pressure to fall to the high left atrial pressure which occurs in severe mitral stenosis.

As the valve cusps become immobile, the loud first heart sound softens and the opening snap disappears. When pulmonary hypertension occurs, the pulmonary component of the second sound is increased in intensity and the mitral diastolic murmur may become quieter because of the reduction of cardiac output.

### INVESTIGATION

#### Chest X-ray

The chest X-ray usually shows a generally small heart with an enlarged left atrium (see Fig. 11.13). Pulmonary venous hypertension (see p. 538) is usually also present. Late in the course of the disease a calcified mitral valve may be seen on a penetrated or lateral view. The signs of pulmonary oedema or pulmonary hypertension may also be apparent when the disease is severe.

#### ECG

In sinus rhythm the ECG shows a bifid P wave due to delayed left atrial activation (Fig. 11.66). This double-humped P wave is best seen in leads II, $V_3$ and $V_4$. A biphasic P wave with a large late negative component is seen in lead $V_1$ (Fig. 11.67). However, atrial fibrillation is frequently present. As the disease progresses, the ECG

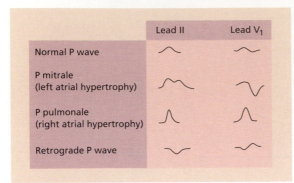

|  | Lead II | Lead V$_1$ |
|---|---|---|
| Normal P wave | | |
| P mitrale (left atrial hypertrophy) | | |
| P pulmonale (right atrial hypertrophy) | | |
| Retrograde P wave | | |

**Fig. 11.66**  A bifid P wave as seen on the ECG in mitral stenosis (P mitrale). Also shown for comparison are other P wave abnormalities.

features of right ventricular hypertrophy (right axis deviation and perhaps tall R waves in lead V$_1$) may develop (Fig. 11.67).

### Echocardiogram (see Fig. 11.24)
The movement of the valve cusps and the rate of diastolic filling of the left ventricle may be measured—severe mitral stenosis produces immobility of the valve cusps and slow filling of the ventricles. The echocardiogram appearances are usually sufficient to allow surgical management to be considered; transoesophageal echocardiography is particularly useful in this situation. CW Doppler is used to estimate peak mitral transvalvular gradient and the valve area (see Fig. 11.24). The presence of tricuspid regurgitation can be used to estimate pulmonary arterial pressure.

### Cardiac catheterization
This is only required if an adequate echocardiogram is impossible to obtain or if coexisting cardiac problems (e.g. mitral regurgitation or coronary artery disease) are

suspected. The typical findings in mitral stenosis are a diastolic pressure that is higher in the left atrium than in the left ventricle (Fig. 11.68). This gradient of pressure is usually proportional to the degree of the stenosis.

### TREATMENT
Mild mitral stenosis may need no treatment other than prompt therapy of attacks of bronchitis. Although infective endocarditis in pure mitral stenosis is uncommon, antibiotic prophylaxis is advised (see p. 10). Early symptoms of mitral stenosis such as mild dyspnoea can usually be treated with low doses of diuretics. The onset of atrial fibrillation requires treatment with digoxin and anticoagulation to prevent atrial thrombus and systemic embolization. If pulmonary hypertension develops or the symptoms of pulmonary congestion persist despite therapy, surgical relief of the mitral stenosis is advised. There are four operative measures.

#### Trans-septal balloon valvotomy
This is a relatively new technique whereby a catheter is introduced into the right atrium via the femoral vein. The interatrial septum is then punctured and the catheter advanced into the left atrium and across the mitral valve. A balloon is passed over the catheter to lie across the valve, and then inflated briefly to split the valve commissures. The procedure is performed under local anaesthesia in the cardiac catheter laboratory. As with other valvotomy techniques, significant regurgitation may result necessitating valve replacement (see below). This procedure is not suitable for heavily calcified or regurgitant valves.

#### Closed valvotomy
This operation is advised for patients with mobile, non-calcified and non-regurgitant mitral valves. The fused cusps are forced apart by a dilator introduced through the apex of the left ventricle and guided into position by

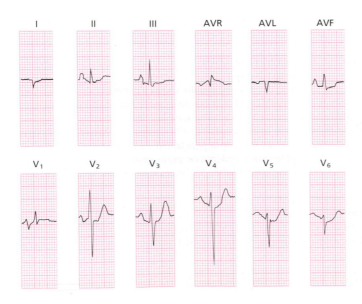

**Fig. 11.67**  A 12-lead ECG of a patient with severe mitral stenosis. Note the right axis deviation (frontal plane axis = +120°), the left atrial conduction abnormality (large terminal negative component of the P wave in V$_1$) and the right ventricular hypertrophy (R wave in V$_1$ and right axis deviation).

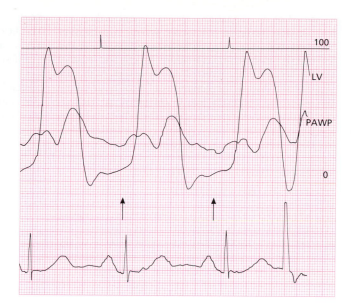

**Fig. 11.68** Simultaneous recordings of the ECG, the left ventricular (LV) and the pulmonary arterial wedge pressure (PAWP). The PAWP is almost equivalent to the left atrial pressure. Thus at end-diastole (the onset of the QRS complex) the PAWP is significantly higher than the LV pressure (arrows). The pressure gradient is due to mitral valve stenosis.

the surgeon's finger inserted via the left atrial appendage. Cardiopulmonary bypass is not needed for this operation. Closed valvotomy may produce a good result for 10 or more years. The valve cusps often re-fuse and eventually another operation may be necessary.

### Open valvotomy

This operation is often preferred to closed valvotomy. The cusps are carefully dissected apart under direct vision. Cardiopulmonary bypass is required. Open dissection reduces the likelihood of causing traumatic mitral regurgitation.

### Mitral valve replacement

Replacement of the mitral valve is necessary if:
● Mitral regurgitation is also present
● There is a badly diseased or badly calcified stenotic valve that cannot be reopened without producing significant regurgitation

Artificial valves (see p. 602) may work successfully for more than 20 years. Anticoagulants are generally necessary to prevent the formation of thrombus, which might obstruct the valve or embolize.

## MITRAL REGURGITATION

Of the many causes of mitral valve regurgitation, rheumatic heart disease (50%) and the prolapsing mitral valve are the most common. Any disease that causes dilatation of the left ventricle may cause mild mitral regurgitation, e.g.:
● Aortic valve disease
● Acute rheumatic fever
● Myocarditis
● Cardiomyopathy
● Hypertensive heart disease
● Ischaemic heart disease

### Other causes

IN HYPERTROPHIC CARDIOMYOPATHY, left ventricular contraction is disorganized and mitral regurgitation often results.

MYOCARDIAL INFARCTION OR INFECTIVE ENDO-CARDITIS — Mitral regurgitation may follow these conditions.

CONNECTIVE TISSUE DISORDERS such as systemic lupus erythematosus — mitral regurgitation may occur.

COLLAGEN ABNORMALITIES such as Marfan's syndrome and Ehlers–Danlos syndrome may be associated with mitral regurgitation.

DEGENERATION OF THE VALVE CUSPS OR MITRAL ANNULAR CALCIFICATION may result in regurgitation.

RUPTURE OF THE CHORDAE TENDINEAE (due to myocardial infarction or trauma) and infective endocarditis may cause very sudden mitral regurgitation.

### PATHOPHYSIOLOGY

Regurgitation into the left atrium produces left atrial dilatation but little increase in left atrial pressure if the regurgitation is long-standing as the regurgitant flow is accommodated by the large left atrium. With acute mitral regurgitation the normal compliance of the left atrium does not allow much dilatation and the left atrial pressure rises. Thus, in acute mitral regurgitation the left atrial *v* wave is greatly increased and pulmonary venous pressure rises to produce pulmonary oedema.

Since a proportion of the stroke volume is regurgitated, the stroke volume increases to maintain the forward cardiac output and the left ventricle therefore enlarges.

### SYMPTOMS

Mitral regurgitation can be present for many years and the cardiac dimensions may be greatly increased before any symptoms occur. The increased stroke volume may be sensed as a 'palpitation'. Dyspnoea and orthopnoea may develop owing to pulmonary venous hypertension occurring as a direct result of the mitral regurgitation and secondarily to left ventricular failure. Fatigue and lethargy develop because of the reduced cardiac output. In the late stages of the disease the symptoms of right heart failure also occur and eventually lead to congestive cardiac failure. Cardiac cachexia may develop. Thromboembolism is less common than in mitral stenosis, but subacute infective endocarditis is much more common.

## SIGNS (see Clinical memo in Fig. 11.65)

The physical signs of uncomplicated mitral regurgitation are:

A LATERALLY DISPLACED, THRUSTING, DIFFUSE APEX BEAT AND A SYSTOLIC THRILL.

A SOFT FIRST HEART SOUND occurs because of the incomplete apposition of the valve cusps and their partial closure by the time ventricular systole begins.

A PAN-SYSTOLIC MURMUR due to regurgitation occurring throughout the whole of systole, which is loudest at the apex but radiates widely over the precordium and into the axilla.

A PROMINENT THIRD HEART SOUND occurs because of the sudden rush of blood back into the dilated left ventricle in early diastole. Sometimes a short mid-diastolic flow murmur may follow the third heart sound.

The signs related to atrial fibrillation, pulmonary hypertension, and left and right heart failure may develop later in the disease. The onset of atrial fibrillation has a much less dramatic effect on symptoms than in mitral stenosis.

## INVESTIGATION

### Chest X-ray

The chest X-ray may show left atrial and left ventricular enlargement. There is an increase in the CTR, and valve calcification may be seen.

### ECG

The ECG shows the features of left atrial delay (bifid P waves) and left ventricular hypertrophy (Fig. 11.69) as manifest by tall R waves in the left lateral leads, e.g. leads I, AVL and $V_6$, and deep S waves in the right-sided precordial leads, e.g. leads $V_1$ and $V_2$. ($SV_1$ plus $RV_5$ or $RV_6$ >35 mm indicates left ventricular hypertrophy.) Left ventricular hypertrophy occurs in about 50% of patients with mitral regurgitation. Atrial fibrillation may be present.

### Echocardiogram

The echocardiogram shows a dilated left atrium and left ventricle. There may be specific features of chordal or papillary muscle rupture. CW Doppler can determine the velocity of the regurgitant jet.

### Cardiac catheterization

This demonstrates a prominent left atrial systolic pressure wave, and when contrast is injected into the left ventricle it may be seen regurgitating into an enlarged left atrium during systole.

## TREATMENT

Mild mitral regurgitation in the absence of symptoms can be managed conservatively following the patient with serial echocardiograms. Prophylaxis against endocarditis is required (see p. 10). Any evidence of progressive cardiac enlargement generally warrants early surgical intervention by either mitral valve repair or replacement. The advantages of surgical intervention are diminished in more advanced disease. In patients who are not considered appropriate for surgical intervention, or in whom surgery will be considered at a later date, management usually involves treatment with ACE inhibitors, diuretics and possibly anticoagulants. Sudden torrential mitral regurgitation, as seen with chordal or papillary muscle rupture or infective endocarditis, may necessitate emergency mitral valve replacement.

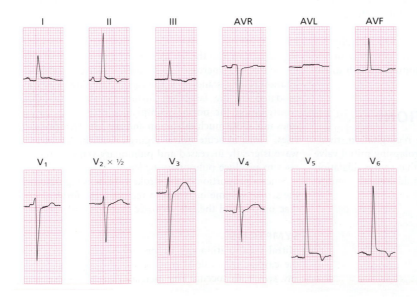

**Fig. 11.69** A 12-lead ECG showing features of left ventricular hypertrophy. Note the size of the S wave seen in $V_1$ (21 mm); S in $V_1$ + R in $V_6$ = >35 mm.

# Prolapsing (billowing) mitral valve

This is also known as Barlow's syndrome or floppy mitral valve. It is due to excessively large mitral valve leaflets, an enlarged mitral annulus, abnormally long chordae or disordered papillary muscle contraction. Histology may demonstrate myxomatous degeneration of the mitral valve leaflets. It is more commonly seen in young women than in men or older women and it has a familial incidence. Its cause is usually unknown but it may be due to Marfan's syndrome, thyrotoxicosis, rheumatic or ischaemic heart disease. It also occurs in association with atrial septal defect and as part of hypertrophic cardiomyopathy. Mild mitral valve prolapse is so common that it should be regarded as a normal variant.

## PATHOPHYSIOLOGY

During ventricular systole, a mitral valve leaflet (most commonly the posterior leaflet) prolapses into the left atrium. This may result in abnormal ventricular contraction, papillary muscle strain and some mitral regurgitation. Usually the syndrome is not haemodynamically serious. Thromboembolism may occur.

## SYMPTOMS

Atypical chest pain is the most common symptom. Usually the pain is left submammary and stabbing in quality. Sometimes it is substernal, aching and severe. Rarely it is similar to typical angina pectoris. Palpitations may be experienced because of the abnormal ventricular contraction or because of the atrial and ventricular arrhythmias that are commonly associated with mitral valve prolapse.

## SIGNS

The most common sign is a mid-systolic click, which is produced by the sudden prolapse of the valve and the tensing of the chordae tendineae that occurs during systole. This may be followed by a late systolic murmur due to some regurgitation. Sometimes, pan-systolic mitral regurgitation occurs. The signs typically fade quickly but return later.

## INVESTIGATION

### Chest X-ray

The chest X-ray is usually normal unless significant mitral regurgitation is present.

### ECG

The ECG is often abnormal with inverted or biphasic T waves in the inferior leads (leads II, III and AVF) and in the left lateral precordial leads (leads $V_5$ and $V_6$). The ST segment may also be slightly depressed in these leads.

### Echocardiogram

The diagnosis is confirmed on M-mode echocardiography, which typically shows posterior movement of one or both mitral valve cusps into the left atrium during systole.

### Cardiac catheterization

Contrast angiograms performed during cardiac catheterization reveal the systolic prolapse of the mitral valve into the left atrium, and mitral regurgitation, if present, is seen. This investigation is not normally required.

## TREATMENT

Usually, β-blockade is effective for the treatment of the atypical chest pain and palpitations. Sometimes more specific antiarrhythmic drug treatment is necessary. When a prolapsing mitral valve is associated with significant mitral regurgitation and atrial fibrillation, anticoagulation is advised to prevent thromboembolism. Very occasionally, mitral valve replacement may be necessary for severe regurgitation, although many surgeons prefer to repair rather than replace such valves. Prophylaxis against endocarditis (see p. 10) is advised if there is significant mitral valve regurgitation.

# AORTIC STENOSIS

There are three causes of aortic valve stenosis:

1 Congenital aortic valve stenosis develops progressively because of turbulent blood flow through a congenitally abnormal (usually bicuspid) aortic valve. Most congenitally abnormal aortic valves occur in men.
2 Rheumatic fever results in progressive fusion, thickening and calcification of a previously normal three-cusped aortic valve. In rheumatic heart disease the aortic valve is affected in about 45% of cases and there is usually associated mitral valve disease.
3 The wear and tear of age may lead to arteriosclerotic degeneration and calcification of the aortic valve. It is not usually severely stenotic and symptoms are not usually present.

Valvular aortic stenosis should be distinguished from other causes of obstruction to left ventricular emptying (Fig. 11.70), which include:

SUPRAVALVULAR OBSTRUCTION—a congenital fibrous diaphragm above the aortic valve

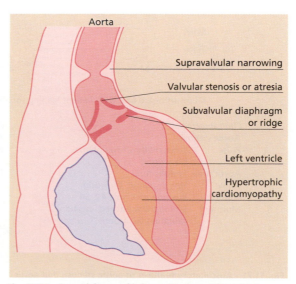

Fig. 11.70 Several forms of left ventricular outflow tract obstruction.

HYPERTROPHIC CARDIOMYOPATHY—septal muscle hypertrophy obstructs left ventricular outflow

SUBVALVULAR AORTIC STENOSIS—a congenital condition in which a fibrous ridge or diaphragm is situated immediately below the aortic valve

## PATHOPHYSIOLOGY

Obstructed left ventricular emptying leads to increased left ventricular pressure and compensatory left ventricular hypertrophy. In turn, this results in relative ischaemia of the left ventricular myocardium, and consequent angina, arrhythmias and left ventricular failure. The obstruction to left ventricular emptying is relatively more severe on exercise. Normally, exercise causes a many-fold increase in cardiac output, but when there is severe narrowing of the aortic valve orifice the cardiac output can hardly increase. Thus, the blood pressure falls, coronary ischaemia worsens, the myocardium fails and cardiac arrhythmias develop particularly on exercise.

## SYMPTOMS

There are usually no symptoms until aortic stenosis is moderately severe (when the aortic orifice is reduced to one-third of its normal size). At this stage, exercise-induced syncope, angina and dyspnoea may develop. When symptoms occur, the prognosis is poor—on average, death occurs within 2–3 years if there has been no surgical intervention.

## SIGNS (see Clinical memo in Fig. 11.71)

Aortic stenosis is characterized by abnormalities of the pulse, precordial pulsation and auscultation.

### Pulse

The carotid pulse is of small volume and is slow rising or plateau in nature (see p. 529).

### Precordial palpation

The apex beat is not usually displaced because hypertrophy (as opposed to dilatation) does not produce noticeable cardiomegaly. However, the pulsation is sustained and obvious—a *heaving apex beat*. A double impulse is sometimes felt because the fourth heart sound or atrial contraction ('kick') may be palpable. A systolic thrill may be felt in the aortic area.

### Auscultation (see Fig. 11.71)

The most obvious auscultatory finding in aortic stenosis is a mid-systolic ejection murmur that is usually 'diamond' shaped (crescendo–decrescendo). The murmur is usually longer when the disease is more severe, as a longer left ventricular ejection time is needed. The intensity of the murmur is not a good guide to the severity of the condition because it is lessened by a reduced cardiac output. The murmur is usually rough in quality and best heard in the aortic area. It radiates widely and is usually easily heard over the clavicles and the carotid arteries.

### Other findings

A SYSTOLIC EJECTION CLICK (see p. 534), unless the valve has become immobile and calcified

SOFT OR INAUDIBLE AORTIC SECOND HEART SOUND when the aortic valve becomes immobile

REVERSED SPLITTING OF THE SECOND HEART SOUND (splitting on expiration) (see p. 533)

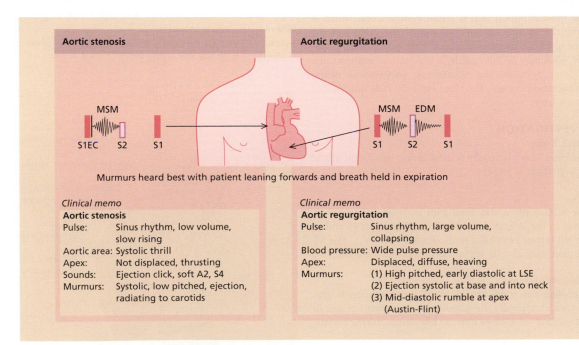

Murmurs heard best with patient leaning forwards and breath held in expiration

*Clinical memo*
**Aortic stenosis**
| | |
|---|---|
| Pulse: | Sinus rhythm, low volume, slow rising |
| Aortic area: | Systolic thrill |
| Apex: | Not displaced, thrusting |
| Sounds: | Ejection click, soft A2, S4 |
| Murmurs: | Systolic, low pitched, ejection, radiating to carotids |

*Clinical memo*
**Aortic regurgitation**
| | |
|---|---|
| Pulse: | Sinus rhythm, large volume, collapsing |
| Blood pressure: | Wide pulse pressure |
| Apex: | Displaced, diffuse, heaving |
| Murmurs: | (1) High pitched, early diastolic at LSE |
| | (2) Ejection systolic at base and into neck |
| | (3) Mid-diastolic rumble at apex (Austin-Flint) |

**Fig. 11.71** Auscultatory features of aortic stenosis and aortic regurgitation. EC, ejection click; EDM, early diastolic murmur; MSM, mid-systolic murmur; S₁, first heart sound.

A PROMINENT FOURTH HEART SOUND (see p. 533), unless coexisting mitral stenosis prevents this Degenerative disease of the aortic valve (aortic sclerosis) results in a loud mid-systolic murmur but, because there is little stenosis, there are no signs of left ventricular hypertrophy or of a slow rising pulse. This murmur can be ignored.

## INVESTIGATION

### Chest X-ray

The chest X-ray usually reveals a relatively small heart with a prominent, dilated, ascending aorta. This occurs because turbulent blood flow above the stenosed aortic valve produces so-called 'poststenotic dilatation'. The aortic valve may be calcified. When heart failure occurs, the CTR increases.

### ECG

The ECG shows left ventricular hypertrophy and left atrial delay. A left ventricular 'strain' pattern due to 'pressure overload' (depressed ST segments and T wave inversion in leads orientated towards the left ventricle, i.e. leads I, AVL, $V_5$ and $V_6$) is common when the disease is severe. Usually, sinus rhythm is present, but ventricular arrhythmias may be recorded.

### Echocardiogram

The echocardiogram readily demonstrates the thickened, calcified and immobile aortic valve cusps. Left ventricular hypertrophy may also be seen. The gradient across the valve can be estimated by CW Doppler (see Fig. 11.23).

### Cardiac catheterization

Cardiac catheterization is used to document the systolic pressure difference (gradient) between the aorta and the left ventricle (Fig. 11.72). A gradient of 50 mmHg or more is usually sufficient to advise surgery. A trivial degree of aortic regurgitation that is undetectable clinically is often demonstrated by contrast aortography. Coronary angiography is important before recommending surgery.

## TREATMENT

Patients with aortic stenosis should not overly exert themselves, and in particular they should not compete in strenuous physical games. Angina is best treated with $\beta$-blockade because vasodilators such as glyceryl trinitrate or isosorbide dinitrate may aggravate exertional syncope. Antibiotic prophylaxis against infective endocarditis is essential (see p. 10).

Irrespective of symptoms, aortic valve replacement with a prosthetic or tissue valve is recommended when aortic stenosis is severe. Cardiopulmonary bypass is necessary to achieve this. Provided that the valve is not severely deformed or heavily calcified, critical aortic stenosis in childhood or adolescence can be treated by valvotomy (performed under direct vision by the surgeon or by balloon dilatation using X-ray visualization). This produces temporary relief from the obstruction. Aortic valve replacement will usually be needed a few years later.

Balloon dilatation (valvuloplasty) has been tried in adults, especially in the elderly, as an alternative to surgery. Generally results are poor and such treatment is reserved for patients unfit for surgery or as a 'bridge' to surgery (i.e. to improve them for surgery).

## AORTIC REGURGITATION

The most common causes of aortic regurgitation are rheumatic fever and infective endocarditis complicating a previously damaged valve. This can be a congenitally abnormal valve (e.g. a bicuspid valve) or one damaged by rheumatic fever. There are numerous other causes and associations (Table 11.33). The majority of patients with aortic regurgitation are men (75%), but rheumatic aortic regurgitation occurs more commonly in women.

### PATHOPHYSIOLOGY

Aortic regurgitation is reflux of blood from the aorta through the aortic valve into the left ventricle during diastole. If net cardiac output is to be maintained, the total volume of blood pumped into the aorta must increase, and consequently the left ventricular size must

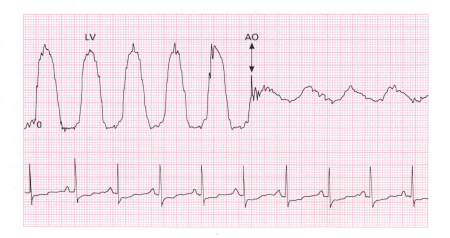

**Fig. 11.72** ECG and pressure trace as a cardiac catheter is withdrawn from the left ventricle (LV) to the aorta (AO). Note that the peak systolic pressure changes from 250 to 130 mmHg (arrow). The 120 mmHg peak-to-peak systolic gradient indicates severe aortic valvular stenosis.

*Acute aortic regurgitation*
Acute rheumatic fever
Infective endocarditis
Dissection of the aorta
Ruptured sinus of Valsalva aneurysm
Failure of prosthetic heart valve

*Chronic aortic regurgitation*
Rheumatic heart disease
Syphilis
Arthritides
    Reiter's syndrome
    Ankylosing spondylitis
    Rheumatoid arthritis
Hypertension (severe)
Bicuspid aortic valve
Aortic endocarditis
Marfan's syndrome
Osteogenesis imperfecta

**Table 11.33**   Causes and associations of aortic regurgitation.

enlarge. Because of the aortic run-off during diastole, diastolic blood pressure falls and coronary perfusion is decreased. In addition, the larger left ventricular size is mechanically less efficient so that the demand for oxygen is greater and cardiac ischaemia develops.

### SYMPTOMS

In aortic regurgitation significant symptoms occur late and do not develop until left ventricular failure occurs. As with mitral regurgitation, a common symptom is 'pounding of the heart' because of the increased left ventricular size and its vigorous pulsation. Angina pectoris is a frequent complaint. Varying grades of dyspnoea occur depending on the extent of left ventricular dilatation and dysfunction. Arrhythmias are relatively uncommon.

### SIGNS (see Clinical memo in Fig. 11.71)

The signs of aortic regurgitation are many and are due to the hyperdynamic circulation, reflux of blood into the left ventricle and the increased left ventricular size.

The pulse is bounding or collapsing (see p. 528). The following signs, which are rare, also indicate a hyperdynamic circulation:

QUINCKE'S SIGN—capillary pulsation in the nail beds
DE MUSSET'S SIGN—head nodding with each heart beat
DUROZIER'S SIGN—systolic bruit over the femoral arteries when the stethoscope is lightly applied
PISTOL SHOT FEMORALS—a sharp bang heard on auscultation over the femoral arteries in time with each heart beat

The apex beat is displaced laterally and downwards and is thrusting in quality.

On auscultation there is a high-pitched diastolic murmur running from the aortic component of the second heart sound (see Fig. 11.71).

It is loudest in early diastole and is heard best at the lower left sternal edge or the cardiac apex.

### INVESTIGATION

#### Chest X-ray

The chest X-ray features are those of left ventricular enlargement and possibly of dilatation of the ascending aorta. The ascending aortic wall may be calcified in syphilis and the aortic valve may be calcified if valvular disease is responsible for the regurgitation.

#### ECG

The ECG appearances are those of left ventricular hypertrophy due to 'volume overload', i.e. tall R waves and deeply inverted T waves in the left-sided chest leads, and deep S waves in the right-sided leads. Normally, sinus rhythm is present.

#### Echocardiogram

The echocardiogram demonstrates vigorous cardiac contraction and a dilated left ventricle. The aortic root may also be enlarged. Diastolic fluttering of the mitral leaflets or septum occurs in severe aortic regurgitation (producing the Austin Flint murmur, see p. 535). The regurgitant jet can be detected by CW Doppler.

#### Cardiac catheterization

During cardiac catheterization, injection of contrast medium into the aorta (aortography) will outline aortic valvular abnormalities and allow assessment of the degree of regurgitation.

### TREATMENT

The underlying cause of aortic regurgitation (e.g. syphilitic aortitis or infective endocarditis) may require specific treatment. The treatment of aortic regurgitation usually requires aortic valve replacement but the timing of surgery is important.

Because symptoms do not develop until the myocardium fails and because the myocardium does not recover fully after surgery, it is important to operate before significant symptoms occur. The timing of the operation is best determined according to haemodynamic, echocardiographic or nuclear angiographic criteria.

Both mechanical prostheses and tissue valves are used. Tissue valves are preferred in the elderly and when anticoagulants must be avoided, but are contraindicated in children and young adults because of the rapid calcification and degeneration of the valves.

Antibiotic prophylaxis against infective endocarditis (see p. 10) is necessary even if a prosthetic valve replacement has been performed.

## TRICUSPID STENOSIS

This uncommon valve lesion, which is seen much more often in women than in men, is usually due to rheumatic heart disease and is frequently associated with mitral and/or aortic valve disease. Tricuspid stenosis is also seen in the carcinoid syndrome.

### PATHOPHYSIOLOGY

Tricuspid valve stenosis results in a reduced cardiac output, which is restored towards normal when the right atrial pressure increases. The resulting systemic venous congestion produces hepatomegaly, ascites and dependent oedema.

## SYMPTOMS

Usually, patients with tricuspid stenosis complain of symptoms due to the associated left-sided rheumatic valve lesions. The abdominal pain (due to hepatomegaly) and swelling (due to ascites) and peripheral oedema that occur are relatively severe when compared with the degree of dyspnoea.

## SIGNS

If the patient remains in sinus rhythm, which is unusual, there is a prominent jugular venous *a* wave. This presystolic pulsation may also be felt over the liver. There is usually a rumbling mid-diastolic murmur, which is heard best at the lower left sternal edge and is louder on inspiration. It may be missed because of the murmur of coexisting mitral stenosis. A tricuspid opening snap may occasionally be heard.

Hepatomegaly, abdominal ascites and dependent oedema may be present.

## INVESTIGATION

### Chest X-ray

On the chest X-ray there may be a prominent right atrial bulge.

### ECG

The enlarged right atrium may be manifest on the ECG by peaked, tall P waves (≥3 mm) in lead 2.

### Echocardiogram

The echocardiogram may show a thickened and immobile tricuspid valve, but this is not so clearly seen as an abnormal mitral valve.

### Cardiac catheterization

This demonstrates a diastolic pressure gradient between the right atrium and the right ventricle. Contrast injection will demonstrate a large right atrium.

## TREATMENT

Medical management consists of diuretic therapy and salt restriction. Tricuspid valvotomy is occasionally possible, but tricuspid valve replacement is often necessary. Other valves usually also need replacement because tricuspid valve stenosis is rarely an isolated lesion.

# TRICUSPID REGURGITATION

Functional tricuspid regurgitation may occur whenever the right ventricle dilates, e.g. in cor pulmonale, myocardial infarction or pulmonary hypertension.

Organic tricuspid regurgitation may occur with rheumatic heart disease, infective endocarditis, carcinoid syndrome, Ebstein's anomaly (a congenitally malpositioned tricuspid valve) and other congenital abnormalities of the atrioventricular valves.

## SYMPTOMS AND SIGNS

The valvular regurgitation gives rise to high right atrial and systemic venous pressure. Patients may complain of the symptoms of right heart failure.

Physical signs include a large jugular venous *cv* wave and a palpable liver that pulsates in systole. Usually a right ventricular impulse may be felt at the left sternal edge, and there is a blowing pan-systolic murmur, best heard on inspiration at the lower left sternal edge. Atrial fibrillation is common.

## TREATMENT

Functional tricuspid regurgitation usually disappears with medical management. Severe organic tricuspid regurgitation may require operative repair of the tricuspid valve (annuloplasty or plication). Very occasionally, tricuspid valve replacement may be necessary. In drug addicts with infective endocarditis of the tricuspid valve, surgical removal of the valve is recommended to eradicate the infection. This is usually well tolerated in the short term. The insertion of a prosthetic valve for this condition is considered on p. 602.

# PULMONARY STENOSIS

This is usually a congenital lesion, but it may rarely result from rheumatic fever or from the carcinoid syndrome. Congenital pulmonary stenosis may be associated with an intact ventricular septum or with a ventricular septal defect (Fallot's tetralogy).

Pulmonary stenosis may be valvular, subvalvular or supravalvular. Multiple congenital pulmonary arterial stenoses are usually due to infection with rubella during pregnancy.

## SYMPTOMS AND SIGNS

The obstruction to right ventricular emptying results in right ventricular hypertrophy which in turn leads to right atrial hypertrophy. Severe pulmonary obstruction may be incompatible with life, but lesser degrees of obstruction give rise to fatigue, syncope and the symptoms of right heart failure. Mild pulmonary stenosis may be asymptomatic.

The physical signs are characterized by a harsh midsystolic ejection murmur, best heard on inspiration, to the left of the sternum in the second intercostal space. This murmur is often associated with a thrill. The pulmonary closure sound is usually delayed and soft. There may be a pulmonary ejection sound if the obstruction is valvular. A right ventricular fourth sound and a prominent jugular venous *a* wave are present when the stenosis is moderately severe. A right ventricular heave may be felt.

## INVESTIGATION

### Chest X-ray

The chest X-ray usually shows a prominent pulmonary artery due to poststenotic dilatation.

### ECG

The ECG demonstrates both right atrial and right ventricular hypertrophy, although it may sometimes be normal even in severe pulmonary stenosis.

### Cardiac catheterization

The passage of a catheter through the right heart allows the level and degree of the stenosis to be established by measuring the systolic pressure gradient.

### TREATMENT

Treatment of severe pulmonary stenosis requires pulmonary valvotomy (balloon valvotomy or direct surgery).

## PULMONARY REGURGITATION

This is the most common acquired lesion of the pulmonary valve. It results from dilatation of the pulmonary valve ring, which occurs with pulmonary hypertension. It is characterized by a decrescendo diastolic murmur beginning with the pulmonary component of the second sound (Graham Steell murmur) that is difficult to distinguish from the murmur of aortic regurgitation. Pulmonary regurgitation usually causes no symptoms and treatment is rarely necessary.

## PROSTHETIC HEART VALVES

There are two groups of prosthetic heart valve: tissue and mechanical. Tissue valves are usually fashioned from a pig aortic valve (xenograft); occasionally a human aortic valve is used (homograft). Mechanical valves are of various types, the most common being a ball-and-cage design (Starr–Edwards valve), a tilting disc (Björk–Shiley valve) or a double tilting disc (St Jude valve). The disadvantage of the mechanical valve over the tissue valve is that formal anticoagulation is required. However, mechanical valves are much harder wearing; a tissue valve tends to degenerate after about 10 years. Unlike a tilting disc valve, the ball of a ball-and-cage valve presents some obstruction to flow through the valve. Although ball-and-cage valves have always been mechanically satisfactory some tilting disc valves have been mechanically insecure. Prosthetic valves may become detached from the valve ring, thrombose, stick, degenerate or become infected. Echocardiography is often helpful, but echoes are scattered from the mechanical valve making assessment of the structure of the valve rather difficult. This is particularly troublesome with the mitral valve, but the advent of transoesophageal echocardiography has largely overcome this problem. Transoesophageal echocardiography is the investigation of choice when prosthetic valve endocarditis is suspected.

## Infective endocarditis

Infective endocarditis is an infection of the endocardium or vascular endothelium. The disease may occasionally occur as a fulminating or acute infection, but more commonly runs an insidious course and is known as subacute (bacterial) endocarditis (SBE). The incidence is 6–7 per 100 000 per year in the UK, but is much more common in developing countries. Endocarditis occurs most commonly on rheumatic or congenitally abnormal valves as well as in mitral valve prolapse and calcified aortic valve disease. It also occurs in association with congenital lesions such as ventricular septal defect or persistent ductus arteriosus. A very similar disease may occur from infection of arteriovenous fistulas. Prosthetic valves or prosthetic vascular material may be similarly infected and this is one of the reasons for the increasing incidence of endocarditis in developed countries. The organisms are often non-virulent.

Virulent organisms may infect normal valves, especially when the victim is generally debilitated or immunologically incompetent.

The term 'infective endocarditis' is preferred because not all the infecting organisms are bacteria.

### AETIOLOGY

Many organisms cause infective endocarditis. At the present time the three most common organisms are:

1 *Streptococcus viridans* (e.g. *Strep. viridans mitis* and *Strep. viridans sanguis*) (50% of cases). These organisms are part of the bacterial flora of the pharynx and upper respiratory tract, and the infection may follow dental extraction or cleaning, tonsillectomy or bronchoscopy.

2 *Enterococcus faecalis* (found in perineal and faecal bacterial flora). Infections with this organism are more usual in older men with prostatic disease, in women with genitourinary infections, or following pelvic surgery.

3 *Staphylococcus aureus*. This organism may cause subacute endocarditis and is responsible for 50% of the acute forms. Patients with central venous catheters used for parenteral feeding, temporary pacemaker electrode catheters or pulmonary artery (Swan–Ganz) catheters are prone to this infection. Cellulitis or skin abscesses are often the origin of the infection, particularly in drug addicts who 'mainline'.

Infective endocarditis can also be caused by:

1 *Staphylococcus epidermidis*, *Histoplasma*, *Brucella*, *Candida* and *Aspergillus*. Infections with these organisms are particularly common in intravenous drug addicts, alcoholics and patients with prosthetic heart valves.

2 *Coxiella burnetii* (the causative organism of Q fever, see p. 45). This may cause a subacute infection.

Although Gram-negative bacteraemia/septicaemia frequently occur, endocarditis with these organisms is unusual.

### PATHOLOGY

Infection occurs along the edges of the heart valves. It is more common on the left side, with mitral and aortic regurgitation being the commonest valve lesions complicated by endocarditis. In drug addicts the valves in the right heart are usually affected.

The endocardium on the low-pressure side of a shunt

such as ventricular septal defect is infected and it is the pulmonary artery that is infected when a persistent ductus arteriosus is present; in both instances the lesions are 'jet lesions' produced on the wall opposite the shunt (Fig. 11.73).

Hypertrophic cardiomyopathy, syphilitic aortic regurgitation, prolapsing mitral valve and arteriosclerotic valve lesions may also be rarely complicated by endocarditis.

The lesion of infective endocarditis is a mass of fibrin, platelets and infecting organisms known as a vegetation. The chance of an organism sticking to a vegetation is increased because of the clumping together of bacteria caused by agglutinating antibodies. These can develop because of repeated infection with the bacterium over a period of years. In acute endocarditis, vegetations may be very large and may embolize. Virulent microorganisms may rapidly destroy the valve cusp, producing ulceration and regurgitation.

The extracardiac manifestations result either from embolization or from the deposition of immune complexes. The latter is thought to be responsible for arthralgia, Roth spots and Janeway lesions, focal glomerulonephritis and acute vasculitis (see below).

Splenic and renal infarcts are produced by emboli. Myocardial infarction can result from coronary emboli, and pulmonary infarction may occur if right-sided lesions embolize.

## PRESENTATIONS
### Subacute endocarditis
The patient presents with fever, night sweats, weight loss, weakness and symptoms due to cardiac failure or embolism. Another important presentation is the combination of renal failure and a heart murmur. It is not usually possible to date the onset of the illness.

### Acute endocarditis
In intravenous drug abusers or following an acute suppurative illness such as pneumonia or meningitis, the development of acute endocarditis is suggested by the persistence of fever and the development of heart murmurs, vasculitis (with petechial haemorrhage) and emboli, including metastatic abscesses. The onset of severe heart failure may indicate chordal rupture or acute valvular destruction.

### Prosthetic endocarditis
There are two varieties: the first develops soon after surgery and is due to infection of the prosthesis at surgery, and the second occurs late and follows a bacteraemia. In both cases it is the valve ring that is infected. This produces myocardial abscesses and damage, for example to the conduction system. Vegetations in the valve may prevent it from opening and closing properly. Emboli are common.

## CLINICAL FEATURES (Table 11.34)
The patients are often elderly. They appear pale (often anaemic) and ill. They are intermittently pyrexial and may complain of myalgia and arthralgia. Some of the following signs and symptoms may be present but endocarditis must always be suspected in a patient with a heart murmur and a fever.

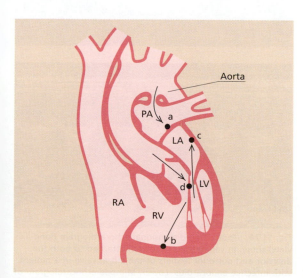

Fig. 11.73 Jet lesions produced in infective endocarditis. a, a lesion in the pulmonary artery (PA) because of a ductus arteriosus. b, a lesion in the right ventricle (RV) due to a ventricular septal defect. c, a lesion in the left atrium (LA) due to mitral regurgitation. d, a lesion in the left ventricle (LV) and on the mitral valve chordae tendineae due to aortic regurgitation. RA, right atrium.

| | Approximate % |
|---|---|
| General systems | |
| Malaise | 95 |
| Clubbing | 10 |
| Cardiac | |
| Murmurs | 90 |
| Cardiac failure | 50 |
| Arthralgia | 25 |
| Pyrexia | 90 |
| Skin lesions | |
| Osler's nodes | 15 |
| Splinter haemorrhages | 10 |
| Janeway lesions | 5 |
| Petechiae | 50 |
| Eyes | |
| Roth spots | 5 |
| Conjunctival splinter haemorrhages | Rare |
| Splenomegaly | 40 |
| Neurological | |
| Cerebral emboli | 20 |
| Mycotic aneurysm | 10 |
| Renal | |
| Haematuria | 70 |

Table 11.34  Clinical features of infective endocarditis.

## Cardiac findings

The signs of any underlying heart disease should be obvious, but occasionally only trivial lesions such as mild aortic regurgitation or a bicuspid aortic valve are present. The development of a new murmur or a change in the character of an existing murmur may warn of the presence of endocarditis.

## Vascular lesions

Small petechial or mucosal haemorrhages occur because of vasculitis. They are usually small and red, usually with a pale centre. They frequently appear on the mucosa of the pharynx and conjunctivae. Sometimes they are seen on the retinae (Roth spots). Small, flat, erythematous, non-tender macules are seen mainly on the thenar and hypothenar eminences (Janeway lesions); these blanch with pressure. Splinter haemorrhages may develop.

Embolic lesions such as hard, painful, tender, subcutaneous swellings occur in the fingers, toes, palms and soles (Osler's nodes).

## Clubbing of the fingers

Mild clubbing of the fingers and toes appears late in the disease, and thus it only occurs in subacute endocarditis. It is rare nowadays because of relatively rapid diagnosis and treatment of the endocarditis.

## Splenomegaly

Slight splenomegaly is common. If a splenic infarct has occurred, the spleen may be painful and tender and a friction rub may be heard over it.

## Renal lesions

Haematuria is common, usually due to infarction as a result of emboli. Renal abscesses and acute glomerulonephritis also occur.

## Arthritis

Arthritis of the major joints is frequently seen.

## Other embolic phenomena

Cerebral emboli can occur, usually to the middle cerebral artery or its branches. Mycotic infected aneurysms are seen and may present after the endocarditis has healed. Peripheral arterial, pulmonary and coronary infarcts may also occur.

## INVESTIGATION

BLOOD. A normochromic normocytic anaemia is usual and C-reactive protein and the ESR are increased. A polymorphonuclear leucocytosis is common and thrombocytopenia can occasionally occur.

LIVER BIOCHEMISTRY is often mildly disturbed with, in particular, an increased serum alkaline phosphatase.

IMMUNOGLOBULINS AND COMPLEMENT. Serum immunoglobulins are increased, but total complement and C3 complement are decreased owing to immune complex formation. Circulating immune complexes are present in more than 70% of cases but are not routinely measured.

URINE. Proteinuria may occur and microscopic haematuria is nearly always present.

BLOOD CULTURES are positive in about three-quarters of cases. At least six sets of samples are usually taken and cultured in aerobic and anaerobic conditions. Special culture techniques may be necessary for unusual microorganisms such as *Brucella* and *Histoplasma*. Serological tests are needed to incriminate *Coxiella* and *Chlamydia*, and may be helpful for *Candida* and *Brucella*.

ECHOCARDIOGRAPHY (particularly using the transoesophageal approach) is used to visualize vegetations (Fig. 11.74), but small vegetations typical of the subacute disease can be missed. Echocardiography is useful to document valvular dysfunction and to identify patients in need of urgent surgery. Vegetations may persist despite treatment.

CHEST X-RAY may show evidence of heart failure or emboli in right-sided endocarditis.

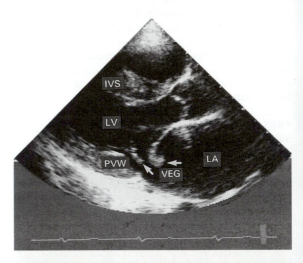

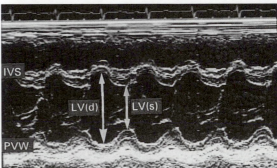

**Fig. 11.74** *Upper*: Two-dimensional echocardiogram (long-axis view) showing vegetations (arrowed) attached to both the anterior and posterior leaflets of the mitral valve in a patient with infective endocarditis. *Lower*: M-mode echocardiogram of the left ventricle in the same patient showing hyperdynamic contraction associated with volume overloading from the associated severe mitral regurgitation. Compare with Fig. 11.22c. IVS, interventricular septum; LV, left ventricle; LV(d) and LV(s), diastolic and systolic left ventricular dimensions; PVW, posterior ventricular wall; LA, left atrium; VEG, vegetation.

ECGs may show evidence of myocardial infarction (emboli) or conduction defects.

## TREATMENT

### Drug therapy

Any underlying infection should be treated (e.g. a dental abscess should be drained). The endocarditis is treated with bactericidal antibiotics chosen on the basis of the results of the blood culture and antibiotic sensitivity assessment. The treatment should continue for 4–6 weeks. Serum levels are measured and 'back titration' is performed to ensure that sufficient bactericidal antibiotic activity is present to inhibit growth of the organism.

*Strep. viridans* is usually treated with i.v. benzylpenicillin 2.4 g 6-hourly daily and low-dose gentamicin 1 mg kg$^{-1}$ 8-hourly for the first 2 weeks because of the additive effects of gentamicin and penicillin against *Strep. viridans*. Oral amoxycillin 6 g daily can replace intravenous therapy after 2 weeks.

*Strep. faecalis* (enterococcus) is managed with penicillin and gentamicin (3 mg kg$^{-1}$ in divided 8-hourly doses). The dosage of penicillin should be higher (up to 24 g daily) than for *Strep. viridans* because *Strep. faecalis* is relatively insensitive to penicillin and ampicillin 8 g daily is often substituted. The exact dose of gentamicin depends on renal function and efficacy, and blood levels should be measured at least twice each week.

It is more difficult to choose antibiotics when the infecting organism has not been isolated. However, in the acute form of the disease this is likely to be *Staphylococcus*, and treatment should include flucloxacillin and fusidic acid. In the subacute form, unless it is highly likely that the infecting organism is *Strep. viridans*, it is usual to begin treatment with a broad-spectrum combination of antibiotics such as gentamicin and ampicillin. The treatment is adjusted if it is not successful.

The recurrence of fever may suggest that the antibiotic therapy is inadequate, but may also signal a drug reaction. The antibiotics may be omitted for 24–72 hours to test this.

### Surgery

There are several situations in which surgery is necessary:

- Extensive damage to a valve
- Early infection of prosthetic material
- Worsening renal failure
- Persistent infection but failure to culture an organism
- Embolization
- Large vegetations
- Progressive cardiac failure

The timing of surgery is important. On the one hand the infection should, if possible, be eradicated before surgery is undertaken, but on the other hand the heart should not be left in a badly compromised haemodynamic state. In general, early surgery is preferable.

## PROGNOSIS

The prognosis is worse when the organism cannot be isolated, when cardiac failure is present, when infection occurs on a prosthetic valve, and when the microorganisms found are resistant to therapy. In general, 70% of those affected are treated effectively, but greater awareness of the subacute form of the disease will improve the success rate.

## PROPHYLAXIS (see p. 10)

Those at risk of developing endocarditis should receive antibiotic therapy before undergoing a procedure likely to result in a bacteraemia. The form of the prophylaxis depends on the procedure and on the likelihood of endocarditis. High-risk patients are those with a prosthetic heart valve or a previous history of endocarditis.

# Congenital heart disease

A congenital cardiac malformation occurs in about 1% of live births. There is an overall male predominance, although some individual lesions (e.g. atrial septal defect and persistent ductus arteriosus) occur more commonly in females. The aetiology of congenital cardiac disease is often unknown but involves:

MATERNAL RUBELLA INFECTION (persistent ductus arteriosus, and pulmonary valvular and arterial stenosis)

MATERNAL ALCOHOL ABUSE (septal defects)

MATERNAL DRUG TREATMENT AND RADIATION

GENETIC ABNORMALITIES, e.g. the familial form of atrial septal defect and congenital heart block

CHROMOSOMAL ABNORMALITIES, e.g. septal defects and mitral and tricuspid valve defects associated with Down's syndrome (trisomy 21) or coarctation of the aorta in Turner's syndrome (45, XO).

Some symptoms and signs are common in congenital heart disease:

CENTRAL CYANOSIS occurs because of right-to-left shunting of blood or because of complete mixing of systemic and pulmonary blood flow.

PULMONARY HYPERTENSION results from large left-to-right shunts. The persistently raised pulmonary flow leads to the development of increased pulmonary artery vascular resistance and consequent pulmonary hypertension. This is known as the Eisenmenger reaction (or the Eisenmenger syndrome when due specifically to a ventricular septal defect). The development of pulmonary hypertension significantly worsens the prognosis.

CLUBBING OF THE FINGERS may occur in congenital cardiac conditions associated with prolonged cyanosis.

PARADOXICAL EMBOLISM of thrombus from the systemic veins to the systemic arterial system may occur when a communication exists between the right and left heart.

REDUCED GROWTH is common in children with cyanotic heart disease.

SYNCOPE is common when severe right or left ventricular outflow tract obstruction is present. Exertional syncope, associated with deepening central cyanosis, may occur in Fallot's tetralogy. Exercise results in increased resistance to pulmonary blood flow but reduced systemic vascular resistance. Thus, the right-to-left shunt increases and cerebral oxygenation falls.

SQUATTING is the posture adopted by children with Fallot's tetralogy. It results in obstruction of venous return of desaturated blood and an increase in the peripheral systemic vascular resistance. This leads to a reduced right-to-left shunt and improved cerebral oxygenation.

The most common congenital lesions are shown in Table 11.35 as well as their occurrence in first-degree relatives.

Genetic factors should be considered in all patients presenting with congenital heart disease, e.g. parents with a child suffering from Fallot's tetralogy stand a 4% chance of conceiving another child with the disease and fetal ultrasound screening of the mother during pregnancy is essential.

## Ventricular septal defect (VSD)

VSD is the most common congenital cardiac malformation (1 in 500 live births). It may occur as an isolated abnormality or in association with other anomalies. Left ventricular pressure is higher than right ventricular pressure; blood therefore moves from left to right and pulmonary blood flow increases. When pulmonary blood flow is very large, obliterative pulmonary vascular changes may cause the pulmonary arterial pressure to equal the systemic pressure (Eisenmenger's syndrome). Consequently, the shunt is reduced or reversed (becoming right-to-left) and central cyanosis may develop.

### CLINICAL FEATURES

A small VSD (maladie de Roger) presents with a loud and sometimes long systolic murmur in an asymptomatic patient. Such VSDs usually close spontaneously. Moderate VSDs produce some fatigue and dyspnoea. Physical signs include cardiac enlargement and a prominent apex beat. There is often a palpable systolic thrill at the lower left sternal edge. A loud 'tearing' pan-systolic murmur is heard at the same position.

Large VSDs are associated with increasing pulmonary hypertension (right ventricular parasternal heave and a loud, pulmonary component of the second heart sound).

The murmur may be soft because the increased right ventricular pressure may be nearly equal to the left ventricular pressure, so that flow across the VSD is small.

### INVESTIGATION

A small VSD produces no abnormal X-ray or ECG findings. On the chest X-ray, larger defects show a prominent pulmonary artery owing to increased pulmonary blood flow. In Eisenmenger's syndrome the radiological signs of pulmonary hypertension (i.e. 'pruned' pulmonary arteries) can be seen. Cardiomegaly occurs when a moderate or a large VSD is present. The ECG shows features of both left and right ventricular hypertrophy. The size and location of the VSD, and its haemodynamic consequences, can be assessed by 2-D echocardiography and CW Doppler (Fig. 11.75).

### TREATMENT

Moderate and large VSDs should be surgically repaired before the development of severe pulmonary hypertension. Infective endocarditis prophylaxis (see p. 10) should be advised.

## Atrial septal defect (ASD)

This congenital condition is often first diagnosed in adults. It is more common in women than in men. There are two types of ASD—ostium secundum and ostium primum. The common form of ASD is ostium secundum. Communication at the level of the atria allows left-to-right shunting of blood. Because the pulmonary vascular resistance is low and the right ventricle is easily distended (i.e. it is compliant), there is a considerable increase in right heart output. Above the age of 30 years there may be an increase in pulmonary vascular resistance, which gives rise to pulmonary hypertension. Atrial arrhythmias, particularly atrial fibrillation, are common at this stage.

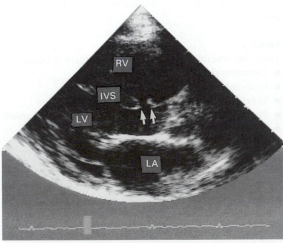

**Fig. 11.75**  Two-dimensional echocardiogram (long-axis view) showing a ventricular septal defect (arrowed). Colour Doppler would provide graphic demonstration of the left to right shunt. RV, right ventricle; IVS, interventricular septum; LV, left ventricle; LA, left atrium.

| | Percentage of congenital lesions | Occurrence in first-degree relatives (%) |
|---|---|---|
| Ventricular septal defect | 39 | 4 |
| Atrial septal defect | 10 | 2 |
| Persistent ductus arteriosus | 10 | 4 |
| Pulmonary stenosis | 7 | |
| Coarctation of the aorta | 7 | 2 |
| Aortic stenosis | 6 | 4 |
| Fallot's tetralogy | 6 | 4 |
| Others | 15 | |

**Table 11.35**  Common congenital lesions.

| Sternal impulse: | Right ventricular heave |
| Sounds: | Loud P$_2$ |
| | Fixed split S$_2$ (A$_2$–P$_2$) |
| Murmurs: | Mid-systolic ejection in |
| | pulmonary area |

**Information box 11.2**   Atrial septal defect.

## CLINICAL FEATURES (Information box 11.2)

Most children with ASDs are asymptomatic, although they are prone to pulmonary infection. Some complain of dyspnoea and weakness. Palpitations due to atrial arrhythmias are not uncommon. Right heart failure may develop in later life.

The physical signs of ASD reflect the volume over-loading of the right ventricle. Therefore, the splitting of the second sound is wide and fixed (see p. 533). The increased flow through the right heart produces a loud ejection systolic pulmonary flow murmur, and sometimes a diastolic tricuspid flow murmur may be heard. A right ventricular impulse can usually be felt.

## INVESTIGATION

THE CHEST X-RAY shows a prominent pulmonary artery and pulmonary plethora (Fig. 11.76). Figure 11.77 shows a more severe case with pulmonary hypertension. There may be noticeable right ventricular enlargement.

THE ECG usually shows some degree of right bundle branch block (because of dilatation of the right ventricle) and right axis deviation.

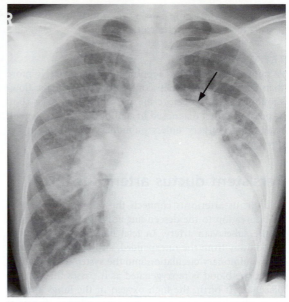

**Fig. 11.77**   A PA chest X-ray from a young woman with an atrial septal defect. The film shows a prominent main pulmonary artery and pulmonary arterial plethora. The heart is increased in size.

THE ECHOCARDIOGRAM demonstrates right ventricular hypertrophy and pulmonary arterial dilatation. The interventricular septum moves abnormally. Sometimes the ASD is part of a major developmental abnormality and may also involve the ventricular septum and the mitral and tricuspid valves. In this case there is left axis deviation on the ECG. Two-dimensional cardiography will define the site and size of the defect (Fig. 11.78).

FLOW DISTURBANCE can be assessed by Doppler.

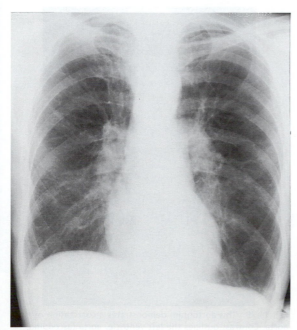

**Fig. 11.76**   The patient from whom this plain chest X-ray was recorded had chronic obstructive pulmonary disease and pulmonary hypertension. Note the very large proximal pulmonary arteries.

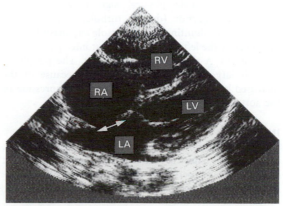

**Fig. 11.78**   Two-dimensional echocardiogram sub-costal four-chamber view (similar to Fig. 11.75, but rotated clockwise), showing an ostium secundum atrial septal defect (arrowed) in a young girl. Colour Doppler can demonstrate the left to right shunt. LA, left atrium; RA, right atrium; LV, left ventricle; RV, right ventricle.

CARDIAC CATHETERIZATION is not always necessary with the advent of echocardiography.

## TREATMENT

A significant ASD (i.e. a pulmonary flow that is more than 50% increased when compared with systemic flow) should be repaired before the age of 10 years or as soon as possible if first diagnosed in adulthood. There is a good result from surgery unless pulmonary hypertension has developed.

# Persistent ductus arteriosus (PDA)

The ductus arteriosus connects the pulmonary artery at its bifurcation to the descending aorta immediately distal to the subclavian artery. In fetal life the ductus diverts blood away from the unexpanded, and hence high-resistance, pulmonary circulation into the systemic circulation, where the blood is reoxygenated as it passes through the placenta. At birth, the high oxygen in the lungs and the reduced pulmonary vascular resistance triggers closure of the duct. If the duct is malformed, i.e. it does not contain sufficient elastic tissue, it will not close. This is more common in females and is sometimes associated with maternal rubella. Premature babies are often born with persistent ducts that are anatomically normal but are immature in that they lack the mechanism to close.

Because aortic pressure exceeds pulmonary artery pressure throughout the cardiac cycle, a persistent duct produces continuous aorta-to-pulmonary artery shunting. This leads to an increased pulmonary venous return to the left heart and an increased left ventricular volume load.

## CLINICAL FEATURES

If the shunt is large, the left heart volume overload results in severe left heart failure. However, there are often no symptoms until later in life when heart failure or infective endocarditis develop.

The characteristic physical sign is a continuous 'machinery' murmur (due to turbulent aortic-to-pulmonary artery shunting in both systole and diastole), best heard below the left clavicle in the first interspace or over the first rib. A thrill may often be felt. The peripheral pulse is large in volume ('bounding') because of the increased left heart blood flow and the decompression of the aorta into the pulmonary artery.

## INVESTIGATION

The aorta and pulmonary arterial system are prominent radiologically. There is both a left atrial abnormality and left ventricular hypertrophy on the ECG. The echocardiogram shows a dilated left atrium and left ventricle.

## TREATMENT

Premature infants with a persistent duct may be treated medically with indomethacin, which inhibits prostaglandin production and stimulates duct closure. In other cases the duct can be ligated surgically with very little risk. Surgery should be performed as soon as possible and not later than 5 years.

# Coarctation of the aorta

Coarctation of the aorta occurs twice as commonly in men as in women. It is also associated with Turner's syndrome. The coarctation is a narrowing of the aorta at, or just distal to, the insertion of the ductus arteriosus (Fig. 11.79). In 80% of cases coarctation of the aorta is associated with a bicuspid (and potentially stenotic) aortic valve.

Severe narrowing of the aorta encourages the formation of a collateral arterial circulation involving the periscapular and intercostal arteries. Decreased renal perfusion can lead to the development of systemic hypertension that persists even after surgical correction.

## CLINICAL FEATURES

Coarctation of the aorta is often asymptomatic for many years. Headaches and nose bleeds (due to hypertension) and claudication and cold legs (due to poor blood flow in the lower limbs) may be present.

Physical examination reveals hypertension in the upper limbs, and weak, delayed (radiofemoral delay) pulses in the legs.

A mid-to-late systolic murmur due to turbulent flow through the coarctation may be heard over the upper precordium or the back. Vascular bruits from the collateral circulation may also be heard.

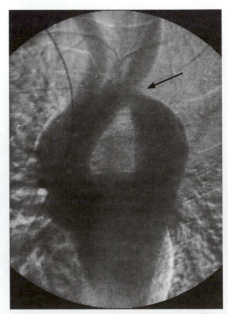

**Fig. 11.79** This aortogram demonstrates a coarctation of the aorta. Contrast outlines the left ventricle, aorta (ascending, arch and descending) and three major arteries arising from the aorta (right subclavian, right carotid and innominate). Immediately after the innominate artery the aorta is very markedly narrowed due to a coarctation of the aorta.

## INVESTIGATION

The chest X-ray may reveal a dilated aorta indented at the site of the coarctation. This is manifested by an aorta (seen in the upper right mediastinum) shaped like a figure '3'. In adults, tortuous and dilated collateral intercostal arteries may erode the undersurfaces of the ribs ('rib notching') (Fig. 11.80). The ECG demonstrates left ventricular hypertrophy. Echocardiography sometimes shows the coarctation and other associated anomalies. Aortography will show the defect and digital vascular imaging allows the coarctation to be visualized after the intravenous injection of contrast. MRI will also demonstrate the coarctation.

## TREATMENT

The treatment is surgical excision of the coarctation and end-to-end anastomosis of the aorta. If the coarctation is extensive, prosthetic vascular grafts may be needed. When surgery is performed in childhood, hypertension usually resolves completely. However, when the operation is performed on adults the hypertension persists in 70% because of previous renal damage.

# Fallot's tetralogy

This is the most common cyanotic congenital heart abnormality in children who survive beyond the neonatal period. It consists of the following four features (Fig. 11.81):

1  A VSD.
2  Right ventricular outflow obstruction. The level of the obstruction may be subvalvular, valvular or supravalvular. The commonest obstruction is subvalvular,

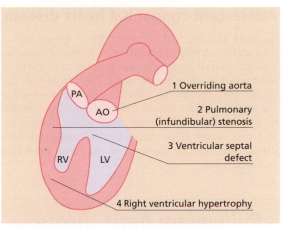

**Fig. 11.81**    The four features of Fallot's tetralogy.

1 Overriding aorta
2 Pulmonary (infundibular) stenosis
3 Ventricular septal defect
4 Right ventricular hypertrophy

either alone (50%) or in combination with valvular stenosis (25%).
3  Positioning of the aorta above the VSD ('overriding aorta').
4  Right ventricular hypertrophy.

This combination of lesions leads to a high right ventricular pressure and right-to-left shunting of blood through the VSD. Thus the patient is centrally cyanosed.

## CLINICAL FEATURES

Children with this condition may present with dyspnoea or fatigue or with hypoxic episodes (Fallot's spells), i.e. deep cyanosis and possible syncope, on exertion. Squatting is common.

Physical signs include a parasternal heave and a systolic ejection murmur, often associated with a thrill in the second left interspace close to the sternum. The second heart sound is usually single because the pulmonary component is too soft to be heard. Central cyanosis is commonly present from birth, and finger clubbing and polycythaemia are obvious after about 1 year. Growth may be retarded.

## INVESTIGATION

The chest X-ray shows a large right ventricle and a small pulmonary artery. The ECG reveals right ventricular hypertrophy and the echocardiogram demonstrates discontinuity between the aorta and the anterior wall of the ventricular septum. Cardiac catheterization is performed to evaluate the size and degree of the right ventricular outflow obstruction.

## TREATMENT

Complete surgical correction of this combination of lesions is possible even in infancy. Often a palliative procedure—an anastomosis between a subclavian artery and a pulmonary artery (Blalock shunt)—is performed on very young infants.

This operation results in an increased blood supply to the lungs. Fallot's spells may need treatment with β-blockade or, when severe, with diamorphine to relax the right ventricular outflow obstruction.

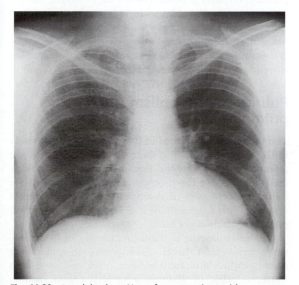

**Fig. 11.80**    PA plain chest X-ray from a patient with coarctation of the aorta. The prominent abnormality on this film is the 'erosion' ('scalloping') of the lower margins of the 5th, 6th and 7th ribs due to collateral flow in the intercostal arteries. On the upper mediastinal border is a small calcified bulge due to calcification of post-stenotic dilatation.

## Adolescent congenital heart disease

As more children with structural heart disease survive into adulthood there is a need for an increased awareness amongst general physicians and cardiologists of the problems posed by these young adults. Both atrial and ventricular arrhythmias are common sequels of long-standing structural heart disease and are often quite resistant to treatment. Sudden cardiac death is not uncommon. End-stage heart failure secondary to congenital heart disease can now be managed by heart or heart–lung transplantation.

# Pulmonary heart disease

## Pulmonary hypertension

An elevated pulmonary arterial pressure, known as pulmonary hypertension, has numerous causes:

CHRONIC LUNG DISEASE, which is diagnosed clinically and by abnormalities of lung function.

INCREASED PULMONARY BLOOD FLOW because of left-to-right shunting through a VSD, ASD or PDA.

LEFT VENTRICULAR FAILURE, MITRAL VALVE DISEASE, LEFT ATRIAL TUMOUR OR THROMBUS, OR PULMONARY VENO-OCCLUSIVE DISEASE, which cause an elevation in the pulmonary arterial pressure secondary to an elevation of the pulmonary venous and pulmonary capillary pressure; the pulmonary wedge pressure is elevated in these cases.

PULMONARY THROMBOEMBOLIC DISEASE.

PRIMARY PULMONARY HYPERTENSION, a rare condition seen predominantly in young women. Its aetiology is unknown but recurrent small pulmonary emboli, pulmonary vasoconstriction due to neural, humoral factors or drugs (e.g. oral contraceptives, *Crotalaria* teas and the appetite suppressant fenfluramine), connective-tissue disease and familial causes have all been suggested.

Pulmonary hypertension leads to enlarged proximal pulmonary arteries, right ventricular hypertrophy and right atrial dilatation. The pulmonary arterial changes depend on the aetiology of the pulmonary hypertension.

Multiple peripheral pulmonary arterial stenoses can produce a syndrome that is similar to pulmonary hypertension, but the pressure in the distal pulmonary bed is normal or low.

### CLINICAL FEATURES

Chest pain, exertional dyspnoea, syncope and fatigue are common symptoms, and sudden death may occur. Other symptoms are due to the cause of the pulmonary hypertension.

On physical examination there is a prominent *a* wave in the jugular venous pulse, a right ventricular (parasternal) heave and a loud pulmonary component to the second heart sound. Other findings include a right ventricular fourth heart sound, a systolic pulmonary ejection click, a mid-systolic ejection murmur and an early diastolic murmur due to pulmonary regurgitation (Graham Steell murmur). If tricuspid regurgitation develops, there is a pan-systolic murmur and a large jugular *v* wave.

### INVESTIGATION

The chest X-ray may show right ventricular enlargement and right atrial dilatation. The pulmonary artery is usually prominent and the enlarged proximal pulmonary arteries taper rapidly. Peripheral lung fields are oligaemic.

The ECG demonstrates right ventricular hypertrophy (right axis deviation, possibly a predominant R wave in lead $V_1$, and inverted T waves in right precordial leads) and a right atrial abnormality (tall peaked P waves in lead II) (Fig. 11.82).

Other investigations are performed to evaluate the cause of pulmonary hypertension. It is particularly important to look for treatable conditions such as left-to-right shunts, mitral stenosis or left atrial tumours with echocardiography. Radioisotope lung scans and sometimes open lung biopsy are performed, e.g. in young patients with severe pulmonary hypertension of unknown cause. Pulmonary angiography is dangerous and is rarely necessary.

### TREATMENT

Treatment is determined by the condition underlying pulmonary hypertension. Primary pulmonary hypertension is treated with anticoagulation (because of the possibility of recurrent thromboembolism). Diuretic treatment may be used for right ventricular failure, but care should be taken to avoid reduction of the left ventricular filling pressure. Hypoxia is avoided by the use of oxygen therapy when necessary. Vasodilators including calcium antagonists such as verapamil and prostacyclins have been tried, but with little long-term success. Usually there is a progressive downhill course. Heart and lung transplantation is recommended for young patients.

## Pulmonary embolism (acute cor pulmonale)

Thrombus, usually formed in the systemic veins or rarely in the right heart, may dislodge and embolize into the pulmonary arterial system. Post-mortem studies indicate that this is a very common condition (microemboli are found in up to 60% of autopsies) but it is not usually diagnosed this frequently in life. Ten per cent of clinical pulmonary emboli are fatal.

Conditions leading to the formation of clot in the systemic veins (and hence predisposing to pulmonary emboli) include prolonged bed rest, pelvic and lower limb fractures, pelvic or abdominal surgery, cardiac failure, pregnancy and childbirth, oral contraceptive drugs, malignant disease, chronic pulmonary disease and hypercoagulable states.

Atrial fibrillation may allow thrombus formation in the right atrium, and septal or right ventricular infarction

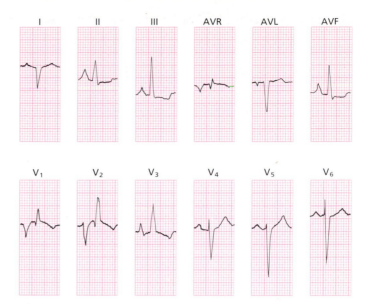

**Fig. 11.82** A 12-lead ECG demonstrating pulmonary hypertension. There is right axis deviation (+120°), right ventricular hypertrophy (dominant secondary R wave [R'] in V₁) and a combination of left and right atrial conduction abnormalities.

may favour thrombosis in the right ventricle. A small proportion (less than 10%) of pulmonary emboli are due to these cardiac causes.

After pulmonary embolism, lung tissue is ventilated but not perfused, resulting in impaired gas exchange. After some hours surfactant is no longer produced by the non-perfused lung, alveolar collapse occurs and hypoxaemia is the result. The haemodynamic consequence of pulmonary embolism is an elevation of pulmonary arterial pressure and a reduction in cardiac output. The zone of lung that is no longer perfused by the pulmonary artery may infarct but often does not do so because oxygen continues to be supplied by the bronchial circulation and the airways.

## CLINICAL FEATURES

A small embolus may present with effort dyspnoea, tiredness, syncope and, occasionally, cardiac arrhythmias.

A medium-sized embolus leading to pulmonary infarction can present with sudden onset of pleuritic pain, cough with haemoptysis, and dyspnoea.

A massive pulmonary embolus presents as a medical emergency: the patient has severe central chest pain and suddenly becomes shocked, pale and sweaty, with marked tachypnoea and tachycardia. Syncope may result if the cardiac output is transiently but dramatically reduced. Death may follow rapidly.

Physical signs vary according to the size of the embolus and the occurrence of pulmonary infarction:

A SMALL EMBOLUS may reveal no abnormal signs apart from a few basal crackles.

LARGE EMBOLI lead to a right ventricular heave, a gallop rhythm, tachycardia and a prominent *a* wave in the jugular venous pulse. The second heart sound may be loud because of pulmonary hypertension or soft if the cardiac output is very reduced. Continuous (systolic and diastolic) murmurs may be generated by turbulent

blood flow around the embolic obstructions.

WITH PULMONARY INFARCTION, a pleural rub and pyrexia may also be present.

DEEP VENOUS THROMBOSIS. Although a clinical deep venous thrombosis is not commonly observed, a detailed investigation of the lower limb and pelvic veins will reveal thrombosis in more than half of the cases.

## INVESTIGATION

The chest X-ray is often normal but the abrupt cut-off of a pulmonary artery or a translucency of an underperfused distal zone is occasionally seen. Later, atelectasis leads to opacities. An infarction may be visualized as a wedge-shaped opacity adjacent to the pleural edge, a pleural effusion and a raised hemidiaphragm. Past infarcts may be seen as opaque linear scars.

The ECG is usually normal except for sinus tachycardia. In relatively severe cases, however, right atrial dilatation produces tall, peaked P waves in lead II, and right ventricular hypertrophy and dilatation give rise to right axis deviation, some degree of right bundle branch block and T wave inversion in the right precordial leads (Fig. 11.83). The classical pattern of an S wave in lead I and a Q wave and inverted T waves in lead III (S1, Q3, T3), which reflects right ventricular 'strain', is not usually present.

If pulmonary infarction has occurred, there will be a polymorphonuclear leucocytosis, an elevated ESR and increased lactate dehydrogenase levels.

Pulmonary embolism usually results in arterial hypoxaemia and hypocapnia.

A pulmonary technetium-99m scintigram may demonstrate underperfused areas (Fig. 11.84). The specificity of this technique is greatly improved when combined with a ventilation scintigram performed after inhalation of radioactive xenon gas (see p. 646). The finding of a non-

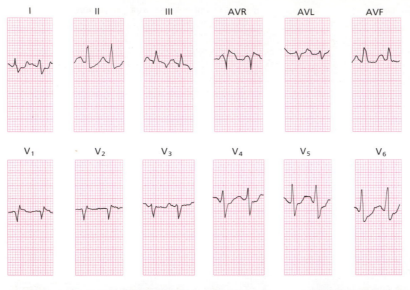

**Fig. 11.83** A 12-lead ECG demonstrating some features of acute pulmonary embolism. There is an S wave in lead I, a Q wave in lead III and an inverted T wave in lead III (the S1, Q3, T3 pattern). There is sinus tachycardia (160 b.p.m.) and an incomplete right bundle branch block pattern (an R wave in AVR and V₁ and an S wave in V₆).

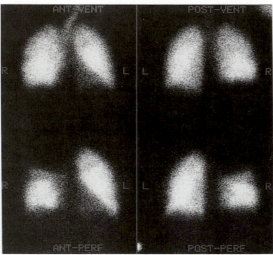

**Fig. 11.84** Ventilation (top) and perfusion (bottom) lung scans which demonstrate absence of perfusion but normal ventilation in the right upper lobe.

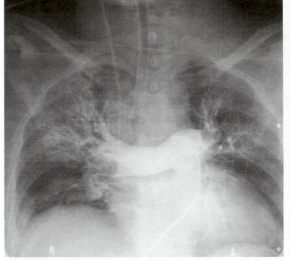

**Fig. 11.85** Contrast injected directly into the main pulmonary artery (pulmonary angiogram) demonstrates a large filling defect in the interlobar segment of the right pulmonary artery and extensive occlusion in the proximal left pulmonary artery.

perfused but ventilated zone is more suggestive of pulmonary embolism.

Pulmonary angiography is sometimes undertaken if surgery is considered in acute massive embolism. The test is performed by injecting contrast material through a catheter inserted into the main pulmonary artery. Filling defects or obstructed vessels can be delineated (Fig. 11.85). Angiography is hazardous but the risk may be reduced if contrast is injected into each pulmonary artery separately. If the patient is *in extremis* and the diagnosis is obvious, surgery should proceed without prior angiography.

## TREATMENT
### Prevention of further emboli
The basis of therapy is intravenous heparin, starting with a bolus of 10 000 U and followed by the continuous infusion of 1000–2000 U hour⁻¹. Oral anticoagulants are usually begun after 48 hours and the heparin is tapered off as the oral anticoagulant becomes effective. Oral anticoagulants are continued for 6 weeks to 6 months, depending on the likelihood of recurrence of venous thrombosis or embolism.

### Dissolution of the thrombus
Fibrinolytic therapy such as streptokinase (250 000 U by i.v. infusion over 30 min, followed by streptokinase 100 000 U i.v. hourly) is often used following a major embolism. It may also be given into the pulmonary artery.

## Surgery

Surgical embolectomy is rarely necessary, but when the haemodynamic circumstances are very severe there may be no alternative. Inferior vena caval interruption or plication, or the insertion of a filter into the inferior vena cava, may occasionally be necessary if anticoagulant or fibrinolytic therapy is contraindicated or fails to prevent recurrences of pulmonary embolism.

## Chronic cor pulmonale

Cor pulmonale is the commonest variety of pulmonary hypertensive heart disease.

### CAUSES

These are listed in Table 11.36.

### PATHOPHYSIOLOGY

Pulmonary vascular resistance is increased because of effective loss of pulmonary tissue and because of pulmonary vasoconstriction caused by hypoxia and acidosis. The increased pulmonary vascular resistance leads to pulmonary hypertension, which initially occurs only during an acute respiratory infection. Eventually, the pulmonary hypertension becomes persistent and progressively more severe. The pulmonary vascular bed is gradually obliterated by muscular hypertrophy of the arterioles and thrombus formation. Right ventricular function is progressively compromised because of the increased pressure load. Hypoxia further impairs right ventricular function, and, as it develops, left ventricular function is also depressed.

### CLINICAL FEATURES

The clinical features are those of pulmonary hypertension and right ventricular failure occurring in patients with chronic chest disease. The dominant clinical picture depends on the type of lung disease.

### TREATMENT

Vigorous therapy of the pulmonary condition may lead to marked improvement of blood gases and consequent improvement of the heart failure. Acute chest infections must be treated promptly. Oxygen therapy over a long period may reduce established pulmonary hypertension, with improvement in overall prognosis (see p. 661). Any heart failure should be treated (see p. 573). Extensive surgical removal of organized thrombus may be considered.

## Atrial myxoma

This is the commonest primary cardiac tumour. A myxoma usually develops in the left atrium and is a polypoid, gelatinous structure attached by a pedicle to the atrial septum. The tumour may obstruct the mitral valve or may be a site of thrombi that then embolize. It is also associated with constitutional symptoms: the patient may present with dyspnoea, syncope or a mild fever. The most important physical signs are a loud first heart sound, a tumour 'plop' (a loud third heart sound produced as the pedunculated tumour comes to an abrupt halt), a mid-diastolic murmur, and signs due to embolization. A raised ESR is usually present.

The diagnosis is easily made by echocardiography because the tumour is demonstrated as a dense space-occupying lesion (Fig. 11.86). Surgical removal usually results in a complete cure.

Myxomas may also occur in the right atrium or in the ventricles. Other primary cardiac tumours include rhabdomyomas and sarcomas.

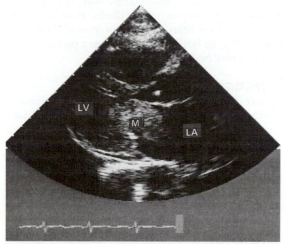

**Fig. 11.86** Two-dimensional echocardiogram (long-axis view) showing an echo-dense mass obstructing the mitral valve orifice. This was removed surgically and proved to be an atrial myxoma. LV, left ventricle; LA, left atrium; M, mass.

## Myocardial disease

Myocardial disease that is not due to a specific heart muscle disorder or a known infiltrative, metabolic/toxic or neuromuscular disorder may be caused by:

Intrinsic lung disease, e.g.
  Chronic bronchitis and emphysema
  Asthma
  Pulmonary fibrosis
Recurrent pulmonary emboli
Skeletal abnormalities, e.g
  Kyphoscoliosis
Hypoventilation, e.g.
  Morbid obesity (Pickwickian syndrome)
Neuromuscular disease, e.g.
  Poliomyelitis
  Myasthenia gravis
Obstruction, e.g.
  Sleep-apnoea syndrome

**Table 11.36**  Causes of cor pulmonale.

- An acute or chronic inflammatory pathology (myocarditis)
- Idiopathic myocardial disease (cardiomyopathy)

## MYOCARDITIS

Myocarditis, whether idiopathic or infective, is the most common form of inflammatory endomyocardial disease. A definitive aetiology with isolation of viruses or bacteria is uncommon. Causative factors include:

VIRUSES, particularly Coxsackie, influenza, rubella, polio, adenovirus and echovirus.

PROTOZOA, e.g. *Trypanosoma cruzi*, which causes Chagas' disease and is endemic in central and South America, and *Toxoplasma gondii*—a common cause of myocarditis in the newborn or in immunologically compromised adults.

RADIATION, CHEMICALS AND DRUGS, e.g. lead poisoning, emetine and chloroquine.

BACTERIAL INFECTION, e.g. diphtheria, which is due to an exotoxin produced by *Corynebacterium, Rickettsia, Chlamydia, Coxiella* (the causative agent of Q fever).

### CLINICAL FEATURES

Patients present with an acute illness, often characterized by fever and cardiac failure. There may be a history of previous respiratory or febrile illness. Physical examination reveals soft heart sounds, a prominent third sound and tachycardia (gallop rhythm). Often a pericardial friction rub may be heard.

### INVESTIGATION

CHEST X-RAY may show some cardiac enlargement, depending on the stage and virulence of the disease.

THE ECG demonstrates ST and T wave abnormalities and arrhythmias. Diphtheritic myocarditis may induce heart block, and Chagas' disease produces both heart block and ventricular tachyarrhythmias.

CARDIAC ENZYMES are elevated.

CARDIAC BIOPSY shows acute inflammation.

VIRAL ANTIBODY TITRES may be increased.

### TREATMENT

General management includes bed rest and the eradication of any acute infection. Therapy is directed towards the management of cardiac failure and the treatment of cardiac arrhythmias. Depending on the aetiology, the prognosis is usually good, although a chronic cardiomyopathy may occasionally ensue.

## CARDIOMYOPATHY

These idiopathic conditions are classified according to their clinical presentation as:

1 Dilated cardiomyopathy—ventricular dilatation

2 Hypertrophic cardiomyopathy—myocardial hypertrophy

3 Restrictive cardiomyopathy—impaired ventricular filling

## Dilated cardiomyopathy (DCM)

DCM is characterized by dilatation and impaired systolic function of the left ventricle and/or right ventricle. The aetiology of idiopathic DCM is unknown. The frequency of the ACE DD genotype (see p. 110) is higher than matched controls suggesting that ACE gene variants may contribute to the pathogenesis. There is also an association with viral (Coxsackie) infection and an immune-mediated pathogenesis is likely. Many cases of systemic heart muscle disease present with clinical features of DCM and they include:

CARDIOVASCULAR DISEASE (ischaemic, rheumatic, congenital, systemic hypertension)

GENERALIZED DISEASE, e.g. haemochromatosis, sarcoidosis

CONNECTIVE TISSUE DISORDERS, e.g. systemic lupus erythematosus, systemic sclerosis

NEUROMUSCULAR DISEASE, e.g. muscular dystrophy, Friedreich's ataxia

GLYCOGEN STORAGE DISEASE, e.g. Pompe's disease

PRIMARY HEART MUSCLE DISEASE, e.g. amyloidosis

ALCOHOL EXCESS

CYTOTOXIC DRUG THERAPY, e.g. doxorubicin, cyclophosphamide

### CLINICAL FEATURES

Symptoms depend on the relative degree of right and left heart failure and the incidence of cardiac arrhythmias and emboli.

Physical signs reflect heart failure, i.e. cardiomegaly, tachycardia, jugular venous pressure elevation, third or fourth heart sounds and basal crackles. Ventricular dilatation leads to functional mitral or tricuspid valvular regurgitation.

### INVESTIGATION

CHEST X-RAY demonstrates generalized cardiac enlargement

THE ECG shows diffuse non-specific ST segment and T wave changes. Conduction disturbances, sinus tachycardia and arrhythmias (such as atrial fibrillation, ventricular premature contractions or ventricular tachycardia) may also be seen.

THE ECHOCARDIOGRAM reveals dilatation of the left ventricle and/or right ventricle with poor global contraction (Fig. 11.87).

CARDIAC BIOPSY shows variable fibrosis and non-specific leucocyte infiltration. Infiltrative disorders (e.g. amyloid) may be detected in specific cases.

### TREATMENT

Management involves the conventional treatment of heart failure and arrhythmias. A history of embolization is an

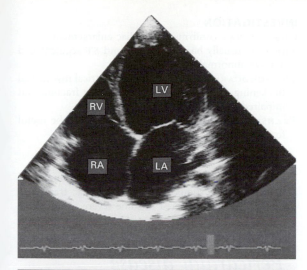

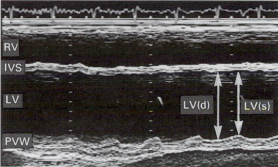

**Fig. 11.87** Two-dimensional (apical four-chamber view) and M-mode echocardiograms in a case of dilated cardiomyopathy. The heart has a 'globular' appearance with all four chambers dilated. The extremely impaired left ventricular function can be appreciated from the M-mode recording. Compare the systolic shortening fraction with that of Figs 11.22 and 11.74. LA, left atrium; RA, right atrium; LV, left ventricle; LV(d) and LV(s), diastolic and systolic left ventricular dimensions; IVS, interventricular septum; PVW, posterior ventricular wall.

indication for anticoagulant treatment. Prolonged bed rest, corticosteroid therapy, the avoidance of alcohol, and nutritional supplements may be indicated in special cases. Metoprolol has been shown to improve haemodynamic and clinical function in some patients. Severe congestive cardiomyopathy in relatively young adults is treated with cardiac transplantation.

## Hypertrophic cardiomyopathy (HCM)

Also known as hypertrophic obstructive cardiomyopathy (HOCM), this is characterized by marked hypertrophy of the left and/or right ventricle, particularly the interventricular septum in the absence of a cardiac or systemic cause. The hypertrophied muscle results in distorted left ventricular contraction and abnormal mitral valve movement during systole. Some degree of mitral regurgitation may develop. Apposition of the anterior cusp of the mitral valve to the hypertrophied septum may cause some

obstruction to left ventricular emptying. About half of the cases of HCM are familial and due to a genetic disorder of cardiac β-myosin heavy chain (βMHC). In the families with a high instance of sudden death, there is an increased frequency of ACE gene polymorphism (DD) (see p. 110). It has been suggested that allele D, which is associated with increased plasma ACE levels, interacts with growth regulators, e.g. c-*myc*. Thus the high frequency of allele D and different βMHC mutations may account for the variable clinical presentations of HCM. The aetiology is unknown in sporadic cases. The failure of hypertrophy to manifest before completion of the adolescent growth phase may make diagnosis difficult in children.

### CLINICAL FEATURES

Patients with this condition may present with syncope or presyncope (typically exertional), angina, cardiac arrhythmias or sudden death. As with other cardiomyopathies, dyspnoea due to left ventricular failure is a common but late presentation. In this case left ventricular failure is not due to the failing contractile function of the myocardium; instead, it is due to the inability of the heart muscle to relax. Thus, left ventricular filling and therefore left ventricular emptying are impaired.

The classical physical findings are:

DOUBLE APICAL PULSATION (forceful atrial contraction produces a palpable fourth heart sound)

JERKY CAROTID PULSE because of rapid ejection and sudden obstruction to left ventricular outflow during asystole

EJECTION SYSTOLIC MURMUR because of left ventricular outflow obstruction late in systole that can be increased by physical manoeuvres, e.g. Valsalva, squatting

PAN-SYSTOLIC MURMUR due to mitral regurgitation

FOURTH HEART SOUND

### INVESTIGATION

CHEST X-RAY is usually unremarkable.

THE ECG demonstrates left ventricular hypertrophy (see Fig. 11.69) and ST and T wave changes.

THE ECHOCARDIOGRAM is diagnostic because it shows septal hypertrophy (greater than the hypertrophy of the posterior wall), abnormal mitral valve movement and a very vigorously contracting ventricle (Fig. 11.88).

### TREATMENT

Firstly, sudden death must be avoided by antiarrhythmic treatment. Long-term amiodarone treatment is effective. Syncope or chest pain may be treated with β-blockade. Vasodilators should be avoided because they may aggravate left ventricular outflow obstruction owing to peripheral venous blood pooling. Occasionally, resection of septal myocardium may be indicated.

## Restrictive cardiomyopathy

Some cardiomyopathies do not present with muscular hypertrophy or ventricular dilatation. Instead, ventricular

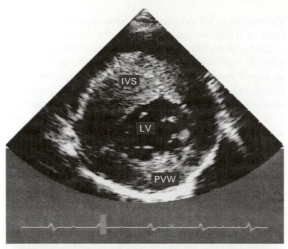

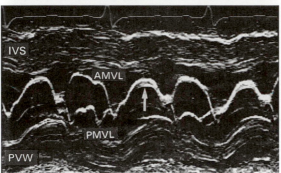

**Fig. 11.88**  Two-dimensional echocardiogram (short-axis view) and M-mode recording of the mitral valve in a case of hypertrophic cardiomyopathy. The grossly thickened interventricular septum is shown, resulting in a small left ventricular cavity. This condition is associated with an abnormal anterior motion of the mitral valve during systole (arrowed). IVS, interventricular septum; LV, left ventricle; PVW, posterior ventricular wall; AMVL, PMVL, anterior and posterior mitral valve leaflets.

filling is restricted (as with constrictive pericarditis).

Conditions associated with this form of cardiomyopathy are amyloidosis, sarcoidosis, Loeffler's endocarditis and endomyocardial fibrosis; in the latter two conditions there is myocardial and endocardial fibrosis associated with eosinophilia. Thrombus formation is common in restrictive cardiomyopathy.

### CLINICAL FEATURES

Dyspnoea, fatigue and embolic symptoms may be the presenting features. Restriction to ventricular filling also results in persistently elevated venous pressures and consequent hepatic enlargement, ascites and dependent oedema.

Physical signs are similar to those of constrictive pericarditis, i.e. a high jugular venous pressure with diastolic collapse (Friedreich's sign) and elevation of the jugular venous pressure with inspiration (Kussmaul's sign). Cardiac enlargement with a third or fourth heart sound is common.

### INVESTIGATION

CHEST X-RAY confirms the cardiac enlargement.

THE ECG usually has low-voltage and ST segment and T wave abnormalities.

THE ECHOCARDIOGRAM shows symmetrical myocardial thickening and a normal systolic ejection fraction, but impaired ventricular filling.

TRANSVENOUS ENDOCARDIAL BIOPSY may be useful for more detailed diagnosis.

### TREATMENT

There is no specific treatment. Cardiac failure and embolic problems should be treated. Cardiac transplantation should be considered in some severe cases.

# Pericardial disease

The normal pericardium lubricates the surface of the heart, prevents sudden deformation or dislocation of the heart, and acts as a barrier to the spread of infection. There are three common presentations of pericardial disease:

1 Acute pericarditis
2 Pericardial effusion
3 Constrictive pericarditis

## Acute pericarditis

Inflammation of the pericardium gives rise to chest pain that is substernal and sharp. It may be referred to the neck or shoulders. It is relieved by sitting forward and made worse by lying down and, like pleurisy, is aggravated by movement and respiration.

Acute pericarditis has numerous aetiologies, but Coxsackie viral infections and myocardial infarction are the commonest causes in the UK. Viral pericarditis can occur in epidemics. Other aetiologies include uraemia, connective tissue disease, trauma, postpericardiotomy, rheumatic fever, tuberculosis and malignancy.

### CLINICAL FEATURES

The cardinal clinical sign is a pericardial friction rub. There is usually a fever when pericarditis is due to viral or bacterial infection, rheumatic fever or myocardial infarction.

### INVESTIGATION

During the first week of the illness the ECG shows ST segment elevation, concave upwards, in all leads facing the epicardial surface, i.e. the anterior, lateral and inferior leads (Fig. 11.89). ST segment depression is only seen in the cavity leads (AVR and $V_1$). Later, the ST segment falls and T wave inversion develops. As the illness improves the T waves become normal.

Cardiac enzymes may be elevated if there is associated myocarditis.

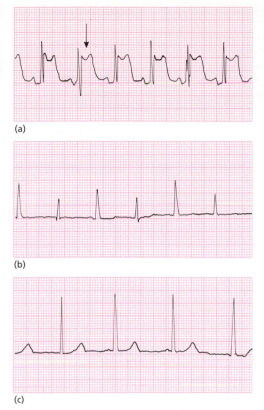

(a)

(b)

(c)

**Fig. 11.89**   ECGs associated with pericarditis.
(a) Acute pericarditis. Note the raised ST segment, concave
upwards (arrow).
(b) Chronic phase of pericarditis associated with a pericardial
effusion. Note the T wave flattening and inversion and the
alternation of the QRS amplitude (QRS alternans).
(c) The same patient after evacuation of the pericardial fluid.
Note that the QRS voltage has increased and the T waves
have returned to normal.

## TREATMENT

Treatment consists of anti-inflammatory medication such
as oral aspirin, naproxen or indomethacin. Occasionally,
if pericarditis is severe or recurrent, systemic corticosteroids may be needed.

### VARIETIES OF PERICARDITIS
#### Viral pericarditis

This tends to affect young adults and is sudden in onset.
Usually, the illness lasts for only a few weeks and the
prognosis is good, although sudden deaths do occur.
However, recurrences do occur.

#### Bacterial pericarditis

Septicaemia or pneumonia may rarely be complicated by
purulent pericarditis. *Staphylococcus* and *Haemophilus
influenzae* account for two-thirds of such cases.

Antibiotics and surgical drainage may be required. This
form of pericarditis, especially when due to *Staphylococcus*, is usually fatal.

#### Tuberculous pericarditis

This is typified by a chronic low-grade fever, especially in
the evening, associated with signs and symptoms of acute
pericarditis, malaise and weight loss. Pericardial aspiration may be required to make the diagnosis. The pericardial effusion is usually serous but may be blood-stained.
Specific antituberculous chemotherapy is needed.

#### Uraemic pericarditis

This is often asymptomatic. It usually develops in the terminal stages of uraemia.

#### Pericarditis following myocardial infarction

A pericardial friction rub and the recurrence of chest pain
and fever occurs in about 20% of patients during the first
few days after myocardial infarction, especially anterior
wall infarction.

#### Dressler's syndrome

This is pericarditis occurring 1 month to 1 year after an
acute myocardial infarction (see p. 589).

#### Malignant pericarditis

Carcinoma of the bronchus, carcinoma of the breast and
Hodgkin's disease are the most common tumours to
infiltrate the pericardium. Leukaemia and malignant
melanoma are also associated with pericarditis.
Pericardiocentesis may be useful in diagnosing the
malignancy.

## Pericardial effusion

Although acute pericarditis is initially dry and fibrinous,
almost all aetiologies of this inflammatory reaction also
induce the formation of a pericardial effusion. The
effusion collects in the closed pericardium. When the
pericardium can distend no more, it may produce mechanical embarrassment to the circulation by preventing
ventricular filling; this is called cardiac tamponade.

### CLINICAL FEATURES

The clinical features include a raised jugular venous
pressure, with sharp diastolic collapse—y descent
(Friedreich's sign), a paradoxical pulse (the blood pressure falls during inspiration), increased neck vein distension during inspiration (Kussmaul's sign) and reduced
cardiac output. Because of the effusion, the apex beat may
not be palpable and heart sounds are soft. Although a
friction rub is often heard, it may be quieter than before
the fluid accumulated as the effusion separates the
visceral from the parietal pericardium.

### INVESTIGATION

The ECG shows reduced voltages, and the chest X-ray
may demonstrate an increasingly large globular heart with
sharp outlines. The pulmonary veins are typically not
distended.

Echocardiography is the most useful technique for
demonstrating a pericardial effusion (see Fig. 11.25).

## TREATMENT

When the effusion collects rapidly and the circulation is embarrassed, the effusion must be tapped. Pericardiocentesis is also indicated when a malignant, tuberculous or a purulent effusion is suspected. In the UK, malignancy is the most common cause of reaccumulation of pericardial effusion. Reaccumulation may require pericardial fenestration, i.e. the creation of a pericardial window, either transcutaneously via a balloon pericardiotomy under local anaesthesia or using a conventional surgical approach.

## Constrictive pericarditis

Following tuberculous pericarditis, haemopericardium, or acute pericarditis due to viral infection, bacterial infection or rheumatic heart disease, the pericardium may become thick, fibrous and calcified. The heart is then encased in a solid shell and cannot fill properly.

### CLINICAL FEATURES

There are signs of systemic venous congestion, i.e. ascites, dependent oedema, hepatomegaly and jugular venous distension, without much breathlessness or pulmonary venous distension. There are also signs of impaired ventricular filling, i.e. Kussmaul's sign, Friedreich's sign and pulsus paradoxus.

Atrial fibrillation is common (30%) and a loud heart sound, called a pericardial knock, due to rapid ventricular filling may be heard. This is an early third heart sound.

Other causes of ascites must be excluded (see p. 266).

### INVESTIGATION

The chest X-ray shows a relatively small heart with obvious calcification seen on the lateral film and using fluoroscopy.

The ECG shows low QRS voltages and T wave inversion, and the echocardiogram will demonstrate the thickened pericardium and the relative immobility of the heart. CT is also good at detecting thickness and calcification of the pericardium.

### TREATMENT

Treatment involves the surgical removal of a substantial proportion of the pericardium. About half the patients do well, but in the others persistent constriction, atrial fibrillation and myocardial disease prevent full recovery.

## *The cardiovascular system in systemic disease*

The heart can be involved in many diseases (Table 11.37).

## *Systemic hypertension*

Blood pressure within a population has a skewed distribution, i.e. there is a single peak frequency of blood press-

| Disease | Cardiac involvement |
|---|---|
| *Endocrine disorders* | |
| Diabetes mellitus | Coronary artery disease |
| Thyrotoxicosis | Atrial fibrillation |
| | Cardiomyopathy |
| Hypothyroidism | Bradycardia |
| | Heart failure |
| | Coronary disease |
| | Pericardial effusion |
| Acromegaly | Cardiomegaly |
| | Hypertension |
| | Cardiac arrhythmias |
| Cushing's syndrome | Hypertension |
| Conn's syndrome | Hypertension |
| Phaeochromocytoma | Hypertension |
| *Connective-tissue disorders* | |
| Systemic lupus erythematosus | Non-infective endocarditis (Libman–Sachs) |
| | Myocarditis |
| | Pericarditis |
| Systemic sclerosis | Myocarditis |
| | Pericarditis |
| | Arrhythmias |
| Polyarteritis nodosa | Hypertension |
| | Pericarditis |
| | Arrhythmias |
| Rheumatoid disease and ankylosing spondylitis | Aortic and mitral regurgitation |
| | Pericarditis |
| *Miscellaneous* | |
| Renal failure | Hypertension |
| | Heart failure |
| | Pericarditis |
| | Infective endocarditis |
| Morbid obesity | Hypertension |
| | Cardiomegaly |
| | Associated with atherosclerotic coronary artery disease |
| Gout | Hypertension |
| Carcinoid syndrome | Pulmonary stenosis |
| | Tricuspid stenosis |
| Alcohol | Cardiomyopathy |
| | Atrial arrhythmias |
| Syphilis | Aortic regurgitation |
| | Coronary arterial stenosis (ostial) |
| | Ascending aortic aneurysm |

**Table 11.37** Cardiac involvement in some systemic disorders.

ure and there are more individuals with high pressures than low pressures. Different populations have different levels of blood pressure, with those of African origin tending to have higher pressure than Caucasians, i.e. the whole distribution is shifted to the left. The distribution curves for systolic and diastolic blood pressure are similar. Risk of mortality and morbidity rises continuously with increasing blood pressure throughout the range. The rise of risk is not linear, however, being steeper at higher pressures.

The level of blood pressure can be said to be abnormal when it is associated with a clear increase in morbidity and mortality. This level varies with age, sex, race and country. For life insurance reasons and for simple clinical purposes, a diastolic blood pressure in a young adult above 100 mmHg and/or 160 mmHg systolic is taken as definitely hypertensive and a diastolic pressure above 95 mmHg is regarded as probably hypertensive. The World Health Organization have used a definition of 160/95 mmHg, and in Framingham (a small town in Massachusetts, USA), where a very detailed population study is being carried out, 160/95 mmHg was deemed abnormal and 140/90 to 160/95 mmHg was regarded as borderline. The significance of a single elevated reading is unclear and for a firm diagnosis the blood pressure should be elevated on more than one examination.

In a proportion of patients the blood pressure increases due to the presence of a doctor ('white coat hypertension'). In patients without probable target organ damage, some weeks or months can be taken to be sure that the blood pressure is elevated. The blood pressure should be taken twice with the patient in the sitting position and this should be repeated three or four times over several months. When target organ damage is present or the blood pressure reading is very high, a more urgent assessment is needed.

If there is any doubt about the validity of blood pressure measurements taken in the clinic, ambulatory blood pressure monitoring offers a non-invasive assessment during normal daily activities and largely circumvents the problem of 'white coat hypertension'.

## CAUSES

In the large majority of cases no cause can be identified, and this form of hypertension is known as primary or essential. A cause of hypertension can be discovered in less than 10% of patients; such cases are known as secondary hypertension.

### Essential hypertension

No single factor has been found to explain essential hypertension; many factors are probably responsible. The blood pressure is determined by the product of the cardiac output and the peripheral vascular resistance.

In the early stages of essential hypertension the increase of blood pressure is due to a small increase in cardiac output. This could be due to sympathetic overactivity. Later in the disease, the cardiac output is normal but the peripheral resistance is increased. It is possible that the initial increase in cardiac output induces vascular changes that then sustain and increase the blood pressure.

The baroreceptor reflexes operate at a higher pressure in hypertension. An increased blood pressure should stimulate a bradycardia via the carotid sinus baroreceptor mechanism. This does not happen in essential hypertension. This abnormal reflex may be due to the hypertension rather than being its cause.

The causes of essential hypertension include the following.

GENETIC FACTORS. Racial and familial tendencies to high blood pressure are found.

ENVIRONMENTAL FACTORS. Numerous factors have been related to the development of hypertension but only the following appear to be important.

OBESITY. Blood pressure rises with increasing obesity. This relationship persists even when errors of blood pressure measurement in obese subjects (cuff artefact, see p. 530) are taken into account.

ALCOHOL INTAKE. Ingestion of alcohol acutely raises blood pressure and alcohol intake tends to be higher in individuals with higher pressures. Reduction or withdrawal of regular alcohol intake reduces blood pressure 5–10 mmHg.

SALT INTAKE. There is much controversy about the role of salt in hypertension. There is some evidence of a relationship between the salt intake of an individual and the level of the blood pressure *within* populations. Similar, but weaker relationships are found between populations. There is less convincing evidence that a moderate reduction of salt intake will reduce blood pressure. Salt intake may increase intravascular volume in the initial stages of the genesis of hypertension, but once peripheral vascular resistance becomes raised, alterations of salt intake may play little part in the regulation of blood pressure.

HUMORAL FACTORS have been implicated in the genesis of hypertension including catecholamines, the renin–angiotensin system, and atrial natriuretic peptide. Convincing evidence is lacking that any of these are involved.

### Secondary hypertension

This should always be considered in patients with hypertension. In particular, a careful search should be made in hypertensive patients presenting under the age of 35 years. The causes of secondary hypertension can be divided into the following.

RENAL CAUSES (see p. 463). Renal diseases are the most common causes of secondary hypertension, accounting for over 80% of cases. Chronic glomerulonephritis, chronic atrophic pyelonephritis and congenital polycystic kidneys are the conditions usually involved. It may be difficult to determine whether renal disease has caused hypertension or whether the hypertension has produced the renal disease.

The mechanism by which renal disease causes hypertension is probably related to salt and water retention. Occasionally, renal artery stenosis due to fibromuscular hyperplasia or atheroma may cause hypertension (renovascular hypertension) owing to excess renin production (see p. 464).

ENDOCRINE CAUSES (see Table 16.39). These include:
- Conn's syndrome
- Adrenal hyperplasia

- Phaeochromocytoma
- Cushing's syndrome
- Acromegaly

CARDIOVASCULAR CAUSES. Renovascular hypertension is discussed above.

Coarctation of the aorta (see p. 608) should be considered in young patients with hypertension and a late systolic murmur.

PREGNANCY. Hypertension in the early stages of pregnancy is usually essential hypertension or due to renal disease.

Pre-eclampsia or toxaemia of pregnancy is diagnosed when hypertension develops in the last 3 months of pregnancy and is associated with oedema and proteinuria. The cause of pre-eclampsia is unknown.

Pre-eclampsia may worsen, with the development of severe hypertension, nausea, vomiting, pulmonary oedema and fits. This condition, known as eclampsia, needs urgent treatment (see p. 624).

DRUGS. Oestrogen-containing contraceptives, other steroids, carbenoxolone, liquorice and vasopressin may all cause hypertension. Paroxysms of severe hypertension may occur in patients taking monoamine oxidase inhibitors who eat cheese or other tyramine-containing foods and those who drink wines.

## PATHOPHYSIOLOGY

An increase in vascular tone initially accounts for the increased peripheral vascular resistance. As the disease progresses, the walls of small arteries thicken and atheroma develops in larger arteries. Malignant hypertension is characterized by fibrinoid necrosis of the vascular wall.

The increased peripheral vascular resistance leads to a greater impedance to left ventricular emptying. Consequently, left ventricular hypertrophy develops.

A reduction in renal perfusion pressure can occur, leading to decreased glomerular filtration and reduced sodium and water excretion. The renal changes are described in more detail on p. 463. The decreased renal perfusion leads to the production of renin, which converts angiotensinogen to angiotensin I. This is changed to angiotensin II, which stimulates the secretion of aldosterone and further contributes to salt and water retention (see Fig. 16.28).

Secondary aldosteronism, which occurs with severe or accelerated hypertension and with the use of diuretics, is characterized by high serum levels of aldosterone and renin. In primary aldosteronism (Conn's syndrome), only the aldosterone is raised. About 10% of patients with essential hypertension have a high plasma renin level, and 25% have a low renin level.

In some cases the pressure rises rapidly and these patients are said to have 'malignant' hypertension. Without treatment death occurs within 1–2 years.

The accelerated rise in blood pressure produces cerebral oedema, left ventricular failure and severe renal impairment, with proteinuria and microscopic haematuria. Retinal haemorrhages, exudates and papilloedema are also seen and are diagnostic of malignant hypertension.

## COMPLICATIONS

Hypertension is a risk factor for developing atheroma and patients may therefore develop thrombotic cerebral vascular disease, coronary artery disease and peripheral vascular disease. The increased pressure in the circulation can result in heart failure, cerebral haemorrhage, renal disease and dissecting aortic aneurysms.

## ASSESSMENT OF PATIENTS

The possible causes and consequences of hypertension are assessed. In uncomplicated or essential hypertension, apart from the high blood pressure there are usually no signs, symptoms or abnormal investigations.

### History

The patient with mild hypertension is usually asymptomatic. Nose bleeds and headaches have been traditionally regarded as possible symptoms, but are probably no commoner than in the general population. There may be a past history of renal disease or a family history of hypertension.

Secondary causes of hypertension are suggested by a specific history, such as attacks of sweating and tachycardia in phaeochromocytoma.

Angina may occur either because of associated coronary artery disease or because of the high oxygen demand from hypertrophied muscle. If cardiac failure develops, breathlessness occurs.

Accelerated or malignant hypertension presents with visual impairment, nausea and vomiting, fits, transient paralysis, severe headaches, impairment of consciousness, or symptoms of acute cardiac failure.

### Examination

In the majority of patients the only sign is the high blood pressure, but in others features of the cause of hypertension may be noted. For example, there may be abdominal bruit due to renovascular obstruction, or delayed femoral pulses due to coarctation of the aorta.

Hypertensive heart disease presents with a loud aortic second sound, a prominent left ventricular apical heave and a fourth heart sound. Sinus tachycardia and a third heart sound develop if cardiac failure occurs.

Examination of the retina may reveal various abnormalities which are known as Keith–Wagener retinal changes. They are graded as follows:

GRADE 1—increased tortuosity of retinal arteries and increased reflectiveness (silver wiring)

GRADE 2—grade 1 plus the appearance of arteriovenous nipping produced when thickened retinal arteries pass over the retinal veins

GRADE 3—grade 2 plus flame-shaped haemorrhages and soft 'cotton wool' exudates

GRADE 4—grade 3 plus papilloedema (bulging and blurring of the edges of the optic disc)

The presence of haemorrhages, exudates or papilloedema

is diagnostic of malignant hypertension which requires urgent treatment.

## INVESTIGATION (see also p. 822)

Routine investigation of a hypertensive patient should always include:

- Chest X-ray
- ECG
- Echocardiogram
- Urinalysis
- Fasting blood lipids
- Urea, creatinine and electrolytes

If the urea or the creatinine level is abnormal, creatinine clearance, intravenous excretion urography, renal ultrasound and other tests of renal function are necessary. If the tests of renal function or an abnormal bruit suggest a renovascular cause, full renal investigation is essential.

If coarctation of the aorta is suspected, digital vascular imaging with intravenous contrast injection or MRI will usually demonstrate the lesion.

If the patient is not taking diuretics, a low serum potassium should suggest an endocrine problem, and aldosterone, cortisol and renin measurements should be performed. A history suggestive of phaeochromocytoma can be investigated with measurement of serum catecholamines or urinary catecholamine metabolites.

The chest X-ray may show a large heart and pulmonary congestion if heart failure has developed, or rib notching in coarctation of the aorta.

The ECG may show left ventricular hypertrophy or signs of myocardial infarction or ischaemia. Very rarely, ECG features of hyperkalaemia (see Fig. 10.6) (e.g. with renal failure) or hypokalaemia may be detected.

## TREATMENT

In the young, the secondary causes of hypertension should be excluded before treatment is commenced. When the blood pressure is only mildly or moderately elevated, it may be difficult to persuade an asymptomatic patient that treatment is necessary. However, there are definite advantages from treating diastolic blood pressures in excess of 100 mmHg. If the diastolic blood pressure is between 90 and 100 mmHg it should be carefully reassessed on several occasions with the patient in a comfortable, relaxed position. If it is truly elevated (above 90 mmHg) it should be actively treated, especially in young men, and particularly so if there is any evidence of retinal, cardiac or renal end-organ damage. There is no evidence to support treating mild to moderate blood pressure elevation in the very old (>80 years). However, patients between 65 and 80 years with a diastolic pressure above 90 mmHg or a systolic blood pressure above 160 mmHg or both do benefit from treatment. The Framingham studies have shown that the systolic blood pressure in this group is as important as the diastolic blood pressure and is the best guide to the risk of peripheral arterial disease. Thus, a man with a systolic pressure of 170 mmHg has twice the risk of dying compared with a man with a systolic pressure of 120 mmHg. Only in the elderly has it been demonstrated that isolated systolic hypertension is associated with an increased risk of cardiovascular events. Nevertheless it is recommended that patients of all ages with a persistent systolic pressure above 160 mmHg should be treated. The thresholds for drug treatment of hypertension which have been recommended by the British Hypertension Society are illustrated in Fig. 11.90.

### General measures

A review of the patient's life-style and diet may suggest modifications that could lead to some reduction of blood pressure, such as:

WEIGHT REDUCTION. Obese patients should lose weight. This leads to a true fall in blood pressure as well as to a reduction of artefactually increased cuff measurements.

REDUCTION OF HEAVY ALCOHOL CONSUMPTION. This also leads to a small reduction in blood pressure of around 5–10 mmHg.

SALT RESTRICTION. This is generally of little effect except in some individuals. Usually, the patient is advised not to add salt at the table.

REGULAR EXERCISE, MEDITATION AND BIOFEEDBACK. These are all techniques that have been claimed to lead to blood pressure reduction. An attempt should be made to reduce stress and anxiety.

Young people should jog for 30 min three times per week and elderly patients should walk longer distances than usual.

Patients should also be told to stop smoking to reduce their overall coronary risk. It is doubtful whether cessation of smoking reduces the blood pressure except in malignant hypertension. Hyperlipidaemia should also be corrected (see p. 858) to reduce the risk of atheroma.

### Drug treatment

A large number of drugs are used to treat hypertension (Table 11.38). This reflects the difficulty in finding a single drug that effectively lowers blood pressure without producing side-effects that may be more troublesome or more dangerous than the hypertension itself. Compliance is a problem as the side-effects of drug therapy are frequent and the immediate benefits of treatment are not obvious to the patient.

### Available drugs

DIURETICS. Loop diuretics (e.g. frusemide 40 mg daily or bumetanide 1–2 mg daily) and thiazide diuretics (e.g. bendrofluazide 5 mg daily or cyclopenthiazide 0.5 mg daily) are equally effective at lowering the blood pressure. Thiazides are usually preferred because the duration of action is longer, the diuresis is not so severe, and they cost less. Loop diuretics are restricted to those with cardiac or renal impairment for whom an additional diuretic effect is required.

Although diuretics may lower blood pressure transiently by sodium and water excretion, they also act by directly dilating arterioles. Oral potassium supplements are often not required. Occasionally, hypokalaemia occurs and this is most effectively treated with a potassium-sparing diuretic.

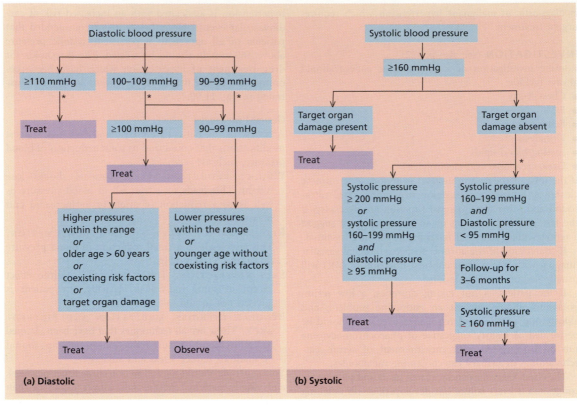

**Fig. 11.90**  Thresholds for treatment of diastolic (a) and systolic (b) hypertension as recommended by the British Hypertension Society. From P. Sever *et al.* (1993) *British Medical Journal* 306: 983–987. *, Repeated measurements.

| Associated disease | Diuretic | β-Blocker | ACE inhibitor | Calcium blocker | α₁-Blocker |
|---|---|---|---|---|---|
| Diabetes | Care[a] | Care[b] | Yes | Yes | Yes |
| Gout | No | Yes | Yes | Yes | Yes |
| Dyslipidaemia | ?[c] | ?[c] | Yes | Yes | Yes |
| Ischaemic heart disease | Yes | Yes | Yes | Yes | Yes |
| Heart failure | Yes | No | Yes | Care[d] | Yes |
| Asthma | Yes | No | Yes | Yes | Yes |
| Peripheral vascular disease | Yes | Care[e] | Care[e] | Yes | Yes |
| Renal artery stenosis | Yes | Yes | No | Yes | Yes |

[a]Diuretics may aggravate diabetes.
[b]β-Blockers may worsen glucose tolerance and aggravate lipid disorders; β-blockers may mask hypoglycaemia.
[c]β-Blockers and diuretics may disturb lipid profile.
[d]Verapamil and diltiazem may exacerbate heart failure.
[e]ACE inhibitors and β-blockers must be used with care in peripheral vascular disease.
ACE, angiotensin-converting enzyme.
ACE inhibitors are now the drugs of choice when diabetes is present, see p. 484.

**Table 11.38**  Advantages and disadvantages of hypotensive drugs with respect to associated conditions (modified from British Hypertension Society).

Potassium-sparing diuretics (e.g. triamterene 150–250 mg daily, spironolactone 50–200 mg and amiloride 5–10 mg daily) are not effective hypotensive agents, with the exception of spironolactone in primary or secondary aldosteronism. These diuretics are combined with others to treat hypokalaemia, which very occasionally occurs in hypertensive patients on diuretics.

Thiazide diuretics may cause hyperuricaemia and may precipitate gout. They may worsen glucose intolerance. Thiazide diuretics increase the serum renin level. Unlike other hypotensives, their effect is not postural.

β-ADRENERGIC ANTAGONISTS (Table 11.39). The mechanism by which β-blockers reduce hypertension is unclear. Although they reduce the force of cardiac contraction and renin production, they probably act predominantly via the central nervous system. β-Blockers also reduce anxiety. Propranolol 80 mg twice daily, atenolol 50–100 mg daily and oxprenolol 80 mg twice daily have been most widely used for the treatment of blood pressure, but there is a wide range of β-blockers with different properties:

CARDIOSELECTIVITY implies a greater effect on $\beta_1$-receptors (cardiac receptors) than on $\beta_2$-receptors. Such a selective effect is preferred when bronchospasm, intermittent claudication or diabetes is present. Metoprolol, atenolol and acebutolol are cardioselective β-blockers.

INTRINSIC SYMPATHOMIMETIC ACTIVITY is necessary if bradycardia complicates therapy with β-blockade. Pindolol has the largest degree of ISA.

POOR LIPID SOLUBILITY (e.g. sotalol) is an advantage if central nervous system side-effects are prominent.

The complications of β-blockade include aggravation of ventricular failure, bradycardia, cold extremities, aching muscles, fatigue, weakness, bad dreams and hallucinations. Non-selective β-blockade may lead to elevation of serum potassium and may mask or prolong the effects of hypoglycaemia. β-Blockers can, however, usefully be used in patients with both hypertension and angina.

VASODILATORS. Dilatation of the peripheral arterioles leads to a fall in blood pressure. There are many mechanisms by which vasodilatation can be achieved.

CALCIUM ANTAGONISTS (see Table 11.25) such as nifedipine (20 mg twice daily), diltiazem (60 mg three times daily), verapamil (120–240 mg daily in divided doses) and amlodipine (5–10 mg once daily) reduce blood pressure predominantly by arteriolar dilatation but also by reducing the force of cardiac contraction. They have proved to be effective antihypertensive agents with only a few side-effects; those that do occur include bradycardia and conduction defects (verapamil and diltiazem), headaches, constipation, flushing and fluid retention. The routine use of calcium antagonists

in the treatment of hypertension has been increasing as they prove to be safe and effective drugs.

$\alpha_1$-ADRENERGIC ANTAGONISTS such as prazosin (500 μg to a maximum of 20 mg daily) and doxazosin (1–4 mg daily) are postsynaptic α-blockers that produce vasodilatation and are very effective hypotensive drugs. Their main complication is marked hypotension following the first dose, especially when the patient is salt-depleted because of previous diuretic therapy. Presynaptic ($\alpha_2$-adrenergic) antagonists such as phentolamine are now used only in combination with β-blockers in the treatment of phaeochromocytoma. Labetolol (300–600 mg daily in divided doses) is a combined β- and α-blocker but it has little advantage over β-blockers.

ACE INHIBITORS (see Table 11.22) such as captopril (50–150 mg daily in divided doses), lisinopril (10–20 mg daily) and enalapril (10–20 mg daily) block the conversion of angiotensin I to angiotensin II, which is a more powerful vasoconstrictor. ACE inhibitors also block the degradation of bradykinin, which is a vasodilator. Their side-effects include first-dose hypotension and cough. A metallic taste, proteinuria, skin rashes and leucopenia occur generally when they are given in very high doses. The use of ACE inhibitors is increasing as they prove to be safe and effective drugs in the treatment of high blood pressure. ACE inhibitors are particularly useful in diabetics with secondary nephropathy where there is some evidence that proteinuria may be attenuated and they are now the drugs of choice. ACE inhibitors should not be used in the presence of renal artery stenosis since in this situation the renin–angiotensin system is critical to the maintenance of renal blood flow. Blockade of the production of angiotensin II may result in loss of renal blood flow and infarction of the kidney.

NON-DIURETIC THIAZIDES, including indapamide (2.5 mg daily in the morning) and diazoxide (250–600 mg i.v. in divided doses), produce vasodilatation but are seldom used. They produce fluid retention and may provoke glucose intolerance.

HYDRALAZINE (up to 150 mg daily in divided doses) and minoxidil (10 mg or more daily; maximum 50 mg) directly dilate the peripheral arterioles, leading to a fall in blood pressure. Hydralazine, when given in doses

| | Cardiac selectivity | Intrinsic sympathomimetic activity | Lipid solubility | Plasma half-life (hours) |
|---|---|---|---|---|
| Acebutalol | + | + | 0 | 5 |
| Atenolol | + | 0 | 0 | 6 |
| Metoprolol | + | 0 | + | 4 |
| Nadolol | 0 | 0 | 0 | 20 |
| Oxprenolol | 0 | ++ | + | 1.5 |
| Pindolol | 0 | +++ | + | 4 |
| Propranolol | 0 | 0 | ++ | 5 |
| Sotalol | 0 | 0 | 0 | 10 |
| Timolol | 0 | 0 | + | 5 |

**Table 11.39** Main properties of β-blockers.

greater than 200 mg daily, may provoke a lupus ery-thematosus-like syndrome, and minoxidil produces fluid retention and an increase in facial and body hair (hypertrichosis) that renders it unsuitable for women. Both drugs are complicated by sinus tachycardia, which may cause uncomfortable palpitations. They are there-fore often combined with β-blockade for the resist-ant case.

SODIUM NITROPRUSSIDE is effective as an arterial and venous dilator when given intravenously. However, it is inconvenient to use because it must be protected from light to prevent degradation. It is occasionally used for the treatment of hypertensive emergencies such as dissecting aneurysm.

CENTRALLY ACTING DRUGS such as methyldopa (a false adrenergic transmitter) (750 mg daily in divided doses) and clonidine (an $\alpha_2$-agonist) (0.1–0.3 mg daily in divided doses) reduce the degree of vasomotor tone. Both drugs are complicated by tiredness, fluid reten-tion and mild postural hypotension. Methyldopa may also cause a dry mouth, impotence, pyrexia and a posi-tive Coombs' test. Very rarely, a haemolytic anaemia may be produced. It can also rarely cause chronic active hepatitis. Clonidine may cause depression and it is important that it is not stopped suddenly because severe rebound hypertension may occur.

DEBRISOQUINE, BETHANIDINE AND GUANETHIDINE block postsynaptic adrenergic neurones and are power-ful hypotensive drugs. Side-effects include marked pos-tural hypotension, bradycardia, diarrhoea, nasal con-gestion, salivary gland pain and inability to ejaculate. Centrally acting drugs and ganglion blockers are rarely used nowadays.

### Stepped care for the control of hypertension

The majority of patients with mild or moderate hyperten-sion can be treated as outpatients. The usual practice is to attempt to reduce the blood pressure to about 150/95 mmHg. If general adjustment to life-style and diet have not led to an adequate fall in the blood pressure, it is conventional to prescribe either a β-blocker or a diuretic. Diuretics (e.g. bendrofluazide 5–10 mg daily) are pre-ferred if heart failure or peripheral vascular disease is pre-sent, but β-blockers (e.g. propranolol 80 mg twice daily or atenolol 100 mg daily) are more suitable if the patient complains of angina. Calcium antagonists such as nifedi-pine 10 mg twice daily have also been used as a first-line therapy.

If single drug treatment is unsuccessful, it is appropri-ate to prescribe both a β-blocker or a calcium antagonist in combination with a diuretic. The combination of β-blockers and diuretics is particularly attractive because some of their side-effects are partially antagonistic. For example, β-blockers lead to potassium retention, aggrava-tion of heart failure and decreased renin secretion, whilst thiazide diuretics induce the opposite changes. If these combined therapies are insufficient, more powerful vaso-dilators such as hydralazine, prazosin or nifedipine are added to the regimen. ACE inhibitors may be used if these prove inadequate and should always be used with associated diabetes. The hypotensive effect of ACE inhibi-tors is increased by their use with a diuretic.

It is essential that the patient understands that high blood pressure does not go away after a single course of treatment. It is necessary to continue treatment for many years or for life. In addition, the patient's blood pressure must be checked at regular intervals. Since treatment is lifelong the physician must attempt to simplify treatment regimens to improve compliance. Evidence suggests that poor treatment is better than no treatment at all.

Hypertension that is unresponsive to treatment is usu-ally due to the patient not taking the drugs prescribed or to the presence of an underlying primary cause such as coarctation or renal artery stenosis. Such underlying causes must be discovered and corrected before therapy will succeed.

### The management of severe or malignant hypertension

Patients with severe hypertension (diastolic pressure >130 mmHg), hypertensive encephalopathy or severe complications of hypertension such as left ventricular fail-ure or aortic dissection should be admitted to hospital for urgent treatment of their hypertension under close supervision. It is unwise to reduce the blood pressure too rapidly because cerebral, myocardial or renal infarction may result. The majority of hypertensive emergencies can be treated by slowly (over about 24 hours) bringing the diastolic blood pressure back to 100–110 mmHg. This can normally be achieved by using oral nifedipine (10–20 mg) and β-blockade, e.g. atenolol 50 mg. When a more rapid fall of blood pressure is needed, e.g. when managing an aortic dissection, intravenous nitroprusside (0.3 $\mu$g kg$^{-1}$ min$^{-1}$) is the agent of choice. Alternatively, chewable nifedipine (5–10 mg), oral captopril (12.5 mg), intra-venous diazoxide (bolus of 50 mg over 1 min) or a labeta-lol infusion (initially 1 mg min$^{-1}$) may be used.

### The management of hypertension during pregnancy

Mild hypertension in pregnancy is usual, but more severe hypertension (>140/90 mmHg), associated with pro-teinuria and peripheral oedema, may be a prelude to eclampsia. Pre-eclampsia is treated with bed rest and hypotensive drugs known to be safe in pregnancy. Methyldopa, propranolol, atenolol, nifedipine and hydralazine are usually used. Full-blown eclampsia is treated as a hypertensive emergency with intravenous hydralazine. If the high pressure cannot be reduced, the pregnancy may need to be terminated, and this univer-sally reduces the high blood pressure unless the patient had prior high blood pressure.

### PROGNOSIS

Patients with untreated malignant or accelerated hyper-tension have a very poor prognosis—more than 90% will die within the first year. Effective reduction in the blood pressure leads to a dramatic improvement of prognosis. In general, the risk from hypertension depends on:
- Level of blood pressure
- Presence of retinal changes
- Presence of cardiac or renal complications

- Sex of the patient (men are more at risk than women)
- Coexistence of coronary disease and risk factors for coronary disease such as high plasma lipids, diabetes and smoking
- Age of the patient (young patients fare worse than the old)

The cause of death in hypertensive patients is usually myocardial infarction, cardiac failure, renal failure or cerebrovascular accident. Effective treatment of moderate hypertension clearly improves the prognosis for each of these causes of death. The treatment of even mild hypertension reduces the likelihood of stroke or cardiac failure.

# Heart disease in the elderly

As the average age of the population increases, cardiac disease predominates. The elderly population are vulnerable to most forms of heart disease, especially coronary artery disease, hypertension, arrhythmias and degenerative pathologies.

## NORMAL FINDINGS IN THE ELDERLY
Diagnosis of mild forms of heart disease may be difficult in the elderly. The wear and tear of age results in some features that would be regarded as abnormal in the young. For example, a fourth heart sound and a systolic aortic ejection murmur are common findings on examining normal elderly adults. The ECG often shows slight PR interval prolongation (to 0.22 s), left axis deviation and T wave flattening. On the chest X-ray there may be some aortic, valvular or coronary arterial calcification, but the cardiac silhouette is usually normal. The echocardiogram may show mild myocardial hypertrophy and buckling of the ventricular septum.

It is particularly difficult to diagnose and define hypertension in the elderly. Cuff blood pressure usually overestimates intravascular pressure if the old arterial wall is stiff (pseudohypertension). Normally blood pressure steadily increases with age, at least up to the age of 70 years, and blood pressure is particularly labile in the elderly. In the very old (>80 years) there is only a weak association between 'hypertension' and diseases such as stroke, myocardial infarction and heart failure.

## DISEASE PRESENTATION IN THE ELDERLY
Cardiac disease may present in unexpected ways in an old person. It is not unusual for significant bradycardia to present as a fractured hip because the fall that caused the fracture resulted from transient asystole. Left heart failure may present as an acute confusional state due to poor cerebral perfusion, rather than with the classical symptom of breathlessness. Myocardial infarction may not cause any chest pain ('silent' myocardial infarction) but may present as weakness or abdominal pain.

## TREATMENT OF THE ELDERLY
The principles of treatment of heart disease in old people are usually no different from those governing treatment in the young. However, it is important to remember that drug pharmacokinetics are changed in the elderly: absorption is reduced, renal and hepatic clearance are delayed, body fat increases and lean body mass decreases. Old people may forget to take their medications or be confused about the correct dose.

Some therapies seem inappropriate or futile in the elderly. For example, it is probably unnecessary to inflict a spartan life-style or rigorous uncomfortable drug therapy on an old person in an attempt to modify the risk of developing coronary disease. However, there are treatments that have emerged in recent years that are extremely useful for old people, for example, hypertension should be treated (see p. 621). Coronary angioplasty, and perhaps mitral/aortic valvuloplasty, can be undertaken in patients too frail to consider for surgery. Cardiac surgery does carry a much greater (approximately two to five times) risk in the elderly but, as with younger patients, the absolute risk is dependent upon the state of the myocardium, the extent of cardiac disease and the condition of other organ systems. Age is no bar to effective treatment of heart disease.

## SPECIFIC HEART PROBLEMS IN THE ELDERLY
There are a few cardiac conditions that are largely confined to the elderly.

AORTIC SCLEROSIS results from fibrosis and calcification on the aortic side of an otherwise normal tricuspid aortic valve. This may result in an obstruction to left ventricular outflow but it is often trivial. Aortic valve replacement may be necessary if the obstruction is severe.

MITRAL ANNULUS CALCIFICATION occurs predominantly in old women. It is diagnosed from the chest X-ray and it is not usually responsible for any symptoms.

ENDOCARDITIS. A non-infective form of endocarditis may occur in the elderly. It is a hypercoagulable state that presents with cachexia, thrombosis and embolization. Anticoagulation may be needed.

LEV'S DISEASE. Disruption of His–Purkinje conduction by fibrosis and calcification is most common in the old when it is known as Lev's disease. It presents with Stokes–Adams attacks and must be treated by pacemaker insertion.

ATRIAL FIBRILLATION is much more common in the old but it is often well tolerated and *may not need any active treatment* for control of heart rate. Anticoagulation should be considered.

# The heart in pregnancy

In pregnancy the cardiac output and blood volume increase from the second month up to the thirtieth week to 30–50% above the normal levels. This, along with the increased metabolic work, produces the physical signs of warm extremities, a tachycardia with a large-volume pulse and a slight rise in venous pressure. The apex beat is displaced, owing partly to cardiomegaly and partly to a raised diaphragm. The increased blood flow produces a pulmonary systolic murmur and a third heart sound. The diastolic blood pressure is lower owing to vasodilatation.

The added burden of pregnancy on the cardiovascular system can make underlying, otherwise latent, disease clinically apparent. Ten per cent of maternal deaths in England and Wales are due to heart disease. This is usually rheumatic or congenital in origin, but any heart disease can be seen in pregnancy. Moderate to severe mitral stenosis can cause breathlessness early in pregnancy and may lead to pulmonary oedema later in pregnancy. Pregnancy should be avoided in severe mitral stenosis or delayed until after valvotomy. Termination may be necessary in a severe case occurring before the sixteenth week. Most cases of congenital heart disease have been corrected by the time women reach the reproductive age. However, patients with small and uncomplicated septal defects usually tolerate pregnancy well. Patients with prosthetic valves are usually on anticoagulant therapy. This may require a change to heparin because warfarin can cause fetal abnormalities. Patients with pulmonary hypertension of any aetiology have an extremely high mortality (up to 50%) either during or immediately after delivery, and termination should be considered.

*Post partum*, or late in pregnancy, a cardiomyopathy of uncertain aetiology is sometimes seen. There is also a rise in thromboembolic complications of cardiac disease owing to the hypercoagulability that exists *post partum*. Sepsis is a risk during delivery, and patients with heart disease may be at risk of developing infective endocarditis.

## Peripheral vascular disease

## ARTERIAL DISEASE

This can be due to a number of pathological processes.

### Arteriosclerosis
This is the term applied to generalized, age-related arterial changes, which are exaggerated in hypertension. In arteries down to 1 mm in diameter these changes initially take the form of compensatory muscular hypertrophy of the media, which is followed by fibrosis and dilatation of the lumen. In hypertensive vessels of this size, atheroma is often superadded.

Smaller arteries show different changes that are usually most marked in the viscera, especially in the kidneys. Here, though there is medial hypertrophy, the predominant change is intimal thickening by concentric layers of connective tissue, with luminal narrowing.

Arterioles undergo hyaline thickening of their walls and luminal narrowing. The narrowing of small vessels in the kidney owing to hypertension causes renal ischaemia, which further promotes hypertension.

In malignant hypertension, arterioles also show fibrinoid necrosis of their walls.

### Mönckeberg's sclerosis
This is a degenerative disease of unknown cause, characterized by dystrophic calcification of the media. It is especially common in the major lower limb arteries of the elderly, and there is an increased incidence of this degeneration in diabetics.

### Cystic medial necrosis or degeneration
This describes mucoid degeneration of the collagen and elastic tissue of the media, often with cystic changes. It occurs mainly in elderly hypertensives. Dissecting aneurysms of the thoracic aorta are often due to this process. Cystic medial degeneration also occurs in inherited defects of collagen tissue formation (e.g. Marfan's syndrome, Ehlers–Danlos syndrome), again resulting in dissecting aneurysms.

### Atheroma
The pathogenesis of this condition is described on p. 578. The different vessels which may be involved are shown in Table 11.40. Atheroma seldom involves arteries of less than 2 mm in diameter. Most arterial disease is due to atheromatous degeneration.

## Chronic ischaemia of the legs

This is due to atheromatous disease involving the aorta, iliac and/or any other peripheral vessels. It consequently occurs over the age of 50 years, chiefly in men who are smokers.

### SYMPTOMS
- Ischaemic, cramp-like pain, usually in the calves during exercise and relieved by rest (intermittent claudication)
- Rest pain
- Non-healing leg ulcers or gangrene

Both limbs are often affected, but usually one is more severely affected than the other.

### SIGNS
- A cold limb with dry skin and lack of hair
- Absent pulses to diseased areas
- Ulceration or gangrene

### INVESTIGATION
X-RAYS may show calcification of the arteries of the leg. DOPPLER ULTRASOUND defines the severity of the lesion.

| |
|---|
| Abdominal aorta and iliac arteries |
| Proximal coronary arteries |
| Femoral and popliteal arteries, and thoracic aorta |
| Internal carotid arteries |
| Vertebrobasilar system |

**Table 11.40** Common sites of clinically significant atherosclerosis in order of frequency.

AORTOGRAPHY by direct injection of contrast medium into the aorta is used. Angiography is also performed via a percutaneous catheter inserted into the brachial artery and digital vascular imaging with an intravenous injection has been used. These investigations show narrowing and stenosis of the arteries.

## MANAGEMENT

### General

RISK FACTORS should be reduced (e.g. smoking should be stopped, diabetes and hypertension should be treated, and weight should be reduced).

THE LIMBS should be kept warm but local heat should not be applied.

FEET. Care should be taken to avoid infection and trauma of the feet. Elderly patients often need regular visits to a chiropodist.

REGULAR EXERCISE should be taken to encourage the development of anastomotic vessels.

LOW-DOSE ASPIRIN should be given.

VASODILATORS should not be used.

ANTICOAGULANTS are of no benefit.

### Surgery

TIMING. Surgery should not be considered for 3 months after symptoms have developed, to allow time for collaterals to develop. In 75% of patients the disease remains static.

AORTO-ILIAC BYPASS grafts give good results, but reconstructive surgery for blockages below the inguinal ligament is less successful.

BALLOON DILATATION via a catheter inserted into the artery is useful for local iliac or femoral stenoses.

AMPUTATION is necessary for severely ischaemic limbs, usually those with gangrene. Rehabilitation may take months in the elderly and is often unsuccessful.

Many of the patients have generalized atheromatous conditions, so that the overall prognosis often dictates the outcome of localized disease; many die from a myocardial infarction.

## Acute ischaemia of the legs

Like chronic ischaemia of the legs, this is mainly due to atheromatous disease with thrombosis, but it can also occur owing to embolism from the heart (e.g. in atrial fibrillation) or from an atheromatous central vessel.

The clinical picture is of an acutely painful, pale, paralysed, pulseless limb.

Treatment is surgical, with removal of the clot. If gangrene develops, amputation is necessary.

## Aortic aneurysms

### Abdominal aneurysms

The commonest aortic aneurysms are abdominal. These are usually due to atheroma.

Asymptomatic aneurysms may be found as a pulsatile mass on examination or as calcification on an X-ray. A CT scan or ultrasound of the abdomen will demonstrate the size of the aneurysm, the thickness of the aortic wall and whether any leak has occurred. An expanding aneurysm may cause epigastric or back pain. Rupture presents with epigastric pain radiating through to the back. A pulsatile mass is felt and the patient is shocked. Treatment of symptomatic aneurysms is surgical. A ruptured aneurysm requires emergency surgery, but even then the mortality is high.

Large, asymptomatic aneurysms should also be treated surgically (except in the very old) because those larger than 5 cm in diameter have a high risk of rupture. Follow-up with ultrasound is required with small aneurysms and surgery offered when aneurysm reaches 5 cm.

### Thoracic aneurysms

Most thoracic aneurysms in the past were due to syphilis, but now many are due to atheromatous disease. The aneurysms may affect all parts of the thoracic aorta—the ascending aorta, the arch and the descending aorta.

Most are asymptomatic, but when large they can give rise to chest pain or to evidence of pressure on other organs, such as the superior vena cava or the oesophagus. They can rupture.

### Dissecting aortic aneurysms

In the majority of cases, the dissection starts in the ascending aorta. Pain, which is severe and central, often radiating to the back, is the major symptom. The pain radiates down the arms and into the neck and can be difficult to distinguish from myocardial infarction.

On examination, the patient is usually shocked and there may be neurological signs owing to the involvement of the spinal vessels. The peripheral pulses may be absent, but this is not invariable.

The diagnosis is suggested by the presence of back pain with no ECG or enzyme changes of myocardial infarction. The chest X-ray may show a wide mediastinum and CT scanning and ultrasonography with transoesophageal echocardiography if available are diagnostic (Fig. 11.91). Aortography is now rarely necessary to confirm the diagnosis.

Half of the patients are hypertensive and this should be controlled immediately. Emergency surgery is necessary for many dissections.

There is an increased risk of dissection in pregnancy.

Patients with Marfan's syndrome are at particular risk of dissection originating at the root of the aorta. Risk can be assessed by measuring the dimension of the aortic root using serial echocardiography. Elective repair of the aneurysmal aortic root is indicated if the dimensions increase rapidly.

## Thromboangiitis obliterans (Buerger's disease)

This disease, involving the small vessels of the lower limbs, occurs in young men who smoke. It is thought by some workers to be indistinguishable from atheromatous disease. However, pathologically there is inflammation of

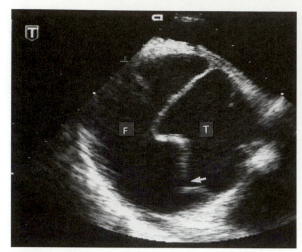 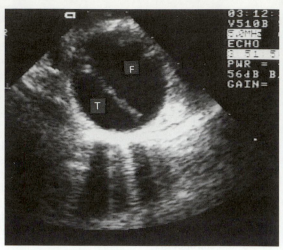

**Fig. 11.91** Two-dimensional transoesophageal echocardiograms from a patient with Marfan's syndrome resulting in dissection of the aorta. From its position in the oesophagus, the transducer can be aimed forward to visualize the greatly enlarged ascending aorta (left), or backwards to show the descending thoracic aorta (right). In both views the dissected intima is seen within the aortic lumen. The main entry point to the false lumen is seen in the ascending aorta (arrowed), just above the aortic valve. T, true lumen; F, false lumen.

the vessels that may indicate a separate disease activity. Clinically it presents with peripheral ischaemia and patients must stop smoking.

## Takayasu's syndrome

This is rare, except in Japan. It is known as 'pulseless disease' or the aortic arch syndrome. It is of unknown aetiology and occurs in young females. There is a vasculitis involving the aortic arch as well as other major arteries. There is also a systemic illness, with pain and tenderness over the affected arteries. Absent peripheral pulses and hypertension are usually found. Corticosteroids help the constitutional symptoms. Heart failure and cerebrovascular accidents eventually occur, but most patients survive for at least 5 years.

## Kawasaki disease (mucocutaneous lymph node syndrome)

This is an uncommon acute febrile illness of early childhood. There is a generalized vasculitis with involvement of the coronary arteries and lymphadenopathy.

## Cardiovascular syphilis

This gives rise to:
● Uncomplicated aortitis
● Aortic aneurysms, usually in the ascending part
● Aortic valvulitis with regurgitation
● Stenosis of the coronary ostia
The diagnosis is confirmed by serology. Treatment is with penicillin. Aneurysms and valvular disease are treated as necessary by the usual methods.

## Connective tissue disorders

These cause vasculitis and can give rise to peripheral vascular disease. They are discussed on p. 406.

## Raynaud's disease and phenomenon

Raynaud's phenomenon consists of spasm of the arteries supplying the fingers or toes and is usually precipitated by cold and relieved by heat. When Raynaud's phenomenon occurs without any underlying disorder, it is then known as Raynaud's disease. This is a common disease affecting 5% of the population and occurring predominantly in young women. The disorder is usually bilateral and fingers are affected more commonly than toes. There is an initial pallor of the skin resulting from vasoconstriction and this is followed by cyanosis due to sluggish blood flow. Redness finally occurs owing to hyperaemia. The duration of the attacks can be variable and can sometimes last for hours. Numbness and burning of the fingers usually occurs and pain can be severe, particularly in the rewarming phase.

Between the attacks the pulses and the digits appear normal, but trophic changes with small areas of gangrene can occur in severe and persistent cases.

### DIAGNOSIS

Primary Raynaud's disease must be differentiated from secondary causes of Raynaud's phenomenon, which are chiefly disorders of connective tissue, particularly systemic sclerosis. It can also occur in cryoglobulinaemia and as a side-effect of drug treatment, especially with β-blocking agents.

### TREATMENT (see p. 1022)

No treatment is usually required for the attacks but any underlying disease must be looked for. The hands and feet should be kept warm, and smoking should be avoided. β-Blockers should be stopped. Nifedipine 10 mg three times daily may be helpful.

# VENOUS DISEASE

## Varicose veins

Varicose veins are a common problem, sometimes giving rise to pain. They are treated by injection or surgery.

## Venous thrombosis

Thrombosis can occur in any vein, but the veins of the leg and the pelvis are the commonest sites.

### Superficial thrombophlebitis
This commonly involves the saphenous veins and is often associated with varicosities. Occasionally the axillary vein is involved, usually as a result of trauma. There is local superficial inflammation of the vein wall, with secondary thrombosis.

The clinical picture is of a painful, tender, cord-like structure with associated redness and swelling.

The condition usually responds to symptomatic treatment with rest, elevation of the limb and analgesics (e.g. non-steroidal anti-inflammatory drugs). Anticoagulants are not necessary, as embolism does not occur from superficial thrombophlebitis.

### Deep-vein thrombosis
A thrombus forms in the vein, and any inflammation of the vein wall is secondary to this.

Thrombosis commonly occurs after periods of immobilization, but it can occur in normal individuals for no obvious reasons. The precipitating factors are discussed on p. 347.

Deep-vein thrombosis occurs in 50% of patients after prostatectomy or following a cerebral vascular accident. In addition, one-third of patients with a myocardial infarct have a deep-vein thrombosis.

Thrombosis can occur in any vein of the leg, but is particularly found in veins of the calf. It is often undetected; autopsy figures give an incidence of over 60% in hospitalized patients.

CLINICAL FEATURES. The major presenting features are:
ASYMPTOMATIC, presenting with clinical features of pulmonary embolism (see p. 611).
PAIN IN THE CALF, often presenting with swelling, redness and engorged superficial veins. The affected calf is often warmer and there may be ankle oedema. Homan's sign (pain in the calf on dorsiflexion of the foot) is often present, but is not diagnostic and occurs with all lesions of the calf.
Thrombosis in the iliofemoral region can present with severe pain, but there are often few physical signs apart from occasional swelling of the thigh and/or ankle oedema.

Complete occlusion, particularly of a large vein, can lead to a cyanotic discoloration of the limb and severe oedema, which can very rarely lead to venous gangrene.

Pulmonary embolism can occur with any deep-vein thrombosis but is more frequent from an iliofemoral thrombosis and is rare with thrombosis confined to veins below the knee. Spread of thrombosis can occur proximally without clinical evidence, so the extent of the thrombosis must be carefully assessed.

INVESTIGATION. Clinical diagnosis is unreliable and confirmation of an iliofemoral thrombosis can usually be made with ultrasound or Doppler ultrasound. Below-knee thromboses can only reliably be detected by venography but whether this is necessary is questionable (see Treatment). A venogram is performed by injecting a vein in the foot with contrast which will detect virtually all thrombi that are present.

TREATMENT. The main aim of therapy is to prevent pulmonary embolism and all patients with thrombi above the knee must be anticoagulated. Anticoagulation of below-knee thrombi is controversial. Bed rest is advised until the patient is fully anticoagulated. The patient should then be mobilized, with an elastic stocking giving graduated pressure over the leg.

Heparin is given normally for 48 hours but how long warfarin should be given is debatable—3 months is the usual recommended period but 4 weeks is long enough if a definite risk factor (e.g. bed rest) has been present. The INR should be at 2–3.0. Anticoagulants do not affect the thrombus that is already present.

Thrombolytic therapy (see p. 348) is occasionally used for patients with a large iliofemoral thrombosis.

PROGNOSIS. Destruction of the deep-vein valves produces a clinically painful, swollen limb that is made worse by standing and is accompanied by oedema and sometimes venous eczema. It occurs in approximately half of the patients with a clinically symptomatic deep-vein thrombosis, and it means that elastic support stockings are then required for life.

PREVENTION. Subcutaneous low-dose heparin (see p. 348) should be given to patients with cardiac failure, a myocardial infarct or surgery to the leg or pelvis.

Early ambulation is indicated as most thromboses occur within the first 72 hours following surgery. Leg exercises should be encouraged and patients should not sit in a chair with their legs immobilized on a stool. An elastic support stocking should be given to patients at high risk, e.g. those with a history of thrombosis or with obesity.

# Further reading

Anderson HV & Willenson JT Thrombolysis in acute myocardial infarction. *New England Journal of Medicine* **329**, 703–709.

Braunwald E (1987) *Heart Disease*, 3rd edn. Philadelphia: WB Saunders.

Fuster V *et al.* (1992) The pathogenesis of coronary artery disease and the acute coronary syndromes. *New England Journal of Medicine* **326**, 242–250 and 310–318.

Hampton JR (1986) *The ECG Made Easy*, 3rd edn. Edinburgh: Churchill Livingstone.

Hurst JW (1990) *The Heart, Arteries and Veins*, 7th edn. New York: McGraw-Hill.

Julian DG, Camm AJ, Fox KS, Hall RJC & Poole-Wilson PA (1995) *Diseases of the Heart*, 2nd edn, in press. London: Baillière Tindall.

Kelly DP & Strauss AW (1994) Inherited cardiomyopathies. *New England Journal of Medicine* **330**, 913–919.

Landau C, Lange R & Hillis LD (1994) Percutaneous transluminal coronary angioplasty. *New England Journal of Medicine* **330**, 981–993.

Severs P *et al.* (1993) Guidelines for the treatment of hypertension. *British Medical Journal* **306**, 983–987.

Sokolow M & McIlroy MB (1986) *Clinical Cardiology*, 4th edn. New York: Lange.

# Structure of the respiratory system

## The nose

The anterior one-third of the nasal cavity is divided into right and left halves by the nasal septum (Fig. 12.1). The nasal vestibule leads to the internal ostium (a) which is the narrowest part of the nasal cavity. This causes a 50% increased resistance to airflow when breathing through the nose rather than through the mouth. The respiratory region (b) is divided by three folds arising from the lateral wall, termed the superior, middle and inferior turbinates. Behind these turbinates are situated the openings of the nasolacrimal duct and the frontal, ethmoidal and maxillary sinuses. The olfactory region for smell is found above the superior turbinate. The nasal cavities communicate with the nasopharynx via the posterior nasal apertures (the choanae (c)), and the eustachian tube opens into this area just above the soft palate.

## The pharynx and larynx

The pharynx is divided by the soft palate into an upper nasopharyngeal and lower oropharyngeal region. There are numerous collections of lymphoid tissue arranged in a circular fashion around the nasopharynx; these include the adenoids. The tonsils lie between the anterior and posterior fauces, separating the mouth from the oropharynx.

The larynx consists of a number of articulated cartilages, vocal cords, muscles and ligaments, all of which serve to keep the airway open during breathing and occlude it during swallowing.

The main motor nerve to the larynx is the recurrent laryngeal nerve. The left recurrent laryngeal nerve leaves the vagus at the level of the aortic arch, hooking round it to run upwards through the mediastinum between the trachea and the oesophagus; it can be affected by disease in these areas. The principal tensor of the vocal cords is the external branch of the superior laryngeal nerve, which can be injured during thyroidectomy.

## The trachea, bronchi and bronchioles

The trachea is 10–12 cm in length. It lies slightly to the right of the midline and divides at the carina into right and left main bronchi. The carina lies under the junction of the manubrium sternum and the second right costal cartilage. The right main bronchus is more vertical than the left and, hence, inhaled material is more likely to pass into it.

The right main bronchus divides into the upper lobe bronchus and the intermediate bronchus, which further subdivides into the middle and lower lobe bronchi. On the left the main bronchus divides into upper and lower lobe bronchi only. Each lobar bronchus further divides into segmental and subsegmental bronchi. There are about 25 divisions in all between the trachea and the alveoli. Of the first seven divisions the bronchi have:
- Walls consisting of cartilage and smooth muscle
- Epithelial lining with cilia and goblet cells
- Submucosal mucus-secreting glands
- Endocrine cells—Kulchitsky or APUD (amine precursor and uptake decarboxylation) containing 5-hydroxytryptamine

In the next 16–18 divisions the bronchioles have:

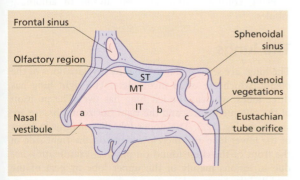

**Fig. 12.1** The anatomy of the nose in longitudinal section. IT, inferior turbinate; MT, middle turbinate; ST, superior turbinate. a, internal ostium; b, respiratory region; c, choanae.

- No cartilage and a muscular layer that progressively becomes thinner
- A single layer of ciliated cells but very few goblet cells
- Granulated Clara cells that produce a surfactant-like substance

The ciliated epithelium is an important defence mechanism. Each cell contains approximately 200 cilia beating at 1000 min$^{-1}$ in organized waves of contraction. Each cilium consists of nine peripheral parts and two inner longitudinal fibrils in a cytoplasmic matrix (Fig. 12.2). Nexin links join the peripheral pairs. Dynein arms consisting of ATPase protein project towards the adjacent pairs. Bending of the cilia results from a sliding movement between adjacent fibrils powered by an ATP-dependent shearing force developed by the dynein arms. Absence of dynein arms leads to immotile cilia. Mucus, which contains macrophages, cell debris, inhaled particles and bacteria, is moved by the cilia towards the larynx at about 1.5 cm min$^{-1}$—the 'mucociliary escalator' (see below).

The bronchioles finally divide within the acinus into smaller respiratory bronchioles that have alveoli arising from the surface (Fig. 12.3). Each respiratory bronchiole supplies approximately 200 alveoli via alveolar ducts. The term 'small airways' refers to bronchioles of less than 2 mm; there are 30 000 of these in the average lung.

## The alveoli

There are approximately 300 million alveoli in each lung. Their total surface area is 40–80 m². The epithelial lining consists largely of type I pneumocytes (Fig. 12.4). These cells have an extremely attenuated cytoplasm, and thus provide only a thin barrier to gas exchange. They are derived from type II pneumocytes. Type I cells are connected to each other by tight junctions that limit the fluid movements in and out of the alveoli.

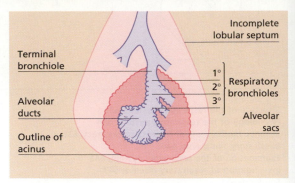

**Fig. 12.3** Branches of a terminal bronchiole ending in the alveolar sacs.

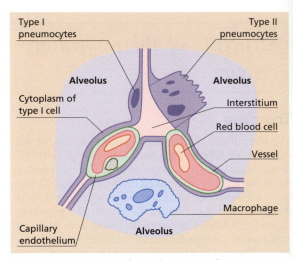

**Fig. 12.4** The structure of alveoli, showing the pneumocytes and capillaries.

Type II pneumocytes are slightly more numerous than type I cells but cover less of the epithelial lining. They are found generally in the borders of the alveolus and contain distinctive lamellar vacuoles, thought to be a source of surfactant. Macrophages are also present in the alveoli and are involved in the defence mechanisms of the lung.

The pores of Kohn are holes in the alveolar wall allowing communication between alveoli of adjoining lobules.

## The lungs

The lungs are separated into lobes by invaginations of the pleura, which are often incomplete. The right lung has three lobes, whereas the left lung has two. The position of the oblique fissures and the right horizontal fissure are shown in Fig. 12.5. The upper lobe lies mainly in front of the lower lobe and therefore signs on the right side in the front of the chest found on physical examination are due to lesions mainly of the upper lobe or part of the middle lobe.

Each lobe is further subdivided into bronchopulmonary segments by fibrous septa that extend inwards from

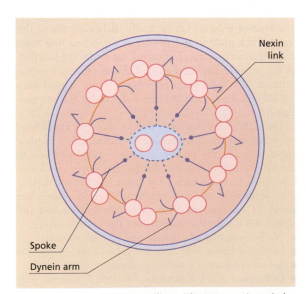

**Fig. 12.2** Cross-section of a cilium. Nine outer microtubular doublets and two central single microtubules are linked by spokes, nexin links and dynein arms.

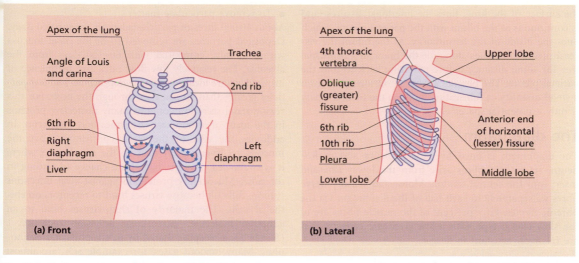

Fig. 12.5   Surface anatomy of the chest. (a) PA; (b) lateral.

the pleural surface. Each segment receives its own segmental bronchus.

The bronchopulmonary segment is further divided into individual lobules approximately 1 cm in diameter and generally pyramidal in shape, the apex lying towards the bronchioles supplying them. Within each lobule a terminal bronchus supplies an acinus and within this struc-

ture further divisions of the bronchioles eventually give rise to the alveoli.

A chest X-ray (Fig. 12.6) illustrates the above features.

## The pleura

The pleura is a layer of connective tissue covered by a simple squamous epithelium. The visceral pleura covers

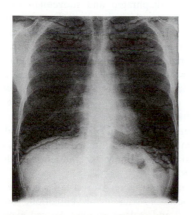

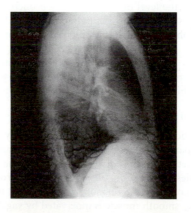

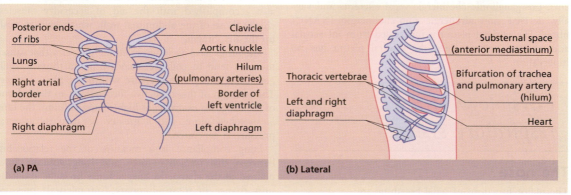

Fig. 12.6   Chest X-rays. (a) PA; (b) lateral.

the surface of the lung, lines the interlobar fissures, and is continuous at the hilum with the parietal pleura, which lines the inside of the hemithorax. At the hilum the visceral pleura continues alongside the branching bronchial tree for some distance before reflecting back to join the parietal pleura. The pleurae are in apposition apart from a small quantity of lubricating fluid, so the pleural cavity is only a potential space.

## The diaphragm

The diaphragm is lined by parietal pleura and peritoneum. Its muscle fibres arise from the lower ribs and insert into the central tendon. Motor and sensory nerve fibres go separately to each half of the diaphragm via the phrenic nerves. Fifty per cent of the muscle fibres are of the slow-twitch type with a low glycolytic capacity that are relatively resistant to fatigue.

## Pulmonary vasculature and lymphatics

The pulmonary artery divides to accompany the bronchi. The arterioles accompanying the respiratory bronchioles are thin-walled and contain little smooth muscle. The pulmonary venules drain laterally to the periphery of the lobules, pass centrally in the interlobular and intersegmental septa, and eventually join to form the four main pulmonary veins.

In addition, a further bronchial circulation arises from the descending aorta. These bronchial arteries supply tissues down to the level of the respiratory bronchiole. The bronchial veins drain into the pulmonary vein, forming part of the physiological shunt observed in normal individuals.

Lymphatic channels lie in the potential interstitial space between the alveolar cells and the capillary endothelium of the pulmonary arterioles.

## Nerve supply to the lung

The innervation of the lung remains incompletely understood. The parasympathetic supply is from the vagus and the sympathetic from the adjacent sympathetic chain. The nerve supplies entwine in a plexus at the nerve root and branches accompany the pulmonary arteries and the airways. Airway smooth muscle is innervated by vagal afferents, postganglionic cholinergic vagal efferents and vagally derived non-adrenergic non-cholinergic (NANC) fibres. The parietal pleura is innervated from intercostal and phrenic nerves whilst the visceral pleura has no innervation.

# Physiology of the respiratory system

## The nose

The major functions of nasal breathing are:
- To heat and moisten the air

- To remove particulate matter

About 10 000 litres of particle-laden air are inhaled daily. Deposited particles are removed from the nasal mucosa within 15 min, compared with 60–120 days from the alveolus. The relatively low flow rates and turbulence of inspired air are ideal for particle deposition, and few particles greater than 10 $\mu$m pass through the nose. For this reason nasal secretion contains many protective proteins in the form of antibodies, lysozymes and interferon. In addition, the cilia of the nasal epithelium move the mucous gel layer rapidly back to the oropharynx where it is swallowed. Bacteria have little chance of settling in the nose. Mucociliary protection against viral infections is more difficult because viruses bind to receptors on epithelial cells. The majority of rhinoviruses bind to an adhesion molecule, intracellular adhesion molecule 1 (ICAM-1), a receptor shared by neutrophils and eosinophils. Many noxious gases, for example $SO_2$, are almost completely removed by nasal breathing.

## Breathing

Lung ventilation can be considered in two parts:
- The mechanical process of inspiration and expiration
- The control of respiration to a level appropriate for the metabolic needs

### MECHANICAL PROCESS

Inspiration is an active process and results from the descent of the diaphragm and movement of the ribs upwards and outwards under the influence of the intercostal muscles. In resting healthy individuals, contraction of the diaphragm is responsible for most of inspiration. Respiratory muscles are similar to other skeletal muscles but are less prone to fatigue. However weakness may play a part in respiratory failure resulting from neurological and muscle disorders and possibly with severe chronic airflow limitation.

Expiration follows passively as a result of gradual lessening of contraction of the intercostal muscles, allowing the lungs to collapse under the influence of their own elastic forces.

Inspiration against increased resistance may require the use of the accessory muscles of ventilation, such as the sternomastoid and scalene muscles. Forced expiration is also accomplished with the aid of accessory muscles, chiefly those of the abdominal wall, which help to push up the diaphragm.

The lungs have an inherent elastic property that causes them to tend to collapse away from the thoracic wall, generating a negative pressure within the pleural space. The strength of this retractive force relates to the volume of the lung; for example, at higher lung volumes the lung is stretched more, and a greater negative intrapleural pressure is generated.

Lung compliance is a measure of the relationship between this retractive force and lung volume. It is defined as the change in lung volume brought about by unit change in transpulmonary (intrapleural) pressure and is measured in litres per kilopascal (litres kPa$^{-1}$). At the end of a quiet expiration, the retractive force exerted by the lungs is balanced by the tendency of the thoracic wall to spring outwards. At this point respiratory muscles are resting and the volume of the lung is known as the *functional residual capacity* (FRC).

Diseases that can affect the movement of the thoracic cage and diaphragm can have a profound effect on ventilation. These include diseases of the thoracic spine such as ankylosing spondylitis and kyphoscoliosis, neuropathies (e.g. the Guillain–Barré syndrome), injury to the phrenic nerves, and myasthenia gravis.

## THE CONTROL OF RESPIRATION
Coordinated respiratory movements result from rhythmical discharges arising in an anatomically ill-defined group of interconnected neurones in the reticular substance of the brain stem known as the respiratory centre. Motor discharges from the respiratory centre travel via the phrenic and intercostal nerves to the respiratory musculature.

The pressures of oxygen and carbon dioxide in arterial blood are closely controlled. In a typical normal adult at rest:
- The pulmonary blood flow of 5 litres min$^{-1}$ carries 11 mmol min$^{-1}$ (250 ml min$^{-1}$) of oxygen from the lungs to the tissues.
- Ventilation at about 6 litres min$^{-1}$ carries 9 mmol min$^{-1}$ (200 ml min$^{-1}$) of carbon dioxide out of the body.
- The normal pressure of oxygen in arterial blood ($P_aO_2$) is between 11 and 13 kPa (83 and 98 mmHg).
- The normal pressure of carbon dioxide in arterial blood ($P_aCO_2$) is 4.8–6.0 kPa (36–45 mmHg).

Neurogenic and chemical factors are involved in the control of ventilation.

### Neurogenic factors
Neural stimuli include:
- Consciously induced changes in rate and depth of breathing
- Impulses from limb receptors, as in exercise, which cause respiratory stimulation
- Impulses arising from pulmonary receptors sensitive to stretch and bronchial irritation
- Juxtapulmonary capillary receptors (J receptors) stimulated by pulmonary congestion
- Impulses arising from receptors in muscles and joints of the chest wall

Abnormal stimuli include:
- Lesions in the pons and midbrain, which give rise to central neurogenic hyperventilation or hypoventilation
- Medullary compression, which leads to respiratory depression

### Chemical stimuli
These cause an increase in ventilation when they stimulate central or peripheral chemoreceptors.
1 Central
   (a) Carbon dioxide. The strongest respiratory stimulant to breathing is a rise in $P_aCO_2$. Sensitivity to

this may be lost in chronic bronchitis, so that in these patients hypoxaemia is the chief stimulus to respiratory drive; treatment with oxygen may therefore reduce respiratory drive and produce a further rise in $P_aCO_2$.
   (b) Hydrogen ion concentration of arterial blood. An increase in [H$^+$] due to metabolic acidosis will increase ventilation with a fall in $P_aCO_2$. In respiratory disease, [H$^+$] and $P_aCO_2$ rise together.
2 Peripheral. A reduced $P_aO_2$ stimulates peripheral chemoreceptors in the carotid and aortic bodies. This stimulus is not strong unless the $P_aO_2$ is below 8 kPa. These chemoreceptors also respond to increases in [H$^+$] and $P_aCO_2$.

The respiratory centre is depressed by severe hypoxaemia and sedatives (e.g. opiates) and stimulated by large doses of aspirin or by pyrexia.

In certain common conditions such as mild asthma, pulmonary embolism and pneumonia there is an increase in ventilation, leading to a reduction in the $P_aCO_2$. These conditions probably cause this effect through stimulation of irritant receptors in the bronchioles and J receptors stimulated deep in the parenchyma of the lung.

Anxiety or hysteria cause hyperventilation, and increased ventilation is also a prominent feature of metabolic acidosis.

Breathlessness on physical exertion is normal and not considered a symptom unless the level of exertion is very light, e.g. walking slowly. Although breathlessness is a very common symptom the sensory and neural mechanisms underlying it remain obscure. The sensation of breathlessness is derived from at least three sources:
1 Changes in lung volume are sensed by receptors in thoracic wall muscles signalling changes in their length.
2 The tension developed by contracting muscles can be sensed by Golgi tendon organs. The tension developed in normal muscle can be differentiated from that developed in muscles weakened by fatigue or disease.
3 Central perception of the sense of effort.

# The airways of the lungs

From the trachea to the periphery, the airways become smaller in size (although greater in number). The cross-sectional area available for airflow increases as the total number of airways increases. The flow of air is maximum in the trachea and slows progressively towards the periphery (as the velocity of airflow depends on the ratio of flow to cross-sectional area). In the terminal airways, gas flow occurs solely by diffusion. The resistance to airflow is very low—0.1–0.2 kPa litre$^{-1}$ in a normal tracheobronchial tree.

Airways expand as lung volume is increased and at full inspiration (total lung capacity, TLC) they are 30–40% larger in calibre than at full expiration (residual volume, RV). In chronic bronchitis and emphysema, which principally affect the smaller airways, the airway narrowing is partially overcome by breathing at a larger lung volume.

## Control of airway tone

This is under the autonomic nervous system. Broncho-motor tone is maintained by vagal efferent nerves and, even in a normal subject, is reduced by atropine or $\beta$-adrenoreceptor agonists. The many adrenoreceptors on the surface of bronchial muscles respond to circulating catecholamines, although sympathetic nerves do not directly innervate them. Airway tone shows a *circadian rhythm*, which is greatest at 04.00 and lowest in the mid-afternoon. Tone can be increased briefly by inhaled stimuli acting on epithelial receptors, which trigger reflex bronchoconstriction via the vagus.

These stimuli include cigarette smoke, inert dust, cold air; airway responsiveness to these increases following respiratory tract infections even in healthy subjects. In asthma, the characteristic increased airway responsiveness is an exaggeration of this normal response and, as the circadian rhythm remains the same, asthmatic symptoms are worst in the early morning.

## Air flow

Movement of air through the airways results from a difference between the pressure in the alveoli and the atmospheric pressure; a positive alveolar pressure occurs in expiration and a negative pressure occurs in inspiration. During quiet breathing the subatmospheric pleural pressure throughout the breathing cycle slightly distends the airways. With vigorous expiratory efforts (e.g. cough), although the central airways are compressed by positive pleural pressures exceeding 10 kPa, the airways do not close completely because the driving pressure for expiratory flow (alveolar pressure) is also increased. *Alveolar pressure $P_{ALV}$ is equal to the elastic recoil pressure of the lung plus the pleural pressure $P_{EL}$.* When there is no airflow (i.e. a pause in breathing) the tendency of the lungs to collapse (the positive recoil pressure) is exactly balanced by an equivalent negative pleural pressure.

As air flows from the alveoli towards the mouth there is a gradual loss of pressure owing to flow resistance (Fig. 12.7). In forced expiration, as mentioned above, the driving pressure raises both the alveolar pressure and the intrapleural pressure. Between the alveolus and the mouth, a point will occur (C in Fig. 12.7) where the airway pressure will equal the intrapleural pressure, and airway compression will occur. However, this compression of the airway is temporary, as the transient occlusion of the airway results in an increase in pressure behind it (i.e. upstream) and this raises the intra-airway pressure so that the airways open and flow is restored. The airways thus tend to vibrate at this point of 'dynamic compression'.

The elastic recoil pressure of the lungs decreases with decreasing lung volume and the 'collapse point' moves upstream (i.e. towards the smaller airways—see Fig. 12.7c). Where there is pathological loss of recoil pressure (as in chronic bronchitis and emphysema), the 'collapse point' starts even further upstream and these patients are often seen to 'purse their lips' in order to increase airway pressure so that their peripheral airways do not collapse. The expiratory airflow limitation is the disordered physiology that underlies chronic airflow limitation. The

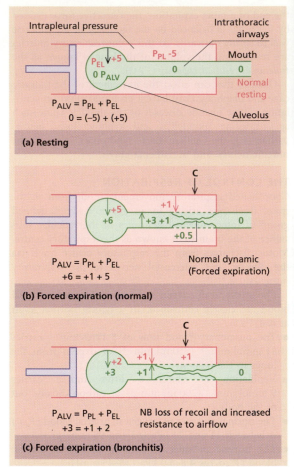

**Fig. 12.7** Diagrams showing the ventilatory forces during (a) resting at functional residual capacity, (b) forced expiration in normal subjects, (c) forced expiration in a patient with chronic bronchitis and emphysema. The respiratory system is represented as a piston with a single alveolus and the collapsible part of the airways within the piston (see text). C, compression point; $P_{ALV}$, alveolar pressure; $P_{EL}$, elastic recoil pressure; $P_{PL}$, pleural pressure.

measurement of the forced expiratory volume in 1 s ($FEV_1$) is a useful clinical index of this phenomenon.

On inspiration the intrapleural pressure is always less than the intraluminal pressure within the intrathoracic airways, so there is no limitation to airflow with increasing effort. Inspiratory flow is limited only by the power of the inspiratory muscles.

## Flow–volume loops

The relationship between maximal flow rates on expiration and inspiration is demonstrated by the maximal flow–volume (MFV) loops. Figure 12.8a shows this in a normal subject.

In subjects with healthy lungs the clinical importance of flow limitation will not be apparent, since maximal flow rates are rarely achieved even during vigorous exercise. However, in patients with severe chronic bronchitis and emphysema, limitation of expiratory flow occurs

**Fig. 12.8** (a and b) Maximal flow–volume loops, showing the relationship between maximal flow rates on expiration and inspiration in (a) a normal subject and (b) a patient with severe airflow limitation. Flow–volume loops during tidal breathing at rest (starting from the functional residual capacity [FRC]) and during exercise are also shown. The highest flow rates are achieved when forced expiration begins at total lung capacity (TLC) and represent the peak expiratory flow rate (PEFR). As air is blown out of the lung, so the flow rate decreases until no more air can be forced out, a point known as the residual volume (RV). Because inspiratory airflow is only dependent on effort, the shape of the maximal inspiratory flow–volume loop is quite different, and inspiratory flow remains at a high rate throughout the manoeuvre. (c and d) Flow–volume loops of patients with large airway (tracheal) obstruction, showing plateauing of maximal expiratory flow high in the lung volume. (c) Extrathoracic tracheal obstruction with a proportionally greater reduction of maximal inspiratory (as opposed to expiratory) flow rate. (d) Intrathoracic large airway obstruction; the expiratory plateau is more pronounced and inspiratory flow rate is less reduced than in (c). In severe airflow limitation the ventilatory demands of exercise cannot be met (cf. a and b) greatly reducing effort tolerance

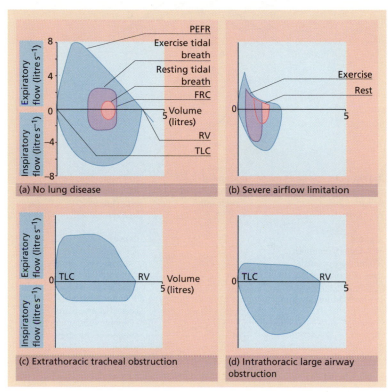

even during tidal breathing at rest (see Fig. 12.8b). To increase ventilation these patients have to breathe at higher lung volumes and also allow more time for expiration by increasing flow rates during inspiration, where there is proportionally much less flow limitation. This explains the clinical phenomenon of a prolonged expiratory time in patients with severe airflow limitation.

The measurement of the volume that can be forced in from RV in 1 s ($FIV_1$) will always be greater than that which can be forced out from TLC in 1 s ($FEV_1$). Thus, the ratio of $FEV_1$ to $FIV_1$ is below 1. The only exception to this occurs when there is significant obstruction to the airways outside the thorax, e.g. a tumour mass in the upper part of the trachea. Under these circumstances expiratory airway narrowing is prevented by the tracheal resistance (a situation similar to pursing the lips) and expiratory airflow becomes more effort-dependent. During forced inspiration this same resistance causes such negative intraluminal pressure that the trachea is compressed by the surrounding atmospheric pressure. Inspiratory flow thus becomes less effort-dependent, and the ratio of $FEV_1$ to $FIV_1$ becomes greater than 1. This phenomenon, and the characteristic flow volume loop, is used to diagnose extrathoracic airways obstruction (Fig. 12.8c).

When obstruction occurs in large airways within the thorax (lower end of trachea and main bronchi), expiratory flow is impaired more than inspiratory flow but a characteristic plateau to expiratory flow is seen (Fig. 12.8d).

# Ventilation and perfusion relationships

For efficient gas exchange it is important that there is a match between ventilation of the alveoli ($\dot{V}_A$) and their perfusion ($\dot{Q}$). There is a wide variation in the $\dot{V}_A/\dot{Q}$ ratio throughout both normal and diseased lung. In the normal lung the extreme relationships between alveolar ventilation and perfusion are:

- Ventilation but no perfusion (physiological dead space)
- Perfusion but no ventilation (physiological shunting)

These and the 'ideal' match are illustrated in Fig. 12.9. In normal lungs there is a tendency for ventilation not to be matched by perfusion towards the apices, with the reverse occurring at the bases.

An increased physiological shunt results in arterial hypoxaemia. The effects of an increased physiological dead space can usually be overcome by a compensatory increase in the ventilation of normally perfused alveoli. In advanced disease this compensation cannot occur,

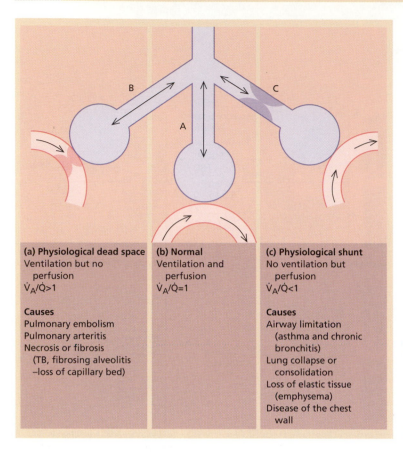

**(a) Physiological dead space**
Ventilation but no
   perfusion
$\dot{V}_A/\dot{Q}>1$

**Causes**
Pulmonary embolism
Pulmonary arteritis
Necrosis or fibrosis
   (TB, fibrosing alveolitis
   –loss of capillary bed)

**(b) Normal**
Ventilation and
   perfusion
$\dot{V}_A/\dot{Q}=1$

**(c) Physiological shunt**
No ventilation but
   perfusion
$\dot{V}_A/\dot{Q}<1$

**Causes**
Airway limitation
   (asthma and chronic
   bronchitis)
Lung collapse or
   consolidation
Loss of elastic tissue
   (emphysema)
Disease of the chest
   wall

**Fig. 12.9** Relationships between ventilation and perfusion: a schematic diagram showing the alveolar–capillary interface. The centre shows normal ventilation and perfusion. On the left there is a block in perfusion (physiological dead space), while on the right there is reduced ventilation (physiological shunting).

leading to increased alveolar and arterial $P\text{co}_2$, together with hypoxaemia.

Hypoxaemia occurs more readily than hypercapnia because of the different ways in which oxygen and carbon dioxide are carried in the blood. Carbon dioxide can be considered to be in simple solution in the plasma, the volume carried being proportional to the partial pressure. Oxygen is carried in chemical combination with haemoglobin in the red blood cell, and the relationship between the volume carried and the partial pressure is not linear (see Fig. 13.5). Alveolar hyperventilation resulting in a low alveolar $P\text{co}_2$ and a high alveolar $P\text{o}_2$ will therefore lead to a marked reduction in the carbon dioxide content of the resulting blood but no increase in the oxygen content. The hypoxaemia of even a small amount of physiological shunting cannot therefore be compensated for by hyperventilation.

The $P_a\text{o}_2$ and $P_a\text{co}_2$ of some individuals who have mild disease of the lung causing slight $\dot{V}_A/\dot{Q}$ mismatch may still be normal. Increasing the requirements for gas exchange by exercise will widen the $V/Q$ mismatch and the $P_a\text{o}_2$ will fall. $\dot{V}/\dot{Q}$ mismatch is by far the commonest cause of arterial hypoxaemia.

## Alveolar stability

The alveoli of the lung are essentially hollow spheres. Surface tension acting at the curved internal surface tends to cause the sphere to decrease in size. The surface tension within the alveoli would make the lungs extremely difficult to distend were it not for the presence of surfactant. The type II cells within the alveolus secrete an insoluble lipoprotein largely consisting of dipalmitoyl lecithin, which forms a thin monomolecular layer at the air–fluid interface. Surfactant reduces surface tension so that alveoli remain stable.

Fluid surfaces covered with surfactant exhibit a phenomenon known as hysteresis, i.e. the surface-tension-lowering effect of the surfactant can be improved by a transient increase in the size of the surface area of the alveoli. During quiet breathing, small areas of the lung undergo collapse, but it is possible to re-expand these rapidly by a deep breath, hence the importance of sighs or deep breaths as a feature of normal breathing. Failure of such a mechanism, which can occur, for example, in patients with fractured ribs, gives rise to patchy basal lung collapse. Surfactant levels may be reduced in a number of diseases that cause damage to the lung (e.g. pneumonia), and may play a central role in the respiratory distress syndrome of the newborn. Severe reduction in perfusion of the lung causes impairment of surfactant activity and may well account for the characteristic areas of collapse associated with pulmonary embolism.

# Defence mechanisms of the respiratory tract

Pulmonary disease often results from a failure of the many defence mechanisms that usually protect the lung in a healthy individual (Fig. 12.10). These can be divided into physical and physiological mechanisms and humoral and cellular mechanisms.

## Physical and physiological mechanisms

HUMIDIFICATION—prevents dehydration of the epithelium.

PARTICLE REMOVAL—over 90% of particles greater than 10 $\mu$m in diameter are removed in the nostril or nasopharynx. Of the remainder, 5–10 $\mu$m particles become impacted in the carina and 1–2 $\mu$m particles are deposited in the distal lungs. Most pollen grain (>20 $\mu$m) particles are deposited in the nose and conjunctiva.

PARTICLE EXPULSION—by coughing, sneezing or gagging.

RESPIRATORY TRACT SECRETIONS.

The mucus of the respiratory tract is a gelatinous substance consisting chiefly of acid and neutral polysaccharides. The mucus consists of a 5 $\mu$m thick gel that is relatively impermeable to water. This floats on a liquid or sol layer that is present around the cilia of the epithelial cells.

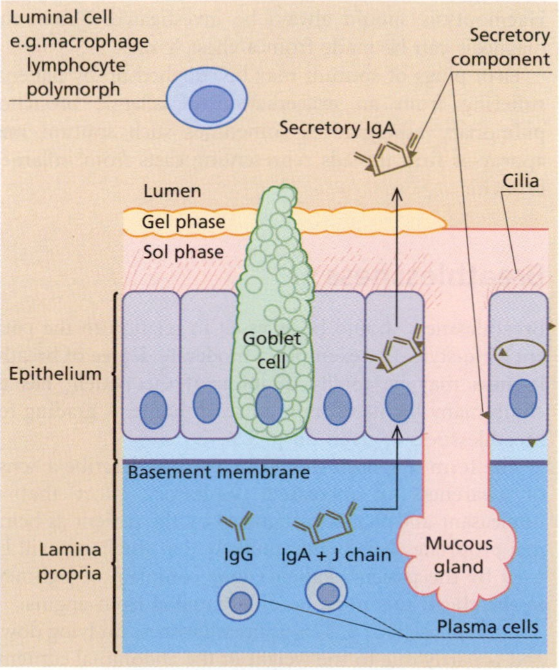

The gel layer is secreted from goblet cells and mucous glands as distinct globules that coalesce increasingly in the central airways to form a more or less continuous mucus blanket. Under normal conditions the tips of the cilia are in contact with the undersurface of the gel phase and coordinate their movement to push the mucus blanket upwards. Whilst it may only take 30–60 min for mucus to be cleared from the large bronchi, there may be a delay of several days before clearance is achieved from respiratory bronchioles. One of the major long-term effects of cigarette smoking is a reduction in mucociliary transport. This contributes to recurrent infection and in the larger airways it prolongs contact with carcinogens.

Congenital defects in mucociliary transport occur. In the 'immotile cilia' syndrome there is an absence of the dynein arms in the cilia themselves, and in cystic fibrosis an abnormal mucus is associated with ciliary dyskinesia. Both diseases are characterized by recurrent infections and eventually with the development of bronchiectasis.

## Humoral and cellular mechanisms

### Non-specific soluble factors

$\alpha_1$-ANTITRYPSIN is present in lung secretions. It inhibits chymotrypsin and trypsin and neutralizes proteases and elastase.

LYSOZYME is an enzyme found in granulocytes that has bacteriocidal properties.

LACTOFERRIN is synthesized from epithelial cells and neutrophil granulocytes and has bacteriocidal properties.

INTERFERON (see p. 139) is produced by most cells in response to viral infection. It is a potent suppressor of lymphocyte function and lowers the threshold for mast cell histamine release. It renders other cells resistant to infection by any other virus.

COMPLEMENT is present in secretions. In association with antibodies, it plays an important cytotoxic role.

### Pulmonary alveolar macrophages

These are derived from precursors in the bone marrow and migrate to the lungs via the bloodstream. They phagocytose particles, including bacteria, and are removed by the mucociliary escalator, lymphatics and bloodstream. They are the dominant cell in the airways and at the level of the alveoli and comprise 90% of all cells obtained by bronchoalveolar lavage.

Macrophages (see p. 133) process antigens and play a part in both cellular and humoral immunity.

### Lymphoid tissue (see p. 133)

The bronchus-associated lymphoid tissue (BALT) consists of lymphocytes present either in aggregates (tonsils and adenoids) or scattered. It forms an important immunological defence mechanism. Lymphocytes become sensitized to antigens, resulting in local production of secretory IgA. IgG and IgE are also present in secretions derived from B lymphocytes in the lamina propria.

**Fig. 12.10**  Defence mechanisms present at the epithelial surface.

# *Respiratory symptoms*

## Runny, blocked nose and sneezing

Nasal symptoms are extremely common. The differentiation between the common cold or allergic rhinitis as a cause of 'runny nose' (rhinorrhoea), nasal blockage and attacks of sneezing is difficult. In allergic rhinitis, symptoms may be seasonal, following contact with grass pollen, or perennial, when the house-dust mite is the important allergen. Colds are frequent during the winter but, if more than three occur, the patient is probably suffering from perennial rhinitis rather than from infection due to a virus. Patients may be able to identify the cause of their symptoms if, for example, they sneeze whilst walking in the park in summer or after making beds.

Nasal secretions are usually thin and runny in rhinitis but thicker and yellow-green in the common cold. Nose bleeds and blood-stained nasal discharge are common occurrences and are not as serious as haemoptysis. Nevertheless, a blood-stained nasal discharge associated with nasal obstruction and pain may be the presenting feature of a nasal tumour. Total nasal blockage with loss of smell is often a feature of nasal polyps.

## Cough

Cough is the commonest manifestation of lower respiratory tract disease. Smokers often have a morning cough with little sputum. Cough is the cardinal feature of chronic bronchitis, while sputum production and coughing, particularly at night, can be symptoms of asthma. Cough also occurs in asthmatics after mild exertion or following a forced expiration. A cough can also occur for psychological reasons.

A worsening cough is the commonest presenting symptom of a bronchial carcinoma. The explosive character of a normal cough is lost when laryngeal paralysis is present—a bovine cough—usually resulting from carcinoma of the bronchus infiltrating the left recurrent laryngeal nerve. Cough may be accompanied by stridor in whooping cough and in the presence of laryngeal or tracheal obstruction.

Despite the popularity of cough mixtures, the correct treatment of this symptom is to identify and treat the underlying cause. Cough may persist in some individuals for many weeks following a respiratory tract infection, perhaps as the result of persisting bronchial inflammation and increased airway responsiveness (see p. 668), a process that may settle with inhaled corticosteroid treatment.

## Sputum

Approximately 100 ml of mucus is produced daily in a healthy, non-smoking individual. This flows at a regular pace up the airways, through the larynx, and is swallowed. Excess mucus is expectorated as sputum. The most common cause of excess mucus production is cigarette smoking.

Mucoid sputum is clear and white but can contain black specks resulting from the inhalation of carbon. Yellow or green sputum is due to the presence of cellular material, including bronchial epithelial cells, or neutrophil or eosinophil granulocytes. Yellow sputum is not necessarily due to infection, as eosinophils in the sputum, as seen in asthma, can give the same appearance. The production of large quantities of yellow or green sputum is characteristic of bronchiectasis.

Blood-stained sputum (haemoptysis) varies from small streaks of blood to massive bleeding. It requires thorough investigation. The following should be borne in mind.

- The commonest cause of haemoptysis is acute infection, particularly in exacerbations of chronic bronchitis and emphysema, but it should not be attributed to this without investigation.
- Other common causes are pulmonary infarction, bronchial carcinoma and tuberculosis.
- In lobar pneumonia, the sputum is rusty in appearance when blood is present.
- Pink, frothy sputum is seen in pulmonary oedema.
- In bronchiectasis, the blood is often mixed with purulent sputum.
- Massive haemoptyses (>200 ml of blood in 24 hours) are usually due to bronchiectasis or tuberculosis (see p. 664).
- Uncommon causes of haemoptyses are idiopathic pulmonary haemosiderosis, Goodpasture's syndrome, microscopic polyarteritis, trauma, blood disorders and benign tumours.

Haemoptysis should always be investigated. Often, the diagnosis can be made from a chest X-ray.

Firm plugs of sputum may be coughed up by patients suffering from an exacerbation of allergic bronchopulmonary aspergillosis; sometimes such sputum may appear as firm threads representing casts from inflamed bronchi.

## Breathlessness

Breathlessness should be assessed in relation to the patient's life-style. For example, a moderate degree of breathlessness may be totally disabling if the patient has to climb many flights of stairs to reach home. A grading for breathlessness is given on p. 526.

The term *dyspnoea* should be used to describe a sense of awareness of increased respiratory effort that is unpleasant and that is recognized by the patient as being inappropriate. It is highly unlikely that this term will be used by the patient. Patients may complain of tightness in the chest; this must be differentiated from angina.

*Orthopnoea* (see p. 526) is breathlessness on lying down and is partly due to the weight of the abdominal contents pushing the diaphragm further into the thorax. Such patients are also made uncomfortable by bending over.

The terms *tachypnoea* and *hyperpnoea* refer, respectively, to an increased rate of breathing and an increased level of ventilation, which may be appropriate to the situation (e.g. during exercise). *Hyperventilation* is overbreathing and results in a lowering of the alveolar and arterial $Pco_2$.

Paroxysmal nocturnal dyspnoea is described on p. 526.

Respiratory diseases can cause breathlessness within minutes or hours or else more slowly over days, weeks or months. The typical causes of breathlessness over differing time periods are:

1 Sudden
   (a) Inhaled foreign body
   (b) Pneumothorax
   (c) Pulmonary embolism
2 Over a few hours
   (a) Asthma
   (b) Pneumonia
   (c) Pulmonary oedema
   (d) Extrinsic allergic alveolitis
3 Intermittent
   (a) Asthma
   (b) Pulmonary oedema
4 Over days
   (a) Pleural effusions
   (b) Carcinoma of the bronchus/trachea
5 Over months or years
   (a) Chronic bronchitis and emphysema
   (b) Cryptogenic fibrosing alveolitis
   (c) Occupational fibrotic lung disease
   (d) Non-respiratory causes—anaemia, hyperthyroidism

## Wheezing

Wheezing is a common complaint and is the result of airflow limitation due to any cause. The symptom of wheezing is *not* diagnostic of asthma; it may be absent in the early stages of this disease, and may also occur in patients with chronic bronchitis and emphysema.

## Chest pain

The commonest type of chest pain encountered in respiratory disease is a localized sharp pain, often referred to as pleuritic. It is made worse by deep breathing or coughing and can be precisely localized by the patient. Localized anterior chest pain may be accompanied by tenderness of a costochondral junction due to costochondritis. Pain in the shoulder tips suggests irritation of the diaphragmatic pleura, whereas central chest pain radiating to the neck and arms is typically of cardiac origin. Retrosternal soreness may occur in patients with tracheitis, and a constant, severe, dull pain may be the result of invasion of the thoracic wall by carcinoma.

# Examination of the respiratory system

## The nose

The anterior part of the nose can be examined using a nasal speculum and light source. In allergic rhinitis the mucosa lining the nasal septum and inferior turbinate appears swollen and a dark red or plum colour. Nasal polyps can also be identified, as can a frequent site of nasal haemorrhage (Little's area).

## The chest (Table 12.1)

Radiology has become an essential part of examination of the chest. Diseases such as tuberculosis or lung cancer may not be detectable on clinical examination but are obvious on the chest X-ray. Conversely, the abnormal physical signs in asthma or chronic bronchitis may be associated with a normal chest X-ray.

### INSPECTION

The patient should be observed carefully, paying particular attention to mental alertness, cyanosis, breathlessness at rest, use of accessory muscles and any deformity or scars on the chest. A coarse tremor or flap of the outstretched hands indicates $CO_2$ intoxication. Prominent veins on the chest may imply obstruction of the superior vena cava. The jugular venous pressure should be assessed.

*Central cyanosis* (see p. 528) is assessed on the colour of the tongue and lips, and indicates a $P_ao_2$ below 6 kPa. *Peripheral cyanosis* is noted on the fingernails and skin of the extremities and in the absence of central cyanosis is due to a reduced peripheral circulation.

*Finger clubbing* is present when the normal angle between the base of the nail and the nail fold is lost. The base of the nail is fluctuant owing to increased vascularity, and there is an increased curvature of the nail in all directions, with expansion of the end of the digit. Some causes of clubbing are given in Table 12.2. Clubbing is not seen in chronic bronchitis.

### PALPATION

The position of the mediastinum should be ascertained by checking whether the trachea is central and whether the cardiac apex is in the fifth intercostal space. The supraclavicular fossa is examined for enlarged lymph nodes. The distance between the sternal notch and the cricoid cartilage (three to four finger breadths in full expiration) is reduced in patients with severe airflow limitation. Movement of the upper and lower parts of the chest should be assessed. Compression of the chest laterally and anteroposteriorly may produce a localized pain suggestive of a rib fracture.

### PERCUSSION

This should be performed symmetrically on both sides for comparison. Liver dullness is usually detected

| Pathological process | Chest wall movement | Mediastinal displacement | Percussion note | Breath sounds | Vocal resonance | Added sounds |
|---|---|---|---|---|---|---|
| Consolidation (i.e. lobar pneumonia) | Reduced on affected side | None | Dull | Bronchial | Increased | Fine crackles |
| **Collapse** | | | | | | |
| Major bronchus | Reduced on affected side | Towards lesion | Dull | Diminished or absent | Reduced or absent | None |
| Peripheral bronchus | Reduced on affected side | Towards lesion | Dull | Bronchial | Increased | Fine crackles |
| **Fibrosis** | | | | | | |
| Localized | Reduced on affected side | Towards lesion | Dull | Bronchial | Increased | Coarse crackles |
| Generalized (e.g. cryptogenic fibrosing alveolitis) | Reduced on both sides | None | Normal | Vesicular | Increased | Fine crackles |
| Pleural effusion (>500 ml) | Reduced on affected side | Away from lesion (in massive effusion) | Stony dull | Vesicular reduced or absent | Reduced or absent | None |
| Large pneumothorax | Reduced on affected side | Away from lesion | Normal or hyperresonant | Reduced or absent | Reduced or absent | None |
| Asthma | Reduced on both sides | None | Normal | Vesicular Prolonged expiration | Normal | Expiratory polyphonic wheeze |
| Chronic bronchitis and emphysema | Reduced on both sides | None | Normal | Vesicular Prolonged expiration | Normal | Expiratory polyphonic wheeze and coarse crackles |

**Table 12.1** Physical signs of respiratory disease.

*Respiratory*
Bronchial carcinoma, especially epidermoid (squamous cell) type—major cause
Chronic suppurative lung disease
　　Bronchiectasis
　　Lung abscess
　　Empyema
Pulmonary fibrosis (e.g. cryptogenic fibrosing alveolitis)
Pleural and mediastinal tumours (e.g. mesothelioma)
Cryptogenic organizing pneumonia

*Cardiovascular*
Cyanotic heart disease
Subacute infective endocarditis

*Miscellaneous*
Congenital—no disease
Cirrhosis
Inflammatory bowel disease

**Table 12.2** Some causes of finger clubbing.

anteriorly at the level of the sixth rib. Liver and cardiac dullness are lost with over-inflated lungs. The percussion note is dull over consolidation and stony dull over a pleural effusion.

## AUSCULTATION

The diaphragm of the stethoscope should be used. The patient is asked to take deep breaths through the mouth.

Inspiration sounds more prolonged than expiration. Healthy lungs filter off most of the high-frequency component, mainly due to turbulent flow in the larynx. Normal breath sounds are harsher anteriorly over the upper lobes (particularly on the right) and described as vesicular. Vesicular sounds may be loud in a thin healthy subject or soft in patients with emphysema. Breath sounds are reduced or absent in a pneumothorax, over a pleural effusion or when the bronchus to a lobe is obstructed by a carcinoma.

BRONCHIAL BREATHING. These abnormal breath sounds are heard best over consolidated or collapsed lung and sometimes over areas of localized fibrosis or bronchiectasis. Such areas conduct the high-frequency hissing component of breath sounds well. Characteristically, the noise heard during inspiration and expiration is equally long but separated by a short silent phase. Bronchial breathing can be imitated by listening over the larynx, particularly if the subject breathes with the vocal cords in a position to sound a whispered 'eee'.

Whispering pectoriloquy (whispered, and therefore higher-pitched, sounds heard distinctly) invariably accompanies bronchial breathing.

ADDED SOUNDS. The terms rhonchi, rales and crepitations are best discarded and replaced with the simple terms wheezes and crackles.

WHEEZE is usually heard during expiration and results from vibrations in the collapsible part of the airways when apposition occurs as a result of the flow-limiting mechanisms. Wheezes are heard in asthma and in chronic bronchitis and emphysema, but are not invariably present. In the most severe cases of asthma a wheeze may not be heard, as the airflow may be insufficient to generate the sound. Wheezes may be monophonic (single large airway obstruction) or polyphonic (narrowing of many small airways).

CRACKLES. These brief crackling sounds are probably produced by opening of previously closed bronchioles, and their timing during breathing is of significance— early inspiratory crackles are associated with diffuse airflow limitation, whereas late inspiratory crackles are characteristically heard in pulmonary oedema, fibrosis of the lung and bronchiectasis. They may be described as fine or coarse but this is of no significance.

PLEURAL RUB. This is a creaking or groaning sound that is usually well localized. It is indicative of inflammation and roughening of the pleural surfaces, which normally glide silently over one another.

VOCAL RESONANCE AND FREMITUS. Healthy lung attenuates high-frequency notes, leaving the booming low-pitched components of speech. Consolidated lung has the reverse effect, transmitting the high frequencies; the spoken word then takes on a bleating quality. Whispered speech can barely be heard over healthy lung, whereas consolidation allows its clear transmission. Sonorous sounds such as 'ninety-nine' are well transmitted across healthy lung to produce vibration that can be felt over the chest wall. Consolidated lung transmits these low-frequency noises less well, and pleural fluid severely dampens or obliterates the vibrations altogether.

## Additional bedside tests

Since so many patients with respiratory disease have airflow limitation, airflow should be routinely measured at the bedside using a peak flow meter. This will provide a much more accurate assessment than any physical sign.

## *Investigation of respiratory disease*

## Routine haematological and biochemical tests

These should include tests for:
- Haemoglobin, to detect the presence of anaemia
- Packed cell volume (PCV) (secondary polycythaemia occurs with chronic bronchitis and emphysema)

- Routine biochemistry

Other blood investigations sometimes required include $\alpha_1$-antitrypsin levels, autoantibodies, and, in asthma, IgE to specific allergens (RAST; radioallergosorbent test) and *Aspergillus* antibodies.

## Sputum

Sputum should be inspected for colour:
- Yellow-green indicates inflammation (infection or allergy)
- Presence of blood suggests neoplasm or pulmonary infarct

Microbiological studies (Gram stain and culture) are not helpful in upper respiratory tract infections or in acute or chronic bronchitis. They are of value in:
- Pneumonia
- Diagnosis of tuberculosis (Ziehl–Nielsen stain)
- Unusual clinical problems
- *Aspergillus* lung disease

## Cytology

This is extremely useful in the diagnosis of bronchial carcinoma. Advantages are:
- Quick result
- Cheap
- Non-invasive

However, its value depends on the production of sputum and the presence of a reliable cytologist. Sputum can be induced following the inhalation of nebulized hypertonic saline (5%). This is unpleasant and for important samples it is better to proceed to transtracheal aspiration or more usually bronchoscopy and bronchial washings (see p. 650).

### Transtracheal aspiration

This technique involves pushing a needle through the cricothyroid membrane, through which a catheter is threaded to a position just above the carina. This procedure induces coughing, and specimens are collected by aspiration or by the introduction and subsequent aspiration of sterile saline. It is an excellent technique (although not often required) for assessing infection in the lower respiratory tract because it obviates any possibility of contamination of the specimen with bacteria from the pharynx and mouth.

## Chest X-ray

The following must be taken into account when viewing films:
CENTRING OF THE FILM. The distance between each clavicular head and the spinal processes must be equal.
PENETRATION.
THE VIEW. Postero-anterior (PA) is the routine film. Antero-posterior (AP) films are only taken in very ill patients who are unable to stand up or be taken to the radiology department; the cardiac outline appears

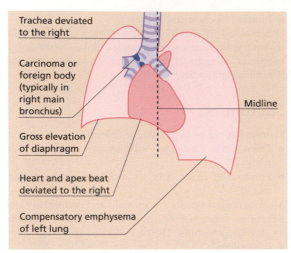

Trachea deviated to the right

Carcinoma or foreign body (typically in right main bronchus)

Midline

Gross elevation of diaphragm

Heart and apex beat deviated to the right

Compensatory emphysema of left lung

**Fig. 12.11** Collapse of the right lung. Diagram showing a raised right diaphragm and compensatory emphysema of the left lung.

bigger and the scapulae cannot be moved out of the way.

The following should be noted:
- The shape and body structure of the chest wall
- Whether the trachea is central
- Whether the diaphragm is elevated or flat
- The shape, size and position of the heart
- The shape and size of the hilar shadows
- The vascular shadowing and the size and shape of any abnormalities of the lungs

### X-ray abnormalities

COLLAPSE AND CONSOLIDATION. A diagram showing the X-ray changes in collapse of a whole lung is given in Fig. 12.11. In collapse of the middle lobe, all that may be detected is a loss of the clear outline of the right atrium, which distinguishes it from collapse of the right lower lobe. In consolidation, the segments or lobes of the lung are opaque but the bronchi are patent, producing an air bronchogram. Causes of collapse are shown in Table 12.3.

PLEURAL EFFUSION. Pleural effusions need to be more than 500 ml to cause much more than blunting of the costophrenic angle. On an erect film they produce a

characteristic shadow with a curved upper edge rising into the axilla. If very large, the whole of one side of the thorax may be opaque, with shift of the mediastinum to the opposite side.

FIBROSIS. Localized fibrosis causes streaky shadowing and the accompanying loss of lung volume causes mediastinal structures to move to the same side. More generalized fibrosis in the lung can lead to a honeycomb appearance (see p. 694), seen as diffuse shadows containing multiple circular translucences a few millimetres in diameter.

ROUND SHADOWS. The causes of round shadows are shown in Table 12.4.

MILIARY MOTTLING. This term describes numerous minute opacities, 1–3 mm in size, which are caused by many pathological processes. The commoner causes are miliary tuberculosis, pneumoconiosis, sarcoidosis, fibrosing alveolitis and pulmonary oedema, though the latter is usually perihilar and accompanied by larger, fluffy shadows. A rare but striking cause of miliary mottling is pulmonary microlithiasis.

## Computed tomography

This technique is carried out by the rotation of an X-ray tube around the patient in a series of complete circles. The signals are detected by an array of scintillation crystals and are processed quantitatively by a computer to produce a two-dimensional image of high resolution for each axial scan or cut. CT gives a numerical indication of the relative densities of particular tissues, but only fat is different enough to be reliably diagnosed. Normal lung

---

*Tumours*
Enlarged tracheobronchial lymph nodes due to:
  Malignant disease
  Tuberculosis

Inhaled foreign bodies (e.g. peanuts) in children, usually in the right main bronchus

Bronchial casts or plugs (e.g. allergic bronchopulmonary aspergillosis)

Retained secretions—postoperatively and in debilitated patients

**Table 12.3**  Causes of collapse of the lung.

---

Carcinoma

Metastatic tumours (usually multiple shadows)

Tuberculoma (may be calcification within the lesion)

Lung abscess (usually with fluid level)

Encysted interlobar effusion (usually in horizontal fissure)

Hydatid cysts (rare and often with a fluid level)

Arteriovenous malformations (usually adjacent to a vascular shadow)

Aspergilloma

Rheumatoid nodules

Rare causes
  Bronchial carcinoid
  Cylindroma
  Chondroma
  Lipoma

Other shadows related to mediastinum
  Pericardium  }
  Oesophagus   } Seen on lateral chest X-ray
  Spinal cord  }

**Table 12.4**  Causes of round shadows in the lung.

is of sufficiently low density (90% air, 10% soft tissue) to allow the trachea and main bronchus to show up on cuts, particularly when the latter are running at right angles or at the same plane rather than in an oblique direction (Fig. 12.12). This is also true for the large pulmonary vessels and for other mediastinal structures to the extent that CT is the radiographic procedure of choice for investigating the mediastinum and hilar regions.

CT is essential in staging of carcinoma of the bronchus and CT scanning should be extended to include the liver, adrenal glands and brain. Although CT will identify enlarged mediastinal lymph nodes, these may not be malignant and require biopsy. Nevertheless, the absence of any lymph node enlargement on CT scanning is a useful indication favouring operability.

High-resolution CT in which the slices are between 1 and 2 mm thick compared to the conventional CT slice of 10 mm has improved the value of the technique for the assessment of interstitial lung disease and can produce diagnostic information. It is of particular value in:

1 Detection of pulmonary involvement and its extent in sarcoidosis, lymphoma, cryptogenic and extrinsic alveolitis, occupational lung disease

2 Bronchiectasis. High-resolution CT has a sensitivity and specificity of greater than 90% compared with bronchograms

3 Distinguishing emphysema from interstitial lung disease or pulmonary vascular disease as a cause of a low gas transfer factor with otherwise normal lung function

4 Diagnosis of lymphangitis carcinomatosa.

## Magnetic resonance imaging (MRI)

This technique has proved less useful than CT because of its poorer imaging of the lung parenchyma. It can produce images in sagittal and coronal as well as transverse planes and for this reason is of value in assessing disease near the lung apex, the spine and the thoraco-abdominal regions. Flowing blood does not provide a signal in MRI. Vascular structures appear as hollow tubes making this technique useful in the differentiation of masses around the aorta or in the hilar regions.

## Radioisotope lung scanning

This technique has been widely used for the detection of pulmonary emboli.

### Perfusion scan

Macro-aggregated human albumin labelled with technetium-99m is injected intravenously. The particles are of such a size that they impact in pulmonary capillaries, where they remain for a few hours. A gamma camera is then used to detect the position of the macro-aggregated human albumin. The resultant pattern indicates the distribution of pulmonary blood flow; cold areas occur where there is defective blood flow (e.g. in pulmonary emboli).

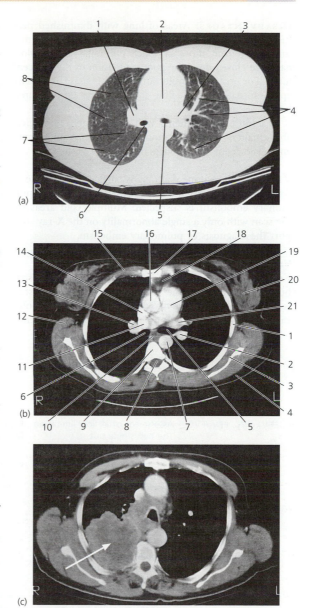

**Fig. 12.12** CT scan of the lung.
(a) Soft-tissue—showing normal lung markings. 1, right hilum; 2, mediastinum; 3, left hilum; 4, lung vessels; 5, L. main bronchus; 6, R. main bronchus; 7, position of oblique fissure; 8, peripheral lung vessels.
(b) Bone setting—showing normal mediastinal structures. 1, rib; 2, descending L. pulmonary artery; 3, scapula; 4, subcutaneous fat; 5, L. main bronchus; 6, R. main bronchus; 7, descending aorta; 8, spinal canal; 9, vertebral body; 10, oesophagus; 11, R. pulmonary artery; 12, muscle; 13, R. superior pulmonary vein; 14, superior vena cava; 15, costal cartilage; 16, ascending aorta; 17, sternum; 18, thymic remnant; 19, pulmonary trunk; 20, breast tissue; 21, L. superior pulmonary vein.
(c) Scan showing a central carcinoma of the bronchus and enlarged lymph nodes.

DISADVANTAGES. Areas of lung with diminished perfusion caused by pulmonary emboli cannot be distinguished from those in which pulmonary blood flow has been closed down by poor ventilation of the adjacent lung. For example, mild asthma can cause a patchy appearance. (NB Peak flow should always be measured before a scan.)

In addition, in patients with an obvious radiological abnormality, a scan cannot differentiate pulmonary embolism from other causes of defective perfusion.

VALUE. Radioisotope scanning is particularly of value in patients whose chest X-ray is normal and in whom pulmonary embolism is suspected. Multiple cold areas on the scan with only a single abnormality on the X-ray support the diagnosis of pulmonary embolism.

### Ventilation–perfusion scan

Xenon-133 gas is inhaled into the lung and its distribution is detected at the same time as a perfusion scan is carried out. Using the two scans, a pulmonary embolus causes a striking diminution of perfusion relative to ventilation. Other lung diseases (e.g. asthma or pneumonia) impair both ventilation and perfusion. Unfortunately, however, a pulmonary embolus often produces substantial changes in the lung substance (e.g. atelectasis) so that such a clear distinction is not always obvious. Nevertheless, this is a better technique than perfusion scan alone.

## Respiratory function tests (Table 12.5)

In practice, airflow limitation can be assessed by use of relatively simple tests that have good intrasubject repeatability. Normal values are required for their interpretation since these tests vary considerably, not only with sex, age and height, but also within individuals of the same age, sex and height. The standard deviation about the mean for a group of individuals is therefore very high; for example, the standard deviation for the peak expiratory flow rate is approximately 50 litre $min^{-1}$ and for the $FEV_1$ it is approximately 0.4 litres. Repeated measurements of lung function are required for assessing the progression of disease in an individual patient.

| Test | Use | Advantages | Disadvantages |
|---|---|---|---|
| PEFR | Monitoring changes in airflow limitation in asthma | Portable Can be used at the bedside | Effort dependent Poor measure of airflow limitation |
| $FEV_1$, FVC, $FEV_1$/FVC | Assessment of airflow limitation The best single test | Reproducible Relatively effort independent | Bulky equipment but smaller portable machines now available |
| Flow–volume curves | Assessment of flow at lower lung volumes Detection of large airway obstruction both intra and extra thoracic (e.g. tracheal stenosis, tumour) | Recognition of patterns of flow–volume curves for different diseases | Sophisticated equipment needed |
| Airways resistance | Assessment of airflow limitation | Sensitive | Technique difficult to perform |
| Lung volumes | Differentiation between restrictive and obstructive lung disease | Essential adjunct to $FEV_1$ | Sophisticated equipment needed |
| Gas transfer | Assessment and monitoring of extent of interstitial lung disease and emphysema | Non-invasive (compared to lung biopsy or radiation from repeated chest X-rays and CT) | Sophisticated equipment needed |
| Blood gases | Assessment of respiratory failure | Can detect early lung disease when measured during exercise | Invasive |
| Pulse oximetry | Postoperative ICU and sleep studies | Continuous monitoring Non-invasive | Measures saturation only |
| *Exercise tests* 6-min walk | Practical assessment for disability and effects of therapy | No equipment required | Time consuming Learning effect At least two walks required |
| Cardiorespiratory assessment | Early detection of lung/heart disease Fitness assessment | Essential in differentiating breathlessness due to lung or heart disease | Expensive and complicated equipment required |

ICU, intensive care unit.

**Table 12.5**  Respiratory function tests and exercise tests.

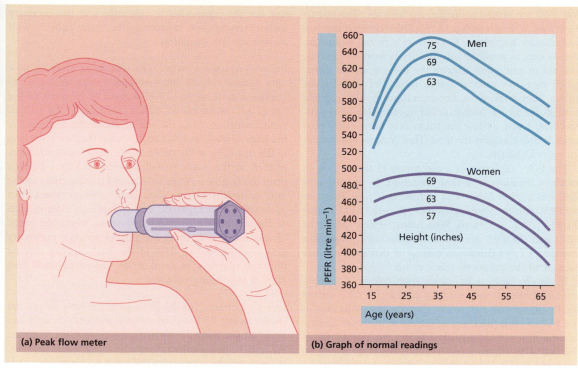

**Fig. 12.13**   Peak flow measurements. (a) Peak flow meter. The lips should be tight around the mouthpiece. (b) Graph of normal readings for men and women.

## Tests of ventilatory function

These tests are mainly used to assess the degree of airflow limitation present during expiration.

PEAK EXPIRATORY FLOW RATE (PEFR). This is an extremely simple and cheap test. Subjects are asked to take a full inspiration to total lung capacity and then blow out forcefully into the mini-Wright peak flow meter (Fig. 12.13), which is held horizontally; the lips must be placed tightly around the mouthpiece. The best of three tests is recorded.

Although reproducible, PEFR is not a good measure of airflow limitation since it only measures the expiratory flow rate in the first 2 ms of expiration and overestimates lung function in patients with moderate airflow limitation. PEFR is best used to monitor progression of disease and its treatment. Regular measurements of peak flow rates on waking, during the afternoon, and before bed demonstrate the wide diurnal variations in airflow limitation that characterize asthma and allow an objective assessment of treatment to be made (Fig. 12.14).

SPIROMETRY. The Vitalograph spirometer measures the $FEV_1$ and the forced vital capacity (FVC). Both the $FEV_1$

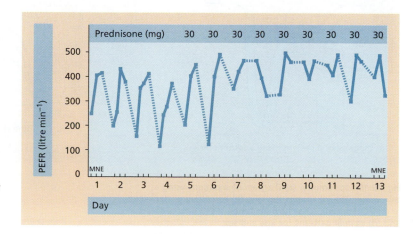

**Fig. 12.14**   Diurnal variability in airflow limitation, showing the effect of steroids. M, morning; N, noon; E, evening.

and FVC are related to height, age and sex. The instrument used is shown in Fig. 12.15a. The technique involves a maximum inspiration followed by a forced expiration (for as long as possible) into the dry bellows spirometer. The act of expiration triggers the moving record chart, which measures volume against time. The record chart moves for a total of 5 s, but expiration should continue until all the air has been expelled from the lungs, as patients with severe airflow limitation may have a very prolonged forced expiratory time. This is demonstrated on the record chart in Fig. 12.15.

The FEV₁ expressed as a percentage of the FVC is an excellent measure of airflow limitation. In normal subjects it is around 75%. With increasing *airflow limitation* the FEV₁ falls proportionately more than the FVC, so that the FEV₁/FVC is reduced. With *restrictive lung disease* the FEV₁ and the FVC are reduced in the same proportion and the FEV₁/FVC remains normal or may even increase because of the enhanced elastic recoil.

In chronic airflow limitation (particularly in emphysema and asthma) the total lung capacity (TLC) is usually increased, yet there is nearly always some reduction in the FVC. This is the result of disease in the small airways causing obstruction to airflow before the normal RV is reached. This trapping of air within the lung (giving an increased RV) is a characteristic feature of these diseases.

OTHER TESTS. Tests such as the measurement of airways resistance in a body plethysmograph are more sensitive but the equipment is expensive and the necessary manoeuvres are too exhausting for many patients with chronic airflow limitation.

FLOW–VOLUME LOOPS. The ability to measure flow rates against volume (flow–volume loops; see Fig. 12.8) enables a more sophisticated analysis to be made of the site of airflow limitation within the lung. At the start of expiration from TLC, the site of maximum resistance is the large airways, and this accounts for the flow reduction in the first 25% of the curve. As the lung volume reduces further, so the elastic pressures within the lung holding open the smaller airways reduce, and disease either of the lung parenchyma or the small airways themselves becomes readily apparent. For example, in diseases such as chronic bronchitis and emphysema, where the brunt of the disease falls upon the smaller airways, expiratory flow rates at 50% or 25% of the vital capacity may be disproportionately reduced when compared with flow rates at larger lung volumes.

LUNG VOLUME. The subdivisions of the lung volume are shown in Fig. 12.16. Tidal volume and vital capacity can be measured using a simple spirometer, but the TLC and RV need to be measured by an alternative technique. TLC is measured by connecting the lungs to a reservoir containing a known amount of non-absorbable gas (helium) that can readily be measured. If the concentration of the gas in the reservoir is known at the start of the test and

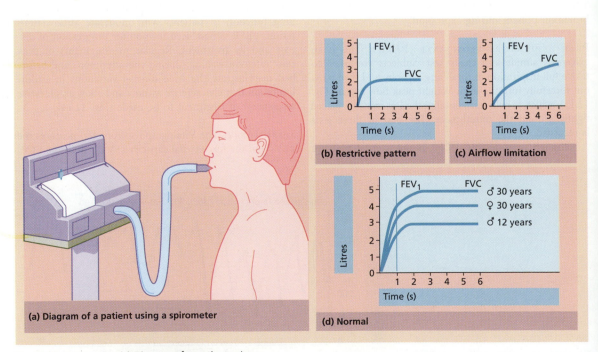

**Fig. 12.15** Spirometry. (a) Diagram of a patient using a spirometer. (b)–(d) Graphs showing (b) restrictive pattern (FEV₁ and FVC reduced), (c) airflow limitation (FEV₁ only reduced), and (d) normal patterns for age and sex.

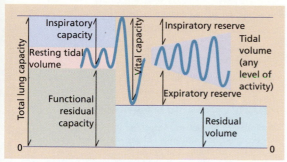

**Fig. 12.16**   The subdivisions of the lung volume.

is measured after equilibration of the gas has occurred (when the patient has breathed in and out of the reservoir), the dilution of the gas will reflect the TLC. This technique is known as *helium dilution*. RV can be calculated by subtracting the vital capacity from the TLC.

The TLC measured using this technique is inaccurate if large cystic spaces are present in the lung, because the helium cannot diffuse into them. Under these circumstances the thoracic gas volume can be measured more accurately using a body plethysmograph. The difference between the two measurements can be used to define the extent of non-communicating air space within the lungs.

**Measurement of blood gases**
This technique is described on p. 727.

The measurement of the partial pressure of both oxygen and carbon dioxide within arterial blood is an extremely useful test in diseases of the respiratory and circulatory systems. It is essential in the management of cases of respiratory failure and severe asthma, when repeated measurements are often the best guide to therapy.

TRANSFER FACTOR. This measures the transfer of gas across the alveolar–capillary membrane and reflects the uptake of oxygen from the alveolus into the red cell. A low concentration of carbon monoxide is inhaled and is avidly taken up in a linear fashion by circulating haemoglobin, the amount of which must be known when the test is performed. In normal lungs the transfer factor is a true measure of the diffusing capacity of the lungs for oxygen and depends on the thickness of the alveolar–capillary membrane. In lung disease the diffusing capacity ($D_{CO}$) also depends on the $V/Q$ relationship as well as on the area and thickness of the alveolar membrane. To control for differences in lung volume, the uptake of carbon monoxide is related to the lung volume; this is known as the transfer coefficient ($K_{CO}$).

Gas transfer is usually reduced in patients with severe degrees of emphysema and fibrosis. Overall gas transfer can be thought of as a relatively non-specific test of lung function but one that can be particularly used in the early detection and assessment of progress of diseases affecting the lung parenchyma (e.g. cryptogenic pulmonary fibrosis, sarcoidosis and asbestosis).

# Exercise tests

The predominant symptom in respiratory medicine is that of breathlessness. The degree of disability produced by breathlessness can be assessed before and after treatment by asking the patient to walk for 6 min along a measured track. This has been shown to be a reproducible and useful test once the patient has undergone an initial training walk to overcome the learning effect. Increasing emphasis is being placed on exercise tests incorporating assessment of both lung and heart function in the investigation of breathlessness. Such tests involve the use of sophisticated equipment enabling measurement of uptake of oxygen ($Vo_2$), work performed, heart rate and blood pressure together with serial ECGs. Correlation of these variables allows:
- The early detection of lung disease
- The detection of myocardial ischaemia
- The distinction between lung and heart disease
- Assessment of fitness

# Pleural aspiration

Diagnostic aspiration is necessary for all but very small effusions. A needle attached to a 20 ml syringe is inserted through an intercostal space over an area of dullness. Fluid is withdrawn and the presence of any blood is noted. Samples are sent for protein estimation, cytology and bacteriological examination, including culture and Ziehl–Nielsen stain for tuberculosis. Large amounts of fluid can be aspirated through a large needle to help relieve extreme breathlessness. Because of the risk of introducing infection into the pleural space with the subsequent development of an empyema (see Practical box 12.2) this technique must be performed using full aseptic precautions.

Pleural aspiration, drainage and biopsy are being increasingly performed under ultrasound guidance or following X-ray localization of the fluid.

# Pleural biopsy

Experienced operators obtain tissue in nearly all patients and, provided multiple specimens are taken, positive results may be expected in up to 80% of cases of tuberculosis and in 60% of cases of malignancy. The technique is illustrated in Fig. 12.17. If tissue is not obtained by blind pleural biopsy, the pleura can be examined by fibreoptic thoracoscopy and any lesions biopsied, yielding further results in a further 80% (see Practical box 12.1).

**Pleural drainage**
This is carried out when large effusions are present producing severe breathlessness or for drainage of an empyema (see Practical box 12.2).

Pleurodesis is performed for recurrent/malignant effusion.

# Mediastinoscopy and scalene node biopsy

This technique is used increasingly in the management of carcinoma of the bronchus. It involves inspection of the

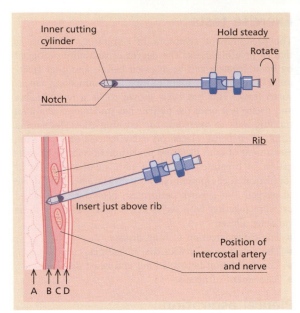

**Fig. 12.17** Technique of pleural biopsy. The biopsy needle is shown penetrating the chest wall. A, lung parenchyma; B, pleural space; C, muscle; D, skin and subcutaneous tissue.

Pleural biopsy is usually performed at the end of the aspiration of fluid

A small skin incision is made, as the end of the Abrams' pleural biopsy needle is fairly blunt

Once in place through the pleura, the back part of the needle is rotated to open the notch; this is kept pointing forward

With lateral pressure the needle is withdrawn so that the notch will snag against the pleura

The needle is held firmly and the hexagonal grip is twisted clockwise to cut the biopsy. To avoid damage to the intercostal vessel or nerve, the notch should never be directed upwards when the biopsy is taken

Several biopsies should be taken at different angles by repeated insertion of the needle

Specimens should be put in sterile saline for culture for tuberculosis and into 10% formol saline for histological examination

**Practical box 12.1**    Pleural biopsy.

Carefully sterilize skin over aspiration site. Sterile gloves, cap, gown and mask must be worn

Anaesthetize the skin, muscle and pleura with 2% lignocaine

Make small incision, then push a 28 French gauge Argyle catheter into the pleural space

Attach to three-way tap and 50 ml syringe

Aspirate up to 1000 ml. Stop aspiration if patient becomes uncomfortable—shock may ensue if too much fluid is withdrawn too quickly

A silastic pigtail catheter can be inserted under X-ray control and attached to tubing and bag for slower aspiration. For drainage and effusions, an 8–12 French gauge pigtail is inserted using the Seldinger technique in which the needle used to enter the pleural space is withdrawn over a control wire along which the catheter is then passed. A 14–16 French gauge pigtail catheter is used for drainage of empyema

*For pleurodesis*
Tetracycline 500 mg or bleomycin 15 units in 30–50 ml sodium chloride 0.9% solution is instilled into the pleural cavity to achieve pleurodesis in recurrent/maligant effusion

**Practical box 12.2**    Pleural drainage.

lesions for cytological examination for malignant cells, and appropriate staining and culture for bacteria including *Mycobacterium* and *Pneumocystis carinii*.

Diffuse parenchymal lung disease can be investigated using transbronchial biopsy. The biopsy forceps are pushed as far as possible to the periphery of the lung, the patient is asked to breathe in, and the jaws of the forceps are closed, removing a small piece of peripheral airway and surrounding lung parenchyma. Biplanar screening allows isolated peripheral lesions to be biopsied in the same way. A histological diagnosis can be made in 95% of central lung cancers but in only 50–75% of peripheral lesions biopsied during fibreoptic bronchoscopy.

Peripheral lesions are best biopsied percutaneously using a fine needle under direct X-ray or CT control.

## Bronchoalveolar lavage

This technique can be used both in patients who have disease confined to one lobe and in those with more diffuse lung disease. The tip of the fibreoptic bronchoscope is lodged in the segmental orifice and 20 ml of 0.9% sterile saline is squirted down the suction port of the bronchoscope and immediately aspirated. This is repeated five times; about 40–60% of the total volume is recovered. Fluid is strained through two layers of surgical gauze and the volume is noted. The cells are then spun down and resuspended at a concentration of $1 \times 10^7$ cells/ml for differential counting. Since there is a considerable overlap in the distribution of cells seen in bronchoalveolar wash specimens in different diseases, this technique has no value in diagnosis. However, it can be used to monitor progression of disease, since improvement is charac-

mediastinal structures using a mediastinoscope inserted by blunt dissection downwards from behind the proximal end of the clavicle. Subsequent biopsy of tissue will reveal the presence or absence of malignant cells in enlarged lymph nodes previously detected by CT, allowing accurate staging of the disease.

## Fibreoptic bronchoscopy (Practical box 12.3)

Central bronchial lesions can be biopsied readily. Washings can be taken from lobes containing more peripheral

This enables the direct visualization of the bronchial tree as far as the subsegmental bronchi under a local anaesthetic.

*Indications*
Lesions requiring biopsy seen on chest X-ray

Haemoptysis

Stridor

Positive sputum cytology for malignant cells with no chest X-ray abnormality

Collection of bronchial secretions for bacteriology, especially tuberculosis

Recurrent laryngeal nerve paralysis of unknown aetiology

Infiltrative lung disease (to obtain a transbronchial biopsy)

Investigation of collapsed lobes or segments and aspiration of mucus plugs

*Procedure*
The patient is starved overnight

Atropine 0.6 mg i.m. is given 30 min before the procedure

Topical anaesthesia (lignocaine 2% gel) is applied to the nose, nasopharynx and pharynx

Intravenous sedation (e.g. diazepam 10 mg or midazolam 2.5–10 mg) may be needed

The bronchoscope is passed through the nose, nasopharynx and pharynx under direct vision to minimize trauma

Lignocaine (2 ml of 4%) is dropped through the instrument onto the vocal cords

The bronchoscope is passed through the cords into the trachea

All segmental and subsegmental orifices should be identified

Biopsies and brushings should be taken of macroscopic abnormalities or occasionally from peripheral lesions under radiographic control

*Disadvantages*
All patients require sedation to tolerate the procedure

Minor and transient cardiac dysrhythmias occur in up to 40% of patients on passage of the bronchoscope through the larynx

Oxygen supplementation is required in patients with $P_aO_2$ below 8 kPa

Fibreoptic bronchoscopy should be performed with care in the very sick and transbronchial biopsies avoided in ventilated patients due to increased risk of pneumothorax

Massive bleeding may occur on accidental biopsy of vascular lesions or carcinoid tumours. Rigid bronchoscopy may be required to allow adequate access to bleeding point and haemostasis

**Practical box 12.3** Fibreoptic bronchoscopy.

terized by a reduction in the number of cells and a return towards the normal proportions of different cell types.

## Skin-prick tests

The tip of a fine needle is placed through a drop of allergen solution on the volar surface of the forearm into the epidermis, which is gently pricked with an upward lifting motion. A separate needle should be used for each allergen. If the patient is sensitive to the allergen, a weal develops and the diameter of the induration (not the erythema) should be measured after 15 min. A weal of at least 2 mm diameter and greater than the reaction to the control solution is a positive test. The results should be interpreted in the light of the history (see p. 654).

Skin tests can be inhibited by concurrent administration of antihistamines, so these should be stopped 48 hours before testing. They are not inhibited by bronchodilators or corticosteroids.

# Smoking

## Epidemiology

General household surveys in the UK have shown a continuing decline in the prevalence of cigarette smoking in men but not women: 44% of men and 34% of women aged 16 and over have smoked tobacco in some form. Manufactured cigarettes were smoked by an equal proportion of both sexes (34%). Cigarette smoking is now commonest between the ages of 16 and 24 years (42% in both sexes). At the age of 15 more girls (27%) than boys (18%) smoke cigarettes. A greater proportion of professional workers than manual workers have given up smoking. In the USA the proportion of adult males who smoke is now only 36% and in women the prevalence is now 29%. Cigarette consumption is rising in Central and Eastern Europe and China in contrast to that in Western Europe and North America.

## Dangers

Cigarette smoking is addictive. Smoking nearly always begins in adolescence for psychosocial reasons and, once it is a regular habit, the pharmacological properties of nicotine play an important part in persistence, conferring some advantage to the smoker's mood. Very few cigarette smokers (less than 2%) can limit themselves to occasional or intermittent smoking. The dangers are listed in Table 12.6.

There is a significant dose–response relationship between the smoking of 0–40 cigarettes daily and lung cancer mortality. Sputum production and airflow limitation increase with daily cigarette consumption, and effort tolerance decreases, partly due to high levels of carboxyhaemoglobin in bronchitis patients. Smoking and asbestos exposure are synergistic in producing bronchial carcinoma, increasing the risk in asbestos workers by up to five to eight times that of non-smokers exposed to asbestos.

Cigarette smokers who change to other forms of tobacco are unlikely to reduce the risk, as they continue to inhale, and some of the highest levels of carboxyhaemoglobin have been found in cigar smokers.

Environmental tobacco smoke—passive smoking—has been shown to cause more frequent and more severe attacks of asthma in children and possibly increases the number of cases of asthma. It is also associated with a small but definite increase in lung cancer.

## Toxic effects

Cigarette smoke contains polycyclic aromatic hydrocarbons and nitrosamines, which are potent carcinogens and mutagens in animals. It causes release of enzymes from neutrophil granulocytes and macrophages that are capable of destroying elastin and leading to lung damage. Pulmonary epithelial permeability increases even in symptomless cigarette smokers, and correlates with the concentration of carboxyhaemoglobin in blood. This altered permeability possibly allows easier access to carcinogens.

## Stopping smoking

If the entire population could be persuaded to stop smoking, the effect on health care in the Western World would be enormous. National campaigns, bans on advertisement and a substantial increase in the cost of cigarettes are the most certain ways of achieving this. Only one in five general practitioners actively encourage their patients to give up smoking, yet simple advice and follow-up can motivate some 50% of their patients to stop. In smoking withdrawal clinics, success rates of 80% can be achieved in the first month, though only 15–20% of patients remain abstinent in the long term. Nicotine chewing gum has been advocated but is probably no better than verbal advice. Nicotine patches are available over the counter and better than placebo in helping smokers stop, though they must not be used by those suffering from heart disease. Chest symptoms usually have to be severe to stop patients from smoking.

## Diseases of the upper respiratory tract

## The common cold (acute coryza)

This highly infectious illness comprises a mild systemic upset and prominent nasal symptoms. It is due to infection by rhinoviruses, the majority of which belong to the picornavirus group and exist in at least 100 different antigenic strains. Infectivity from close personal contact (nasal mucus on hands) or droplets is high in the early stages of the infection, and spread is facilitated by overcrowding and poor ventilation. On average, individuals suffer two to three colds per year but the incidence lessens with age, presumably as a result of accumulating immunity to the causative virus strains. The incubation is from 12 hours to an upper limit of 5 days. The clinical features are tiredness, slight pyrexia, malaise and a sore nose and pharynx. Profuse, watery nasal discharge, eventually

---

Lung cancer
Chronic bronchitis and emphysema
Carcinoma of the oesophagus
Ischaemic heart disease
Peripheral vascular disease
Bladder cancer
An increase in abnormal spermatozoa
Memory problems

*Maternal smoking*
A decrease in birthweight of the infant
An increase in fetal and neonatal mortality
An increase in asthma

*Passive smoking*
Risk of asthma, pneumonia and bronchitis in infants of
    smoking parents
An increase in cough and breathlessness in smokers
    and non-smokers with chronic bronchitis, emphysema
    and asthma
Increased cancer risk

**Table 12.6**  The dangers of cigarette smoking.

becoming thick and mucopurulent, persists for up to a week. Sneezing is present in the early stage. Secondary bacterial infection occurs only in a minority.

## Sinusitis

Sinusitis is an infection of the paranasal sinuses that often complicates upper respiratory tract infections, e.g. coryza and allergic rhinitis. Acute infections are usually caused by *Streptococcus pneumoniae* and *Haemophilus influenzae*. Symptoms include frontal headache and facial pain and tenderness, usually with nasal discharge, but are often difficult to differentiate from symptoms of the common cold.

Treatment is with antibiotics. Many strains of *H. influenzae* are now resistant to amoxycillin so co-amoxiclav or cefaclor are preferred. In addition nasal treatment with decongestants such as xylometazoline or anti-inflammatory therapy with topical corticosteroids such as fluticasone propionate nasal spray should be given to reduce swelling of the mucosa and unblock the sinus openings. Rare complications include local and cerebral abscesses. Chronic sinusitis can be a cause of headaches, but often these headaches are due to tension.

## Rhinitis

Rhinitis is present if sneezing attacks, nasal discharge or blockage occur for more than an hour on most days for:
● A limited period of the year (seasonal rhinitis)
● Throughout the whole year (perennial rhinitis)

### Seasonal rhinitis

This is often called hay fever and is the most common of all allergic diseases. It is better described as seasonal allergic rhinitis. Worldwide prevalence rates vary from 2% to 10%. Prevalence is maximum in the second decade, when up to 20% of young people suffer symptoms in June and July.

Nasal irritation, sneezing and watery rhinorrhoea are the most troublesome symptoms but many also suffer from itching of the eyes and soft palate and occasionally even itching of the ears due to the common innervation of the pharyngeal mucosa and the ear. In addition, approximately 20% suffer from attacks of asthma. The common seasonal allergens are shown in Fig. 12.18.

### Perennial rhinitis

Patients with perennial rhinitis rarely have symptoms that affect the eyes or throat. Half have symptoms predominantly of sneezing and watery rhinorrhoea, whilst the other half complain mostly of nasal blockage. The patient may lose the sense of smell and taste. A swollen mucosa can obstruct drainage from the sinuses, causing sinusitis in half of the patients. Perennial rhinitis is most frequent in the second and third decade, decreasing with age, and can be divided into four main types.

PERENNIAL ALLERGIC RHINITIS. The major cause of this is an allergen called Der p1 contained in the faecal

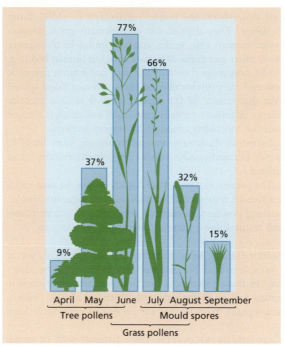

**Fig. 12.18** Seasonal allergic rhinitis: bar graph showing the proportion of patients whose symptoms are worst in the month or months indicated. The causative agents are also shown.

particles of the house-dust mite *Dermatophagoides pteronyssinus*; these particles are approximately 20 μm in diameter (Fig. 12.19), not dissimilar in size to pollen grains. The house-dust mite itself is <0.5 mm in size, invisible to the naked eye (Fig. 12.19), and is found in

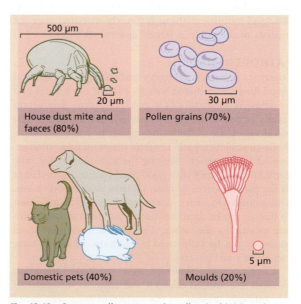

**Fig. 12.19** Common allergens causing allergic rhinitis and asthma—the house-dust mite, faeces of house-dust mites, pollen grains, domestic pets and moulds. Percentages are those of positive skin-prick tests to these allergens in patients with allergic rhinitis.

dust throughout the house, particularly in older, damp dwellings. They depend for nourishment upon desquamated human skin scales and are found in abundance (4000 mites per gram of surface dust) in human bedding.

The next most common allergens come from domestic pets and are proteins derived from urine or saliva spread over the surface of the animal as well as skin protein. Allergy to urinary protein from small mammals is a major cause of morbidity amongst laboratory workers.

Industrial dust, vapours and fumes are more likely to cause occupationally related perennial rhinitis than asthma.

The presence of perennial rhinitis makes the nose more reactive to non-specific stimuli such as cigarette smoke, washing powders, household detergents, strong perfumes and traffic fumes; these are *not* acting as allergens.

PERENNIAL NON-ALLERGIC RHINITIS WITH EOSINOPHILIA. No extrinsic allergic cause can be identified in these patients, either from the history or on skin testing but, as in patients with perennial allergic rhinitis, eosinophilic granulocytes are present in nasal secretions.

VASOMOTOR RHINITIS. These patients with perennial rhinitis have no demonstrable allergy or eosinophilia in nasal secretions. They may be suffering from non-specific nasal hyperreactivity due to an imbalance of the autonomic nervous system innervating the erectile tissue (sinusoids) in the nasal mucosa.

NASAL POLYPS. These are round, smooth, soft, semi-translucent, pale or yellow, glistening structures attached to the sinus mucosa by a relatively narrow stalk or pedicle and occur in patients with both allergic and vasomotor rhinitis. They cause nasal obstruction, loss of smell and taste and mouth breathing, but rarely sneezing, since the mucosa of the polyp is largely denervated.

## PATHOGENESIS

Sneezing, increased secretion and changes in mucosal blood flow are mediated both by efferent nerve fibres and by released mediators (see p. 671). Mucus production results largely from parasympathetic stimulation, whilst blood vessels are under both sympathetic and parasympathetic control. Sympathetic fibres maintain tonic contraction of blood vessels, keeping the sinusoids of the nose partially constricted with good nasal patency. Stimulation of the parasympathetic system dilates these blood vessels. This stimulation varies spontaneously in a cyclical fashion so that air intake alternates slowly over several hours from one nostril to the other. The erectile cavernous nasal sinusoids can be influenced by emotion, which, in turn, can affect nasal patency.

Allergic rhinitis develops as a result of interaction between the inhaled allergen and adjacent molecules of IgE antibody present on the surface of mast cells found in nasal secretions and within the nasal epithelium. Release of preformed mediators, in particular histamine, causes an increase in permeability of the epithelium, allowing allergen to reach IgE-primed mast cells in the lamina propria. Sneezing results from stimulation of afferent nerve endings and begins within minutes of the allergen entering the nose. This is followed by nasal secretion and eventually nasal blockage at a maximum of 15–20 min after contact with the allergen.

Although the mast cell contains or can generate many other potent vasomotor and chemotactic factors (see Fig. 12.32), the exact role for each of these has still to be evaluated. It is likely that histamine plays a more important role in the development of allergic rhinitis than of asthma, since antihistamines are a useful and effective treatment for allergic rhinitis but are of little value in the everyday management of asthma. More mast cells are present in the nasal mucosa of individuals with rhinitis compared with those without rhinitis, and increase as allergen stimulation continues, accounting for the increasing responsiveness of the nose to lower amounts of grass pollen as the season progresses. The mechanisms for recruitment of mast cells under these circumstances probably involves the release of interleukin-3 from T lymphocytes.

## DIAGNOSIS AND INVESTIGATION

A DETAILED HISTORY is mandatory for the diagnosis of allergic factors in rhinitis.

SKIN-PRICK TESTING indicates that the mechanisms leading to allergic rhinitis (or asthma) are present in human skin. It does not necessarily mean that the particular allergen producing the weal causes the respiratory disease. However, if there is a positive clinical history for that allergen, a causative role is likely.

SPECIFIC SERUM IgE ANTIBODY against the particular allergen provides the same information as the skin-prick test.

## TREATMENT
### Allergen avoidance
Removal of a household pet or total enclosure of industrial processes releasing sensitizing agents can lead to cure of rhinitis and, indeed, asthma.

Pollen avoidance is impossible. Contact may be diminished by wearing sunglasses, driving with the car windows shut, avoiding walks in the countryside (particularly in the late afternoon when the number of pollen grains is highest at ground level), and keeping the bedroom window shut at night. These measures are rarely sufficient in themselves to control symptoms. Exposure to pollen is generally lower at the seaside, where sea breezes keep pollen grains inland.

The house-dust mite infests most areas of the house, but particularly the bedroom. Mite counts are extremely low in hospitals where carpets are absent, floors are cleaned frequently and mattresses and pillows are covered in plastic sheeting that can be wiped down. Such conditions need to be reproduced in the home if mite counts are to be reduced to levels that can diminish symptoms. Avoidance is best achieved by enclosing bedding in fabric specifically designed to prevent the passage of mite allergen though allowing water vapour through. This is both comfortable and reduces symptoms. Acaricides are less effective.

### Antihistamines

Antihistamines remain the commonest therapy for rhinitis, and many can be purchased directly over the counter in the UK. They are particularly effective against sneezing, but are less effective against rhinorrhoea and have little influence on nasal blockage. The first generation sedative antihistamines should not be used. Second generation drugs such as astemizole (10 mg daily), cetirizine (10 mg once daily) and terfenadine (60 mg twice daily) are highly specific for $H_1$ receptors; they do not cross the blood–brain barrier and are therefore not associated with sedation. The recommended dose of terfenadine and astemizole must not be exceeded nor must they be prescribed with erythromycin or ketoconazole (which reduce their hepatic metabolism) since fatal cardiac arrhythmias may occur. Although rarely sufficient for the treatment of rhinitis, antihistamines will control itching in the eyes and palate.

### Decongestants

Drugs with sympathomimetic activity ($\alpha$-adrenergic agents) are widely used for the treatment of nasal obstruction. They may be taken orally or more commonly as nasal drops or sprays (e.g. ephedrine nasal drops). Xylometazoline and oxymetazoline are widely used because they have a prolonged action and tachyphylaxis does not develop. Secondary nasal hyperaemia can occur some hours later as a rebound effect and rhinitis medicamentosa can develop if patients subsequently take increasing quantities of the local decongestant to overcome this phenomenon. Local decongestants may be the only effective treatment for vasomotor rhinitis, but patients must be warned about rebound nasal obstruction and must use the drug carefully. Usually, such preparations should only be prescribed for a limited period to open the nasal airways for administration of other therapy, particularly topical corticosteroids.

### Anti-inflammatory drugs

These drugs, previously considered to act primarily by preventing release of mediators from mast cells and called therefore anti-allergic compounds, are now known to influence a number of aspects of inflammation including mast cell and eosinophil activation and nerve function, and are best labelled anti-inflammatory drugs. Sodium cromoglycate applied topically in spray or powder form is of limited value in the treatment of allergic rhinitis, though is very effective in the management of allergic conjunctivitis.

### Corticosteroids

The most effective treatment for rhinitis is the use of small doses of topically administered corticosteroid preparations (e.g. beclomethasone spray twice daily or fluticasone propionate spray once daily). The amount used is insufficient to cause systemic effects and the effect is primarily anti-inflammatory. Preparations should be started prior to the beginning of seasonal symptoms. The combination of a topical corticosteroid with a non-sedative antihistamine taken regularly is particularly effective.

Seasonal and perennial rhinitis respond readily to a short course (2 weeks) of treatment with oral prednisolone 5–10 mg daily if other therapy has failed. Nasal polyps respond well to such oral doses of corticosteroids and their recurrence may be prevented by continuous application of topical corticosteroids.

## Pharyngitis

Only about one-third of sore throats are due to infection with a haemolytic streptococcus and this proportion appears to be falling. The commonest viruses causing pharyngitis are those of the adenovirus group, which consists of about 32 serotypes. Endemic adenovirus infection causes the common sore throat, in which the oropharynx and soft palate are reddened and the tonsils are inflamed and swollen. Within 1 or 2 days the tonsillar lymph nodes enlarge. Occasionally, localized epidemics occur, particularly in schools in the summer-time, with episodes of fever, conjunctivitis, pharyngitis and lymphadenitis of the neck glands; these are due to adenovirus serotype 8. These diseases are self-limiting, and symptomatic treatment is all that is required.

More persistent and severe tonsillitis requires antibiotic therapy. The bacteria causing this are now predominantly *H. influenzae* and *Staphylococcus aureus* many producing $\beta$-lactamase and therefore resistant to penicillin/ amoxycillin. Treatment should be with co-amoxiclav 250 mg three times daily or cefaclor 250 mg three times daily.

## Acute laryngotracheobronchitis

Acute laryngitis is an occasional but striking complication of upper respiratory tract infections, particularly those caused by viruses of the parainfluenza group and the measles virus. Inflammatory oedema extends to the vocal cords and the epiglottis, causing considerable narrowing of the airway; in addition, there may be associated tracheitis or tracheobronchitis. Children under the age of 3 years are most severely affected. The voice becomes hoarse, the cough assumes a barking quality (croup) and there is audible laryngeal stridor. Progressive airways obstruction may occur, with recession of the soft tissue of the neck and abdomen during inspiration, and in severe cases central cyanosis may occur. Inhalation of steam may be helpful; in severe cases endotracheal intubation may be necessary. Oxygen and adequate fluids should be given. Rarely, a tracheostomy may be required.

## Acute epiglottitis

*H. influenzae* type B can cause life-threatening infection of the epiglottis, a condition that is rare over the age of 5 years. The young child becomes extremely ill with a high fever, and severe airflow obstruction may rapidly occur. This is a life-threatening emergency and requires urgent endotracheal intubation and intravenous ceftazidime (25–150 mg kg$^{-1}$ in children). Chloramphenicol (50–100 mg kg$^{-1}$ in children) can also be used. The epiglottis, which is red and swollen, should not be inspected until facilities to maintain the airways are available. Other manifestations of *H. influenzae* type b (Hib) are meningitis, septic arthritis and osteomyelitis. All can be prevented by immunization with a purified polyribosylribitol phosphate from the capsule of Hib linked to a non-toxic diphtheria toxin PRP-T to increase immunogenicity. It is highly effective when given to infants at 2, 3 and 4 months with primary immunization against diphtheria, tetanus and pertussis (DTP) reducing death rates from Hib infections virtually to zero.

## Influenza (see p. 55)

The influenza virus belongs to the orthomyxovirus group and exists in two main forms—A and B. Influenza B is associated with localized outbreaks of milder nature, whereas influenza A is the cause of worldwide pandemics. Influenza A has a capacity to develop new antigenic variants at irregular intervals. Human immunity develops against the haemagglutinin (H) antigen and the neuraminidase (N) antigen on the viral surface. Major shifts in the antigenic make-up of influenza A viruses provide the necessary conditions for major pandemics, whereas minor antigenic drifts give rise to less severe epidemics because immunity in the population is less blunted.

The most serious pandemic of influenza occurred in 1918, and was associated with more than 20 million deaths worldwide. More recently, in 1957, a major shift in the antigenic make-up of the virus led to the appearance of influenza A2 type H2–N2, which caused a worldwide pandemic. A further pandemic occurred in 1968 owing to the emergence of Hong Kong influenza type H3–N2, and minor antigenic drifts have caused outbreaks around the world ever since.

### CLINICAL FEATURES

The incubation period of influenza is usually 1–3 days. The illness starts abruptly with a fever, shivering and generalized aching in the limbs. This is associated with severe headache, soreness of the throat and a persistent dry cough that can last for several weeks. Influenza viruses can cause a prolonged period of debility and depression that may take weeks or months to clear; this is known as the postviral syndrome.

### COMPLICATIONS

Secondary bacterial infection, particularly with *Strep. pneumoniae* and *H. influenzae*, is common following influenza virus infection. Rarer, but more serious, is the development of pneumonia caused by *Staph. aureus*, which has a mortality of up to 20%. Postinfectious encephalomyelitis rarely occurs after infection with influenza virus.

### DIAGNOSIS

Laboratory diagnosis of all cases is not necessary. Definitive diagnosis can be established by demonstrating a four-fold increase in the complement-fixing antibody or the haemagglutinin antibody when measured before and after an interval of 1–2 weeks. Viral cultures are still a research procedure.

### TREATMENT

Treatment is bed rest and aspirin, together with antibiotics for individuals with chronic bronchitis, or heart or renal disease.

### PROPHYLAXIS

Protection by influenza vaccines is only effective in up to 70% of people and is of short duration, usually lasting for only a year. Influenza vaccine should not be given to individuals who are allergic to egg protein as some are manufactured in chick embryos. New vaccines have to be prepared to cover each change in viral antigenicity and are therefore in limited supply at the start of an epidemic. Routine vaccination is reserved for susceptible people with chronic heart, lung or kidney disease, and the elderly. In pandemics key hospital and health service personnel are also vaccinated.

Amantadine hydrochloride 100–200 mg daily may attenuate influenza A infection and should be reserved for individuals with chronic respiratory or cardiovascular disease who have not previously been immunized.

## Inhalation of foreign bodies

Children inhale foreign bodies, frequently peanuts, more commonly than adults. In the adult, inhalation often occurs after an excess of alcohol or under general anaesthesia (loose teeth or dentures).

When the foreign body is large it may impact in the trachea. The person chokes and then becomes silent; death occurs unless the material is quickly removed (see Emergency box 12.1).

Impaction usually occurs in the right main bronchus and produces:

● Choking
● Persistent monophonic wheeze

*Emergency*

The Heimlich manoeuvre is used to expel the obstructing object:

**Stand behind patient**

Encircle your arms around the upper part of the abdomen just below the patient's rib cage

Give a sharp, forceful squeeze, forcing the diaphragm sharply into the thorax. This should expel sufficient air from the lungs to force the foreign body out of the trachea

*Non-emergency*

Fibreoptic bronchoscopy should be performed

**Emergency box 12.1**   Treatment of inhaled foreign bodies (Heimlich manoeuvre).

- Later, persistent suppurative pneumonia
- Lung abscess (common)

# Diseases of the lower respiratory tract

## Acute bronchitis

Acute bronchitis in previously healthy subjects is often viral. Bacterial infection with organisms such as *Strep. pneumoniae* and *H. influenzae* is a common sequel to viral infections, and is more likely to occur in individuals who are cigarette smokers and in those with chronic bronchitis and emphysema.

The illness begins with an irritating, unproductive cough, together with discomfort behind the sternum. This may be associated with tightness in the chest, wheezing and shortness of breath. The cough becomes productive, the sputum being yellow or green. There is a mild fever and a neutrophil leucocytosis; wheeze with occasional crackles can be heard on auscultation. In otherwise healthy adults the disease improves spontaneously in 4–8 days without the patient becoming seriously ill. Treatment with antibiotics may be given, e.g. amoxycillin 250 mg three times daily, though it is not known whether this hastens recovery in otherwise healthy individuals.

## Chronic bronchitis and emphysema

### Definitions

Chronic bronchitis is defined on the basis of the *history* as:

- Cough productive of sputum on most days for at least 3 months of the year for more than 1 year

Emphysema, on the other hand, is defined *pathologically* as:

- Dilatation and destruction of the lung tissue distal to the terminal bronchioles

Clinical observations led to the suggestion that there were two distinct types of patient:

THE TYPE A FIGHTER is *pink and puffing* in that, although very breathless, arterial tensions of oxygen and carbon dioxide are relatively normal and there is no cor pulmonale. These individuals were thought to be suffering predominantly from emphysema with little bronchitis.

THE TYPE B NON-FIGHTER, on the other hand, is *blue and bloated*, he does not appear to be breathless, but has marked arterial hypoxaemia, carbon dioxide retention, secondary polycythaemia and cor pulmonale. These patients were thought to be suffering predominantly from chronic bronchitis.

Although this is an attractive concept and has some clinical usefulness, it is not supported by post-mortem studies that have shown no difference in the degree of mucous gland hyperplasia (i.e. bronchitis) or in the amount of emphysema in patients with type A compared with type B disease.

Autopsy studies have also shown that substantial numbers of centri-acinar emphysematous spaces are found in the lungs of 50% of British smokers over the age of 60 years and are unrelated to the diagnosis of significant respiratory disease before death.

Alternative terms such as chronic obstructive pulmonary disease (COPD), chronic obstructive lung disease (COLD) or chronic obstructive airways disease (COAD) are unhelpful and should be replaced by the term 'chronic bronchitis and emphysema', as both these conditions coexist to a greater or lesser degree in each patient.

As the common tests for 'airway obstruction', the $FEV_1$ and PEFR, actually measure airflow limitation (caused by both loss of elastic recoil and/or narrowing of airways), the term 'chronic airflow limitation' is the preferred terminology to describe the functional and physiological problem in chronic bronchitis and emphysema.

### EPIDEMIOLOGY AND AETIOLOGY

Chronic bronchitis and emphysema have a prevalence, diagnosed on history, of 17% in men and 8% in women in the age group 40–64 years. In the USA similar prevalence figures have been obtained and many developing countries are showing an increased prevalence.

There is no doubt that cigarette smoking is a major factor in the development of chronic bronchitis and emphysema. Not only are these diseases virtually confined to cigarette smokers, they are also related to the number of cigarettes smoked per day. The risk of death from chronic bronchitis and emphysema in patients smoking 30 cigarettes daily is 20 times that of a non-smoker. The bronchitis mortality amongst male doctors in relation to the number of cigarettes smoked is shown in Fig. 12.20.

Climate and air pollution are of less importance; nevertheless, there is a great increase in mortality from chronic bronchitis and emphysema during periods of heavy

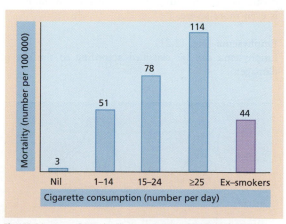

**Fig. 12.20** Bronchitis death rates per 100 000 British male doctors according to their smoking habits. (From Doll R & Peto R (1976) *British Medical Journal* **2**, 1525.)

atmospheric pollution. The effect of urbanization, social class and occupation may also play a part in aetiology, but these effects are difficult to separate from that of smoking.

The socio-economic burden of chronic bronchitis and emphysema is considerable. In the UK chronic bronchitis and emphysema cause approximately 18 million lost working days for men and 2.1 million lost working days for women per year, accounting for some 7% of all days of sickness absence from work. Nevertheless, the number of patients discharged from hospitals in the UK with this disease has been steadily falling; the death rate has also fallen in the last 20 years from 200 to 70 per 100 000.

## PATHOPHYSIOLOGY
### Chronic bronchitis
The most consistent pathological finding in chronic bronchitis is hypertrophy of the mucus-secreting glands of the bronchial tree. The hypertrophy of these mucous glands is evenly distributed throughout the lung, and is mainly seen in the larger bronchi. In addition, the number of the mucus-secreting goblet cells increases. This leads to increased mucus production and the regular expectoration of sputum.

In more advanced cases, the bronchi themselves are obviously inflamed and pus is seen in the lumen. Microscopically there is infiltration of the walls of the bronchi and bronchioles with acute and chronic inflammatory cells. The epithelial layer may become ulcerated and, when the ulcers heal, squamous epithelium may replace the columnar cells. The inflammation leads to widespread narrowing in the peripheral airways.

The small airways are particularly affected early in the disease, initially without the development of any significant breathlessness. This initial inflammation of the small airways is reversible and accounts for the improvement in airway function if smoking is stopped early.

Further progression of the disease leads to progressive squamous cell metaplasia, and fibrosis of the bronchial walls. The physiological consequences of these changes is the development of airflow limitation. If the airway narrowing is combined with emphysema (causing loss of the elastic recoil of the lung) the resulting airflow limitation is even more severe.

### Emphysema (Fig. 12.21)
Emphysema can be classified according to the site of damage:

IN CENTRI-ACINAR EMPHYSEMA distension and damage of lung tissue is concentrated around the respiratory bronchioles, whilst the more distal alveolar ducts and alveoli tend to be well preserved. This form of emphysema is extremely common; when of modest extent, it is not necessarily associated with disability. Severe centri-acinar emphysema is associated with substantial airflow limitation.

PAN-ACINAR EMPHYSEMA is less common. Here, distension and destruction appear to involve the whole of the acinus, and in the extreme form the lung becomes a mass of bullae. Severe airflow limitation and $V_A/Q$ mismatch occur. This type of emphysema occurs in $\alpha_1$-antitrypsin deficiency (see p. 659).

IN IRREGULAR EMPHYSEMA there is scarring and damage affecting the lung parenchyma patchily without particular regard for acinar structure.

Emphysema can lead to expiratory airflow limitation (see p. 636) and air trapping. The loss of lung elastic recoil results in an increase in TLC while the loss of alveoli with emphysema results in decreased gas transfer.

$V/Q$ mismatch occurs partly because of damage and mucus plugging of smaller airways from chronic bronchitis and also because of the rapid expiratory closure of the smaller airways due to loss of elastic recoil from emphysema. This leads to a fall in $P_aO_2$ and a subsequent rise in $P_aCO_2$.

$CO_2$ is normally the major stimulant of the respiratory centre. In the face of a prolonged high $P_aCO_2$ this sensitivity is diminished and hypoxaemia becomes the chief drive to respiration. In this situation an attempt to abolish hypoxaemia by administration of oxygen can result in an increase in $P_aCO_2$ by decreasing the respiratory drive.

## PATHOGENESIS
### Cigarette smoking
Bronchoalveolar washes have shown that smokers have neutrophil granulocytes present within the lumen of the lung that are absent in non-smokers. Additionally, the small airways of smokers are infiltrated by granulocytes. These granulocytes are capable of releasing elastases and proteases, which possibly help to produce emphysema. It is suggested that an imbalance between protease and antiprotease activity may produce the damage. $\alpha_1$-Antitrypsin is a major serum antiprotease which can be inactivated by cigarette smoke (see below).

The hypertrophy of mucous glands in the larger air-

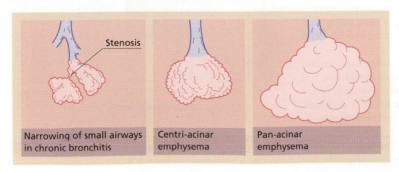

Narrowing of small airways in chronic bronchitis

Centri-acinar emphysema

Pan-acinar emphysema

**Fig. 12.21** The pathological features of chronic bronchitis and emphysema.

ways is thought to be a direct response to persistent irritation resulting from the inhalation of cigarette smoke. The smoke has an adverse effect on surfactant, favouring overdistension of the lungs.

### Infections

Infections are frequent and are often the precipitating cause of acute exacerbations of the disease. However, the role of infection in the development of the progressive airflow limitation that characterizes disabling chronic bronchitis and emphysema is far less clear. Nevertheless, release of enzymes from the excess neutrophil granulocytes found in infections probably adds to the lung damage.

### $\alpha_1$-Antitrypsin (see p. 271)

$\alpha_1$-Antitrypsin is produced in the liver, secreted into the blood and diffuses into the lung. Here it functions as an antiprotease that inhibits neutrophil elastase, a proteolytic enzyme capable of destroying alveolar wall connective tissue. More than 75 allelles of $\alpha_1$-antitrypsin gene have been described. The three main phenotypes are MM (normal), MZ (heterozygous deficiency) and ZZ (homozygous deficiency); these groups are defined by the serum level of $\alpha_1$-antitrypsin. About 1 child in 5000 in Britain is born with the homozygous deficiency, but not all develop chest disease. Those who do develop breathlessness under the age of 40 years have radiographic evidence of basal emphysema and are usually, but not always, cigarette smokers. Hereditary deficiency of $\alpha_1$-antitrypsin accounts for about 2% of emphysema cases and a few develop liver disease (see p. 271).

## CLINICAL FEATURES

### Symptoms

The characteristic symptoms of chronic bronchitis and emphysema are cough with the production of sputum, wheeze and breathlessness following many years of a smoker's cough. Colds seem to 'go down to the chest' and frequent infective exacerbations occur, giving purulent sputum. Symptoms can be worsened by factors such as cold, foggy weather and atmospheric pollution. With advanced disease, breathlessness becomes severe even after mild exercise such as dressing.

### Signs

In mild disease there are no signs apart from 'wheeze' throughout the chest. In severe disease, the patient is tachypnoeic, with prolonged expiration. The accessory muscles of respiration are used and there may be intercostal indrawing on inspiration and pursing of the lips on expiration (see Fig. 12.7). Chest expansion is poor, the lungs are hyperinflated, and there is loss of the normal cardiac and liver dullness.

The 'pink puffer' is always breathless and is not usually cyanosed. Rarely oedema or heart failure may be seen.

The 'blue bloater' is oedematous, deeply cyanosed, with hypoventilation and often little respiratory effort. These patients are likely to have hypercapnia, which gives the following physical findings:

- Peripheral vasodilatation
- A bounding pulse
- Later, a coarse flapping tremor of the outstretched hands

More severe hypercapnia leads to:

- Confusion
- Progressive drowsiness and coma with papilloedema

There is often considerable overlap between these two clinical patterns.

## COMPLICATIONS

### Respiratory failure

The latter stages of chronic bronchitis and emphysema are characterized by the development of respiratory failure. For practical purposes this is said to occur when there is either a $P_a o_2$ of less than 8 kPa (60 mmHg) or a $P_a co_2$ of more than 7 kPa (55 mmHg) (see Chapter 13).

The persistence of chronic alveolar hypoxia and hypercapnia leads to constriction of the pulmonary arterioles and subsequent pulmonary arterial hypertension.

### Cor pulmonale

Patients may develop cor pulmonale (see p. 613), which is defined as heart disease secondary to disease of the lung. It is characterized by pulmonary hypertension, right ventricular hypertrophy, and eventually right heart failure. On examination, the patient is centrally cyanosed (owing to the lung disease) and, when heart failure develops, breathlessness and ankle oedema occur. Initially a prominent parasternal heave may be felt due to right ventricular hypertrophy and a loud pulmonary second sound may be heard. In very severe pulmonary hypertension there is incompetence of the pulmonary valve. With right heart failure, tricuspid incompetence may develop with a greatly elevated jugular venous pressure (JVP), ascites and upper abdominal discomfort due to swelling of the liver.

## DIAGNOSIS

This is usually clinical. There is a history of breathlessness and sputum production in a lifetime smoker. It is unwise to make a diagnosis of chronic bronchitis and emphysema in the absence of cigarette smoking unless there is a family history of lung disease suggestive of a deficiency of $\alpha_1$-antitrypsin.

In clinical practice, emphysema is often incorrectly diagnosed on signs of overinflation of the lungs (e.g. loss of liver dullness on percussion), since this may occur with other diseases such as asthma. Furthermore, centri-acinar emphysema may be present without signs of overinflation. Some elderly men develop a barrel-shaped chest due to osteoporosis of the spine and a consequent decrease in height. This should not be attributed to emphysema.

In a number of patients the airflow limitation is reversible and the distinction between asthma and chronic bronchitis and emphysema can be difficult.

## INVESTIGATION

LUNG FUNCTION TESTS show evidence of airflow

limitation (see Figs 12.8 and 12.15). The ratio of the $FEV_1$ to the FVC is reduced and the PEFR is low. Lung volumes may be normal or increased, and the gas transfer coefficient of carbon monoxide is low when significant emphysema is present.

ON CHEST X-RAY the diagnosis of chronic bronchitis and emphysema is not always possible as the chest X-ray can be normal, even when the disease is advanced. The classic features are the presence of bullae, severe overinflation of the lungs with low, flattened diaphragms, and a large retrosternal air space on the lateral film. There may also be a deficiency of blood vessels in the peripheral half of the lung fields compared with relatively easily visible proximal vessels.

THE HAEMOGLOBIN LEVEL AND PCV may be elevated.

BLOOD GASES are often normal. In the advanced case there is evidence of hypoxaemia and hypercapnia.

SPUTUM EXAMINATION is unnecessary in the ordinary case as *Strep. pneumoniae* or *H. influenzae* are the only common organisms to produce acute exacerbations. Occasionally *Moraxella catarrhalis* may be the causative bacterium.

ELECTROCARDIOGRAM. In cor pulmonale the P wave is taller (P pulmonale) and there may be right bundle branch block (RSR' complex) and the changes of right ventricular hypertrophy.

$\alpha_1$-ANTITRYPSIN. Measurement of serum $\alpha_1$-antitrypsin levels (normal range 20–48 mmol litre$^{-1}$).

## TREATMENT

The single most important aspect in the management of chronic bronchitis and emphysema is to persuade the patient to stop smoking. Even at a late stage of the disease this may slow down the rate of deterioration and prolong the time before disability and death occur (Fig. 12.22). Accompanying heart failure should be treated (see p. 572).

### Drug therapy

Drug therapy is used both for the short-term management of exacerbations and for the long-term relief of symptoms. In some cases the therapy is similar to that used in asthma (see p. 673).

BRONCHODILATORS. Many patients feel less breathless following the inhalation of a $\beta$-adrenoceptor agonist such as salbutamol (200 $\mu$g 4–6-hourly). More prolonged and greater bronchodilatation results from the use of the anticholinergic agents ipratropium bromide 40 $\mu$g four times daily or oxitropium bromide 200 $\mu$g twice daily. Objective evidence of improvement in the peak flow or $FEV_1$ may be small, but with severe disability it may be of considerable help. Long-acting preparations of theophylline are of little benefit.

CORTICOSTEROIDS. In symptomatic patients with chronic bronchitis and emphysema, a trial of corticosteroids is always indicated, since a proportion of patients have a large, unsuspected, reversible element to their disease and airway function may improve considerably. Prednisolone 30 mg daily should be given for 2 weeks, with measurements of lung function before and after the treatment period. If there is objective evidence of a substantial degree of improvement in airflow limitation (>15%), prednisolone should be gradually reduced and replaced by inhaled corticosteroids (beclomethasone 100–500 $\mu$g three times daily). The long-term value of regular inhaled corticosteroids in all patients with chronic bronchitis and emphysema awaits evaluation.

ANTIBIOTICS. Prompt antibiotic treatment shortens exacerbations and should always be given in acute episodes as they may prevent subsequent further lung damage. Patients can be given a supply of antibiotics to keep at home to start as soon as their sputum turns yellow or green. Amoxycillin-resistant *H. influenzae* has become an increasing problem, occurring in 10–20% of isolates from sputum. Resistance to cefaclor 250 mg 8-hourly is significantly less frequent and it has become the antibiotic of choice.

Long-term treatment with antibiotics remains controversial. They were once thought to be of no value, but

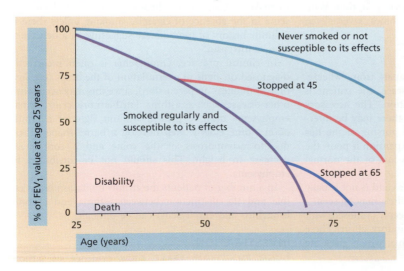

**Fig. 12.22** Influence of smoking on airflow limitation. (From Fletcher CM & Peto R (1977) *British Medical Journal* **1**, 1645.)

Figure labels:
% of $FEV_1$ value at age 25 years
Age (years)
Never smoked or not susceptible to its effects
Stopped at 45
Smoked regularly and susceptible to its effects
Stopped at 65
Disability
Death

eradication of infection and keeping the lower respiratory tract free of bacteria may help to prevent deterioration in lung function.

DIURETIC THERAPY. This is necessary for all oedematose patients.

$\alpha_1$-ANTITRYPSIN REPLACEMENT. Weekly or monthly infusions of $\alpha_1$-antitrypsin has been recommended for patients with levels of this compound below 11 mol litre$^{-1}$ (310 mg litre$^{-1}$) and abnormal lung function. Whether this modifies the long-term progression of the disease has still to be determined.

MUCOLYTICS AND VACCINES. There is little evidence that mucolytics are of any benefit, though it is vital that patients are encouraged to cough up sputum, initially with the help of a physiotherapist. Symptomatic treatment with steam inhalations may help to liquefy the sputum so that it can be more easily coughed up. Influenza vaccines should be given yearly to patients with disabling chronic bronchitis and emphysema.

### Treatment of respiratory failure

There are many causes of respiratory failure (Fig. 12.23) but by far the most common is chronic bronchitis and emphysema. In this type II respiratory failure the $P_a{CO_2}$

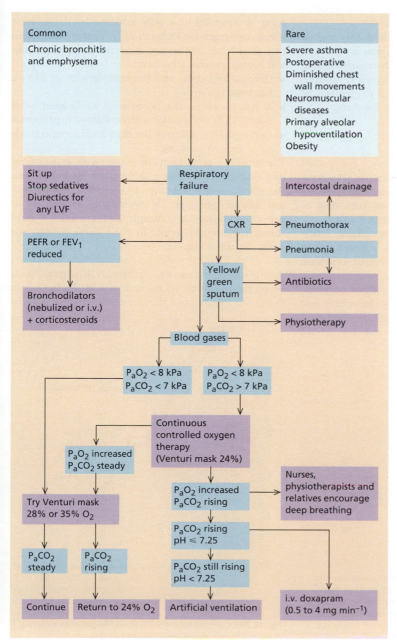

**Fig. 12.23** Algorithm for the treatment of respiratory failure. LVF, left ventricular failure.

is elevated and the $P_a o_2$ is reduced. It is important to realize that whereas hypercapnia is intoxicating, hypoxaemia is potentially lethal. The primary aim of the management of respiratory failure is to improve the $P_a o_2$ by continuous oxygen therapy. This nearly always leads to a rise in the $P_a co_2$ (see p. 728). Small increases in $P_a co_2$ can be tolerated but not if the pH falls dramatically. The pH should not be allowed to fall below 7.25; under such circumstances, increased ventilation must be achieved either by the use of a respiratory stimulant or by artificial ventilation.

Figure 12.24 shows a fixed-performance mask (Venturi mask) for the administration of oxygen. This style of mask is used when only low concentrations of oxygen can be given. It should be compared with the variable-performance face mask (see Fig. 13.16).

Initially, 24% oxygen is given, which is only slightly greater than the concentration of oxygen in air but, because of the shape of the oxygen–haemoglobin dissociation curve, this small increase in oxygen is valuable. Gradually, the concentration of inspired oxygen can be increased if there is no dramatic rise in the $P_a co_2$.

### Additional measures

These include:

REMOVAL OF RETAINED SECRETIONS. The patient should be encouraged to cough to remove secretions. Physiotherapy is helpful. If this fails, bronchoscopy and/or aspiration via an endotracheal tube may be necessary. A tracheostomy is only rarely required.

RESPIRATORY STIMULANTS. Doxapram, 0.5–4 mg $min^{-1}$ by slow i.v. infusion, may help in the short term to arouse the patient and to stimulate coughing, with clearance of some secretions.

ASSISTED VENTILATION (see p. 728). This is occasionally used for patients with chronic bronchitis and emphysema with severe respiratory failure when there is a definite precipitating factor and the overall

prognosis is reasonable. This can be a difficult ethical problem.

Corticosteroids, antibiotics and bronchodilators should also be administered (see above).

### Further management at home

Two controlled trials (chiefly in men) have indicated that the continuous administration of oxygen at 2 litres $min^{-1}$ via nasal prongs to achieve an oxygen saturation of greater than 90% for large proportions of the day and night can prolong life. Survival curves from these two studies are shown in Fig. 12.25. Only 30% of those not receiving long-term oxygen therapy survived for more than 5 years. A fall in pulmonary artery pressure was achieved if oxygen was given for 15 hours daily, but substantial improvement in mortality was only achieved by the administration of oxygen for 19 hours daily. These results suggest that long-term continuous domiciliary oxygen therapy will benefit patients who have:

- Chronic bronchitis and emphysema with an $FEV_1$ of less than 1.5 litres
- A $P_a o_2$ on air on two occasions 3 weeks apart of less than 7.3 kPa (55 mmHg) with or without hypercapnoea
- Carboxyhaemoglobin of less than 3%, i.e. patients who have stopped smoking

The provision of 19 hours of oxygen daily at a flow rate of 1–3 litre $min^{-1}$, using a 28% oxygen mask to increase the arterial oxygen saturation to over 90%, needs 20 oxygen cylinders per week. This is extremely expensive. Oxygen concentrators are cheaper and are now available through the health service in the UK for patients who fulfill the above criteria.

ADDITIONAL THERAPY. Pulmonary hypertension can be partially relieved by the use of oral $\beta$-adrenoceptor

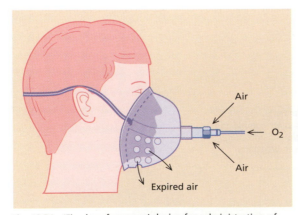

**Fig. 12.24** 'Fixed-performance' device for administration of oxygen to spontaneously breathing patients (Venturi mask). Oxygen is delivered through the injector of the Venturi mask at a given flow rate. A fixed amount of air is entrapped and the inspired oxygen can be accurately predicted. Masks are available to deliver 24%, 28% and 35% oxygen.

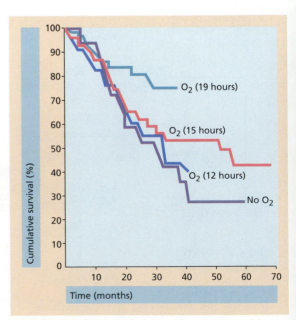

**Fig. 12.25** Cumulative survival curves for patients receiving oxygen. Oxygen doses are in hours per day.

stimulants such as salbutamol (4 mg three times daily), but whether this is useful in the long term is unknown.

The sensation of breathlessness can be reduced by the use of either promethazine 125 mg daily or dihydrocodeine 1 mg kg$^{-1}$ by mouth. Reduced breathlessness and increased exercise tolerance also result from the combined administration of dihydrocodeine and oxygen delivered from a portable cylinder.

EXERCISE TRAINING. A modest increase in exercise capacity with diminution in the sense of breathlessness and improved general well-being can result from exercise training. Regular training periods can be instituted at home; climbing stairs or walking fixed distances combined with regular clinic visits for encouragement. Breathing exercises are probably of less value. Quality of life though not life expectancy or decline in lung function can be improved by a multidisciplinary approach emphasizing physiotherapy, exercise, education and smoking cessation.

### PROGNOSIS

In general, 50% of patients with severe breathlessness die within 5 years (Fig. 12.25), but even in the severe group stopping smoking helps the prognosis.

## Nocturnal hypoxia

It has been shown that patients with chronic bronchitis and emphysema who show severe arterial hypoxaemia also suffer from profound nocturnal hypoxaemia with a $P_aO_2$ as low as 2.5 kPa (19 mmHg), particularly during the rapid eye movement (REM) phase of sleep.

Because patients with chronic bronchitis and emphysema are already hypoxic, the fall in $P_aO_2$ produces a much larger fall in oxygen saturation (owing to the steepness of the oxyhaemoglobin dissociation curve) and desaturation of up to 50% occurs. The mechanism is alveolar hypoventilation due to:

- Inhibition of intercostal and accessory muscles in REM sleep
- Shallow breathing in REM sleep, which reduces ventilation, particularly in severe chronic bronchitis and emphysema
- An increase in upper airway resistance due to a reduction in muscle tone

These nocturnal hypoxaemic episodes are associated with a further rise in pulmonary arterial pressure, and the majority of deaths in patients with chronic bronchitis and emphysema occur during the night, possibly due to cardiac arrhythmias. These patients additionally show severe secondary polycythaemia, partly as a result of the severe nocturnal hypoxaemia.

Each episode of desaturation is usually terminated by arousal from sleep, so that normal sleep is reduced and the patient suffers from daytime sleepiness. Patients with arterial hypoxaemia should never be given sleeping tablets, which will further depress respiratory drive. Treatment is with nocturnal administration of oxygen and ventilatory support.

VENTILATORY SUPPORT. Positive pressure ventilation can be administered non-invasively through a tightly fitting nasal mask with bilevel positive airway pressure—inspiratory to provide inspiratory assistance and expiratory to prevent alveolar closure, each adjusted independently. The use of these devices to maintain adequate ventilation during sleep and allow respiratory muscles to rest at night, though effective in chronic chest wall (e.g. kyphoscoliosis) or neuromuscular disease (e.g. previous poliomyelitis) has not led to improvement in respiratory function, respiratory muscle strength, exercise tolerance or breathlessness in patients with chronic bronchitis and emphysema.

## Obstructive sleep apnoea

This condition occurs most often in overweight middle-aged men and affects 1–2% of the population. It can occur in children particularly with enlarged tonsils.

The major symptoms and their frequency are:

- Loud snoring (95%)
- Daytime sleepiness (90%)
- Unrefreshed sleep (40%)
- Restless sleep (40%)
- Morning headache (30%)
- Nocturnal choking (30%)
- Reduced libido (20%)
- Morning drunkenness (5%)
- Ankle swelling (5%)

Apnoeas occur when the airway at the back of the throat is sucked closed when breathing in during sleep. When awake this tendency is overcome by the action of opening muscles of the upper airway—the genioglossus and palatal muscles, which become hypotonic during sleep (Fig. 12.26). Partial narrowing results in snoring, occlusion in apnoea and critical narrowing in hypopnoeas. Patients are woken by the struggle to breathe against the blocked throat. The awakenings are so brief that the patient remains unaware of them but is woken thousands of times per night leading to daytime sleepiness and impaired performance. Important contributory factors are obesity, a small pharyngeal opening and chronic airflow limitation.

Correctable factors occur in about one-third of cases and include:

- Encroachment on pharynx: obesity, acromegaly, enlarged tonsils
- Nasal obstruction: nasal deformities, rhinitis, polyps, adenoids
- Respiratory depressant drugs: alcohol, sedatives, strong analgesics

The diagnosis can usually be made by non-invasive ear or finger oximetry, best performed at home, accompanied by observation of the pattern of the snore–silence–snore cycle by the patient's family. Arterial oxygen saturation falls significantly in a cyclical manner. However, false-negative or equivocal results may occur in 50% necessitating full polysomnographic studies. These involve:

- Electroencephalography to record patterns of sleep and arousal

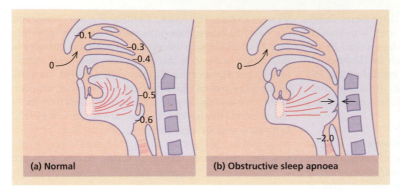

**Fig. 12.26** Section through head, showing pressure changes (kPa) in (a) the normal situation and (b) obstructive sleep apnoea. There is a pressure drop during inspiration as air is sucked through the turbinates and in patients with obstructive sleep apnoea this is sufficient to collapse the pharynx, obstructing inspiration.

- Recording of thoracoabdominal movements to assess breathing
- Oronasal flow
- Oximetry

The diagnosis of sleep apnoea/hypopnoea is made if there are more than 15 apnoeas or hypopnoeas in any 1 hour of sleep.

Management consists of correction of treatable factors (see above) with, if necessary, continuous nasal positive airway pressure delivered by a nasal mask during sleep. Such systems raise the pressure in the pharynx by about 1 kPa, keeping the walls apart.

## Bronchiectasis

Bronchiectasis may be defined simply as dilatation of the bronchi.

Bronchial walls become inflamed, thickened and irreversibly damaged. The mucociliary transport mechanism is impaired and frequent bacterial infections ensue. Clinically, the disease is characterized by cough productive of large amounts of sputum.

### AETIOLOGY

Bronchial obstruction followed by infection plays a major role. In the past bronchiectasis frequently followed pneumonia in childhood.

Bronchiectasis is still a rare complication of whooping cough and measles in the Western world. Localized bronchiectasis also rarely results from tuberculous enlargement of lymph nodes at the hilum of the lung, particularly around the origin of the middle-lobe bronchus. Bronchial obstruction in children from other causes (e.g. inhaled peanuts) can give rise to gross suppurative lung disease and residual bronchiectasis.

Progressive bronchiectasis has been described in non-smoking patients of both sexes, with no other underlying cause. This syndrome is known as chronic bronchial sepsis.

Cystic fibrosis (see p. 665) also leads to bronchiectasis, as over 75% of children with cystic fibrosis now survive to adult life. Occasionally cystic fibrosis may present with bronchiectasis in adults. Bronchiectasis can also be associated with other congenital abnormalities, e.g. Kartagener's syndrome, which is characterized by sinusitis and transposition of viscera with bronchiectasis, associated with 'immotile cilia'. Immunoglobulin deficiencies particularly IgA or $IgG_4$ can lead to recurrent infections and bronchiectasis.

### CLINICAL FEATURES

Patients with mild bronchiectasis only produce yellow or green sputum after an infection, often viral. Localized areas of the lung may be particularly affected, when sputum production will depend on position. As the condition worsens, the patient suffers from persistent halitosis, recurrent febrile episodes with malaise, and episodes of pneumonia. Clubbing occurs, and coarse crackles can be heard over the infected areas, usually the bases of the lungs. When the condition is severe there is continuous production of foul-smelling, thick, khaki-coloured sputum. Haemoptysis, either as blood-stained sputum or as a massive haemorrhage, can occur. Breathlessness may result from airflow limitation.

### INVESTIGATION

THE CHEST X-RAY may be quite normal or may show dilated bronchi with thickened bronchial walls and sometimes multiple cysts containing fluid.

HIGH-RESOLUTION CT SCANNING can show bronchial wall thickening and is the investigation of choice (Fig. 12.27).

BRONCHOGRAMS. This investigation is uncomfortable

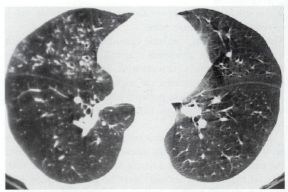

**Fig. 12.27** CT scan showing bronchiectasis in the right middle lobe. Note dilated bronchi with thickened wall and adjacent artery giving a signet ring appearance.

for the patient and is only required if the diagnosis is in doubt or where there is reason to believe that the disease may be localized and therefore amenable to surgical treatment. The left lower lobe and lingula are the commonest sites for localized disease.

SPUTUM EXAMINATION with culture and sensitivity of the organisms is essential for adequate treatment. The major pathogens are *Staph. aureus, Pseudomonas aeruginosa, H. influenzae* and anaerobes. Other pathogens include *Strep. pneumoniae* and *Klebsiella pneumoniae*. *Aspergillus fumigatus* can be isolated from 10% of sputum specimens in cystic fibrosis, but the role of this organism is uncertain.

SINUS X-RAYS.

SERUM IMMUNOGLOBULINS.

SWEAT ELECTROLYTES
CILIAL MOTILITY STUDIES } where appropriate.

## TREATMENT

### Postural drainage

Postural drainage is of vital importance and patients must be trained by physiotherapists to tip themselves into appropriate positions at least three times daily for 10–20 min. Most patients find that lying over the side of the bed with head and thorax down is the most effective position.

### Antibiotics

Experience from the treatment of cystic fibrosis suggests that bronchopulmonary infections should be eradicated if progression of the disease is to be halted. In mild cases, intermittent chemotherapy with cefaclor 500 mg three times daily or ciprofloxacin 500 mg twice daily may be the only therapy needed. Flucloxacillin 500 mg 6-hourly is the best treatment if *Staph. aureus* is isolated. Chloramphenicol is a useful drug in persistent infection.

If the sputum remains yellow or green despite regular physiotherapy and intermittent chemotherapy, or if lung function deteriorates despite treatment with bronchodilators, it is likely that there is infection with *Ps. aeruginosa*. Treatment requires parenteral or aerosol chemotherapy at regular 3-monthly intervals. Ceftazidime 2 g intravenously 8-hourly or by inhalation (1 g twice daily) has been shown to be effective. Ciprofloxacin 500 mg twice daily orally is equally effective. These drugs are replacing older drug regimens involving tobramycin or gentamicin together with tircarcillin or azlocillin. High sputum levels of some antibiotics can be achieved by inhalation. A treatment regimen of carbenicillin 1 g and gentamicin 80 mg given by a compressor-driven nebulizer twice daily was found to be of benefit in young adult patients with chronic *Pseudomonas* infection but many physicians prefer intravenous therapy with ceftazidime.

### Bronchodilators

Bronchodilators are useful in patients with demonstrable airflow limitation.

### Surgery

Unfortunately, bronchiectasis is rarely sufficiently localized for surgery to be of any value.

## COMPLICATIONS

The incidence of complications has fallen with antibiotic therapy. Pneumonia, pneumothorax, empyema and metastatic cerebral abscess can occur. Severe, life-threatening haemoptysis can also occur, particularly in patients with cystic fibrosis.

MASSIVE HAEMOPTYSIS originates from the high pressure systemic bronchial arteries and has a mortality of 25%. Other causes include pulmonary tuberculosis, aspergilloma, lung abscess and infection, and primary and secondary malignant tumours.

Bed rest and antibiotic treatment is essential together with blood transfusion if required. Urgent fibreoptic bronchoscopy is necessary to detect the source of bleeding. If the haemoptysis does not settle rapidly the affected area must be surgically resected. Bronchial artery embolization is the treatment of choice in those not fit for surgery.

# Cystic fibrosis

Cystic fibrosis (CF) is due to an alteration in the viscosity and tenacity of mucus production at epithelial surfaces. The classical form of the syndrome includes bronchopulmonary infection and pancreatic insufficiency, with a high sweat sodium and chloride concentration. It is an autosomally recessive inherited disorder with a carrier frequency in Caucasians of 1 in 22 (see p. 123). There is a gene mutation on the long arm of chromosome 7 (7q 21.3 → 7q 22.1). A specific deletion in the coding region (the codon for phenylalanine at position 508 in the amino acid sequence [$\Delta F_{508}$]) has been found resulting in a defect in a transmembrane regulator protein (see p. 125) now called the cystic fibrosis transmembrane conductance regulator (CFTR) which probably represents a critical chloride channel (Fig. 12.28). The mutation alters the secondary and tertiary structure of the protein leading to a failure of opening of the chloride channel in response to elevated cyclic AMP in epithelial cells. This results in a decreased excretion of chloride into the airway lumen and a threefold increase in the reabsorption of sodium into the epithelial cells. With less excretion of salt there is less excretion of water and increased viscosity and tenacity of airway secretions. A possible reason for the high salt content of sweat is that there is a CFTR-independent mechanism of chloride secretion in the sweat gland with an impaired reabsorption of sodium chloride in the distal end of the duct.

The frequency of $\Delta F_{508}$ mutation in CF is 70% in the USA and UK, <50% in southern Europe and 30% in Ashkenazic families. The identification of this transmembrane regulator protein will allow more accurate detection of carriers of the mutant gene.

## CLINICAL FEATURES

Although the lungs of babies born with CF are structurally normal at birth, respiratory symptoms are usually the presenting feature. CF is now the commonest cause of recurrent bronchopulmonary infection in childhood, and

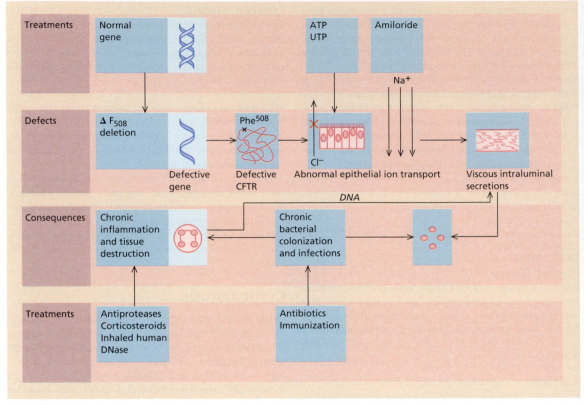

**Fig. 12.28**  Cystic fibrosis—abnormalities and recent therapeutic advances (see text).

is an important cause in early adult life. Finger clubbing is almost universal, haemoptysis is frequent and breathlessness occurs in the later stages as airflow limitation develops. Older children may also develop nasal polyps.

Puberty and skeletal maturity are delayed in most patients with the disease. Males are almost always infertile owing to failure of development of the vas deferens and epididymis. Females are able to conceive, but often develop secondary amenorrhoea as the disease progresses.

About 85% of patients have symptomatic steatorrhoea owing to pancreatic dysfunction (see p. 290). Children may be born with meconium ileus due to the viscoid consistency of meconium in CF and later in life develop the meconium ileus equivalent (MIE) syndrome, an important cause of small intestinal obstruction unique to CF.

Cholesterol gallstones appear to occur with increased frequency and cirrhosis develops in about 5% of older patients.

### DIAGNOSIS

The diagnosis of CF in older children and adults may be difficult. It depends on the clinical history together with:
- A family history of the disease.
- A high sweat sodium concentration over 60 mmol litre$^{-1}$. (Meticulous technique by laboratories performing regular sweat analysis is essential, but the test

is still difficult to interpret in adults.)
- Absent vas deferens and epididymis.
- Decreased immunoreactive trypsin (p. 290).

### TREATMENT

Antibiotic treatment for the respiratory disease is described under bronchiectasis on p. 665 and treatment of pancreatic insufficiency is described on p. 290. The understanding of the basic abnormality in CF has led to dramatic changes in treatment—potential treatments to improve hydration of secretions include blocking of Na$^+$ reabsorption with amiloride or stimulating Cl$^-$ secretion with a triphosphate nucleotide (adenosine or uridine triphosphates, ATP and UTP) which stimulate nucleotide receptors by a pathway independent of cAMP. Viscosity of secretions is contributed to by macromolecules such as DNA from dead inflammatory cells. Human DNase capable of degrading DNA has been cloned, sequenced and expressed by recombinant techniques. Inhalation of this material has been shown to improve FEV$_1$ by 20%. Similarly, inhaled or oral corticosteroids and antiproteases such as inhaled $\alpha_1$-antitrypsin help to reduce inflammation and improve lung function.

So far tested only in experimental animals is the delivery to the epithelium of the normal CFTR gene using as a vector a replication-deficient adenovirus containing normal human CFTR complementary DNA which is trophic for epithelial cells. Successful trials in CF patients would herald a new era of treatment.

## PROGNOSIS AND COUNSELLING

The prognosis has consistently improved; 90% of children now survive into their teens and the mean survival is 29 years. The long-term outlook is uncertain, but progressive respiratory failure almost inevitably occurs. Of particular concern is the finding in sputum of *Pseudomonas cepacia* a plant pathogen previously considered a harmless commensal. Its acquisition can be associated with accelerated disease and rapid death. Multiple antibiotic resistance is common and spread is from person to person. Drastic strategies have been introduced to limit transmission which include rigid segregation of both inpatients and outpatients and the instruction to CF sufferers not to socialize together. Groups formed for mutual support and education have been disrupted leading to considerable distress. Genetic screening is available to identify carriers of the $\Delta F_{508}$ deletion allowing 75% of couples at risk to be identified. Screening for the carrier state should be offered to persons or couples with a family history of CF together with counselling (see p. 123).

## Lung transplantation

Indications for this treatment are patients under 60 years with a life expectancy of less than 18 months, no underlying cancer and no serious systemic disease. The main diseases treated by transplantation are:

- Pulmonary fibrosis
- Primary pulmonary hypertension
- Cystic fibrosis
- Bronchiectasis
- Emphysema—particularly $\alpha_1$-antitrypsin deficiency
- Eisenmenger's syndrome

Since donor material is limited, single lung transplantation is preferred to double lung or heart–lung transplantation and can be successfully undertaken in pulmonary fibrosis, pulmonary hypertension and emphysema. Bilateral lung transplantation is required in infective conditions to prevent spill-over of bacteria from the diseased lung to a single lung transplant. Eisenmenger's syndrome requires heart–lung transplant.

## COMPLICATIONS AND TREATMENT

1 Early; post-transplant pulmonary oedema needs diuretics and respiratory support by ventilation
2 Infections, particularly within first 3 months:
   (a) Bacterial pneumonia—antibiotics
   (b) Cytomegalovirus—ganciclovir
   (c) Herpes simplex—acyclovir
   (d) *P. carinii*—prophylactic co-trimoxazole
3 Immunosuppression is with cyclosporin, azathioprine and prednisolone
4 Rejection:
   (a) Early—first few weeks: high-dose i.v. corticosteroids
   (b) Late—3 months: in obliterative bronchiolitis high-dose i.v. corticosteroids are sometimes effective

Prognosis is improving rapidly with 2-year survival of 75% and 5-year survival of almost 50%.

## Chronic cough

Pathological coughing results from two mechanisms:

1 Stimulation of sensory nerves in the epithelium by secretions, foreign bodies, cigarette smoke and tumours
2 Sensitization of the cough reflex in which there is an abnormal increase in the sensitivity of the cough receptors demonstrable by inhalation of the tussive agents capsaicin or low chloride solutions

Sensitization of the cough reflex presents clinically as a persistent tickling sensation in the throat with paroxysms of coughing induced by changes in air temperature, aerosol sprays, perfumes and cigarette smoke. It is found in association with viral infections, oesophageal reflux, postnasal drip, cough variant asthma, idiopathic cough, and in 15% of patients taking angiotensin converting enzyme (ACE) inhibitors. The association with the latter implicates neuroactive peptides—prostaglandins $E_2$ and $F_{2\alpha}$ and bradykinin. In the absence of chest X-ray abnormalities, investigations should include:

- ENT examination and sinus CT for postnasal drip
- Lung function tests and histamine bronchial provocation testing for cough variant asthma
- Ambulatory oesophageal pH monitoring for oesophageal reflux
- CT scan of thorax for interstitial lung disease
- *V/Q* scans for recurrent pulmonary embolism
- Fibreoptic bronchoscopy for inhaled foreign body or tumour
- ECG, echocardiography and exercise testing for cardiac causes
- Hyperventilation testing and psychiatric appraisal

Appropriate treatment for any of the conditions discovered can relieve symptoms. In the absence of any pathology management of cough is difficult. Morphine treatment will depress the sensitized cough reflex but its unwanted effects limit its use long term. Nebulized bupivocaine is of value. Demulcent preparations and cough sweets provide temporary relief only.

# *Asthma*

Asthma is a common chronic inflammatory condition of the lung airways whose cause is incompletely understood. Symptoms are cough, wheeze, chest tightness and shortness of breath, often worse at night. It has three characteristics:

1 Airflow limitation which is usually reversible spontaneously or with treatment. In chronic asthma inflammation may lead to irreversible airflow limitation.
2 Airway hyperresponsiveness to a wide range of stimuli (see below).

3 Inflammation of the bronchi with eosinophils, T lymphocytes and mast cells with associated plasma exudation, oedema, smooth muscle hypertrophy, mucus plugging and epithelial changes.

The underlying pathology in preschool children may be different in that they may not exhibit appreciable bronchial hyperreactivity. There is no evidence that chronic inflammation is the basis for the episodic asthma associated with viral infections.

## PREVALENCE

In many countries, the prevalence of asthma is increasing, particularly in the second decade of life where this disease affects 10–15% of the population. There is also a geographical variation, with asthma being common in, for example, New Zealand, but being much rarer in Far Eastern countries such as China and Malaysia. Long-term follow-up in developing countries suggests that the disease may become more frequent as individuals become more 'Westernized'. Studies of occupational asthma suggest that a high percentage of the work-force, perhaps up to 20%, may become asthmatic if exposed to potent sensitizers.

## CLASSIFICATION

Asthma can be divided into:
- Extrinsic—implying a definite external cause
- Intrinsic or cryptogenic—when no causative agent can be identified

EXTRINSIC ASTHMA occurs in atopic individuals who show positive skin-prick reactions to common inhaled allergens. Positive skin tests to inhalant allergens are shown in 90% of children with asthma, whereas only 50% of adults show this phenomenon. Eczema is often seen in childhood (see p. 997).

INTRINSIC ASTHMA often starts in middle age. Nevertheless, many show positive skin tests and on close questioning give a history of respiratory symptoms compatible with childhood asthma.

This classification is of little value in clinical practice. Non-atopic individuals may develop asthma in middle age from extrinsic causes such as sensitization to occupational agents or aspirin intolerance, or because they were given β-adrenoreceptor-blocking agents for concurrent hypertension or angina. Extrinsic causes must be considered in all cases of asthma and, where possible, avoided.

## AETIOLOGY AND PATHOGENESIS

There are two major factors involved in the development of asthma and many other stimuli that can precipitate attacks (Fig. 12.29).

### Atopy and allergy

The term 'atopy' was used by clinicians at the beginning of the century to describe a group of disorders, including asthma and hay fever, that appeared:
- To run in families

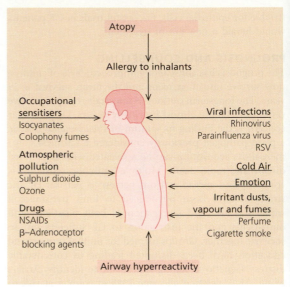

**Fig. 12.29**  Causes of asthma. RSV, respiratory syncytial virus.

- To have characteristic wealing skin reactions to common allergens in the environment
- To have circulating antibody in their serum that could be transferred to the skin of non-sensitized individuals

The term is now best used to describe those individuals who readily develop antibodies of IgE class against common materials present in the environment. Such antibodies are present in 30–40% of the population, and there is a link between serum IgE levels and both the prevalence of asthma and airway responsiveness to histamine or methacholine. Genetic and environmental factors affect serum IgE levels. Whilst the precise location of the genes controlling IgE production remains to be determined, early childhood exposure to allergens and maternal smoking have an important influence on IgE production.

The allergens involved are similar to those in rhinitis, though the particle size of pollens (>20 $\mu$m) means that they are much more likely to cause conjunctivitis, rhinitis and pharyngitis than asthma. Allergens from the faecal particles of the house-dust mite are the most important extrinsic cause of asthma worldwide. The fungal spores from *A. fumigatus* give rise to a complex series of lung disease, including asthma (see p. 692).

### Increased responsiveness of the airways of the lung (airway hyperreactivity)

Bronchial reactivity can be demonstrated by asking the patient to inhale gradually increasing concentrations either of histamine or methacholine (*bronchial provocation tests*). This induces a transient episode of airflow limitation in susceptible individuals (approximately 20% of the population); the dose of the agonist (provocation dose) necessary to produce a 20% fall in $FEV_1$ is known as the $PD_{20}FEV_1$. Patients with clinical symptoms of asthma respond to very low doses of methacholine, i.e. they have a low $PD_{20}FEV_1$ (<11 $\mu$mol). In general, the greater the degree of hyperreactivity, the more persistent the symptoms and the greater the need for treatment.

Some patients also react to methacholine but at higher doses and include those with:

- Attacks of asthma only on extreme exertion
- Wheezing or prolonged periods of coughing following a viral infection
- Cough variant asthma
- Problems with asthma only during the pollen season
- Allergic rhinitis, but not complaining of any lower respiratory symptoms until specifically questioned
- Some subjects with no respiratory symptoms

Although the degree of hyperreactivity can itself be influenced by allergic mechanisms (see p. 670 and Fig. 12.32), its pathogenesis and mode of inheritance remain to be elucidated.

## PATHOGENESIS AND PRECIPITATING FACTORS
### Occupational sensitizers

Over 200 materials encountered at the work-place are known to give rise to occupational asthma. The important causes are recognized occupational diseases in the UK and patients in insurable employment are therefore eligible for statutory compensation provided they apply within 10 years of leaving the occupation in which the asthma developed (Table 12.7). The development of asthma following exposure to some of these materials is linked to the development of specific IgE antibody in serum in some cases, whilst in others the cause has yet to be determined.

The proportion of employees developing occupational asthma depends primarily upon the level of exposure. Proper enclosure of industrial processes or appropriate ventilation can greatly reduce the risk. Atopic individuals develop occupational asthma more rapidly when exposed to agents causing the development of specific IgE anti-

| Cause | Source |
|---|---|
| *Non-IgE related* | |
| Isocyanates | Polyurethane varnishes Industrial coatings |
| Colophony fumes | Soldering Electronics industry |
| *IgE related* | |
| Allergens from animals and insects | Laboratories |
| Allergens from flour and grain | Farmers Millers Grain handlers |
| Proteolytic enzymes | Manufacture (but not use) of 'biological' washing powders |
| Complex salts of platinum | Metal refining |
| Acid anhydrides and polyamine hardening agents | Industrial coatings |

**Table 12.7** Occupational asthma in the UK.

body. Non-atopic individuals can also develop asthma when exposed to such agents, but usually after a longer period.

### Non-specific factors

The characteristic feature of bronchial hyperreactivity in asthmatics means that as well as reacting to specific antigens their airways will also respond to a wide variety of non-specific stimuli.

COLD AIR AND EXERCISE. Most asthmatics experience an attack of wheezing after prolonged and continuous exercise. Typically, the attack does not occur during the exercise period but at its conclusion. The inhalation of cold, dry air will also precipitate an attack. In both cases the wheezing is thought to be precipitated by the cooling and drying of the epithelial lining of the bronchi. Exercise and cold air provocation tests can be performed.

ATMOSPHERIC POLLUTION AND IRRITANT DUSTS, VAPOURS AND FUMES. Many patients with asthma experience worsening of symptoms on contact with cigarette smoke, car exhaust fumes, strong perfumes or high concentrations of dust in the atmosphere. Further minor epidemics of the disease have occurred during periods of heavy atmospheric pollution in industrial areas, caused by the presence of high concentrations of sulphur dioxide, ozone and nitrogen dioxide in the air.

EMOTION. It is well known that emotional factors may influence asthma, but there is no evidence that patients with the disease are any more psychologically disturbed than their non-asthmatic peers.

DRUGS. Non-steroidal anti-inflammatory drugs (NSAIDs), particularly aspirin, have an important role in the development and precipitation of attacks in approximately 5% of patients with asthma. This effect is almost universal in those individuals who have both nasal polyps and asthma. The precise mechanism involved is unknown but it is thought that treatment with these drugs leads to an imbalance in the metabolism of arachidonic acid. NSAIDs inhibit arachidonic acid metabolism via the cyclooxygenase pathway, preventing the synthesis of prostaglandins. It is suggested that under these circumstances arachidonic acid is preferentially metabolized via the lipoxygenase pathway, resulting in the production of leukotrienes, previously known as the slow-reacting substances for anaphylaxis (Fig. 12.30).

The airways of the lung have a direct parasympathetic innervation that tends to produce bronchoconstriction. There is no direct sympathetic innervation of the smooth muscle of the bronchi, and antagonism of parasympathetically induced bronchoconstriction is critically dependent upon circulating adrenaline acting through $\beta_2$-receptors on the surface of smooth muscle cells. Inhibition of this effect by $\beta$-adrenoreceptor-blocking drugs such as propranolol leads to bronchoconstriction and airflow limitation, but only in asthmatic subjects. The so-called selective $\beta_1$-adrenoceptor-blocking drugs such as atenolol may

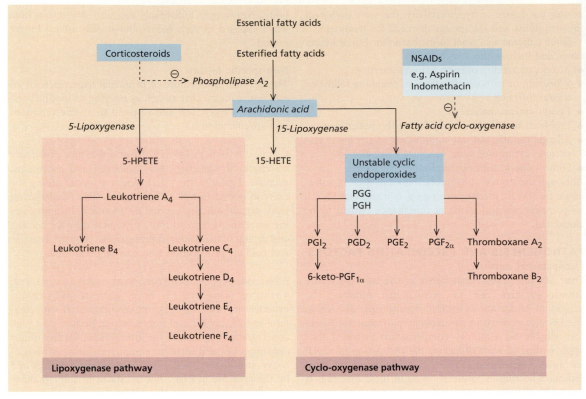

**Fig. 12.30** Arachidonic acid metabolism and the effect of drugs.

still induce attacks of asthma; their use in asthmatic patients for hypertension or angina should be questioned and calcium antagonists such as nifedipine should be used if appropriate.

### Allergen-induced asthma

The experimental inhalation of allergen by atopic asthmatic individuals leads to the development of four types of reaction, as illustrated in Fig. 12.31.

The commonest reaction is *immediate asthma*, in which airflow limitation begins within minutes of contact with the allergen, reaches its maximum in 15–20 min and subsides by 1 hour.

Many asthmatics subsequently develop a more prolonged and sustained attack of airflow limitation that responds poorly to inhalation of bronchodilator drugs such as salbutamol—the *late-phase reaction*.

The combination of an immediate reaction followed by a late reaction is known as a *dual asthmatic response*.

The inhalation of some materials, particularly occupational sensitizers such as the isocyanates, usually causes the development of an *isolated late reaction* with no preceding immediate response.

The development of the late-phase reaction is associated with an increase in the underlying level of airway hyperreactivity such that individuals may show continuing episodes of asthma on subsequent days—*recurrent asthmatic reactions.*

The pathogenesis of asthma is complex and not fully understood. It involves a number of cells, mediators, nerves and vascular leakage that can be activated by several different mechanisms, of which exposure to allergens is the most important (Fig. 12.32).

MAST CELLS (see p. 133). These are increased in both the epithelium and surface secretions of asthmatics and can generate and release powerful smooth muscle and vasoactive mediators, such as histamine, prostaglandin $D_2$ ($PGD_2$) and leukotriene $C_4$ ($LTC_4$), which cause the immediate asthmatic reaction. Since potent $\beta_2$-adreno-ceptor agonists such as salbutamol have little effect on airway inflammation or hyperreactivity but inhibit mast cell mediator release, many other factors are now considered important in the pathogenesis of late and recurrent asthmatic reactions leading to more severe asthma.

EPITHELIUM. Epithelial cells are shed during exacerbations of asthma (they can readily be identified in sputum), causing increased permeability to inhaled allergens, exposure of afferent nerve endings, loss of the putative epithelial-derived relaxant factor, possibly nitric oxide, and neutral endopeptidase capable of breaking down sensory neuropeptides, and generation of chemoattractant factors such as 15-hydroxyeicosatetraenoic acid (15-HETE). Epithelial cells can also produce cytokines, particularly granulocyte macrophage colony stimulating

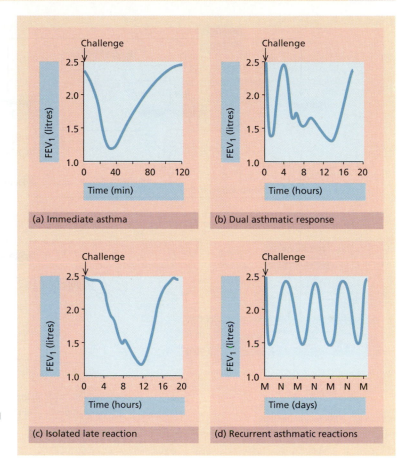

**Fig. 12.31** Different types of asthmatic reactions following challenge with allergen. (a) Immediate asthma. (b) Dual asthmatic response. (c) Isolated late reaction. (d) Recurrent asthmatic reactions. M, midnight; N, noon.

factor (GM-CSF), tumour necrosis factor-$\alpha$ (TNF-$\alpha$) and interleukin 8 (IL-8), all capable of initiating and enhancing inflammation.

BASEMENT MEMBRANE. Recently biopsy studies have shown that the sub-basement membrane region, the lamina reticularis, is widened even in the mildest asthmatics owing to increased deposition of collagen types III and V and fibronectin, indicating that inflammation occurs at the earliest stages of the disease.

NERVES. Damage or loss of epithelial cells exposes C-fibre afferent nerve endings that can release the sensory neuropeptides substance P, neurokinin A and calcitonin gene-related peptide, contributing towards broncho-constriction, microvascular leakage and mucus secretion.

MACROPHAGES AND LYMPHOCYTES. These cells are abundant in the mucous membranes of the airways and the alveoli. Macrophages may play a particularly important role in the initial uptake and presentation of allergens to lymphocytes. They can release prostaglandins, thromboxanes, leukotriene B$_4$ (LTB$_4$) and platelet activating factor (PAF). T-helper lymphocytes (CD4) show evidence of activation and the release of their cytokines may play an important part in the migration and activation

of mast cells (IL-3) and eosinophils (IL-5). In addition production of IL-4 leads to the switching of antibody production by B lymphocytes to IgE. The activity of both macrophages and lymphocytes is influenced by cortico-steroids but not $\beta_2$-adrenoceptor agonists.

EOSINOPHILS. These cells are found in large numbers in the bronchial secretions of asthmatics. When activated, they release LTC$_4$, PAF and basic proteins such as major basic protein (MBP) and eosinophil cationic protein (ECP) that are toxic to epithelial cells. Both the number and activation of eosinophils is rapidly decreased by corticosteroids.

MEDIATORS. The exact role of the many potent smooth muscle and vasoactive mediators, including LTC$_4$, LTD$_4$, thromboxanes and the sensory neuropeptides, as well as the chemoattractants LTB$_4$ and PAF, remains unknown and awaits the introduction of effective and specific antagonists. Studies with potent selective H$_1$ antagonists have shown that histamine plays only a small role in the pathogenesis of the persisting airflow limitation of asthma.

## CLINICAL FEATURES
Patients suffering from asthma exhibit virtually identical symptoms to those suffering from airflow limitation

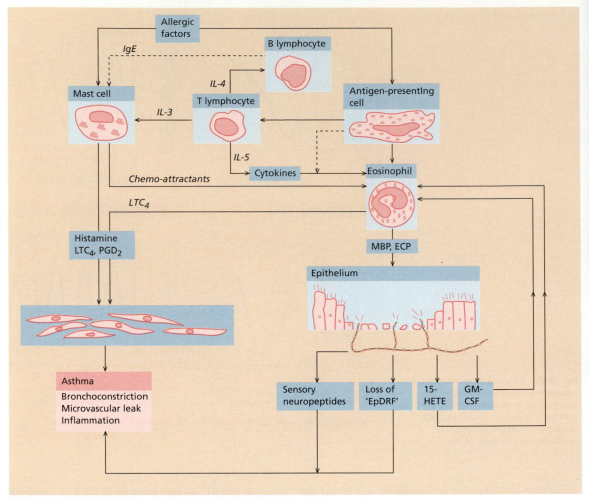

**Fig. 12.32**  Pathogenesis of asthma. ECP, eosinophil cationic protein; EpDRF, epithelial derived relaxant factor; MBP, major basic protein.

caused by chronic bronchitis and emphysema. Wheezing attacks and episodic shortness of breath are almost universal. Symptoms are usually worst during the night. Cough is a frequent symptom that sometimes predominates and is often misdiagnosed as being due to bronchitis. Nocturnal cough can be a presenting feature.

There is a tremendous variation in the frequency and duration of the attacks. Some patients may have only one or two attacks a year that last for a few hours, whilst others may have attacks lasting for weeks. Some patients can have chronic symptoms. Attacks may be precipitated by all the factors illustrated in Fig. 12.29; the signs of asthma are listed in Table 12.1.

### INVESTIGATION
There is no single satisfactory diagnostic test for all asthmatic patients.

### Lung function tests
The diagnosis of asthma is based on the demonstration of a greater than 15% improvement in $FEV_1$ or PEFR following the inhalation of a bronchodilator. However, this is often not present if the asthma is in remission or in very severe chronic disease, when little reversibility can be demonstrated.

### Peak flow charts
Measurements of PEFR on waking, in the middle of the day, and before bed are particularly useful in demonstrating the variable airflow limitation that characterizes the disease. An example is shown in Fig. 12.14. This technique is also of help in the longer-term assessment of the patient's disease and its response to treatment. Peak flows need to be measured over several days and preferably over a weekend or short holiday if the effect of work exposure is also being studied.

### Exercise tests
These have been widely used in the diagnosis of asthma in children. Ideally, the child should run for 6 min on a treadmill at a work-load sufficient to increase the heart

rate above 160 beats per minute. A negative test does not rule out asthma.

### Histamine or methacholine bronchial provocation tests (see p. 668)

This test indicates the presence of airway hyperreactivity, a feature found in all asthmatics, and can be particularly useful in investigating those patients whose main symptom is cough. The test should not be performed on individuals who have poor lung function ($FEV_1$ <1.5 litres).

### Trial of corticosteroids

Prednisolone 30 mg orally should be given daily for 2 weeks to all patients who present with severe airflow limitation. A substantial improvement (>15%) confirms the presence of an asthmatic element and that the administration of steroids will prove beneficial to the patient. The dose is slowly reduced over several weeks and is replaced by inhaled corticosteroids in those who will benefit.

### Blood and sputum tests

Patients with asthma may have an increase in the number of eosinophils in peripheral blood (>$0.4 \times 10^9$/litre). This is rarely helpful in the diagnosis. The presence of large numbers of eosinophils, particularly when present in clumps in sputum, is helpful in the differential diagnosis of asthma from chronic bronchitis and emphysema.

### Chest X-ray

There are no diagnostic features of asthma on the chest X-ray. A chest X-ray may be helpful in excluding a pneumothorax, which can occur as a complication, or in detecting the pulmonary shadows associated with allergic bronchopulmonary aspergillosis.

### Skin tests

Skin-prick tests should be performed in all cases of asthma to help identify extrinsic causes. Experimentally, the inhalation of an allergen that gives rise to a large weal on skin testing will almost always produce an attack of asthma in patients with the disease, but whether this occurs in everyday life depends on the concentrations encountered in the atmosphere.

### Allergen provocation tests

These are seldom, if ever, required in the clinical investigation of patients. An exception is the investigation of food allergy causing asthma. This diagnosis is difficult; blind oral challenges with the food disguised in opaque gelatine capsules are necessary to confirm or refute a causative link (see p. 172).

## MANAGEMENT

Asthma is an extremely common disease producing considerable morbidity. The aim of treatment must be:
- To abolish symptoms
- To restore normal or best possible long-term airway function
- To reduce the risk of severe attacks
- To enable normal growth to occur in children
- To minimize absence from school/work

This involves:
- Patient and family participation
- Avoidance of identified causes where possible
- Use of lowest effective dose of convenient medications minimizing short-term and long-term side-effects

Many asthmatics belong to self-help groups whose aim is to further their understanding of the disease and to foster self-confidence and fitness.

### Control of extrinsic factors

Measures must be taken to avoid causative allergens such as the house-dust mite, pets, moulds and foods (see allergic rhinitis), particularly in childhood.

Avoidance of the house-dust mite is now possible with effective and comfortable covers for bedding and changes to living accommodation. Active and passive smoking should be avoided as should $\beta$-blockers both in tablet and eyedrop form.

Individuals intolerant to aspirin may benefit, though are rarely cured, by avoiding salicylates. Other agents, e.g. preservatives and colouring materials such as tartrazine, should be avoided if shown to be a causative factor. Fifty per cent of individuals sensitized to occupational agents may be cured if they are kept permanently away from exposure. The remaining 50% continue to have symptoms as severe as when exposed to materials at work. This is particularly so if they had been symptomatic for a long time before the diagnosis was made.

This underlines two points:
1 The importance of the rapid identification of extrinsic causes of asthma and their removal wherever possible (e.g. the family pet)
2 Once extrinsic asthma is initiated, it may become self-perpetuating

### Drug treatment

The mainstay of asthma therapy is the use of therapeutic agents delivered as aerosols or powders directly into the lungs (Practical box 12.4). The advantages of this method of administration are obvious. Drugs are delivered direct to the lung and the first-pass metabolism in the liver is avoided; both these factors mean that much lower doses are necessary and unwanted effects are slight.

Both national and international guidelines have been published on the step-wise treatment of asthma (Information box 12.1) based on three important factors:
1 Asthma self-management with regular asthma monitoring using mini peak flow meters and individual treatment plans discussed with each patient
2 The appreciation that asthma is an inflammatory disease and that anti-inflammatory therapy should be started even in mild cases
3 A diminution in the role of bronchodilators, e.g. salbutamol since they are not anti-inflammatory and regular treatment with these drugs on their own may be associated with worsening of asthma and even asthma deaths

$\beta_2$-ADRENOCEPTOR AGONISTS. The newer bronchodilator preparations contain $\beta$-adrenoceptor agonists

*Use of an inhaler*
The canister is shaken

The patient exhales to functional residual capacity (not
residual volume), i.e. normal expiration

The aerosol nozzle is placed to the open mouth

The patient simultaneously inhales rapidly and activates
the aerosol

Inhalation is completed

The breath is held for 10 s if possible

Even with good technique only 15% of the contents is
inhaled and 85% is deposited on the wall of the
pharynx and ultimately swallowed

*Spacers*
These are plastic conical spheres inserted between the
patient's mouth and the inhaler. They are designed to
reduce particle velocity so that less drug is deposited in
the mouth. Spacers also diminish the need for
coordination between aerosol activation and
inhalation. They are useful in children and in the
elderly

**Practical box 12.4**   Inhaled therapy.

that, unlike isoprenaline, are selective for the $\beta_2$-adreno-
ceptors of the respiratory tract and do not stimulate the
$\beta_1$-adrenoceptors of the myocardium. These drugs are
potent bronchodilators in that they cause relaxation of
bronchial smooth muscle. Such treatment is very effective
in relieving symptoms but does little for the underlying
inflammatory nature of the disease. Inhalants such as salbutamol (100 $\mu$g) or terbutaline (250 $\mu$g) should be prescribed as two puffs as required.

Salmeterol (50–100 $\mu$g), a highly selective and potent
$\beta_2$-adrenoceptor agonist, is effective by inhalation for up
to 12 hours, reducing the need for administration to twice
daily. Only the mildest asthmatics with intermittent
attacks should rely upon this treatment alone. Some

patients use nebulizers at home for self-administration of
salbutamol or terbutaline. Such treatment is very effective
owing to the high dose delivered, but patients must not
rely on repeated home administration of nebulized $\beta_2$-
adrenoceptor agonists for worsening asthma, and must
be encouraged to seek medical advice urgently if their
condition does not improve. Tablets of $\beta_2$-adrenoceptor
agonists are less effective than when the drug is inhaled.
To help those who cannot coordinate activation of the
aerosol and inhalation, new devices that are breath-
activated have been developed.

ANTICHOLINERGIC BRONCHODILATORS. Muscarinic
receptors are found in the respiratory tract; large airways
contain mainly M3 receptors whereas the peripheral lung
tissue contains M3 and M1 receptors. Non-selective muscarinic antagonists such as atropine were used for relief
of bronchoconstriction. Currently ipratropium bromide
20–40 $\mu$g three or four times daily or oxitropium bromide (200 $\mu$g twice daily) by aerosol inhalation are used
and may be additive to $\beta_2$-adrenoceptor stimulants.

ANTI-INFLAMMATORY DRUGS. The exact mode of
action of sodium cromoglycate and nedocromil sodium
remains unknown but this class of drugs appears to prevent activation of inflammatory cells, possibly by blocking
a specific chloride channel which in turn prevents calcium
influx. These drugs are particularly effective in patients
with milder asthma. Sodium cromoglycate is taken regularly either in the form of a Spincap containing 20 mg or
in aerosol form from a metered-dose inhaler delivering
5 mg per puff. The dose should be two puffs four times
daily from an inhaler, or one Spincap three or four times
daily. Nedocromil sodium is taken as an aerosol at a dose
of 4 mg (2 puffs) two to four times daily.

INHALED CORTICOSTEROIDS. All patients who have
regular persisting symptoms in spite of treatment with as-
required $\beta_2$-adrenoceptor agonists, sodium cromoglycate

| Step | PEFR | Treatment |
|------|------|-----------|
| **1** Occasional symptoms less frequent than daily | 100% predicted | As-required bronchodilators<br>If used more than once daily move to step 2 |
| **2** Daily symptoms | ≤80% predicted | Anti-inflammatory drugs<br>Sodium cromoglycate or low-dose inhaled corticosteroids up to 800 $\mu$g. Not controlled move to step 3 |
| **3** Severe symptoms | 50–80% predicted | High-dose inhaled corticosteroids up to 2000 $\mu$g daily |
| **4** Severe symptoms uncontrolled with high-dose inhaled corticosteroids | 50–80% predicted | Add regular long-acting $\beta_2$-agonists e.g. salmeterol |
| **5** Severe symptoms deteriorating | ≤50% predicted | Add prednisolone 40 mg daily |
| **6** Severe symptoms deteriorating in spite of prednisolone | ≤30% predicted | Hospital admission |
| Short-acting bronchodilator treatment taken at any step on as-required basis | | |

**Information box 12.1**   The step-wise management of asthma.

or nedocromil need regular treatment with inhaled corticosteroids. Beclomethasone dipropionate is available in doses of 50, 100 and 250 μg per puff, budesonide is available in doses of 200 μg per metered inhalation and fluticasone propionate as a Dischaler 50, 100 and 250 μg per inhalation. Fluticasone propionate is twice as potent as beclomethasone dipropionate with considerably less bioavailability, indicating that fluticasone may become the inhaled steroid of choice when used at high doses. High-dose beclomethasone, budesonide and fluticasone should be reserved for patients who have not responded to lower dose inhaled corticosteroids. The unwanted effects of inhaled corticosteroids are oral candidiasis, which may develop in 5% of patients, and hoarseness due to the effect of corticosteroids on the laryngeal muscles. In children inhaled steroids at doses greater than 400 μg daily have been shown to retard growth at least in the short term. Asthma itself retards growth. Catch-up growth may occur when asthma improves and doses of inhaled steroids can be reduced.

ORAL CORTICOSTEROIDS. Use of oral corticosteroids is necessary for those individuals not controlled on inhaled corticosteroids. The dose should be kept as low as possible to avoid side-effects. The effect of short-term treatment with prednisolone 30 mg daily is shown in Fig. 12.14. Some patients require continuing treatment with oral corticosteroids. Studies suggest that treatment with low doses of methotrexate (15 mg weekly) can significantly reduce the dose of prednisolone needed to control the disease in some patients and cyclosporin also improves lung function in some steroid-dependent asthmatics.

ANTIBIOTICS. There is no evidence that antibiotics are helpful in the management of patients who suffer from properly diagnosed asthma. However, wheezing frequently occurs in exacerbations of chronic bronchitis and emphysema associated with infected sputum.

Yellow or green sputum containing eosinophils and bronchial epithelial cells may be coughed up in acute exacerbations of asthma. This is not due to bacterial infection and antibiotics are not required.

**Management of severe asthma** (Emergency box 12.2)
Although this condition is often called 'status asthmaticus', it is better considered as severe asthma that has not been controlled by the patient's use of medication. Patients with severe asthma have:
- Inability to complete a sentence in one breath.
- Tachycardia ≥ 110 beats per minute.
- Pulsus paradoxus (>10 mmHg). In very severe asthma no paradoxus is detected.
- Wheezing. Chest may be silent in severe asthma owing to insufficient airflow.

PEFR should be measured in all patients presenting with severe asthma, and if below 30% predicted or approximately 150 litre min$^{-1}$ (in adults), the patient should be taken to hospital and started on 40–60% oxygen.

Treatment is commenced with 5 mg of nebulized sal-

---

*At home*

The patient is assessed. Tachycardia with pulsus paradoxicus and cyanosis indicate a severe attack

If the PEFR is less than 150 litre min$^{-1}$ (in adults), an ambulance should be called. All doctors should carry peak flow meters

Nebulized salbutamol 5 mg or terbutaline 10 mg is administered

Hydrocortisone sodium succinate 200 mg i.v. is given

Oxygen 40–60% is given if available

Prednisolone 60 mg orally

*At hospital*

The patient is reassessed

Oxygen 40–60% is given

The PEFR is measured using a low-reading peak flow meter, as an ordinary meter only measures from 60 litre min$^{-1}$ upwards

Nebulized salbutamol 5 mg or terbutaline 10 mg is repeated and administered 4-hourly

Add nebulized ipratropium bromide 0.5 mg to nebulized salbutamol/terbutaline

Hydrocortisone 200 mg i.v. is given 4-hourly for 24 hours. Prednisolone is continued at 60 mg orally daily for 2 weeks

Arterial blood gases are measured; if the $P_a\text{CO}_2$ is greater than 7 kPa, ventilation should be considered

A chest X-ray is performed to exclude pneumothorax

One of the following intravenous infusions is given if no improvement is seen:
    Salbutamol 3–20 μg min$^{-1}$, or
    Terbutaline 1.5–5 μg min$^{-1}$

**Emergency box 12.2**  Treatment of severe asthma.

---

butamol or 10 mg terbutaline with oxygen as the driving gas. A chest X-ray is taken to exclude a pneumothorax. If no improvement occurs with nebulized therapy, 250 μg of salbutamol or terbutaline should be administered by i.v. infusion over 10 min. Intravenous aminophylline is now not used for severe asthma because of its narrow therapeutic index. Hydrocortisone 200 mg i.v. should be administered 4-hourly for 24 hours and 60 mg of prednisolone should be given orally daily. Patients who do not respond to this regimen may require ventilation.

Patients should be kept in hospital for at least 5 days, since the majority of sudden deaths occur 2–5 days after admission. Oral corticosteroids can be reduced from 60 mg to 30 mg once improvement occurs. Further reduction should be gradual on an outpatient basis until an appropriate maintenance dose or substitution by inhaled corticosteroid aerosols can be achieved.

If the PEFR is greater than 150 litre min$^{-1}$, patients may improve dramatically on nebulized therapy and may not require hospital admission. Their regular treatment should be increased, probably to include treatment for 2 weeks with 30 mg of prednisolone followed by a gradual reduction in the oral dose and substitution by an inhaled corticosteroid preparation.

## PROGNOSIS

Although asthma often improves in children as they reach their teens, it is now realized that the disease frequently returns in the second, third and fourth decades. Overall, in adults, there is a tendency for asthma to improve with age.

# Diseases of the lung parenchyma

## PNEUMONIAS

Pneumonia may be defined as an inflammation of the substance of the lungs. It is usually caused by bacteria. Clinically it presents as an acute illness characterized in the majority of cases by the presence of cough, purulent sputum and fever together with physical signs or radiological changes compatible with consolidation of the lung.

The advent of antibiotics might have been expected to decrease dramatically the mortality from pneumonia. However, mortality statistics obtained from death certificates show the reverse. This is because the dramatic

decrease in deaths from pneumonia in children under 10 years has been counterbalanced by an increase in deaths from pneumonia in individuals over the age of 70 years.

## CLASSIFICATION

Pneumonia can be classified both anatomically and on the basis of the aetiology.

### Site

Pneumonias are either localized, e.g. affecting the whole of one lobe, or diffuse, when they primarily affect the lobules of the lung, often in association with the bronchi and bronchioles, a condition referred to as 'bronchopneumonia'.

### Aetiology

An aetiological factor can be discovered in approximately 75% of patients. The term 'atypical pneumonias' was used to describe pneumonia caused by agents such as *Mycoplasma*, influenza A virus, *Chlamydia* and *Coxiella burnetii*. These types of pneumonia alone account for almost one-fifth of the cases of pneumonia (Table 12.8) and the term 'atypical' should be dropped. Pneumonias may also result from:

- Chemical causes, e.g. aspiration of vomit (see p. 681)
- Radiotherapy (see p. 696)
- Allergic mechanisms (see p. 691)

*Mycobacterium tuberculosis* is an important cause of pneumonia; it is considered separately, since both its

| Infecting agent | Frequency as a cause of pneumonia (%) | Clinical circumstances |
|---|---|---|
| *Streptococcus pneumoniae* | 50 | Community pneumonia patients usually previously fit |
| *Mycoplasma pneumoniae* | 6 | As above |
| Influenza A virus (usually with a bacterial component) | 5 | As above |
| *Haemophilus influenzae* | 5 | Pre-existing lung disease: chronic bronchitis and emphysema |
| *Chlamydia pneumoniae* | 5 | Community-acquired pneumonia |
| *Chlamydia psittaci* | 3 | Contact with birds (though not inevitable) |
| *Staphylococcus aureus* | 2 | Children, intravenous drug abusers, associated with influenza virus infections |
| *Legionella pneumophila* | 2 | Institutional outbreaks (hospitals and hotels), sporadic, endemic |
| *Coxiella burnetti* | 1 | Abattoir and animal-hide workers |
| *Pseudomonas aeruginosa* | <1 | Cystic fibrosis |
| *Pneumocystis carinii*<br>*Actinomyces israelii*<br>*Nocardia asteroides*<br>Cytomegalovirus<br>*Aspergillus fumigatus* | <1 | AIDS, lymphomas, leukaemias, use of cytotoxic drugs and corticosteroids |
| Anaerobic organisms | <1 | Inhalation pneumonia, alcohol abuse, postoperative |
| None isolated | 20 | — |

**Table 12.8**  The aetiology of pneumonia in the UK.

mode of presentation and its treatment are very different from the infective agents.

### Precipitating factors

- *Strep. pneumoniae*—often follows influenza or para-influenza viral infection
- Hospitalized 'ill' patients—often infected with Gram-negative organisms
- Cigarette smoking
- Alcohol excess
- Bronchiectasis (e.g. in cystic fibrosis)
- Bronchial obstruction (e.g. carcinoma)—occasionally associated with infection with 'non-pathogenic' organisms
- Immunosuppression (e.g. AIDS or treatment with cytotoxic agents)—organisms include *P. carinii, Mycobacterium avium intracellulare*, cytomegalovirus
- Intravenous drug abuse—frequently associated with *Staph. aureus* infection
- Inhalation from oesophageal obstruction—often associated with infection with anaerobes

### CLINICAL PRESENTATION

The clinical presentation varies according to the immune state of the patient and the infecting agent. In the commonest type of pneumonia—caused by *Strep. pneumoniae*—there is often a preceding history of a viral infection. The patient rapidly becomes more ill with a high temperature (up to 39.5°C), pleuritic pain and a dry cough. A day or two later, rusty-coloured sputum is produced and at about the same time the patient may develop labial herpes simplex. The patient breathes rapidly and shallowly, the affected side of the chest moves less, and signs of consolidation may be present together with a pleural rub.

### INVESTIGATION

Chest X-ray confirms the area of consolidation (Fig. 12.33) but radiological changes lag behind the clinical course so that X-ray changes may be minimal at the start of the illness. Conversely, consolidation may remain on the chest X-ray for several weeks after the patient is clinically cured. The chest X-ray should always return to normal by 6 weeks, except in patients with severe airflow limitation. Persistent changes on the chest X-ray after this time suggest a bronchial abnormality, usually a carcinoma, with persisting secondary pneumonia. Chest X-rays should rarely be repeated more frequently than at weekly intervals during the acute illness and then at 6 weeks after discharge from hospital.

In *Strep. pneumoniae* pneumonia, there is often a white blood cell count that is greater than $15 \times 10^9$/litre (90% polymorphonuclear leucocytosis) and an erythrocyte sedimentation rate (ESR) greater than 100 mm hour$^{-1}$.

The individual features of different pneumonias are given below. The *overall investigation* and *management* is shown in Fig. 12.34 and discussed on p. 681.

## *Mycoplasma* pneumonia

This is a common cause of pneumonia. It often occurs in patients in their teens and twenties, frequently amongst those living in boarding institutions. Generalized features such as headaches and malaise often precede the chest symptoms by 1–5 days. Cough may not be obvious initially and physical signs in the chest may be scanty.

On chest X-ray, usually only one of the lower lobes is involved but sometimes there may be dramatic shadowing in both lower lobes. There is frequently no correlation between the X-ray appearances and the clinical state of the patient.

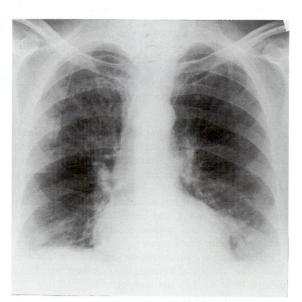

(a)    (b)

**Fig. 12.33** Chest X-rays to show (a) lobar pneumonia and (b) diffuse pneumonia.

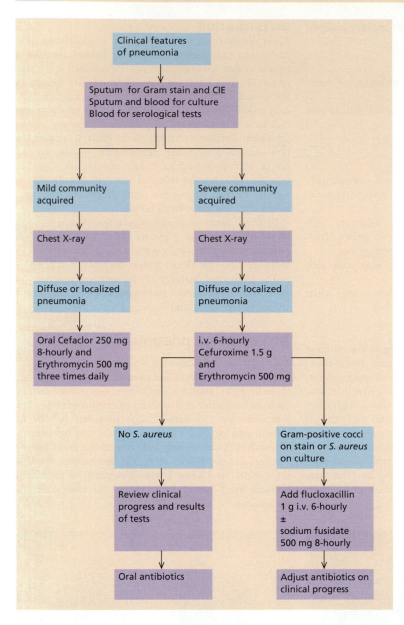

**Fig. 12.34** Algorithm for the management of pneumonia (see also p. 681). CIE, counter-immunoelectrophoresis.

The white blood cell count is not raised. Cold agglutinins occur in half of the cases. The diagnosis is confirmed by a rising antibody titre. Treatment is with erythromycin 500 mg four times daily for 7–10 days. Tetracycline is effective.

Although most patients recover in 10–14 days, the disease can be protracted, with cough and X-ray appearance lasting for weeks and relapses occurring. Lung abscesses and pleural effusions are rare.

Extrapulmonary complications can occur at any time during the illness and occasionally dominate the clinical picture. Most are rare but they include:

- Myocarditis and pericarditis
- Rashes and erythema multiforme
- Haemolytic anaemia and thrombocytopenia
- Myalgia and arthralgia

- Meningo-encephalitis and other neurological abnormalities
- Gastrointestinal symptoms (e.g. vomiting, diarrhoea)

## Viral pneumonia

Viral pneumonia is uncommon in adults, bacteria being the usual cause of the pneumonia *per se*. Influenza A virus or adenovirus infection can occasionally produce pneumonia.

## Other pneumonias

### *Haemophilus influenzae*

*H. influenzae* is frequently identified in the yellow-green sputum produced during exacerbation of chronic bronchitis. It is therefore not surprising that this organism may be the cause of pneumonia in people suffering from chronic bronchitis and emphysema. The pneumonia can be diffuse or confined to one lobe. There are no special features to separate it from other bacterial causes of pneumonia. It responds well to treatment with oral cefaclor 250 mg 8-hourly.

## Chlamydia psittaci (see p. 46)
Typically the individual has been working with infected birds, especially parrots, but a history of contact is not always elicited. The incubation period is 1–2 weeks and the disease may pursue a very low-grade course over several months. Symptoms include malaise, high fever, cough and muscular pains. The liver and spleen are occasionally enlarged and scanty 'rose spots' may be seen on the abdomen. The chest X-ray shows segmental or a diffuse pneumonia. Occasionally the illness presents with a high, swinging fever and dramatic prostration with photophobia and neck stiffness that can be confused with meningitis. The diagnosis is confirmed by the demonstration of a rising titre of complement-fixing antibody. Erythromycin or tetracycline are the antibiotics of choice.

## Chlamydia pneumoniae
Chlamydia pneumoniae has only recently been recognized as a respiratory pathogen in man. Outbreaks have been reported in institutions and within families suggesting person-to-person spread without any avian or animal reservoir. Serological tests on patients admitted to hospital with community-acquired pneumonia suggest that 5–10% may be the result of C. pneumoniae infection. Since this infection has only recently been recognized it may account for a substantial number of previous pneumonias in which no organism had been isolated. In general, disease is mild with 50% of C. pneumoniae infections presenting as pneumonia, 28% as acute bronchitis, 10% with a 'flu-like illness and 12% with upper respiratory illnesses. Type-specific microimmunofluorescence tests are required to distinguish C. pneumoniae from C. psittaci and C. trachomatis. Treatment is with erythromycin or tetracycline.

## Staphylococcus aureus
Staph. aureus normally only causes a pneumonia after a preceding influenzal viral illness. The infection starts in the bronchi, leading to patchy areas of consolidation in one or more lobes, which break down to form abscesses. These may appear as cysts on the chest X-ray.

Pneumothorax, effusion and empyemas are frequent. Septicaemia develops with metastatic abscesses in other organs.

Fulminating staphylococcal pneumonia occurring in influenza epidemics can lead to death in hours. All patients with this type of pneumonia are very ill; intravenous antibiotics must be administered promptly, but are not always effective.

Areas of pneumonia (septic infarcts) are also seen in staphylococcal septicaemia. This is frequently seen in intravenous drug abusers and also in patients with central catheters being used for parenteral nutrition. The infected puncture site is the source of the Staphylococcus. Pulmonary symptoms are often few but breathlessness and cough occur and the chest X-ray reveals areas of consolidation. Abscess formation is frequent.

Diagnosis and treatment are shown in Fig. 12.34.

## Coxiella burnetii (Q-fever) (see p. 45)
The patient develops systemic symptoms of fever, malaise and headache, often associated with multiple lesions on the chest X-ray. The illness may run a chronic course and is occasionally associated with endocarditis. Diagnosis is made by an increase in the titre of complement-fixing antibody, and erythromycin or tetracycline is the usual treatment.

## Legionella pneumophila (see p. 35)
Three epidemiological patterns of this disease are recognized:
1 Outbreaks amongst previously fit individuals staying in hotels, institutions or hospitals where the shower facilities or cooling systems have been contaminated with the organism
2 Sporadic cases occurring in many parts of the world where the source of the infection is unknown
3 Outbreaks occurring in immunocompromised patients and in middle-aged and elderly male smokers
Legionella grows well in water up to 40°C in temperature, and the infection is almost certainly spread by the aerosol route. Adequate chlorination and temperature control of the water supply are important factors in the prevention of the disease.

The incubation period is 2–10 days. Males are affected twice as commonly as females. The infection may be mild, but the characteristic picture is of malaise, myalgia, headache and a fever with rigors and a pyrexia of up to 40°C. Half of the patients have gastrointestinal symptoms, with nausea, vomiting, diarrhoea and abdominal pain. Patients may be acutely ill, with mental confusion and other neurological signs. Haematuria occurs and occasionally renal failure.

The patient is tachypnoeic with initially a dry cough that later may become productive and purulent. The chest X-ray usually shows unilateral lobar and then multilobar shadowing, sometimes with a small pleural effusion. Cavitation is rare.

A strong presumptive diagnosis of L. pneumophila infection is possible in the majority of patients if they have three of the four following features:
1 A prodromal virus-like illness
2 A dry cough, confusion or diarrhoea
3 Lymphopenia without marked leucocytosis
4 Hyponatraemia
Hypoalbuminaemia and abnormal levels of liver enzymes are common in this disease. The diagnosis is confirmed by a change in antibody titre, but the quickest way is by the direct immunofluorescent staining of the organism in the pleural fluid, sputum or bronchial washings. A Gram

stain does not detect the organism. Culture is possible but takes up to 3 weeks.

The organism is sensitive to erythromycin, which is the antibiotic of choice. Rifampicin is also being used. Mortality can be up to 30% in elderly patients but most patients recover spontaneously.

Prevention is important with chlorination and sealing of water supplies.

### Gram-negative bacteria

These are the cause of many hospital-acquired pneumonias but they are occasionally responsible for cases in the community.

*Klebsiella pneumoniae*. Pneumonia due to *Klebsiella* usually occurs in the elderly with a history of heart or lung disease, diabetes, alcohol excess or malignancy. The onset is often sudden, with severe systemic upset. The sputum is purulent, gelatinous or blood-stained. The upper lobes are more commonly affected and the consolidation is often extensive. There is often swelling of the infected lobe so that on the lateral chest X-ray there is bulging of the fissures. The organism can be found in the sputum or in the blood. Treatment is dependent on the sensitivity of the organism, but a cephalosporin or chloramphenicol is usually required. The mortality is high, partly owing to the presence of an underlying condition.

*Pseudomonas aeruginosa*. Pneumonia due to this organism is of considerable significance in patients with cystic fibrosis, since it correlates with a worsening clinical condition and mortality. It is also seen in patients with neutropenia following cytotoxic chemotherapy. The isolation of *P. aeruginosa* must be interpreted with care because the organism grows well on bacterial culture medium and may simply represent contamination from the upper airways. Pseudomonal and other Gram-negative infections respond well to treatment with the 4-quinolone antibiotic ciprofloxacin (100–200 mg i.v. over 30–60 min twice daily) or ceftazidime (2 g bolus i.v. 8-hourly). The combination of tobramycin 3–5 mg kg$^{-1}$ i.v. or i.m. daily in 8-hourly doses together with carbenicillin 5 g i.v. 4–6-hourly is now less commonly used. These antibiotics can however be inhaled direct into the lung via nebulizers and are still used in patients with CF (see p. 665).

Modifications may have to be made in the light of sensitivity testing. Tobramycin is nephrotoxic and also produces vestibular damage, so that blood levels should be monitored. Azlocillin and ticarcillin are also available.

*Moraxella catarrhalis*. This organism, previously known as *Branhamella catarrhalis*, has been found to be associated with exacerbations of chronic bronchitis and occasionally with fatal pneumonia. Some strains produce a β-lactamase capable of destroying amoxycillin. The exact role of this organism in bronchopulmonary infection remains to be determined.

### Anaerobic bacteria

Infections with these organisms usually occur in those with an underlying condition, e.g. diabetes, and are often associated with aspiration. *Bacteroides* is the commonest organism and is sensitive to metronidazole. The prognosis depends largely on the precipitating cause.

## Pneumonias due to opportunistic infections

These are commonly becoming recognized in the immunocompromised patient.

### *Pneumocystis carinii*

This is by far the commonest opportunistic infection, accounting for 80% of the cases of pneumonia in patients with acquired immunodeficiency syndrome (AIDS) (see p. 101) particularly when the CD4 lymphocyte count is ≤200/mm$^3$. It is also seen in patients receiving immunosuppressive therapy. In the developing world, however, *Pneumocystis carinii* pneumonia (PCP) is not infrequently found in malnourished children.

It is likely that infection with the organism occurs by inhalation, perhaps in childhood, and the organism may remain latent for many years, being reactivated when immunosuppression occurs. Clinically the pneumonia is associated with a high fever, breathlessness and dry cough. In patients with AIDS, the clinical features are described on p. 101.

The typical radiographic appearance of PCP is of a diffuse bilateral alveolar and interstitial shadowing beginning in the perihilar regions and spreading out in a butterfly pattern. A variety of typical chest X-ray appearances are now well recognized including a localized infiltrate, nodule, cavity or a pneumothorax. In patients receiving aerosolized pentamidine for prophylaxis, infiltrate may be localized to the upper zones. Investigation includes induction of sputum with hypertonic saline or fibreoptic bronchoscopy with bronchoalveolar lavage; the diagnosis can be made in 90% of cases by staining using indirect immunofluorescence with monoclonal antibodies.

Shadowing on the chest X-ray in AIDS patients, though most commonly due to *P. carinii* can result from:
- Cytomegalovirus
- *M. avium intracellulare*
- *M. tuberculosis*
- *L. pneumophila*
- *Cryptococcus*
- Pyogenic bacteria
- Kaposi's sarcoma
- Lymphoid interstitial pneumonia
- Non-specific interstitial pneumonitis

TREATMENT is with oral trimethoprim–sulphamethoxazole 120 mg kg$^{-1}$ daily in divided doses or i.v. pentamidine 4 mg kg$^{-1}$ daily.

The mortality partly depends on the underlying condition; with treatment it is approximately 25%.

### *Actinomyces israeli* (see p. 36)

The clinical picture is that of severe pneumonia, lung abscess or empyema.

### Nocardia asteroides

This produces a similar picture to *Actinomyces*, though of greater severity. The chest X-ray often shows irregular opacities in one or both lungs, particularly in the mid-zones.

### Cytomegalovirus (see p. 48)

Bronchitis and pneumonia may occur but these are usually a more minor part of the generalized systemic illness.

### Aspergillus fumigatus (see p. 691)

This fungus gives rise to a widespread invasion of lung tissue in patients who are immunocompromised. It is a serious pneumonia that is usually rapidly fatal.

### Mycobacterium avium intracellulare (MAI)

This bacterium causes lung disease in patients with AIDS primarily as part of disseminated disease when CD4 lymphocyte counts are $\leq 100/mm^3$ with the pulmonary complications being of less significance than the extra-pulmonary involvement. Therapeutic regimens include combinations of ciprofloxacin, clofazimine, rifampicin and ethambutol. Clarithromycin and azithromycin may prove to be particularly efficacious.

### Cryptococcus

Infection with this fungus is usually disseminated but pulmonary involvement includes intrathoracic lymph node enlargement and effusions.

### Kaposi's sarcoma

Intrathoracic involvement usually follows cutaneous manifestations and includes nodules or infiltrates in the lungs with lymph node enlargement and endobronchial lesions. Haemorrhage can accompany any of these lesions.

### Lymphatic interstitial pneumonia

Infiltration with lymphocytes, plasma cells and immunoblasts characterizes this disease which is more common in children than in adults. It is thought to be a viral pneumonia and causes diffuse reticulonodular infiltrates on the chest X-ray. Corticosteroid therapy appears to be of benefit.

## Rare causes of pneumonia

Pneumonia may be seen in the course of infection by *Bordetella pertussis*, typhoid and paratyphoid bacillus, brucellosis, leptospirosis and a number of viral infections including measles, chickenpox and glandular fever. It is not usually a major feature. Details of these infections are described in Chapter 1.

## Aspiration pneumonia

The acute aspiration of gastric contents into the lungs can produce an extremely severe and sometimes fatal illness due to the intense destructiveness of gastric acid—the Mendelson syndrome. It can complicate anaesthesia, particularly during pregnancy.

In the absence of a tracheo-oesophageal fistula, aspiration only occurs during periods of impaired consciousness (e.g. during sleep), in reflux oesophagitis or oesophageal stricture, or in bulbar palsy. Because of the bronchial anatomy, the most usual site for spillage is the posterior segment of the right lower lobe. The persistent pneumonia is often due to anaerobes and it may progress to lung abscess or even bronchiectasis. It is vital to identify any underlying problem, since appropriate corrective measures can lead to resolution of the pulmonary problems.

## Cryptogenic organizing pneumonia (COP)

This condition is an organizing pneumonia of unknown aetiology although probably not infective. It is characterized by the presence of buds of connective tissue in alveolar ducts and respiratory bronchioles and the absence of any detectable microorganism. Clinical features are a short history of cough and breathlessness with fever, sometimes pleuritic chest pain and a raised ESR, normal white blood count and patchy or confluent shadows bilaterally on the chest X-ray. Finger clubbing is prominent. Lung function tests show a restrictive defect. Diagnosis is important because the disease responds rapidly to corticosteroid treatment.

## Diffuse pneumonia (bronchopneumonia)

Diffuse pneumonia is very common. It is differentiated from severe bronchitis by signs of bronchial breathing or patchy shadows on the chest X-ray (see Fig. 12.33).

Widespread diffuse pneumonia is a common terminal event, largely resulting from an inability of patients dying from other conditions (e.g. cancer) to cough up retained secretions, allowing infection to develop throughout the lungs. Treatment in this situation is rarely appropriate.

## General management of pneumonia

This is shown in the algorithm given in Fig. 12.34.

Sputum should always be sent for culture. In *mild* cases treatment should be started immediately with oral cefaclor and erythromycin (see below).

More severe cases need to be admitted to hospital and a chest X-ray performed. Other investigations required are:

- Sputum—Gram stain and culture
- White blood-cell count is raised above $15 \times 10^9$/litre (with a high neutrophil count) in more than 50% of patients with pneumococcal pneumonia but only in 10% of cases of *Legionella* or *Mycoplasma* pneumonia
- Blood culture

Treatment should be started immediately (without waiting for the result of these investigations). In more than 20% of cases, more than one organism is involved.

Further investigations may be necessary for the diagnosis of certain types of pneumonia:

- *Mycoplasma* antibodies (IgM and IgG)—in acute and convalescent samples. Cold agglutinins present in 50%.
- *Legionella* and *Chlamydia* antibodies—immunofluorescent tests.
- Pneumococcal antigen—counterimmunoelectrophoresis (CIE) of sputum, urine and serum (three to four times more sensitive than sputum or blood cultures).

A high percentage of organisms causing pneumonia (e.g. *Mycoplasma pneumoniae*, *H. influenzae* and *L. pneumophila*) will not respond to penicillin or ampicillin/amoxycillin. These drugs should no longer be prescribed and should be replaced by a combination of bactericidal antibiotics that cover the commonest organisms. Treatment is commenced with cefuroxime 750 mg to 1.5 g i.v. 6-hourly together with erythromycin 500 mg i.v. 6-hourly. The purpose of this programme is to treat pneumonia with sufficient doses of appropriate antibiotics at the earliest stage. The treatment can always be modified and reduced in the light of clinical progress and subsequent bacteriological and serological findings. The chances of identifying a causative organism are greatly decreased in individuals who have received antibiotics in the week prior to their admission to hospital.

The overall mortality for pneumonia is currently 5% but for pneumonia due to *Staph. aureus* it is in excess of 25%. Patients who die from pneumonia usually have not received the appropriate antibiotics in sufficient doses before or during the early stages of hospital admission. Severe community-acquired pneumonia has a high mortality particularly in those over 65 years. The presence of a respiratory rate $\geq$30 min$^{-1}$, a diastolic blood pressure $\leq$60 mmHg and a blood urea >7 mmol litre$^{-1}$ indicates a poorer prognosis and the need for intensive care. In spite of treatment in the intensive care unit approximately 50% of such patients will die.

### General measures

These include care of the mouth and skin. Fluids should be encouraged, to avoid dehydration. The patient is normally nursed sitting up or in the most comfortable position. Cough should normally be encouraged, but if it is unproductive and distressing, suppressants such as codeine linctus can be given. Physiotherapy is needed to help and encourage the patient to cough.

Pleuritic pain may require analgesia, but powerful analgesia (e.g. opiates) should be used with care because they cause respiratory depression.

In severe hypoxia, oxygen therapy should be given; however, since the hypoxia is often due to a physiological shunt (see p. 638), it may make little difference to the hypoxaemia.

### Severe hospital-acquired pneumonias

These should be treated in the same way as severe community-acquired pneumonias once appropriate samples for culture and sensitivities have been taken. Gram-negative bacteria are common and treatment should include i.v. ciprofloxacin or ceftazidime. Immunosuppressed patients may require very high-dose broad-spectrum antibiotics as well as antifungal and antiviral agents.

## Complications of pneumonia

### Lung abscess

This term is used to describe severe localized suppuration in the lung associated with cavity formation on the chest X-ray, often with the presence of a fluid level, and not due to tuberculosis.

Causes of lung abscesses are many, but the commonest is aspiration, particularly amongst alcohol abusers following aspiration pneumonia. Lung abscesses also frequently follow the inhalation of a foreign body into a bronchus and occasionally occur when the bronchus is obstructed by a bronchial carcinoma.

Abscesses may develop during the course of specific pneumonias, particularly when the infecting agent is *Staph. pyogenes* or *K. pneumoniae*. Septic emboli, usually staphylococci, result in multiple lung abscesses. Infarcted areas of lung may occasionally cavitate and rarely become infected. Amoebic abscesses may occasionally develop in the right lower lobe following transdiaphragmatic spread from an amoebic liver abscess.

The clinical features are those of persisting and worsening pneumonia associated with the production of large quantities of sputum, which is often foul-smelling owing to the growth of anaerobic organisms. There is usually a swinging fever. Chronic or subacute lung abscesses follow an inadequately treated pneumonia. Fever, malaise and weight loss occur. The chest signs may be few but clubbing often develops. The patient is often anaemic with a high ESR.

### Empyema

Empyema means the presence of pus within the pleural cavity. This usually arises after the rupture of a lung abscess into the pleural space or from bacterial spread from a severe pneumonia. Typically an empyema cavity becomes infected with anaerobic organisms and the patient is severely ill with a high fever and a neutrophil granulocytosis.

### Investigation

Bacteriological investigation of lung abscess and empyema is best conducted on specimens obtained by transtracheal aspiration, bronchoscopy or percutaneous transthoracic aspiration.

### Treatment

Although anaerobic organisms are found in up to 70% of lung abscesses and empyemas, there is usually a mixed flora, often with aerobes, particularly *Strep. milleri*. Anaerobic cocci, black-pigmented bacteroids and fusobacteria are the commonest anaerobes found.

Antibiotics should be given to cover both aerobic and anaerobic organisms; prolonged courses are often necessary. Treatment should be cefuroxime 1 g i.v. 6-hourly, erythromycin 500 mg i.v. 8-hourly and metronidazole

500 mg i.v. 8-hourly for 5 days, followed by oral cefaclor and metronidazole for a prolonged period depending on bacterial sensitivities. Abscesses occasionally require surgery.

Empyemas should be treated by prompt tube drainage (see p. 650) or rib resection and drainage of the empyema cavity followed by appropriate antibiotic treatment for up to 6 weeks.

# TUBERCULOSIS (see p. 36)

Tuberculosis is on the increase particularly where immunosuppressive drugs have altered the host defence mechanisms, or in AIDS. In developing countries, it still remains a problem partly because of inadequately supervised treatment.

## EPIDEMIOLOGY

For the last 20 years tuberculosis was thought to be under control, but it is now the world's leading cause of death from a single infectious disease due to:

- Inadequate programmes for disease control
- Multiple drug resistance
- Co-infection with HIV
- Rapid rise in the world's population of young adults—the age group with the highest mortality from tuberculosis

Although the risk of contracting tuberculosis is between 20 and 50 times greater in the developing countries compared to the Western World even there the disease is on the increase. In the last 5 years there has been a 12% increase in the USA, a 33% increase in Switzerland and a 25% increase in Italy.

In the UK, there has been no decline in the number of cases with 7000 new cases per year.

In the UK the incidence of tuberculosis in immigrants from the Asian subcontinent and West Indies is 40 and four times as common, respectively, as in the native White population. This has led to great variation in the frequency of the disease in different areas of the UK. It is a notifiable disease.

## PATHOLOGY

The first infection with *M. tuberculosis* is known as primary tuberculosis. It is usually subpleural, often in the mid to upper zones. Within an hour of reaching the lung, tubercle bacilli reach the draining lymph nodes at the hilum of the lung and a few escape into the bloodstream.

The initial reaction comprises exudation and infiltration with neutrophil granulocytes. These are rapidly replaced by macrophages that ingest the bacilli. These interact with T lymphocytes with the development of cellular immunity that can be demonstrated 3–8 weeks after the initial infection by the development of a positive reaction in the skin to an intradermal injection of protein from tubercle bacilli (tuberculin).

At this stage the classical pathology of tuberculosis can be seen. Granulomatous lesions consist of a central area of necrotic material of a cheesy nature, called caseation, surrounded by epithelioid cells and Langhans' giant cells with multiple nuclei, both cells being derived from the macrophage. Lymphocytes are present and there is a varying degree of fibrosis. Subsequently the caseated areas heal completely and many become calcified. It is now known that at least 20% of these calcified primary lesions contain tubercle bacilli, initially lying dormant but capable of being activated by depression of the host defence system. Reactivation leads to typical post-primary pulmonary tuberculosis with cavitation, usually in the apex or upper zone of the lung. 'Post-primary tuberculosis' refers to all forms of tuberculosis that occur after the first few weeks of the primary infection when immunity to the mycobacterium has developed.

## CLINICAL FEATURES AND INVESTIGATION

Primary tuberculosis is symptomless in the great majority of individuals. Occasionally there may be a vague illness, sometimes associated with cough and wheeze. A small transient pleural effusion or erythema nodosum (see p. 1005) may occasionally occur, both representing allergic manifestations of the infective process.

Enlargement of lymph nodes compressing the bronchi can give rise to collapse of segments or lobes of the lung. Apart from cough and a monophonic wheeze, the individual remains remarkably well and the collapse disappears as the primary complex heals. Occasionally, persistent collapse can give rise to subsequent bronchiectasis, often in the middle lobe (Brock's syndrome).

The manifestations of primary and post-primary tuberculosis are shown in Fig. 12.35, together with the times when they usually occur. Extrapulmonary manifestations are summarized on p. 37. Miliary tuberculosis can occur within 3 years of the primary infection, or can occur much later as a manifestation of reactivation or, rarely, reinfection with tubercle bacillus.

Reactivation in the lung, or indeed in any extrapulmonary location, can occur as immunity wanes, usually with age and chronic ill-health and all manifestations as shown in Fig. 12.35.

### Miliary tuberculosis

This disease is the result of acute diffuse dissemination of tubercle bacilli via the bloodstream. It can be a difficult diagnosis to make, especially in older people, where it is particularly covert. This form of disseminated tuberculosis is universally fatal without treatment.

It may present in an entirely non-specific manner with the gradual onset of vague ill-health, loss of weight and then fever. Occasionally the disease presents as tuberculosis meningitis. Usually there are no abnormal physical signs in the early stages, although eventually the spleen and liver become enlarged. Choroidal tubercles are seen in the eyes. These lesions are about one-quarter of the diameter of the optic disc and are yellowish and slightly shiny and raised in nature, later becoming white in the centre. There may be one or many in each eye.

The chest X-ray may be entirely normal in miliary tuberculosis as the tubercles are not visible until the miliary shadows are 1 or 2 mm in diameter; they have a hard outline. The lesions can increase in size up to 5–10 mm.

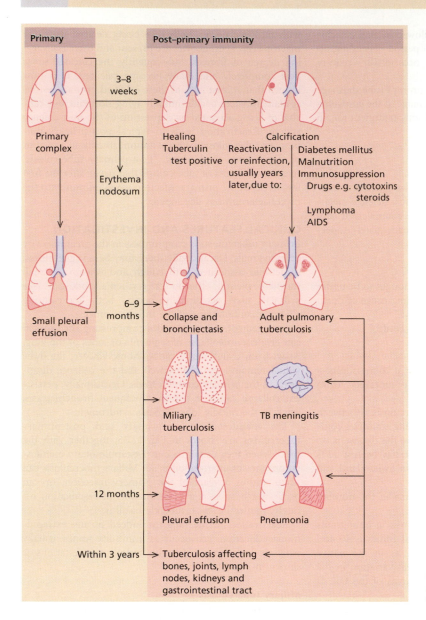

**Fig. 12.35** The manifestations of primary and post-primary tuberculosis.

Sarcoidosis and staphylococcal or *Mycoplasma* pneumonia can mimic the chest X-ray appearance of miliary tuberculosis.

The Mantoux test is positive but is occasionally negative in people with very severe disease. Transbronchial biopsies are frequently positive before any abnormality is visible on the chest X-ray. CT scanning may reveal lung parenchymal abnormalities at an earlier stage.

Biopsy and culture of liver and bone marrow may be necessary in patients presenting with a pyrexia of unknown origin (PUO). In the past, a trial of anti-tuberculous therapy was often used in individuals with a PUO. The fever should settle within 2 weeks of starting chemotherapy if it is due to tuberculosis. This approach is still occasionally used in susceptible individuals when a diagnosis cannot be confirmed.

**Pulmonary tuberculosis**

Typically there is gradual onset of symptoms over weeks or months. Tiredness, malaise, anorexia and loss of weight together with a fever and cough remain the outstanding features of pulmonary tuberculosis. Drenching night sweats are now rather uncommon and are more usually due to anxiety. Sputum in tuberculosis may be mucoid, purulent or blood-stained. Many patients suffer a dull ache in the chest and it is not uncommon for patients to complain of recurrent colds.

A pleural effusion or pneumonia can be the presenting feature of tuberculosis. Physical examination is of little value. Finger clubbing is only present if the disease is advanced and associated with considerable production of purulent sputum. There are often no physical signs in the chest even in the presence of extensive radiological changes, though occasionally persistent crackles may be heard. Physical signs of an associated effusion, pneumonia or fibrosis may be present.

An abnormal chest X-ray is often found with no symptoms, but the reverse is extremely rare—pulmonary tuberculosis is unlikely in the absence of any radiographic abnormality. The chest X-ray (Fig. 12.36) typically shows patchy or nodular shadows in the upper zones, loss of volume, and fibrosis with or without cavitation. Calcification may be present. The X-ray appearances alone may strongly suggest tuberculosis, but every effort must be made to obtain microbiological evidence. A single X-ray does not give an indication of the activity of the disease. Very similar chest X-ray appearances occur in histoplasmosis and other fungal infections of the lung, including cryptococcosis, coccidioidomycosis and aspergillosis.

### Lymph node tuberculosis manifestation

The patient presents with a tender lump, usually supraclavicular or in the anterior triangle of the neck. This form of tuberculosis is discussed on p. 37.

### Tuberculosis in patients with AIDS

Intrathoracic lymphadenopathy and diffuse or miliary infiltrates is common in patients with AIDS, and cavitation less common than in patients without AIDS. Disseminated tuberculosis is particularly frequent, occurring in over one-third of cases.

### DIAGNOSIS

CHEST X-RAY.

STAINING. The sputum is stained with Ziehl–Nielsen (ZN) stain for acid and alcohol-fast bacilli (AAFB).

CULTURE. The sputum is cultured on Dover's or Lowenstein–Jensen medium for 4–8 weeks. Cultures to determine the sensitivity of the bacillus to antibiotics take a further 3–4 weeks.

FIBREOPTIC BRONCHOSCOPY with washings from the affected lobes is useful if no sputum is available. This has replaced techniques such as gastric washings.

BIOPSIES of the pleura, lymph nodes and solid lesions within the lung (tuberculomas) may be required to make the diagnosis.

The slow growth of *M. tuberculosis* in culture has hindered the ability to make a rapid definitive diagnosis. Newer techniques are being developed which should play an increasing role in rapid diagnosis. Radiolabelled DNA probes specific for various mycobacterial species can identify organisms in culture. The sensitivity of these methods has been enhanced by amplifying target DNA using the polymerase chain reaction. This allows direct testing of sputum and other fluids providing a laboratory diagnosis within 48 hours; it is still being evaluated.

### PREVENTION

### BCG vaccination

Vaccination with BCG (Bacille Calmette–Guérin) has been given to schoolchildren in the UK since 1954. BCG is a bovine strain of *M. tuberculosis* that lost its virulence after growth in the laboratory for many years. Early trials showed that it decreases the risk of developing tuberculosis by about 70%. With the continuing decrease in the incidence of tuberculosis it is becoming less cost-effective to administer this vaccine, and the procedure is being stopped in certain areas of the UK. However, in other areas with a high immigrant population, the vaccine is being administered 6 weeks after birth rather than at the traditional age of 13 years. This is to prevent the disease from developing in young children, where it can progress extremely rapidly and in whom any delay in diagnosis can be fatal. BCG is only given to individuals who are tuberculin-negative; those with positive tests are further screened by a chest X-ray. BCG should be given at a dose of 0.1 ml intradermally to children and adults, but at a dose of 0.05 ml to infants. The practice of BCG vaccination in the UK, thereby producing cellular immunity and a positive tuberculin test, is an important reason why the Mantoux test is of little value in clinical practice for subsequent diagnosis of active disease.

### Contact tracing

Tuberculosis is spread from person to person and effective tracing of close contacts has helped to limit spread of the disease as well as to identify diseased individuals at an early stage. Screening procedures involve screening all close family members or other individuals who share the same kitchen and bathroom facilities. Occasionally, close contacts at work or school may also be screened. Contacts who are ill should be thoroughly investigated for tuberculosis. If they are well, a chest X-ray is taken and a tuberculin test is performed (Practical box 12.5).

In adults, even if the tuberculin test is positive, provided the chest X-ray is negative nothing more need be done. In patients with HIV infection, who have not had BCG, chemoprophylaxis with isoniazid is often given. In

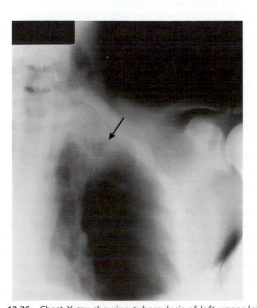

**Fig. 12.36**  Chest X-ray showing tuberculosis of left upper lobe with cavitation.

Mainly used for:

Contact tracing
BCG vaccination programmes

It is rarely of any value in the diagnosis of tuberculosis

Patients are tested with:

Purified protein derivative (PPD) of *Myobacterium tuberculosis* or
Old tuberculin (OT)

The test is based on cell-mediated immunity with the development of induration and inflammation at the site of infection due to infiltration with mainly T lymphocytes. In patients with AIDS the test may be falsely negative due to impairment of delayed hypersensitivity

*The Mantoux Test*

This is used for individual patients

0.1 ml of a 1 : 1000 strength PPD (equivalent to 10 tuberculin units) is injected intradermally
The induration is measured (not the erythema) after 72 hours. The test is positive if the induration is 10 mm or more in diameter

*The Tine Test*

This is a simple test used for large-scale screening

Four pointed needles mounted on a plastic base are used
The tips of the needles are covered with OT and are pressed firmly into the skin once
The presence of papules that are confluent with each other after 72 hours indicates a positive result

**Practical box 12.5**   Tuberculin testing.

children, a positive tuberculin test is usually taken as evidence of infection, and treatment is instituted. If the tuberculin test is negative in children and young adults (<35 years) it is repeated at 6 weeks, and if it remains negative then BCG is administered. If it has become positive (without BCG), this is again taken as an indication of active disease and the individual is treated.

Children under the age of 1 year who have a family member with tuberculosis are given chemoprophylaxis with a daily dose of isoniazid 5–10 mg kg$^{-1}$ for 6 months together with immunization with a strain of BCG that is resistant to isoniazid.

In general, much greater emphasis is placed on contact tracing and investigation of those under the age of 35 years and in some immigrant groups (Irish and Asian) in whom the disease is more virulent and prevalent.

## TREATMENT

Bed rest does not affect the outcome of the disease. Some patients will require hospitalization for a brief period; these include ill patients, those in whom the diagnosis is uncertain and, most importantly, those individuals from whom it is essential to gain cooperation. The most important factor in the successful treatment of tuberculosis lies in the continual self-administration of drugs for

6 months; lack of patient compliance is a major reason why 5% of patients do not respond to treatment. *In vitro* resistance to one or more of the antituberculous drugs occurs in less than 1% of patients in the UK.

Long stay in hospital is now only required for persistently uncooperative patients, many of whom are homeless and abuse alcohol.

### Six-month regimen

This is now standard practice for patients with pulmonary and lymph node disease: daily administration of rifampicin 600 mg and isoniazid 300 mg. (For those whose body weight is below 55 kg, rifampicin is reduced to 450 mg daily.) These are given as combination tablets and are taken 30 min before breakfast, since the absorption of rifampicin is influenced by food. This is supplemented for the first 2 months by pyrazinamide at a dose of 1.5 g (body weight <55 kg) or 2.0 g daily. Studies have indicated that pyrazinamide is of particular value in treating mycobacteria present within macrophages and for this reason it may have a very valuable effect on preventing subsequent relapse.

### Longer regimens

Treatment of bone tuberculosis should be continued for a total of 9 months and of tuberculous meningitis for 12 months. The drugs used are the same as for pulmonary tuberculosis with pyrazinamide prescribed for the first 2 months only.

### Drug-resistant organisms

The development of resistance after initial drug sensitivity (secondary drug resistance) occurs in patients who do not comply with the treatment regimens. Primary drug resistance is seen in immigrants and those exposed to others infected with resistant organisms. Multidrug resistance occurring particularly in patients with HIV infection is a major therapeutic problem with a high mortality. Nosocomial transmission of multidrug-resistant tuberculosis to health care workers and to other patients is recognized and poses a major public health problem. The drug treatment of suspected drug resistance in HIV-positive and HIV-negative patients is:

● With multiple drug resistance use at least three drugs to which the organism is sensitive.
● With resistance to one of the four main drugs, use the other three.

Therapy should be continued for up to 2 years and in HIV-positive patients for at least 12 months after negative cultures.

### Unwanted effects of drug treatment

RIFAMPICIN. This drug induces liver enzymes, which may be transiently elevated in many patients. The drug should only be stopped if the serum bilirubin becomes elevated, which is extremely rare. Thrombocytopenia has been reported. Rifampicin stains body secretions pink and the patients should be warned of the change in colour of their urine, tears and sweat. Induction of liver enzymes means that concomitant drug treatment may be made less effective (see Chapter 14) and oral contraception should not be used.

ISONIAZID. This gives rise to very few unwanted effects. At high doses it may produce a peripheral neuropathy but this is extremely rare when the normal dose of 200–300 mg is given daily. Nevertheless, it is customary to prescribe pyridoxine 10 mg daily to prevent this effect (see Fig. 3.5) Occasionally, isoniazid gives rise to allergic reactions in the form of a skin rash and fever, with hepatitis occuring in less than 1% of cases. The latter, however, may be fatal if the drug is continued.

PYRAZINAMIDE. The main unwanted effect of this drug is severe hepatic toxicity, though recent experience suggests that this is much rarer than initially thought using present dosage schedules. Gout due to hyperuricaemia may occur.

ETHAMBUTOL. This drug can cause a dose-related retrobulbar neuritis that presents with colour blindness for green, reduction in visual acuity and a central scotoma. It usually reverses provided that the drug is stopped when symptoms develop; patients should therefore be warned of its effects. Because of this problem ethambutol is rarely used unless resistance of *M. tuberculosis* is present to one or more of the other drugs.

All patients should be seen by an ophthalmologist prior to treatment.

STREPTOMYCIN. The main unwanted effect of streptomycin is irreversible damage to the vestibular nerve. It is more likely to occur in the elderly and in those with renal impairment. Allergic reactions to streptomycin are more common than to rifampicin, isoniazid and pyrazinamide. This drug is only used if patients are very ill and not responding adequately to therapy.

### Follow-up

Patients should be seen regularly for the duration of chemotherapy and once more after 3 months, since relapse, though very unlikely, usually occurs within this period of time.

### Chemoprophylaxis

Patients who have any chest X-ray changes compatible with previous tuberculosis and who are about to undergo long-term treatment that has an immunosuppressive effect, such as renal dialysis or treatment with corticosteroids, should receive chemoprophylaxis with isoniazid 200–300 mg daily.

## Other mycobacteria

*M. kansasii* occurs in water and milk, though not in soil. Disease caused by this mycobacterium has mainly been described in Europe and the USA. It rarely causes a relatively benign type of human pulmonary disease, usually in middle-aged males. Men working in dusty jobs (e.g.

miners) appear to be especially at risk, as are those who have underlying chronic bronchitis and emphysema. *M. avium intracellulare* is an important cause of pulmonary infection in AIDS patients (see p. 103).

# GRANULOMATOUS LUNG DISEASE

A granuloma is a mass or nodule composed of chronically inflamed tissue formed by the response of the mononuclear phagocyte system (macrophage/histiocyte) to a slowly soluble antigen or irritant. If the foreign substance is inert (e.g. an inhaled dust), the phagocytes turn over slowly; if the substance is toxic or reproducing, the cells turn over faster, producing a granuloma.

A granuloma is characterized by epithelioid multinucleate giant cells, as seen in tuberculosis. Granulomas may be caused by:

- Tuberculosis (see p. 683)
- Fungal and helminthic infections
- Hypersensitivity reactions
- Neoplasms

They are also found in disorders with no known cause, such as sarcoidosis.

## Sarcoidosis

Sarcoidosis is a multisystem granulomatous disorder, commonly affecting young adults and usually presenting with bilateral hilar lymphadenopathy, pulmonary infiltration and skin or eye lesions. The diagnosis is confirmed on the histological evidence of widespread, non-caseating, epithelioid granulomas in more than one organ. Poisoning with beryllium can rarely produce a clinical and histological picture identical to sarcoidosis, though contact with this element is now strictly controlled.

### EPIDEMIOLOGY AND AETIOLOGY

Sarcoidosis is a common disease that is often detected by mass X-ray studies. There is great geographical variation. The prevalence in the UK is approximately 19 in 100 000 of the population. It is common in the USA but is uncommon in Japan. The course of the disease is much more severe in American Blacks than in Whites. There is no relation with any histocompatibility antigen, but cases of sarcoidosis are seen within families, possibly suggesting an environmental factor. Other aetiological factors suggested are an atypical mycobacterium or fungus, the Epstein–Barr virus and occupational, genetic, social or other environmental factors (a higher incidence occurs in rural rather than in urban populations); none have been substantiated.

### IMMUNOPATHOLOGY

TYPICAL SARCOID GRANULOMAS consist of focal accumulations of epithelioid cells, macrophages and lymphocytes, mainly T cells.

DEPRESSED CELL-MEDIATED REACTIVITY to tuberculin and other antigens such as *Candida albicans* is present.

OVERALL LYMPHOPENIA—circulating T lymphocytes are low but B cells are slightly increased.

BRONCHOALVEOLAR LAVAGE shows a great increase in the number of cells; lymphocytes (particularly CD4 helper cells) are greatly increased.

ALVEOLAR MACROPHAGES—the number is increased but they represent a reduced percentage of the total number of cells.

TRANSBRONCHIAL BIOPSIES show infiltration of the alveolar walls and interstitial spaces with mononuclear cells, mainly T cells, prior to granuloma formation.

It seems likely that the decrease in circulating T lymphocytes and changes in delayed hypersensitivity responses are the result of sequestration of lymphocytes within the lung. There is no evidence to suggest that patients with sarcoidosis suffer from an overall defect in cellular immunity, since the frequency of fungal, viral and bacterial infections is not increased and there is no substantiated evidence of a greater risk of developing malignant neoplasms.

## CLINICAL FEATURES

The peak incidence is in the third and fourth decades, with a female preponderance. Sarcoidosis can affect many different organs of the body. The commonest presentation is with respiratory symptoms or abnormalities found on chest X-rays (50%). Fatigue or weight loss occurs in 5%, peripheral lymphadenopathy in 5% and a fever in 4%. A chest X-ray may be negative in up to 20% of non-respiratory cases, though lesions may be detected later.

BILATERAL HILAR LYMPHADENOPATHY is a characteristic feature of sarcoidosis. It is often symptomless and simply detected on a routine chest X-ray. Occasionally, the bilateral hilar lymphadenopathy is associated with a dull ache in the chest, malaise and a mild fever.

Although the chest X-ray may not show any evidence of infiltration in the lung fields, evidence from CT scanning (Fig. 12.37), transbronchial biopsies and bronchoalveolar lavage indicate that the lung parenchyma is nearly always involved.

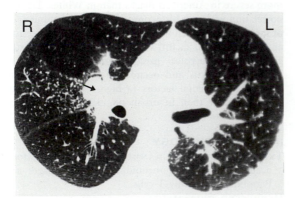

**Fig. 12.37** CT scan in sarcoidosis. Note enlarged glands at the hilum (arrow) and nodular shadowing, particularly in right middle lobe.

The differential diagnosis of the bilateral hilar lymphadenopathy includes:

LYMPHOMA—though it is rare for this only to affect the hilar lymph nodes.

PULMONARY TUBERCULOSIS—though it is rare for the hilar lymph nodes to be symmetrically enlarged.

CARCINOMA OF THE BRONCHUS with malignant spread to the contralateral hilar lymph nodes—again it is rare for this to give rise to a typical symmetrical picture.

In the early stages it may be difficult to distinguish enlarged lymph nodes on the chest X-ray from the pulmonary arteries, and lymph node enlargement is not always symmetrical. It is for these reasons that, in the absence of additional erythema nodosum (see below), histological confirmation of the disease process is advisable.

### Pulmonary infiltration

This type of sarcoidosis may be progressive and may lead to increasing effort dyspnoea and eventually cor pulmonale and death. The chest X-ray shows a mottling in the mid-zones proceeding to generalized fine nodular shadows. Eventually, widespread pulmonary line shadows develop, reflecting the underlying fibrosis. A honeycomb appearance can occasionally occur. Pulmonary function tests show a typical restrictive lung defect (see below).

It is possible to have a normal chest X-ray with abnormal lung function tests; conversely, lung infiltration may be present on the X-ray with lung function tests in the normal range.

### Extrapulmonary manifestations

Skin and ocular sarcoidosis are the commonest extrapulmonary presentations.

SKIN SARCOIDOSIS. This is seen in 10% of cases; apart from erythema nodosum, a chilblain-like lesion known as lupus pernio is seen, as are nodules (see p. 1022). Sarcoidosis is the commonest cause of erythema nodosum (see p. 1006). The association of bilateral symmetrical hilar lymphadenopathy with erythema nodosum only occurs in sarcoidosis.

ANTERIOR UVEITIS. This is common and may present with misting of vision, pain and a red eye, but posterior uveitis may simply present as progressive loss of vision. Although ocular sarcoidosis accounts for about 5% of uveitis presenting to ophthalmologists, evidence of asymptomatic uveitis may be found in up to 25% of patients with sarcoidosis. Conjunctivitis may occur and retinal lesions have been recognized recently.

Keratoconjunctivitis sicca and lacrimal gland enlargement may also occur. Uveoparotid fever is a syndrome of bilateral uveitis and parotid gland enlargement together with occasional development of facial nerve palsy and is sometimes seen with sarcoidosis.

METABOLIC MANIFESTATIONS. It is rare for sarcoidosis to present with problems of calcium metabolism, though hypercalcaemia is found in 10% of established cases. Hypercalcaemia and hypercalciuria can lead to the development of renal calculi and nephrocalcinosis. The cause of the hypercalcaemia has been shown to be high circulating 1,25-dihydroxy vitamin $D_3$, with the 1$\alpha$-hydroxylation occurring in sarcoid macrophages in the lung in addition to that taking place in the kidney.

THE CENTRAL NERVOUS SYSTEM. Involvement of the CNS is rare (2%) but can lead to severe neurological disease (see p. 930).

BONE AND JOINT INVOLVEMENT. Arthralgia without erythema nodosum is seen in 5% of cases. Bone cysts are found, particularly in the digits, with associated swelling. In the absence of swelling, routine X-rays of the hands are unnecessary.

HEPATOSPLENOMEGALY. Sarcoidosis is a cause of hepatosplenomegaly, though it is rarely of any clinical consequence.

CARDIAC INVOLVEMENT. Cardiac involvement is rare (3%). Ventricular dysrhythmias, conduction defects and cardiomyopathy with congestive cardiac failure may be seen.

## INVESTIGATION

CHEST X-RAY (see above).

FULL BLOOD COUNT. Mild normochromic, normocytic anaemia with raised ESR.

SERUM BIOCHEMISTRY — raised serum calcium and hypergammaglobulinaemia.

TRANSBRONCHIAL BIOPSY is the most useful investigation. Positive results are seen in 90% of cases of pulmonary sarcoidosis with or without X-ray evidence of lung involvement. The test provides positive histological evidence of a granuloma in approximately one-half of patients with clinically extrapulmonary sarcoidosis in whom the chest X-ray is normal.

THE KVEIM TEST, which involved an intradermal injection of sarcoid tissue, was regularly used for confirmation of the diagnosis. It should not now be used because of the risk of transmission of infection. It is less sensitive and less specific than transbronchial biopsy which has superseded it.

TUBERCULIN TEST is negative in 80% of patients with sarcoidosis; it is of no diagnostic value.

SERUM LEVEL OF ACE is two standard deviations above the normal mean value in over 75% of patients with untreated sarcoid. Raised (but lower) levels are also seen in patients with lymphoma, pulmonary tuberculosis, asbestosis and silicosis, rendering the test of no diagnostic value. However, it is a simple test and is of use in assessing the activity of the disease and therefore as a guide to treatment with corticosteroids. Reduction of serum ACE during treatment with corticosteroids has not, however, yet been proved to reflect resolution of the disease.

LUNG FUNCTION TESTS show a restrictive lung defect with pulmonary infiltration. There is a decrease in TLC, a decrease in both $FEV_1$ and FVC and a decrease in gas transfer.

## TREATMENT

Both the need to treat and the value of corticosteroid therapy are contested in many aspects of this disease.

Hilar lymphadenopathy on its own with no evidence of chest X-ray involvement of the lungs or decrease in lung function tests does not require treatment. Persisting infiltration on the chest X-ray or abnormal lung function tests are unlikely to improve without corticosteroid treatment. If the disease is not improving spontaneously 6 months after diagnosis, treatment should be started with prednisolone 30 mg for 6 weeks, reducing to alternate day treatment with prednisolone 15 mg for 6–12 months. Although there are no controlled trials that have proved the efficacy of such treatment, it is difficult to withhold corticosteroids when there is continuing deterioration of the disease.

Topical or systemic prednisolone should be given for patients suffering from involvement of the eyes or the presence of persistent hypercalcaemia. The erythema nodosum of sarcoidosis will respond rapidly to a short course of prednisolone 5–15 mg for 2 weeks.

Myocardial sarcoidosis and neurological manifestations are also treated with prednisolone, and uveoparotid fever responds rapidly to steroids.

## PROGNOSIS

Sarcoidosis is a much more severe disease in certain racial groups, particularly American Blacks, where death rates of up to 10% have been recorded. It is probable that the disease is fatal in less than 1 in 20 individuals in the UK, most often as a result of respiratory failure and cor pulmonale but, rarely, from myocardial sarcoidosis and renal damage.

The chest X-ray provides a guide to prognosis. The disease remits by 2 years in over two-thirds of patients with hilar lymphadenopathy alone, in approximately one-half with hilar lymphadenopathy plus chest X-ray evidence of pulmonary infiltration, but in only one-third of patients with X-ray evidence of infiltration without any demonstrable lymphadenopathy.

# Histiocytosis X

## CLINICAL FEATURES

There are three variants of this disease, all characterized by the presence of granulomas consisting predominantly of characteristic histiocytes intermingled with eosinophilic and neutrophilic granulocytes, giant cells and lymphocytes. Electron microscopic studies have shown that the histiocytes contain granules characteristic of Langerhan cells. Fibrosis may occur early, with the development of multiple small cysts producing a honeycomb appearance.

### Eosinophilic granuloma

This is the commonest variant in adults. It presents with increasing effort dyspnoea and cough. The chest X-ray shows diffuse bilateral mottling with translucencies with thick walls, and gas transfer is decreased. Recurrent pneumothorax occurs. The granulomas can also be found in bones.

### Letterer–Siwe disease

This is usually a fatal disease of infancy that occurs under the age of 3 years. It is a widespread disease with skin lesions, lymphadenopathy, hepatosplenomegaly and bone lesions.

### Hand–Schüller–Christian disease

This usually begins under the age of 5 years. It is characterized by defects in bone, exophthalmos and diabetes insipidus. Pulmonary lesions show diffuse nodular shadows with hilar lymphadenopathy simulating sarcoidosis.

### PROGNOSIS

Both Hand–Schüller–Christian disease and eosinophilic granuloma may recover spontaneously; survival for 20 years has been reported for both conditions.

### TREATMENT

Treatment is with corticosteroids and cyclophosphamide, though there is no evidence as yet that this treatment substantially alters the outcome.

## Wegener's granulomatosis

This disease of unknown aetiology is characterized by lesions involving the upper respiratory tract, the lungs and the kidneys. Often the disease starts with severe rhinorrhoea with subsequent nasal mucosal ulceration followed by cough, haemoptysis and pleuritic pain. Occasionally there may be involvement of the skin and nervous system. A chest X-ray usually shows single or multiple nodular masses or pneumonic infiltrates with cavitation. The most remarkable radiographic feature is the migratory pattern, with large lesions clearing in one area and new lesions appearing in another.

The typical histological changes are usually best seen in the kidneys, where there is a necrotizing glomerulonephritis.

This disease responds well to treatment with cyclophosphamide 150–200 mg daily. A variant of Wegener's granulomatosis called 'mid-line granuloma' particularly affects the nose and paranasal sinuses and is particularly mutilating; it has a poor prognosis.

### Anti-neutrophil cytoplasmic antibodies (ANCA) (see p. 383 and p. 451)

ANCA is found in the acute phase of vasculitides associated with neutrophil infiltration of the vessel wall and may be found in a wide range of diseases. cANCA is more specific for Wegener's granulomatosis (greater than 90%) but only in the active stage. cANCA positivity is found in only one-third of inactive or treated cases. pANCA is closely associated with a number of vasculitic syndromes,

Churg–Strauss syndrome and microscopic polyarteritis; 10–15% of cases of progressive glomerulonephritis with anti-glomerular basement membrane (GBM) antibodies are pANCA positive and these are the most likely to suffer pulmonary haemorrhage.

# RESPIRATORY MANIFESTATIONS OF SYSTEMIC CONNECTIVE TISSUE DISEASE

## Rheumatoid disease (see p.387)

The features of respiratory involvement in rheumatoid disease are illustrated in Fig. 12.38.

Pleural adhesions, thickening and effusion are the commonest lesions. The effusion is often unilateral and tends to be chronic. It has a low glucose content but this can occur in any chronic pleural effusion.

Rheumatoid diffuse fibrosing alveolitis can be considered as a variant of the cryptogenic form of the disease (see p. 694). The clinical features and gross appearance are the same but the disease is often more chronic.

Rheumatoid nodules showing the typical histological appearances are rare in the lung. On the chest X-ray these appear as single or multiple nodules ranging in size from a few millimetres to a few centimetres. The nodules frequently cavitate. They usually produce no symptoms but can give rise to a pneumothorax or pleural effusion.

Obliterative disease of the small bronchioles is rare. It is characterized by progressive breathlessness and irreversible airflow limitation. Corticosteroids may prevent progression.

Involvement of the cricoarytenoid joints gives rise to dyspnoea, stridor, hoarseness and occasionally severe obstruction necessitating tracheostomy. Caplan's syndrome is due to a combination of dust inhalation and the disturbed immunity of rheumatoid arthritis. It occurs

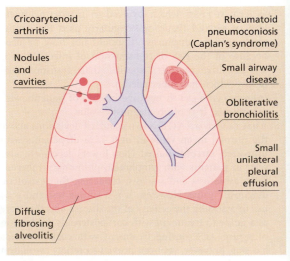

**Fig. 12.38** The respiratory manifestations of rheumatoid disease.

particularly in coal-worker's pneumoconiosis but it can occur in individuals exposed to other dusts, such as silica and asbestos. Typically the lesions appear as rounded nodules 0.5–5 cm in diameter, though sometimes they become incorporated into large areas of fibrosis that are indistinguishable radiologically from progressive massive fibrosis. There may be little evidence of simple pneumoconiosis prior to the development of the nodule.

These lesions may precede the development of the arthritis. Rheumatoid factor is always present in the serum.

## Systemic lupus erythematosus (see p. 400)

The commonest respiratory manifestation of this disease, occurring in up to two-thirds of cases, is the development of pleurisy, with or without an effusion. Effusions are usually small and bilateral. Basal pneumonitis is often present, perhaps as a result of poor movement of the diaphragm, or restriction of chest movements due to pleural pain. Pneumonia also occurs, either due to infection or to the disease process itself. Unlike rheumatoid arthritis, diffuse pulmonary fibrosis is rare.

## Systemic sclerosis

Autopsy studies have indicated that there is almost always some evidence of diffuse fibrosis of alveolar walls and obliteration of capillaries and the alveolar space. Severe changes result in nodular then streaky shadowing on the chest X-ray, followed by cystic changes, ending up with a honeycomb lung. Function tests indicate a restrictive lesion and poor gas transfer.

Pneumonia may occur due to inhalation from the dilated oesophagus. Breathlessness may be worsened by restriction of chest wall movement due to thickening and contraction of the skin and trunk.

## PULMONARY INFILTRATION WITH EOSINOPHILIA (PIE)

The common types and characteristics of these diseases are shown in Table 12.9. They range from very mild, simple, pulmonary eosinophilias to the often fatal polyarteritis nodosa.

## Simple and prolonged pulmonary eosinophilia

Simple pulmonary eosinophilia is a relatively mild illness with a slight fever and cough and usually lasting for less than 2 weeks. It is probably due to a transient allergic reaction in the alveolus. Many allergens have been implicated, including *Ascaris lumbricoides*, *Ankylostoma braziliense* and *Trichuris trichiura* as well as drugs such as *p*-aminosalicylic acid, aspirin, penicillin, nitrofurantoin and sulphonamides. Often, no allergen is identified. No treatment is required and the disease is self-limiting. Occasionally, however, the disease becomes more prolonged, with a high fever lasting for over a month. There is usually an eosinophilia in the blood and this condition is called *prolonged pulmonary eosinophilia*. Similar allergens are thought to be involved, with the addition of *Strongyloides stercoralis*. In both conditions the chest X-ray shows either localized or diffuse opacities. Corticosteroid therapy is indicated, with resolution of the disease over the ensuing weeks.

## Asthmatic bronchopulmonary eosinophilia

This is characterized by the presence of asthma, transient fleeting shadows on the chest X-ray, and blood or sputum eosinophilia. By far the commonest cause worldwide is allergy to *A. fumigatus* (see below), although *Candida albicans* may be an allergen in a small number of patients. In many, the appropriate allergen has still to be identified.

## Diseases caused by *Aspergillus fumigatus*

The various types of lung disease caused by *A. fumigatus* are illustrated in Fig. 12.39.

The spores of *A. fumigatus* (5 μm in diameter) are readily inhaled and are present in the atmosphere throughout the year, though they are at their highest concentration in the late autumn. They can be grown from

| Disease | Symptoms | Blood eosinophils (%) | Multisystem involvement | Duration | Outcome |
|---|---|---|---|---|---|
| Simple pulmonary eosinophilia | Mild | 10 | None | <1 month | Good |
| Prolonged pulmonary eosinophilia | Mild/moderate | >20 | None | >1 month | Good |
| Asthmatic bronchopulmonary eosinophilia | Moderate/severe | 5–20 | None | Years | Fair |
| Tropical pulmonary eosinophilia | Moderate/severe | >20 | None | Years | Fair |
| Hypereosinophilic syndrome | Severe | >20 | Always | Months/years | Poor |
| Polyarteritis nodosa | Severe | >20 | Always | Months/years | Poor/fair |

**Table 12.9** Common types and characteristics of pulmonary infiltration with eosinophilia.

the sputum in up to 15% of patients with chronic lung disease in whom they do not produce disease. They are an important cause of extrinsic asthma in atopic individuals.

**Allergic bronchopulmonary aspergillosis** (Fig. 12.39)
In allergic bronchopulmonary aspergillosis *Aspergillus* actually grows in the walls of the bronchi and eventually produces proximal bronchiectasis. There are episodes of eosinophilic pneumonia throughout the year, particularly in late autumn and winter. The episodes present with a wheeze, cough, fever and malaise. They are associated with expectoration of firm sputum plugs containing the fungal mycelium, which results in the clearing of the pulmonary infiltrates on the chest X-ray. Occasionally the large mucus plugs obliterate the bronchial lumen, causing collapse of the lung.

Repeated episodes of eosinophilic pneumonia left untreated can result in progressive pulmonary fibrosis that is often seen in the upper zones and can give rise to a similar chest X-ray appearance to that produced by tuberculosis.

The peripheral blood eosinophil count is usually raised, and total levels of IgE are extremely high (both that specific to *Aspergillus* and non-specific). Skin-prick testing with protein allergens from *A. fumigatus* gives rise to positive immediate skin tests. Sputum may show eosinophils and mycelia, and precipitating antibodies are usually found in the serum.

Lung function tests show a decrease in lung volumes and gas transfer in more chronic cases but in all cases evidence of reversible airflow limitation can be demonstrated.

Treatment for this allergic pneumonia is with prednisolone 30 mg daily, which readily causes clearing of the pulmonary infiltrates. Frequent episodes of the disease can be prevented by long-term treatment with prednisolone, but doses as high as 10–15 mg daily are usually required. Moderately severe asthma itself requires continuous treatment with oral corticosteroids. Inhaled corticosteroids do not influence the occurrence of pulmonary infiltrates but are useful for the asthmatic element of the disease.

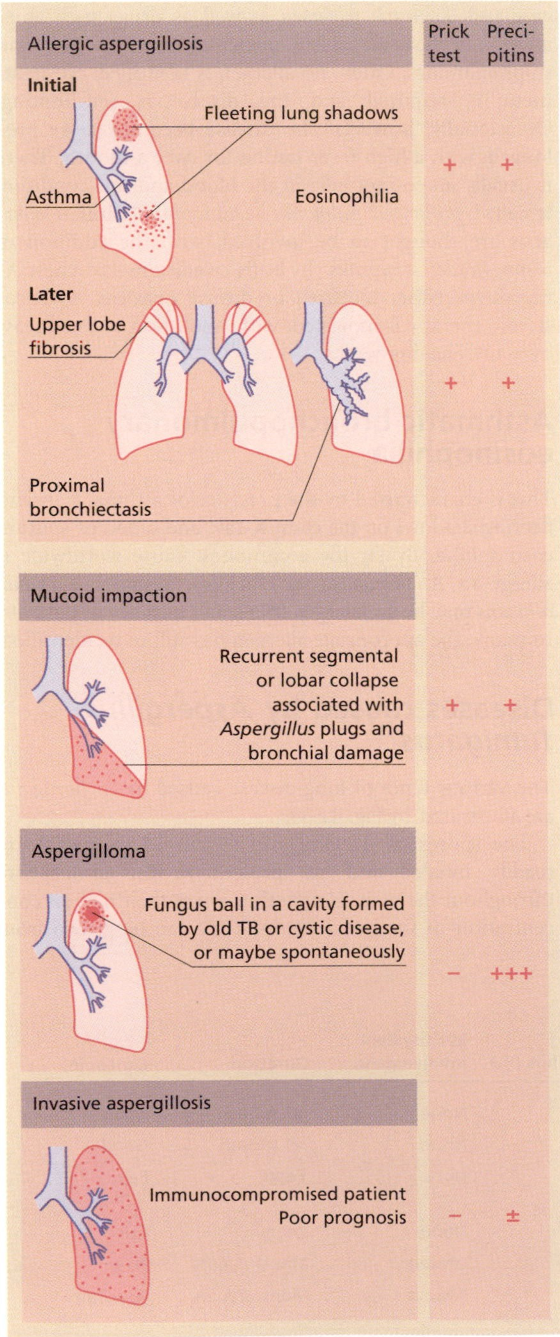

**Aspergilloma and invasive aspergillosis** (Fig. 12.39)
This is a totally separate disease from allergic bronchopulmonary aspergillosis. It simply represents the growth within previously damaged lung tissue of *A. fumigatus*, which forms a ball of mycelium within lung cavities. The typical appearance on the chest X-ray is of a round lesion with an air 'halo' above it. The continuing antigenic stimulation gives rise to large quantities of precipitating antibody in the serum. The aspergilloma itself causes little trouble, though occasionally massive haemoptysis may occur, requiring resection of the damaged area of lung containing the aspergilloma. Although treatment with antifungal agents, such as amphotericin (250 $\mu$g kg$^{-1}$ i.v.), has been tested in both allergic bronchopulmonary aspergillosis and aspergilloma, this has had little success, though it remains the only treatment for invasive aspergillosis, when it is often combined with flucytosine (200 mg kg$^{-1}$ i.v. daily in four doses).

# Tropical pulmonary eosinophilia

This condition presents with cough and wheeze together with fever, lassitude and weight loss. The typical appearance of the chest X-ray is of bilateral hazy mottling that is frequently uniformly distributed in both lung fields. The individual shadows may be as large as 5 mm or may

| | Prick test | Precipitins |
|---|---|---|
| **Allergic aspergillosis** | | |
| Initial — Fleeting lung shadows, Asthma, Eosinophilia | + | + |
| Later — Upper lobe fibrosis, Proximal bronchiectasis | + | + |
| **Mucoid impaction** — Recurrent segmental or lobar collapse associated with *Aspergillus* plugs and bronchial damage | + | + |
| **Aspergilloma** — Fungus ball in a cavity formed by old TB or cystic disease, or maybe spontaneously | − | +++ |
| **Invasive aspergillosis** — Immunocompromised patient, Poor prognosis | − | ± |

**Fig. 12.39** Diseases caused by *Aspergillus fumigatus*.

become more confluent, giving the appearance of pneumonia. It is found in many tropical countries, but particularly in the Asian subcontinent, due to an allergic reaction to microfilaria, probably from *Wuchereria bancrofti*.

The disease is characterized by a very high eosinophil count in peripheral blood. The filarial complement fixation test is positive in almost every case. The treatment of choice is diethylcarbamazine at a dose of $5 \, mg \, kg^{-1}$ body weight for 10–14 days; this usually produces a good response.

## The hypereosinophilic syndrome

This disease is characterized by eosinophilic infiltration in various organs, sometimes associated with an eosinophilic arteritis. The heart muscle is particularly involved, but pulmonary involvement in the form of pleural effusion or interstitial lung disease occurs in about 40% of cases. Typical features are fever, weight loss, recurrent abdominal pain, persistent non-productive cough and congestive cardiac failure. Corticosteroid treatment may be of value in some cases.

## Polyarteritis nodosa (see p. 406)

This is a rare disease characterized by foci of necrotizing arteritis that sooner or later affect many organs in the body. The lungs are rarely involved, except in the variant of polyarteritis nodosa known as the Churg–Strauss syndrome (see below).

The upper respiratory tract may be involved, with nasal obstruction and rhinorrhoea. The chest X-ray may show consolidation that is ill-defined and transgresses anatomical boundaries. These shadows may disappear and reappear over periods of 2–12 weeks, and some may represent intra-alveolar haemorrhage or pulmonary infarcts. pANCA is usually negative in the serum. The overall 5-year survival for polyarteritis nodosa is 80% with corticosteroids and immunosuppressive therapy.

Microscopic polyarteritis involves the kidneys and the lungs, resulting in recurrent haemoptysis. pANCA is usually positive in the serum (see p. 405).

## Allergic granulomatosis (Churg–Strauss syndrome)

The pathology of this condition is dominated by an eosinophilic infiltration and it occurs in patients usually in their fourth decade who have a previous history of rhinitis and asthma. It may simply represent an unusual progression of allergic disease in a subset of predisposed individuals. It is characterized by a high blood eosinophil count, vasculitis of small arteries and veins, and extravascular granulomas. The lungs, peripheral nerves and skin are most often affected and renal failure is much less common than in generalized polyarteritis nodosa. Transient patchy pneumonia-like shadows may occur as in polyarteritis nodosa, but sometimes these can be massive

and bilateral. Skin lesions include tender subcutaneous nodules as well as petechial or purpuric lesions. The disease responds well to corticosteroids. pANCA can be positive.

# GOODPASTURE'S SYNDROME AND IDIOPATHIC PULMONARY HAEMOSIDEROSIS

## Goodpasture's syndrome (see also p. 451)

The disease often starts with an upper respiratory tract infection followed by cough and intermittent haemoptysis, tiredness and eventually anaemia, though massive bleeding may occur. The chest X-ray shows transient blotchy shadows due to intrapulmonary haemorrhage. These features usually precede the development of an acute glomerulonephritis by several weeks or months. The course of the disease is variable; some spontaneously improve while others proceed to renal failure. The disease usually occurs in individuals over 16 years of age. It is thought to be due to a type II cytotoxic hypersensitivity reaction, the hypothesis being that there may be a shared antigen between a virus and the basement membrane of both kidney and lung. Anti-GBM antibodies are found in the serum and pANCA may be positive. An association with influenza A2 virus has been reported. Treatment is with corticosteroids, but plasmapheresis to remove the antibodies has led to dramatic improvement in some cases.

## Idiopathic pulmonary haemosiderosis

This is a similar disease to Goodpasture's syndrome, but the kidneys are less frequently involved. Most cases occur in children under 7 years of age. Characteristically, haemosiderin-containing macrophages are found in the sputum. The child develops a chronic cough and anaemia and the chest X-ray shows diffuse shadows due to intrapulmonary bleeding, and eventually miliary nodulation. There is an association with a sensitivity to cows' milk, and an appropriate diet is usually tried. The prognosis in general is poor and treatment with corticosteroids or azathioprine is usually given.

# PULMONARY FIBROSIS AND HONEYCOMB LUNG

Pulmonary fibrosis is the end result of many diseases of the respiratory tract. It may be:

LOCALIZED, e.g. following unresolved pneumonia.

BILATERAL, e.g. in tuberculosis.

WIDESPREAD, e.g. in cryptogenic fibrosing alveolitis, due to drugs (busulphan, bleomycin and cyclophosphamide) or in industrial lung disease. Sometimes with widespread fibrosis a typical radiological appearance is seen that is known as honeycomb lung. This

*Localized*
Systemic sclerosis
Sarcoidosis
Tuberculosis
Asbestosis
Berylliosis

*Diffuse*
Cryptogenic fibrosing alveolitis
Rheumatoid lung
Histiocytosis X
Tuberose sclerosis
Neurofibromatosis

**Table 12.10**   The main causes of honeycomb lung.

refers to the presence, often diffusely in both lungs, of cysts between 0.5 and 2 cm in diameter that are thick-walled and do not fill with opaque material on bronchography. The cystic air spaces probably represent dilated and thickened terminal and respiratory bronchioles. The main causes are shown in Table 12.10.

## Cryptogenic fibrosing alveolitis (CFA)

This relatively rare disorder of unknown aetiology causes diffuse fibrosis throughout the lung fields, usually in late middle age. The cardinal features are progressive breathlessness and cyanosis, which eventually lead to respiratory failure, pulmonary hypertension and cor pulmonale. Gross clubbing occurs in two-thirds of cases and bilateral fine end-inspiratory crackles are heard on auscultation. Rarely, an acute form known as the Hamman–Rich syndrome occurs. The chest X-ray appearance initially is of ground-glass appearance, progressing to obvious small nodular shadows with streaky fibrosis and finally a honeycomb lung.

A number of autoimmune diseases are seen in association with this condition. For example, chronic active hepatitis occurs in 5–10% of cases.

Similar lung changes are also seen in rheumatoid arthritis, systemic sclerosis and Sjögren's syndrome, often associated with Raynaud's phenomenon.

CFA has also been reported in association with coeliac disease, ulcerative colitis and renal tubular acidosis.

### PATHOGENESIS
Histologically there are two main features:
1  Cellular infiltration and thickening and fibrosis of the alveolar walls
2  Increased cells within the alveolar space (mainly shed type II pneumocytes and macrophages)
The pathogenesis of damage and fibrosis is complex and several factors are involved (Fig. 12.40).

### INVESTIGATION
CT SCAN shows characteristic changes (Fig. 12.41).
RESPIRATORY FUNCTION TESTS show a restrictive ventilatory defect—the lung volumes are reduced, the $FEV_1$ and FVC ratio is normal to high (with both values being reduced) and gas transfer is reduced. Peak flow rates may be normal.
BLOOD GASES show an arterial hypoxaemia with normal $P_aco_2$.
THE ESR is high.
BRONCHOALVEOLAR LAVAGE shows increased numbers of cells (particularly neutrophils).
ANTINUCLEAR FACTOR is positive in one-third of patients.
RHEUMATOID FACTOR is positive in 50% of patients.
IN YOUNGER PATIENTS histological confirmation may be necessary, requiring a transbronchial lung biopsy or even an open lung biopsy to obtain a larger specimen.

### DIFFERENTIAL DIAGNOSIS
The diagnosis of CFA can be made in an elderly person presenting with the above signs and laboratory test results. In younger people the differential diagnosis includes extrinsic allergic alveolitis, bronchiectasis, chronic left heart failure, sarcoidosis, industrial lung disease and lymphangitis carcinomatosa.

### PROGNOSIS AND TREATMENT
The median survival time for patients with CFA is approximately 5 years although mortality is very high with the acute form. Treatment with prednisolone (30 mg daily) is usually prescribed for disabling disease, though its benefit has still to be proved by appropriate controlled trials. Azathioprine or cyclophosphamide may also be used. Supportive treatment includes oxygen therapy.

## Extrinsic allergic alveolitis

In this disease there is a widespread diffuse inflammatory reaction in both the small airways of the lung and alveoli. It is due to the inhalation of a number of different antigens, as illustrated in Table 12.11. By far the commonest of these diseases worldwide is farmer's lung, which affects up to 1 in 10 of the farming community in poor, wet areas around the world. In Western countries the incidence is almost certainly declining as more mechanized farming procedures are introduced.

### PATHOGENESIS
Histologically there is an initial infiltration of the small airways and alveolar walls with neutrophils followed by lymphocytes and macrophages, leading to the development of non-caseating granulomas. These comprise multinucleated giant cells, occasionally containing the inhaled antigenic material. The major allergic response to the inhaled antigens is through cellular immunity, though there is evidence in some cases of an additional immediate hypersensitivity reaction involving specific IgE antibody and the deposition of immune complexes. All these mechanisms can attract and activate alveolar macrophages, so that continued antigenic exposure results in the development of pulmonary fibrosis.

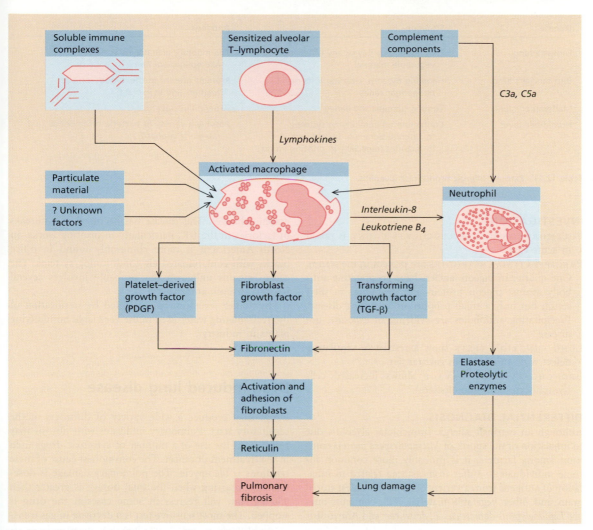

**Fig. 12.40** Pathogenesis of pulmonary fibrosis. Macrophages can be activated by several factors e.g. soluble immune complexes and sensitized T-lymphocytes resulting in the release of various cytokines leading to fibrosis.

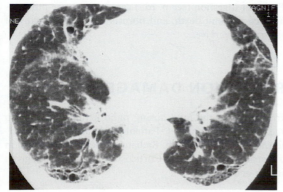

**Fig. 12.41** CT scan showing cryptogenic fibrosing alveolitis.

## CLINICAL FEATURES

The typical history is that of the onset of fever, malaise, cough and shortness of breath several hours after exposure to the causative antigen. For example, a farmer forking hay in the morning may only notice symptoms during the late afternoon and evening that resolve by the following morning. On examination the patient may have a fever, tachypnoea and coarse end-inspiratory crackles and wheezes throughout the chest. Cyanosis may be severe even at rest. Continuing exposure leads to a chronic illness characterized by severe weight loss, effort dyspnoea and cough, and the features of fibrosing alveolitis (see p. 694).

The chest X-ray shows fluffy nodular shadowing with the subsequent development of streaky shadows, particularly in the upper zones, and, in very advanced cases, honeycomb lung.

| Disease | Situation | Antigens |
|---------|-----------|----------|
| Farmer's lung | Forking mouldy hay or any other mouldy vegetable material | Thermophilic actinomycetes and *Micropolyspora faeni* |
| Bird fancier's lung | Handling pigeons, cleaning lofts or budgerigar cages | Proteins present in the 'bloom' on the feathers and in excreta |
| Maltworker's lung | Turning germinating barley | *Asperigillus clavatus* |
| Humidifier fever | Contaminated humidifying systems   In air conditioners of humidifiers   In factories (especially in printing works) | Possibly a variety of bacteria or amoebae (e.g. *Naegleria gruberi*) |

**Table 12.11**  Extrinsic allergic bronchiolar alveolitis.

## INVESTIGATION

POLYMORPHONUCLEAR LEUCOCYTE COUNT is raised in acute cases.

PRECIPITATING ANTIBODIES are present in the serum. One-quarter of pigeon fanciers have precipitating antibody against pigeon protein and droppings in their serum but only a small proportion have lung disease. Precipitating antibodies are evidence of *exposure*, not disease.

LUNG FUNCTION TESTS show a restrictive ventilatory defect with a decrease in gas transfer.

BRONCHOALVEOLAR LAVAGE shows increased cells (lymphocytes and granulocytes).

## DIFFERENTIAL DIAGNOSIS

Although an extrinsic allergic bronchiolar alveolitis due to inhalation of the spores of *Micropolyspora faeni* is common among farmers, it is probably more common for these individuals to suffer from asthma related to inhalation of antigens from a variety of mites that infest stored grain and other vegetable material. The common ones are *Lepidoglyphus domesticus*, *L. destructor* and *Acarus siro*. Symptoms of asthma resulting from inhalation of these allergens are often mistaken for farmer's lung.

Pigeon fancier's lung is quite common, but alveolitis from budgerigars is very rare.

## MANAGEMENT

Prevention is the aim. This can be achieved by change in work practice, with the use of silage for animal fodder and the drier storage of hay and grain. It is difficult to control pigeon fancier's lung, since individuals remain addicted to their hobby.

Prednisolone, initially in large doses of 30–60 mg daily, is necessary to cause regression of the early stages of the disease. Established fibrosis will not resolve and in some patients the disease may progress inexorably to respiratory failure in spite of intensive therapy. Farmer's lung is a recognized occupational disease in the UK and sufferers are entitled to compensation depending on their degree of disability.

## Humidifier fever

Humidifier fever may present with the typical features of extrinsic allergic bronchiolar alveolitis without any radiographic changes. This disease has occurred in outbreaks in factories in the UK, particularly in printing works. In North America it is more commonly found in office blocks with contaminated air-conditioning systems. The cause remains unknown but probably involves several bacteria or even amoebae.

Humidifier fever can be prevented by sterilization of the recirculating water used in the very large humidifying plants in industry.

## Drug-induced lung disease

Drugs may produce a wide variety of disorders of the respiratory tract. Pulmonary infiltrates with fibrosis may result from the use of a number of cytotoxic drugs used in the treatment of cancer. The commonest cause of these reactions is bleomycin. The pulmonary damage is dose-related, occurring when the total dosage is greater than 450 mg, but will regress in some cases if the drug is stopped. The most sensitive test is a decrease in gas transfer and therefore gas transfer should be measured repeatedly during treatment with the drug. The use of corticosteroids may help resolution.

Some of the most important drugs affecting the respiratory tract are shown in Table 12.12, together with the types of reaction they produce. The list is not exhaustive; for example, over 20 different drugs are known to produce a systemic lupus erythematosus-like syndrome, sometimes complicated by pulmonary infiltrates and fibrosis. Paraquat ingestion (see p. 755) can cause severe pulmonary oedema and death, and fibrosis develops in many of those who survive.

## RADIATION DAMAGE

Irradiation of the lung during radiotherapy can cause a radiation pneumonitis. Patients complain of breathlessness and a dry cough. Radiation pneumonia results in a restrictive lung defect. Corticosteroids should be given in the acute stage.

| Disease | Drugs |
|---|---|
| Asthma ± rhinitis | Penicillins |
| | Sulphonamides |
| | Cephalosporins |
| | Aspirin |
| | NSAIDs |
| | Tartrazine |
| | Iodine-containing contrast media |
| | Non-selective $\beta$-adrenoceptor-blocking drugs (e.g. propranolol) |
| | Suxamethonium |
| | Thiopentone |
| Diffuse lung injury infiltrate and/or fibrosis | Amiodarone |
| | Hexamethonium |
| | Nitrofurantoin |
| | Paraquat |
| | Continuous oxygen |
| | Cytotoxic agent—many, particularly busulphan, CCNU, bleomycin |
| Pulmonary eoinophilia | Antibiotics |
| | Penicillin |
| | Tetracycline |
| | Sulphonamides |
| | NSAIDs |
| | Anti-epileptic |
| | Phenytoin |
| | Carbamazepine |
| | Others |
| | Chlorpropamide |
| Opportunistic pulmonary infections | Corticosteroids |
| | Azathioprine |
| | Other cytotoxic drugs |
| Respiratory depression | Sedatives |
| | Opiates |
| SLE-like syndrome including pulmonary infiltrates, effusions and fibrosis | Hydralazine |
| | Procainamide |
| | Isoniazid |
| | p-Aminosalicylic acid |
| Cough | ACE inhibitors |

CCNU, chloroethyl-cyclohexyl-nitrosourea (lomustine); NSAIDs, non-steroidal anti-inflammatory drugs; SLE, systemic lupus erythematosus.

**Table 12.12** Drug-induced respiratory disease.

# Occupational lung disease

Exposure to dusts, gases, vapours and fumes at work can lead to the development of the following types of lung disease:
- Acute bronchitis and even pulmonary oedema from irritants such as sulphur dioxide, chlorine, ammonia or the oxides of nitrogen
- Pulmonary fibrosis due to mineral dust
- Occupational asthma (see Table 12.7)

- Extrinsic allergic bronchiolar alveolitis (see Table 12.11)
- Bronchial carcinoma due to industrial agents (e.g. asbestos, polycyclic hydrocarbons, radon in mines)

The degree of fibrosis that follows inhalation of mineral dust varies. While iron (siderosis), barium (baritosis) and tin (stannosis) lead to dramatic dense nodular shadowing on the chest X-ray, their effect on lung function and symptoms is minimal. Exposure to silica or asbestos, on the other hand, leads to extensive fibrosis and disability. Coal dust has an intermediate fibrogenic effect and accounts for 90% of all compensated industrial lung diseases. Lung fibrosis from exposure to asbestos has become an increasing problem. The term pneumoconiosis means the accumulation of dust in the lungs and the reaction of the tissue to its presence. The term is not wide enough to encompass all occupational lung disease and is now generally used in relation to coal dust and its effects on the lung.

## Coal-worker's pneumoconiosis

Improved conditions and contraction of the coal industry have led to a considerable reduction in the number of cases of pneumoconiosis to about 2 per 1000 wage earners. The disease is caused by dust particles approximately 2–5 $\mu$m in diameter that are retained in the small airways and alveoli of the lung. The incidence of the disease is related to total dust exposure, which is highest at the coal face, particularly if ventilation and dust suppression are poor. Two very different syndromes result from the inhalation of coal.

### Simple pneumoconiosis

This simply reflects the deposition of coal dust in the lung. It produces a fine micronodular shadow on the chest X-ray and is by far the commonest type of pneumoconiosis. It is graded on the chest X-ray appearance according to standard categories set by the International Labour Office (see below). Considerable dispute remains about the effects of simple pneumoconiosis on respiratory function and symptoms, many arguing that the development of the latter is largely due to chronic bronchitis and emphysema, commonly related to cigarette smoking.

Categories of simple pneumoconiosis are as follows:

1 Small round opacities are definitely present but are few in number.
2 Small round opacities are numerous but normal lung markings are still visible.
3 Small round opacities are very numerous and normal lung markings are partly or totally obscured.

The importance of simple pneumoconiosis is that it may lead to the development of progressive massive fibrosis (PMF) (see below). This virtually never occurs on a background of category 1 simple pneumoconiosis but occurs in 30% of those with category 3. Usually category 2 simple pneumoconiosis, which carries a 7% risk of developing PMF, must be present before benefit may be awarded for disability.

**Progressive massive fibrosis**

The lesions in this disease are round fibrotic masses several centimetres in diameter, almost invariably in the upper lobes and sometimes having necrotic central cavities. The pathogenesis of PMF is still not understood, though it seems clear that some fibrogenic promoting factor is present in individuals developing the disease. This was thought to be *M. tuberculosis*, but is now thought to be immune complexes, analogous to the development of large fibrotic nodules in coal miners with rheumatoid arthritis (Caplan's syndrome). The development of both rheumatoid factor and antinuclear factor in the serum of patients with PMF is common, as it is in those suffering from asbestosis and silicosis. Pathologically there is apical destruction and disruption of the lung, resulting in emphysema and airway damage. Lung function tests show a mixed restrictive and obstructive ventilatory defect with loss of lung volume, irreversible airflow limitation and reduced gas transfer.

The patient with PMF suffers considerable effort dyspnoea, usually with a cough. The sputum can be black. The disease can progress (or even develop) after exposure to coal dust has ceased. Eventually respiratory failure may intervene.

## Silicosis

This disease is uncommon though it may still be encountered in workers in foundries where sand used in moulds has to be removed from the metal casts (fettling), in sand blasting, and amongst stone-masons, pottery and ceramic workers.

Silicosis is caused by the inhalation of silica (silicon dioxide). This dust is highly fibrogenic. For example, a coal miner can remain healthy with 30 g of coal dust in his lungs but would be dead if he had inhaled 3 g of silica. Silica seems particularly toxic to alveolar macrophages and readily initiates the fibrogenic mechanism (see Fig. 12.40). The chest X-ray appearances and clinical features of the disease are similar to those of PMF. The chest X-ray appearance is distinctive: thin streaks of calcification are seen around the hilar lymph nodes ('eggshell' calcification).

## Asbestosis

Asbestos is a mixture of silicates of iron, magnesium, nickel, cadmium and aluminium, and has the unique property of occurring naturally as a fibre. It possesses remarkably resistant properties to heat, acid and alkali, hence its widespread use. Asbestos is mined in southern Africa, Canada and the former USSR. World production is 4 million tons, of which 90% is chrysotile, 6% crocidolite and 4% amosite in type.

Chrysotile or white asbestos is the softest asbestos fibre. Each fibre is often as long as 2 cm but only a few micrometres thick. It is less fibrogenic than crocidolite.

Crocidolite (blue asbestos) is particularly resistant to chemical destruction. It exists in straight fibres up to 50 $\mu$m in length and 1–2 $\mu$m in width. It is now known that this type of asbestos is by far the most important in the development of all types of asbestosis and particularly of mesothelioma. This may be due to the fact that it is readily trapped in the lung. Its long, thin shape means that it can be inhaled, but subsequent rotation against the long axis of the smaller airways, particularly in turbulent airflow during expiration, causes the fibres to impact. Crocidolite is also particularly resistant to macrophage and neutrophil enzymic destruction. Exposure to asbestos occurred particularly in naval shipbuilding yards and in power stations but its ubiquitous use meant that light exposure was common. Up to 50% of urban dwellers had evidence of asbestos bodies (asbestos fibre covered in protein secretions) in their lungs at post mortem. New regulations in the UK prevent the use of crocidolite and severely restrict the use of chrysotile, and enforce careful dust control measures. These changes should eventually abolish the problem.

There is an important synergistic relationship between asbestosis and cigarette smoking and the development of bronchial carcinoma, usually adenocarcinoma; the risk is increased fivefold. There is also an increased risk in non-smokers and it is also present in workers exposed to asbestos who do not have clinically recognized asbestosis but who do have pleural plaques or thickening. Workers will continue to be exposed to blue asbestos in the course of demolition or in the replacement of insulation, and it should be remembered that there is a considerable time lag between exposure and development of the disease, particularly mesothelioma (20–40 years).

The diseases caused by asbestos are summarized in Table 12.13. Bilateral-diffuse pleural thickening, asbestosis, mesothelioma and asbestos-related carcinoma of the bronchus are all eligible for industrial injuries benefit in the UK, but account for only one-quarter of the number of cases of compensation compared to coal-worker's pneumoconiosis. Asbestosis is the disease most frequently compensated (900 cases per year). This progressive disease is characterized by breathlessness and is accompanied by finger clubbing and bilateral basal end-inspiratory crackles. Fibrosis not detectable on chest X-ray may be revealed on CT scan. No treatment is known to alter the progress of the disease, though corticosteroids are often prescribed.

The number of cases of mesothelioma presenting for compensation has increased fivefold in the last decade to over 400 cases per year. Often open lung biopsy is needed to obtain sufficient tissue for diagnosis. No treatment influences the universally fatal outcome. Although pleural effusions are the commonest presentation of mesothelioma, occasionally they may have a benign origin and may regress spontaneously.

## Byssinosis

This disease occurs worldwide but is declining rapidly in areas where the numbers of people employed in cotton mills are falling. In the UK the disease is confined to areas of Lancashire and Northern Ireland. The symptoms start on the first day back at work after a break (Monday

| | Exposure | Chest X-ray | Lung function | Symptoms | Outcome |
|---|---|---|---|---|---|
| Asbestos bodies | Light | Normal | Normal | None | Evidence of asbestos exposure only |
| Pleural plaques | Light | Pleural thickening (parietal pleura) and calcification (also in diaphragmatic pleura) | Mild restriction | Rare, occasional mild effort dyspnoea | No other sequelae |
| Bilateral diffuse | Light/moderate | Bilateral diffuse thickening (of both parietal and visceral pleura) more than 5 mm thick and extending over more than one-quarter of the chest wall | Restrictive ventilatory defect | Effort dyspnoea | May progress in absence of further exposure |
| Mesothelioma | Light (20–40 year interval from light exposure to disease) | Pleural effusion, usually unilateral | Restrictive ventilatory defect | Pleuritic pain, increasing dyspnoea | Median survival 2 years |
| Asbestosis | Heavy (5–10 year interval from exposure to disease) | Diffuse bilateral streaky shadows, honeycomb lung | Severe restrictive ventilatory defect and reduced gas transfer | Progressive dyspnoea | Poor, progression in some cases after exposure ceases |
| Asbestos related carcinoma of the bronchus | | The features of asbestosis, bilateral diffuse pleural thickening or bilateral pleural plaques plus those of bronchial carcinoma | | | Fatal |

**Table 12.13** The effects of asbestos on the lung.

sickness) with improvement as the week progresses. Tightness in the chest, cough and breathlessness occur within the first hour in dusty areas of the mill, particularly in the blowing and carding rooms where raw cotton is cleaned and the fibres are straightened.

The exact nature of the disease and its aetiology remain disputed. Two important features are that pure cotton does *not* cause the disease, and that cotton dust has some effect on airflow limitation in all those exposed. Individuals with asthma are particularly badly affected by exposure to cotton dust. The most likely aetiology is endotoxins from bacteria present in the raw cotton causing constriction of the airways of the lung. There are no changes on the chest X-ray and there is considerable dispute as to whether the progressive airflow limitation seen in some patients with the disease is due to the cotton dust or to other effects such as cigarette smoking or coexistent asthma.

## Berylliosis

Beryllium–copper alloy has a high tensile strength and is resistant to metal fatigue, high temperature and corrosion. It is used in the aerospace industry, in atomic reactors and in many electrical devices.

Although beryllium is inhaled into the lungs, it causes a systemic poisoning that gives rise to a clinical picture similar to sarcoidosis. The major chronic problem is that of progressive dyspnoea with pulmonary fibrosis. However, strict control of levels in the working atmosphere have made the disease a rarity.

## Lung cysts

These may be congenital, bronchogenic cysts or may result from a sequestrated pulmonary segment. Hydatid disease causes fluid-filled cysts. Thin-walled cysts are due to lung abscesses, which are particularly found in staphylococcal pneumonia, tuberculous cavities, septic pulmonary infarction, primary bronchogenic carcinoma, cavitating metastatic neoplasm, or paragonimiasis caused by the lung fluke *Paragonimus westermani*.

## Tumours of the respiratory tract

Bronchial carcinoma accounts for 95% of all primary tumours of the lung. Alveolar cell carcinoma accounts for

2% of lung tumours and other less malignant or benign tumours account for the remaining 3%.

# BENIGN TUMOURS

### Pulmonary hamartoma
This is the most common benign tumour of the lung and is usually seen as a very well-defined round lesion 1–2 cm in diameter in the periphery of the lung. Growth is extremely slow, but the tumour may reach several centimetres in diameter. Rarely it arises from a major bronchus and causes obstruction.

### Bronchial carcinoid
This rare tumour resembles intestinal carcinoid tumour and is locally invasive, eventually spreading to mediastinal lymph nodes and finally to distant organs. It is a highly vascular tumour that projects into the lumen of a major bronchus causing recurrent haemoptysis. It grows slowly and eventually blocks the bronchus, leading to lobar collapse. Rarely, it gives rise to the carcinoid syndrome (see p. 214).

### Cylindroma, chondroma and lipoma
These are extremely rare tumours that may grow in the bronchus or trachea, causing obstruction.

# TRACHEAL TUMOURS

Primary tumours of the trachea are very rare—the relative incidence compared to laryngeal and bronchial tumours is 1 : 75 and 1 : 180 respectively. The majority are malignant. Benign tumours are extremely rare but include squamous papilloma, leiomyoma, haemangiomas and tumours of neurogenic origin.

### DIAGNOSIS AND TREATMENT
These tumours are diagnosed in the same way as bronchial carcinoma. Tracheal tumours cause severe and rapidly progressive dyspnoea and stridor. Flow–volume curves show typical and dramatic reductions in inspiratory flow (extrathoracic tracheal tumours) (see p. 637). Laser treatment provides rapid and effective destruction of tumour with temporary relief of symptoms. Radiotherapy is often given and occasionally surgery may be possible. The prognosis is very poor.

# MALIGNANT TUMOURS

## Bronchial carcinoma

This is the most common malignant tumour in the Western World and is now the third most common cause of death in the UK after heart disease and pneumonia. Mortality rates worldwide are highest in Scotland, closely followed by England and Wales. In the UK, 35 000 people die each year from bronchial carcinoma, with a male-to-female ratio of 3.5 : 1. Although the rising mortality from this disease has levelled off in men, it continues to rise in women, accounting for 1 in 8 of all deaths from malignant disease in women, second only to carcinoma of the breast.

The strength of the association between cigarette smoking and bronchial carcinoma overshadows any other aetiological factors (Table 12.14) but there is a higher incidence of bronchial carcinoma in urban compared with rural areas, even when allowance is made for cigarette smoking. Passive smoking (the inhalation of other people's smoke by non-smokers) increases the risk of bronchial carcinoma by a factor of 1.5. Occupational factors include exposure to asbestos, and an association is also claimed for workers in contact with arsenic, chromium, iron oxide, petroleum products and oils, coal tar, products of coal combustion, and radiation. Tumours associated with occupational factors are mostly adenocarcinomas and appear to be less related to cigarette smoking.

### CELL TYPES
Bronchial carcinoma is divided into small-cell carcinoma and non-small-cell carcinoma, a division based on the characteristics of the disease and its response to treatment. Studies of mean doubling times of carcinomas indicate that development from the initial malignant change to presentation takes many years; for adenocarcinoma it takes approximately 15 years, for squamous carcinoma 8 years and for small-cell carcinoma 3 years.

### Non-small-cell carcinoma
SQUAMOUS OR EPIDERMOID CARCINOMA is the commonest carcinoma in this group, accounting for approximately 40% of all carcinomas. It occasionally cavitates, and widespread metastases occur relatively late.

LARGE-CELL CARCINOMA represents a less well-differentiated tumour that metastasizes early. It accounts for 25% of all tumours.

ADENOCARCINOMA arises peripherally from mucous glands in the small bronchi and often produces a subpleural mass. Invasion of the pleura and the mediastinal lymph nodes is common, as are metastases to the brain

| | |
|---|---:|
| Non-smokers | 10 |
| Ex-smokers | 43 |
| Continuing smokers | |
|    Any tobacco | 104 |
|    Pipe/cigar | 58 |
|    Cigarette | 140 |
| Number of cigarettes | |
|    1–14 | 78 |
|    15–24    per day | 127 |
|    25 or more | 251 |

**Table 12.14**  Death rates from lung cancer (age standardized) per 100 000 according to tobacco consumption in male British doctors.

and bones. Adenocarcinoma accounts for approximately 10% of all bronchial carcinomas and frequently arises in or around scar tissue. It is the commonest bronchial carcinoma associated with asbestos and is proportionally more common in non-smokers, in women, in the elderly, and in the Far East.

ALVEOLAR CELL CARCINOMA (BRONCHIOLAR CARCINOMA) accounts for only 1–2% of lung tumours and occurs either as a peripheral solitary nodule or as diffuse nodular lesions of multicentric origin. Occasionally this tumour is associated with expectoration of very large volumes of mucoid sputum.

### Small-cell carcinoma
This tumour, often called oat-cell carcinoma, accounts for 20–30% of all lung cancers. It arises from endocrine cells (Kulchitsky cells). These cells are members of the APUD system, which explains why many polypeptide hormones are secreted by these tumours. Some of these polypeptides act in an autocrine fashion, i.e. they feed back on the cells and cause cell growth. Small-cell carcinoma is now considered to be a systemic disease. Although the tumour is rapidly growing and highly malignant, it is the only one of the bronchial carcinomas that responds to chemotherapy.

### CLINICAL FEATURES
The frequencies of the common symptoms of lung cancer on presentation are shown in Table 12.15. Chest pain and discomfort are often described as fullness and pressure in the chest. Sometimes the pain may be pleuritic owing to invasion of the pleura or ribs.

Commonly there are no abnormal physical signs. Enlarged supraclavicular lymph nodes are frequently found with small-cell carcinoma. There may be signs of a pleural effusion or of lobar collapse. Signs of an unresolved pneumonia or of associated underlying disease (e.g. diffuse pulmonary fibrosis in asbestosis) may be present.

### Direct spread
The tumour may directly involve the pleura and ribs. Carcinoma in the apex of the lung can erode the ribs and involve the lower part of the brachial plexus (C8, T1 and T2), causing severe pain in the shoulder and down the inner surface of the arm (Pancoast's tumour). The sympathetic ganglion may also be involved, producing Horner's syndrome (see p. 883). Further extension may involve the recurrent laryngeal nerve as it passes down the aortic arch, causing unilateral vocal cord paresis with hoarseness and a bovine cough, and rarely the tumour may cause spinal cord compression.

Bronchial carcinoma can also directly invade the phrenic nerve, causing paralysis of the diaphragm. It can involve the oesophagus, producing progressive dysphagia, and the pericardium, producing pericardial effusion and malignant dysrhythmias. It can also involve the superior vena cava, producing superior vena caval obstruction leading to early morning headache, facial congestion and oedema involving the upper limbs; the jugular veins are distended, as are the veins on the chest that form a collateral circulation with veins arising from the abdomen.

### Metastatic complications
Bony metastases are common, giving rise to severe pain and pathological fractures. There is frequent involvement of the liver. Secondary deposits in the brain present as a change in personality, epilepsy or a focal neurological lesion. Carcinoma of the bronchus is a cause of secondary deposits in the adrenal gland.

### Non-metastatic extrapulmonary manifestations
Although approximately 10% of small-cell tumours are thought to produce ectopic hormones at some stage, clinically important extrapulmonary manifestations are relatively rare apart from finger clubbing (Table 12.16).

Hypertrophic pulmonary osteoarthropathy (HPOA) (see also p. 411) occurs in approximately 3% of all bronchial carcinomas, particularly squamous-cell carcinomas and adenocarcinomas. Symptoms include joint stiffness and severe pain in the wrists and ankles, sometimes associated with gynaecomastia. X-rays show the characteristic proliferative periostitis at the distal ends of long bones, which have an onion-skin appearance. HPOA is invariably associated with clubbing of the fingers. It may regress after resection of the lung tumour or as a result of vagotomy at thoracotomy.

### INVESTIGATION
#### Chest X-ray
This is the most valuable screening test for bronchial carcinoma. It is a relatively insensitive test, however, since the tumour mass needs to be between 1 and 2 cm in size to be recognized reliably. CT scanning can identify small tumour masses (see Fig. 12.12), but is at present too time-consuming and expensive to replace the chest X-ray.

About 70% of all bronchial carcinomas arise centrally, the rest peripherally (particularly adenocarcinomas). At the time of clinical presentation the chest X-ray will demonstrate over 90% of carcinomas. A small proportion arise within the main bronchus or trachea or else present with metastatic or non-metastatic complications but with no detectable mass on the chest X-ray.

| Symptom | Frequency (%) |
|---|---|
| Cough | 41 |
| Chest pain | 22 |
| Cough and pain | 15 |
| Coughing blood | 7 |
| Chest infection | |
| Malaise | |
| Weight loss | |
| Shortness of breath | <5 each |
| Hoarseness | |
| Distant spread | |
| No symptoms | |

**Table 12.15** The frequency of the common presenting symptoms of bronchial carcinoma.

*Metabolic* (universal at some stage)
Loss of weight
Lassitude
Anorexia

*Endocrine* (10%) (usually small-cell carcinoma)
Ectopic adrenocorticotrophin syndrome
Syndrome of inappropriate secretion of antidiuretic hormone (SIADH)
Hypercalcaemia (usually squamous cell carcinoma)
Rarer—hypoglycaemia, thyrotoxicosis, gynaecomastia

*Neurological* (2–16%)
Encephalopathies—including subacute cerebellar degeneration
Myelopathies—motor neurone disease
Neuropathies—peripheral sensorimotor neuropathy
Muscular disorders—polymyopathy, myasthenic syndrome (Eaton–Lambert syndrome)

*Vascular and haematological* (rare)
Thrombophlebitis migrans
Non-bacterial thrombotic endocarditis
Microcytic and normocytic anaemia
Disseminated intravascular coagulopathy
Thrombotic thrombocytopenic purpura
Haemolytic anaemia

*Skeletal*
Clubbing (30%)
Hypertrophic osteoarthropathy (± gynaecomastia) (3%)

*Cutaneous* (rare)
Dermatomyositis
Acanthosis nigricans
Herpes zoster

**Table 12.16** Non-metastatic extrapulmonary manifestations of bronchial carcinoma (percentage of all cases).

Bronchial carcinoma can appear as round shadows on a chest X-ray (see p. 644). Characteristically the edge of the tumour has a fluffy or spiked appearance, though sometimes it may be entirely smooth with cavitation, particularly when the tumour is epidermoid in type. Carcinoma can also cause collapse of the lung.

Carcinoma causing partial obstruction of a bronchus interrupts the mucociliary escalator, and bacteria are retained within the affected lobe. This gives rise to the so-called secondary pneumonia that is commonly seen on a chest X-ray of a patient presenting with bronchial carcinoma.

The hilar lymph nodes on the side of the tumour are frequently involved in carcinoma of the lung. A large pleural effusion may also be present.

Carcinoma can spread through the lymphatic channels of the lung to give rise to lymphangitis carcinomatosa (Fig. 12.12d); this is usually unilateral and associated with striking dyspnoea. The chest X-ray shows streaky shadowing throughout the lung. This appearance may be seen in both lungs, particularly when it is due to metastatic spread, usually from tumours below the diaphragm (the stomach and colon) and from the breast.

## Computed tomography

CT is particularly useful for identifying pathological changes in the mediastinum (e.g. enlarged lymph nodes (see Fig. 12.12), local spread of the tumour) and for identifying secondary spread of carcinoma to the opposite lung by detecting masses too small to be seen on the chest X-ray. Lymph nodes larger than 1.5 cm are considered pathological, although whether they are due to metastatic tumour, reactive hyperplasia or previous lung disease (e.g. tuberculosis) can only be determined by biopsy. A normal CT scan prior to surgery excludes the need for mediastinoscopy and node biopsy. CT scanning should be extended to include the liver, adrenal glands and the brain to identify distant metastases if present.

## Magnetic resonance imaging

This may have some advantages over CT in mediastinal lesions when they are near to major vessels.

## Fibreoptic bronchoscopy (see p. 650)

This technique is used to obtain cytological specimens from peripheral lesions as well as to obtain biopsy evidence of any tumours seen. If the carcinoma involves the first 2 cm of either main bronchus, the tumour is inoperable. Widening and loss of the sharp angle of the carina indicates the presence of enlarged mediastinal lymph nodes, either malignant or reactive. They can be biopsied by passage of a needle through the bronchial wall. Vocal cord paresis on the left indicates involvement of the recurrent laryngeal nerve and inoperability.

## Transthoracic fine-needle aspiration biopsy

This involves the direct aspiration through the chest wall of peripheral lung lesions under appropriate X-ray or CT screening. Specimens can be obtained from 75% of peripheral lesions that could not be biopsied transbronchially. Pneumothorax occurs in 25% of patients, occasionally requiring drainage. Mild haemoptysis occurs in 5%. Implantation metastases do not occur.

## TREATMENT

Unlike some other cancers, there has been no improvement in survival from carcinoma of the bronchus apart from small cell cancer (see below). Only 20% of patients are alive 1 year after diagnosis and only 6–8% after 5 years (cf. 50% for breast or cervix).

## Surgery

The only treatment of any value for non-small-cell cancer of the lung is surgery. Only 20% of all cases are suitable for resection and only 25–30% survive for 5 years. The mortality of thoracotomy in patients over 65 years with metastatic disease exceeds the expected 5-year survival rate and should therefore be avoided.

PREOPERATIVE ASSESSMENT. Radionuclide scanning for detection of metastatic disease in liver and bone is rarely positive in the absence of symptoms or abnormal enzyme tests (serum alkaline phosphatase) and is therefore unnecessary. A normal chest CT scan indicates no mediastinal spread of the tumour and favours curative resection.

Because of their common aetiology, chronic bronchitis and emphysema are frequently present. An $FEV_1$ of less than 1.5 litres is not compatible with an active life following pneumonectomy, although the surgery itself can be successfully accomplished. This also applies when the gas-transfer test is reduced by 50%.

### Radiation therapy for cure

High-dose radiotherapy (6500 rad; 65 Gy) can produce results that are as good as those of surgery in patients who are fit and who have slowly growing squamous carcinoma. It is the treatment of choice if the tumour is inoperable for reasons such as poor lung function.

Radiation pneumonitis (defined as an acute infiltrate precisely confined to the radiation area and occurring within 3 months of radiotherapy) develops in 10–15%. Radiation fibrosis, a fibrotic change occurring within 1 year or so of radiotherapy and not precisely confined to the radiation area, occurs to some degree in all cases. These complications are usually of little importance.

### Symptomatic radiation treatment

Bone pain, haemoptysis and the superior vena cava syndrome respond favourably to irradiation in the short term.

### Chemotherapy

This is not effective for the treatment of non-small-cell cancer of the lung. In small-cell cancer, single or combination chemotherapy has resulted in a fivefold increase in median survival from 2 to 10 months. A small number of patients enjoy several years of remission. Good results have been achieved with the combination of mitomycin, ifosfamide and cisplatin (see p. 375). The unwanted effects are greater than with single-agent chemotherapy with etoposide alone, which should be reserved for elderly patients and those with additional medical or physical disabilities.

### Laser therapy, endobronchial irradiation and tracheobronchial stents

This is used in the palliation of inoperable lung cancer. The techniques are complementary and considerable skill is required both in deciding which single or combination of therapies is required and in their execution.

Tracheobronchial narrowing from intraluminal tumour or extrinsic compression causes disabling breathlessness, intractable cough and complications which may lead to death including infection, haemoptysis and respiratory failure. A neodymium–Yag (Nd–Yag) laser passed through a fibreoptic brochoscope can be used to vaporize inoperable fungating intraluminal carcinoma involving short segments of trachea or main bronchus. Benign tumours, strictures and vascular lesions can also be effectively treated with immediate relief of symptoms.

Endobronchial irradiation (brachytherapy) is useful for the treatment of both intraluminal tumour and malignant extrinsic compression. A radioactive source is afterloaded into a catheter placed adjacent to the carcinoma under fibreoptic bronchoscope control. Radiation dose falls rapidly with distance from the source minimizing damage to adjacent normal tissue. Reduction in endoscopically assessed tumour size occurs in 70–95% of cases.

Tracheobronchial stents made of silicone or as expandable metal springs are now available for insertion into strictures caused by tumour or from external compression or when there is weakening and collapse of the tracheobronchial wall.

### Terminal care (see p. 376)

Patients dying of cancer of the lung need attention to their overall well-being. They must not be ignored simply because they cannot be cured. A lot can be done to make the patient's remaining life symptom-free and as active as possible.

Daily treatment with prednisolone (up to 15 mg daily) may improve appetite. Morphine or diamorphine must be given regularly for pain, either in the form of a sustained-release morphine sulphate tablet twice daily or else as regular elixirs or injections. Many patients benefit from a continuous subcutaneous injection of opiates given by a pump. Candidiasis and other infections in the mouth are common and must be looked for and treated. Patients taking opiates are frequently constipated, so regular laxatives should be prescribed. Short courses of palliative radiotherapy for bone pain, severe cough or haemoptysis are helpful.

Both the patient and the relatives require counselling, a task that should be shared between nurses, social workers, hospital chaplains and doctors.

### SCREENING FOR LUNG CANCER

Screening programmes (yearly chest X-ray, 4-monthly sputum cytology) have been tried in high-risk groups but the success rate is minimal, underlining the need for prevention.

# Secondary tumours

Metastases in the lung are very common and usually present as round shadows 1.5–3 cm in diameter. They may be detected on chest X-ray in patients already diagnosed as having carcinoma. The primary is usually in the

- Kidney
- Prostate
- Breast
- Bone
- Gastrointestinal tract
- Cervix or ovary

They nearly always develop in the parenchyma and are often relatively asymptomatic even when the chest X-ray shows extensive pulmonary metastases. It is rare for metastases to develop in the bronchi, when they may present with haemoptysis.

Carcinoma, particularly of the stomach, pancreas and breast, can involve mediastinal glands and spread along the lymphatics of both lungs (lymphangitis carcinomatosa), which can lead to progressive and severe breathlessness. On the chest X-ray, bilateral lymphadeno-pathy is seen together with streaky basal shadowing fanning out over both lung fields.

Occasionally a pulmonary metastasis may be detected as a *solitary round shadow* on chest X-ray in an asymptomatic patient. The commonest primary tumour to do this is a renal carcinoma. The differential diagnosis includes:

- Primary bronchial carcinoma
- Tuberculoma
- Benign tumour of the lung
- Hydatid cyst

Single pulmonary metastases can be removed surgically but, as CT scans usually show the presence of small metastases undetected on chest X-ray, surgery is seldom performed.

# Disorders of the chest wall and pleura

## Trauma

Trauma to the thoracic wall can be due to penetrating wounds and can lead to pneumothoraces or haemothoraces.

### RIB FRACTURES

Rib fractures can be caused by trauma or coughing (particularly in the elderly), and can occur in patients with osteoporosis. Pathological rib fractures may be due to metastatic spread from carcinoma of the bronchus, breast, kidney, prostate and thyroid. Ribs can also become involved by a mesothelioma. Fractures may not be readily visible on a PA chest X-ray, and lateral X-rays and oblique views may be necessary.

Pain may prevent adequate chest expansion and coughing and this can lead to pneumonia.

Treatment is with adequate analgesia using oral agents or by local infiltration or an intercostal nerve block.

More than one fracture in one rib can lead to a flail segment with paradoxical movement, i.e. part of the chest wall moves inwards during inspiration. This can produce inefficient ventilation and may require intermittent positive-pressure ventilation.

### RUPTURE OF THE TRACHEA OR A MAJOR BRONCHUS

Rupture of the trachea or even a major bronchus can occur during deceleration injuries, leading to pneumothorax, surgical emphysema, pneumomediastinum and haemoptysis. Surgical emphysema is caused by air leaking into the subcutaneous connective tissue; this can also occur after the insertion of an intercostal drainage tube. A pneumomediastinum occurs when air leaks from the lung inside the parietal pleura and extends along the bronchial walls.

### RUPTURE OF THE OESOPHAGUS

Rupture of the oesophagus from external injury, endoscopic procedures, bougienage or necrotic carcinoma may lead to the serious complication of mediastinitis. This requires vigorous antibacterial chemotherapy.

### LUNG CONTUSION

This causes widespread fluffy shadows on the chest X-ray due to intrapulmonary haemorrhage. This may give rise to adult respiratory distress syndrome or shock lung (see p. 733).

## Kyphoscoliosis

Kyphoscoliosis may be congenital, idiopathic, due to disease of the vertebrae such as tuberculosis or osteomalacia, or due to neuromuscular disease such as Friedreich's ataxia or poliomyelitis. The respiratory effects of severe kyphoscoliosis are often more pronounced than might be expected and respiratory failure and death often occur in the fourth or fifth decade. The abnormality should be corrected at an early stage if possible. Bilevel positive airway pressure ventilation delivered through a tightly fitting nasal mask is the treatment of choice for respiratory failure (see p. 729).

## Ankylosing spondylitis (see p. 394)

Limitation of chest wall movement is often well compensated by diaphragmatic movement and the respiratory effects of this disease are relatively mild. It is associated with upper lobe fibrosis of unknown aetiology.

## Pectus excavatum and carinatum

Pectus excavatum causes few problems other than embarrassment due to the deep vertical furrow in the chest, which can be corrected surgically. The heart is seen to lie well to the left on the chest X-ray. Pectus carinatum (pigeon chest) is often the result of rickets. No treatment is required.

## Dry pleurisy

'Dry pleurisy' is the term used to describe pleurisy when there is inflammation but no appreciable effusion. The localized inflammation produces sharp localized pain, made worse on deep inspiration, coughing and occasionally on twisting and bending movements. Common causes are pneumonia, pulmonary infarct and carcinoma. Rarer causes are rheumatoid arthritis and systemic lupus erythematosus.

EPIDEMIC MYALGIA (BORNHOLM DISEASE) is due to infection by Coxsackie B virus. This illness is common in young adults in the late summer and autumn and is characterized by an upper respiratory tract illness followed by pleuritic pain in the chest and upper abdomen with tender muscles. The chest X-ray remains normal and the illness clears within 1 week.

# Pleural effusion

A pleural effusion is an excessive accumulation of fluid in the pleural space. It can be detected on X-ray when 300 ml or more of fluid is present and clinically when 500 ml or more is present. The chest X-ray appearances range from the obliteration of the costophrenic angle to dense homogeneous shadows occupying part or all of the hemithorax. Fluid below the lung (a subpulmonary effusion) can simulate a raised hemidiaphragm. Fluid in the fissures may resemble an intrapulmonary mass. The physical signs are shown in Table 12.1.

## DIAGNOSIS
This is by pleural aspiration (see p. 649). The fluid that accumulates may be a transudate or an exudate.

TRANSUDATES. Effusions that are transudates can be bilateral. The protein content is less than 30 g litre$^{-1}$ and the lactic dehydrogenase is less than 200 IU litre$^{-1}$. Causes include:
- Heart failure
- Hypoproteinaemia (e.g. nephrotic syndrome)
- Constrictive pericarditis
- Hypothyroidism
- Ovarian tumours producing right-sided pleural effusion—Meigs' syndrome

EXUDATES. The protein content of exudates is greater than 30 g litre$^{-1}$ and the lactic dehydrogenase is greater than 200 IU litre$^{-1}$. Causes include:
- Bacterial pneumonia (common)
- Carcinoma of the bronchus (common) ⎫
- Pulmonary infarction (common) ⎬ Fluid may be blood-stained
  ⎭
- Tuberculosis
- Connective-tissue disease
- Post-myocardial infarction syndrome (rare)
- Acute pancreatitis (high amylase content) (rare)
- Mesothelioma (rare)
- Sarcoidosis (very rare)
- Yellow-nail syndrome (effusion due to lymph-oedema) (rare)
- Familial Mediterranean fever (rare)

Pleural biopsy (see p. 649) may be necessary to diagnose the cause of the effusion. Treatment is of the underlying condition.

## MALIGNANT PLEURAL EFFUSIONS
Malignant pleural effusions that reaccumulate and are symptomatic can be aspirated to *dryness* followed by the instillation of a sclerosing agent such as tetracycline or bleomycin. Effusions should be drained slowly since rapid shift of the mediastinum causes severe pain and occasionally shock. This treatment produces only temporary relief.

# Chylothorax

This is due to the accumulation of lymph in the pleural space, usually resulting from leakage from the thoracic duct due to trauma or to infiltration by carcinoma.

# Empyema

This is the presence of pus in the pleural space and can be a complication of pneumonia (see p. 682).

# Pneumothorax

'Pneumothorax' means air in the pleural space. It may occur due to trauma to the chest or may be spontaneous. Pneumothorax may be localized if the visceral pleura has previously undergone adhesion to the parietal pleura, or generalized if the whole hemithorax contains air. Normally the pressure in the pleural space is negative but this is lost once a communication is made with atmospheric pressure; the elastic recoil pressure of the lung then causes it to partially deflate. If the communication between the airways and the pleural space remains (an open pneumothorax), a bronchopleural fistula is created. Once the communication between the lung and the pleural space is obliterated, air will be reabsorbed at a rate of 1.25% of the total radiographic volume of the hemithorax per day. Thus, a 50% collapse of the lung will take 40 days to reabsorb completely once the pneumothorax is closed.

It has been postulated that a valvular mechanism may develop through which air can be sucked during inspiration but not expelled during expiration. The intrapleural pressure remains positive throughout breathing, the lung deflates further, the mediastinum shifts, and venous return to the heart decreases, with increasing respiratory and cardiac embarrassment. This tension pneumothorax is very rare unless the patient is on positive ventilation.

### Spontaneous pneumothorax
This usually occurs in young males, the male-to-female ratio being 6 : 1. It is caused by the rupture of a pleural bleb, usually apical, and is thought to be due to congenital defects in the connective tissue of the alveolar walls. Both lungs are affected with equal frequency. Often these patients are tall and thin.

In patients over 40 years of age, the usual cause is underlying chronic bronchitis and emphysema. Rarer causes include bronchial asthma, carcinoma, a lung abscess breaking down and leading to bronchopleural fistula, and severe pulmonary fibrosis with cyst formation.

The sudden onset of unilateral pleuritic pain or increasing breathlessness are the usual presenting features. If the pneumothorax enlarges, the patient becomes more breathless and may develop pallor and tachycardia. There may be few physical signs if the pneumothorax is small. The characteristic features and management are shown in Fig. 12.42. The main aim is to get the patient back to active life as soon as possible.

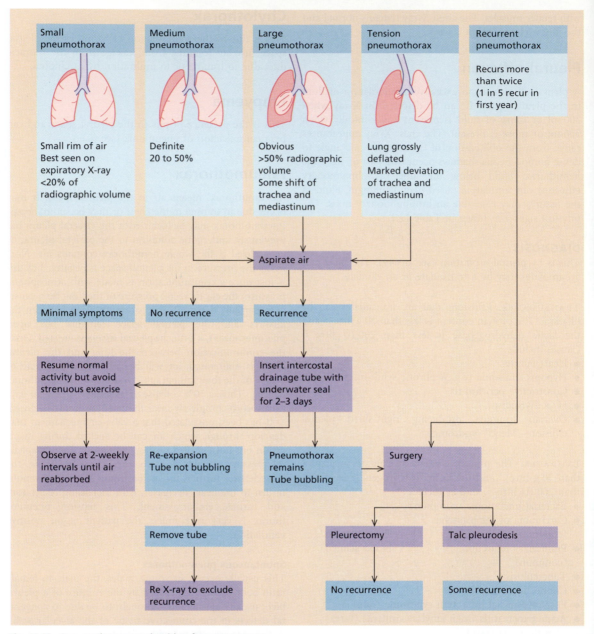

**Fig. 12.42**   Pneumothorax: an algorithm for management.

Infiltrate 2% lignocaine down to the pleura in the
second intercostal space in the mid-clavicular line

Push a 3–4 cm 16 French gauge cannula through the
pleura

Connect cannula to a three-way tap and 50 ml syringe

Aspirate up to 2.5 litres air—stop if resistance to suction
felt or patient coughs excessively

Repeat chest X-ray (in exspiration) in the X-ray
department

**Practical box 12.6**   Simple aspiration.

The procedure for simple aspiration is shown in
Practical box 12.6.

## Disorders of the diaphragm

### Diaphragmatic fatigue

The diaphragm can become fatigued if the force of contraction during inspiration exceeds 40% of the force it
can develop in a maximal static effort. When this occurs

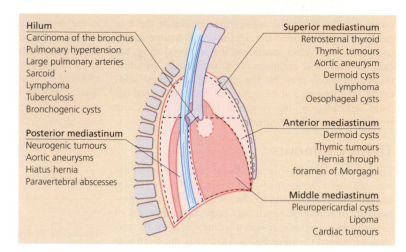

**Hilum**
Carcinoma of the bronchus
Pulmonary hypertension
Large pulmonary arteries
Sarcoid
Lymphoma
Tuberculosis
Bronchogenic cysts

**Posterior mediastinum**
Neurogenic tumours
Aortic aneurysms
Hiatus hernia
Paravertebral abscesses

**Superior mediastinum**
Retrosternal thyroid
Thymic tumours
Aortic aneurysm
Dermoid cysts
Lymphoma
Oesophageal cysts

**Anterior mediastinum**
Dermoid cysts
Thymic tumours
Hernia through
foramen of Morgagni

**Middle mediastinum**
Pleuropericardial cysts
Lipoma
Cardiac tumours

**Fig. 12.43**  Subdivisions of the mediastinum and mass lesions.

acutely in patients with exacerbations of chronic airflow limitation or CF or in quadriplegics, positive-pressure ventilation is required followed by attempts to increase the strength and endurance of the diaphragm by breathing against a resistance for 30 min a day.

UNILATERAL DIAPHRAGMATIC PARALYSIS is common and symptomless. The affected diaphragm is usually elevated and moves paradoxically on inspiration. A sniff causes the paralysed diaphragm to rise, the unaffected diaphragm to descend. Causes include:

- Surgery
- Carcinoma of the bronchus with involvement of the phrenic nerve
- Neurological, including poliomyelitis, herpes zoster
- Trauma to cervical spine, birth injury, subclavian vein puncture
- Infection: tuberculosis, syphilis, pneumonia

BILATERAL DIAPHRAGMATIC WEAKNESS or paralysis causes breathlessness in the supine position and is a cause of sleep apnoea leading to daytime headaches and somnolence. Tidal volume is decreased and respiratory rate increased. Vital capacity is substantially reduced when lying down, and sniffing causes a paradoxical inward movement of the abdominal wall best seen in the supine position. Causes include viral infections, multiple sclerosis, motor neurone disease, poliomyelitis, Guillain–Barré syndrome, quadriplegia after trauma and rare muscle diseases. Treatment is either diaphragmatic pacing or night-time assisted ventilation.

COMPLETE EVENTRATION OF THE DIAPHRAGM (invariably left-sided) is a congenital condition in which muscle is replaced by fibrous tissue. It presents as marked elevation of the left hemidiaphragm, sometimes associated with gastrointestinal symptoms. Partial eventration, usually on the right, causes a hump (often anteriorly) on the diaphragmatic shadow on X-ray.

HERNIAS occur through the diaphragm, the commonest being through the oesophageal hiatus, but occasionally anteriorly, through the foramen of Morgani, posterolaterally through the foramen of Bochdalek or at any site following traumatic tears.

HICCUPS —see p. 175.

## Mediastinal lesions

The mediastinum is defined as the region between the pleural sacs. It is additionally divided as shown in Fig. 12.43. Tumours affecting the mediastinum are rare. Masses are detected very accurately on CT scan (Fig 12.44).

### Retrosternal or intrathoracic thyroid

The commonest mediastinal tumour is a retrosternal or intrathoracic thyroid, which is nearly always an extension of the thyroid present in the neck. Enlargement of the thyroid by a colloid goitre or malignant disease and,

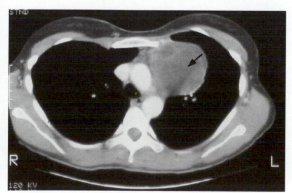

**Fig. 12.44**  CT scan of a dermoid cyst in the mediastinum.

rarely, in thyrotoxicosis causes displacement of the trachea and oesophagus to the opposite side. Symptoms of compression develop insidiously before producing the cardinal feature of dyspnoea. Very occasionally an intrathoracic thyroid may be the cause of dysphagia and, rarely, of hoarseness of the voice and vocal cord paralysis from stretching of the recurrent laryngeal nerve. The treatment is surgical removal.

## Thymic tumours

The thymus is large in childhood and occupies the superior and anterior mediastinum. It involutes with age but may be enlarged both by cysts, which are rarely symptomatic, or tumours, which may cause the symptoms of myasthenia gravis or may lead to compression of the trachea or, rarely, the oesophagus. Surgery is the treatment of choice. Approximately half of the patients presenting with a thymic tumour have myasthenia gravis.

## Pleuro-pericardial cysts

These cysts, which may be up to 10 cm in diameter, are filled with clear fluid and are usually situated anteriorly in the cardiophrenic angle on the right in 70% of cases. Infection only rarely occurs; malignant change does not occur. The diagnosis is usually made by needle aspiration. No treatment is required, but these patients should be followed up as an increase in cyst size suggests an alternative pathology; surgical excision is then advisable.

# Further reading

Davies RJ & Ollier S (1989) *Allergy: the Facts.* Oxford: Oxford University Press.

Miller AC & Harvey JE (1993) Guidelines for the management of spontaneous pneumothorax. *British Medical Journal* **307**, 114–116.

Weinberger SE (1993) Medical Progress: Recent advances in pulmonary medicine. *New England Journal of Medicine* **328**, 1389–1397 and 1462–1470.

## Introduction

Intensive care medicine (or 'critical care medicine') is concerned predominantly with the management of patients with acute life-threatening conditions ('the critically ill') in a specialized unit. It also encompasses the resuscitation and transport of those who become acutely ill, or are injured, either elsewhere in the hospital or in the community. As well as emergency cases, intensive care units admit high-risk patients electively after major surgery (Table 13.1).

An intensive care unit is fully equipped with monitoring and technical facilities, including an adjacent laboratory for the rapid determination of blood gases and simple biochemical data such as serum potassium and blood glucose. Patients can receive continuous expert nursing care and the constant attention of appropriately trained medical staff. These conditions and facilities are not available on a general ward. Teamwork and a multidisciplinary approach is central to the provision of intensive care and is most effective when directed and coordinated by a committed specialist. In the UK about 1% of the acute beds in the hospital are usually allocated to intensive care, but elsewhere in the developed world the proportion is often much higher.

In all critically ill patients, the immediate objective is to preserve life and prevent, reverse or minimize damage to vital organs such as the brain and the kidneys. This is achieved by supporting cardiovascular and respiratory function in order to maximize delivery of oxygen to the tissues.

This chapter concentrates on cardiovascular and respiratory problems. Many patients have failure of other organs such as the kidney and liver as well; treatment of these is dealt with in more detail in the appropriate chapters. Feeding the critically ill patient is discussed further in Chapter 3.

*Emergency surgical*
Acute intra-abdominal catastrophe
  Ruptured/leaking abdominal aortic aneurysm
  Perforated viscus, especially with faecal soiling of
    peritoneum (often complicated by septic shock)

Trauma (often complicated by hypovolaemic and
  later septic shock)
  Multiple injuries
  Massive blood loss
  Severe head injury

*Elective surgical*
  Extensive/prolonged procedure, e.g.
    oesophagogastrectomy
  Major head and neck surgery
  Coexisting cardiovascular or respiratory disease

*Emergency medical*
Respiratory failure
  Exacerbation of chronic bronchitis
  Pneumonia (may be complicated by septic shock)

Drug overdose

Postcardiopulmonary resuscitation (may be
  complicated by cardiogenic shock)

**Table 13.1** Some common indications for admission to intensive care.

# Oxygen delivery

Oxygen delivery (oxygen flux) is defined as the total amount of oxygen delivered to the tissues per unit time. It is dependent on the volume of blood flowing through the microcirculation per minute (i.e. the total cardiac output—$\dot{Q}_t$) and the amount of oxygen contained in that blood (i.e. the arterial oxygen content—$C_aO_2$). Oxygen is transported in combination with haemoglobin or dissolved in plasma. The amount combined with haemoglobin is determined by the oxygen capacity of the haemoglobin (usually taken as 1.34 ml $O_2$ per gram of haemoglobin) and its percentage saturation with oxygen ($SO_2$), while the volume dissolved in plasma depends on the partial pressure of oxygen ($PO_2$). Except when hyperbaric oxygen is administered, the amount of dissolved oxygen in plasma is sufficiently small to be ignored for most practical purposes.

Clinically, however, the concept of oxygen flux provides little information about the relative flow to individual organs. Furthermore, some organs have high oxygen requirements relative to their blood flow and may become hypoxic even if the overall oxygen flux is apparently adequate.

# CARDIAC OUTPUT

Cardiac output is the product of heart rate and stroke volume, and is affected by changes in either (Fig. 13.1).

## Heart rate

### Increased heart rate

When heart rate increases, the duration of systole remains essentially unchanged, whereas diastole, and thus the time available for ventricular filling, becomes progressively shorter, and the stroke volume eventually falls. In the normal heart this occurs at rates greater than about 160 beats per minute, but in those with cardiac pathology, especially when this restricts ventricular filling (e.g. mitral stenosis), stroke volume may fall at much lower heart rates. Furthermore, tachycardias cause a marked increase in myocardial oxygen consumption and this may precipitate ischaemia in areas of the myocardium that have reduced coronary perfusion.

### Decreased heart rate

When the heart rate falls, a point is reached at which the increase in stroke volume is insufficient to compensate for the bradycardia and again cardiac output falls.

Alterations in heart rate are often caused by disturbances of rhythm (e.g. artrial fibrillation, complete heart block or junctional arrhythmias), in which ventricular filling is not augmented by atrial contraction and stroke volume therefore falls.

## Stroke volume

Three factors determine the stroke volume: pre-load, myocardial contractility and after-load (see p. 569).

### Pre-load

This is defined as the tension of the myocardial fibres at the end of diastole, just before the onset of ventricular contraction, and is therefore related to the degree of stretch of the fibres (Fig. 13.2). As the end-diastolic volume of the ventricle increases, tension in the myocardial fibres is increased and stroke volume rises (Fig. 13.3).

Myocardial oxygen consumption ($\dot{V}_m o_2$) increases only slightly with an increase in pre-load and this is therefore the most efficient way of improving cardiac output.

### Myocardial contractility

This refers to the ability of the heart to perform work, independent of changes in pre-load and after-load.

The state of myocardial contractility determines the response of the ventricles to changes in pre-load and

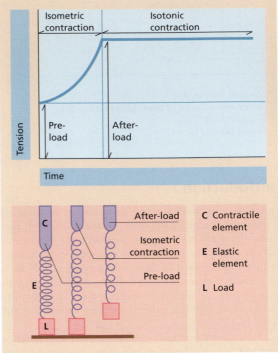

**Fig. 13.2** The relationship between myocardial tension and contraction. 'Pre-load' is the tension of the myocardial fibres prior to the onset of systole and depends on the degree to which they are passively stretched. During isometric contraction, the tension in the contractile elements increases. The tension required to open the aortic valve and eject blood from the ventricle is 'after-load'.

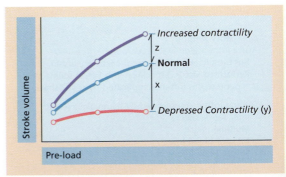

**Fig. 13.3** Ventricular function (Starling curve). As pre-load is increased, stroke volume rises. If the ventricle is overstretched, stroke volume will fall (x). In myocardial failure, the curve is depressed and flattened (y). Increasingly contractility shifts the curve upwards and to the left (z).

after-load. Contractility is often reduced in intensive care patients, either as a result of pre-existing myocardial damage, e.g. ischaemic heart disease, or the acute disease process itself. Changes in myocardial contractility alter the slope and position of the Starling curve; the resulting worsening ventricular performance is manifested as a depressed, flattened curve (Fig. 13.3).

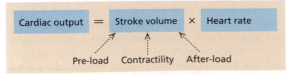

**Fig. 13.1** The determinants of cardiac output.

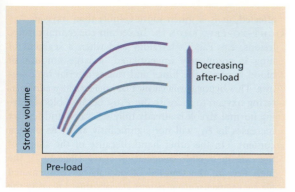

**Fig. 13.4** The effect of changes in after-load on the ventricular function curve. At any given pre-load, decreasing after-load increases the stroke volume.

### After-load

This is defined as the myocardial wall tension developed during systolic ejection (Fig. 13.2). In the case of the left ventricle the resistance imposed by the aortic valve, the peripheral vascular resistance and the elasticity of the major blood vessels are important determinants of after-load.

*Decreasing* the after-load can increase the stroke volume achieved at a given pre-load (Fig. 13.4), whilst also reducing the ventricular wall tension and the myocardial oxygen consumption. The reduction in wall tension may lead to an increase in coronary blood flow, thereby improving the myocardial oxygen supply–demand ratio. Excessive reductions in after-load will cause hypotension.

An *increase* in after-load, on the other hand, can cause a fall in stroke volume and is a potent cause of increased $V_mO_2$. Right ventricular after-load is normally negligible

because the resistance of the pulmonary circulation is very low.

## OXYGENATION OF THE BLOOD

Oxygen content ($C_aO_2$) is dependent on the amount of haemoglobin present per unit volume of blood, its oxygen capacity and its percentage saturation with oxygen. For this reason, maintenance of an 'adequate' haemoglobin concentration is essential in critically ill patients. Tissue oxygenation is, however, also dependent on blood flow. This is in turn determined not only by the cardiac output and its distribution, but also by the viscosity of the blood. The latter depends largely on the packed cell volume (PCV) and it is generally considered that the optimal balance between oxygen-carrying capacity and tissue flow is achieved at a PCV of approximately 30–35%.

## Oxyhaemoglobin dissociation curve

The saturation of haemoglobin with oxygen is determined by the partial pressure of oxygen ($P_{O_2}$) in the blood, the relationship between the two being described by the oxyhaemoglobin dissociation curve (Fig. 13.5). The sigmoid shape of this curve is important clinically for a number of reasons:

- Falls in $P_aO_2$ may be tolerated provided that the percentage saturation remains above 90%.
- Increasing the $P_aO_2$ to above normal has only a minimal effect on oxygen content unless hyperbaric oxygen is administered (when the amount of oxygen in solution in plasma becomes significant).
- Once on the steep 'slippery slope' of the curve, a small decrease in $P_aO_2$ can cause large falls in oxygen content, while increasing $P_aO_2$ only slightly (e.g. by adminis-

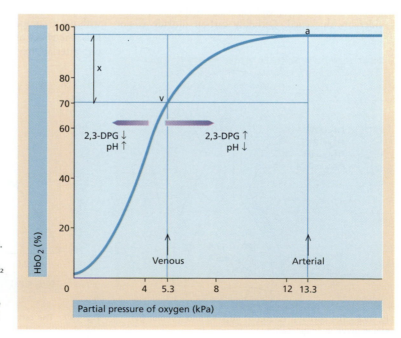

**Fig. 13.5** The oxyhaemoglobin dissociation curve: a, arterial point; v, venous point; x, arteriovenous oxygen content difference. The curve will move to the right in the presence of acidosis (metabolic or respiratory), pyrexia or an increased red cell 2,3-DPG concentration. For a given arteriovenous oxygen content difference, the mixed venous $P_{O_2}$ will then be higher. Furthermore, if the mixed venous $P_{O_2}$ is unchanged, the arteriovenous oxygen content difference increases and more oxygen is off-loaded to the tissues (see p. 296).

tering 28% oxygen to a patient with chronic bronchitis) can lead to useful increases in oxygen saturation.

The $P_{a}O_2$ is in turn influenced by the alveolar oxygen tension ($P_{A}O_2$), the efficiency of pulmonary gas exchange, and the partial pressure of oxygen in mixed venous blood ($P_{\bar{v}}O_2$).

### Alveolar oxygen tension

The partial pressures of inspired gases are shown in Fig. 13.6. By the time the inspired gases reach the alveoli they are fully saturated with water vapour at body temperature (37°C), which has a partial pressure of 6.3 kPa (47 mmHg) and contains $CO_2$ at a partial pressure of approximately 5.3 kPa (40 mmHg). The $P_{A}O_2$ is thereby reduced to approximately 13.4 kPa (100 mmHg).

The clinician can influence $P_{A}O_2$ by administering oxygen or increasing the barometric pressure (i.e. administering hyperbaric oxygen). Because of the reciprocal relationship between the partial pressures of oxygen and carbon dioxide in the alveoli, a small increase in $P_{A}O_2$ can be produced by lowering the $P_{A}CO_2$ (e.g. using mechanical ventilation).

### Pulmonary gas exchange

In *normal* subjects there is a small alveolar–arterial oxygen difference ($P_{A-a}O_2$). This is due to:

- A small (0.133 kPa, 1 mmHg) pressure gradient across the alveolar membrane
- A small amount of blood (2% of total cardiac output) bypassing the lungs via the bronchial and thebesian veins
- A small ventilation/perfusion mismatch

*Pathologically* there are three causes of a $P_{A-a}O_2$ difference:

DIFFUSION DEFECT. This is not an important cause of hypoxaemia even in conditions such as fibrosing alveolitis, in which the alveolar capillary membrane is considerably thickened. Certainly carbon dioxide is not affected, as it is much more soluble than oxygen.

RIGHT-TO-LEFT SHUNTS. In certain congenital cardiac lesions, e.g. Fallot's tetralogy and when a segment of lung is completely unventilated, a large amount of blood bypasses the lungs and causes arterial hypoxaemia. This hypoxaemia cannot be corrected by administering oxygen to increase the $P_{A}O_2$, because blood leaving normal alveoli is already fully saturated and further increases in $P_{O_2}$ will not significantly affect its oxygen content. On the other hand, because of the shape of the carbon dioxide dissociation curve (Fig. 13.7), the high $P_{CO_2}$ of the shunted blood can be compensated for by overventilating patent alveoli, thus lowering the $CO_2$ content of the effluent blood. Indeed, many patients with acute right-to-left shunts hyperventilate in response to the hypoxia or stimulation of mechanoreceptors in the lung, so that the $P_{a}CO_2$ is normal or low.

VENTILATION/PERFUSION ($\dot{V}/\dot{Q}$) MISMATCH. This is discussed in more detail in Chapter 12. Diseases of the lung parenchyma result in a $\dot{V}/\dot{Q}$ mismatch, producing an increase in alveolar dead space and hypoxaemia. The former can be compensated for by increasing overall ventilation. In contrast to the hypoxia resulting from a true right-to-left shunt (see above), that due to areas of low $\dot{V}/\dot{Q}$ can be partially corrected by administering oxygen and thereby increasing the $P_{A}O_2$ even in poorly ventilated areas of lung.

### Mixed venous $P_{O_2}$ ($P_{\bar{v}}O_2$)

This is the partial pressure of oxygen in pulmonary arterial blood that has been thoroughly mixed during its passage through the heart. If $P_{a}O_2$ remains constant, the $P_{\bar{v}}O_2$ will fall if more oxygen has to be extracted from each unit volume of blood arriving at the tissues. A fall in $P_{\bar{v}}O_2$ therefore indicates that either oxygen delivery has fallen or that tissue oxygen requirements have increased without a compensatory rise in cardiac output. If $P_{\bar{v}}O_2$ falls, the effect of a given degree of pulmonary shunting on arterial oxygenation will be exacerbated. Thus,

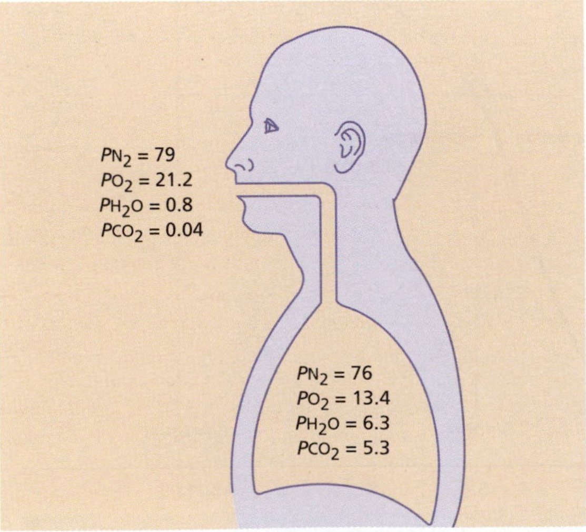

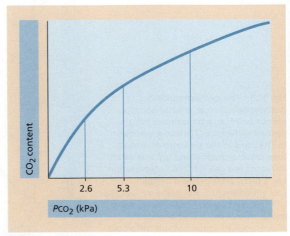

**Fig. 13.6** The partial pressures of inspired and alveolar gas (values given in kilopascals).

$PN_2 = 79$
$PO_2 = 21.2$
$PH_2O = 0.8$
$PCO_2 = 0.04$

$PN_2 = 76$
$PO_2 = 13.4$
$PH_2O = 6.3$
$PCO_2 = 5.3$

**Fig. 13.7** The carbon dioxide dissociation curve. Note that in the physiological range the curve is essentially linear.

worsening arterial hypoxaemia does not necessarily indicate a deterioration in pulmonary function but may instead reflect a fall in cardiac output and/or a rise in oxygen consumption.

The $P_{\bar{v}}O_2$ is also influenced by the position of the oxyhaemoglobin dissociation curve (see Fig. 13.5), a factor not incorporated in the concept of oxygen flux. Thus, if the arteriovenous oxygen content difference remains constant, a shift of the curve to the right, which occurs with acidosis, hypercarbia, pyrexia and a rise in red cell 2,3-diphosphoglycerate (2,3-DPG) levels, may cause the $P_{\bar{v}}O_2$ to rise. If the $P_{\bar{v}}O_2$ remains unchanged, more oxygen will be unloaded at tissue level. A shift of the curve to the left, on the other hand, will cause a fall in the $P_{\bar{v}}O_2$. It might be argued, then, that under certain circumstances an acidosis may be beneficial in terms of tissue oxygenation, provided that it is not severe enough to interfere with cardiac function. It is probable though, that shifts of the dissociation curve are of little clinical significance.

# Acute disturbances of haemodynamic function (shock)

Shock is difficult to define. The term is used to describe acute circulatory failure with inadequate or inappropriately distributed tissue perfusion resulting in generalized cellular hypoxia.

## Causes
The causes are shown in Table 13.2. Very often shock can result from a combination of these factors.

# PATHOPHYSIOLOGY
## Sympatho-adrenal response to shock (Fig. 13.8)

Hypotension stimulates the baroreceptors, and to a lesser extent the chemoreceptors, causing increased sympathetic nervous activity. Later this is augmented by the release of catecholamines from the adrenal medulla. The resulting vasoconstriction, together with increased myocardial contractility and heart rate, helps to restore blood pressure and cardiac output.

Reduction in perfusion of the renal cortex stimulates the juxtaglomerular apparatus to release renin. This converts angiotensinogen to angiotensin I, which is in turn converted in the lungs to the potent vasoconstrictor angiotensin II. Angiotensin II also stimulates secretion of aldosterone by the adrenal cortex, causing sodium and water retention. This helps to restore the circulating volume.

## Neuroendocrine response to shock

RELEASE OF PITUITARY HORMONES: adrenocorticotrophic hormone (ACTH), growth hormone (GH), vasopressin (antidiuretic hormone, ADH) and $\beta$-endorphin. (Endogenous opioid peptides such as $\beta$-endorphin, dynorphin and the enkephalins may be partly responsible for some of the cardiovascular changes.)

RELEASE OF CORTISOL, which causes fluid retention and antagonizes insulin.

RELEASE OF GLUCAGON, which raises blood sugar.

## Release of mediators

The presence of severe infection (often with bacteraemia or endotoxaemia) or of large areas of devitalized tissue (e.g. following trauma or major surgery) can trigger a massive inflammatory response with systemic activation of leucocytes and release of a variety of potentially damaging 'mediators'. Although clearly beneficial when targeted against local areas of infection or necrotic tissue, dissemination of this response can produce widespread tissue damage.

### Microorganisms and their toxic products
In septic shock the inflammatory cascade is triggered by the presence of microorganisms, their toxic products (e.g. endotoxin) or both in the bloodstream. Endotoxin is a lipopolysaccharide derived from the cell wall of Gram-negative bacteria which is thought to be a particularly important trigger of septic shock.

### Activation of complement cascade
One of the many functions of the complement system is to attract and activate leucocytes, which then marginate on to endothelium and release inflammatory mediators such as proteases and toxic oxygen radicals; these can produce local tissue damage. For example, the free radical superoxide ($O_2^-$) can participate in a number of chemical reactions, yielding hydrogen peroxide ($H_2O_2$) and hydroxyl radicals ($OH^-$), which can damage cell membranes, interfere with the function of a number of enzyme systems and increase capillary permeability.

### Cytokines
Macrophage and lymphocyte-derived cytokines such as the interleukins (ILs) and tumour necrosis factor (TNF)

| |
|---|
| Cardiogenic (e.g. ischaemic cardiac damage) |
| Mechanical<br>Obstruction to outflow (e.g. pulmonary embolus)<br>Restricted cardiac filling (e.g. cardiac tamponade) |
| Peripheral circulation<br>Hypovolaemic<br>  Exogenous losses (e.g. haemorrhage, burns)<br>  Endogenous losses (e.g. sepsis, anaphylaxis)<br>Normovolaemic<br>  Dilatation<br>  Sequestration          (e.g. sepsis,<br>  Arteriovenous shunting    anaphylaxis)<br>  Maldistribution of flow |

**Table 13.2**  Causes of shock.

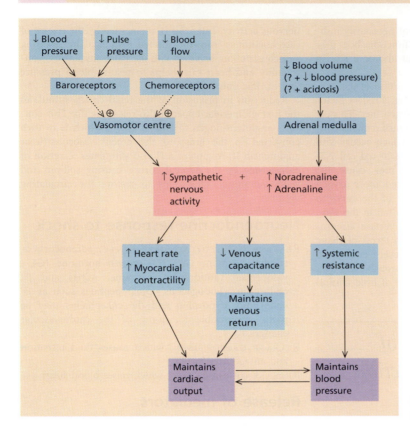

Fig. 13.8   The sympatho-adrenal response to shock.

are involved in the pathogenesis of shock. TNF release initiates many of the responses to endotoxin and acts synergistically with IL-1, in part through induction of cyclo-oxygenase, platelet activating factor (PAF) and nitric oxide synthase (see below).

**Platelet-activating factor**
This vasoactive lipid is released from various cell populations, such as leucocytes and macrophages, in shock. Its effects, which are caused both directly and through the secondary release of other mediators, include hypotension, increased vascular permeability and platelet aggregation.

**Products of arachidonic acid metabolism**
(see Fig. 12.30)
Arachidonic acid, derived from the increased breakdown of membrane phospholipid, is metabolized to form prostaglandins and leukotrienes, which are important inflammatory mediators. Prostaglandins currently thought to be of importance in shock include:
● Prostacyclin, which is a vasodilator and inhibits platelet aggregation
● Thromboxane $A_2$, which causes pulmonary vasoconstriction and activates platelets
● Prostaglandin $F_{2\alpha}$, which may be responsible for the early phase of pulmonary hypertension commonly seen in experimental septic shock
Leukotrienes have a variety of effects including a

reduction in cardiac output, vasoconstriction, increased vascular permeability and platelet activation.

**Lysosomal enzymes**
These are released in response to hypoxia, ischaemia, sepsis and acidosis. As well as being directly cytotoxic, they can cause myocardial depression and coronary vasoconstriction. Furthermore, lysosomal enzymes can convert inactive kininogens, which are usually combined with $\alpha_2$-globulin, to vasoactive kinins such as bradykinin. These substances can cause vasodilatation and increased capillary permeability, as well as myocardial depression. They can also activate clotting mechanisms.

**Endothelium-derived vasoactive mediators**
Endothelial cells synthesize a number of mediators which contribute to the regulation of blood vessel tone and the fluidity of the blood; these include prostacyclin, endothelin-1 and endothelium-derived relaxing factor (EDRF). The latter has now been identified as nitric oxide (NO) which is synthesized from L-arginine under the influence of NO synthases. Increased NO production is responsible for the sustained vasodilatation and hyporeactivity to adrenergic agonists which is seen in septic shock and may also be involved in severe haemorrhagic/traumatic shock. Endothelin-1 is a potent vasoconstrictor, but its role in shock is not yet well understood.

**Endothelial leucocyte adhesion molecule**

This molecule is expressed on endothelial cells after exposure to inflammatory mediators, including TNF, and is involved in the adhesion of polymorphonuclear cells to the endothelium. This is considered to be one of the earliest steps in the cascade of events leading to tissue damage and adhesion molecules may therefore play an important role in the pathogenesis of organ failure.

## Microcirculatory changes

Since shock is a syndrome caused by inadequate tissue perfusion, the final common pathway for the pathophysiological changes is the microcirculation.

In the *early stages of septic shock* there is vasodilatation, maldistribution of flow, arteriovenous shunting and increased capillary permeability with interstitial oedema. Although these microvascular abnormalities may largely account for the reduced oxygen extraction often seen in septic shock there may also be a primary defect of cellular oxygen utilization. Initially, before hypovolaemia supervenes, or when therapeutic replacement of circulating volume has been adequate, cardiac output is usually high and peripheral resistance low. Vasodilatation and increased capillary permeability also occur in anaphylactic shock.

In the initial stages of *other forms of shock*, and sometimes when hypovolaemia supervenes in sepsis and anaphylaxis, increased sympathetic activity causes constriction of both precapillary arterioles and, to a lesser extent, the postcapillary venules. This helps to maintain the systemic blood pressure. In addition, the hydrostatic pressure within the capillaries falls and fluid is mobilized from the extravascular space into the intravascular compartment. If shock persists, the accumulation of metabolites, such as lactic acid and carbon dioxide, combined with the release of vasoactive substances, causes relaxation of the precapillary sphincters, while the postcapillary venules, which are more sensitive to hypoxic damage, become relatively unresponsive to these substances and remain constricted. Blood is therefore sequestered within the dilated capillary bed and fluid is forced into the extravascular spaces, causing interstitial oedema, haemoconcentration, and an increase in viscosity.

This reduction in flow through the microcirculation, combined with the increase in viscosity, makes the blood highly coagulable. There is also systemic activation of the clotting cascade and platelet aggregation with clot formation occurring within the capillary bed. Plasminogen is converted to plasmin, which breaks down these clots, liberating fibrin/fibrinogen degradation products (FDPs). The cells that are supplied by capillaries blocked by this process of disseminated intravascular coagulation (DIC) (see p. 345) inevitably become hypoxic and eventually die. Tissue ischaemia is further exacerbated as capillaries are compressed by interstitial oedema. In this way vital organs may suffer serious damage. Finally, because clotting factors and platelets are consumed in DIC, they are unavailable for haemostasis elsewhere and a coagulation defect results—hence the alternative name for DIC of 'consumption coagulopathy'. This process occurs earlier and is more severe in septic shock.

The capillary endothelium can be damaged by a number of factors (particularly in septic shock), including DIC, microemboli, release of vasoactive compounds, complement, and activated leucocytes. Capillary permeability is thereby increased and fluid is lost into the extravascular space, causing further hypovolaemia, interstitial oedema and organ dysfunction.

## Metabolic changes

Gluconeogenesis and triglyceride formation are stimulated by increased glucagon and catecholamine levels, whilst glucagon increases hepatic mobilization of glucose from glycogen. Catecholamines inhibit insulin release and reduce peripheral glucose uptake. Combined with elevated circulating levels of other insulin antagonists such as cortisol and GH these changes ensure that the majority of shocked patients are hyperglycaemic. Occasionally hypoglycaemia is precipitated by depletion of hepatic glycogen stores and inhibition of gluconeogenesis.

Muscle proteolysis is initiated to provide energy and hepatic protein synthesis is preferentially augmented to produce the 'acute phase reactants' (see p. 132).

Once the supply of oxygen to the cells is insufficient for continuation of the tricarboxylic acid (TCA) cycle, production of energy in the form of ATP becomes dependent on anaerobic metabolism. Under these circumstances, glucose is metabolized in the normal way to pyruvate but is then converted to lactate instead of entering the Krebs cycle. The $H^+$ ions released cause a metabolic acidosis. This pathway is relatively inefficient in terms of energy production. Eventually, because of the reduced availability of ATP, the sodium pump fails, cells swell due to accumulation of salt and water, and potassium losses increase. In the final stages, release of lysosomal enzymes may contribute to cell death.

## Multiple organ failure (MOF)

Impaired tissue perfusion, microcirculatory abnormalities, and defective oxygen utilization precipitated by dissemination of the inflammatory response with the systemic release of 'mediators' (see above) can damage vital organs. The most severely ill patients may develop MOF, which is almost invariably associated with persistent or recurrent sepsis. Following severe shock, damage to the mucosa of the gastrointestinal tract may allow bacteria or endotoxin within the gut lumen to gain access to the circulation, thereby perpetuating the generalized inflammatory response. Sequential failure of organs occurs progressively over weeks, although the pattern of organ dysfunction is variable. In most cases the lung is the first organ to be affected with the development of the adult respiratory distress syndrome (ARDS) (see below) in association with cardiovascular instability and deteriorating renal function. Secondary pulmonary infection is common in ARDS, acting as a further stimulus to the inflammatory response. Later, liver and renal failure develop (see also p. 725). Characteristically, these patients initially have a hyperdynamic circulation with vasodilatation and a high cardiac output. Eventually, however, cardiovascular collapse supervenes and is the usual terminal event.

Treatment is supportive and prevention of organ damage in those at risk is therefore crucial. Aggressive resuscitation is essential and activation of macrophages must be prevented or minimized by early excision of devitalized tissue and drainage of infection. Preservation of the integrity of the gut mucosal barrier is also necessary by aggressive haemodynamic support in order to maximize splanchnic perfusion. Early enteral feeding may also be beneficial. Early recognition of organ dysfunction and prompt intervention may reverse organ impairment and improve outcome.

The mortality of MOF is extremely high; factors affecting outcome include the number of organs that fail and the duration of organ failure.

## CLINICAL SIGNS

Although many clinical features are common to all types of shock there are certain important respects in which they differ (Information box 13.1):

**Hypovolaemic shock**
1  Inadequate tissue perfusion:

*Hypovolaemic shock*
Low central venous pressure (CVP) and pulmonary artery
    occlusion pressure (PAOP)
Low cardiac output
Increased systemic vascular resistance

*Cardiogenic shock*
Clinical signs usually associated with very low cardiac
    output
Increased systemic vascular resistance
CVP and PAWP usually high

*Cardiac tamponade*
Parallel increase in CVP and PAOP
Low cardiac output
Increased systemic vascular resistance

*Pulmonary embolism*
Low cardiac output
High CVP, high pulmonary artery pressure but low PAWP
Increased systemic vascular resistance

*Anaphylaxis*
Low systemic vascular resistance
Low CVP and PAOP
High cardiac output

*Septic shock*
Low systemic vascular resistance
Low CVP and PAWP
Cardiac output usually high
Myocardial depression—low ejection fraction. Stroke
    volume maintained by ventricular dilatation. Cardiac
    output increased by tachycardia

**Information box 13.1** Haemodynamic changes in shock.

(a)  Skin—cold, pale, blue, slow capillary refill
(b)  Kidneys—oliguria, anuria
(c)  Brain—confusion and restlessness
2  Increased sympathetic tone:
(a)  Tachycardia, narrowed pulse pressure
(b)  Sweating
(c)  Blood pressure—may be maintained initially (despite up to a 25% reduction in circulating volume if the patient is young and fit), but later hypotension supervenes
3  Metabolic acidosis and tachypnoea

*Additional clinical features* may occur in the following types of shock.

**Cardiogenic shock**
1  Signs of myocardial failure, e.g. raised jugular venous pressure (JVP), pulsus alternans, 'gallop' rhythm, basal crackles, pulmonary oedema

**Mechanical shock**
1  Elevated JVP
2  Pulsus paradoxus and muffled heart sounds in cardiac tamponade
3  Kussmaul's sign (JVP rises on inspiration) in cardiac tamponade
4  Signs of pulmonary embolism (if present) (see p. 610)

**Anaphylactic shock** (see p. 738)
1  Signs of profound vasodilatation:
(a)  Warm peripheries
(b)  Low blood pressure
2  Erythema, urticaria, angio-oedema, pallor, cyanosis
3  Bronchospasm, rhinitis
4  Oedema of the face, pharynx and larynx
5  Pulmonary oedema
6  Hypovolaemia due to capillary leak
7  Nausea, vomiting, abdominal cramps, diarrhoea

**Septic shock**
1  Pyrexia and rigors, or hypothermia (unusual)
2  Nausea, vomiting
3  Vasodilatation, warm peripheries
4  Bounding pulse
5  Rapid capillary refill
6  Hypotension
7  Occasionally signs of cutaneous vasoconstriction
8  Other signs:
(a)  Jaundice
(b)  Coma (rare)
(c)  Coagulopathy
The diagnosis of septicaemia is easily missed. In the elderly, the classical signs may not be present and, for example, mild confusion, tachycardia and tachypnoea may be the only clues, sometimes associated with unexplained hypotension, a reduction in urine output, a rising plasma creatinine and glucose intolerance.

## MONITORING

Invasive monitoring is unnecessary in straightforward cases, such as a fit young man with moderate traumatic

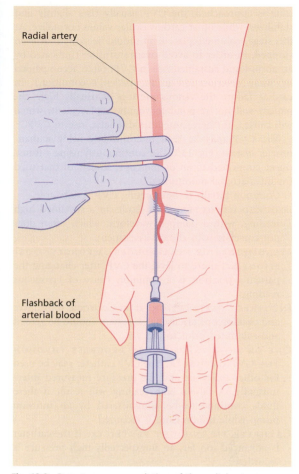

**Fig. 13.9**   Percutaneous cannulation of the radial artery.

haemorrhage, but will be required in the more seriously ill patients and in those who fail to respond to initial treatment (see later). Clinical assessment must never be neglected.

## Clinical indices of tissue perfusion

Pale, cold skin, delayed capillary refill and the absence of visible veins in the hands and feet indicate poor perfusion. Skin temperature measurements can help clinical evaluation as vasoconstriction is an early compensatory response.

Urinary flow is a sensitive indicator of renal perfusion and haemodynamic performance.

## Blood pressure

Alterations in blood pressure are often interpreted as reflecting changes in cardiac output. However, if there is vasoconstriction with a high peripheral resistance, the blood pressure may be normal, even when the cardiac output is reduced. Conversely the vasodilated patient may be hypotensive despite a very high cardiac output.

The absolute level of blood pressure is also important, since hypotension may jeopardize perfusion of vital organs. The adequacy of blood pressure in an individual patient must always be assessed in relation to the pre-morbid value.

Blood pressure is traditionally measured with a sphygmomanometer, but automated instruments using a microphone to detect Korotkoff's sounds or continuous monitoring with an intra-arterial cannula, usually in the radial artery (Practical box 13.1), can be used (Fig. 13.9).

## Central venous pressure (CVP)

This provides a fairly simple method of assessing the adequacy of a patient's circulating volume and the contractile state of the myocardium. The absolute value of the CVP is not as important as its response to a fluid challenge (the infusion of 100–200 ml of fluid over 1–3 min) (Fig. 13.10). The hypovolaemic patient will initially respond to transfusion with little or no change in CVP, together with some improvement in cardiovascular function (falling heart rate, rising blood pressure and increased peripheral temperature). As the normovolaemic state is approached, the CVP usually rises slightly and stabilizes, while other cardiovascular values normalize. At this stage, volume replacement should be slowed, or even stopped, in order to avoid overtransfusion (indicated by an abrupt and sustained rise in CVP, often accompanied by some deterioration in the patient's condition). In cardiac failure the venous pressure is usually high; the patient will not respond to volume replacement, which will cause a further, sometimes dramatic, rise in CVP.

The CVP may be read intermittently using a manometer system (Fig. 13.11) or continuously using a transducer connected to an oscilloscope, similar to that used for intra-arterial monitoring.

Common pitfalls in interpreting CVP results are:

BLOCKED CATHETER. This results in a sustained high reading, with a damped waveform which often does not correlate with clinical assessment.

MANOMETER OR TRANSDUCER WRONGLY POSITIONED. Failure to level the CVP after changing the patient's position is a common cause of erroneous readings.

INCORRECT CALIBRATION. If an electronic transducer and oscilloscope are used, the system should be zeroed and calibrated prior to use.

ONE OR MORE INFUSIONS IN PROGRESS THROUGH THE CVP CATHETER. The CVP catheter may be used for other infusions and the pressure measured intermittently. A falsely high reading will result if these fluids continue to be administered by an infusion pump while the pressure is recorded.

CATHETER TIP IN RIGHT VENTRICLE. If the catheter is advanced too far, an unexpectedly high pressure is recorded.

The catheter should be positioned in the superior vena cava. It is usually inserted via a percutaneous puncture

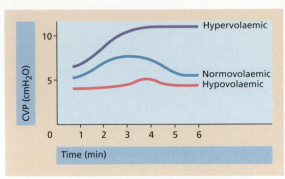

**Fig. 13.10** The effects of rapid administration of a 'fluid challenge' to patients with a central venous pressure within the normal range. (From Sykes MK (1963) Venous pressure as a clinical indication of adequacy of transfusion. *Annals of the Royal College of Surgeons of England* **33**, 185–197. With permission.)

of a subclavian or internal jugular vein   (Practical box 13.2) (Fig. 13.12).

## Left atrial pressure

In uncomplicated cases careful interpretation of the CVP is an adequate guide to the filling pressures of both sides of the heart. In many critically ill patients, however, this is not the case and there is a disparity in function between the two ventricles. Most commonly, left ventricular performance is worst, so that the left ventricular function curve is displaced downward and to the right (Fig. 13.13). This situation is encountered in some patients with clinically significant ischaemic heart disease and has also been reported in major trauma, sepsis, peritonitis, hepatic failure, valvular heart disease and after cardiac surgery. High

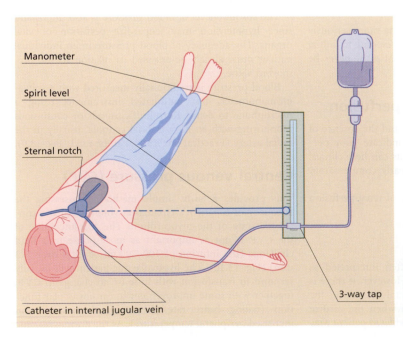

**Fig. 13.11** Central venous pressure measurement using a manometer system. The reading must be referred to the level of the right atrium (indicated by the axillary fold or, provided the patient is supine, the sternal notch) using a spirit level.

1  The procedure is explained to the patient.
2  The patient is placed head-down to distend the central veins (this facilitates cannulation and minimizes the risk of air embolism but may exacerbate respiratory distress and is dangerous in those with raised intracranial pressure).
3  The skin is cleaned. Sterile precautions are taken throughout the procedure.
4  Local anaesthetic (1% plain lignocaine) is injected intradermally to raise a weal at the apex of a triangle formed by the two heads of sternomastoid with the clavicle at its base.
5  A small incision is made through the weal.
6  The cannula is inserted through the incision and directed laterally downwards and backwards until the vein is punctured just beneath the skin and deep to the lateral head of sternomastoid.
7  It is checked that venous blood is easily aspirated using a syringe attached to the cannula.
8  The cannula is threaded off the needle into the vein.
9  The CVP manometer line is connected.
10  If the catheter is in a large vein, venous blood will flow back when the giving-set tap is open and the infusion bottle is on the floor.
11  The CVP is measured. The fluid level in the manometer should then fall rapidly and fluctuate with respiration.
12  A chest X-ray should be taken to verify that the tip of the catheter is in the superior vena cava and to exclude pneumothorax.

*Possible complications*
Accidental arterial puncture (carotid or subclavian)
Damage to thoracic duct on left
Air embolism
Pneumothorax
Thrombosis
Catheter-related sepsis

**Practical box 13.2**   Procedure for cannulation of the internal jugular vein.

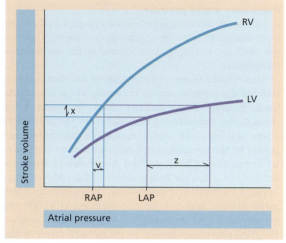

**Fig. 13.13**   Left ventricular (LV) and right ventricular (RV) function curves in a patient with left ventricular dysfunction. Since the stroke volume of the two ventricles must be the same (except perhaps for a few beats during a period of circulatory adjustment), left atrial pressure (LAP) must be higher than right atrial pressure (RAP). Moreover, an increase in stroke volume (x) produced by a small rise in RAP (v) will be associated with a marked increase in LAP (z).

right ventricular filling pressures, with normal or low left atrial pressures, are less common but may occur in right ventricular ischaemia and in situations where the pulmonary vascular resistance (i.e. right ventricular after-load) is raised, such as acute respiratory failure and pulmonary embolism.

If there is a disparity in ventricular function after cardiac surgery, then the left atrium can be cannulated directly. If the thorax is not open, however, some other means of determining left ventricular filling pressure must be devised.

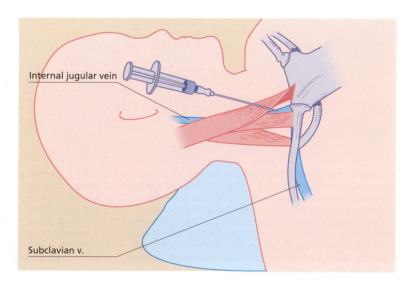

**Fig. 13.12**   Cannulation of the right internal jugular vein with a catheter-over-needle device.

## Pulmonary artery pressure

A 'balloon flotation catheter' enables prompt and reliable catheterization of the pulmonary artery, without the need for screening, and minimizes the incidence of arrhythmias.

These 'Swan–Ganz' catheters can be inserted centrally through the femoral vein or via a vein in the antecubital fossa. Passage of the catheter from the major veins, through the chambers of the heart, into the pulmonary artery and into the wedge position is monitored and guided by the pressure waveforms recorded from the distal lumen (Fig. 13.14). A chest X-ray should always be obtained to check the final position of the catheter. Once in place, the balloon is deflated and the pulmonary artery mean, systolic and end-diastolic pressures (PAEDP) can be recorded. The pulmonary artery occlusion pressure (PAOP—previously known as pulmonary artery wedge pressure PAWP) is measured by reinflating the balloon, thereby propelling the catheter distally until it impacts in a medium-sized pulmonary artery. In this position there is a continuous column of fluid between the distal lumen of the catheter and the left atrium, so that PAOP is usually a reflection of left atrial pressure.

The technique is generally safe—the majority of complications are related to user inexperience. Pulmonary artery catheters should preferably be removed within 72 hours, since the incidence of complications then increases progressively (Table 13.3).

| Complication | Comments |
|---|---|
| Arrhythmias | May occur during passage of catheter through right ventricle<br>Usually benign<br>Can often be prevented with lignocaine |
| Sepsis | May occur at insertion site<br>Septicaemia or endocarditis may develop |
| Knotting | May occur when catheter coils in right ventricle |
| Valve trauma | Occurs if catheter withdrawn with balloon inflated or due to valves repeatedly closing on catheter |
| Thrombosis/embolism | |
| Pulmonary infarction | May occur if catheter remains in 'wedge' position |
| Pulmonary artery rupture | Usually fatal<br>May occur if balloon is inflated when catheter already 'wedged' |
| Balloon rupture/ leak/embolism | Rare |

**Table 13.3**  Some complications of Swan–Ganz catheters.

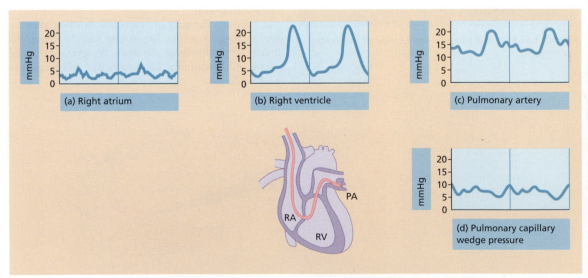

**Fig. 13.14** Passage of a Swan–Ganz catheter through the chambers of the heart into the 'wedge' position. (a) Once in the thorax, marked respiratory oscillations are seen. The catheter should be advanced further towards the lower superior vena cava/right atrium, where oscillations become more pronounced. The balloon should then be inflated and the catheter advanced. (b) When the catheter is in the right ventricle, there is no dicrotic notch and the diastolic pressure is close to zero. The patient should be returned to the horizontal, or slightly head-up, position before advancing the catheter further. (c) When the catheter reaches the pulmonary artery a dicrotic notch appears and there is elevation of the diastolic pressure. The catheter should be advanced further with the balloon inflated. (d) Reappearance of a venous waveform indicates that the catheter is 'wedged'. The catheter is deflated to obtain the pulmonary artery pressure. The balloon is inflated intermittently to obtain the pulmonary capillary wedge pressure (also known as pulmonary capillary occlusion pressure).

# Cardiac output

The only quantitatively accurate methods for measuring cardiac output are invasive. Of these, the thermodilution technique is most commonly used clinically. This uses a modified pulmonary artery catheter with a lumen opening in the right atrium and a thermistor located a few centimetres from its tip. A known volume (usually 10 ml) of ice-cold 5% dextrose is injected as a bolus into the right atrium. This mixes with, and cools, the blood passing through the heart and the transient fall in temperature is continuously recorded by the thermistor in the pulmonary artery. The cardiac output is computed from the total amount of indicator (i.e. cold) injected, divided by the average concentration, i.e. the amount of cooling, and the time taken to pass the thermistor.

# MANAGEMENT (Emergency box 13.1)

Delays in making the diagnosis and initiating treatment, as well as inadequate resuscitation, contribute to the development of MOF and must be avoided.

A patent airway must be maintained and oxygen is given. If necessary, an oropharyngeal airway or an endotracheal tube is inserted. The latter has the advantage of preventing aspiration of gastric contents. *Very rarely* emergency tracheostomy is indicated (see below).

The underlying cause of shock should be corrected, e.g. haemorrhage should be controlled or infection eradicated. In patients with septic shock, every effort must be made to identify the source of infection and isolate the causative organism. As well as a thorough history and clinical examination, X-rays, ultrasonography and CT scanning may be required to locate the origin of the infection. Appropriate samples (urine, sputum, cerebrospinal fluid, pus drained from abscesses) should be sent to the laboratory for microscopy, culture and sensitivities. Several blood cultures should be performed and 'blind' antibiotic therapy should be commenced. If an organism is isolated, the therapy can be adjusted appropriately.

The choice of antibiotic depends on the source of infection—whether this was acquired in hospital or in the community. Abscesses must be drained and infected indwelling catheters removed.

Whatever the aetiology of the haemodynamic abnormality, tissue blood flow must be restored by achieving and maintaining an adequate cardiac output, as well as ensuring that arterial blood pressure is sufficient to maintain perfusion of vital organs.

# Pre-load and volume replacement

Optimizing pre-load is the most efficient way of increasing cardiac output. Volume replacement is obviously essential in hypovolaemic shock but is also required in anaphylactic and septic shock because of vasodilatation, sequestration of blood and loss of circulating volume due to capillary leak.

In mechanical shock, high filling pressures may be required to maintain an adequate stroke volume. Even

---

**Ensure adequate oxygenation and ventilation**

1  Maintain patent airway
     May need: oropharyngeal airway, endotracheal tube, tracheostomy (rarely)

2  Administer oxygen

3  Support respiratory function
     May need: CPAP (p. 731), mechanical ventilation

*Monitor:*  respiratory rate
             blood gases
             chest X-ray

**Restore cardiac output and blood pressure**

1  Expand circulating volume using:
     Blood
     Colloids
     Crystalloids
   *rapidly via one or more large bore i.v. cannulae*

2  Support cardiovascular function
     May need: inotropic support, vasodilators, intra-aortic balloon counterpulsation

*Monitor:*  skin colour
             capillary refill time
             peripheral temperature
             urine flow
             blood pressure (usually intra-arterial)
             ECG
             CVP in most cases
             Swan–Ganz catheter (in selected cases)

**Investigate**
All cases
  HB, PCV
  WBC
  Blood glucose
  Platelets, coagulation
  Urea, creatinine, electrolytes
  Liver biochemistry
  Blood gases
  Acid–base state

Selected cases
  Blood cultures
  Blood lactate
  Fibrinogen degradation products

**Treat underlying cause**
For example: control haemorrhage, treat infection (antibiotics, remove indwelling catheters, surgical exploration, drainage)

**Treat complications**
For example; coagulopathy, renal failure

**Administer analgesia**
Small divided doses of opiates i.v.

**Emergency box 13.1**  Management of shock. Patients require intensive nursing care (see p. 735).

---

in cardiogenic shock, careful volume expansion may, on occasions, lead to a useful increase in cardiac output. On the other hand, patients with severe cardiac failure, in whom ventricular filling pressures may be markedly elevated, often benefit from measures to reduce pre-load (and after-load) such as the administration of diuretics and vasodilators (see below).

*The circulating volume must be replaced quickly* (in minutes not hours) to reduce tissue damage and prevent acute renal failure. Fluid is administered via wide-bore intravenous cannulae to allow large volumes to be given quickly and the effect is continuously monitored.

Care must be taken to prevent volume overload, which leads to cardiac dilatation, a reduction in stroke volume, and a rise in left atrial pressure with a risk of pulmonary oedema. Pulmonary oedema is more likely in very ill patients because of a low colloid osmotic pressure (usually due to a low serum albumin) and disruption of the alveolar–capillary membrane (e.g. in ARDS). The development of pulmonary oedema can also be influenced by other unquantifiable factors, such as the hydrostatic and oncotic pressures within the interstitial spaces. Since the pulmonary lymphatics remove excess fluid, pulmonary oedema will only occur when this mechanism is overwhelmed or impaired. Left ventricular filling pressures should therefore not be allowed to rise to more than 15–18 mmHg in the critically ill. In general, however, many more patients are undertransfused rather than overtransfused.

### Choice of fluid for volume replacement

BLOOD. This is conventionally given for haemorrhagic shock as soon as it is available. In extreme emergencies, uncrossmatched group O negative blood can be used, but an emergency crossmatch can be performed in about 30 min and is as safe as the standard procedure. Donor blood is often separated into its various components for storage, necessitating the transfusion of packed red cells to maintain haemoglobin and plasma, or a plasma substitute, for volume replacement.

*Complications* of blood transfusion are discussed on p. 331. Special problems arise when large volumes of stored blood are transfused rapidly. These include:

TEMPERATURE CHANGES. Bank blood is stored at 4°C and transfusion may result in hypothermia, peripheral venoconstriction (which slows the rate of the infusion) and arrhythmias. Some therefore recommend that if possible blood should be warmed prior to the transfusion.

COAGULOPATHY. Stored blood has essentially no effective platelets and is deficient in clotting factors. Large transfusions can therefore produce a coagulation defect. This may need to be treated by replacing clotting factors with fresh frozen plasma and the administration of platelet concentrates.

METABOLIC ACIDOSIS/ALKALOSIS. Stored blood is now preserved in citrate/phosphate/dextrose (CPD) solution, which is less acidic than the acid/citrate/dextrose (ACD) solution used previously. Metabolic acidosis attributable solely to blood transfusion is rare and in any case rarely requires correction. A metabolic alkalosis often develops 24–48 hours after a large blood transfusion, probably mainly due to metabolism of the citrate; this will be exacerbated if the preceding acidosis has been corrected with intravenous sodium bicarbonate.

HYPOCALCAEMIA. Stored blood is anticoagulated with citrate, which binds calcium ions. This can reduce total body ionized calcium levels and cause myocardial depression. This is uncommon in practice, but if necessary can be corrected by administering 10 ml of 10% calcium chloride intravenously. Routine treatment with calcium is not recommended.

INCREASED OXYGEN AFFINITY. In stored blood, the red cell 2,3-DPG content is reduced, so that the oxyhaemoglobin dissociation curve is shifted to the left. The oxygen affinity of haemoglobin is therefore increased and oxygen delivery is impaired. This effect is less marked with blood stored in CPD. Red cell levels of 2,3-DPG are substantially restored within 12 hours of transfusion.

HYPERKALAEMIA. Plasma potassium levels rise progressively as blood is stored. However, hyperkalaemia is rarely a problem as prewarming of the blood increases red cell metabolism—the sodium pump becomes active and potassium levels fall.

MICROEMBOLISM. Microaggregates in stored blood may be filtered out by the pulmonary capillaries. This process is thought by some to contribute to ARDS.

RED CELL CONCENTRATES. Nutrient additive solutions, i.e. saline, adenine, glucose and mannitol (SAGM), are now available which allow red cell storage in the absence of plasma (see p. 333).

Because of the complications of blood transfusion, in particular the risk of disease transmission, as well as their expense, the use of crystalloid solutions, plasma, plasma substitutes and oxygen-carrying solutions for volume replacement is assuming greater importance.

CRYSTALLOID SOLUTIONS. Although crystalloid solutions, e.g. saline, are cheap, convenient to use and free of side-effects, the administration of large volumes of these fluids to critically ill patients should, in general, be avoided. They are rapidly lost from the circulation into the extravascular spaces and volumes of crystalloid two to four times that of colloid are required to achieve an equivalent haemodynamic response. Although volume replacement with predominantly crystalloid solutions is advocated by some for the uncomplicated, previously healthy patient with traumatic or perioperative hypovolaemia, a more reasonable approach is to use crystalloids initially but to use colloids in addition if there is continued need for volume replacement in excess of about 1 litre.

COLLOIDAL SOLUTIONS. These produce a greater, and more sustained increase in plasma volume, with associated improvements in cardiovascular function and oxygen transport. They also increase colloid osmotic pressure.

*Human albumin solution* (HAS) is a natural colloid (see p. 334) and is not generally used for routine volume replacement, particularly if volume losses are continuing since other cheaper solutions are equally effective in the short term. Some recommend administration of HAS at a later stage in those who are hypoalbuminaemic.

*Dextrans* are polymolecular polysaccharides in either 5% dextrose or normal saline. They are commercially available as low molecular weight dextran (dextran 40; mol. wt 40 000) and dextran 70, and have a powerful osmotic effect. They interfere with crossmatching and have a small rate of allergic reactions (0.07–1.1%). Normally a dose of 1.5 g dextran per kilogram of body weight should not be exceeded because of the risk of renal damage. In practice dextrans are rarely used in the UK because of the availability of other agents.

*Polygelatin solutions* (Haemaccel, Gelofusine) have an average molecular weight of 35 000, which is iso-osmotic with plasma. They are cheap. Large volumes can be administered, since coagulation defects do not occur and renal function is not impaired. However, because they readily cross the glomerular basement membrane, their half-life in the circulation is approximately 4 hours and they can promote an osmotic diuresis. Allergic reactions occur in up to 10% of cases. These solutions are particularly useful during the acute phase of resuscitation, especially when volume losses are continuing but in many patients colloids with a longer half-life will be required later to achieve haemodynamic stability.

*Hydroxyethyl starch* (HES) has a mean molecular weight of approximately 450 000 and a half-life of about 6 hours. Volume expansion is equivalent to, or slightly greater than, the volume infused. The incidence of allergic reactions is approximately 0.1%. Although more expensive than gelatins, HES is a valuable volume expander.

OXYGEN-CARRYING BLOOD SUBSTITUTES are being developed, e.g. fluorocarbon emulsions.

*Haemoglobin solutions* also have potential as oxygen-delivering resuscitation fluids, but their use is limited by their short intravascular retention time and their high affinity for oxygen.

# Myocardial contractility and inotropic agents

Myocardial contractility can be impaired by hypoxaemia and hypocalcaemia, as well as by some drugs (e.g. *β*-blockers, antiarrhythmics and sedatives). Severe lactic acidosis can depress myocardial contractility and may limit the response to inotropes. Attempted correction of acidosis with intravenous sodium bicarbonate, however, generates additional carbon dioxide which diffuses across cell membranes producing or exacerbating intracellular acidosis. Other disadvantages of bicarbonate therapy include sodium overload and a left shift of the oxyhaemoglobin dissociation curve. Also ionized calcium levels may be reduced and, combined with the fall in intracellular pH, may be responsible for impairing myocardial performance. Treatment of lactic acidosis should therefore concentrate on correcting the cause, while acidosis may be most safely controlled by hyperventilation. Bicarbonate should only be administered to correct extreme and persistent metabolic acidosis (see p. 519).

When a patient remains hypotensive despite adequate volume replacement, and perfusion of vital organs is jeopardized, pressor agents may be administered to improve cardiac output and blood pressure. In some cases inotropic agents are given to redistribute blood flow (e.g. dopamine can be used to increase renal perfusion — see below). There is evidence that survival of patients with septic or traumatic shock (as well as following major surgery and in those with ARDS) is associated with supranormal values for cardiac output, oxygen delivery and oxygen consumption. Some now advocate that in the most severely ill patients, and in those who fail to respond to simple measures, treatment should be directed at increasing these variables until they equal or exceed the median values found in survivors.

It must be remembered, however, that all inotropes increase myocardial oxygen consumption, particularly if a tachycardia develops, and that this can lead to an imbalance between myocardial oxygen supply and demand, with the development or extension of ischaemic areas. For this reason such agents should be used with caution, particularly in cardiogenic shock following myocardial infarction and those known to have ischaemic heart disease.

All inotropic agents should be administered via a large central vein, and their effects carefully monitored.

Some of the currently available inotropes are considered here (see also p. 574).

### Adrenaline

*Adrenaline* stimulates both *α*- and *β*-adrenergic receptors, but at low doses *β* effects seem to predominate. This produces a tachycardia, with an increase in cardiac index and a fall in peripheral resistance. At higher doses, *α*-mediated vasoconstriction develops. If this produces a useful increase in perfusion pressure, urine output may increase and renal failure may be avoided. However, as the dose is further increased, cardiac output may actually fall, accompanied by marked vasoconstriction, tachycardia and a metabolic acidosis. A reduction in renal blood flow then occurs, with oliguria and a risk of acute renal failure. Prolonged high-dose administration may eventually cause peripheral gangrene. For these reasons the minimum effective dose should be used for as short a time as possible. The addition of low-dose dopamine to the regimen may help to preserve renal function (see below). Despite its disadvantages, adrenaline remains a useful potent inotrope and is used when other agents have failed. When haemodynamic monitoring is not available adrenaline is probably the agent of choice in septic shock, and should probably be combined with low-dose dopamine.

### Noradrenaline

This is predominantly an *α*-adrenergic agonist. It can be of value in those with severe hypotension associated with a low systemic resistance, for example in septic shock. There is a risk of producing excessive vasoconstriction with impaired organ perfusion and increased after-load.

Noradrenaline administration must therefore be accompanied by full haemodynamic monitoring, including determination of cardiac output (see above) and calculation of the peripheral resistance.

### Isoprenaline

This $\beta$-adrenergic stimulant has both inotropic and chronotropic effects. It reduces peripheral resistance by dilating skin and muscle blood vessels and diverts flow away from vital organs such as the kidneys. The increase in cardiac output produced by isoprenaline is mainly due to the tachycardia, and this, together with the development of arrhythmias, seriously limits its value. There are now few indications for isoprenaline in the critically ill adult.

### Dopamine

This is a natural precursor of noradrenaline which acts on D1 and D2 dopamine receptors, as well as $\alpha$- and $\beta$-adrenergic receptors. Its main action (at a dose of 3–10 $\mu g\,kg^{-1}\,min^{-1}$) is on $\beta_1$-adrenoreceptors on cardiac muscle, increasing cardiac contractility without increasing rate. The dosage, however, is critical.

In LOW DOSES (1–3 $\mu g\,kg^{-1}\,min^{-1}$) dopaminergic vasodilatory receptors in the renal, mesenteric, cerebral and coronary circulations are activated. D1 receptors are located on postsynaptic membranes and mediate vasodilatory effects whilst D2 receptors are presynaptic and potentiate these vasodilatory effects by preventing the release of noradrenaline. This results in an increase in renal plasma flow and glomerular filtration rate with an improved urinary output. It also increases hepatic blood flow. ·

In MEDIUM DOSES (3–10 $\mu g\,kg^{-1}\,min^{-1}$) activation of $\beta_1$-adrenoreceptors occurs with an increase in heart rate, myocardial contractility and cardiac output.

In HIGH DOSES (>20 $\mu g\,kg^{-1}\,min^{-1}$) dopamine increases noradrenaline and therefore activates $\alpha_1$-adrenergic receptors leading to vasoconstriction. This causes an increase in after-load and raises the ventricular filling pressures.

### Dopexamine

This analogue of dopamine is a vasodilator ($\beta_2$-agonist) that does not stimulate $\alpha$-receptors. It is a positive inotrope and increases renal blood flow, but in septic shock may exacerbate hypotension by further reducing systemic vascular resistance. It is likely to be most useful in those with low cardiac output and peripheral vasoconstriction.

### Dobutamine

Dobutamine is closely related to dopamine with predominant $\beta_1$ activity and less $\alpha$ constricting activity, but equal positive 'inotropic' effect.

● It has no specific effect on the renal vasculature although urine output often increases as cardiac output and blood pressure improve.

● It reduces systemic resistance and improves cardiac performance, thereby decreasing both after-load and ventricular filling pressures.

● It produces a greater improvement in cardiac output than dopamine for a given increase in myocardial oxygen consumption.

For these reasons, dobutamine is probably the agent of choice in patients with cardiogenic shock and cardiac failure.

### Enoximone

This agent, active both orally (see Fig. 11.52) and intravenously, is a phosphodiesterase inhibitor with inotropic and vasodilator properties. Enoximone may, however, cause profound vasodilatation and precipitate or worsen hypotension due to profound vasodilatation. It is sometimes useful in the management of acute cardiac failure.

### Summary

Many still consider dopamine to be the inotrope of choice in most critically ill patients, largely because of its effects on splanchnic blood flow, although others favour dopexamine as a means of increasing cardiac output and organ blood flow. Dobutamine is equally popular and is particularly indicated in patients in whom the vasoconstriction caused by dopamine could be dangerous (i.e. patients with cardiac disease and septic patients with fluid overload or myocardial failure). The combination of dobutamine and noradrenaline is currently popular for the management of patients who are shocked with a low systemic resistance. Dobutamine is given to achieve an optimal cardiac output, while noradrenaline is used to restore an adequate blood pressure by reducing vasodilatation. However this combination can only be used safely when guided by full haemodynamic monitoring.

Adrenaline, because of its potency, remains a useful agent in those patients unresponsive to other measures, particularly after cardiac surgery, and is a cheap, effective agent for the management of septic shock.

## Diuretic therapy (see p. 503)

Diuretics increase salt and water excretion by the kidneys, thereby decreasing ventricular filling pressure (pre-load). This is the major form of therapy in sodium retention with fluid overload.

## Vasodilator therapy (see also p. 573)

In selected cases, after-load reduction may be used to increase stroke volume and decrease myocardial oxygen requirements by reducing the systolic ventricular wall tension. Vasodilatation also decreases heart size and the diastolic ventricular wall tension so that coronary blood flow is improved. The relative magnitude of the falls in pre-load and after-load depends on the pre-existing haemodynamic disturbance, concurrent volume replacement and the agent selected (see below).

Vasodilator therapy is most beneficial in patients with cardiac failure in whom the ventricular function curve is flat (see Fig. 13.4) and falls in pre-load have only a limited effect on stroke volume. This form of treatment may therefore sometimes be useful in cardiogenic shock and in the management of patients with pulmonary oedema associated with low cardiac output. Vasodilators may also be valuable in shocked patients who remain vasoconstricted and oliguric despite restoration of an adequate blood pressure.

Such therapy is potentially dangerous and should be guided by continuous haemodynamic monitoring, including pulmonary artery catheterization or direct measurement of left atrial pressure. The circulating volume must be adequate before treatment is started. Falls in pre-load should be prevented, except in those with cardiac failure, in order to avoid serious reductions in cardiac output and blood pressure. If diastolic pressure is allowed to fall, coronary blood flow may be jeopardized and, particularly if a reflex tachycardia develops in response to the hypotension, myocardial ischaemia may be precipitated.

### α-Adrenergic antagonists

These predominantly dilate arterioles and therefore mainly influence after-load.

Phenoxybenzamine is unsuitable for use in the critically ill because of its slow onset (1–2 hours to maximum effect) and prolonged duration of action (2–3 days).

Phentolamine is very potent with a rapid onset and short duration of action (15–20 min). It can be used for short-term control of blood pressure in a hypertensive crisis, but can produce a marked tachycardia.

### Vasodilators acting directly on the vessel wall

These agents are those most commonly used to achieve vasodilatation in the critically ill.

HYDRALAZINE. This predominantly affects arterial resistance vessels. It therefore reduces after-load and blood pressure, while cardiac output and heart rate usually increase. Hydralazine is usually given as an intravenous bolus to control acute increases in blood pressure, particularly after cardiac surgery.

SODIUM NITROPRUSSIDE (SNP). This dilates arterioles and venous capacitance vessels, as well as the pulmonary vasculature by donating nitric oxide. SNP therefore reduces the after-load and pre-load of both ventricles and can improve cardiac output and the myocardial oxygen supply–demand ratio. It has been suggested that SNP can exacerbate myocardial ischaemia by producing a 'steal' phenomenon in the coronary circulation.

The effects of SNP are rapid in onset and spontaneously reversible within a few minutes of discontinuing the infusion.

A large overdose of SNP can cause cyanide poisoning, with intracellular hypoxia caused by inhibition of cytochrome oxidase, the terminal enzyme of the respiratory chain. This is manifested as a metabolic acidosis and a fall in the arteriovenous oxygen content difference.

NITROGLYCERINE (NTG) AND ISOSORBIDE DINITRATE (ISDN). These are both predominantly venodilators. They can therefore cause marked reductions in pre-load, which may be associated with falls in cardiac output and compensatory vasoconstriction. For the reasons discussed above, they are of most value in those with cardiac failure in whom pre-load reduction may reduce ventricular wall tension and improve coronary perfusion without adversely affecting cardiac performance. Furthermore, these agents may reverse myocardial ischaemia by increasing and redistributing coronary blood flow. They are therefore often used in preference to SNP in patients with cardiac failure and/or myocardial ischaemia. Both NTG and ISDN reduce pulmonary vascular resistance by donating nitric oxide, an effect that can occasionally be exploited in patients with a low cardiac output secondary to pulmonary hypertension.

## Mechanical support of the myocardium

Intra-aortic balloon counterpulsation (IABCP) is the most widely used technique for mechanical support of the failing myocardium. It is discussed on p. 553.

## Adjunctive therapy in shock

Attempts have been made to identify agents that would prevent the release, or inhibit the effects, of the various mediators released in shock. For example, non-steroidal anti-inflammatory drugs (NSAIDs) (which inhibit cyclo-oxygenase) have been used to limit prostaglandin production, naloxone has been used to block the effects of endogenous opioid peptides, PAF antagonists are available and monoclonal antibodies to some of the cytokines or their receptors, as well as endotoxin itself, have been developed and investigated. Recently there has been considerable interest in the ability of NO synthase inhibitors to reverse the vasodilatation associated with some forms of circulatory shock. Other approaches have included administration of prostacyclin and removal of mediators by plasma exchange/haemofiltration. In the future naturally occurring cytokine antagonists or their soluble receptors may prove useful. At present, however, the role of these various adjunctive therapies in clinical practice remains unclear.

In animal studies very large doses of steroids have been shown to reduce mortality in septic shock, but clinical trials in humans have shown that steroids are of no benefit and their administration to such patients is no longer recommended.

## Renal failure

Acute renal failure is a common and serious complication of critical illness which adversely affects the prognosis.

The importance of preventing renal failure by rapid and effective resuscitation, as well as the avoidance of nephrotoxic drugs (especially NSAIDs), cannot be overemphasized. Shock and sepsis are the commonest causes of acute renal failure in the critically ill but it remains important to diagnose the cause of renal dysfunction and exclude reversible pathology, especially obstruction (see Chapter 9).

Oliguria is usually the first indication of renal impairment and should prompt immediate attempts to optimize cardiovascular function, particularly by expanding the circulating volume. Low-dose dopamine may be used to enhance renal blood flow. If these measures fail to reverse oliguria some recommend administration of diuretics such as frusemide or mannitol (see Chapter 9).

If oliguria persists, it is important to reduce crystalloid intake and review drug doses. Dialysis is indicated for fluid overload, electrolyte disturbances (especially hyperkalaemia), acidosis and, to a lesser extent, uraemia.

Intermittent haemodialysis has a number of disadvantages in the critically ill. In particular it is frequently complicated by hypotension and it may be difficult to remove sufficient volumes of fluid. Peritoneal dialysis is also frequently unsatisfactory in these patients and is contraindicated in those who have undergone intra-abdominal surgery. The use of continuous haemofiltration, usually with dialysis, is therefore preferred (see Chapter 9).

# Respiratory failure

## Types and causes

The respiratory system consists of a gas exchanging organ (the lungs) and a ventilatory pump (respiratory muscles/thorax) either or both of which can fail and precipitate respiratory failure.

Respiratory failure occurs when pulmonary gas exchange is sufficiently impaired to cause hypoxaemia with or without hypercarbia. In practical terms respiratory failure is present when the $P_a o_2$ is <8 kPa (60 mmHg) or the $P_a co_2$ is >7 kPa (55 mmHg).

It can be divided into:
- Type I respiratory failure, in which the $P_a o_2$ is low and the $P_a co_2$ is normal or low
- Type II respiratory failure, in which the $P_a o_2$ is low and the $P_a co_2$ is high

TYPE I or 'acute hypoxaemic' respiratory failure occurs with diseases that damage lung tissue, with hypoxaemia due to right-to-left shunts or $\dot{V}/\dot{Q}$ mismatch. Common causes include pulmonary oedema, pneumonia, ARDS and, in the chronic situation, pulmonary fibrosing alveolitis.

TYPE II or 'ventilatory failure' occurs when alveolar ventilation is insufficient to excrete the volume of carbon dioxide being produced by tissue metabolism. Inadequate alveolar ventilation is due to reduced ventilatory effort, inability to overcome an increased resistance to ventilation, failure to compensate for an increase in dead space and/or carbon dioxide production, or a combination of these factors. The most common cause is chronic bronchitis and emphysema. Other causes include chest-wall deformities, respiratory muscle weakness (e.g. Guillain–Barré syndrome) and depression of the respiratory centre.

Deterioration in the mechanical properties of the lungs and/or chest wall increases the work of breathing and the oxygen consumption/carbon dioxide production of the respiratory muscles. The concept that respiratory muscle fatigue (either acute or chronic) is an important factor in the pathogenesis of respiratory failure is controversial.

## MONITORING

A clinical assessment of respiratory distress should be made on the following criteria:
- The use of accessory muscles of respiration
- Tachypnoea
- Tachycardia
- Sweating
- Pulsus paradoxus
- Inability to speak
- Signs of carbon dioxide retention (see p. 659)
- Asynchronous respiration (a discrepancy in the rate of movement of the abdominal and thoracic compartments)
- Paradoxical respiration (abdominal and thoracic compartments move in opposite directions)
- Respiratory alternans (breath-to-breath alteration in the relative contribution of intercostal/accessory muscles and the diaphragm)

This can be supplemented by measuring tidal volume and vital capacity. Blood gas analysis should be performed to guide oxygen therapy and to provide an objective assessment of respiratory function.

The most sensitive clinical indicator of increasing respiratory difficulty is a rising respiratory rate. Tidal volume is a less sensitive indicator.

Minute ventilation rises initially in acute respiratory failure and falls precipitously only at a late stage when the patient is exhausted. Vital capacity is often a better guide to deterioration and is particularly useful in patients with respiratory inadequacy due to neuromuscular problems, e.g. the Guillain–Barré syndrome, in which the vital capacity decreases as weakness increases.

### Pulse oximetry

Lightweight oximeters which measure the changing amount of light transmitted through pulsating arterial blood and provide a continuous, non-invasive assessment of $S_a o_2$ can be applied to an ear lobe or finger. These devices are reliable, easy to use and do not require calibration, although it is important to appreciate that pulse oximetry is not a very sensitive guide to changes in oxygenation.

# Blood gas analysis

Automation of measurements can give a false impression of reliability and accuracy and may lead to an uncritical acceptance of the results. Errors can result from malfunction of the analyser or incorrect sampling techniques. Care must be taken over the following.

1 The sample should be analysed immediately or the syringe should be immersed in iced water (the end having first been sealed with a plastic cap) to prevent the continuing metabolism of white cells causing a reduction in $Po_2$ and a rise in $Pco_2$.

2 The sample must be adequately anticoagulated to prevent clot formation within the analyser. However, excessive dilution of the blood with heparin, which is acidic, will significantly reduce its pH. Heparin (1000 i.u. $ml^{-1}$) should just fill the dead space of the syringe, i.e. approximately 0.1 ml. This will adequately anticoagulate a 2 ml sample.

3 Air almost inevitably enters the sample. The gas tensions within these air bubbles will equilibrate with those in the blood, thereby lowering the $Pco_2$, and, usually, raising the $Po_2$ of the sample. However, provided the bubbles are ejected immediately by inverting the syringe and expelling the air that rises to the top of the sample, their effect is insignificant.

Normal values of blood gas analysis are shown in Table 13.4. The interpretation of the results of blood gas analysis can be considered in two separate parts:

● Disturbances of acid–base balance
● Alterations in oxygenation

Interpretation of results requires a knowledge of the history, the age of the patient, the inspired oxygen concentration and any other relevant treatment (e.g. the administration of sodium bicarbonate, and the ventilator settings for those on mechanical ventilation).

## Disturbances of acid–base balance

The physiology of acid–base control is discussed on p. 514. Acid–base disturbances can be described in relation to the diagram illustrated in Fig. 10.6, which shows $P_aco_2$ plotted against arterial [$H^+$].

Both acidosis and alkalosis can occur, each of which may be either metabolic (primarily affecting the bicarbonate component of the system) or respiratory (primarily affecting $Pco_2$). Compensatory changes may also be apparent. In clinical practice, arterial [$H^+$] values *outside* the range 18–126 nmol $litre^{-1}$ (pH 6.9–7.7) are very rarely encountered.

| | | |
|---|---|---|
| $H^+$ | 35–45 nmol $litre^{-1}$ | (pH 7.35–7.45) |
| $Po_2$ | 10–13.3 kPa | (75–100 mmHg) |
| $Pco_2$ | 4.8–6.1 kPa | (36–46 mmHg) |
| Plasma $HCO_3^-$ | 22–26 mmol $litre^{-1}$ | |
| $O_2$ saturation | 95–100% | |

**Table 13.4** Normal values for measurements obtained when blood gas analysis is performed.

RESPIRATORY ACIDOSIS. This is caused by retention of carbon dioxide. The $P_aco_2$ and [$H^+$] rise. A chronically raised $P_aco_2$ is compensated by renal retention of bicarbonate and the [$H^+$] returns towards normal. A constant arterial bicarbonate concentration is then usually established within 5 days. This represents a primary respiratory acidosis with a compensatory metabolic alkalosis (see p. 516). Common causes of respiratory acidosis include ventilatory failure and chronic bronchitis and emphysema (type II respiratory failure where there is a high $P_aco_2$ and a low $P_ao_2$—see Chapter 12).

RESPIRATORY ALKALOSIS. In this case the reverse occurs and there is a fall in $P_aco_2$ and [$H^+$], often with a small reduction in bicarbonate concentration. If hypocarbia persists, some degree of renal compensation may occur, producing a metabolic acidosis, although in practice this is unusual. A respiratory alkalosis is often produced, intentionally or unintentionally, when patients are artificially ventilated; it may also be seen with hypoxaemic (type I) respiratory failure (see Chapter 12), spontaneous hyperventilation and in those living at high altitudes.

METABOLIC ACIDOSIS. This may be due to excessive acid production, most commonly lactic acid during an episode of shock or following cardiac arrest. A metabolic acidosis may also develop in chronic renal failure and following the loss of large amounts of alkali, e.g. from the gut or from the kidney in renal tubular acidosis.

Respiratory compensation for a metabolic acidosis is usually slightly delayed because the blood–brain barrier initially prevents the respiratory centre from sensing the increased blood [$H^+$]. Following this short delay, however, the patient hyperventilates and 'blows off' carbon dioxide to produce a compensatory respiratory alkalosis. There is a limit to this respiratory compensation, since values for $P_aco_2$ less than about 1.4 kPa (11 mmHg) are, in practice, never achieved. It should also be noted that respiratory compensation cannot occur if the patient's ventilation is controlled or if their respiratory centre is depressed, for example by drugs or head injury.

METABOLIC ALKALOSIS. This can be caused by loss of acid, e.g. from the stomach with nasogastric suction or in high intestinal obstruction, or excessive administration of absorbable alkali. Overzealous treatment with intravenous sodium bicarbonate is frequently implicated.

Respiratory compensation for a metabolic alkalosis is often slight and it is rare to encounter a $P_aco_2$ >6.5 kPa (50 mmHg), even with severe alkalosis.

## Alterations in oxygenation

When interpreting the $P_ao_2$ it is important to remember that it is the oxygen content of the arterial blood that matters and that this is determined by the percentage saturation of haemoglobin with oxygen. The relationship between the latter and the $Po_2$ is determined by the oxyhaemoglobin dissociation curve. In general, if the saturation is greater than 90%, oxygenation can be considered to be adequate. It must be remembered, however, that on the steep portion of the oxygen dissociation curve small falls in $P_a o_2$ will cause significant reductions in oxygen content. $P_a o_2$ is also influenced by factors other than pulmonary function, including alterations in $P_{\bar{v}} o_2$ caused by changes in the metabolic rate and/or cardiac output.

## MANAGEMENT

Conventional management of patients with respiratory failure includes the administration of supplemental oxygen, the control of secretions, the treatment of pulmonary infection, the control of airways obstruction and measures to limit pulmonary oedema. Correction of abnormalities which may lead to respiratory muscle weakness, such as hypophosphataemia and malnutrition, is also important.

## Oxygen therapy

### Methods of oxygen administration

Oxygen is initially given via a face mask. In the majority of patients (except patients with chronic bronchitis and chronically elevated $P_a co_2$) the concentration of oxygen given is not important and oxygen can therefore be given by a simple face mask or nasal cannula (Fig. 13.15). With these devices the inspired oxygen concentration varies from about 35 to 55%, with oxygen flow rates of between 6 and 10 litres min$^{-1}$. Nasal cannulae are often preferred because they are less claustrophobic and do not interfere with feeding or speaking, but they can cause ulceration of the nasal or pharyngeal mucosa. Figure 13.15 should be compared with the fixed performance mask shown in Fig. 12.24, with which the oxygen concentration can be controlled. It is vital to use this latter type of mask in patients with chronic bronchitis and emphysema with chronic type II failure.

### Oxygen toxicity

Experimentally, mammalian lungs have been shown to be damaged by continuous exposure to high concentrations of oxygen; oxygen toxicity in humans is less well proven. Nevertheless, it is reasonable to assume that high concentrations of oxygen might damage the lungs and so the lowest inspired oxygen concentration compatible with adequate arterial oxygenation should be used. Long-term administration of 50% oxygen or less, or of 100% oxygen for less than 24 hours, is probably safe. *Dangerous hypoxia should never be tolerated through a fear of oxygen toxicity.*

## Respiratory support

If, despite the above measures, the patient continues to deteriorate or fails to improve, the institution of some form of respiratory support should be considered.

Some of the techniques of respiratory support currently available are shown in Table 13.5. Negative-pressure ventilation is now seldom used, but is occasionally employed for long-term ventilation of patients with chronic respir-

| Technique | Comments |
|---|---|
| Intermittent positive-pressure ventilation (IPPV) | May be given with positive end-expiratory pressure (PEEP) |
| Continuous positive airway pressure (CPAP) | Given via an endotracheal tube or mask |
| Intermittent mandatory ventilation (IMV) | May be given with PEEP |
| High-frequency jet ventilation (HFJV) | May be useful in those with lung leak e.g. bronchopleural fistula |
| Low volume pressure limited inverse-ratio mechanical ventilation with low level PEEP | May achieve improved oxygenation whilst minimizing peak airway pressure |
| Extracorporeal respiratory assistance | Reduces ventilation requirements and 'rests' the lungs |

**Table 13.5**  Techniques for respiratory support.

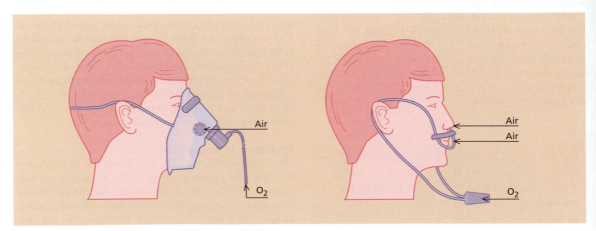

**Fig. 13.15**  Methods of administering supplemental oxygen to the unintubated patient. Simple face mask (left). Nasal cannulae (right).

atory failure due to neuromuscular disease or skeletal deformity. The patient's body is enclosed in an airtight 'tank' within which a negative pressure is created intermittently by a separate pump. Cuirass ventilators encase only the thorax.

## INTERMITTENT POSITIVE-PRESSURE VENTILATION (IPPV)

IPPV has a number of important advantages over negative-pressure ventilation. In particular, the airway is secured and protected and secretions can be aspirated more easily. In addition, IPPV can be used more successfully in those with diseases involving the lung parenchyma. Furthermore, access to and movement of the patient is relatively unrestricted.

A number of refinements and modifications of IPPV have been developed, including IPPV with positive end-expiratory pressure (PEEP), intermittent mandatory ventilation (IMV), and low volume pressure limited inverse-ratio ventilation. Other techniques include high-frequency jet ventilation (HFJV) and extracorporeal respiratory assistance. These will be discussed later in this chapter.

The rational use of IPPV depends on a clear understanding of its potential beneficial effects, as well as its dangers.

### Beneficial effects

These include:

IMPROVED CARBON DIOXIDE ELIMINATION. By adjusting the volume of ventilation, the $P_a\text{co}_2$ can be returned to within normal limits.

RELIEF FROM EXHAUSTION. Artificial ventilation removes the work of breathing and relieves the extreme exhaustion that may be present in patients with respiratory failure. In some cases, if ventilation is not instituted, this exhaustion may culminate in respiratory arrest.

EFFECTS ON OXYGENATION. In those with severe pulmonary parenchymal disease, the lungs may be very stiff and the work of breathing is therefore greatly increased. Under these circumstances the institution of IPPV may significantly reduce total body oxygen consumption; consequently $P_{\bar{v}}\text{o}_2$, and thus $P_a\text{o}_2$, may improve. Because ventilated patients are connected to a leak-free circuit it is possible to administer high concentrations of oxygen (up to 100%) accurately and to apply a positive end-expiratory pressure. In selected cases the latter may reduce shunting and increase $P_a\text{o}_2$ (see below).

### Indications

ACUTE RESPIRATORY FAILURE with signs of severe respiratory distress (e.g. respiratory rate >40 min$^{-1}$, inability to speak, patient exhausted) persisting despite maximal therapy. Confusion, restlessness, agitation, a decreased conscious level, a rising $P_a\text{co}_2$ and extreme hypoxaemia are further indications. Care should be taken before ventilating patients with chronic lung disease as patients previously severely incapacitated will

be difficult to wean off the ventilator and also relapse early. The most important criteria are the patient's previous exercise tolerance and ability to lead an independent existence.

ACUTE VENTILATORY FAILURE due, for example, to myasthenia gravis or Guillain–Barré syndrome. Artificial ventilation should be instituted when the vital capacity has fallen to 10–15 ml kg$^{-1}$. This will avoid complications such as atelectasis and infection as well as preventing respiratory arrest. The tidal volume and respiratory rate are relatively insensitive in the above conditions and change late in the course of the disease. A high $P_a\text{co}_2$ (particularly if rising) is an indication for urgent artificial ventilation.

OTHER INDICATIONS include:
- Prophylactic postoperative ventilation in poor risk patients
- Head injury—to avoid hypoxia and hypercarbia which increase cerebral blood flow and intracranial pressure, hyperventilation to reduce intracranial pressure
- Trauma—chest injury and lung contusion
- Severe left ventricular failure with pulmonary oedema (see p. 576)
- Coma with breathing difficulties, e.g. following drug overdose

### Institution

IPPV requires endotracheal intubation. If the patient is conscious the procedure must be fully explained before anaesthesia is induced. Intubating patients in severe respiratory failure is an extremely hazardous undertaking and *should only be performed by experienced staff*. In extreme emergencies it may be preferable to ventilate the patient by hand using an oropharyngeal airway, a face mask and a self-inflating bag until experienced help arrives. The patient is usually hypoxic and hypercarbic, with increased sympathetic activity, and the stimulus of laryngoscopy and intubation can precipitate dangerous arrhythmias and even cardiac arrest. If possible, therefore, the ECG and oxygen saturation should be monitored, and the patient preoxygenated with 100% oxygen before intubation. In some deeply comatose patients, no sedation will be required, but in the majority of patients a short-acting intravenous anaesthetic agent followed by muscle relaxation will be necessary.

The complications of endotracheal intubation are given in Table 13.6.

Endotracheal tubes can now safely be left in place for several weeks and tracheostomy is therefore less often performed. Tracheostomy may be required for the long-term control of excessive bronchial secretions, particularly in those with a reduced conscious level, and/or to maintain an airway and protect the lungs in those with impaired pharyngeal and laryngeal reflexes.

A life-threatening obstruction of the upper respiratory tract that cannot be bypassed with an endotracheal tube should have a cricothyroidotomy, which is safer, quicker and easier to perform. Tracheostomy performed under these circumstances can be extremely hazardous. Other

| Complication | Comments |
|---|---|
| *Immediate* | |
| Tube in one or other bronchus (usually the right) | Avoid by checking both lungs are being inflated, i.e. both sides of the chest move and air entry is heard on auscultation. X-ray to check position of tube and to exclude lung collapse |
| Tube in oesophagus | Gives rise to hypoxia and abdominal distension |
| *Early* | |
| Migration of the tube out of trachea | |
| Leaks around the tube | |
| Obstruction of tube due to kinking or secretions | A dangerous complication. The patient becomes distressed, cyanosed and has poor chest expansion. The following should be performed immediately:<br>• Manual inflation with 100% oxygen<br>• Endotracheal suction<br>• Check position of tube<br>• Deflate cuff<br>• Check tube for 'kinks'<br>If no improvement, ventilate with face mask and then insert new endotracheal tube |
| *Late* | |
| Mucosal oedema and ulceration | |
| Damage to the cricoarytenoid cartilages | |
| Tracheal narrowing and fibrosis | |

**Table 13.6**  Complications of endotracheal intubation.

indications are head and neck injuries, including burns to the face and upper airway.

Tracheostomy has a mortality rate of up to 3%. Complications of tracheostomy are shown in Table 13.7.

Minitracheostomy involves inserting a small diameter tube percutaneously into the trachea via the cricothyroid membrane using a guide wire. It can be performed under local anaesthesia. This technique facilitates the clearance of copious secretions in those who are unable to cough effectively but can protect their airway.

As for endotracheal intubation (Table 13.6), plus:

*Early*
Surgical complications
  Pneumothorax
  Haemorrhage
Tube misplaced in pretracheal subcutaneous tissues
Subcutaneous emphysema

*Intermediate*
Erosion of tracheal cartilages (may cause tracheo-oesophageal fistula)
Erosion of innominate artery (may lead to fatal haemorrhage)
Infection

*Late*
Tracheal stenosis at level of stoma, cuff or tube tip
Collapse of tracheal rings at level of stoma

**Table 13.7**  Complications of tracheostomy.

**Dangers of IPPV**

General dangers include:

COMPLICATIONS of endotracheal intubation or tracheostomy.

DISCONNECTION OR MECHANICAL FAILURE. These are unusual but dangerous. A method of manual ventilation, e.g. a self-inflating bag, and oxygen must always be available by the bedside.

BAROTRAUMA. Overdistension of the lungs during IPPV can rupture alveoli and cause air to dissect centrally along the perivascular sheaths. This pulmonary interstitial air can sometimes be seen on chest X-ray as linear or circular perivascular collections or subpleural blebs. Other complications are pneumothorax, pneumomediastinum, pneumoperitoneum and subcutaneous emphysema. Intra-abdominal air originating from the alveoli is probably always associated with pneumomediastinum.

The incidence of barotrauma is greatest in those patients who require high inflation pressures, with or without a positive end-expiratory pressure, and the risk of pneumothorax is increased in those with destructive lung disease (e.g. staphylococcal pneumonia, emphysema), asthma or fractured ribs.

A tension pneumothorax can be rapidly fatal in ventilated patients with respiratory failure. Suggestive signs include the development or worsening of hypoxia, fighting the ventilator, an unexplained increase in inflation pressure, as well as hypotension and tachycardia, sometimes accompanied by a rising CVP. Examination may reveal unequal chest expansion, mediastinal shift (deviated trachea, displaced apex beat) and a hyperresonant hemithorax. Although, traditionally, breath sounds are diminished over the pneumothorax, this sign can be extremely misleading in ventilated patients. If there is time, the diagnosis can be confirmed by chest X-ray.

Other dangers of IPPV include:

RESPIRATORY COMPLICATIONS. IPPV is frequently complicated by a deterioration in gas exchange due to $\dot{V}/\dot{Q}$ mismatch and collapse of peripheral alveoli. The latter can largely be prevented by using large tidal volumes (10–15 ml kg$^{-1}$) and reducing the respiratory rate (usually to 10–12 min$^{-1}$) to avoid hypocarbia or by the application of PEEP (see below). Secondary pulmonary infection is a common complication of IPPV and high inflation pressure may contribute to 'ventilation induced' lung injury.

CARDIOVASCULAR COMPLICATIONS. The intermittent application of positive pressure to the lungs and thoracic wall impedes venous return and distends alveoli, thereby 'stretching' the pulmonary capillaries and causing a rise in pulmonary vascular resistance. Both these mechanisms can produce a fall in cardiac output.

In *normal subjects*, the fall in cardiac output is prevented by constriction of capacitance vessels, which restores venous return. Hypovolaemia, pre-existing pulmonary hypertension, right ventricular failure and autonomic dysfunction (as may be present in those with Guillain–Barré syndrome, acute spinal cord injury or diabetes) will exacerbate the haemodynamic disturbance. Expansion of the circulating volume, on the other hand, can often restore cardiac output.

In *patients with heart failure*, cardiac output and blood pressure are usually unaffected, or even increased by positive pressure ventilation. Therefore, IPPV should be used without hesitation in patients with cardiogenic pulmonary oedema who have severe respiratory distress and exhaustion.

GASTROINTESTINAL COMPLICATIONS. Initially, many artificially ventilated patients will develop abdominal distension associated with an ileus. The cause is unknown, although the use of non-depolarizing neuromuscular blocking agents and opiates may in part be responsible.

SALT AND WATER RETENTION. IPPV, particularly with PEEP, causes increased ADH secretion and possibly a reduction in circulating levels of atrial natriuretic peptide. Combined with a fall in cardiac output and a reduction in renal cortical blood flow, these can cause salt and water retention. This fluid retention is often particularly noticeable in the lungs.

## Positive end-expiratory pressure (PEEP)

A positive airway pressure can be maintained at a chosen level throughout expiration by attaching a threshold resistor valve to the expiratory limb of the circuit. PEEP should be considered if it proves impossible to achieve adequate oxygenation of arterial blood (more than 90% saturation) using conventional positive-pressure venti-

lation without raising the inspired oxygen concentration to potentially dangerous levels (conventionally 50%). PEEP is not, however, a panacea for all patients who are hypoxic and, indeed, it may often be detrimental, not least because the use of levels of PEEP in excess of 5 cmH$_2$O is associated with an increased risk of barotrauma. Most recommend that pressures in excess of 15–20 cmH$_2$O should not be exceeded.

The primary effect of PEEP is to re-expand underventilated lung units thereby reducing shunt and increasing the $P_a\text{o}_2$.

Unfortunately, the inevitable rise in mean intrathoracic pressure that follows the application of PEEP may further impede venous return, increase pulmonary vascular resistance and thus reduce cardiac output. This effect is probably least when the lungs are stiff. The fall in cardiac output can be ameliorated by expanding the circulating volume, although in some cases inotropic support may be required. Thus, although arterial oxygenation is often improved by the application of PEEP, a simultaneous fall in cardiac output can lead to a reduction in total oxygen delivery.

## OTHER TECHNIQUES FOR RESPIRATORY SUPPORT

### Continuous positive airway pressure (CPAP)

The application of CPAP achieves for the spontaneously breathing patient what PEEP does for the ventilated patient. Oxygen and air are delivered under pressure via an endotracheal tube or via a tightly fitted face mask. Not only can it improve oxygenation but the lungs become less stiff, breathing becomes easier and vital capacity improves.

### Intermittent mandatory ventilation

This technique allows the patient to breathe spontaneously between the 'mandatory' tidal volumes delivered by the ventilator. It is important that these mandatory breaths are timed to coincide with the patient's own inspiratory effort (synchronized IMV:SIMV). SIMV can be used with or without PEEP or CPAP. It was originally introduced as a technique for weaning patients from artificial ventilation but is now used extensively as an alternative to conventional IPPV. Spontaneous respiration may be assisted during SIMV by applying a constant preset airway pressure at the start of inspiration ('pressure support'). The level of pressure support can be reduced as the patient improves.

### High-frequency jet ventilation

Adequate oxygenation and CO$_2$ elimination can be achieved by injecting gas into the trachea at rates of up to several thousand breaths per minute. In clinical practice rates of between 60 and 300 breaths per minute are usually employed.

Potential advantages of HFJV are largely related to the low peak airway pressures; for example the risk of barotrauma is reduced. Moreover, HFJV can be used to ventilate patients with large air leaks due, for example, to a bronchopleural fistula or lung lacerations. The place of

HFJV in the management of patients with acute respiratory failure is less clear.

### Low volume, pressure limited inverse-ratio mechanical ventilation

A constant preset inspiratory pressure is delivered for a prescribed time, generating low tidal volumes and reducing peak inspiratory pressure. Respiratory rate is increased in order to achieve adequate carbon dioxide removal. When combined with a prolonged inspiratory time and low level PEEP this technique may provide optimal oxygenation whilst minimising the high peak airway pressures which are thought to exacerbate pulmonary damage. Hypercarbia is inevitable but should be accepted ('permissive hypercarbia').

### Extracorporeal respiratory assistance

Recently there has been renewed interest in the use of extracorporeal gas exchange to reduce ventilation requirements and 'rest' the lungs. Carbon dioxide is removed using low flow veno-venous bypass through a membrane lung. The combination of normal pulmonary perfusion and minimum ventilation may reduce barotrauma and provide optimal conditions for lung healing. The indications for the use of this demanding technique are at present unclear.

## WEANING

The respiratory muscles eventually become weak and uncoordinated as they perform no work during conventional mechanical ventilation. Moreover, there is usually some persisting abnormality of lung function. Thus, in patients who have been artificially ventilated for any length of time, spontaneous respiration usually has to be resumed gradually.

### Critical illness neuropathy

This recently recognized acquired polyneuropathy has most often been described in association with persistent sepsis and MOF. It is characterized by a primary axonal degeneration involving both motor and sensory nerves. Clinically the initial manifestation is often difficulty in weaning the patient from respiratory support. There is muscle wasting, the limbs are weak and flaccid and deep tendon reflexes are reduced or absent. Cranial nerves are relatively spared.

Nerve conduction studies confirm axonal damage. The cerebrospinal fluid (CSF) protein concentration is normal or minimally elevated. These findings differentiate critical illness neuropathy from Guillain–Barré syndrome in which nerve conduction studies show evidence of demyelination and CSF protein is usually high (see Chapter 18).

The cause of critical illness neuropathy is not known and there is no specific treatment. With resolution of the underlying critical illness, complete recovery can be anticipated between 1 and 6 months, although weaning from respiratory support and rehabilitation are likely to be prolonged.

### Criteria for weaning patients from artificial ventilation

Clinical assessment is of paramount importance when deciding whether a patient can be weaned from the ventilator. The patient's conscious level, psychological state, metabolic function, the effects of drugs, cardiovascular performance and mechanical factors must all be taken into account. Objective criteria are based on an assessment of pulmonary gas exchange (blood gas analysis), lung mechanics and muscular strength.

### Techniques for weaning

Patients who have received artificial ventilation for less than 24 hours, e.g. elective IPPV after major surgery, can usually resume spontaneous respiration immediately and no weaning process is required. This procedure can also be adopted for those who have been ventilated for longer periods but who clearly fulfil the objective criteria for weaning.

The *traditional* method of weaning in difficult cases is to allow the patient to breathe entirely spontaneously for a short time, following which IPPV is reinstituted. The periods of spontaneous breathing are gradually increased and the periods of IPPV are reduced. Initially it is usually advisable to ventilate the patient throughout the night. This method can be stressful and tiring both for patients and staff, although some patients do not tolerate IMV (see below) and the traditional method of weaning may then be necessary.

SIMV can be used to provide a smoother, more controlled method of weaning; it may also enable weaning to commence at an earlier stage than is possible using the conventional method. There is no evidence, however, that SIMV enables patients who could not be weaned using conventional methods to resume spontaneous respiration, and in some cases the weaning process may be unnecessarily prolonged.

The application of CPAP can prevent the alveolar collapse, hypoxaemia and fall in compliance that might otherwise occur when patients start to breathe spontaneously. It is therefore often used during weaning with IMV and in spontaneously breathing patients prior to extubation, particularly when they were previously receiving IPPV with PEEP.

### Extubation

This should not be considered until patients can cough, swallow, protect their own airway and are sufficiently alert to be cooperative. Patients are assessed on their ability to breathe spontaneously via the endotracheal tube over a period of time. In those who have undergone prolonged artificial ventilation, this period may need to be 24–48 hours, or even longer, while patients ventilated for less than 12–24 hours can often be extubated within 10–15 min. During this 'trial of spontaneous respiration' the patient should be closely observed for any signs of respiratory distress.

# Adult respiratory distress syndrome

## Definition and causes

This syndrome was originally described in 1967 as acute respiratory distress in adults characterized by severe dyspnoea, tachypnoea, cyanosis refractory to oxygen therapy, a reduction in lung compliance and diffuse alveolar infiltrates seen on the chest X-ray. ARDS can therefore be defined as diffuse pulmonary infiltrates, refractory hypoxaemia, stiff lungs and respiratory distress. A PAWP less than 16 mmHg is often included in the definition in an attempt to exclude cardiogenic pulmonary oedema. ARDS can occur as a non-specific reaction of the lungs to a wide variety of insults, including shock (especially septic shock), sepsis, fat embolism, trauma, burns, pancreatitis, cardiopulmonary bypass, lung contusion, inhalation of smoke or toxic gases, Goodpasture's syndrome, amniotic fluid embolism and aspiration pneumonia. By far the commonest predisposing factor is sepsis and 20–40% of patients with severe sepsis will develop ARDS. Pneumonia is a common complication of ARDS.

## PATHOPHYSIOLOGY

ARDS can be considered as the earliest manifestation of a generalized inflammatory reaction and is therefore usually associated with the development of MOF.

### Non-cardiogenic pulmonary oedema

This is the cardinal feature of ARDS and is the first and clinically most evident sign of a generalized increase in vascular permeability caused by the microcirculatory changes and release of inflammatory mediators described previously (see p. 713). The pulmonary epithelium is also damaged in the early stages of ARDS, reducing surfactant production and lowering the threshold for alveolar flooding.

### Pulmonary hypertension

This is a common feature of ARDS. Initially, mechanical obstruction of the pulmonary circulation may occur as a result of vascular compression by interstitial oedema and subsequently oedema of the vessel wall itself. Later, constriction of the pulmonary vasculature may develop in response to increased autonomic nervous activity and circulating substances such as catecholamines, 5-hydroxytryptamine, thromboxane, FDPs, complement and activated leucocytes. Those vessels supplying alveoli with low oxygen tensions constrict (the 'hypoxic vasoconstrictor response'), diverting pulmonary blood flow to better oxygenated areas of lung, thus limiting the degree of shunt.

### Haemorrhagic intra-alveolar exudate

This is rich in platelets, fibrin, fibrinogen and clotting factors; fibrin and fibronectin are deposited along the alveolar ducts with the incorporation of cellular debris. This exudate may inactivate surfactant and stimulate inflammation, as well as promoting hyaline membrane formation.

### Fibrosis

Within 7 days of the onset of ARDS, formation of a new epithelial lining is underway and activated fibroblasts accumulate in the interstitial spaces. Subsequently, interstitial fibrosis progresses, with loss of elastic tissue and obliteration of the lung vasculature, together with lung destruction and emphysema.

### Physiological changes

Shunt and dead space increase, compliance falls and there is evidence of airflow limitation. Although the lungs in ARDS are diffusely injured, the pulmonary lesions, when identified as densities on a CT scan, are predominantly located in dependent regions. This is probably explained by the effects of gravity on the distribution of extravascular lung water and areas of lung collapse.

## CLINICAL PRESENTATION

The first sign of the development of ARDS is often an unexplained tachypnoea, followed by increasing hypoxaemia, dyspnoea and laboured breathing. Fine crackles are heard throughout both lung fields. Later, the chest X-ray shows bilateral, diffuse shadowing with an alveolar pattern and air bronchograms that may then progress to the picture of complete 'white-out'.

## MANAGEMENT

This is based on treatment of the underlying condition (e.g. eradication of sepsis) and supportive measures (such as mechanical ventilation).

Pulmonary oedema formation should be limited by minimizing left ventricular filling pressure with fluid restriction, the use of diuretics and, if these measures fail to prevent fluid overload, by haemofiltration. The aim should be to achieve a consistently negative fluid balance. If possible plasma oncotic pressure should be maintained by administering colloidal solutions with a long half-life. In patients with ARDS, however, colloids are unlikely to be retained within the vascular compartment; once they enter the interstitial space, the transvascular oncotic gradient is lost and the main determinants of interstitial oedema formation become the microvascular hydrostatic pressure and lymphatic drainage. There is therefore some controversy concerning the relative merits of colloids or crystalloids for volume replacement in patients likely to develop ARDS, or in whom the condition is established. Cardiovascular support and the reduction of oxygen requirements are also important.

The administration of high-dose steroids to patients with established ARDS does not appear to improve outcome and current evidence suggests that prophylactic administration to those at risk of developing ARDS is of no value. Moreover, there is a suggestion that steroids may have an adverse effect on the prognosis of ARDS and their use is no longer recommended.

### Inhaled nitric oxide

This vasodilator, when inhaled, can improve $\dot{V}/\dot{Q}$ matching and oxygenation by increasing perfusion of ventilated lung units, as well as reducing pulmonary hypertension. Its role in the management of ARDS has yet to be established.

### Prostacyclin

Although this agent reduces pulmonary and systemic vascular resistance, and consequently improves cardiac output, its use may be complicated by hypotension and a deterioration in gas exchange. Outcome does not seem to be improved.

## PROGNOSIS

Despite the treatment outlined, the mortality from established severe ARDS remains high at more than 50% overall. Prognosis is, however, very dependent on aetiology; when ARDS occurs in association with septic shock mortality rates may be as high as 90%, whereas in ARDS associated with fat embolism around 90% may survive. Approximately 40% of uncomplicated cases die, but the mortality rises with increasing age and failure of other organs such as kidneys and liver. Many of those dying with ARDS now do so as a result of MOF and haemodynamic instability rather than impaired gas exchange.

## Brain death

Brain death means 'the irreversible loss of the capacity for consciousness combined with the irreversible loss of the capacity to breathe'. Both these are essentially functions of the brain stem. Death, if thought of in this way, can arise either from causes outside the brain (i.e. respiratory and cardiac arrest) or from causes within the head. With the advent of artificial ventilation it became possible to support such a dead patient temporarily, although in all cases cardiovascular failure eventually supervenes and progresses to asystole.

Before considering a diagnosis of brain death it is essential that certain preconditions and exclusions are fulfilled.

### Preconditions
- The patient must be in apnoeic coma (i.e. unresponsive and on a ventilator, with no spontaneous respiratory efforts).
- Irremediable structural brain damage due to a disorder that can cause brain stem death must have been diagnosed with certainty (e.g. head injury, intracranial haemorrhage).

### Exclusions
- The possibility that unresponsive apnoea is the result of poisons, sedative drugs or neuromuscular blocking agents must be excluded.
- Hypothermia must be excluded as a cause of coma. The central body temperature should be more than 35°C.
- There must be no significant metabolic or endocrine disturbance that could produce or contribute to coma. There should be no profound abnormality of the plasma electrolytes, acid–base balance, or blood glucose levels.

## DIAGNOSTIC TESTS FOR THE CONFIRMATION OF BRAIN DEATH

*All brain stem reflexes are absent in brain death.*

*The following tests should not be performed in the presence of seizures or abnormal postures.*
- The pupils should be fixed and unresponsive to bright light. Both direct and consensual light reflexes should be absent. The size of the pupils is irrelevant, although most often they will be dilated.
- Corneal reflexes should be absent.
- Oculocephalic reflexes should be absent, i.e. when the head is rotated from side to side, the eyes move with the head and therefore remain stationary relative to the orbit. In a comatose patient whose brain stem is intact, the eyes will rotate relative to the orbit (i.e. doll's eye movements will be present).
- There are no vestibulo-ocular reflexes on caloric testing (see p. 890).
- There should be no motor responses within the cranial nerve territory to painful stimuli applied centrally or peripherally. Spinal reflexes may be present.
- There must be no gag or cough reflex in response to pharyngeal, laryngeal or tracheal stimulation.
- Spontaneous respiration should be absent. The patient should be ventilated with 5% $CO_2$ in 95% $O_2$ for 10 min and then disconnected from the ventilator for a further 10 min. Oxygenation is maintained by insufflation with 100% oxygen at high flow rates via a catheter placed in the endotracheal tube. The patient is observed for any signs of spontaneous respiratory efforts. A blood gas sample should be obtained during this period to ensure that the $P_a\text{co}_2$ is sufficiently high to stimulate spontaneous respiration (>6.7 kPa [50 mmHg]).

The examination should be performed (and repeated after a few hours) by two doctors of senior status a minimum of 6 hours after the onset of coma or, if due to cardiac arrest, at least 24 hours after restoration of an adequate circulation.

It is not necessary to perform confirmatory tests such as EEG and carotid angiography, as these may be misleading.

In suitable cases, and provided the patient was carrying a donor card and/or the consent of relatives has been obtained, the organs of those in whom brain stem death has been established may be used for transplantation. In all cases in the UK the coroner's consent must be obtained.

# General aspects of intensive care

## Overall patient management

These critically ill patients require multidisciplinary care with:

- Intensive skilled nursing care (patient/nurse ratio 1:1).
- Regular physiotherapy.
- Careful management of pain and distress with analgesics and sedation as necessary.
- Constant reassurance and support. Critically ill patients easily become disorientated and psychologically disturbed.
- Nutritional support (see p. 169). Enteral nutrition should always be used if possible.
- $H_2$-receptor antagonists or sucralfate (to prevent stress-induced ulceration). They are generally used, but are probably unnecessary in the fed patient.
- TED stockings and subcutaneous heparin to prevent venous thrombosis.
- Care of the mouth, prevention of constipation and of pressure sores.

## RESULTS, COSTS AND PATIENT SELECTION

For many critically ill patients, intensive care is undoubtedly life-saving and resumption of a normal life-style is to be expected.

In the most seriously ill patients, however, immediate mortality rates are high, a significant number die soon after discharge from the intensive care unit, and the quality of life for some of those who do survive may be poor. Moreover, intensive care is expensive, particularly for those with the worst prognosis.

Inappropriate use of intensive care facilities has other implications. The patient may experience unnecessary suffering and loss of dignity, while relatives may also have to endure considerable emotional pressures. In some cases treatment may simply prolong the process of dying, or sustain life of dubious quality, and in others the risks of interventions may outweigh the potential benefits.

Both for a humane approach to the management of critically ill patients and to ensure that limited resources are used appropriately, it is therefore important to avoid admitting patients who cannot benefit from intensive care and to limit further aggressive therapy when the prognosis is clearly hopeless.

Currently decisions to limit therapy, or not to resuscitate in the event of cardiorespiratory arrest, are made jointly by the medical staff of the unit, the primary physician or surgeon and the nurses, normally in consultation with the patient's family.

## SCORING SYSTEMS

A variety of scoring systems have been developed that can be used to evaluate the severity of a patient's illness. These have included an assessment of the severity of the acute disturbance of physiological function (acute physiology, age, chronic health evaluation—APACHE) and a measure of the therapeutic effort expended on a patient (therapeutic intervention scoring system—TISS). Other systems have been designed for particular categories of patient (e.g. the injury severity score for trauma victims). The APACHE score is widely applicable and has been extensively validated. It can accurately quantify the severity of illness and predict the overall mortality for large groups of critically ill patients, and is therefore useful when auditing a unit's clinical activity, for comparing results nationally or internationally and as a means of characterizing groups of patients in clinical studies. Although the APACHE methodology can also be used to estimate individual risks of mortality, no scoring system has yet been devised that can predict with certainty the outcome in an individual patient; they must not, therefore, be used in isolation as a basis for limiting or discontinuing treatment.

# Further reading

Barton R & Cerra FB (1989) The hypermetabolism multiple organ failure syndrome. *Chest* **96**, 1153–1160.

Forrester JS, Ganz W, Diamond G, McHugh T, Chonette DW & Swan HJC (1972) Thermodilution cardiac output determination with a single flow-directed catheter. *American Heart Journal* **83**, 306–311.

Hinds CJ & Watson JD (1994) *Intensive Care: A Concise Textbook.* London: Baillière Tindall.

Jennett B (1982) Brain death. *Intensive Care Medicine* **8**, 1–3.

Knaus WA, Wagner DP, Draper EA, Zimmerman JE, Bergner M, Bastos PG *et al.* (1991) The APACHE III Prognostic System. Risk prediction of hospital mortality for critically ill hospitalized adults. *Chest* **100**, 1619–1636.

Parrillo JE, Parker MM, Natanson C, Suffredini AF, Danner RL, Cunnion RE & Ognibene FP (1990) Septic shock in humans. Advances in the understanding of pathogenesis, cardiovascular dysfunction and therapy. *Annals of Internal Medicine* **113**, 227–242.

Ridley S, Jackson R, Findlay J & Wallace P (1990) Long-term survival after intensive care. *British Medical Journal* **301**, 1127–1130.

Stauffer JL, Olson DE & Petty TL (1981) Complications

and consequences of endotracheal intubation and tracheostomy. A prospective study of 150 critically ill adult patients. *American Journal of Medicine* **70**, 65–76.

Wiener-Kronish JP, Gropper MA & Matthay MA (1990) The adult respiratory distress syndrome: definition and prognosis, pathogenesis and treatment. *British Journal of Anaesthesia* **65**, 107–129.

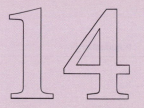

# 14

# Adverse drug reactions and poisoning

# ADVERSE DRUG REACTIONS

## The size of the problem

Any substance that possesses useful therapeutic effects may also produce unwanted, toxic or adverse effects. The incidence of adverse drug reactions in the population is not really known. A survey of 1160 patients given a variety of drugs showed that the incidence of adverse reactions increased with age from about 3% in patients 10–20 years of age to about 20% in patients 80–89 years of age. It has been estimated that about 0.5% of patients who die in hospital do so as a result of their treatment rather than the condition for which they were admitted.

# Classification

Adverse drug reactions can be classified in several ways. They may be divided into reactions due to:
- Overdosage
- Intolerance
- Side-effects
- Secondary effects
- Idiosyncrasy
- Hypersensitivity

Another system of classification divides them into two types:
1 Type A: the results of an exaggerated but otherwise normal pharmacological action of a drug
2 Type B: totally aberrant effects not expected from the known pharmacological actions of a drug
In this chapter adverse drug reactions are divided into three types (Table 14.1):
1 Dose-dependent
2 Dose-independent

3 Pseudoallergic
The mechanisms underlying many drug reactions, however, are unclear and these reactions cannot at present be classified easily, e.g. hepatotoxicity and analgesic nephropathy.

## Dose-dependent reactions

These occur in all patients given sufficiently large doses of any drug. The effects produced may be subdivided into two further groups:
1 Reactions that are predictable, being exaggerated therapeutic actions, e.g. depression of cardiac contractility by lignocaine or quinidine, or central nervous depression by barbiturates or narcotics
2 Reactions that appear to be unrelated to their therapeutic effects, e.g. the ototoxicity produced by streptomycin
The first group, being predictable, can be anticipated and looked for without much difficulty. The second unpredictable group poses serious problems of recognition and quantification, particularly with a new drug.

Factors that influence the dose at which these dose-dependent effects appear are described on p. 739.

## Dose-independent reactions

These occur in only a small proportion of patients and tend to be limited to certain well-defined manifestations. The possibility, however, of new syndromes occurring must never be overlooked. These reactions usually occur in patients who have previously been exposed and sensitized to the drug itself, to another drug of the same chemical class, or to one of another class of drugs that shares similar antigenic properties. For example, exposure to one form of penicillin usually produces a state of hypersensitivity to other penicillin derivatives, and, in a small proportion of patients, also to cephalosporin derivatives which share cross-antigenicity with the 6-amino-penicillanic acid nucleus.

Most drugs are of relatively low molecular weight and only become antigenic when they are combined covalently and irreversibly with other substances of high

|                               | Dose-independent | Dose-dependent | Pseudoallergic |
|-------------------------------|------------------|----------------|----------------|
| All patients                  | Yes              | No             | No             |
| All drugs                     | Yes              | No             | No             |
| Previous exposure necessary   | No               | Yes            | No             |
| Treatment                     | Reduce dose      | Stop drug      | Avoid drug     |
|                               |                  |                | Reduce dose    |

**Table 14.1** Comparison between dose-dependent, dose-independent and pseudoallergic reactions.

molecular weight, usually proteins. The drug is then said to be a *hapten*. Sometimes it is a metabolite of the drug or an impurity produced during manufacture that acts as the hapten. The most common of these dose-independent reactions are acute hypersensitivity reactions. These are due to the release of histamine and other mediators following the interaction of antigen with antibody (IgE) produced by B lymphocytes and bound to the cell membranes of mast cells or circulating basophils. The released substances cause rashes, oedema and the more serious effects of bronchospasm, peripheral vasodilatation and cardiovascular collapse—the anaphylactic reaction (see p. 716 and Emergency box 14.1).

Circulating antigen–antibody complexes (immune complexes) cause the serum sickness syndrome. They are deposited for example in the basement membrane of the renal glomerulus.

Delayed hypersensitivity reactions, such as contact dermatitis, are due to the formation of sensitized T lymphocytes, which activate a cell-mediated immune response.

Other forms of dose-independent reactions include various blood dyscrasias. These may involve the production of antibodies to circulating blood elements, leading to:

THROMBOCYTOPENIC PURPURA (e.g. with quinine)
HAEMOLYTIC ANAEMIA (e.g. with methyldopa)
DEPRESSION OF BONE MARROW FUNCTION, either selective (e.g. agranulocytosis) or total (aplastic anaemia). For example, chloramphenicol is a very effective antibiotic, but about one person in every 20 000 develops a fatal aplastic anaemia that is unrelated to the dose administered and which cannot at present be predicted by any pre-dose screening test. The exact mechanism of this aplasia is unknown.

## Pseudoallergic reactions

In some susceptible patients, substances mimic the allergic reactions described under dose-independent reactions but without the same immunological mechanisms occurring. Unlike allergic reactions they occur on first contact with a drug rather than after previous sensitizing exposure. Susceptibility to such a reaction appears to be determined by genetic and environmental factors. These reactions are produced by compounds that are able to release histamine and other mediators directly from mast cells without involving an antigen–antibody reaction. Examples are:

- Itching, bronchospasm and vasodilatation due to histamine release by morphine
- The flushing, urticaria, angio-oedema, conjunctivitis, rhinitis, bronchial asthma, hypotension and even fatal shock produced by aspirin

It is probable that reactions to many other drugs are also due to this mechanism (Table 14.2). An interesting

Anaphylaxis usually follows injections or occasionally insect bites.

*Clinical features*
Bronchospasm
Laryngeal spasm
Breathlessness
Cyanosis
Hypotension
Nausea, vomiting, diarrhoea

*Treatment*
Lay patient head down
Ensure airway free
Monitor blood pressure

Give:

Adrenaline (1 : 1000) i.m. 0.5–1.0 mg every 15 min
Intravenous fluids
Oxygen by variable concentration mask
Chlorpheniramine 10–20 mg slow i.v. infusion over 24 hours
Hydrocortisone 100 mg i.v. every 4 hours
In severe cases, continue prednisolone 20 mg every 6 hours

**Emergency box 14.1** Anaphylaxis.

Aspirin and other non-steroidal anti-inflammatory drugs
Barbiturates
Anaesthetics (intravenous)
Neuromuscular blocking drugs
Morphine
Chlorpropamide/alcohol interaction (p. 745)
Sodium cromoglycate
Polypeptides, γ-globulin
Dextrans and other colloids
Radiographic contrast media
Cremophor (solvent for some intravenous drugs)
Tartrazine
Intravenous compounds vitamins B and C

**Table 14.2** Agents that are believed to be capable of producing pseudoallergic reactions through release of histamine and other mediators.

example is the anaphylactic response produced by aspirin in one patient with urticaria pigmentosa and generalized mastocytosis.

If use of the particular drug to which the pseudoallergic reaction occurs cannot be avoided, its dose should be kept as low as possible, or, in the case of intravenous administration, it should be given by slow infusion rather than rapid injection. Sometimes it is possible to desensitize a patient by starting with a small dose of the drug and gradually increasing it under supervision.

# Factors influencing dose-dependent adverse drug reactions

## Formulation

The active agent represents only a small proportion of the total weight of a tablet or capsule. Similarly, drugs for injection require solubilization or suspension in a fluid vehicle of varying complexity. Other constituents of dosage forms, called *excipients*, are not necessarily inert, and may play an important part in facilitating or hindering the absorption of a drug. The proportion of an administered drug dose that reaches its site of action in the systemic circulation is known as its bioavailability. If the drug is given intravenously its bioavailability is 100%.

The dose-dependent adverse effects of many drugs are related to higher blood levels than those necessary for their therapeutic action (Fig. 14.1). A formulation that results in such high blood levels may, therefore, produce unacceptable effects. In the case of a poorly soluble drug, its physical form may be important in determining its dissolution rate and, therefore, its rate of absorption. For example, when the particle size of digoxin was reduced

by a manufacturer, many patients experienced digitalis toxicity because the rate and extent of absorption was increased. Similarly, the influence of a change of the excipient on a drug's bioavailability was seen in Australia when a manufacturer of phenytoin capsules changed from using the relatively water-insoluble calcium sulphate to the much more soluble lactose. This led to an increase in the bioavailability of phenytoin, which was even more marked because of the 'saturation kinetics' that phenytoin exhibits (see p. 743).

Modification of the physical form of a drug, and changes in other constituents, permits the development of 'controlled release' formulations. These produce sustained levels within the therapeutic range and prevent early peak blood levels that enter the toxic range (see Fig. 14.1). This effect is particularly useful in drugs with a short half-life.

## Route of administration

Parenteral administration of a drug may produce higher peak levels than are produced by oral administration, and may therefore produce more marked concentration-related adverse effects. For example, the intravenous administration of many drugs, particularly as bolus injections, may cause unwanted cardiac or central nervous effects. Intrathecal penicillin can produce encephalopathy and convulsions due to the toxic effects of high concentrations on the central nervous system; this route is nowadays seldom used.

Adverse reactions may occur owing to accidents during administration; for example, arterial rather than venous injection of thiopentone results in vascular spasm, arterial thrombosis and gangrene.

## Pregnancy

Some drugs given in the first 3 months of pregnancy may cause congenital abnormalities and are said to be teratogenic. The best known example of a teratogenic drug is thalidomide, which resulted in bizarre and therefore easily recognizable abnormalities such as absent or grossly abnormal limbs (amelia, phocomelia). Stilboestrol administration during pregnancy produced adenosis and adenocarcinoma of the vagina in the female offspring when they reached their late teens or early twenties. This was recognized because of the normally relatively low incidence of this carcinoma in this age group. Low-grade teratogens that cause only minor deformities infrequently are likely to be unrecognized or demonstrated only with difficulty. Other drugs that are known or suspected to be teratogenic are given in Table 14.3.

Drugs given after the period of organogenesis may affect the growth or function of normally formed fetal tissues or organs. The more important of these drugs are given in Table 14.4.

## Age

Some drugs produce specific adverse effects at the extremes of life.

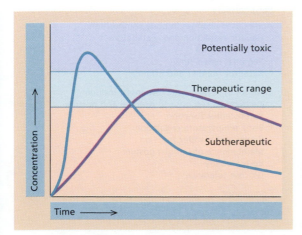

**Fig. 14.1** Relationships between blood drug concentration, its effect and time after oral administration.

*Definite or strongly suspected teratogens*
Thalidomide
Anticonvulsants
Antineoplastic drugs
Folic acid antagonists
Alcohol
Warfarin
Lithium
Oestrogens
Stilboestrol
Androgenic steroids
Etretinate
Angiotensin-converting enzyme inhibitors
Isotretinoin
Podophyllum resin
Organic mercury

*Possible teratogens*
Inhalational anaesthetics
Vitamin A
Progestogens
Live vaccines (some)
Radiographic dyes
Penicillamine
Progesterones (high doses)

**Table 14.3**  Agents known or suspected to be teratogenic in humans.

| Drug | Effect |
|---|---|
| *Antibacterial drugs* | |
| Tetracyclines | Dental discoloration |
| Aminoglycosides | Eighth nerve damage |
| Novobiocin | Jaundice, kernicterus |
| Sulphonamides | |
| *Antithyroid drugs* | |
| Iodides | |
| Carbimazole | Neonatal hypothyroidism, goitre |
| Lithium | |
| Povidone-iodine | |
| *Anticoagulants* | |
| Warfarin | Fetal and neonatal haemorrhage |
| *Hypoglycaemics* | |
| Sulphonylureas | Fetal and neonatal hypoglycaemia |
| *Cardiovascular drugs* | |
| β-Agonists | Fetal tachycardia, delayed labour |
| β-Antagonists | Fetal and neonatal bradycardia, |
| Reserpine | impaired adrenergic responses |
| *Central nervous system drugs* | |
| Narcotics | |
| Alcohol | Central nervous depression, |
| Barbiturates | withdrawal syndromes |
| Benzodiazepines | |
| *Corticosteroids and sex hormones* | Fetal and neonatal adrenal suppression, virilization of female fetus |
| *Non-steroidal anti-inflammatory drugs* | |
| Aspirin | Premature closure of fetal ductus |
| Indomethacin | arteriosus, delayed labour, increased blood loss |

**Table 14.4**  Drugs that may have unwanted effects on the fetus during intrauterine life if given to the mother.

### Neonates

In the neonatal period, drug-metabolizing enzymes may be deficient for at least a month after birth, particularly in the premature neonate. Neonates have problems in effectively metabolizing vitamin K analogues, sulphonamides, barbiturates, morphine and curare. One of the most dramatic examples is the production of the 'grey baby' syndrome by chloramphenicol in premature infants. This consists of circulatory collapse and muscular hypotonia and is thought to be due to a combination of defective hepatic conjugation of chloramphenicol and accumulation of unconjugated drug because of immature renal excretion.

In addition to hepatic immaturity, newborn infants have a relatively lower glomerular filtration rate and renal plasma flow than adults, which results in reduced excretion of drugs such as aminoglycosides and digoxin.

### The elderly

Adverse drug reactions occur commonly in the elderly (Table 14.5). They receive more drugs on average because of their increased incidence of disease conditions, and are therefore more likely to experience drug interactions. They are also more susceptible to most dose-related adverse drug reactions.

Reduced hepatic drug extraction and metabolism occurs with increasing age. This contributes to the increased incidence of adverse effects in older patients following the administration of central depressant drugs such as sedatives, tranquillizers and hypnotics. Age-related changes in the sensitivity of the central nervous system to the effects of these compounds may also be involved.

Polypharmacy

Age-related changes in body composition
  Hepatic extraction and metabolism
  Renal clearance
  Regional blood flow
  Receptor number and affinity

Changes in homeostatic responses, including:
  Tachycardia response to exercise and posture
  Baroreceptor function
  Body temperature regulation
  Bowel and bladder function
  Maintenance of upright posture
  Body stability
  Glucose tolerance

Compliance

Disease

**Table 14.5**  Some factors which influence drug response in elderly patients.

Glomerular filtration rate falls with age, leading to the accumulation of drugs principally excreted unchanged by the kidney. In view of this, doses of digoxin, lithium and aminoglycosides have to be reduced in elderly patients.

Increasing age is also associated with changes in body composition, as well as with a general tendency to a decrease in body weight. Both of these may influence the distribution and tissue levels of administered drugs.

## Differences in enzyme activity

Differences in enzyme activity between individuals may be either inherited or acquired.

### Inherited

There are marked differences in the rates of drug metabolism between individuals. Some of these are known to be due to polymorphic genetic control of the metabolic pathways involved (Table 14.6).

Other examples include the exacerbation of acute intermittent porphyria by barbiturates and the occurrence of a rare familial resistance to coumarin anticoagulants.

### Acquired enzyme inhibition

Many adverse drug reactions occur due to the administration of drugs which cause inhibition of enzymes.

MONOAMINE OXIDASE. This is a widely distributed enzyme that is responsible for the intercellular degradation of, amongst other monoamines, adrenaline, noradrenaline, dopamine and 5-hydroxytryptamine (serotonin). Its inhibition by monoamine oxidase inhibitors (MAOIs) may, therefore, give rise to serious adverse effects from the following agents if taken concurrently (Fig. 14.2):

INDIRECTLY ACTING SYMPATHOMIMETIC AMINES such as ephedrine and phenylpropanolamine, whose pressor and cardiac actions are due to the release of noradrenaline from adrenergic nerve terminals, are potentiated by monoamine oxidase inhibition.

FOODS THAT CONTAIN TYRAMINE, such as cheeses, wines, meat and yeast products. Tyramine is an indirectly acting amine with similar actions to phenylpropanolamine.

MONOAMINE-REUPTAKE INHIBITING (TRICYCLIC) ANTIDEPRESSANTS can cause serious central nervous stimulation, convulsions and circulatory collapse if given together with an MAOI.

ANTIHYPERTENSIVE DRUGS such as reserpine, guanethidine and bethanidine release noradrenaline from its neuronal stores and so can produce serious hypertension if given with an MAOI.

PETHIDINE may produce severe narcotic effects with coma and hyperthermia in patients receiving MAOIs, possibly owing to raised levels of cerebral 5-hydroxytryptamine.

Reversible inhibition of monooxidase type A (RIMA, see p. 973) drugs are now available causing less adverse effects.

XANTHINE OXIDASE. Inhibition of xanthine oxidase by allopurinol can lead to reduced breakdown of purines such as 6-mercaptopurine and azathioprine, with an increased risk of their dose-dependent adverse effects, for example on the bone marrow.

ALDEHYDE DEHYDROGENASE. This is inhibited by disulfiram, resulting in an accumulation of acetaldehyde after ingestion of alcohol, with the resulting 'antabuse' reaction of flushing, hypotension, headache, sweating, nausea, vomiting and even cardiovascular collapse. This forms the basis of one approach to the management of alcohol dependence (see p. 985). A similar reaction may occur with the antimicrobial drug metronidazole.

Competition by drugs for hepatic drug-metabolizing pathways is not uncommon and is recognized as a basis

| Deficient enzyme | Drugs involved | Adverse effects |
|---|---|---|
| Cholinesterase | Succinylcholine | Prolonged neuromuscular blockade, apnoea |
| N-Acetyltransferase | Isoniazid | Peripheral neuropathy |
| | Procainamide Phenelzine Hydralazine | Systemic lupus erythematosus |
| Glucose-6-phosphate dehydrogenase (see Table 6.13) | Primaquine Sulphonamides Nitrofurantoin Quinine Chloramphenicol | Haemolysis |
| Glutathione peroxidase | Sulphonamides | Haemolysis |
| Methaemoglobin reductase | Sulphonamides Nitrites | Methaemoglobinaemia |
| Mixed function oxidase (cytochrome P450) | Debrisoquine Phenformin (withdrawn) Metoprolol | Hypotension Lactic acidosis Bradycardia, marked β-blockade |

Table 14.6  Adverse drug reactions associated with inherited enzyme deficiencies.

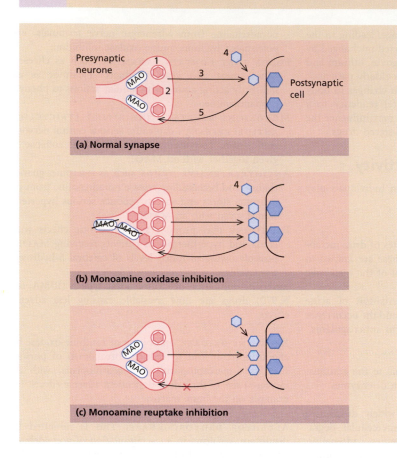

**Fig. 14.2** Mechanism by which monoamine oxidase inhibitors and monoamine reuptake inhibitors influence indirectly and directly acting sympathomimetic amines.
1. Granular store of catecholamine;
2. free cytoplasmic catecholamine;
3. catecholamine released into synaptic cleft by nerve impulse or indirectly acting amine such as ephedrine or tyramine;
4. exogenously administered, directly acting amine such as noradrenaline;
5. reuptake of catecholamine into the neurone, terminating its action.
(a) Normal synapse;
(b) monoamine oxidase inhibition leads to increased catecholamine release by nerve impulse and potentiation of the effect, or sympathomimetic amine;
(c) monoamine reuptake inhibition, e.g. tricyclics, leads to increased effects of transmitter or administered amine.

for adverse drug interactions. For example, cimetidine increases the anticoagulant effect of warfarin, the sedative effect of diazepam and the β-adrenoreceptor blocking action of propranolol by inhibiting their hepatic metabolism. Sulphonamides decrease phenytoin metabolism so that toxic levels may be reached.

### Acquired enzyme induction

The activity of hepatic drug-metabolizing enzymes may be increased by a large number of common substances, including insecticides, pesticides, polycyclic aromatic hydrocarbons, and some drugs such as barbiturates, phenytoin, carbamazepine and rifampicin. Such enzyme induction results in increased drug metabolism and breakdown, reducing the therapeutic activity of certain drugs. Examples include oral anticoagulants, corticosteroids and the contraceptive pill. The importance of enzyme induction lies in the exaggerated effects that can occur if the inducing drug is discontinued and the drug whose metabolism was being induced, e.g. warfarin, continues to be given in an increased dosage.

## Protein binding

Many drugs are loosely bound to plasma and tissue proteins. The free unbound fraction is pharmacologically active. This fraction is increased in conditions in which hypoproteinaemia occurs (see Table 14.7). Competition between drugs for common binding sites can lead to a transient increase in free levels of one following its displacement by another, but the clinical importance of this is uncertain because increased clearance of the free fraction occurs, which tends to re-establish the original equilibrium between free and bound drug levels.

## Route and kinetics of metabolism

Adverse reactions are particularly likely to occur where the relationship between drug dose and blood level is non-linear, so that relatively small increments in the dose given may lead to unexpectedly large increases in the blood level. Such a relationship is typical of saturation kinetics, in which hepatic metabolizing pathways become saturated or exhausted at a certain dose. Above this dose, proportionately more unchanged drug enters the systemic circulation. An important example of this phenomenon is seen with phenytoin (Fig. 14.3).

Some adverse effects are due not to the parent compound but to highly reactive metabolites. For example, when paracetamol is taken in overdose the capacity of hepatic conjugating mechanisms is exceeded and a hepatotoxic metabolite is formed and accumulates.

| Disease | Mechanism | Drugs involved | Effects |
|---|---|---|---|
| Liver disease; renal disease; cancer | Reduced serum albumin | Acidic drugs, e.g. aspirin | Increased free drug, risk of increased toxicity |
| Acute and chronic inflammation, myocardial infarction, surgery, trauma, cancer | Increased $\alpha_1$-acid glycoprotein | Basic drugs, e.g. $\beta$-antagonists, anti-arrhythmics | Reduced free drug, possibility of reduced therapeutic and toxic effects |
| Renal disease; cardiac failure | Reduced renal excretion | Digoxin, aminoglycosides, lithium | Increased therapeutic and toxic effects |
| Chronic liver disease; cardiac failure | Reduced hepatic uptake and clearance | Centrally acting drugs, steroids, warfarin, propranolol, tolbutamide, theophylline, lignocaine | Increased therapeutic and toxic effects |
| Cardiac failure | Reduced gastrointestinal perfusion and drug absorption | Digoxin | Possibility of reduced absorption and therapeutic effects, but importance uncertain |

**Table 14.7**  Influence of disease on drug toxicity through changes in pharmacokinetics.

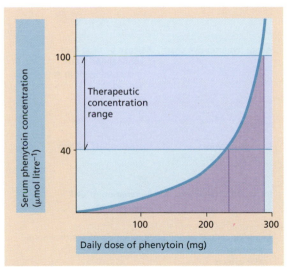

**Fig. 14.3**  Saturation kinetics as exhibited by phenytoin. The measurements were obtained from one patient on several maintenance doses of phenytoin and show a curvilinear relationship between dose and serum concentration. Note the relatively small dose range compatible with a therapeutic concentration.

## Excretion

Many drugs are excreted by the kidney, while others are reabsorbed. Changes in urinary pH affect elimination; for example, the excretion of the acidic drug aspirin is increased, whereas that of the basic drug mexiletine is reduced, by alkalinization of the urine. This may be important clinically in patients who have a persistently high urine pH from renal disease or a vegetarian diet. Competition for renal tubular excretion also occurs, e.g. penicillin competes with probenecid.

## Local factors

The therapeutic action of some drugs is markedly dependent on the local physiological environment at its site of action. A good example is the effect of myocardial potassium concentration on the cardiac actions of digitalis glycosides, hypokalaemia leading to enhancement of their action, with the risk of toxicity. Another example is the influence of changes in sodium and potassium status on the response to lithium.

## Drug interactions

Drugs can interact within the body in many ways that may lead to adverse effects. Some important examples are given in Table 14.8.

## Patient compliance

Patient compliance is also a factor in adverse reactions. Compliance is influenced by the drug formulation, frequency of dosage, number of drugs prescribed, and by the patient's age and ability to comprehend instructions.

## Influence of disease on adverse drug reactions

Disease processes may increase the risk and severity of adverse drug reactions in three ways.

1 Disease may lead to changes in the pharmacokinetics of a drug. A reduction in protein binding or reduced renal or hepatic clearance will potentiate the effects of certain drugs (Table 14.7).

| Drug A *may interact with* | Drug B | Potential results | Mechanism |
|---|---|---|---|
| *Reduced hepatic excretion* Carbamazepine Phenytoin Diazepam Propranolol Theophylline Coumarin anticoagulants | Cimetidine Sodium valproate Chloramphenicol Ciprofloxacin Sulphonamides Tolbutamide Indomethacin Clofibrate Tamoxifen | Potentiation of drug A | Inhibition of hepatic enzymes by drug B |
| *Reduced renal excretion* Penicillins Cephalosporins Dapsone | Probenecid | Increased plasma levels of drug A | Reduced tubular secretion of drug A |
| Mexiletine Amphetamine | Antacids (systemically absorbed) | Increased plasma levels of drug A | Reduced excretion of drug A in alkaline urine |
| *Inhibition of neuronal uptake* Monoamine reuptake inhibiting antidepressants, e.g. imipramine, amitriptyline Fenfluramine | Noradrenaline Adrenaline Phenylephrine | Potentiation of pressor action of drug B | Inhibition by drug A of neuronal uptake of drug B (see Fig. 14.2) |
| *Inhibition of monoamine oxidase* MAOIs, e.g. phenelzine | Amphetamine Ephedrine Phenylpropanolamine Pseudoephedrine Fenfluramine Levodopa Tyramine-containing food and wines | Acute hypertensive crisis | Release by drug B of monoamine stores increased by drug A (see Fig. 14.2) |
| | Pethidine and other narcotics Fluoxetine | Central nervous excitation and coma | Increased 5HT activity |
| *Summation of effects* Barbiturates | Alcohol | Increased CNS depression | Summation of CNS depression |
| Benzodiazepines | Other CNS depressants | | |
| Monoamine reuptake inhibiting antidepressants, e.g. imipramine, amitriptyline | Anticholinergics Antihistamines Antiparkinsonian drugs | Excessive central and peripheral atropine-like effects | Summation of anticholinergic actions |
| | Monoamine oxidase inhibitors, e.g. phenelzine | Central nervous excitation, coma | Increased central monoamine activity |
| Thiazide and loop diuretics | Corticosteroids Carbenoxolene | Hypokalaemia | Renal potassium loss |
| Angiotensin-converting enzyme inhibitors, e.g. captopril, enalapril | Potassium-sparing diuretics | Hyperkalaemia | Potassium retention |
| Antiarrhythmic drugs | β-Adrenoceptor blocking drugs, particularly propranolol | Myocardial depression | Summation of myocardial depression |
| Antihypertensive drugs | Vasodilators Alcohol Fenfluramine Levodopa Bromocriptine | Hypotension | Summation of hypotensive effects |
| Loop diuretics | Aminoglycosides Cephaloridine Cephalothin | Increased nephrotoxicity and ototoxicity | Uncertain |

**Table 14.8**  Some clinically important drug interactions leading to adverse effects.

| Drug A *may interact with* | Drug B | Potential results | Mechanism |
|---|---|---|---|
| *Others* | | | |
| Digoxin | Thiazide and loop diuretics | Toxicity of drug A | Hypokalaemia |
| | Quinidine | Toxicity of drug A | Clearance of drug A reduced |
| | Amiodarone | | by drug B |
| | Nifedipine | | |
| | Verapamil | | |
| Lithium | Haloperidol | Involuntary movements | Uncertain |
| Competitive neuromuscular blocking drugs, e.g. tubocurarine | Aminoglycosides Propranolol Lithium Quinidine | Potentiation of drug A | Uncertain |
| Metronidazole Chlorpropamide | Alcohol | Flushing, hypotension | Uncertain |
| Alcohol | Disulfiram | 'Antabuse' reaction: flushing, hypotension, tachycardia, arrhythmias | Inhibition by drug B of metabolism of drug A producing acetaldehyde accumulation |
| Azathioprine 6-Mercaptopurine | Allopurinol | Toxicity of drug A | Xanthine oxidase inhibition by drug B |

5HT, 5-hydroxytryptamine; MAOIs, monoamine oxidase inhibitors.

**Table 14.8**　Continued.

2 Changes in receptor density and function may occur. For example, there is evidence that the enhanced bronchoconstrictor effects of $\beta$-adrenoceptor antagonists in asthmatic patients may be due to a reduction ('down-regulation') in $\beta$-receptor number produced by long-term treatment with $\beta$-agonists such as salbutamol. The sensitivity of patients with myasthenia gravis to the neuromuscular blocking effects of streptomycin, neomycin or kanamycin may be due to drug-induced changes in cholinergic receptors.

3 Some inherited diseases are associated with enhanced drug toxicity (Table 14.9).

There are also several examples of disease-related enhanced drug toxicity the nature of which is not yet understood (Table 14.10).

# Monitoring adverse drug reactions

Clinical trials of new drugs are conveniently classified into:

PHASE 1: in which the drug is given to a small number

| Inherited disease | Drug | Reaction |
|---|---|---|
| Haemophilia and von Willebrand's disease | Salicylates | Prolongs bleeding time |
| Hereditary myopathies, myotonia congenita | Halothane Caffeine Succinylcholine Potassium chloride | Malignant hyperthermia (malignant hyperpyrexia) |
| Osteogenesis imperfecta | Halothane Succinylcholine | Pyrexia |
| Periodic paralysis | Potassium chloride Insulin Adrenaline Ethanol Liquorice derivatives | Paralysis |
| Familial dysautonomia | Cholinergic and adrenergic agonists | Denervation supersensitivity |

**Table 14.9**　Some examples of enhanced drug toxicity associated with inherited diseases.

| Disease | Drug | Reaction |
|---------|------|----------|
| Glandular fever (infectious mononucleosis) | Ampicillin Amoxycillin | Rash |
| Hypothyroidism Respiratory failure | CNS depressants | Enhanced CNS depression and respiratory failure |
| Burns Renal failure Polyneuropathy | Succinylcholine | Release of potassium producing cardiac arrhythmias |
| Rheumatoid arthritis and other connective tissue diseases | Salicylates | Hepatotoxicity (rare) |
| Cystic fibrosis | Isoprenaline Theophylline | Bronchospasm |
| Renal failure | Clofibrate Benzodiazepines Monoamine reuptake inhibiting antidepressants (tricyclic) | Severe myopathy Fatal dialysis dementia |

**Table 14.10**  Some examples of drug toxicity associated with disease states, the nature of which is not yet understood.

of normal volunteers in closely controlled and supervised conditions to study its kinetics and pharmacological effects.

PHASE 2: in which the drug is given to a relatively small number of patients with the disease for which its use is proposed. The therapeutic efficacy, correct dosage and pharmacokinetics of the drug are determined by comparing the data with those for normal subjects to obtain some evidence of its safety.

PHASE 3: in which the clinical evaluation of the drug is extended to large numbers of patients (perhaps hundreds). Trials include comparisons with placebos and with established treatments.

PHASE 4: (postmarketing surveillance, PMS): in which long-term assessment of the safety and efficacy of the drug is made in thousands of patients, following the licensing of the drug for marketing.

Experience has shown that careful observation of patients in phase 2 and phase 3 clinical trials is only likely to detect those adverse reactions that occur in 1% or more of patients exposed to a drug. Adverse reactions with an incidence of less than 1% require detection in phase 4 (PMS) studies.

Several countries have developed systems for collecting information about suspected adverse drug reactions. In the UK two systems are of particular interest—the prescription event monitoring and yellow card system.

## Prescription event monitoring (PEM)

The PEM scheme involves identifying doctors and their patients as the prescriptions for a particular drug pass through the central Prescription Pricing Authority office. Relevant prescriptions are photocopied and the copies are sent in confidence to the Drug Surveillance Research Unit in Southampton. Each 'test' drug under investigation is matched with a 'control' drug that is chemically or pharmacologically similar and already marketed for the same

indications. Similar numbers of patients receiving each drug are selected and a simple questionnaire is sent to their general medical practitioners, requesting information on age, new diagnoses or events that have come to the doctor's attention, and reasons for any referral to a consultant or admission to hospital. PEM should be able to identify adverse drug reactions that have an incidence of 1 in 3000 or greater.

## Yellow card system

The voluntary yellow card system has been the most productive to date in the UK for identifying important adverse drug reactions. Yellow reply-paid cards are supplied to doctors and dentists, who are encouraged to use them to report any suspected adverse drug reactions to the government's advisory Committee on Safety of Medicines. Although the rate of reporting is low, this system has drawn attention to the association of oral contraceptives and thromboembolism, hepatitis and methyldopa, jaundice and halothane, and extrapyramidal effects and metoclopramide. At present, only this system is potentially capable of detecting risk at all levels of incidence.

When suspicion has been aroused through the yellow card system, the existence or otherwise of a true association between a reported event and the implicated drug must be demonstrated epidemiologically by case control or cohort studies, and by clinical pharmacological and toxicological studies of the possible mechanisms involved.

The problems associated with long-term surveillance of many thousands of patients must not be underestimated. Such studies are costly in both time and money, and it is difficult to maintain the integrity of the study cohort, the interest and commitment of the doctors, and the compliance of the patients.

# *Reduction of adverse drug reactions*

The incidence of adverse drug reactions can be reduced by:

- The development and marketing of safer drugs by the pharmaceutical industry
- Tighter control by drug-regulatory authorities within government on the licensing, promotion and marketing of drugs

In addition, the doctor must think carefully about every drug he or she prescribes.

The hazards of adverse drug reaction can be substantially reduced by:

- Understanding the mechanisms underlying the reactions
- Excluding a history of adverse reaction
- Individualizing drug dosage

Prescribing manuals and therapeutic textbooks give recommended ranges of drug doses. The choice of dose for an individual patient, however, depends on a large variety of factors, including genetic and environmental factors, most of which are still only poorly understood. The prescribing doctor must, therefore, determine the optimum drug dose for the patient from the advised range given by considering the factors already discussed and on the basis of his or her own experience. In some cases the dose can be decided by monitoring its therapeutic effect; for example, prothrombin time can be measured when using an oral anticoagulant drug, or blood sugar when using insulin or an oral hypoglycaemic drug. In addition, for drugs with a narrow therapeutic ratio (i.e. the ratio of the dose necessary to produce a therapeutic effect to that necessary to produce a toxic effect), or whose kinetics are not linear, titration of the dose to obtain a desirable blood level may be of value. Such control is called 'therapeutic drug monitoring', and is particularly helpful with digoxin, gentamicin, lithium and phenytoin, whose potentially toxic concentrations are relatively close to the therapeutic range (Table 14.11).

## Maintaining a low threshold of suspicion

Most important of all is that all prescribing doctors should be continually aware of the possibility that any clinical or life event (e.g. an accident) may be associated in some way with a patient's treatment. The lower the threshold of suspicion on the part of the doctor, the lower the risk of serious long-term adverse drug reactions in the patient.

# POISONING

In most hospitals in the Western World the commonest reason for acute admission of young people to a medical ward is acute poisoning. Such poisoning is usually by self-administration of prescribed or over-the-counter medicines. Occasionally, however, toxic agents are accidentally ingested or inhaled at home or work or are administered with criminal intent. The types of poisoning are shown in Information box 14.1.

Self-poisoning is usually a cry for help and some 30% of patients admitted with overdose state that they are

---

*Self-poisoning* refers to the deliberate ingestion of an overdose of a drug or some other substance not meant for consumption

*Suicide* is the term applied to all patients who die whether it was their intention to kill themselves or not

*Accidental poisoning* occurs mostly in children below 5 years of age, but can occur in adults, e.g. from the accidental inhalation of a gas, ingestion of fluid from a wrongly labelled bottled, stings and bites, or eating poisonous foods (such as mushrooms)

*Non-accidental poisoning* is the deliberate administration of a poison to a child

*Homicidal poisoning*

**Information box 14.1**    Types of poisoning.

---

| Drug | Therapeutic plasma concentration range | Toxic levels | Optimum time for sampling after dose (hours) |
|---|---|---|---|
| Carbamazepine | 21–42 $\mu$mol litre$^{-1}$ | >42 $\mu$mol litre$^{-1}$ | >8 |
| Digoxin | 1.3–2.6 nmol litre$^{-1}$ | >2.6 nmol litre$^{-1}$ | >8 |
| Gentamicin | Trough <2 mg litre$^{-1}$ | >2 mg litre$^{-1}$ | 6–8 (immediately pre-dose) |
| | Peak 5–10 mg litre$^{-1}$ | >12 mg litre$^{-1}$ | >1 |
| Lithium | 0.6–1.0 mmol litre$^{-1}$ | >1.5 mmol litre$^{-1}$ | >10 |
| Phenytoin | 40–80 $\mu$mol litre$^{-1}$ | >80 $\mu$mol litre$^{-1}$ | >10 |
| Theophylline | 55–110 $\mu$mol litre$^{-1}$ | >110 $\mu$mol litre$^{-1}$ | >4 |

**Table 14.11**    Drugs for which plasma concentration monitoring may be helpful.

unaware of the toxic effects of the drug. The patient often takes whatever drug is easily available at home. Doctors should therefore always prescribe limited amounts of drugs, and it is advisable to keep only small amounts of tablets, preferably foil-wrapped, in the home. Patients should be advised about the potential danger of drugs that should be kept out of reach of children.

The majority of cases (80%) of self-poisoning do not require intensive medical management but all require a sympathetic and caring approach to their problems. Both the patient and the family may require psychiatric help (see p. 974) and the social services should be contacted to help with social and domestic problems.

In England and Wales there are over 100 000 hospital admissions each year for self-poisoning, the commonest being with benzodiazepines and anti-depressants, followed by paracetamol and then aspirin. In 1992 there were 3947 deaths from poisoning with medicinal agents and non-medicinal substances. Most deaths occur outside hospital where the commonest causes are from carbon monoxide poisoning from vehicle exhaust fumes and faulty appliances using natural gas.

Information from other continents is difficult to compare, but in Asia and Africa it seems that poisoning is a significant medical problem, with children being a particularly vulnerable group. In Cairo, over half of the enquiries at the poisons reference centre involve the poisoning of children. The proportion of accidental poisoning in Asia and Africa is higher than in Europe and North America. Snake bite is an important cause of mortality in Asia and Africa.

The number of admissions from self-poisoning is increasing. However, as a result of good supportive care and the reduced availability of coal gas and barbiturates, the mortality of patients has declined and is now well under 1%. Studies of the drugs involved reveal that:

ACUTE OVERDOSES usually involve more than one drug.

ALCOHOL is the most commonly implicated second 'drug' in mixed self-poisonings; 60% of men and 45% of women consume some alcohol at the same time as the drug.

THERE IS A POOR CORRELATION BETWEEN THE DRUG HISTORY AND THE TOXICOLOGICAL FINDINGS. Therefore, patients' statements about the type and amount of drug ingested should not be relied on.

THE USE OF MINOR TRANQUILLIZERS AND ANTI-DEPRESSANTS IS INCREASING; barbiturates are now virtually unavailable in the UK.

### HISTORY

Eighty per cent of adults are conscious on arrival at hospital and the diagnosis of self-poisoning can usually be made easily from the history. In the unconscious patient a history from friends or relatives is helpful, and the diagnosis can often be inferred from tablet bottles or a suicide note brought by the ambulance attendants.

It should be emphasized that in any patient with an altered conscious level, drug overdose must always be considered in the differential diagnosis.

### EXAMINATION

On arrival at hospital the patient must be assessed urgently in the accident and emergency department. The following should be evaluated:

1 Level of consciousness—a useful practical grading is:
   (I)   Drowsy but responds to commands
   (II)  Unconscious but responds to mild stimulation
   (III) Unconscious but responds only to maximal painful stimuli (sternal rubbing)
   (IV)  Unconscious and no response
   Alternatively the Glasgow Coma Scale (see p. 901) should be used
2 Respiratory effort and cyanosis
3 Blood pressure and pulse rate
4 Pupil size and reaction to light (NB opiates constrict)
5 Evidence of head injury or drug addiction

If the patient is unconscious the following should also be checked:
- Presence or absence of cough and gag reflex
- Temperature—measured with a low-reading rectal thermometer

The physical signs that may aid identification of the agents responsible for poisoning are shown in Fig. 14.4.

# Principles of management

Most patients with self-poisoning require only general care and support of the vital systems. However, for a few drugs additional therapy is required.

Blood and urine samples should always be taken on admission for the determination of drug levels, as these are invaluable for the management of certain poisons and are helpful in legal problems. Drug screens of blood and urine are occasionally indicated in the seriously ill, unconscious patient in whom the cause of coma is unknown.

Routine haematological and biochemical investigations are of value, particularly in the differential diagnosis of coma.

## Care of the unconscious patient (see also p. 903)

In all cases the patient should be nursed in the lateral position with the lower leg straight and the upper leg flexed; in this position the risk of aspiration is reduced. A clear passage for air should be ensured by the removal of any obstructing object, vomit or dentures, and by backward elevation of the mandible. Nursing care of the mouth and pressure areas should be instituted. Catheterization of the bladder is usually unnecessary as bladders can be emptied by gentle suprapubic pressure. Insertion of venous cannulae and intravenous fluids are usually unnecessary unless the patient has been unconscious for more than 24 hours.

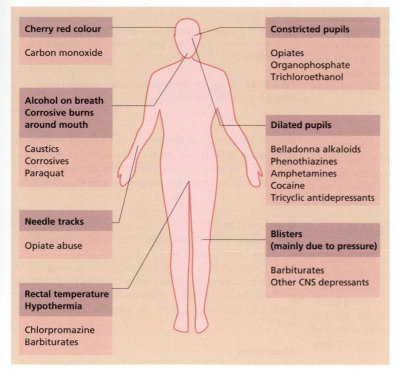

**Cherry red colour**

Carbon monoxide

**Alcohol on breath**
**Corrosive burns around mouth**

Caustics
Corrosives
Paraquat

**Needle tracks**

Opiate abuse

**Rectal temperature**
**Hypothermia**

Chlorpromazine
Barbiturates

**Constricted pupils**

Opiates
Organophosphate
Trichloroethanol

**Dilated pupils**

Belladonna alkaloids
Phenothiazines
Amphetamines
Cocaine
Tricyclic antidepressants

**Blisters**
**(mainly due to pressure)**

Barbiturates
Other CNS depressants

**Fig. 14.4** Physical signs in poisoning.

## Respiratory support

If respiratory depression is minimal, oxygen (approximately 60%) should be administered via a mask. A nasopharyngeal or oropharyngeal airway should be inserted and constant monitoring with a Wright spirometer is mandatory to detect any further depression of ventilation.

Loss of the cough or gag reflex is the prime indication for intubation. The gag reflex is assessed by positioning the patients on their side and making them gag using a sucker. In most patients the reflexes are depressed sufficiently to allow intubation without the use of sedatives or relaxants. The complications of endotracheal tubes are discussed on p. 730.

If ventilation remains inadequate, intermittent positive-pressure ventilation (IPPV) should be instituted (see p. 729). Blood gas analysis is useful to confirm the need for IPPV. Hypoxaemia is common in the unconscious patient, particularly after the ingestion of opiates and barbiturates, and can easily go undetected without blood gas analysis.

## Cardiovascular support

Hypotension (blood pressure below 80 mmHg) is a common feature of drug overdose and is caused by the physiological effects listed in Table 14.12. The classic features of shock—tachycardia and pale cold skin—may be present, but vasodilatation may also be seen, e.g. with barbiturate overdose.

In the majority of cases, hypotension is mild and elevation of the feet is the only treatment required. In patients with more severe hypotension, volume expanders such as dextran should be used. In severely hypotensive patients, the measurement of central venous pressure (CVP) is helpful. Urine output (aiming for $0.5 \, ml \, kg^{-1} \, hour^{-1}$) is also an important longer-term guide to the adequacy of the circulation, as many vasodilated overdose patients are adequately perfused with a systolic blood pressure of as low as 90–100 mmHg. Some hypotensive patients may need to be catheterized in order to monitor urine output.

If a patient fails to respond to the above measures, intensive therapy is required (see p. 721).

Arrhythmias are commonly seen with tricyclic antidepressants. All shocked patients should have ECG monitoring. Known arrhythmogenic factors such as hypoxia, acidosis and hypokalaemia should be corrected.

## Special problems

### Hypothermia

Defined as a rectal temperature of below 35°C, this is a common problem, especially in older patients or those

---

An expanded venous bed due to venous vasodilatation
Hypovolaemia due to inadequate fluid intake in prolonged coma
Institution of IPPV in an already hypovolaemic patient
Myocardial depression due to the direct effect of the drug, exaggerated by hypoxia, acidosis and hypothermia

---

IPPV, intermittent positive-pressure ventilation.

**Table 14.12** Causes of hypotension after drug overdose.

poisoned with chlorpromazine or a similar neuroleptic. Hypothyroidism should always be excluded. Hypothermia is compounded by drug-induced vasodilatation and environmental exposure. The patient should be covered with a 'space blanket' and given intravenous and intragastric fluids at normal body temperature. Inspired gases should also be warmed to 37°C.

### Rhabdomyolysis

Rhabdomyolysis can occur from pressure necrosis in drug-induced coma or it may complicate heroin abuse without coma. The risk of renal failure from myoglobinaemia is potentiated by dehydration and acidosis.

### Convulsions

These may occur in serious tricyclic antidepressant poisoning, and in antihistamine, anticonvulsant or phenothiazine poisoning. Diazepam 10 mg i.v. is the standard treatment for fits of any cause. The patient should also receive a loading dose of phenytoin (1 g administered intravenously over 4 hours via a central vein) and a maintenance dose of 100 mg 8-hourly if the fits are not immediately controlled. Persistent fits must be controlled rapidly, as they may otherwise result in severe hypoxia, brain damage and laryngeal trauma.

### Stress bleeding

Measures to prevent stress ulceration of the stomach should be started on admission in all patients who are unconscious and require intensive care. Administration of antacid by intragastric tube is usually adequate although $H_2$ antagonists are often used.

## SPECIFIC MANAGEMENT

Many techniques have been developed to decrease drug absorption and increase drug elimination, but most of these manoeuvres are only helpful with a few drugs. These, as well as antidotes to specific drugs, are described below.

## Decreasing drug absorption

Vigorous attempts to empty the gastrointestinal tract are indicated when drugs that cause potentially fatal complications other than coma or respiratory depression have been ingested. Examples of such drugs are aspirin, paracetamol, colchicine, organophosphates, iron salts and tricyclic antidepressants. It is important to remember that the risk of aspiration into the lungs associated with the use of gastric lavage may well cause more problems than the effects of the drugs themselves. Gastric lavage does not remove stomach contents completely.

### Induced emesis

Induced emesis may be useful in small children as they are more difficult to lavage. It is rarely used in adults, as only small amounts of drug are recovered.

Paediatric ipecacuanha emetic mixture (*not* the undi-

Salicylates
Basic drugs such as quinidine or tricyclic antidepressants, where gastric emptying is delayed
Paracetamol

**Table 14.13** Drugs for which gastric lavage is useful more than 4 hours after ingestion.

luted fluid extract) is the emetic of choice. The dose is 10 ml for a child and is given to children over 6 months old. Other emetics such as apomorphine, saline, copper sulphate and mustard are dangerous and should not be used.

### Gastric lavage

This procedure is of use only when a large quantity of drug has been taken. The earlier gastric lavage is performed, the greater the amount of drug that is retrieved. It is of little value after 4 hours except for the drugs shown in Table 14.13. Lavage is contraindicated for some poisons, e.g. corrosives, petrol or paraffin (Practical box 14.1).

### Absorbents

If administered promptly (within 4 hours) and in sufficient quantity, activated charcoal significantly reduces the gastrointestinal absorption of many drugs. The ratio of charcoal to the amount of poison to be absorbed is about 10 : 1 and hence is most useful when relatively small doses of drugs are toxic, as with tricyclic antidepressants, and when emesis, gastric lavage and aspiration are contraindicated. It can be administered by mouth or down a nasogastric tube.

### Skin decontamination

Absorption should be minimized for those poisons which are absorbed through the skin by removal of contami-

Should be performed by an experienced nurse and doctor

The main danger is from pulmonary aspiration, and it is vital that the tracheobronchial tree is protected either by an intact cough reflex or by a cuffed endotracheal tube

The patient should be positioned lying on the left side, with the head over the end or side of the bed so that the mouth and throat are at a lower level than the larynx and trachea

A wide-bore tube (Jacques' gauge 30) is lubricated with glycerine or Vaseline and passed into the stomach. Aspiration is performed first, and then followed by lavage using 300 ml of water at body temperature for the first washing

This process should be repeated at least three or four times, using up to 500 ml of water on each occasion

An aliquot of the washing should be saved in case it is needed for drug analysis

**Practical box 14.1** Technique of gastric lavage.

nated clothing and careful washing of the skin with soapy water.

## Increasing drug elimination

### Forced alkaline diuresis
This potentially lethal technique is rarely necessary, as few drugs are excreted in their unchanged form. Its benefits have been shown to be outweighed by its serious complications unless monitoring of fluid balance and urine pH is scrupulous. It is mainly used in salicylate poisoning, which is discussed below.

### Peritoneal dialysis
The use of this technique is limited by its low efficacy but it may be indicated for patients severely poisoned by ethylene glycol.

### Haemodialysis
This technique may be useful for patients with severe poisoning by lithium salts or methyl or ethyl alcohols. Rarely, patients with severe salicylate poisoning (blood salicylate level >900 mg litre$^{-1}$ or 6.5 mmol litre$^{-1}$) refractory to forced alkaline diuresis may be helped by haemodialysis.

### Haemoperfusion
This involves the passage of heparinized blood through devices containing absorbent particles, such as activated charcoal or resins, to which drugs are adsorbed. Its use should be considered in patients severely poisoned with certain drugs (e.g. theophylline, short- and medium-acting barbiturates and glutethimide) who fail to improve despite the use of adequate supportive measures.

## Antagonizing the effects of poisons

These techniques will be considered under the individual drugs. Specific antidotes are available for a small number of drugs. Antidotes act in a number of ways:

INTERACTION WITH POISON TO FORM AN INERT COMPLEX THAT IS THEN EXCRETED, e.g. desferrioxamine in iron overdose

ACCELERATION OR DETOXIFICATION OF A POISON, e.g. methionine, N-acetylcysteine in paracetamol poisoning

PREVENTION OF THE FORMATION OF A MORE TOXIC COMPOUND, e.g. ethanol used as a competitive substrate for the metabolizing enzyme to prevent formation of toxic metabolites in methanol poisoning

COMPETITION WITH THE POISON FOR ESSENTIAL RECEPTORS, e.g. naloxone in opiate poisoning

BLOCKADE OF RECEPTORS THROUGH WHICH THE TOXIC EFFECTS ARE MEDIATED, e.g. atropine used to block cholinergic receptors in organophosphate poisoning

## Specific drug problems

In this section only specific treatment regimens will be discussed. The general principles of management of self-poisoning will always be required.

## ANALGESICS

Analgesic poisoning is common in some areas, accounting for one-third of all cases of self-poisoning admitted to hospital. Salicylate poisoning has decreased over the past decade, while paracetamol poisoning has increased.

Combinations of aspirin or paracetamol and narcotic analgesics such as codeine or dextropropoxyphene are frequently taken. Co-proxamol, a combination of paracetamol and dextropropoxyphene can cause severe respiratory depression and is a major cause of death.

Accidental poisoning with analgesics has decreased since the introduction of child-resistant bottles.

## Salicylates

Salicylates are well absorbed from the stomach and small intestine. They are metabolized to form salicyluric acid and salicyl phenolic glucuronides, a process that is saturated at therapeutic dosage. At high doses, renal excretion becomes important. Overdosage stimulates the respiratory centre, directly increasing the depth and rate of respiration and thereby producing a respiratory alkalosis. Compensatory mechanisms include renal excretion of bicarbonate and potassium, which results in a metabolic acidosis. Salicylates also interfere with carbohydrate, fat and protein metabolism, as well as with oxidative phosphorylation. This gives rise to increased lactate, pyruvate and ketone bodies, all of which contribute to the acidosis.

Symptoms and signs of salicylate poisoning include tinnitus, nausea and vomiting, overbreathing, hyperpyrexia and sweating with a tachycardia. Alternatively, the patient may appear completely well, even with high blood levels of salicylate. The ingestion of 10–20 g of aspirin by an adult (or one-tenth of this amount for a child) is likely to cause moderate or severe toxicity.

With severe intoxication (salicylate levels 800–1000 mg litre$^{-1}$; 5.6–7.2 mmol litre$^{-1}$), confusion delirium, convulsions and coma result. Coma is common in children. It should be remembered that consciousness is not impaired unless the blood salicylate level is very high or, more commonly, another drug has been taken.

Cerebral and pulmonary oedema are serious complications, and may be exacerbated by forced diuresis.

### TREATMENT
Aspirin delays gastric emptying and gastric lavage should be performed up to 12 hours after the ingestion in all but the mildest cases and in severe cases up to 24 hours. Activated charcoal in repeated doses should be given.

Intravenous fluids may be necessary to correct dehydration and hypokalaemia. Occasionally intramuscular vitamin K is required to correct hypoprothrombinaemia. Making the urine alkaline is also effective in increasing urine salicylate excretion.

Forced alkaline diuresis is used if the blood level exceeds 500 mg litre$^{-1}$ (3.6 mmol litre$^{-1}$) in adults, 300 mg litre$^{-1}$ (2.2 mmol litre$^{-1}$) in children. Increasing the pH of the urine from 7 to 8 increases the renal excretion of salicylic acid by about a factor of 10. In the first hour, 1500 ml of fluid should be given as 500 ml 5% dextrose, 500 ml 1.4% sodium bicarbonate and then 500 ml 5% dextrose again. Sufficient potassium should be mixed with each 500 ml bag to keep the serum potassium level above 3.5 mmol litre$^{-1}$. If less than 200 ml of urine is produced in the first hour, diuresis should be discontinued. The urine pH should be measured regularly (every 15 or 30 min) and kept at between 7.5 and 8.5. The plasma pH and arterial blood gases should be monitored at least 2-hourly to ensure that pH does not rise above 7.6; the plasma electrolytes should also be measured. If facilities are not available for constant observation by medical and nursing staff, alkaline diuresis may be more dangerous than the salicylate poisoning itself and should not be used.

## Paracetamol (see also p. 256)

Self-poisoning with paracetamol is common and the outcome can often be fatal. Paracetamol is converted to a toxic metabolite, N-acetyl-p-benzoquinonimine, which is normally inactivated by conjugation with reduced glutathione. After a large overdose, glutathione is depleted and the toxic metabolite binds covalently with sulphydryl groups on liver cell membranes causing necrosis. Marked liver necrosis can occur with as little as 10 g (20 tablets), and death with 15 g. The prothrombin time (the The International Normalized Ratio, INR) is the best guide to the severity of the damage.

The clinical features in the first 24 hours include nausea and vomiting, but the patient is fully conscious. Most patients recover within 48 hours, but some develop liver failure, which usually becomes apparent in 72–96 hours. Acute renal failure can occur, sometimes in the absence of severe liver damage.

### MANAGEMENT (Fig. 14.5)

Treatment depends on the interval between overdose and presentation and on the plasma concentration of paracetamol. Blood for paracetamol level should be taken immediately.

Within 4 hours of ingestion, gastric lavage should be considered in adults who have taken a single dose of 7.5 g or more, and in children after a single dose of 150 mg kg$^{-1}$ or more.

The antidote of choice is acetylcysteine given intravenously; it provides sulphydryl groups that increase the availability of hepatic glutathione. The decision to give treatment is based on the plasma paracetamol concentration, measured 4 hours after the overdose, or later by referring to a graph of log concentration against time,

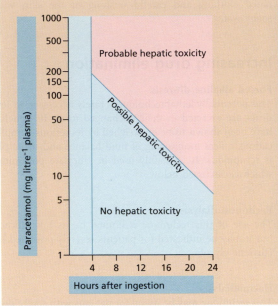

**Fig. 14.5** Nomogram for paracetamol. See text for explanation.
Cautions for the use of this chart:
**1** Units of measurement used must be the same as in this normogram.
**2** Serum levels drawn before 4 hours may not represent peak levels.
**3** The graph should be used only in relation to a single acute ingestion.

with a line joining 200 mg litre$^{-1}$ (1.32 mmol litre$^{-1}$) at 4 hours and 50 mg litre$^{-1}$ (0.33 mmol litre$^{-1}$) at 12 hours (Fig. 14.5). If the concentration is above, on, or even slightly below, the line, treatment should be given. Care must be taken concerning the units in which the results of estimations are reported.

Some patients, including chronic alcoholics and those taking enzyme-inducing drugs such as phenytoin and carbamazepine, are at greater risk of liver damage and should be treated at concentrations of paracetamol half as great as those indicated by the standard treatment graph.

For maximum protective action, treatment should be started within 8 hours. If a potentially toxic dose of paracetamol has been taken, treatment must be given at once. Therapy with acetylcysteine can be stopped if the concentration of paracetamol is subsequently found to be below the treatment line.

Acetylcysteine is given as an intravenous infusion diluted with 5% glucose solution with an initial dose of 150 mg kg$^{-1}$ in 200 ml over 15 min followed by 50 mg kg$^{-1}$ in 500 ml in 4 hours, and then 100 mg kg$^{-1}$ in 1 litre in the following 16 hours. Occasionally, patients develop a pseudoallergic reaction with wheezing, flushing and hypotension, and if this occurs the infusion should be suspended. Intravenous hydrocortisone and chlorpheniramine should be injected and the infusion restarted at a lower rate when the reaction has subsided.

Oral methionine is an alternative and is significantly

cheaper than acetylcysteine but absorption and efficacy is unreliable if the patient is vomiting. The benefit of methionine in patients presenting late has not been determined. The dose is 2.5 g by mouth every 4 hours for a total of four doses.

Pregnant women should be treated in the same way as other patients and there is no evidence that either acetylcysteine or methionine are teratogenic or fetotoxic.

Concentrations of paracetamol are not a reliable guide to the value of treatment in patients who present more than 16 hours after ingestion of the drug. The benefit of treatment with acetylcysteine after 24 hours has been established only in patients who have evidence of encephalopathy but it is worth treating all patients who have taken a potentially dangerous overdose (more than 150 mg kg$^{-1}$) and who present 16–24 hours later. Treatment can be stopped 24 hours after ingestion if the patient is asymptomatic, if the plasma paracetamol level is below 10 mg litre$^{-1}$ and if the INR is normal.

The risk of severe liver damage is assessed from measurement of the INR, serum creatinine concentration and blood pH. A poor prognosis is indicated by an INR above 3, raised serum creatinine concentration or a blood pH below 7.3 recorded more than 24 hours after overdose. If any of these abnormalities are present, advice should be sought from a specialist liver or poisons treatment unit.

### Further treatment

In patients who present within 8 hours of the overdose, the INR and serum creatinine should be measured about 24 hours after the overdose or when treatment with the antidote is complete. Patients with normal values can be discharged. For patients presenting after 8 hours, the INR and serum creatinine should be measured after completion of treatment and at 48 hours after overdose. Patients should remain in hospital until it is clear that the tests are not dangerously abnormal and the values are returning towards normal.

If a combination of paracetamol and dextropropoxyphene has been ingested, naloxone should be given intravenously in an initial dose of 0.8–2 mg and repeated at 2–3 min intervals up to a total of 10 mg if necessary. If this combination is taken with alcohol, then death from respiratory depression may occur rapidly.

In patients who present after 16 hours it is important to monitor and maintain fluid and electrolyte balance and glucose levels and to monitor for signals of encephalopathy. Haemorrhage should be treated with fresh frozen plasma. Patients with incipient or established hepatic failure may be candidates for haemoperfusion or liver transplantation. Those who develop severe hepatic damage and then recover do not develop long-term sequelae and can be treated with normal therapeutic doses of paracetamol.

## Non-steroidal anti-inflammatory drugs (NSAIDs)

Self-poisoning with NSAIDs has increased, particularly as ibuprofen is available without prescription. Overdoses will produce a variety of effects including nausea, vomiting, headache, tinnitus and gastrointestinal bleeding. Severe poisoning causes widespread metabolic abnormalities, hepatic and renal damage, and convulsions occur with mefenamic acid. Treatment is with gastric lavage leaving 50 g activated charcoal in the stomach, oral activated charcoal 50 g every 4 hours, intravenous cimetidine 200–600 mg 6-hourly and diazepam for convulsions.

## Opiates

Opiates produce respiratory depression leading to coma. Pin-point pupils are seen. Naloxone 0.8–2 mg i.v. is a competitive antagonist but, as it is short-acting, repeated injections may be required.

# PSYCHOTROPIC DRUGS

## Benzodiazepines

Benzodiazepines are commonly taken in cases of self-poisoning, accounting for 40% of all drug overdosages in the UK. On their own they are remarkably safe but they potentiate the CNS-depressant effects of other drugs taken with them, such as barbiturates or ethanol. Benzodiazepines produce drowsiness, ataxia, dysarthria, nystagmus and sometimes coma. Mild hypotension and respiratory depression may occur. Most patients recover within 24 hours. Deaths from benzodiazepines alone are rare. Flumazenil, a benzodiazepine antagonist, is only useful for severe respiratory depression but the patient should be carefully monitored.

## Antidepressants

### Monoamine oxidase inhibitors

Self-poisoning with MAOIs is uncommon and has a lower toxicity than with tricyclic antidepressants. Symptoms do not usually develop for at least 12 hours after the overdose, when catecholamine levels in the tissues have risen. The clinical features include CNS overactivity, with agitation, hallucinations and muscle rigidity. Facial grimacing and writhing movements of the limbs and trunk may occur. There is usually dilatation of the pupils, tachycardia, a rising blood pressure and profuse sweating, although hypotension may occur. Muscle tone may be exaggerated and convulsions are common. Hyperpyrexia also occurs.

Gastric lavage is performed (see p. 750).

### Tricyclic antidepressants

Most of the features of self-poisoning with these agents are due to the anticholinergic effects of the drugs. Clinical features include a decrease in the level of consciousness, but deep coma does not usually occur. Convulsions, increased muscle tone, hyperreflexia and extensor plantar responses sometimes occur. The pupils are usually fixed and dilated and there may be ophthalmoplegia and gaze paralysis. Urinary retention may be present. Cardiovascular effects include hypotension and sinus tachycardia. More serious tachyarrhythmias and conduction defects are uncommon and are thought to be due to the quinidine-like action of these drugs. Ventricular arrhythmias are a cause of death in the first few hours following overdose.

If more than 15 tablets have been taken within 4 hours of admission or if the patient is unconscious, gastric lavage should be performed, followed by instillation of a single large dose of activated charcoal. Cardiac arrhythmias may need treatment but often this is not necessary. Anti-arrhythmic therapy is often not effective; correction of any accompanying acidosis and hypoxia is more important.

Most patients recover consciousness within 24 hours, while most cardiac abnormalities settle within 12 hours.

Antidepressants such as mianserin produce only mild clinical effects, with drowsiness, hypotension and sinus tachycardia, which are less severe than with the tricyclic antidepressants.

## Antipsychotics

### Lithium
Self-poisoning with this agent usually occurs in patients on long-term maintenance therapy. It is sometimes accidental owing to:

IMPAIRMENT OF LITHIUM ELIMINATION BY THE KIDNEY, owing to the administration of a diuretic

OTHER FACTORS AFFECTING WATER AND ELECTROLYTE BALANCE, such as nausea, vomiting, diarrhoea or exposure to high temperatures

In acute overdoses there is a delayed onset of symptoms of more than 12 hours due to the slow entry of lithium into the tissues.

Clinical features include nausea, vomiting, diarrhoea, coarse tremor, apathy and decreased consciousness. There may be restlessness and ataxia with increased muscle tone and rigidity. Electrolyte disturbances, such as hypokalaemia, occur with ECG changes. Acute renal failure is a rare complication. Coma is associated with a bad prognosis.

Serum lithium concentrations correlate poorly with the severity of acute lithium poisoning but, nevertheless, levels in excess of 2 mmol litre$^{-1}$ can be fatal.

Intravenous fluids are necessary to maintain a good urinary output. Forced diuresis should not be used but peritoneal or haemodialysis may be helpful in severe cases (when levels >5 mmol litre$^{-1}$ are detected).

### Phenothiazine
Clinical features include hypotension, hypothermia, CNS and respiratory depression, arrhythmias and dyskinesia. The latter can be treated with benztropine 2 mg i.v.

## CARDIORESPIRATORY DRUGS

These may be taken deliberately or sometimes accidentally by the elderly, often when one tablet is mistaken for another.

## β-Adrenoceptor blocking drugs

A small overdose of these drugs produces a bradycardia, but a large overdose can produce convulsions, hallucinations, coma, severe bradycardia, hypoglycaemia and hypotension. Atropine 0.6–1.2 mg i.v. is given. Glucagon in a bolus dose of 10 mg i.v. followed by an infusion of 3 mg hour$^{-1}$ should be used for severe hypotension. This agent activates adenyl cyclase, promoting formation of cAMP, which is a direct β-stimulant of the heart. If this is unavailable, isoprenaline 2 mg diluted in 500 ml normal saline or 5% dextrose at a rate of 20–40 drops per minute should be given.

## Digoxin

Self-poisoning with this agent is uncommon but chronic poisoning in patients on digoxin is frequent. Clinical features include nausea, vomiting and cardiac arrhythmias, such as heart block and various tachyarrhythmias, including ventricular tachycardia.

Treatment is supportive. Cardiac abnormalities are treated, and hypokalaemia should be corrected.

Digoxin-specific antibody is available for life-threatening overdosage and can be used for severe digitoxin as well as digoxin poisoning.

## Theophylline

Overdosage causes vomiting, restlessness, agitation, tachycardia and dilated pupils. Convulsions, arrhythmias, gastric haemorrhage and hypokalaemia are seen in severe cases. Gastric lavage is performed and activated charcoal given with intravenous diazepam to control convulsions.

## Other

Self-poisoning by cardiorespiratory drugs is becoming more frequent. Overdosage results in an exaggerated pharmacological effect and treatment should be aimed at counteracting this, e.g. an overdose of salbutamol is treated with a β-blocker.

# Household and industrial poisons

Virtually all substances found in the home have been ingested either by adults because of poorly labelled bottles or accidentally by children. Occasionally household agents are deliberately taken. Many kitchen products contain bleaches (sodium hypochlorite or hydrogen peroxide), acids or alkalis and the main problem after poisoning with them is their corrosive action on the gut. There is an immediate burning pain in the lips, mouth, throat, retrosternal area and stomach, and ulceration may follow. Vomiting may occur, with blood in severe cases.

The major long-term complication is oesophageal stricture. Poisoning with sodium hypochlorite should be treated with sufficient water or milk to dilute it. Gastric lavage is contraindicated unless very substantial quantities have been taken. Alkalis should not be neutralized.

Some household products contain solvents, e.g. acetone in nail varnish remover or toluene in paints, which may be sniffed accidentally or intentionally (see p. 759).

## PARAQUAT

Over the last few years, accidental poisoning with paraquat has become less common in the developed world and deliberate self-poisoning now accounts for most cases. However in some developing countries it is the commonest single cause of poisoning. Paraquat is found in commonly used brands of weedkiller as an aqueous 20% solution (Gramoxone) or 2.5% solution (Weedol). A dose of 1.5 g may be fatal. Clinical features include ulcers in the mouth and oesophagus, diarrhoea and vomiting, epistaxis, pulmonary oedema, and later pulmonary fibrosis, respiratory failure and renal failure. Treatment is with gastric lavage with Fuller's earth or bentonite and purging with magnesium sulphate. Haemodialysis or haemoperfusion may be useful in removing the paraquat if started early.

The outcome can be predicted by relating the plasma paraquat concentration to the number of hours that have elapsed since ingestion. It is doubtful whether any treatment affects the outcome.

## CARBON MONOXIDE

Carbon monoxide poisoning is a worldwide problem. Domestic gas in the UK (except in Northern Ireland) does not contain carbon monoxide, but the combustion of any fuel gas in the absence of adequate oxygen and ventilation may lead to domestic carbon monoxide poisoning. The other common sources of carbon monoxide are the exhaust fumes of petrol engines and from certain gas appliances that use propane and butane gases.

Carbon monoxide combines readily with haemoglobin to form carboxyhaemoglobin, thus preventing the formation of oxyhaemoglobin. The clinical features of carbon monoxide poisoning include mental impairment, including coma in severe cases. Headache, nausea and vomiting, and the classic pink colour of the skin due to the carboxyhaemoglobin are seen. More severe toxicity produces widespread effects, including myocardial damage and respiratory distress. Treatment consists of removing the patient from the carbon monoxide source, and giving as high a concentration of oxygen as possible. Hyperbaric oxygen should be considered if the victim is unconscious or has a blood carboxyhaemoglobin level in excess of 10%.

## DISC BATTERIES

Batteries more than 20 mm in diameter can lodge in the oesophagus and a chest X-ray should always be performed. Batteries should be removed by endoscopy because they may break open liberating mercury and manganese, which have corrosive effects. Most batteries will pass through the gut in 48 hours but, if they do not and are seen on X-ray to be disintegrating, they should be surgically removed.

## INSECTICIDES

Carbamates and organophosphate insecticides are used extensively in the home and agricultural market. They may be ingested accidentally, inhaled, or absorbed through the skin when protective clothing is not worn. These agents are potent inhibitors of cholinesterase and produce an accumulation of acetylcholine. Carbamate poisoning is generally less severe and of shorter duration.

The clinical features are due to the muscarinic and nicotinic effects of acetylcholine. They include nausea, vomiting, hypersalivation, muscle weakness, bronchospasm, and respiratory failure; convulsions may also occur. The plasma cholinesterase activity will be low.

Treatment involves washing any contaminated skin. Atropine 2 mg i.v. is given repeatedly to obtain full atropinization. Pralidoxime mesylate 1 g i.v., a cholinesterase reactivator, is used in severe cases but its benefit has not been established.

Chlorphenoxyphenol poisoning may require treatment with alkaline diuresis.

## CYANIDE

Cyanide is found in a wide range of industrial compounds, e.g. rodenticide and fertilizers. Hydrogen cyanide is also released from polyurethane foams.

Ingestion or inhalation of this agent produces rapid onset of dizziness and headache, followed by acute shortness of breath, shock and eventual coma. Cyanosis is not present and the skin colour is red. There may be an odour of bitter almonds. Cyanide inhibits cytochrome oxidase, preventing cellular respiration, which leads to hypoxia, metabolic acidosis and frequently death. Treatment is urgent; oxygen is given and an intravenous combination of sodium nitrite (300 mg over 3 min) and sodium thiosulphate (12.25 g over 10 min). This is followed by 300 mg of dicobalt edetate intravenously over 1 min and 300 mg given a minute later if no recovery occurs. 50% Dextrose 50 ml i.v. should also be given after the dicobalt edetate.

## METHANOL, ETHANOL AND ETHYLENE GLYCOL

These agents are all chiefly metabolized by alcohol dehydrogenase in the liver. In poisoning, there is increased lactate formation, which increases the metabolic acidosis found after methanol (due to formate) or ethylene glycol ingestion (due to glycolate).

Minor poisoning with methanol causes headache, breathlessness and photophobia. In severe poisoning there is papilloedema and eventually optic atrophy and blindness. Poisoning with methanol is treated with gastric lavage and correction of acidosis with bicarbonate infusion. Ethanol infusion and haemodialysis are used to remove methanol in patients who have taken more than 30 g of methanol and who have a blood level of methanol greater than 500 mg litre$^{-1}$ (15.6 mmol litre$^{-1}$). Intravenous folinic acid may prevent ocular toxicity.

Ethanol poisoning produces severe depression of consciousness and hypoglycaemia, particularly in children. Treatment usually only consists of gastric lavage with an endotracheal tube in position. The use of fructose is no longer advised and peritoneal dialysis or haemodialysis is only indicated for very severe cases. Chlormethiazole, used for alcohol withdrawal, is dangerous if the patient takes alcohol and should therefore be used as an inpatient therapy only.

Poisoning with ethylene glycol (antifreeze) causes gastrointestinal upset and neurological involvement, including coma, followed by cardiorespiratory collapse and acute renal failure. Treatment is by gastric lavage and correction of the acidosis with intravenous sodium bicarbonate and of the hypocalcaemia with intravenous calcium solutions. Ethanol is given orally or intravenously to maintain an ethanol blood level of 1000 mg litre$^{-1}$ in severe cases to inhibit the metabolism of ethylene glycol. Haemodialysis is indicated in patients who have taken more than 50 g of ethylene glycol or who have plasma levels >500 mg litre$^{-1}$ (8.1 mmol litre$^{-1}$).

## HEAVY METALS

## Mercury

Chronic mercury poisoning causes tremor (hatters' shakes), excessive salivation, scanning speech, anxiety and depression. In the hatters' trade, rabbit fur was stirred in vats of hot mercuric nitrate to make felt, and inhalation of the vapour led to signs of chronic mercury poisoning.

Acute mercury poisoning is seen after the ingestion of mercuric salts (e.g. mercuric chloride), inhalation of mercuric vapours or the ingestion of mercuric oxide in 'button' batteries. It is treated by induced emesis, lavage and injections of dimercaprol or penicillamine.

## Lead

Acute lead poisoning is rare. Chronic lead poisoning, however, commonly occurs.

#### Occupational lead poisoning

This is a notifiable disease in the UK and work with lead is covered by strict regulations. Most lead poisoning occurs in scrap metal or smelting workers. Blood levels in these workers should be lower than 800 $\mu$g litre$^{-1}$ (4 mmol litre$^{-1}$).

#### Domestic lead poisoning

This usually occurs in children owing to the ingestion of old lead-based paint around the home. Most toys have lead-free paint. Chronic ingestion of water from lead pipes and acute accidental ingestion of fluid from car batteries are other frequent causes of lead poisoning.

After absorption, lead interferes with haem and globin synthesis (see p. 303). It also binds to bone, and in patients suffering from chronic exposure small amounts of lead can be found in many tissues.

### CLINICAL FEATURES

ANOREXIA, NAUSEA AND VOMITING
A BLUE LINE ON THE GUMS
CONSTIPATION AND SEVERE ABDOMINAL COLIC
DENSE METAPHYSEAL BANDS at the growing end of long bones, particularly the wrist and knee in children (lead lines)
ANAEMIA, with erythrocytes showing basophil stippling
PERIPHERAL NERVE LESIONS giving wrist drop and foot drop, with muscle involvement
LEAD ENCEPHALOPATHY, with eventual seizures and impairment of consciousness.

The diagnosis is made on the basis of the clinical features. The blood level of lead is very variable; levels above 800 $\mu$g litre$^{-1}$ (4 mmol litre$^{-1}$) are toxic.

### TREATMENT

It is most important to remove the source of lead intoxication. Sodium calcium edetate (calcium EDTA), D-penicillamine and dimercaprol have all been used for treatment.

## Iron

Poisoning with iron tablets is often accidental in children. Symptoms include nausea, vomiting, abdominal pain, diarrhoea and haematemesis due to a direct corrosive effect. In severe cases, hypotension, hepatic damage and coma can occur. Treatment is urgent and a serum iron concentration should be sent off as an emergency. Administer gastric lavage and intragastric desferrioxamine 5–10 g and 2 g i.m. 12-hourly or a slow i.v. infusion of 15 mg kg$^{-1}$ hour$^{-1}$ (maximum 80 mg kg$^{-1}$ in 24 hours).

## Arsenic

Acute poisoning with arsenic causes vomiting, abdominal pain and diarrhoea. It is treated with rehydration and dimercaprol. Chronic poisoning causes excess salivation, weakness, anorexia and polyneuritis. There is a 'raindrop' pigmentation of the skin. Arsenic accumulates in the hair and the nails.

# Venomous animals

## Snakes

The adder (*Vipera berus*) is the only poisonous snake native to the UK. However, a number of dangerous snakes are kept as pets, and worldwide venomous snakes still cause significant mortality. There are three types of venomous snake:

1 Viperidae have long erectile fangs. They are subdivided into two types:
   (a) Viperinae (true vipers, e.g. Russell's viper [dabora], European adder), which are found in all parts of the world except America and the Asian Pacific.
   (b) Crotalinae (pit-vipers, e.g. rattlesnakes, Malayan pit-viper), which are found in Asia and America. They have small heat-sensitive pits between the eyes and the nostrils.
   The venom of both of these classes of snake is vasculotoxic.
2 Elapidae (cobras, mambas, kraits, coral-snakes) are found in all parts of the world except Europe. They have short, unmoving fangs and the venom produces neurotoxic features. Venom from the Asian cobra and the African spitting cobra also produces local tissue necrosis.
3 Hydrophiidae (sea-snakes) are found in Asian Pacific coastal waters. They have short fangs and flattened tails. The venom is myotoxic.

## CLINICAL FEATURES
### Viperidae
Russell's viper is the most important cause of snake-bite mortality in India, Pakistan and Burma. There is local swelling at the site of the bite, which may become massive. Local tissue necrosis may occur, particularly with cobra bites. Evidence of systemic involvement occurs within 30 min, including vomiting, evidence of shock and hypotension; haemorrhage due to incoaguable blood can be fatal.

### Elapidae
There is not usually any swelling at the site of the bite, except with Asian cobras and the African spitting cobra—here the bite is painful and is followed by local tissue necrosis. Vomiting occurs first followed by shock and then neurological symptoms and muscle weakness, with paralysis of the respiratory muscles in severe cases. Cardiac muscle can also be involved.

### Hydrophidae
Systemic features are muscle involvement, myalgia and myoglobinuria, which can lead to acute renal failure. Cardiac and respiratory paralysis may occur.

## MANAGEMENT
A firm pressure bandage should be placed over the bite and the limb immobilized. This greatly delays the spread of the venom.

Arterial tourniquets should not be used and incision or excision of the bite area should not be performed. The type of snake should be identified if possible.

In about 50% of cases no venom has been injected by the snake bite and antivenoms are not generally indicated (unless systemic effects are present) as they can cause sev-

ere allergic reactions. Nevertheless, careful observation for 12–24 hours is necessary and antivenom must always be given when indicated, as the mortality of snake bite is 10–15% with certain snakes.

General supportive measures should be given as necessary, as for all poisoning. These include diazepam for anxiety and intravenous fluids with volume expanders for hypotension. Treatment of acute respiratory, cardiac and renal failure is instituted as necessary.

Specific measures, i.e. antivenoms, can rapidly neutralize venom, but only if an amount in excess of the amount of venom is given. Antivenoms cannot reverse the effects of the venom so they must be given early. They do minimize some of the local effects and may prevent necrosis at the site of the bite. Antivenoms should be administered intravenously by slow infusion, the same dose being given to children and adults.

Allergic reactions are frequent, and adrenaline (1 in 1000 solution) should be available. Antivenoms are usually rapidly effective. In severe cases the antivenom infusion should be continued even with allergic reactions, with subcutaneous injections of adrenaline being given as necessary. Large quantities of antivenom may be required. Some forms of neurotoxicity, such as those induced by the death adder, respond to anticholinesterase therapy with neostigmine and atropine.

Local wounds often require little treatment. If necrosis is present, antibiotics should be given together with initially minimal surgical treatment. Skin grafting may be required later. Antitetanus prophylaxis must be given.

Antivenoms must be kept readily available in all snake-infested areas.

# Scorpions

Scorpion stings are a serious problem in the tropics and cause 1000 deaths per year in Mexico. The poison glands are situated in the end of the tail.

Severe pain occurs immediately at the site of puncture, followed by swelling. This should be treated by a firm pressure bandage to avoid the spread of the neurotoxic venom. Signs of systemic involvement include vomiting, respiratory depression and haemorrhage. Treatment is supportive. Antivenom is available in certain countries.

# Spiders

The black widow spider (*Latrodectus mactans*) is found in North America and the tropics and occasionally in Mediterranean countries. The bite quickly becomes painful and generalized muscle pain, sweating, headache and shock occur due to absorption of rapidly acting neurotoxins. No systemic treatment is required except in cases of severe systemic toxicity, when specific antivenom should be given where this is available. Intravenous calcium gluconate may help the muscle spasms.

*Loxosceles* causes many bites in Central and South America. *L. reclusa*, the brown recluse spider, is also found in the southern USA. Spiders are often found in bedrooms, so that patients are often bitten at night. There is a burning pain at the site of the bite, followed by a necrotic ulcer in some cases. Systemic effects, which include fever, vomiting and haemolysis, are rare. No treatment is indicated except in severe cases, when an antivenom should be given if available.

*Phoneutria nigriventer*, the banana spider, and *Atrax robustus*, the Sydney funnel-web spider, can both give nasty bites, which are occasionally fatal.

## Insects

Insect stings, e.g. from wasps and bees, and bites, e.g. from ants, produce pain and swelling at the puncture site. Death occurs (12 per year in the UK) and is usually due to anaphylaxis, which requires urgent treatment (see p. 738). Patients who have severe local reactions to stings or a mild anaphylactic reaction should carry a Medi-jet syringe for self-administration of adrenaline should a further sting occur. Desensitization can be carried out, but the course is prolonged and often needs to be repeated.

## Marine animals

There are many poisonous fish that can be dangerous. They are usually found in tropical waters but cases have been described worldwide. Stringrays and scorpion fish are two examples that sting by injecting venom through barbed spines. There is immediate severe local pain and swelling, which may be followed by tissue necrosis. Systemic effects include diarrhoea, vomiting, hypotension, cardiac arrhythmias and convulsions. Treatment is supportive. Care should always be taken in waters where these fish are known to be present.

Venomous Coelenterata include jellyfish, sea anemones and the Portuguese man-of-war. The tentacles contain toxin that, following a sting, produces painful wheals at the site of contact. These wheals may become necrotic. Rarely there are systemic side-effects, including abdominal pain, diarrhoea and vomiting, hypotension and convulsions. Treatment consists of removing the tentacles, having first applied acetic acid (vinegar) to them. Alcohol compounds should not be used.

### Molluscs

Only the octopus and cone-shells are venomous to humans. The blue-ringed octopus, which is found in Australia, has saliva which contains the neurotoxin tetrodotoxin. This flows into the wounds from the beak of the octopus and can cause serious systemic effects.

In cone-shells the venom is found in association with their radular teeth. A bite initially produces local numbness, which can then spread over the body and may eventually lead to paralysis.

### Seafood poisoning

This can occur with fish and shellfish. In some cases it is attributable to toxins, but most poisonings occur as a result of pathogens such as *Salmonella* or hepatitis A virus. Ichthyosarcotoxic fish contain toxins in their blood, skin and muscle and are the commonest cause of poisoning.

CIGUATERA. Poisoning occurs chiefly with the reef-dwelling fish from around the Pacific and Caribbean. The fish contain ciguatoxins from the plankton *Gambier discus*. Most cases of poisoning are due to the red snapper, grouper, barracuda and amberjack fish but many other species may be responsible. The poisonous fish cannot be distinguished from identical fish that do not contain the poison. The toxin is unaffected by cooking.

Symptoms occur from a few minutes to 30 hours after ingestion of the fish. They include numbness and paraesthesia of the lips, abdominal pain, nausea, vomiting and diarrhoea. Visual blurring, photophobia, metallic taste in the mouth, myositis and eventual hypotension and shock can also occur.

Treatment is symptomatic, but symptoms can last for up to 2 weeks.

SCROMBOID FISH. Fish such as tuna, mackerel and skipjack contain a high degree of histidine. This is decarboxylated by bacteria to histamine and, particularly if the fish are allowed to spoil, large amounts can accumulate in the fish, producing flushing, burning, pruritus, headache, urticaria, nausea, vomiting and bronchospasm 2–3 hours after ingestion. Treatment is symptomatic; care should be taken only to eat fresh fish.

Tetrodotoxin-containing puffer-fish are found in both sea and freshwater areas of Asia, India and the Caribbean. Symptoms that follow ingestion are circumoral paraesthesia, malaise and hypotension, with more severe cases producing ataxia and neuromuscular paralysis. The mortality is 50–60%.

SHELLFISH. Bivalve molluscs, e.g. mussels, oysters, scallops and clams, can acquire the neurotoxin saxitoxin from the dinoflagellate *Gonyaulax*. These protozoa colour the sea red and molluscs should never be taken from such areas. Symptoms are similar to those caused by tetrodotoxin, but are usually less severe. Treatment is symptomatic.

# Plants

Many plants are known to be poisonous, but in practice it is unusual for severe poisoning to occur. Children are the usual victims. Only two people are known to have died from plant poisoning in the UK since the early 1970s. The commonest effects of nettles and poison ivy are dermatitis followed by vomiting. Poisonous plants commonly ingested include hemlock, laburnum, deadly nightshade and green potatoes. Deadly nightshade (*Atropa belladonna*) contains hyoscyamine and hyoscine. When ingested these cause the anticholinergic effects of a dry mouth, nausea and vomiting, eventually leading to blurring of the vision, hallucinations, confusion and hyperpyrexia.

# Mushrooms

There are many poisonous mushrooms that can be confused with edible fungi and be eaten by mistake. Nevertheless, apart from transient nausea, vomiting and diarrhoea, which can occur with many species, very severe reactions are rare.

Fatal mushroom poisoning is almost invariably due to *Amanita phalloides* (the death-cap mushroom). This fungus contains phallotoxins and amatoxins, both of which interfere with cell metabolism. Toxicity is increased if the mushrooms are eaten raw, as some toxins are inactivated by heat. In general, the sooner the symptoms occur, the less serious the poisoning, depending on the type of mushroom ingested. Within 2 hours, nausea, vomiting, diarrhoea and sweating occur. After about 6 hours, patients complain of headache and dizziness, and severe vomiting occurs at about 12 hours. After 72 hours, the more serious complications of hepatocellular and renal failure may occur, which have a high mortality.

The diagnosis is made by obtaining a careful history, with identification of the mushroom if possible. Amatoxins can be measured in the blood by radioimmunoassay.

Treatment should include gastric aspiration and lavage and general support. There is some evidence that haemodialysis may be of some value.

Other mushrooms that are poisonous include:

FLY AGARIC (*Amanita muscaria*), which contains a little muscarine and other hallucinogenic substances

INK CAP (*Coprinus atramentarius*), which contains a dehydrogenase inhibitor with a disulfiram-like effect, producing flushing, swelling, a rash on the face and hands, and cardiovascular effects, particularly after alcohol

FALSE BLUSHER (*Amanita pantherina*), which produces similar features to deadly nightshade because of its atropine-like effects

# Drug abuse (see p. 985)

## Solvents

Solvent abuse has become a common problem, particularly in teenagers who inhale volatile organic solvents such as toluene in glues ('glue sniffing'). Many other solvents, such as aerosols (hair lacquer), antifreeze and petrol, can also be misused. Solvents are applied to a piece of cloth or put into a plastic bag and inhaled, often until consciousness is lost. The patient presents either in the acute intoxicated state or as a chronic abuser with excoriation and rashes over the face and a peripheral neuropathy. Sudden death can occur and is probably due to cardiac arrhythmias. Stigmata of solvent abuse include sores or a rash around the nose and mouth and glue on the clothing.

## Other drugs

Drug addicts frequently overdose themselves and are commonly admitted to hospital with the signs of opiate injection. Tell-tale injection sites and pin-point pupils are important clues. Naloxone is given in the same dosage as for co-proxamol overdose (see p. 753).

### Cannabis

Cannabis is usually smoked and often taken casually. Initially there is euphoria, followed by drowsiness and sleep. Redness of the conjunctivae and pupil dilatation are seen. No specific treatment is required.

### Amphetamines

Amphetamines are taken for their stimulatory effect. In overdose there is confusion, delirium, hallucinations and violent behaviour. Cardiac arrhythmias can be a major problem. Treatment is with sedatives, such as diazepam. Forced acid diuresis may be used but is rarely required.

### Cocaine

Cocaine can be taken by injection, inhalation or ingestion. It produces excitement, over-alertness, euphoria and restlessness. This is followed by delirium, tremor, convulsions, pyrexia and cardiac arrhythmias, which may cause cardiac failure. Respiratory failure may also occur.

Treatment is symptomatic and supportive. There is no specific antidote. $\beta$-Blockers should not be used to treat hypertension or tachycardia.

### Ecstasy

This drug is also known as MDMA (3,4-methylenedioxymethamphetamine) and is a semi-synthetic hallucinogenic drug whose initial effects are sympathomimetic and may cause tachyarrhythmias, hyperpyrexia, clonic movements and convulsions, coagulopathy, rhabdomyolysis and renal failure. Treatment consists of gastric lavage, chlorpromazine, $\alpha$- and $\beta$-adrenergic blockade, intravenous fluids and passive cooling.

# Poison information services

Information on poisoning can be obtained from the poisons information services at the following numbers:

## Poisons Information Service

Belfast 0232 240503
Birmingham 021 554 3801

Cardiff 0222 709901
Dublin 010 3531 379964
Edinburgh 031 229 2477
031 229 2441 (Viewdata)
Leeds 0532 430715
0532 316838
London 071 635 9191
071 955 5095
Newcastle 091 232 5131

Laboratory analysis may help in the diagnosis and management of some cases. Information on the available services can be obtained from the Poisons Information Service in London or the local services in each country.

# Further reading

Ballantine B, Marrs T & Turner P (1993) *General and Applied Toxicology*. Basingstoke: Macmillan.

Crome P (1982) Antidepressant overdosage. *Drugs* **23**, 431–461.

Davies DM (ed) (1986) *Textbook of Adverse Drug Reactions*, 3rd edn. Oxford: Oxford University Press.

Henry J & Volans G (1984) *ABC of Poisoning*. Part 1. *Drugs*. London: British Medical Association.

Kallos P & West GB (1983) Pseudo-allergic reactions in man. In: Turner P & Shand DG (eds) *Recent Advances in Clinical Pharmacology*, Vol. 3, pp. 235–252. Edinburgh: Churchill Livingstone.

Prescott LF (1983) Paracetamol overdose—pharmacological considerations and clinical management. *Drugs* **25**, 270–314.

Silverstone T & Turner P (1994) *Drug Treatment in Psychiatry*, 5th edn. London: Routledge.

Turner P, Richens A & Routledge P (1986) *Clinical Pharmacology*, 5th edn. Edinburgh: Churchill Livingstone.

Vale JA & Meredith TJ (1985) *Concise Guide to the Management of Poisoning*, 3rd edn. Edinburgh: Churchill Livingstone.

# Heat

In health, the core temperature of humans is maintained by the thermoregulatory centre in the hypothalamus at a constant 37°C. Heat is produced by cellular metabolism, and is lost through the skin by vasodilatation and sweating and in air expired from the lungs. Sweating occurs when the ambient temperature is greater than 32.5°C and during exercise. The evaporation of sweat is an important mechanism in keeping the skin cool and the body temperature down.

## Acclimatization

Acclimatization to a hotter climate takes 1–2 weeks. There is a gradual increase in sweating, and the sweat has a lower salt content. This process allows increased evaporation.

## Heat cramps

These are painful cramps in the muscles (usually of the legs) after exercise. They often occur in fit young people who are well acclimatized when they take vigorous exercise in hot weather. The symptoms are thought to be the result of a low extracellular sodium caused by replenishment of water but not salt during prolonged sweating. The cramps respond to salt and water replacement and can be prevented by increasing dietary salt intake.

## Heat exhaustion

This usually occurs in subjects who are not acclimatized and who undertake heavy exercise. It typically occurs in troops who are suddenly landed in a hot climate without prior acclimatization. Heat exhaustion is caused by water depletion, or salt and water depletion, due to sweating. Water loss can be as high as 5–6 litres per day, and up to 20 g of salt can be lost.

Common symptoms are giddiness, generalized fatigue, weakness and syncope. Many patients are not seriously affected, but they may go on to develop hypotension, a rise in body temperature to 38–40°C, and signs of volume depletion. Dehydration and delirium can eventually occur. Sweating usually continues until the late stages. The serum sodium can be high in water depletion, but is normal or low if both water and salt are depleted.

### TREATMENT

The patient is removed from the heat and cooled using cold sponging and fans.

Oral rehydration with both salt and water may be all that is required; 25 g of sodium chloride and 5 litres of water in the first 24 hours is given, with adequate replacements thereafter. In severe heat exhaustion, intravenous fluid is required. Isotonic saline is usually given, depending on the level of sodium in the serum. Careful monitoring is required and any subsequent potassium loss must be corrected.

## Heat stroke

Heat stroke is an acute life-threatening situation when the body temperature is above 41°C. The patient suffers from headache, nausea, vomiting and weakness. The skin is hot. Sweating is often absent, but this is not invariable, even in severe heat stroke. Neurological involvement leads to confusion, delirium and eventually coma.

Heat stroke occurs in hot, humid climates with little cooling wind, even without exercise. Patients are usually unacclimatized; in some, sweating is limited owing to prickly heat (i.e. inflammation of the sweat glands after prolonged exposure to high temperatures). Old age, diabetes and alcohol are all further precipitating factors.

The diagnosis is clinical. The patient must be rapidly removed from the hot area, and then cooled with sponging and ice if available.

Unconscious patients need to be managed in intensive care (see p. 709) and rapid cooling with ice packs started. Fluids may be required, but these must be given with care as hypovolaemia is not present in many patients.

Prompt treatment is essential and can lead to a rapid and complete recovery; any delay may be fatal.

### COMPLICATIONS
- Shock
- Cerebral oedema

● Renal and hepatic failure

Treatment of the complications is described in the appropriate chapters.

## Malignant hyperpyrexia

This is discussed on p. 954.

## *Cold*

Hypothermia is defined as a fall in the core (i.e. rectal) temperature to below 35°C. It is frequently lethal when the core temperature falls below 32°C.

*Frostbite* is local cold injury that occurs when tissue freezes.

## Hypothermia

Hypothermia occurs in a variety of clinical settings:

IN THE HOME ENVIRONMENT. Hypothermia may occur in cold climates when there is poor heating, inadequate clothing and poor nutrition. Depressant drugs (e.g. hypnotics), alcohol, hypothyroidism or intercurrent illness may also contribute. Hypothermia is commonly seen in the poor and elderly, the latter having a diminished ability to feel cold and often a decrease in the insulating fat layer. Infants and neonates become hypothermic very rapidly at normal room temperature because of their relatively large surface area and lack of subcutaneous fat.

DURING EXPOSURE TO EXTREMES OF TEMPERATURE OUTSIDE. Hypothermia is a prominent cause of death in climbers, skiers, Arctic and Antarctic travellers and in wartime. Wet, cold conditions and windchill, physical exhaustion and inadequate clothing are common contributory factors.

FOLLOWING IMMERSION IN COLD WATER. Dangerous hypothermia can develop after several hours' immersion at temperatures of 15–20°C. Below 12°C the patient's limbs become anaesthetized and paralysed and take some hours to recover after the patient is rescued.

### CLINICAL FEATURES

Mild hypothermia (32–35°C) causes shivering and initially a feeling of intense cold. The subject is alert and usually takes appropriate action to rewarm, e.g. huddling, extra clothing or exercise. As the core temperature falls, severe hypothermia (below 32°C) initially causes impairment of judgement (including awareness of the cold) and later leads to altered consciousness and coma. Death follows, usually from ventricular fibrillation.

### DIAGNOSIS

If a thermometer is available (which must be low reading), the diagnosis is straightforward. If not, a rapid clinical assessment should be made. The hypothermic

patient feels cold to the touch—the abdomen, groin and axillae are cold and clammy. If consciousness is impaired (i.e. if the patient is uncooperative, sleepy or in a coma), the core temperature is almost certainly below 32°C; this is a medical emergency.

### SEQUELAE

The pulse rate and volume fall, and respiration becomes shallow and slow. Muscle stiffness develops and the tendon reflexes are depressed. The systemic blood pressure falls. As coma ensues, the pupillary and other brain-stem reflexes are lost (the pupils are fixed and may be dilated in severe hypothermia).

Metabolic changes are variable, with either metabolic acidosis or alkalosis occurring. Arterial oxygen tension readings may appear normal since they are measured at room temperature, but these measurements are falsely high as the arterial $Po_2$ falls 7% per °C fall in temperature.

Ventricular arrhythmias (tachycardia and fibrillation) or asystole are the usual cause of death and may occur during treatment. 'J' waves—rounded waves above the isoelectric line immediately after the QRS complex—are pathognomonic of hypothermia. Prolongation of the PR interval, QT interval and QRS complex also occur.

### MANAGEMENT

The principles of management of this serious emergency are to rewarm the patient gradually while correcting metabolic abnormalities and treating cardiac arrhythmias. Hypothyroidism must always be looked for (see p. 803).

If the patient is awake, with a temperature above 32°C, rewarming can be achieved by placing the patient in a warm room, using 'space blankets', and giving warm fluids orally. Outdoors, the same result can be achieved by adding extra clothing, huddling with the subject, and using a warmed sleeping bag. Rewarming may take several hours. Alcohol should be avoided—it may add to confusion, boost confidence factitiously, cause peripheral vasodilatation (and further heat loss) or precipitate hypoglycaemia.

#### Severe hypothermia

In severe hypothermia, the patient may appear dead. (Hypothermia should always be excluded before brain death is diagnosed.) Warming should take place gradually, aiming at an increase in temperature of 1°C per hour. The patient should be covered with a 'space blanket' and placed in a warm room. Direct surface heat from an electric blanket is also helpful. Any underlying condition should be treated promptly. Drug overdose should always be excluded.

Warmed intravenous fluids are given slowly and metabolic disturbances are corrected. Hypothyroidism, if present, should be treated with triiodothyronine 10 μg i.v. 8-hourly. Various methods of artificial rewarming have been suggested—warm humidified air by inhalation, gastric or peritoneal lavage, or haemodialysis—but in practice these are rarely used. The cardiac rhythm should be monitored and arrhythmias corrected.

Careful monitoring of all vital functions is required;

appropriate treatment and intensive care are given as necessary.

## PREVENTION

Prevention of hypothermia is particularly important in the elderly, who should be advised to try to improve general heating and insulation in the house. Heat should be provided in the bedrooms, and the use of safe electric blankets advised. Financial help will be needed by many patients. Constant supervision should be given during cold spells, when warm food and extra blankets must be provided.

## Frostbite

The formation of ice crystals in the skin and superficial tissues begins when the temperature there falls to −3°C; ambient temperatures generally have to be below −6°C for this to occur.

## RECOGNITION

Frostbitten tissue is pale, greyish and initially doughy to the touch. Later it freezes hard, when it looks (and feels) like meat taken from a deep freeze. This condition may occur when working or exercising in low temperatures and typically develops without the patient's knowledge. Hands and feet that have 'lost their feeling' are an important feature when the temperature is below −5°C, as frostbite may then develop insidiously.

## MANAGEMENT

The frostbitten patient should, if possible, be transported (or walk, even on frostbitten feet) to a place of safety before treatment commences. Warming using the body heat of a companion or by immersion in water at 39–42°C should be continued until obvious thawing occurs. This may be painful. Blisters will form within several days and, depending on the degree of frostbite, a blackened carapace or shell develops as the blisters regress or burst. Dry, non-adherent dressings and strict aseptic precautions are essential. Frostbitten tissues are anaesthetized and are at risk from infection and further trauma. Recovery takes place over many weeks. Surgery may be required, but should be avoided in the early stages, as it is difficult to predict the eventual amount of recovery.

## *High altitudes*

The partial pressure of ambient (and hence alveolar and arterial) oxygen falls in a near-linear relationship to altitude (Fig. 15.1).

Below 3000 m there are few important clinical effects. Commercial aircraft are pressurized to 2750 m and the resulting hypoxia causes breathlessness only in those with severe cardiorespiratory disease. The incidence of thromboembolism is, however, slightly greater than at sea level

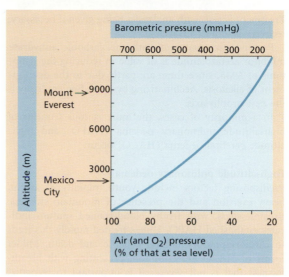

**Fig. 15.1** Diagram to show the decrease in oxygen and barometric pressure with increasing altitude.

in sedentary travellers on long flights.

Above 3000–3500 m, hypoxia causes a spectrum of related clinical syndromes that affect visitors to high altitudes, principally climbers, trekkers, skiers and troops (Table 15.1). These conditions, which often coexist, occur largely during the acclimatization process. This may last some weeks, but enables man to live (permanently if necessary) at altitudes up to about 5600 m. At greater heights, although man can survive for days or weeks, deterioration due to chronic hypoxia is inevitable.

It has now been demonstrated on several occasions that ascent to the highest of the world's summits is possible without the use of supplementary oxygen. At the summit of Everest the barometric pressure is 34 kPa (253 mmHg). This enables an acclimatized mountaineer to have an alveolar $P_{O_2}$ of 4.0–4.7 kPa (30–35 mmHg)—near the physiological limits of man.

## Acute mountain sickness (AMS)

This term is used to describe the malaise, nausea, headache and lassitude that are common above 3500 m. Following arrival at this altitude there is usually a latent interval of 6–36 hours before the onset of symptoms.

| Condition | Incidence (%) | Usual altitude (m) |
|---|---|---|
| Acute mountain sickness | 70 | 3500–4000 |
| Acute pulmonary oedema | 2 | 4000 |
| Acute cerebral oedema | 1 | 4500 |
| Retinal haemorrhages | 50 | 5000 |
| Deterioration | 100 | 5600 |
| Chronic mountain sickness | Rare | 4500 |

**Table 15.1** Conditions caused by sustained hypoxia.

Treatment is rest, with analgesics being given if necessary; recovery is almost invariable.

Prophylactic treatment with the carbonic anhydrase inhibitor acetazolamide is of value in reducing the symptoms of AMS, since these are partly due to the development of alkalosis. Acclimatizing by ascending gradually is the best prophylaxis.

In a minority of cases, the more serious sequelae of high-altitude pulmonary oedema (HAPO) and high-altitude cerebral oedema (HACO) occur.

### High-altitude pulmonary oedema

Predisposing factors include youth, rapidity of ascent, heavy exertion and the presence of mountain sickness. Breathlessness, with frothy blood-stained sputum indicates established HAPO. Unless treated rapidly this leads to cardiorespiratory failure, collapse and death. Milder forms of HAPO are common, presenting with breathlessness that is not severe; it is important to recognize them.

### High-altitude cerebral oedema

Cerebral oedema is a poorly understood sequel of hypoxia. It is probably the result of the abrupt increase in cerebral blood flow that occurs even at modest altitudes of 3500–4000 m. Headache is usual, and is accompanied by varying disturbances of cerebral function; drowsiness, ataxia, nystagmus and papilloedema are common. Coma and death follow if the condition progresses.

#### TREATMENT

Any but the milder forms of AMS require urgent treatment. Oxygen should be given if it is available, and descent to a lower altitude should take place as quickly as possible. Dexamethasone or betamethasone are effective treatments in HAPO or HACO. Diuretics are of little value.

## Retinal haemorrhages

Small 'flame' haemorrhages in the nerve fibre layer of the retina are common above 5000 m. They are usually symptomless unless they cover the macula, when there is painless loss of central vision. Recovery is usual.

## Deterioration

Prolonged residence between 5600 and 7000 m leads to a syndrome of weight loss, anorexia and listlessness after several weeks. Above 7500 m deterioration develops more quickly, although it is possible to survive for a week or more at altitudes over 8000 m.

## Chronic mountain sickness

This rare syndrome occurs in long-term residents of high altitudes after several decades. It has been described clearly only in the Andes, but may occur in Tibet and elsewhere in central Asia.

Polycythaemia, drowsiness, cyanosis, finger clubbing, congested cheeks and ear lobes, and right ventricular enlargement occur. The condition is gradually progressive.

By way of contrast, coronary artery disease and hypertension are rare in the native populations of high altitudes.

# Diving

The increases in ambient pressure to which a diver is exposed at various depths are summarized in Table 15.2.

Various methods are used to supply air to the diver. With the simplest, e.g. a snorkel, the limiting factor, which occurs below 0.5 m, is the respiratory effort required to suck air into the lungs. At greater depths this 'forced negative-pressure ventilation' ultimately results in pulmonary capillary damage and haemorrhagic pulmonary oedema. Scuba tanks, the method commonly used for sporting diving down to 50 m, carry compressed air at a pressure balanced with the water pressure.

Divers who work at great depths for commercial purposes or for underwater exploration breathe helium/oxygen or nitrogen/oxygen mixtures delivered by hose from the surface.

A wide variety of complex medical problems may affect divers at all depths. These are summarized below.

## PROBLEMS DURING COMPRESSION (i.e. DESCENT)

### Barotrauma

Barotrauma of the middle ear ('squeeze') is the commonest disorder in divers. This is caused by an inability to equalize the pressure in the middle ear usually as a result of Eustachian tube blockage. Deafness occurs with eventual rupture of the tympanic membrane followed by acute vertigo.

Paranasal sinus barotrauma ('squeeze') is due to dysfunction of the nasal or paranasal sinus with blockage of the sinus ostea. Pain over the frontal sinus occurs.

| Sea depth (m) | Pressure | |
| | Absolute (atmospheres) | mmHg |
| --- | --- | --- |
| 0 | 1 | 760 |
| 10 | 2 | 1520 |
| 50 | 6 | 4560 |
| 90 | 10 | 7600 |

Table 15.2   Pressure in relation to sea depth.

Treatment of both conditions is with decongestants. It can be prevented by avoiding diving when the airways are blocked, e.g. with a respiratory tract infection.

## Nitrogen narcosis

When compressed air is breathed below 30 m the narcotic effects of nitrogen cause impairment of cerebral function with changes of mood and performance that may be life-threatening. The condition reverses rapidly on ascent.

Nitrogen narcosis is avoided by replacing air with helium/oxygen mixtures, which can enable divers to descend to 700 m.

At these great depths neurological disturbances occur that are believed to be the result of the direct effects of pressure on neurones. Tremor, hemiparesis and psychological changes may occur.

## Oxygen narcosis

Pure oxygen cannot be used for diving because oxygen becomes toxic to the lungs when the alveolar oxygen pressure exceeds 1.5 atmospheres absolute (5 m of water) and to the nervous system at around 10 m of water.

In the lungs, linear atelectasis appears and there is endothelial cell damage with exudation and pulmonary oedema. In the nervous system there is initially a feeling of apprehension, nausea and sweating, followed by muscle twitching and generalized convulsions, which may be fatal underwater.

## PROBLEMS DURING DECOMPRESSION (i.e. ASCENT)

Decompression sickness ('the bends') occurs on returning to the surface and is caused by the release of inert gases, usually nitrogen or helium, which form bubbles in the tissues as the ambient pressure falls. It only occurs when the diver ascends too rapidly. Decompression tables are available for calculating the time needed to come to the surface safely from any given depth.

## Decompression sickness

This can take a mild form (type 1 'non-neurological bends'), with skin irritation, mottling or joint pain only, or be more serious (type 2 'bends'), in which a variety of neurological features appear. Patients with type 2 'bends' may develop cortical blindness, hemiparesis, sensory disturbances or cord lesions. If nitrogen bubbles occur in the pulmonary vessels, divers experience retrosternal discomfort, dyspnoea and cough ('the chokes'). These symptoms develop within minutes or hours of a dive.

Treatment is with oxygen. In addition, all but the mildest forms of decompression sickness (i.e. skin mottling alone) require recompression, usually in a pressure chamber.

A long-term problem is aseptic necrosis caused by infarction due to nitrogen bubbles lodging in nutrient arteries supplying bone. It is seen in 5% of deep-sea divers. Neurological damage may also persist.

## Lung rupture, pneumothorax and surgical emphysema

These emergencies occur principally when divers 'breath-hold' while making emergency ascents after losing their gas supply. Following lung rupture the patient notes severe dyspnoea, cough and haemoptysis. Pneumothorax and emphysema usually respond to 100% oxygen. Air embolism may occur and should be treated with recompression and hyperbaric oxygen.

---

# *Ionizing radiation*

Ionizing radiation is either penetrating (X-rays, $\gamma$-rays or neutrons) or non-penetrating ($\alpha$ or $\beta$ particles). Penetrating radiation affects the whole body, while non-penetrating radiation only affects the skin. All radiation effects, however, depend on the type of radiation, the distribution of dose and the dose rate.

Absorption of doses greater than 100 rads of $\gamma$-radiation, e.g. following survival from a nuclear explosion or nuclear power plant accident, causes acute radiation syndromes of varying severity. Long-term effects also occur, sometimes decades after exposure, as radiation increases the rate of mutagenesis.

Radiation dosage is measured in joules per kilogram ($J\,kg^{-1}$); $1\,J\,kg^{-1}$ is also known as 1 gray (1 Gy). This is equivalent to 100 rads. Radioactivity is measured in becquerels (Bq); 1 Bq is equal to the amount of radioactive material in which there is one disintegration per second. 1 curie (Ci) is equal to $3.7 \times 10^{10}$ Bq.

Radiation differs in the density of ionization it causes. Therefore a dose equivalent called a sievert (Sv) is used. This is the absorbed dose weighted for the damaging effect of the radiation. The annual background radiation is approximately 2.5 mSv.

Excessive exposure to ionizing radiation occurs following accidents in hospitals, industry, nuclear power plants and strategic nuclear explosions.

## Mild acute radiation sickness

Nausea, vomiting and malaise follow doses of approximately 1 Gy (75–125 rad). Lymphopenia occurs within several days, followed 2–3 weeks later by a fall in all white cells and platelets. There is a late risk of leukaemia and solid tumours.

## Severe acute radiation sickness

Many systems are affected; the extent of the damage depends on the dose of radiation received. The effects of radiation are summarized in Table 15.3.

*Acute effects*
Haemopoietic syndrome
Gastrointestinal syndrome
CNS syndrome
Radiation dermatitis

*Delayed effects*
Infertility
Teratogenesis
Cataract
Neoplasia
   Acute myeloid leukaemia
   Thyroid
   Salivary glands
   Skin
   Others

**Table 15.3** The effects of radiation.

### Haemopoietic syndrome

Absorption of doses between 2 and 10 Gy (200–1000 rad) is followed by early and transient vomiting in some individuals, followed by a period of relative well-being. Lymphocytes are particularly sensitive to radiation damage and severe lymphopenia develops over several days. A decrease in granulocytes and platelets occurs 2–3 weeks later as no new cells are being formed by the damaged marrow. Thrombocytopenia with bleeding develops and frequent, overwhelming infections occur, with a very high mortality.

### Gastrointestinal syndrome

Absorption of doses greater than 6 Gy (600 rad) causes vomiting several hours after exposure. This then stops, only to recur some 4 days later accompanied by severe diarrhoea. Owing to radiation inhibition of cell division, the villous lining of the intestine becomes denuded. Intractable bloody diarrhoea follows, with dehydration, secondary infection and death.

### CNS syndrome

Exposures above 30 Gy (3000 rad) are followed rapidly by nausea, vomiting, disorientation and coma; death due to severe cerebral oedema follows in 36 hours.

### Radiation dermatitis

Skin erythema, purpura, blistering and secondary infection occur. Total loss of body hair is a bad prognostic sign and usually follows an exposure of at least 5 Gy (500 rad).

### Late effects of radiation exposure

The survivors of the nuclear bombing of Hiroshima and Nagasaki have provided information on the long-term effects of radiation. The risk of developing acute myeloid leukaemia or cancer, particularly of the skin, thyroid and salivary glands, increases. Infertility, teratogenesis and cataract are also late sequelae of radiation exposure.

### TREATMENT

Acute radiation sickness is a medical emergency. Hospitals should be immediately informed of the type and length of exposure so that suitable arrangements can be made to receive the patient. The initial radiation dose absorbed can be reduced by removing clothing contaminated by radioactive materials.

Treatment of radiation sickness is largely supportive and consists of prevention and treatment of infection, haemorrhage and fluid loss. Storage of the patient's white cells and platelets for future use should be considered, if feasible.

Accidental ingestion or exposure to bone-seeking radioisotopes (e.g. strontium-90 and caesium-137) should be treated with chelating agents (e.g. EDTA) and massive doses of oral calcium. Radioiodine contamination should be treated immediately with potassium iodide 133 mg daily. This will block 90% of radioiodine absorption by the thyroid if given immediately before exposure.

## Electric shock

Electric shock may produce clinical effects in three ways:
1 *Pain and psychological sequelae.* The common 'electric shock' is usually a painful, but harmless, stimulus that is an unpleasant and frightening experience. It produces no lasting neurological damage or cutaneous evidence of damage.
2 *Disruption of specific biological processes.* Ventricular fibrillation, muscular contraction and spinal cord damage follow a major shock. These are seen typically following a lightning strike.
3 *Electrical burns.* These are either superficial burns (e.g. lightning may cause a fern-shaped burn), or necrosis of subcutaneous tissues due to the heat generated by the electricity.

## Smoke

Smoke consists of particles of carbon in hot air and gases. These particles are mainly coated with organic acids and aldehydes. Use was widespread of synthetic materials (e.g. polyvinyl chloride) that release other substances, such as carbon monoxide and hydrochloric acid, on combustion. Respiratory symptoms may be immediate or delayed. Patients are dyspnoeic and tachypnoeic. Laryngeal stridor may require intubation. Hypoxia and pulmonary oedema can be fatal. Treatment is to remove the subject from the smoke and give oxygen. Intensive care may be required.

## Noise

The intensity of sound is expressed in terms of the square of the sound pressure. The bel is a ratio and is equivalent to a 10-fold increase in sound intensity; a decibel (dB) is one-tenth of a bel. Sound is made up of a number of frequencies ranging from 30 hertz (Hz) to 20 kHz, with most being between 1 and 4 kHz. When measuring sound, these different frequencies must be taken into account. In practice a scale known as A-weighted sound is used; sound levels are reported as dB(A). A hazardous sound source is defined as one with an overall sound pressure greater than 90 dB(A).

Repeated prolonged exposure to loud noise, particularly in the frequency range of 2–6 kHz, causes first temporary and later permanent hearing loss due to damage to the organ of Corti, with destruction of hair cells and, eventually, the auditory neurones. This is a common occupational problem, not only in industry and the armed forces, but also in the home (e.g. from electric drills and sanders), in sport (e.g. motor racing) and in entertainment (pop stars, their audiences and disc jockeys).

Serious noise-induced hearing loss is almost wholly preventable by personal protection (ear muffs, ear plugs); little treatment can be offered once deafness becomes established.

# Drowning and near drowning

Drowning is a common cause of accidental death, accounting for over 100 000 deaths annually worldwide. Approximately 40% of drownings occur in children under 5 years of age. Exhaustion, alcohol, drugs and hypothermia all contribute to the overall problem. In addition, drowning can also occur following an epileptic attack or after a myocardial infarct whilst in the water.

### 'Dry' drowning
Between 10 and 15% of drownings occur without aspiration of water into the lungs. Laryngeal spasm is thought to occur with anoxia occurring due to apnoea.

### 'Wet' drowning
Aspiration of fresh water affects the pulmonary surfactant with alveolar collapse and ventilation–perfusion mismatch leading to hypoxaemia. Aspiration of hypertonic sea water pulls additional fluid into the lungs with further ventilation–perfusion mismatch. In practice, however, there is little difference between salt-water and freshwater drowning as in both groups severe hypoxaemia occurs leading to death in some. Severe metabolic acidosis develops in the majority of survivors.

In patients who aspirate more than 22 ml kg$^{-1}$ of water, electrolyte and volume changes do occur, but very few of such patients have survived.

## EMERGENCY TREATMENT OF NEAR DROWNING
It must be remembered that patients can survive up to 30 min underwater without suffering brain damage and if the water is near 0°C this time can be much longer. The exact reasons for this are not clearly understood, but it is probably related to the protective role of the diving reflex. It has been shown experimentally that submersion in water causes a reflex slowing of the pulse and vasoconstriction. In addition, hypothermia decreases oxygen consumption of both the heart and brain.

Patients should be turned to one side and the mouth cleared of any debris. Mouth-to-mouth respiration should be immediately started together with cardiac resuscitation if this is appropriate (see p. 551).

Mouth-to-mouth resuscitation should always be attempted, even in the absence of a pulse and the presence of fixed dilated pupils, as patients can frequently make a dramatic recovery.

All patients should be subsequently admitted to hospital for intensive monitoring. Intensive care therapy may be required, and patients are liable to develop the adult respiratory distress syndrome (ARDS).

## PROGNOSIS
The prognosis is good if the patient is fully conscious on admission to hospital but poor if the patient is still in a coma.

# Ultraviolet light

Ultraviolet (UV) light consists of UVB (wavelength 290–320 nm) and UVA (320–400 nm). Wavelengths 100–290 nm are stopped by the ozone layer.
- UVB causes sunburn.
- UVA and UVB cause skin ageing and skin cancer.
Sunscreens absorb UV energy but many preparations only absorb UVB.

The sun protection factor (SPF) is a guide to the sunscreen performance, but there is no worldwide standard and often the protective effect is only against UVB. With a normal skin, a water-resistant sunscreen of 8–10 containing p-aminobenzoic acid is recommended to avoid sunburn.

# Motion sickness

This common problem, particularly in children, is caused by repetitive stimulation of the labyrinth of the ear. It occurs frequently at sea and in cars, but may occur on horseback or on less usual forms of transport such as camels or elephants. Nausea, sweating, dizziness, vertigo and profuse vomiting occur, accompanied by an irresistible desire to stop moving.

Prophylactic antihistamines or vestibular sedatives (hyoscine or cinnarizine) are of some value.

kers' perception of their environment and some of the symptoms of this syndrome may well be psychological in nature.

# Sick building syndrome

The World Health Organization has defined the sick building syndrome as an excess of work-related irritation of the skin and mucous membranes (usually eyes, nose and throat) and other symptoms including headache, fatigue and difficulty in concentrating reported by workers in modern office buildings.

In 25% of cases a specific cause has been found, such as contamination of humidification systems, but in the remainder the symptoms have been attributed to reduced rates of ventilation with outdoor air. Increasing the supply of outdoor air does not, however, lower affected wor-

# Further reading

Bennett P & Elliot D (1993) *The Physiology and Medicine of Diving*, 4th edn. London: WB Saunders.

Melamed Y, Shupak A & Bitterman H (1992) Medical problems associated with underwater diving. *New England Journal of Medicine* 326(1): 30.

Modell JH (1993) Drowning. *New England Journal of Medicine* 328: 253–256.

Nelson RN, Rund DA & Keller MD (1985) *Environmental Emergencies*. Philadelphia: WB Saunders.

Simon H (1993) Hyperthermia. *New England Journal of Medicine* 329(7): 483–487.

# 16 *Endocrinology*

## Introduction

Hormones are chemical messengers produced by a variety of specialized secretory cells. They may be transported to a distant site of action (the classical 'endocrine' effect) or may act directly upon nearby cells ('paracrine' activity). In the hypothalamus, elsewhere in the brain and in the gastrointestinal tract there are many such cells secreting hormones, some of which have true endocrine or paracrine activity, while others behave more like neurotransmitters. The distinction between neurotransmitters that act across synaptic clefts, intercellular factors acting across gap junctions and classical endocrine and paracrine activity is becoming increasingly blurred. There are also many chemical messengers involved in cell regulation such as cytokines, growth factors and interleukins.

## Synthesis, storage and release of hormones

Hormones may be of several chemical structures: polypeptide, glycoprotein, steroid or amine. In the case of polypeptides, neural or endocrine stimulation of the specific mRNA increases the synthesis of its hormone product. This is often in the form of a precursor molecule that may itself be biologically inactive. This 'prohormone' may be further processed before being packaged into granules, in the Golgi apparatus. These granules are then transported to the plasma membrane before release. This release may be in a brief spurt caused by the sudden stimulation of granules often induced by an intracellular $Ca^{2+}$-dependent process, or it may be 'constitutive' (immediate and continuous secretion).

## Plasma transport

Most hormones are secreted into the systemic circulation but, in the hypothalamus, they are released into the pituitary portal system. Much higher concentrations of the releasing factors thus reach the pituitary than occur in the systemic circulation.

Many hormones are bound to proteins within the circulation. Only the free (unbound) hormone is available to the tissues and thus biologically active. The binding serves to buffer against very rapid changes in plasma levels of the hormone. This principle is important in interpreting many tests of endocrine function, which often measure total rather than free hormone since binding proteins are frequently altered in disease states. Binding proteins comprise both specific, high-affinity proteins of limited capacity, such as thyroxine-binding globulin (TBG) and other less-specific low-affinity ones, such as prealbumin and albumin. The most important and clinically relevant binding proteins are shown in Table 16.1.

## Hormone action and receptors

Hormones act at the cell surface and/or within the cell. Many hormones bind to specific cell-surface receptors where they trigger internal messengers (Fig. 16.1a). Cell surface receptors are a family of 'G proteins' which bind the hormone on the cell surface and then activate so-called 'second messengers' via GTP. The second messengers include cyclic AMP for adrenocorticotrophic hormone (ACTH), luteinizing hormone (LH), follicle stimulating hormone (FSH) and parathyroid hormone (PTH), a calcium-phospholipid system for thyrotrophin releasing hormone (TRH), vasopressin and angiotensin II, and

| Hormone | Binding protein(s) |
|---|---|
| Thyroxine ($T_4$) | Thyroxine-binding globulin (TBG) |
| | Thyroxine-binding prealbumin (TBPA) |
| | Albumin |
| Tri-iodothyronine ($T_3$) (less bound than $T_4$) | Thyroxine-binding globulin (TBG) |
| | Albumin |
| Cortisol | Cortisol-binding globulin (CBG) |
| Testosterone Oestradiol | Sex hormone-binding globulin (SHBG) |
| Insulin-like growth factor 1 (IGF-1) | IGF-binding proteins 1–6 (IGF-BP 1–6) |

**Table 16.1** Plasma hormones with important binding proteins.

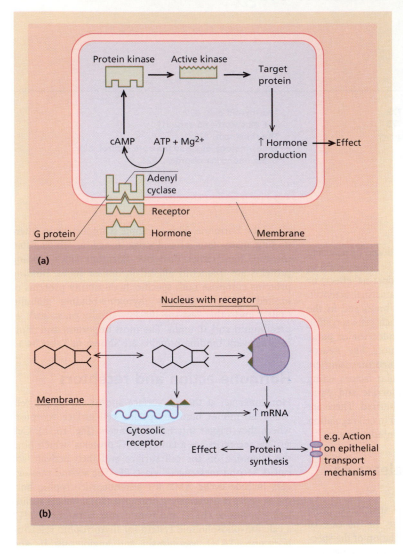

**Fig. 16.1**  (a) Binding of hormone to cellular surface receptor with subsequent release of a second messenger, here cAMP, which initiates intracellular mechanisms of an active kinase acting on a target protein to increase mRNA production and thus hormone production and 'effect'.
(b) Direct entry of steroid and thyroid hormones into the cell with subsequent binding to a cytosolic or core protein to initiate mRNA production and the subsequent hormone 'effect'.

tyrosine kinase for insulin and insulin-like growth factor-1 (IGF-1). These then cause rapid alterations in cell-membrane ion transport or slower responses such as DNA, RNA and protein synthesis. Some hormones act by activation of the membrane-bound phosphoinositide pathways.

Others, especially steroids, enter most cells of the body where they act on intracellular protein receptors, often altering the activity of intracellular enzymes by phosphorylation or dephosphorylation.

Steroid hormone–receptor complexes are usually transported into the nucleus (Fig. 16.1b), where they interact with DNA to regulate gene transcription, and thus protein synthesis. The characteristics of different hormone systems are shown in Table 16.2.

The sensitivity and/or number of receptors for a hormone is often decreased after prolonged exposure to a high hormone concentration, the receptors thus becoming less sensitive ('down-regulation') e.g. angiotensin II receptor, $\beta$-adrenoceptor. The reverse is true when

stimulation is absent or minimal, the receptors showing increased numbers or sensitivity ('up-regulation').

Abnormal receptors are an occasional, though very rare, cause of endocrine disease (see p. 774).

## Control and feedback

Most hormone systems are controlled by some form of feedback; an example is the hypothalamic–pituitary–thyroid axis (Fig. 16.2).

1  TRH is secreted in the hypothalamus and travels via the portal system to the pituitary where it stimulates the thyrotrophs to produce thyroid-stimulating hormone (TSH).

2  TSH is secreted into the systemic circulation where it stimulates increased thyroidal iodine uptake and thyroxine ($T_4$) and tri-iodothyronine ($T_3$) synthesis and release.

3  Serum levels of $T_4$ and $T_3$ are thus increased by TSH; in addition, the conversion of $T_4$ to $T_3$ (the more active

|  | Peptides and catecholamines | Steroids and thyroid hormones |
|---|---|---|
| Protein binding: | No | Yes |
| Changes in plasma concentrations: | Rapid changes | Slow fluctuations |
| Plasma half-life: | Short (seconds to minutes) | Long (minutes to days) |
| Type of receptors: | Cell membrane | Intracellular |
| Mechanism: | Activate preformed enzymes | Stimulate protein synthesis |
| Secretion: | Secretory granules<br>Constitutive plus bursts | Direct passage rapidly<br>Related to secretion rate |
| Speed of effect: | Rapid (seconds to minutes) | Slow (hours to days) |

**Table 16.2**   Characteristics of different hormone systems.

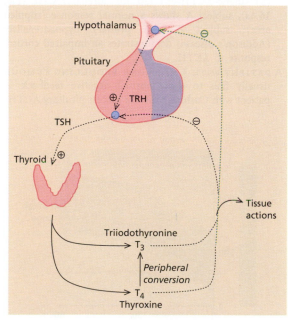

**Fig. 16.2**   The hypothalamic–pituitary–thyroid feedback system. The green line indicates probable negative feedback at hypothalamic level.

hormone) in peripheral tissues is stimulated by TSH.

4 $T_4$ and $T_3$ then enter cells where they bind to nuclear receptors and promote increased metabolic and cellular activity.

5 Blood levels of $T_3$ and $T_4$ are sensed by receptors in the pituitary and possibly the hypothalamus. If they rise above the normal range, TRH and TSH production is suppressed, leading to less $T_4$ and $T_3$ secretion.

6 Peripheral $T_3/T_4$ levels thus fall to normal.

7 If, however, $T_3$ and $T_4$ levels are low (e.g. post thyroidectomy), increased amounts of TRH and thus TSH are secreted, stimulating the remaining thyroid to produce more $T_3$ and $T_4$; blood levels of $T_4/T_3$ may be restored to normal, although at the expense of increased TSH drive, reflected by a high TSH level ('compensated euthyroidism').

This is known as a 'negative feedback' system, referring to the effect of $T_4$ and $T_3$ on the pituitary and hypothalamus. There are also positive feedback systems, classically seen in the regulation of the normal menstrual cycle.

## Patterns of secretion

Hormone secretion may be continuous or intermittent. The former is shown by the thyroid hormones, where $T_4$ has a half-life of 7–10 days and $T_3$ of about 6–10 hours. Levels over the day, month and year show very little variation. In contrast, secretion of the gonadotrophins, LH and FSH, is normally pulsatile, with major pulses released every 2 hours or so. Continuous infusion of LH to produce a steady equivalent level does *not* produce the same result (e.g. ovulation in the female) as the intermittent pulsatility, and may indeed produce down-regulation and amenorrhoea. Thus the long-acting superactive gonadotrophin releasing hormone (GnRH) analogue buserelin produces down-regulation of the GnRH receptors and subsequent very low androgen or oestrogen levels, which are clinically valuable both in carcinoma of the prostate in men and in infertility in women.

Pulsatile GnRH administration on the other hand can produce normal menstrual cyclicity, ovulation and fertility in women with hypothalamic amenorrhoea but intact pituitary LH and FSH stores.

### Biological rhythms

The most important rhythms are circadian and menstrual.

Circadian changes mean changes over the 24 hours of the day–night cycle and is best shown for the glucocorticoid cortisol axis. Figure 16.3 shows plasma cortisol levels measured over 24 hours—levels are highest in the early morning and lowest overnight. Additionally, cortisol release is pulsatile, following the pulsatility of pituitary ACTH. Thus 'normal' cortisol levels (stippled areas) vary during the day and great variations can be seen in samples taken only 30 min apart (Fig. 16.3). The circadian (light–dark) rhythm is seen in reverse with the pineal hormone, melatonin, which shows high levels during dark, though there is no clear clinical role for this.

The menstrual cycle is the best example of a longer (28-day) biological rhythm (see p. 784).

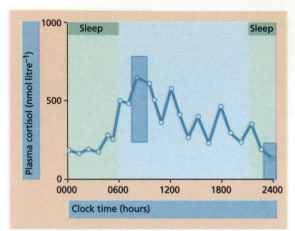

**Fig. 16.3** Plasma cortisol levels during a 24-hour period. Note both the pulsatility and the shifting baseline. Normal ranges for 0900 and 2400 are shown by the boxes.

### Other regulatory factors

STRESS. Though difficult to define, stress can produce rapid increases in ACTH and cortisol, growth hormone (GH), prolactin, adrenaline and noradrenaline. These can occur within seconds or minutes.

SLEEP. Secretion of GH and prolactin is increased during sleep, especially the rapid eye movement (REM) phase.

## Testing endocrine function

Ideally, cellular levels of hormones would be measured, but this is currently impossible. Body fluids are the normal substitute and are usually an excellent approximation, but it must be remembered that they do not always reflect the current tissue action of the relevant hormone.

### Blood levels

Assays for all important hormones are now available. Obviously the time, day and condition of measurement may make great differences to hormone levels. The method and timing of samples will depend upon the characteristics of the endocrine system involved.

BASAL LEVELS are especially useful for systems with long half-lives, e.g. $T_4$ and $T_3$. These vary little over the short term and random samples are therefore satisfactory.

BASAL SAMPLES may also be satisfactory if interpreted with respect to normal ranges for the time of day/month, diet or posture concerned. Examples are FSH, oestrogen and progesterone and aldosterone. All relevant details must be recorded or the data may prove uninterpretable.

STRESS-RELATED HORMONES (e.g. catecholamines, prolactin, GH, ACTH and cortisol) may require samples to be taken via an indwelling needle some time after venepuncture; otherwise, high levels may be artefactual.

### Urine collections

24-Hour collections have the advantage of providing an 'integrated mean' of a day's secretion but are often incomplete or wrongly timed. They also vary with sex and body size or age. Written instructions should be provided.

Saliva is sometimes used for steroid estimations, especially in children.

### Stimulation and suppression tests

These are valuable in instances of hormone deficiency or excess:

WHERE SECRETORY CAPACITY OF A GLAND IS DAMAGED, maximal stimulation by the trophic hormone will give a diminished output. Thus, in the Synacthen (SYNthetic-ACTH-en) test for adrenal reserve (Fig. 16.4a), subject A shows a normal response (stippled area); subject B with primary hypoadrenalism (Addison's disease) demonstrates an impaired cortisol response to ACTH.

A PATIENT WITH A HORMONE-PRODUCING TUMOUR usually fails to show normal negative feedback. A patient with Cushing's disease (excess pituitary ACTH)

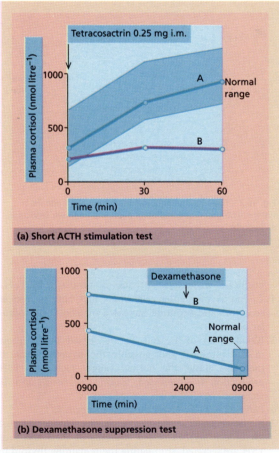

**(a) Short ACTH stimulation test**

**(b) Dexamethasone suppression test**

**Fig. 16.4** (a) Short ACTH stimulation test showing a normal response in a healthy subject (A) and a decreased response in a patient with Addison's disease (B). (b) Dexamethasone suppression tests in a normal subject (A) and a patient with Cushing's disease (B), showing inadequate suppression.

will thus fail to suppress ACTH and cortisol production when given a dose of synthetic steroid, as would normal subjects. Figure 16.4b shows the response of a normal subject (A) given 1 mg dexamethasone at midnight; cortisol is suppressed the following morning. Subject B with Cushing's disease shows inadequate suppression.

The detailed protocol for each test must be followed exactly, since even slight differences in technique will produce variations in results. Details of commoner tests are given in the Appendix.

### Measurement of hormone concentrations

Circulating levels of most hormones are very low ($10^{-9}$–$10^{-12}$ mol litre$^{-1}$) and cannot be measured by simple chemical techniques. Radioimmunoassay (RIA), previously by far the most common technique in endocrine assays, is being rapidly supplanted by immunoradiometric type assays (IRMA). These are increasingly being automated and using non-radioactive end-points such as colorimetric. Other techniques include high pressure liquid chromatography (HPLC).

RIA has limitations; in particular the immunological activity of a hormone, as used in developing the antibody, may not necessarily correspond to biological activity, and the increasing stringency of Health and Safety requirements has led to a search for methods not involving radioactivity.

RIA is, however, widely being replaced by IRMAs. These rely on highly specific antibodies (usually monoclonal) that are themselves labelled rather than labelling the hormone concerned. Usually employing a solid-phase system, the principles are otherwise similar to those of RIA, requiring incubation and separation of bound and free fractions, except that the 'signal' is obviously proportional to the amount of substance present (i.e. this is a saturation analysis). The label need not be a radioactive label, but may involve a fluorimetric, colorimetric, chemiluminescent or enzymatic end-point.

# An introduction to endocrine disease

## EPIDEMIOLOGY

The commonest endocrine disorders, excluding diabetes mellitus (Chapter 17), are:

THYROID DISORDERS, affecting four to eight new patients per primary care physician per year. Most common problems are thyrotoxicosis, primary hypothyroidism and goitre.

SUBFERTILITY, affecting 5–10% of all couples, often with an endocrine component, and increasingly treatable.

MENSTRUAL DISORDERS AND EXCESSIVE HAIR GROWTH IN YOUNG WOMEN, particularly polycystic ovary syndrome.

OSTEOPOROSIS, especially in postmenopausal women, is of increasing importance in fracture of the femur and premature death and disability.

PRIMARY HYPERPARATHYROIDISM, affecting about 0.1% of the population.

CHILDREN WITH SHORT STATURE OR DELAYED PUBERTY.

While most other endocrine conditions are very uncommon, they often affect young people and are usually curable or completely controllable with appropriate therapy. Hormones are also widely used therapeutically:

ORAL CONTRACEPTIVE PILL, the choice of perhaps 25–30% of women aged 18–35 years using contraception

HORMONE REPLACEMENT THERAPY (HRT) (oestrogens ± progestogens) for postmenopausal women (see p. 786)

---

**Body size and shape**

Short stature
Tall stature
Excessive weight or weight gain
Loss of weight

**'Metabolic' effects**

Tiredness
Weakness
Increased appetite
Decreased appetite
Polydipsia/thirst
Polyuria/nocturia
Tremor
Palpitation
Anxiety

**Local effects**

Swelling in the neck
Carpal tunnel syndrome
Bone or muscle pain
Protrusion of eyes
Visual loss (acuity and/or fields)
Headache

**Reproduction/sex**

Loss or absence of libido
Impotence
Oligomenorrhoea/amenorrhoea
Subfertility
Galactorrhoea
Gynaecomastia
Delayed puberty
Precocious puberty

**Skin**

Hirsuties
Hair thinning
Pigmentation
Dry skin
Excess sweating

**Information box 16.1** Common presenting complaints in endocrine disease.

CORTICOSTEROID THERAPY is widely used in non-endocrine disease such as asthma (see p. 675).

## SYMPTOMS

Common endocrine presenting symptoms are shown in Information box 16.1, which demonstrates the many effects that hormonal abnormalities can produce.

Hormones produce widespread effects upon the body; focal symptoms are less common than with other systems. Many endocrine symptoms are diffuse and vague, and the differential diagnosis is often wide.

## HISTORY AND EXAMINATION

A detailed history including the past, family and social history should be taken (Information box 16.2).

Physical signs are listed under the relevant systems. A full drug history is mandatory as endocrine problems are quite often iatrogenic (Table 16.3).

# Specific points about endocrine disease

As with other systems, endocrine diseases may be congenital or acquired and can be caused by a variety of pathologies. However, several forms of illness are commoner than in other systems.

### Autoimmune disease

Organ-specific autoimmune diseases have now been shown for every major endocrine organ (Table 16.4).

| Drug[a] | Effect |
|---|---|
| *Drugs inducing endocrine disease* | |
| Chlorpromazine<br>Metoclopramide<br>Oestrogens | Increase prolactin, causing galactorrhoea |
| Iodine<br>Amiodarone | Hyperthyroidism |
| Lithium<br>Amiodarone | Hypothyroidism |
| Chlorpropamide | Inappropriate ADH secretion |
| Ketoconazole<br>Metyrapone,<br>  aminoglutethimide | Hypoadrenalism |
| *Drugs simulating endocrine disease* | |
| Sympathomimetics<br>Amphetamines | Mimic thyrotoxicosis or phaeochromocytoma |
| Liquorice<br>Carbenoxolone | Mineralocorticoid activity; can simulate aldosteronism |
| Purgatives | Hypokalaemia |
| Diuretics | Secondary aldosteronism |
| ACE inhibitors | Hypoaldosteronism |
| *Exogenous hormones or stimulating agents*<br>Use, abuse or misuse, by patient or doctor, of the following: | |
| Steroids | Cushing's syndrome<br>Diabetes |
| Thyroxine | Thyrotoxicosis factitia |
| Vitamin D preparations<br>Milk and alkali<br>  preparations | Hypercalcaemia |
| Insulin<br>Sulphonylureas | Hypoglycaemia |

[a]Drugs causing gynaecomastia are listed in Table 16.15. Amiodarone may cause both hypothyroidism and hyperthyroidism.

**Table 16.3**   Drugs and endocrine disease.

---

**Past history**

Necessary details may include:
Previous pregnancies (ease of conception, postpartum haemorrhage)
Relevant surgery (e.g. thyroidectomy, orchidopexy)
Radiation (e.g. to neck, gonads, thyroid)
Drug exposure (e.g. chemotherapy, sex hormones, oral contraceptives)
In childhood, developmental milestones and growth

**Family history**

Family history of:
   Autoimmune disease
   Endocrine disease
   Essential hypertension
   Diabetes

Family details of:
   Height
   Weight
   Body habitus
   Hair growth
   Age of sexual development

**Social history**

Detailed records of alcohol intake (e.g. in subfertility, obesity)
Drug abuse (e.g. cannabis and subfertility)
Full details of occupation, e.g. access to drugs, chemicals
Diet, e.g. salt, liquorice, iodine

**Information box 16.2**   Past, family and social history.

---

They are characterized by the presence of specific antibodies in the serum, often present years before clinical symptoms are evident. The conditions are usually commoner in women and have a strong genetic component, often with an identical-twin concordance rate of 50% and with HLA associations (see individual diseases). Several of the autoantigens have now been identified (Table 16.4).

### Endocrine tumours

Hormone-secreting tumours occur in all endocrine organs, most commonly pituitary, thyroid and parathyroid. Fortunately, they are more commonly benign than malignant. While often considered to be 'autonomous', that is independent of the physiological control mechanisms, many do show evidence of feedback occurring at a higher 'set-point' than normal (e.g. ACTH secretion from a pituitary basophil adenoma).

| Organ and frequency if known | Antibody | Antigen if known | Clinical syndrome |
|---|---|---|---|
| *Stimulating* | | | |
| Thyroid 1 in 100 | Thyroid-stimulating immunoglobulin (TSI, TSAb) | TSH receptor | Graves' disease, neonatal thyrotoxicosis |
| | Thyroid growth immunoglobulin | | Goitre |
| *Destructive* | | | |
| Thyroid 1 in 100 | Thyroid microsomal antibody Thyroglobulin | Peroxidase enzyme | Primary hypothyroidism (myxoedema) |
| Adrenal 1 in 20 000 | Adrenal cortex | 21-hydroxylase enzyme | Primary hypoadrenalism (Addison's disease) |
| Pancreas 1 in 500 | Islet cell | ? GAD | Type I (insulin-dependent) diabetes |
| Stomach | Gastric parietal cell Intrinsic factor | | Pernicious anaemia |
| Skin | Melanocyte | | Vitiligo |
| Ovary 1 in 500 | Ovary | | Primary ovarian failure (not all autoimmune) |
| Testis | Testis | | Primary testicular failure |
| Parathyroid | Parathyroid chief cell | | Primary hypoparathyroidism |
| Pituitary | Pituitary-specific cells | | Selective hypopituitarism, e.g. GH deficiency, hyperprolactinaemia |

Population frequencies are approximate and refer to northern Europe. GAD, glutamic acid decarboxylase; GH, growth hormone.
NB Other related diseases include myasthenia gravis and autoimmune liver disease.

**Table 16.4** Types of autoimmune disease.

The molecular basis of some of these tumours is now understood, e.g. an abnormal G protein in prolactinomas and abnormalities on chromosome 11 in multiple endocrine neoplasia (MEN) type 1 tumours and on chromosome 10 in MEN type 2A (see p. 824).

### Enzymatic defects
The biosynthesis of most hormones involves many stages. Deficient or abnormal enzymes can lead to absent or reduced production of the terminal hormone. In general, severe deficiencies present early in life with obvious signs; partial deficiencies usually present later with mild signs or are only evident under stress. An example of an enzyme deficiency is congenital adrenal hyperplasia (CAH). Again the molecular basis is now known for several abnormalities, particularly for CAH where the coding gene is on the short arm of chromosome 6, and affected patients have defects such as point mutations or deletions.

### Receptor abnormalities
Hormones work by activating cellular receptors. There are rare conditions in which hormone secretion and control are normal but the receptors are defective: thus, if androgen receptors are defective, normal levels of androgen will not produce masculinization (e.g. testicular feminization). There are also a number of rare syndromes of diabetes and insulin resistance from receptor abnor-

malities (Chapter 17); other examples include nephrogenic diabetes insipidus and pseudohypoparathyroidism.

# Central control of endocrine function

## Anatomy

Many peripheral hormone systems are controlled by the hypothalamus and pituitary. The hypothalamus is sited at the base of the brain around the third ventricle and above the pituitary stalk, which leads down to the pituitary itself, carrying the hyophyseal–pituitary portal blood supply.

The important anatomical relationships of the hypothalamus and pituitary (Fig. 16.5) include the optic chiasm just above the pituitary fossa; any expanding lesion from the pituitary or hypothalamus can thus produce visual field defects by pressure on the chiasm. The pituitary is itself encased in a bony box; any lateral, anterior or posterior expansion must cause bony erosion. Upward expansion of the gland through the diaphragma sellae is

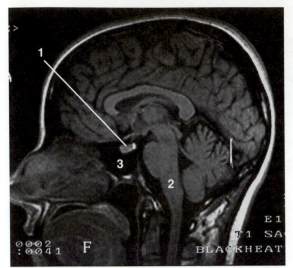

**Fig. 16.5** MRI of a sagittal section of the brain showing the pituitary fossa (1) and its important anatomical relationships. 2, Medulla; 3, Sphenoid sinus. By kind permission of Dr Martin Jeffree.

termed 'suprasellar extension'. The normal fossa is of very variable size but a true lateral X-ray should show a well-defined outline with a single floor. The commonest cause of apparent abnormality is a poorly aligned film.

Embryologically, the anterior pituitary is formed from Rathke's pouch (endodermal) which meets an outpouching of the third ventricular floor to become the posterior pituitary.

## Physiology

### Hypothalamus

This contains many vital centres for such functions as appetite, thirst, thermal regulation and sleep/waking. It acts as an integrator of many neural and endocrine inputs to control the release of releasing factors. Amongst other important influences it plays a role in the circadian rhythm, menstrual cyclicity, stress, exercise and mood.

From the hypothalamus the portal system runs down the stalk through which releasing factors are transported to the pituitary.

### Anterior pituitary

Releasing or inhibitory hormones (Table 16.5) produced in the hypothalamus travel down the portal system and stimulate or inhibit specific cells within the pituitary. These cells then stimulate or inhibit the synthesis and release of trophic hormones, which in turn stimulate the peripheral glands. This pattern is illustrated in Fig. 16.6. Many hormones are under dual control of stimulatory and inhibitory hypothalamic factors. For example:

GROWTH HORMONE RELEASE is stimulated by growth hormone releasing hormone (GHRH) but inhibited by somatostatin (growth hormone release inhibitory hormone, GHRIH).

TSH RELEASE is stimulated by TRH but partially inhibited by somatostatin.

SOME HORMONES have a dual stimulatory control, e.g. corticotrophin releasing factor (CRF) and vasopressin are endogenous stimulators of ACTH release. Uniquely, prolactin is under predominant inhibitory dopaminergic control with some stimulatory TRH control (Fig. 16.6).

### Posterior pituitary

This, in contrast, acts merely as a storage organ. Antidiuretic hormone (ADH, vasopressin) and oxytocin, both nonapeptides, are synthesized in the supraoptic and paraventricular nuclei in the anterior hypothalamus. They are then transported along a single axon and stored in the posterior pituitary. This means that damage to the stalk or pituitary alone does not prevent synthesis and release of ADH and oxytocin. ADH is discussed on p. 820; oxytocin produces milk ejection and uterine myometrial contraction.

Synthetic hypothalamic hormones and their antagonists are now available for testing of endocrine function and for treatment.

### Endorphins and the ACTH families of peptides

Some but not all of the endorphins (ENDogenous mORPHINe) are derived from part of the ACTH precursor molecular (Fig. 16.7). This scheme demonstrates some of the complex processing of pituitary peptides including the role of a 'prohormone', proopiomelanocortin, from which the major hormone, ACTH, is split. Pigmentation in humans is due to ACTH and β-lipotrophin, not from α- and β-melanocyte stimulating hormone (MSH) which are not found in humans.

The endorphins have opioid activity and are thought to be mediators of stress-induced analgesia. They have also been found within the gut but their physiological role remains uncertain. The hypothalamus also contains large amounts of other neuropeptides such as natriuretic factor, bombesin and vasoactive intestinal peptide (VIP) that can also alter pituitary hormone secretion.

# Presentations of hypothalamic and pituitary disease

## Pituitary space-occupying lesions and tumours (Table 16.6)

Pituitary tumours are the commonest cause of pituitary disease and, as with most endocrine disease, problems may be caused by excess hormone secretion, by local effects of a tumour or inadequate production of hormone by the remaining normal pituitary, hypopituitarism.

| Hypothalamic hormones | Pituitary hormones | Peripheral hormones |
|---|---|---|
| Gonadotrophin-releasing hormone (GnRH, LHRH) (decapeptide) | Luteinizing hormone (LH) Follicle-stimulating hormone (FSH) (Two-chain ($\alpha$, $\beta$) peptides MW 32 000) | Oestrogens/androgens (steroid ring) |
| Prolactin inhibiting factor (PIF) (dopamine) | Prolactin (PRL) (single chain peptide MW 23 000) | — |
| Growth hormone-releasing hormone (GHRH) (40 amino acids) Somatostatin (GHRIH) (cyclic peptide, 14 amino acids) | Growth hormone (GH) | Insulin-like growth factor (IGF-1 or somatomedin C) (small peptides MW 5000–9000) |
| Thyrotrophin-releasing hormone (TRH) (tripeptide) | Thyroid-stimulating hormone (TSH) (two-chain ($\alpha$, $\beta$) peptide MW 28 000) | Thyroxine, tri-iodothyronine ($T_4$, $T_3$—thyronines) |
| Corticotrophin-releasing factor (CRF) (41 amino acids) | Adrenocorticotrophic hormone (ACTH) (single chain peptide, 39 amino acids MW 4500) | Cortisol (steroid ring) |
| Vasopressin, antidiuretic hormone (ADH) (nonapeptide) | — | — |
| Oxytocin (nonapeptide) | — | — |

NB The $\alpha$ chains of LH, FSH and TSH are identical. MW, molecular weight.
Biochemical structure and abbreviation shown in parentheses.

**Table 16.5** Nomenclature and biochemistry of hypothalamic, pituitary and peripheral hormones.

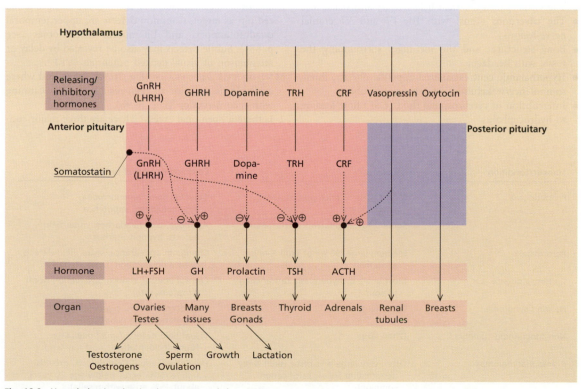

**Fig. 16.6** Hypothalamic releasing hormones and the pituitary trophic hormones. +, stimulation; –, inhibition. See text for abbreviations.

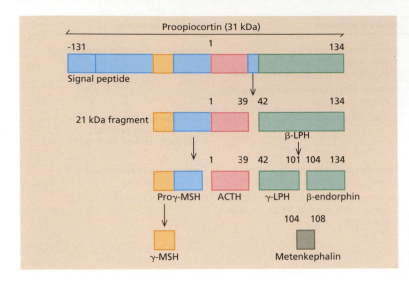

**Fig. 16.7** Processing of the ACTH precursor molecule (proopiocortin) illustrating some of the products. MSH, melanocyte-stimulating hormone (see text); LPH, lipotrophin.

## INVESTIGATION

Investigation of a possible or proven tumour thus follows three lines:

1 Is there a tumour? How big is it and what local anatomical effects is it exerting? Pituitary and hypothalamic space-occupying lesions, hormonally active or not, can cause symptoms by infiltration of, or pressure on:

- The visual pathways, with field defects and visual loss
- The cavernous sinus, with III, IV and VI cranial nerve lesions
- Bony structures and the meninges surrounding the fossa, with headache
- Hypothalamic centres: altered appetite, obesity, thirst, somnolence/wakefulness or precocious puberty
- Interruption of cerebrospinal fluid (CSF) flow leading to hydrocephalus

- Rarely, invasion of the sphenoid sinus causing CSF rhinorrhoea

Investigations include:

LATERAL SKULL X-RAYS may show enlargement of the fossa. This is a common incidental finding and requires further investigation (Fig. 16.8).

VISUAL FIELDS. These should be plotted formally by automated computer perimetry, Goldmann perimetry and/or by confrontation at the bedside using a small red pin as target. Common defects are upper temporal quadrantanopias and bitemporal hemianopias (see p. 881). Subtle defects may also be revealed by delay or attenuation of visual evoked potentials (VEP).

MRI OF THE PITUITARY (Fig. 16.9a), when and where available, is superior to high-resolution CT scanning with reconstruction (Fig. 16.9b).

2 Is there a hormonal excess? There are three major con-

| Tumour/condition | Usual size | Commonest clinical presentation |
|---|---|---|
| Prolactinoma | Most <10 mm (microprolactinoma) | Galactorrhoea, amenorrhoea, hypogonadism, impotence |
| | Some >10 mm (macroprolactinoma) | As above, plus headaches, visual field defects, hypopituitarism |
| Acromegaly | Medium-large (90%+ of skull X-rays abnormal) | Change in appearance, visual field defects, chance observation, hypopituitarism |
| Cushing's disease | Most small, or hyperplasia rather than tumour | Central obesity, chance observation (local symptoms rare) |
| Nelson's syndrome | Often large | Postadrenalectomy, pigmentation, sometimes local symptoms |
| Non-functioning tumours | Often large | Visual field defects (small ones often found incidentally at post mortem) |
| Craniopharyngiomas | Often very large and cystic (skull X-ray abnormal in 50%+, calcification common) | Headaches, visual field defects, growth failure (50% occur below age 20 years, about 15% arise within sella) |

**Table 16.6** Characteristics of pituitary tumours.

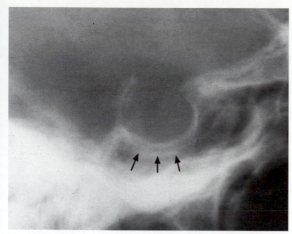

**Fig. 16.8** Lateral skull X-ray showing double floor (arrows) and enlargement of the pituitary fossa in a patient with acromegaly.

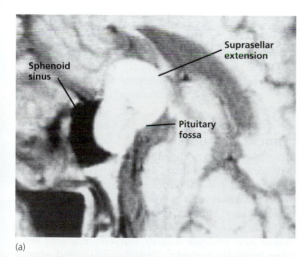

(a)

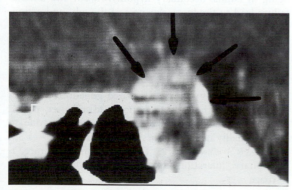

(b)

**Fig. 16.9** (a) MRI of pituitary fossa showing tumour with suprasellar extension. (b) CT scan (sagittal reconstruction) showing a pituitary tumour with suprasellar extension (arrows show upper border).

ditions that may be caused by tumour or hyperplasia.

(a) GH excess, leading to acromegaly or gigantism. These are usually acidophil adenomas.

(b) Prolactin excess (prolactinoma or hyper-prolactinaemia). Histologically these are chromo-phobe adenomas; many of these appear to result from an abnormal G protein in the pituitary receptor (see p. 769).

(c) Cushing's disease and Nelson's syndrome (excess ACTH secretion)—basophil adenomas or hyper-plasia.

The clinical features of acromegaly and Cushing's disease or hyperprolactinaemia are usually, but not always, obvious. Hyperprolactinaemia may be clinically 'silent'. Tumours producing LH, FSH or TSH are very rare. Some apparently 'non-functioning' tumours, which are common and usually chromophobe aden-omas, may produce the α-subunit of LH, FSH and TSH (see Table 16.9).

3 Is there a deficiency of any hormone? Clinical examin-ation may give clues; thus, short stature in a child with a pituitary tumour is likely to be due to GH deficiency. A slow, lethargic adult with pale skin is likely to be TSH and/or ACTH deficient. Milder deficiencies may not be obvious, and require specific testing (see Table 16.6).

The differential diagnosis of apparent pituitary adenomas additionally includes craniopharyngioma, a usually cystic hypothalamic tumour arising from Rathke's pouch that often mimicks an intrinsic pituitary lesion. Though pre-senting at any age, it is the commonest tumour in chil-dren and is often calcified.

Less common are cysts of Rathke's pouch, meningi-omas, gliomas, chondromas, pinealomas and carotid artery aneurysms masquerading as tumours. Secondary deposits occasionally present as apparent pituitary tumours, often presenting as diabetes insipidus.

**TREATMENT** (Table 16.7)

This depends on the type and size of tumour and is dis-cussed in more detail in the relevant sections (acromegaly see p. 799, prolactinoma see p. 794). In general therapy has three aims:

1 *Removal/control of tumour*

(a) Surgery—usually via the trans-sphenoidal route is the treatment of choice. Large tumours are removed via the open transfrontal route. Radio-therapy is given if the tumour is incompletely removed.

(b) Radiotherapy—external three-beam technique, or occasionally via implant of yttrium needles. Used when surgery is impracticable as it rarely abolishes tumour mass.

(c) Medical—octreotide or bromocriptine sometimes shrinks specific types of tumour.

2 *Reduction of excess hormone secretion.* Usually obtained by surgical removal but sometimes by medical treat-ment, e.g. bromocriptine or octreotide alone. Prolactinomas respond with significant tumour shrink-age to bromocriptine (see p. 794). Acromegaly, how-

|  | Advantages | Disadvantages |
|---|---|---|
| *Surgical* | | |
| Trans-sphenoidal adenomectomy or hypophysectomy | Relatively minor procedure | Limited value if significant suprasellar extension<br>Needs considerable expertise<br>Risks of CSF leakage/meningitis |
| Transfrontal | Good access to suprasellar region | Major procedure<br>Danger of frontal lobe damage<br>High chance of subsequent hypopituitarism |
| *Radiotherapy* | | |
| External (40–50 Gy) | Non-invasive<br>Prevents recurrence | Slow action<br>May not be effective |
| Yttrium implantation | High local dose | Later hypopituitarism<br>Great expertise needed |
| *Medical* | | |
| Bromocriptine (for prolactinomas and acromegaly) | Non-invasive<br>Reversible | Not curative, long term<br>Significant side-effects in minority |
| Octreotide (for acromegaly) | Non-invasive<br>Reversible | Expensive |

**Table 16.7**  Comparisons of primary treatment for pituitary tumours.

ever, responds less well (see p. 800). ACTH secretion usually cannot be controlled by medical means.

3 *Replacement of hormone deficiencies* (as detailed in Table 16.10).

Small tumours producing no significant symptoms, pressure or endocrine effects may be observed with regular clinical, visual field, imaging and endocrine assessments.

# Hypopituitarism

## PATHOPHYSIOLOGY

Deficiency of hypothalamic releasing hormones or of pituitary trophic hormones may be either selective or multiple. There are, for example, rare congenital isolated deficiencies of LH/FSH and ACTH, some of which may be autoimmune in nature.

Multiple deficiencies usually result from tumour growth or other destructive lesions. With the latter there is generally a progressive loss of anterior pituitary function in the order shown from left to right in Fig. 16.6. GH and gonadotrophins, LH before FSH, are usually first affected. Rather than prolactin deficiency, hyperprolactinaemia occurs relatively early because of loss of tonic inhibitory control by dopamine. TSH and ACTH are usually last to be affected. Panhypopituitarism refers to deficiency of all anterior pituitary hormones; it is most commonly caused by pituitary tumours, surgery or radiotherapy.

Vasopressin and oxytocin secretion will *only* be significantly affected if the hypothalamus is involved, either by a hypothalamic tumour or by major suprasellar extension of a pituitary lesion.

## CAUSES

Disorders causing hypopituitarism are listed in Table 16.8; pituitary and hypothalamic tumours are the commonest.

## CLINICAL FEATURES

Symptoms and signs depend upon the extent of hypothalamic and/or pituitary deficiencies. Loss of libido, amenorrhoea and impotence are symptoms of gonadotrophin and thus gonadal deficiencies, while hyperprolactinaemia may cause galactorrhoea and hypogonadism. GH deficiency is clinically 'silent' except in children, though new evidence suggests markedly impaired well-being in adults. Secondary hypothyroidism and adrenal failure lead to tiredness, slowness of thought and action, and mild hypotension. Long-standing panhypopituitarism may give the classical picture of pallor with hairlessness ('alabaster skin').

Particular syndromes related to hypopituitarism include:

KALLMANN'S SYNDROME (isolated gonadotrophin deficiency, which leads to hypogonadism); see p. 787. One sex-linked form has been shown to be due to abnormality of a cell adhesion molecule.

SHEEHAN'S SYNDROME. This situation, now rare, is pituitary infarction following postpartum haemorrhage.

PITUITARY APOPLEXY. A pituitary tumour may infarct or haemorrhage into itself. This may produce severe headache sometimes followed by acute life-threatening hypopituitarism.

THE 'EMPTY SELLA' SYNDROME. This is sometimes

Congenital
Isolated deficiency of pituitary hormones (e.g. Kallmann's
  syndrome)

Infective
Basal meningitis (e.g. tuberculosis)
Encephalitis
Syphilis

Vascular
Pituitary apoplexy
Sheehan's syndrome (postpartum necrosis)
Carotid artery aneurysms

Immunological
Pituitary antibodies

Neoplastic
Pituitary or hypothalamic tumours
Craniopharyngioma
Meningiomas
Gliomas
Pinealoma
Secondary deposits, especially breast

Traumatic
Skull fracture through base
Surgery, especially transfrontal

Infiltrations
Sarcoidosis
Histiocytosis X
Haemochromatosis

Others
Radiation damage
Fibrosis
Chemotherapy
Empty sella syndrome

'Functional'
Anorexia nervosa
Starvation
Emotional deprivation

**Table 16.8**  Causes of hypopituitarism.

due to a defect in the diaphragma and extension of the subarachnoid space (cisternal herniation) or may follow spontaneous infarction of a tumour. All or most of the sella turcica may be devoid of apparent pituitary tissue, but, despite this, pituitary function is usually normal, the pituitary being eccentrically placed and flattened against the floor or roof of the fossa.

## INVESTIGATION

Each axis of the hypothalamic–pituitary system may require separate investigation. The presence of normal gonadal function (ovulatory/menstruation or normal libido/erections) suggests that multiple defects of anterior pituitary function are unlikely.

Tests range from the simple basal levels, e.g. $T_4$ for the

| Axis | Tests for end-organ product | Feedback hormone | Tests for pituitary reserve | Tests for hypothalamic feedback |
|---|---|---|---|---|
| *Anterior pituitary* | | | | |
| HP–ovarian | Plasma oestradiol | LH | LHRH test | Clomiphene test |
| | Plasma progesterone | FSH | | |
| | Ultrasound (pelvic) | Inhibin | | |
| HP-testicular | Plasma testosterone | LH | LHRH test | Clomiphene test |
| | Sperm count | FSH | | |
| | | Inhibin | | |
| Growth | Plasma GH/IGF-1 | IGF-1 | GHRH test | Insulin tolerance test, sleep sampling, response to exercise arginine, clonidine |
| Breast | Plasma prolactin | — | TRH test | — |
| Thyroid | Plasma $T_4$/$T_3$ | TSH | TRH test | — |
| Adrenal | Plasma cortisol | ACTH | CRF test | Basal 0900 cortisol Short Synacthen Insulin tolerance test |
| *Posterior pituitary* | | | | |
| Thirst | Plasma and urine osmolalities | Vasopressin response to small amounts of hypertonic saline (300 mmol litre⁻¹) | | |

See text for abbreviations.

**Table 16.9**  Tests for hypothalamic–pituitary (HP) function.

thyroid axis, to stimulatory tests for the pituitary, and tests of feedback for the hypothalamus (Table 16.9). The insulin tolerance test is now less widely used, as basal 0900 h cortisol levels above 500 nmol litre$^{-1}$ reliably indicate an adequate reserve and levels below 100 nmol litre$^{-1}$ predict an inadequate response. The intravenous Synacthen test, though indirect, has proved to be an adequate indicator of hypothalamic–pituitary adrenal status.

## TREATMENT

Steroid and thyroid hormones are essential for life. Both may be given as oral replacement drugs, aiming to restore the patient to clinical and biochemical normality (Table 16.10). Sex hormone production may be replaced with androgens and oestrogens for symptomatic control; if necessary, human chorionic gonadotrophin (HCG, mainly LH) and metrotrophin (Pergonal) or urofollitrophin (Metrodin, mainly FSH) can be given if fertility is desired. Pulsatile GnRH (luteinizing hormone releasing hormone, LHRH) therapy is sometimes used where there is residual pituitary function but is expensive and time-consuming.

GH therapy may be given if necessary in the growing child and also produces substantial changes in body composition, work capacity and psychological well-being in acquired GH deficiency in the adult; long-term safety is not yet established and therapy may cost £4000–10 000 per annum—at present it is only used in clinical trials.

Two important warnings are necessary:

1  Thyroid replacement should not commence until normal glucocorticoid function has been demonstrated or replacement steroid therapy initiated.
2  Glucocorticoid deficiency may mask impaired urine concentrating ability, diabetes insipidus only becoming apparent after steroid replacement.

## Weight, exercise and stress

These are important factors in hypothalamic–pituitary function. Anorexia nervosa, the 'slimming disease' commonly affecting young females, is associated with major functional hypopituitarism (see p. 987). This often presents as amenorrhoea, without which the diagnosis is extremely unlikely. Anorexia is an extreme example, but more marginal degrees of underweight are a cause of secondary amenorrhoea and oligomenorrhoea, and are often unrecognized as a cause of subfertility. Similar effects are seen in female athletes undergoing heavy training with menstrual irregularity that invariably reverts to normal when training stops.

Stress, though difficult to define, also affects endocrine function, especially menstruation. Emotional deprivation in childhood is an important cause of growth retardation and may be mediated by reduced GH secretion.

# Reproduction and sex

Normal physiology of the female and male reproductive systems will first be considered, followed by their common disorders.

## Embryology

Until 8 weeks the sexes share a common development, with a primitive genital tract including the Wolffian and Müllerian ducts. There are additionally a primitive perineum and primitive gonads. In the *presence* of a Y chromosome the potential testis develops while the ovary regresses. In the *absence* of a Y chromosome, the potential

| Axis | Usual replacement | Additional therapy |
|------|-------------------|--------------------|
| Gonadal | Males: testosterone 250–500 mg i.m. every 3–4 weeks or oral or implant<br>Females: cyclical oestrogen/progestogen oral or patch or implant | HCG plus FSH (Pergonal) to produce testicular development, spermatogenesis or ovulation; used for infertility<br>(Pulsatile LHRH used in both sexes) |
| Breast (prolactin) | Bromocriptine 3–15 mg daily as replacement inhibition | — |
| Growth | None usually given in adult though GH has effects on muscle mass/well-being | For growth in children, GH injections |
| Thyroid | Thyroxine 0.1–0.2 g daily | |
| Adrenal | Hydrocortisone 15–40 mg daily<br>Prednisolone 5–10 mg daily<br>(Normally no need for mineralocorticoid replacement) | ACTH (tetracosactrin) to prevent or reverse adrenal suppression |
| Thirst | Desmopressin (DDAVP) 10–20 $\mu$g one to three times daily by nasal spray or now by tablet, 0.1–0.2 mg three times daily | Carbamazepine, thiazides or chlorpropamide are sometimes useful in mild diabetes insipidus |

HCG, human chorionic gonadotrophin (mainly LH).

**Table 16.10**  Replacement therapy for hypopituitarism.

ovary develops and related ducts form a uterus and the upper vagina. Production of Müllerian inhibitory factor from the early 'testis' produces atrophy of the Müllerian duct, while, under the influence of testosterone and dihydrotestosterone, the Wolffian duct differentiates into an epididymus, vas deferens, seminal vesicles and prostate. Androgens induce transformation of the perineum to include a penis, penile urethra and scrotum containing the testes, which descend in response to androgenic stimulation. At birth testicular volume is 0.5–1 ml.

## Definitions

Relevant terminology is shown in Information box 16.3.

## PHYSIOLOGY

### The male

An outline of the hypothalamic–pituitary–testicular axis is shown in Fig. 16.10a.

1 Pulses of LHRH (GnRH) are released from the hypothalamus and stimulate LH and FSH release from the pituitary.
2 LH stimulates testosterone production from Leydig cells of the testis.
3 Testosterone acts systemically to produce male secondary sexual characteristics, anabolism and the maintenance of libido. It also acts locally within the testis to aid spermatogenesis. Both testosterone and oestrogen

| | |
|---|---|
| Menarche | Age at first period |
| Primary amenorrhoea | Failure to begin spontaneous menstruation by age 16 years |
| Secondary amenorrhoea | Absence of menstruation for 3 months in a woman who has previously had cycles |
| Oligomenorrhoea | Irregular long cycles; often used for any length of cycle above 32 days |
| Dyspareunia | Pain or discomfort in the female during intercourse |
| Libido | Sexual interest or desire; often difficult to assess and is greatly affected by stress, tiredness and psychological factors |
| Menstruation | Onset of spontaneous (usually regular) uterine bleeding in the female |
| Impotence | Inability of the male to achieve or sustain an erection adequate for satisfactory intercourse |
| Azoospermia | Absence of sperm in the ejaculate |
| Oligospermia | Reduced numbers of sperm in the ejaculate; normal values are disputed |
| Virilization | Occurrence of male secondary sexual characteristics in the female |

**Information box 16.3**  Definitions in reproductive medicine.

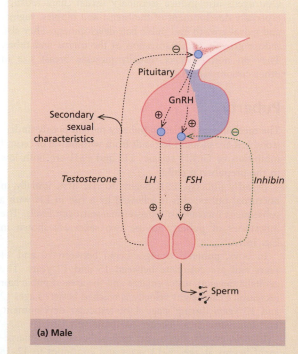

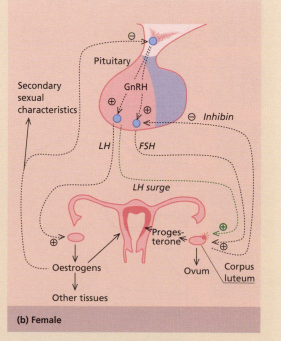

**Fig. 16.10**  (a) Male and (b) female hypothalamic–pituitary–gonadal axes. Note the close parallels. The green lines indicate probable feedback.

circulate largely bound to sex hormone-binding globulin (SHBG) (see p. 769).

4 FSH stimulates the Sertoli cells in the seminiferous tubules to produce mature sperm and the feedback hormone inhibin.

5 Testosterone feeds back on the hypothalamus/pituitary to inhibit LHRH secretion.

6 Inhibin causes feedback on the pituitary to decrease FSH secretion.

The secondary sexual characteristics of the male for which testosterone is necessary are the growth of pubic, axillary and facial hair, enlargement of the external genitalia, deepening of the voice, sebum secretion, muscle growth and frontal balding.

### The female

The female situation is more complex (Figs 16.10b and 16.11).

1 In the adult female, higher brain centres impose a menstrual cycle of 28 days upon the activity of hypothalamic GnRH.

2 Pulses of GnRH, at about 2-hour intervals, stimulate release of pituitary LH and FSH.

3 LH stimulates ovarian androgen production.

4 FSH stimulates follicular development and aromatase activity (an enzyme required to convert ovarian androgens to oestrogens). FSH also stimulates inhibin from ovarian stromal cells. Inhibin, in turn, inhibits FSH release.

5 Although many follicles are 'recruited' for development in early folliculogenesis, by day 8–10 a 'leading' follicle is selected for development into a mature Graafian follicle.

6 Oestrogens show a double feedback action on the pituitary, initially inhibiting gonadotrophin secretion (negative feedback), but later high-level exposure results in increased GnRH secretion and increased LH sensitivity to GnRH (positive feedback), which leads to the mid-cycle LH surge inducing ovulation from the leading follicle (Fig. 16.11).

7 The follicle then differentiates into a corpus luteum, which secretes both progesterone and oestradiol during the second half of the cycle (luteal phase).

8 Oestrogen initially and then progesterone cause uterine endometrial proliferation in preparation for possible implantation; if implantation does not occur, the corpus luteum regresses and progesterone secretion and inhibin levels fall allowing increased GnRH and FSH secretion so that the endometrium is shed (menstruation).

9 If implantation and pregnancy follow, human chorionic gonadotrophin (HCG) production from the corpus luteum maintains corpus luteum function till 10–12 weeks, by which time the placenta will be making sufficient oestrogens and progesterone to support itself.

10 Oestrogen circulates largely bound to SHBG (see p. 769).

Oestrogens also induce secondary sexual characteristics, especially development of the breast and nipples, vaginal and vulval growth and pubic hair development. They also induce growth and maturation of the uterus and tubes. They do not, however, usually increase breast size in other circumstances.

## Puberty

The mechanisms initiating puberty remain poorly understood but are thought to result from withdrawal of central inhibition of GnRH release. LH and FSH are both low in the prepubertal child.

In early puberty, FSH begins to rise first, initially in nocturnal pulses; this is followed by a rise in LH with a subsequent increase in testosterone/oestrogen levels. The milestones of puberty in the two sexes are shown in Fig. 16.12.

In boys, pubertal changes begin between 10 and 14 years and are complete between 15 and 17 years. The genitalia develop, testes enlarge and the area of pubic hair increases. Peak height velocity is reached between ages 12 and 17 years during stage 4 of testicular development. Full spermatogenesis occurs comparatively late.

In girls, events start a year earlier. Breast bud enlargement begins at ages 9–13 years and continues to 12–18 years. Pubic hair growth commences at ages 9–14 years and is completed at 12–16 years. Menarche occurs relatively late (age 11–15 years) but peak height velocity is

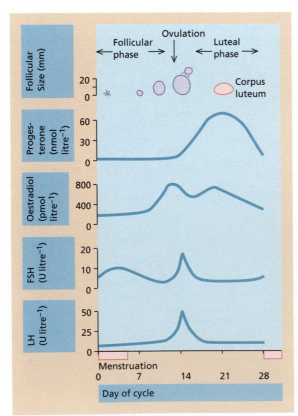

**Fig. 16.11** Hormonal and follicular changes during the normal menstrual cycle.

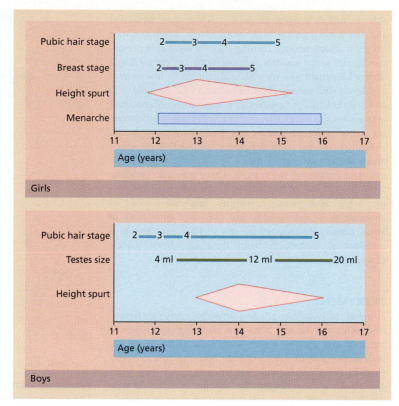

**Fig. 16.12** The age of development of features of puberty. Stages and testicular size show mean ages and all vary considerably between individuals. The same is true of height spurt, shown here in relation to other data. The ages of menarche show approximate 5th, 50th and 95th centiles. Numbers 2 to 5 indicate stages of development.

reached much earlier than in boys (age 10–13 years). Growth is completed earlier than in boys.

**Precocious puberty**

Development of menarche (girls) or secondary sexual characteristics (boys) before the age of 9 years is premature, and may take the following forms:

IDIOPATHIC (TRUE) PRECOCITY, commoner in girls. This is a diagnosis of exclusion with no apparent cause for premature breast or pubic hair development, and an early growth spurt; it may be normal and run in families. Treatment has been with cyproterone acetate, an anti-androgen with progestational activity, but long-acting LHRH analogues causing suppression of gonadotrophin release with reduced sex hormone production have largely superseded cyproterone: these may be given by nasal spray, by subcutaneous injection or preferably by implant.

CEREBRAL PRECOCITY. Many causes of hypothalamic disease, especially tumours, may present in this way. In boys this must be rigorously excluded.

FORBES–ALBRIGHT SYNDROME, usually in girls, with precocity, polyostotic fibrous dysplasia and skin pigmentation (*café-au-lait*).

PREMATURE THELARCHE is early breast development alone, usually transient between ages 2 and 4 years. It may regress or persist till puberty.

PREMATURE ADRENARCHE is early development of pubic hair without significant other changes, usually after age 5 years and commoner in girls.

**Delayed puberty**

Over 95% of children show signs of pubertal development by age 14 years. In its absence, investigation should begin by age 15 years. Causes of hypogonadism (below) are clearly relevant but most cases represent constitutional delay:

IN CONSTITUTIONAL DELAY, pubertal development, bone age and stature should be in parallel. A family history may confirm that other family members did the same.

IN BOYS, testicular volume >5 ml indicates the onset of puberty. A rising serum testosterone is an earlier clue.

IN GIRLS, the breast bud is the first sign. Ultrasound allows accurate assessment of ovarian and uterine development.

BASAL LH/FSH LEVELS may identify the site of a defect, and LHRH tests can indicate the stage of early puberty.

IF ANY PROGRESSION AT ALL IS EVIDENT CLINICALLY, observation is usually indicated.

LOW-DOSE SHORT-TERM SEX HORMONE THERAPY to induce puberty is possible when delay is great and problems are serious (e.g. severe teasing at school). Specialist assessment is advisable.

## The menopause

The menopause, or cessation of periods, naturally occurs about the age of 45–55 years. During the late forties, FSH initially, and then LH concentrations begin to rise, probably as follicle supply diminishes. Oestrogen levels fall and the cycle becomes disrupted. Most women notice irregular scanty periods coming on over a variable period, though in some sudden amenorrhoea or menorrhagia occur. Eventually the menopausal pattern of low oestradiol levels with grossly elevated LH and FSH (usually >50 and >25 U litre$^{-1}$, respectively) is established. Menopause may also occur surgically, with radiotherapy to the ovaries and with ovarian disease (e.g. premature menopause).

Features of oestrogen deficiency are hot flushes, which occur in most women and can be disabling, vaginal dryness and atrophy of the breasts. There may also be vague symptoms of loss of libido, loss of self-esteem, non-specific aches and pains, irritability, depression, loss of concentration and weight gain. Women show loss of bone density (osteoporosis, see p. 426) and the premenopausal protection from ischaemic heart disease disappears.

## TREATMENT

Some of the usual hazards of oestrogens apply (see below) but most physicians are now treating symptomatic patients much more widely and some recommend the widespread use of HRT, though still much less widely than in the USA. Current evidence suggests that, when given with a progestogen, the benefits of HRT far outweigh the small risks, unless there are clear contraindications. The overall benefits may be summarized as follows:

SYMPTOMATIC IMPROVEMENT in many, but not all, menopausal symptoms for the majority of women. Oestrogen-deficient symptoms respond well to oestrogen replacement, the vaguer symptoms generally, but not always, less well. Vaginal symptoms respond to local oestrogen preparations.

REDUCTION IN ISCHAEMIC HEART DISEASE and cerebrovascular disease mortality—blood pressure falls in the majority.

PROTECTION AGAINST FRACTURES OF WRIST, SPINE AND HIP, secondary to osteoporosis, at least where HRT is used before the age of 60 years when loss of bone mass is maximal. This is due to predominant protection of trabecular rather than cancellous bone.

In HRT oestrogen should be given cyclically with a progestogen (if the uterus is present) to prevent endometrial carcinoma from unopposed oestrogen action.

Apart from individual risks from oestrogen therapy (e.g. migraine, thrombosis)—and even with these the effect of HRT may not parallel those of the 'pill': the oestrogen dose is much smaller and does not guarantee contraception—the main concerns have been induction of cancer of the uterus or breast. Given with a progestogen, the risk of uterine cancer is not significantly increased, while the data on breast carcinoma are conflicting. There is of course the inconvenience of withdrawal bleeds, unless a hysterectomy has been performed. The preferred route of administration has been oral, but oestrogen implants and skin patches are now also widely used. The length of treatment with HRT is controversial.

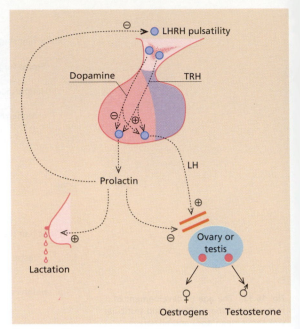

**Fig. 16.13** The control of prolactin secretion.

### Premature menopause

The commonest cause of early menopause in the twenties and thirties is ovarian failure which is usually autoimmune in nature. HRT should be given, as the risk of osteoporosis and premature ischaemic heart disease far outweigh the risks.

### The ageing male

In the male there is no sudden 'change of life'. However, there is a progressive loss in sexual function with reduction in morning erections and frequency of intercourse.

The age of onset varies widely but overall testicular volume diminishes and gonadotrophin levels gradually rise. If premature hypogonadism is present for any reason, replacement testosterone therapy should be given to prevent osteoporosis (see p. 427). A new agent, finasteride, which is an inhibitor of 5α-reductase, is now used in benign prostatic hypertrophy. It prevents the conversion of testosterone to dihydrotestosterone which causes local prostatic hyperplasia.

## Physiology of prolactin secretion

The hypothalamic–pituitary control of prolactin secretion is illustrated in Fig. 16.13.

It is under tonic dopamine inhibition, while other factors known to increase prolactin secretion (e.g. TRH) are probably of less importance. Prolactin stimulates milk secretion but also reduces gonadal activity. It decreases LHRH pulsatility at hypothalamic level and, to a lesser extent, blocks the action of LH on the ovary or testis, producing hypogonadism. These actions may be clinically important.

**Information box 16.4**   Sexual and menstrual disorders.

# Disorders of sex and reproduction

## CLINICAL FEATURES

A detailed history and examination of all systems is required (Information box 16.4).

### Tests of gonadal function

The patient and partner are their own best assay for gonadal endocrine function. A man having regular satisfactory intercourse or a woman with regular ovulatory periods is most unlikely to have significant endocrine disease, assuming the history is accurate (check with the partner!). When symptoms are present, much can be deduced by basal measurements of the gonadotrophins, oestrogens/testosterone and prolactin:

- LOW TESTOSTERONE OR OESTRADIOL WITH HIGH GONADOTROPHINS indicates primary gonadal disease.
- LOW LEVELS OF LH/FSH AND TESTOSTERONE/OESTRADIOL imply hypothalamic–pituitary disease.
- CONFIRMATION OF NORMAL FEMALE REPRODUCTIVE ENDOCRINOLOGY requires the demonstration of ovulation—this is achieved by measurement of luteal phase serum progesterone and/or by serial ovarian ultrasound in the follicular phase.
- COMPLETE DEMONSTRATION OF NORMAL MALE AND FEMALE FUNCTION requires a pregnancy—in the male, in the first instance there should be a healthy sperm count ($20–200 \times 10^6$/ml), good motility ($>60\%$ Grade I) and few abnormal forms ($<20\%$).
- HYPERPROLACTINAEMIA can be confirmed or excluded by direct measurement of preferably two to three samples. Levels may increase with stress; ideally, a cannula should be inserted and samples taken through it 30 min later.
- THE CLOMIPHENE TEST examines hypothalamic negative feedback. Clomiphene is a competitive oestrogen antagonist that binds to, but does not activate, oestrogen receptors, thus inducing a rise in gonadotrophin secretion in the normal subject.

More detailed tests are indicated in Table 16.11.

## DISORDERS IN THE MALE

### Hypogonadism

#### CLINICAL FEATURES

Male hypogonadism may be a presenting complaint or an incidental finding, e.g. during investigation for sub-

| Test | Uses/comments |
|---|---|
| *Male* | |
| Basal testosterone (serum) | Normal levels exclude hypogonadism |
| Sperm count | Normal count excludes any deficiency |
| | Motility and abnormal sperms should be noted |
| *Female* | |
| Basal oestradiol (serum) | Normal levels exclude hypogonadism |
| Luteal phase progesterone (days 18–24) | If $>30$ nmol litre$^{-1}$, suggests ovulation |
| Ultrasound of ovaries | To confirm ovulation |
| *Both sexes* | |
| Basal LH/FSH (serum) | Demonstrates state of feedback system for hormone production (LH) and germ cell production (FSH) |
| LHRH test | Shows adequacy (or otherwise) of LH and FSH stores in pituitary |
| HCG test (testosterone or oestradiol measured) | Response shows potential of ovary or testis; failure demonstrates primary gonadal problem |
| Clomiphene test (LH and FSH measured) | Tests hypothalamic negative feedback system; clomiphene is oestrogen antagonist |
| Postcoital test | Demonstrates state of sperm and sperm–mucus interaction |

**Table 16.11**   Tests of gonadal function.

General
Maintenance of libido
Deepening of voice
Fronto-temporal balding
Facial, axillary and limb hair

Pubic hair
Maintenance of male pattern

Testes and scrotum
Maintenance of testicular size/consistency
Rugosity of scrotum
Maintenance of erectile and ejaculatory function
Stimulation of spermatogenesis

Skeletal
Epiphyseal fusion
Maintenance of muscle bulk

**Table 16.12** Physiological effects of androgens, which may be absent or decreased in androgen deficiency.

Reduced gonadotrophins (hypothalamic–pituitary disease)
Hypopituitarism
Selective gonadotrophic deficiency (Kallmann's syndrome)

Hyperprolactinaemia

Primary gonadal disease (congenital)
Anorchia/Leydig cell agenesis
Chromosome abnormality (e.g. Klinefelter's syndrome)
Enzyme defects
$5\alpha$-Reductase deficiency

Primary gonadal disease (acquired)
Testicular torsion
Castration
Local testicular disease
Chemotherapy/radiation toxicity
Renal failure
Cirrhosis/alcohol
Sickle cell disease

Androgen receptor deficiency

**Table 16.13**  Causes of male hypogonadism.

fertility. The testes may be small and soft. Except with subfertility, the complaints are usually of androgen deficiency (Table 16.12) rather than deficiency of semen production. Sperm only makes up a very small proportion of seminal fluid volume.

Causes of male hypogonadism are shown in Table 16.13.

## INVESTIGATION

Testicular disease may be initially apparent but basal levels of testosterone, LH and FSH should be measured. These will allow the distinction between primary gonadal (testicular) failure and hypothalamic–pituitary disease to be made. Biopsy of the testes may be indicated, though rarely yields a treatable cause.

Skull radiology, pituitary CT scan, prolactin levels and other pituitary function tests may be needed. Depending on the causes, semen analysis, chromosomal analysis (e.g. to exclude Klinefelter's syndrome) and bone age estimation may be required.

## TREATMENT

The cause can rarely be reversed. Replacement therapy should be commenced (Table 16.14). Primary gonadal failure should be treated with androgens. Patients with hypothalamic–pituitary disease may be given LH and

FSH (Pergonal) or pulsatile LHRH if fertility is required, otherwise they should receive androgen replacement.

Special instances of hypogonadism include:

CRYPTORCHIDISM. By the age of 5 years both testes should be in the scrotum. After that age the germinal epithelium is increasingly at risk; lack of descent by puberty is associated with infertility. Surgical exploration and orchidopexy are usually undertaken but a short trial of HCG occasionally induces descent: an HCG test with a testosterone response 72 hours later excludes anorchia. Intra-abdominal testes have an increased risk of developing malignancy; if presentation is after puberty, orchidectomy is advised.

KLINEFELTER'S SYNDROME (seminiferous tubule dysgenesis). This chromosomal disorder (47XXY) affecting 1 in 1000 males involves loss of both Leydig cells and seminiferous tubular dysgenesis. Patients usually present with poor sexual development, small or undescended testes, gynaecomastia or infertility. They are sometimes mentally retarded. Clinical examination shows small pea-size but firm testes, usually gynae-

| Preparation | Dose | Remarks |
|---|---|---|
| Testosterone mixed esters | 250–500 mg i.m. every 3–6 weeks | Injection can be painful<br>Aggression if excessive dosage<br>Usual maintenance therapy |
| Testosterone propionate | 50–100 mg i.m. every 1–2 weeks | Frequent injections needed as half-life is short<br>Good initial therapy |
| Testosterone undecanoate | 80–240 mg daily, orally in divided doses | Variable dose, irregular absorption<br>Very expensive |
| —— | | |

NB Mesterolone and methyltestosterone are no longer advised; they are weakly active and can cause cholestasis.

**Table 16.14**  Androgen replacement therapy.

comastia and often signs of androgen deficiency. Confirmation is by chromosomal analysis. Treatment is androgen replacement therapy, though if the patient is mentally subnormal this should be used carefully. No treatment is possible for the abnormal seminiferous tubules and infertility.

ISOLATED DEFICIENCY OF LHRH OR LH/FSH (Kallmann's syndrome). Also known as hypogonadotrophic hypogonadism, this is often associated with decreased sense of smell (anosmia), and sometimes with other bony (cleft-palate), renal and cerebral abnormalities (e.g. colour blindness). It is often familial and is usually X-linked; the genetic defect has recently been identified. Management is that of secondary hypogonadism; fertility is possible.

OLIGOSPERMIA OR AZOOSPERMIA. These may be secondary to androgen deficiency and corrected by replacement but more often they result from primary testicular diseases in which case they are rarely treatable.

AZOOSPERMIA WITH NORMAL TESTICULAR SIZE AND LOW FSH LEVELS suggests a vas deferens block.

Physiological
  Neonatal
  Pubertal
  Old age
Hyperthyroidism
Liver disease
Oestrogen-producing tumours (testis, adrenal)
HCG-producing tumours (testis, lung)
Starvation/refeeding
Carcinoma of breast
Drugs
  Oestrogenic
    Oestrogens
    Digitalis
    Cannabis
    Diamorphine
  Antiandrogens
    Spironolactone
    Cimetidine
    Cyproterone
  Others
    Gonadotrophins
    Cytotoxics

**Table 16.15**  Causes of gynaecomastia.

## Lack of libido and impotence

Many patients with impotence have no definable organic cause. A careful history of physical disease, related symptoms, stress and psychological factors, together with drug and alcohol abuse, must be taken. The presence of nocturnal emissions and frequent satisfactory morning erections largely excludes endocrine disease as a cause.

True erectile difficulty may be psychological, neurogenic, vascular, endocrine or related to drugs. Vascular disease may be more common than realized and is often associated with vascular problems elsewhere. The endocrine causes are those of hypogonadism (above) and can be excluded by normal testosterone, gonadotrophin and prolactin levels. Autonomic neuropathy, most commonly from diabetes mellitus, is a common partial, if not total, identifiable cause (see Chapter 17). Many drugs can be responsible—cannabis, diuretics, metoclopramide, bethanidine/guanethidine, methyldopa and $\beta$-blockers all produce impotence.

Psychogenic impotence is frequently a diagnosis of exclusion, though complex tests of penile vasculature and function are now available in some centres.

Apart from cessation of the offending drug, methods of treatment include vacuum condoms, intracavernosal injections of papaverine and phentolamine, penile implants and vacuum expanders; specialist advice is essential.

If no organic disease is found, or if there is clear evidence of psychological problems, the couple should receive psychosexual counselling.

## Gynaecomastia

Gynaecomastia is development of breast tissue in the male. Causes are shown in Table 16.15.

Pubertal gynaecomastia occurs in perhaps 50% of normal boys, often asymmetrically. It usually resolves spontaneously within 6–18 months but after this duration may require surgical removal, as fibrous tissue will have been laid down. The cause is thought to be relative oestrogen excess.

In the older male, gynaecomastia requires a full assessment to exclude potentially serious underlying disease, such as bronchial carcinoma and testicular tumours (e.g. Leydig cell tumour). Drug effects are common (especially digoxin and spironolactone) and once these are excluded most cases have no definable cause. Surgical removal is occasionally necessary.

## DISORDERS IN THE FEMALE

## Hypogonadism

Impaired ovarian function, whether primary or secondary, will lead both to oestrogen deficiency and abnormalities of the menstrual cycle. The latter is very sensitive to disruption, cycles becoming anovulatory and irregular before disappearing altogether. Symptoms will depend on the age at which the failure develops. Thus, before puberty, primary amenorrhoea will occur, possibly with delayed puberty; if after puberty, secondary amenorrhoea and possibly hypogonadism will result.

### Oestrogen deficiency

The physiological effects of oestrogens and symptoms/signs of deficiency are shown in Table 16.16.

## Amenorrhoea

Absence of periods or markedly irregular infrequent periods (oligomenorrhoea) are a common presentation, often the earliest, of female gonadal disease. Important

| Physiological effect | Consequence of deficiency |
|---|---|
| *Breast* | |
| Development of connective and duct tissue | |
| Nipple enlargement and areolar pigmentation | Small, atrophic breasts |
| *Pubic hair* | |
| Maintenance of female pattern | Thinning and loss of pubic hair |
| *Vulva and vagina* | |
| Vulval growth | Atrophic vulva |
| Vaginal glandular and epithelial proliferation | Atrophic vagina |
| Vaginal lubrication | Dry vagina and dyspareunia |
| *Uterus and tubes* | |
| Myometrial and tubal hypertrophy | |
| Endometrial proliferation | Small, atrophic uterus and tubes |
| *Skeletal* | |
| Epiphyseal fusion | Eunuchoidism (if prepubertal) |
| Maintenance of bone mass | Osteoporosis |

**Table 16.16**   Effects of oestrogens and consequences of oestrogen deficiency.

factors in clinical assessment of such patients are shown in Information box 16.5.

PREGNANCY. This must *always* be considered.

GENITAL TRACT ABNORMALITIES, such as imperforate hymen, should be remembered, especially in primary amenorrhoea.

WEIGHT-RELATED AMENORRHOEA. A minimum body weight is necessary for regular menstruation. While anorexia nervosa is the extreme form (see p. 987), this condition is common and may be seen at weights within the 'normal' range. Many of these subjects may have additional minor endocrine disease (e.g. polycystic ovarian disease) but restoration of body weight to above the 50th centile is often helpful. Similar problems occur with intensive physical training in athletes and dancers.

HYPOTHALAMIC AMENORRHOEA. Some dispute the existence of this condition, linking all amenorrhoea to low weight or increased stress. A few patients, however, do appear to have defective cycling mechanisms without apparent explanation.

HYPOTHYROIDISM results in increased TRH which stimulates prolactin secretion.

SEVERE ILLNESS, even in the absence of weight loss.

AFTER STOPPING THE CONTRACEPTIVE PILL.

### INVESTIGATION

Basal levels of FSH, LH, oestrogen and prolactin allow initial distinction between primary gonadal and hypothalamic–pituitary causes (Table 16.17). Ovarian biopsy is necessary to confirm the diagnosis of primary ovarian failure. Subsequent investigations are also shown in Table 16.17.

### TREATMENT

Treatment is that of the cause wherever possible (e.g. hypothyroidism, low weight, stress, excessive exercise).

Primary ovarian disease is rarely treatable except in the rare condition of 'resistant' ovary, where high-dose Pergonal can occasionally lead to folliculogenesis. Hyperprolactinaemia should be corrected (see below). Polycystic ovarian syndrome is discussed in detail below.

## Hirsuties

### PATHOPHYSIOLOGY

The extent of hair growth varies between individuals, families and races, being more extensive in the Mediterranean and Asian populations. Soft vellous hair on the

**History**

? Pregnant
Age of onset
Age of menarche, if any
Sudden or gradual onset
General health
Weight, absolute and changes in recent past
Stress (job, life-style, exams, relationships)
Excessive exercise
Drugs
Hirsuties, acne, virilization
Headaches/visual symptoms
Sense of smell
Past history of pregnancies
Past history of gynaecological surgery

**Examination**

General health
Body shape and skeletal abnormalities
Weight and height
Hirsuties and acne
Evidence of virilization
Maturity of secondary sexual characteristics
Galactorrhoea
Normality of vagina, cervix and uterus

**Information box 16.5**   Clinical assessment of amenorrhoea.

| Diagnosis | Biochemical markers | Possible secondary tests |
|---|---|---|
| *Ovarian failure* | | |
| Ovarian dysgenesis[a] | High FSH | Repeat FSH |
| Premature ovarian failure[a] | High LH | Karyotype (see p. 116) |
| Steroid biosynthetic defect[a] | | Laparoscopy/biopsy of ovary |
| (Ovariectomy) | | Serum oestradiol |
| (Chemotherapy) | | HCG stimulation |
| | | |
| *Partial ovarian failure* | | Serum oestradiol |
| Resistant ovary syndrome | High FSH | Serum testosterone, androgens, SHBG |
| Polycystic ovarian syndrome[a] | High LH | Ultrasound of ovary |
| | | Serum prolactin |
| | | Laparoscopy and biopsy of ovary |
| | | |
| *Gonadotrophin failure* | | |
| Hypothalamic–pituitary disease[a] | Low FSH | X-ray pituitary fossa |
| Kallmann's syndrome[a] | Low LH | Serum oestradiol |
| Anorexia[a] | | LHRH test |
| Weight loss[a] | | Clomiphene test |
| General illness[a] | | Serum thyroxine |
| Hypothyroidism[a] | | Serum prolactin |
| | | |
| *Hyperprolactinaemia* | | |
| Prolactinoma[a] | High prolactin | Repeat prolactin (if >2000 mU litre$^{-1}$ then tumour probable) |
| Idiopathic hyperprolactinaemia[a] | | Pituitary fossa X-ray |
| Hypothyroidism[a] | | MRI or CT scan of pituitary fossa |
| Polycystic ovarian disease[a] | | Serum thyroxine |
| Drugs | | |
| | | |
| *Others (Cycle defect? Other endocrine disease?)* | | |
| Hypothalamic cause[a] | Normal FSH | Serum thyroxine |
| Weight gain/loss[a] | Normal LH | Serum testosterone, SHBG |
| Mild polycystic disease | Normal prolactin | Laparoscopy and biopsy of ovary |
| Cushing's syndrome | | |
| Thyrotoxicosis | | |
| Post-pill amenorrhoea | | |
| | | |
| *Androgen excess* | | |
| Gonadal tumour | High androgen | Androgen measurement (testosterone, androstenedione) |
| | | |
| *Uterine/vaginal abnormality* | | |
| Imperforate hymen[a] | | Examination under anaesthesia plus endometrial biopsy |
| Absent uterus[a] | | Progestogen challenge |
| Lack of endometrium | | |

[a]These conditions may present as primary amenorrhoea.

**Table 16.17**  Differential diagnosis and investigation of amenorrhoea.

face and elsewhere is not sex-hormone dependent, nor is hair on the forearm or lower leg. Hair in the beard, moustache, breast, chest, axilla, abdominal midline, pubic and thigh areas is sex-hormone dependent. Any excess in the latter regions is thus usually a mark of increased ovarian or adrenal androgen production. Hair has a long growing cycle with spontaneous variations and clinical changes are therefore slow.

Oestrogens are converted to androgens in adipose tissue, which presumably explains the frequent coexistence of hirsuties and obesity without definable endocrine disease.

## CLINICAL FEATURES
The complaint is common and often accompanied by severe anxiety and social stress. Important questions are:

AGE AND SPEED OF ONSET. Rapid progression and pre-pubertal or late onset suggest a more serious cause.

ACCOMPANYING VIRILIZATION (clitoromegaly, frontal balding, male phenotype, greasy skin, acne). This implies substantial androgen excess.

MENSTRUATION. The greater the disruption the more likely a serious cause.

## CAUSES AND INVESTIGATION
These are summarized in Table 16.18.

## TREATMENT
The underlying cause should be removed in the rare instances where this is possible (e.g. drugs, adrenal or ovarian tumours). Other therapy is either local or systemic.

| Condition | Clinical presentation | Menstruation | Investigation (results) |
|---|---|---|---|
| *Hirsuties without virilization* | | | |
| Familial | Family history often present Long history, beginning after menarche | Normal | Normal |
| Idiopathic | Long history, beginning after menarche | Normal | Normal |
| Polycystic ovarian syndrome (mild) | Long history, beginning after menarche Sometimes acne or greasy skin | Normal to chaotic | Androgens (↑) SHBG (↓) LH (↑) Ultrasound of ovary |
| Late-onset congenital adrenal hyperplasia | Often before menarche Often short stature Sometimes acne or greasy skin | Variable | 17-Hydroxyprogesterone (↑) |
| *Hirsuties with virilization* | | | |
| Polycystic ovarian syndrome (severe) | Long history, beginning after menarche | Chaotic or amenorrhoea | Androgens (↑) SHBG (↓) LH (↑) Ultrasound of ovary |
| Ovarian neoplasms | Short history, any adult age | Usually amenorrhoea | Ultrasound of ovary Laparoscopy and biopsy of ovary |
| Congenital adrenal hyperplasia | Infancy or childhood | — | 17-Hydroxyprogesterone (↑) Pregnanetriol (↑) ACTH (↑) |
| Adrenal tumours | Any age | Usually amenorrhoea | CT scan of adrenal |

Drugs causing hirsuties include androgens, phenytoin, diazoxide, minoxidil, cyclosporin and some progestogens.

**Table 16.18**  Conditions causing hirsuties.

### Local therapy

Plucking, bleaching, depilatory cream or wax and shaving may all help and are underused. Waxing is of especial value where the 'bikini area' is causing the concern. Electrolysis is slow and expensive.

### Systemic therapy

Oestrogens (e.g. oral contraceptives) reduce free androgens by increasing SHBG levels when these are low. Prednisolone given in a reverse circadian manner (5 mg at night, 2.5 mg in the morning) may rarely improve hirsuties in polycystic ovarian syndrome when given alone, though is more effective in restoring regular menstruation.

Cyproterone acetate (50–200 mg daily) is an antiandrogen but is also teratogenic and a weak glucocorticoid and progestogen. Given continuously it produces amenorrhoea, and so is normally given for days 1–14 of each cycle. In women of childbearing age, contraception is essential.

Other agents of doubtful efficacy include spironolactone, bromocriptine and cimetidine.

## Polycystic ovarian syndrome

### PATHOPHYSIOLOGY

This very common condition, originally known in its severe form as the Stein–Leventhal syndrome, is charac-terized by multiple ovarian cysts and by excess androgen production from the ovaries and adrenals, although whether the basic defect is in the ovary, adrenal or pituitary, remains unknown. The ovarian cysts represent arrested follicular development.

### CLINICAL FEATURES

It is a common cause of amenorrhoea/oligomenorrhoea, hirsuties or acne, usually beginning shortly after menarche. It is sometimes associated with marked obesity, but weight may be normal. Mild virilization occurs in severe cases.

Recent studies have shown an association of polycystic ovarian syndrome with menstrual disturbance and hypertension and hyperlipidaemia; it appears that insulin resistance may form part of the mechanism of the syndrome.

### INVESTIGATION

The most accurate investigation is ovarian ultrasound (Fig. 16.14), although a skilled observer is necessary and some apparently normal women show the abnormality. The typical ultrasonic features are those of a thickened capsule, multiple 3–5 mm cysts and a hyperechogenic stroma. Biochemically there are increased free androgens, though total testosterone may be normal. SHBG is low. The LH : FSH ratio is usually raised (>2 : 1) but the FSH

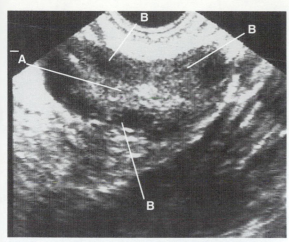

**Fig. 16.14** Polycystic ovary on a transvaginal scan showing hyperechogenic areas in the centre (A) surrounded by multiple peripheral cystic structures (B). (Courtesy of Dr Li-Chang Cheng.)

*Physiological*
Sleep (REM) phase
Pregnancy
Suckling
Nipple stimulation
Stress
Coitus

*Pathological*
Production by tumours
    Prolactinomas
    Occurs in some acromegalics
Interference with stalk
    Any hypothalamic/pituitary tumour
Idiopathic hyperprolactinaemia
Polycystic ovarian syndrome
Primary hypothyroidism
Chest wall injury
Renal failure
Liver failure

*Drug-induced*
Dopamine antagonists (e.g. metoclopramide and phenothiazines)
Oestrogens
Opiates
Cimetidine
Methyldopa
Reserpine

**Table 16.19**   Causes of hyperprolactinaemia.

is normal or low. Mild hyperprolactinaemia is common but rarely exceeds 1500 mU litre$^{-1}$.

## TREATMENT

This depends upon whether the aim is to produce fertility, regularize periods or reduce hirsuties.

REVERSE CIRCADIAN RHYTHM, prednisolone (2.5 mg in the morning, 5 mg on retiring) to suppress pituitary production of ACTH upon which adrenal androgens partly depend. Regular ovulatory cycles often ensue; hirsuties seldom respond to this treatment alone, but acne frequently does. Steroid instruction and a card must be supplied.

OESTROGENS/ORAL CONTRACEPTIVES FOR HIRSUTIES (see above).

CYPROTERONE as above.

For fertility, in addition to prednisolone:

CLOMIPHENE 50–200 mg daily from days 2–6 of cycle (or tamoxifen 10–40 mg daily) plus HCG 5000 U i.m. on day 12/13. This can occasionally cause ovarian hyperstimulation and specialist supervision is essential.

WEDGE RESECTION OR LASER SURGERY OF THE OVARY — rarely.

## Hyperprolactinaemia

Mildly increased prolactin levels (400–600 mU litre$^{-1}$) may be physiological, pathological or secondary to drug therapy (Table 16.19), while higher levels require a diagnosis. Not all patients with galactorrhoea have hyperprolactinaemia, but the other causes are poorly understood ('normoprolactinaemic galactorrhoea').

### CLINICAL FEATURES

Hyperprolactinaemia *per se* usually presents with:
- Galactorrhoea, spontaneous or expressible (60% of cases)
- Oligomenorrhoea or amenorrhoea
- Decreased libido in both sexes
- Decreased potency
- Subfertility
- Symptoms or signs of oestrogen or androgen deficiency — in the long term osteoporosis may result, especially in women
- In the peripubertal patient, as delayed or arrested puberty

Additionally, headaches and/or visual field defects may be present if there is a pituitary tumour (more common in men).

### INVESTIGATION

Once physiological and drug causes have been excluded:

AT LEAST THREE PROLACTIN LEVELS SHOULD BE MEASURED. Mean levels of >2000–3000 mU litre$^{-1}$ suggest a prolactinoma (see p. 778)

A GOOD QUALITY SKULL X-RAY should be obtained.

VISUAL FIELDS should be checked.

ANTERIOR PITUITARY FUNCTION should be assessed if there is any clinical evidence of hypopituitarism or radiological evidence of tumour. Hypothyroidism must be excluded.

MRI OF THE PITUITARY is necessary (if available) if there is an obvious tumour, and desirable if not. MRI is more sensitive than CT though the latter should be used if MRI is not available.

Macroprolactinoma refers to tumours above 10 mm in diameter, microprolactinoma to smaller ones. The size of tumour may affect the choice of treatment.

## TREATMENT

Treatment is dependent upon circumstances and facilities. Hyperprolactinaemia should be reduced with bromocriptine, a dopamine agonist. Initial doses should be small (e.g. 1 mg) and taken *during food*, beginning at bedtime. The dose should be gradually increased, usually to 2.5 mg three times daily, judged on clinical response and prolactin levels. Maintenance doses are 2.5–15 mg daily in divided doses. Side-effects include nausea and vomiting, dizziness and syncope, constipation and cold peripheries. Newer agents include lisuride.

If a tumour is present this is likely to shrink with bromocriptine. Definitive therapy is controversial and will depend upon the size of the tumour, the patient's wish for fertility and local facilities.

TRANS-SPHENOIDAL SURGERY often restores normo-prolactinaemia but there is a considerable late recurrence rate (50% at 5 years). Bromocriptine may produce hardening of the tumour and surgery should not be delayed beyond 2–3 months' treatment.

RADIOTHERAPY is only slowly effective and can sometimes cause eventual hypopituitarism. It should, however, be used after surgery in larger tumours, especially where families are complete.

SMALL TUMOURS in asymptomatic patients without hypogonadism may need only observation.

RARELY, TUMOURS ENLARGE DURING PREGNANCY to produce headaches and visual defects. Bromocriptine should be restarted.

MICROPROLACTINOMAS. There is some evidence that some microprolactinomas may not recur after several years of dopamine agonist therapy.

## ORAL CONTRACEPTION

The combined oestrogen–progestogen pill is widely used for contraception and has a low failure rate ($<1$ per 100 woman-years). 'Pills' contain 20–50 $\mu$g of oestrogen, usually ethinyloestradiol, together with a variable amount of one of several progestogens.

The mechanism of action is twofold:

1 Suppression by oestrogen of gonadotrophins, thus preventing follicular development, ovulation and luteinization

2 Progestogen effects on cervical mucus, making it hostile to sperm, and on tubal motility and the endometrium

Side-effects of these preparations are shown in Information box 16.6; most of the serious ones are rare and are less common on modern 20–30 $\mu$g oestrogen pills. While some problems require immediate cessation of the pill, the importance of other milder side-effects must be judged against the hazards of pregnancy occurring with inadequate contraception, especially if other effective methods are not practicable or acceptable. It is clear, however, that the hazards of the combined pill are greater in women over 35 years, especially in smokers and those with other risk factors for cardiovascular disease (e.g. hypertension, hyperlipidaemias). The 'mini-pill' (progestogen only) is less effective but is often suitable

where oestrogens are contraindicated (Information box 16.6). A progesterone antagonist, mifepristone, has recently been introduced which, in combination with a prostaglandin analogue, induces abortion of pregnancy up to 9 weeks' gestation. It prevents progesterone-induced inhibition of uterine contraction.

## SUBFERTILITY

This term, kinder than infertility, is defined as the inability of a couple to conceive after 1 year of unprotected intercourse. Investigation requires the combined skills of gynaecologist, endocrinologist and, ideally, andrologist.

---

**General**
Weight gain
Loss of libido
Pigmentation (chloasma)
Breast tenderness
Increased growth rate of some malignancies

**Cardiovascular**
Increased blood pressure[a]
Deep vein thrombosis[a]
Myocardial infarction
Stroke

**Gastrointestinal**
Nausea and vomiting
Abnormal liver biochemistry[a]
Gallstones increased
Hepatic tumours

**Nervous system**
Headache
Migraine[a]
Depression[a]

**Malignancy**
Possible increase in cancer of the breast

**Gynaecological**
Amenorrhoea
'Spotting'
Cervical erosion

**Haematological**
Increased clotting tendency

**Endocrine/metabolic**
Impaired glucose tolerance
Worsened lipid profile

**Drug interactions (reduced contraceptive effect due to enzyme induction)**
Antibiotics
Barbiturates
Phenytoin
Carbamazepine
Rifampicin

[a]Common reasons for stopping oral contraceptives.

**Information box 16.6**  Adverse effects and drug interactions of oral contraceptives.

Both partners must be considered and every aspect of the physiology critically examined.

## CAUSES (Fig. 16.15)

MALE FACTOR. About 30–40% of couples have a major identifiable male factor.

FEMALE FACTORS. Female tubal problems account for perhaps 20%; a similar proportion have ovulatory disorders.

UNCOMMON CAUSES. Inadequate intercourse, hostile cervical mucus and vaginal factors are uncommon (5%).

'IDIOPATHIC'—15% have no apparent explanation.

BOTH PARTNERS. A significant proportion have both male and female problems.

## CLINICAL ASSESSMENT

Both partners should be seen, not just the woman, and the following factors checked:

THE MAN: previous testicular damage (e.g. orchitis, trauma, undescended testes), urethral symptoms and venereal problems, local surgery and use of alcohol and drugs. A semen analysis early in the investigations is essential.

THE WOMAN: previous pelvic infection, regularity of periods, previous surgery, alcohol intake and smoking. Adequacy of body weight (see p. 782).

TOGETHER: frequency and adequacy of intercourse, use of lubricants.

Examination should include an assessment of secondary sexual characteristics, body habitus and general health. In men, size and consistency of the testes are important, plus exclusion of a varicocele. In women, vaginal examination allows a check on the uterus and ovaries.

## INVESTIGATION

Appropriate tests for particular defects are shown in Fig. 16.15.

## TREATMENT

Counselling of both partners is essential. Any defect(s) found should be treated if possible. Ovulation can usually be induced by exogenous hormones if simpler measures fail, while *in vitro* fertilization (IVF) and similar techniques are becoming more widely used, especially where there is tubal blockage, oligospermia or 'idiopathic subfertility'.

# DISORDERS OF SEXUAL DIFFERENTIATION

An individual's sex can be defined in several ways:

CHROMOSOMAL SEX. The normal female is 46XX, the normal male 46XY. The Y chromosome confers male sex; if it is not present, development follows female lines.

GONADAL SEX. This is obviously determined predominantly by chromosomal sex but requires normal embryological development.

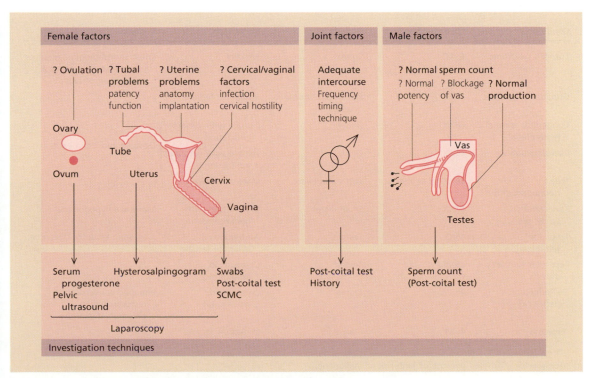

**Fig. 16.15** The major factors involved in subfertility and their investigation. SCMC, sperm–cervical mucus contact test.

PHENOTYPIC SEX—the normal physical appearance and characteristics of male and female body shape. This in turn is a manifestation of gonadal sex and subsequent sex hormone production.

SOCIAL SEX (GENDER)—heavily dependent on phenotypic sex and normally assigned on appearance of the external genitalia at birth.

SEXUAL ORIENTATION—heterosexual, homosexual (male/male or female/female) or bisexual (both sexes). Recent studies suggest that there may be some element of genetic determination of homosexuality.

Disorders of sexual differentiation are rare but may affect chromosomal, gonadal, endocrine and phenotypic development (Table 16.20).

# The growth axis

## Physiology and control of growth hormone (Fig. 16.16)

GH is the pituitary factor responsible for stimulation of body growth in humans. Its secretion is stimulated by GHRH, released into the portal system from the hypothalamus; it is also under inhibitory control by GHRIH (somatostatin). GH stimulates the hepatic production of an intermediate (IGF-1, previously known as somatomedin C) that actually stimulates growth. Plasma levels

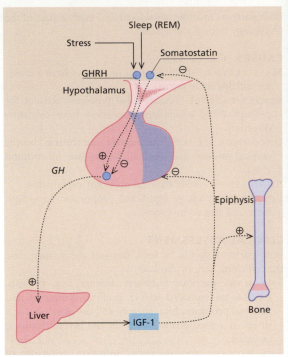

**Fig. 16.16** The control of growth hormone (GH) and insulin-like growth factor-1 (IGF-1) secretion and action.

| Condition | Chromosomes | Gonads | Phenotype | Remarks |
|---|---|---|---|---|
| Turner's syndrome | 45XO | Streak | Female | Often morphological features (short stature, web neck, coarctation of aorta) |
| Gonadal dysgenesis | 46XY | Streak or minimal testes[a] | Immature female | |
| Congenital adrenal hyperplasia | 46XX | Ovary | Female with variable virilization | Obvious androgen excess |
| Virilizing tumour | 46XX | Ovary | Female with variable virilization | |
| True hermaphroditism | 46XX/XY or mosaic | Testis and ovary | Male or ambiguous | |
| Klinefelter's syndrome | 47XXY | Small testes | Male, often with gynaecomastia | Many are hypogonadal |
| Testicular feminization | 46XY | Testes[a] | Ambiguous or infantile female | Androgen receptor defective |
| Testicular synthetic defects | 46XY | Testes[a] | Cryptorchid, ambiguous | |
| 5α-Reductase deficiency | 46XY | Testes | Cryptorchid, ambiguous | Impaired conversion of testosterone to dihydrotestosterone |
| Anorchia | 46XY | Absent | Immature female | |

[a]Gonadectomy advised because of high risk of malignancy.

**Table 16.20** Disorders of sexual differentiation.

of IGF-1, however, reflect local growth activity poorly, partly as there are multiple IGF-binding proteins (IGF-BP). The metabolic actions of the system are:
- Increasing collagen and protein synthesis
- Promoting retention of calcium, phosphorus and nitrogen, necessary substrates for anabolism
- Opposing the action of insulin

GH release is intermittent and mainly nocturnal, especially during REM sleep. The frequency and size of GH pulses increase during the growth spurt of adolescence and decline thereafter. Acute stress and exercise both stimulate GH release while, in the normal subject, hyperglycaemia suppresses it.

## Normal growth

Factors other than GH involved in linear growth in the human are:

GENETIC. Children of two short parents will probably be short.

NUTRITIONAL. Adequate nutrients must be available; impaired growth can result from inadequate dietary intake or small-bowel disease (e.g. coeliac disease).

GENERAL HEALTH. Any serious systemic disease in childhood is likely to reduce growth (e.g. renal failure).

INTRAUTERINE GROWTH RETARDATION. These infants often grow poorly in the long term, while infants with simple prematurity usually catch up.

EMOTIONAL DEPRIVATION AND PSYCHOLOGICAL FACTORS. These can impair growth by complex, poorly understood mechanisms, possibly involving temporarily decreased GH secretion.

The relevant aspects of history and examination in the assessment of problems are shown in Information box 16.7.

## Assessment of growth

Charts showing ranges of height and weight for normal British children are available (Fig. 16.17); other national data are available. Height must be measured very carefully, ideally at the same time of day on the same instrument by the same observer.

In general, there are three overlapping phases of growth: infantile (0–2 years), which appears largely substrate (food) dependent; childhood (age 2 years to puberty), which is largely GH dependent; and the adolescent 'growth spurt', dependent on GH *and* sex hormones.

More important than current height is height velocity, which requires at least two measurements some months apart and, ideally, multiple serial measurements. This is a rate of current growth (cm per year), while attained height is largely dependent upon previous growth.

Standard deviation scores (SDS) based on the degree of deviation from age–sex norms are widely used by experts—these and growth velocities are far more sensitive than simple charts in assessing growth.

The approximate future height of a child ('mid-

### History

Pregnancy records
Rate of growth (home/school records, e.g. heights on kitchen door)
Comparison with peers at school and siblings
Change in appearance (old photos)
Change in shoe/glove/hat size or frequency of 'growing out'
Age of appearance of pubic hair, breasts, menarche

### Physical signs

Evidence of systemic disease
Body habitus, size, relative weight, proportions (span versus height)
Skin thickness, interdental separation
Facial features
Spade hands/feet
Grading of secondary sexual characteristics

**Information box 16.7**  Assessment of problems of growth and development.

parental height') can be simply predicted from the parental heights. For a boy, this is

[(Maternal height +13 cm (5 inches) + Paternal height)/2]

and for a girl

[(Paternal height −13 cm (5 inches) + Maternal height)/2].

Thus, with a father of 5 ft 10 inches and mother of 5 ft 1 inch, the predicted heights are 5 ft 8 inches for a son and 5 ft 3 inches for a daughter.

## GROWTH FAILURE—SHORT STATURE

When children or their parents complain of short stature particular attention should focus on:
- Intrauterine growth retardation, weight and gestation at birth
- Possible systemic disorder—any system but especially small-bowel disease
- Evidence of skeletal, chromosomal or other congenital abnormalities
- Endocrine status—particularly primary hypothyroidism
- Dietary intake and use of drugs, especially steroids for asthma
- Emotional, psychological, family and school problems

School, general practitioner, clinic and home records of height and weight should be obtained if possible to allow growth-velocity calculation. If unavailable, such data must be obtained prospectively.

A child with normal growth velocity is unlikely to have significant endocrine disease. However, low growth velocity without apparent systemic cause requires further investigation. Sudden cessation of growth suggests major physical disease; if no gastrointestinal, respiratory, renal or skeletal abnormality is apparent, then a cerebral tumour or hypothyroidism are likeliest.

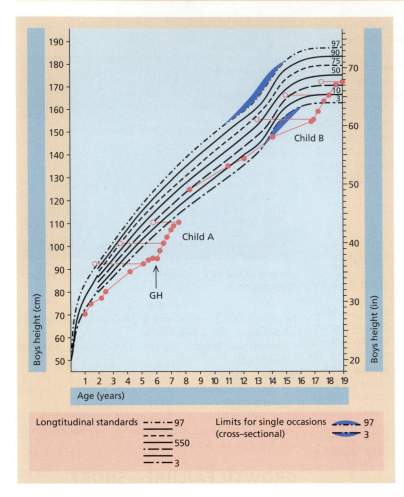

**Fig. 16.17**  A height chart for boys. Child A illustrates the course of a child with hypopituitarism, initially treated with cortisol and thyroxine, but showing growth only after growth hormone treatment. Child B shows the course of a child with constitutional growth delay without treatment. The open circles (○) show the data corrected for bone age. (Based on a Tanner–Whitehouse chart, reproduced by permission of Castlemead Publications. New updated charts will be published in 1994–5 with slightly greater heights than previously.)

Consistently slow-growing children require full endocrine assessment.

Features of the commoner causes of growth failure are given in Table 16.21. Where constitutional delay is clearly shown and symptoms require intervention then very low dose sex steroids in 3–6 month courses will usually induce acceleration of growth.

### INVESTIGATION

Systemic disease having been excluded, the following should be undertaken:

THYROID FUNCTION TESTS: serum TSH and $T_4$ to exclude hypothyroidism.

GH STATUS: basal levels are of little value, though urinary GH measurements may prove to be of some value in screening. Overnight repeated sampling is optimal but the GH response to Bovril, exercise, clonidine, arginine and insulin are all used; a normal peak response is >20 mU litre$^{-1}$. The 'gold standard' test has been the insulin tolerance test (ITT), but this *should only be performed in specialist centres* for safety reasons.

ASSESSMENT OF BONE AGE: non-dominant hand and wrist X-rays allow assessment of bone age by comparison with standard charts (Tanner, Greulich and Pyle).

### TREATMENT

SYSTEMIC ILLNESS should be treated.

PRIMARY HYPOTHYROIDISM: replace with thyroxine 0.05–0.2 mg daily (see p. 804).

GH INSUFFICIENCY: human GH (collected from pituitaries) was previously used but was withdrawn as cases of Creutzfeld–Jakob disease were reported. It has been superseded by very expensive recombinant GH, which is given as nightly injection in doses of 10–20 U m$^{-2}$ of body surface area. Treatment should be supervised in expert centres.

The place of GH treatment in so-called 'short normal' children has still not been adequately defined. In Turner's syndrome (see p. 796) large doses of GH are needed combined with oxandrolone, a growth-stimulating synthetic sex steroid.

## GROWTH HORMONE EXCESS— GIGANTISM AND ACROMEGALY

GH stimulates skeletal and soft-tissue growth. GH excess therefore produces gigantism in children (if acquired before epiphyseal fusion) but acromegaly in adults.

| Cause | Family history | Growth pattern, clinical features and puberty | Bone age | Remarks |
|-------|----------------|-----------------------------------------------|----------|---------|
| Constitutional delay | Often present | Slow from birth, immature but appropriate with late but spontaneous puberty | Moderate delay | Often difficult to differentiate from GH deficiency; growth velocity measurement vital |
| Familial short stature | Positive | Slow from birth, clinically normal with normal puberty | Normal | Need heights of all family members |
| GH insufficiency | Rare | Slow growth, immature often overweight, delayed puberty | Moderate delay increasing with time | Early investigation and treatment vital; increased suspicion if child is plump |
| Primary hypothyroidism | Rare | Slow growth, immature and delayed puberty | Marked delay | Measure TSH, T$_4$ in all cases of short stature; clear clinical signs not obvious |
| Small-bowel disease | Sometimes | Slow, immature, usually thin for height, delayed puberty | Delayed | Diarrhoea and/or macrocytosis/anaemia; occasionally no gastrointestinal symptoms |

**Table 16.21**  Clinical features of common causes of short stature.

# Tall stature

The commonest causes are hereditary (two tall parents!), idiopathic (constitutional) or early development. It can occasionally be due to thyrotoxicosis. Other causes include chromosomal abnormalities (e.g. Klinefelter's syndrome, Marfan's syndrome) or metabolic abnormalities. GH excess is a very rare cause and is usually clinically apparent.

# Acromegaly

This is due to a pituitary tumour in almost all cases. Hyperplasia due to GHRH excess is rare.

## CLINICAL FEATURES

Symptoms and signs of acromegaly are shown in Fig. 16.18. One-third of patients present with changes in appearance, one-quarter with visual field defects or headaches; in the remainder the diagnosis is made by an alert observer in another clinic, e.g. diabetic, hypertension, dental, dermatology.

## INVESTIGATIONS

GH LEVELS are normally very low ($<1$ mU litre$^{-1}$) in adults except during stress or as occasional spikes but, unless levels are always below 1 mU litre$^{-1}$, one cannot exclude the diagnosis.

GLUCOSE TOLERANCE TEST is diagnostic. Acromegalics fail to suppress GH below 2 mU litre$^{-1}$ and some show a paradoxical rise; about 25% of acromegalics have a diabetic glucose tolerance test.

IGF-1 LEVELS. A single plasma level of IGF-1 reflects mean 24-hour GH levels and is useful in diagnosis.

LATERAL SKULL X-RAYS: abnormal in 90% as the tumours are relatively large.

VISUAL FIELDS: field defects are common.

HIGH-RESOLUTION CT SCANS are virtually never normal; MRI often gives even better definition of tumour extent and anatomy, particularly where surgery is contemplated.

PITUITARY FUNCTION: partial or complete anterior hypopituitarism is common.

PROLACTIN: mild to moderate hyperprolactinaemia occurs in 30% of patients.

## MANAGEMENT AND TREATMENT

Untreated acromegaly results in markedly reduced survival with most deaths from heart failure, coronary artery disease and hypertension related causes. Treatment is therefore indicated in all except the elderly or those with minimal abnormalities. The general pros and cons of surgery, radiotherapy and medical treatment are discussed on p. 779.

Preferred treatment is controversial and complete cure is often slow, if possible at all. The choice lies between:

TRANS-SPHENOIDAL SURGERY with subsequent radiotherapy if excision is incomplete or if GH has not been normalized after surgery. Many authorities would give postoperative radiotherapy in nearly all cases, as the tumours frequently recur.

TRANSFRONTAL SURGERY for big tumours with pressure effects. Postoperative radiotherapy is again usually given as excision is virtually never complete.

EXTERNAL RADIOTHERAPY (takes 1–10+ years to be

| Symptoms | Signs | |
|---|---|---|
| Change in appearance | Visual field defects | Prominent supraorbital |
| Increased size of hands/feet | Broad nose | ridge |
| Headaches | **Large tongue** | Prognathism |
| Visual deterioration | Goitre | **Interdental separation** |
| Tiredness | | |
| Weight gain | | |
| Amenorrhoea/ | | |
| oligomenorrhoea | Galactorrhoea | **Thick greasy skin** |
| in women | Hirsuties | |
| Galactorrhoea | | |
| Impotence or poor libido | Carpal tunnel syndrome | **Tight rings** |
| Deep voice | **Spade-like hands** | |
| Goitre | **and feet** | |
| Breathlessness | | |
| Excessive sweating | Proximal myopathy | Heart failure |
| Pain/tingling in hands | Arthropathy | Hypertension |
| Polyuria/polydipsia | | |
| Muscular weakness | | Glycosuria |
| Joint pains | | |
| | | |
| Old photographs are | | |
| frequently useful | | (plus possible signs of |
| Symptoms of | | hypopituitarism) |
| hypopituitarism may be | Oedema | |
| present as well | | |

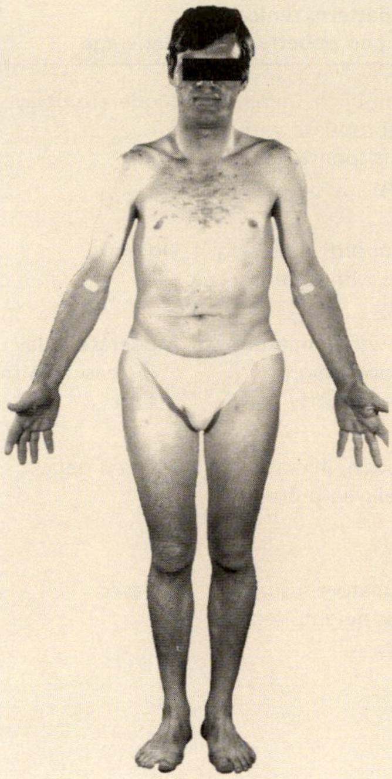

**Fig. 16.18** The signs of acromegaly. Bold type indicates signs of greater discriminant value.

effective), possibly plus bromocriptine or octreotide.

OCTREOTIDE. The synthetic analogue of somatostatin (GHRIH, p. 796) called octreotide is now the treatment of choice in resistant cases, and as a short-term treatment while other modalities become effective. It has to be given by subcutaneous injection in doses of 50–200 $\mu$g 8-hourly but is associated with mild steatorrhoea and an increased incidence of gallstones. It is extremely expensive.

BROMOCRIPTINE ALONE, usually reserved for the elderly and frail. It can be given to shrink tumours prior to definitive therapy or to control symptoms and persisting GH secretion. It is probably only effective in mixed growth-hormone producing (somatotroph) and prolactin producing (mammotroph) tumours. The dose is 10–60 mg daily (higher than for prolactinomas) but should start slowly (see Hyperprolactinaemia). It has largely been replaced by octreotide.

Progress can be assessed by mean GH levels and by IGF-1 measurements.

When present hypopituitarism should be corrected (see p. 782) and concurrent diabetes and/or hypertension should be treated conventionally; both usually improve with treatment of the acromegaly. It is not yet clear by how much the cardiac prognosis is improved by energetic treatment. There appears to be an excess of large bowel carcinoma in acromegaly.

# The thyroid axis

The metabolic rate of many tissues is controlled by the thyroid hormones, and overactivity and underactivity of the gland pose the commonest of all endocrine problems.

## Anatomy

The gland consists of two lateral lobes connected by an isthmus. It is closely attached to the thyroid cartilages and to the upper end of the trachea, and thus moves on swallowing. It is often palpable in normal women.

Embryologically it originates from the base of the tongue and descends to the middle of the neck. Remnants of thyroid tissue can sometimes be found at the base of the tongue (lingual thyroid) and along the line of descent. The gland has a rich blood supply from superior and inferior thyroid arteries.

The thyroid consists of follicles lined by cuboidal epithelioid cells. Inside is the colloid, which is an iodinated glycoprotein, thyroglobulin, synthesized by the follicular cells. Each follicle is surrounded by basement membrane, between which are parafollicular cells containing calcitonin-secreting C cells.

## Biochemistry

The thyroid hormones, $T_4$ and $T_3$ are synthesized within the gland (Fig. 16.19).

More $T_4$ than $T_3$ is produced but $T_4$ is converted in some peripheral tissues (liver, kidney and muscle) to the more active $T_3$ by 5′-monodeiodination; an alternative 3′-monodeiodination yields the inactive reverse $T_3$ ($rT_3$). The latter step occurs particularly in severe non-thyroidal illness (see below).

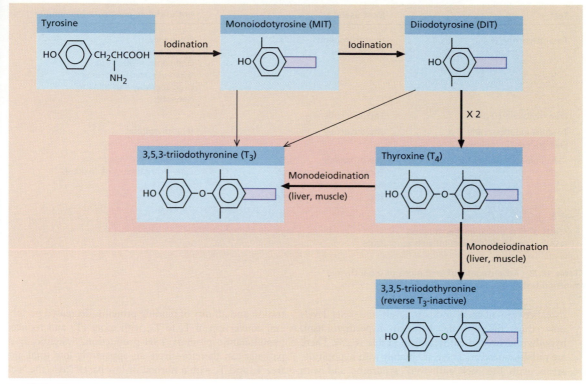

**Fig. 16.19** The synthesis and metabolism of the thyroid hormones. The shaded areas denote the side-chain shown for tyrosine.

In plasma, more than 99% of all $T_4$ and $T_3$ is bound to hormone-binding proteins (thyroxine-binding globulin, TBG; thyroid-binding prealbumin, TBPA; and albumin). Only free hormone is available for tissue action, where $T_3$ binds to specific nuclear receptors within the cell. Factors affecting TBG are shown in Table 16.22.

*Increased TBG*
Hereditary
Pregnancy
Oestrogen therapy
Oral contraceptive use
Hypothyroidism
Phenothiazines
Acute viral hepatitis

*Decreased TBG*
Hereditary
Androgens
Corticosteroid excess
Thyrotoxicosis
Nephrotic syndrome
Major illness
Malnutrition
Chronic liver disease

*Drugs causing altered binding*
Non-steroidal anti-inflammatory drugs
Phenytoin

**Table 16.22** Factors affecting thyroxine-binding globulin (TBG) levels.

**Deficiency**

Globally dietary iodine deficiency is an important cause of thyroid disease as it is an essential requirement for thyroid hormone synthesis. The recommended daily intake of iodine should be at least 140 $\mu$g and dietary supplementation of salt and bread has reduced the number of areas where 'endemic goitre' still occurs (see below).

## Physiology of the hypothalamic–pituitary–thyroid axis (Fig. 16.2)

1 TRH is released in the hypothalamus and stimulates release of TSH from the pituitary.
2 TSH stimulates the TSH receptor in the thyroid to increase synthesis of both $T_4$ and $T_3$ and also to release stored hormone, producing increased plasma levels of $T_4$ and $T_3$.
3 $T_4$ and $T_3$ feed back on the pituitary and perhaps hypothalamus to reduce TRH and TSH secretion.

## Thyroid function tests

RIAs for total $T_4$, free $T_4$, total $T_3$, free $T_3$ and IRMAs (see p. 773) for TSH are widely available. There are only minor significant circadian rhythms, and measurements may be made at any time. Particular uses of the tests are summarized in Table 16.23.

Tests include:

TSH MEASUREMENT. IRMAs for TSH now differen-

| Test | Most useful in | Not useful or possibly misleading in |
|------|----------------|--------------------------------------|
| Total thyroxine (T$_4$) | Hypothyroidism[a]<br>Thyrotoxicosis[a] | Pregnancy<br>Oestrogen therapy<br>Oral contraceptive use<br>'Sick euthyroid' syndrome<br>Drug therapy, e.g. NSAIDs<br>Neonates |
| Free thyroxine (fT$_4$) | Thyrotoxicosis | |
| Total tri-iodothyronine (T$_3$)<br>Free tri-iodothyronine (fT$_3$) | Thyrotoxicosis[a] | Hypothyroidism |
| TSH (immunoradiometric assay) | Thyrotoxicosis<br>Primary hypothyroidism[a]<br>Neonatal screening[a]<br>Hypothalamic–pituitary disease | 'Sick euthyroid' syndrome<br>Early in treatment of toxicosis |

[a]Tests of first choice in this situation.
NSAIDs, non-steroidal anti-inflammatory drugs.

**Table 16.23** Advantages and limitations of usual thyroid function tests.

tiate between normal and low levels and TSH levels now thus discriminate between hyperthyroidism, hypothyroidism and euthyroidism (Table 16.23). There are pitfalls, however. These are mainly with hypopituitarism, with the 'sick euthyroid' syndrome and with dysthyroid eye disease, all of which may give 'false' (i.e. misleading, not incorrect) low results implying hyperthyroidism. As a single test of thyroid function it is the most sensitive in most circumstances but many laboratories prefer to perform at least two tests—serum T$_3$ or free T$_3$ where hyperthyroidism is suspected, serum T$_4$ or free T$_4$ where hypothyroidism is likely.

THYROID HORMONE UPTAKE TESTS (THUT) are now used much less. There are many forms of this measurement of free protein-binding sites, used to calculate the 'free thyroxine index' (FTI). Depending on the method of calculation, high values may imply hypothyroidism or hyperthyroidism; check with your laboratory. TBG is sometimes measured directly.

'FREE' T$_4$ TESTS attempt to measure only the unbound active hormone. They thus avoid the need for THUT and calculation of the FTI. Though not perfect, many of them are adequate for clinical use.

TRH TEST. This has been rendered almost obsolete except for investigation of hypothalamic–pituitary dysfunction.

Primary hypothyroid patients show a high basal TSH level with an excessive rise; hyperthyroid subjects show suppression with a minimal increment of TSH. Flat responses are also seen in pituitary disease, with solitary autonomous nodules, Graves' eye disease and excessive thyroxine replacement, and in patients on steroids or with Cushing's syndrome.

**Problems in interpretation of thyroid function tests**
There are three major areas of difficulty.

SERIOUS ACUTE OR CHRONIC ILLNESS. Thyroid function is affected in several ways, with reduced concentration and affinity of binding proteins, decreased peripheral conversion of T$_4$ to T$_3$, with more rT$_3$ and reduced hypothalamic–pituitary TSH production. Systemically ill patients can therefore have an apparently low total and free T$_4$ and T$_3$ with a normal or low basal TSH (the 'sick euthyroid' syndrome). Levels are usually only mildly below normal and the tests should be repeated after resolution of the underlying illness.

PREGNANCY AND ORAL CONTRACEPTIVES. These lead to greatly increased TBG and thus to high or high-normal total T$_4$ and high THUT levels. The normal physiological changes during pregnancy are not fully understood but rarely cause clinical problems.

DRUGS. Many drugs affect thyroid function tests by interfering with protein binding. The commonest are listed in Table 16.22. Basal TSH should be measured.

## Antithyroid antibodies

Serum antibodies to the thyroid are common and may be either destructive or stimulating; both occasionally coexist in the same patient.

1 Destructive antibodies may be directed against the microsomes or against thyroglobulin; the antigen for thyroid microsomal antibodies is the peroxidase enzyme. They may be detected by haemagglutination techniques and are found in up to 20% of the normal population, especially older women, but only 10–20% of these develop overt hypothyroidism.

2 TSH receptor antibodies (TRAb). These IgG antibodies can be measured in two ways:

(a) By the inhibition of binding of TSH to its receptors (TSH-binding inhibitory immunoglobulin, TBII).

(b) By demonstrating that they stimulate the release of cyclic AMP (thyroid-stimulating immunoglobulin/antibody TSI, TSAb).

These antibodies are seen in Graves' disease (p. 807). Long-acting thyroid stimulator (LATS) assay and LATS-protector (LATS-P) assay also demonstrate TSH antibodies but bear little correlation to clinical thyroid disease. These latter tests have been superseded by the above.

# HYPOTHYROIDISM

## PATHOPHYSIOLOGY

Underactivity of the thyroid may be primary, from disease of the thyroid, or secondary to hypothalamic–pituitary disease (reduced TSH drive) (Table 16.24).

### Causes of primary hypothyroidism

ATROPHIC (AUTOIMMUNE) HYPOTHYROIDISM. This is the commonest cause of hypothyroidism and is associated with microsomal autoantibodies leading to lymphoid infiltration of the gland and eventual atrophy and fibrosis. It is six times more common in females and the incidence increases with age. The condition is associated with other autoimmune disease such as pernicious anaemia. In some instances the condition shows intermittent hypothyroidism with recovery.

HASHIMOTO'S THYROIDITIS. This form of autoimmune thyroiditis, again commoner in women and commonest in late middle age, produces atrophic changes with regeneration, leading to goitre formation. This is usually firm and rubbery but may range from soft to hard. Thyroid microsomal antibodies are again present, often in very high titres. Patients may be hypothyroid or euthyroid, though may go through an initial toxic phase, 'Hashitoxicity'. Thyroxine therapy may shrink the goitre even when the patient is not hypothyroid, though this may take a long time.

IODINE DEFICIENCY. In mountainous areas (the Alps, Himalayas, South America, Central Africa) dietary iodine deficiency still exists, in some areas as 'endemic goitre' where goitre, occasionally massive, is common. The patients may be euthyroid or hypothyroid depending on the severity of iodine deficiency. The mechanism is thought to be borderline hypothyroidism leading to TSH stimulation and thyroid enlargement in the face of continuing iodine deficiency.

DYSHORMONOGENESIS. This rare condition is due to genetic defects in the synthesis of thyroid hormones; patients develop hypothyroidism with a goitre. One particular familial form is associated with sensorineural deafness (Pendred's syndrome).

## CLINICAL FEATURES (Fig. 16.20)

Hypothyroidism may produce many symptoms. The classical picture of the slow, dry-haired, thick-skinned, deep-voiced patient with weight gain, cold intolerance, bradycardia and constipation makes the diagnosis easy; the term 'myxoedema' refers to the accumulation of mucopolysaccharide in subcutaneous tissues. Milder symptoms are, however, more common.

Special difficulties in diagnosis may arise:

CHILDREN WITH HYPOTHYROIDISM may not show classical features but often have a slow growth velocity, poor school performance and sometimes arrest of pubertal development.

YOUNG WOMEN WITH HYPOTHYROIDISM may not show obvious signs. Hypothyroidism should be excluded in all patients with oligomenorrhoea/amenorrhoea, menorrhagia, infertility and hyperprolactinaemia.

AMONG THE ELDERLY, many of the clinical features are difficult to differentiate from normal ageing.

## INVESTIGATION OF PRIMARY HYPOTHYROIDISM (Table 16.23)

TSH is now the investigation of choice; a high TSH level confirms primary hypothyroidism. A low total or free $T_4$ level confirms the hypothyroid state and is especially important if there is any evidence of hypothalamic and pituitary disease, when TSH may be low or normal.

Thyroid and other organ-specific antibodies may be present. Other abnormalities include:

ANAEMIA. This is usually normochromic and normocytic in type but it may be macrocytic (sometimes this is due to associated pernicious anaemia) or microcytic (in women, due to menorrhagia).

INCREASED ASPARTATE TRANSFERASE LEVELS, from muscle and/or liver.

INCREASED CREATINE KINASE LEVELS.

| Primary |
|---|
| Congenital |
|   Agenesis |
|   Ectopic thyroid remnants |
| |
| Defects of hormone synthesis |
|   Iodine deficiency |
|   Dyshormonogenesis |
|   Antithyroid drugs |
|   Other drugs, e.g. lithium, amiodarone |
| |
| Autoimmune |
|   Atrophic thyroiditis |
|   Hashimoto's thyroiditis |
| |
| Infective |
|   Post subacute thyroiditis |
| |
| Post surgery |
| |
| Post irradiation |
|   ¹³¹I therapy |
|   External neck irradiation |
| |
| Infiltration |
|   Tumour |
| |
| Peripheral resistance to thyroid hormone |
| |
| Secondary |
| Hypopituitarism |
| Isolated TSH deficiency |

Table 16.24 Causes of hypothyroidism.

| Symptoms | Signs | |
|---|---|---|
| Tiredness/malaise | **Mental slowness** | Large tongue |
| Weight gain | Psychosis/dementia | |
| Anorexia | Ataxia | Periorbital oedema |
| Cold intolerance | Poverty of movement | Deep voice |
| Poor memory | Deafness | (Goitre) |
| Change in appearance | | |
| Depression | 'Peaches and | Dry skin |
| Psychosis | cream' complexion | Mild obesity |
| Coma | **Dry thin hair** | |
| Deafness | Loss of eyebrows | Myotonia |
| Poor libido | | Muscular hypertrophy |
| Goitre | Hypertension | Proximal myopathy |
| Puffy eyes | Hypothermia | Slow-relaxing reflexes |
| Dry, brittle, | Heart failure | |
| unmanageable hair | **Bradycardia** | Anaemia |
| Dry, coarse skin | **Pericardial effusion** | |
| Arthralgia | | |
| Myalgia | Cold peripheries | |
| Constipation | Carpal tunnel syndrome | |
| Menorrhagia or | Oedema | |
| oligomenorrhoea | | |
| in women | | |
| | | |
| A history from a relative | | |
| is often revealing | | |
| Symptoms of other | | |
| autoimmune disease | | |
| may be present | | |

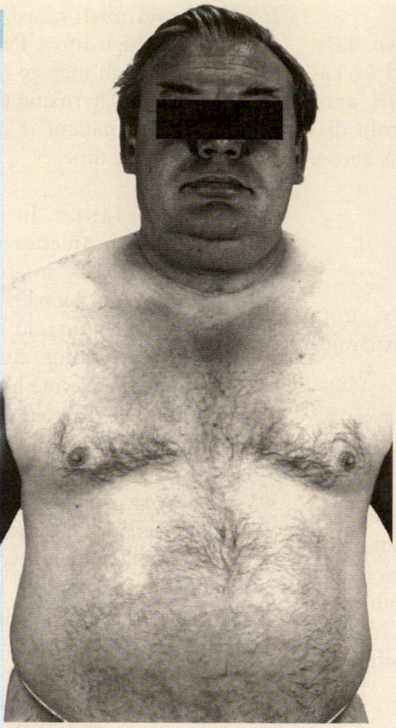

**Fig. 16.20** The signs of hypothyroidism. The bold type indicates signs of greater discriminant value.

HYPERCHOLESTEROLAEMIA.

HYPONATRAEMIA due to an increase in ADH and impaired free water clearance.

### TREATMENT

Replacement therapy with $T_4$ is given for life. The starting dose will depend upon the age and fitness of the patient, especially cardiac performance. In the young and fit, 100 $\mu$g daily is suitable, while 50 $\mu$g daily is more appropriate for the old or frail. $T_3$ offers no significant advantage over $T_4$.

Patients with ischaemic heart disease require even lower initial doses, especially if the hypothyroidism is severe and long-standing. Most physicians would then begin with 25 $\mu$g daily and perform serial ECGs, increasing the dose at 2–6 week intervals if angina does not occur or worsen and the ECG does not deteriorate. Some, however, would use $T_3$ beginning with 2.5 $\mu$g 8-hourly, doubling the dose every 48 hours up to 10 $\mu$g three times daily. If progress is satisfactory, $T_4$ (100 $\mu$g daily) is then started and $T_3$ is discontinued 5 days later.

Adequacy of replacement should be assessed clinically and by thyroid function tests (TSH and possibly $T_4$) after at least 6 weeks on a steady dose; the aim is to restore TSH to within the normal range. If serum TSH remains high, the dose of $T_4$ should be increased in 25-$\mu$g increments and the tests repeated 6 weeks later. This stepwise progression should be continued until TSH becomes normal. The usual maintenance dose is 100–200 $\mu$g given as a single daily dose; excessive replacement is probably dangerous.

Clinical improvement on $T_4$ may not begin for 2 weeks, though is quicker on $T_3$, and full resolution of symptoms may take 6 months. The importance of lifelong therapy must be emphasized and the possibility of other autoimmune endocrine disease developing, especially Addison's disease, should be considered.

## Borderline hypothyroidism or compensated euthyroidism

Patients are frequently seen with low normal serum $T_4$ levels and slightly raised TSH levels. Sometimes this follows surgery or radioiodine therapy when it can reasonably be seen as 'compensatory'. Most physicians would now treat with $T_4$ where the TSH is above twice normal, or when possible symptoms are present, but would simply repeat the tests (and measure thyroid antibodies) 3–6 months later where TSH is only marginally raised.

## Myxoedema coma

Though very rare, severe hypothyroidism, especially in the elderly, may present with confusion or even coma.

Hypothermia is often present and the patient may have severe cardiac failure, hypoventilation, hypoglycaemia and hyponatraemia.

The mortality was previously at least 50% and patients require full intensive care. Optimal treatment is controversial and data lacking; most physicians would advise $T_3$ orally or intravenously in doses of 2.5–5 $\mu$g every 8 hours, then increasing as above. Large intravenous doses should not be used.

Additional measures, though unproven, should include:

- Oxygen (by ventilation if necessary)
- Monitoring of cardiac output and pressures via Swan–Ganz catheter
- Gradual rewarming
- Hydrocortisone 100 mg i.v. 8-hourly
- Dextrose infusion to prevent hypoglycaemia

**'Myxoedema madness'**

Depression is common but occasionally with severe hypothyroidism in the elderly the patient may become frankly demented or psychotic, sometimes with striking delusions. This may occur shortly after starting $T_4$ replacement.

## Screening for hypothyroidism

The incidence of congenital hypothyroidism is approximately 1 : 3500 births. Untreated, severe hypothyroidism leads to permanent neurological and intellectual damage ('cretinism'). Routine screening of the newborn using a blood-spot, as in the Guthrie test, to detect a high TSH level as an indicator of primary hypothyroidism is efficient; cretinism is prevented if $T_4$ is started within the first few months of life.

Screening of elderly patients is controversial but there is little doubt that the incidence of unsuspected thyroid disease in those over 65 years is 1–3%. With this and undiagnosed hyperthyroidism many physicians believe in screening of all elderly hospital attenders.

## GOITRE (THYROID ENLARGEMENT)

Goitre is more common in women than in men and may be either physiological or pathological.

### CLINICAL FEATURES

Most commonly a goitre is noticed as a cosmetic defect by the patient or by friends or relatives. The majority are painless but pain or discomfort can occur in acute varieties. Goitres can produce dysphagia and difficulty in breathing, implying oesophageal or tracheal compression.

Clinical examination should record the size, shape, consistency and mobility of the gland as well as whether its lower margin can be demarcated (thus implying the absence of retrosternal extension). A bruit may be present. Associated lymph nodes should be sought and the tracheal position determined if possible. Examination should never omit an assessment of the patient's clinical thyroid status.

There is a WHO grading of goitre:

GRADE 0      No palpable or visible goitre
GRADE 1      Palpable goitre

1A      Goitre detectable only on palpation
1B      Goitre palpable and visible with neck extended
GRADE 2      Goitre visible with neck in normal position
GRADE 3      Large goitre visible from a distance

Specific enquiry should be made about any medication, especially iodine-containing preparations, and possible exposure to radiation.

### ASSESSMENT

Two facts are essential about any goitre: its pathological nature and the patient's thyroid status.

The nature can often be judged clinically. Goitres are usually separable into diffuse and nodular types, the causes of which differ (Table 16.25).

Particular points of note are:

PUBERTY AND PREGNANCY may produce a diffuse increase in size of the thyroid.

IN GRAVES' DISEASE (autoimmune hyperthyroidism) the gland is again diffusely enlarged, often somewhat firm and frequently associated with a bruit.

ACUTE TENDERNESS in a diffuse swelling, sometimes with severe pain, is suggestive of an acute viral thyroiditis (de Quervain's). This is usually associated with a systemic viral illness and may produce transient clinical hyperthyroidism with an increase in serum $T_4$ (see p. 807).

PAIN in a goitre may be caused by thyroiditis, bleeding into a cyst or (rarely) a thyroid tumour.

SIMPLE GOITRE: in this instance no clear cause is found

Physiological
   Puberty
   Pregnancy

Autoimmune
   Graves' disease
   Hashimoto's disease

Thyroiditis
   Acute (de Quervain's thyroiditis)
   Chronic fibrotic (Riedel's thyroiditis)

Iodine deficiency (endemic goitre)

Dyshormonogenesis

Goitrogens (e.g. sulphonylureas)

Multinodular goitre

Diffuse goitre
   Colloid
   Simple

Cysts

Tumours
   Adenomas
   Carcinoma
   Lymphoma

Miscellaneous
   Sarcoidosis
   Tuberculosis

**Table 16.25**   Causes and types of goitre.

for enlargement of the thyroid, which is usually smooth and soft. It may be associated with thyroid growth-stimulating antibodies.

NODULAR GOITRES may have multiple or solitary nodules. Commonest is the multinodular goitre, especially in older patients. The patient is usually euthyroid but may be hyperthyroid. Multinodular goitre is the commonest cause of tracheal and/or oesophageal compression and may cause laryngeal nerve palsy. It may also extend retrosternally.

SOLITARY NODULES present a difficult problem. A history of pain, rapid enlargement or associated lymph nodes in such a situation suggests the possibility of thyroid carcinoma. The majority of such nodules are, however, cystic or benign and, indeed, may simply be the largest solitary nodule of a multinodular goitre. Risk factors for malignancy include previous irradiation, long-standing iodine deficiency and occasional familial cases. Solitary toxic nodules (Plummer's syndrome) are quite uncommon and may be associated with $T_3$ production.

FIBROTIC GOITRE (Riedel's thyroiditis): this rare condition, usually producing a 'woody' gland, is associated with other midline fibrosis and is often difficult to distinguish from carcinoma, being irregular and hard.

EXCESSIVE DOSES OF CARBIMAZOLE OR PROPYLTHIOURACIL will induce goitre.

IODINE DEFICIENCY AND DYSHORMONOGENESIS (see above) can also cause goitre.

MALIGNANCY. Rarely the thyroid is the site of a metastatic deposit or the site of origin of a lymphoma.

## INVESTIGATION

Clinical findings will dictate appropriate initial tests:

THYROID FUNCTION TESTS—TSH plus $T_4$ or $T_3$ (see Table 16.23)

CHEST AND THORACIC INLET X-RAYS where appropriate to detect tracheal compression and large retrosternal extensions

### Additional investigations

FINE NEEDLE ASPIRATION (FNA). In patients with a solitary nodule or a dominant nodule in a multinodular goitre, there is a 5% chance of malignancy; in view of this, FNA should be performed. This can be done in the outpatient clinic. Cytology in expert hands can usually differentiate the suspicious or definitely malignant nodule.

ULTRASOUND with high resolution is a sensitive method for delineating nodules and can demonstrate whether they are cystic or solid. Unfortunately, even cystic lesions can be malignant and therefore FNA is the preferred technique.

THYROID SCAN ($^{125}$I or $^{131}$I) is useful to distinguish between functioning (hot) or non-functioning (cold) nodules. A hot nodule is virtually never malignant; however a cold nodule is malignant in 10% of cases. FNA has therefore reduced the need for imaging and will reduce the necessity for surgery.

## TREATMENT

During puberty and pregnancy a goitre associated with euthyroidism rarely requires intervention. If euthyroid, the patient should be reassured that spontaneous resolution is likely. In other situations the patient should be rendered euthyroid.

Indications for surgical intervention are:

THE POSSIBILITY OF MALIGNANCY. A history of rapid growth, pain, cervical lymphadenopathy or previous irradiation to the neck are worrying features. FNA should be performed. Surgery may be necessary.

PRESSURE SYMPTOMS on the trachea or, more rarely, oesophagus. The possibility of retrosternal extension should be excluded.

COSMETIC REASONS. A large goitre is often a considerable anxiety to the patient even though functionally and anatomically benign.

# THYROID CARCINOMA

The different types of thyroid carcinoma, their characteristics and treatment are listed in Table 16.26. The tumour is relatively uncommon, being responsible for 400 deaths annually in the UK.

Particular points are:

PAPILLARY AND FOLLICULAR CARCINOMAS may take up iodine, shown by scanning. Such patients after total thyroidectomy may be given a therapeutic radioiodine dose, which will be taken up by remaining thyroid tissue or metastatic lesions. Replacement $T_4$ will subsequently be needed and should suppress TSH, which may otherwise stimulate any residual differentiated car-

| Cell type | Frequency | Behaviour | Spread | Prognosis |
|---|---|---|---|---|
| Papillary | 70% | Occurs in young people, slow-growing | Local, sometimes lung/bone secondaries | Good, especially in young |
| Follicular | 20% | Commoner in females | Metastases to lung/bone | Good if resected |
| Anaplastic | <5% | Aggressive | Locally invasive | Very poor |
| Lymphoma | <2% | Variable | Sometimes responsive to radiotherapy | |
| Medullary cell | 5% | Often familial | Local and metastases | Poor |

Table 16.26  Types of thyroid malignancy.

cinoma. Lungs and bone are the commonest sites of metastases, while local invasion is often a problem. The measurement of thyroglobulin in plasma has been used as a tumour marker for the presence of neoplastic tissue.

ANAPLASTIC CARCINOMAS AND LYMPHOMA do not respond to radioactive iodine.

MEDULLARY CARCINOMA, often associated with MEN (see p. 824), is usually treated by total thyroidectomy. The patient's family should be screened for this and other endocrine neoplastic conditions.

# HYPERTHYROIDISM

Hyperthyroidism is common, affecting perhaps 2–5% of all females at some time and with a sex ratio of 5 : 1, most often between ages 20 and 40 years. Nearly all cases are caused by intrinsic thyroid disease; a pituitary cause is extremely rare (Table 16.27).

## Graves' disease

PATHOGENESIS. This is the commonest cause of hyperthyroidism and is due to an autoimmune process. Serum IgG antibodies bind to the thyroid TSH receptor stimulating thyroid hormone production, behaving like TSH. These TSH receptor antibodies can be measured in serum (see p. 802). There is an association with HLA-B8, Dw3 and 50% concordance is seen amongst monozygotic twins with a 5% concordance rate in dizygotic twins.

*Yersinia enterocolitica* as well as *Escherichia coli* and other Gram-negative organisms contain TSH binding sites. This raises the possibility that the initiating event in the pathogenesis may be an infection in a genetically susceptible individual.

Associated with the thyroid disease in many cases are eye changes (see below) and other signs such as vitiligo and pretibial myxoedema. Rarely lymphadenopathy and splenomegaly may occur. Graves' disease is also associated with other autoimmune disorders such as pernicious anaemia and myasthenia gravis.

---

Graves' disease
Solitary toxic nodule/adenoma
Toxic multinodular goitre
Acute thyroiditis
   Viral
   Autoimmune
   Post irradiation
Thyrotoxicosis factitia (secret $T_4$ consumption)
Exogenous iodine
Drugs—amiodarone
Metastatic differentiated thyroid carcinoma
TSH-secreting tumours (e.g. pituitary)
HCG-producing tumours
Hyperfunctioning ovarian teratoma (struma ovarii)

---

Only the first three are common.
HCG, human chorionic gonadotrophin.

**Table 16.27**   Causes of hyperthyroidism.

The natural history is one of fluctuation, many patients showing a pattern of alternating relapse and remission; perhaps only 40% of subjects have a single episode. Many patients eventually become hypothyroid.

## Toxic solitary adenoma/nodule (Plummer's disease)
This is the cause of about 5% of cases of hyperthyroidism. It does not usually remit after a course of antithyroid drugs.

## Toxic multinodular goitre
This commonly occurs in older women; again antithyroid drugs are rarely successful in inducing a remission.

## De Quervain's thyroiditis
This is transient thyrotoxicosis from an acute inflammatory process, probably viral in origin. Apart from the toxicosis there is usually fever, malaise and pain in the neck with tachycardia and local thyroid tenderness. Thyroid function tests show initial thyrotoxicosis, the erythrocyte sedimentation rate (ESR) is raised and thyroid scans show *suppression* of uptake in the acute phase, though hypothyroidism, usually transient, may then follow after a few weeks. Treatment of the acute phase is with aspirin, using short-term prednisolone in severely symptomatic cases.

## CLINICAL FEATURES OF HYPERTHYROIDISM
The symptoms of hyperthyroidism affect many systems; they and relevant signs are shown in Fig. 16.21.

Symptomatology and signs vary with age and with the underlying aetiology. Important points are:

THE EYE SIGNS, PRETIBIAL MYXOEDEMA AND THYROID ACROPACHY only occur in Graves' disease. Pretibial myxoedema is an infiltration on the shin, essentially only occurring with eye disease (see below). Thyroid acropachy is very rare and consists of clubbing, swollen fingers and periosteal new bone formation.

IN THE ELDERLY a frequent presentation is with atrial fibrillation, other tachycardias and/or heart failure, often with few other signs. Thyroid function tests are mandatory in any patient with unexplained atrial fibrillation.

CHILDREN frequently present with excessive height or excessive growth rate, or with behavioural problems such as hyperactivity. They may also show weight gain rather than loss.

SO-CALLED 'APATHETIC THYROTOXICOSIS' in some elderly patients presents with a clinical picture more like hypothyroidism. There may be very few signs and a high degree of clinical suspicion is essential.

## DIFFERENTIAL DIAGNOSIS
Thyrotoxicosis is often clinically obvious but treatment should never be instituted without biochemical confirmation.

Differentiation of the mild case from anxiety states may be difficult; useful positive clinical markers are eye signs, proximal myopathy and wasting. The hyperdynamic cir-

| Symptoms | | Signs | |
| --- | --- | --- | --- |
| Weight loss | | Irritability | **Exophthalmus** |
| Increased appetite | | Psychosis | Lid lag |
| Irritability/behaviour change | | **Hyperkinesis** | Conjunctival oedema |
| Restlessness | | Tremor | Ophthalmoplegia |
| Malaise | | | **Goitre, bruit** |
| Muscle weakness | | Systolic hypertension | |
| Tremor | | Cardiac failure | |
| Choreoathetosis | | **Tachycardia or atrial** | |
| Breathlessness | | **fibrillation** | Weight loss |
| Palpitation | | **Warm vasodilated** | |
| Heat intolerance | | **peripheries** | |
| Vomiting | | | |
| Diarrhoea | | | Proximal muscle wasting |
| Eye complaints* | | | (shoulder and hips) |
| Goitre | | Onycholysis | **Proximal myopathy** |
| Oligomenorrhoea | | Palmar erythema | |
| Loss of libido | | | |
| Gynaecomastia | | | |
| Onycholysis | | | |
| Tall stature (in children) | | Thyroid acropachy | |
| | | **Pretibial myxoedema** | |
| *Only in Graves' disease | | | |

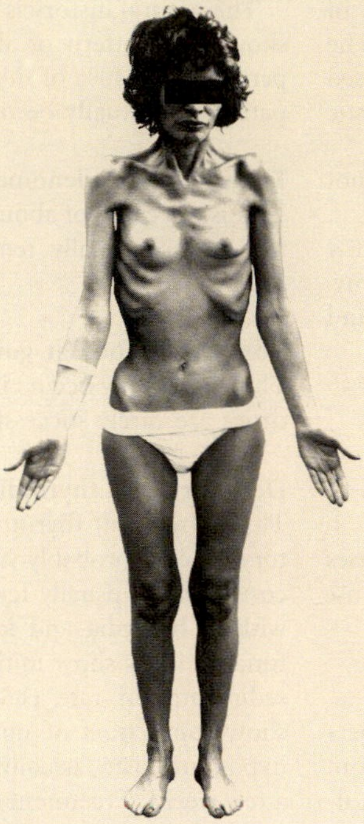

**Fig. 16.21**   The signs of hyperthyroidism. The bold type indicates signs of greater discriminant value.

culation with warm peripheries seen with thyrotoxicosis can be compared with the clammy hands of anxiety.

## INVESTIGATION

Serum TSH is suppressed ($<0.1$ mU litre$^{-1}$) though most physicians also like to confirm the diagnosis with a raised serum $T_3$ or $T_4$; the former is more sensitive as there are occasional cases of '$T_3$ toxicosis'. Microsomal (directed against thyroid peroxidase) and thyroglobulin antibodies are present in most cases of Graves' disease.

TSH receptor antibodies are not measured routinely, but are present: TSI 80% positive, TBII 60–90% in Graves' disease.

The TRH test is now very rarely necessary. A normal TSH rise excludes the diagnosis; a flat response is characteristic but not diagnostic.

## TREATMENT

Three possibilities are available: antithyroid drugs, surgery and radioiodine. Practices and beliefs differ widely within and between countries; it also depends on patient preference and local expertise. Some general guidelines are:

PATIENTS WITH LARGE GOITRES, SINGLE OR MULTIPLE NODULAR GOITRES are unlikely to remit after a course of antithyroid drugs.

RADIOIODINE is now more widely used in the UK for those under the age of 40 years as has previously happened elsewhere; theoretical risks of carcinogenesis were not proven.

PATIENTS WITH DYSTHYROID EYE DISEASE may show worsening of eye problems after radioiodine, though this can often be prevented by steroid or early $T_4$ administration.

PATIENTS WHO DEMONSTRATE POOR COMPLIANCE with drug therapy should probably undergo surgery.

PATIENT PREFERENCE, with informed discussion of the alternatives, must be given great weight.

### Antithyroid drugs

Carbimazole is most often used in the UK. Occasionally propylthiouracil is also used. Methimazole, the active metabolite of carbimazole, is used in the USA.

These drugs inhibit the formation of thyroid hormones and also have minor other actions; carbimazole/ methimazole is also an immunosuppressive agent. Initial doses and side-effects are detailed in Table 16.28.

Though thyroid hormone synthesis is reduced very quickly, the long half-life of $T_4$ (7 days) means that clinical benefit is not apparent for 10–20 days. As many of the manifestations of hyperthyroidism are mediated via the sympathetic system, $\beta$-blockers are used to provide rapid partial symptomatic control; they also decrease peripheral conversion of $T_4$ to $T_3$. Drugs preferred are those without intrinsic sympathomimetic activity (Table 16.28). They should not be used alone for hyperthyroidism except when the condition is self-limiting, e.g. subacute thyroiditis.

Subsequent management is either by gradual dose titration or a 'block and replace' regimen.

| Drug | Usual starting dose | Side-effects | Remarks |
|---|---|---|---|
| *Antithyroid drugs* | | | |
| Carbimazole | 10–20 mg 8-hourly | Rash, nausea, vomiting, arthralgia, agranulocytosis (0.1%), jaundice | Active metabolite is methimazole Mild immunosuppressive activity |
| Propylthiouracil | 100–200 mg 8-hourly | Rash, nausea, vomiting, agranulocytosis | Blocks conversion of $T_4$ to $T_3$ |
| *β-Blockers for symptomatic control* | | | |
| Propranolol | 40–80 mg 6 to 8-hourly | Avoid in asthma; use with care in heart failure | Use β-blocking agents without intrinsic sympathomimetic activity |
| Nadolol | 40–240 ,g daily | Usual β-blocker side-effects | May need higher doses in hyperthyroidism as metabolism is increased |

**Table 16.28** Drugs used in the treatment of thyrotoxicosis.

GRADUAL DOSE TITRATION

1 Review after 4–6 weeks and reduce dose of carbimazole depending on clinical state and $T_4/T_3$ levels. TSH levels may remain suppressed for long periods.
2 When clinically *and* biochemically euthyroid, stop β-blockers.
3 Review after 2–3 months and, if controlled, reduce carbimazole. Once-daily dosage is now possible.
4 Gradually reduce dose to 5 mg daily over 12–18 months if thyrotoxicosis remains controlled.
5 When euthyroid on 5 mg daily carbimazole, discontinue.
6 About 50% of patients will relapse, mostly within the following 2 years. Long-term antithyroid therapy is then used or surgery or radiotherapy is considered (see below).
7 Propylthiouracil is used in similar fashion but doses required are tenfold higher (50–500 mg daily).

'BLOCK AND REPLACE' REGIMEN. With this policy, full doses of antithyroid drugs, usually carbimazole 30–45 mg daily, are given to suppress the thyroid completely while replacing thyroid activity with $T_4$ 0.1 mg daily. This is continued usually for 18 months, the claimed advantages being the avoidance of over- or under-treatment and the better use of the immunosuppressive action. Against this there is no 'feel' for whether the patient is likely to relapse as with the titration method.

TOXICITY (Table 16.28). The major side-effect is agranulocytosis that occurs in approximately 1 in 1000 patients within 3 months of treatment. All patients must be warned to seek immediate medical attention if they develop unexplained fever or sore throat; this is best done with a written sheet. If toxicity occurs on carbimazole, propylthiouracil may be used and vice versa; side-effects are only occasionally repeated on the other drug.

**Surgery—subtotal thyroidectomy**
Thyroidectomy should only be performed in patients who have previously been rendered euthyroid. Conventional practice is to stop the antithyroid drug 10–14 days before operation and to give potassium iodide (60 mg three times daily), which reduces the vascularity of the gland.
    Particular indications for surgery are:
● Patient choice.
● A large goitre is unlikely to respond to antithyroid medication.
Indications for either surgery or radioiodine are:
● Persistent drug side-effects (also suitable for radioiodine)
● Poor compliance with drug therapy
● Recurrent hyperthyroidism after drugs
The operation should only be performed by experienced surgeons to reduce the chance of complications:
EARLY POSTOPERATIVE BLEEDING causing tracheal compression and asphyxia is a rare emergency requiring immediate removal of all clips/sutures to allow escape of the blood/haematoma.
LARYNGEAL NERVE PALSY (1%); vocal chord movement should be checked preoperatively. Mild hoarseness is more common and thyroidectomy is best avoided in serious singers!
TRANSIENT HYPOCALCAEMIA in up to 10% but with permanent hypoparathyroidism in less than 1%.
RECURRENT HYPERTHYROIDISM (less than 5%).
HYPOTHYROIDISM — about 10% of patients are hypothyroid within 1 year and this percentage increases with time. It is likeliest if microsomal antibodies are positive. Automated computer thyroid registers with annual TSH screening are used in some regions.

**Radioactive iodine**
Iodine-131 in an empirical dose (usually $18–40 \times 10^{10}$ Bq) accumulates in the thyroid and destroys the gland by local radiation. Early discomfort in the neck and immediate worsening of hyperthyroidism are sometimes seen; again patients must be rendered euthyroid before treatment though they have to stop antithyroid drugs about 5 days before radioiodine.

    If worsening occurs, the patient should not receive carbimazole for 2–3 days after radioiodine, as it will prevent radioiodine uptake by the gland. They should receive propranolol (Table 16.28) until carbimazole can be restarted if necessary; euthyroidism normally returns in 2–3 months.

Apart from the immediate problems above, a major complication is the progressive incidence in subsequent hypothyroidism affecting the majority of subjects over the following 20 years. Though 75% of patients are rendered euthyroid in the short term, a small proportion remain hyperthyroid; increasing the radioiodine dose reduces recurrence but increases the rate of hypothyroidism. Again, long-term surveillance of thyroid function is necessary with frequent tests in the first year after therapy.

## Special situations in hyperthyroidism

### Thyroid crisis
This rare condition, with a mortality of 10%, is a rapid deterioration of thyrotoxicosis with hyperpyrexia, severe tachycardia and extreme restlessness. It is usually precipitated by stress, infection, surgery in an unprepared patient or radioiodine therapy. With careful management it should no longer occur.

Treatment is urgent. Propranolol in full doses is started immediately together with potassium iodide, antithyroid drugs, corticosteroids (which suppress many of the manifestations of hyperthyroidism) and full supportive measures.

### Hyperthyroidism in pregnancy and neonatal life
Maternal hyperthyroidism during pregnancy is uncommon and usually mild. Diagnosis can be difficult because of misleading thyroid function tests, although TSH is largely reliable. The pathogenesis is almost always Graves' disease. TSI crosses the placenta to stimulate the fetal thyroid. Carbimazole also crosses the placenta, but $T_4$ does so poorly. The smallest dose of carbimazole necessary is used and the fetus must be monitored (see below). The paediatrician should be informed and the infant checked immediately after birth — overtreatment with carbimazole can cause fetal goitre.

If necessary (high doses needed, poor patient compliance or drug side-effects), surgery can be performed, preferably in the second trimester. Radioactive iodine is absolutely contraindicated.

### The fetus and maternal Graves' disease
Any mother with a history of Graves' disease may have circulating TSI. Even if she has been treated (e.g. by surgery), the immunoglobulin may still be present to stimulate the fetal thyroid, and the fetus can thus become hyperthyroid, while the mother remains euthyroid.

Any such patient should therefore be monitored during pregnancy. Fetal heart rate provides a direct biological assay of thyroid status, and monitoring should be performed at least monthly. Rates above 160 $min^{-1}$ are strongly suggestive of fetal hyperthyroidism and maternal treatment with carbimazole and/or propranolol may be used. To prevent the mother becoming hypothyroid, $T_4$ may be given as this does not easily cross the placenta. Sympathomimetics, used to prevent premature labour, are contraindicated as they may provoke fatal tachycardia in the fetus.

Thyrotoxicosis may also develop in the neonatal period as TSI has a half-life of approximately 3 weeks. Manifestations in the newborn include irritability, failure to thrive and persisting weight loss, diarrhoea and eye signs. Thyroid function tests are difficult to interpret as neonatal normal ranges vary with age.

Untreated neonatal thyrotoxicosis is probably associated with hyperactivity in later childhood.

## THYROID EYE DISEASE

This is also known as dysthyroid eye disease or ophthalmic Graves' disease.

### PATHOPHYSIOLOGY
The evidence suggests that the exophthalmos of Graves' disease is due to specific antibodies that cause retro-orbital inflammation with swelling and oedema of the extraocular muscles leading to limitation of movement. This leads to proptosis which can sometimes be unilateral, and increased pressure on the optic nerve may cause optic atrophy. Histology shows a focal oedema and glycosaminoglycan deposition followed by fibrosis.

While often associated with Graves' hyperthyroidism, it need not be so and patients may be hyperthyroid, euthyroid or hypothyroid. TSH receptor antibodies are almost invariably found in the serum but their role in the pathogenesis in unclear.

### CLINICAL FEATURES
The clinical appearances are characteristic (Fig. 16.22). Proptosis and limitation of eye movements (by 'tight' muscles) are direct effects of the inflammation, while conjunctival oedema, lid lag and corneal scarring are secondary to the proptosis and lack of eye cover. The ability to close the eyes completely is important, as otherwise corneal damage may occur. Visual impairment from optic nerve pressure may occur. Eye manifestations often do not parallel the clinical course of Graves' disease — in particular the degree of toxicosis. Only 5–10% threaten sight, but the discomfort and cosmetic problems cause great patient anxiety. There is a grading system (see Fig. 16.22).

### INVESTIGATIONS
Few investigations are necessary if the appearances are characteristic and bilateral. TSH and $T_3$ or $T_4$ should be measured.

The exophthalmos should be measured to allow progress to be monitored. If appearances or measurements are markedly discrepant in the two eyes, other retro-orbital space-occupying lesions should be considered: CT or MRI of the orbits will exclude other causes and show enlarged muscles and oedema.

### TREATMENT
If patients are thyrotoxic this should be normalized, but hypothyroidism must be avoided as this may exacerbate

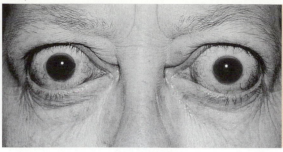

**Fig. 16.22** The signs of thyroid eye disease.

Grade 0 No signs or symptoms

Grade 1 Only signs, no symptoms

Grade 2 Soft tissue involvement

Grade 3 Proptosis (measured with exophthalmometer)

Grade 4 Extraocular muscle involvement

Grade 5 Corneal involvement

Grade 6 Sight loss with optic nerve involvement

the eye problem: an increased incidence of eye problems after radioiodine treatment reflects this. Direct treatment may be either local or systemic:

METHYLCELLULOSE EYEDROPS are given to aid lubrication. Some patients gain relief by sleeping upright.

SYSTEMIC STEROIDS (prednisolone 30–120 mg daily) usually reduce inflammation if more severe symptoms are present. Pulse intravenous methylprednisolone may be more rapidly effective in severe cases.

IRRADIATION OF THE ORBITS (20 Gy in divided doses) is also used in severe instances, with steroid cover.

LATERAL TARSORRHAPHY will protect the cornea if lids cannot be closed.

SURGICAL DECOMPRESSION of the orbit(s) is occasionally needed.

CORRECTIVE EYE MUSCLE SURGERY may improve diplopia due to muscle changes, but should be deferred till the situation has been stable for 6 months. Plastic surgery around the eyes may also be of value.

# The glucocorticoid axis

## ADRENAL ANATOMY AND FUNCTION

The human adrenals, weighing only 8–10 g together, comprise an outer cortex with three zones (reticularis, fasciculata and glomerulosa) producing steroids and an inner medulla that synthesizes, stores and secretes catecholamines (see Adrenal medulla, p. 824).

The adrenal steroids are grouped into three classes based on their predominant physiological effects:

GLUCOCORTICOIDS. These are named after their effects on carbohydrate metabolism; major actions are listed in Table 16.29.

MINERALOCORTICOIDS. Their predominant effect is on the extracellular balance of sodium and potassium in the distal tubule of the kidney: aldosterone is the predominant mineralocorticoid in humans (about 50%); corticosterone makes a small contribution. The weak mineralocorticoid activity of cortisol is also important since it is present in considerable excess. Aldosterone is produced solely in the zona glomerulosa.

ANDROGENS. Although secreted in considerable quantities, most have only relatively weak intrinsic androgenic activity until metabolized peripherally to testosterone or dihydrotestosterone.

*Increased or stimulated*
Gluconeogenesis
Glycogen deposition
Protein catabolism
Fat deposition
Sodium retention
Potassium loss
Free water clearance
Uric acid production
Circulating neutrophils

*Decreased or inhibited*
Protein synthesis
Host response to infection
Lymphocyte transformation
Delayed hypersensitivity
Circulating lymphocytes
Circulating eosinophils

**Table 16.29** The actions of glucocorticoids.

The relative potency of common steroids is shown in Table 16.30.

## BIOCHEMISTRY

All steroids have the same basic skeleton (Fig. 16.23a) and the chemical differences between them are slight. The major biosynthetic pathways are also shown in Fig. 16.23b.

## PHYSIOLOGY

Glucocorticoid production by the adrenal is under hypothalamic–pituitary control (Fig. 16.24). Corticotrophin releasing factor (CRF) is secreted in the hypothalamus in

| Steroid | Glucocorticoid effect[a] | Mineralocorticoid effect[a] |
|---|---|---|
| Cortisol (hydrocortisone) | 1 | 1 |
| Prednisolone | 4 | 0.7 |
| Dexamethasone | 40 | 2 |
| Aldosterone | 0.1 | 400 |
| Fludrocortisone | 10 | 400 |

[a]Cortisol is arbitrarily defined as 1.

**Table 16.30** Glucocorticoid and mineralocorticoid potency of equal amounts of common steroids.

response to circadian rhythm, stress and other stimuli. It travels down the portal system to stimulate ACTH release from the anterior pituitary corticotrophs. Circulating ACTH stimulates cortisol production in the adrenal. The cortisol secreted (or any other synthetic corticosteroid) feeds back on the hypothalamus and pituitary to inhibit further CRF/ACTH release. The set-point of this system clearly varies through the day according to the circadian rhythm, and is usually overridden by severe stress.

Following adrenalectomy or Addison's disease, cortisol secretion will be absent or reduced; ACTH levels will therefore rise.

Mineralocorticoid secretion is mainly controlled by the renin–angiotensin system (see p. 822).

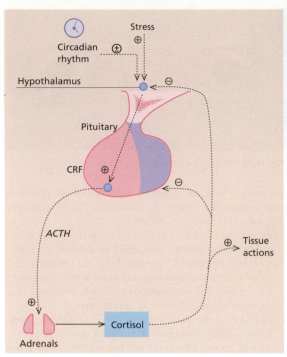

**Fig. 16.24** Control of the hypothalamic–pituitary–adrenal axis. CRF, corticotrophin-releasing factor.

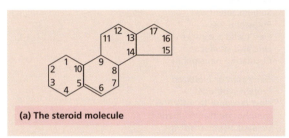

**(a) The steroid molecule**

**Fig. 16.23** (a) The steroid molecule.

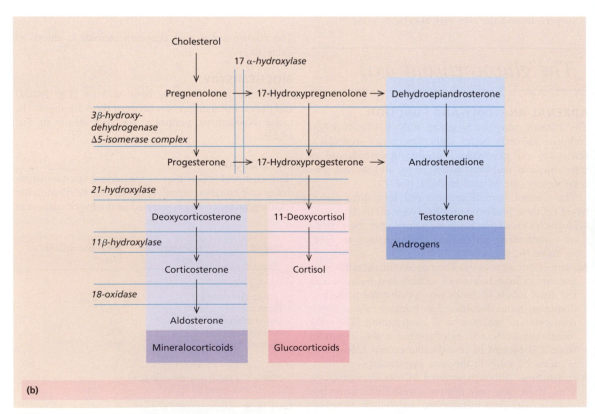

**(b)**

**Fig. 16.23** (b) The major steroid biosynthetic pathways.

## INVESTIGATION OF GLUCOCORTICOID ABNORMALITIES

### Basal levels

ACTH and cortisol are released episodically. The following precautions are therefore necessary when taking a blood sample:

- Sampling time should be accurately recorded.
- Stress should be minimized.
- Sampling should be delayed for 48 hours after admission if Cushing's syndrome is suspected.
- Appropriate reference ranges (for time and assay method) should be used.

Suppression and stimulation tests are used in instances of excess and deficient cortisol production respectively.

### Dexamethasone suppression tests

Administration of synthetic glucocorticoid to a normal subject produces prompt feedback suppression of CRF and ACTH levels and thus of endogenous cortisol secretion (prednisolone and dexamethasone are not measured by most cortisol assays). Three forms of the test, used in the diagnosis and differential diagnosis of Cushing's syndrome, are available (Table 16.31).

### ACTH stimulation tests

Synthetic ACTH (tetracosactrin, which consists of the first 24 amino acids of human ACTH) is given to stimulate adrenal cortisol production. Details are given in Table 16.31.

# Addison's disease—primary hypoadrenalism

## PATHOPHYSIOLOGY AND CAUSES

In this uncommon condition there is destruction of the entire adrenal cortex. Glucocorticoid, mineralocorticoid and sex steroid production are therefore *all* reduced. This differs from hypothalamic–pituitary disease, in which mineralocorticoid secretion remains largely intact, being predominantly stimulated by angiotensin II.

Adrenal sex steroid production is also largely independent of pituitary action. In Addison's disease reduced cortisol levels lead, through feedback, to increased CRF and ACTH production, the latter being responsible for the hyperpigmentation.

| |
|---|
| Autoimmune disease ($\approx$ 80%) |
| Tuberculosis ($\approx$20%) |
| Surgical removal |
| Haemorrhage/infarction |
|    Meningococcal septicaemia |
|    Venography |
| Infiltration |
|    Malignant destruction |
|    Amyloid |
| Drugs, e.g. rifampicin |
|    ketoconazole |
| AIDS |
| Schilder's disease (adrenal leucodystrophy) |

**Table 16.32** Causes of primary hypoadrenalism.

| Test | Protocol | Measure | Normal test result | Use |
|---|---|---|---|---|
| *Dexamethasone* | | | | |
| Overnight | Take 1–2 mg on going to bed on day 0 | Plasma cortisol at 0900 on day 1 | Plasma cortisol <100 nmol litre$^{-1}$ | Screening test only. Confirm with 'low-dose' test |
| 'Low-dose' 48 h | 0.5 mg 6-hourly $\times$ 8 doses from 0900 on day 0 | Plasma cortisol at 0900 on days 0 and +2 | Plasma cortisol <50 nmol litre$^{-1}$ at end of test | For diagnosis of Cushing's syndrome May not suppress in obesity and depression |
| 'High-dose' | 2 mg 6-hourly $\times$ 8 doses from 0900 on day 0 | Plasma cortisol at 0900 on days 0 and +2 (24 hour urinary steroids on days 0 and +2) | Plasma cortisol on day +2 <50% of that on day 0 | Differential diagnosis of Cushing's syndrome; pituitary-dependent disease suppresses in about 90% |
| *ACTH (Synacthen)* | | | | |
| Short | Tetracosactrin 0.25 mg i.m. at time 0 | Plasma cortisol at time 0, +30 and +60 min | Basal cortisol >170 nmol litre$^{-1}$ Cortisol at +30 min >580 nmol litre$^{-1}$. Rise >190 nmol litre$^{-1}$ | To exclude primary adrenal failure |
| Long | Depot tetracosactrin 1 mg i.m. at time 0 | Plasma cortisol at time 0, +1, +2, +3, +4, +5, +8 and +24 hours | Maximum >1000 nmol litre$^{-1}$. Rise must be >580 nmol litre$^{-1}$ | To demonstrate/exclude adrenal suppression |

**Table 16.31** Details of dexamethasone suppression and ACTH (Synacthen) tests.

| Symptoms | Signs |
|---|---|
| Weight loss<br>Anorexia<br>Malaise<br>Weakness<br>Fever<br>Depression<br>Impotence/amenorrhoea<br>Nausea/vomiting<br>Diarrhoea<br>Confusion<br>Syncope from postural<br>  hypotension<br>Abdominal pain<br>Constipation<br>Myalgia<br>Joint or back pain<br><br>Features of other<br>  autoimmune disease<br>  (e.g. vitiligo) are<br>  quite common. | **Buccal pigmentation**<br><br>**Postural hypotension**<br><br>**Pigmentation, especially of new scars**<br>General wasting<br><br>Loss of weight<br>Dehydration<br><br><br><br>Loss of body hair<br><br><br><br><br><br>(Vitiligo) |

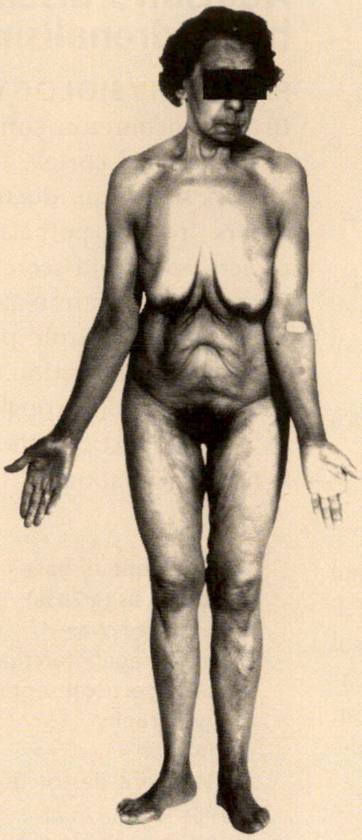

**Fig. 16.25** The signs of primary hypoadrenalism (Addison's disease). The bold type indicates signs of greater discriminant value.

Primary hypoadrenalism shows a marked female preponderance and is now most often caused by autoimmune disease (≈80%) rather than tuberculosis (≈20%). All other causes are rare (Table 16.32). Autoimmune adrenalitis results from the destruction of the adrenal cortex by organ-specific autoantibodies. There is an association with other autoimmune conditions, e.g. pernicious anaemia, hypoparathyroidism, thyroiditis, premature ovarian failure, type 1 diabetes mellitus.

### CLINICAL FEATURES
These are shown in Fig. 16.25. The symptomatology of Addison's disease is often vague—non-specific complaints of weakness, tiredness, weight loss and anorexia predominate.

Important features are:

PIGMENTATION (dull, slaty, grey-brown) in the mouth (opposite the molars), hand and all flexural regions is the predominant sign. It is particularly significant if it occurs in a recent scar. It is caused by the direct action of ACTH on melanocytes.

POSTURAL SYSTOLIC HYPOTENSION, due to hypovolaemia and sodium loss, is usually present even if supine blood pressure is normal.

### INVESTIGATION
Once Addison's disease is suspected, investigation is urgent. If the patient is seriously ill or very hypotensive, hydrocortisone 100 mg should be given intramuscularly, ideally *after* a blood sample is taken for later measurement of plasma cortisol, or an ACTH stimulation test can be performed immediately. Full investigation should be delayed until emergency treatment has improved the patient's condition.

Otherwise, tests are as follows:

SINGLE CORTISOL MEASUREMENTS are of virtually no value.

THE SHORT ACTH STIMULATION TEST should be performed (see Table 16.31). An absent or impaired cortisol response is seen, confirmed if necessary by a long ACTH stimulation test to exclude adrenal suppression by steroids.

A 0900 PLASMA ACTH LEVEL — a high level (>80 ng litre$^{-1}$) with low or low-normal cortisol confirms primary hypoadrenalism.

ELECTROLYTES AND UREA: these classically show hyponatraemia, hyperkalaemia and a high urea but can be normal.

BLOOD GLUCOSE may be low, with symptomatic hypoglycaemia.

ADRENAL ANTIBODIES are present in many cases of autoimmune adrenalitis.

CHEST AND ABDOMINAL X-RAYS may show evidence of tuberculosis and/or calcified adrenals.

SERUM ALDOSTERONE is reduced with high plasma renin activity.

HYPERCALCAEMIA AND ANAEMIA (after rehydration) are sometimes seen. They resolve on treatment.

### TREATMENT
Long-term treatment is with replacement glucocorticoid and mineralocorticoid; tuberculosis must be treated if

| Drug | Dose |
|------|------|
| *Glucocorticoid* | |
| Cortisol | 30 mg daily: 20 mg on waking, 10 mg at 1800 |
| *or* Prednisolone | 7.5 mg daily: 5 mg on waking, 2.5 mg at 1800 |
| *or* Dexamethasone | 0.75 mg daily: 0.5 mg on waking, 0.25 mg at 1800 |
| *Mineralocorticoid* | |
| Fludrocortisone | 0.05–0.4 mg daily |

**Table 16.33** Average replacement steroid dosages for adults with primary hypoadrenalism.

present or suspected. Replacement dosage details are shown in Table 16.33.

Adequacy of glucocorticoid dose is judged by:

- Clinical well-being and restoration of normal, but not excessive, weight
- Normal cortisol levels during the day while on replacement hydrocortisone (this cannot be used for synthetic steroids)

Fludrocortisone replacement is assessed by:

- Restoration of serum electrolytes to normal
- Blood pressure response to posture (it should not fall >10 mmHg systolic after 2 min standing)
- Suppression of plasma renin activity to normal

**Patient advice**

All patients requiring replacement steroids should:

CARRY A STEROID CARD.

WEAR A MEDIC-ALERT BRACELET; this gives details of their condition so that emergency replacement therapy can be given if found unconscious.

KEEP AN (UP-TO-DATE) AMPOULE OF HYDROCORTISONE at home in case oral therapy is impossible, and the general practitioner has to be called.

**Acute hypoadrenalism**

The major deficiencies are of salt, steroid and glucose.

ASSUMING NORMAL CARDIOVASCULAR FUNCTION, 1 litre of normal saline should be given over 30–60 min with 100 mg of intravenous hydrocortisone.

DEXTROSE should be infused if there is hypoglycaemia.

SUBSEQUENT SALINE REQUIREMENTS may be for several litres within 24 hours (assessing with central venous pressure line if necessary) plus hydrocortisone, 100 mg i.m. 6-hourly, until the patient is clinically stable.

ORAL REPLACEMENT MEDICATION is then started, initially hydrocortisone about 20 mg 8-hourly or equivalent, reducing to 20 mg + 10 mg or equivalent over a few days.

FLUDROCORTISONE is unnecessary acutely as the high cortisol doses provide sufficient mineralocorticoid activity—it should be introduced later.

# Secondary hypoadrenalism

This may arise from hypothalamic–pituitary disease or from long-term steroid therapy leading to hypothalamic–pituitary–adrenal suppression.

Most patients with the former have panhypopituitarism (see p. 780) and need $T_4$ replacement as well as cortisol; in this case hydrocortisone must be started *before* $T_4$.

The commonest cause of hypoadrenalism is long-term corticosteroid medication for non-endocrine disease. The hypothalamic–pituitary axis and the adrenal may both be suppressed and the patient may have vague symptoms of feeling unwell. The long ACTH stimulation test should demonstrate a delayed cortisol response. Weaning off steroids is often a long and difficult business.

# Cushing's syndromes

Cushing's syndrome is the term used to describe the clinical state of increased free circulating glucocorticoid. It occurs most often following the therapeutic administration of synthetic steroids (see below); all the spontaneous forms of the syndrome are rare.

## PATHOPHYSIOLOGY AND CAUSES

Causes of Cushing's syndrome are usually subdivided into two groups (Table 16.34):

1 Increased circulating ACTH from the pituitary (≈60% of cases), known as Cushing's disease, or an ectopic tumour (≈15%) with consequential glucocorticoid excess
2 A primary excess of endogenous or exogenous glucocorticoid hormone alone, with subsequent (physiological) suppression of ACTH

## CLINICAL FEATURES

The predominant clinical features of Cushing's syndrome are those of glucocorticoid excess and are illustrated in Fig. 16.26.

Particular points include:

PIGMENTATION only occurs with ACTH-dependent causes.

A CUSHINGOID APPEARANCE can be caused by excess alcohol consumption (pseudo-Cushing's syndrome)—the pathophysiology is poorly understood.

IMPAIRED GLUCOSE TOLERANCE or frank diabetes are common, especially in the ectopic ACTH syndrome.

*ACTH-dependent disease*
Pituitary-dependent (Cushing's disease)
Ectopic ACTH-producing tumours
ACTH administration

*Non-ACTH-dependent causes*
Adrenal adenomas
Adrenal carcinomas
Glucocorticoid administration

*Others*
Alcohol-induced pseudo-Cushing's syndrome

**Table 16.34** Causes of Cushing's syndrome.

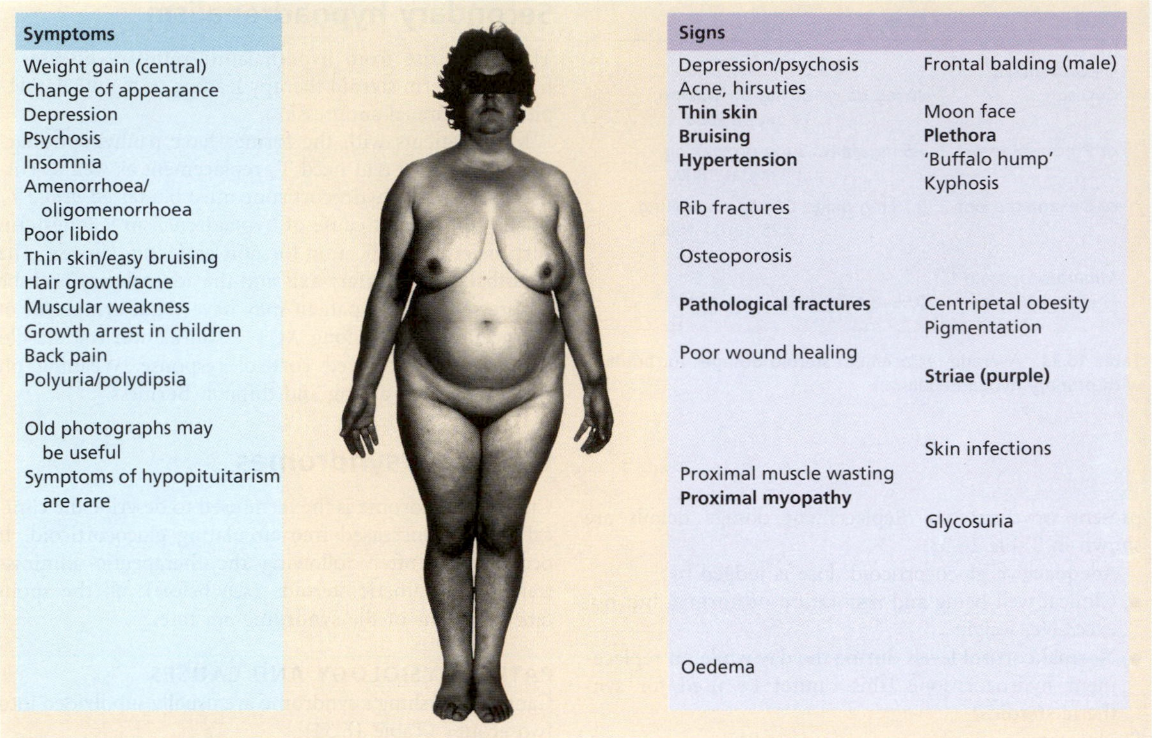

| Symptoms | Signs | |
|---|---|---|
| Weight gain (central) | Depression/psychosis | Frontal balding (male) |
| Change of appearance | Acne, hirsuties | |
| Depression | **Thin skin** | Moon face |
| Psychosis | **Bruising** | **Plethora** |
| Insomnia | **Hypertension** | 'Buffalo hump' |
| Amenorrhoea/ | | Kyphosis |
| oligomenorrhoea | Rib fractures | |
| Poor libido | | |
| Thin skin/easy bruising | Osteoporosis | |
| Hair growth/acne | | |
| Muscular weakness | **Pathological fractures** | Centripetal obesity |
| Growth arrest in children | | Pigmentation |
| Back pain | Poor wound healing | |
| Polyuria/polydipsia | | **Striae (purple)** |
| | | |
| Old photographs may | | Skin infections |
| be useful | Proximal muscle wasting | |
| Symptoms of hypopituitarism | **Proximal myopathy** | |
| are rare | | Glycosuria |
| | | |
| | Oedema | |

**Fig. 16.26** The signs of Cushing's syndrome. The bold type indicates signs of most value in discriminating Cushing's syndrome from simple obesity and hirsuties.

HYPOKALAEMIA due to the mineralocorticoid activity of cortisol is common with ectopic ACTH secretion.

## DIAGNOSIS

There are two phases to the investigation:
1 Confirmation of the presence or absence of Cushing's syndrome
2 Differential diagnosis of its cause

### Confirmation

Confirmation rests on demonstrating inappropriate cortisol secretion, not suppressed by exogenous glucocorticoids: difficulties occur with obesity and depression where cortisol dynamics are often abnormal. Random cortisol measurements are of no value.

Investigations to confirm the diagnosis include:

24-HOUR URINARY FREE CORTISOL MEASUREMENTS. Repeatedly normal values (corrected for body mass) render the diagnosis most unlikely.

48-HOUR LOW-DOSE DEXAMETHASONE TEST (see Table 16.31). Patients with Cushing's syndrome fail to suppress plasma or urinary cortisol levels. The overnight dexamethasone test is unreliable but has occasional value in excluding the diagnosis.

CIRCADIAN RHYTHM. After 48 hours in hospital, cortisol samples are taken at 0900 and 2400 hours (without warning the patient). Normal subjects show a pronounced circadian variation (see Fig. 16.3); those with Cushing's syndrome have high evening cortisol levels, though the 0900 value may be normal.

INSULIN TOLERANCE TEST. This is useful in depression or obesity, when abnormal circadian and suppression responses are seen. The normal rise of cortisol with hypoglycaemia does not occur in patients with Cushing's syndrome.

### Differential diagnosis of the cause

This can be extremely difficult. The classical ectopic ACTH syndrome is distinguished by a short history, pigmentation and weight loss, unprovoked hypokalaemia, clinical or chemical diabetes and plasma ACTH levels above 200 ng litre$^{-1}$. Severe hirsuties/virilization suggests an adrenal tumour.

Biochemical and radiological procedures for diagnosis include:

ADRENAL CT SCAN. Adrenal adenomas and carcinomas causing Cushing's syndrome are relatively large and always detectable by CT scan. Carcinomas are distinguished by large size, irregular outline and signs of infiltration or metastases.

PITUITARY CT OR MRI. Of less value than the adrenal scan; only a minority of tumours of significant size are detected with confidence by CT, and indeed over 80% of skull X-rays are normal. MRI may be superior.

PLASMA POTASSIUM LEVELS. All diuretics must be stopped. Hypokalaemia is common with ectopic ACTH secretion.

HIGH-DOSE DEXAMETHASONE TEST (see Table 16.31).

Failure of urinary or plasma cortisol suppression suggests an ectopic source of ACTH or an adrenal tumour. The metyrapone test has been shown to be of little value.

PLASMA ACTH levels. Low or undetectable ACTH levels ($<10$ ng litre$^{-1}$) on two or more occasions are a reliable indicator of non-ACTH-dependent disease.

CRF TEST. Exaggerated ACTH responses to exogenous CRF suggest pituitary-dependent Cushing's disease.

CHEST X-RAY is mandatory to demonstrate a carcinoma of the bronchus or a bronchial carcinoid. Lesions may be very small; if ectopic ACTH is suspected, whole-lung and mediastinal CT scanning should be performed.

Further investigations may involve selective catheterization of the inferior petrosal sinus to measure ACTH for pituitary lesions, or blood samples taken throughout the body in a search for ectopic sources. Bronchoscopy, cytology and regional arteriograms are occasionally necessary.

## TREATMENT

Untreated Cushing's syndrome has a very bad prognosis, with death from hypertension, myocardial infarction, infection and heart failure. Whatever the underlying cause, cortisol hypersecretion should be controlled prior to surgery or radiotherapy. Considerable morbidity and mortality is otherwise associated with operating on unprepared patients. The usual drug is metyrapone, an 11-hydroxylase blocker, which is given in doses of 750 mg to 4 g daily in three to four divided doses. Plasma cortisol should be monitored, aiming to reduce the mean level during the day to 300–400 nmol litre$^{-1}$, equivalent to normal production rates. Aminoglutethimide is sometimes used, but trilostane has been abandoned.

Choice of treatment depends upon the cause.

### Cushing's disease (pituitary-dependent hyperadrenalism)

Treatment options are surgery, radiotherapy and medical control; the choice remains controversial.

Trans-sphenoidal removal of the tumour, by an experienced surgeon, is the treatment of choice. Selective surgery nearly always leaves the patient ACTH deficient immediately postoperatively, even after CRF, and this is considered a good prognostic sign. Transfrontal surgery is very rarely necessary because most tumours are small, though they are occasionally locally invasive.

Yttrium implantation of radioactive needles in the fossa produces good results in some centres but it is not generally available.

External irradiation alone is very slow, only effective in 20–50% and of little value except in those unfit for, or unwilling to, have surgery. Children, however, respond much better to radiotherapy, 80% being cured.

Medical therapy to reduce ACTH (e.g. bromocriptine, cyproheptadine) is rarely effective and bilateral adrenalectomy is now very little used, though remains an effective last resort.

### Other causes

Adrenal adenomas should be resected after achievement of clinical remission with metyrapone. Contralateral adrenal suppression may last for years.

Carcinomas are highly aggressive and the prognosis is poor. In general, if there are no widespread metastases, tumour bulk should be reduced surgically and the adrenolytic drug op'DDD given; new preparations have reduced the side-effects of nausea/vomiting and ataxia. Some would also give radiotherapy to the tumour bed after surgery.

Ectopic tumour sources should be removed if possible. Otherwise chemotherapy/radiotherapy should be used, depending on the tumour. Control of the Cushing's syndrome with metyrapone is beneficial for symptoms.

If the source is not clear, cortisol hypersecretion should be controlled with medical therapy until a diagnosis can be made.

### Nelson's syndrome

This rare syndrome is of increased pigmentation associated with an enlarging pituitary tumour occurring after bilateral adrenalectomy. The tumour may be locally invasive but most physicians believe it can be prevented by pituitary radiotherapy soon after adrenalectomy, though the latter is now rarely used.

### Incidental adrenal tumours ('Incidentalomas')

With the advent of abdominal CT scanning, unsuspected adrenal masses have been discovered in $\approx$1% of scans. These obviously include the described adrenal tumours but cysts, myelolipomas and metastases are also seen. If found functional tests to exclude secretory activity should be performed; if none is found then most authorities recommend removal of large ($>4$–5 cm) and functional tumours but observation of smaller lesions.

# Congenital adrenal hyperplasia (CAH)

## PATHOPHYSIOLOGY

This condition, comprising six major types, results from an autosomal recessive deficiency of an enzyme in the cortisol synthetic pathways, most commonly 21-hydroxylase which occurs in about 1 in 15 000 births. The 21-hydroxylase deficiency has been shown to be due to defects on chromosome 6 near the HLA-region affecting a cytochrome P450 enzyme (P450$_{C21}$).

As a result, cortisol secretion is reduced and feedback leads to increased ACTH secretion to maintain adequate cortisol—this in turn leads to diversion of the steroid precursors into the androgenic steroid pathways (Fig. 16.27). Thus, 17-hydroxyprogesterone, androstenedione and testosterone levels are increased, leading to virilization. Rarely, aldosterone synthesis is impaired with resultant salt wasting.

The other forms affect 11$\beta$-hydroxylase, 17$\alpha$-hydroxylase, 3$\beta$-hydroxysteroid dehydrogenase (see Fig. 16.23b) and a cholesterol side chain cleavage enzyme.

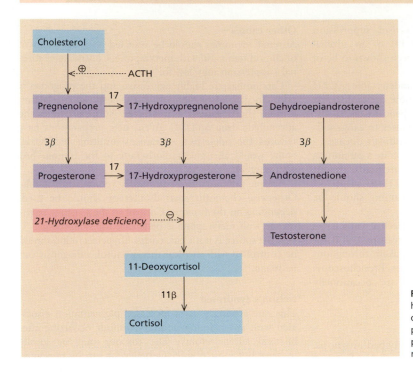

**Fig. 16.27**  Effects of congenital adrenal hyperplasia (21-hydroxylase deficiency) on steroid biosynthesis. Precursors and products present in excess appear in purple boxes. Those present in normal or reduced quantity appear in blue boxes.

## CLINICAL FEATURES

If severe, this presents at birth with sexual ambiguity or adrenal failure. In the female, clitoral hypertrophy, urogenital abnormalities and labioscrotal fusion are common, but the syndrome may be unrecognized in the male. Some cases include salt-losing states. Precocious puberty with hirsuties is a later presentation, while some milder cases only present in adult life, usually accompanied by primary amenorrhoea. Hirsutism developing before menarche is suggestive of CAH.

## INVESTIGATION

Expert advice is essential in the confirmation and differential diagnosis of $P450_{C21}$ deficiency.

- 17-Hydroxyprogesterone levels are increased (see Fig. 16.27).
- Urinary pregnanetriol excretion is increased.
- Basal ACTH levels are raised.

## TREATMENT

Replacement of glucocorticoid activity and mineralocorticoid activity if deficient is as for primary hypoadrenalism (see above). Correct dosage is often difficult to establish in the child but should ensure normal 17-hydroxyprogesterone and ACTH levels while allowing normal growth; excessive replacement leads to stunting of growth.

## Uses and problems of therapeutic steroid therapy

Apart from their use as therapeutic replacement for endocrine deficiency states, synthetic glucocorticoids are widely used for many non-endocrine conditions (Information box 16.8).

Short-term use (e.g. for acute asthma) carries little risk of significant side-effects except for the simultaneous suppression of immune responses. The danger lies in their continuance, often through medical oversight or patient default.

Long-term therapy with synthetic or natural steroids will, in most respects, mimic endogenous Cushing's syndrome. Exceptions are the relative absence of hirsuties, acne, hypertension and severe sodium retention, as the synthetic steroids have low androgenic and mineralocorticoid activity.

Excessive doses of steroids may also be absorbed from skin when strong dermatological preparations are used but inhaled steroids very rarely cause Cushing's syndrome, although they may cause adrenal suppression.

The major hazards are detailed in Information box 16.9; in the long term many are of such severity that the clinical need for high-dose steroids should be continually and critically assessed.

### Supervision of steroid therapy

All patients receiving steroids should carry a steroid card and know that:

LONG-TERM STEROID THERAPY MUST NEVER BE STOPPED SUDDENLY. Doses should be reduced very gradually, with most being given in the morning at the time of withdrawal—this minimizes adrenal suppression. Many authorities believe that 'alternate day therapy' produces less suppression.

DOSES NEED TO BE INCREASED in times of serious intercurrent illness (defined as presence of a fever),

**Respiratory disease**
Asthma
Chronic bronchitis and emphysema
Sarcoidosis
Hay fever (usually topical)

**Cardiac disease**
Postmyocardial infarction syndrome

**Renal disease**
Some nephrotic syndromes
Some glomerular nephritides

**Gastrointestinal disease**
Ulcerative colitis
Crohn's disease
Chronic active hepatitis

**Obstetrics**
Prevention/treatment of ARDS (see p. 733)

**Rheumatological disease**
Systemic lupus erythematosus
Polymyalgia rheumatica
Temporal arteritis
Vasculitides

**Neurological disease**
Cerebral oedema

**Skin disease**
Topical steroids
e.g. pemphigus, eczema

**Tumours**
Hodgkin's lymphoma
Other lymphomas

**Transplantation**
Immunosuppression

**Information box 16.8**   Some therapeutic uses of glucocorticoids.

**Physiological**
Adrenal and/or pituitary suppression

**Pathological**
*Cardiovascular*
Increased blood pressure

*Gastrointestinal*
Peptic ulceration exacerbation (possibly)
Pancreatitis

*Renal*
Polyuria
Nocturia

*Central nervous*
Depression
Euphoria
Psychosis
Insomnia

*Endocrine*
Weight gain
Glycosuria/hyperglycaemia/diabetes
Impaired growth
Amenorrhoea

*Bone and muscle*
Osteoporosis
Proximal myopathy and wasting
Aseptic necrosis of the hip
Pathological fractures

*Skin*
Thinning
Easy bruising

*Eyes*
Cataracts

*Increased susceptibility to infection*
(signs and fever are frequently masked)
Septicaemia
Tuberculosis
Skin, e.g. fungi

**Information box 16.9**   Adverse effects of corticosteroid therapy.

| Procedure | Premedication | Intraoperative and postoperative | Resumption of normal maintenance |
|---|---|---|---|
| Simple procedures (e.g. gastroscopy, simple dental extractions) | Hydrocortisone 100 mg i.m. | — | Immediately if no complications |
| Minor surgery (e.g. varicose veins, hernias) | Hydrocortisone 100 mg i.m. | Hydrocortisone 20 mg oral 6-hourly or 50 mg i.m. every 6 hours for 24 hours if not eating | After 24 hours if no complications |
| Major surgery (e.g. hip replacement, vascular surgery) | Hydrocortisone 100 mg i.m. | Hydrocortisone 50–100 mg i.m. every 6 hours for 72 hours | After 72 hours if normal progress and no complications perhaps double normal dose for next 2–3 days |
| Gastrointestinal tract surgery or major thoracic surgery (not eating or ventilated) | Hydrocortisone 100 mg i.m. | Hydrocortisone 100 mg i.m. every 6 hours for 72 hours or longer if still unwell | When patient eating normally again; until then higher doses (up to 50 mg 6-hourly) may be needed |

**Table 16.35**   Steroid cover for operative procedures.

accident and stress. Double doses should be taken during these times.

OTHER PHYSICIANS, ANAESTHETISTS AND DENTISTS *must* be told about steroid therapy.

**Steroids and surgery**

Any patient receiving steroids or who has recently received them and may still be suppressed requires careful control of steroid medication around the time of surgery. Details are shown in Table 16.35.

# The thirst axis

Thirst and water regulation is largely controlled by ADH (vasopressin), which is synthesized in the hypothalamus, and then migrates in neurosecretory granules along axonal pathways to the posterior pituitary. Pituitary damage alone *without hypothalamic involvement* does not therefore lead to ADH deficiency as the hormone can still 'leak' from the damaged end of the intact axon.

Changes in plasma osmolality are sensed by osmoreceptors in the anterior hypothalamus. Vasopressin secretion is suppressed at levels below 280 mosmol kg$^{-1}$, thus allowing maximal water diuresis. Above this level, plasma vasopressin increases in direct proportion to plasma osmolality. At the upper limit of normal (295 mosmol kg$^{-1}$) maximum antidiuresis is achieved and thirst is experienced at about 298 mosmol kg$^{-1}$.

Other factors affecting vasopressin release are shown in Table 16.36.

At normal concentrations the kidney is the predominant site of action. Via a cyclic AMP mechanism it allows the collecting tubule to become permeable to water, thus permitting reabsorption of hypotonic luminal fluid. At high concentrations vasopressin also causes vasoconstriction.

Disorders of vasopressin secretion or activity include:

- Deficiency as a result of hypothalamic disease (diabetes insipidus)
- Inappropriate excess of the hormone
- 'Nephrogenic' diabetes insipidus—a condition in which the renal tubules are insensitive to vasopressin, an example of a receptor abnormality

While all these are uncommon, they need to be distinguished from the occasional patient with 'hysterical water drinking' and those whose renal tubular function has been impaired by electrolyte abnormalities, such as hypokalaemia or hypercalcaemia.

## Diabetes insipidus (DI)

### CLINICAL FEATURES

Deficiency of vasopressin leads to polyuria, nocturia and compensatory polydipsia. Daily urine output may reach as much as 10–15 litres, leading to dehydration that may be very severe if the thirst mechanisms are impaired or the patient is denied fluid.

Causes of DI are listed in Table 16.37. The commonest is hypothalamic–pituitary surgery, following which tran-

| *Increased by:* |
| Increased osmolality |
| Hypovolaemia |
| Hypotension |
| Nausea |
| Hypothyroidism |
| Angiotensin II |
| Adrenaline |
| Cortisol |
| Nicotine |
| Antidepressants |
| |
| *Decreased by:* |
| Decreased osmolality |
| Hypervolaemia |
| Hypertension |
| Ethanol |
| $\alpha$-Adrenergic stimulation |

**Table 16.36**  Factors affecting vasopressin release.

| *Cranial diabetes insipidus* |
| Congenital |
| Idiopathic |
| Tumours |
|     Craniopharyngioma |
|     Pituitary with suprasellar extension |
|     Hypothalamic tumour, e.g. glioma |
|     Metastases, especially breast |
|     Lymphoma/leukaemia |
| Infections |
|     Tuberculosis |
|     Meningitis |
|     Cerebral abscess |
| Infiltrations |
|     Sarcoidosis |
|     Histiocytosis X |
| Post surgical |
|     Transfrontal |
|     Trans-sphenoidal |
| Trauma |
|     Base of skull fracture |
| Post radiotherapy (to head) |
| Vascular |
|     Haemorrhage/thrombosis |
|     Sheehan's syndrome |
| |
| *Nephrogenic diabetes insipidus* |
| Idiopathic |
| Renal tubular acidosis |
| Hypokalaemia |
| Hypercalcaemia |
| Drugs, e.g. |
|     Lithium |
|     Demethylchlortetracycline (demeclocycline) |
|     Glibenclamide |

**Table 16.37**  Causes of diabetes insipidus.

sient DI is common, frequently remitting after a few days or weeks. Primary overdrinking (polydipsia) is a common differential diagnosis.

DI may be masked by simultaneous cortisol deficiency—cortisol replacement allows a water diuresis and DI then becomes apparent.

DIDMOAD syndrome (Wolfram syndrome) is a rare recessive disorder comprising diabetes insipidus, diabetes mellitus, optic atrophy and deafness.

### BIOCHEMISTRY

- High or high-normal plasma osmolality with low urine osmolality (in primary polydipsia plasma osmolality tends to be low)
- Resultant high or high-normal plasma sodium
- Failure of urinary concentration with fluid deprivation
- Restoration of urinary concentration with vasopressin or an analogue

The latter two points may be studied with a formal water-deprivation test (see Appendix). In normal subjects, plasma osmolality remains normal while urine osmolality rises above 700 mosmol kg$^{-1}$. In DI, plasma osmolality rises while the urine remains dilute, only concentrating after exogenous vasopressin is given (cranial DI) or not concentrating after vasopressin if renal DI is present. This test can give equivocal results and measurement of vasopressin during the test is helpful.

### TREATMENT

Synthetic vasopressin (desmopressin, DDAVP) is the treatment of choice. It is given intranasally as a spray 10–20 $\mu$g once to three times daily or intramuscularly 2–4 $\mu$g daily. Response is variable and must be monitored carefully with fluid input/output charts and plasma osmolality measurements. An oral preparation, 0.1–0.2 mg daily, is now available with shorter action than the spray.

Alternative agents in mild DI, probably working by sensitizing the tubules to endogenous vasopressin, include thiazide diuretics, carbamazepine 200–400 mg daily or chlorpropamide (200–350 mg daily). These are rarely used, especially with the risk of hypoglycaemia from chlorpropamide.

## Nephrogenic diabetes insipidus

In this condition, renal tubules are resistant to normal or high levels of plasma vasopressin. It may be inherited as a sex-linked recessive or can be acquired as a result of renal disease, drug ingestion, hypercalcaemia or hypokalaemia. Wherever possible the cause should be reversed.

## Other causes of polyuria and polydipsia

Diabetes mellitus, hypokalaemia and hypercalcaemia are diagnoses to be considered. In the case of diabetes mellitus the cause is an osmotic diuresis secondary to glycosuria and this leads to dehydration and an increased perception of thirst due to hypertonicity of the extracellular fluid.

Primary or hysterical polydipsia is a relatively common cause of thirst and polyuria. It is a psychiatric disturbance characterized by the excessive intake of water. Plasma sodium and osmolality fall as a result and the urine produced is appropriately dilute. Vasopressin levels become virtually undetectable. Prolonged primary polydipsia may lead to the phenomenon of 'renal medullary washout', with a fall in the concentrating ability of the kidney.

Characteristically the diagnosis is made by a water-deprivation test. A low plasma osmolality is usual at the start of the test, and since vasopressin secretion and action can be stimulated, the patient's urine becomes concentrated (albeit 'maximum' concentrating ability may be impaired); the initially low urine osmolality gradually increases with the duration of the water deprivation.

## Syndrome of inappropriate antidiuretic hormone (SIADH)

### CLINICAL FEATURES

The presentation is usually vague, with confusion, nausea, irritability and, later, fits and coma. There is no oedema. Mild symptoms usually occur with plasma sodium levels below 125 mmol litre$^{-1}$ and serious manifestations are likely below 115 mmol litre$^{-1}$.

The syndrome must be distinguished from those causing similar dilutional hyponatraemia from excess infusion of dextrose/water solutions or diuretic administration (thiazides or amiloride, see p. 503).

### DIAGNOSIS

The usual features are:

- Dilutional hyponatraemia due to excessive water retention
- Low plasma osmolality with higher 'inappropriate' urine osmolality
- Continued urinary sodium excretion >30 mmol litre$^{-1}$
- Absence of hypokalaemia (or hypotension)
- Normal renal and adrenal and thyroid function

The causes are listed in Table 16.38.

### TREATMENT

The underlying cause should be corrected where possible. For symptomatic relief:

FLUID INTAKE should be restricted to 500–1000 ml daily.

PLASMA OSMOLALITY AND SODIUM AND BODY WEIGHT should be measured frequently.

IF WATER RESTRICTION IS POORLY TOLERATED OR INEFFECTIVE, demethylchlortetracycline (600–1200 mg daily) may be given; this inhibits the action of vasopressin on the kidney causing a reversible form of nephrogenic diabetes insipidus. It may, however, cause photosensitive rashes.

WHEN THE SYNDROME IS VERY SEVERE, hypertonic saline (300 mmol litre$^{-1}$ slowly i.v.) is rarely given and frusemide may be used. These should be used with extreme caution by specialists.

*Tumours*
Small-cell carcinoma of lung
Prostate
Thymus
Pancreas
Lymphomas

*Pulmonary lesions*
Pneumonia
Tuberculosis
Lung abscess

*CNS causes*
Meningitis
Tumours
Head injury
Subdural
Cerebral abscess
SLE vasculitis

*Metabolic causes*
Alcohol withdrawal
Porphyria

*Drugs*
Chlorpropamide
Carbamazepine
Cyclophosphamide
Vincristine

---

SLE, systemic lupus erythematosus.

**Table 16.38**   Causes of the syndrome of inappropriate ADH secretion (SIADH).

*Excessive renin, and thus angiotension II, production*
Renal artery stenosis
Other local renal disease
Renin-secreting tumours

*Excessive production of catecholamines*
Phaeochromocytoma

*Excessive GH production*
Acromegaly

*Excessive aldosterone production*
Adrenal adenoma (Conn's syndrome)
Idiopathic adrenal hyperplasia
Dexamethasone-suppressible hyperaldosteronism

*Excessive production of other mineralocorticoids*
Cushing's syndrome (massive excess of cortisol, a weak mineralocorticoid)
Congenital adrenal hyperplasia (in some cases)
Tumours producing other mineralocorticoids, e.g. corticosterone

*Exogenous 'mineralocorticoids'*
Liquorice ingestion
Abuse of mineralocorticoid preparations

**Table 16.39**   Endocrine causes of hypertension.

- Those with unusual symptoms (e.g. sweating attacks or weakness)

## The renin–angiotensin–aldosterone axis

### Biochemistry and actions
The renin–angiotensin–aldosterone system is illustrated in Fig. 16.28.

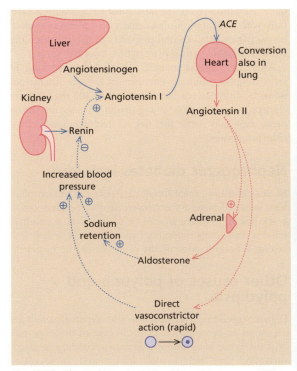

**Fig. 16.28**   The renin–angiotensin–aldosterone system. ACE, angiotensin converting enzyme.

# Endocrinology of blood pressure control

The control of blood pressure (BP) is complex involving neural, cardiac, hormonal and many other mechanisms.

BP is dependent upon cardiac output and peripheral resistance. Although cardiac output can be increased in endocrine disease (e.g. thyrotoxicosis), the main role of hormonal mechanisms is control of peripheral resistance and of circulating blood volume. The oral contraceptive pill is a common endocrine cause of hypertension.

## When to investigate for secondary hypertension

Endocrine causes account for less than 5% of all hypertension (Table 16.39). It is impracticable and unnecessary to screen all hypertensive patients for secondary causes. The highest chances of detecting such causes are in:
- Subjects under 35 years old, especially those without a family history of hypertension
- Those with accelerated (malignant) hypertension
- Those with indications of renal disease (proteinuria, unequal renal sizes)
- Those with hypokalaemia before diuretic therapy
- Those resistant to conventional antihypertensive therapy

Angiotensinogen, an $\alpha_2$-globulin of hepatic origin, circulates in plasma. The enzyme, renin, is secreted by the kidney in response to decreased renal perfusion pressure or flow; it cleaves the decapeptide angiotensin I from angiotensinogen. Angiotensin I is inactive but is further cleaved by converting enzyme (present in lung and vascular endothelium) into the active peptide, angiotensin II, which has two major actions:

1 It causes powerful vasoconstriction (within seconds).
2 It stimulates the adrenal zona glomerulosa to increase aldosterone production.

Aldosterone causes sodium retention and urinary potassium loss (hours to days).

The vasoconstrictor action of angiotensin II is short term, while the sodium retention induced by aldosterone increases total body sodium and BP in the longer term.

As BP increases and sodium is retained, the stimuli to renin secretion are reduced. Dietary sodium excess will tend to suppress renin secretion, whereas sodium deprivation or urinary sodium loss will increase it.

## Atrial natriuretic factors/peptides (ANP)

These peptides are secreted from atrial granules. They produce marked effects on the kidney, increasing sodium and water excretion and glomerular filtration rate and lowering BP, plasma renin activity and plasma aldosterone.

They appear to play a significant role in cardiovascular and fluid homeostasis but there is no evidence of primary defects in their secretion causing disease.

Analogues that break down ANP as well as inhibiting the aminopeptidases are under development and might prove of value in producing a sodium diuresis.

## RENIN (AND ANGIOTENSIN) DEPENDENT HYPERTENSION

Many forms of unilateral and bilateral renal diseases are associated with hypertension. The classic example is renal artery stenosis: the major hypertensive effects of this and other situations such as renin-secreting tumours are directly or indirectly due to angiotensin II.

Renin inhibitors have been produced and are under clinical trial. They appear to produce much the same effects as angiotensin-converting enzyme inhibitors and hold promise as antihypertensive agents, though none are yet available for clinical use.

## Renal artery stenosis

This is discussed on p. 463.

## DISORDERS OF ALDOSTERONE SECRETION

## Primary hyperaldosteronism

### PATHOPHYSIOLOGY
This rare condition (<1% of all hypertension) is caused by excess aldosterone production leading to sodium retention, potassium loss and the combination of hypokalaemia and hypertension.

### CAUSES (Table 16.39)
Adrenal adenomas (Conn's syndrome) account for 60% of cases; 30% are due to bilateral adrenal hyperplasia, which may be secondary to excess of a pituitary aldosterone-stimulating factor that is as yet unidentified.

### CLINICAL FEATURES
The usual presentation is with hypertension and hypokalaemia ($<3.5$ mmol litre$^{-1}$), although 20% of patients have initial potassium levels of 3.5–4.2 mmol litre$^{-1}$. The few symptoms are non-specific; muscle weakness, nocturia and tetany are rarely seen. The hypertension may be severe and associated with renal and retinal damage.

Adenomas, often very small, are commoner in young females, while bilateral hyperplasia rarely occurs before age 40 years and is commoner in males.

### INVESTIGATION
The characteristic features are:
HYPOKALAEMIA. A high-salt diet should be given for several days before testing and diuretics must be stopped 3 weeks before investigation; plasma samples must be separated quickly. Bethanidine or prazosin may be used for temporary control of blood pressure as they do not alter renin or aldosterone secretion.
URINARY POTASSIUM LOSS. Levels over 30 mmol daily during hypokalaemia are inappropriate.
ELEVATED PLASMA ALDOSTERONE LEVELS that are not suppressed with saline infusion (300 mmol over 4 hours) or fludrocortisone administration.
SUPPRESSED PLASMA RENIN ACTIVITY—$\beta$-blockers and other drugs may interfere with renin activity.
Once a diagnosis of aldosteronism is established, differentiation of adenoma from hyperplasia involves adrenal CT or MRI (not infallible as tumours may be very small), complex biochemical testing, adrenal scintillation scanning (now rarely needed) and venous catheterization.

### TREATMENT
An adenoma should be surgically removed; BP falls in 70% of patients. Those with hyperplasia should be treated with the aldosterone antagonist spironolactone (100–400 mg daily); side-effects include nausea, rashes and gynaecomastia. Amiloride (10–40 mg daily) is a less effective alternative, used especially as spironolactone in long term use has been linked with tumour development in animals. Calcium channel blockers are also effective.

## Secondary hyperaldosteronism

This situation arises when there is excess renin (and hence angiotensin II) stimulation of the zona glomerulosa. Common causes are accelerated hypertension and renal artery stenosis, when the patient will be hypertensive. Causes associated with normotension include congestive cardiac failure and cirrhosis, where excess aldosterone production contributes to sodium retention.

Spironolactone is of value in both situations. Angiotensin-converting enzyme (ACE) inhibitors, e.g. captopril, enalapril or lisinopril, are effective in heart failure, both symptomatically and in increasing life expectancy (see p. 574).

## Hypoaldosteronism

Except as part of primary hypoadrenalism (Addison's disease, see p. 813), this is very uncommon. Causes include hyporeninaemic hypoaldosteronism, aldosterone biosynthetic defects and drugs (e.g. ACE inhibitors, heparin).

## THE ADRENAL MEDULLA

The major catecholamines, noradrenaline and adrenaline, are produced in the adrenal medulla (Fig. 16.29) although most noradrenaline is derived from sympathetic neuronal release. While noradrenaline and adrenaline undoubtedly produce hypertension when infused, they probably play little part in BP regulation in normal humans.

## Phaeochromocytoma

Phaeochromocytomas, tumours of the sympathetic nervous system, are very rare (less than 1 in 1000 cases of hypertension); 90% arise in the adrenal, while 10% occur elsewhere in the sympathetic chain; 25% are multiple and 10% are malignant, though this cannot be determined on simple histological examination. Some are associated with MEN syndromes (see below). Most tumours release both noradrenaline and adrenaline but large tumours produce almost entirely noradrenaline.

### CLINICAL FEATURES

The clinical features are those of catecholamine excess and are frequently, but not necessarily, intermittent (Table 16.40). The diagnosis should particularly be considered when cardiovascular instability has been demonstrated and in severe hypertension in pregnancy.

### DIAGNOSIS

The possibility needs to be considered quite frequently in patients with hypertension. Specific tests are:

MEASUREMENT OF URINARY METABOLITES (preferably metanephrines rather than vanillylmandelic acid (VMA) — Fig. 16.29) is a useful screening test; normal levels on three 24-hour collections of metanephrines virtually exclude the diagnosis. Many drugs and dietary vanilla interfere with these tests.

IF HIGH METANEPHRINES OR VMAs ARE FOUND, plasma catecholamines are estimated.

URINARY CATECHOLAMINES are measured in some centres.

CT SCANS, initially of the abdomen, are helpful to localize the tumours which are often large.

MRI usually shows the lesion clearly.

SCANNING WITH [$^{131}$I]METAIODOBENZYLGUANIDINE produces specific uptake in sites of sympathetic activity with about 90% success. It is particularly useful in extra-adrenal tumours.

### TREATMENT

Tumours should be removed if this is possible. Medical preoperative and perioperative treatment is vital and includes complete α- and β-blockade with phenoxybenzamine (20–80 mg daily initially in divided doses), then propranolol (120–240 mg daily), plus transfusion of whole blood to re-expand the contracted plasma volume. The α-blockade *must* precede the β-blockade. Labetolol is not recommended. Surgery in the unprepared patient is fraught with dangers of both hypertension and hypotension; expert anaesthetic help is vital and sodium nitroprusside should be available in case sudden severe hypertension develops.

When operation is not possible, combined α- and β-blockade can be used long term.

Patients should be kept under clinical and biochemical review after tumour resection as about 10% recur or develop a further tumour.

## Other endocrine disorders

## DISEASES OF MANY GLANDS

### Multiple gland failure

This is caused by autoimmune disease as detailed in Table 16.4 (see p. 775). Commonest are the associations of primary hypothyroidism and type 1 diabetes, and either of these with Addison's disease or pernicious anaemia.

### Multiple endocrine neoplasia

This is the name given to the simultaneous or metachronous recurrence of tumours involving a number of endocrine glands (Table 16.41). They are inherited in an autosomal dominant manner and are thought to arise from the expression of a recessive oncogenic mutation, which has now been isolated.

Affected persons may pass on the mutation to their offspring in the germ cell, but for the disease to become evident a somatic mutation must also occur, e.g. deletion or loss of a normal homologous chromosome. The defect in MEN 1 is on the long arm of chromosome 11 near an area containing a number of oncogenes that encode for proteins with fibroblastic growth factor activity. The gene for MEN 2a is on chromosome 10 close to the retinol binding gene.

Screening unaffected members of a family shows that a significant number of affected individuals are unrecognized, especially with hypercalcaemia.

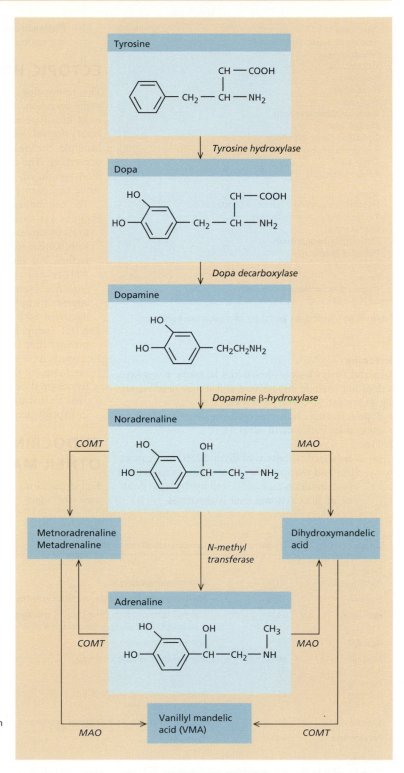

**Fig. 16.29** The synthesis and metabolism of catecholamines. COMT, catechol-O-methyl transferase; MAI, monoamine oxidase.

## MANAGEMENT

Treatment is surgical.

TYPE 1. All four parathyroid glands are removed (as all may be involved) followed by vitamin D (1,25-dihydrocalciferol) replacement therapy. Pancreatic tumours are often multiple and recurrence after partial pancreatectomy is invariable. Other tumours are treated surgically if necessary.

TYPE 2. Tumours may also be recurrent or bilateral and a careful follow-up is necessary.

*Symptoms*
Anxiety or panic attacks
Palpitations
Tremor
Sweating
Headache
Flushing
Nausea and/or vomiting
Weight loss
Constipation or diarrhoea
Raynaud's phenomenon
Chest pain
Polyuria/nocturia

*Signs*
Hypertension—intermittent or constant
Tachycardia plus arrhythmias
Bradycardia
Orthostatic hypotension
Pallor or flushing
Glycosuria
Fever
(Signs of hypertensive damage)

**Table 16.40**  Symptoms and signs of phaeochromocytoma.

### Screening

A careful family history should first be taken. If negative, it does not exclude involvement and it may need repeating at regular (1–5 year) intervals.

1  *Type 1.* Fasting calcium estimation (if elevated, look for other manifestations of MEN 1).
2  *Type 2*
   (a)  Medullary carcinoma of thyroid (MCT). Pentagastrin and calcium infusion test with measurement of calcitonin to pick up 'C' cell hyperplasia: doubling of the calcitonin level is abnormal.

(b)  Phaeochromocytoma. VMA and metanephrine estimations.

## ECTOPIC HORMONE SECRETION

This terminology refers to hormone synthesis, and normally secretion, from a neoplastic non-endocrine cell, most usually seen in tumours that have some degree of embryological resemblance to specialist endocrine cells. Multiple theories have been advanced to explain the occurrence. The clinical effects may be those of the hormone produced, with or without manifestations of systemic malignancy.

The commonest situations seen are:

HYPERCALCAEMIA OF MALIGNANT DISEASE, often from squamous cell tumours of lung and breast, often with bone metastases. It is mediated by many different factors, but very rarely by PTH itself (see p. 431); a PTH-related protein (PTHrP) with considerable sequence homology has recently been isolated and appears to be the most frequent cause. Treatment is discussed on p. 432.

SIADH (see p. 821). Again, this is commonest from a primary lung tumour.

ECTOPIC ACTH SYNDROME (see p. 815). Small-cell carcinoma of the lung, carcinoid tumours and medullary thyroid carcinomas are the commonest causes.

PRODUCTION OF INSULIN-LIKE ACTIVITY may result in hypoglycaemia (see p. 853).

## ENDOCRINE TREATMENT OF OTHER MALIGNANCIES

Endocrine forms of treatment for malignancy have been used for many years, for example oophorectomy for

| Organ | Frequency | Tumours/manifestations |
|---|---|---|
| **Type 1** | | |
| Parathyroid | 95% | Adenomas/hyperplasia |
| Pituitary | 70% | Adenomas—prolactinoma, ACTH or growth hormone secreting (acromegaly) |
| Pancreas | 50% | Islet cell tumours (secreting insulin, glucagon, somatostatin, VIP, pancreatic polypeptide) Zollinger–Ellison syndrome |
| Adrenal | 40% | Non-functional adenoma |
| Thyroid | 20% | Adenomas—multiple or single |
| | | |
| **Type 2a** | | |
| Adrenal | Most | Phaeochromocytoma (70% bilateral) Cushing's syndrome |
| Thyroid | Most | Medullary carcinoma (calcitonin producing) |
| Parathyroid | 60% | Hyperplasia |
| | | |
| **Type 2b** | | |
| Type 2a with Marfanoid phenotype and intestinal and visceral ganglioneuromas | | |
| Neuromas also present around lips and tongue | | |

VIP, vasoactive intestinal polypeptide.

**Table 16.41**  Multiple endocrine neoplasia syndromes.

breast cancer and orchidectomy for prostatic malignancy. Newer more acceptable therapies include the anti-oestrogen tamoxifen for breast carcinoma and the LHRH analogues, buserelin and goserelin, for prostatic cancer.

# Further reading

Besser GM & Cudworth AG (1987) *Clinical Endocrinology—An Illustrated Text*. London: Gower.

DeGroot LJ, Reed Larsen P, Refetoff S & Stanbury JB (1984) *The Thyroid and Its Disorders*, 5th edn. New York: Wiley.

Greenspan FS (1991) *Basic and Clinical Endocrinology*, 3rd edn. Los Altos: Lange Medical Publishers.

Griffin JE (1992) *Textbook of Endocrine Physiology*, 2nd edn. Oxford: Oxford University Press.

Grossman A (1992) *Clinical Endocrinology*. Oxford: Blackwell Scientific Publications.

Hall R, Anderson J, Smart GA & Besser GM (eds) (1989) *Fundamentals of Clinical Endocrinology*, 4th edn. London: Pitman Medical.

Wilson JB & Foster DW (eds) (1992) *Textbook of Endocrinology*, 8th edn. Brighton: W.B. Saunders.

**Subject journals**

*Baillière's Clinical Endocrinology and Metabolism*—a series of up-to-date reviews of specific topics. London: Baillière Tindall.

*Clinical Endocrinology*, Blackwell Scientific, Oxford—mainly original papers in clinical endocrinology with concise clinical reviews.

*Endocrine Reviews*, Williams & Wilkins, Baltimore—largely very detailed and lengthy reviews of basic endocrinology.

*Endocrinology*, Williams & Wilkins, Baltimore—original papers in basic endocrinology.

*Journal of Clinical Endocrinology and Metabolism*, Williams & Wilkins, Baltimore—original papers in clinical endocrinology with some clinical reviews.

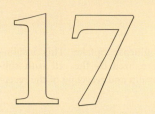

# Diabetes mellitus and other disorders of metabolism

## Diabetes mellitus

### Introduction

Diabetes mellitus is a group of metabolic disorders characterized by chronic hyperglycaemia due to relative insulin deficiency, or resistance or both. It is common and affects approximately 30 million people worldwide. Diabetes is usually irreversible and, although patients can have a reasonably normal life-style, its late complications result in reduced life expectancy and considerable uptake of health resources. Macrovascular disease leads to an increased prevalence of coronary artery disease, peripheral vascular disease and stroke, while microvascular damage results in diabetic retinopathy and contributes to nephropathy.

#### Insulin secretion

Insulin is the key hormone involved in the storage and controlled release within the body of the chemical energy available from food. It is synthesized in the β cells of the pancreatic islets in the form of proinsulin, which is stored in secretory granules close to the cell membrane. A biochemically inert peptide fragment known as connecting (C) peptide breaks off from proinsulin in the secretory process, so that equimolar quantities of insulin and C-peptide are released into the circulation. Insulin enters the portal circulation and is carried to the liver, its prime target organ. About 50% of secreted insulin is extracted and degraded in the liver; the residue is broken down by the kidney. C-peptide is only partially extracted by the liver (and hence provides a useful index of the rate of insulin secretion), but is mainly degraded by the kidney.

#### An outline of glucose metabolism

Blood glucose levels are closely regulated in health and rarely stray outside the range of 3.5–8.0 mmol litre$^{-1}$ (63–44 mg dl$^{-1}$), despite the varying demands of food, fasting and exercise. The principal organ of glucose homeostasis is the liver, which absorbs and stores glucose (as glycogen) in the postabsorptive state and releases it into the circulation between meals to match the rate of glucose utilization by peripheral tissues. The liver also manufactures glucose (6 carbons) from 3-carbon molecules derived from breakdown of fat and protein by the process of gluconeogenesis.

GLUCOSE PRODUCTION. About 200 g of glucose is produced and utilized each day. More than 90% is derived from the liver, three-quarters from glycogen and one-quarter from gluconeogenesis. The remaining 5–10% derives from renal gluconeogenesis.

GLUCOSE UTILIZATION. The brain is the major consumer of glucose. Its requirement is 1 mg kg$^{-1}$ body weight per minute, or 100 g daily in a 70 kg man. Glucose uptake by the brain is obligatory and is not dependent on insulin, and the glucose used is oxidized to carbon dioxide and water.

Other tissues, such as muscle and fat, are facultative glucose consumers. The effect of insulin peaks associated with meals is to lower the threshold for glucose entry into cells; at other times, energy requirements are largely met by fatty-acid oxidation. Glucose taken up by muscle is stored as glycogen or broken down to lactate, which re-enters the circulation and becomes an important substrate for hepatic gluconeogenesis. Glucose is used by fat tissue as a source of energy and as a substrate for triglyceride synthesis; lipolysis releases fatty acids from triglyceride together with glycerol, another substrate for hepatic gluconeogenesis.

HORMONAL REGULATION. Insulin is the major regulator of intermediary metabolism, although its actions are modified in important respects by other hormones. Dose–response curves for the production and utilization of glucose are shown in Fig. 17.1.

At low insulin levels, glucose production is maximal and utilization is minimal; at high levels the situation is reversed. At intermediate plasma insulin levels of 40–50 mU litre$^{-1}$, hepatic glucose production is largely suppressed but peripheral utilization remains low. This observation forms the theoretical basis for the low-dose insulin regimen used to treat diabetic ketoacidosis (see below).

The effect of counter-regulatory hormones (glucagon, adrenaline, cortisol and growth hormone) is to shift the dose–response curves to the right, resulting in greater production of glucose and less utilization for a given level of insulin.

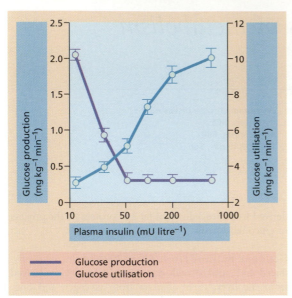

**Fig. 17.1** The effect of different insulin levels on glucose production and glucose utilization. Hepatic glucose production rises as insulin levels fall. Conversely, peripheral uptake of glucose is promoted at high insulin levels.

*The insulin receptor* is a glycoprotein (400 kDa) which straddles the cell membrane of many target cells. It consists of a dimer with two α subunits, which include the binding sites for insulin, and two β subunits, which traverse the cell membrane and initiate at least some of the intracellular actions of insulin (Fig. 17.2). The DNA sequence coding for the receptor has been isolated and sequenced and is located on the short arm of chromosome 19.

Insulin molecules bind to these receptors forming a complex that promotes glucose uptake. This insulin–receptor complex is internalized by the cell with subsequent degradation of insulin and recycling of the receptor to the cell surface.

## TYPES OF DIABETES

Diabetes may be primary or secondary (Table 17.1). Although insulin-dependent diabetes mellitus (IDDM, type I diabetes) and non-insulin-dependent diabetes mellitus (NIDDM, type II diabetes) represent two distinct diseases from the epidemiological point of view, clinical distinction may sometimes be difficult. The two disease processes should, in clinical terms, be visualized as opposite ends of a continuous spectrum (Table 17.2).

## Insulin-dependent diabetes mellitus (type I diabetes)

### EPIDEMIOLOGY

Approximately one person in 300 in the UK is treated with insulin, but some of these would be considered to have NIDDM by the criteria shown in Table 17.2. IDDM is most common in populations of European extraction, and within Europe there is a marked increase in incidence as one moves north. The highest incidence occurs in northern Scandinavia, but there is an unexplained hot-spot in the island of Sardinia which has the second highest rate in the world. The frequency of IDDM in various countries is shown in Fig. 17.3.

The incidence in childhood is maximal at 10–13 years of age. Presentation is more common in the spring and autumn than in the summer, and it has been suggested

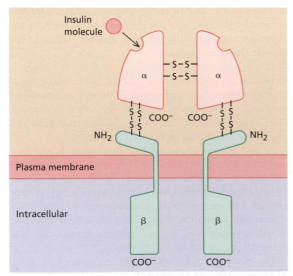

**Fig. 17.2** The insulin receptor consists of α and β subunits linked by disulphide bridges. The β subunits straddle the cell membrane and initiate some of the intracellular actions of insulin.

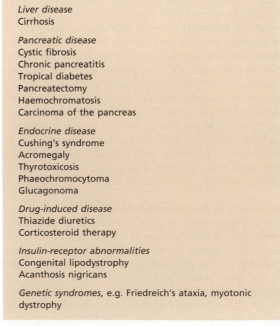

*Liver disease*
Cirrhosis

*Pancreatic disease*
Cystic fibrosis
Chronic pancreatitis
Tropical diabetes
Pancreatectomy
Haemochromatosis
Carcinoma of the pancreas

*Endocrine disease*
Cushing's syndrome
Acromegaly
Thyrotoxicosis
Phaeochromocytoma
Glucagonoma

*Drug-induced disease*
Thiazide diuretics
Corticosteroid therapy

*Insulin-receptor abnormalities*
Congenital lipodystrophy
Acanthosis nigricans

*Genetic syndromes*, e.g. Friedreich's ataxia, myotonic dystrophy

**Table 17.1** Causes of secondary diabetes.

| | IDDM (type I) | NIDDM (type II) |
|---|---|---|
| Epidemiology: | Patients are:<br>  Younger<br>  Usually lean<br>  European extraction (most commonly)<br><br>Seasonal incidence<br><br>? Viral aetiology | Patients are:<br>  Older<br>  Often overweight<br>  All racial groups (increasing incidence in<br>    immigrants to the UK) |
| Heredity | HLA-DR3 or DR4 in >90%<br><br>30–35% concordance in identical twins | No HLA links<br>Glucokinase gene abnormalities in some families<br><br>90% concordance in identical twins |
| Pathogenesis | Autoimmunity:<br>  Islet cell antibody<br>  Insulin autoantibodies<br>  Insulitis<br>  Associations with other organ-specific<br>    autoimmune diseases<br>  Antibodies to insulin and GAD (glutamic acid<br>    decarboxylase)<br>  Immunosuppression following diagnosis delays<br>    β cell destruction | No evidence of immune disturbance |
| Clinical | Insulin deficiency<br><br>May develop ketoacidosis<br><br>Always need insulin | Partial insulin deficiency, insulin resistance<br><br>May develop non-ketotic hyperosmolar state<br><br>Sometimes need insulin |

**Table 17.2**  The spectrum of diabetes: a comparison of insulin-dependent diabetes mellitus (IDDM) and non-insulin-dependent diabetes mellitus (NIDDM).

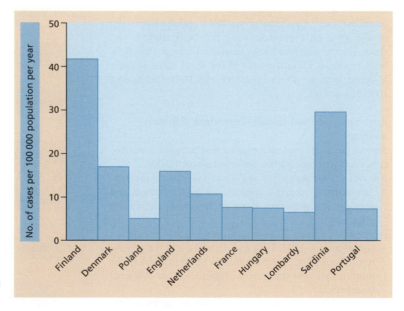

**Fig. 17.3**  The incidence of insulin-dependent diabetes mellitus (type I diabetes) in different European countries 1989–90 (EURODIAB ACE Study).

that this might be related to the greater prevalence of viral infections at these times. The incidence of IDDM is rising, in Europe, with an approximate doubling over the past 20–30 years.

## AETIOLOGY
### Genetic susceptibility
IDDM is not genetically predetermined, but an increased susceptibility to the disease may be inherited.

### Identical twins
The identical twin of a patient with IDDM has a 30–35% chance of developing the disease. This implies that non-genetic factors must also be involved.

### Inheritance
The child of an insulin-dependent diabetic patient has an increased chance of developing IDDM. This risk, curiously, is greater with a diabetic father (between 1 in 20

and 1 in 40) than with a diabetic mother (1 in 40–80). If one child in a family has IDDM, each sibling has a 1 in 20 risk of developing diabetes. If a sibling is HLA-identical, the risk rises to 1 in 6.

HLA SYSTEM. More than 90% of IDDM patients carry HLA-DR3 and/or DR4 compared with 40% of the general population. The relative risk conferred by DR3 is about 7, DR4 about 9, but the highest risk of 14 is with DR3/DR4 heterozygote. Since the risk is additive a model based on two susceptibility genes (one associated with DR3 and one with DR4) has been proposed. Stronger associations have been reported with the DQ region. Most people have two alleles with aspartic acid at position 57 on the HLA-DQ $\beta$ chain which confer resistance to the development of diabetes. Substitution of aspartate at position 57 by another amino acid considerably increases susceptibility to IDDM as do alleles coding for arginine at position 52 on the $\alpha$ chain. These DQ polymorphisms determine the degree of autoimmune response against the pancreatic islet cells but other genes, probably interacting with environmental factors, are necessary for the development of diabetes.

In contrast, individuals with HLA-DR2 have a considerably reduced risk (0.12 times normal) of developing diabetes. The reasons for this protective effect are unclear.

THE INSULIN GENE. Associations between IDDM and other chromosomes (apart from chromosome 6) have been described. A polymorphous DNA region close to the insulin gene on chromosome 11 has been studied, and short, intermediate and long insertions (see p. 109) have been reported. Homozygosity of the short (class I) allele is found in some 80% of patients with IDDM as against 40% of controls.

### Autoimmunity and insulin-dependent diabetes mellitus

Several pieces of evidence suggest that autoimmune processes are involved in the pathogenesis of IDDM.

ASSOCIATION WITH OTHER AUTOIMMUNE DISEASE. Autoimmune thyroid disease, Addison's disease and pernicious anaemia are more common in patients and their relatives.

IMMUNOGENETIC ASSOCIATIONS. The association between HLA-DR3, DR4 and diabetes, and the protective effect of DR2 might represent idiosyncrasies in the immune process that result in increased (or reduced) susceptibility.

THE INSULITIS PROCESS. Autopsies of patients who died soon after diagnosis are characterized by infiltration of the pancreatic islets by mononuclear cells. A similar pattern occurs in other autoimmune diseases, e.g. thyroiditis.

IMMUNE ABNORMALITIES AT DIAGNOSIS. About 70% of newly presenting patients have islet-cell antibodies. These react with human islets and can be detected by immunofluorescence. They usually become undetectable within a few years of diagnosis. In such patients increased numbers of activated T lymphocytes may

also be present in the circulation at diagnosis.

Of newly diagnosed patients with IDDM, 80% have antibodies to the enzyme glutamic acid decarboxylase (GAD). Pancreatic $\beta$ cells have high levels of this enzyme and the GAD autoantigen may be critical for the initiation of $\beta$ cell destruction.

IMMUNOSUPPRESSION with agents such as cyclosporin at or soon after diagnosis prolongs $\beta$-cell survival.

### Environmental factors

A viral aetiology has been suspected for many years. This is based on the seasonal incidence of the condition, anecdotal associations, and analysis of viral antibody titres at diagnosis. IgM antibodies to Coxsackie B4 have been reported in 20–30% of new cases. However, in view of the long prodromal period (see below), it seems likely that viruses precipitate rather than initiate the onset of diabetes.

### The diabetes prodrome

Prospective study of first-degree relatives of children with diabetes has revealed that islet-cell antibodies may appear in the circulation months or even years before diagnosis. Insulin antibodies have also been reported in this period,

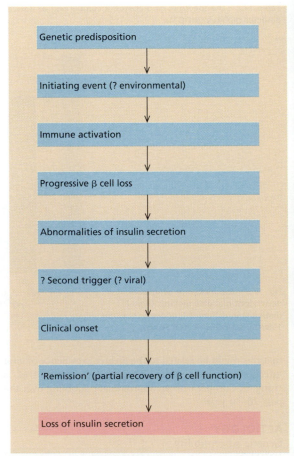

Genetic predisposition

Initiating event (? environmental)

Immune activation

Progressive $\beta$ cell loss

Abnormalities of insulin secretion

? Second trigger (? viral)

Clinical onset

'Remission' (partial recovery of $\beta$ cell function)

Loss of insulin secretion

**Fig. 17.4**  The possible sequence of events leading to the development of insulin-dependent diabetes mellitus.

and abnormalities of insulin secretion in response to intravenous glucose may develop.

The sequence of events leading to diagnosis may be as shown in Fig. 17.4. Better understanding of this sequence may in time permit strategies of prevention to be tested.

# Non-insulin-dependent diabetes mellitus (type II diabetes)

## EPIDEMIOLOGY

Unlike IDDM this is relatively common in all populations enjoying an affluent life-style. Large differences in prevalence have been reported. The disease may be present in a subclinical form for years before diagnosis, and the incidence increases markedly with age and degree of obesity. The onset may be accelerated by the stress of pregnancy, drug treatment or intercurrent illness. Estimates of prevalence using the WHO criteria would suggest an overall prevalence of around 2% in the UK. NIDDM is twice as prevalent in people of Afro-Caribbean ancestry and three to five times more prevalent in people from South Asia than in white Europeans.

The rates shown in Table 17.3 have been reported in various populations.

Epidemiological surveys suggest that indolent well-fed populations are two to twenty times as likely to develop NIDDM as lean populations of the same race.

## AETIOLOGY
### Genetics
Identical twins of a patient with NIDDM have an almost 100% chance of developing diabetes and about 25% of other patients have a first-degree relative with NIDDM. Certain families exist in which diabetes appears to travel as an autosomal dominant characteristic, but NIDDM is almost certainly a polygenic disorder. Some families show abnormalities of the gene which codes for the enzyme glucokinase on chromosome 7. The defect differs from one family to another and more than 20 mutations have been described so far. Studies in other family groups have shown linkage between the inheritance of diabetes and markers on chromosomes 3 and 20. The next decade is likely to see the identification of many of the gene abnormalities which predispose to NIDDM.

### Immunology
There is no evidence of immune involvement in its pathogenesis.

| Group | Age (years) | Rate (%) |
|---|---|---|
| USA | 20–74 | 6.9 |
| USA—Mexican immigrants | 25–65 | 17.0 |
| USA—Pima Indians | 25+ | 25.5 |
| Malta | 15+ | 7.7 |
| Indonesia | 15+ | 1.7 |
| New Guinea (highlands) | 20+ | 0.0 |

**Table 17.3** Prevalence of non-insulin-dependent diabetes mellitus in various populations (WHO criteria).

### Insulin secretion and action
Patients with NIDDM, unlike those with IDDM, retain about 50% of their $\beta$-cell mass at autopsy.

Abnormalities of insulin secretion develop early in the course of the disease. Normal subjects have a biphasic insulin response to intravenous glucose. In NIDDM the first-phase insulin response to intravenous glucose is lost, and insulin secretion in response to oral glucose is delayed and exaggerated. The majority of patients manifest reduced insulin secretion relative to the prevailing glucose concentration, and progressive $\beta$-cell loss occurs in many patients, although not to the extent seen in IDDM. It is not known whether this is due to 'exhaustion' of surviving $\beta$ cells or to some independent process of damage. Islet amyloid deposits are commonly seen in NIDDM, destroying the cells and interfering with glucose and hormone transport. The amyloid deposits are derived from islet amyloid polypeptide (IAPP), which may oppose the action of insulin, possibly explaining the insulin resistance that is also present. Obesity is present in 80% of patients with NIDDM, but insulin resistance may also be marked in lean individuals.

# Impaired glucose tolerance

If an oral glucose tolerance test (Practical box 17.1) is administered at random to a large population, 1–2% will be found to have unsuspected diabetes. A much larger group—5% or more (depending on the age, race and nutritional state of the population)—fall into an intermediate category now referred to as impaired glucose tolerance (IGT). The criteria for this category are given below. Follow-up shows that some (2–4% yearly) go on to develop diabetes, but that the abnormality does not progress in the majority. Obesity and lack of regular physical exercise make progression to frank diabetes more likely. Classification is complicated by the poor reproducibility of the oral glucose tolerance test and the group is certainly heterogeneous. Some are obese, some have liver disease, and others are on medication that impairs glucose tolerance; individuals in this category have a risk of cardiovascular disease that is twice that of people with normal glucose tolerance, but do not develop the specific microvascular complications of diabetes.

# Tropical diabetes

A distinct variety of diabetes has been described. This is found only in developing countries on or near the equator. The following features have been described:
- Onset is before the age of 30 years.
- There is a history of severe malnutrition.
- There is insulin dependence, sometimes with severe but fluctuating insulin resistance.
- Ketoacidosis does not develop when insulin is withdrawn.

There are two main variants:

FIBROCALCULOUS PANCREATIC DIABETES. This is associated with exocrine pancreatic deficiency, pancreatic fibrosis (often leading to calcification) and the

After an overnight fast, 75 g of glucose is taken in 250–350 ml of water. Blood samples are taken in the fasting state and 2 hours after the glucose has been given.
    A specific enzymatic glucose assay must be used.

*Note:* The concentration of glucose measured in plasma is 10% greater than that of whole blood.

**Diabetes**
This is present when the fasting *blood* glucose is over 6.7 mmol litre$^{-1}$ and/or when the 2-hour value is over 10 mmol litre$^{-1}$. Corresponding values for *plasma* glucose are 7.8 mmol litre$^{-1}$ and 11.1 mmol litre$^{-1}$.

**Impaired glucose tolerance**
This is present when the fasting blood glucose is below 6.7 mmol litre$^{-1}$ and when the 2-hour value is between 6.7 and 10 mmol litre$^{-1}$. Corresponding values for *plasma* glucose are 7.8 and 11.1 mmol litre$^{-1}$. Impaired glucose tolerance can only be diagnosed using the oral glucose tolerance test.

Intermediate sampling times (e.g. 30 min and 60 min) are not needed for the diagnosis of diabetes by WHO criteria. However, simultaneous blood and urine glucose measurements can be used to define a low renal threshold for glucose.
    Diabetes can usually be diagnosed on the basis of fasting or random blood glucose measurements (see text). *The glucose tolerance test should be reserved for borderline cases only.*

**Practical box 17.1**   The oral glucose tolerance test.

presence of stones in the pancreatic duct. There may be a history of recurrent abdominal pain, and in 75% of cases there is evidence of pancreatic calcification on plain abdominal X-ray. Most populations in which this condition arises are subject to malnutrition and have a diet based on cassava. Cyanates are present in the cassava root and may be a factor in the pancreatic damage.

PROTEIN-DEFICIENT PANCREATIC DIABETES. This form appears to be a direct consequence of malnutrition. The main differences from the fibrocalculous variant are that exocrine pancreatic function is unimpaired and there is no evidence of pancreatic fibrosis or calcification. Abdominal pain is not a feature.

In both forms of tropical diabetes, insulin secretion is preserved, although impaired; this is the likely explanation for the observed resistance to ketosis.

# CLINICAL PRESENTATION OF DIABETES

## Acute presentation
Young people often present with a brief 2–4 week history and report the classic triad of symptoms:

POLYURIA, due to the osmotic diuresis that results when blood glucose levels exceed the renal threshold

THIRST, due to the resulting loss of fluid and electrolytes

WEIGHT LOSS, due to fluid depletion and the accelerated breakdown of fat and muscle secondary to insulin deficiency

Ketoacidosis may be the presenting feature if these early symptoms are not recognized and treated.

## Subacute presentation
The clinical onset may be over several months, particularly in older patients. Thirst, polyuria and weight loss are usual features but medical attention is sought for such symptoms as lack of energy, visual blurring due to glucose-induced changes in refraction, or pruritus vulvae or balanitis due to *Candida* infection.

## Complications
Complications may be the presenting feature. These include:

● Staphylococcal skin infections
● Retinopathy noted during a visit to the optician
● A polyneuropathy causing tingling and numbness in the feet
● Impotence
● Arterial disease, resulting in myocardial infarction or peripheral gangrene

## Asymptomatic diabetes
Glycosuria or a raised blood glucose may be detected on routine examination (e.g. for insurance purposes) in individuals who have no symptoms of ill health.

# Physical examination

This is often unrewarding in younger patients, but evidence of weight loss and dehydration may be present, and the breath may smell of ketones. Older patients may present with established complications, and the presence of the characteristic retinopathy is diagnostic of diabetes.

# INVESTIGATION OF DIABETES

The diagnosis is usually simple. Blood glucose is so closely controlled by the body that even small deviations become important.

1 In *symptomatic* patients, a single elevated blood glucose, measured by a reliable method, indicates diabetes.

2 In *asymptomatic* or *mildly symptomatic* patients, the diagnosis is made on:

(a) One, preferably two, fasting venous *blood* glucose levels above 6.7 mmol litre$^{-1}$ (120 mg dl$^{-1}$); the equivalent venous *plasma* level is 7.8 mmol litre$^{-1}$ (140 mg dl$^{-1}$), or

(b) One, preferably two, random values above 10 mmol litre$^{-1}$ (180 mg dl$^{-1}$) in venous whole blood or 11.1 mmol litre$^{-1}$ (200 mg dl$^{-1}$) in venous plasma.

**3** A glucose tolerance test (GTT) is unnecessary when the criteria above are satisfied, and should be reserved for true borderline cases.

**4** Glycosuria is measured using sensitive glucose-specific dipstick methods. Glycosuria is not diagnostic of diabetes but indicates the need for further investigation. About 1% of the population have renal glycosuria. This is an inherited low renal threshold for glucose, transmitted either as a Mendelian dominant or recessive trait.

#### Other investigations

No further tests are needed to diagnose diabetes. Other routine investigations include screening the urine for proteinuria, a full blood count, urea and electrolytes, liver biochemistry and a fasting blood sample for cholesterol and triglycerides. The latter test is useful to exclude an associated hyperlipidaemia but should only be performed after blood glucose has been brought under control.

It is important to remember that diabetes may be *secondary* to other conditions (see Table 17.1), may be *precipitated* by underlying illness and be *associated* with autoimmune disease or hyperlipidaemia. Hypertension is present in one-third of European patients with NIDDM and 50% of Afro-Caribbeans.

## TREATMENT OF DIABETES

#### Guidelines to therapy

All patients with diabetes require diet therapy. Good glycaemic control is unlikely to be achieved with insulin or oral therapy when diet is neglected, especially when the patient is also overweight.

Insulin is always indicated in a patient who has been in ketoacidosis, and is usually indicated in patients who present under the age of 40 years. Insulin is also indicated in older patients following primary or secondary failure of oral therapy (see below). Tablets should be avoided in younger patients and are contraindicated in pregnancy.

In older patients the approach to therapy is empirical. Diet alone should be tried in the first instance, and dietary knowledge and compliance should always be reassessed with care before proceeding to the next step. This is of particular importance in the obese patient who fails to lose weight.

When diet fails to achieve satisfactory control, thin patients are usually treated with a sulphonylurea drug, and obese patients with a biguanide. Primary failure of treatment occurs when these agents (alone or in combination) never achieve the desired level of control. Other patients may show a good initial response followed by progressive loss of control over the succeeding months or years; this is referred to as secondary failure of treatment.

Since this approach is largely empirical, it is not surprising that practice differs from one country to another. For example, metformin (the only biguanide in common use) is very widely employed in France, tends to be used less in the UK, and is not licensed in the USA. Criteria of control also vary, so that what is classed as primary failure at one centre may be seen as a success in another. The most widespread error in management is procrastination; the patient whose control is inadequate on tablets should start insulin without undue delay.

### Diet

The diet for a diabetic patient is no different from the diet considered healthy for the population as a whole.

#### Carbohydrate

This should consist of unrefined carbohydrate rather than simple sugars such as sucrose. Carbohydrate is absorbed relatively slowly from fibre-rich foods, preventing the rapid swings in circulating glucose seen when refined sugars are ingested. For example, the glucose peak seen after eating an apple is much flatter than that seen after drinking the same amount of carbohydrate as apple juice.

#### Calories

Calories should be tailored to the needs of the patient. The total amount of carbohydrate in the diet should provide 50–55% of the total calories with fat 30–35% and protein 15%.

THE OVERWEIGHT DIABETIC PATIENT is started on a reducing diet of approximately 1000–1600 kcal daily (4000–6000 kJ).

THE LEAN PATIENT is put on an isocaloric diet.

PATIENTS WHO ARE UNDERWEIGHT because of untreated diabetes require energy supplementation.

#### Prescribing a diet

Most people find it extremely difficult to modify their eating habits, and repeated advice and encouragement are needed if this is to be achieved. A diet history is taken, and the diet prescribed should involve the least possible interference with the life-style of the patient. It is important to stress that patients on insulin or oral agents should eat the same amount at the same time each day. Patients on insulin require snacks between meals and at bedtime to buffer the effect of injected insulin. Alcohol is not forbidden, but its energy content should be taken into account. Patients on insulin should be warned to avoid alcoholic binges since these may precipitate severe hypoglycaemia.

#### The role of patient education and community care

The care of diabetes is based on self-management by the patient, who is helped and advised by those with specialized knowledge. The quest for improved glycaemic control has made it clear that whatever the technical expertise applied, the outcome depends on willing cooperation by the patient. This in turn depends on an understanding of the risks of diabetes and the potential benefits of glycaemic control and other measures such as maintaining a lean weight, stopping smoking and taking care of the feet.

If accurate information is not supplied, misinformation from friends and other patients will take its place. For this reason, many patients have exaggerated fears of, for example, blindness (about 1 patient in 20 is blind after 30 years of diabetes), death during hypoglycaemia (extremely rare), or the risk of passing diabetes on to their children (2–5% of offspring develop IDDM).

Organized training programmes involving all healthcare workers including nurse specialists, dietitians and chiropodists are now a recognized part of good diabetes care.

## Tablet treatment (Table 17.4)

### Sulphonylureas

These have two main actions:
1 They increase basal and stimulated insulin secretion.
2 They reduce peripheral resistance to insulin action.

The effects upon insulin secretion are most marked in the early stages of treatment, but the peripheral effects are more important for maintenance therapy. The sulphonylureas should be avoided in young ketotic patients, who require early insulin therapy, and are contraindicated in pregnancy. Insulin should be substituted during major surgery or severe intercurrent illness.

These drugs have similar actions and potency. All should be used with care in patients with liver disease, and only those primarily excreted by the liver should be given to patients with renal impairment. Sulphonylureas all encourage weight gain and are not the first choice in obese patients. Tolbutamide is the safest drug in the very elderly because of its short duration of action. Chlorpropamide has the disadvantages of a long duration of action and a wider range of side-effects, and is now less widely used.

DRUG INTERACTIONS (see p. 746). All sulphonylureas bind to circulating albumin and may be displaced by other drugs, such as sulphonamides, that compete for their binding sites. Their clinical effect may be reduced by thiazide diuretics or steroid therapy.

SIDE-EFFECTS. Hypoglycaemia is the most common and dangerous side-effect. Because the action of many sulphonylureas persists for more than 24 hours, recurrent or prolonged hypoglycaemia is likely, and hospital admission is usually necessary. Skin rashes and other sensitivity reactions may occur.

Chlorpropamide use is often associated with a facial flush when alcohol is taken. It may also cause a cholestatic jaundice and a syndrome of inappropriate antidiuretic hormone (ADH) secretion in 2–4% of patients.

### Biguanides

Metformin acts by reducing glucose absorption from the gut and by increasing insulin sensitivity. Unlike the sulphonylureas it does not induce hypoglycaemia in normal volunteers. It is usually reserved for patients in middle or old age, particularly for the overweight since it does not promote weight gain. It may be given in combination with sulphonylureas when a single agent has proved to be ineffective.

Its side-effects include anorexia, epigastric discomfort and diarrhoea. Lactic acidosis has occurred in patients with severe hepatic or renal disease, and metformin is contraindicated when these are present.

## Other drugs

Acarbose, an $\alpha$-glucosidase inhibitor, inhibits intestinal amylase, sucrase and maltase activity, thereby reducing carbohydrate absorption. It is being used in NIDDM patients who are inadequately controlled on diet alone or on diet with oral hypoglycaemic agents. Its long-term value is unproven.

## Insulin treatment

### Injections

The needles used to inject insulin are very fine and sharp. Even though most injections are virtually painless, patients are understandably apprehensive and treatment begins with a lesson in injection technique. Insulin is either drawn up into special plastic insulin syringes marked in units (100 U in 1 ml), or is administered by a pen injection device. Injections are given at 90° to the skin of the thighs or abdomen, and the needle is usually

| | Duration of action (hours) | Excretion/metabolism | Dose range per 24 hours |
|---|---|---|---|
| *Sulphonylureas* | | | |
| Tolbutamide | 6–8 | Hepatic | 1–2 g in divided doses |
| Chlorpropamide | 36–48 | Renal | 100–500 mg |
| Glibenclamide | 12–20 | Hepatic and renal | 2.5–20 mg |
| Gliclazide | 10–12 | Hepatic and renal | 40–320 mg in divided doses |
| Tolazamide | 12–24 | Hepatic | 100–750 mg |
| Gliquidone | 5 | Hepatic | 15–60 mg |
| Glipizide | 5–12 | Hepatic | 2.5–40 mg daily |
| | | | |
| *Biguanides* | | | |
| Metformin | 12–20 | Unchanged in urine | 1–2 g in 2–3 doses |

**Table 17.4** Drugs used in non-insulin-dependent diabetes mellitus.

inserted to its full length. Most patients starting insulin injection prefer pen devices when given a choice.

ADVANTAGES OF PEN INJECTION DEVICES
- Useful in the visually impaired (audible clicks, clear numbering)
- Easy to use
- Convenient to carry around
- Can be used discreetly in public places (e.g. restaurants)
- Some psychological benefit in 'needle phobias'
- Available free in the UK

DISADVANTAGES OF PEN INJECTION DEVICES
- Zinc insulins cannot be used because they aggregate in the pen cartridges.
- Pen needles are not yet available on prescription.
- Pens produced by one manufacturer cannot be used with insulin from another.

The injection site used should be changed regularly to prevent areas of lipohypertrophy. The rate of insulin absorption depends on local subcutaneous blood flow, and is accelerated by exercise, local massage or a warm environment. Absorption is more rapid from the abdomen than from the arm, and is slowest from the thigh. All these factors can influence the shape of the insulin profile.

All patients need careful training for a life with insulin, but routine hospital admission to begin insulin treatment is unnecessary where facilities for community support exist.

### Choice of insulin

SPECIES. Insulin is found in every creature with a backbone, and the central part of the molecule shows few species differences. (For example, fish insulin produces hypoglycaemia in humans.) Small differences in the amino acid sequence may alter the antigenicity of the molecule. Beef insulin differs from human insulin by three amino acids and pork from human by one. Both may induce antibody formation, beef more readily than pork.

Human insulin is produced by DNA coding of cultured yeast or bacterial cells to produce proinsulin, with subsequent enzymatic cleavage to insulin.

All forms of injected insulin, even human, may result in antibody formation, but insulin antibodies usually have little clinical importance. Human insulin has largely replaced the other varieties, mainly as the result of market forces. Some patients report altered perception of hypoglycaemia on human insulins. This effect has not been reproduced in double blind trials, but such patients should be offered the opportunity to try a different species of insulin.

PURITY. Insulins used in the Western World are now of very high purity, but older products are still widely distributed elsewhere.

FORMULATION (Table 17.5). There are two main types of insulin:
1 Insulin prepared in a clear solution (soluble or crystalline). These insulins are short-acting and are the only insulins to be used in emergencies such as ketoacidosis or for surgical operations.
2 Insulins premixed with retarding agents (either protamine or zinc) that precipitate crystals of varying size according to the conditions employed. These insulins are intermediate or long acting.

### Clinical use

In normal subjects a sharp increase in insulin occurs after meals; this is superimposed on a constant background of

| | Eli Lilly | Novo-Nordisk | |
|---|---|---|---|
| | | **Manufacturer** | |
| Soluble | Humulin S | Human Velosulin | Human Actrapid |
| Zinc | Humulin Zn | — | Human Semitard (amorphous zinc) |
| | Humulin Lente | | Human Ultratard (crystalline zinc) |
| | | | Human Monotard (amorphous 30%, crystalline 70%) |
| Protamine (Isophane) | Humulin I | Human Insulatard | Human Protaphane |
| Soluble: Protamine mixtures (% soluble) | | | |
| 10% | Humulin M1 | — | — |
| 20% | Humulin M2 | — | — |
| 30% | Humulin M3 | Human Mixtard 30/70 | Human Actraphane |
| 40% | Humulin M4 | — | — |
| 50% | — | Human Initard 50/50 | — |

All produced by recombinant DNA technology.

**Table 17.5** Human insulin preparations.

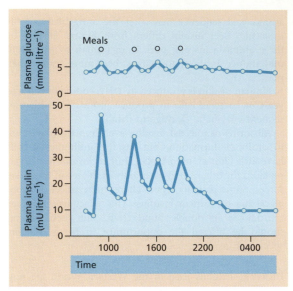

**Fig. 17.5**  Glucose and insulin profiles in normal subjects.

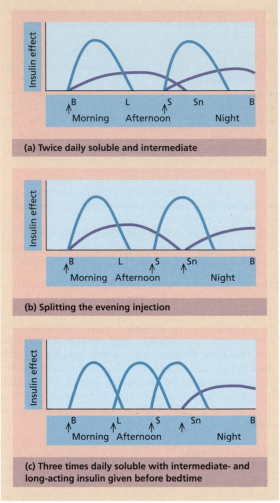

**(a) Twice daily soluble and intermediate**

**(b) Splitting the evening injection**

**(c) Three times daily soluble with intermediate- and long-acting insulin given before bedtime**

**Fig. 17.6**  Insulin regimens. Profiles of soluble insulins are shown as blue lines and intermediate- or long-acting insulin as purple lines. The arrows indicate when the injections are given. (a) Twice daily soluble and intermediate. (b) Splitting the evening injection. (c) Three times daily soluble with additional intermediate or long-acting insulin given before bedtime. B, breakfast; L, lunch; S, supper; Sn, snack (bedtime).

secretion (Fig. 17.5). Insulin therapy attempts to reproduce this pattern. In order to achieve this, a common strategy is to give intermediate-acting insulin to control the afternoon and night blood sugar level, and short-acting insulins morning and evening to match meal times (Fig. 17.6a).

Ideal control is often hard to achieve for four reasons:
1  In normal people, insulin is secreted directly into the portal circulation and passes directly to the liver in high concentration. The insulin injected by diabetics passes into the systemic circulation before passage to the liver.
2  Subcutaneous soluble insulin takes 60–90 min to achieve peak plasma levels—the onset and offset of action are too slow.
3  The absorption of subcutaneous insulin into the circulation is variable; the longer acting the preparation, the more erratic the absorption.
4  Basal insulin levels are constant in the normal state, but injected insulin invariably peaks and declines, with resulting swings in metabolic control.

Individuals vary and therapy must be tailored accordingly. One approach to therapy is outlined here.
YOUNG PATIENTS are started on two injections daily of an intermediate insulin at a dose of 8–10 U twice daily. Some recovery of endogenous insulin secretion may occur over the first few months (the 'honeymoon period') and the insulin dose may need to be reduced. Requirements rise thereafter and a multiple injection regimen is then appropriate for most younger patients. This is flexible and usually highly acceptable.
PATIENTS WITH NIDDM. Twice-daily injections of premixed soluble and isophane insulins, e.g. Mixtard, are effective in the majority of patients with NIDDM.
OLDER PATIENTS may sometimes manage adequately on a single daily injection.
If glycaemic control is inadequate with the standard approach, the alternatives are multiple insulin injections

or continuous subcutaneous insulin infusion (CSII). Both methods require a planned approach to life, with special attention to diet and exercise and frequent blood-glucose testing.

MULTIPLE INJECTIONS. The introduction of 'pen injection' devices has made this approach much more acceptable to patients. Two variants are shown diagrammatically in Fig. 17.6b,c. Multiple injection regimens and infusion devices have the advantage of flexibility concerning meal times, which is of great value to patients with busy jobs, shift workers and those who travel regularly. The amount eaten at each meal can be chosen at meal time and an appropriate dose of insulin given. With twice daily regimens, the size and timing of meals is fixed more rigidly.

INFUSION DEVICES. CSII is delivered by a small pump strapped around the waist that infuses a constant trickle of insulin via a needle in the subcutaneous tissues. Meal-time doses are delivered when the patient touches a button on the side of the pump.

This approach is particularly useful in the overnight period. Disadvantages include the nuisance of being attached to a gadget, skin infections, and the risk of ketoacidosis if the flow of insulin is broken (since these patients have no protective reservoir of depot insulin). Infusion pumps should only be used by specialized centres able to offer a round-the-clock service to their patients.

## Social implications

Patients starting on insulin need to inform the driving licence authority and their insurance companies. They are also wise to inform their employers. Certain types of work are unsuitable for insulin-treated patients, including driving heavy goods or public service vehicles, working at heights, piloting an aircraft or working close to dangerous machinery in motion. Certain professions such as the police and the armed forces are barred to all diabetic patients but there are few other limitations, although a considerable amount of ill-informed prejudice still exists.

## Complications

AT THE INJECTION SITE. Shallow injections result in intradermal insulin delivery and painful, reddened lesions or even scarring. Injection site abscesses occur but are extremely rare.

Local allergic responses sometimes occur early in therapy but usually resolve spontaneously. Generalized allergic responses are exceptionally rare.

Lipodystrophies that may occur include lipoatrophy, a local allergic response now virtually abolished by the use of highly purified insulins, and lipohypertrophy, occurring as a result of overuse of a single injection site with any type of insulin.

INSULIN RESISTANCE. The most common cause of mild insulin resistance is obesity. Occasional unstable patients require massive insulin doses, often with a fluctuating requirement. There are often associated behavioural problems. Insulin resistance associated with antibodies directed against the insulin receptor has been reported in patients with acanthosis nigricans.

WEIGHT GAIN. Patients who are non-compliant with their diet and predisposed to weight gain may show progressive weight gain on treatment, especially if the insulin dose is increased inappropriately.

HYPOGLYCAEMIA. This is the most common complication of insulin therapy and is a major cause of anxiety for patients and relatives. Symptoms develop when the blood glucose level is below 2.5 mmol litre$^{-1}$ and typically develop over a few minutes, with most patients experiencing 'adrenergic' features of sweating, tremor and a pounding heart beat. Physical signs include pallor and a cold sweat. Many patients with long-standing diabetes report loss of these warning symptoms and are at a greater risk of drifting into severe hypoglycaemia. Such patients appear pale, drowsy or detached, signs that their relatives quickly learn to recognize. Behaviour is clumsy or inappropriate, and some become irritable or even aggressive. Others slip rapidly into hypoglycaemic coma. Occasionally, patients develop convulsions during hypoglycaemic coma, especially at night. It is important not to confuse this with idiopathic epilepsy, especially since patients with frequent hypoglycaemia often have abnormalities on the EEG. Another presentation is with a hemiparesis that resolves within a few minutes when glucose is administered.

Hypoglycaemia is a common problem. Virtually all patients experience intermittent symptoms and one in three will go into a coma at some stage in their lives. A minority suffer attacks that are so frequent and severe as to be virtually disabling.

Hypoglycaemia results from an imbalance between injected insulin and a patient's normal diet, activity and basal insulin requirement. The times of greatest risk are before meals and during the night. Irregular eating habits, unusual exertion and alcohol excess may precipitate episodes; others appear to be due simply to variation in insulin absorption.

A further problem is that diabetic patients have an impaired ability to counter-regulate glucose levels after hypoglycaemia. The glucagon response is invariably deficient, even though the $\alpha$ cells are preserved and respond normally to other stimuli. The adrenaline response may also fail in patients with a long duration of diabetes.

Nocturnal hypoglycaemia is commonly caused by attempts to compensate for the slight increase in insulin requirements from 4 a.m. (the 'dawn phenomenon'). This is related to the nocturnal peak of growth hormone secretion. Since injected insulin inevitably peaks and declines, increasing the evening dose of insulin to combat fasting hyperglycaemia increases the risk of hypoglycaemia in the early hours of the morning. It was widely believed that this hypoglycaemia caused a rebound hyperglycaemia (the 'Somogyi effect') owing to an unbalanced counter-regulatory response, but in practice fasting hyperglycaemia is usually due to insulin deficiency.

The diagnosis of hypoglycaemia is simple and can usually be made on clinical grounds. Patients should carry a card or wear a bracelet or necklace identifying themselves as diabetic, and these should be looked for in unconscious patients. If real doubt exists, it will do no harm to administer glucose whilst a laboratory blood glucose result is awaited.

Any form of rapidly absorbed carbohydrate will relieve the early symptoms, and patients should always carry glucose or sweets. Drowsy patients will often be able to take carbohydrate in liquid form, e.g. a spoonful of sugar in water. Milk should be avoided since fat delays gastric emptying and slows recovery. Unconscious patients should be given intravenous glucose (50 ml of 50% dextrose solution) followed by a flush of normal saline to preserve the vein, or intramuscular glucagon (1 mg). Glucagon acts by mobilizing hepatic glycogen, and works almost as rapidly as glucose. It is simple to administer and can be given at home by relatives. Glycogen reserves should be replenished with oral glucose once the patient revives.

## Measuring control

The 'artificial pancreas' is a system of blood glucose control that works by continuous blood glucose analysis. This is fed into a computer, which delivers an appropriate amount of insulin into the circulation. Patients on insulin need to devise their own simplified form of this feedback loop.

### Urine tests
Urine tests (dipstix) are simple to perform, and it can usually be assumed that a patient with consistently negative tests and no symptoms of hypoglycaemia is well controlled. Even so, the correlation between urine tests and simultaneous blood glucose is poor for three reasons:
1 Changes in urine glucose lag behind changes in blood glucose.
2 The mean renal threshold is around 10 mmol litre$^{-1}$ but the range is wide (7–13 mmol litre$^{-1}$). The threshold also rises with age.
3 Urine tests can give no guidance concerning blood glucose levels below the renal threshold.
Urinary ketones may also be measured by a dipstick test. This is rarely helpful in routine outpatient management, but can be useful in special situations such as intercurrent infections. Heavy ketonuria can inhibit some dipstick tests for glucose.

### Blood glucose testing
This provides the best assessment of day-to-day control. The fasting blood glucose concentration is a useful guide to therapy in NIDDM.

A random blood glucose test (e.g. in the clinic) is of limited value, but patients may easily be taught to provide their own profiles by testing finger-prick blood samples with reagent strips and reading these with the aid of a visual scale or reflectance meter. It has been amply demonstrated that most patients are willing and able to provide reasonably accurate results provided they have been properly taught.

Blood is taken from the side of a fingertip (*not* from the tip, which is densely innervated) using a special lancet, e.g. Monolet, which can be fitted to a spring-loaded device. Patients are asked to take regular profiles (e.g. four daily samples on 2 days each week) and to note these in a diary or record book. Home blood glucose monitoring is essential for good diabetic control. Patients are encouraged to adjust their insulin dose as appropriate and should ideally be able to obtain advice over the telephone when needed.

### Glycosylated haemoglobin (HbA$_1$ or HbA$_{1c}$)
Glycosylation of haemoglobin occurs as a two-step reaction, resulting in the formation of a covalent bond between the glucose molecule and the terminal valine of the $\beta$-chain of the haemoglobin molecule. The rate at which this reaction occurs is related to the prevailing glucose concentration. Glycosylated haemoglobin is expressed as a percentage of the normal haemoglobin (normal range approximately 4–8% depending on technique of measurement). This test provides an index of the average blood glucose concentration over the life of the haemoglobin molecule (approximately 6 weeks). The figure will be misleading if the life-span of the red cell is reduced or if an abnormal haemoglobin or thalassaemia is present. Although the glycosylated haemoglobin test provides a rapid assessment of the level of glycaemic control in a given patient, blood glucose testing is needed before the clinician can know what to do about it.

Glycosylated plasma proteins ('fructosamine') may also be measured as an index of control. Glycosylated albumin is the major component and fructosamine measurement relates to glycaemic control over the preceding 1–3 weeks. The technique is cheaper and quicker than glycosylated haemoglobin measurement and lends itself to automation. It is useful in patients with haemoglobinopathy and in pregnancy (when haemoglobin turnover is changeable). Correlation between the two tests is weak. This may reflect the greater interindividual variation in plasma proteins than in haemoglobin. It is also less reliable and measurement of HbA$_{1c}$ is often preferred.

### Does good glycaemic control matter?
The answer to this question involves a number of separate issues.
1 *Is poor control associated with an increased risk of microvascular complications?* Retrospective studies have repeatedly shown that those with the worst control have the highest rate of complications.
2 *Is this increased risk reversible?* There are many difficulties in answering this question:
   (a) The gestation of diabetic complications is lengthy, often 10–20 years.
   (b) Control was difficult to quantify before HbA$_{1c}$ tests were introduced.
   (c) Good control is difficult to achieve, so comparisons have usually been between 'poor and worse' control rather than between 'good and bad'.
   (d) Some patients are easier to bring into good control than others, so the groups selected as 'well' or 'poorly' controlled in previous studies were not strictly comparable.
Studies in experimental animals strongly suggest that improved control is protective and this has now been confirmed in humans. The Diabetes Control and Complications Trial (DCCT) in the USA compared standard versus intensive insulin therapy in a prospective controlled trial of young patients with IDDM. Even on intensive therapy, mean blood glucose levels were 40% above the non-diabetic range, but this level of control reduced the risk of progression to retinopathy, nephropathy or neuropathy over the 7 years of the study by some 60%. Near-normoglycaemia should, therefore, be the goal for all young patients with IDDM. Unwanted

effects of this policy include weight gain and a 2–3 fold increase in the risk of severe hypoglycaemia. Control should be less strict in those with a history of recurrent severe hypoglycaemia. It remains unclear whether equally stringent standards should be applied in patients with NIDDM, particularly since a protective effect upon progression of macrovascular disease has yet to be demonstrated. A large trial in patients with NIDDM is due to report shortly and should allow this question to be answered.

3  *Can established complications be halted or reversed by intensive insulin therapy?* Insulin infusion devices have made near-normal blood glucose control possible for closely supervised groups of patients. Studies in patients with established retinopathy or nephropathy have shown that patients with early retinopathy benefit from 2–3 years of intensive therapy, but that patients with more advanced retinal changes or proteinuria do not. Retinopathy may show a transient deterioration when strict control is first established. These observations suggest that microvascular lesions may be self-perpetuating once a threshold level of damage has been reached.

4  *Is macrovascular disease influenced by control?* Patients with impaired glucose tolerance have an increased rate of large vessel disease but rarely develop microvascular lesions. This might be because large arteries are more sensitive to elevated glucose levels, but it has also been suggested that hyperinsulinaemia (present in many patients with NIDDM and a common consequence of insulin treatment) is a cause of accelerated atherogenesis. At present there is little evidence that good glycaemic control protects against arterial disease.

# DIABETIC METABOLIC EMERGENCIES

The main terms used are defined in Table 17.6.

## Diabetic ketoacidosis

### CAUSES
Diabetic ketoacidosis is the hallmark of IDDM. Its main causes can be grouped as follows:
- Previously undiagnosed diabetes
- Interruption of insulin therapy
- The stress of intercurrent illness

The majority of cases reaching hospital could have been *prevented* by earlier diagnosis, better communication between patient and doctor, and better patient education.

The most common error of management is for patients to reduce or omit insulin because they feel unable to eat owing to nausea or vomiting. This is a factor in at least 25% of all hospital admissions. Insulin should never be stopped.

### PATHOGENESIS
Ketoacidosis is a state of uncontrolled catabolism associated with insulin deficiency. Insulin deficiency is a necessary precondition since only a modest elevation in insulin levels is sufficient to inhibit hepatic ketogenesis. Even so, stable patients do not readily develop ketoacidosis when insulin is withdrawn. Other factors include counter-

| | |
|---|---|
| Ketonuria | Detectable ketone levels in the urine; it should be appreciated that ketonuria occurs in fasted non-diabetics and may be found in relatively well-controlled patients with insulin-dependent diabetes mellitus |
| Ketosis | Elevated plasma ketone levels in the absence of acidosis |
| Diabetic ketoacidosis | A metabolic emergency in which hyperglycaemia is associated with a metabolic acidosis due to greatly raised (>5 mmol litre⁻¹) ketone levels |
| Non-ketotic hyperosmolar state | A metabolic emergency in which uncontrolled hyperglycaemia induces a hyperosmolar state in the absence of significant ketosis |
| Lactic acidosis | A metabolic emergency in which elevated lactate levels induce a metabolic acidosis. In diabetic patients it is rare and associated with biguanide therapy |

**Table 17.6**  Terms used in uncontrolled diabetes.

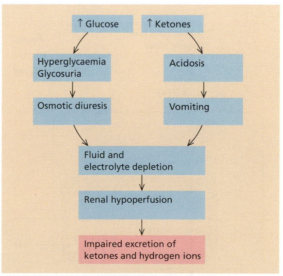

**Fig. 17.7**  Dehydration occurs during ketoacidosis as a consequence of two parallel processes. Hyperglycaemia results in osmotic diuresis, and hyperketonaemia results in acidosis and vomiting. Renal hypoperfusion then occurs and a vicious circle is established as the kidney becomes less able to compensate for the acidosis.

regulatory hormone excess and fluid depletion. The combination of insulin deficiency with excess of its hormonal antagonists leads to the parallel processes shown in Fig. 17.7.

In the absence of insulin, hepatic glucose production accelerates and peripheral uptake by tissues such as muscle is reduced. Rising glucose levels lead to an osmotic diuresis, loss of fluid and electrolytes, and dehydration. Plasma osmolality rises and renal perfusion falls.

In parallel, rapid lipolysis occurs, leading to elevated circulating free fatty-acid levels. The free fatty acids are broken down to fatty acyl-CoA within the liver cells, and this in turn is converted to ketone bodies within the mitochondria (Fig. 17.8).

Accumulation of ketone bodies produces a metabolic acidosis. This is typically associated with nausea and vomiting, leading to further loss of fluid and electrolytes. The excess ketones are excreted in the urine but also appear in the breath, producing a distinctive smell similar to that of acetone. Respiratory compensation for the acidosis leads to hyperventilation, graphically described as 'air hunger'. Progressive dehydration impairs renal excretion of hydrogen ions and ketones, aggravating the acidosis. As the pH falls below 7.0 ([$H^+$] >100 nmol litre$^{-1}$), pH-dependent enzyme systems in many cells function less effectively. Untreated, severe ketoacidosis is invariably fatal.

### CLINICAL FEATURES

The features of ketoacidosis are those of uncontrolled diabetes with acidosis, and include prostration, hyperventilation (Kussmaul respiration), nausea, vomiting and, occasionally, abdominal pain. The latter is sometimes so severe as to cause confusion with a surgical acute abdomen.

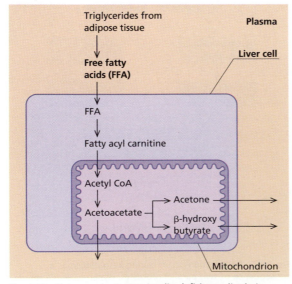

**Fig. 17.8** Ketogenesis. During insulin deficiency, lipolysis accelerates and free fatty acids taken up by liver cells form the substrate for ketone formation (acetoacetate, acetone and β-hydroxybutyrate) within the mitochondrion.

Some patients are mentally alert at presentation, but confusion and stupor are common. Up to 5% present in coma. Evidence of marked dehydration is present and the eyeball is lax to pressure in severe cases. Hyperventilation is present but becomes less marked in very severe acidosis owing to respiratory depression. The smell of ketones on the breath allows an instant diagnosis to be made by those able to detect the odour. The skin is dry and the body temperature is often subnormal, even in the presence of infection; in such cases, pyrexia may develop later.

### DIAGNOSIS

This is confirmed by demonstrating hyperglycaemia with ketonaemia or heavy ketonuria, and acidosis. No time should be lost and treatment is started as soon as the first blood sample has been taken.

Hyperglycaemia is demonstrated by dipstick, while a blood sample is sent to the laboratory for confirmation. Ketonaemia is confirmed by centrifuging a blood sample and testing the plasma with a dipstick that measures ketones. An arterial blood sample is taken for blood gas analysis.

Further investigations are detailed below.

### MANAGEMENT

The principles of management are as follows (Information box 17.1).

REPLACE THE FLUID LOSSES.

REPLACE THE ELECTROLYTE LOSSES. Potassium levels need to be monitored with great care to avoid the cardiac complications of hypokalaemia or hyperkalaemia.

RESTORE THE ACID–BASE BALANCE. A patient with healthy kidneys will rapidly compensate for the metabolic acidosis once the circulating volume is restored. Bicarbonate is seldom necessary, although it is usual for this to be given as isotonic 1.26% bicarbonate solution (not 8.4% which is grossly hyperosmolar) if the pH is below 7.0 ([$H^+$] >100 nmol litre$^{-1}$).

REPLACE THE DEFICIENT INSULIN. Modern treatment is with low doses of insulin, which lower blood glucose by suppressing hepatic glucose output rather than by stimulating peripheral uptake, and are therefore much less likely to produce hypoglycaemia. Soluble insulin is given as an intravenous infusion where facilities for adequate supervision exist, or as hourly intramuscular injections. The subcutaneous route is avoided because subcutaneous blood flow is reduced in shocked patients.

MONITOR BLOOD GLUCOSE CLOSELY. Hourly measurement is needed in the initial phases of treatment.

REPLACE THE ENERGY LOSSES. When plasma glucose falls to near-normal values (12 mmol litre$^{-1}$), saline infusion should be replaced with 5% dextrose containing 20 mmol KCl litre$^{-1}$. The insulin infusion rate is reduced and adjusted according to blood glucose.

SEEK THE UNDERLYING CAUSE. Physical examination may reveal a source of infection, e.g. a perianal abscess. Two common markers of infection are misleading: fever is unusual even when infection is present and

**Information box 17.1** Guidelines for the diagnosis and management of diabetic ketoacidosis.

polymorpholeucocytosis is present even in the absence of infection. Relevant investigations include a chest X-ray, urine and blood cultures, and an ECG (to exclude myocardial infarction). If infection is suspected, broad-spectrum antibiotics are started once the appropriate cultures have been taken.

## Problems of management

HYPOTENSION. This may lead to renal shutdown. Plasma expanders (or whole blood) are therefore given if the systolic blood pressure is below 80 mmHg. A central venous pressure line is useful in this situation. A bladder catheter is inserted if no urine is produced within 2 hours, but routine catheterization is unnecessary.

COMA. The usual principles apply (see p. 903). It is essential to pass a nasogastric tube to prevent aspiration since gastric stasis is common and the rare, but fatal, complication of acute gastric dilatation may result.

CEREBRAL OEDEMA. This rare, but feared, complication has mostly been reported in children or young adults. Excessive rehydration and use of hypertonic fluids such as 8.4% bicarbonate may sometimes be responsible. The mortality is high.

HYPOTHERMIA. Severe hypothermia with a core temperature below 33°C may occur and may be overlooked unless a rectal temperature is taken with a low-reading thermometer.

LATE COMPLICATIONS. These include stasis pneumonia and deep-vein thrombosis, and occur especially in the comatose or elderly patient.

COMPLICATIONS OF THERAPY. These include hypoglycaemia and hypokalaemia. Overenthusiastic fluid replacement may precipitate pulmonary oedema in older patients. Hyperchloraemic acidosis may develop in the course of treatment since patients have lost a large variety of negatively charged electrolytes, which are replaced with chloride. The kidneys usually correct this spontaneously within a few days.

### Subsequent management

Intravenous fluids and insulin are continued until the patient feels able to eat and keep food down. The drip is then taken down and a similar amount of insulin is given as three or four soluble subcutaneous doses per day until a maintenance regimen can be restarted.

Sliding-scale regimens are often unnecessary and may even delay the establishment of stable blood glucose levels.

The treatment of diabetic ketoacidosis is incomplete without a careful enquiry into the causes of the episode and advice as to how to avoid its recurrence.

## Non-ketotic hyperosmolar state

This condition, in which severe hyperglycaemia develops without significant ketosis, is the metabolic emergency characteristic of uncontrolled NIDDM. Patients present in middle or later life, often with previously undiagnosed diabetes. Common precipitating factors include consumption of glucose-rich fluids (e.g. Lucozade), concurrent medication such as thiazide diuretics or steroids, and intercurrent illness.

Non-ketotic coma and ketoacidosis represent two ends of a spectrum rather than two distinct disorders. The biochemical differences (shown in Information box 17.2)

**Examples of blood values**

| | Severe ketoacidosis | Non-ketotic hyperosmolar coma |
|---|---|---|
| $Na^+$ (mmol litre$^{-1}$) | 140 | 155 |
| $K^+$ (mmol litre$^{-1}$) | 5 | 5 |
| $Cl^-$ (mmol litre$^{-1}$) | 100 | 110 |
| $HCO_3^-$ (mmol litre$^{-1}$) | 5 | 30 |
| Urea (mmol litre$^{-1}$) | 8 | 15 |
| Glucose (mmol litre$^{-1}$) | 30 | 50 |
| Arterial pH | 7.0 | 7.35 |

The *osmolality* can be measured directly, or can be calculated approximately from the formula:

Osmolality = 2($Na^+ + K^+$) + glucose + urea

The normal range is 285–300 mosmol litre$^{-1}$

For example, in the example of severe ketoacidosis given above:

Osmolality = 2(140 + 5) + 30 + 8 = 328 mosmol litre$^{-1}$

and in the example of non-ketotic hyperosmolar coma:

Osmolality = 2(155 + 5) + 50 + 15 = 385 mosmol litre$^{-1}$

The *anion gap* is calculated as ($Na^+ + K^+$) − ($Cl^- + HCO_3^-$) (see p. 516). The normal anion gap is less than 17.

In the example of ketoacidosis the anion gap is 40, and in the example of non-ketotic hyperosmolar coma the anion gap is 20. Mild hyperchloraemic acidosis may develop in the course of therapy. This will be shown by a rising plasma chloride and persistence of a low bicarbonate even though the anion gap has returned to normal.

**Information box 17.2** Electrolyte changes in diabetic ketoacidosis and non-ketotic hyperosmolar state.

may partly be explained as follows:

AGE. The extreme dehydration characteristic of non-ketotic coma may be related to age. Old people experience thirst less acutely, and more readily become dehydrated. In addition, the mild renal impairment associated with age results in increased urinary losses of fluid and electrolytes.

THE DEGREE OF INSULIN DEFICIENCY is less severe in non-ketotic coma. Endogenous insulin levels are sufficient to inhibit hepatic ketogenesis, whereas glucose production is unrestrained.

### CLINICAL PRESENTATION

The characteristic clinical features are dehydration and stupor or coma. Impairment of consciousness is directly related to the degree of hyperosmolality. Evidence of underlying illness such as pneumonia or pyelonephritis may be present, and the hyperosmolar state may predispose to stroke, myocardial infarction or arterial insufficiency in the lower limbs.

### INVESTIGATION AND TREATMENT

These are according to the guidelines for ketoacidosis with some exceptions. Many patients are extremely sensitive to insulin and the glucose concentration may plum-

met. The resultant change in osmolality may cause cerebral damage. It is sometimes useful to infuse insulin at a rate of 3 U hour$^{-1}$ for the first 2–3 hours, increasing to 6 U hour$^{-1}$ if glucose is falling too slowly. Normal saline is the standard fluid for replacement. Avoid half-normal saline (0.45%) except in exceptional circumstances, since rapid dilution of the blood may cause more cerebral damage than a few hours of exposure to hypernatraemia.

### PROGNOSIS

The reported mortality is around 20–30%, mainly because of the advanced age of the patients and the frequency of intercurrent illness. Unlike ketoacidosis, non-ketotic hyperglycaemia is not an absolute indication for subsequent insulin therapy, and survivors may do well on diet and oral agents.

## Lactic acidosis

Lactic acidosis may occur in diabetic patients on biguanide therapy. Phenformin, the agent responsible in the great majority of reported cases, has now been withdrawn in the UK. The risk in patients taking metformin is extremely low provided that the therapeutic dose is not exceeded and the drug is withheld in patients with advanced hepatic or renal dysfunction.

Patients present with a severe metabolic acidosis, usually without significant hyperglycaemia or ketosis, and treatment is by rehydration and infusion of isotonic 1.26% bicarbonate. The mortality is in excess of 50%.

## COMPLICATIONS OF DIABETES

When insulin was introduced it was assumed that it would provide complete and adequate replacement therapy, just as thyroxine does in hypothyroidism.

Time proved that insulin-treated patients still have a considerably reduced life expectancy. Those diagnosed before the age of 20 years have only a 60–70% chance of living past the age of 45 years, although there are recent indications of improved survival. The excess deaths are mainly due to diabetic nephropathy, but there is also a considerable excess cardiovascular mortality. Heart disease, peripheral vascular disease and stroke are the major causes of death in patients over the age of 50 years.

**Macrovascular complications**

Diabetes is a risk factor (Table 17.7) in the development of atherosclerosis. This risk is related to that of the background population. For example, Japanese diabetics are much less likely to develop atherosclerosis than patients in Europe but are much more likely to develop it than non-diabetic Japanese. The excess risk to diabetics compared with the general population increases as one moves down the body:

STROKE is twice as likely.

MYOCARDIAL INFARCTION is three to five times as likely and women with diabetes lose their premeno-

Duration of diabetes
Age
Systolic hypertension
Hyperinsulinaemia due to insulin resistance associated
   with obesity and syndrome X
Hyperlipidaemia, particularly hypertriglyceridaemia
Proteinuria (including microalbuminuria)

Other factors are the same as for the general
population

**Table 17.7**   Diabetic risk factors for macrovascular
complications.

pausal protection from coronary artery disease.
AMPUTATION OF A FOOT for gangrene is 50 times as
   likely.
Diabetes is additive with other risk factors for large-vessel
disease. In other words, the diabetic who smokes or is
obese, hypertensive or hyperlipidaemic adds the risks
conferred by these conditions to that of diabetes itself.

### Insulin resistance

Hyperinsulinaemia due to insulin resistance associated
with obesity is sometimes known as 'syndrome X'. Con-
fusingly the same term is used by cardiologists for a rare
variant of angina. Syndrome X includes glucose intolerance, hypertension, central obesity and dyslipoproteinae-
mia (increased very low density lipoprotein and reduced
high-density lipoprotein). It is found in patients with
NIDDM and carries a high risk of coronary artery disease.

### Microvascular complications

In contrast to macrovascular disease, which is prevalent
in Western populations as a whole, microvascular disease
is specific to diabetes. Small blood vessels throughout the
body are affected but the disease process is of particular
danger in three sites:

● Retina
● Renal glomerulus
● Nerve sheath

Diabetic retinopathy, nephropathy and neuropathy tend
to manifest 10–20 years after diagnosis in young patients.
They present earlier in older patients, probably because
these have had unrecognized diabetes for months or even
years prior to diagnosis.

## Diabetic eye disease

Diabetes can affect the eyes in a number of ways. The
most common and characteristic form of involvement is
diabetic retinopathy. About one in three young patients
is likely to develop visual problems, and in the UK 5%
have in the past become blind after 30 years of diabetes;
diabetes is the commonest cause of blindness in the
population as a whole up to the age of 60 years.

   Other forms of eye disease may also occur:
THE LENS may be affected by reversible osmotic changes
in patients with acute hyperglycaemia—causing
blurred vision—or by cataracts.

NEW VESSEL FORMATION IN THE IRIS (rubeosis
   iridis) may develop as a late complication of diabetic
   retinopathy and can cause glaucoma.
EXTERNAL OCULAR PALSIES, especially of the sixth
   nerve, can occur (a mononeuritis).

### The natural history of retinopathy

Diabetes causes increased thickness of the basement
membrane and increased permeability of the retinal capillaries. Aneurysmal dilatation may occur in some vessels
while others become occluded. These changes are first
detectable by fluorescein angiography: a fluorescent dye
is injected into an arm vein and photographed in transit
through the retinal vessels. This technique is not necessary to screen effectively for retinal disease. After 20 years
of IDDM, almost all patients have some retinopathy—
60% progress to proliferative retinopathy (Fig. 17.9).
After 20 years of NIDDM >80% have some retinopathy,
20% have proliferative changes (Fig. 17.10).

BACKGROUND RETINOPATHY. The first abnormality
visible through the ophthalmoscope is the appearance of
dot 'haemorrhages', which are actually due to capillary
microaneurysms. Leakage of blood into the deeper layers
of the retina produces the characteristic 'blot' haemorrhage, while exudates of fluid rich in lipids and protein
give rise to hard exudates. These have a bright yellow-
white colour and are often irregular in outline with a
sharply defined margin.

   These changes rarely develop in young patients with a
duration of diabetes under 10 years, but by 20 years virtually all eyes will at least manifest the occasional dot
haemorrhage on careful ophthalmoscopy. In contrast,
retinopathy may be present at diagnosis or shortly thereafter in older patients.

   Background retinopathy does not in itself constitute a

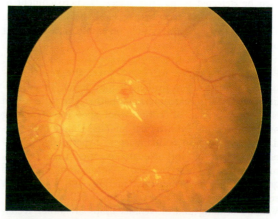

**Fig. 17.9**   Background retinopathy and maculopathy. Dot and
blot haemorrhages are visible together with hard exudates
forming ring-like structures in areas of ischaemia. These areas
partially surround, and one hard exudate encroaches upon,
the macula. The visual acuity has fallen swiftly from 6/6 to
6/12. Focal laser photocoagulation is indicated to prevent
further deterioration of macular vision.

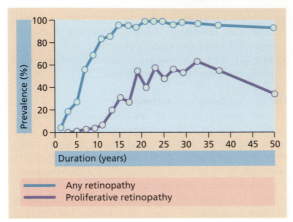

**Fig. 17.10**  Prevalance of retinopathy in relation to duration of the disease in patients with insulin-dependent diabetes mellitus diagnosed under the age of 33 years. Almost all have background change and 60% progress to proliferative retinopathy. (From *Ophthalmology* (1984) **102**, 520. With permission.)

threat to vision but may progress to two other distinct forms of retinopathy: maculopathy or proliferative retinopathy. Both are the consequence of damage to retinal blood vessels and resultant retinal ischaemia.

DIABETIC MACULOPATHY. This may lead to blindness in the absence of proliferation and particularly affects the older patient with NIDDM. Macular oedema is the first feature of maculopathy and may in itself result in permanent macular damage if not treated early. The first, and only, sign of this is deteriorating visual acuity and the condition cannot be diagnosed with standard ophthalmoscopy. This is why it is essential to screen patients with diabetes regularly for changes in visual acuity. In most cases, however, maculopathy does not generate sufficient oedema to cause early loss of acuity. The process may then be detected in its later stages as encroachment of hard exudates and haemorrhages on the macular area. These changes are easily visible on ophthalmoscopy, but only through fully dilated pupils.

PREPROLIFERATIVE RETINOPATHY. Progressive retinal ischaemia leads to further changes which herald proliferative, sight-threatening retinopathy. The earliest sign is the appearance of 'cotton-wool spots', representing oedema resulting from retinal infarcts. Unlike hard exudates they may also occur in severe hypertensive retinopathy. The term 'soft exudate' is often used synonymously but is best avoided. Cotton-wool spots are greyish-white, have indistinct margins and a dull matt surface, unlike the glossy appearance of hard exudates. Venous beading and/or venous loops are other recognized preproliferative changes.

PROLIFERATIVE RETINOPATHY. Hypoxia is thought to be the signal for formation of new vessels. These lie superficially or grow forward into the vitreous, resembling fronds of seaweed. They branch repeatedly, are frag-

ile, bleed easily (because they lack the normal supportive tissue) and may give rise to a fibrous-tissue reaction.

With advanced retinopathy, haemorrhages can be preretinal or into the vitreous. A vitreous haemorrhage presents as a loss of vision in one eye, sometimes noticed on waking, or as a floating shadow affecting the field of vision. Ophthalmoscopy gives the appearance of a featureless, grey haze. Partial recovery of vision is the rule, as the blood is reabsorbed, but repeated bleeds may occur.

Loss of vision may also result from fibrous proliferation associated with new vessel formation. This may give rise to traction bands that contract with the course of time, producing retinal detachment.

### Cataracts

Senile cataracts develop some 10–15 years earlier in diabetic patients than in the remainder of the population.

Juvenile or 'snowflake' cataracts are much less common. These are diffuse, rapidly progressive cataracts associated with very poorly controlled diabetes. They should be distinguished from temporary lens changes that occasionally appear during hyperosmolar coma and resolve when the coma is brought under control.

### Examination of the eye

Careful systematic examination of the eye is essential. Visual acuity and eye movements are tested, and the pupils are dilated with a quick-acting mydriatic such as tropicamide 0.5%. Dilating drugs should not be used in patients with a history of glaucoma, except with the advice of an ophthalmologist.

The examination begins at arm's length. At this distance, cataracts are silhouetted against the red reflex of the retina. The ophthalmoscope is advanced until the retina is in focus. The examination begins at the optic disc, moves through each quadrant in turn, and ends with the macula (since this is least comfortable for the patient). The ophthalmoscope is then adjusted to the +10 dioptre lens for examination of the cornea, anterior chamber and lens. The location of abnormalities should always be sketched in the notes for future reference.

### Management of diabetic eye disease

There is no specific medical treatment for background retinopathy, but patients are advised not to smoke and hypertension should be treated. Rapid progression may occur in pregnant patients and in those with nephropathy, and these groups need frequent monitoring. All patients with retinopathy should be examined regularly by a diabetologist or ophthalmologist. Early referral to an ophthalmologist is essential in the following circumstances:

- Deteriorating visual acuity
- Hard exudates encroaching on the macula
- Preproliferative changes (cotton-wool spots or venous beading)
- New vessel formation

The ophthalmologist may perform fluorescein angiography to define the extent of the problem. Maculopathy and proliferative retinopathy are treatable by retinal laser photocoagulation; in the latter condition early effective therapy reduces the risk of visual loss by about 50%. The value of photocoagulation is particularly marked in those with disc (as against peripheral) new vessels. In one trial only 15% of treated, as against 50% of untreated, eyes with disc new vessels progressed to legal blindness. Treatment in this case is by panretinal photocoagulation with 2000–5000 laser burns to each eye.

## The diabetic kidney

The kidney may be damaged by diabetes in three main ways:

1 Glomerular damage
2 Ischaemia due to hypertrophy of afferent and efferent arterioles
3 Ascending infection

### Diabetic glomerulosclerosis

Clinical nephropathy secondary to glomerular disease usually manifests 15–25 years after diagnosis and affects 30–40% of patients diagnosed under the age of 30 years. It is the leading cause of premature death in young diabetic patients. Older patients may also develop nephropathy, but the proportion affected is much smaller.

The earliest functional abnormality in the diabetic kidney is renal hypertrophy associated with a raised glomerular filtration rate; this appears soon after diagnosis and is related to poor glycaemic control.

The initial structural lesion in the glomerulus is thickening of the basement membrane. Associated changes may result in disruption of the protein cross-linkages that make the membrane an effective filter. In consequence, a progressive leak of protein into the urine occurs. The earliest evidence of this is 'microalbuminuria' (i.e. amounts of urinary albumin so small as to be undetectable by dipsticks (see p. 440)), which in turn may, after some years, progress to intermittent albuminuria followed by persistent proteinuria. Light-microscopic changes of glomerulosclerosis become manifest; both diffuse and nodular glomerulosclerosis can occur. The latter is sometimes known as the *Kimmelstiel–Wilson lesion*. At a later stage still, the glomerulus is replaced by hyaline material.

At the stage of persistent proteinuria, the plasma creatinine is normal but the average patient is only some 8–10 years from end-stage renal failure. The proteinuria may become so heavy as to induce a transient nephrotic syndrome, with peripheral oedema and hypoalbuminaemia.

Patients with nephropathy typically show a normochromic normocytic anaemia and a raised erythrocyte sedimentation rate (ESR). Hypertension is a common development and may itself damage the kidney still further. A rise in plasma creatinine is a late feature that progresses inevitably to renal failure, although the rate of progression may vary widely between individuals.

The natural history of this process is shown in Fig. 17.11. A curious feature is that almost all patients with long-established diabetes have abnormalities on renal biopsy but only a proportion develop the features of a progressive renal disease.

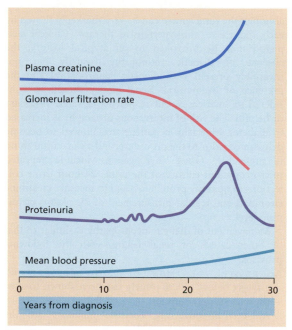

**Fig. 17.11** Schematic representation of the natural history of nephropathy. The typical onset is 15 years after diagnosis. Intermittent proteinuria leads to persistent proteinuria. In time, the plasma creatinine rises as the glomerular filtration rate falls.

### Ischaemic lesions

Arteriolar lesions, with hypertrophy and hyalinization of the vessels, affect both afferent and efferent arterioles. The appearances are similar to those of hypertensive disease but are not necessarily related to the blood pressure in patients with diabetes.

### Infective lesions

Urinary tract infections are more common in women but not men with diabetes. Ascending infection may occur because of bladder stasis due to autonomic neuropathy, and infections more easily become established in damaged renal tissue. Autopsy material frequently reveals interstitial changes suggestive of infection, but ischaemia may produce similar changes and the true frequency of pyelonephritis in diabetes remains uncertain.

Untreated infections in diabetics can result in renal papillary necrosis, in which renal papillae are shed in the urine, but this complication is rare.

### Diagnosis and management of diabetic nephropathy

The urine of all diabetic patients should be checked regularly for the presence of protein. Many centres also screen for microalbuminuria since there is some evidence that meticulous glycaemic control or early antihypertensive treatment at this stage may delay the onset of frank proteinuria. Once proteinuria is present, other possible causes for this should be considered (see below), but once these are excluded, a presumptive diagnosis of diabetic nephropathy can be made. For practical purposes this implies inevitable progression to end-stage renal failure, although the time course can be very markedly slowed by early aggressive antihypertensive therapy. Clinical suspicion may be provoked by an atypical history, the absence of diabetic retinopathy (usually but not invariably present with diabetic nephropathy) and the presence of haematuria. Renal biopsy should be considered in such cases, but in practice is rarely necessary or helpful. The risk of intravenous urography is increased in diabetes, especially if patients are allowed to become dehydrated prior to the procedure, and a renal ultrasound is preferable. Other investigations include repeated microscopy and culture of the urine, 24-hour urine collections to quantify protein loss and to measure creatinine clearance, and regular measurement of the plasma creatinine level.

Management of diabetic nephropathy is similar to that of other causes of renal failure, with the following provisos:

AGGRESSIVE TREATMENT OF BLOOD PRESSURE with a target below 140/90 mmHg has been shown to slow the rate of deterioration of renal failure considerably. Angiotensin-converting enzyme inhibitors are the drugs of choice (see p. 622).

ORAL HYPOGLYCAEMIC AGENTS partially excreted via the kidney (e.g. chlorpropamide) must be avoided.

INSULIN SENSITIVITY INCREASES and drastic reductions in dosage may be needed.

DIABETIC RETINOPATHY tends to progress rapidly and frequent ophthalmic supervision is essential.

Management of end-stage disease is made more difficult by the fact that patients often have other complications of diabetes such as blindness, autonomic neuropathy or peripheral vascular disease. Vascular shunts tend to calcify rapidly and hence chronic ambulatory peritoneal dialysis may be preferable to haemodialysis. The failure rate of renal transplants is somewhat higher than in non-

diabetic patients. A segmental pancreatic graft is sometimes performed at the same time as a renal graft. Although pancreatic grafts have a limited viability, owing to progressive fibrosis within the graft, they may give the patient a year or so of freedom from insulin injections.

Diabetic nephropathy is becoming less common as diabetic care improves.

## Diabetic neuropathy

Diabetes can damage peripheral nervous tissue in a number of ways. The vascular hypothesis postulates occlusion of the vasa nervorum as the prime cause. This seems likely in isolated mononeuropathies but the diffuse symmetrical nature of the common forms of neuropathy implies a metabolic cause. Since hyperglycaemia leads to increased formation of sorbitol and fructose in Schwann cells, accumulation of these sugars may disrupt function and structure.

The earliest functional change in diabetic nerves is delayed nerve conduction velocity; the earliest histological change is segmental demyelination, due to damage to Schwann cells. In the early stages axons are preserved, implying prospects of recovery, but at a later stage irreversible axonal degeneration develops.

The following varieties of neuropathy may occur (Fig. 17.12):

1 Symmetrical mainly sensory polyneuropathy (distal)
2 Acute painful neuropathy
3 Mononeuropathy and multiple mononeuropathy:
   (a) Cranial nerve lesions
   (b) Isolated peripheral nerve lesions
4 Diabetic amyotrophy
5 Autonomic neuropathy

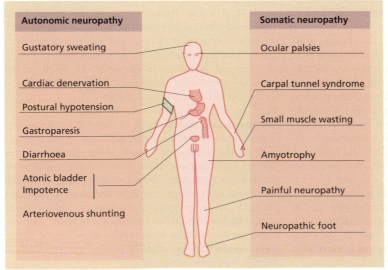

**Fig. 17.12** The neuropathic man.

## Symmetrical mainly sensory polyneuropathy

This is often unrecognized by the patient in its early stages. Early clinical signs are loss of vibration sense, pain sensation (deep before superficial) and temperature sensation in the feet. At later stages patients may complain of a feeling of 'walking on cotton wool' and can lose their balance when washing the face or walking in the dark owing to impaired proprioception. Involvement of the hands is less common and results in a 'stocking and glove' sensory loss. Complications include unrecognized trauma, beginning as blistering due to an ill-fitting shoe or a hot water bottle, and leading to ulceration.

SEQUELAE OF NEUROPATHY. Involvement of motor nerves to the small muscles of the feet gives rise to interosseous wasting. Unbalanced traction by the long flexor muscles leads to a characteristic shape of the foot, with a high arch and clawing of the toes, which in turn leads to abnormal distribution of pressure on walking, resulting in callus formation under the first metatarsal head or on the tips of the toes and perforating neuropathic ulceration.

Neuropathic arthropathy (Charcot's joints) may sometimes develop in the ankle. The hands show small-muscle wasting as well as sensory changes but it is important to differentiate these signs and symptoms from those of the carpal tunnel syndrome, which occurs with increased frequency in diabetes and may be amenable to surgery.

## Acute painful neuropathy

A diffuse, painful neuropathy is rare. The patient describes burning or crawling pains in the feet, shins and anterior thighs. These symptoms are typically worse at night, and pressure from bedclothes may be intolerable. It may present at diagnosis or develop after sudden improvement in glycaemic control (e.g. when insulin is started). It usually remits spontaneously after 3–12 months if good control is maintained. A more chronic form, developing later in the course of the disease, is sometimes resistant to almost all forms of therapy. Neurological assessment is difficult because of the hyperaesthesia experienced by the patient, but muscle wasting is not a feature and objective signs can be minimal.

## Mononeuropathy and multiple mononeuropathy

CRANIAL NERVE LESIONS. Isolated or multiple palsies of nerves to the external eye muscles, especially the third and sixth nerves, are more common in diabetes. A characteristic feature of diabetic third nerve lesions is that pupillary reflexes are retained owing to sparing of pupillomotor fibres. Full spontaneous recovery is the rule.

ISOLATED PERIPHERAL NERVE LESIONS. Manifestations may be sensory, motor, or mixed, and multiple nerves may be involved ('mononeuritis multiplex'). The onset is usually abrupt and sometimes painful; recovery is typically slow and incomplete. Lesions are more likely to occur at common sites for external pressure palsies or nerve entrapment, e.g. the median nerve in the carpal tunnel.

## Diabetic amyotrophy

This condition is usually seen in older men with diabetes. Presentation is with painful wasting, usually asymmetrical, of the quadriceps muscles. The wasting may be very marked and knee reflexes are diminished or absent. The affected area is often extremely tender. Extensor plantar responses sometimes develop and CSF protein content is elevated. Diabetic amyotrophy is usually associated with periods of poor glycaemic control and may be present at diagnosis. It often resolves in time with careful control of the blood glucose.

## Autonomic neuropathy

Asymptomatic autonomic disturbances can be demonstrated on laboratory testing in many patients, but symptomatic autonomic neuropathy is rare. It affects both the sympathetic and parasympathetic nervous system and can be disabling.

THE CARDIOVASCULAR SYSTEM. Vagal neuropathy results in tachycardia at rest and loss of sinus arrhythmia. At a later stage the heart may become denervated (resembling a transplanted heart). Cardiovascular reflexes such as the Valsalva manoeuvre are impaired.

Postural hypotension occurs owing to loss of sympathetic tone to peripheral arterioles. A warm foot with a bounding pulse is sometimes seen in a polyneuropathy as a result of peripheral vasodilatation.

GASTROINTESTINAL TRACT. Vagal damage can lead to gastroparesis, often asymptomatic, but sometimes leading to intractable vomiting. Diarrhoea often occurs at night accompanied by urgency and incontinence. Diarrhoea and steatorrhoea may occur owing to bacterial overgrowth and treatment is with antibiotics.

BLADDER INVOLVEMENT. Loss of tone, incomplete emptying, and stasis (predisposing to infection) can occur, and may ultimately result in an atonic, painless, distended bladder.

IMPOTENCE. This is common. The first manifestation is incomplete erection which may in time progress to total impotence; retrograde ejaculation also occurs. However, impotence in diabetes is not always due to autonomic neuropathy. Other causes include anxiety, depression, alcohol excess, drugs, primary or secondary gonadal failure and inadequate vascular supply due to atheroma in pudendal arteries. Treatment should ideally include sympathetic counselling of both partners. Some patients may benefit from intracavernous injection of papaverine (see p. 789) or the use of vacuum devices to produce an erection which is then maintained by slipping a tight rubber band over the base of the penis until intercourse is complete.

# The diabetic foot

Many amputations in diabetes could be delayed or prevented by more effective patient education and medical supervision. Ischaemia, infection and neuropathy combine to produce tissue necrosis. Although these factors may coexist, it is important to distinguish between the ischaemic and the neuropathic foot (Table 17.8).

### Management of the diabetic foot

Many diabetic foot problems are avoidable, so patients need to learn the principles of foot care and should be advised concerning appropriate footwear and the risks of smoking. Older patients should visit a chiropodist regularly and should not cut their own toe-nails.

Once tissue damage has occurred in the form of ulceration or gangrene, the aim is preservation of viable tissue. The two main threats are:

INFECTION. This rapidly takes hold in a diabetic foot, and early effective antibiotic treatment is essential. Collections of pus are drained and excision of infected bone is needed if osteomyelitis develops and does not respond to appropriate antibiotic therapy. Regular X-rays of the foot are needed to check on progress.

ISCHAEMIA. The blood flow to the feet is assessed clinically or with the Doppler ultrasound stethoscope. Femoral arteriography may be performed, since localized areas of occlusion may be amenable to bypass surgery or angioplasty.

Foot problems are the major cause of hospital bed occupancy by diabetic patients. Good liaison between surgeon and physician is essential if this period in hospital is to be used efficiently. When irreversible arterial insufficiency is present, it is often quicker and kinder to opt for an early major amputation rather than subject the patient to a debilitating sequence of conservative procedures.

# Infections

There is no evidence that diabetic patients with good glycaemic control are more prone to infection than normal subjects. However, poorly controlled diabetes entails increased susceptibility to the following infections:

1 *Skin*
   (a) Staphylococcal infections (boils, abscesses, carbuncles)
   (b) Mucocutaneous candidiasis
2 *Urinary tract*
   (a) Urinary tract infections (in women)
   (b) Pyelonephritis
   (c) Perinephric abscess
3 *Lungs*
   (a) Staphylococcal and pneumococcal pneumonia
   (b) Gram-negative bacterial pneumonia
   (c) Tuberculosis

One reason why poor control lends to infection is that chemotaxis and phagocytosis by polymorphonuclear leucocytes is impaired at high blood glucose concentrations.

Conversely, infections may lead to loss of glycaemic control, and are a common cause of ketoacidosis. Insulin-treated patients need to increase their dose by up to 25% in the face of infection, and non-insulin-treated patients may need insulin cover while the infection lasts. Patients should be told never to omit their insulin dose, even if they are nauseated and unable to eat; instead they should test their blood glucose frequently and seek urgent medical advice.

## Skin and joints (see p. 1023 and p. 412)

Joint contractures in the hands are a common consequence of childhood diabetes. The sign may be demonstrated by asking the patient to join the hands as if in prayer; the metacarpophalangeal and interphalangeal joints cannot be apposed. Thickened, waxy skin can be noted on the backs of the fingers. These features may be due to glycosylation of collagen and are not progressive. The condition is sometimes referred to as diabetic cheiroarthropathy.

Osteopenia in the extremities is also described in IDDM but rarely leads to clinical consequences.

# SPECIAL SITUATIONS

## Surgery

Smooth control of diabetes minimizes the risk of infection and balances the catabolic response to anaesthesia and surgery. The procedure for insulin-treated patients is simple:

1 Long acting and/or intermediate insulin should be stopped the day before surgery with soluble insulin substituted.
2 Whenever possible, diabetic patients should be first on the morning theatre list.
3 An infusion of glucose, insulin and potassium is given during surgery. The insulin can be injected into the glucose solution or administered by syringe pump. A standard combination is 16 U of soluble insulin with 10 mmol KCl in 500 ml of 10% dextrose, infused at 100 ml hour$^{-1}$.
4 Postoperatively, the infusion is maintained until the patient is able to eat. Other fluids needed in the peri-

| | Ischaemia | Neuropathy |
|---|---|---|
| Symptoms: | Claudication<br>Rest pain | Usually painless<br>Sometimes painful<br>neuropathy |
| Inspection: | Dependent rubor<br>Trophic changes | High arch<br>Clawing of toes<br>No trophic changes |
| Palpation: | Cold<br>Pulseless | Warm<br>Bounding pulses |
| Ulceration: | Painful<br>Heels and toes | Painless<br>Plantar |

**Table 17.8** Distinguishing features between ischaemia and neuropathy in the diabetic foot.

operative period must be given through a separate intravenous line and must not interrupt the glucose/insulin/potassium infusion. Glucose levels are checked every 2–4 hours and potassium levels are monitored. The amount of insulin and potassium in each infusion bag is adjusted either upwards or downwards according to the results of regular monitoring of the blood glucose and serum potassium concentrations.

The same approach is used in the emergency situation, with the exception that a separate variable rate insulin infusion may be needed to bring blood glucose under control before surgery.

Non-insulin-treated patients should stop medication 2 days before the operation. Patients with mild hyperglycaemia (fasting blood glucose below 8 mmol litre$^{-1}$) can be treated as non-diabetic. Those with higher levels are treated with soluble insulin prior to surgery, and with glucose, insulin and potassium during and after the procedure, as for insulin-treated patients.

## Pregnancy and diabetes

Modern management has transformed the outcome of pregnancy in women with diabetes. Thirty years ago one pregnancy in three ended with the death of the fetus or neonate. Today, the results in specialized centres approach those of non-diabetic pregnancy. This improvement is due to meticulous glycaemic control and careful medical and obstetric management. When the pregnancy is planned, optimal glycaemic control is sought prior to conception.

### Glycaemic control in pregnancy
The patient should perform daily home blood glucose profiles; the renal threshold falls in pregnancy and urine tests are therefore of little or no value. Insulin requirements rise, and intensified insulin regimens may become necessary. The aim is to maintain blood glucose and Hb A$_{1c}$ or fructosamine levels within the normal range.

### General management
The patient is seen at intervals of 2 weeks or less at a clinic managed jointly by obstetrician and physician. Circumstances permitting, the aim should be outpatient management with a spontaneous vaginal delivery at term. Retinopathy and nephropathy may deteriorate during pregnancy. Expert fundoscopy and urine testing for protein should be undertaken at booking, 28 weeks and before delivery.

### Obstetric problems associated with diabetes
Poorly controlled diabetes is associated with macrosomia, hydramnios, pre-eclampsia and intrauterine death. Ketoacidosis in pregnancy carries a 50% fetal mortality, but maternal hypoglycaemia is relatively well tolerated.

### Neonatal problems
Maternal diabetes, especially when poorly controlled, is associated with fetal macrosomia. The infant of a diabetic mother is more susceptible to hyaline membrane disease than non-diabetic infants of similar maturity. In addition, neonatal hypoglycaemia may occur. The mechanism is as follows: maternal glucose crosses the placenta, but insulin does not; the fetal islets hypersecrete to combat maternal hyperglycaemia, and a rebound to hypoglycaemic levels occurs when the umbilical cord is severed.

These complications are due to hyperglycaemia in the third trimester. Poor glycaemic control in the first trimester carries an increased risk of congenital malformations, particularly of the cardiovascular and central nervous systems.

### Gestational diabetes
This term refers to glucose intolerance that develops in the course of pregnancy and remits following delivery.

The condition is typically asymptomatic and is demonstrated biochemically on the basis of random testing in each trimester and by oral glucose tolerance testing if the plasma glucose concentration is 7 mmol litre$^{-1}$ or more. Since the renal threshold for glucose falls during normal pregnancy and glucose tolerance deteriorates, the condition may easily be misdiagnosed.

Treatment is with diet in the first instance, but most patients require insulin cover during the pregnancy. Insulin does not cross the placenta. Oral agents are avoided because of the potential risk to the fetus as they do cross the placenta.

Gestational diabetes has been associated with a higher frequency of obstetric problems, fetal macrosomia and neonatal hypoglycaemia. It is likely to recur in subsequent pregnancies. Gestational diabetes is often the harbinger of NIDDM in later life.

Not all diabetes presenting in pregnancy is gestational. True IDDM may develop, and swift diagnosis is essential to prevent the development of ketoacidosis. Hospital admission is required if the patient is symptomatic, or has ketonuria or a markedly elevated blood glucose level.

## Brittle diabetes

There is no precise definition for this term, which is used to describe patients with recurrent ketoacidosis and/or recurrent hypoglycaemic coma. Of these, the largest group is made up of those who experience recurrent severe hypoglycaemia.

### Recurrent severe hypoglycaemia
This affects 1–3% of insulin-dependent patients. Most are adults who have had diabetes for more than 10 years. By this stage endogenous insulin secretion is negligible in the great majority of patients. Pancreatic $\alpha$ cells are still present in undiminished numbers, but the glucagon response to hypoglycaemia is virtually absent. Long-term patients are thus subject to fluctuating hyperinsulinaemia due to erratic absorption of insulin from injection sites, and lack a major component of the hormonal defence against hypoglycaemia. In this situation adrenaline secretion becomes vital, but this too may become impaired in the course of diabetes. Loss of adrenaline secretion has been attributed to autonomic neuropathy, but this is unlikely to be the sole cause; central adaptation to recurrent hypoglycaemia may also be a factor.

The following factors may also predispose to recurrent hypoglycaemia:

OVERTREATMENT WITH INSULIN. Frequent biochemical hypoglycaemia lowers the glucose level at which symptoms develop. Symptoms often reappear when overall glucose control is relaxed.

AN UNRECOGNIZED LOW RENAL THRESHOLD FOR GLUCOSE. Attempts to render the urine sugar-free will inevitably produce hypoglycaemia.

EXCESSIVE INSULIN DOSES. A common error is to increase the *dose* when a patient needs more frequent injections to overcome a problem of *timing*.

ENDOCRINE CAUSES. These include pituitary insufficiency, adrenal insufficiency and premenstrual insulin sensitivity.

ALIMENTARY CAUSES. These include exocrine pancreatic failure and diabetic gastroparesis.

RENAL FAILURE. The kidneys are important sites for the clearance of insulin which tends to accumulate if renal function is lost.

PATIENT CAUSES. Patients may be unintelligent, uncooperative or may manipulate their therapy.

### Recurrent ketoacidosis

This usually occurs in adolescents or young adults, and the most severe form is more common in girls. Although metabolic decompensation may develop very rapidly, it is often impossible to pin-point an underlying abnormality. Many theories exist concerning the causes of this condition, but all agree that it is heterogeneous. The following categories have been suggested:

IATROGENIC. Inappropriate insulin combinations may be a cause of swinging glycaemic control. For example, a once-daily regimen may cause hypoglycaemia during the afternoon or evening and pre-breakfast hyperglycaemia due to insulin deficiency.

INTERCURRENT ILLNESS. Unsuspected infections, including urinary tract infections and tuberculosis, may be present. Thyrotoxicosis can also manifest as unstable glycaemic control.

PSYCHOSOCIAL CAUSES. These certainly form the largest category. It has been suggested that neuroendocrine mechanisms such as catecholamine secretion might mediate the metabolic disturbance. Other patients undoubtedly manipulate their illness, whether consciously or unconsciously.

UNKNOWN AETIOLOGY. The most 'brittle' patients of all are usually female, aged 15–25 years and often overweight, and typically suffer from amenorrhoea. The insulin requirement is variable but is often high. Sophisticated 'cheating' has been detected in some of these patients, but this should never be assumed without convincing proof.

# Hypoglycaemia

Hypoglycaemia develops when hepatic glucose output falls below the rate of glucose uptake by peripheral tissues. Hepatic glucose output may be reduced by:

- The inhibition of hepatic glycogenolysis and gluconeogenesis by insulin
- Depletion of hepatic glycogen reserves by malnutrition, fasting, exercise or advanced liver disease
- Impaired gluconeogenesis (e.g. following alcohol ingestion)

In the first of these categories, insulin levels are raised, the liver contains adequate glycogen stores, and the hypoglycaemia can be reversed by injection of glucagon. In the other two situations, insulin levels are low and glucagon is ineffective.

Peripheral glucose uptake is accelerated by high insulin levels and by exercise, but these conditions are normally balanced by increased glucose output. Insulin or sulphonylurea therapy for diabetes accounts for the vast majority of cases of severe hypoglycaemia encountered in an accident and emergency department.

The commonest symptoms and signs of hypoglycaemia are neurological. The brain consumes about 50% of the total glucose produced by the liver. This high energy requirement is needed to generate ATP used to maintain the potential difference across axonal membranes.

## Insulinomas

Insulinomas are pancreatic islet cell tumours that secrete insulin. Most are sporadic but some patients have multiple tumours arising from neural crest tissue (multiple endocrine neoplasia). Some 95% of these tumours are benign. The classic presentation is with fasting hypoglycaemia, but early symptoms may also develop in the late morning or afternoon. Recurrent hypoglycaemia is often present for months or years before the diagnosis is made, and the symptoms may be atypical or even bizarre; the presenting features in one series are given in Table 17.9. Common misdiagnoses include psychiatric disorders, particularly pseudodementia in elderly people, epilepsy and cerebrovascular disease.

### DIAGNOSIS

Whipple's triad remains the basis of clinical diagnosis. This is satisfied when:

1 Symptoms are associated with fasting or exercise
2 Hypoglycaemia is confirmed during these episodes
3 Glucose relieves the symptoms

A fourth criterion—demonstration of inappropriately high insulin levels during hypoglycaemia—may usefully be added to these.

In practice, the diagnosis is confirmed by the demonstration of hypoglycaemia in association with inappropri-

| Diplopia |
| Sweating, palpitations, weakness |
| Confusion or abnormal behaviour |
| Loss of consciousness |
| Grand mal seizures |

**Table 17.9**  Presenting features of insulinoma.

ate and excessive insulin secretion. Hypoglycaemia is demonstrated by:

MEASUREMENT OF OVERNIGHT FASTING (16 HOURS) GLUCOSE AND INSULIN LEVELS ON THREE OCCASIONS. About 90% of patients with insulinomas will have low glucose and non-suppressed (normal or elevated) insulin levels.

PERFORMING A PROLONGED 72 HOUR SUPERVISED FAST if overnight testing is inconclusive and symptoms persist.

Autonomous insulin secretion is demonstrated by lack of the normal feedback suppression during hypoglycaemia. This may be shown by measuring insulin, C-peptide or proinsulin during a spontaneous episode of hypoglycaemia.

Many patients also have an abnormal (diabetic) glucose tolerance test, but this has no diagnostic value.

### TREATMENT

The most effective therapy is surgical excision of the tumour. Insulinomas are often very small and difficult to localize. Highly selective angiography and contrast-enhanced CT scanning are used in the first instance. Highly selective angiography is very operator dependent and referral to a skilled operator is warranted if initial attempts at localization fail. 'Blind' laparotomy runs the risk that the surgeon may be unable to find the insulinoma and resorts to partial pancreatectomy, with unpleasant consequences if the tumour remains in the unexcised pancreas. Localization is also possible using a rapid insulin assay on blood sampled at different levels from the pancreatic vein.

Medical treatment with diazoxide is useful when the insulinoma is malignant, in patients in whom a tumour cannot be located, and in elderly patients with mild symptoms. Symptoms may remit on treatment with the somatostatin analogue octreotide.

## Hypoglycaemia with other tumours

Hypoglycaemia may develop in the course of advanced neoplasia and cachexia, and has been described in association with many tumour types. Certain massive tumours, especially sarcomas, may produce hypoglycaemia due to secretion of insulin-like growth factor 1. True ectopic insulin secretion is extremely rare.

## Postprandial hypoglycaemia

If frequent *venous* blood glucose samples are taken following a prolonged glucose tolerance test, about one in four subjects will have at least one value below 3 mmol litre$^{-1}$. The arteriovenous glucose difference is quite marked during this phase, so that very few are truly hypoglycaemic in terms of arterial (or capillary) blood glucose content. Failure to appreciate this simple fact led some authorities to believe that postprandial (or reactive) hypoglycaemia was a potential 'organic' explanation for a variety of complaints that might otherwise have been

considered psychosomatic. An epidemic of false 'hypoglycaemia' followed, particularly in the USA. Later work showed a poor correlation between symptoms and biochemical hypoglycaemia. Even so, a number of otherwise normal people occasionally become pale, weak and sweaty at times when meals are due, and report benefit from advice to take regular snacks between meals.

True postprandial hypoglycaemia may develop in the presence of alcohol, which 'primes' the $\beta$ cells to produce an exaggerated insulin response to carbohydrate. The person who substitutes alcoholic beverages for lunch is particularly at risk. Postprandial hypoglycaemia sometimes occurs after gastric surgery, owing to rapid gastric emptying and mismatching of food and insulin. This is referred to as 'dumping' but it is now rarely encountered (see p. 194).

## Hepatic and renal causes of hypoglycaemia

The liver can maintain a normal glucose output despite extensive damage, and hepatic hypoglycaemia is uncommon. It is particularly a problem with fulminant hepatic failure.

The kidney has a subsidiary role in glucose production (via gluconeogenesis in the renal cortex), and hypoglycaemia is sometimes a problem in terminal renal failure.

Hereditary fructose intolerance occurs in 1 in 20 000 live births and can cause hypoglycaemia (see p. 863).

## Endocrine causes of hypoglycaemia

Endocrine disorders resulting in deficiencies of hormones antagonistic to insulin are rare but well-recognized causes of hypoglycaemia. These include hypopituitarism, isolated adrenocorticotrophic hormone (ACTH) deficiency and Addison's disease.

## Drug-induced hypoglycaemia

Many drugs have been reported to produce isolated cases of hypoglycaemia, but usually only when other predisposing factors are present. The following are among the more important:

SULPHONYLUREAS may be used in the treatment of diabetes or may be taken by non-diabetics in suicide attempts.

QUININE may produce severe hypoglycaemia in the course of treatment for falciparum malaria.

SALICYLATES may cause hypoglycaemia following accidental ingestion by children, but this complication is very rare in adults.

PROPRANOLOL has been reported to induce hypoglycaemia in the presence of strenuous exercise or starvation.

PENTAMIDINE may cause hypoglycaemia when used in the treatment of resistant *Pneumocystis* pneumonia in people with AIDS.

## Alcohol-induced hypoglycaemia

Alcohol inhibits gluconeogenesis. Alcohol-induced hypoglycaemia was first described in poorly nourished chronic alcoholics but may also present in binge drinkers and in children who have taken relatively small amounts of alcohol, since they have a diminished hepatic glycogen reserve. The clinical presentation is with coma and hypothermia.

## Factitious hypoglycaemia

This is a relatively common variant of self-induced disease and is much more common than an insulinoma. Hypoglycaemia is produced by surreptitious self-administration of insulin or sulphonylureas. Many patients in this category have been extensively investigated for an insulinoma. Measurement of C-peptide levels during hypoglycaemia should identify patients who are injecting insulin; sulphonylurea abuse can be detected by chromatography of plasma or urine.

## *Disorders of lipid metabolism*

## PHYSIOLOGY

Lipids are insoluble in water, and are transported in the bloodstream as macromolecular complexes. In these complexes, lipids (principally triglyceride, cholesterol and cholesterol esters) are surrounded by a stabilizing coat of phospholipid. Proteins (called apoproteins) embedded into the surface of these 'lipoprotein' particles exert both a stabilizing function and allow the particles to be recognized by receptors in the liver and the peripheral tissues. The structure of a chylomicron (one type of lipoprotein particle) is illustrated in Fig. 17.13.

The genes for all the major apoproteins and that for the low-density lipoprotein (LDL) receptor have been isolated, sequenced and their chromosomal sites mapped. Production of abnormal apoproteins is known to produce, or predispose to, several types of lipid disorder, and it is likely that others will be discovered. Genetic abnor-malities which affect the LDL receptor cause familial hypercholesterolaemia.

Five principal types of lipoprotein particles are found in the blood (Fig. 17.14). They are structurally different and can be separated in the laboratory by their density and electrophoretic mobility. The larger particles give postprandial plasma its cloudy appearance.

### Chylomicrons

Chylomicrons are synthesized in the small intestine postprandially. They contain triglyceride and a small amount of cholesterol, and provide the main mechanism for transporting the digestion products of dietary fat to the liver and peripheral tissues. Each newly formed chylomicron contains several different apoproteins (B-48, A-I, A-II), and acquires apoproteins C-II and E by transfer from high-density lipoprotein (HDL) particles in the bloodstream. Apoprotein C-II binds to specific receptors in the peripheral tissues and the liver and allows the endothelial enzyme, lipoprotein lipase, to remove triglyceride from the particle. The remaining chylomicron remnant particle, which contains most of the original cholesterol, is taken up by the liver by mechanisms which are still not fully understood, possibly mediated by apoprotein E.

### Very low density lipoprotein (VLDL) particles

These are synthesized and secreted by the liver and contain most of the endogenously synthesized triglyceride

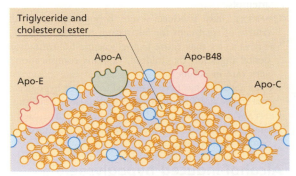

**Fig. 17.13** Schematic diagram of the surface of a chylomicron particle (75–1200 nm) showing the apoprotein lying in the membrane.

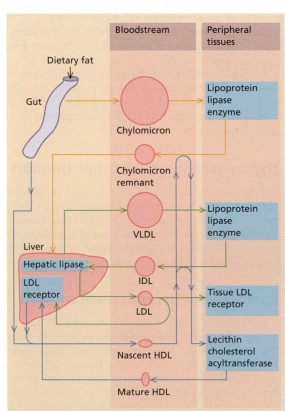

**Fig. 17.14** Schematic representation of the sites of origin, interaction between and fate of the major lipoprotein particles.

and a smaller quantity of cholesterol. Apoprotein B-100 is an essential component. Apoproteins C and E are later incorporated into VLDL by transfer from HDL particles. As they pass round the circulation VLDL particles bind through apoprotein C allowing triglyceride to be progressively removed by lipoprotein lipase. This leaves a particle, now depleted of triglyceride and apoprotein C, called an intermediate-density lipoprotein (IDL) particle.

### Intermediate-density lipoprotein particles

These also contain apoprotein B-100 and can bind to the hepatocyte through apoprotein E. Once bound, IDL particles can be catabolized, or have further triglyceride removed (by the enzyme hepatic lipase) producing LDL particles.

### Low-density lipoprotein particles

LDL particles are the main carrier of cholesterol, and deliver it both to the liver and to peripheral cells. The surface of the LDL particle contains a single apoprotein B-100, and also apoprotein E. The apoprotein B-100 is the principal ligand for the LDL receptor. This receptor lies within coated pits on the surface of the hepatocyte. Once bound to the receptor, the coated pit invaginates and fuses with liposomes which destroy the LDL particle (Fig. 17.15). The number of hepatic LDL receptors regulates the circulating LDL concentration. The circulating LDL concentration is also regulated by controlling the activity of the rate-limiting enzyme in the cholesterol synthetic pathway, hydroxymethylglutaryl coenzyme A (HMG-CoA) reductase. Not all the cholesterol synthesized by the liver is packaged immediately into lipoprotein particles. Some is converted into bile salts. Both bile salts and cholesterol are excreted in the bile: both are then reabsorbed through the terminal ileum and recirculated (enterohepatic circulation).

### High-density lipoprotein particles

HDL particles are produced in both the liver and intestine. The nascent particles are disc shaped, seemingly inert and contain E apoproteins. They are modified by acquiring some surface components of chylomicron and VLDL particles as these are broken down into smaller particles. The materials gained by the nascent HDL particles include phospholipids, and the A and C apoproteins. The more mature HDL particles take up cholesterol from cell membranes in the peripheral tissues. As it is taken up the enzyme lecithin–cholesterol acyltransferase (LCAT), activated by the apoprotein A on the particle's surface, esterifies the sequestered cholesterol. The HDL particle is then capable of transporting this cholesterol away from the periphery to the liver (reverse cholesterol transport) where it binds through apoprotein E. HDL particles carry 20–30% of the total quantity of cholesterol in the blood.

When a laboratory measures fasting serum lipids, the majority of the total cholesterol concentration consists of LDL particles with a 20–30% contribution from HDL particles. The triglyceride concentration largely reflects the circulating number of VLDL particles, since chylomicrons are not normally present in the fasted state. If the patient is not fasted the total triglyceride concentration will be raised due to the presence of triglyceride-rich chylomicrons as well as VLDL particles.

# EVIDENCE FOR A RELATIONSHIP BETWEEN LIPOPROTEIN CONCENTRATIONS, ATHEROMA AND CARDIOVASCULAR RISK

### LDL cholesterol

EPIDEMIOLOGICAL LINKS BETWEEN CHOLESTEROL AND CORONARY HEART DISEASE. Population studies have repeatedly demonstrated a strong association between both total and LDL cholesterol concentration and coronary heart risk. There is a strong link between mean fat consumption, mean serum cholesterol concentration and the prevalence of coronary heart disease between countries. The exception is France where the cardiovascular risk is only moderate—perhaps due to high alcohol consumption. Studies of migrants, particularly of Japanese men migrating to Hawaii, have shown that as diet changes, and cholesterol concentrations rise, so does the cardiovascular risk. Such studies show the importance of the environment rather than the genetic make-up of a population.

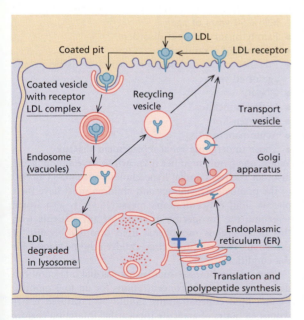

**Fig. 17.15** Receptor-mediated endocytosis. LDL receptors are formed in the endoplasmic reticulum and transported via the Golgi apparatus to the cell surface. LDLs bind to these receptors, are internalized and taken up by the endosome. The receptor is recycled back to the surface, while the LDL is broken down by the lysosomes, freeing cholesterol needed for membrane synthesis.

The Multiple Risk Factor Intervention Trial (MRFIT) screened one-third of a million American men for various cardiovascular risk factors and then followed them for 6 years. Data from this study have shown that although cardiovascular risk rises progressively as total cholesterol concentration increases (Fig. 17.16), the risk increase is modest for individuals with no other cardiovascular risk factors. With each additional risk factor (see Table 18.25), the effect produced by the same difference in cholesterol concentration becomes greatly magnified. The Framingham Study has reproduced these findings in a separate population.

ANIMAL AND BIOCHEMICAL STUDIES. Diverse laboratory studies have shown a strong link between dietary fat intake, resultant elevation of LDL cholesterol concentrations and the development of atheroma.

PATIENTS WITH MONOGENIC INHERITED LIPID DISORDERS. Young men with the monogenic disorder familial hypercholesterolaemia are normal apart from considerably elevated LDL cholesterol concentrations, yet they die of premature cardiovascular disease, and only 20–30% reach retirement age.

PREVENTION TRIALS. Two large well-controlled primary prevention studies (the Lipid Research Clinics Trial and the Helsinki Heart Study) have shown an increasing improvement in cardiovascular risk with increasing duration of treatment for hyperlipidaemia. (Intervention trials are discussed more fully below.)

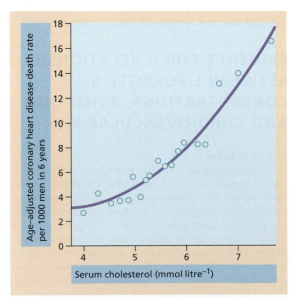

**Fig. 17.16** The Multiple Risk Factor Intervention Trial: relationship between levels of serum cholesterol and risks of fatal coronary artery disease in a longitudinal study of more than 361 000 men screened for entry into the trial. (From Stamler J, Wentworth D & Neaton JD (1986) *Journal of the American Medical Association* **256**, 2823.)

### HDL cholesterol

Epidemiological studies have shown that HDL particles appear to protect against atheroma. This effect may be due to the ability of the particle to transport cholesterol from the peripheral tissues to the liver. HDL particles have important effects on the function of platelets and of the haemostatic cascade. These properties may favourably influence thrombogenesis.

### VLDL particles

There is a weaker independent link between raised concentrations of (triglyceride-rich) VLDL particles and cardiovascular risk. The evidence is only epidemiological so there is a weaker case for the treatment of hypertriglyceridaemia when it occurs alone.

### Chylomicrons

Excess chylomicrons do not confer an excess cardiovascular risk, but raise the total plasma triglyceride concentration.

## Screening

Most patients with hyperlipidaemia are asymptomatic and have no clinical signs. Many are discovered whilst screening high-risk individuals.

### Whose lipids should be measured?

There are great doubts as to whether blanket screening of plasma lipids is warranted. Selective screening of people at high risk of cardiovascular disease should be undertaken including those with:

- Family history of coronary heart disease (especially below 50 years of age)
- Family history of lipid disorders
- Presence of a xanthoma
- Presence of xanthelasma or corneal arcus before the age of 40 years
- Obesity
- Diabetes mellitus
- Hypertension
- Acute pancreatitis
- Those undergoing renal replacement therapy

Where one family member is known to have a monogenic disorder such as familial hypercholesterolaemia (1 in 500 of the population), siblings and children must have their plasma lipid concentrations measured. It is also worth screening the prospective partners of any patients with this heterozygous monogenic lipid disorder because of the small risk of producing children homozygous for the condition.

Acute severe illnesses such as myocardial infarction can derange plasma lipid concentrations for up to 3 months. Plasma lipid concentrations should be measured either within 48 hours of an acute myocardial infarction (before derangement has had time to occur) or 3 months later.

Serum cholesterol concentration does not change significantly after a meal and as a screening test a random blood sample is sufficient. If the total cholesterol concentration is raised above 6.5 mmol litre$^{-1}$, HDL cholesterol, triglyceride, and LDL cholesterol concentrations should be quantitated on a fasting sample. If a test for hypertriglyceridaemia is needed, a fasting blood sample is mandatory.

## SECONDARY HYPERLIPIDAEMIA

If a lipid disorder has been detected it is vital to carry out a clinical history, examination and simple special investigations to detect causes of secondary hyperlipidaemia (Table 17.10), which may need treatment in their own right. The biochemical tests needed are for thyroid stimulating hormone, fasting blood glucose concentration, urea and electrolyte concentrations and liver biochemistry.

## CLASSIFICATION, CLINICAL FEATURES AND INVESTIGATION OF PRIMARY HYPERLIPIDAEMIAS

As the genetic basis of lipid disorders becomes clearer the genetic classification of Goldstein and colleagues is proving of greater clinical relevance than the Fredrickson (WHO) classification (based on the pattern of lipoproteins found in plasma). The lack of direct correspondence between these two systems of classification can be confusing. For clarity we have used the genetic classification and not the Fredrickson classification. This has the advantage that the genetic disorders may be grouped by the results of simple lipid biochemistry into causes of hypertriglyceridaemia alone, hypercholesterolaemia alone or of combined hyperlipidaemia.

### Hypertriglyceridaemia alone (without hypercholesterolaemia)

The majority of cases will be due to multiple genes acting together to produce a modest excess circulating concentration of VLDL particles, such cases being termed *polygenic hypertriglyceridaemia*. In a proportion of cases there will be a family history of a lipid disorder or its effects (pancreatitis). Such cases are often classified as *familial hypertriglyceridaemia*. The defect underlying the vast majority of such cases is not understood. The only clinical feature is a history of attacks of pancreatitis or retinal vein thrombosis in some individuals.

LIPOPROTEIN LIPASE DEFICIENCY AND APOPROTEIN C-II DEFICIENCY are rare diseases which produce

greatly elevated triglyceride concentrations due to the persistence of chylomicrons (and not VLDL particles) in the circulation. The chylomicrons persist because the triglyceride within cannot be metabolized if the enzyme lipoprotein lipase is defective or because they cannot gain access to the normal enzyme due to deficiency of the apoprotein C-II on the surface of the chylomicron particles. The disorder is unlikely to be confused clinically with cases of polygenic or familial hypertriglyceridaemia as the patients present in childhood with eruptive xanthomas, lipaemia retinalis and retinal vein thrombosis, pancreatitis and hepatosplenomegaly. If the disorder is not identified in childhood it can present in adults with gross hypertriglyceridaemia resistant to simple measures. The most important test is to confirm the presence of chylomicrons in fasting plasma stored overnight (chylomicrons float like cream). This is confirmed by plasma electrophoresis or ultracentrifugation. An abnormality of apoprotein C can be deduced if the hypertriglyceridaemia improves temporarily after infusing fresh frozen plasma, and lipoprotein lipase deficiency is likely if it does not.

### Hypercholesterolaemia (without hypertriglyceridaemia)

The monogenic disorder of heterozygous *familial hypercholesterolaemia* is present in 1 in 500 of the normal population. The average general practitioner would therefore be expected to have four such patients on his or her list, but because of clustering within families the prevalence is lower in some general practice lists and much higher in others. Surprisingly, most individuals with this disorder remain undetected. Patients may have no physical signs, in which case the diagnosis is made on the presence of very high plasma cholesterol concentrations which are unresponsive to dietary modification and are associated with a typical family history. Diagnosis can be more easily made if typical clinical features are present. These include xanthomatous thickening of the Achilles tendons and xanthomas over the extensor tendons of the fingers. Xanthelasma may be present, but is not diagnostic of familial hypercholesterolaemia. The genetic defect of this disorder is the underproduction or malproduction of the LDL cholesterol receptor in the liver. Many different monogenic lesions producing various abnormalities of the receptor have been described in different families.

Homozygous familial hypercholesterolaemia is very rare indeed. Affected children have no LDL receptors in the liver. They have a hugely elevated LDL cholesterol concentration, and massive deposition of lipid in arterial walls, the aorta and the skin. The natural history is for death from ischaemic heart disease in late childhood or adolescence. Plasmapheresis has been used to regularly remove LDL cholesterol with some success in these patients. Liver transplantation offers the possibility of cure, but the numbers of patients having undergone this procedure is small. The possibility of gene therapy offers a glimmer of hope on the horizon for affected individuals.

Patients who have raised serum cholesterol concentrations, but do not have familial hypercholesterolaemia

| |
|---|
| Hypothyroidism |
| Diabetes mellitus (when poorly controlled) |
| Obesity |
| Renal impairment |
| Nephrotic syndrome |
| Dysglobulinaemia |
| Hepatic dysfunction |
| Drugs: oral contraceptives in susceptible individuals, retinoids, thiazide diuretics, corticosteroids, opDDD (used in the treatment of Cushing's syndrome) |

**Table 17.10**   Causes of secondary hyperlipidaemia.

exist in the right hand tail of the normal distribution of cholesterol concentration, and are deemed to have *polygenic hypercholesterolaemia*. The precise nature of the polygenic variation in plasma cholesterol concentration remains unknown.

## Combined hyperlipidaemia (hypercholesterolaemia and hypertriglyceridaemia)

The most common patient group is a *polygenic combined hyperlipidaemia*.

FAMILIAL COMBINED HYPERLIPIDAEMIA is relatively common affecting 1 in 200 of the general population. The genetic basis for the disorder has not yet been characterized. It is diagnosed by finding raised cholesterol and triglyceride concentrations in association with a typical family history.

REMNANT HYPERLIPIDAEMIA is a rare cause of combined hyperlipidaemia. It is due to accumulation of LDL remnant particles and is associated with an extremely high risk of cardiovascular disease. It may be suspected in a patient with raised total cholesterol and triglyceride concentrations by finding xanthomas in the palmar creases (diagnostic) and the presence of tuberous xanthomas typically over the knees and elbows. Remnant hyperlipidaemia is almost always due to the inheritance of a variant of the apoprotein E allele (apoprotein E2) together with an aggravating factor such as another primary hyperlipidaemia. When suspected clinically the diagnosis can be confirmed using ultracentrifugation of plasma, or phenotyping apoprotein E.

## MANAGEMENT OF HYPERLIPIDAEMIA (Table 17.11)

### Hypertriglyceridaemia (without hypercholesterolaemia)

A serum triglyceride concentration below 2.0 mmol litre$^{-1}$ is normal. In the range 2.0–6.0 mmol litre$^{-1}$ no specific intervention will be needed unless there are many coincident cardiovascular risk factors, and in particular a strong family history of early cardiovascular death. In general, patients should be advised that they have a minor lipid problem, offered advice on weight reduction if obese, and advice on correcting other cardiovascular risk factors.

If the triglyceride concentration is above 6.0 mmol litre$^{-1}$ there is a risk of pancreatitis and retinal vein thrombosis. Patients should be advised to reduce their weight if overweight and start a formal lipid-lowering diet (see below). A proportion of individuals with hypertriglyceridaemia have livers which respond to even moderate degrees of alcohol intake by allowing accumulation or excess production of VLDL particles. If hypertriglyceridaemia persists lipid measurements should be repeated before and after a 6 week interval of complete abstinence from alcohol. If a considerable improvement results, lifelong abstinence may prove necessary. Other drugs, including thiazides, oestrogens and glucocorticoids, can have a similar effect to alcohol in susceptible patients.

If the triglyceride concentration remains elevated above 6.0 mmol litre$^{-1}$, despite the above measures, drug therapy is warranted. A fibric acid derivative is the agent of first choice. Nicotinic acid may be used in addition but its side-effects are often a problem. Fish oil capsules (Maxepa) which contain $\omega$-3 ($n$-3) long-chain fatty acids are also effective in lowering triglyceride concentrations.

The severe hypertriglyceridaemia associated with the rare disorders of lipoprotein lipase deficiency and apoprotein C-II deficiency may require restriction of dietary fat to 10–20% of total energy intake and the introduction of medium-chain triglycerides, which are not absorbed via chylomicrons.

### Hypercholesterolaemia (without hypertriglyceridaemia)

Individuals with polygenic hypercholesterolaemia require a graded approach (see Table 17.11) and most will not need drug therapy. Perimenopausal women with hypercholesterolaemia should be offered female hormone replacement therapy as the risk of cardiovascular disease rises sharply after the menopause and hormone replacement therapy reduces this risk even in normocholesterolaemic women. A small number of women respond

| Cholesterol concentration 6.5–7.8 mmol litre$^{-1}$ | Take age, overall cardiovascular risk profile and cardiovascular status into account. Prescribe lipid-lowering diet, with advice on reduction of body weight if patients are obese. Monitor the response and re-emphasize the importance of diet as necessary. Consider adding drug therapy if the response is inadequate, particularly in young patients with a poor family history or a constellation of other risk factors |
|---|---|
| Cholesterol concentration >7.8 mmol litre$^{-1}$ | Full investigation is required to characterize the lipoprotein disorder by measurement of cholesterol subfractions. Prescribe a formal lipid-lowering diet with calorie restriction is if patient is overweight. Monitor the response. The aim is to reduce the serum cholesterol concentration below 6.5 mmol litre$^{-1}$. Drug therapy is required for those with an inadequate response to diet |

**Table 17.11**   The graded management for hypercholesterolaemia. (Adapted from Lewis B (1988) *Journal of the Royal College of Physicians of London* **22**, 28–31.)

adversely to exogenous oestrogens with a rise in lipids and, therefore, measurement of the fasting lipids is necessary shortly after starting treatment.

Individuals with familial hypercholesterolaemia will require treatment with both diet and drugs (Table 17.12).

FIBRATES raise HDL concentrations (beneficial) and reduce LDL cholesterol concentrations by 10–15% and are useful in patients with modest hypercholesterolaemia. Gemfibrozil has been demonstrated to reduce the incidence of cardiovascular events in a carefully performed large randomized double-blind placebo-controlled trial (Helsinki Heart Study) of patients with moderate hypercholesterolaemia, whereas the benefit of the other fibrates on outcome has not been investigated.

BILE ACID BINDING RESINS produce an 8–15% reduction in LDL cholesterol concentration. Cholestyramine has been shown to reduce the incidence of cardiovascular events in hypercholesterolaemic patients in a carefully performed randomized double-blind placebo-controlled trial (Lipid Research Clinics Trial). The safety profile of these drugs is good and their long-term safety is established. They are particularly useful when a lipid-lowering agent needs to be given to women of childbearing age. They have a synergistic effect when given with an HMG-CoA reductase inhibitor. This combination can reduce LDL cholesterol concentrations by 50–60%.

HMG-CoA REDUCTASE INHIBITORS reduce LDL cholesterol concentrations by 30–40%. There are no trial data showing an influence on outcome. In severe hypercholesterolaemia it is often combined with a bile acid binding resin (see above). Concurrent therapy with HMG-CoA reductase inhibitors and fibrates is usually avoided, in view of their overlapping side-effects, but in very severe cases such mixed therapy has been undertaken under very close supervision.

PROBUCOL is now used only rarely as a fourth-line agent.

## Combined hyperlipidaemia (hypercholesterolaemia and hypertriglyceridaemia)

Treatment is the same for all varieties of combined hyperlipidaemia. For any given cholesterol concentration the hypertriglyceridaemia found in the combined hyperlipidaemias increases the cardiovascular risk considerably. Treatment is aimed to reduce serum cholesterol below 6.5 mmol litre$^{-1}$ and triglycerides below 2.0 mmol litre$^{-1}$. Therapy is with diet in the first instance and with drugs if an adequate response has not occurred. Fibric acid derivatives are the treatment of choice since these reduce both cholesterol and triglyceride concentrations, and also have the benefit of raising cardioprotective HDL concentrations. The combination of fibric acid derivative and bile acid binding resin is of considerable use when a fibr-

ate alone produces an insufficient reduction in LDL cholesterol. Nicotinic acid can be used in addition, although its unwanted effects render it a third-line agent.

## The lipid-lowering diet

Studies have shown that dietitians helping patients adjust their own diet to meet the nutritional targets set out below produce a better lipid-lowering effect than issuing of standard diet sheets and advice from a doctor. The main elements of a lipid-lowering diet are:

REDUCTION OF TOTAL FAT INTAKE. Dairy products and meat are the principal sources of saturated fat in the diet. Intake of these products should therefore be reduced, and fish and poultry should be substituted. Visible fat and skin should be removed before cooking and preparing meat dishes. Meat products including pâtés, sausages and reconstituted meats (such as luncheon meat) should be avoided since the concentration of fat is unknown and often high. Baking and grilling of meats reduces the fat content and is preferred to frying. Low-fat or cottage cheese and skimmed or semi-skimmed milk should be substituted for the standard full-fat varieties. Pastries and cakes contain large quantities of fat and should be avoided. The overall aim should be to decrease fat intake such that it is providing approximately 30% of the total energy intake in the diet. Further reduction in fat intake is unacceptable to many patients.

SUBSTITUTION OF MONOUNSATURATES AND POLYUNSATURATES. Monounsaturated oils, particularly olive oil, and polyunsaturated oils such as sunflower, safflower, corn and soya oil should be used in cooking instead of saturated fat-rich alternatives.

REDUCTION IN DIETARY CHOLESTEROL INTAKE. Liver, offal and fish roes should be avoided. Although eggs and prawns are rich in cholesterol their total contribution to the body's cholesterol pool is small and they can still be part of a balanced lipid-lowering diet.

INCREASE FIBRE (non-starch polysaccharides, NSPs) content. Food high in soluble fibre, such as pulses, legumes, root vegetables, leafy vegetables, and unprocessed cereals, help reduce circulating lipid concentrations, and should be substituted in the diet in the place of higher fat alternatives.

REDUCE ALCOHOL CONSUMPTION. Excess alcohol is an important cause of secondary hyperlipidaemia, and may worsen primary lipid disorders.

ACHIEVE IDEAL BODY WEIGHT. Treatment of obesity is particularly important in the management of hyperlipidaemia both because it will exacerbate the lipid disorder itself, and also because obesity is an independent cardiovascular risk factor.

## Prevention trials

Since relatively few deaths will occur in a group of middle-aged subjects, approximately 20 000 high-risk patients need to be studied for at least 5 years in a prevention trial to demonstrate whether treating hyper-

| Drug | Mechanism of action | Contraindications and adverse reactions | Expected lipid-lowering effect | Long-term safety |
|---|---|---|---|---|
| Fibric acid derivatives, e.g. gemfibrozil, bezafibrate, fenofibrate, ciprofibrate | Complex and not fully understood<br>1 Limit substrate availability for hepatic triglyceride synthesis<br>2 Modulate LDL/ligand interaction<br>3 Promote action of lipoprotein lipase<br>4 Stimulate reverse transport of cholesterol | *Contraindications*<br>Severe hepatic or renal impairment, gallbladder disease, pregnancy<br>*Adverse effects*<br>Reversible myositis, nausea, predispose to gallstones, non-specific malaise, impotence | Reduction of LDL cholesterol by 10–15% and triglycerides by 25–35%. HDL cholesterol concentrations increase by 0–15% (newer agents often have greater beneficial effect on HDL) | No knowledge of effect on developing fetus. Avoid in women of childbearing age. Medium-term safety appears good but there is little really long-term experience |
| Bile acid binding resins, e.g. cholestyramine, colestipol (several times more expensive than most fibrates) | Bind bile acids in the gut preventing enterohepatic circulation. This promotes liver to convert cholesterol to bile acids. Also stimulates formation of hepatic LDL receptors which take up more cholesterol from the circulation | *Adverse effects*<br>Gastrointestinal adverse effects predominate: nausea, flatulence, abdominal bloating, alteration in bowel habit. Palatability is a problem for some<br>*Counselling*<br>Other drugs bind to resins and should be taken 1 hour before or 4 hours afterwards | 8–15% reduction in LDL. Little or no effect on HDL cholesterol. 5–15% rise in triglyceride concentration | Not systemically absorbed. Safety profile is good and theoretically resins are of low risk in women of childbearing age. Fat-soluble vitamin supplements may be required in children, pregnancy and breastfeeding |
| HMG-CoA reductase inhibitors, e.g. simvastatin, fluvastatin, pravastatin (several times more expensive than most fibrates) | Inhibit the rate-limiting step in cholesterol synthesis | *Contraindications*<br>Active liver disease, pregnancy, lactation<br>*Adverse effects*<br>Derangement of liver biochemistry tests (recommended to measure liver biochemistry before and periodically during treatment). Myositis. Interferes with cyclosporin elimination and raises its blood concentration | 30–40% reduction in LDL cholesterol. Little effect on triglycerides or HDL cholesterol | Undetermined |
| Nicotinic acid and derivatives, e.g. nicotinic acid, nicofuranose, acipimox | Unclear. Probably inhibits lipid synthesis in the liver by reducing free fatty acid concentrations due to an inhibitory effect on lipolysis in fat tissue | *Contraindications*<br>Pregnancy, breastfeeding<br>*Adverse effects*<br>Value limited by frequent side-effects: headache, flushing, dizziness, nausea, malaise, itching, abnormal liver biochemistry. Glucose intolerance, hyperuricaemia, activation of peptic ulcers, hyperpigmentation may occur | Reduce LDL and triglycerides by 5–10%. Modest HDL increase | Medium-term safety known but marred by the adverse effects listed |

**Table 17.12** Drugs used in the management of hyperlipidaemia.

| Drug | Mechanism of action | Contraindications and adverse reactions | Expected lipid-lowering effect | Long-term safety |
|---|---|---|---|---|
| Probucol | Unclear | *Contraindications* History of cardiac arrhythmias <br><br> *Adverse effects* Nausea, vomiting, flatulence, diarrhoea, abdominal discomfort. Ventricular arrhythmias in some patients | Reduces LDL cholesterol by 5–10%. Little effect on triglyceride concentrations. Reduces HDL cholesterol: this has been seen as disadvantageous. However, regression of xanthomata clearly documented in severe hyperlipidaemia | Medium-term safety known but marred by the adverse effects listed and by concern over its inhibitory effect on HDL concentrations |
| ω-3 Marine triglycerides | Reduce hepatic VLDL secretion | Occasional nausea and belching | Reduces triglycerides in severe hypertriglyceridaemia. No favourable change in other lipids, and may aggravate hypercholesterolaemia in a few patients | No long-term experience |

**Table 17.12** (*cont.*)   Drugs used in the management of hyperlipidaemia.

cholesterolaemia produces a reduction in death rate. No such large well-designed trial has been performed.

During a 5–10 year period of follow-up many more middle-aged subjects will develop non-fatal cardiovascular disease than will die. Thus if cardiovascular end-points, and not death, are used in cholesterol-lowering trials, much smaller numbers of patients (approximately 4000) need be recruited to have a reasonable chance of showing a real effect if one exists. The two best controlled primary intervention studies (the Helsinki Heart Study and the Lipid Research Clinics Trial) each used different drug therapies in 4000 patients in two different countries and both demonstrated a significant improvement in cardiovascular risk with treatment of hypercholesterolaemia. Furthermore the improvement in cardiovascular risk

increased progressively year by year (Fig. 17.17). These two well-designed trials provide the strongest evidence that cholesterol-lowering therapy is worthwhile.

Both these studies were of insufficient size to examine mortality as an end-point, and this was appreciated when they were designed. Despite this limitation some critics erroneously state that 'the trials showed that treating hypercholesterolaemia has no effect on mortality'!

Unfortunately, although well-designed trials have been undertaken, many poorly constructed trials with inconclusive results litter the literature and some hint at an increase in mortality due to violent death and suicide in treated patients. Overall, however, the weight of evidence favouring the judicious treatment of lipid disorders is great.

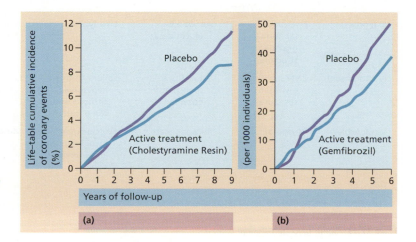

**Fig. 17.17** Follow-up study of coronary events in controls and patients treated for hypercholesterolaemia in two study groups: (a) Lipid Research Clinics Study; (b) Helsinki Heart Study.

## OTHER LIPID DISORDERS

### Hypolipidaemia

Low lipid levels can be found in severe protein–energy malnutrition. They are also seen occasionally with severe malabsorption and in intestinal lymphangiectasia.

### Abetalipoproteinaemia

This is described on p. 213.

### Familial α-lipoprotein deficiency (Tangier disease)

One of the two HDL apoproteins, apoprotein A-I, is deficient in homozygotes with this very rare disease, so that there is little HDL in plasma. Tangier disease is inherited as an autosomal recessive. The serum cholesterol is low, but serum triglycerides are normal or high. Cholesterol accumulates in reticuloendothelial tissue, although the mechanism is uncertain, producing enlarged and orange-coloured tonsils and hepatosplenomegaly. There are also corneal opacities and a polyneuropathy.

## Inborn errors of carbohydrate metabolism

### Glycogen storage disease

All mammalian cells can manufacture glycogen, but the main sites of its production are the liver and muscle. Glycogen is a high-molecular-weight glucose polymer. In glycogen storage disease there is either an abnormality in the molecular structure or an increase in glycogen concentration owing to a specific enzyme defect. Almost all these conditions are autosomal recessive in inheritance and present in infancy, except for McArdle's disease, which presents in adults.

Table 17.13 shows the classification and clinical features of some of these diseases. New specific enzyme defects, e.g. liver phosphorylase, phosphorylase kinase, are being recognized.

### Galactosaemia

Galactose is normally converted to glucose. However, a deficiency of the enzyme galactose-1-phosphate uridyl-

| Type | Affected tissue | Enzyme defect | Clinical features | Tissue needed for diagnosis[a] | Outcome |
|------|-----------------|---------------|-------------------|-------------------------------|---------|
| I (Von Gierke) | Liver, intestine, kidney | Glucose-6-phosphatase | Hepatomegaly, hypoglycaemia, stunted growth, obesity, hypotonia | Liver | If patients survive initial hypoglycaemia, prognosis is good; hyperuricaemia is a late complication |
| II (Pompé) | Liver, muscle, heart | Lysosomal α-glucosidase | Heart failure, cardiomyopathy | Leucocytes, liver, muscle | Death in first 6 months; juvenile and adult variants seen |
| III (Forbes) | Liver, muscle (abnormal glycogen structure) | Amylo-1,6-glucosidase | Like type I | Leucocytes, liver, muscle | Good prognosis |
| IV (Anderson) | Liver (abnormal glycogen structure) | 1,4-α-Glucan branching enzyme | Failure to thrive, hepatomegaly, cirrhosis and its complications | Leucocytes, liver, muscle | Death in first 3 years |
| V (McArdle) | Muscle only | Phosphorylase | Muscle cramps and myoglobinuria and exercise (in adults) | Muscle | Normal life span; exercise must be avoided |

[a]Tissue obtained is used for the biochemical assay of the enzyme.

Table 17.13 Some glycogen storage diseases.

transferase results in accumulation of galactose-1-phosphate in the blood. This deficiency, inherited as an autosomal recessive, results in hypoglycaemia and acidosis in the neonate. Progressive hepatosplenomegaly, cataracts, renal tubular defects and mental retardation occur.

Treatment is with a galactose-free diet, which, if started early, results in normal development. Untreated patients die within a few days. Prenatal diagnosis and diagnosis of the carrier state are possible by measurement of the level of galactose-1-phosphate in the blood.

Galactokinase deficiency also results in galactosaemia and early cataract formation.

## Defects of fructose metabolism

Absorbed fructose is chiefly metabolised in the liver to lactic acid or glucose. Three defects of metabolism occur; all are inherited as autosomal recessive traits:

FRUCTOSURIA is due to fructokinase deficiency. It is a benign condition.

FRUCTOSE INTOLERANCE is due to fructose-1-phosphate aldolase deficiency. Fructose-1-phosphate accumulates after fructose ingestion, resulting in symptoms of hypoglycaemia. Hepatomegaly and renal tubular defects occur but are reversible on a fructose-free diet. Intelligence is normal and there is an absence of dental caries.

FRUCTOSE-1,6-DIPHOSPHATE DEFICIENCY leads to a failure of gluconeogenesis, and to hepatomegaly.

## Pentosuria

Pentosuria is due to L-xylulose reductase deficiency. It has no clinical significance.

# Inborn errors of amino acid metabolism

Inborn errors of amino acid metabolism are chiefly inherited as autosomal recessive conditions. The major ones are shown in Table 17.14.

# Amino acid transport defects

Amino acids are filtered by the glomerulus but 95% of the filtered load is reabsorbed in the proximal convoluted tubule by an active transport mechanism.

Aminoaciduria results from:
- Abnormally high plasma amino acid levels (e.g. phenylketonuria)
- Any inherited disorder that damages the tubules secondarily (e.g. galactosaemia)

- Tubular reabsorptive defects, either generalized (e.g. Fanconi syndrome) or specific (e.g. cystinuria)
- Amino acid transport defects can be congenital or acquired.

# GENERALIZED AMINOACIDURIAS

## Fanconi syndrome

This occurs in a juvenile form (De Toni–Fanconi–Debré syndrome); in adult life it is often acquired due to, for example, heavy metal poisoning, drugs or some renal diseases. There is defective tubular reabsorption of:
- Most amino acids
- Glucose
- Urate
- Phosphate, resulting in hypophosphataemic rickets
- Bicarbonate, with failure to transport hydrogen ions, causing a renal tubular acidosis that then produces a hyperchloraemic acidosis

Other abnormalities include:
- Potassium depletion, primary or secondary to the acidosis
- Polyuria
- Increased excretion of immunoglobulins and other low-molecular-weight proteins

Various combinations of the above abnormalities have been described.

The juvenile form begins at the age of 6–9 months, with failure to thrive, vomiting and thirst. There is also acidosis, dehydration and vitamin D-resistant rickets.

In the adult, the disease is similar to the juvenile form, but osteomalacia is a major feature.

Treatment is with large doses of vitamin D (e.g. 1–2 $\mu$g of 1$\alpha$-hydroxycholecalciferol with regular blood calcium monitoring).

## Lowe's syndrome (oculocerebrorenal dystrophy)

In this syndrome there is generalized aminoaciduria combined with mental retardation, hypotonia, congenital cataracts and an abnormal skull shape.

# SPECIFIC AMINOACIDURIAS

## Cystinuria

There is defective tubular reabsorption and jejunal absorption of cystine and the dibasic amino acids lysine, ornithine and arginine. Inheritance is either completely or incompletely recessive, so that heterozygotes who have increased excretion of lysine and cystine only can occur. Cystine absorption from the jejunum is impaired but, nevertheless, cystine in peptide form can be absorbed. Cystinuria leads to urinary stones and is responsible for approximately 1–2% of all urinary calculi. The disease often starts in childhood, although most cases present in adult life.

| Disease | Enzyme defect | Incidence | Biochemical and clinical features | Treatment | Prognosis |
|---|---|---|---|---|---|
| Albinism | Tyrosinase | 1 in 13 000 | Amelanosis—whitish hair, pink-white skin, grey-blue eyes<br>Nystagmus, photophobia, strabismus | Symptomatic | Good |
| Alkaptonuria | Homogentisic acid oxidase | 1 in 100 000 | Homogentisic acid polymerizes to produce a black-brown product that is deposited in cartilage and other tissue (ochronosis)<br>Urine darkens on standing<br>Sweat stains clothing<br>Arthritis | None | Good |
| Homocystinuria | | | Homocystine is excreted in urine | — | — |
|   Type I | Cystathionine synthetase | | Mental handicap<br>Marfan-like syndrome<br>Thrombotic episodes | — | — |
|   Type II | Methylene tetrahydrofolate reductase | | Survivors have mental retardation | — | Mainly die as neonates |
| Phenylketonuria | Phenylalanine-4-hydroxylase | 1 in 20 000 | Brain damage with mental retardation and epilepsy<br>Phenylpyruvate and its derivatives excreted in urine | Diet low in phenylalanine in first few months of life prevents damage | — |
| Histidinaemia | Histidine deaminase | Very rare | Mental retardation | — | — |
| 'Maple syrup' disease | Branched-chain ketoacid decarboxylase | Very rare | Failure to thrive<br>Fits, neonatal acidosis and severe cerebral degeneration<br>Valine, isoleucine and their derivatives are excreted in urine<br>A milder form is seen | — | Early death |
| Oxalosis (hyperoxaluria) | Glyoxylic acid dehydrogenase | Very rare | Nephrocalcinosis, renal stones, renal failure due to deposition of calcium oxalate | — | Death occurs in first two decades |

There are many other enzyme defects producing, for example, alaninaemia, ammonaemia, argininaemia, citrullinaemia, isovaleric acidaemia, lysinaemia, ornithinaemia or tyrosinaemia.

**Table 17.14**   The major inborn errors of amino acid metabolism.

Treatment is with a high fluid intake in order to keep the urinary cystine concentration low. Patients are encouraged to drink up to 3 litres over 24 hours and to drink even at night. Penicillamine should be used for patients who cannot keep the cystine concentration of their urine low.

The condition cystinosis (see p. 866) must not be confused with cystinuria.

## Hartnup's disease

There is defective tubular reabsorption and jejunal absorption of most neutral amino acids but not their pep-tides. The resulting tryptophan malabsorption produces nicotinamide deficiency (see p. 163). Patients can be asymptomatic, but others develop evidence of pellagra, with cerebellar ataxia, psychiatric disorders and skin lesions. Treatment is with nicotinamide and often brings about considerable improvement.

## Tryptophan malabsorption syndrome (blue diaper syndrome)

This is due to an isolated transport defect for tryptophan; the tryptophan excreted oxidizes to a blue colour on the baby's diaper.

## Familial iminoglycinuria

This occurs when there is defective tubular reabsorption of glycine, proline and hydroxyproline. It seems to have few clinical effects.

## Methionine malabsorption syndrome

This is due to failure to absorb and excrete methionine, and results in diarrhoea, vomiting and mental retardation. Patients characteristically have an oast-house smell.

# Lysosomal storage diseases

Lysosomal storage diseases are due to inborn errors of metabolism which are mainly inherited in an autosomal recessive manner.

## Glucosylceramide lipidoses: Gaucher's disease

This is the most prevalent lysosomal storage disease and is due to a deficiency in glucocerebrosidase, a specialized lysosomal acid $\beta$-glucosidase. This results in accumulation of glucosylceramide in the lysosomes of the reticuloendothelial system, particularly the liver, bone marrow and spleen. Several mutations have been characterized in the glucocerebrosidase gene, the commonest being a single base change causing the substitution of arginine to serine; this is seen in 70% of Jewish patients. The typical Gaucher cell, a glucocerebroside-containing reticuloendothelial histiocyte, is found in the bone marrow. There are three clinical types, the commonest presenting in adult life with an insidious onset of hepatosplenomegaly. There is a high incidence in Ashkenazi Jews (1 in 3000 births), and patients have a characteristic pigmentation on exposed parts, particularly the forehead and hands. The clinical spectrum is variable with patients developing anaemia, evidence of hypersplenism and pathological fractures due to bone involvement. Nevertheless, many have a normal life-span.

Acute Gaucher's disease presents in infancy or childhood with rapid onset of hepatosplenomegaly with neurological involvement due to Gaucher cells in the brain. The outlook is poor.

Some patients with non-neuropathic Gaucher's disease show considerable improvement with infusion of L-glucerase (mannose-terminated placental glucocerebrosidase).

## Sphingomyelin cholesterol lipidoses: Niemann–Pick disease

The disease is due to a deficiency of lysosomal sphingomyelinase which results in the accumulation of sphingomyelin cholesterol and glycosphingolipids in the reticuloendothelial macrophages and many organs, particularly the liver, spleen, bone marrow and lymph nodes. The disease usually presents within the first 6 months of life with mental retardation and hepatosplenomegaly. Typical foam cells are found in the marrow, lymph nodes, liver and spleen.

## The mucopolysaccharidoses (MPS)

These are a group of disorders caused by the deficiency of lysosomal enzymes required for the catabolism of glycosaminoglycans (mucopolysaccharides).

The catabolism of dermatan sulphate, heparan sulphate, keratin sulphate or chondroitin sulphate may be affected either singularly or together.

Accumulation of glycosaminoglycans in the lysosomes of various tissues results in the disease. Ten forms of MPS have been described; all are chronic but progressive and a wide spectrum of clinical severity can be seen within a single enzyme defect. The MPS types show many clinical features though in variable amounts with dysostosis, abnormal facies, poor vision and hearing and joint dysmobility (either stiff or hypermobile) being frequently seen. Mental retardation is present in, for example, Hurler (MPS IH) and San Filippo A (MPS IIIA) types, but normal intelligence and life-span are seen in Scheie (MPS IS).

## The GM$_2$ gangliosidoses

In these conditions there is accumulation of GM$_2$ gangliosides in the central nervous system and peripheral nerves. It is particularly common (1 : 2000) in Ashkenazi Jews. *Tay–Sachs disease* is the severest form where there is a progressive degeneration of all cerebral function, with fits, epilepsy, dementia and blindness and death usually occurs before 2 years of age. The macula has a characteristic cherry spot appearance.

## Fabry's disease

This X-linked recessive condition is due to a deficiency of the lysosomal hydrolase $\alpha$-galactosidase, causing an accumulation of glycosphingolipids with terminal $\alpha$-galactosyl moieties in the lysosomes of various tissues including the liver, kidney, blood vessels and the ganglion cells of the nervous system. The patients present with peripheral nerve involvement, but eventually most patients develop renal problems in adult life.

## Diagnosis

Many of the sphingolipidoses can be diagnosed by demonstrating the enzyme deficiency in the appropriate tissue.

Prenatal diagnosis is becoming possible in a number of the conditions by obtaining specimens of amniotic cells (see p. 124). Carrier states can also be identified, so that sensible genetic counselling can be given.

# Cystinosis

In cystinosis, cystine accumulates in the reticuloendothelial cells. It is inherited in an autosomal recessive manner. The exact mechanism is unknown but it is thought to be a defect of cystine transport across the lysosomal membrane. Three forms are recognized: the infantile form is usually fatal in the first year owing to renal failure; the intermediate form presents in early/young adult life with fever and renal problems; and the adult form is benign. The generalized aminoaciduria seen in these patients often causes confusion with the Fanconi syndrome. Corneal deposits of cystine are seen.

# Amyloidosis

This is a disorder of protein metabolism in which there is extracellular deposition of insoluble fibrillar protein, either localized or widely distributed throughout the body.

Characteristically the amyloid protein consists of $\beta$-pleated sheets that are responsible for the insolubility and resistance to proteolysis. A smaller part of the protein is the amyloid P component (AP), which is derived from normal circulatory glycoprotein and is related to the acute-phase reactant, C-reactive protein (CRP).

Amyloid in tissues appears as an amorphous, homogeneous substance that stains pink with haematoxylin and eosin and stains red with Congo red, which also shows a green fluorescence in polarized light.

## Hereditary systemic amyloidosis

In the Portuguese type I neuropathic amyloidosis, fibrils composed of prealbumin formed into $\beta$ sheets are found, producing a polyneuropathy.

In *familial Mediterranean fever*, renal amyloidosis is a common serious complication. Deposition of amyloid A (AA) fibrils occurs.

## Local amyloidosis

Deposits of amyloid fibrils of various types can be localized to various organs or tissues, e.g. skin, heart and brain. An amyloid syndrome due to $\beta_2$-microglobulin deposition as amyloid fibrils is seen in patients on chronic dialysis (see p. 490).

## Senile amyloid

Amyloid deposits are frequently found in the elderly. In particular, cerebral deposits of the A4 protein are found, and this protein is also seen in the brains of patients with Down's syndrome and Alzheimer's disease (see p. 964).

Apoprotein E (involved in LDL transport, see p. 855) interacts directly with $\beta$-A4 protein in senile plaques and neurofibrillary tangles in the brain. The gene for apoprotein E is on chromosome 19 and may be an important susceptibility factor in the aetiology of Alzheimer's disease.

## Immunocyte-related amyloidosis

In this variety, the deposits consist of amyloid light (AL) chain fragments. The molecular weights of these fragments range from 5000 to 25 000. The amyloidosis is usually associated with lymphoproliferative diseases of the B-cell lineage, e.g. myeloma, Waldenström's macroglobulinaemia or non-Hodgkin's lymphoma.

### CLINICAL FEATURES

The clinical features are related to the organs involved, patients presenting with heart failure, nephrotic syndrome, purpura or bleeding, peripheral neuropathy or weight loss. Weakness and paraesthesia of the hand may occur due to the carpal tunnel syndrome. On examination, a characteristic feature is macroglossia, which only occurs in this form of amyloidosis. Hepatomegaly and occasionally splenomegaly are seen.

### INVESTIGATION

The diagnosis is made on the presence of the characteristic histological features mentioned above in a biopsy of the rectum or gums. The bone marrow may show plasma cells in primary amyloidosis or a lymphoproliferative disorder. A paraproteinaemia and light chains in the urine may be seen as a result of associated conditions.

### TREATMENT

Treatment is symptomatic or of the associated cause.

## Reactive systemic amyloidosis

In reactive systemic amyloidosis, the amyloid (AA) is composed of protein A (molecular weight 8500), which is a precursor of the normal serum component serum amyloid A (SAA), an acute-phase reactant. Overproduction of SAA as well as its degradation to AA determines whether amyloidosis occurs. This type of amyloidosis, which used to be known as secondary amyloidosis, involves the spleen, liver, kidney and adrenal glands. It is associated with long-standing chronic infections (e.g. tuberculosis), inflammation (e.g. rheumatoid arthritis), malignancy (e.g. Hodgkin's disease), and also occurs in familial Mediterranean fever.

Clinically there is hepatosplenomegaly. Hepatic failure and renal failure with renal-vein thrombosis or the nephrotic syndrome may develop.

# The porphyrias

This heterogeneous group of rare inborn errors of metabolism is caused by abnormalities of enzymes involved in

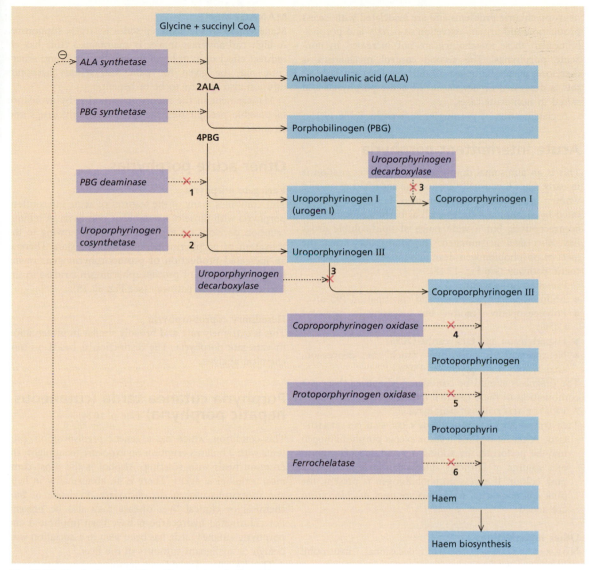

**Fig. 17.18** Porphyrin metabolism. The numbers indicate the blocks occurring in forms of porphyria. 1, acute intermittent porphyria; 2, congenital (erythropoietic) porphyria; 3, porphyria cutanea tarda; 4, hereditary coproporphyria; 5, variegate porphyria; 6, erythropoietic protoporphyria.

the biosynthesis of haem, resulting in overproduction of the intermediate compounds called porphyrins (Fig. 17.18).

Structurally, porphyrins consist of four pyrrole rings. These pyrrole rings are formed from the precursors glycine and succinyl-CoA, which are converted to δ-aminolaevulinic acid (δ-ALA) in a reaction catalysed by the enzyme δ-ALA synthetase. Two molecules of δ-ALA condense to form a pyrrole ring.

Porphyrins can be divided into uroporphyrins, coproporphyrins or protoporphyrins depending on the structure of the side-chain. They are termed type I if the structure is symmetrical and type III if it is asymmetrical.

Both uroporphyrins and coproporphyrins can be excreted in the urine.

The sequence of enzymatic changes in the production of haem is shown in Fig. 17.18. The chief rate-limiting step is the enzyme δ-ALA synthetase, as an increase in this enzyme results in an overproduction of porphyrins. Haem provides a negative feedback mechanism on this enzyme.

In porphyria the excess production of porphyrins occurs either in the liver (hepatic porphyrias) or in the bone marrow (erythropoietic porphyria), but porphyrias can also be classified in terms of clinical presentation as acute or non-acute. Acute porphyrias usually produce neuropsychiatric problems and are associated with excess production and urinary excretion of δ-ALA and porphobilinogen; these metabolites are not increased in non-acute porphyrias. The second control mechanism is therefore porphobilinogen deaminase (see Fig. 17.18); this is depressed or normal in the acute porphyrias and raised in non-acute cases.

A classification of porphyrias is given in Table 17.15.

## Acute intermittent porphyria

This is an autosomal dominant disorder. Presentation is in early adult life, usually around the age of 30 years, and women are affected more than men. It may be precipitated by alcohol and drugs such as barbiturates and oral contraceptives, but a wide range of lipid-soluble drugs have also been incriminated. The abnormality lies at the level of porphobilinogen deaminase in the haem biosynthetic pathway (see Fig. 17.18).

Presentation is with:

- Abdominal pain, vomiting and constipation (90%)
- Polyneuropathy (motor, but occasionally sensory) (70%)
- Hypertension and tachycardia (70%)
- Neuropsychiatric disorders (such as depression, anxiety and frank psychosis) (50%)

The diagnosis should be considered whenever there is a combination of these cardinal features or:

A FAMILY HISTORY of porphyria.

THE URINE TURNS RED-BROWN OR RED ON STANDING. A classic bedside test for excess porphobilinogen may be performed by adding one volume of urine to one volume of Ehrlich's aldehyde, which produces a pink colour. If excess porphobilinogen is present, the pink colour persists when two volumes of chloroform are added.

### Other investigations

NORMAL BLOOD COUNT; occasional neutrophil leucocytosis

ABNORMAL LIVER BIOCHEMICAL TESTS—elevated bilirubin and transferases

BLOOD UREA often raised

SCREENING. Family members should be screened to detect latent cases. Urinalysis is not adequate and measurement of erythrocyte porphobilinogen deaminase and ALA synthetase is extremely sensitive.

## MANAGEMENT

Management of the acute episodes is largely supportive. A high carbohydrate intake is maintained (this has an indirect effect on porphyrin overproduction), and a narcotic may be given for pain. Intravenous haematin infusion also appears to be of benefit.

Management in the remission period is by avoidance of possible precipitating factors, particularly drugs and alcohol.

## Other acute porphyrias

### Variegate porphyria

This combines many of the features of acute intermittent porphyria with those of a cutaneous porphyria. A bullous eruption develops on exposure to sunlight owing to the activation of porphyrins deposited in the skin. There is an increased production of protoporphyrinogens owing to an abnormality of protoporphyrinogen oxidase in the haem biosynthetic pathway (see Fig. 17.18).

### Hereditary coproporphyria

This is extremely rare and broadly similar in presentation to variegate porphyria. The distinction is based on biochemical analysis.

## Porphyria cutanea tarda (cutaneous hepatic porphyria) (see p. 1024)

This condition, which has a genetic predisposition, presents with a bullous eruption on exposure to sunlight; the eruption heals with scarring. Alcohol is the most common aetiological agent. There is an abnormality in hepatic uroporphyrinogen decarboxylase. Evidence of biochemical or clinical liver disease may also be present. Polychlorinated hydrocarbons have been implicated and porphyria cutanea tarda has been seen in association with benign or malignant tumours of the liver.

The diagnosis depends on demonstration of increased levels of urinary uroporphyrin. Histology of the skin shows subepidermal blisters with perivascular deposition of periodic acid–Schiff-staining material. The serum iron and transferrin saturation are often raised. The liver biopsy shows mild iron overload as well as features of alcoholic liver disease.

Remission can be induced by venesection; this should be repeated if the urinary uroporphyrin rises in the

|  | Hepatic | Erythropoietic |
|---|---|---|
| Acute: | Acute intermittent porphyria Variegate porphyria Hereditary coproporphyria | |
| Non-acute: | Porphyria cutanea tarda | Congenital porphyria Erythropoietic protoporphyria |

**Table 17.15** The classification of porphyrias.

remission phase. Chloroquine may also have a useful role in promoting urinary excretion of uroporphyrins.

## Erythropoietic porphyrias

### Congenital porphyria

This is extremely rare and is transmitted as an autosomal recessive trait. Its victims show extreme sensitivity to sunlight and develop disfiguring scars. Dystrophy of the nails, blindness due to lenticular scarring, and brownish discoloration of the teeth also occur.

### Erythropoietic protoporphyria

This is commoner than congenital porphyria and is inherited as an autosomal dominant trait. It presents with irritation and burning pain in the skin on exposure to sunlight. Hepatic involvement may also occur. Diagnosis is made by fluorescence of the peripheral red blood cells and by increased protoporphyrin in the red cells and stools. Oral $\beta$-carotene provides effective protection against solar sensitivity; the reason for this is not known.

## Further reading

The Diabetes Control and Complications Trial Research Group (1993) The effect of intensive treatment of diabetes on the development and progression of long-term complications in insulin-dependent diabetes mellitus. *New England Journal of Medicine* **329**: 977–986.

Ferner RE, Alberti KGMM (1989) Sulphonylureas in the treatment of non-insulin dependent diabetes. *Quarterly Journal of Medicine* **73**, 987–995.

Galton DJ, Krone W (1991) *Hyperlipidaemia in Practice*. London: Gower Medical Publishing.

Kohner EM (1989) Diabetic retinopathy. *British Medical Bulletin* **45**: 148–173.

Scriver CR, Beaudet AL, Sly WS & Valle D (1989) *The Metabolic Basis of Inherited Disease*, 6th edn. New York: McGraw-Hill.

Tattersall RB, Gale EAM (eds) (1990) *Diabetes Clinical Management*. Edinburgh: Churchill Livingstone.

Ward JD (1989) Diabetic neuropathy. *British Medical Bulletin* **45**: 111–126.

# 18 Neurological diseases and diseases of voluntary muscle

## Introduction

The wide range of neurological conditions seen in the UK is summarized in Table 18.1. The pattern of practice has changed much in the last 40 years with the disappearance of poliomyelitis, and (almost) of neurosyphilis, the treatment for Parkinson's disease, the use of newer anticonvulsants and now, the emergence of AIDS. Despite clinical neurology being primarily concerned with the organic conditions of Table 18.1, 'neurological' symptoms may be the presenting features of common psychological illness (e.g. depression or anxiety) which require sympathy, interpretation and therapy.

## Neurology in developing countries

Low standards of nutrition, hygiene and education, with widespread economic hardship, contribute to different patterns of disease. Common neurological conditions of the Indian subcontinent, South East Asia and Africa include:

- Leprosy
- Tuberculosis (meningitis, tuberculoma)
- Meningococcal meningitis
- Tetanus
- Rabies
- Cerebral malaria
- Multiple vitamin deficiencies
- Cysticercosis
- Neurological complications of AIDS (Africa and South East Asia)

Of these, only tuberculosis and meningococcal infection are seen commonly in Europe. AIDS, however, is increasing.

Prevalence rates often differ widely from annual incidence rates; these will be mentioned under the individual diseases.

| Disorder | Rate |
|---|---|
| Herpes zoster | 440 |
| Back pain and sciatica | 300 |
| Stroke | 150 |
| Epilepsy and single seizures | 50 |
| Dementia | 50 |
| Polyneuropathy | 40 |
| Transient ischaemic attacks | 30 |
| Bell's palsy | 25 |
| Parkinson's disease | 20 |
| Alcohol abuse (neurological complications) | 20 |
| Meningitis | 15 |
| Encephalitis | 15 |
| Subarachnoid haemorrhage | 15 |
| Metastatic brain tumour | 15 |
| Benign brain tumour | 10 |
| Primary malignant brain tumour | 5 |
| Metastatic cord tumour | 5 |
| Trigeminal neuralgia | 4 |
| Multiple sclerosis | 3 |
| Motor neurone disease | 2 |
| All primary muscle disease | 1.5 |
| Intracranial abscess | 1 |
| Benign spinal cord tumour | 1 |
| Huntington's disease | 0.4 |
| Myasthenia gravis | 0.4 |

Table 18.1 Neurological diseases: annual incidence rates per 100 000 population in the UK.

## Symptoms

There are two essential questions in any neurological diagnosis:

1 What is/are the site(s) of the lesion(s)?
2 What is the likely pathology?

Most of the diagnoses in neurology are made on a detailed history alone. The method of recording the details is beyond the scope of this chapter, but an important point is that the history should read chronologically and portray the story of the disease. A summary should conclude the history.

# HEADACHE

Headache at some time is an almost universal experience. It varies from an infrequent and trivial nuisance to a symptom of serious disease.

## Mechanism of headache

Pain receptors are found in the vessels at the base of the brain (both arterial and venous) and in the meninges. These receptors are also present in extracranial vessels, the muscles of the scalp, neck and face, the paranasal sinuses, the eyes and the teeth. The brain substance itself is almost devoid of pain receptors.

The pain of headache is mediated by mechanical and chemical (e.g. 5-hydroxytryptamine, histamine) stimulation of receptors: nerve impulses are carried centrally via the fifth and ninth cranial nerves and via the upper cervical sensory roots.

## Pressure headaches

Intracranial mass lesions displace the meninges and the basal vessels. When these structures are physically moved by changes in cerebrospinal fluid (CSF) pressure (e.g. coughing), pain is exacerbated. Cerebral oedema, which accumulates around mass lesions, causes further shift. Headache is typically worse after lying down for some hours (as cerebral oedema increases).

Any headache, however mild, that is present on waking and which is made worse by coughing, straining or sneezing may well be due to displacement or dilatation of the intracranial vessels and may be due to a mass lesion. These are often called 'the headaches of raised intracranial pressure'. Vomiting often accompanies them.

## Headache of subacute onset

The onset and progression of a headache over days or weeks with or without the features of 'pressure headaches' should always raise the suspicion of an intracranial mass lesion or serious intracranial disease.

Encephalitis (see p. 927) and viral meningitis (see p. 925) should be considered. Giant-cell arteritis causes headache, with scalp tenderness, particularly over the age of 60 years.

## The single episode of severe headache

This common emergency is caused principally by:
● Subarachnoid haemorrhage
● Migraine
and, occasionally,

● Meningitis

Particular attention should be paid to the suddenness of onset (suggestive of a subarachnoid haemorrhage), neck stiffness and vomiting (meningeal irritation) and rashes and fever (meningitis).

## Recurrent headaches

Migraine (see p. 935) and tension headache (see p. 934) are the commonest causes of recurrent pain. Sinusitis, glaucoma and migrainous neuralgia should also be considered. Hangover headache is usually obvious! Malignant hypertension occasionally causes a patient to seek medical advice because of headache. Headaches are not caused by essential hypertension.

Intermittent hydrocephalus due to an intraventricular tumour is a rare cause of recurrent prostrating headache with weakness of the lower limbs.

'Eyestrain' from refractive error is an unusual cause of headache.

## Headache following head injury

Subdural haematoma (see p. 911) should be considered, whether or not the headaches are suggestive of a mass lesion. The vast majority of post-traumatic headaches (see p. 938), which last days, weeks or months are not, however, associated with any serious intracranial cause.

## Chronic headaches

Almost all recurring headaches with a history going back for several years or more are due to muscle tension and/or migraine (see p. 935). Depression usually accompanies them.

# DIZZINESS, VERTIGO AND BLACKOUTS

'Dizziness' is a word patients use for a wide variety of complaints ranging from a vague feeling of unsteadiness to severe, acute vertigo. It is also frequently used to describe the light-headedness that is felt in anxiety and 'panic attacks', during palpitations, and in syncope or chronic ill-health. Therefore, the site of this symptom must be determined, i.e. whether it is perceived in the limbs, the chest or the head.

Vertigo (an illusion of movement) is a more definite symptom. It is usually a sensation of rotation in which the patient feels that their surroundings are spinning or moving. Vertigo indicates disease of the labyrinth, vestibular pathways or their central connections.

Like dizziness, 'blackouts' is a vague, descriptive term implying either altered consciousness, visual disturbance or falling. Epilepsy, syncope, hypoglycaemia and other conditions must be considered (see p. 916). However, commonly no sinister cause is found. A careful history, particularly from an eye-witness, is essential.

Spasticity
Parkinson's disease
Cerebellar ataxia
Sensory loss (joint position)
Distal weakness
Proximal weakness
Apraxia of gait

**Table 18.2**  Common neurological causes of difficulty in walking.

# DIFFICULTY WALKING

This is a common presenting complaint in neurological disease; the main causes are given in Table 18.2. Arthritis and muscle pain also alter the gait, making it stiff and slow. The recognition of an abnormal gait is important in diagnosis.

## Spasticity

Spasticity (see p. 893) with or without pyramidal weakness causes stiffness and jerkiness of gait, which is maintained on a narrow base. The toes catch level ground, causing wearing down and scuffing of the toes of the shoes. The pace shortens. Clonus may be noticed as involuntary extensor jerking of the legs.

When the problem is predominantly unilateral and weakness is marked (in a hemiparesis), the weaker leg drags stiffly and is circumducted.

## Parkinson's disease (see p. 918)

Here there is muscular rigidity in both the extensors and the flexors of the limbs. Power remains normal. The gait slows; the pace shortens to a shuffle. The base remains narrow. Falls occur. A stoop is apparent and swinging of the arms is diminished. The gait is 'festinant', i.e. hurried, as small rapid steps are taken. There is particular difficulty in initiating movement and in turning quickly. Sometimes when the patient stops or is halted, a few rapid, small and unsteady backward steps are taken; this is known as retropulsion.

## Cerebellar ataxia

In disease of the lateral lobes of the cerebellum the stance becomes broad-based, unstable and tremulous. The gait tends to veer towards the side of the more affected cerebellar lobe (see p. 897).

In disease of the cerebellar vermis (a midline structure), the trunk becomes unsteady and there is a tendency to fall backwards (truncal ataxia).

## Sensory ataxia

The ataxia of peripheral sensory lesions (e.g. polyneuropathy, see p. 945) is due to diminution of the sense of proprioception (joint position). The patient cannot perceive accurately the position of the legs. The gait becomes broad-based and high-stepping or 'stamping'.

The ataxia is made worse by removal of additional sensory input, e.g. in the dark or when the eyes are closed. This is the basis of a positive Romberg's test, which was first described in the sensory ataxia of tabes dorsalis (see p. 928).

# Weakness of the lower limbs

With distal weakness the affected leg is lifted over obstacles. When the dorsiflexors of the foot are weak, such as in a common peroneal nerve palsy (see p. 945), the foot, having been lifted, returns to the ground with a visible and audible 'slap'.

Weakness of proximal lower limb muscles (e.g. polymyositis, muscular dystrophy) leads to difficulty in rising from the sitting position. Once upright, the patient walks with a waddling gait, the pelvis being ill-supported by each lower limb as it carries the full weight of the body.

# Apraxia of gait

In frontal-lobe disease (e.g. tumours, hydrocephalus, infarction) the central organization of walking is disturbed. The patient is able to move the legs normally while sitting or lying but cannot walk in an organized way. This is known as 'apraxia of gait'—a failure of the skilled movement of walking. Urinary incontinence and a degree of dementia are often present.

# *Neurological examination*

The following headings summarize the essential elements of the clinical examination:

1  State of consciousness, arousal
2  Appearance, attitude, insight
3  Mental state (see p. 960)
4  Orientation in time and place
5  Recall of recent and distant events/memory
6  Level of intellect
7  Language and speech/cerebral dominance
8  Disorders of higher function (e.g. apraxia)
9  Gait
10  Romberg's test
11  The skull—shape, circumference, bruits
12  The neck—stiffness, palpation and auscultation of carotid arteries
13  *The cranial nerves*—see individual nerves
14  *The motor system*
   (a)  Upper limbs:
      (i)  Wasting and fasciculation
      (ii)  Posture of the outstretched arms—drift, rebound, tremor
      (iii)  Tone—if increased, is it spasticity or 'extrapyramidal' rigidity?

(iv)  Power—weakness may be graded roughly into 'slight', 'moderate' or 'severe' or numerically (0–5) (Table 18.3)

(v)  Tendon reflexes: + or ++, normal; +++, increased; 0, absent even with reinforcement

(b)  Thorax and abdomen:

(i)  Respiration

(ii)  Abdominal reflexes and muscles

(c)  The lower limbs:

(i)  Wasting and fasciculation

(ii)  Tone, power and tendon reflexes

(iii)  Plantar responses

15  Coordination and fine movements

16  *The sensory system.* First, the patient is asked whether or not the feeling in the limbs, face and trunk is entirely normal.

(a)  Posterior columns:

(i)  Light touch

(ii)  Vibration (using a 128 Hz tuning fork)

(iii)  Joint position

(iv)  Two-point discrimination (normal: 0.5 cm on fingertips, 2 cm on soles)

(b)  Spinothalamic tracts:

(i)  Pain (pin prick)—using a split orange-stick

(ii)  Temperature

Chart areas of abnormal sensation

## Short neurological examination

A detailed neurological examination is time-consuming and is not necessary in all patients, particularly those without symptoms suggestive of neurological disease. A short examination will detect the majority of defects (Practical box 18.1).

## *Investigation*

The history and examination remain most valuable 'tests' in neurology, but computed tomography (CT), magnetic resonance imaging (MRI), and other non-invasive tests have revolutionized the management of patients.

---

**Look at the patient:**
General demeanour
Speech
Gait
Arm swinging

**Examine head:**
Fundi
Pupils
Eye movements
Facial movements
Tongue

**Examine upper limbs:**
Posture of outstretched arms
Wasting, fasciculation
Power, tone
Coordination
Reflexes

**Examine lower limbs:**
Power (hip flexion, ankle dorsiflexion), tone
Reflexes
Plantar responses

**Assess sensation:**
Ask the patient

**Practical box 18.1**  Short neurological examination.

---

| Test | Yield |
|------|-------|
| Urinalysis | Glycosuria (polyneuropathy), ketones (coma), Bence-Jones proteins (cord compression) |
| Blood | Raised MCV (B$_{12}$ deficiency), high ESR (giant-cell arteritis) |
| Serum electrolytes | Hyponatraemia, hypokalaemia (weakness) |
| Blood glucose | Hypoglycaemia (coma), diabetes mellitus (coma) |
| Serum calcium | Hypocalcaemia (tetany) |
| Chest X-ray | Bronchial carcinoma, spinal or rib lesions, thymoma |

ESR, erythrocyte sedimentation rate.

**Table 18.4**  The value of some investigations in neurological disease.

## PRELIMINARY INVESTIGATION

Examples of helpful routine investigations are given in Table 18.4.

## SPECIALIZED TESTS

### Skull X-rays

Plain X-rays should not be done unnecessarily. Examples of diagnostically important changes are:

---

| Grade | Definition |
|-------|------------|
| 0 | No contraction |
| 1 | Flicker of contraction |
| 2 | Active movement with gravity eliminated |
| 3 | Active moment against gravity |
| 4 | Active movement against gravity and resistance |
| 5 | Normal power |

**Table 18.3**  Grades of muscle weakness (Medical Research Council).

FRACTURES AND LESIONS OF THE VAULT OR BASE OF SKULL (e.g. metastases)

ENLARGEMENT OR DESTRUCTION OF THE SELLA TURCICA (e.g. intrasellar tumour, raised intracranial pressure)

INTRACRANIAL CALCIFICATION (e.g. tuberculoma, oligodendroglioma, wall of an aneurysm, cysticercosis)

PINEAL CALCIFICATION (to show midline shift)

## Spinal X-rays

These show fractures and degenerative, destructive and congenital bone lesions.

## Computed tomography

### Method

This technique uses a collimated X-ray beam moving synchronously with detectors across a slice of brain between 2 mm and 13 mm thick. The transmitted X-irradiation from an element, or pixel of that slice ($<1$ mm$^2$) is processed by computer and a numerical value (the Hounsfield number) is assigned to its density (air = $-1000$ units; water = 0; bone = $+1000$ units).

The difference in X-ray attenuation between bone, brain and CSF makes it possible to distinguish normal and infarcted tissue, tumour, extravasated blood and oedema. Examples of normal CT scans are shown in Fig. 18.1.

The image can be enhanced with intravenous contrast media to show areas of increased blood supply and oedema more clearly. Additional information about the subarachnoid space and the cerebral ventricles is obtained by scanning after the intrathecal injection of water-soluble contrast media (e.g. metrizamide) or air. In general, lesions greater than 1 cm in diameter can be visualized on CT scans.

The method is safe (apart from occasional systemic reactions to contrast); the irradiation involved is small.

### Uses

CT scanning is used for the diagnosis of:
- Cerebral tumours
- Intracerebral haemorrhage and infarction
- Subdural and extradural haematoma
- Subarachnoid haemorrhage
- Lateral shift of midline structures and displacement of the ventricular system
- Cerebral atrophy
- Pituitary lesions
- Spinal lesions (with CT myelography)

The CT scan can also be used to show that a brain is anatomically normal with a high degree of accuracy.

### Limitations

LESIONS UNDER 1 CM IN DIAMETER may be missed.

LESIONS WITH ATTENUATION CLOSE TO THAT OF BONE may be missed if they are near the skull.

LESIONS WITH ATTENUATION SIMILAR TO THAT OF BRAIN may be difficult to diagnose (e.g. 'isodense' subdural haematoma).

THE RESULTS ARE POOR WHEN THE PATIENT CANNOT COOPERATE—a general anaesthetic may occasionally be necessary.

## Magnetic resonance imaging

This technique makes use of the properties of protons aligned in a strong magnetic field. The protons are bombarded with radiofrequency waves at right angles to generate images. The equipment is expensive and still restricted to specialized units.

MRI scanning can distinguish between white matter and grey matter (Fig. 18.2) in the brain. Brain tumours, syringomyelia, the lesions of multiple sclerosis (MS) and lesions in the posterior fossa and at the foramen magnum are demonstrated well. In the spinal cord the technique can visualize tumours, cord compression and vascular malformations and is replacing myelography.

## Cerebral angiography and digital imaging

This demonstrates the cerebral arterial and venous systems. Contrast is injected intra-arterially or intravenously.

Carotid and vertebral arteriography is used for the demonstration of aneurysms, arteriovenous malformations and venous occlusion. Films of the aortic arch and the carotid and vertebral arteries demonstrate occlusion, stenoses and atheromatous plaques. Spinal angiography is used to investigate arteriovenous malformations of the cord.

Conventional arteriography is invasive and requires a general anaesthetic; it should rarely be performed outside a specialist centre. It carries a mortality of around 1% and a 1% risk of stroke.

Digital subtraction angiography (DSA), using a computerized subtraction technique is superseding traditional angiography. Contrast is injected intravenously or intra-arterially. No anaesthetic is necessary.

## Myelography

A water-soluble radiopaque dye is injected into the lumbar (or rarely cervical) subarachnoid space and viewed by conventional X-rays or CT. This is used in the diagnosis of tumours of the spinal cord and other causes of cord compression.

Radiculography is an examination confined to the lumbar region to show the anatomy of nerve roots.

## Isotope brain and bone scanning

A radioisotope, usually [$^{99m}$Tc]pertechnate is injected intravenously to detect:
- Vascular tumours
- Arteriovenous malformations
- Cerebral infarcts

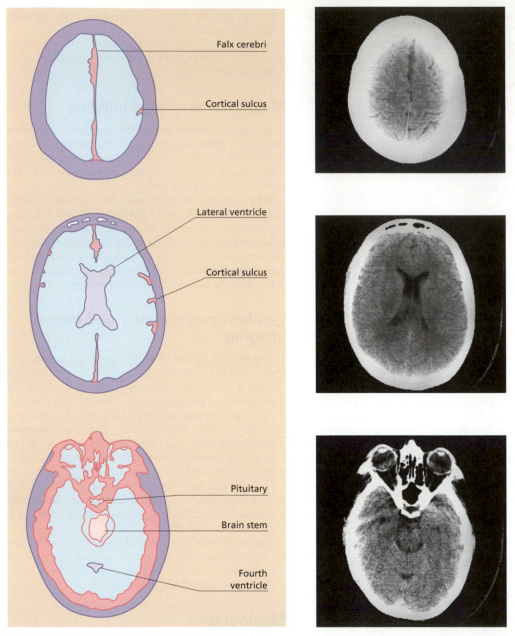

**Fig. 18.1** Normal CT head scan: transverse sections at three levels.

● Subdural haematoma

Isotope brain scanning is safe, non-invasive and cheap but has largely been overtaken by CT scanning because of the high incidence of false-negative isotope scans.

Isotope bone scanning is useful for detecting vertebral lesions (e.g. metastases).

## Electroencephalography

The electroencephalogram (EEG) is recorded from scalp electrodes on 16 channels simultaneously for 10–30 min.

The main value of the EEG is in the diagnosis of epilepsy and diffuse brain diseases.

### Epilepsy (see p. 912)

Spikes, or spike and wave abnormalities occur, but it should be emphasized that patients with epilepsy may have a normal EEG between fits.

### Diffuse brain disorders

Slow-wave EEG abnormalities are seen in encephalitis, dementia and metabolic states (e.g. hypoglycaemia and hepatic coma).

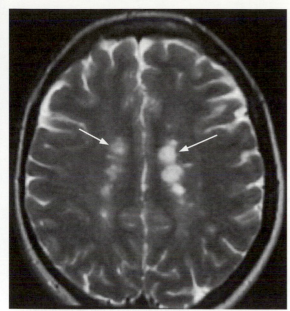

**Fig. 18.2** Multiple areas of high signal on T2 weighted images in the peri-ventricular white matter in a patient with multiple sclerosis.

**Brain death** (see p. 734)
The EEG is isoelectric (i.e. flat). An EEG is no longer necessary to confirm the diagnosis of brain death in the UK.

## Electromyography and nerve conduction studies

### Electromyography
A concentric needle electrode is inserted into voluntary muscle. The amplified recording is viewed on an oscilloscope and heard through a speaker. The following can be demonstrated:
- Normal interference pattern
- Denervation and reinnervation
- Myopathic, myotonic or myasthenic changes (see p. 951)

### Peripheral nerve conduction
Four measurements are of principal value in the diagnosis of neuropathies and nerve entrapment:
1 Mean conduction velocity (motor and sensory) (Fig. 18.3)
2 Distal motor latency
3 Sensory action potentials
4 Muscle action potentials

## Cerebral-evoked potentials

Visual-evoked potentials record the time taken for the response to a retinal stimulus to travel to the occipital cortex. Their value is chiefly in documenting previous retrobulbar neuritis (see p. 882), which causes a permanent delay in the latency despite clinical recovery of vision.

Similar techniques exist for the measurement of auditory and somatosensory potentials (from an arm or leg).

## Lumbar puncture (Practical box 18.2)

### Examination of the CSF
The indications for lumbar puncture are:
DIAGNOSIS OF MENINGITIS AND ENCEPHALITIS
DIAGNOSIS OF MS AND NEUROSYPHILIS
INTRATHECAL INJECTION OF CONTRAST MEDIA AND DRUGS
DIAGNOSIS OF SUSPECTED SUBARACHNOID HAEMORRHAGE (sometimes)
MEASUREMENT OF CSF PRESSURE (e.g. in benign intracranial hypertension, see p. 934)
REMOVAL OF CSF THERAPEUTICALLY (e.g. in benign intracranial hypertension)
DIAGNOSIS OF MISCELLANEOUS CONDITIONS (e.g. certain polyneuropathies, sarcoidosis, intrathecal neoplastic involvement)

## Biopsy

### Muscle
Biopsy is useful in the diagnosis of inflammatory and dystrophic disorders of muscle (see p. 951).

### Peripheral nerve
Biopsy, usually of the sural nerve, is carried out to aid diagnosis in certain polyneuropathies, e.g. due to vasculitides.

### Brain
Brain biopsy (e.g. of a non-dominant frontal lobe) is undertaken to diagnose inflammatory and degenerative brain diseases.

CT-guided stereotactic biopsy of intracranial mass lesions is being used increasingly. It is less traumatic and more accurate than conventional biopsy through a skull burr hole or craniotomy.

## Psychometric assessment

Formal psychometric testing is used to assess intellectual function. Preservation of the verbal IQ (a measure of past attainments) in the presence of deterioration of the performance IQ (a measure of present abilities) is a useful indicator of dementia. Low subtest scores (e.g. for block design, speech or constructional skills) indicate impaired function of specific regions of the brain. The main limitation of these techniques is that depression and lack of concentration can also impair scores.

## Miscellaneous tests

Certain specialized tests are employed in the diagnosis of individual (and often rare) neurological diseases. Examples are:
SERUM ENZYMES LIBERATED FROM MUSCLE —greatly

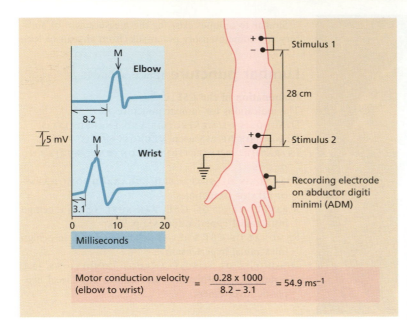

Motor conduction velocity (elbow to wrist) $= \dfrac{0.28 \times 1000}{8.2 - 3.1} = 54.9 \text{ ms}^{-1}$

**Fig. 18.3** Measurement of motor conduction velocity of the ulnar nerve. A recording electrode on the abductor digiti minimi records the muscle action potential (M) from the ulnar nerve at the elbow (stimulus 1) and at the wrist (stimulus 2). From these values the motor conduction velocity can be calculated.

---

Lumbar puncture should not be performed in the presence of raised intracranial pressure or when an intracranial mass lesion is a possibility.

**Technique**

The patient is placed on the edge of the bed in the left lateral position with the knees and chin as close together as possible

The third and fourth lumbar spines are marked. The fourth lumbar spine usually lies on a line joining the iliac crests

Using sterile precautions, 2% lignocaine is injected into the dermis by raising a bleb in either the third or fourth lumbar interspace

The special lumbar puncture needle is pushed through the skin in the midline. It is pressed steadily forwards and slightly towards the head

When the needle is felt to penetrate the dura mater, the stylet is withdrawn and a few drops of CSF are allowed to escape

The CSF pressure can now be measured by connecting a manometer to the needle. The patient's head must be on the same level as the sacrum. Normal CSF pressure is 60–150 mmH$_2$O. It rises and falls with respiration and the heart beat

Specimens of CSF are collected in three sterilized test tubes and sent to the laboratory. An additional sample in which the sugar level can be measured, together with a simultaneous blood sample for blood sugar measurement, should be taken when relevant (e.g. in meningitis)

Patients are usually asked to lie flat after the procedure to avoid a headache that may develop but this is probably of little value

Analgesics may be required

**Contraindications for lumbar puncture**

Suspicion of a mass lesion in the brain or spinal cord. Caudal herniation of the cerebellar tonsils ('coning') may occur if an intracranial mass is present and the pressure below is reduced by removal of CSF. This is extremely dangerous (see p. 933)

Any cause of raised intracranial pressure

Local infection near the site of puncture

Congenital lesions in the lumbosacral region (e.g. meningomyelocele)

Platelet count below $40 \times 10^9$/litre and other clotting abnormalities, including anticoagulant drugs

Unconscious patients and those with papilloedema must have a CT scan before lumbar puncture

These contraindications are relative, i.e. there are circumstances when lumbar puncture is carried out in spite of them.

The composition of the normal CSF is shown in Table 18.5.

**Practical box 18.2**  Lumbar puncture.

| Appearance | Crystal clear Colourless |
|---|---|
| Pressure | 60–150 mm of $H_2O$ with patient recumbent |
| Cell count | 5 per $mm^3$ No polymorphs Mononuclear cells only |
| Protein | 0.2–0.4 g litre$^{-1}$ |
| Glucose | $\frac{2}{3}$ to $\frac{1}{2}$ of blood glucose |
| IgG | <15% of total CSF protein |
| Oligoclonal bands | Absent |

**Table 18.5**  The normal CSF.

raised in many primary muscle diseases (see p. 951). Creatine phosphokinase is the enzyme usually assayed in most laboratories.

SERUM COPPER AND CAERULOPLASMIN in Wilson's disease (see p. 270).

ANTIBODIES TO ACETYLCHOLINE RECEPTOR PRO-TEIN in myasthenia gravis (see p. 952).

# Functional anatomy

The functional unit of the nervous system is the neurone, with its cell body and axon, which terminates at a synapse. The specificity, size and type of each group of neurones varies greatly. For example, an α motor neurone of the anterior horn cell of the lumbar spinal cord has an axonal length of over 1 m and innervates several hundred to 2000 muscle fibres—to form the motor unit. By contrast, a spinal or intracerebral internuncial neurone may have an axon under 100 μm in length and terminate solely on one or other neuronal cell body.

It is now generally agreed that transmission at most if not all synapses is mediated by chemical neurotransmitters. These transmitters are released by action potentials passing down the axon. They then react with the receptors on the postsynaptic cell body, increasing its ionic permeability and propagating a further action potential within it.

This combination of electrical activity in the axon and chemical release at the synapse is the basis of all neurological function.

Important neurotransmitter substances are:
- Acetylcholine
- Noradrenaline
- Adrenaline
- 5-Hydroxytryptamine
- γ-Aminobutyric acid (GABA)
- Opioid peptides
- Prostaglandins
- Histamine
- Dopamine
- Glutamate

The exact role of these neurotransmitters in pathogenesis is being evaluated, but it is now thought that a wide variety of acute and chronic neurological disease may be mediated, at least in part, by a final common pathway of neuronal injury involving excessive stimulation of glutamate receptors. Effective glutamate antagonists are being used in clinical trials (see p. 941).

# The cerebral cortex

## CEREBRAL LOCALIZATION

This subject causes everyone considerable difficulty. The following paragraphs summarize the areas of principal clinical importance in general medicine.

## The dominant hemisphere

The concept of cerebral dominance arose with the observation that right-handed stroke (and other) patients with acquired language disorders had destructive lesions within the left hemisphere. Almost all right-handed people have language function in the left hemisphere; so do over 70% of those who are apparently left-handed.

Destructive lesions within the left frontotemporoparietal region cause disorders of:
SPOKEN LANGUAGE—known as aphasia or dysphasia
WRITING—known as agraphia
READING—known as alexia (or acquired dyslexia)

Developmental dyslexia describes children who have delayed and disorganized reading and writing ability with normal intelligence.

## The non-dominant hemisphere

Disorders in right-handed patients with right hemisphere lesions are more difficult to define but comprise abnormalities of perception of internal and external space. Examples of this are losing the way in familiar surroundings, failing to put on clothing correctly ('dressing apraxia') or failure to draw simple shapes ('constructional apraxia').

## APHASIA AND DYSARTHRIA

Aphasia (or dysphasia) is a loss or defect in language and is caused by left frontotemporoparietal lesions.

Dysarthria is simply disordered articulation. Any lesion that produces paralysis, slowing or incoordination of the muscles of articulation or local discomfort will cause dysarthria. Examples are upper and lower motor lesions of the lower cranial nerves, cerebellar lesions, Parkinson's disease and local lesions of the mouth, larynx, pharynx and tongue. Many aphasic patients are also somewhat dysarthric.

## Some varieties of aphasia

**Broca's aphasia (expressive aphasia, anterior aphasia)**
A lesion in the left frontal lobe causes reduced fluency of speech with comprehension relatively preserved.

The patient makes great efforts to initiate speech. Language is reduced to a few disjointed words and there is failure to construct sentences.

Patients who recover from this form of aphasia say that they knew what they wanted to say, but 'could not get the words out'.

**Wernicke's aphasia (receptive aphasia, posterior aphasia)**
A left temporoparietal lesion leaves language that is fluent but the words themselves are incorrect. This varies from the insertion of a few incorrect or non-existent words into fluent speech (when it may be difficult to recognize aphasia) to a profuse outpouring of jargon, i.e. rubbish with wholly non-existent words. This may be so bizarre as to be confused with psychotic behaviour.

Patients who have recovered from Wernicke's aphasia say that when aphasic they found the speech of others like a wholly unintelligible foreign language, and though they knew they were speaking could neither stop themselves nor understand what they said.

**Nominal aphasia (anomic aphasia or amnestic aphasia)**
This describes difficulty naming familiar objects. When it occurs in a severe and isolated form it is caused by a left posterior temporal/inferior parietal lesion. Naming difficulty is, however, an early sign in all types of aphasia.

**Global aphasia (central aphasia)**
This is the expressive disturbance characteristic of Broca's aphasia and the loss of comprehension of Wernicke's. It is due to widespread damage to the areas concerned with speech and is the commonest form of aphasia after a severe left hemisphere infarct. Writing and reading are also affected.

## CLINICAL FEATURES OF LOCAL CEREBRAL LESIONS

Focal lesions of the cerebral cortex cause symptoms and signs by three processes:
1 Destruction or suppression of function of cortical neurones and surrounding structures (Table 18.6)
2 Synchronous discharge of neurones by irritative lesions which cause partial (focal) seizures that may become generalized seizures (Table 18.7)
3 Displacement of the intracranial contents (see p. 933) and surrounding cerebral oedema

## MEMORY AND ITS DISORDERS

(see p. 964)

Disorders of memory follow damage to the medial surface of the temporal lobe and its brain stem connections,

| Site of lesion | Disorder |
|---|---|
| Either frontal region | Intellectual impairment<br>Personality change<br>Urinary incontinence<br>Monoparesis or hemiparesis |
| Left frontal region | Broca's aphasia |
| Left temporoparietal region | Acalculia<br>Alexia<br>Agraphia<br>Wernicke's aphasia<br>Right–left disorientation<br>Homonymous field defects |
| Right temporal region | Confusional states<br>Failure to recognize faces<br>Homonymous field defects |
| Either parietal region | Contralateral sensory loss or neglect<br>Constructional apraxia[a]<br>Agraphaesthesia[b]<br>Failure to recognize surroundings<br>Limb apraxia<br>Homonymous field defects |
| Right parietal region | Dressing apraxia<br>Failure to recognize faces<br>Neglect of left limbs |
| Occipital lobes and occipitoparietal region | Visual field defects (see p. 881)<br>Visuospatial defects<br>Disturbances of visual recognition |

[a]Inability to draw or construct shapes and patterns.
[b]Inability to recognize shapes drawn on the palm.

**Table 18.6** Principal disorders seen with a destructive lesion of the cortex in a right-handed individual.

| Site of lesion | Effects |
|---|---|
| Frontal region | Partial seizures—focal motor seizures of contralateral limbs<br>Conjugate deviation of head and eyes away from the lesion |
| Temporal region | Formed visual hallucinations<br>Complex partial seizures<br>Memory disturbances (e.g. *déjà vu*) |
| Parietal region | Partial seizures—focal sensory seizures of contralateral limbs<br>Crude visual hallucinations (e.g. shapes in one part of the field) |
| Occipital region | Visual disturbances (e.g. flashes) |

**Table 18.7** Effects of an irritative lesion of the cortex.

Alcohol (Wernicke–Korsakoff syndrome)
Head injury (severe)
Anoxia
Posterior cerebral artery occlusion (bilateral)
Herpes simplex encephalitis
Chronic sedative and solvent abuse
Bilateral invasive tumours
Arsenic poisoning
Following hypoglycaemia

**Table 18.8**  Causes of amnestic syndrome.

including the hippocampi, fornices and mammillary bodies. Bilateral lesions are usually necessary to cause amnesia.

It is characteristic of all organic disorders of memory that more recent events are recalled poorly in contrast to the relative preservation of distant memories.

Memory loss is a part of dementia of any cause and occurs in a wide variety of clinical situations (Table 18.8).

## The cranial nerves

### THE OLFACTORY NERVE (FIRST CRANIAL NERVE)

This sensory nerve arises from olfactory (smell) receptors in the nasal mucosa. Branches pierce the cribriform plate and synapse in the olfactory bulb. The olfactory tract then passes to the olfactory cortex in the anteromedial surface of the temporal lobe.

Loss of the sense of smell (anosmia) occurs with head injury and tumours of the olfactory groove (e.g. meningioma, frontal glioma).

The sense of smell is often lost, sometimes permanently, after upper respiratory viral infections. It is diminished in nasal obstruction.

### THE OPTIC NERVE (SECOND CRANIAL NERVE) AND THE VISUAL SYSTEM

The optic nerve carries axons from the ganglion cells of the retina to the lateral geniculate bodies. The visual pathway is shown in Fig. 18.4. It should be noted that the lens causes the image on the retina to be inverted. Thus, an object in the lower part of the visual field is projected to the upper retina and an object in the temporal half of the visual field is projected to the nasal half of the retina.

At the optic chiasm, fibres travelling in the nasal portions of the optic nerves cross to the opposite sides, where they join uncrossed temporal fibres from the lateral portion of each optic nerve. One optic tract thus carries fibres from the temporal side of the ipsilateral retina and the nasal side of the contralateral retina.

From the lateral geniculate body, fibres pass in the

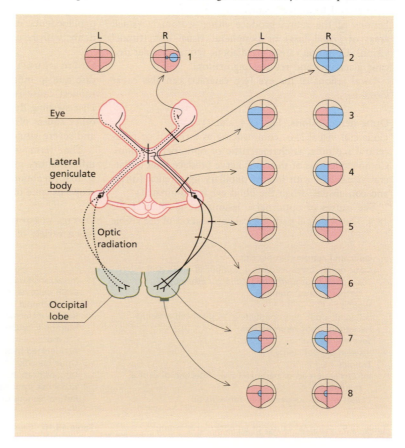

**Fig. 18.4**  The visual pathway
1, Paracentral scotoma—retinal lesion.
2, Mononuclear field loss—optic nerve lesion. 3, Bitemporal hemianopia—chiasmal lesion. 4, Homonymous hemianopia—optic tract lesion.
5, Homonymous quadrantanopia—temporal lesion. 6, Homonymous quadrantanopia—parietal lesion.
7, Homonymous hemianopia—occipital cortex or optic radiation.
8, Homonymous hemianopia—occipital pole lesion.

optic radiation to the visual cortex of the occipital lobe.

The visual field projected to each optic tract, radiation and cortex is called 'homonymous', to indicate the different (i.e. bilateral) origins of each pathway. (A homonym is the same word used to denote different things.)

Field defects are 'hemianopic' when half the field is affected, and 'quadrantanopic' when a quadrant is affected. 'Congruous' denotes symmetry and 'incongruous' lack of symmetry.

## Visual acuity

This should be tested with a Snellen test chart and corrected for refractive errors with lenses or a pinhole. The corrected visual acuity should be recorded. The normal acuity should be 6/6 to 6/9 in both eyes.

Blindness can be due to:

- Ocular causes, e.g. glaucoma, macular degeneration or diabetes
- Central (neurological) causes, e.g. optic nerve lesions, chiasmal compression

## Visual field defects

These should be charted by confrontation with white and red headed pins and, if abnormal or in doubt, recorded in detail with a Goldmann (or similar) screen. The common defects are shown in Fig. 18.4.

**Retinal and local eye lesions** (Fig. 18.4, site 1)
Lesions of the retina produce either scotomata (small areas of visual loss) or peripheral visual loss (tunnel vision). Common causes are diabetic retinal vascular disease, glaucoma and retinitis pigmentosa.

Local lesions of the eye (e.g. cataract) can also cause visual loss.

**Optic nerve lesions** (Fig. 18.4, site 2)
Unilateral visual loss, commencing as a central or paracentral scotoma, is characteristic of optic nerve lesions. Complete lesions of the optic nerve produce total unilateral visual loss with loss of pupillary light reflex (direct and consensual) when the blind eye is illuminated.

The causes of optic nerve lesions are given in Table 18.9. The principal pathological appearances of the visible part of the nerve (the disc) seen on fundoscopy are:

- Disc swelling (papilloedema)
- Pallor (optic atrophy)

PAPILLOEDEMA (TABLE 18.10). This means swelling of the papilla—the optic disc. The earliest ophthalmoscopic signs are redness of the disc followed by blurring and heaping up of its margins (the nasal margin first). There is loss of the normal, visible, spontaneous pulsation of the retinal veins. The physiological cup becomes obliterated and the disc engorged, with dilatation of its vessels and the retinal veins. Small haemorrhages surround the disc.

True disc oedema should be distinguished from various conditions that simulate it. Marked hypermetropic (long-sighted) refractive errors make the disc appear pink, distant and ill-defined. Opaque (myelinated) nerve fibres near the disc and hyaline bodies (drusen) can be mistaken for disc swelling.

In difficult cases fluorescein angiography is diagnostic. In papilloedema, fluorescein injected intravenously leaks from the disc capillaries and may be seen and photographed.

Early papilloedema from causes other than optic neuritis (see below) often produces few visual symptoms, the patient's complaints being those of the underlying disease.

As disc oedema develops there is enlargement of the blind spot and blurring of the vision. As the disc becomes engorged its arterial blood flow is reduced and, in severe papilloedema, infarction of the nerve occurs, often suddenly, with resulting blindness.

OPTIC NEURITIS. Optic neuritis is swelling of the optic disc due to inflammation of the optic nerve. The commonest cause is demyelination (e.g. multiple sclerosis). Disc swelling due to optic neuritis is distinguished from other causes of disc oedema by the occurrence of early and severe visual loss.

The term retrobulbar neuritis implies that the inflammatory process is 'behind the bulb' (i.e. the eye), so that no abnormality may be seen with the ophthalmoscope in spite of visual impairment.

OPTIC ATROPHY. Disc pallor (optic atrophy) may follow a variety of pathological processes, including infarc-

---

Optic and retrobulbar neuritis
Optic nerve compression (e.g. tumour or aneurysm)
Toxic optic neuropathy (e.g. tobacco, ethambutol, methyl alcohol, quinine)
Syphilis
Ischaemic optic neuropathy (e.g. in giant-cell arteritis)
Hereditary optic neuropathies
Severe anaemia
Vitamin $B_{12}$ deficiency
Trauma
Infective—spread of paranasal sinus infection or orbital cellulitis
Causes of papilloedema (see Table 18.10)

**Table 18.9** Principal causes of an optic nerve lesion.

---

Intracranial mass lesions
Brain oedema, e.g. encephalitis, trauma
Subarachnoid haemorrhage
Benign intracranial hypertension
Metabolic causes, e.g. $CO_2$ retention, chronic anoxia, hypocalcaemia
Accelerated hypertension
Optic neuritis
Disc infiltration, e.g. leukaemia
Ischaemic optic neuropathy
Retinal venous obstruction (thrombosis, orbital lesions)

**Table 18.10** Causes of papilloedema.

tion of the nerve, demyelinating optic neuritis (in MS), optic nerve compression, syphilis, vitamin $B_{12}$ deficiency and toxins (e.g. quinine and methyl alcohol).

Optic atrophy is described as consecutive or secondary when it follows papilloedema. The degree of visual loss depends upon the underlying pathology.

### Lesions of the optic chiasm (Fig. 18.4, site 3)

Bi-temporal hemianopic field defects occur when a lesion compresses the central part of the chiasm. Common causes are:

- Pituitary neoplasm
- Craniopharyngioma
- Secondary neoplasm

### Lesions of the optic tract and optic radiation (Fig. 18.4, sites 4, 5 and 6)

Homonymous hemianopia or quadrantanopia are the typical field defects caused by unilateral compression or infarction of these structures. Optic tract lesions are rare.

Temporal lobe lesions (due to tumour or infarction) cause upper quadrantanopic defects; parietal lobe lesions cause lower quadrantanopic defects.

### Lesions of the occipital cortex (Fig. 18.4, sites 7 and 8)

Homonymous hemianopic defects are caused by unilateral posterior cerebral artery infarction. The macular region (at the occipital pole) is spared because it has a separate blood supply from the middle cerebral artery.

Damage to one occipital pole causes a small, congruous, scotomatous, homonymous hemianopia (site 8).

Widespread bilateral occipital lobe damage by tumour, trauma or infarction causes the syndrome of 'cortical blindness' (Anton's syndrome). The patient is blind but characteristically lacks insight into the degree of visual loss and may deny it. The pupillary responses are normal (see also p. 908).

## The pupils

Sympathetic impulses from fibres in the nasociliary nerve stimulate the dilator muscle of the pupil (dilator pupillae).

Preganglionic sympathetic fibres to the eye (and face) originate in the hypothalamus, pass uncrossed through the midbrain and lateral medulla and emerge finally from the spinal cord at T1 (close to the lung apex). Postganglionic fibres begin in the superior cervical ganglion. These pass to the pupil in the nasociliary nerve from a plexus surrounding the internal carotid artery. Those fibres to the face (sweating and pilo-erection) form a plexus surrounding the external carotid artery. This arrangement is of clinical importance in Horner's syndrome.

Parasympathetic impulses from the ciliary ganglion in the short ciliary nerves to the sphincter muscle of the pupil (sphincter pupillae) cause the pupil to constrict.

An outline of the arrangement of parasympathetic fibres to the pupils and the mechanism of the light reflex is shown in Fig. 18.5.

### The light reflex

Afferent fibres in each optic nerve (some crossing in the chiasm, see Fig. 18.5) pass to both lateral geniculate bodies and relay to the Edinger–Westphal nuclei via the pretectal nucleus.

Efferent (parasympathetic) fibres from each Edinger–Westphal nucleus pass via the third nerve to the ciliary ganglion and thence to the pupil.

Light constricts the pupil of the eye being tested (direct reflex) and the contralateral pupil (consensual reflex).

### The convergence reflex

Fixation on a near object requires convergence of the ocular axes and is accompanied by pupillary constriction.

The afferent fibres in each optic nerve, which pass through both lateral geniculate bodies, also relay to the convergence centre. This centre receives 1a spindle afferent fibres from the extraocular muscles—principally the medial recti, which are innervated by the third nerve. The efferent route is from the convergence centre to the Edinger–Westphal nucleus, ciliary ganglion and pupils. Voluntary or reflex fixation on a near object is thus accompanied by appropriate convergence and pupillary constriction.

### Clinical abnormalities of the pupils

DEGENERATIVE CHANGES IN OLD AGE. The pupil tends to become small (3–3.5 mm) in old age (senile miosis) and may be irregular; a bright light is necessary to demonstrate constriction and the convergence reflex is sluggish. A slight difference between the size of the pupils is common (physiological anisocoria) but the changes may cause confusion with the Argyll Robertson pupil.

THE ARGYLL ROBERTSON PUPIL. This is a small, irregular (3 mm or less) pupil that is fixed to light, but constricts on convergence. The lesion is believed to be in the area surrounding the aqueduct.

The Argyll Robertson pupil is (almost) diagnostic of neurosyphilis. Similar changes are occasionally seen in diabetes mellitus.

THE MYOTONIC PUPIL (HOLMES–ADIE PUPIL). This is a dilated pupil seen most commonly in young women. It is usually unilateral. There is no reaction (or a very slow reaction) to a bright light and also an incomplete constriction to convergence. The condition is due to denervation in the ciliary ganglion.

The myotonic pupil is of no pathological significance but is often associated with diminished or absent tendon reflexes.

HORNER'S SYNDROME. This syndrome is due to interruption of sympathetic fibres to one eye. It presents as unilateral pupillary constriction with slight relative ptosis and enophthalmos. The conjunctival vessels may be injected. There is loss of sweating of the same side of the face or body; the extent depends upon the level of the lesion. The syndrome indicates a lesion of the sympath-

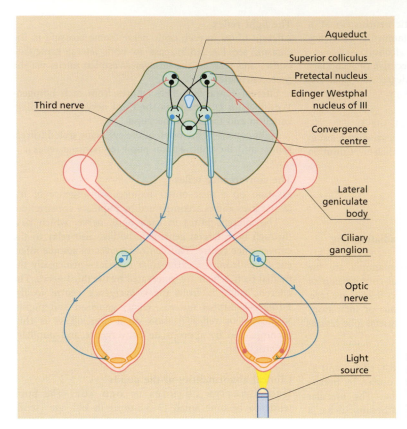

**Fig. 18.5** The pupils: afferent and parasympathetic efferent pathways. Some fibres concerned with the pupillary light reflex can bypass the lateral geniculate body and go to the pretectal nucleus.

etic pathway on the same side. Causes of Horner's syndrome are given in Table 18.11.

The level of the lesion is indicated by the distribution of the loss of sweating:

CENTRAL LESIONS affect sweating over the entire half of the head, arm and upper trunk.

LESIONS OF THE NECK PROXIMAL TO THE SUPERIOR CERVICAL GANGLION cause diminished sweating on the face.

LESIONS DISTAL TO THE SUPERIOR CERVICAL GANGLION do not affect sweating at all.

Pharmacological tests may indicate the level of the lesion. For example, a lesion distal to the superior cervical ganglion causes denervation hypersensitivity of the pupil, which dilates when 1 : 1000 adrenaline is instilled. This dose has little effect on the normal pupil or a proximal lesion. In clinical practice the test is of limited value.

Other abnormalities of the pupils seen in coma are discussed on p. 902.

## THE OCULAR MOVEMENTS AND THIRD, FOURTH AND SIXTH CRANIAL NERVES

The control of eye movement can be divided into:
1 The central upper motor neurone mechanisms, which drive the normal yoked parallel movements of the eyes (conjugate gaze)
2 The oculomotor, abducens and trochlear nerves and the muscles they supply

### Conjugate gaze

Fast voluntary and reflex eye movements originate in each frontal lobe. Fibres pass in the anterior limb of the

---

*Hemisphere and brain stem lesions*
Massive cerebral infarction
Pontine glioma
Lateral medullary syndrome
'Coning' of the temporal lobe

*Cervical cord lesions*
Syringomyelia
Cord tumours

*T1 root lesions*
Bronchial neoplasm (apical)
Apical tuberculosis
Cervical rib
Brachial plexus trauma

*Sympathetic chain in the neck*
Following thyroid/laryngeal surgery
Carotid artery occlusion
Neoplastic infiltration
Cervical sympathectomy

*Miscellaneous*
Congenital
Migrainous neuralgia (usually transient)

**Table 18.11**   Causes of Horner's syndrome.

internal capsule and cross in the pons to end in the centre for lateral gaze (paramedian pontine reticular formation (PPRF)) (Fig. 18.6a), which is close to each sixth nerve nucleus. It also receives fibres from:

THE IPSILATERAL OCCIPITAL CORTEX. These pathways are concerned with movements to track or pursue objects within the visual fields.

BOTH VESTIBULAR NUCLEI. These pathways are concerned with the relationship between eye movements and the position of the head and neck (doll's head reflexes, see p. 903).

Lateral eye movements are coordinated from the centre of lateral gaze through the medial longitudinal fasciculus (MLF) (Fig. 18.6b). Fibres from the centre pass to both the ipsilateral sixth nerve nucleus and, having crossed the midline, the opposite third nerve nucleus via the MLF. Each sixth nerve nucleus (supplying the lateral rectus) and the opposite third nerve nucleus (supplying the medial rectus and others) are thus linked. The eyes move with parallel axes and at the same velocity.

## Abnormalities of conjugate lateral gaze

A destructive lesion of one side of the brain allows the eyes to be driven laterally by the intact opposite pathway.

A destructive frontal-lobe lesion (e.g. an infarct) causes failure of conjugate lateral gaze to the side opposite to the lesion (Fig. 18.6a). In an acute lesion the eyes are often deviated past the midline to the side of the lesion and therefore look *towards the normal limbs*. There is usually a contralateral hemiparesis.

An irritative frontal-lobe lesion (e.g. an epileptic focus), by stimulating the opposite lateral gaze centre, drives the eyes away from the side of the lesion.

A unilateral destructive brain stem lesion involving the centre causes failure of horizontal conjugate gaze towards the side of the lesion. There is usually a hemiparesis and the eyes are deviated towards the paralysed limbs.

### Doll's head reflexes and skew deviation
These are of diagnostic value in coma (see p. 903).

### Internuclear ophthalmoplegia
Internuclear ophthalmoplegia (INO) is one of the commoner complex brain stem signs that involve the oculomotor system. It is due to a lesion within the MLF.

It is a common sign in MS. When present bilaterally it is almost pathognomonic of MS. Unilateral lesions are also caused by small brain stem infarcts. In a right INO there is a lesion of the right MLF (see Fig. 18.6b). On attempted left lateral gaze the right eye fails to adduct. The left eye develops coarse nystagmus in abduction.

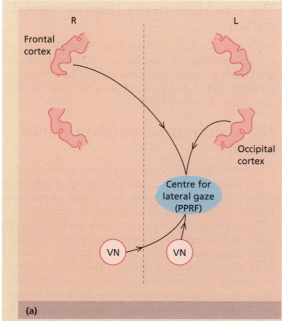
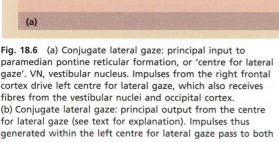
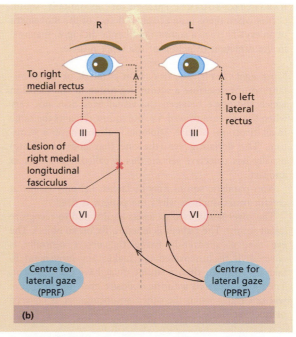

**Fig. 18.6**  (a) Conjugate lateral gaze: principal input to paramedian pontine reticular formation, or 'centre for lateral gaze'. VN, vestibular nucleus. Impulses from the right frontal cortex drive left centre for lateral gaze, which also receives fibres from the vestibular nuclei and occipital cortex.
(b) Conjugate lateral gaze: principal output from the centre for lateral gaze (see text for explanation). Impulses thus generated within the left centre for lateral gaze pass to both the ipsilateral VI nerve nucleus (lateral rectus muscle, abduction) and via the medial longitudinal fasciculus to neurones in the contralateral right III nerve nucleus (medial rectus muscle, adduction). Thus voluntary gaze to the left is initiated in the right frontal cortex. (From Bannister R (1985) *Brain's Clinical Neurology*, 6th edn. Oxford: Oxford University Press.) For lesion of right medial longitudinal fasciculus see text.

The side of the lesion is on the side of impaired adduction, not on the side of the nystagmus.

## Abnormalities of vertical gaze

A failure of up-gaze is caused by an upper brain stem lesion, such as a supratentorial mass pressing from above, or a tumour of the brain stem (e.g. a pinealoma). When the pupillary convergence reflex fails, this combination is called Parinaud's syndrome.

Defective up-gaze also occurs in certain degenerative disorders (e.g. progressive supranuclear palsy, see p. 920).

Impairment of up-gaze also occurs as part of normal ageing.

## Weakness of the extraocular muscles (diplopia)

Diplopia (double vision) implies that there is weakness of one or more of the extraocular muscles.

The cause is usually a lesion of the third, fourth or sixth cranial nerves (or a combination of these) or their nuclei, or disease of the neuromuscular junction (myasthenia gravis) or the ocular muscles.

### Squint (strabismus)

This is the appearance of the eyes when the visual axes fail to meet at the fixation point.

PARALYTIC SQUINT. Paralytic or 'incomitant' squint occurs when there is an acquired defect of the movement of an eye. There is a squint (and hence diplopia) maximal in the direction of action of the weak muscle.

NON-PARALYTIC SQUINT. Non-paralytic or 'concomitant' squint describes a squint beginning in childhood in which the angle between the visual axes does not vary when the eyes are moved, i.e. the squint remains the same in all directions of gaze. Diplopia is almost never a symptom. The deviating eye (the one that does not fixate) usually has defective vision; this is called 'amblyopia ex anopsia'.

Non-paralytic squint may be latent, i.e. only visible at certain times, such as when the patient is tired.

The *cover test* is used to assess squint and to recognize latent squint. The patient is asked to fix on an object. The eye that is apparently fixing the object centrally is covered. If the uncovered eye makes any movement to take up fixation, then a squint must have been present. The test is repeated with the opposite eye—the fixing eye will not move when the other, squinting, eye is covered or uncovered.

## The oculomotor nerve (third cranial nerve)

The nucleus of the third nerve lies ventral to the aqueduct in the midbrain. Efferent fibres to four external ocular muscles (the superior, inferior and medial recti, and the inferior oblique), the levator palpebrae superioris and the

| |
|---|
| Aneurysm of the posterior communicating artery |
| 'Coning' of the temporal lobe (see p. 933) |
| Infarction of the nerve |
|   In diabetes mellitus |
|   Atheroma |
| Midbrain infarction |
| Midbrain tumour |

**Table 18.12**  Common causes of an oculomotor nerve lesion.

sphincter pupillae (parasympathetic) enter the orbit through the superior orbital fissure.

The common causes of an oculomotor nerve lesion are given in Table 18.12. Signs of such a lesion are:
- Unilateral complete ptosis
- The eye facing 'down and out'
- Fixed and dilated pupil

'Sparing of the pupil' means that the parasympathetic fibres which run in a discrete bundle on the superior surface of the nerve are undamaged by the lesion and the pupil reacts normally.

In diabetes, infarction of the nerve usually spares the pupil. In a third nerve palsy the eye can still abduct (sixth nerve) and 'intort' (fourth nerve). When a patient with a right third nerve lesion attempts to converge and look downwards, the conjunctival vessels of the right eye can be seen to twist clockwise; this is 'intortion' and indicates that the trochlear nerve is intact.

## The trochlear nerve (fourth cranial nerve)

The trochlear nerve supplies the superior oblique muscle.

An isolated fourth nerve lesion is a rarity. The head is tilted away from the side of the lesion. The patient complains of diplopia when attempting to look down and away from the affected side.

## The abducens nerve (sixth cranial nerve)

The abducens nerve supplies the lateral rectus muscle.

In a sixth nerve lesion there is a convergent squint with diplopia maximal on looking to the side of the lesion. The eye cannot be abducted beyond the midline.

There are many causes of a sixth nerve lesion. The nerve may be involved in the brain stem, e.g. MS. In raised intracranial pressure it is compressed against the tip of the petrous temporal bone. The nerve sheath may be infiltrated by tumours, particularly nasopharyngeal carcinoma. An isolated sixth nerve palsy due to infarction may occur in diabetes mellitus. A sixth nerve lesion is a common sequel of head injury.

## THE TRIGEMINAL NERVE (FIFTH CRANIAL NERVE)

The trigeminal nerve is mainly sensory but contains some motor fibres.

Sensory fibres (Fig. 18.7 and see Figs 18.10 and 18.11)

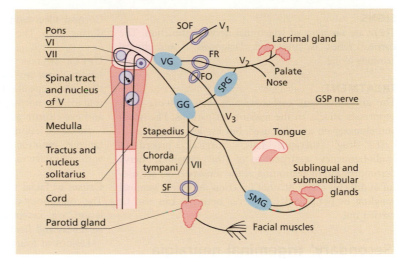

**Fig. 18.7** Fifth and seventh cranial nerves and their relationships. FO, foramen ovale; FR, foramen rotundum; GG, geniculate ganglion; GSP, greater superficial petrosal; SF, stylomastoid foramen; SMG, submandibular ganglion; SOF, superior orbital fissure; SPG, sphenopalatine ganglion; VG, Gasserian ganglion.

from the three divisions—ophthalmic ($V_1$), maxillary ($V_2$) and mandibular ($V_3$)—pass to the trigeminal ganglion at the apex of the petrous temporal bone. From here central fibres enter the brain stem. Ascending fibres transmitting the sensation of light touch enter the nucleus in the pons. Descending fibres carrying pain and temperature sensation form the spinal tract of the fifth nerve and end in the spinal nucleus in the medulla and upper cervical cord.

Motor fibres arise in the upper pons and join the mandibular branch to supply the muscles of mastication.

### Signs of a trigeminal nerve lesion

Diminution of the corneal reflex is often the first sign of a fifth nerve lesion.

A complete fifth nerve lesion causes unilateral sensory loss on the face, tongue and buccal mucosa. The jaw deviates to the side of the lesion when the mouth is opened.

Central (brain stem) lesions of the lower trigeminal nuclei (e.g. in syringobulbia, see p. 939) produce a characteristic circumoral sensory loss.

When the spinal tract (or spinal nucleus) alone is involved, the sensory loss is restricted to pain and temperature sensation, i.e. 'dissociated' (see p. 898).

### Causes of trigeminal nerve lesions

BRAIN STEM. Lesions at this site involve the nuclei and central connections, and include:
- Brain stem glioma
- MS
- Infarction
- Syringobulbia

CEREBELLOPONTINE ANGLE. Here the nerve is compressed by:
- Acoustic neuroma
- Meningioma
- Secondary neoplasm

APEX OF THE PETROUS TEMPORAL BONE. Infection from chronic middle-ear disease involves the nerve at this

site. The combination of this with pain and a sixth nerve lesion is called Gradenigo's syndrome.

CAVERNOUS SINUS. Here the trigeminal ganglion is compressed by:
- Aneurysm of internal carotid artery
- Extension of a pituitary neoplasm
- Cavernous sinus thrombosis
- Secondary neoplasm

The trigeminal ganglion is infected in ophthalmic herpes zoster (see p. 928), the commonest lesion of the ganglion.

PERIPHERAL BRANCHES OF THE TRIGEMINAL NERVE. These are affected by neoplastic infiltration of the skull base.

## Trigeminal neuralgia

Trigeminal neuralgia ('tic douloureux') is a condition of unknown cause, seen most commonly in old age. It is almost always unilateral.

### SYMPTOMS

Severe paroxysms of knife-like or electric-shock-like pain, lasting seconds, occur in the distribution of the fifth nerve. The pain tends to commence in the mandibular division ($V_3$) and spreads to the maxillary ($V_2$) and (rarely) to the ophthalmic division ($V_1$). It occurs many times a day.

Each paroxysm is stereotyped, brought on by stimulation of a specific 'trigger zone' in the face. Washing, shaving, a cold wind or eating are examples of the trivial stimuli that may provoke the pain. The face may be screwed up in agony (hence 'tic'—an involuntary movement).

The pain characteristically does not occur at night. Spontaneous remissions last for months or years before recurrence.

## SIGNS

There are no signs of trigeminal nerve dysfunction. The corneal reflex is preserved. Diagnosis is on clinical grounds alone.

## TREATMENT

The anticonvulsant carbamazepine 600–1200 mg daily suppresses attacks in the majority of patients. Phenytoin and clonazepam are also used, but are less effective.

If drug therapy fails, surgical procedures (radiofrequency extirpation of the ganglion, nerve decompression or sectioning of the sensory root) are useful in difficult cases. Alcohol injection into the trigeminal ganglion or peripheral fifth nerve branches can also be carried out.

## 'Secondary' trigeminal neuralgia

Trigeminal neuralgia also occurs in MS (see p. 922), with lesions of the cerebellopontine angle (see below) and with tumours of the fifth nerve (e.g. neuroma). These lesions are usually accompanied by physical signs (e.g. a depressed corneal reflex).

## Idiopathic trigeminal neuropathy

A chronic and isolated fifth nerve lesion may sometimes develop without any apparent cause. When sensory loss is severe, trophic changes (facial scarring and corneal ulceration) occur.

## Postherpetic neuralgia (see p. 928)

This may occur in the distribution of one division of the trigeminal nerve, commonly the first.

# THE FACIAL NERVE (SEVENTH CRANIAL NERVE)

This nerve is largely motor in function, supplying the muscles of facial expression. The nerve carries sensory taste fibres from the anterior two-thirds of the tongue via the chorda tympani. The complex arrangement of the nerves to the face, their nuclei and connections is shown in Fig. 18.7.

The facial nerve arises from the seventh nerve nucleus in the pons and leaves the skull through the stylomastoid foramen.

Part of each facial nucleus supplying the upper face (principally the frontalis muscle) receives some supranuclear fibres from each hemisphere.

### Unilateral facial weakness

LOWER MOTOR NEURONE (LMN) LESIONS. A unilateral LMN lesion causes weakness of all the muscles of facial expression on the same side. The face, especially the angle of the mouth, falls, and dribbling occurs from the corner of the mouth. There is weakness of frontalis and of eye closure since the upper facial muscles are weak.

Corneal ulceration may occur if the cornea is exposed during sleep. The platysma muscle is also weak.

UPPER MOTOR NEURONE (UMN) LESIONS. UMN lesions cause weakness of the lower part of the face on the side opposite the lesion. The frontalis muscle is spared; the normal furrowing of the brow is preserved, and eye closure and blinking are not affected.

In UMN lesions there is relative preservation of spontaneous 'emotional' movement (e.g. smiling) compared with voluntary movement.

### Causes of facial weakness

The commonest cause of facial weakness is a supranuclear lesion, e.g. cerebral infarction, leading to UMN facial weakness and hemiparesis.

Lesions at four other levels may be recognized by the associated signs.

PONS. The sixth nerve nucleus is encircled by the seventh nerve fibres and is therefore often involved in pontine lesions of the seventh nerve, causing a lateral rectus palsy.

If there is accompanying damage to the neighbouring centre for lateral gaze (see p. 885) and corticospinal tract, there is the combination of:
● LMN facial weakness
● Failure of conjugate lateral gaze (towards the lesion)
● Contralateral hemiparesis
Causes include pontine tumours (e.g. glioma), demyelination and vascular lesions.

The facial nucleus is affected in poliomyelitis (see p. 929) and in motor neurone disease (see p. 940); the latter usually causes bilateral weakness.

CEREBELLOPONTINE ANGLE. The fifth, sixth and eighth nerves are affected with the seventh nerve in lesions in the cerebellopontine angle. Causes are acoustic neuroma and meningioma.

WITHIN THE PETROUS TEMPORAL BONE. The geniculate ganglion (a sensory ganglion for taste) lies at the genu of the facial nerve (see Fig. 18.7). Fibres join the facial nerve in the chorda tympani and carry taste from the anterior two-thirds of the tongue. The (motor) nerve to the stapedius muscle leaves the facial nerve distal to the genu.

Lesions within the petrous temporal bone cause:
● Loss of taste on the anterior two-thirds of the tongue
● Hyperacusis (an unpleasantly loud distortion of noise) due to paralysis of the stapedius muscle
Causes include:
● Bell's palsy
● Trauma
● Infection of the middle ear
● Herpes zoster (Ramsay Hunt syndrome)
● Tumours (e.g. glomus tumour)

WITHIN THE FACE. Branches of the facial nerve pierce the parotid gland and supply the muscles of facial expression. The nerve can be damaged here by parotid gland tumours, mumps (epidemic parotitis), sarcoidosis (see p. 687) and trauma.

The nerve is also affected in polyneuritis (e.g. Guillain–Barré syndrome, see p. 946), usually bilaterally.

Weakness of the muscles of the face also occurs in primary muscle disease and disease of the neuromuscular junction. Weakness is usually bilateral. Causes include:

- Dystrophia myotonica (see p. 954)
- Facio-scapulo-humeral dystrophy (see p. 953)
- Myasthenia gravis (see p. 952)

## Bell's palsy

This is a common, acute, isolated facial nerve palsy believed to be due to a viral infection that causes swelling of the nerve within the petrous temporal bone.

### SYMPTOMS

The patient notices marked unilateral facial weakness, sometimes with loss of taste on the anterior two-thirds of the tongue. Pain behind the ear is common at onset. The diagnosis is made on clinical grounds. No other cranial nerves are involved.

### MANAGEMENT AND COURSE

Spontaneous improvement usually occurs towards the end of the second week. Thereafter, continuing recovery occurs but this may take 12 months to become complete. About 15% of patients are left with a severe, unsightly, residual weakness.

Electrophysiological tests are of some help in predicting the outcome. After the third week, the absence of an evoked potential from muscle (the nerve is stimulated over the parotid gland) indicates that recovery is unlikely.

Steroids (e.g. prednisolone 60 mg daily, reducing to nil over 10 days) or adrenocorticotrophic hormone (ACTH) reduce the proportion of patients left with a severe deficit, provided the drugs are given at the onset.

A tarsorrhapy (suturing of the upper to the lower lid) may be necessary if there is prolonged corneal exposure. Adhesive tape is a useful temporary measure.

Cosmetic surgery and/or reinnervation (e.g. anastomosis of the lingual nerve to the facial nerve) are sometimes indicated after a year has elapsed from the initial attack if there is severe residual paralysis.

The condition occasionally recurs and is very rarely bilateral.

## Ramsay Hunt syndrome

This is herpes zoster (shingles) of the geniculate ganglion.

There is a facial palsy (identical to Bell's palsy) with herpetic vesicles in the external auditory meatus (which receives a sensory twig from the facial nerve) and sometimes in the soft palate. Deafness may occur.

Treatment for shingles should be given (see p. 1015).

## HEMIFACIAL SPASM

This is an irregular clonic spasm of the facial muscles, usually occurring in middle-aged women. It varies in severity from a mild inconvenience to a severe and disabling condition when it affects all the facial musculature of one side.

The causes are:

- Idiopathic
- Acoustic neuroma
- Paget's disease of the skull
- Following Bell's palsy
- Pressure from aberrant vessels in the cerebellopontine angle

### SIGNS

There are clonic spasms of the facial muscles on one side. A mild LMN facial weakness is common.

### MANAGEMENT

Mild cases require no treatment. In severe cases various destructive or decompressive procedures on the facial nerve in the cerebellopontine angle are helpful. Local injection of botulinum toxin reduces the movements for some months. Drugs are of no value.

## Myokymia

Facial myokymia is a rare, continuous, fine, sinuous movement of the lower face that is seen in brain stem lesions (e.g. MS, brain stem glioma).

The term myokymia is also used to describe the innocent twitching around the eye that commonly occurs in fatigue.

# THE VESTIBULOCOCHLEAR NERVE (EIGHTH CRANIAL NERVE)

This nerve has two parts—cochlear and vestibular.

## Cochlear nerve

Auditory fibres from the spiral organ (of Corti) in the cochlea pass to the cochlear nuclei in the pons. Fibres from these nuclei cross the midline and pass upwards through the medial lemnisci to the medial geniculate bodies and the temporal gyri.

The symptoms of a cochlear nerve lesion are deafness and tinnitus. The signs are of hearing loss, with bone conduction decreased as well as air conduction. This is called sensorineural or perceptive deafness.

## Vestibular nerve

Vestibular fibres from the three semicircular canals, the saccule and the utricle pass to the vestibular nuclei in the pons. Vestibular nerve fibres also pass directly to the cerebellum.

The vestibular nuclei are connected to the spinal cord, the cerebellum, the nuclei of the ocular muscles and the centre for lateral gaze, the spinal muscles and the temporal lobe.

The maintenance of balance and posture depends in part upon impulses passing between the neck and spinal muscles and the vestibular system.

The main symptom of a vestibular lesion is vertigo. Vomiting frequently accompanies acute vertigo of any cause. Nystagmus is the principal physical sign, often with loss of balance.

## Vertigo

Vertigo, the definite illusion of movement of the subject or surroundings, indicates a disturbance of vestibular, brain stem or, rarely, cortical function. The principal causes are given in Table 18.13.

Deafness and tinnitus accompanying vertigo indicate that its origin is from the ear or the eighth cranial nerve.

### Nystagmus

Nystagmus is a rhythmic oscillation of the eyes. It is a sign of disease of either the ocular or the vestibular system and its connections. Nystagmus is described as either 'pendular' or 'jerk'.

For true nystagmus to be present it must be sustained and demonstrable within binocular gaze.

PENDULAR NYSTAGMUS. Pendular movement means movements to and fro which are similar both in velocity and amplitude. Pendular nystagmus is almost always binocular, horizontal and present in all directions of gaze.

It is seen when there is poor visual fixation (e.g. long-standing, severe visual impairment) or as a congenital lesion, when it is sometimes associated with head-nodding. It very rarely occurs in 'neurological' diseases.

JERK NYSTAGMUS. Jerk nystagmus (the usual nystagmus of neurological disease) has a fast and a slow component to the rhythmic movement. It is seen in vestibular, brain stem, cerebellar and (very rarely) cortical lesions.

The direction of the nystagmus is named after the fast component, which can be thought of as a reflex attempt to correct the slower component.

Considerable difficulties exist when attempts are made to use the direction of jerk nystagmus alone as a localizing sign, although it is both a common and valuable indication of abnormality. The following are useful starting points:

| |
|---|
| Ménière's disease |
| Drugs (e.g. gentamicin, anticonvulsant intoxication) |
| Toxins (e.g. ethyl alcohol) |
| 'Vestibular neuronitis' |
| Multiple sclerosis |
| Migraine |
| Acute cerebellar lesions |
| Cerebellopontine angle lesions |
| Partial seizures (temporal lobe focus) |
| Brain stem ischaemia or infarction |
| Benign positional vertigo |

**Table 18.13** Principal causes of vertigo.

HORIZONTAL OR ROTARY NYSTAGMUS may be either of peripheral (middle ear) or central (brain stem and its connections) origin. In peripheral lesions it is usually transient (minutes or hours); in central lesions it is long-lasting (weeks, months or more).

VERTICAL NYSTAGMUS is caused only by central lesions.

DOWN-BEAT NYSTAGMUS, a rarity, is caused by lesions around the foramen magnum.

## Investigation of vestibulocochlear nerve lesions

AUDIOMETRY is of value in distinguishing sensorineural deafness from conductive deafness.

CALORIC TESTS are used to assess function of the labyrinth. These record the evoked nystagmus when first ice cold, then warm, water is run into the external meatus. Decreased or absent nystagmus indicates ipsilateral labyrinth, eighth nerve or brain stem involvement. In the normal caloric test:

ICE COLD WATER IN THE LEFT EAR causes nystagmus with the fast movement to the right

WARM WATER IN THE LEFT EAR causes nystagmus with the fast movement to the left

The right ear would give opposite responses.

AUDITORY EVOKED POTENTIALS record the response from a repetitive 'click' stimulus. The level of the lesion may be detected by abnormalities in the response.

## Lesions of the eighth nerve and its connections

Lesions at five levels can be recognized by the associated signs.

### Cortex

Vertigo sometimes occurs as an aura in a partial seizure of temporal lobe origin.

Deafness is very rare in cortical lesions.

### Pons

Vertigo is common with demyelinating or vascular lesions of the brain stem that involve the vestibular nuclei and their connections. A sixth or seventh nerve lesion, an internuclear ophthalmoplegia or contralateral hemiparesis help localization. Nystagmus is frequently present.

Deafness is very rare in pontine lesions.

### Cerebellopontine angle

Perceptive deafness occurs. Sixth, seventh and fifth nerve lesions develop, followed by cerebellar signs (ipsilateral) and later 'pyramidal' signs (contralateral). Nystagmus is usually present.

Causes include acoustic neuroma, meningioma and secondary neoplasm.

**Petrous temporal bone**

A seventh nerve lesion may be present. Causes include trauma, middle ear infection and Paget's disease of bone.

**End-organ disease**

The main causes are:

- Ménière's disease
- Drugs (e.g. gentamicin)
- Noise
- Middle-ear infection
- Intrauterine rubella
- Congenital syphilis
- Mumps
- 'Vestibular neuronitis'

## Ménière's disease

This condition is characterized by recurrent attacks of the three symptoms—vertigo, tinnitus and deafness. It is associated with a dilatation of the endolymph system of unknown cause.

### SYMPTOMS

The sudden, unprovoked attacks of vertigo with vomiting and loss of balance last from minutes to hours. Tinnitus and deafness accompany an attack but may be over-shadowed by the degree of vertigo. The attacks are recurrent over months or years. Ultimately deafness develops and the vertigo ceases.

### SIGNS

Nystagmus often accompanies an attack. Sensorineural deafness may be found.

### MANAGEMENT

Medical treatment with vestibular sedatives (e.g. cinnarizine or prochlorperazine) is unsatisfactory. Each attack is, however, self-limiting. Betahistine 8 mg three times daily is sometimes helpful.

Recurrent severe attacks may require surgery (e.g. ultrasound destruction of the labyrinth or vestibular nerve section).

## Vestibular neuronitis

This common but poorly understood syndrome describes an acute attack of severe vertigo with nystagmus, often with vomiting, but without loss of hearing. It is believed to follow or accompany viral infections that affect the labyrinth.

The disturbance lasts for several days or weeks but is self-limiting and rarely recurs. Treatment is with vestibular sedatives. The condition is sometimes followed by benign positional vertigo. Very similar symptoms may be caused by demyelination or vascular lesions within the brain stem.

## Benign positional vertigo and positional nystagmus

Positional vertigo is vertigo precipitated by head movements, usually into a particular position. It may occur when turning in bed or on sitting up. The vertigo is transient, lasting seconds or minutes.

Vertigo can be produced by moving the patient's head suddenly (Hallpike's test). There is a latent interval of a few seconds, followed by nystagmus.

The syndrome of benign positional vertigo sometimes follows 'vestibular neuronitis', head injury or ear infection. It usually lasts for some months. There are no sequelae, although the condition sometimes recurs. Treatment is with vestibular sedatives.

Positional nystagmus (and vertigo) that is without a latent interval and does not fatigue is occasionally seen with neoplasms of the posterior fossa.

# THE GLOSSOPHARYNGEAL AND VAGUS NERVES (NINTH AND TENTH CRANIAL NERVES)

## The glossopharyngeal nerve

This mixed nerve arises in the medulla and leaves the skull through the jugular foramen with the vagus and accessory nerves.

Its sensory fibres supply all sensation to the tonsillar fossa and pharynx (the afferent pathway of the gag reflex), and taste to the posterior third of the tongue.

Motor fibres supply the stylopharyngeus muscle, autonomic fibres supply the parotid gland, and a sensory branch supplies the carotid sinus.

Isolated lesions are most unusual, since lesions at the jugular foramen also affect the vagus and sometimes the accessory nerves.

### Glossopharyngeal neuralgia

This is a rare, severe, paroxysmal neuralgia. Pain involves the pharynx and is triggered by swallowing.

## The vagus nerve

This mixed nerve supplies the striated muscle of the pharynx (efferent pathway of the gag reflex), the larynx (including the vocal cords via the recurrent laryngeal nerves) and the upper oesophagus.

There are some sensory fibres from the larynx.

Parasympathetic fibres supply the heart and abdominal viscera.

## Ninth and tenth nerve lesions

A unilateral lesion of the ninth nerve causes diminished sensation on one side of the pharynx. A unilateral tenth nerve lesion causes unilateral failure of voluntary and reflex elevation of the soft palate, which is drawn to the side opposite the lesion. Individual lesions of these nerves are unusual.

Bilateral combined lesions of the ninth and tenth nerves cause weakness of elevation of the palate, depression of palatal sensation and loss of the gag reflex.

The cough is depressed and the vocal cords are paralysed. The patient complains of difficulty in swallowing, choking (particularly with fluids) and hoarseness.

The causes of ninth and tenth nerve lesions are given in Table 18.14.

**Lesions of the recurrent laryngeal nerves**
Unilateral paralysis of this important branch of each vagus causes hoarseness (dysphonia) and depression of the forceful, explosive part of the cough reflex. Bilateral acute lesions, e.g. postoperatively, are a serious emergency and cause respiratory obstruction.

The left recurrent laryngeal nerve (which loops beneath the aorta) is more commonly affected than the right.

Causes of recurrent laryngeal nerve lesions include:
- Mediastinal tumours
- Aneurysm of the aorta
- Trauma or surgery to the neck

# THE ACCESSORY NERVE (ELEVENTH CRANIAL NERVE)

This motor nerve to the trapezius and sternomastoid muscles arises in the medulla and leaves the skull through the jugular foramen with the ninth and tenth nerves.

A lesion of the eleventh nerve causes weakness of the sternomastoid (rotation of the head and neck to the opposite side) and the trapezius (shoulder shrugging). The principal causes are shown in Table 18.14.

# THE HYPOGLOSSAL NERVE (TWELFTH CRANIAL NERVE)

The motor nerve to the tongue arises in the medulla and leaves the skull through the anterior condylar foramen.

## Twelfth nerve lesions

A LMN lesion of the twelfth nerve leads to unilateral weakness, wasting and fasciculation of the tongue. When protruded the tongue deviates towards the weaker side.

| Site | Pathology |
|------|-----------|
| Brain stem | Infarction |
| | Syringobulbia |
| | Motor neurone disease (motor fibres) |
| | Poliomyelitis (motor fibres) |
| Jugular foramen | Carcinoma of nasopharynx |
| | Glomus tumour |
| | Internal jugular vein thrombosis |
| Neck and nasopharynx | Carcinoma of nasopharynx |
| | Metastases |
| | Polyneuropathy |

**Table 18.14** Principal causes of lesions of the ninth, tenth and eleventh cranial nerves.

Some causes of a hypoglossal nerve (or nucleus) lesion are:
1 In the brain stem:
  (a) Motor neurone disease
  (b) Syringobulbia
  (c) Poliomyelitis
2 At the skull base:
  (a) Trauma
  (b) Tumours
  (c) Nasopharyngeal carcinoma
  (d) Glomus tumour
3 In the neck:
  (a) Trauma
  (b) Tumours

Bilateral supranuclear (UMN) lesions cause the tongue movements to be slow; in addition the tongue cannot be protruded very far. There is no fasciculation.

# BULBAR AND PSEUDOBULBAR PALSY

## Bulbar palsy

A bulbar palsy describes weakness of LMN type of the muscles supplied by the lower cranial nerves whose nuclei lie in the medulla (the 'bulb'). The weakness is caused by lesions of the lower cranial nerve nuclei, the (ninth to twelfth) cranial nerves themselves or the muscles they supply.

The symptoms, signs and causes of a bulbar palsy are mentioned under the sections on the ninth to twelfth cranial nerves. Isolated lesions of these nerves are rare.

## Pseudobulbar palsy

In pseudobulbar palsy, bilateral supranuclear (UMN) lesions of the lower cranial nerves cause weakness and poverty of movement of the tongue and the pharyngeal musculature. Signs of a pseudobulbar palsy are a stiff, slow, spastic tongue (which is not wasted) and dysarthria with a 'gravelly' spastic voice that is slow and sounds 'dry'. The gag reflex and palatal reflex are preserved. The jaw jerk is exaggerated. Emotional lability (inappropriate laughing or crying) often accompanies pseudobulbar palsy. The principal causes are:
MOTOR NEURONE DISEASE, in which there are often both upper UMN and LMN lesions
MULTIPLE SCLEROSIS, in which it occurs mainly as a late event
CEREBROVASCULAR DISEASE, in which it may occur with multi-infarct dementia
Severe difficulty with swallowing, dysarthria and a slow-moving tongue also occur in the late stages of Parkinson's disease and this should be distinguished from both pseudobulbar and bulbar palsy.

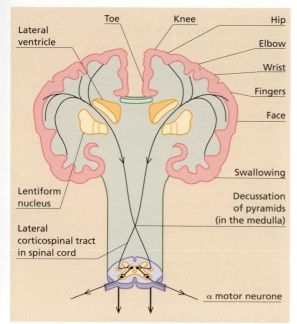

**Fig. 18.8** The crossed corticospinal ('pyramidal') tracts. The cortical representation of various parts of the body are shown.

# The motor system

## THE CORTICOSPINAL TRACTS

The corticospinal tracts originate from the neurones of the fifth layer of the cortex and terminate on the motor nuclei of the cranial nerves and anterior horn cells of the spinal cord. The pathways of importance (Fig. 18.8) in clinical diagnosis decussate in the medulla and pass to the contralateral halves of the cord as the crossed lateral corticospinal tracts. This is the 'pyramidal' system, disease of which causes UMN lesions.

A small proportion of the corticospinal outflow remains uncrossed (the anterior corticospinal tracts).

## Characteristics of upper motor neurone lesions (Table 18.15)

### Drift of the upper limb
In the normal individual the outstretched upper limbs are held symmetrically, even when the eyes are closed. In a

Drift of upper limb
Weakness with a characteristic distribution
Increase in tone of the spastic type
Exaggerated tendon reflexes
An extensor plantar response
Loss of abdominal reflexes
No muscle wasting
Normal electrical excitability of muscle

**Table 18.15** Signs of an upper motor neurone lesion.

'pyramidal' lesion, the affected upper limb drifts downwards, medially and tends to pronate and flex slightly. This important sign may occur early, before weakness is evident.

### Weakness
A UMN ('pyramidal') lesion above the decussation causes weakness of the contralateral limbs, i.e. a hemiparesis. In an acute, severe lesion such as an infarct of the internal capsule, this weakness will be dense, but in partial lesions there is a characteristic pattern of weakness in the limbs: in the upper limb the flexors are stronger than the extensors, and in the lower limb the extensors are stronger than the flexors. In the upper limb the weaker movements are thus shoulder abduction and elbow extension; in the forearm and hand, the wrist and finger extensors and abductors are weaker than their antagonists. In the lower limb the weaker movements are flexion and abduction of the hip, flexion of the knee, and dorsiflexion and eversion of the ankle.

When the UMN lesion is below the decussation, the hemiparesis is on the same side as the lesion.

### Increase in tone (spasticity)
An acute lesion of one pyramidal tract causes a flaccid paralysis (and areflexia). An increase in tone follows within several days owing to loss of the inhibitory effect of the corticospinal pathway and an increase in spinal reflex activity. This increase in tone affects all muscle groups on the affected side but is most easily detected in the stronger muscles. It is characterized by changing resistance to passive movement; the change may be sudden—the 'clasp-knife' effect. The tendon reflexes are exaggerated and clonus can commonly be demonstrated.

### Changes in superficial reflexes
The plantar response becomes extensor. In a severe lesion (e.g. an infarct of the internal capsule causing hemiplegia) this response can be elicited from a wide area of the affected limb. As recovery occurs the area that is sensitive becomes smaller until only the posterior third of the lateral aspect of the sole is receptive. The stimulus may have to be unpleasant (an orange-stick is the correct instrument to use). For the response to be certainly extensor, the dorsiflexion of the great toe should be accompanied by fanning of the toes.

The abdominal (and cremasteric reflexes) are abolished on the affected side.

The signs of a pyramidal lesion may be minimal. Weakness, spasticity or changes in superficial reflexes may predominate. The absence of one group of signs does not exclude a UMN lesion.

## Clinical patterns of upper motor neurone disorders

Two main patterns of clinical features occur in UMN (pyramidal) disorders: hemiparesis and paraparesis.

Hemiparesis means weakness of the limbs of one side;

it is usually (but by no means always) caused by a lesion within the brain. Paraparesis means weakness of both lower limbs and is characteristically diagnostic of a spinal cord lesion.

The terms hemiplegia and paraplegia strictly indicate total paralysis but the terms are often used loosely to describe severe weakness.

### Hemiparesis

The level of a unilateral lesion of the corticospinal tracts may be determined by the accompanying features.

MOTOR CORTEX. Weakness localized to one contralateral limb (monoplegia) or part of a limb is characteristic of an isolated lesion of the motor cortex. There may be a defect in higher cortical function (e.g. aphasia). Focal epilepsy may occur.

INTERNAL CAPSULE. Since the corticospinal fibres are tightly packed in the internal capsule, occupying about 1 cm², a small lesion causes a large deficit. For example, an infarct of a small branch of the middle cerebral artery (see p. 906) causes a sudden, dense, contralateral hemiplegia that includes the face.

PONS. A pontine lesion is rarely confined to the corticospinal tract alone. Adjacent structures such as cranial nerve nuclei (e.g. of the sixth or seventh nerve) are involved, causing ipsilateral cranial nerve lesions with contralateral hemiparesis.

SPINAL CORD. A lesion of one lateral corticospinal tract in the cord causes an ipsilateral UMN lesion and is indicated by a reflex level in the upper limbs (e.g. absent biceps jerk) or the presence of a Brown-Séquard syndrome (see p. 898). A spinal cord cause of a hemiparesis is unusual.

### Paraparesis

Paraparesis (or tetraparesis, when the four limbs are involved) indicates bilateral damage to the corticospinal tracts. Spinal cord disease is the usual cause, but bilateral cerebral lesions can cause a similar picture (Table 18.16).

## THE EXTRAPYRAMIDAL SYSTEM AND THE CONTROL OF MOVEMENT

The extrapyramidal system is a general term for the basal ganglia. In disorders of this system, the commonest of which is Parkinson's disease, there is a combination of:

REDUCTION IN MOVEMENT, i.e. bradykinesia (slow movement) or akinesia (no movement)
INVOLUNTARY MOVEMENTS (tremor, chorea, dystonia or athetosis)
RIGIDITY

## Anatomy and physiology

### Structure

The corpus striatum, consisting of the caudate nucleus, globus pallidus and putamen (the latter two forming the

*Spinal lesions*
Spinal cord compression (see Table 18.47)
Multiple sclerosis
Myelitis (e.g. VZV)
Motor neurone disease
Subacute combined degeneration of the cord
Syringomyelia
Syphilis
Familial or sporadic paraparesis
Vascular disease of the cord
Non-metastatic manifestation of malignancy
Tropical spastic paraparesis (HTLV-1)

*Cerebral lesions[a]*
Parasagittal cortical lesions
  Meningioma
  Venous sinus thrombosis
Hydrocephalus
Multiple cerebral infarction

———

[a]All are rare causes of a paraparesis.
HTLV-1, human T-cell leukaemia virus 1; VZV, varicella zoster virus.

**Table 18.16**   Causes of a spastic paraparesis.

lentiform nucleus) lies close to the substantia nigra, thalami and subthalamic nuclei. There are interconnections between these structures and the cerebral cortex, the cerebellum and the reticular formation, the cranial nerve nuclei (particularly the vestibular nerve) and the spinal cord.

The overall function of this complex system is the initiation and modulation of movement. The system modulates cortical motor activity by a series of hypothetical servo loops.

It is now clear that in many basal ganglia disorders there are substantial and specific changes in neurotransmitter profile rather than discrete anatomical lesions.

In Parkinson's disease there is reduction of:
DOPAMINE (to 10% of normal) in the putamen and substantia nigra.
NORADRENALINE AND 5-HYDROXYTRYPTAMINE (to 40% of normal) in the putamen.
GLUTAMIC ACID DECARBOXYLASE (GAD) in substantia nigra and cerebral cortex. GAD is the enzyme responsible for synthesizing GABA.
Cholinergic activity is relatively well preserved in Parkinson's disease.

Changes in the neurotransmitter profile are associated with characteristic clinical patterns. For example:
IN PARKINSON'S DISEASE an increase in dopamine activity (due to levodopa therapy) relieves rigidity. In excess (in both normal people and those with Parkinson's disease), levodopa therapy causes chorea.
IN HUNTINGTON'S DISEASE (chorea) there is a marked reduction in acetylcholine and GABA activity in the striatum. Dopamine activity is normal.
IN NORMAL people an increase in acetylcholine activity or a decrease in dopamine activity causes rigidity and

bradykinesia (parkinsonism). For example, reserpine (which depletes neurones of dopamine) and phenothiazines or butyrophenones (which block dopaminergic neurones) cause or exacerbate parkinsonism.

Clinically, extrapyramidal disorders are classified broadly into the akinetic-rigid syndromes (see p. 918), in which poverty of movement predominates, and the dyskinesias, in which there are a variety of involuntary movements.

# THE CEREBELLUM

The cerebellum receives afferent fibres from:
- Proprioceptive organs in joints and muscles
- The vestibular nuclei
- The basal ganglia
- The corticospinal system

Efferent fibres pass from the cerebellum to:
- Each red nucleus
- The vestibular nuclei
- The basal ganglia
- The anterior horn cells

Each lateral lobe of the cerebellum coordinates movement of the ipsilateral limb. The vermis (a midline structure) is concerned with maintenance of axial (midline) posture and balance.

## Cerebellar lesions

Expanding mass lesions within the cerebellum produce hydrocephalus, causing severe headaches, vomiting and papilloedema. 'Coning' of the cerebellar tonsils through the foramen magnum and respiratory arrest occur, often within hours. Very rarely 'tonic seizures' of the limbs occur with cerebellar masses.

### Lateral cerebellar lobes
A lesion within one cerebellar lobe (e.g. a tumour or infarction) causes disruption of the normal sequence of movements (dyssynergia) on the side of the lesion.

POSTURE AND GAIT. The outstretched arm is held still in the early stages of a cerebellar lesion but there is rebound overshoot when the limb is pressed downwards by the examiner and released. Gait is ataxic with a broad base; the patient falters towards the side of the lesion.

TREMOR AND ATAXIA. Movement is imprecise in direction, in force and in distance (dysmetria).

Rapid alternating movements (tapping, clapping or rotary movements of the hand) are clumsy and disorganized (dysdiadochokinesis).

'Intention tremor' (action tremor, with past-pointing) is seen when the 'finger–nose–finger' and 'heel—shin' tests are performed.

NYSTAGMUS (see p. 890). Coarse horizontal nystagmus appears with cerebellar lobar lesions. Its direction is towards the side of the lesion.

DYSARTHRIA. Speech is affected (usually with bilateral lesions). A halting, jerking dysarthria results—the 'scanning speech' of cerebellar lesions.

OTHER SIGNS. Titubation—rhythmic tremor of the head in either to and fro ('yes–yes') movements or rotary ('no–no') movements—also occurs, mainly when cerebellar connections are involved (e.g. in essential tremor and MS).

Hypotonia and depression of reflexes are also sometimes seen with cerebellar disease, but are usually of little value as localizing signs. 'Pendular', i.e. slow, reflexes also occur.

### Midline cerebellar lesions
Lesions of the cerebellar vermis have a dramatic effect on the equilibrium of the trunk and axial musculature. Truncal ataxia causes difficulty in standing and sitting unsupported, with a rolling, broad, ataxic gait.

Lesions of the flocculonodular region cause vertigo, vomiting and ataxia of gait if they extend to the roof of the fourth ventricle.

Table 18.17 summarizes the main causes of cerebellar disease.

## TREMOR

Tremor is an oscillation, regular and sinusoidal, of a part or parts of the body. Different varieties are outlined below.

| Tumours | Haemangioblastoma |
| | Medulloblastoma |
| | Secondary neoplasm |
| | Compression by acoustic neuroma |
| Vascular lesions | Haemorrhage |
| | Infarction |
| | Arteriovenous malformation |
| Infection | Abscess |
| | AIDS |
| | Kuru |
| Developmental | Arnold–Chiari malformation |
| | Basilar invagination |
| | Cerebral palsy |
| Toxic and metabolic | Anticonvulsant drugs |
| | Chronic alcohol abuse |
| | Following carbon monoxide poisoning |
| | Lead poisoning |
| Inherited | Friedreich's ataxia |
| | Ataxia telangiectasia |
| | Essential tremor |
| Miscellaneous | Multiple sclerosis |
| | Hydrocephalus |
| | Postinfective cerebellar syndrome of childhood |
| | Hypothyroidism |
| | Non-metastatic manifestation of malignancy |
| | Cerebral oedema of chronic hypoxia |

Table 18.17   Principal causes of cerebellar syndromes.

### Postural tremor

Everyone has a physiological tremor of the outstretched hands at 8–12 Hz. This is increased with anxiety, hyperthyroidism and certain drugs (lithium, sodium valproate and sympathomimetics) or in mercury poisoning. A coarse, postural tremor is seen in chronic alcohol abusers and in benign essential tremor (usually at 5–8 Hz). Postural tremor does not worsen on movement.

### Intention tremor

Tremor that is exacerbated by action, with past-pointing and accompanying slowness and incoordination of rapid alternating movement (dysdiadochokinesis), occurs in cerebellar lobe disease and with lesions of cerebellar connections. Titubation (tremor of the head) and nystagmus may be present.

### Rest tremor

This is present at rest, is between 4 and 7 Hz and is not made worse by action. It occurs primarily in Parkinson's disease and is sometimes described as 'pill-rolling' between the thumb and index finger.

### Other tremors

Tremor is seen following lesions of the red nucleus (e.g. infarction, demyelination) and rarely with frontal-lobe lesions.

## LOWER MOTOR NEURONE LESIONS

The LMN is the motor pathway from the anterior horn cell (or cranial nerve nucleus) via a peripheral nerve to the motor end plate.

The motor unit consists of a single anterior horn cell, the single fast-conducting α motor nerve fibre that leaves the spinal cord via the anterior root, and the group of muscle fibres (100–2000) being supplied via the mixed peripheral nerve. Anterior horn cell activity is modulated by the impulses from:
- The corticospinal tracts
- The extrapyramidal system (basal ganglia and cerebellum)
- Afferent fibres from the posterior roots

### Signs of lower motor neurone lesion

Voluntary muscle depends upon the motor unit for all movement and also for its metabolic integrity. Signs follow rapidly if the LMN is interrupted at any point in its course (Table 18.18). Wasting appears within 3 weeks of the development of an LMN lesion. Fasciculation occurs and is due to visible contractions of single motor units.

### Causes of a lower motor neurone lesion

Examples of LMN lesions at various levels are:
ANTERIOR HORN CELL—poliomyelitis, motor neurone disease

| Signs |
|---|
| Weakness |
| Wasting |
| Hypotonia |
| Reflex loss |
| Fasciculation |
| Fibrillation potentials (detected electromyographically, see p. 877) |
| Contractures of muscle |
| 'Trophic' changes in skin and nails |

**Table 18.18**  Signs of a lower motor neurone lesion.

SPINAL ROOT—cervical and lumbar root lesions, neuralgic amyotrophy
PERIPHERAL (OR CRANIAL) NERVE—nerve trauma or compression, polyneuropathy

## THE SPINAL REFLEX ARC

The components of the spinal reflex arc are illustrated in Fig. 18.9. The stretch reflex is the physiological basis for the tendon reflexes. For example, in the knee jerk, a tap on the patellar tendon activates stretch receptors in the quadriceps. Impulses in first-order sensory neurones pass directly to LMNs (L3 and L4), which activate the quadriceps, causing a contraction.

Loss of a tendon reflex is caused by a lesion anywhere along the spinal reflex path. The reflex lost indicates the level of the lesion (Table 18.19).

### Reinforcement

Distraction of the patient's attention, clenching the teeth or pulling of the interlocked fingers increases the activity

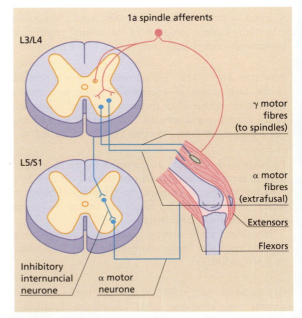

**Fig. 18.9**  The knee jerk: an example of a spinal reflex arc.

| Spinal level | Reflex |
|--------------|--------|
| C5–6 | Supinator |
| C5–6 | Biceps |
| C7 | Triceps |
| L3–4 | Knee |
| S1 | Ankle |

**Table 18.19** Spinal levels of tendon reflexes.

of the stretch reflex. Such 'reinforcement' manoeuvres should be carried out before a reflex is recorded as absent.

## The sensory system

## Peripheral nerves and spinal roots

Peripheral nerves carry all modalities of sensation from either free or specialized nerve endings to the dorsal root ganglia and thus to the cord.

The sensory distribution of the spinal roots (dermatomes) is shown in Fig. 18.10.

### The spinal cord (Fig. 18.11)

#### Posterior columns
For clinical purposes, the sensory modalities of vibration sense, joint position, light touch and two-point discrimination travel uncrossed in the posterior columns to the gracile and cuneate nuclei in the medulla. Axons from second-order neurones cross the midline in the brain stem to form the medial lemniscus and pass to the thalamus.

#### Spinothalamic tracts
Fibres carrying pain and temperature sensation synapse in the dorsal horn of the cord, cross the cord and pass as the spinothalamic tracts to the thalamus and reticular formation.

### The sensory cortex

The projection of fibres from the thalamus to the sensory cortex of the parietal region is shown in Fig. 18.11. Connections also exist between the thalamus and the motor cortex.

### LESIONS OF THE SENSORY PATHWAYS

Paraesthesiae, numbness and pain are the principal symptoms of lesions of the sensory pathways below the level

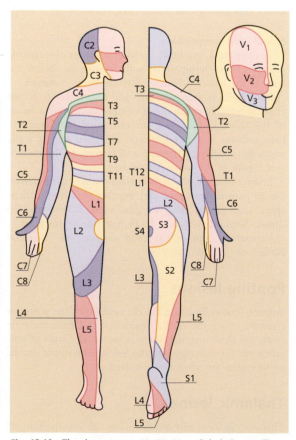

**Fig. 18.10** The dermatomes. V₁, V₂, V₃, ophthalmic, maxillary and mandibular branches of trigeminal nerve.

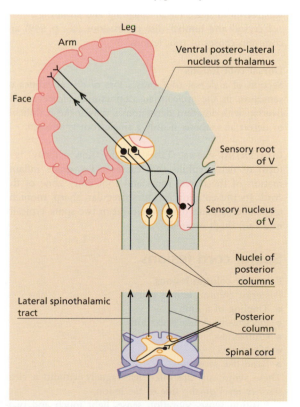

**Fig. 18.11** The principal sensory pathways. The posterior columns remain uncrossed until the medulla. The spinothalamic tracts cross close to their entry into the spinal cord.

of the thalamus. The quality and distribution of the symptoms may suggest the site of the lesion.

## Peripheral nerve lesions

The symptoms are felt in the distribution of the affected peripheral nerve (see p. 944).

Section of a nerve is followed by complete sensory loss. Nerve entrapment (see p. 944) causes numbness, pain and tingling. Tapping the site of compression sometimes causes a sharp, electric-shock-like pain in the distribution of the nerve (Tinel's sign).

### Neuralgia

Neuralgia refers to local pain of great severity in the distribution of a damaged nerve. Examples are:
- Trigeminal neuralgia (see p. 887)
- Postherpetic neuralgia (see p. 928)
- Causalgia

## Spinal root lesions

### Root pain

The pain of root compression is referred to the myotome supplied by that root and there is also a tingling discomfort in the dermatome. The pain is made worse by manoeuvres that either stretch the nerve root (as in straight leg raising) or increase the pressure in the spinal subarachnoid space (as in coughing and straining).

Cervical and lumbar disc protrusions (see p. 949) are common causes of root lesions.

### Dorsal root lesions

Section of a dorsal root causes loss of all modalities of sensation in the appropriate dermatome. However, the overlap with adjacent dermatomes may make it difficult to detect anaesthesia if only a single root is affected.

LIGHTNING PAINS. Tabes dorsalis (now a rarity) is a form of neurosyphilis that causes a low-grade inflammation of the dorsal roots and root entry zone of the cord. Its presentation includes irregular, sharp, momentary stabbing pains that involve one or two spots, typically in a calf, thigh or ankle.

## Spinal cord lesions

### Posterior column lesions

Posterior column lesions cause:
- Tingling of a limb
- Electric-shock-like sensations
- Clumsiness
- Numbness
- Band-like sensations

These symptoms are often felt vaguely without a clear sensory level on the side of the lesion.

Position sense, vibration sense, light touch and two-point discrimination are lost below the level of the lesion. Loss of position sense produces sensory ataxia (see p. 873).

LHERMITTE'S PHENOMENON. This is an electric-shock-like sensation radiating down the trunk and limbs that is produced by neck flexion. It indicates a cervical cord lesion. Lhermitte's sign is common in acute exacerbations of MS (see p. 922). It also occurs in cervical spondylotic myelopathy (see p. 949), subacute combined degeneration of the cord (see p. 948) and radiation myelopathy (see p. 939).

### Spinothalamic tract lesions

Pure spinothalamic lesions cause isolated contralateral loss of pain and temperature sensation below the level of the lesion. This is called 'dissociated sensory loss', i.e. pain and temperature are 'dissociated' from light touch, which is preserved.

The spinal level is modified by the lamination of fibres within the spinothalamic tracts. Fibres from the lower spinal roots lie superficially and are therefore damaged first by compressive lesions from outside the cord. As an external compressive lesion (e.g. a midthoracic extradural meningioma; Fig. 18.12) enlarges, the spinal sensory level ascends as deeper fibres become involved. Conversely, a central lesion of the cord (e.g. a syrinx, see p. 939) affects the deeper fibres first.

Symptoms of spinothalamic tract lesions are the absence of pain (resulting in painless burns and minor injuries) or the loss of temperature sensation. Perforating ulcers and neuropathic joints may follow.

### Spinal cord compression

This important syndrome causes a progressive spastic paraparesis (or tetraparesis) with sensory loss below the level of the lesion. Sphincter disturbance is common.

Root pain is frequent but not invariable. It is felt characteristically at the site of compression. With a lesion of the thoracic cord (e.g. an extradural meningioma), pain radiates in a band around the chest and is made worse by coughing, straining and jarring, as the meningeal sheath of the nerve is stretched.

Involvement of one spinothalamic tract (contralateral loss of pain and temperature) together with one corticospinal tract (ipsilateral 'pyramidal' signs) is known as the Brown-Séquard syndrome or hemisection of the cord.

Paraparesis and spinal cord disease are discussed further on pp. 940 and 938.

## Pontine lesions

Pontine lesions lie above the decussation of the posterior columns. Since the medial lemniscus and spinothalamic tracts are close together, there is loss of all forms of sensation on the side opposite the lesion. The upper cranial nerve nuclei are often also involved.

## Thalamic lesions

Thalamic lesions may produce loss of sensation to all modalities of sensation on the opposite side of the body; this is an unusual clinical picture.

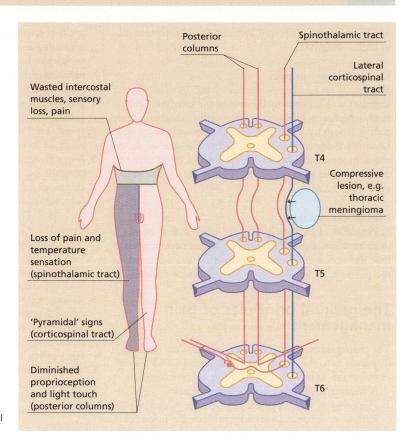

**Fig. 18.12** The clinical features of spinal cord compression.

Labels in figure:
Posterior columns
Spinothalamic tract
Lateral corticospinal tract
Wasted intercostal muscles, sensory loss, pain
T4
Compressive lesion, e.g. thoracic meningioma
Loss of pain and temperature sensation (spinothalamic tract)
T5
'Pyramidal' signs (corticospinal tract)
Diminished proprioception and light touch (posterior columns)
T6

---

Spontaneous pain may also occur. Thalamic pain, sometimes called the 'thalamic syndrome', is usually caused by a small thalamic infarct. The patient develops a hemiparesis that recovers partially. There remains a constant deep-seated pain that affects the paretic limbs. It is often very severe. Movement does not change the pain, which continues night and day. Extreme anguish is usual and the secondary depression that follows may lead to suicide.

## Cortical lesions

Pain is not a feature of destructive cortical lesions.

Irritative phenomena (e.g. partial seizures) in the parietal cortex cause tingling sensations in the affected part.

Sensory loss, neglect of one side and subtle disorders of sensation may occur with lesions of the parietal cortex.

## PAIN

Pain is an unpleasant and unique physical and psychological experience. Acute pain serves a biological purpose, causes sympathetic hyperactivity and is self-limiting. Chronic pain may last for months, much longer than the time required for healing, and autonomic adaptation takes place.

## The physiology of pain

Pain perception is mediated by free nerve endings, the terminations of finely myelinated A$\delta$ and of non-myelinated C fibres. Chemicals released locally as a result of injury either produce pain by direct stimulation or by sensitizing the nerve endings. A$\delta$ fibres give rise to the perception of sharp, immediate pain which is followed after an interval by the slower-onset, duller, more diffuse and prolonged pain mediated by the slower conducting C fibres.

Most sensory input enters the spinal cord via the dorsal spinal roots. Within the spinal cord, sensory input ascends either in the dorsal (posterior) column or in the spinothalamic tract. The cells of the grey matter in the spinal cord are arranged in laminae labelled I to X from dorsal to ventral. A$\delta$ fibres terminate in laminae I and V and excite second-order neurones which send fibres to the contralateral side via the anterior commissure and up the anterolateral column in the direct spinothalamic tract. C fibres mostly terminate in the substantia gelatinosa (laminae II and III). A series of short fibres give rise to long axons which pass through the anterior commissure to the contralateral side and up the spinoreticulothalamic tract. The spinothalamic tracts carry impulses which localize pain while thalamic pathways mediate the emotional components.

The sympathetic nervous system has an important role in modulating pain.

### The gate theory of pain

The gate theory proposes that the distribution of afferent impulses is monitored by the cells of the substantia gelatinosa, which acts like a gate determining whether or not sufficient activity is allowed through to fire the secondary neurones deeper in the dorsal horn. The gate is dominated by descending influences from the brain that can override spinal cord regulatory mechanisms and alter the setting of the gate.

### Endogenous opiates

Enkephalins and endorphins are neurotransmitters at inhibitory synapses (Table 18.20). It has been suggested that the action of endogenous opiates may account for the phenomena of placebo and acupuncture analgesia.

## The general principles of pain management (see also p. 376)

The management of chronic pain depends on reaching a diagnosis as to the cause of the pain by a detailed history, examination and the appropriate use of investigations.

A treatment plan has several components:

1 *Psychological.* The appreciation of pain is always subjective. A chronic pain may profoundly influence a patient's life-style. Depression is almost universally associated with chronic benign pain, whereas overall only 15–20% of cancer patients are clinically depressed. Antidepressant drugs and modification of life style have a place in treatment.

2 *Analgesics.* Analgesic drugs should be prescribed according to the analgesic ladder (see p. 376). Inadequate analgesia following optimal use of a drug from one group indicates the need for prescription from the group one step higher. The prescription should be for regular doses with extra 'as required' doses for breakthrough pain. Medication should be given orally except in cases of gastrointestinal dysfunction or if the patient is comatose. The effect of any prescription should be reviewed regularly at a time interval suited to the severity of the pain.

3 *Co-analgesics.* Co-analgesics are drugs which have a primary indication other than pain but in some conditions are effective either alone or when added to conventional analgesics. Examples are the non-steroidal anti-inflammatory drugs used in bone pain; tricyclic

antidepressants and anticonvulsants used in deafferentation pain (see p. 377). Calcium channel blockers (nifedipine) can improve sympathetically mediated pain. Muscle relaxants, antibiotics and steroids by injection are analgesic when used in specific situations.

4 *Stimulation.* Acupuncture, ultrasound, massage, transcutaneous electrical nerve stimulation (TENS) and spinal cord stimulation all achieve analgesia by an effect on large myelinated nerve fibres.

5 *Nerve blocks.* Pain pathways can be blocked either temporarily by local anaesthetic or permanently using chemicals such as phenol or radiofrequency.
  (a) Somatic system blocks:
      (i)   Peripheral—nerve and plexus blocks.
      (ii)  Central—epidurals and spinals.
  (b) Sympathetic blocks:
      (i)   Central—epidurals and spinals.
      (ii)  Peripheral—sympathetic ganglia and nerve endings.

6 *Ablative neurosurgical techniques*, e.g. dorsal rhizotomy, sympathectomy, cordotomy, should only be performed when physical and pharmacological therapies have failed. These may be carried out percutaneously or by open procedure.

Chronic and recurrent pain is disabling and distressing to the patient. Multidisciplinary pain relief clinics are often helpful in providing specific and supportive therapy but the management of pain should be part of the skills of all doctors.

## Control of the bladder and sexual function

Afferent fibres (T12–S4) record changes in pressure within the bladder and tactile sensation in the genitalia.

The efferent pathways are shown in Table 18.21.

## Disorders of micturition

Bilateral UMN lesions cause frequency of micturition and incontinence. The bladder is small and unusually sensitive to small changes in intravesical pressure.

LMN lesions (which must be bilateral to cause urinary symptoms) cause a flaccid, atonic bladder, which overflows without warning.

Frontal-lobe lesions (e.g. dementia, hydrocephalus) cause a disturbance of awareness of micturition, resulting in incontinence particularly in an ageing population.

## Impotence

Failure of erection of the penis (or clitoris) and ejaculation is caused by bilateral upper or lower motor lesions.

| Peptide | Receptor |
| --- | --- |
| Enkephalins | δ receptors |
| Dynorphins | κ receptors |
| Endorphins | μ receptors |

**Table 18.20** Opioid peptides and their receptors.

| Type of nerve supply | Source | Structure/function supplied |
|---|---|---|
| Parasympathetic | S2–S4 | Detrusor muscle contraction<br>Genitalia (penile erection, engorgement of clitoris) |
| Somatic | Pudendal nerves | External sphincter |
| Sympathetic | T12–L2 | Trigone<br>Ejaculation, orgasm |

**Table 18.21** Efferent nerve supply of the bladder and genitalia.

Depression is also a common cause of impotence. Endocrine aspects of impotence are discussed on p. 789.

# Unconsciousness and coma

The central reticular formation, which extends from the brain stem to the thalamus, influences the state of arousal. This complex process involves interactions between the reticular formation, the cortex and brain stem, and all sensory pathways.

## Disturbed consciousness

### Definitions

CONSCIOUSNESS means awareness of oneself and the surroundings in a state of wakefulness.

CLOUDING OF CONSCIOUSNESS is reduced wakefulness or awareness.

SLEEP is a state of mental and physical inactivity from which the subject can be roused.

STUPOR is an abnormal, sleepy state from which the patient can be aroused by stimuli that may need to be repeated or vigorously applied.

CONFUSION is the state of altered consciousness in which patients are bewildered and misinterpret the world around them.

DELIRIUM is a state of high arousal (seen typically in delirium tremens, see p. 984) in which there is confusion and often hallucinations.

COMA is a state of unrousable unresponsiveness. A grading system for coma used particularly in patients with head injury is shown in Table 18.22. An alternative grading system is given on p. 750.

## Causes of coma

Altered consciousness is produced by three types of process affecting the brain stem, reticular formation and cerebral cortex.

1 *Diffuse brain dysfunction.* Generalized metabolic (e.g. uraemia) or toxic (e.g. septicaemia) disorders can depress brain function.

2 *Direct effect on the brain stem.* Lesions of the brain stem itself damage the reticular activating system.

3 *Indirect effect on the brain stem.* Mass lesions above the

|  | Score |
|---|---|
| *Eye opening (E)* | |
| Spontaneous | 4 |
| To speech | 3 |
| To pain | 2 |
| Nil | 1 |
| *Motor response (M)* | |
| Obeys | 6 |
| Localizes | 5 |
| Withdraws | 4 |
| Abnormal flexion | 3 |
| Extensor response | 2 |
| Nil | 1 |
| *Verbal response (V)* | |
| Orientated | 5 |
| Confused conversation | 4 |
| Inappropriate words | 3 |
| Incomprehensible sounds | 2 |
| Nil | 1 |

Coma score = E + M + V (minimum = 3; maximum = 15)

**Table 18.22** Glasgow Coma Scale.

tentorium cerebelli compress or damage the ascending reticular activating system in the brain stem.

It is important to understand that single focal brain lesions of the cerebral hemispheres do not produce coma unless they compress the brain stem. Oedema frequently surrounds hemisphere lesions, contributing greatly to their effects.

Other coma-like states include the 'locked-in syndrome', a state of unresponsiveness due to massive brain stem infarction. The patient is unable to communicate or move (except sometimes the eyes) but has a functioning cerebral cortex. The 'chronic vegetative state', a sequel of head injury for example, implies loss of sentient behaviour, i.e. the patient perceives little or nothing but lies awake, breathing spontaneously: widespread cerebral damage is present.

Unresponsiveness of psychological origin may cause difficulty in the differential diagnosis of apparent coma.

The principal causes of coma and stupor are shown in Table 18.23. A common cause of coma is self-poisoning but in malarial zones cerebral malaria is frequently seen.

*Diffuse brain dysfunction*
Drug overdose, alcohol
CO poisoning, anaesthetic gases
Hypoglycaemia, hyperglycaemia
Hypoxic/ischaemic brain injury
Hypertensive encephalopathy
Renal failure
Hepatic failure
Respiratory failure with $CO_2$ retention
Hypercalcaemia, hypocalcaemia
Hypoadrenalism, hypopituitarism and hypothyroidism
Hyponatraemia, hypernatraemia
Metabolic acidosis
Hypothermia, hyperpyrexia
Trauma—following closed head injury
Epilepsy—following a generalized seizure
Encephalitis, cerebral malaria
Subarachnoid haemorrhage
Metabolic rarities, e.g. porphyria

*Direct effect on brain stem*
Brain stem haemorrhage or infarction
Brain stem neoplasm
Brain stem demyelination
Wernicke–Korsakoff syndrome
Trauma

*Indirect effect on brain stem*
Hemisphere tumour, infarction, abscess, haematoma,
  encephalitis or trauma
Cerebellar lesions

**Table 18.23**   Principal causes of coma and stupor.

## THE UNCONSCIOUS PATIENT

## Immediate assessment

Immediate action, which takes only seconds, is essential
(Table 18.24).

A history should then be obtained from accompanying
relatives, friends, ambulance drivers or the police. Many
patients with diabetes mellitus, epilepsy or hypoadrenalism, and those who take corticosteroids, wear or carry
identifying discs or cards; these should be looked for.

## Further examination

1  The depth of coma should be recorded (see Table
18.22).
2  A full general and neurological examination should
then be carried out.

| Examine | Action |
|---|---|
| Airway | Clear, and intubate if necessary |
| Pulse (? absent) | ⎫ Perform cardiopulmonary |
| Pupils (? fixed, dilated) | ⎬ resuscitation if appropriate |
| For presence of trauma | If head injury present, anticipate deterioration |

**Table 18.24**   Immediate action in patients with coma (see also
p. 751).

## GENERAL EXAMINATION
### Temperature
This is raised in infection and hyperpyrexia and low in
hypothermia.

### Skin
The following should be noted:
COLOUR (cyanosis, jaundice, purpura, rashes,
  pigmentation)
TEXTURE (coarse and dry in hypothyroidism)
PRESENCE OF INJECTION SITES (diabetics, drug
  addicts)

### Breath
Alcohol or ketones may be smelt. In hepatic failure and
uraemia a distinct fetor is present.

### Respiration
Depressed but regular respiration occurs in most states
of stupor and coma. The presence of particular types of
respiration may point to the diagnosis:
CHEYNE–STOKES RESPIRATION (periodic respiration)
  is alternating hyperpnoea and apnoea. In neurological
  disease it implies bilateral cerebral dysfunction, usually
  deep in the hemispheres or in the upper brain stem,
  and may be a sign of incipient 'coning'. It may occur
  in metabolic comas, particularly if there is $CO_2$ retention from pulmonary disease.
KUSSMAUL (ACIDOTIC) RESPIRATION is deep-sighing
  hyperventilation that occurs principally in diabetic
  ketoacidosis and uraemia.
CENTRAL NEUROGENIC (PONTINE) HYPERVENTIL-
  ATION describes the sustained, rapid, deep breathing
  seen in patients with pontine lesions.
ATAXIC RESPIRATION is the shallow, halting respiration
  that occurs when the medullary respiratory centre is
  damaged. It is frequently a preterminal event.
VOMITING, HICCUP AND EXCESSIVE YAWNING may
  indicate a lesion in the lower brain stem in a stuporose patient.

## NEUROLOGICAL EXAMINATION
### Head and neck
The patient should be examined for evidence of trauma
and neck stiffness.

### Pupils
The size of the pupils and their reaction to light should
be recorded. The following patterns may be seen:
DILATATION OF ONE PUPIL, which becomes fixed to
  light, indicates herniation of the uncus of the temporal
  lobe ('coning') and compression of the third nerve.
  This is a potential neurosurgical emergency.
'PIN-POINT' LIGHT-FIXED PUPILS occur with pontine
  lesions (e.g. a pontine haemorrhage) that interrupt the
  sympathetic pathways.
MID-POSITION OR SLIGHTLY DILATED PUPILS (4–
  6 mm) fixed to light and sometimes irregular are seen
  when damage to the midbrain interrupts the pupillary
  light reflex.

HORNER'S SYNDROME (ipsilateral pupillary constriction and ptosis, see p. 883) occurs with lesions of the hypothalamus and also in 'coning'.

FIXED, DILATED PUPILS are a cardinal sign of brain death. They also occur in deep coma of any cause, but particularly coma due to barbiturate intoxication or hypothermia.

MID-POINT PUPILS that react to light are characteristic in coma of metabolic origin and coma due to most CNS-depressant drugs.

Other pupillary changes due to drugs are described on p. 751.

NB No mydriatic drugs should be given to the unconscious patient.

### Fundi
Papilloedema or retinal haemorrhage should be recorded.

### Ocular movements
In most cases of coma the eyes are slightly divergent. Slow, roving eye movements, usually horizontal, are seen in light coma.

VESTIBULO-OCULAR REFLEXES. Passive head rotation causes conjugate ocular deviation in the direction opposite to the induced head movement (doll's head reflex). This reflex is lost in very deep coma and is absent in brain stem lesions. It is absent in brain death.

A slow tonic deviation of the eyes towards the irrigated ear is seen when ice-cold water is run into the external auditory meatus; this is known as the caloric or vestibulo-ocular reflex and indicates that the brain stem is intact. In coma, this test is used mainly in the diagnosis of brain death (see p. 734).

ABNORMALITIES OF CONJUGATE GAZE (see p. 885). Sustained conjugate lateral gaze occurs towards the side of a destructive hemisphere lesion ('the eyes look towards the normal limbs') because damage to supranuclear pathways prevents contralateral gaze. In a pontine brain stem lesion, sustained conjugate lateral gaze occurs away from the side of the lesion, 'towards the paralysed limbs'.

Rarely, an irritative lesion in the frontal region (e.g. an epileptic focus) may drive the eyes away from the affected hemisphere, i.e. conjugate deviation may occur away from the side of the lesion.

Skew deviation (where one eye is deviated upwards and the other down) is a rare sign. It indicates a brain stem lesion.

SPONTANEOUS EYE MOVEMENTS. Spontaneous eye movements (other than roving eye movements) are distinctly unusual in coma of any cause.

The sudden, brisk, downward-'diving' eye movement seen in pontine (or cerebellar) haemorrhage is known as ocular 'bobbing'.

### Motor responses
Impairment of consciousness makes it difficult to recognize focal neurological signs. The following should be looked for:

RESPONSE TO VISUAL THREAT IN A STUPOROSE PATIENT—asymmetry indicates hemianopia.

TONE—the only evidence of a hemiparesis may be abnormal flaccidity on the affected side.

RESPONSE TO PAINFUL STIMULI—this may be asymmetrical.

THE FACIAL APPEARANCE—drooping of one side of the face, unilateral dribbling, or blowing in and out of the paralysed cheek may occur.

ASYMMETRY OF THE TENDON REFLEXES.

ASYMMETRY OF THE PLANTAR RESPONSES. Both are, however, frequently extensor in coma of any cause.

ASYMMETRY OF DECEREBRATE AND DECORTICATE POSTURING.

## INVESTIGATION
In many instances the cause of coma will be evident from the history and examination (e.g. head injury, cerebral haemorrhage, self-poisoning), and appropriate investigations should be carried out.

If the cause is still unclear, further investigations will be necessary.

### Blood and urine
DRUGS SCREEN, e.g. salicylates, diazepam

ROUTINE BIOCHEMISTRY, e.g. urea, electrolytes, glucose, calcium, liver biochemistry

METABOLIC AND ENDOCRINE STUDIES, e.g. thyroid function tests, serum cortisol

BLOOD CULTURES

Rarities such as cerebral malaria or porphyria should also be considered.

### CT head scan
This may indicate an otherwise unsuspected mass lesion or intracranial haemorrhage.

### CSF examination
Lumbar puncture should only be performed in coma after careful assessment of the case. It is contraindicated if an intracranial mass lesion is a possibility. A CT scan is often necessary to exclude this. CSF examination is likely to alter therapy only if undiagnosed meningo-encephalitis is present.

## MANAGEMENT
The unconscious patient needs careful nursing, meticulous attention to the airway and frequent observation to detect any change in vital function. Longer-term management requirements are:

SKIN: turning, skin care, avoidance of pressure sores, removal of rings

ORAL HYGIENE: mouth washes, suction

EYE CARE: taping of lids, prevention of corneal damage, irrigation

FLUIDS: intragastric or i.v. fluids

CALORIES: liquid diet through a fine intragastric tube, 3000 kcal (1255 kJ) daily

SPHINCTERS: catheterization only if necessary (Paul's

tubing if possible); avoidance of constipation (evacuate rectum manually if necessary)

### PROGNOSIS

The outlook depends upon the cause of coma. A cause must be established before decisions are made about withdrawing supportive care.

## Brain death

This is described on p. 734.

## *Cerebrovascular disease*

Stroke is the third commonest cause of death in developed countries. The incidence of strokes is 1–2 per 1000 population per annum in Europe and the USA but is higher in the Afro-Caribbean population. It is uncommon below the age of 40 years and is slightly more common in males. However, 16% of women compared with 8% of men die of a stroke. This difference is due to the higher mean age of stroke onset and the greater life expectancy in women. The incidence of stroke is decreasing in the age range 30–60 years as hypertension is recognized and treated. In the elderly population, stroke remains a major cause of morbidity and mortality.

Cerebrovascular disease comprises:
- Thromboembolic infarction
- Primary intracranial haemorrhage
- Subarachnoid haemorrhage
- Subdural and extradural haemorrhage and haematoma
- Cortical venous and dural venous sinus thrombosis

### Definitions

STROKE. This is a focal neurological deficit due to a vascular lesion. It is usually of rapid onset and, by definition, lasts longer than 24 hours if the patient survives. Hemiplegia due to middle cerebral arterial thromboembolism is a common example.

A COMPLETED STROKE is when the neurological deficit has reached its maximum, usually within 6 hours of onset.

A STROKE 'IN-EVOLUTION' is when symptoms and signs are getting worse, usually within 24 hours of onset.

A MINOR STROKE. These patients recover without a significant deficit usually within 1 week.

TRANSIENT ISCHAEMIC ATTACK (TIA). This is a focal deficit lasting less than 24 hours. There is complete clinical recovery. The attack is usually of sudden onset. TIAs have a tendency to recur.

These definitions, although valuable, clinically are arbitrary. The clinical picture of 'stroke' may also be caused by tumour, abscess, subdural haematoma or, rarely, by demyelination.

### Pathophysiology

Difficulties occur in the diagnosis of cerebrovascular disease because similar clinical events can be caused by different pathological processes.

COMPLETED STROKE. A completed stroke is caused by three processes:
1 Embolism from a distant site and subsequent brain infarction
2 Thrombosis of a cerebral vessel and subsequent brain infarction
3 Haemorrhage into the brain
The underlying risk factors and predisposing pathology are shown in Table 18.25.

TRANSIENT ISCHAEMIC ATTACKS. TIAs are usually caused by the passage of microemboli into the brain. Less commonly, they may be caused by a fall in cerebral perfusion (e.g. due to a cardiac dysrhythmia, postural hypotension or decreased flow through atheromatous vertebral arteries) but this is usually prevented by autoregulation. Small areas of brain infarction following thrombosis or even haemorrhage may occasionally cause a clinical TIA.

Thromboembolism from vascular disease outside the brain is the cause of:
- 70% of all strokes and
- 90% of TIAs

The principal sources of emboli are atheromatous plaques within the great vessels, the carotid and vertebral systems, or from the heart. The latter are associated with atrial fibrillation often secondary to valvular disease, or mural thrombi formed after myocardial infarction.

---

*Risk factors*
Hypertension
Diabetes mellitus
Obesity
Family history
Cigarette smoking
Hyperlipidaemia
Oral contraceptives
Alcohol
Age

*Predisposing causes*
Extracranial atheroma
Intracranial atheroma
Heart disease, e.g. mitral stenosis
Low cerebral perfusion, e.g. hypotension
Berry aneurysms
Arteriovenous malformation
Miscellaneous:
   Hyperviscosity, e.g. polycythaemia
   Arteritis, e.g. SLE
   Trauma
   Bleeding disorders
   Metabolic diseases, e.g. homocystinuria (very rare)

SLE, systemic lupus erythematosus.

**Table 18.25** Risk factors and predisposing causes in cerebrovascular disease.

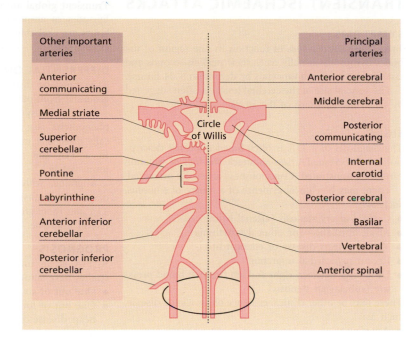

**Fig. 18.13** The arteries supplying the brain.

Other important arteries
- Anterior communicating
- Medial striate
- Superior cerebellar
- Pontine
- Labyrinthine
- Anterior inferior cerebellar
- Posterior inferior cerebellar

Circle of Willis

Principal arteries
- Anterior cerebral
- Middle cerebral
- Posterior communicating
- Internal carotid
- Posterior cerebral
- Basilar
- Vertebral
- Anterior spinal

## Vascular anatomy

An understanding of normal arterial anatomy and the likely sites of atheromatous plaques and stenotic lesions is important.

The circle of Willis (Fig. 18.13) is supplied by the two internal carotid arteries and by the basilar artery, which is formed by the union of the two vertebral arteries. Proximal to the circle, atheromatous plaques and stenoses are common at the following five sites (see Fig. 18.15):

1 The origins of the common carotid arteries
2 The origins of the internal carotid arteries
3 Within the carotid syphon (in the cavernous sinus)
4 Within the subclavian vessels
5 The origins of vertebral arteries

The distribution of the anterior, middle and posterior cerebral arteries, which supply the cerebrum, is shown in Fig. 18.14.

AUTOREGULATION. The smooth muscle of small intracerebral arteries responds directly to changes in pressure gradient across the vessel wall. In the normal situation, constant cerebral blood flow (CBF) can be maintained with systolic blood pressures between 80 and 170 mmHg (i.e. the CBF is independent of perfusion pressure).

In disease states, CBF autoregulation may fail. The contributory causes are:

SEVERE HYPOTENSION (systolic blood pressure <75 mmHg)

SEVERE HYPERTENSION (systolic blood pressure >180 mmHg)

INCREASE IN BLOOD VISCOSITY (polycythaemia, hyperviscosity syndromes)

RAISED INTRACRANIAL PRESSURE

CHANGES IN ARTERIAL $Po_2$ AND $Pco_2$

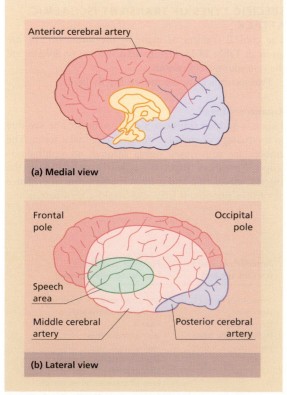

Anterior cerebral artery

**(a) Medial view**

Frontal pole

Occipital pole

Speech area

Middle cerebral artery

Posterior cerebral artery

**(b) Lateral view**

**Fig. 18.14** The distribution of the three major cerebral arteries. (a) Medial view. (b) Lateral view.

# TRANSIENT ISCHAEMIC ATTACKS

## SYMPTOMS

TIAs cause sudden loss of function in one region of the brain. Symptoms usually reach their peak in seconds and last for minutes or hours (but by definition <24 hours).

The general site of the cerebral lesion is often suggested by the clinical pattern of the attack.

## SIGNS

The diagnosis of a TIA is often based upon the description of the event. During an attack the loss of function can be demonstrated. Consciousness is usually preserved.

There may be clinical evidence of a source of embolus, such as:

- Carotid artery stenosis (arterial bruit)
- Atrial fibrillation (or other dysrhythmia)
- Valvular heart disease or endocarditis
- Recent myocardial infarction
- Difference between right and left brachial blood pressure (subclavian stenosis)

There may be other clinical evidence of associated disease, such as:

- Atheroma
- Hypertension
- Postural hypotension
- Bradycardia or low cardiac output
- Diabetes mellitus
- Rare—arteritis, polycythaemia

## SPECIFIC TYPES OF TRANSIENT ISCHAEMIC ATTACK

The clinical features of many of the forms of TIA are given in Table 18.26. Hemiparesis, vertigo or aphasia are the commonest complaints.

Two examples are mentioned briefly here.

### Amaurosis fugax

This is a sudden transient loss of vision in one eye due to the passage of emboli through the retinal arteries. The emboli are sometimes visible through an ophthalmoscope. Amaurosis fugax is suggestive of a TIA in the anterior circulation and is often the first clinical evidence of carotid stenosis. It may also herald a hemiparesis.

### Transient global amnesia

Episodes of amnesia with confusion lasting for several hours are probably caused by ischaemia in the posterior circulation.

## DIFFERENTIAL DIAGNOSIS

TIAs must be distinguished (usually on wholly clinical grounds) from other causes of transient loss of function.

Focal epilepsy is usually accompanied by 'irritative phenomena' (e.g. jerking of the limbs) and characteristically there is a 'march' of events, with some progression. In a TIA the maximum deficit is usually apparent immediately.

Migraine, with a focal prodrome, sometimes causes diagnostic confusion. Headache is distinctly unusual in a TIA and there are usually no visual disturbances suggestive of migraine.

## PROGNOSIS

A TIA is an important prognostic event. Prospective studies have shown that 5 years after the TIA:

- One out of six patients will have suffered a stroke
- One out of four patients will have died (usually from heart disease or stroke)

A TIA in the anterior circulation is generally of more serious prognostic significance than a TIA in the posterior circulation.

## INVESTIGATION AND MANAGEMENT (see p. 909)

# CEREBRAL INFARCTION

Major cerebral infarction from thromboembolism typically produces a stroke, but small infarcts may present as TIAs or may even be symptomless. The clinical picture is very variable and depends on the site and extent of the infarct. It is no longer usual to attempt to subdivide the site into the precise distribution of a single branch vessel. Nevertheless, the site of cerebral infarction may be inferred from the pattern of the physical signs (e.g. cortex, internal capsule, brain stem).

## SYMPTOMS AND SIGNS

The commonest stroke is the hemiplegia caused by infarction of the internal capsule following thromboembolism of a branch of the middle cerebral artery. A similar picture is caused by internal carotid occlusion (Fig. 18.15).

The signs are those of an acute UMN lesion of one side, including the face. Aphasia is usual when the dominant hemisphere is affected. The limbs are at first flaccid and areflexic. Headache is unusual and consciousness is not lost.

After a variable period the reflexes recover and become exaggerated and an extensor plantar response appears. Weakness is maximal at first, and recovers gradually over the course of days, weeks or months.

### Brain stem infarction

Infarction in the brain stem causes complex patterns of dysfunction depending on the site of the lesion and its

| Anterior circulation (carotid system) | Posterior circulation (vertebrobasilar system) |
|---|---|
| Amaurosis fugax | Diplopia, vertigo, vomiting |
| Aphasia | Choking and dysarthria |
| Hemiparesis | Ataxia |
| Hemisensory loss | Hemisensory loss |
| Hemianopic visual loss | Hemianopic visual loss |
| | Transient global amnesia |
| | Tetraparesis |
| | Loss of consciousness (rare) |

**Table 18.26**  Features of transient ischaemic attacks.

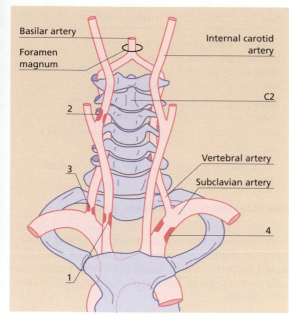

**Fig. 18.15** The principal sites of atheroma in extracerebral vessels: (1) common carotid artery; (2) internal carotid artery; (3) vertebral artery; (4) subclavian artery.

| Clinical feature | Structure involved |
|---|---|
| Hemiparesis or tetraparesis | Corticospinal tracts |
| Sensory loss | Medial lemniscus and spinothalamic tracts |
| Diplopia | Oculomotor system |
| Facial numbness | Fifth nerve nuclei |
| Facial weakness (LMN) | Seventh nerve nucleus |
| Nystagmus, vertigo | Vestibular connections |
| Dysphagia, dysarthria | Ninth and tenth nerve nuclei |
| Dysarthria, ataxia, hiccups, vomiting | Brain stem and cerebellar connections |
| Horner's syndrome | Sympathetic fibres |
| Altered consciousness | Reticular formation |

LMN, lower motor neurone.

**Table 18.27** Features of brain stem infarction.

relationship to the cranial nerve nuclei, long tracts and brain stem connections (Table 18.27).

THE LATERAL MEDULLARY SYNDROME, formerly called posterior inferior cerebellar artery (PICA) thrombosis, or Wallenberg's syndrome, is the most widely recognized syndrome of brain stem infarction. It is caused by PICA or vertebral artery thromboembolism (Fig. 18.16). There is sudden vertigo, vomiting and ipsilateral ataxia, with contralateral loss of pain and temperature sensation (Table 18.28).

COMA may be caused by bilateral brain stem infarction that damages the reticular formation.

| Ipsilateral | Contralateral |
|---|---|
| Facial numbness (V) | Spinothalamic sensory loss |
| Diplopia (VI) | Hemiparesis (mild, unusual) |
| Nystagmus | |
| Ataxia | |
| Horner's syndrome | |
| IX and X nerve lesions | |

**Table 18.28** Features of the lateral medullary syndrome.

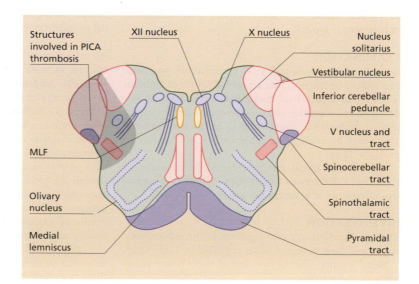

**Fig. 18.16** A cross-section of medulla showing posterior inferior cerebellar artery (PICA) thrombosis. MLF, medial longitudinal fasciculus.

THE 'LOCKED-IN SYNDROME' is caused by upper brain stem infarction; despite being conscious, the patient cannot speak, swallow or move the limbs.

PSEUDOBULBAR PALSY (see p. 347) may be caused by brain stem infarction.

### Other types of infarction

LACUNAR INFARCTION. Lacunes are small ($<1.5$ cm$^3$) areas of infarction seen at post mortem in patients with hypertension. Pure motor stroke, pure sensory stroke, sudden unilateral ataxia and sudden dysarthria with a clumsy hand are typically caused by single lacunar infarcts. Lacunar infarction may be symptomless.

MULTI-INFARCT DEMENTIA. Multiple lacunes or larger infarcts cause the picture of generalized intellectual loss that is sometimes seen in patients with cerebrovascular disease. The condition tends to occur with a stepwise progression with each subsequent infarct. The final picture is of dementia, pseudobulbar palsy and a shuffling gait with small steps. There may be confusion clinically with Parkinson's disease, and this syndrome has been called 'atherosclerotic parkinsonism' in the past.

HEMIANOPIC VISUAL LOSS OR CORTICAL BLINDNESS (Anton's syndrome, see p. 883). This may follow infarction of the posterior cerebral arteries.

WEBER'S SYNDROME. This consists of an ipsilateral third nerve paralysis with a contralateral hemiplegia due to a lesion in one half of the midbrain. Paralysis of upward gaze, due to a lesion localized in the region of the red nucleus, may also occur.

WATERSHED INFARCTION. This describes the multiple cortical infarcts that occur during prolonged episodes of very low cerebral perfusion (e.g. following massive myocardial infarction or hypotensive therapy). The border zones between the areas supplied by the anterior, middle and posterior cerebral arteries are damaged. A syndrome of cortical visual loss and memory and intellectual impairment is typical.

### EXAMINATION

In addition to the neurological examination, particular care should be taken to find a possible source of embolus (e.g. carotid bruit, atrial fibrillation, valve lesion or evidence of endocarditis) and to determine whether hypertension or postural hypotension is or has been present. There may be evidence of other emboli or a history of previous TIAs.

The brachial blood pressure should be measured in each arm; a difference of more than 20 mmHg is suggestive of stenosis of a subclavian artery.

### INVESTIGATION

The usual preliminary investigations in thromboembolic stroke and their potential yields are listed in Table 18.29.

Blood cultures should be taken if there is any possibility of endocarditis.

| Test | Yield |
|---|---|
| Urinalysis, blood glucose | Diabetes mellitus |
| Haemoglobin, platelets | Polycythaemia |
| White cell count | Infection |
| ESR, CRP | Inflammation |
| Serology for syphilis | Possible neurosyphilis |
| Chest X-ray | Neoplasms |
| ECG | Recent infarct, dysrhythmia |

CRP, C-reactive protein; ESR, erythrocyte sedimentation rate.

**Table 18.29**  Preliminary investigation in stroke.

Autoantibody studies, e.g. antinuclear factor (ANF), double-stranded DNA (dsDNA), cardiolipin antibodies, should be performed in young patients to exclude diseases such as systemic lupus erythematosus (SLE) if clinically relevant.

### Further investigation of thromboembolic stroke

CT SCANNING. This is now widely available and is indicated in virtually all patients with a stroke or TIA. CT scanning will usually demonstrate the site of a lesion and distinguish between a haemorrhage (see p. 910) and infarction. An infarct which appears as a low-density area without a mass effect is not usually visible in the first few hours. Detection increases over the succeeding few days and 90% of all infarcts are detected at 1 week. It will also rule out or show unexpected mass lesions, e.g. subdural haematoma, tumour or abscess.

MRI SCANNING usually becomes abnormal within a few hours. Haematomas are detected better than with CT.

CAROTID DOPPLER AND DUPLEX SCANNING. These ultrasound studies are of value in screening for carotid artery disease: in skilled hands they are highly effective in demonstrating internal carotid artery stenosis, the principal surgical target in stroke patients.

ANGIOGRAPHY (conventional carotid arteriography or DSA) is valuable in anterior circulation TIAs to diagnose surgically accessible arterial stenoses (mainly internal carotid artery stenosis).

There is a high probability of finding a carotid stenosis when there is a loud localized carotid bruit in the neck.

The majority of normotensive young patients (below 60 years) with TIA or stroke in the anterior circulation who recover well should be considered for angiography, though the yield in terms of internal carotid (and other accessible) arterial stenoses is under 5%. In more elderly patients, the risks of the procedure and the relatively poor results of vascular surgery in preventing further stroke usually make further investigation unwise.

Vertebral and arch angiography are rarely performed following posterior circulation TIAs and strokes unless there is a clinical suggestion of subclavian artery disease.

LUMBAR PUNCTURE is no longer a routine investigation in stroke. It is indicated only in special circumstances (e.g. when blood syphilitic serology is positive).

## IMMEDIATE MANAGEMENT

The initial decision whether to admit a stroke patient to hospital depends upon the clinical state and facilities available at home. Often the practical difficulties of caring for the disabled for what may be a prolonged period determine these immediate decisions. In practice, many TIAs and mild strokes can be managed at home and specialist advice sought when necessary. Patients admitted to stroke units fare better than those admitted to a general ward.

The management of the unconscious patient is described on p. 903. Immediate supportive measures and nasogastric fluids are given. Frequent turning to avoid bed sores is necessary.

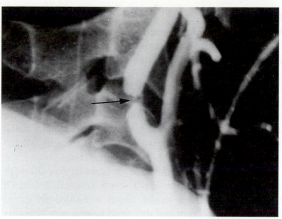

**Fig. 18.17**  Carotid arteriogram showing a tight stenosis of internal carotid artery (arrow).

## LONG-TERM MANAGEMENT

### Medical therapy

All risk factors (see Table 18.25) should be identified and, if possible, treated.

HYPERTENSIVE THERAPY. The control of high blood pressure is the single most important factor in the prevention of stroke. Hypertension is often seen in the acute stage of a stroke and hypotensive agents are not immediately necessary. Sustained or severe hypertension needs treatment (see p. 620), but the pressure must be lowered slowly to avoid a sudden fall in cerebral perfusion pressure.

ANTICOAGULANTS are used when there is atrial fibrillation, other paroxysmal dysrhythmias or when there are certain cardiac valve lesions (uninfected) or cardiomyopathies. They can also be used in 'stroke in evolution'. Anticoagulants are potentially dangerous in the 2 weeks following cerebral infarction because of the risk of provoking cerebral haemorrhage. There are wide differences in clinical practice regarding their use.

ANTIPLATELET THERAPY (see p. 347). Aspirin (300 mg daily) has been shown to reduce the incidence of stroke in patients who have had a TIA, although the exact dose is under review. Ticlopidine (250 mg twice daily), a platelet antiaggregant has also been shown to be effective but further studies are required.

OTHER MEASURES. Polycythaemia should be treated (see p. 328). Baclofen (a GABA agonist) is sometimes helpful in the management of severe spasticity following stroke (see p. 940).

### Surgical approaches

INTERNAL CAROTID ENDARTERECTOMY. This is considered in symptomatic patients who are shown to have internal carotid artery stenosis (Fig. 18.17) that narrows the arterial lumen by more than 70%. In these patients, the risk of further TIA/stroke is reduced by approxi-

mately 75% following successful surgery. The procedure however has a mortality around 3%. It is not currently recommended for asymptomatic cases.

EXTRACRANIAL–INTRACRANIAL BYPASS. Anastomosis of the superficial temporal artery (external carotid) through a burr hole to a cortical branch of the middle cerebral artery (internal carotid) was widely advocated in the decade 1975–85 when there had been internal carotid occlusion. Trials suggest no overall benefit.

## REHABILITATION

### Physiotherapy and speech therapy

Skilled physiotherapy is of particular value in the first few months following the stroke. It is helpful in relieving spasticity, preventing contractures and teaching stroke patients to use walking aids. The effect of physiotherapy on the longer-term outcome is inadequately researched.

Speech therapy is frequently recommended in aphasia. It is possible that the spontaneous return of speech is hastened as much by normal conversation with a relative as by a therapist, though the trained therapist has a vital understanding of the problems and frustration of the aphasic patient.

Both physiotherapy and speech therapy have an undoubted psychological role. Stroke is frequently a devastating event and, particularly when it occurs during working life, radically alters the pattern of the patient's remaining years. Many patients become unemployable and cannot lead independent lives. The financial consequences to the sufferer are usually considerable. The loss of self-esteem makes secondary depression common.

Following recovery from stroke, various aids and modifications may be necessary at home, for example stair rails, portable lavatories, bath rails, hoists, sliding boards, wheelchairs, tripods, modification of doorways and sleep arrangements, stair lifts and kitchen modifications. A visit to the patient's home with the occupational therapist and their primary care physician to discuss these problems is valuable.

## PROGNOSIS

Between one-third and one-half of patients will die in the first month following a stroke. This early mortality is lower for thromboembolic infarction (under one-quarter) than for intracerebral haemorrhage (around three-quarters). A poor outcome is likely when there is coma, a defect in conjugate gaze and a severe hemiplegia. Recurrent strokes are common (10% in the first year) and, in addition, many patients die subsequently of a myocardial infarction. Of initial survivors, 30–40% are alive after 3 years.

Gradual improvement usually follows stroke, although the patient may be left with a severe residual deficit. Of those who survive a stroke, about one-third return to independent mobility and one-third have severe disability requiring permanent institutional care.

If, in general, there is sufficient language to be intelligible at 3 weeks, the outlook for recovery of fluent speech is good. Many stroke patients are, however, left with word-finding difficulties.

# PRIMARY INTRACRANIAL HAEMORRHAGE

## Intracerebral haemorrhage

### AETIOLOGY

Rupture of microaneurysms (Charcot–Bouchard aneurysms, 0.8–1.0 mm in diameter) is the principal cause of primary intracerebral haemorrhage. This occurs typically in patients with hypertension and occurs at well-defined sites—basal ganglia, pons, cerebellum and subcortical white matter. Saccular ('berry') aneurysms and arteriovenous malformations also bleed into the brain.

### RECOGNITION

Clinically, there is no entirely reliable way of distinguishing between haemorrhage and infarction, as both produce a focal deficit. Cerebral haemorrhage, however, tends to be accompanied by a severe headache and to cause a more severe general deficit (e.g. coma) than a thromboembolic stroke.

On CT an intracerebral haemorrhage is almost always immediately visualized (cf. thrombosis, see p. 908). It appears as a high-density lesion sometimes with blood in the ventricular or subarachnoid space.

### MANAGEMENT

The general management of cerebral haemorrhage is as for cerebral infarction, although the immediate prognosis is not as good. Only when an intracerebral haematoma behaves as an expanding mass lesion causing deepening coma and coning should urgent surgical removal be considered. Anticoagulant drugs are of course contraindicated.

## Cerebellar haemorrhage

It is important to recognize cerebellar haemorrhage because it causes an acute hydrocephalus. There is head-ache and rapid reduction of consciousness with signs of brain stem origin (e.g. nystagmus, ocular palsies). The gaze deviates to the side of the lesion. Emergency surgery may be necessary to remove a cerebellar haematoma.

# SUBARACHNOID HAEMORRHAGE

The term subarachnoid haemorrhage (SAH) describes spontaneous rather than traumatic arterial bleeding into the subarachnoid space.

## INCIDENCE

SAH accounts for 10% of cerebrovascular disease and has an annual incidence of 15 per 100 000.

## CAUSES

The causes of SAH are shown in Table 18.30. It is unusual to find any contributing disease.

**Saccular ('berry') aneurysms** (Fig. 18.18)
Saccular aneurysms form on the circle of Willis and its adjacent branches. The common sites of aneurysms are:
JUNCTION OF THE POSTERIOR COMMUNICATING ARTERY AND THE INTERNAL CAROTID ARTERY — posterior communicating artery aneurysm
JUNCTION OF THE ANTERIOR COMMUNICATING ARTERY AND THE ANTERIOR CEREBRAL ARTERY — anterior communicating artery aneurysm
BIFURCATION OF THE MIDDLE CEREBRAL ARTERY — middle cerebral artery aneurysm
Other sites are on the basilar artery, the PICA, the intracavernous internal carotid artery and the ophthalmic artery. Saccular aneurysms are an incidental finding in 1% of autopsies and may be multiple.

Aneurysms cause symptoms either by spontaneous rupture (when there is usually no preceding history) or by pressure effects on surrounding structures, e.g. a posterior communicating aneurysm may cause a painful third nerve palsy (see p. 886).

**Arteriovenous malformation (AVM)**
This is a lesion of developmental origin, usually within the hemisphere. An AVM may cause epilepsy, which is

| | |
|---|---|
| Saccular ('berry') aneurysms | 70% |
| Arteriovenous malformation | 10% |
| No lesion found | 20% |
| *Rare associations* | |
| Bleeding disorders | |
| Mycotic aneurysms (endocarditis, see p. 604) | |
| Acute bacterial meningitis | |
| Brain tumours (e.g. metastatic melanoma) | |
| Arteritis (e.g. systemic lupus erythematosus) | |
| Spinal subarachnoid haemorrhage from a spinal arteriovenous malformation | |
| Coarctation of the aorta | |
| Marfan's syndrome, Ehlers–Danlos syndrome | |
| Polycystic kidneys | |

**Table 18.30**   Causes of subarachnoid haemorrhage.

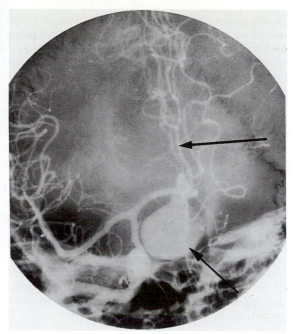

**Fig. 18.18** Carotid arteriogram showing a large aneurysm of the anterior communicating artery (bottom arrow). The top arrow indicates the anterior cerebral arteries.

often focal. Once an AVM has ruptured to cause an SAH there is a tendency to rebleed at a rate of 10% per year.

### CLINICAL FEATURES
The onset is sudden with a devastating headache, often occipital. This is usually followed by vomiting and often by loss of consciousness. The patient remains comatose or drowsy for several hours to several days. Less-severe headaches may cause diagnostic difficulties.

On examination, there is neck stiffness and a positive Kernig's sign. Papilloedema is sometimes present and may be accompanied by retinal haemorrhages and sub-hyaloid haemorrhage (massive retinal haemorrhage tracking beneath the hyaloid membrane).

### INVESTIGATION
CT scanning shows subarachnoid or intraventricular blood. The CSF is yellow (xanthochromic) several hours after SAH. Lumbar puncture is not necessary if the diagnosis is made by CT.

Carotid and vertebral angiography is usually performed in all patients who are potentially fit for surgery (i.e. those who are young—below 55–60 years—and not in coma) to establish the site of the bleeding.

### DIFFERENTIAL DIAGNOSIS
SAH must be differentiated from severe migraine. This is sometimes difficult. Acute meningitis may also cause a very abrupt headache.

### COMPLICATIONS
Blood clot in the subarachnoid space can lead to obstruction of CSF flow and hydrocephalus. This can be

asymptomatic but can be a cause of deteriorating conscious level a few days or weeks after the initial event. Diagnosis is by CT and a drainage procedure may be required.

### MANAGEMENT
Nearly half the cases of SAH are either dead or moribund before they reach hospital. Of the remainder, a further 10–20% die in the early weeks in hospital from further bleeding.

Patients who are comatose or who have severe neurological deficits have a poor prognosis. In others, where angiography demonstrates aneurysm, a direct neurosurgical approach to clip the neck of the aneurysm is carried out. In selected cases the results of surgery are excellent.

The immediate treatment of patients with SAH is bed rest and supportive measures. Hypertension should be controlled. Dexamethasone and antifibrinolytic agents are often prescribed, but their place in therapy is dubious. Nimodipine, a calcium-channel blocking agent, has been shown to reduce the mortality.

Severe spasm of the intracranial arteries sometimes complicates SAH and is a poor prognostic sign.

It is usual to refer all cases of SAH to a specialist centre for a decision about angiography and possible surgery.

## SUBDURAL AND EXTRADURAL HAEMORRHAGE AND HAEMATOMA

These conditions are of great neurosurgical importance as both may cause death unless treated promptly.

**Subdural haematoma (SDH)** (see Fig. 18.20b, p. 931)
SDH occurs when blood accumulates in the subdural space following rupture of a vein. It is almost always due to head injury, which may be minor, but the latent interval between injury and symptoms may be weeks or months. Chronic SDH is common in the elderly and in patients with alcohol abuse.

Headache, drowsiness and confusion are common; the symptoms are indolent and often fluctuate. Focal deficits such as hemiparesis or sensory loss may develop and epilepsy may occur. Stupor and coma gradually ensue.

**Extradural haemorrhage** (see Fig. 18.20a)
This follows a tear of a branch of a middle meningeal artery, usually underlying a linear skull fracture. Blood accumulates rapidly over minutes or hours in the extradural space. The most characteristic picture is of a head injury with a brief duration of unconsciousness followed by a 'lucid interval' of recovery. The patient then develops a progressive hemiparesis and stupor, and rapid transtentorial 'coning', with first an ipsilateral dilated pupil, followed by bilateral fixed dilated pupils, tetraplegia and death.

An acute subdural haemorrhage presents in a similar way.

## MANAGEMENT

The diagnosis of extradural or subdural haemorrhage or haematoma is confirmed by CT scan and/or arteriography. MRI scanning is also used.

Surgical drainage is carried out. If it is performed early, the outlook is excellent. When far from specialist help (e.g. in wartime or at sea), drainage should be carried out when the diagnosis is suspected on clinical grounds alone; this procedure has been life-saving.

In the elderly, some SDHs resolve spontaneously and can be monitored with serial CT scans.

## CORTICAL VENOUS AND DURAL VENOUS SINUS THROMBOSIS

These are unusual complications of skull and paranasal (air) sinus infection, dehydration or severe intercurrent illness. There is also an association with pregnancy and the contraceptive pill.

### Cortical venous thrombosis

The venous infarct caused by the thrombosis leads to focal signs (e.g. hemiparesis) and epilepsy. There is often a fever.

### Dural venous sinus thromboses

CAVERNOUS SINUS THROMBOSIS. This causes ocular pain, proptosis and chemosis. An external and internal ophthalmoplegia with papilloedema develop.

LATERAL AND SAGITTAL SINUS THROMBOSIS. This causes raised intracranial pressure with headache, papilloedema and often epilepsy.

## MANAGEMENT

Treatment and investigation is directed at the underlying cause of the thrombosis. Anticonvulsants are used in epilepsy and antibiotics in infection. Anticoagulants are sometimes used.

## *Epilepsy and other causes of recurrent loss of consciousness*

## EPILEPSY

An epileptic seizure is a convulsion or transient abnormal event experienced by the subject due to a paroxysmal discharge of cerebral neurones. Epilepsy, by definition, is the continuing tendency to have such seizures, even if a long interval separates attacks. A generalized convulsion or *grand mal* fit is the commonest recognized event.

### INCIDENCE

Epilepsy is a common condition. Some 3% of the population have two or more seizures during their lives. In Britain approximately 65 people suffer from their first seizure each day. Around one-quarter of a million people in Britain take anticonvulsants. In Asia the prevalence is similar to that in Western nations; the condition is said to be over twice as common in Africa.

### PATHOPHYSIOLOGY

The spread of electrical activity between cortical neurones is normally restricted. Synchronous discharge of neurones in normal brain takes place in small groups only; these limited discharges are responsible for the normal rhythms of the EEG.

During a seizure, large groups of neurones are activated repetitively and 'hypersynchronously'. There is a failure of inhibitory synaptic contact between neurones. This causes high-voltage spike-and-wave activity on the EEG.

Epileptic activity confined to one area of the cortex is associated with specific symptoms and signs (partial seizures). This activity may remain focal or may spread to cause paroxysmal activity in both hemispheres and a generalized convulsion. This spread is called secondary generalization of a partial seizure.

### Seizure threshold

Each individual has a threshold for seizure activity. Experimentally some chemicals (e.g. pentylenetetrazol, a gas) induce seizures in all subjects. Individuals who are more likely than others in the population to have seizures in response to various stimuli, for example flashing lights, are said to have a 'low seizure threshold', although this is a concept, not an actual measurement.

### CLASSIFICATION

Epilepsy is classified according to the clinical type of seizure (Table 18.31).

### Generalized seizures

Generalized implies abnormal electrical activity which is widespread in the brain, and is primarily of constitutional origin, i.e. developmental.

TONIC–CLONIC SEIZURES (GRAND MAL SEIZURES, GENERALIZED CONVULSIONS). Following a vague warning, the body enters a rigid tonic phase that lasts for up to a minute. Subjects may utter a cry and fall, sometimes injuring themselves. The tongue may be bitten and there may be incontinence of urine or faeces.

This is followed by a convulsion (the clonic phase) in which the muscles jerk rhythmically. This lasts a few seconds to a few minutes. Seizures are usually self-limiting, leaving the patient drowsy or in coma for several hours.

TYPICAL ABSENCES (PETIT MAL). This type of generalized epilepsy is almost invariably a disorder of childhood, and by definition an attack is accompanied by 3-Hz spike-and-wave in the EEG. The child ceases activity, stares and pales slightly. The eyelids may twitch. The attack lasts for a few seconds only. A few jerks may occur.

After an attack, the child carries on as if nothing had

*Generalized seizures*

1   Absence seizures[a]
    (a) Typical absences with 3-Hz spike-and-wave
        discharge (*petit mal*)
    (b) Atypical absences with other EEG changes

2   Myoclonic seizures

3   Tonic–clonic seizures (*grand mal*, major
    convulsions)[a]

4   Tonic seizures

5   Akinetic seizures

*Partial seizures*
These start by activation of a group of neurones in one
part of one hemisphere. They are also called focal
seizures

1   Simple partial seizures (no impairment of
    consciousness),[a] e.g. Jacksonian seizures

2   Complex partial seizures (with impairment of
    consciousness)[a]

3   Partial seizures evolving to tonic–clonic seizures[a]

4   Apparent generalized tonic–clonic seizures, with
    EEG but not clinical evidence of focal onset[a]

———

[a]Common varieties of epilepsy.

Table 18.31   Classification of epilepsy.

happened. Typical absence attacks are never due to identifiable local lesions. Children with typical absence attacks may in adult life develop generalized seizures.

The term *petit mal* should not be used to describe the absence attacks of partial seizures (see below).

## Partial seizures (focal seizures)

'Partial' or 'focal' implies an area of brain, e.g. a temporal lobe, which generates abnormal electrical activity that may spread. An acquired lesion, e.g. a tumour, is a cause of such activity. The seizure frequently has clinical features that provide evidence of its site of origin.

When these features precede a *grand mal* fit, the warning they give to the patient or relatives is called the 'aura' and the seizure is said to become secondarily generalized.

JACKSONIAN (MOTOR SEIZURES). These simple partial seizures originate in the motor cortex. Jerking movements typically begin at the angle of the mouth or in the thumb and index finger, spreading to involve the limbs on the side opposite the epileptic focus. The clinical evidence of this spread of activity is called the 'march' of the seizure. Conjugate gaze (see p. 885) may deviate away from a frontal lobe focus (an 'adversive seizure'). Paralysis of the affected limbs may follow for several hours (Todd's paralysis).

TEMPORAL LOBE SEIZURES. These complex partial seizures are associated with strange disturbances of smell or feelings of unreality (*jamais vu*) or undue familiarity (*déja vu*) with the surroundings. Visual hallucinations (visions or faces) may be seen. Absence attacks or vertigo may occur.

Many other types of partial seizure are known, e.g. autonomic disturbances with piloerection or flushing, sensory disturbances (parietal cortex), crude visual shapes (occipital cortex) or strange sounds (auditory cortex).

## AETIOLOGICAL AND PRECIPITATING FACTORS
(Table 18.32)

A cause for epilepsy is found in under one-quarter of patients. A number of secondary factors may trigger seizures in those with a low seizure threshold.

### Family history

About 30% of patients with epilepsy have a history of seizures in first-degree relatives. Usually the mode of inheritance is uncertain; a low seizure threshold appears to run in some families. Generalized typical absence seizures (*petit mal*) are sometimes inherited as an autosomal dominant trait with variable penetrance.

### Trauma and surgery

Perinatal trauma (causing cerebral contusion and haemorrhage) and fetal anoxia are common causes of seizures in childhood. Hypoxic damage to the medial temporal lobes (medial temporal sclerosis) is another cause.

Head injury is sometimes followed by epilepsy within the first week ('early' epilepsy) or many months or years later ('late' epilepsy). To cause epilepsy, the injury must (almost always) be sufficient to cause coma. The presence of early epilepsy, a depressed skull fracture, cerebral contusion, a dural tear or intracranial haematoma increases the incidence of late post-traumatic epilepsy.

Surgery to the cerebral hemispheres is followed by seizures in about 10% of patients.

### Pyrexia

High fevers in children under 5 years are sometimes associated with generalized seizures ('febrile convulsions'). In the majority there is no tendency for the seizures to recur in adult life.

### Intracranial mass lesions

All mass lesions affecting the cerebral cortex may cause epilepsy—either partial or secondary generalized seizures. If the onset of seizures is in adult life, the chance of an unsuspected mass lesion being present is around 3%.

Family history
Trauma and surgery to the head
Pyrexia in children
Intracranial mass lesions
Cerebral infarction
Drugs, alcohol and drug withdrawal
Encephalitis
Metabolic abnormalities
Degenerative brain disorders
Photosensitivity and auditory stimuli

Table 18.32   Aetiological and precipitating factors in epilepsy.

Hydrocephalus, of any cause, may be associated with seizures.

### Cerebral infarction

Seizures may follow cerebral infarction, especially in the elderly.

### Drugs, alcohol and drug withdrawal

Phenothiazines, monoamine oxidase inhibitors, tricyclic antidepressants, amphetamines, lignocaine and nalidixic acid may occasionally provoke fits either in overdose or in therapeutic doses in individuals with a low seizure threshold.

Chronic alcohol abuse is a common cause of seizures. These occur either while drinking or during periods of abstention. Alcohol-induced hypoglycaemia can also provoke attacks.

Withdrawal of anticonvulsant drugs (especially phenobarbitone) and withdrawal of benzodiazepines may provoke seizures.

### Encephalitis and other inflammatory conditions of the brain

Seizures are frequently the presenting feature of encephalitis, chronic meningitis (e.g. tuberculosis), cerebral abscess, cortical venous thrombosis and neurosyphilis.

### Metabolic abnormalities

Seizures may occur with the following metabolic abnormalities:

- Hypocalcaemia
- Hypoglycaemia
- Hyponatraemia
- Acute hypoxia
- Porphyria
- Uraemia
- Hepatic failure

### Degenerative brain disorders

Seizures can occur in Alzheimer's disease and in many rarer degenerative diseases. Epilepsy is three times more common in patients with MS than in the general population.

### Photosensitive and other types of reflex epilepsy

Seizures are sometimes precipitated by flashing lights or a flickering television screen. This photosensitivity can be seen on the occipital recording of the EEG. Very rarely other stimuli provoke attacks.

## DIAGNOSIS AND INVESTIGATION

The history from a witness of the attack is of prime importance.

### Electroencephalogram

This is the single most useful test in the *diagnosis* of epilepsy.

DURING A SEIZURE the EEG is almost invariably abnormal, because epileptic activity reaches the surface of the brain.

EEG EVIDENCE OF SEIZURE ACTIVITY is shown typically by a cortical spike focus (e.g. in a temporal lobe) or by generalized spike-and-wave activity.

IN PETIT MAL, 3-Hz spike-and-wave activity is seen. It is always present during an attack and is frequently seen in the interictal intervals (i.e. between attacks).

A NORMAL EEG BETWEEN ATTACKS does not exclude epilepsy. Many people suffering from epilepsy have normal interictal EEG activity. In addition, an abnormal interictal EEG does not prove that an attack was epileptic.

EEG TELEMETRY, with video recordings of attacks has greatly added to the value of this investigation in the study of attacks of disturbed consciousness whose nature is uncertain.

### CT scanning and/or MRI

This should be performed on all patients other than children even though the diagnostic yield of treatable lesions is extremely low for both EEG or imaging tests.

### Other investigations

Routine investigations (blood picture, serum biochemistry, chest X-ray) may indicate an underlying metabolic or structural cause. Such tests are normal in idiopathic epilepsy.

## TREATMENT

### Emergency measures

The emergency treatment of a seizure is simply to ensure that patients harm themselves as little as possible and that the airway is patent in a prolonged seizure and in post-ictal coma. Wooden mouth gags, tongue forceps and physical restraint frequently cause injury rather than prevent it.

Most seizures last only minutes. A prolonged seizure (longer than 3 min) or repeat seizures outside hospital are best treated with rectal diazepam solution (10 mg).

If there is any suspicion of hypoglycaemia, blood should be taken for the measurement of glucose, and intravenous glucose should be given.

### Long-term anticonvulsant drugs

Anticonvulsant drugs are indicated in recurrent seizures. Opinions differ as to whether treatment is necessary following the first attack. Phenytoin, carbamazepine and sodium valproate are the most effective drugs prescribed. Phenobarbitone, primidone and the benzodiazepine clonazepam are also used. There are differences in opinion about the most appropriate drugs for each particular variety of seizure: one suggested scheme is given in Table 18.33.

Phenytoin has the advantage of being cheap and effective. The therapeutic level of phenytoin in serum is well defined and this should be monitored in the majority of patients (Table 18.34). The therapeutic serum levels of other anticonvulsants are less clearly defined and routine estimations are not usually performed.

It is preferable to try to use one drug alone in the treatment of epilepsy, although a second (or third) drug may

| Type of seizure | Drug |
|---|---|
| Generalized tonic–clonic seizures | Phenytoin |
| Generalized absence (*petit mal*) seizures | Sodium valproate |
| Partial seizures | Carbamazepine Sodium valproate |

**Table 18.33**  Suggested scheme for the use of anticonvulsant drugs.

| Drug | Adult daily dose (mg) | Therapeutic level (µmol litre⁻¹) |
|---|---|---|
| Phenytoin | 300 | 40–80 |
| Carbamazepine | 200 × 3 | 20–50[a] |
| Sodium valproate | 200 × 3 | 200–700[a] |

——
[a]Poorly defined.

**Table 18.34**  Therapeutic levels of anticonvulsant drugs.

| Drug | Non-dose related side-effects |
|---|---|
| Phenytoin | Rashes Blood dyscrasias Lymphadenopathy Systemic lupus erythematosus |
| Carbamazepine | Rashes Blood dyscrasias, particularly severe leucopenia |
| Sodium valproate | Anorexia Hair loss Liver damage |

**Table 18.35**  Some idiosyncratic unwanted effects of anticonvulsant drugs.

be needed in resistant cases. Alternatively, vigabatrin and lamotrigine can also be used in resistant cases.

UNWANTED EFFECTS. Intoxication with all anticonvulsants causes a syndrome of ataxia, nystagmus and dysarthria.

Chronic administration of phenytoin can cause gum hypertrophy, hypertrichosis, osteomalacia, folate deficiency, polyneuropathy and encephalopathy. The more common idiosyncratic (i.e. non-dose-related) side-effects are summarized in Table 18.35.

The question of withdrawal of drug therapy is often raised by the patients. Unfortunately, withdrawal can be socially disastrous for patients in preventing them from driving. Careful discussion with an experienced physician is important: withdrawal should not be considered until the patient has been free of all fits for at least 2 years.

### Status epilepticus

This is when seizures follow each other without recovery of consciousness. It is a medical emergency with a mortality of 10–15%. When *grand mal* seizures follow one another there is a serious risk of death from cardiorespiratory failure. Several treatment regimes are available. Immediate intravenous injection of diazepam 10 mg followed by intravenous infusion of 200 mg litre⁻¹ over 24 hours is the first line of treatment. Chlormethiazole 0.8% should be given by intravenous infusion if status epilepticus continues or returns. Phenytoin i.v., phenobarbitone i.v., clonazepam i.v. are also used. Ventilatory support must be available when status is treated.

'Status' can also occur in absence seizures and in focal epilepsy. 'Epilepsy partialis continua' is a continuous seizure of a small part of the body, e.g. a finger, without loss of consciousness. It is often due to a cortical neoplasm or, in the elderly, a cortical infarct.

### Neurosurgical treatment

Several surgical approaches have been used in epilepsy. The most important is amputation of the anterior temporal lobe (usually of the non-dominant side) in those with partial seizures or partial seizures that are secondarily generalized. Indications include poor control on drug therapy and a clearly defined focus of abnormal electrical activity.

### Pregnancy and epilepsy

Fits are sometimes more frequent mainly because of poor absorption and poor compliance with drug therapy. Regular monitoring of drug levels is required. Breast feeding is only contraindicated with patients on phenobarbitone or primidone. There is a small increased risk of fetal abnormalities. Higher doses of the contraceptive pill may be required in those taking enzyme-inducing drugs such as phenytoin.

### The social consequences of epilepsy

The great majority of patients with epilepsy can be managed by a general practitioner or as an outpatient, and have infrequent seizures that alter the pattern of their lives relatively little. In the small minority who have exceedingly frequent seizures, treatment in hospital or residential care is necessary.

There remains, however, a considerable social stigma attached to the diagnosis, an important fact to be considered when the nature of attacks of disturbed consciousness is uncertain. Employers are reluctant to take on patients who have seizures.

Present trends are to encourage both adults and children with epilepsy to lead lives as unrestricted as possible, though with simple, sensible provisos such as avoiding swimming alone and dangerous sports such as rock-climbing or solo canoeing. It is also wise to advise on simple domestic matters, e.g. that the bathroom door should remain unlocked.

### Driving and epilepsy

Those who have suffered from more than one seizure are unable to hold a driving licence in the UK unless they satisfy the following criteria whether on or off treatment.

1  They shall have been free from any form of epileptic attack whilst awake for a period of 2 years prior to the issue of a licence.

2  In the cases of attacks whilst asleep, the attacks must have occurred only whilst asleep and the patient must not have had an attack for 3 years prior to the issue of a licence.

The rules for those holding Public Service Vehicle and Heavy Goods Vehicle licences (PSV and HGV) are stricter: any attack after the age of 3 years automatically bars an applicant indefinitely from holding such a licence.

It is the duty of a doctor to inform patients of these regulations: the patient should then write to the licensing authorities. Similar strict regulations exist for potential aircraft pilots, sea captains and other similar activities. The correct diagnosis of an attack at any age has therefore become of major social and legal importance.

## OTHER CAUSES OF RECURRENT ATTACKS OF DISTURBED CONSCIOUSNESS AND FALLS

(Table 18.36)

Episodes of transient disturbance of consciousness and falls are common clinical problems. It is usually possible to distinguish between a 'fit' (a seizure), a 'faint' (syncope) and other types of attack from the history given by the patient and the account of an eye witness.

| |
| --- |
| Syncope (situational or vasovagal) |
|   'Faint' |
|   Cough |
|   Effort |
|   Micturition |
|   Carotid sinus |
| Epilepsy |
| Narcolepsy and cataplexy |
| Transient ischaemic attacks |
| Psychogenic attacks |
| Panic attacks |
| Hyperventilation |
| Night terrors   }  in children |
| Breath holding  } |
| Choking |
| Cardiac arrhythmias |
| Postural hypotension |
| Hypoglycaemia |
| Hypocalcaemia |
| Vertigo |
| Drop attacks |
| Hydrocephalus |

**Table 18.36** Causes of attacks of disturbed consciousness and falling.

## Syncope ('fainting', vasovagal attacks) and related disorders (see p. 527)

Sudden reflex bradycardia and peripheral and splanchnic vasodilatation leading to loss of consciousness occurs commonly in response to prolonged standing, fear, venesection or pain. This is also known as neurocardiogenic syncope. It almost never occurs in the recumbent posture. The subject falls to the ground and is unconscious for less than 2 minutes. Recovery is rapid. A few jerking movements are uncommon, but do occur. Incontinence of urine is exceptional.

This is the 'simple faint' from which the majority of the population suffer at some time, particularly in childhood, in youth or in pregnancy.

Syncope may occur after micturition in men (particularly at night) and when the venous return to the heart is obstructed by breath-holding and severe coughing.

The syndrome of carotid sinus syncope is believed to be due to excessive sensitivity of the sinus to external pressure. It may occur in elderly patients who lose consciousness on touching of the neck.

Postural hypotension occurs in patients with impaired autonomic reflexes, e.g. in the elderly, in autonomic neuropathy, or with ganglion-blocking drugs used in hypertension, with phenothiazines, levodopa or tricyclic antidepressants. A tilt test will show hypotension as the patient is raised to the vertical and is useful in diagnosis.

Transient cerebral ischaemia in the posterior cerebral circulation is a cause of episodes of loss of consciousness in patients with cervical spondylosis in which vertebral artery compression occurs.

Cardiac arrhythmias (cardiac syncope, Stokes–Adams attacks—see p. 527) are important causes of recurrent episodes of loss of consciousness, particularly in the elderly. There is sometimes a preceding warning of palpitations (either fast or slow). The loss of consciousness is sudden and accompanied by pallor. Exceptionally, there are convulsive movements ('anoxic convulsions'). Flushing may occur when the patient recovers. The usual cardiac arrhythmias that cause loss of consciousness are paroxysmal bradycardias (e.g. in complete heart block) or tachycardias (e.g. ventricular tachycardias, ventricular fibrillation). Supraventricular tachycardias are unusual causes of loss of consciousness.

Effort syncope (syncope on exertion) is of cardiac origin (e.g. aortic stenosis, hypertrophic obstructive cardiomyopathy).

### INVESTIGATION

Syncope and related conditions where cerebral blood flow is impaired can usually be distinguished from epilepsy on the clinical history alone.

Cardiac monitoring may sometimes be necessary to detect an arrhythmia. Tilt testing (see p. 541) is useful in neurocardiogenic syncope.

## MANAGEMENT

The immediate management of syncope, or impending syncope, is to lie the patient down, to elevate the lower limbs and to record the pulse. In the rare circumstances where cerebral blood flow cannot be restored, e.g. in a dentist's chair, syncope may be followed by cerebral infarction.

## Drop attacks

These sudden episodes of weakness of the lower limbs with falling but without loss of consciousness occur in middle-aged women. They are believed to be due to sudden changes in tone in the lower limbs, presumably of brain stem origin. Previously they have been regarded as forms of TIA, from which they are distinct.

## Panic attacks, night terrors, psychogenic attacks and hyperventilation

Panic attacks are usually associated with an autonomic disturbance, e.g. tachycardia, sweating and piloerection. Consciousness is usually preserved. Hyperventilation (see below) is common.

Night terrors are sudden episodes seen in children who awake as if from a dream in a state of terror.

Psychogenic attacks cause considerable difficulty in diagnosis. Attacks resembling *grand mal* fits may occur but more usually there are bizarre and irregular limb movements.

The alkalosis accompanying hyperventilation leads to a feeling of light-headedness, which may be accompanied by circumoral and peripheral tingling and tetany (e.g. carpopedal spasm) (see p. 430).

## Hypoglycaemia (see also p. 852)

Hypoglycaemia causes attacks in which the patient either feels unwell or may lose consciousness, sometimes with a convulsion. There is often some warning, with hunger, shaking and sweating. There is prompt relief with intravenous (or oral) glucose.

Hypoglycaemic attacks unrelated to diabetes are rare. Most patients who feel unwell after fasting or in the early morning have no serious organic disease.

## Hypocalcaemia

A *grand mal* fit may accompany hypocalcaemia (see p. 430).

## Vertigo

Acute episodes of vertigo may cause prostration: consciousness is sometimes lost for a few seconds.

## Choking

Sudden prostration sometimes follows choking, particularly when a large bolus of meat obstructs the larynx. The patient goes blue, is speechless and may die in the attack if the obstruction is not relieved.

Treatment involves immediately grasping the patient around the abdomen and squeezing hard in an effort to eject the food (Heimlich manoeuvre, see p. 656).

## SLEEP AND ITS DISTURBANCES

Sleep is required on a regular basis. The reason for this is unclear; it is postulated that the laying down of memory is one important component. Complex pathways between the cortex and reticular formation are involved in the production and maintenance of sleep. During a normal night's sleep, there are periods of deep sleep associated with rapid eye movement (REM). Dreaming occurs during REM sleep.

In insomnia, sleep is fitful. Less time than usual is spent in REM sleep. Sleep requirement falls to as little as 4 hours a night in old age. Insomnia, particularly early morning waking, is a common symptom of depression (see p. 970). In practice, insomnia itself is rarely a feature of serious organic neurological disease but in the elderly nocturnal confusion and/or nightmares are caused by drugs and organic brain disease.

In sleep apnoea, the normal short periods of apnoea seen during REM sleep are prolonged. This occurs with brain stem lesions and with upper airways obstruction, when it is accompanied by snoring. The latter is particularly important in patients with chronic bronchitis and emphysema, who may become severely hypoxic (see p. 663).

## Narcolepsy and cataplexy

Narcoleptic attacks are periods of irresistible sleep in inappropriate circumstances. They may occur when there is little distraction, after meals, while travelling in a vehicle, or without obvious cause. Genetically, narcolepsy is strongly associated with HLA-DR2 and HLA-DQwl antigens

Cataplexy is a sudden loss of tone in the lower limbs with preservation of consciousness. Attacks are set off by sudden surprise or emotion.

The two conditions are related and may be accompanied by hypnagogic hallucinations (terrifying hallucinations on falling asleep), hypnopompic hallucinations (on waking) and sleep paralysis (a frightening inability to move whilst drowsy). The EEG is normal in these attacks.

Treatment is with methylphenidate, other amphetamine-like drugs, or small doses of tricyclic antidepressants.

# *Parkinson's disease and other movement disorders*

Disorders of movement can be classified broadly into akinetic–rigid syndromes, where there is loss of movement with increase in muscle tone, and dyskinesias, where there are added movements outside voluntary control. Both are due to disorders of neurotransmitters of the extrapyramidal system.

Parkinson's disease is much the commonest of these conditions. A classification of movement disorders is given in Table 18.37.

# AKINETIC–RIGID SYNDROMES

## Idiopathic Parkinson's disease

In 1817, James Parkinson, a physician in Hoxton, London, described the clinical appearance of patients with the 'shaking palsy'. The disease is common and worldwide, with prevalence increasing sharply with age to about 1 in 200 in those over 70 years. The condition is clinically distinct from other 'parkinsonian' syndromes.

There are few clues as to its cause:

NICOTINE. Some epidemiological studies suggest the disease is less prevalent in tobacco smokers than in lifelong abstainers.

MINUTE DOSES OF A PYRIDINE COMPOUND (MPTP) (see p. 920) cause a severe parkinsonian syndrome. The significance of this to idiopathic Parkinson's disease is not clear.

SURVIVORS OF ENCEPHALITIS LETHARGICA, which is presumed to be a viral disease, develop parkinsonism. However, it is not thought that the idiopathic disease is related to this or to another infective agent.

The condition is not inherited.

### PATHOLOGY

In the pars compacta of the substantia nigra there is progressive cell degeneration and the appearance of eosinophilic inclusion bodies (Lewy bodies). Degeneration also occurs in other brain stem nuclei. Biochemically there is loss of dopamine (and melanin) in the striatum that correlates well with the areas of cell loss and also with the degree of akinesia. The underlying cause of these biochemical changes remains obscure (see p. 894).

---

*Akinetic–rigid syndromes*
Idiopathic Parkinson's disease
Drug-induced parkinsonism, e.g.
    phenothiazines
MPTP-induced parkinsonism
Postencephalitic parkinsonism
'Parkinsonism plus'
Childhood akinetic–rigid syndromes

*Dyskinesias*
Essential tremor
Chorea
Hemiballismus
Myoclonus
Tic or 'habit spasms'
Torsion dystonias

———

MPTP, 1-methyl-4-phenyl-1,2,3,6-tetrahydropyridine.

**Table 18.37**  A classification of movement disorders.

### CLINICAL FEATURES

There is a combination of tremor, rigidity and akinesia, together with important changes in posture.

#### Symptoms

The commonest symptoms are tremor and slowness of movement. Patients also complain that the limbs feel stiff and ache and that fine movements are difficult. The slowness of movement causes the characteristic symptoms of difficulty in rising from a chair or getting into or out of bed. Writing becomes small (micrographia) and spidery, with a tendency to tail off at the end of a line. Other evidence of the disease often comes from relatives who have noted slowness and an impassive facial expression.

#### Signs

TREMOR. This is a characteristic 4–7 Hz rest tremor that is usually decreased by action and increased by emotion. 'Pill-rolling' movements of the fingers and thumbs may be seen. The shaking is sometimes unilateral or more prominent on one side.

RIGIDITY. Stiffness of the limbs develops that can be felt throughout the range of movement and is equal in opposing groups of muscles (in contrast to the selective increase in tone found in spasticity). This 'lead-pipe' rigidity is often more marked on one side and is present in the neck and axial muscles (where it is difficult to examine).

The rigidity is usually more easily felt when a joint is moved slowly and gently. Simultaneous active movement of the opposite limb increases the tone of the side under examination. When combined with tremor, the smooth plasticity of the increase in tone is broken up into a jerky resistance to passive movement, a phenomenon known as 'cogwheeling'.

AKINESIA. The poverty and slowing of movement (bradykinesia) is an additional handicap, distinct from rigidity. There is difficulty in initiating movement. Rapid finger movements (such as piano-playing movements) become indistinct, slow and tremulous. The immobility of the face gives a mask-like facies with the appearance of depression. The frequency of spontaneous blinking is reduced, causing a 'serpentine stare'.

POSTURAL CHANGES. A stoop is characteristic and the gait is shuffling, festinant and with poor arm swinging. The posture is sometimes called 'simian' to describe the forward flexion, immobility of the arms and lack of facial expression. The patient sits with the trunk bent forward and motionless, without gesture or animation, but the limbs are tremulous. Balance is impaired, but despite this the gait remains on a narrow base. Falls are common as the usual corrective righting reflexes fail, the sufferer falling stiffly 'like a telegraph pole'.

SPEECH. Speech is altered to a monotonous slurring dysarthria, due to the combination of akinesia, tremor and rigidity. Dribbling is frequent, and dysphagia occurs as the disease progresses.

GASTROINTESTINAL SYMPTOMS. These include heartburn, dysphagia, constipation and weight loss.

OTHER FINDINGS. Urinary difficulties are common, especially in men. The skin is greasy and sweating is excessive.

Power remains normal until advanced akinesia makes its assessment difficult. There is no sensory loss, although patients often complain of discomfort in the limbs. The reflexes are normal (though they may be asymmetrical, following an asymmetrical increase in tone). The plantar responses are flexor.

Cognitive function is preserved, at least in the early stages. Dementia sometimes occurs in the late stages.

### Natural history

Parkinson's disease progresses over a period of years, beginning as a mild inconvenience but slowly overtaking the patient. Remissions are unknown except for rare and remarkable short-lived periods of release. These tend to occur at times of great emotion, fear or excitement, when the sufferer is released for seconds or minutes and able to move quickly.

The rate of progression is very variable, with a benign form running over several decades. Usually the course is over 10–15 years, with death resulting from bronchopneumonia.

### DIFFERENTIAL DIAGNOSIS

There is no laboratory test for the disease. The diagnosis is made on clinical grounds alone. The condition must be distinguished from other akinetic–rigid syndromes. Hypothyroidism and depression also cause slowing of movement.

Certain diffuse or multifocal brain diseases cause some features of 'parkinsonism' (i.e. the slowing, rigidity and tremor). Alzheimer's disease, multi-infarct dementia, and the sequelae of repeated head injury (e.g. in boxers, see p. 938) or hypoxia are the commoner examples.

### TREATMENT

Older treatments with anticholinergic drugs altered the disease little, and frequently caused mental confusion. Benzhexol is still used in mild cases and as an adjunct to other therapy. Amantadine, originally introduced as an antiviral agent, is also sometimes helpful.

### Levodopa

The introduction of levodopa in the late 1960s was a revolutionary therapeutic approach, apparently replacing the lost neurotransmitter dopamine. Today levodopa is usually combined with a peripheral decarboxylase inhibitor—benserazide (co-beneldopa, as Madopar) or carbidopa (co-careldopa, as Sinemet). This combined therapy reduces the peripheral side-effects, principally nausea, of levodopa and its metabolites.

Treatment is commenced gradually (co-beneldopa 125 mg or co-careldopa '110' one tablet three times daily) and increased until either an adequate improvement has taken place or side-effects limit further increase in dose.

The great majority of patients with idiopathic Parkinson's disease (but not other parkinsonian syndromes) improve initially with levodopa. The response in severe, previously untreated disease may be dramatic.

UNWANTED EFFECTS OF LEVODOPA THERAPY. Nausea and vomiting within an hour of treatment are the commonest symptoms of the dose being too large. Confusion and visual hallucinations also occur. Chorea occurs in acute overdose.

As there are considerable problems with long-term treatment, levodopa therapy should not be started until necessary. Sometimes the drug appears to become ineffective, even with increasing doses. The disease progresses and the patient suffers from severe episodes of 'freezing' and falls. Fluctuation in the response to levodopa may also occur. The duration of action of the drug contracts, and the patient begins to suffer from a 'chronic levodopa syndrome', fluctuating between dopa-induced dyskinesias (chorea and dystonic movements) and severe and sometimes sudden immobility (on–off syndrome).

These are major and often insoluble problems in management. Approaches to treatment of the complications include the following:

THE INTERVAL BETWEEN LEVODOPA DOSES can be shortened and the individual doses reduced.

SELEGILINE—a type B monoamine oxidase inhibitor—inhibits the catabolism of dopamine in the brain. This sometimes has the effect of smoothing out the response to levodopa.

BROMOCRIPTINE, a directly acting dopaminergic agonist, is sometimes used.

'DRUG HOLIDAYS'—periods of drug withdrawal—are sometimes helpful. They require close supervision since severe rigidity and akinesia follow the withdrawal of levodopa.

### Psychiatric aspects

Depression is common in Parkinson's disease as the symptoms become worse and unresponsive to treatment. It is particularly difficult to treat, since type A monoamine oxidase inhibitor antidepressants (e.g. phenelzine) are absolutely contraindicated with levodopa, and tricyclic antidepressants (e.g. amitriptyline) have extrapyramidal side-effects.

All antiparkinsonian drugs, particularly in high doses, may cause confusion with visual hallucinations, which may exacerbate an associated dementia.

### Neurosurgery

Stereotactic placement of small lesions in the ventrolateral nucleus of the thalamus was commonly used in the two decades preceding the development of levodopa. The procedure was effective in reducing tremor but poor for relieving akinesia; it is now rarely performed.

Attempts to transplant fetal or autologous dopamine-containing tissue (adrenal medulla) to the cerebral ventricles or basal ganglia, though technically feasible, have not produced any major clinical improvement in patients with Parkinson's disease despite some early claims.

**Physiotherapy and physical aids**

Skilled and determined physiotherapy can improve the gait and help the patient to overcome particular problems.

Sensible guidance should be given about:

CLOTHING—avoiding zips, fiddly buttons and lace-up shoes.

CUTLERY—using built-up handles.

CHAIRS—high, upright chairs are easier to rise from than deep, comfortable armchairs.

RAILS—should be fitted near the lavatory and bath.

SHOES—should be easy to put on and have smooth soles.

FLOORING—patients' feet sometimes 'stick' to carpets and rugs and they prefer to walk on vinyl or linoleum.

WALKING AIDS are often a hindrance in the early stages but later a frame or a tripod may be helpful.

## Drug-induced parkinsonism

Reserpine, phenothiazines and butyrophenones induce a parkinsonian syndrome, with slowness and rigidity but usually little tremor. Methyldopa and tricyclic antidepressants also cause some slowing of movement. These syndromes tend not to progress. They respond poorly to levodopa. They disappear when the drug is stopped.

**Other movement disorders due to neuroleptic drugs**

Neuroleptic drugs (i.e. phenothiazines and butyrophenones) also produce other varieties of movement disorder. Three are described here.

AKATHISIA. This is a restless, repetitive and irresistible need to move.

ACUTE DYSTONIC REACTIONS. These sometimes follow, unpredictably, single doses of these drugs, even those used as antiemetics or vestibular sedatives (such as prochlorperazine and metoclopramide). Spasmodic torticollis, trismus and oculogyric crises (i.e. episodes of sustained upward gaze) may occur. These acute dystonias respond promptly to the intravenous injection of an anticholinergic drug (e.g. benztropine 1–2 mg).

CHRONIC TARDIVE DYSKINESIAS. These disabling disorders consist of mouthing and smacking of the lips, grimaces and contortion of the face and neck. They tend to occur some 6 months after commencing neuroleptic therapy and may be made temporarily worse when the offending drug is stopped. Only about half of the cases eventually recover.

## Postencephalitic parkinsonism

An epidemic of an encephalitic illness (encephalitis lethargica) occurred in 1918–1930 that left in its wake a severe extrapyramidal syndrome of parkinsonism with added dystonic movement disorders. Many of the survivors were permanently disabled. Occasionally, sporadic cases of the disease have been recorded recently in the UK; a recent epidemic may have occurred in Bulgaria.

## MPTP-induced parkinsonism

MPTP (1-methyl-4-phenyl-1,2,3,6-tetrahydropyridine) is an impurity produced inadvertently when opiate analgesics are synthesized illicitly. A few cases of a severe and largely irreversible parkinsonian syndrome have followed ingestion of minute quantities of MPTP. The relevance of this to idiopathic Parkinson's disease is not clear.

## 'Parkinsonism plus'

This describes rare disorders in which there is parkinsonism and evidence of a separate pathology.

Progressive supranuclear palsy is the commonest disorder and consists of axial rigidity, dementia and signs of parkinsonism together with a striking inability to move the eyes vertically or laterally.

Other examples of 'Parkinsonism plus' are the rare multiple system atrophies, e.g. olivopontocerebellar degeneration and primary autonomic failure (Shy–Drager syndrome).

## Akinetic–rigid syndromes in children

A group of extremely rare disorders cause an akinetic–rigid syndrome in those under 20 years of age. The most important are Wilson's disease and athetoid cerebral palsy.

**Wilson's disease**

This is a rare and treatable disorder of copper metabolism that is inherited as an autosomal recessive disease. There is deposition of copper in the brain (particularly in the basal ganglia), in the cornea and in the liver (see p. 270). It is most important that all young patients with cirrhosis are screened for this condition, as the neurological damage is irreversible unless early treatment is instituted.

Children with the disease have an akinetic–rigid syndrome and/or dyskinesias followed by progressive intellectual impairment.

DIAGNOSIS AND TREATMENT (see p. 270)

**Athetoid cerebral palsy**

Writhing movements of the limbs, sometimes with an increase in tone, are seen in cerebral palsy following kernicterus. This is now much less common following the prophylactic treatment of rhesus haemolytic disease.

# DYSKINESIAS

## Benign essential tremor

This common condition, often inherited as an autosomal dominant trait, causes tremor at 5–8 Hz that is usually worse in the upper limbs. The head is often tremulous (titubation) and also the trunk. Pathologically there is patchy neuronal loss in the cerebellum and cerebellar connections. Tremor is seen when the hands adopt a posture, such as holding a glass or a spoon. Oscillations are not usually present at rest nor do they worsen on movement.

Essential tremor may be seen at any age but occurs most frequently in the elderly. It is slowly progressive but rarely produces a severe disability. Writing is shaky and untidy but there is no micrographia. Anxiety exacerbates the tremor, sometimes dramatically.

Treatment is often unnecessary. Many of those affected are reassured to find they do not have Parkinson's disease, with which the condition is often confused.

Small doses of alcohol and β-adrenergic blockers such as propranolol often reduce the tremor. The anticonvulsant primidone also helps some patients. Sympathomimetics (e.g. salbutamol) make the tremor worse.

Though usually postural, in some cases the tremor may occur at rest (i.e. like Parkinson's disease) or be cerebellar (i.e. with past pointing).

## Chorea

Chorea consists of jerky, quasi-purposive and sometimes explosive movements, following each other but flitting from one part of the body to another. The causes of chorea are listed in Table 18.38; the commoner conditions are outlined below.

### Huntington's disease
Relentlessly progressive chorea and dementia in middle life are the hallmarks of this inherited disease.

The prevalence of the disease is about 1 in 20 000. It occurs worldwide. Inheritance is as an autosomal dominant trait with full penetrance; the children of an affected parent have a 50% chance of inheriting the disease. The family history of the disease in previous generations is often concealed, either by design or default. A mutation has been identified at the distal short arm of chromosome 4 with a sequence of randomly repeated trinucleotides (CAG). The messenger RNA for the gene is expressed in many tissues and its protein product has been termed huntingtin.

Huntington's disease
Sydenham's chorea
Benign hereditary chorea
Abetalipoproteinaemia (see p. 213) and chorea

Choreas associated with:
Drugs—phenytoin, levodopa, alcohol
Thyrotoxicosis, pregnancy and oral contraceptive pill
Systemic lupus erythematosus
Polycythaemia vera
Encephalitis lethargica
Stroke (basal ganglia)
Rarities (tumour, trauma, subdural haematoma, carbon monoxide poisoning)

**Table 18.38** Causes of chorea.

PATHOLOGY. There is cerebral atrophy with marked loss of small neurones in the caudate nucleus and putamen. Three important changes in neurotransmitters occur:
1 There is reduction in the enzymes synthesizing acetylcholine and GABA in the striatum.
2 There is depletion of GABA, angiotensin-converting enzyme and met-enkephalin in the substantia nigra.
3 Somatostatin levels are high in the corpus striatum.
These changes may be secondary to the cell damage. In contrast to Parkinson's disease, dopamine and tyrosine hydroxylase activity are normal.

MANAGEMENT AND COURSE. There is steady progression, of both the dementia and chorea. No treatment arrests the disease, although phenothiazines may reduce the chorea by causing drug-induced parkinsonism. Tetrabenazine or sulpiride may help to control the chorea. Death usually occurs between 10 and 20 years after the onset.

Mutation analysis, which is accurate and specific, is becoming available for presymptomatic testing. This raises ethical problems and centres performing these tests have adopted a common protocol for counselling.

### Sydenham's chorea (St Vitus' dance)
Thomas Sydenham described this transient chorea of adolescence and childhood in 1686. Fewer than half of the cases follow within 3 months of rheumatic fever (see p. 591). It may recur, or appear, in adult life during pregnancy (chorea gravidarum) or in those taking oral contraceptives. In each case there is a diffuse mild encephalitis.

The onset of the chorea is usually gradual. Irritability, insolence and inattentiveness herald the onset of fidgety movements, which are sometimes predominantly unilateral. A minority of patients are confused. Although rheumatic heart disease is sometimes found, the child usually does not have a fever or other features of rheumatic fever. The antistreptolysin-O (ASO) titre and erythrocyte sedimentation rate (ESR) are usually normal.

Recovery occurs spontaneously within weeks or months.

## Hemiballismus

Hemiballismus (also called hemiballism) describes violent swinging movements of one side of the body caused usually by infarction or haemorrhage in the contralateral subthalamic nucleus.

## Myoclonus

Myoclonus is the sudden, involuntary jerking of a single muscle or a group of muscles. It occurs in a wide range of disorders and is sometimes provoked by a sudden stimulus such as a loud noise.

### Benign essential myoclonus
Nocturnal myoclonus, i.e. sudden jerking of a limb or the body on falling asleep, is extremely common and not pathological.

'Paramyoclonus multiplex' is widespread, random muscle jerking usually occurring in adolescence. Fits do not occur.

### Myoclonic epilepsy
Muscle jerking is a feature of many different forms of epilepsy.

### Progressive myoclonic epilepsy
These very rare conditions include various familial and metabolic disorders where myoclonus accompanies a progressive encephalopathy.

An example is Lafora body disease, a syndrome of myoclonus, epilepsy and dementia, with mucopolysaccharide inclusion bodies in neurones, liver cells and intestinal mucosa.

### Static myoclonic encephalopathy
Myoclonus may follow a severe brain insult such as severe cerebral anoxia following cardiac arrest.

## Tics

Repetitive twitching movements of the face, neck or hand are part of our normal motor gestures. Patients or their relatives seek advice about them when they become too frequent or irritating. Simple transient tics, e.g. sniffing or a particular facial grimace, are common in childhood, but may persist into adult life.

The rare Gilles de la Tourette syndrome is the occurrence of multiple tics accompanied by sudden explosive barking and grunting with the utterance of sexually related obscenities. The condition develops in childhood or adolescence, in either sex, and is usually lifelong. This is thought to be due to an organic disorder of the basal ganglia. Treatment with haloperidol is sometimes helpful.

## Torsion dystonias

Dystonia implies a movement caused by a prolonged muscular contraction when a part of the body is thrown into spasm. A classification of these unusual conditions is given in Table 18.39.

### Dystonia musculorum deformans
This rare disease is frequently inherited (there are various modes of transmission) and commences in childhood as dystonic spasms of the limbs that affect gait and posture. It is gradually progressive, spreading to all parts of the body over one or two decades. Intellect is not impaired. Spontaneous remissions occasionally occur.

### Spasmodic torticollis
Dystonic spasms gradually develop around the neck, usually in the third to fifth decade. They cause the head to turn (torticollis) or to be drawn backwards (retrocollis) or forwards (antecollis).

Minor dystonic movements can also affect the trunk or limbs. A curious feature is that some patients have a 'trigger area', often on the jaw. Gentle pressure at this site relieves the involuntary movement.

Various psychiatric explanations have been advanced for this and other movement disorders, but it is now felt that they are organic conditions. Torticollis may remit but many cases remain for life.

### Writer's cramp
This is a specific inability to perform a previously highly developed skilled movement, especially writing, due to a curious dystonic posturing. It occurs particularly in those who spend many hours each day writing, and is thus seen less frequently now than in former years. Other skilled functions of the hand are normal and there are no other neurological signs. Prolonged rest sometimes seems to help the condition but it may become a major disability.

### Blepharospasm and oromandibular dystonia
These related conditions consist of spasms of forced blinking or involuntary movement of the mouth and tongue, e.g. lip-smacking and protrusion of the tongue and jaw. Speech may be affected.

### TREATMENT
All dystonic movement disorders are particularly difficult to treat. Butyrophenones (e.g. haloperidol and sulpiride) are sometimes helpful. Blepharospasm and spasmodic torticollis can be helped by minute subcutaneous injections of botulinum toxin.

---

*Generalized dystonia*
Dystonia musculorum deformans
Drug-induced dystonia (e.g. metoclopramide)
Symptomatic dystonia (e.g. after encephalitis lethargica
    or in Wilson's disease)
Paroxysmal dystonia (very rare, familial, with marked
    fluctuation)

*Focal dystonia*
Spasmodic torticollis
Writer's cramp
Oromandibular dystonia
Blepharospasm
Hemiplegic dystonia (e.g. following stroke)

**Table 18.39**  A classification of dystonias.

# Multiple sclerosis

MS is a common disease of unknown cause in which there are multiple areas of demyelination within the brain and spinal cord. These are 'disseminated in time and place' (hence the old name 'disseminated sclerosis'). An acquired defect in the oligodendroglial cells that produce myelin is responsible.

The commonest age of onset is between 20 and 35 years, the disease being commoner in women. In the UK MS causes disability of varying degree in over 50 000 people.

## PREVALENCE

The disease occurs worldwide, but the prevalence varies widely, being directly proportional to the distance from the equator. At 50–65° N (roughly Land's End to Iceland) the prevalence is 60–100 per 100 000 people; at latitudes less than 30° N the prevalence is less than 10 per 100 000; and at the equator it is a rarity. In the Southern Hemisphere the variation is similar, with progressive increase in prevalence away from the equator.

## AETIOLOGY

The cause of the disease is unknown.

### Familial incidence and HLA linkage

First-degree relatives of a patient have an increased chance of developing MS, although there is no clear-cut pattern of inheritance. There is an increased concordance amongst monozygotic twins.

In Caucasians in northern Europe and the USA, there is a positive association between MS and antigens HLA-A3, B7 and DR2.

### Infection

Although efforts to transmit MS experimentally have been uniformly unsuccessful, there is an abnormal immune response in MS patients, with an increase in the titres of serum and CSF antibodies to many common viruses, particularly measles.

Certain epidemic transmissible zoonoses, such as scrapie, a demyelinating disease in sheep, are pathologically similar to MS. Human T-cell leukaemia virus 1 (HTLV-1) infection in humans (tropical spastic paraparesis) is an example of a viral demyelinating disease.

### Diet

It has been suggested that MS is related to the consumption of large quantities of animal fats. Surveys in Norway have shown that MS is distinctly uncommon in coastal fishing communities compared with agricultural areas. However, the role of diet is particularly difficult to evaluate.

## PATHOLOGY

The essential features are plaques of demyelination, initially 2–10 mm in size (Fig. 18.19). These lesions are perivenular and have a predilection for the following sites within the brain and spinal cord:
- Optic nerves
- Brain stem and its cerebellar connections
- Cervical cord
- Periventricular region

Plaques rarely destroy large groups of neighbouring anterior horn cells (so that muscle wasting is unusual) and never occur in the myelin sheaths of peripheral nerves. Remyelination seldom occurs and the mechanism of the remission of symptoms is unclear.

## CLINICAL FEATURES

No single group of signs or symptoms is diagnostic of MS. Despite this, the disease is often recognizable on

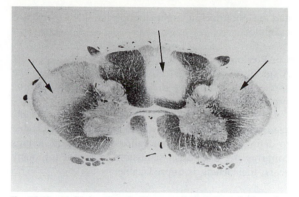

Fig. 18.19   Multiple sclerosis. Cross-section of the spinal cord showing demyelination (arrows) in the posterior column and lateral corticospinal tracts. (Courtesy of Professor W.I. Macdonald).

clinical grounds. There are two patterns:
1. Relapsing and remitting MS with lesions occurring in different parts of the CNS at different times
2. Chronic progressive MS (approximately 20%)

Common presentations of MS are described below.

### Optic neuropathy (ON)

SYMPTOMS. The patient complains of blurring of vision in one eye. Mild ocular pain is usual. The symptoms progress, usually over days, to produce severe visual loss. Recovery occurs, typically within a month. Bilateral ON occasionally occurs.

SIGNS. The signs of ON depend upon the site of the plaque. When the lesion is in the optic nerve head there is disc swelling (optic neuritis). If the lesion is several millimetres proximal to the disc there are often no ophthalmoscopic features ('the doctor sees nothing and the patient sees nothing'); this is known as retrobulbar neuritis.

Optic neuritis is easily distinguished from papilloedema of other causes by the presence of early visual loss.

A relative afferent pupillary defect is often present in the early stages. This persists after recovery.

SEQUELAE. There are usually no residual symptoms, but small scotomata and defects in colour vision can be demonstrated. Following the attack, disc pallor appears (optic atrophy), first in the temporal region and then spreading to affect the whole disc. The visual evoked responses (VER) remain abnormal (see below).

### Brain stem demyelination

An acute episode affecting the brain stem causes diplopia, vertigo, facial numbness or dysphagia. 'Pyramidal' signs in the limbs occur when the corticospinal tracts are involved.

A typical picture is sudden diplopia and vertigo with nystagmus, but without tinnitus or deafness. This lasts for some weeks before recovery. Diplopia in MS may be caused by many different lesions—a sixth nerve lesion and an internuclear ophthalmoplegia (INO) are two examples.

### Cord lesion

A spastic paraparesis is caused by demyelination in the cord. There is difficulty in walking and sensory disturbance. Urinary symptoms are common.

In the initial episode it may be impossible to decide, even with specialized tests, whether or not a lesion is due to demyelination. The appearance of subsequent lesions confirms the diagnosis. Remissions may last for many years; their length is unpredictable.

### Unusual presentations

Epilepsy occurs more commonly in MS patients than in the general population. So, too, does trigeminal neuralgia (see p. 887). Tonic spasms or brief spasms of a limb are other unusual symptoms of this disease.

### End-stage multiple sclerosis

In the later stages of the disease the patient is severely disabled with a combination of spastic tetraparesis, ataxia, optic atrophy, nystagmus, brain stem signs, pseudobulbar palsy and incontinence of urine. Dementia is common. Death follows from uraemia and/or bronchopneumonia.

### DIFFERENTIAL DIAGNOSIS

Few other neurological diseases of young people follow a similar relapsing and remitting course. Thromboembolism causes symptoms that are characteristically more sudden in onset. Other degenerative conditions, such as Friedreich's ataxia, are gradually progressive, without remissions.

Initially individual plaques (e.g. in the optic nerve, brain stem or cord) may cause diagnostic difficulty; they must be distinguished from compressive, inflammatory, mass or vascular lesions.

CNS sarcoidosis, SLE and Behçet's syndrome may mimic the relapsing pattern of MS.

### INVESTIGATION

MRI of the brain is now the first-line investigation. Multiple plaques are visible, principally in the periventricular region and brain stem (see Fig. 18.2). The lesions are rarely visible on CT scan. Examination of the peripheral blood and urine is unhelpful and there are no features on plain X-rays.

Table 18.40 summarizes the changes seen in the CSF. The appearance and pressure of the fluid and the level of glucose are normal, and serological tests for syphilis are negative. The presence of oligoclonal bands of IgG indicate the production of immunoglobulin (to unknown antigens) within the CNS. This investigation is now being superseded by MRI.

### Electrophysiological tests

Delay in the visual-evoked response (VER) follows optic neuropathy. As some attacks are subclinical, a delayed VER may provide evidence of a second lesion within the CNS in, for example, an undiagnosed cord lesion.

Brain stem and somatosensory evoked potentials are also sometimes measured.

Peripheral nerve studies are normal. EEG recordings are unhelpful.

## MANAGEMENT AND PROGNOSIS

Once diagnosed, practical decisions need to be taken about employment, home and plans for the future in the face of a potentially disabling disease for which there is no curative treatment. It is now usual practice to inform patients of the diagnosis.

There is no method of predicting the course of MS but there is wide variation in its severity. Many MS patients live self-sufficient, productive lives while others are gravely disabled.

Wise counsel and honesty, tempered with reassurance of the benign course of many cases of MS, is important.

Many forms of therapy have been suggested for MS, including cryotherapy, pyrotherapy, vaccines, purified protein derivative (PPD), transfer factor, electrical stimulation, gluten-free diets, sunflower seed oil, arsenicals and hyperbaric oxygen. None of these has been shown to benefit patients.

Short courses of ACTH and corticosteroids are used widely in exacerbations and do sometimes appear to reduce temporarily the effect of a relapse. They do not influence the outlook in the long term. Immunosuppressants (azathioprine, cyclophosphamide) are also used, but there is no agreement about their value. Recently $\beta$ interferon has been shown to reduce the attack rate by a third and reduces the number of lesions seen on MRI.

In any chronic neurological disease, treatment of intercurrent infections is important. Urinary infection frequently exacerbates the symptoms.

Muscle relaxants (e.g. baclofen, benzodiazepines and dantrolene) reduce the pain and discomfort of spasticity, particularly when there are flexor spasms of the lower limbs. Prevention of bed sores is vital.

| Constituent | Normal | MS | Comments |
|---|---|---|---|
| Cell count | <5/mm³ | 5–60/mm³ | Rarely up to 100/mm³, typically mononuclear cells |
| Total protein | 0.2–0.4 g litre⁻¹ | 0.4–1.0 g litre⁻¹ | Normal in 40% of cases |
| IgG | <15% of total protein | >15% of total protein | Normal in 60% of cases |
| Oligoclonal IgG | Negative | Positive | Bands present in 80% of cases |

Table 18.40   The CSF in multiple sclerosis (MS).

## Other measures

There is much that should be done for a patient with any chronic neurological disease. Practical advice at work, on walking aids, wheelchairs, car conversions, alterations in houses and gardens can be given. Support in a wide range of areas from fear and reactive depression to the sexual difficulties of the disabled is also helpful. Liaison between family practitioner, physiotherapist, occupational therapist and social worker is important.

# Infective and inflammatory disease

## MENINGITIS

Meningitis (inflammation of the meninges) may be caused by:

- Bacteria
- Viruses
- Fungi
- Other organisms
- Malignant cells
- Drugs and contrast media
- Blood (following SAH)

The term is usually restricted to inflammation due to infective agents (Table 18.41). Microorganisms reach the meninges either by direct extension from the ears, nasopharynx, a cranial injury or congenital meningeal defect, or by spread via the bloodstream.

Immunocompromised patients (AIDS patients and those receiving cytotoxic drugs) are at an increased risk of meningitis, which may be caused by unusual organisms.

## PATHOLOGY

In acute bacterial meningitis the pia-arachnoid is congested with polymorphs. A layer of pus forms that may organize to form adhesions, causing cranial nerve palsies and hydrocephalus. In tuberculous infection the brain is covered in a viscous grey-green exudate; numerous tubercles are found on the meninges. Cerebral oedema is common in bacterial meningitis.

In viral meningitis there is a predominantly lymphocytic inflammatory reaction in the CSF without the formation of pus or adhesions. There is no cerebral oedema unless viral encephalitis develops.

## CLINICAL FEATURES (Table 18.42)

### Meningitic syndrome

There is intense malaise, fever, rigors, severe headache, photophobia and vomiting. The patient is irritable and often prefers to lie still.

Neck stiffness and a positive Kernig's sign appear within a few hours. In milder cases (and many viral meningitides) there are few other signs, but it is most unreliable to rely on the clinical impression alone when assessing the severity of the infection.

In uncomplicated meningitis, consciousness is not impaired, although the patient may be delirious with a high fever. Papilloedema may occur. The appearance of drowsiness, lateralizing signs and cranial nerve lesions indicate a complication such as a venous sinus thrombosis (see p. 912), severe cerebral oedema or hydrocephalus, or an alternative diagnosis such as a cerebral abscess (see p. 930) or encephalitis (see p. 927).

---

**Bacteria**
Neisseria meningitidis[a]
Haemophilus influenzae[a]
Streptococcus pneumoniae[a]
Staphylococcus aureus
Listeria monocytogenes
Gram-negative bacilli
Mycobacterium tuberculosis
Treponema pallidum

**Viruses**
Enteroviruses
    Echo
    Coxsackie
    Polio
Mumps
Herpes simplex
HIV
Epstein–Barr virus

**Fungi**
Cryptococcus neoformans
Candida
(Coccidioides immitis, Histoplasma capsulatum, Blastomyces dermatitidis in USA)

---

[a]These organisms account for 70% of acute bacterial meningitis outside the neonatal period. A wide variety of infective agents are responsible for the remaining 30% of cases.

**Table 18.41**  Infective causes of meningitis in the UK.

| Clinical feature | Probable cause |
|---|---|
| Petechial rash | Meningococcal infection |
| Skull fracture<br>Ear disease<br>Congenital CNS lesion | Pneumococcal infection |
| Previous antibiotics | Partially treated bacterial infection |
| Immunocompromised patients | HIV infection<br>Unusual organisms |
| Rash or pleurodynia | Enterovirus infection |
| International travel | Poliomyelitis<br>Malaria |
| Occupational history (working with drains, canals, polluted river water), recreational swimming: prostration, myalgia, conjunctivitis and jaundice | Leptospirosis |

**Table 18.42**  Clinical clues in meningitis.

## Specific varieties of meningitis

Particular attention should be paid to rashes and associated clinical features (see Table 18.42), and a search should be made for infected foci.

ACUTE BACTERIAL MENINGITIS. The onset is sudden, with rigors and a high fever. A petechial rash, often sparse, is strong evidence of meningococcal meningitis. Septicaemia may present with acute septicaemic shock.

VIRAL MENINGITIS. This is almost always a benign, self-limiting condition lasting 4–10 days. Headache may follow for some weeks but there are no serious sequelae.

TUBERCULOUS MENINGITIS. Tuberculosis causes a chronic meningitis commencing with vague headache, lassitude, anorexia and vomiting. Meningitic signs may appear only after some weeks. Drowsiness, focal signs and seizures may occur. A similar picture occurs in cryptococcal meningitis, the commonest fungal meningitis in Europe.

MALIGNANT MENINGITIS. Malignant cells sometimes cause a subacute or chronic meningitic process. Meningitis, cranial nerve palsies, paraparesis and root lesions are seen, often in complex patterns. The CSF shows increased cells and protein and often a low glucose. Treatment is with intrathecal cytotoxic agents. The prognosis is poor.

## DIFFERENTIAL DIAGNOSIS

Acute meningitis may resemble SAH, severe migraine and other causes of a sudden severe headache. Meningitis should be considered in all patients who have headache and fever.

## MANAGEMENT

Meningitis is an emergency that has a high mortality even in countries with highly developed systems of health care. Although viral meningitis is a self-limiting condition, untreated bacterial meningitis is lethal; in most series the death rate is around 15% even with treatment.

If meningococcal (or other acute bacterial) meningitis is diagnosed clinically, particularly in children, immediate treatment with intravenous benzylpenicillin should be started with subsequent urgent investigations. In this acute illness, minutes count.

If there is no suggestion of an intracranial mass lesion (when CT scanning should be performed), immediate lumbar puncture should be carried out. Typical changes in the CSF are shown in Table 18.43. CSF pressure is characteristically elevated. Blood should be taken for culture and glucose levels as well as for routine tests. Chest and skull films should be taken if possible.

Gram-staining of the CSF may demonstrate organisms (e.g. Gram-positive intracellular diplococci—pneumococcus; Gram-negative cocci—meningococcus). Ziehl–Nielsen stain demonstrates acid-fast bacilli (tuberculosis), though these organisms are rarely numerous. Indian ink stains fungi.

Many serological tests are now available for CSF. Syphilitic serology should always be carried out.

The clinical picture and CSF examination should allow at least a presumptive diagnosis of the cause of the meningitis to be made within several hours of presentation. Patients with impaired consciousness should be nursed as described on p. 903. General management includes diazepam for convulsions and analgesics for headache.

## Treatment of bacterial meningitis

It is often possible to distinguish between viral, pyogenic, tuberculous and other organisms from the clinical setting and immediate examination of the CSF. If bacterial meningitis is suspected, high doses of antibiotics are started immediately. There should be close liaison with a microbiologist. In children, dexamethasone should also be given as this reduces the frequency of complications particularly deafness.

In a pyogenic meningitis in an adult (where the organism is unknown), intravenous benzylpenicillin 2 g 2-hourly and intravenous chloramphenicol 75 mg kg$^{-1}$ have been given. Because of resistant organisms it is now recommended that immediate i.v. cefotaxime is used instead. If the diagnosis of pneumococcal or meningococcal infection has been made, penicillin alone or cefotaxime are used. Chloramphenicol alone or third-generation cephalosporins should be used in *Haemophilus* infections.

Tuberculous meningitis is treated for at least 9 months with antituberculous drugs; rifampicin, isoniazid and pyrazinamide is the usual combination (see p. 686).

It is no longer necessary to use intrathecal antibiotics.

Local infection (e.g. an infected paranasal sinus) should also be treated, surgically if necessary. Surgical repair of

|  | Normal | Viral | Pyogenic | Tuberculosis |
|---|---|---|---|---|
| Appearance | Crystal clear | Clear/turbid | Turbid/purulent | Turbid/viscous |
| Mononuclear cells | <5/mm³ | 10–100/mm³ | <50/mm³ | 100–300/mm³ |
| Polymorph cells | Nil | Nil$^a$ | 200–3000/mm³ | 0–200/mm³ |
| Protein | 0.2–0.4 g litre$^{-1}$ | 0.4–0.8 g litre$^{-1}$ | 0.5–2.0 g litre$^{-1}$ | 0.5–3.0 g litre$^{-1}$ |
| Glucose | >½ blood glucose | >½ blood glucose | <½ blood glucose | <⅓ blood glucose |

$^a$Some polymorph cells may be seen in the early stages of viral meningitis.

**Table 18.43** Typical changes in the CSF in meningitis.

depressed skull fracture or meningeal tear may be necessary.

Polyvalent vaccines are available against recurrent pneumococcal meningitis (e.g. when there is a CSF leak following skull fracture) and against some strains of meningococci (see p. 23). In meningococcal outbreaks rifampicin prophylaxis should be given to contacts and family members as well as to the patient.

## Differential diagnosis of CSF pleocytosis

Difficulties occur in meningitis when a raised, often mixed (lymphocyte and polymorph, i.e. pleocytic) picture is found but no infecting organism. This is sometimes called 'aseptic meningitis'. The conditions listed in Table 18.44 should be considered.

## ENCEPHALITIS

Encephalitis is inflammation of brain parenchyma. It is caused by a wide variety of viruses and may also occur in bacterial and other infections.

## Acute viral encephalitis

In many cases a viral aetiology is presumed but not confirmed serologically or by culture. The usual organisms cultured from cases of viral encephalitis in adults in the UK are Echo, Coxsackie, mumps and herpes simplex viruses.

Adenovirus, varicella zoster, influenza, measles and other viruses are rarer causes.

### CLINICAL FEATURES
Many of these infections cause a mild self-limiting illness with headache and drowsiness. In a minority there is a more serious illness accompanied by focal signs, seizures and coma. Herpes simplex virus (HSV-1) accounts for many of these severe infections in Britain and has a mortality of around 20% even with treatment. In the Far East the Japanese B arbovirus is a more usual, and epidemic, cause of severe encephalitis, with a high mortality.

Partially treated bacterial meningitis
Viral meningitis
Tuberculosis or fungi
Neoplastic meningitis
Parameningeal foci (e.g. paranasal sinus)
Syphilis
Intracranial abscess
Cerebral venous or arterial infection
Following subarachnoid haemorrhage
Encephalitis, including AIDS
Rare causes (e.g. cerebral malaria, sarcoidosis, Behçet's
    syndrome, Lyme disease)

**Table 18.44**  Causes of CSF pleocytosis.

### DIFFERENTIAL DIAGNOSIS
This includes:
- Bacterial meningitis complicated by cerebral oedema and/or cerebral venous thrombosis
- Cerebral abscess
- Acute disseminated encephalomyelitis
- Toxic confusional states in febrile illnesses and in septicaemia

### INVESTIGATION
Investigation in severe cases includes CT scanning (which characteristically shows areas of oedema), EEG (which shows slow-wave changes and/or 'periodic complexes') and viral serology of blood and CSF.

Brain biopsy is now seldom performed in the UK.

### TREATMENT
Suspected herpes simplex encephalitis is immediately treated with intravenous acyclovir, the active form of which inhibits DNA synthesis. Phosphorylation of this drug is dependent upon the presence of viral thymidine kinase; thus the drug is specific for herpesvirus infections. If the patient is in coma the outlook is poor whether or not drugs are given.

Supportive measures are required for comatose patients. Seizures are treated with anticonvulsants.

Prophylactic immunization is possible against Japanese B encephalitis and sometimes advised particularly for travellers to the Far East in endemic areas.

## Acute disseminated encephalomyelitis (ADE)

This follows many common viral infections (e.g. measles, varicella zoster, mumps and rubella) and rarely after immunization against rabies, influenza or pertussis. The clinical syndrome is often similar to acute viral encephalitis, with added focal brain stem and/or spinal cord lesions due to demyelination, but in which viral particles are not usually present. The prognosis is variable. Mild cases recover completely but in severe cases (those in coma) mortality is around 25% and the survivors often have permanent brain damage. Treatment is supportive, with steroids and anticonvulsants.

## MYELITIS

Myelitis means inflammation of the spinal cord causing paraparesis or tetraparesis. It occurs with varicella zoster or as part of a postinfective encephalomyelitis. Poliomyelitis is a specific enterovirus infection of anterior horn cells (see p. 50).

Transverse myelitis is described on p. 939).

## HERPES ZOSTER (SHINGLES)

This is a recrudescence of infection with varicella zoster virus within the dorsal root ganglia, the original infection having been acquired in an attack of chickenpox many years previously. The viruses causing chickenpox and shingles are identical.

### CLINICAL FEATURES

The skin changes are described on p. 1015.

In the cranial nerves, herpes zoster has a predilection for the fifth and seventh nerve. 'Ophthalmic herpes' is infection of the first division of the fifth nerve and may lead to corneal scarring and secondary panophthalmitis. 'Geniculate herpes' (the Ramsay Hunt syndrome, see p. 889) leads to facial palsy accompanied by vesicles on the pinna, external auditory meatus and fauces.

The local complications of shingles are secondary bacterial infection, very rarely purpura and necrosis in the affected segment ('purpura fulminans'), generalized herpes zoster, and postherpetic neuralgia.

A myelitis, meningo-encephalitis or motor radiculopathy may be caused by varicella zoster.

Treatment with acyclovir is given (see p. 1015).

#### Postherpetic neuralgia

Postherpetic neuralgia is pain in the zone of the previous eruption; it occurs in some 10% of patients (often elderly). It is a burning, continuous pain responding poorly to all analgesics. Depression is almost universal. Treatment is unsatisfactory but there is a trend towards gradual recovery over 2 years.

## NEUROSYPHILIS

Syphilis is described on p. 91.

Tertiary neurological disease is now rare but a wide variety of syndromes still occur, particularly in those who may have had many sexual partners.

For practical purposes, negative serological tests for syphilis in blood exclude the disease.

The main syphilitic syndromes are described below.

#### Asymptomatic neurosyphilis

This is the term used to describe positive CSF serology without signs.

#### Meningovascular syphilis

This presents as:

SUBACUTE MENINGITIS often with cranial nerve palsies and papilloedema

A FOCAL FORM (a gumma), is an expanding intracranial mass which causes epilepsy, raised pressure and focal deficits, e.g. hemiplegia

PARAPARESIS caused by a spinal meningovasculitis

#### Tabes dorsalis

This is a complex syndrome in which demyelination occurs in the dorsal roots. Many of the features are due to 'de-afferentation'. The elements of the syndrome are:

- Lightning pains (see p. 898)
- Ataxia, loss of reflexes, widespread sensory loss and some muscle wasting
- Neuropathic joints (Charcot's joints)
- Argyll Robertson pupils
- Ptosis and optic atrophy

#### General paralysis of the insane (GPI)

The grandiose title indicates that this is a syndrome of madness and weakness. The dementia is often similar to that associated with Alzheimer's disease (see p. 965). Progressive dementia, brisk reflexes, extensor plantar reflexes and tremor occur. Death follows within 3 years of the onset.

Argyll Robertson pupils are usually present. Seizures may occur.

#### Other forms

Mixtures of the syndromes described above occur.

In congenital neurosyphilis (acquired *in utero*), there are features of both tabes dorsalis and GPI in childhood; this is known as taboparesis.

In secondary syphilis, a self-limiting meningeal reaction occurs that may be symptomless or may cause a subacute meningitis.

### TREATMENT

Benzylpenicillin 1 g daily by injection for 10 days in primary infection eliminates the risk of future tertiary syphilis. Established neurological disease can be arrested but not usually reversed with penicillin. Parenteral penicillin for 2–3 weeks is given for all forms of neurosyphilis. Allergic reactions (Jarisch–Herxheimer reactions) may occur; high-dose steroid cover is usually given with penicillin to reduce their severity.

## AIDS AND THE NERVOUS SYSTEM

Individuals with HIV infection frequently present with or develop neurological disease. In addition, HIV-infected patients have a high rate of cerebrovascular disease. There is a variety of clinical neurological pictures, which may be confusing.

#### Meningitis

ACUTE ASEPTIC MENINGITIS. This is believed to be a primary HIV meningitis. Spontaneous recovery is usual.

CHRONIC MENINGITIS. This may occur with HIV itself, fungi (e.g. *Cryptococcus neoformans* or *Aspergillus*), tuberculosis, *Listeria monocytogenes*, *Escherichia coli* or other organisms. Treatment is typically difficult and unsuccessful.

#### Diffuse encephalopathies

AIDS–DEMENTIA COMPLEX. This is a diffuse, progressive, usually fatal HIV-related dementia, sometimes associated with a cerebellar syndrome, thought to be due to a primary cerebral HIV infection.

ENCEPHALITIS. Cytomegalovirus, herpes simplex, *Toxoplasma* and other organisms cause a severe and often fatal encephalitis.

CNS LYMPHOMA AND PROGRESSIVE MULTIFOCAL LEUCOENCEPHALOPATHY (see p. 930). These are progressive late complications of HIV infection. They are usually fatal.

**Paraparesis**
This occurs in AIDS in the following patterns.

ACUTE HIV TRANSVERSE MYELITIS. This is believed to be a primary HIV myelitis. Spontaneous recovery is usual.

MYELOPATHY DUE TO INFECTION, e.g. with herpes simplex or zoster, cytomegalovirus.

CNS LYMPHOMA. Lymphomatous masses cause cord compression or malignant meningitis.

**AIDS-related neuropathy**
Three patterns occur:
1 Mononeuropathy, e.g. a common peroneal nerve lesion
2 Mononeuritis multiplex (see p. 945)
3 Polyneuropathy (see p. 945)

**MANAGEMENT OF AIDS** (see p. 104)

# OTHER INFECTIONS

The nervous system is involved in many infective diseases.

**Rabies** (see p. 57)
Rabies is transmitted to humans from infected animals via penetrating wounds. The rabies virus multiplies in the wound and migrates via the peripheral nerves and dorsal root ganglia to the CNS. A fatal encephalitis follows in which, at autopsy, characteristic neuronal inclusion bodies (Negri bodies) are observed.

**Tetanus** (see p. 24)
Tetanus may follow even a trivial wound. There is liberation of a powerful toxin that travels within motor nerves to reach the CNS, where it binds irreversibly with certain sialic acid-containing gangliosides. The toxin blocks inhibition of spinal reflexes, resulting in spasms.

**Botulism** (see p. 25)
The paralytic symptoms of botulism are caused by a presynaptic block in neuromuscular transmission.

**Lyme disease** (see p. 43)
This produces a chronic radiculopathy. A paraparesis can occur.

**Leprosy** (see p. 37)
In tuberculoid leprosy a mononeuritis multiplex is seen. The infected nerves become large and palpable as hard cords. The peripheral nerves are also affected in lepromatous leprosy.

**Poliomyelitis** (see p. 50)
In this condition there is invasion of the anterior horn cells by the pathogenic virus. Many infections are subclinical but in a minority there is serious paralytic disease involving the respiratory muscles and sometimes causing a bulbar palsy.

Other examples of infection involving the CNS are summarized in Table 18.45. See also individual viral infections in Chapter 1.

# MISCELLANEOUS CONDITIONS

**Progressive rubella encephalitis**
Some 10 years after the primary infection there is rarely a progressive syndrome of mental impairment, fits, optic

| Organism | Disease | CNS manifestation |
|---|---|---|
| *Rickettsia* | Typhus<br>Scrub typhus<br>Rocky mountain spotted fever | Meningo-encephalitis |
| *Plasmodium falciparum* | Malaria | Meningo-encephalitis |
| *Toxoplasma gondii* | Toxoplasmosis | Meningo-encephalitis (e.g. in AIDS) |
| *Naegleria fowleri* (a freshwater amoeba) | | Meningo-encephalitis |
| *Entamoeba histolytica* | Amoebiasis | Brain abscess |
| *Trypanosoma rhodesiense*<br>*Trypanosoma gambiense* | Trypanosomiasis | Subacute encephalitis |
| *Echinococcus granulosus* | Hydatid disease | Intracranial cysts |
| *Taenia solium* | Cysticercosis | Multiple intracranial cysts |
| *Schistosoma mansoni* | Schistosomiasis | Encephalopathy<br>Cord lesions |
| *Strongyloides stercoralis* | Strongyloidiasis | Meningo-encephalitis |

**Table 18.45** Miscellaneous CNS infections.

atrophy, cerebellar and pyramidal signs. There is evidence of local antibody production against rubella viral antigen within the CNS.

### Subacute sclerosing panencephalitis (SSPE)

The persistence of measles antigen in the CNS is believed to be the cause of this rare late sequel to measles infection. Progressive mental deterioration, fits, myoclonus and pyramidal signs occur, usually in a child. Diagnosis is confirmed by demonstrating a high titre of measles antibody in the blood and CSF.

### Creutzfeld–Jakob disease (CJD)

This is a slowly progressive dementia characterized pathologically by 'spongiform encephalopathy'. It occurs worldwide and is transmitted by an agent resistant to many of the usual sterilization processes. This is an example of a 'prion' (proteinaceous infectious particles) or 'slow' virus disease. Infection has been transmitted from post-mortem and surgical specimens and corneal grafts, and to the recipients of human growth hormone (which was obtained from human pituitary glands removed at autopsy). The pathology of CJD is very similar to bovine spongiform encephalopathy of cattle.

The condition has a long incubation period, sometimes up to several years. Death is almost invariable within 2 years from the onset of symptoms.

### Kuru

This is a dementia and cerebellar ataxia occurring in the highlands of New Guinea. It is believed to have been spread by ritual cannibalism. Spongiform change occurs in the brain (very similar to that in CJD). This obscure condition is also believed to be transmitted by a slow virus.

### Progressive multifocal leucoencephalopathy

This is an opportunistic infection with the papovaviruses JC and SV-40 (and others) in patients who are immunocompromised. Multifocal demyelinating hemisphere lesions develop that contain virus particles. Death is usual after several years.

### Reye's syndrome (see also p. 277)

This is a severe encephalitic illness, usually of children, accompanied by fatty infiltration of the liver and hypoglycaemia. A viral cause has been postulated but other factors, including aspirin therapy, have also been implicated.

### Mollaret's meningitis

This term is used to describe recurrent episodes of 'aseptic meningitis' over many years. A viral cause is postulated. Some of these patients are helped by treatment with the mitotic poison colchicine.

### Vogt–Koyanagi–Harada syndrome

This is a recurrent inflammatory disease of cells of neural crest origin, causing uveitis, meningo-encephalitis, vitiligo, deafness and alopecia.

### ME: myalgic encephalomyelitis (epidemic neuromyasthenia) (see p. 963)

Headache, fever, lassitude, torpor, myalgia and depression sometimes follow viral infection (e.g. hepatitis, infectious mononucleosis, Coxsackie infections). It is particularly difficult to distinguish between organic and psychological elements in these cases and there is wide variation of opinion about causation.

### Sarcoidosis (see p. 687)

This condition may cause a chronic meningo-encephalitis with sarcoid lesions within the brain and spinal cord, a peripheral neuropathy, cranial nerve palsies (particularly bilateral seventh nerve palsies) or, rarely, a myopathy.

### Behçet's syndrome (see p. 413)

The three principal features are recurrent oral and genital ulceration, inflammatory ocular disease and neurological syndromes. Brain stem and cord lesions, aseptic meningitis, encephalitis and cerebral venous thrombosis also occur.

## ABSCESSES WITHIN THE NERVOUS SYSTEM

### Brain abscess (Fig. 18.20c)

A focal area of infection within the cerebrum or cerebellum presents as an expanding mass lesion (see p. 932). The usual organisms are streptococci (aerobic, anaerobic and microaerophilic species), *Bacteroides* spp., staphylococci and enterobacteria. Mixed infections are common. Fungi can also cause brain abscesses. Multiple abscesses may develop. A parameningeal (e.g. ear, nose, paranasal sinus, skull fracture) or distant (e.g. lung, heart, abdomen) focus of infection may be present. Frequently no cause is found.

### Tuberculoma

Tubercle bacilli cause chronic caseating intracranial granulomas—tuberculomas—which are the commonest single intracranial masses in areas such as India where tuberculosis is common. Tuberculomas either present as mass lesions or occur in the course of tuberculous meningitis. They may also be symptomless and appear on skull X-rays as areas of intracranial calcification.

#### CLINICAL FEATURES

Headache, focal signs (e.g. hemiparesis, aphasia, hemianopia), epilepsy and raised intracranial pressure occur. Fever, leucocytosis and a raised ESR are usual in cerebral abscess but are not always present. The presentation may thus be remarkably similar to many cerebral neoplasms. The symptoms may be indolent, developing over weeks, particularly in the cerebral hemispheres. Cerebellar abscesses tend to develop more acutely.

#### MANAGEMENT

Urgent CT or MRI scanning is essential. The search for a focus of infection should include a detailed examination

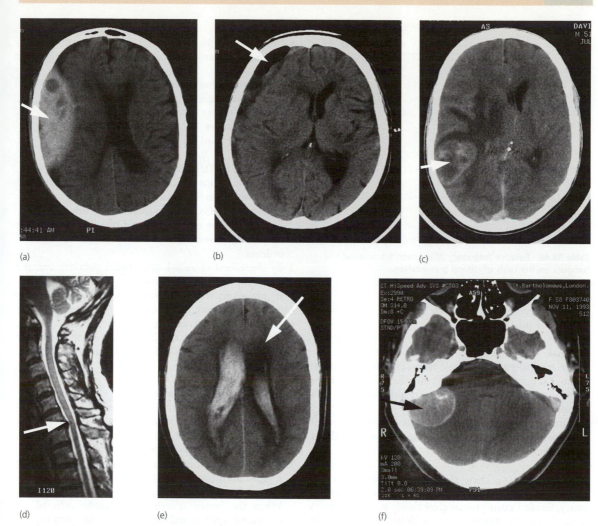

(a)                          (b)                          (c)

(d)                          (e)                          (f)

**Fig. 18.20** Appearances of various conditions in CT or MRI modality. (a) Extradural haemorrhage (CT). (b) Subdural haematoma (CT). (c) Parietal (cube) abscess (CT). (d) Cervical spinal cord showing minor disc protrusion (MRI). (e) Intraventricular haemorrhage (CT). (f) Cerebello-pontine angle meningioma (CT).

of the skull, ears and paranasal sinuses.

Lumbar puncture is contraindicated in suspected brain abscess prior to scanning.

Treatment should be carried out with liaison between neurosurgeon and microbiologist. Surgical decompression may be necessary if antibiotics are unsuccessful. Despite treatment, the mortality of abscess remains high, at around 25%, and epilepsy is common in survivors.

## Subdural empyema

This is usually secondary to local infection. The features are similar to those of a cerebral abscess.

## Intracranial epidural abscess

Rarely, a collection of pus tracks along the intracranial epidural space, causing sequential cranial nerve lesions, typically without evidence of raised pressure. There is usually evidence of local infection. Drainage is necessary.

## Spinal epidural abscess

*Staphylococcus aureus* is the usual organism responsible. It reaches the spine via the bloodstream, e.g. from a boil. There is fever and usually back pain followed by paraparesis or root lesions. Emergency myelography, decompression and antibiotics are indicated.

## *Intracranial tumours*

Primary intracranial tumours account for approximately 10% of all neoplasms. The commoner varieties of tumours are outlined in Table 18.46; around one-quarter are metastases (see Fig. 18.20e).

Differences between overall annual incidence rates (see Table 18.1) and presentation as clinical problems (Table 18.46) are accounted for by the fact that small meningi-

| Tumour | Relative frequency (%) |
|---|---|
| *Primary malignant (glioma)* <br> Astrocytoma <br> Oligodendroglioma | 40 |
| *Benign* <br> Meningioma <br> Neurofibroma | 30 |
| *Metastases* <br> Bronchus <br> Breast <br> Stomach <br> Prostate <br> Thyroid <br> Kidney | 25 |

**Table 18.46** Relative frequency of common intracranial tumours on the basis of clinical presentation.

omas and cerebral metastases are commonly found unexpectedly at post mortem.

### Gliomas
These are malignant, intrinsic tumours that originate in neuroglia, usually within the cerebral hemispheres. Their cause is unknown. They are occasionally associated with neurofibromatosis.

Primary intracranial malignant tumours virtually never metastasize outside the CNS and spread only by direct extension.

ASTROCYTOMAS. These gliomas arise from astrocytes. They are classified into grades I-IV, depending on malignancy. Grade I astrocytomas grow slowly over many years while grade IV tumours cause death within several months.

Cystic astrocytomas occur in childhood, usually within the cerebellum. They are relatively benign.

OLIGODENDROGLIOMAS. These arise from oligodendroglia and grow slowly, usually over several decades. Calcification is common.

### Meningiomas (see Fig. 18.20d)
These benign tumours arise from the arachnoid membrane and may grow to a large size, usually over years. When close to the skull they erode bone. They often occur along the intracranial venous sinuses, which they may invade. They are rare below the tentorium.

### Neurofibromas
These arise from Schwann cells and occur principally in the cerebellopontine angle, where they arise from the eighth nerve sheath (see p. 890).

Other less common neoplasms include:
- Cerebellar haemangioblastoma
- Ependymoma of the fourth ventricle
- Colloid cyst of the third ventricle

- Pinealoma
- Chordoma of the skull base
- Glomus tumour—a vascular neoplasm of the jugular bulb
- Medulloblastoma—a cerebellar tumour of childhood
- Craniopharyngioma (see p. 778)

**Pituitary tumours**
These are discussed on p. 776.

## CLINICAL FEATURES
Mass lesions within the cranium produce symptoms and signs in three coexisting ways:
1 By the direct effects of the mass on surrounding structures, which are either destroyed or suffer impairment of function from infiltration, pressure or cerebral oedema
2 By the effects of raised intracranial pressure and the shift of intracranial contents
3 By provoking either generalized or partial seizures
Although neoplasms, either secondary or primary, are the commonest lesions to cause these effects, cerebral abscess, tuberculoma, subdural and intracranial haematoma may also produce symptoms and signs that may be clinically indistinguishable.

### Direct effects of mass lesions
These will depend upon the site of the mass and its speed of growth. The hallmark of a mass lesion is a progressive deterioration of function.

Three examples of possible effects are given below:
1 A left frontal meningioma (see Fig. 18.20d) will cause a vague disturbance of personality, apathy and impairment of intellectual function over several months. When the frontal speech area becomes affected, an expressive aphasia will develop. As the corticospinal pathways become involved, a right hemiparesis will follow.
2 A right parietal glioma involving the fibres of the optic radiation will cause a left homonymous field defect. Cortical sensory loss and a left hemiparesis may follow. Partial seizures causing episodes of numbness of the left limbs may develop.
3 A left eighth nerve sheath neurofibroma (an 'acoustic neuroma') (see Fig. 18.20f) growing in the cerebellopontine angle will cause progressive perceptive deafness (VIII), vertigo (VIII), numbness of the left side of the face (V) and facial weakness (VII), followed by cerebellar ataxia as the cerebellar connections are compressed.
The direct effects are commonly those that first bring the patient to seek medical attention. The rate of progression will vary greatly from a few days or weeks to several years in the case of a slowly enlarging mass. Since cerebral oedema surrounds many mass lesions it is often difficult on clinical grounds to distinguish its effect from that of the mass itself.

### Raised intracranial pressure
The triad of headache, vomiting and papilloedema is an important, though relatively unusual, presentation of a

mass lesion. These symptoms usually imply that obstruction to CSF pathways has occurred. Typically this picture is produced early by masses within the posterior fossa and as a later event with lesions above the tentorium.

Shift of the intracranial contents produces symptoms and signs that coexist with the direct effects of an expanding mass:

DISTORTION OF THE UPPER BRAIN STEM, as midline structures are displaced either caudally or laterally by a hemisphere mass (see Fig. 18.20), leads to impairment of consciousness (drowsiness progressing to stupor and coma).

COMPRESSION OF THE MEDULLA by herniation of the cerebellar tonsils caudally through the foramen magnum (an example of 'coning') causes impairment of consciousness, respiratory depression, bradycardia, decerebrate posturing and death.

FALSE LOCALIZING SIGNS APPEAR ('false' only because they are not related directly to the site of the mass).

Three examples of false localizing signs are:

1 A sixth nerve lesion, first on the side of a mass and later bilaterally, is caused as the nerve is compressed during its long intracranial course.

2 A third nerve lesion develops as the uncus of the temporal lobe herniates caudally, compressing the third nerve against the petroclinoid ligament and stretching it by downward displacement of the posterior communicating artery. The first sign of this is dilatation of the pupil as the parasympathetic fibres in the nerve are compressed.

3 Hemiparesis on the same side (i.e. 'the one you don't expect') as a hemisphere tumour is caused by compression of the brain stem (the contralateral cerebral peduncle) on the free edge of the tentorium.

These false localizing signs are of importance in clinical neurology because their development indicates that a shift of the brain is taking place. Urgent surgical intervention may be necessary.

### Seizures

Partial seizures, simple or complex, which may evolve to generalized tonic–clonic seizures, are characteristic features of many hemisphere masses, whether malignant or benign. The site of origin of a partial seizure is frequently of localizing value (see p. 913). Generalized tonic–clonic seizures with EEG (but not clinical) evidence of a focal onset also occur.

### INVESTIGATION

CT scan is the investigation of choice when the diagnosis of a tumour is suspected.

### CT scan

It is important to emphasize that CT indicates only the site of a mass and not its nature. Cerebral abscess, cerebral infarction, benign and malignant tumours have characteristic, but not entirely diagnostic, appearances. Contrast enhancement adds to the discriminating ability of CT and should be used when a mass is suspected.

### MRI

MRI is often more discriminating than other noninvasive tests, particularly for posterior fossa tumours.

### EEG

The EEG may show electrical abnormalities in the region of a mass (but it may be normal): it is rarely of major value in management. The main exception is with cerebral abscess, where the EEG shows characteristic marked slow wave changes.

### Technetium brain scan

This is sometimes useful to confirm the site of a lesion shown on CT, but the test discriminates poorly and misses many tumours. Very occasionally this test shows a lesion that has been missed by CT.

### Skull films

Plain X-rays of the skull are discussed on p. 874. In pituitary and parasellar lesions they do give important information about changes in the dorsum sellae and clinoid processes. In hemisphere lesions, plain films are frequently abnormal but the test has little value as a screening process.

### 'Routine' tests

Since the proportion of cerebral tumours that prove to be metastases is high, 'routine' tests such as a chest X-ray are of great importance.

### Specialized neuroradiology

Angiography, ventriculography and other contrast studies may sometimes be necessary to define the site or the blood supply of a mass.

### Lumbar puncture

*Lumbar puncture is contraindicated when the differential diagnosis includes any mass lesion.*

Examination of CSF rarely yields diagnostically useful information in this situation, and the procedure may be followed by immediate herniation of the cerebellar tonsils. If there are pressing reasons for the procedure it should be carried out after careful assessment of the consequences and after a CT scan has been performed.

### TREATMENT

Surgical exploration and either biopsy or removal of the mass is usually carried out to ascertain its nature. Some benign tumours can be removed in their entirety.

Radiotherapy is usually recommended for gliomas and for radiosensitive metastases. Chemotherapy is of little value in the majority of primary brain tumours.

Cerebral oedema surrounding a tumour is rapidly reduced by corticosteroids; dexamethasone or betamethasone are used by injection in an emergency. Intravenous mannitol may also be used as an osmotic diuretic.

Epilepsy is treated with anticonvulsants.

With all malignant brain tumours the overall outlook is poor, with less than 50% survival at 1 year. Meningiomas are, however, often removed in their entirety and thus cured.

# Hydrocephalus

Hydrocephalus means that there is an excessive amount of CSF within the cranium. Although this also occurs in cerebral atrophy, in practice the term hydrocephalus is used to describe different syndromes in which there is, or has been, obstruction to CSF outflow with consequent high pressure and dilatation of the cerebral ventricles. Exceptionally an increase in CSF production occurs.

## Infantile hydrocephalus

Enlargement of the head in infancy is diagnosed in about 1 in 2000 live births. There are several causes:

ARNOLD-CHIARI MALFORMATION. There is elongation of the medulla and abnormal cerebellar tissue (the tonsils) in the cervical canal. Associated spina bifida is common. Syringomyelia may develop.

DANDY–WALKER SYNDROME. There is cerebellar hypoplasia and obstruction to the outflow foramina of the fourth ventricle.

STENOSIS OF THE AQUEDUCT OF SYLVIUS (Fig. 18.21). This may be either congenital or acquired following neonatal meningitis or haemorrhage.

## Hydrocephalus in adult life

Infantile hydrocephalus not infrequently becomes symptomatic only in adult life. The features are of headache,

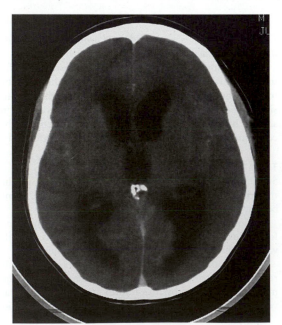

**Fig. 18.21** Hydrocephalus on CT scan. Stenosis of the aqueduct of Sylvius causing gross ventricular dilatation.

vomiting, papilloedema, ataxia and bilateral pyramidal signs.

Hydrocephalus in adults also occurs with:

TUMOURS OF THE POSTERIOR FOSSA AND BRAIN STEM. These obstruct the aqueduct or fourth ventricular outflow.

SUBARACHNOID HAEMORRHAGE, HEAD INJURY OR MENINGITIS (PARTICULARLY TUBERCULOUS). The hydrocephalus is often a transient phenomenon.

TUMOURS OF THE THIRD VENTRICLE. A colloid cyst of the third ventricle causes enlargement of the lateral ventricles, headache and papilloedema.

NORMAL-PRESSURE HYDROCEPHALUS. In this syndrome enlarged cerebral ventricles occur without cortical atrophy. It presents with dementia, urinary incontinence and apraxia, usually in the elderly. The CSF pressure is characteristically normal. It is currently thought that this syndrome is the late result of previous episodes of high pressure, though usually of unknown cause.

PAPILLOMA OF THE CHOROID PLEXUS. This is an extremely rare neoplasm that secretes CSF.

Ventriculo-atrial or ventriculo-peritoneal shunting may be necessary when hydrocephalus is diagnosed.

## Idiopathic (or benign) intracranial hypertension

This syndrome consists of marked papilloedema without other signs in patients who are subsequently shown to have neither a mass lesion nor an increase in ventricular size. It occurs mainly in obese young women with vague menstrual irregularities. Steroid therapy is sometimes thought to be a cause and many other drugs have been occasionally implicated. Other causes of papilloedema should be excluded.

The condition is benign only in that it is not fatal. Infarction of the optic nerve occurs (with consequent blindness) when the papilloedema is severe and long-standing. Surgical decompression or shunting may be necessary. Thiazide diuretics appear to reduce the intra-cranial pressure in this condition. Weight reduction is important.

# Headache, migraine and facial pain

## 'Tension headache'

The vast majority of chronic and recurrent headaches are believed, on no good evidence, to be due to 'tension' within the scalp muscles. What is certain is that they are, in terms of pathology, innocent. 'Tight band' sensations, pressure behind the eyes, and throbbing and bursting sensations are common.

There may be obvious precipitating factors such as worry, noise, concentrated visual effort or fumes. Depression is also a frequent underlying cause. Tension headaches are often attributed to cervical spondylosis, refractive errors or high blood pressure; the evidence for these is poor. Similar headaches also follow head injuries, which may be minor.

There are no abnormal physical signs other than tenderness and tension in the nuchal and scalp muscles.

## MANAGEMENT
This involves:
- Firm reassurance
- Avoiding the causes
- Analgesics
- Physical treatments—massage, relaxation
- Antidepressants—when indicated

Investigation may be needed to confirm the benign nature of the problem.

# Migraine

Migraine means recurrent headaches associated with visual and gastrointestinal disturbance; despite the origin of the word, it does not invariably mean unilateral headache.

## INCIDENCE
About 10% of any population sampled admit to these symptoms.

## MECHANISMS
The cause of migraine is unknown. The headache, often throbbing, is believed to be due to vasodilatation or oedema of blood vessels, with stimulation of nerve endings near affected extracranial and meningeal arteries. The release of vasoactive substances such as nitric oxide are thought to play a role. In addition, the serum level of 5-hydroxytryptamine rises at the onset of the prodromal symptoms and falls during the headache.

Cerebral symptoms and signs (e.g. tingling of limbs, aphasia, weakness) are caused by ischaemia and/or depression of cortical function.

Definite precipitating factors are unusual. Some patients complain of symptoms at times of relaxation (e.g. weekend migraine). Others find that chocolate (high in phenylethylamine) and cheese (high in tyramine) precipitate attacks. Migraine is common around puberty, at the menopause and premenstrually, and sometimes increases in severity or frequency with the contraceptive pill, in pregnancy and with the development of hypertension.

There is no reason to suppose that migraine is associated with any major intracranial lesion. However, since migraine is such a common symptom complex, an intracranial mass lesion and migraine sometimes both occur in the same patient by coincidence.

Rarely, migraine follows head injuries.

## CLINICAL PATTERNS
There are several types of migraine, the attacks varying from intermittent headaches barely distinguishable from tension headaches to discrete episodes that mimic thromboembolic cerebral ischaemia. The distinction between the variants is somewhat artificial.

The attack itself may be divided into:
- Prodromal symptoms
- Headache and associated symptoms

Prior to the attack some patients experience a feeling of well-being.

### Migraine with aura (classical)
Prodromal symptoms are usually visual and are related to ischaemia in the distribution of the intracranial arteries. There are unilateral patchy scotomata (when the retinal vessels are involved), unilateral blindness (involvement of the ophthalmic artery) and sometimes hemianopic field loss (involvement of the posterior cerebral artery). Teichopsia (flashes) and fortification spectra (jagged lines resembling battlements) are common.

Transient aphasia sometimes occurs, together with tingling, numbness or vague weakness of one side. The patient feels nauseated.

The prodrome lasts for 15 min to 1 hour or more. Headache follows. This is occasionally hemicranial ('splitting the head') but often begins locally and becomes generalized. Nausea increases and vomiting follows. The patient is irritable and prefers to be in a darkened room. The superficial temporal artery (either or both) is engorged and pulsating.

After several hours the attack ceases. There is sometimes a diuresis towards the end of an attack. Sleep often follows.

### Migraine without aura (common)
This is the usual variety of migraine. Prodromal visual symptoms are vague. There is recurrent headache accompanied by nausea and malaise. Distinction from tension headache may be impossible.

### Basilar migraine
The prodromal symptoms are due to ischaemia in the posterior cerebral circulation. Circumoral tingling, numbness of the tongue, vertigo, diplopia, transient blindness, syncope, dysarthria and ataxia occur.

### Hemiplegic migraine
This is a rarity in which classical migraine is accompanied by hemiparesis. Recovery occurs within 24 hours. Exceptionally, cerebral infarction follows.

### Ophthalmoplegic migraine
This is a third (or exceptionally a sixth) nerve palsy occurring in a migraine attack. The condition is rare and is difficult to distinguish from other causes of a third nerve palsy (see p. 886) without investigation.

### Facioplegic migraine
This rarity is unilateral facial weakness occurring during a migraine attack.

## DIFFERENTIAL DIAGNOSIS

The sudden onset of headache may be similar to meningitis or SAH.

The hemiplegic, visual and hemisensory symptoms must be distinguished from thromboembolic TIAs (see p. 906). In TIAs the maximum deficit is present immediately and headache is unusual.

Unilateral tingling or numbness should be distinguished from sensory epilepsy (partial seizures). In the latter a distinct 'march' of symptoms is usual.

## MANAGEMENT
### General measures
These include:

REASSURANCE and relief of anxiety.

AVOIDANCE OF PRECIPITATING DIETARY FACTORS (rarely helpful).

PATIENTS ON ORAL CONTRACEPTIVES — a change in brand or stopping of the drug may help. Severe hemiplegic symptoms are an indication for stopping these drugs.

### During the attack
Paracetamol or other simple analgesics should be given, with antiemetics (e.g. metoclopramide) if necessary.

The 5-hydroxytryptamine ($5HT_1$) agonist sumatriptan is of considerable value either by self-administered subcutaneous injection or orally in recurrent severe attacks. It should not be taken until 24 hours after ergotamine. Ergotamine tartrate (1–2 mg orally or rectally, 360 $\mu$g by aerosol or 0.25–0.5 mg by injection) is sometimes, though not often, helpful if given early in attack. Ergotamine should not be used in patients with a history of vascular disease.

### Prophylaxis
It is particularly difficult to discern the true (as opposed to placebo) effects of prophylactic drugs in migraine. When drugs are necessary, the following are used:

PIZOTIFEN (a 5-hydroxytryptamine antagonist) 0.5 mg at night for several days, increasing to 1.5 mg at night. Common side-effects are slight weight gain and drowsiness.

PROPRANOLOL 10 mg three times daily, increasing to 40–80 mg three times daily.

METHYSERGIDE (a 5-hydroxytryptamine antagonist) 2–6 mg daily. An occasional side-effect is retroperitoneal fibrosis, which precludes its use for longer than 6 months.

## Facial pain

The face is richly supplied with pain-sensitive structures — the teeth, gums, sinuses, temporomandibular joints, jaw and eyes — disease of which causes facial pain. Facial pain is also caused by some specific neurological conditions; these are mentioned below.

### Trigeminal neuralgia
This is described on p. 887.

### Trigeminal nerve lesions
These are described on p. 887.

### Postherpetic neuralgia
This is described on p. 928.

### Migrainous neuralgia (cluster headache)
This condition, which is distinct from migraine despite its name, causes recurrent bouts of excruciating pain that wake the patient at night and are centred around one eye. It affects adults in the third and fourth decades and is more common in men. Alcohol sometimes precipitates an attack.

The pain lasts for several hours. Vomiting occurs. The face and nostril feel congested. A transient ipsilateral Horner's syndrome is common during the attack.

Despite the pain there are no serious sequelae. Treatment of the attack with analgesics is unhelpful. Prophylactic drugs for migraine are of little value. Lithium carbonate sometimes has a dramatic effect in preventing attacks: the drug level should be monitored carefully.

### Atypical facial pain
Facial pain for which no cause can be found is seen in the elderly, mainly in women. It is believed to be a somatic equivalent of depression. Tricyclic antidepressants are sometimes helpful.

### Other causes
Facial pain occurs in usual variants of migraine and in giant-cell arteritis (see below).

## Giant-cell arteritis (cranial arteritis, temporal arteritis) (see p. 406)

This important syndrome is a granulomatous arteritis of unknown aetiology occurring chiefly in those over the age of 60 years and affecting in particular the extradural arteries. Other forms of arteritis, e.g. SLE (see p. 400) and polyarteritis nodosa (see p. 406) can present with similar features but with a more generalized arteritis affecting intracranial arteries and vasa nervorum of the cranial nerves. Giant-cell arteritis is closely related to polymyalgia and these can occur in the same patient.

### CLINICAL FEATURES
#### Headache
Headache is almost invariable. It is felt over the inflamed superficial, temporal or occipital arteries. Touching the skin over the inflamed vessel (e.g. combing the hair) causes pain. The arterial pulsation is soon lost and the artery becomes hard, tortuous and thickened. The skin over the vessels may be red. Rarely, gangrenous patches appear in the scalp.

#### Facial pain
Pain in the face, jaw and mouth occurs and is caused by inflammation of the facial, maxillary and lingual branches

of the external carotid artery. Pain is characteristically worse on eating (jaw claudication). Opening the mouth and protruding the tongue is difficult. A painful, ischaemic tongue occasionally occurs.

### Visual problems

Visual loss due to inflammation and occlusion of the ciliary and/or central retinal artery occurs in 25% of untreated cases. The patient complains of sudden uniocular visual loss, either partial or complete, which is painless. Amaurosis fugax (see p. 906) may precede total visual loss, which is usually permanent.

When the ciliary vessels are affected, the optic disc becomes swollen and pale (see p. 882). The retinal branch vessels are usually normal. If the central retinal artery is occluded, there is sudden unilateral blindness, pallor of the disc and retinal ischaemia.

### Systemic features

Generalized limb pains, proximal limb girdle pain and tenderness, without joint effusion, i.e. polymyalgia rheumatica (see p. 406), occurs in half the cases. Weight loss, sweating and malaise also occur.

### Rare complications

Brain stem ischaemia, cortical blindness, ischaemic neuropathy of peripheral nerves, cranial nerve lesions, and involvement of the aorta, coronary, renal and mesenteric arteries are sometimes seen.

### INVESTIGATION

The ESR is greatly elevated, 60–100 mm hour$^{-1}$ being common, although very rarely the ESR is normal. Plasma $\alpha_2$-globulins are raised and the albumin is occasionally reduced. Normochromic normocytic anaemia occurs.

The diagnosis is usually confirmed by biopsy of a superficial temporal artery. A 1 cm (or greater) segment should be excised because the characteristic granulomatous changes within the walls (lymphocytes, plasma cells, multinucleate giant cells, destruction of the internal elastic lamina) may be patchy.

### TREATMENT

The diagnosis should be established without delay because of the risk of blindness. High doses of steroids (prednisolone, initially 60–100 mg daily) should be started immediately in a patient with typical features even before the biopsy. The dose is reduced as the ESR falls. A characteristic of the condition is that the headache subsides within hours of the first large dose of steroid.

It is usually possible to stop steroid treatment after some months to several years.

# Head injury

There are 200–300 admissions annually for head injury per 100 000 population in most Western countries: 10 people per 100 000 die annually and the prevalence of survivors with a major persisting handicap is of the order of a 100 per 100 000. Road traffic accidents and alcohol abuse are the principal aetiological factors in this major cause of morbidity and mortality.

### Skull fractures

Linear skull fracture of the vault or base is an indication of the severity of injury, but is not necessarily associated with any neurological sequelae. Healing takes place and surgical intervention is usually unnecessary.

Depressed skull fracture of the vault is followed by a high incidence of post-traumatic epilepsy (see p. 913). Surgical elevation and debridement are usually necessary.

The principal local complications of skull fracture are:

RUPTURE OF A MENINGEAL ARTERY, causing an extradural haematoma (see p. 911).

TEARING OF DURAL VEINS, causing SDH (see p. 911) or CSF rhinorrhoea and otorrhoea with its risk of meningitis.

### Brain damage

Older classifications attempted to separate 'concussion', in which transient coma was followed by complete recovery, from brain contusion after which there were prolonged coma and focal signs. There is little pathological support for this. The mechanisms of brain damage following trauma are complex and interrelated. They involve:

- Direct axonal and neuronal damage
- Raised intracranial pressure
- Brain oedema
- Brain ischaemia
- Brain hypoxia

### CLINICAL COURSE

In a mild injury a patient is first stunned or dazed for a few seconds or minutes. Loss of consciousness is transient and following this the patient is alert, and there is no amnesia. The period of loss of consciousness indicates severity; over several hours it is regarded as indicating severe brain injury. The Glasgow Coma Scale (see p. 901) can be used to assess the degree of coma and brain damage as well as indicating prognosis; a low score implies a severe injury and 50% of such patients die or remain in a vegetative state.

Recovery may take a long period of time, depending on the severity of the injury. During early recovery patients are often restless and lethargic and they may have mild focal neurological deficits. Gradually patients become more alert to their surroundings.

### LATE SEQUELAE

These are common causes of morbidity and have important social and medicolegal consequences. They include the following:

PROLONGED AND INCOMPLETE RECOVERY occurs in many patients with severe head injuries. These patients are left with impairment of higher cerebral function, hemiparesis and other deficits.

POST-TRAUMATIC EPILEPSY may occur (see p. 913).

'CHRONIC TRAUMATIC ENCEPHALOPATHY' follows repeated (and often minor) injuries. This 'punch drunk' syndrome is dementia and presents with extrapyramidal and pyramidal signs. It is seen mainly in professional boxers.

THE 'POST-TRAUMATIC SYNDROME' describes the vague complaints of headache, dizziness and malaise that follow even minor head injuries. Depression is prominent. Symptoms may be prolonged.

BENIGN POSITIONAL VERTIGO (see p. 891) is a transient sequel of head injury.

CHRONIC SUBDURAL HAEMATOMA (see p. 911).

HYDROCEPHALUS (see p. 934).

## MANAGEMENT

Patients with head injury require skilled, prolonged and energetic supportive therapy.

Acute management of the unconscious patient is described on p. 903.

## REHABILITATION

Patients left with severe neurological deficits will require rehabilitation in specialized units. Recovery requires not only intensive physiotherapy but also the overall care of their mental state. Many patients are depressed and have behavioural problems and they and their families need long-term support and counselling.

## Diseases of the spinal cord

The cord extends from C1 (its junction with the medulla) to the vertebral body of L1 (the conus medullaris).

The blood supply is via the anterior spinal artery and a plexus on the posterior cord. This network is supplied by the vertebral arteries, the thyrocervical trunk and several branches from the lumbar and intercostal vessels.

## Spinal cord compression

The principal features of cord compression are of radicular pain at the site of compression, spastic paraparesis or tetraparesis and sensory loss which rises to the level of compression.

For example, in compression at the level of T6 a band of pain radiates around the chest wall and is characteristically worse on coughing or straining. A spastic paraparesis develops either over many months, days or hours, depending upon the underlying pathology. Numbness commencing distally in the lower limbs rises to the level of compression (the 'sensory limb'). Compression of the cord is a potential medical emergency. It is sometimes difficult to distinguish chronic cord compression from other causes of paraparesis and tetraparesis on clinical grounds alone. This is because pain and the sensory level may be absent (Table 18.47 and see Table 18.16).

| |
|---|
| Spinal cord neoplasms (see Table 18.48) |
| Disc and vertebral lesions |
|    Trauma |
|    Chronic degenerative |
| Inflammatory |
|    Epidural abscess |
|    Tuberculosis |
|    Granuloma |
| Vertebral neoplasms |
|    Metastases |
|    Myeloma |
| Epidural haemorrhage |
| Rarities |
|    Paget's disease |
|    Epithelial, endothelial and parasitic cysts |
|    Aneurysmal bone cyst |
|    Vertebral angioma |
|    Haematomyelia, arachnoiditis |
|    Osteoporosis |

**Table 18.47**  Causes of spinal cord compression.

**Spinal cord neoplasms** (Table 18.48)

Extramedullary tumours (extradural and intradural) cause cord compression gradually over weeks to months, with local or referred root pain and a sensory level (see p. 898).

Intramedullary tumours (e.g. glioma) typically have a very slowly progressive course over several years. Sensory disturbances similar to syringomyelia (see p. 939) may appear.

**Disc and vertebral lesions**

Central cervical disc protrusion and lumbar disc protrusion are considered on p. 949.

| |
|---|
| *Extradural* |
| Metastases |
|    Bronchus |
|    Breast |
|    Prostate |
|    Lymphoma |
|    Thyroid |
|    Melanoma |
| *Extramedullary* |
| Meningioma |
| Neurofibroma |
| Ependymoma |
| Arteriovenous malformation |
| *Intramedullary* |
| Glioma |
| Ependymoma |
| Haemangioblastoma |
| Lipoma |
| Arteriovenous malformation |
| Teratoma |

**Table 18.48**  Principal spinal cord neoplasms.

## Epidural abscess

This is described on p. 931.

## Epidural haemorrhage and haematoma

These are rare sequelae of anticoagulant therapy, bleeding disorders and trauma. A rapidly progressive cord lesion develops.

## Tuberculosis

Spinal tuberculosis is a frequent cause of cord compression in countries where tuberculosis is common (e.g. India, Pakistan, Bangladesh and Africa). There is destruction of vertebral bodies and disc spaces, with spread of infection along the extradural space. Cord compression and paraparesis follow (Pott's paraplegia).

### MANAGEMENT

Early recognition of the syndrome is vital. Surgical exploration is frequently necessary and, if this is not performed sufficiently early, irreversible paraplegia may follow.

Plain spinal films show degenerative bone disease and destruction of vertebrae by infection or neoplasm. Routine tests, e.g. chest X-ray, may indicate a primary neoplasm or infection.

MRI can identify most lesions and is beginning to replace myelography. Investigations should, if possible, be done promptly in a centre equipped to carry out neurosurgical exploration. The signs of cord compression may increase after lumbar puncture.

The results following the early removal of benign tumours are excellent.

## Transverse myelitis

This broad term is used to describe acute inflammation of the cord and paraplegia occurring with viral infection, MS and other inflammatory and vascular disorders (e.g. syphilis, radiation myelopathy, anterior spinal artery occlusion). Myelography or MRI is usually required to exclude a compressive lesion.

### Anterior spinal artery occlusion

Cord infarction, causing an acute paraparesis or tetraparesis (or tetraplegia) may occur in any thrombotic or embolic vascular disease (e.g. endocarditis, shock, atheroma, diabetes mellitus, syphilis, polyarteritis nodosa). It sometimes occurs during surgery to the posterior mediastinum, and follows dissection of the aorta and trauma. It occasionally occurs as an isolated event.

### Radiation myelopathy

A mild paraparesis and sensory loss sometimes develops within several weeks to a year of radiotherapy if the cord has been damaged. Particular care is usually taken to shield the cord during radiotherapy.

## Metabolic and toxic cord disease

Subacute combined degeneration of the cord due to vitamin $B_{12}$ deficiency (see pp. 948 and 304) is the most important example of metabolic disease causing spinal cord damage.

Cord lesions may also be seen in severe malnutrition, when they are probably due to multiple B-vitamin deficiencies.

### Lathyrism

This is an endemic, spastic paraparesis of central India caused by the toxin $\beta$-($N$)-oxalylaminoalanine. It occurs when excessive quantities of a drought-resistant pulse, *Lathyrus sativa*, are consumed.

## Syringomyelia and syringobulbia

Fluid-filled cavities within the spinal cord (myelia) and brain stem (bulbia) are the essential features of these conditions.

### AETIOLOGY

A history of birth injury may be obtained and bony anomalies at the foramen magnum, spina bifida (see p. 942), Arnold–Chiari malformation (see p. 942) or hydrocephalus (see p. 934) are often seen.

It is believed that in the presence of an anatomical abnormality at the foramen magnum, the normal pulsatile CSF pressure waves are transmitted to the delicate tissues of the cervical cord and brain stem, with secondary cavity formation. The cavity, or syrinx, is in continuity with the central canal of the cord.

### PATHOLOGICAL ANATOMY

The expanding cavity gradually destroys:

- Second-order spinothalamic neurones in the cervical cord
- Anterior horn cells
- Lateral corticospinal tracts

The vestibular system, trigeminal nuclei, sympathetic system and twelfth nerve nuclei may also be affected.

### CLINICAL FEATURES

Patients usually present in the third to fourth decade.

Pain in the upper limbs is common. This may be exacerbated by exertion or coughing. Spinothalamic (pain and temperature) sensory loss in the upper limbs leads to painless burns. Difficulty in walking may occur.

The signs of a cavity in the cervical region are:

AREAS OF DISSOCIATED SENSORY LOSS, i.e. pain and temperature but not touch (posterior column). These may extend in a bizarre distribution over the trunk and upper limbs.

LOSS OF UPPER LIMB REFLEXES.

WASTING of the small muscles of the hand.

SPASTIC PARAPARESIS. This may initially be mild and symptomless.

Neuropathic joints, trophic skin changes and ulcers may follow.

When the cavity extends through the foramen magnum into the brain stem (syringobulbia), there is atrophy and fasciculation of the tongue, nystagmus, Horner's syndrome, hearing loss and impairment of facial sensation.

## MANAGEMENT AND COURSE

The condition is intermittently progressive over several decades.

Investigation shows widening of the cervical canal on plain films and, frequently, ventricular enlargement on CT scan. An MRI scan (the investigation of choice) demonstrates the intrinsic cavity. Myelography (which is sometimes followed by deterioration) shows widening of the cord and herniation of the cerebellar tonsils through the foramen magnum.

There is no curative treatment. Decompression of the foramen magnum sometimes reduces the rate of deterioration.

## Paraplegia (see p. 894)

### MANAGEMENT

The patient who becomes paraplegic from any cause demands skilled and prolonged nursing care. Particular problems are discussed below.

### Bladder

Intermittent (or continuous) catheterization is usually necessary initially. A reflex emptying bladder develops in permanent paraplegia, avoiding the need for catheterization and some of the risks of urinary stasis, infection, and renal and bladder calculi.

### Bowel

Constipation and faecal impaction must be avoided. Manual evacuation is necessary following acute paraplegia, but reflex emptying later develops.

### Skin care

The risk of pressure sores is great. Meticulous attention must be paid to cleanliness and to turning the patient every 2 hours. The sacrum, iliac crests, greater trochanters, heels and malleoli should be inspected frequently. Ripple mattresses and water beds are useful.

If pressure sores develop, plastic surgical repair should be considered.

### The lower limbs

Passive physiotherapy is helpful in avoiding contractures. Severe spasticity (with spasms either in flexion or extension) may be helped by dantrolene sodium, baclofen or diazepam.

### General considerations

The general health and morale of the patient should be considered carefully and regularly. Any intercurrent infection (urinary or respiratory) is potentially hazardous and should be recognized and treated early, as chronic renal failure is the single most common cause of death in paraplegia.

### Rehabilitation

Many patients with traumatic paraplegia or tetraplegia return to partial self-sufficiency and a wheelchair existence. Specialist advice from a skilled rehabilitation unit is necessary. Lightweight, specially adapted wheelchairs are often recommended. The patients have demanding practical, psychological and social needs but with guidance and help can often return to an active role in society.

## Other causes of cord lesions

- MS
- Motor neurone disease
- Familial or sporadic paraparesis
- Non-metastatic manifestation of malignancy (see p. 950)
- Neurosyphilis

Rarities, e.g. sarcoidosis (see p. 687), Behçet's syndrome (see p. 413)

# Degenerative diseases

The term 'degenerative' underlines a present lack of understanding of the aetiology of this group of progressive diseases of the nervous system.

## Motor neurone disease (MND)

In this disease there is progressive degeneration of motor neurones in the spinal cord, in the somatic motor nuclei of the cranial nerves and within the cortex. The condition is sporadic and of entirely unknown cause. Though not familial, recent work has assigned the gene for the condition to chromosome 21. The prevalence is about 6 in 100 000, with a slight male predominance. The onset is in middle life. The sensory system is not involved.

### CLINICAL FEATURES

There are three patterns:
1 Progressive muscular atrophy
2 Amyotrophic lateral sclerosis
3 Progressive bulbar palsy
Although useful as a means of understanding the disease, these are not distinct aetiological or pathological variants; the three merge later in the course of the condition.

### Progressive muscular atrophy

Wasting often begins in the small muscles of one hand and spreads inexorably throughout the arm. Although it may begin unilaterally, wasting soon follows on the opposite side.

Fasciculation is common. It is due to the spontaneous firing of abnormally large motor units formed by the branching fibres of surviving axons that are striving to innervate muscle fibres that have lost their nerve supply. Cramps may occur but pain does not.

The physical signs are of wasting and weakness, with fasciculation that is often widespread. Tendon reflexes are lost when the reflex arc is interrupted (by anterior horn cell loss) but are often preserved or exaggerated because of the loss of motor neurones in the corticospinal tracts.

### Amyotrophic lateral sclerosis (ALS)

'Lateral sclerosis' means disease of the lateral corticospinal tracts (i.e. a spastic paraparesis). 'Amyotrophy' means atrophy of muscle (which would be unusual in most other forms of spastic tetraparesis or paraparesis). The clinical picture is thus of a progressive spastic tetraparesis or paraparesis with added LMN signs and fasciculation. ALS is the term usually given to MND in the USA.

### Progressive bulbar palsy

Here the brunt of the onset of the disease falls upon the lower cranial nerve nuclei and their supranuclear connections. Dysarthria, dysphagia, nasal regurgitation of fluids and choking are common symptoms. For reasons unknown, this form of the disease is more common in women than in men. The characteristic features are of a bulbar and pseudobulbar palsy, i.e. a mixture of UMN and LMN signs in the lower cranial nerves, e.g. a wasted fibrillating tongue with a spastic weak palate.

### COURSE

The ocular movements are not affected. There are never cerebellar or extrapyramidal signs. Awareness is preserved and dementia is unusual. Sphincter disturbance occurs late, if at all.

Remission is unknown. The disease progresses, spreading gradually and causes death, often from bronchopneumonia. Survival for more than 3 years is most unusual, although there are rare 'benign' forms of the condition in which survival is prolonged.

### MANAGEMENT

There are no specific diagnostic tests and the diagnosis can often be made on clinical grounds alone. Cervical radiculopathy and myelopathy and the rare (almost extinct) syphilitic cervical pachymeningitis may sometimes cause diagnostic difficulty. Bulbar myasthenia gravis may sometimes appear similar in the early stages.

Denervation may be confirmed by electromyography, which characteristically shows chronic partial denervation with preserved motor conduction velocity. The CSF is usually normal (the protein may be slightly raised).

No treatment has been shown to influence the course of this disease although recently Riluzole, a glutamate antagonist, has been shown to help, particularly in patients with disease of bulbar onset. Management of patients with MND, who are often well-informed and aware of the outlook, is particularly difficult.

## Spinal muscular atrophies

These are a group of rare genetically determined disorders of the motor neurone that give rise to slowly progressive, usually symmetrical, muscle wasting and weakness. An acute infantile type (Werdnig–Hoffman disease), a chronic childhood type (Kugelberg–Weilander disease)

and adult forms are recognized. Clinically these conditions may be confused with muscular dystrophies (see p. 953), hereditary neuropathies or MND.

## Dementia (see p. 964)

This is a diffuse deterioration in mental function produced by a number of pathological processes. The commonest is Alzheimer's disease. Dementia is discussed on p. 964.

# *Congenital and inherited diseases*

## CEREBRAL PALSY

This term describes disorders apparent at birth or in childhood due to brain damage in the neonatal period leading to non-progressive deficits.

Mental retardation, varying from severe intellectual impairment to mild learning disorders, is common in all forms of cerebral palsy, but severe physical disability is not necessarily associated with a severe defect in higher cerebral function.

### CAUSES

The precise cause of brain damage in an individual child may be difficult to determine. The following may be responsible:

HYPOXIA *in utero* and/or during parturition
TRAUMA, during parturition or in the neonatal period
PROLONGED CONVULSIONS OR COMA (e.g. febrile convulsions, hypoglycaemia) in infancy
KERNICTERUS
CEREBRAL HAEMORRHAGE AND INFARCTION

### CLINICAL FEATURES

Failure to achieve normal developmental milestones is often the earliest feature. More specific motor syndromes become apparent later in childhood or, rarely, in adult life.

#### Spastic diplegia

This is spasticity (predominantly of the lower limbs) with 'scissoring' of the gait.

#### Athetoid cerebral palsy

This is described on p. 920.

#### Infantile hemiparesis

Hemiparesis may be noted at birth or during childhood. Hemiatrophy of the limbs (and atrophy of the contralateral hemisphere) is usual. Seizures are common.

### Congenital ataxia

This is incoordination and hypotonia of the trunk and limbs.

## DYSRAPHISM

Failure of normal fusion of the fetal neural tube leads to this group of congenital anomalies.

### Anencephaly

Anencephaly is absence of the brain and cranial vault, and is incompatible with life.

### Meningo-encephalocele

This is an extrusion of brain and meninges through a midline skull defect that varies from a minor protrusion to a massive defect.

### Spina bifida

In spina bifida there is failure of fusion of the neural tube, usually in the lumbosacral region. Several varieties occur.

SPINA BIFIDA OCCULTA. This is failure of fusion of the vertebral arch only. There are rarely neurological abnormalities and a bony anomaly is seen on X-ray. It occurs in 3% of the population. A dimple or a tuft of hair may overlie the lesion.

MENINGOMYELOCELE AND MYELOCELE WITH SPINA BIFIDA. Meningomyelocele consists of elements of the cord and lumbosacral roots contained within a meningeal sac that herniates through a defect in the vertebrae. In severe cases the lower limbs and sphincters are paralysed. The defect is visible at birth.

Meningocele is a meningeal defect alone.

Hydrocephalus is commonly associated with these abnormalities. Meningitis may follow if a sinus connects the spinal canal with the overlying skin.

## BASILAR IMPRESSION OF THE SKULL (PLATYBASIA)

This is usually a congenital anomaly in which there is invagination of the foramen magnum and skull base upwards. The lower cranial nerves, medulla, upper cervical cord and roots are affected. It is often complicated by the Arnold–Chiari malformation, in which aberrant cerebellar tissue extends through the foramen magnum.

The condition also occurs in Paget's disease and rarely in osteomalacia.

## NEUROECTODERMAL SYNDROMES

These are disorders in which organs derived from ectoderm show a tendency to form tumours and hamartomas, with lesions in the skin, eye and nervous system.

## Neurofibromatosis (von Recklinghausen's disease)

This is characterized by multiple skin neurofibromas and pigmentation. The neurofibromas arise from the neurilemmal sheath. One new case occurs in every 3000 live births. The mode of inheritance is autosomal dominant.

**CLINICAL FEATURES** (see p. 1025)

Clinically neurofibromatosis can be divided into type 1 (or peripheral) and type 2 (bilateral acoustic or central). The predisposing gene for type 1 has been localized to chromosome 17 and for type 2 to the long arm of chromosome 22. The main application for these genetic markers will be for antenatal diagnosis and genetic counselling, although the severity of the disease itself will not be predictable.

### Skin tumours

Subcutaneous, soft, sometimes pedunculated, tumours appear. They may be multiple.

### Skin pigmentation

Multiple *café-au-lait* patches—pale brown macules 1–20 cm in diameter—are found. These are common in the normal population, but more than five patches is abnormal.

### Neural tumours

Many neural tumours occur more frequently in von Recklinghausen's disease than in the general population, including:

- Cutaneous neurofibroma
- Eighth nerve sheath neurofibroma
- Spinal cord and nerve root neurofibroma
- Meningioma
- Glioma (including optic nerve glioma)
- Plexiform neuroma (massive cutaneous overgrowth)

Rarely, the benign tumours undergo sarcomatous change.

### Associated abnormalities

These include:

- Scoliosis
- Orbital haemangioma
- Local gigantism of a limb
- Phaeochromocytoma and ganglioneuroma
- Renal artery stenosis
- Pulmonary fibrosis
- Obstructive cardiomyopathy
- Fibrous dysplasia of bone

**TREATMENT**

Surgery may be necessary for cosmetic reasons. Tumours causing pressure within the nervous system require excision, if this is feasible.

## Tuberose sclerosis (epiloia)

This is a rare autosomal dominant condition whose principal features are adenoma sebaceum, epilepsy and mental retardation (often severe).

**Adenoma sebaceum**

These are reddish nodules (angiofibromas) that develop on the cheeks in childhood.

**Other lesions**

Other lesions include shagreen patches, amelanotic naevi, retinal phakomas (glial masses), renal tumours, glial overgrowth in brain and gliomas. Cardiac rhabdomyomas, hamartomas of lung and kidney, and polycystic kidneys may also occur.

## Sturge–Weber syndrome (encephalofacial angiomatosis)

There is an extensive port-wine naevus on one side of the face (usually in the distribution of a division of the fifth nerve) and a leptomeningeal angioma.

Epilepsy is common. Familial occurrence is exceptional.

## Von Hippel–Lindau syndrome (retinocerebellar angiomatosis)

This is the occurrence in families (dominant inheritance with variable penetrance) of retinal and cerebellar haemangioblastomas or, less commonly, haemangioblastomas of the cord and cerebrum. Renal, adrenal and pancreatic cysts (and haemangioblastomas) may also be found. Polycythaemia sometimes occurs.

There are numerous other disorders related to these conditions, for example ataxia telangiectasia (see p. 943) and Osler–Weber–Rendu syndrome (see p. 341).

## SPINOCEREBELLAR DEGENERATIONS

The classification of this large group of rare inherited disorders is complex. Three conditions will be mentioned here.

## Friedreich's ataxia

This is a progressive degeneration of dorsal root ganglia, spinocerebellar tracts, corticospinal tracts and Purkinje cells of the cerebellum. Difficulty in walking occurs around the age of 12 years and is progressive. The clinical findings are:

● Ataxia of gait and trunk
● Nystagmus (in 25%)
● Dysarthria
● Absent joint position and vibration sense in lower limbs
● Absent reflexes in lower limbs
● Optic atrophy (in 30%)
● Pes cavus
● Cardiomyopathy with T-wave inversion and left ventricular hypertrophy, arrhythmias.

Death is usual before the age of 40.

## Hereditary spastic paraparesis

Isolated progressive paraparesis runs in some families. The inheritance is variable. Additional features including cerebellar signs, pes cavus, wasted hands and optic atrophy are sometimes seen. The conditions are usually mild and progress slowly over many years.

## Ataxia telangiectasia (see p. 147)

This is a rare, autosomal recessive condition that produces a progressive ataxic syndrome in childhood and early adult life.

There is striking telangiectasia of the conjunctiva, nose, ears and skin creases. There are also defects in cell-mediated immunity and antibody production. A defect in DNA repair has been demonstrated. Death is usual by the third decade, either from infection or from the development of lymphoreticular malignancy.

## PERONEAL MUSCULAR ATROPHY AND OTHER INHERITED NEUROPATHIES

These disorders are classified within a large and complex group—the hereditary motor and sensory neuropathies (HMSN).

## Peroneal muscular atrophy

Peroneal muscular atrophy (Charcot–Marie–Tooth disease) is a common clinical syndrome in which there is distal limb wasting and weakness that slowly progresses over many years, mostly in the legs, with variable loss of sensation and reflexes. In advanced cases the distal wasting below the knees is so marked that the legs resemble 'inverted champagne bottles'. Mild cases have only pes cavus and clawing of the toes and may pass unnoticed.

Three forms are recognized:

1 HMSN type I—a demyelinating neuropathy
2 HMSN type II—an axonal neuropathy
3 Distal spinal muscular atrophy

Both autosomal dominant and recessive inheritance is seen in different families. In HMSN type I with dominant inheritance (the commonest form), linkage has been demonstrated for the locus on the long arm of chromosome 1.

Optic atrophy, deafness, retinitis pigmentosa and spastic paraparesis are sometimes seen in variants of these conditions.

## HMSN type III

This was formerly known as the 'hypertrophic neuropathy of Déjérine–Sottas'. It is an autosomal recessive demyelinating sensory neuropathy of childhood leading to severe incapacity during adolescence. It is notable because the CSF protein may be greatly elevated to

10 g litre$^{-1}$ or more, and the CSF pathways are obstructed by greatly hypertrophied nerve roots.

# Diseases of the peripheral nerves

The different nerve fibre types within a peripheral nerve are shown in Table 18.49. All are myelinated except the C fibres, which carry impulses from painful stimuli.

Two pathological processes affect peripheral nerves—axonal (the axon itself) degeneration and demyelination (the myelin sheath). Neuropathies are classified broadly into which of the two processes predominate. Wallerian degeneration refers to the changes seen after section of a nerve.

### Axonal degeneration
Axonal degeneration occurs after a nerve has been sectioned or its axon severely damaged. Within 7–10 days the axon and the myelin sheath distal to the injury degenerate and are inexcitable electrically. When a motor nerve is damaged there is atrophy of the muscle fibres in the motor units it supplies. Denervation may be detected by recording fibrillation potentials on electromyography.

Regeneration occurs by axonal growth down the nerve sheath and axonal sprouting from the stump. Growth takes place at a rate of up to 1 mm daily. In a chronic neuropathic process (e.g. MND or polyneuropathy), sprouts from the terminal axons of normal motor axons reinnervate the denervated muscle fibres; giant polyphasic units are then seen on electromyography.

### Demyelination
Here damage to the myelin sheath (the axon itself is initially preserved) causes conduction block or marked slowing of conduction; this can be used to distinguish demyelination from axonal degeneration. Local demyelination is caused by pressure (compression and entrapment neuropathies) or by inflammation (e.g. Guillain–Barré syndrome).

## Definitions

NEUROPATHY means a pathological process affecting a peripheral nerve or nerves.

MONONEUROPATHY is a process affecting a single nerve, and multiple mononeuropathy (or mononeuritis multiplex) is a process affecting several or multiple nerves.

POLYNEUROPATHY is a diffuse, symmetrical disease process, usually progressing proximally. It is either acute, subacute or chronic. Its course may be progressive, relapsing or towards recovery. Polyneuropathy may be motor, sensory, sensorimotor (mixed) or autonomic.

RADICULOPATHY means a disease process affecting the nerve roots.

## MONONEUROPATHIES

### Peripheral nerve compression and entrapment (Table 18.50)

Damage to a nerve by compression is either acute (e.g. due to a tourniquet or other sustained pressure) or chronic (entrapment neuropathy). In both, demyelination predominates, but some axonal degeneration occurs.

| Nerve | Site of entrapment or compression |
|---|---|
| Median | Carpal tunnel |
| Ulnar | Cubital tunnel |
| Radial | Spiral groove of humerus |
| Posterior interosseous | Supinator muscle |
| Lateral cutaneous of thigh ('meralgia paraesthetica') | Inguinal ligament |
| Common peroneal | Neck of fibula |
| Posterior tibial | Flexor retinaculum (tarsal tunnel) |

Table 18.50   Nerve compression and entrapment.

| Type | Fibre diameter (μm) | Conduction velocity (m s$^{-1}$) | Function |
|---|---|---|---|
| Aα | 10–18 | 90 | Primary spindle afferents α Motor neurones |
| Aγ | 4–8 | 30 | γ Afferents. Motor to muscle spindles |
| Aδ | 2–6 | 30 | Fast pain |
| C | 1–2 | <1 | Slow pain and temperature afferents Autonomic postganglionic |

Table 18.49   Fibre types in peripheral nerves.

Acute compression usually affects nerves which are exposed anatomically (e.g. the common peroneal nerve at the head of the fibula).

Entrapment occurs where a nerve passes through relatively tight anatomical passages (e.g. the carpal tunnel).

These conditions are diagnosed largely from the clinical features. Diagnosis is confirmed by nerve conduction studies and electromyography. The commoner conditions are mentioned below.

## Median nerve compression at the wrist (carpal tunnel syndrome)

This common syndrome is sometimes seen in:
- Hypothyroidism
- Diabetes mellitus
- Pregnancy and obesity
- Rheumatoid arthritis
- Acromegaly

The condition is, however, usually idiopathic. It causes nocturnal tingling and pain in the hand (and sometimes forearm) followed by weakness of the thenar muscles. Wasting of abductor pollicis brevis develops, with sensory loss of the palm and radial three-and-a-half fingers. Tinel's sign may be positive, i.e. tapping on the carpal tunnel will reproduce the pain.

Treatment with a splint at night or a local steroid injection in the wrist gives temporary relief. When the condition occurs in pregnancy (due to fluid retention) it is often self-limiting. Surgical decompression of the carpel tunnel is a simple and definitive treatment.

## Ulnar nerve compression

This typically occurs at the elbow, where the nerve is compressed in the cubital tunnel. It follows fracture of the ulna or prolonged or recurrent pressure on the nerve at this site.

Wasting of the ulnar-innervated muscles develops (hypothenar muscles and interossei) together with sensory loss in the ulnar one-and-a-half fingers.

Decompression and transposition of the nerve at the elbow may be necessary.

The deep (solely motor) branch of the ulnar nerve may be damaged in the palm by recurrent pressure from tools (e.g. screwdrivers), crutches or cycle handlebars.

## Radial nerve compression

The radial nerve is compressed acutely against the humerus, e.g. when the arm is draped over a hard chair for several hours ('Saturday night palsy'). Wrist drop and weakness of finger extension and of the brachioradialis muscle follow. Recovery is usual within 1–3 months.

## Meralgia paraesthetica

Burning, tingling and numbness on the anterolateral aspect of the thigh is caused by entrapment of the lateral cutaneous nerve of the thigh beneath the inguinal ligament.

Many of the patients are obese; weight reduction helps to relieve the symptoms. Division of the inguinal ligament is not usually effective.

## Common peroneal nerve palsy

When the common peroneal nerve is compressed against the head of the fibula (owing to prolonged squatting, wearing plaster casts, prolonged bed rest or coma) there is foot drop and weakness of eversion. A patch of numbness on the anterolateral border of the shin or dorsum of the foot may be found. Recovery is usual (but not invariable) within several months.

## Multiple mononeuropathy (mononeuritis multiplex)

Multiple mononeuropathy occurs in:
- Diabetes mellitus
- Leprosy (still the commonest worldwide)
- Connective tissue disease (polyarteritis nodosa, SLE, giant-cell arteritis, rheumatoid arthritis)
- Sarcoidosis
- Malignancy
- Amyloidosis
- Neurofibromatosis
- AIDS

Diagnosis is largely clinical, supported by electrical studies. Treatment is that of the underlying disease.

## POLYNEUROPATHIES

Although many toxins and disease processes are known to be associated with polyneuropathy (see below), the cause of the majority of cases remains undetermined. The commonest presentation is a chronic or subacute sensorimotor neuropathy. A classification of polyneuropathy is given in Table 18.51.

## Idiopathic chronic sensorimotor neuropathies

The patient complains of a progressive symmetrical numbness and tingling in the hands and feet, which spreads proximally in a 'glove and stocking' distribution. There is distal weakness, which also ascends. Rarely the

Idiopathic chronic sensorimotor neuropathies
Postinfective neuropathy (Guillain–Barré syndrome)
Drugs/toxic, metabolic and vitamin-deficiency neuropathies
Neoplastic neuropathies
Neuropathies in connective tissue diseases
Autonomic neuropathies
Hereditary sensorimotor neuropathies

**Table 18.51** Classification of polyneuropathy.

cranial nerves may be affected. Tendon reflexes involving affected nerves are lost. The symptoms may progress over many months, remain static or remit at any stage. Autonomic features are sometimes seen.

Investigation (nerve conduction studies, electromyography) of the neuropathy shows either axonal degeneration or demyelination, or features of both of these processes. Some cases of demyelinating (not axonal) chronic sensorimotor neuropathy respond to steroid or immunosuppressive therapy.

## Postinfective polyneuropathy (Guillain–Barré syndrome, acute inflammatory neuropathy)

### CLINICAL FEATURES

This demyelinating neuropathy, which is the commonest recognizable acute neuropathy has an autoallergic basis. It follows 1–3 weeks after a viral infection that is often trivial. The patient complains of weakness of distal limb muscles or distal numbness. This ascends over several days or weeks. In mild cases there is little disability, but in some 20% of cases the respiratory and facial muscles are affected and the patient may become paralysed.

Weakness, areflexia and sensory loss are found (i.e. an ascending weakness).

Autonomic features (see below) are sometimes seen. There is a rare proximal form of the condition that initially affects the ocular muscles and in which ataxia is found (Miller–Fisher syndrome).

### DIAGNOSIS

This is established on clinical grounds and is confirmed by nerve conduction studies, which show the slowing of conduction or conduction block seen in demyelinating neuropathies. The CSF contains a normal cell count and sugar level but the protein is frequently raised to 1–3 g litre$^{-1}$.

The differential diagnosis includes other paralytic illnesses such as poliomyelitis, botulism or primary muscle disease.

### TREATMENT AND COURSE

High dosage intravenous γ-globulin reduces the duration and severity and should be given to all patients.

Supportive treatment is essential, with particular attention being paid to compensating for weakness of the respiratory and bulbar muscles. Ventilation may be necessary.

Corticosteroids are sometimes used to treat the Guillain–Barré syndrome but are not of proven value. Plasmapheresis has been shown to be of proven benefit in shortening the period of disability.

Recovery, though gradual over many months, is usual but may be incomplete.

## Diphtheria

Demyelinating neuropathy is sometimes caused by the exotoxin of *Corynebacterium diphtheriae*. Palatal weakness followed by pupillary paralysis and a sensorimotor neuropathy occur several weeks after faucial infection. The condition is now rare in countries where immunization against diphtheria is practised.

## Metabolic, toxic and vitamin-deficiency neuropathies

The commoner of these neuropathies are shown in Table 18.52. All are due to impairment of normal metabolism of the axon, myelin or both.

### METABOLIC NEUROPATHIES

#### Diabetes mellitus

Several varieties of neuropathy occur in diabetes mellitus:
1 Symmetrical sensory polyneuropathy
2 Acute painful neuropathy
3 Mononeuropathy and multiple mononeuropathy
   (a) Cranial nerve lesions
   (b) Isolated peripheral nerve lesions, e.g. median
4 Diabetic amyotrophy
5 Autonomic neuropathy
These are discussed in more detail on p. 848.

#### Uraemia

Progressive sensorimotor neuropathy occurs in chronic uraemia. The response to dialysis is variable but the neuropathy usually improves after renal transplantation.

#### Thyroid disease

A mild chronic sensorimotor neuropathy is sometimes seen in both hyperthyroidism and hypothyroidism.

#### Porphyria

Acute intermittent porphyria is a rare metabolic disorder (see p. 866) in which there are episodes of a severe, mainly proximal, neuropathy, sometimes associated with abdominal pain, confusion and later coma. Alcohol and barbiturates may precipitate attacks.

#### Amyloidosis

This is described on p. 866.

#### Refsum's disease

This is a rare condition inherited as an autosomal recessive trait. There is a sensorimotor polyneuropathy with

| Metabolic | Toxic |
|---|---|
| Diabetes mellitus | Drugs |
| Uraemia | Alcohol |
| Hepatic disease | Industrial toxins |
| Thyroid disease | |
| Porphyria | *Vitamin deficiency* |
| Amyloid disease | B$_1$ (thiamine) |
| Malignancy | B$_6$ (pyridoxine) |
| Refsum's disease | Nicotinic acid |
| | B$_{12}$ |

**Table 18.52** Toxic, metabolic and vitamin-deficiency neuropathies.

ataxia, retinal damage and deafness. It is due to a defect in the metabolism of phytanic acid.

## TOXIC NEUROPATHIES

### Alcohol

A polyneuropathy, mainly in the lower limbs, occurs in chronic alcoholics. Calf pain is common. The response to abstention is variable. Thiamine should be given.

### Drugs

Many drugs have been reported to be associated with a polyneuropathy. The more important ones are shown in Table 18.53.

### Industrial toxins

A wide variety of industrial toxins have been shown to cause polyneuropathy:

LEAD POISONING causes a motor neuropathy.

ACRYLAMIDE (PLASTICS INDUSTRY), TRICHLOR-ETHYLENE (A SOLVENT), HEXANE AND OTHER FAT-SOLUBLE HYDROCARBONS (e.g. those inhaled in glue-sniffing, see p. 985) cause a progressive polyneuropathy.

ARSENIC AND THALLIUM cause a polyneuropathy.

## VITAMIN-DEFICIENCY NEUROPATHIES

Vitamin deficiencies are an important cause of disease of the nervous system because they are potentially reversible if treated early (and progressive if not). They occur in malnutrition, when they are commonly multiple.

### Thiamine (vitamin $B_1$)

Deficiency causes the clinical syndrome of beri-beri (see p. 162). The principal features are polyneuropathy, an amnesic syndrome (Wernicke–Korsakoff psychosis) and cardiac failure. Alcohol abuse is the commonest cause in Western countries. Other neurological consequences of alcohol are summarized in Table 18.54.

WERNICKE–KORSAKOFF SYNDROME. This important syndrome is an acute or gradual encephalopathy associated with alcohol abuse and other causes of thiamine deficiency. The typical triad comprises ocular signs, ataxia and a confusional state, but the condition occurs in partial forms. It is due to ischaemic damage to the brain stem and its connections. Clinical features include:

OCULAR SIGNS. Nystagmus, bilateral lateral rectus palsies, conjugate gaze palsies, fixed pupils and, rarely, papilloedema are found.

ATAXIA. There is a broad-based gait, cerebellar signs in the limbs and vestibular paralysis (absent response to caloric stimulation).

CONFUSION. Apathy, decreased awareness or restlessness, amnesia, stupor and coma occur.

Hypothermia and hypotension due to hypothalamic damage are rare findings.

The condition is underdiagnosed. Erythrocyte transketolase activity is reduced but is of limited practical value because the measurement is rarely available.

Thiamine (i.m. or i.v.) should be given immediately if the diagnosis is in question: it is harmless, the condition is not. Untreated Wernicke–Korsakoff syndrome commonly leads to a severe irreversible amnesic syndrome and residual brain stem signs.

### Pyridoxine (vitamin $B_6$)

Deficiency causes a mainly sensory neuropathy (see p. 164). It may be precipitated during isoniazid therapy for tuberculosis in those who acetylate the drug slowly.

| Drug | Neuropathy | Mode/site of action |
|---|---|---|
| Phenytoin<br>Chloramphenicol<br>Procarbazine | Sensory | Axon |
| Isoniazid | Sensory | Pyridoxine metabolism |
| Dapsone<br>Gold<br>Amphotericin | Motor | Axon |
| Nitrofurantoin<br>Vincristine<br>Chlorambucil<br>Disulfiram<br>Cisplatin | Sensorimotor | Axon |
| Perhexiline (not available in UK) | Sensorimotor | Myelin |

**Table 18.53** Drug-associated neuropathies.

Acute intoxication
  Disturbance of balance, gait and speech
  Coma
  Head injury and its sequelae

Alcohol withdrawal
  'Morning shakes'
  Tremor of arms and legs
  Delirium tremens

Thiamine deficiency
  Polyneuropathy
  Wernicke–Korsakoff syndrome

Epilepsy
  Acute intoxication
  Alcohol withdrawal
  Hypoglycaemia

Cerebellar degeneration

Cerebral infarction

Cerebral atrophy

Dementia

Central pontine myelinolysis

Marchiafava–Bignami syndrome (a rare degeneration of the corpus callosum)

**Table 18.54** Effects of ethyl alcohol on the nervous system (see also Table 3.15 and p. 173)

**Vitamin B$_{12}$**

Deficiency causes disease of the brain, spinal cord and peripheral nerves.

SUBACUTE COMBINED DEGENERATION OF THE CORD. This syndrome of the spinal cord is a sequel of Addisonian pernicious anaemia and rarely other causes of vitamin B$_{12}$ deficiency (see p. 306). It is frequently associated with a polyneuropathy.

The patient complains initially of numbness and tingling of the extremities. The signs are of distal sensory loss (particularly posterior column) with absent ankle jerks (due to the neuropathy) combined with evidence of cord disease (exaggerated knee-jerk reflexes, extensor plantar responses). Optic atrophy and retinal haemorrhage may occur. In the later stages sphincter disturbance, weakness and dementia are seen.

Macrocytosis and megaloblastic changes in the bone marrow are invariable in subacute combined degeneration of the cord. The cause of the B$_{12}$ deficiency should be established (see p. 305). Treatment with parenteral B$_{12}$ reverses the peripheral nerve damage but has little effect on the CNS (cord and brain) signs.

## Neoplastic neuropathy

Polyneuropathy is sometimes seen as a non-metastatic manifestation of malignancy (see p. 950).

In myeloma and other dysproteinaemic states polyneuropathy occurs, probably owing to impaired perfusion of nerve trunks or to demyelination associated with allergic reactions within peripheral nerves.

POEMS SYNDROME is characterized by a chronic inflammatory demyelinating *P*olyneuropathy, *O*rganomegaly (hepatomegaly 50%), *E*ndocrinopathy (gynaecomastia and atrophic testes), an *M* protein band on electrophoresis with less than 5% of plasma cells in the bone marrow and *S*kin hyperpigmentation. Chemotherapy is used.

## Neuropathies associated with connective tissue diseases

Neuropathy occurs in SLE, polyarteritis nodosa, rheumatoid disease and giant-cell arteritis owing to microinfarction of peripheral nerves. This presents either as a multiple mononeuropathy or a symmetrical sensorimotor neuropathy.

## Autonomic neuropathy

Autonomic neuropathy causes postural hypotension, retention of urine, impotence, diarrhoea (or occasionally constipation), diminished sweating, impaired pupillary responses and cardiac arrhythmia.

Many varieties of neuropathy affect autonomic function to a mild, and often subclinical, degree. Occasionally, when there is damage to small myelinated and non-myelinated B and C fibres, the clinical features of the autonomic neuropathy predominate. This situation may occur in diabetes mellitus, in amyloidosis and in the Guillain–Barré syndrome.

## Hereditary sensorimotor neuropathies

These are described on p. 943.

# PLEXUS LESIONS AND RADICULOPATHY

The common conditions that cause nerve root or lumbar or brachial plexus lesions are summarized in Table 18.55.

## Cervical rib (thoracic outlet syndrome)

A fibrous band or cervical rib extending from the tip of the transverse process of C7 to the first rib stretches the lower roots of the brachial plexus (C8 and T1). There is pain along the ulnar border of the forearm, and sensory loss initially in the distribution of T1 with wasting of the thenar muscles, principally the abductor pollicis brevis muscle. Horner's syndrome may occur. The rib or band can be excised.

In other patients the rib or band causes subclavian artery or venous occlusion. The neurological and vascular problems rarely occur together.

## Neuralgic amyotrophy

This is a condition in which severe pain in the muscles of the shoulder is followed by wasting, usually of the infraspinatus, supraspinatus, deltoid and serratus anterior muscles (a 'brachial plexus neuropathy'). The cause is unknown but, since the condition follows viral infection or immunization in some cases, an allergic basis is postulated.

Recovery of the wasted muscles occurs over some months.

## Malignant infiltration

Metastatic disease of nerve roots of the brachial or lumbosacral plexus causes a painful radiculopathy.

| |
|---|
| *Plexus* |
| Trauma |
| Malignant infiltration |
| Cervical rib |
| Neuralgic amyotrophy |
| |
| *Nerve root* |
| Trauma |
| Herpes zoster |
| Meningeal inflammation (e.g. syphilis) |
| Tumours (neurofibroma, metastases) |
| Cervical and lumbar spondylosis |

**Table 18.55** Principal causes of plexus and nerve root lesions.

A common example is an apical bronchial neoplasm (Pancoast's tumour) that causes a T1 lesion and involves the sympathetic outflow. There is wasting of the small muscles of the hand, pain and sensory loss in areas supplied by T1 and ipsilateral Horner's syndrome. This condition also occasionally occurs in apical tuberculosis.

## Cervical and lumbar spondylosis (see Table 8.23)

Spondylosis describes the degenerative changes within vertebrae and intervertebral discs that occur during ageing or secondarily to trauma or rheumatoid disease. The changes are common in the lower cervical and lower lumbar region.

Several, often related, factors are important in producing signs and symptoms, including:

- Osteophytes—local overgrowth of bone
- Congenital narrowing of the spinal canal
- Disc degeneration with posterior or lateral disc protrusion
- Ischaemic changes in the cord and nerve roots

The commoner clinical syndromes will be described. In all these syndromes MRI is now the investigation of choice, if available, replacing myelography.

### Lateral cervical disc protrusion (Fig. 18.22)

The patient complains of pain in the upper limb. A C7 protrusion is the commonest lesion. There is root pain (see p. 898), which radiates into the affected myotome (scapula, triceps and forearm extensors in a C7 lesion) and a sensory disturbance (tingling, numbness) in the affected dermatome. There is weakness and, later, wasting of muscles innervated by the affected root (triceps and finger extensors in a C7 lesion) and reflexes using this root will be lost (the triceps jerk in a C7 lesion).

Although the initial pain is often severe, most cases recover with rest and analgesics. It is usual to immobilize the neck in a collar. Plain X-rays of the cervical spine (oblique views) show encroachment into the exit foraminae by osteophytes. In cases where recovery is delayed,

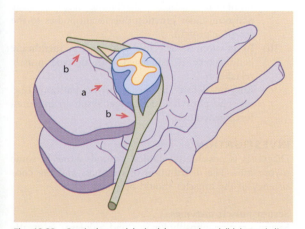

**Fig. 18.22**   Cervical spondylosis: (a) central and (b) lateral disc protrusion.

root compression may be demonstrated with MRI or myelography and surgical root decompression performed.

### Central cervical disc protrusion (cervical myelopathy)

Posterior disc protrusion (see Fig. 18.22), which is common at C4/5, C5/6 and C6/7 levels, causes spinal cord compression (see p. 898). Congenital narrowing of the canal, osteophytic bars and ischaemia are contributory factors.

The patient complains of difficulty in walking. Frequently there are no symptoms in the neck. A spastic paraparesis (or tetraparesis) is found, with variable sensory loss. A reflex level in the upper limbs and evidence of lateral disc protrusion may coexist.

Plain films may show narrowing of the sagittal diameter of the spinal canal and osteophytes but the changes correlate poorly with signs and symptoms. MRI or myelography is necessary to demonstrate the level and extent of cord compression.

Cervical laminectomy or anterior fusion of the vertebral bodies with removal of the disc may be necessary when the cord compression is severe or progressive. The results of surgery are often disappointing. Recovery of the 'pyramidal' signs is unusual, although progression may be halted.

A collar should be fitted. Manipulation of the neck should be avoided.

### Thoracic disc protrusion

Central protrusion of a thoracic disc is a rare cause of paraparesis.

### Lateral lumbar disc protrusion

The L5 and S1 roots are commonly compressed by lateral prolapse of the L4/5 and L5/S1 discs, respectively. There is low back pain and 'sciatica' (pain radiating down the buttock and lower limb). The onset may be acute and follow lifting a heavy weight, or may be subacute and apparently unrelated to exercise.

Straight leg raising is limited. There may be loss of reflexes (ankle jerk in an S1 root lesion or knee jerk in an L4/5 lesion) and weakness of plantar flexion (S1) or extension of the great toe (L5). Sensory loss may be found in the affected dermatome.

Plain films of the lumbar spine show narrowing of the disc space, osteophytes or a narrow canal. Unsuspected malignancy or infection may be demonstrated.

Most cases resolve with rest and analgesics. In the minority, MRI or myelography is necessary and laminectomy is indicated when a root lesion is shown.

### Central lumbar disc protrusion (cauda equina syndrome)

A central disc protrusion causes a lesion of the cauda equina with back pain, weakness of the lower limbs, sacral numbness, retention of urine, impotence and areflexia. Many nerve roots are involved.

The onset is either acute (a cause of an acute flaccid paraparesis) or chronic, when intermittent claudication occurs.

Neoplasms in the lumbosacral region cause a similar picture.

The condition should be suspected if a patient with back pain develops retention of urine. Urgent MRI or myelography followed by decompression is indicated.

### Spinal stenosis

Narrowing of the lumbar spinal canal produces back pain (see p. 418) and is an important cause of buttock claudication. Congenital narrowing of the cervical canal predisposes to cervical myelopathy from minor disc protrusion.

# Non-metastatic manifestations of malignancy

Many neurological syndromes may accompany malignancy. Clinical pictures include:

- Sensorimotor neuropathy
- Cerebellar syndrome
- Dementia and encephalopathy
- Myasthenic–myopathic syndrome (Eaton–Lambert syndrome)
- Progressive multifocal leucoencephalopathy
- Mononeuritis multiplex
- Cranial polyneuropathy
- MND variants
- Spastic paraparesis

The cause of most of these remains obscure. The clinical importance is that the neurological syndrome sometimes precedes clinical recognition of the neoplasm, which is often a small-cell carcinoma of the bronchus or a lymphoma. The neurological signs may recede if the tumour is resected or treated.

# Diseases of voluntary muscle

Weakness is the predominant feature of a myopathy. Its distribution and pattern is of diagnostic importance. A classification of muscle disease is given in Table 18.56. Only the more common conditions are mentioned below.

### PATHOPHYSIOLOGY

Muscle fibres are affected by:

1 Acute inflammation and fibre necrosis (e.g. polymyositis)
2 Chronic degeneration of muscle fibres (e.g. Duchenne muscular dystrophy)
3 Regeneration and fibre hypertrophy

**Acquired myopathies**

*Inflammatory myopathy*
Polymyositis
  Alone
  With skin lesions (dermatomyositis)
  With collagen disease
  With malignancy
Viral, bacterial and parasitic infection
Sarcoidosis

*Metabolic and endocrine myopathy, due to:*
Corticosteroids/Cushing's syndrome
Thyroid disease
Calcium metabolism disorders
Hypokalaemia
Ethanol
Drugs

*Myasthenic disorders*
Myasthenia gravis
Myasthenic–myopathic (Eaton–Lambert) syndrome

**Genetically determined myopathies**

*Muscular dystrophies*
Duchenne muscular dystrophy
Facio-scapulo-humeral dystrophy
Limb girdle dystrophy

*Myotonias*
Dystrophia myotonica
Myotonia congenita

*Periodic paralyses*
Hypokalaemic
Hyperkalaemic
Normokalaemic

*Specific metabolic myopathies, e.g.*
Myophosphorylase deficiency
Other defects of glycogen and fatty acid metabolism
Mitochondrial disease (ragged red muscle fibres)
Malignant hyperpyrexia

**Table 18.56** Classification of muscle disease.

4 Complex immune and metabolic disorders. For example:
  (a) In myasthenia gravis, there is a reduction in the number of available acetylcholine receptors at the neuromuscular junction due to antibodies to the receptor protein.
  (b) In myotonias, defective chloride ion membrane conductance is associated with delayed muscle relaxation.
  (c) Enzyme defects in the glycolytic pathway (e.g. myophosphorylase deficiency) result in impaired force generation.

### INVESTIGATION

Diagnosis is possible on clinical grounds alone in some myopathies. The distribution of weakness and the consistency of the muscles should be noted.

#### Serum muscle enzymes

Serum creatine phosphokinase (and aldolase) is greatly elevated in many dystrophies (e.g. Duchenne muscular dystrophy) and in inflammatory disorders of muscle (e.g. polymyositis). These enzymes are normal in myasthenia, and are usually normal in myotonias and chronic partial denervation.

### Electromyography

When a muscle is weak the normal interference pattern is reduced. An electromyogram is useful to distinguish between primary muscle disease and denervation (e.g. MND). The principal abnormalities are:

MYOPATHY. Short duration 'spiky' polyphasic muscle action potentials are seen. Spontaneous fibrillation is occasionally recorded.

DENERVATION. Fibrillation potentials of about 1 ms in duration and 50–200 $\mu$V in amplitude are seen, and are evidence of reinnervation.

OTHER CHANGES. Myotonic discharges (in myotonias) consist of high-frequency activity that varies repeatedly to cause a characteristic sound on the loudspeaker.

In myasthenia gravis a characteristic decrement in the evoked muscle action potential follows stimulation of the motor nerve. The reverse is seen (an increment in repetitive response) in the rare myasthenic–myopathic syndrome (Eaton–Lambert syndrome), which may accompany carcinoma of the bronchus.

### Muscle biopsy

Information about muscle fibre types (type 1, slow; type 2, fast), denervation, inflammation, dystrophic changes and muscle histochemistry is obtained by muscle biopsy. Electron microscopy is sometimes necessary.

In chronic partial denervation, 'fibre type grouping', i.e. groups of atrophic fibres of the same fibre type, is seen. Hypertrophic fibres also occur. In acute denervation, small angulated fibres are seen scattered randomly between normal fibres. In dystrophies and myositis, the muscle fibres are diffusely abnormal, the nuclei become central, and invasion by inflammatory cells and/or necrosis occurs.

Considerable experience is required to assess these changes accurately.

# INFLAMMATORY MYOPATHIES

## Polymyositis

This group of disorders is characterized by non-suppurative inflammation of skeletal muscle. The muscles are weak and usually painful. In many cases there are skin changes (dermatomyositis, see p. 404) or other connective tissue diseases (see p. 400).

### CLINICAL FEATURES

'Polymyositis alone' is a rare disease, most common in the fourth and fifth decades. Symptoms are of difficulty in rising from a chair, climbing stairs or lifting. Weakness is typically proximal. The weak muscles ache and are sometimes tender and indurated.

As the disease progresses there may be widespread weakness and wasting, with dysphagia, respiratory muscle weakness and cardiac involvement.

### INVESTIGATION

Preliminary investigations show a raised ESR and a mild normochromic normocytic anaemia. ANF is sometimes positive. The serum creatine phosphokinase is usually (but not always) elevated.

The electromyogram shows myopathic changes. Occasionally fibrillation potentials occur and may cause diagnostic difficulty.

Muscle biopsy shows inflammatory changes with infiltration of the muscle by mononuclear cells.

### DIFFERENTIAL DIAGNOSIS

Muscular dystrophies rarely progress as rapidly as polymyositis and there is no muscle pain. Pseudohypertrophy does not occur in polymyositis and there is no family history.

MND is always eventually accompanied by upper motor neurone signs, and prominent fasciculation is common.

### TREATMENT

Corticosteroids and/or azathioprine or cyclophosphamide reduce the symptoms in about 75% of cases. Only rarely does the disease progress to cause grave disability or death from respiratory failure or cardiac involvement.

## Other inflammatory myopathies

Muscle pain and weakness occur in trichinosis due to the ingestion of pork infected with *Trichinella spiralis*.

Acute myositis also occurs with Coxsackievirus infections (see p. 51) and in several other infections.

Tropical pyomyositis of Central Africa is suppurative inflammation of muscle caused by staphylococci and other organisms.

An inflammatory myopathy may occur in sarcoidosis.

# METABOLIC AND ENDOCRINE MYOPATHIES

### Corticosteroids and Cushing's syndrome

Proximal muscle weakness occurs with prolonged high-dose steroid therapy (particularly with $9\alpha$-fluorinated steroids such as dexamethasone and triamcinolone) and in Cushing's syndrome. Selective type-2 fibre atrophy is seen on muscle biopsy.

### Thyroid disease (see p. 800)

Several muscle diseases may occur:

THYROTOXICOSIS is sometimes accompanied by a severe proximal myopathy. There is also an association between thyrotoxicosis and myasthenia gravis, and between thyrotoxicosis and hypokalaemic periodic paralysis. Both associations are seen more frequently in South East Asia.

IN OPHTHALMIC GRAVES' DISEASE, there is swelling and lymphocytic infiltration of the extraocular muscles (see p. 807).

HYPOTHYROIDISM is sometimes associated with muscle pain and stiffness, resembling myotonia. A true proximal myopathy also occurs.

### Disorders of calcium metabolism

Proximal myopathy may occur in osteomalacia of any cause (see p. 425).

### Hypokalaemia

Acute hypokalaemia (e.g. in diuretic therapy) causes a severe flaccid paralysis (periodic paralysis, see p. 510) that is reversed by correcting the electrolyte disturbance.

Chronic mild hypokalaemia (also commonly caused by diuretics) gives rise to a mild, mainly proximal, weakness.

### Alcohol

Severe myopathy with muscle pain, necrosis and myoglobinuria occurs in acute alcoholic excess. (A similar syndrome occurs in diamorphine and amphetamine addicts.) A subacute proximal myopathy occurs with chronic alcohol abuse.

### Drugs

Many drug-induced muscle disorders have been described (Table 18.57). Most respond to drug withdrawal.

## DISORDERS OF THE NEUROMUSCULAR JUNCTION

## Myasthenia gravis

This acquired condition is characterized by weakness and fatiguability of proximal limb, ocular and bulbar muscles. The heart is not affected.

The cause is unknown. IgG antibodies to acetylcholine receptor protein are found. Immune complexes (IgG and complement) are deposited at the postsynaptic membranes causing interference with and later destruction of the acetylcholine receptor.

Thymic hyperplasia is found in 70% of myasthenic

patients below the age of 40 years. In 10% of patients a thymic tumour is found, the incidence increasing with age; antibodies to striated muscle can be demonstrated in these patients. Young patients without a thymoma have an increased association with HLA-B8, DR3.

There is an association between myasthenia gravis and thyroid disease, rheumatoid disease, pernicious anaemia and SLE. Myasthenia gravis is sometimes caused by D-penicillamine treatment in rheumatoid disease.

The prevalence is about 4 in 100 000. It is twice as common in women as in men, with a peak incidence around the age of 30 years.

### CLINICAL FEATURES

Fatiguability is the single most important feature. The proximal limb muscles, the extraocular muscles, and the muscles of mastication, speech and facial expression are those commonly affected in the early stages. Respiratory difficulties may occur.

Complex extraocular palsies, ptosis and a typical fluctuating proximal weakness are found. The reflexes are initially preserved but may be fatiguable. Muscle wasting is sometimes seen late in the disease.

### INVESTIGATION

The clinical picture of fluctuating weakness may be diagnostic but many cases are initially diagnosed as 'hysterical'.

### Tensilon (edrophonium) test

Edrophonium (an anticholinesterase) 10 mg i.v. is injected as a bolus after a test dose of 1–2 mg. Improvement in weakness occurs within seconds and lasts for 2–3 min when the test is positive. To be certain it is wise to have an observer present and to perform a control test using an injection of saline.

Occasionally the test itself causes bronchial constriction and syncope. It should not therefore be carried out where there are no facilities for resuscitation.

### Serum acetylcholine receptor antibodies

These are present in 90% of cases of generalized myasthenia gravis. The antibodies are found in no other condition.

### Nerve stimulation

There is a characteristic decrement in the evoked muscle action potential following stimulation of the motor nerve.

### Other tests

Preliminary tests may show a mediastinal mass on chest X-ray that can be confirmed by mediastinal CT scanning.

Routine peripheral blood studies are normal (the ESR is not raised). Autoantibodies to striated muscle, intrinsic factor or thyroid may be found. Rheumatoid factor and antinuclear antibody tests may be positive.

Muscle biopsy is usually not performed but ultrastructural abnormalities can be seen.

| Disorder | Drugs responsible |
|---|---|
| Subacute proximal myopathy | Diamorphine |
| | Clofibrate |
| | Chloroquine |
| | Lithium |
| | Quinine |
| Myasthenic syndromes | D-Penicillamine |
| | Lithium |
| | Propranolol |
| Malignant hyperpyrexia | Psychotropic drugs |
| | General anaesthetics |

**Table 18.57** Drug-induced muscle disorders.

## COURSE AND MANAGEMENT

The severity of myasthenia gravis fluctuates but most cases have a protracted course. It is important to recognize respiratory impairment, dysphagia and nasal regurgitation; emergency assisted ventilation may be required in myasthenic crises.

Exacerbations are usually unpredictable but may be brought on by infections, by aminoglycosides or other drugs. Enemas (magnesium sulphate) may provoke severe weakness.

### Oral anticholinesterases

Pyridostigmine (60 mg tablet) is the most widely used drug. Its duration of action is 3–4 hours. The dose (usually 4–16 tablets daily) is determined by the patient's response. This drug prolongs the action of acetylcholine by inhibiting the action of the enzyme cholinesterase.

Overdose of anticholinesterase causes severe weakness (cholinergic crisis).

Colic and diarrhoea may occur with anticholinesterases. Oral atropine 0.5 mg with each dose may reduce this.

Although anticholinesterases are of value in treating the weakness, they do not alter the natural history of the disease.

### Thymectomy

Thymectomy offers long-term benefit, though the reason is uncertain. It improves the prognosis, particularly in patients below 40 years with positive receptor antibodies and in those who have had the disease for less than 10 years.

Following thymectomy, some 60% of non-thymoma cases improve. If a thymoma is present, surgery is necessary to remove a potentially malignant tumour, but it is unusual for the myasthenia to improve.

### Immunosuppressant drugs

Corticosteroids are used when there is an incomplete response to anticholinesterases. There is improvement in 70% of cases, although this may be preceded by an initial relapse.

Azathioprine (and sometimes plasmapheresis) is combined with prednisolone in steroid-resistant cases.

## Myasthenic–myopathic syndrome (Eaton–Lambert syndrome)

This is a rare non-metastatic manifestation of small-cell carcinoma of the bronchus. There is defective acetylcholine release at the neuromuscular junction. Proximal muscle weakness, sometimes involving the ocular and bulbar muscles, is found, with absent reflexes. Weakness tends to improve after muscular contraction (unlike myasthenia gravis).

## Other myasthenic syndromes

Other rare myasthenic syndromes occur, for example congenital myasthenia.

# MUSCULAR DYSTROPHIES

These are progressive, genetically determined disorders of skeletal and sometimes cardiac muscle.

## Duchenne muscular dystrophy (DMD)

This is inherited as an X-linked recessive disorder, but one-third of cases arise by spontaneous mutation. It occurs in 1 in 3000 male infants. Recently the DMD locus has been localized to the Xp21 region of the X chromosome and the disease is characterized by the absence of the gene product—the protein dystrophin, which is a rod-shaped cytoskeletal protein found in muscle. DMD is usually obvious by the fourth year, and causes death by the age of 20 years.

### CLINICAL FEATURES

The boy has difficulty in running and in rising to an erect position, when he has to 'climb up his legs with his hands' (Gowers' sign).

There is initially a proximal limb weakness with pseudohypertrophy of the calves. The myocardium is affected. The boy becomes severely disabled by 10 years.

### INVESTIGATION

The diagnosis is often made on clinical grounds alone.

The creatine phosphokinase is grossly elevated (100–200 times the normal level). Muscle biopsy shows characteristic variation in fibre size, fibre necrosis, regeneration and replacement by fat, and on immunochemical staining an absence of dystrophin. The electromyogram shows a myopathic pattern.

### MANAGEMENT

There is no curative treatment. Passive physiotherapy helps to prevent contractures in the later stages of the disease. A trial of prednisolone therapy has shown a short-term improvement in muscle strength and function.

### Carrier detection

A female with an affected brother has a 50% chance of carrying the gene. In carrier females, 70% have a raised creatine phosphokinase level and the remainder usually have electromyographic abnormalities or changes on biopsy. Accurate carrier and prenatal diagnosis can be made using cDNA probes that are co-inherited with the DMD locus.

Genetic advice explaining the inheritance of the condition and counselling about abortion should be given. Determination of the fetal sex by amniocentesis and selective abortion of a male fetus is sometimes carried out. Many proven carrier females choose not to have offspring.

## Limb girdle and facio-scapulo-humeral dystrophy

These milder dystrophies are summarized in Table 18.58. There are many other varieties of muscular dystrophy.

|  | Limb girdle | Facio-scapulo-humeral |
| --- | --- | --- |
| Inheritance: | Autosomal recessive | Autosomal dominant |
| Onset: | 10–20 years | 10–40 years |
| Muscles affected: | Shoulder and pelvic girdle | Face, shoulder and pelvic girdle |
| Progress: | Severe disability within 20–25 years | Normal life expectancy, slow progression |
| Pseudohypertrophy: | Rare | Very rare |

**Table18.58**  Limb girdle and facio-scapulo-humeral dystrophies.

# MYOTONIAS

These conditions are characterized by myotonia, i.e. continued muscle contraction after the cessation of voluntary effort. The electromyogram is characteristic (see p. 951). The myotonias are important because patients tolerate general anaesthetics poorly. The commonest two of these rare conditions are mentioned below.

## Dystrophia myotonica

This autosomal dominant condition causes progressive distal muscle weakness, with ptosis, weakness and thinning of the face and sternomastoids. Myotonia is usually present. The muscle disease is part of a larger syndrome comprising:
- Cataracts
- Frontal baldness
- Intellectual impairment (mild)
- Cardiomyopathy and conduction defects
- Small pituitary fossa and hypogonadism
- Glucose intolerance
- Low serum IgG

The onset of obvious clinical disease is usually between 20 and 50 years. The condition is gradually progressive. Phenytoin or procainamide sometimes helps the myotonia.

## Myotonia congenita (Thomsen's disease)

This is an autosomal dominant disorder. An isolated myotonia, usually mild, occurs in childhood and persists throughout life. The myotonia is accentuated by rest and by cold. Diffuse muscle hypertrophy occurs and the patient appears to have well-developed muscles.

# PERIODIC PARALYSES

These are rare membrane disorders characterized by intermittent flaccid muscle weakness and alterations in serum potassium.

## Hypokalaemic periodic paralysis

This condition, usually inherited as an autosomal dominant trait, is characterized by generalized weakness (including the speech and bulbar muscles) that often starts after a heavy carbohydrate meal or after a period of rest after exertion. Attacks last for several hours. It is often first noted in the teenage years and tends to remit after the age of 35 years. The serum potassium is usually below 3.0 mmol litre$^{-1}$ in an attack. The weakness responds to the administration of potassium chloride.

Similar weakness also occurs in hypokalaemia due to diuretics, and may occur during thyrotoxicosis.

## Hyperkalaemic periodic paralysis

This condition, usually inherited as an autosomal dominant trait, is characterized by sudden attacks of weakness that are sometimes precipitated by exercise. Attacks start in childhood and tend to remit after the age of 20 years. They last from 30 min to 2 hours. Myotonia may occur. The serum potassium is raised.

The attacks are terminated by intravenous calcium gluconate or chloride.

A very rare normokalaemic, sodium-responsive periodic paralysis also occurs.

# SPECIFIC METABOLIC MYOPATHIES

This is a large group of rare, genetically determined muscle diseases. Two of these diseases will be mentioned here.

## Myophosphorylase deficiency (McArdle's syndrome)

This is an autosomal recessive disorder in which there is a lack of skeletal muscle myophosphorylase. The disorder causes easy fatiguability and severe cramp on exercise, with myoglobinuria.

There is no rise in venous lactate during ischaemic exercise; this forms the basis of a test for the condition.

## Malignant hyperpyrexia

Widespread skeletal muscle rigidity and hyperpyrexia developing as a sequel to general anaesthesia is due to a genetic defect in the calcium release channel of the sarcoplasmic reticulum. Sudden death during or after anaesthesia may occur in this rare condition, which is sometimes inherited as an autosomal dominant trait. Dantrolene is useful in controlling the rigidity.

# Further reading

Brain (1986) *Aids to the Examination of the Peripheral Nervous System*, 3rd edn. London: Baillière Tindall.

Bannister R (1992) *Brain and Bannister's Clinical Neurology*, 7th edn. Oxford: Oxford University Press.

Patten J (1977) *Neurological Differential Diagnosis*. London: Harold Starke.

Hopkins AP (1993) *Clinical Neurology, a Modern Approach*. Oxford: Oxford University Press.

*Lancet* (1990) Epilepsy Octet Recent reviews.

*Lancet* (1993) Stroke Octet. **339**.

Swash M (1989) *Hutchinson's Clinical Methods*, 19th edn. London: Baillière Tindall.

# Psychological medicine

## Introduction and general aspects

Psychiatry is the branch of medicine that is concerned with the study and treatment of disorders of mental function. A substantial proportion of patients seen by a doctor suffer from psychiatric illness rather than organic disease. Some of these psychiatric problems occur as a consequence of individual social circumstances that may be difficult to alter. Physical and psychiatric disorders often coincide because:

- Patients with psychiatric problems can present with physical manifestations (e.g. abdominal pain in the irritable bowel syndrome).
- Chronic or severe physical ill-health can result in a psychiatric disorder (e.g. depression in the setting of chronic pain).
- Psychiatric symptoms can be part of a physical disease complex (e.g. depression in hypothyroidism).
- Patients with established psychiatric disorders can also develop physical disease.

For these reasons, the psychological aspects of disease cannot be the exclusive preserve of psychiatrists but must be the concern of all doctors.

### EPIDEMIOLOGY

In primary care in the UK approximately 15% of attenders suffer from psychiatric ill-health. Most of the illnesses are minor mood disorders, taking the form of various combinations of depression and anxiety, and about two-thirds are short-lived in nature and clear within 6 months. However, about 5% of primary care consultations involve patients suffering from major depression requiring energetic treatment. The major psychoses—schizophrenia and manic-depressive illness—are much less common in this setting. The general hospital physician and surgeon will tend to see psychiatric disorders that are associated with physical disease or caused by certain physical treatments as well as disorders related to alcohol and other forms of drug use and abuse.

About 25% of all those referred to psychiatric departments are aged 65 years and over; this includes patients with disorders such as depression and confusional states, which may be reversible, and dementias, which usually are not. It has been estimated that in England about half a million people over 65 years suffer from moderate or severe dementia, and about one-quarter of these are aged 85 years or more.

### COMMUNITY PSYCHIATRY

During the nineteenth century the rise of psychiatry resulted in a remarkable growth in mental asylums. Today these mental hospitals are being closed and patients are being discharged to community-based facilities, e.g. hostels, supervised accommodation and rehabilitation facilities. This *community care* has led to the integration of psychiatry into the community, but there is some anxiety that chronic psychiatric patients end up sleeping rough or occupying low-grade accommodation. Thus the closure of mental hospitals must be accompanied by the simultaneous development of community facilities linked to a hospital inpatient service.

## The psychiatric interview

The interview is of prime importance in making a psychiatric diagnosis:

- It is a technique for obtaining information.
- It serves as a standard situation in which to assess the patient's emotions and attitudes.
- The first interview serves to establish an understanding with the patient that will be the basis of any subsequent therapeutic relationship.

## The psychiatric history

The history records data from several sources. These include the patient's complaints, recent and remote past history and their present life situation up to the time of referral or admission.

The history consists of:

REASON FOR REFERRAL—a brief statement of why and how the patient came to the attention of the doctor

COMPLAINTS—as reported by the patient

PRESENT ILLNESS—a detailed account of the illness from the earliest time at which a change was noted until the patient came to the attention of the doctor, and the degree to which the illness is recognized by the patient (insight)

FAMILY HISTORY—this should focus on the family atmosphere in the patient's childhood, early stresses (including death or separation) and the occurrence of mental illness in family members

PERSONAL HISTORY—a short biography that covers childhood and school, jobs held and lost, marriage and divorce, children, and the present housing, social and financial situation

PERSONALITY—this consists of a person's attitudes and beliefs, moral values and standards, leisure activities and interests and usual reaction to stress and setback

MEDICAL HISTORY—this includes health during childhood, menstrual history, previous mental health and the use and abuse of alcohol, tobacco and drugs

Supplementary information should be obtained from a close relative or friend who can provide corroboration and additional details.

# SYMPTOMS AND SIGNS OF A PSYCHIATRIC DISORDER

## Appearance and general behaviour

Facial appearance, posture and movement provide information about a patient's mood. Patients with retarded depression sit with shoulders hunched, immobile, and with the gaze directed at the floor. Agitated depressives are often tremulous and restless, adjusting their clothing and pacing up and down, while manic patients are often overactive and disinhibited.

Certain uncommon disorders of behaviour are encountered, mainly in schizophrenia. These include the following:

STEREOTYPY is repetition of movements that do not appear to have a purpose; the movement may be repeated in a regular sequence (e.g. rocking backwards and forwards).

MANNERISMS are repeated movements that appear to have some functional significance (e.g. saluting).

NEGATIVISM is when patients do the opposite of what is asked and actively resist efforts to persuade them to comply.

ECHOPRAXIA is when patients automatically imitate the interviewer's movements despite being asked not to do this.

## Speech

Disorders of thinking are usually recognized from the patient's speech.

### Disorders of the stream of thought

There are abnormalities in the amount and speed of the thoughts experienced. At one extreme, there is *pressure of thought*, in which ideas arise in remarkable abundance and variety and pass rapidly through the mind. *Poverty of thought* is the opposite experience, when there appears to be a lack or absence of any thoughts whatsoever and

patients report their minds to be blank or starved of ideas. Pressure of thought characteristically occurs in mania, and poverty of thought in depression; either may be experienced in schizophrenia. The stream of thought can also be suddenly interrupted. Minor degrees of this phenomenon are not uncommon, especially in normal people who are tired or tense.

Severe thought blocking, in which there is a particularly abrupt and complete interruption of the stream of thought, strongly suggests schizophrenia. Patients often describe the experience as a sudden and complete emptying of their minds and may interpret the experience in an unusual way (e.g. as having had their thoughts removed by some alien person, presence or machine).

### Disorders of the form of thought

These include flight of ideas, perseveration, and loosening of associations.

FLIGHT OF IDEAS. The patient's thoughts and speech move quickly from one topic to another, such that one train of thought is not completed before another appears. It is often accompanied by *clang associations* (the tendency to use two or more words with a similar sound), *punning* (the use of one word with two or more different meanings), rhyming, and responding to distracting cues in the immediate surroundings. Flight of ideas is characteristic of mania.

PERSEVERATION. This is the persistent and inappropriate repetition of the same thoughts or actions. It is often associated with dementia but can occur in other conditions.

LOOSENING OF ASSOCIATIONS. This is manifested by a loss of the normal structure of thinking. The most striking impression is an extreme lack of clarity. There are several forms. *Knight's move* or *derailment* denotes transition from one topic to another, either between sentences or within a sentence, with no logical relationship between the two topics and no evidence of flight of ideas as described above. When this abnormality is extreme and disrupts not merely the connections between sentences but also the finer grammatical structure of speech, it is termed *word salad* or *verbigeration*. One effect of loosened associations is sometimes termed talking past the point; the patient always seems to get near to talking about the matter in hand but never quite gets there.

## Mood

In psychiatric disorders, mood may be altered in three ways:
1 Its nature may be changed.
2 It may fluctuate more than usual.
3 It may be inconsistent either with the patient's thoughts and actions or with occurrences in the patient's immediate environment.

### Changes in the nature of mood

Changes in the nature of mood may be towards depression, anxiety or elation.

DEPRESSION may mean the symptom of feeling sad, melancholic or low in spirits, or it may mean the syndrome of depression as characterized by low mood, lack of enjoyment, reduced energy and changes in appetite, sleep and libido.

ANXIETY is a common symptom of worry or apprehension that is often accompanied by physical symptoms such as palpitations, trembling, butterflies in the stomach and hyperventilation.

ANXIETY AND DEPRESSION can occur separately or together and may be associated with an obvious cause or may appear to arise without reason.

ELATION refers to a subjective feeling of high spirits, vitality and even ecstasy, which may or may not be accompanied by exuberant behaviour, increased energy and overactivity.

PHOBIA is an intense fear of a specific object, activity or situation coupled with a wish to avoid it. The fear is irrational in that it is out of all proportion to the real danger. The patient recognizes that it is an exaggerated fear but finds it difficult to control. Objects that provoke such fear include insects, spiders and other animals (e.g. dogs, cats and horses) or natural phenomena such as lightning or the dark. Situations that provoke phobic reactions include open spaces (agoraphobia), closed spaces such as lifts and underground trains (claustrophobia), high places, and crowds.

### Changes in the fluctuation of mood

These may result in a total loss of emotion or an inability to experience pleasure. The former is termed *apathy*. When the normal variation of mood is reduced rather than lost, the mood is described as *blunted*. Emotions that are changeable in a rapid, abrupt and excessive way are termed *labile* emotions.

### Inconsistent or inappropriate mood

This occurs when the normal emotional expression of the person fails to match his thoughts and actions. For example, a patient may laugh when describing the death of a close and loved relative. Such incongruity needs to be distinguished from laughter that indicates that someone is ill at ease when talking about a distressing subject.

Changes of mood are found in a variety of psychiatric disorders, including depression, mania, anxiety, organic psychoses and schizophrenia.

## Thought content

Thought content refers to the worries and preoccupations manifested by the patient and elicited on interview. Abnormal beliefs and experiences are, of course, part of the thought content, but are regarded as sufficiently important to be discussed separately (see below).

An *obsession*, is a recurrent, persistent thought, impulse or image that enters the mind despite the individual's effort to resist it. The individual recognizes that the obsession is self-generated and is not implanted by anyone nor arises from elsewhere.

A *compulsion* is a repetitive and seemingly purposeful action performed in a stereotyped way, referred to as a compulsive ritual. Compulsions are accompanied by a subjective sense that they must be carried out and by an urge to resist. Common obsessions concern dirt, contamination, orderliness and dread of illness, while corresponding compulsions would be repeated hand-washings and checkings.

## Abnormal beliefs and interpretations of events

The main form of abnormal belief is the *delusion* (Information box 19.1). Delusions can be:

PRIMARY or autochthonous, i.e. they appear suddenly and with full conviction but without any preceding or related mental events. For example, a patient on being offered a cup of tea suddenly believes that this indicates that the Russians have landed at Dover.

SECONDARY, i.e. derived from some preceding morbid experience, such as a depressed mood or an auditory hallucination.

Delusions are classified according to their content, and include persecutory delusions (also called paranoid delusions), delusions of reference, guilt, worthlessness or nihilism, religious delusions, and delusions of grandeur, jealousy or control. These are further defined when discussed in relation to specific conditions.

Particular delusions concerning thought control can occur. Patients who have delusions of *thought insertion* believe that some of their thoughts are not their own but have been implanted by some outside force or agency. The same or other patients may believe that thoughts are taken out of their minds by external forces or agencies (*thought withdrawal*), while in delusions of *thought broadcasting* patients believe that their unspoken thoughts are known to other people through radio, television, telepathy or in some other way. Feelings and actions may also be interpreted by the individual as being under the influence or control of some external, usually alien, power. Such *passivity* experiences, occurring in the absence of clear-cut brain diseases, are regarded as diagnostic of schizophrenia. Patients may merely assert that their behaviour is controlled from without and may be unable to give any further explanation. This is usually described as an *experience of passivity*. Patients may develop secondary delusions that explain this alien control as a result of witchcraft, hypnosis, radio waves, television—so-called

This is defined as an abnormal belief arising from distorted judgements and that is:

Held with absolute conviction
Not amenable to reason or modifiable by experience
Not shared by those of a common cultural or social background
Experienced as a self-evident truth of great personal significance
False

**Information box 19.1**   Delusion.

This is defined as a thorough conviction of a sensation when no external object to excite or provoke such a sensation is present. It is:

A false perception and not a distortion
Perceived as inhabiting objective space
Perceived as having qualities of normal perceptions
Perceived alongside normal perceptions
Independent of the individual's will

**Information box 19.2**   Hallucination.

*delusions of passivity.* The disturbances of thought control discussed above are examples of passivity experiences involving the thought processes.

Delusions should be distinguished from *overvalued* ideas, i.e. deeply held personal convictions that are understandable when the individual's background is known. *Ideas of reference* that fall short of delusions are held by people who are particularly self-conscious. Such individuals cannot help feeling that people take particular notice of them in public places, pass comment about them and/or observe things about them that they would prefer were ignored. Such a feeling is not delusional in that individuals who experience it realize that it originates within themselves and that they are no more noticeable or noteworthy than anyone else, but nevertheless cannot dismiss the feeling.

## Abnormal experiences referred to the environment, body or self

*Illusions* are misperceptions of external stimuli and are most likely to occur when the general level of sensory stimulation is reduced.

*Hallucinations* (Information box 19.2) are perceptions that are experienced in the absence of any external stimulus to the sense organs in the outside world (and are not within one's mind as in imagery). Normal people occasionally experience hallucinations, mainly auditory in type, particularly when tired and during the transition between sleeping and waking.

Hallucinations can be *elementary* (e.g. bangs, whistles) or *complex* (e.g. faces, voices, music), and may be auditory, visual, tactile, gustatory, olfactory or of deep sensation.

A change in self-awareness such that the person concerned feels unreal is termed *depersonalization.* In this state the person feels detached or remote from self-experience and unable to feel emotion. The individual is aware of the subjective nature of this alteration. The feeling that the external environment has become unreal and/or remote is termed *derealization.* Both these phenomena occur in healthy people when they are tired, after sensory deprivation and during the use of hallucinogenic drugs, and also occur in certain conditions such as anxiety, depression, schizophrenia and temporal lobe epilepsy.

## Cognitive state (Table 19.1)

There are four processes involved in normal memory:
REGISTRATION —the ability to add new material to the existing memory stores
RETENTION —the ability to retain the memory
RECALL —the ability to bring it back into awareness
RECOGNITION —the feeling of familiarity indicating that a particular person, event or object has been encountered before
Some patients describe the recognition of a situation, person or event as having been encountered before when it is in fact novel—the so-called *déjà vu* experience, whereas

| Function | Questions |
|---|---|
| Orientation | What is the time/day/month/year? |
| | Where are you? What is this place? |
| | Whom do you recognize? |
| Concentration | Repeat months of the year backwards |
| | Take 7 serially from 100 (serial 7s) |
| | Repeat a span of digits (e.g. 5-figure: 43701; 6-figure: 732156) |
| *Memory* | |
| Short-term | Recall test name and address after 2 and 5 min |
| Medium/long-term | Current affairs (e.g. name of the prime minister, occupant of the throne, events in the news) |
| | Dates of World War II |
| Intelligence | Simple arithmetic sums |
| | Meanings of words |
| | Meanings of proverbs |
| | Ability to read and write |
| Higher cortical function | Spatial awareness—drawing 3D objects |
| | Naming of objects |
| | Right–left discrimination (Touch your left ear with your right hand) |

**Table 19.1**  Assessment of cognitive functions.

others report the reverse experience (*jamais vu*) when there is failure to recognize a situation, person or event that has been encountered before. *Déjà vu* experiences occur in healthy people as well as in anxiety states. Both types of experience can occur in epilepsy (see p. 913).

Patients with Wernicke–Korsakoff syndrome, who have extreme difficulty in remembering recent and past events, sometimes report remembering past events that have not actually taken place; this is known as *confabulation*. Failure of memory is termed *amnesia*.

Consciousness can be defined as the awareness of the self and the environment. Attention, concentration and memory are impaired and orientation is disturbed in any condition in which a disorder of consciousness occurs. This subject is considered on p. 901.

## Defence mechanisms

These are a series of subconscious mental processes. The individual is unaware of employing them although may become aware of such motives through self-analysis or demonstration by another person. The defence mechanisms described below are amongst the commonest used and are useful in understanding many aspects of behaviour.

REPRESSION is the exclusion from awareness of memories, emotions and/or impulses that would cause anxiety and distress if allowed to enter consciousness.

DENIAL, a related concept, is believed to be employed when patients behave as though unaware of something that they might reasonably be expected to know. One example would be a patient who, despite being told that a close relative has died, continues to behave as though the relative were still alive.

REGRESSION is the unconscious adoption of patterns of behaviour appropriate to an earlier stage of development. It is often seen in ill people who become childlike and highly dependent in relation to their doctor and nursing care.

PROJECTION involves the unconscious attribution to another person of thoughts or feelings that are in fact one's own.

REACTION FORMATION refers to the unconscious adoption of behaviour opposite to that which reflects the individual's true feelings and intentions.

DISPLACEMENT involves the transferring of emotion from a situation or object with which it is properly associated to another that gives less distress.

RATIONALIZATION refers to the unconscious process whereby a false but acceptable explanation is provided for behaviour that in fact has other, much less acceptable, origins.

SUBLIMATION refers to the unconscious diversion of unacceptable outlets into acceptable outlets.

IDENTIFICATION refers to the unconscious process of taking on some of the characteristics or behaviours of another person, often to reduce the pain of separation or loss.

## Summary of symptoms and signs

When the full psychiatric history is taken and the patient's mental state has been assessed, it is important to provide a concise assessment of the case which is termed a *formulation*. In addition to summarizing the essential features, the formulation includes a differential diagnosis, a discussion of possible causal factors, identification of outstanding issues to be clarified, an outline of further investigations needed and concludes with a concise plan of treatment and a statement of the likely prognosis.

# CAUSES OF A PSYCHIATRIC DISORDER

A single psychiatric disorder may result from several causes.

## Predisposing factors

These are factors, often operating from early life, that determine a person's vulnerability to psychological distress. Such causes include:

- Genetic endowment
- Environment *in utero*
- Personality
- Childhood trauma

There is evidence for a strong genetic factor in the psychoses, and a weaker genetic factor in the neurotic disorders. Intrauterine disturbances may result in minor organic damage to the brain and central nervous system (CNS), which in turn may render the individual liable to develop a serious mental disorder in later life in response to particular kinds of stress.

Personality results from the interaction of genetic endowment, uterine development, early childhood experience and various physical, psychological and social influences manifesting themselves up to and including adolescence. Certain personalities are believed to be particularly prone to develop certain disorders. For example, individuals who manifest certain obsessional traits as part of their personality have an increased risk of developing depressive and obsessional illnesses, while anxious, apprehensive individuals are prone to develop a variety of neurotic disorders. When taking the history, particular care should be taken to assess whether the individual's personality was well developed and mature prior to the development of the illness, as this will be a major factor in determining the outcome of treatment and the prognosis.

## Precipitating factors

These are factors that occur shortly before the onset of a disorder and that appear to have caused it. They may be physical, psychological or social in nature. Whether they produce a disorder depends partly on their severity and partly on the presence of predisposing factors.

PHYSICAL precipitating factors include physical diseases (e.g. hypothyroidism, tumours, metabolic disorders) or drugs (e.g. steroids, hypotensives, alcohol).

PSYCHOLOGICAL factors include loss of self-esteem due to a setback or misfortune such as marital infidelity or financial disaster.

SOCIAL factors include moving house, job difficulties and family disturbances.

Occasionally, the same factor can act in more than one way. A head injury can induce psychological disturbances either through physical changes in the central nervous system or through the stress it provokes in the individual, while marital breakdown may lead to overindulgence in alcohol with secondary impairment of mental processes and psychiatric illness.

## Perpetuating factors

These are factors that prolong the course of a disorder after it has occurred. For example, some psychiatric disorders lead to secondary demoralization. A medical student who suffers a depressive illness may well find it difficult to accept the diagnosis, may feel weak and flawed, and may withdraw from social activities. Such a response could prolong the original disorder.

## PSYCHIATRIC ASPECTS OF PHYSICAL DISEASE

Psychological and physical symptoms commonly occur together; surveys have shown that they tend to cluster in some people, while others remain relatively free from illnesses. The commonest presentation of psychiatric ill-health in physically ill patients is as affective disorders or acute organic brain syndromes. The relationship between psychological and physical symptoms may be understood in one of three ways:

1 Psychological distress and disorder can provoke and precipitate physical disease.

2 Physical distress and disease can cause psychological ill-health (Table 19.2), as can the medication given for the disease.

3 Physical and psychological symptoms and disorders coexist because both are common, particularly in the elderly.

Physically ill patients often respond to their illness by feeling depressed, anxious, angry and/or unable to cope. Such reactions are very often transient and require little in the way of management other than recognition, reassurance and support. Sometimes, however, they persist after the acute stage of the physical illness has passed. Certain factors also increase the risk of a psychiatric disorder occurring in the setting of physical disease (Table 19.3). Treatment is the same as for physically healthy, psychiatrically ill patients, but care must be taken when prescribing psychotropic drugs to avoid drug interactions.

| Symptom | Examples of physical disease |
|---|---|
| Depression | Carcinoma |
| | Infection |
| | Thyroid disorders |
| | Adrenal disorders |
| | Diabetes mellitus |
| Anxiety | Hyperthyroidism |
| | Phaeochromocytoma |
| | Hypoglycaemia |
| | Partial seizures |
| | Alcohol/drug withdrawal |
| Irritability | Head injury |
| | Premenstrual tension |
| | Early dementia |
| | Hypoglycaemia |
| Fatigue | Anaemia |
| | Sleep disorders |
| | Infections |
| | Carcinoma |
| Behavioural disturbance | Epilepsy |
| | Toxic confusional states |
| | Dementia |
| | Porphyria |
| | Hypoglycaemia |

**Table 19.2** Psychiatric symptoms commonly associated with physical diseases.

*Patient*
Previous history of psychiatric illness
History of difficulty in coping with stress
Disturbed personal, family or social circumstances

*Setting*
Intensive care units
Coronary care units
Renal dialysis units

*Physical illness*
Carcinoma
Endocrine disorders
Infections
Metabolic disorders
Head injury
Mutilating surgery

*Physical treatment*
Drugs (e.g. steroids)
Radiotherapy

**Table 19.3** Factors increasing the risk of psychiatric illness in physically ill patients.

PAIN is one symptom that can be thought of as both physical and psychological. It is the commonest medical symptom, can cause considerable psychological distress and can arise from psychological disturbance. The main sites of psychologically determined pain are the head, the neck, the lower back, the abdomen and the genitalia.

Psychologically determined pain is often continuous for lengthy periods and responds poorly to analgesics. It is often described by the patient as waxing and waning in response to emotional stress and, despite its severity, does not necessarily wake the patient from sleep. A particularly dramatic form of chronic, atypical pain is facial pain; antidepressant therapy has been found to be effective in up to 50% of such patients. Another common painful condition in which depression is often present but is masked by the physical symptoms is the irritable bowel syndrome.

### Chronic fatigue syndrome

The cardinal symptoms are fatigue, poor concentration and memory, irritability, alteration in sleep and muscular aches. This syndrome, previously known as myalgic encephalomyelitis (ME), has been attributed to an infection, usually viral. There is, however, no good evidence of any infective cause of this condition at present and laboratory investigations are normal; many patients are depressed.

## CLASSIFICATION OF PSYCHIATRIC DISORDERS

The concept of mental illness is complicated. The diagnosis is only made when:

- There is a recognizable disturbance in one or more psychological functions, e.g. perception, emotion, thought.
- The disturbance is not under the comprehensive control of the individual concerned.
- The disturbance usually (though not invariably) causes distress to the affected individual.
- The disturbance usually (though not invariably) requires expert, professional assessment and treatment for recovery.

Particular problems in psychiatry are posed by such conditions as sexual disorders, drug and alcohol dependence and personality disorders. In 1980, the third edition of the *Diagnostic and Statistical Manual* of the American Psychiatric Association (DSM III) was published (revised 1987). This scheme has five axes. The two main axes are:

- Psychiatric syndromes
- Personality disorders

The others are:

- Physical disorders
- Severity of psychological stressors
- Highest level of adaptive functioning

The most recent revision of the *International Classification of Disease and Related Health Problems* (ICD-10) published by the World Health Organization includes a detailed classification of 300 psychiatric and behavioural disorders.

A simple classification of psychiatric disorders is shown in Table 19.4.

PSYCHOSIS is the term usually applied to a psychiatric disorder that significantly impairs insight, involves a substantial break with reality, exercises a major impact on the individual's personality and functioning, and which may require specialized, inpatient treatment. Certain

*Organic disorders (F00–F09)*

*Functional psychosis*
Schizophrenia (F20–29)
Manic-depressive disorder (F30–39)

*Neurotic disorders*
Phobic anxiety neurosis (F40)
Obsessive-compulsive disorder (F42)
Dissociative (conversion) disorders (F44)
Stress and adjustment reactions (F43)
Hypochondriacal disorders (F45)

*Personality disorders (F60–69)*

*Alcohol and drug abuse and dependence (F10–19)*

*Eating disorders (F50)*

———

The three-character codes refer to the diagnostic categories of the latest edition (the 10th) of the *International Classification of Diseases,* produced by the World Health Organization.

**Table 19.4** A classification of psychiatric disorders.

symptoms that by definition involve an impairment of reality, such as delusions, hallucinations and formal thought disorder, are often termed psychotic symptoms.

NEUROSIS is the term applied to psychiatric disorders in which psychotic symptoms and features are absent, the patient's personality is relatively undamaged, and contact with reality is unimpaired. Neuroses can be thought of as exaggerated forms of the normal reactions to stressful events. Anxiety, depression, irritability and physical symptoms lacking an organic cause are experienced by many people in response to stressful circumstances and events.

## *Organic psychiatric disorders*

Organic brain diseases result from structural pathology, as in senile dementia, or from disturbed CNS function, as in fever-induced delirium. A classification of organic brain syndromes, derived from the American classification, DSM III, is shown in Table 19.5.

Delirium
Dementia
Amnestic syndrome
Organic delusional syndrome
Organic affective syndrome
Intoxication and withdrawal syndromes

**Table 19.5** Classification of organic brain syndromes.

# Delirium

Delirium, also termed toxic confusional state, is an acute or subacute condition in which impairment of consciousness is accompanied by abnormalities of perception and mood. The impairment of consciousness can range from mild befuddlement to serious disorientation and confusion. The degree of impairment classically fluctuates, so that there are intermittent lucid periods. Confusion is usually worse at night. During the acute phase, thought and speech are incoherent, memory is impaired and misperceptions occur. Transient hallucinations, usually visual, and delusions may occur and, as a consequence, the patient may be frightened, suspicious, restless and unco-operative. A large number of diseases may be accompanied by delirium; this is particularly so in elderly patients. Some causes of delirium are listed in Table 19.6. Delirium usually clears within a few days as the underlying illness resolves. If the delirium runs a subacute course, more permanent disorders of cognition, memory or personality may occur.

## INVESTIGATION AND TREATMENT

Investigation and treatment of the underlying physical disease should be undertaken. The patient should be carefully nursed and rehydrated. Pain relief should be adequate and sedation provided if necessary. If a high fever is present, the temperature should be reduced with fans, ice-packs and antipyretic drugs. All current drug therapy should be reviewed and, where possible, stopped. Benzodiazepines are the drugs of choice in the management of minor restlessness, but in severe delirium haloperidol is probably a more effective choice, the daily dose usually ranging between 10 and 60 mg. If necessary, the first dose of 2–10 mg can be administered intramuscularly.

## MANAGEMENT OF THE DISTURBED OR VIOLENT PATIENT

Psychotic, organically impaired and intoxicated patients may be frightened, aggressive, confused and difficult to manage. It is important that those involved in their acute management refrain from threatening behaviour, appear in control (even if they do not feel it!) and avoid being drawn into a confrontation.

When evaluating a disturbed patient in the emergency department, a crucial question is: Could this behaviour be the result of an organic disturbance? Organic psychiatric disorders, particularly those associated with drugs and alcohol, are important causes of behavioural and thought disturbances in emergency clinic attenders. Some organic disorders initially showing signs and symptoms of psychosis, such as poisoning, meningitis and hypoxia, may be life-threatening. Treatment is with chlorpromazine in doses of 25–50 mg orally; i.m. haloperidol causes less hypotension and is an alternative.

# Dementia

Dementia is a syndrome due to disease of the brain in which there is a disturbance of multiple higher cortical functions, including memory, thinking, orientation, comprehension, calculation, learning capacity, language and judgement. However, consciousness is not clouded. There is often an associated deterioration in emotional control, social behaviour and motivation. Presenile dementia and early onset dementia are terms used for patients under 70 years of age and senile dementia for older patients; there is, however, no clinical difference.

About 25% of the elderly population suffer from a psychiatric disability, mainly anxiety and depression. However, dementia affects about 10% of those aged over 65 years and 20% of those over 80 years of age—a total of 650 000 people in England and Wales.

The causes of dementia are shown in Table 19.7; 70% are due to Alzheimer's disease.

DIFFERENTIAL DIAGNOSIS. This includes a depressive disorder which may exhibit many of the features of an early dementia, especially memory impairment, slowed thinking, and lack of spontaneity; delirium; mild or moderate retardation; iatrogenic mental disorders due to medication (Table 19.8).

## Alzheimer's disease

This is a primary degenerative cerebral disease of unknown aetiology. A relationship between the ingestion or

---

*Systemic infection*
Any infection, particularly with high fever (e.g. malaria, septicaemia)

*Metabolic disturbance*
Hepatic failure
Renal failure
Disorders of electrolyte balance
Hypoxia

*Vitamin deficiency*
Thiamine (Wernicke–Korsakoff syndrome, beriberi)
Nicotinic acid (pellagra)
Vitamin $B_{12}$

*Endocrine disease*
Hypoglycaemia

*Brain damage*
Trauma
Tumour
Abscess
Subarachnoid haemorrhage

*Drug intoxication*
Anticonvulsant
Anticholinergic
Anxiolytic/hypnotic
Opiates
Industrial poisons, e.g. DDT, trichloroethylene

*Drug/alcohol withdrawal*

---

DDT, dichlorodiphenyl trichloroethane.

**Table 19.6**   Some causes of delirium.

| Condition | Diagnostic features |
|---|---|
| Alzheimer's disease | Clinical history, CT scan |
| Hypothyroidism | Serum TSH and $T_4$ |
| Subacute combined degeneration of cord | MCV, blood picture, vitamin $B_{12}$ assay |
| Pellagra | Dietary history |
| Hypoparathyroidism | Serum calcium level |
| Multiple cerebral infarction | CT scan |
| Alcohol (Wernicke–Korsakoff syndrome) | Clinical history |
| Intracranial mass, hydrocephalus (including subdural haematoma) | Clinical features, CT scan |
| Chronic traumatic encephalopathy | Clinical history, CT scan |
| Huntington's disease | Family history, chorea |
| Multiple sclerosis | Clinical features, evoked potentials, CSF, MRI scan |
| Spongiform encephalopathy | EEG, ?cerebral biopsy |
| Progressive supranuclear palsy | Clinical features |
| General paralysis of the insane | Syphilitic serology |
| Poisoning by: | |
|   Drugs (chronic barbiturate intoxication) | |
|   Carbon monoxide | Drug levels and clinical history |
|   Heavy metals (organic mercurials, manganese) | |
| Following prolonged anoxia or hypoglycaemia | Clinical findings |
| Chronic hepatic encephalopathy | Clinical features, liver biochemistry |
| AIDS encephalopathy | HIV serology |
| Uraemia, dialysis | Raised blood urea |
| Rare metabolic disorders, e.g. Wilson's disease | Serum copper level, caeruloplasmin level |

MCV, mean corpuscular volume; $T_4$, thyroxine; TSH, thyroid stimulating hormone.

**Table 19.7**  Principal causes of dementia in adults and the features on which the diagnosis is made or excluded.

| Feature | Delirium | Dementia | Acute functional psychosis |
|---|---|---|---|
| Onset | Sudden | Insidious | Sudden |
| 24-h course | Fluctuating | Stable | Stable |
| Consciousness | Reduced | Clear | Clear |
| Attention | Globally impaired | Globally impaired | Variably affected |
| Cognition | Globally impaired | Globally impaired | May be selectively impaired |
| Hallucinations | Usually visual | Often absent | Mainly auditory |
| Delusions | Fleeting, poorly systematized | Often absent | Sustained, systematized |
| Orientation | Usually impaired | Often impaired | May be impaired |
| Psychomotor | Increased, reduced or shifting | Often normal | Varies from retardation to hyperactivity |
| Speech | Often slow, rapid or incoherent perseveration | Difficulty finding words | Normal, slow or rapid |
| Involuntary movements | Often asterixis or coarse tremor | Often absent | Usually absent |
| Physical illness or drug toxicity | One or both are present | Often absent | Usually absent |

After Lipowski ZJ (1989) *New England Journal of Medicine* **320**, 578–581.

**Table 19.8**  Clinical features of delirium, dementia and acute functional psychosis.

accumulation of aluminium ions has been suggested, but is not proven.

CLINICAL FEATURES. The onset is insidious and it develops slowly over a period of years. The onset can be in middle adult life or even earlier but the incidence is higher in later life. In cases with onset before the age of 65–70 years there is a likelihood of a family history of a similar dementia, a more rapid course and prominence of features of temporal and parietal lobe damage. Patients with Down's syndrome are at a high risk of developing Alzheimer's disease.

There are characteristic pathologic changes in the brain including:

NEURONAL REDUCTION in the hippocampus, substantia innominata, locus ceruleus and temporoparietal and frontal cortex.

NEUROFIBRILLARY TANGLES composed of paired helical filaments.

ARGENTOPHIL PLAQUES consisting largely of amyloid protein A4. The gene for the precursor protein of A4 (pro-A4) is localized close to the defect on chromosome 21 causing familial Alzheimer's disease. The significance of these findings is unclear.

GRANULOVACUOLAR BODIES.

Neurochemical changes have been found including a marked reduction in the enzyme choline acetyltransferase, in acetylcholine and in other neurotransmitters and neuromodulators.

**Vascular dementia** (multi-infarct dementia)

This is the second most common cause of dementia and is distinguished from Alzheimer's disease by its history of onset, clinical features and subsequent course. There is usually a history of transient ischaemic attacks with brief impairment of consciousness, fleeting pareses or visual loss. The dementia may follow a succession of acute cerebrovascular accidents or, less commonly, a single major stroke.

**Pick's disease**

This is a dementia in which the cortical atrophy is initially restricted to the frontotemporal region. The cause is unknown.

**DIAGNOSIS**

The presence of dementia is usually diagnosed clinically (see examination of mental state, p. 960), but it can be confirmed by psychometric testing, e.g. Wechsler Scale.

Secondary causes are infrequent, but they must be excluded by appropriate tests (Table 19.7) in all patients as some causes are potentially reversible.

CT or MRI scan will confirm the presence of cortical atrophy and exclude other lesions, e.g. brain tumours.

**MANAGEMENT**

In most cases there is no specific treatment, but conditions such as anxiety and depression often need therapy.

The patient should be kept in the community as long as possible, institutional care being used only in the later stages. Carers must be given support and patients are often admitted to hospital for short periods to give carers respite.

## Amnestic syndrome

The amnestic syndrome (see p. 880) is characterized by a marked impairment of memory occurring in clear consciousness and not as part of a delirium or dementia. Long-term memory is affected but the typical feature is impairment of short-term memory. Often the patient is blandly unconcerned and commonly displays confabulation. One of the commonest causes is severe thiamine deficiency secondary to chronic alcohol abuse but other, less common causes are shown in Table 18.8.

## Organic delusional syndrome

The organic delusional syndrome is characterized by a mental state dominated by delusions that are often accompanied by a persistent and distressing misperception of the environment, sometimes referred to as *delusional tone*. The delusions are very often persecutory but may also be hypochondriacal, pathologically jealous, grandiose or erotic.

## Organic affective syndrome

The organic affective syndrome consists of marked mood changes that result from organic brain damage. There are depressive and manic phases, often occurring suddenly, or there may be a persistently dysphoric state. There is no significant intellectual loss, delusions or hallucinations, and a family history of an affective disorder is uncommon.

## Intoxication and withdrawal syndromes

These are discussed on p. 984.

# *Schizophrenia*

The term schizophrenia was coined by the Swiss psychiatrist Eugen Bleuler in 1908 as a 'rending (disconnection) or splitting of the psychic functions'. The normal integration of emotional and cognitive functions is ruptured in schizophrenia. The annual prevalence of the condition ranges between 2 and 4 per 1000. The lifetime risk of contracting schizophrenia is 1%, but for first-degree relatives of sufferers it is 12%. High rates have been reported in the north-west of the former Yugoslavia and among the Tamils of south India.

**CAUSES**

No one cause has been identified to date. A number of possible causes have been implicated and are the subject of research. Biological causes are indicated in Table 19.9. Psychological theories suggest that schizophrenics have an impaired ability to handle the amount and speed of incoming perceptual stimuli and/or that some schizophrenics have a left hemisphere limbic dysfunction. A popular social theory suggests that disturbances in family relationships or communication are the cause, but the evidence is poor. Studies of so-called *expressed emotion* suggest that schizophrenic patients are particularly vulnerable to highly expressed emotions, and such family atmospheres increase the chances of relapse in treated patients as do intensive psychotherapy and social demands.

## CLINICAL FEATURES

The illness can begin at any age but is rare before puberty; the peak age of onset is in late adolescence and the early twenties. The overall sex incidence is about equal. Schizophrenia is probably not a specific condition but rather a number of clinical syndromes. The symptoms that have been considered as diagnostic of the condition have been termed *first-rank* symptoms and were described by the German psychiatrist Kurt Schneider. They consist of:

- Auditory hallucinations—patients hear their own thoughts spoken aloud and/or hear one or several voices referring to themselves in the third person or referring to them by name, and/or hear voices commenting on their behaviour
- Thought withdrawal, insertion and interruption
- Thought broadcasting
- Delusional perceptions
- External control of emotions
- Somatic passivity and feelings—patients believe that thoughts or acts are due to the influence of others

The World Health Organization's *International Pilot Study of Schizophrenia* has shown that the presence of any one of these symptoms, in the absence of physical disease, is highly discriminating for the diagnosis in a variety of countries and cultures. Other symptoms of acute schizophrenia include behavioural disturbances, thought disorder, hallucinations, delusions and mood abnormalities.

Chronic schizophrenia is characterized by thought disorder and the so-called *negative* symptoms of underactivity, lack of drive, social withdrawal and emotional emptiness. Motor disturbances can occur but they are extremely rare. Such disorders are often described as catatonic and include stupor, excitement, mannerisms, stereotypies and automatic obedience. Delusions in chronic schizophrenia are often held with little emotional response (the so-called *systematized* delusions) and may be *encapsulated* from the rest of the patient's beliefs and behaviour.

## DIFFERENTIAL DIAGNOSIS

Schizophrenia must be distinguished from:
- Organic psychiatric disorders
- Affective disorders
- Personality disorders

The most important organic disorders, particularly in young patients, are drug-induced psychoses and temporal-lobe epilepsy. Some of the drugs that can produce psychosis are listed in Table 19.10.

In older patients, any acute brain syndrome as well as dementia can present in a schizophrenia-like manner. A helpful diagnostic point is that clouding of consciousness and disturbances of memory do not occur in schizophrenia and visual hallucinations are unusual.

Affective disorders present with a more sustained disturbance of mood and any delusions and hallucinations that are detected are usually understandable in terms of the mood disturbance. First-rank symptoms are not normally a feature of affective disorders. Differentiating insidiously arising schizophrenia from a personality disorder in a young person can be exceptionally difficult and the passage of time may be needed for the condition to be clarified.

## COURSE AND PROGNOSIS (Table 19.11)

The prognosis of schizophrenia is highly variable. The patient's psychosocial environment appears important in

---

*Genetic*
40% risk for children of two affected parents
50% risk for monozygotic twin of affected individual
Possible locus on chromosome 5

*Dopamine*
Dopamine agonists (e.g. amphetamine) exacerbate the condition
The therapeutic potency of neuroleptics is directly related to their ability to block dopamine receptors in the brain
Withdrawal of dopamine antagonists causes rebound of symptoms in some patients
Post-mortem studies show increased dopamine binding sites in the brains of affected patients

*Brain damage* (e.g. *in utero* from long-acting virus)
Enlargement of lateral ventricles and widening of cerebral fissures and sulci on CT scans of a subgroup of patients

*Other*
Disturbance in transmethylation
Abnormalities in monoamine oxidase function

**Table 19.9**  Possible biological causes of schizophrenia

---

Glucocorticoids
Anticholinergic agents
Sympathomimetic central stimulants
Phenytoin
Carbamazepine
Disulfiram
Metronidazole
Cardiac glycosides
Hallucinogens, e.g. LSD, mescaline, ecstasy
Amantadine

LSD, lysergic acid diethylamide.

**Table 19.10**  Drugs causing psychosis.

|  | Good factors | Bad factors |
|---|---|---|
| Premorbid state | No family history of schizophrenia | Family history of schizophrenia |
|  | Stable personality | Withdrawn, solitary, eccentric personality |
|  | Warm personal relationships | Poor work record; poverty of relationships |
|  | Stable home relationships | Stormy domestic situation |
| Features of illness | Identifiable precipitating factor or life event | No obvious triggering factor or life event |
|  | Acute onset | Insidious onset |
|  | Few first-rank symptoms | Many first-rank symptoms |
|  | Disturbance of mood | No mood disturbance |
|  | Initiative, interest and motivation maintained | Blunting of emotional responses; initiative, motivation and interest impaired |
|  | Prompt treatment | Treatment delayed |

**Table 19.11**  Prognostic factors in schizophrenia.

that in an understimulating environment negative symptoms worsen, whereas in an excessively stimulating environment positive symptoms may emerge or worsen. Some patients only suffer acute episodes that leave them relatively unimpaired; others insidiously develop chiefly negative symptoms. The most common presentation and course is an initial acute episode of floridly positive symptoms followed by the emergence and persistence of negative symptoms.

A review of treatment studies suggests that between 15 and 25% of schizophrenics recover completely, another two-thirds will have relapses and may develop mild to moderate negative symptoms, while about 1 in 10 will become seriously disabled.

## TREATMENT
The best results are obtained by combining drug and social treatments.

### Antipsychotic (neuroleptic) drugs
These act by blocking D1 and D2 dopamine receptors, so reducing psychomotor excitement and controlling many of the symptoms of schizophrenia without causing disinhibition, confusion or sleep. Such drugs are most effective against acutely occurring, positive symptoms and least effective in the management of chronic, negative symptoms. Complete control of positive symptoms can take up to 3 months and premature discontinuation of treatment can result in prompt relapse.

The phenothiazines are the most extensively used group of neuroleptics. Chlorpromazine (100–1000 mg daily) is the drug of choice when a more sedating drug is required. Trifluoperazine is used when sedation is undesirable. Fluphenazine decanoate is used as a long-term prophylactic to prevent relapse (25–100 mg i.m. every 1–4 weeks). Promazine or thioridazine are useful in the elderly when it is desirable to reduce the risk of extrapyramidal and anticholinergic side-effects.

As antipsychotic drugs block both D1 and D2 dopamine receptors, they usually produce extrapyramidal side-effects. This limits their use in the maintenance therapy of many patients. They also block adrenergic and cholinergic receptors and thereby cause a number of unwanted effects (Table 19.12).

In patients manifesting good prognostic features and responding well to drugs, treatment may be discontinued under supervision after several months. Poor prognosis schizophrenia, on the other hand, usually requires regular maintenance therapy for many months or even years.

Clozapine, a new and atypical neuroleptic drug, is

**Common effects**
*Extrapyramidal*
Acute dystonia
Parkinsonism
Akathisia
Tardive dyskinesia

*Autonomic*
Hypotension
Failure of ejaculation

*Anticholinergic*
Dry mouth
Urinary retention
Constipation
Blurred vision

*Metabolic*
Weight gain

**Rare effects**
*Hypersensitivity*
Cholestatic jaundice
Leucopenia
Skin reactions

**Others**
Precipitation of glaucoma
Galactorrhoea
Amenorrhoea
Cardiac arrhythmias
Seizures
Retinal degeneration (with thioridazine in high doses)

**Table 19.12**  Unwanted effects of neuroleptic drugs.

being used in patients with intractable schizophrenia (approximately 20% of patients) who have failed to respond to at least two conventional antipsychotic drugs. This new drug is a dibenzodiazepine with a higher affinity for D1 than D2 receptors. Hitherto, a drug's antipsychotic potency has been related to the blockade of the D2 receptors. It is claimed that clozapine has dramatic therapeutic effects on negative symptoms, cognitive function and quality of life, but control trials are still in progress. However, this drug is expensive and produces severe agranulocytosis in 1–2% of patients. Therefore it can only be prescribed to registered patients by doctors and pharmacists registered with the Clozaril patient-monitoring service. The starting dose is 25 mg per day with a maintenance dose of 150–300 mg daily. White cell counts should be monitored weekly for 18 weeks and then 2-weekly for the length of treatment.

### Psychological treatment

This consists of reassurance, support and a good doctor–patient relationship. Psychotherapy of an intensive or exploratory kind is contraindicated.

### Social treatment

Social treatment involves attention being paid to the patient's environment and social functioning. Patients with any degree of residual impairment and negative symptoms usually require rehabilitation in a structured work and social environment. Parents and relatives need advice concerning the optimum amount of emotional and social stimulation to be provided for the patient. Some patients can manage a normal job, whereas others require a sheltered workshop. A very small number of severely disabled patients require long-term residential medical and nursing care.

The treatment of most psychiatric conditions is *multidisciplinary*, that is to say, in addition to the active involvement of psychiatrists and psychiatric nurses, other professionals including psychologists, psychiatric social workers, community psychiatric nurses, occupational therapists and counsellors play important therapeutic roles. This is particularly true in the case of the major psychoses. While psychiatrists and psychiatric nurses are crucially involved in the hospital management of such conditions, community psychiatric nurses play important roles in maintaining patients within the community. Psychologists, in addition to their skills in assessing the psychological status of patients, deliver cognitive, behavioural and other forms of therapy while occupational therapists work within hospital and community settings to assess and improve patient's social and occupational skills.

## Manic-depressive disorder

The central feature of this disorder is an abnormality of mood, either depression or elation or both. Mood is best considered in terms of a continuum ranging from severe depression at one extreme to severe mania at the other, with normal, stable mood at the centre (Fig. 19.1).

Manic-depressive disorders are divided into bipolar manic-depression, in which patients suffer attacks of both depression and mania, and unipolar disorders, in which there is either mania alone or, more commonly, depression alone. First-degree relatives of patients suffering from bipolar illness have an increased risk of manic-depressive illness but not those of patients with unipolar illness.

*Depression* is classically divided into endogenous depression and reactive depression, although the validity of this distinction is doubtful.

The criteria of *endogenous* depression include:
● Pervasive and unresponsive depression
● Early morning waking
● Diurnal variation of mood (worse in the morning)
● Profoundly depressive ideas (e.g. guilt, suicidal feelings)
● The lack of an obvious precipitating cause
● A stable premorbid personality

The criteria of *reactive* depression include:
● A fluctuating depression responsive to environmental change
● Self-pity rather than self-blame
● A clear precipitating cause
● A vulnerable or predisposed personality
● Absence of the criteria of endogenous depression

A mixture of both types is a commoner presentation than a pure form of either.

### CLINICAL FEATURES

The clinical features of mania reflect a marked elevation of mood (Table 19.13). The term hypomania refers to a

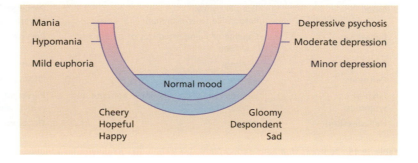

**Fig. 19.1** Continuum of normal and abnormal mood.

| | |
|---|---|
| Mood | Elevated, infectious, labile |
| Talk | Fast, pressurized, flight of ideas, punning, rhyming |
| Energy | Excessive, restless, distractible |
| Ideation | Grandiose, self-confident, delusions of wealth, power, influence or of religious significance, persecutory delusions |
| Cognition | Formal testing difficult, disturbance of retrieval of memories |
| Physical | Insomnia, mild to moderate weight loss |
| Behaviour | Disinhibition, increased sexual interest, excessive drinking or spending |
| Hallucinations | Fleeting auditory or, more rarely, visual |

**Table 19.13** Clinical features of mania.

| | |
|---|---|
| Mood | Depressed, miserable, unhappy |
| Talk | Impoverished, slow, monotonous, incomplete |
| Energy | Lacking, retarded (in some cases agitation), apathetic |
| Ideation | Feelings of futility, guilt, self-reproach, unworthiness, hypochondriacal preoccupations, worrying, suicidal thoughts, delusions of guilt, nihilism, persecution |
| Cognition | Verbal memory impaired, pseudodementia in elderly patients |
| Physical | Early waking, appetite and weight loss, constipation, loss of libido, impotence, fatigue, bodily aches and pains |
| Behaviour | Retardation or agitation, poverty of movement and expression |
| Hallucinations | Auditory—often abusive, hostile, critical |

**Table 19.14** Clinical features of depression.

mild form of mania characterized by euphoria, overactivity and disinhibition. It can be difficult to distinguish this from simple exuberance, enthusiasm and good humour.

At the opposite pole of the affective continuum, major depressive illness is also characterized by disturbances of mood, talk, energy and ideation (Table 19.14). The mood may be described by the patient in physical terms, e.g. like a weight in the head, a tightness of the chest, or a feeling of almost physical pain. Depressed patients describe the world as grey, themselves as lacking a zest for living, and their bodies as devoid of pleasure and feeling. Anxiety is common, obsessional symptoms may emerge and, in the severer forms, delusions of guilt, persecution and of bodily disease are not uncommon. In severe depression apparent organic impairment, detectable on cognitive testing, can result in disorientation.

Depression is a common experience. It occurs in the setting of physical disease, social stress, personal problems and life crises. It is important to distinguish the more severe and potentially life-threatening major form, requiring energetic treatment, from the less severe minor form, which, with simple support, sympathy and reassurance, usually lifts (Table 19.15).

The aetiological factors in manic-depressive disorders are listed in Table 19.16.

## DIFFERENTIAL DIAGNOSIS
This is shown in Table 19.17.

Occasionally, doctors are called upon to distinguish between normal grief following a separation or bereavement, and depressive illness. A number of symptoms that commonly occur in depressive illness also follow bereavement, most notably sleep disturbance, appetite and weight loss, and tearfulness. However, a number of distinguishing features can usually be identified (Table 19.18).

Two conditions presenting in women and characterized by disturbance of mood may well be related to

| | Minor | Major |
|---|---|---|
| Mood | Transiently low<br>Responsive to environment | Persistently low<br>Unresponsive to environment |
| Behaviour | Capable of being lifted out of gloom and sadness | Persistently agitated and/or retarded |
| Suicidal feelings | Fleeting | Persistent |
| Delusions | Absent | Often present |
| Physical symptoms | Vague aches and pains, some appetite and sleep loss | Persistent bowel changes, appetite and weight loss, sleep disturbance and early waking |
| Hallucinations | Absent | Occasionally present |

**Table 19.15** Features that help distinguish major from minor depression.

**Biological**
*Genetic*
10–15% of first-degree relatives have an affective disorder (risk in community is 1–2%)
68% of monozygotic twins reared together or apart are concordant for manic-depressive disorder
23% of dizygotic twins are concordant
Possible links with genetic markers

*Biochemical*
Imbalance in neurotransmitters (e.g. monoamine neurotransmitters are depleted in depression, but increased in mania)
Loss of diurnal rhythm of plasma cortisol in depression
Hormonal factors (e.g. depression is more common after childbirth, in premenstrual phase, with use of oral
  contraceptives, the menopause and post-hysterectomy)
Electrolytes—intracellular sodium is high in affective disorders

**Psychological**
*Maternal deprivation*
Psychoanalysis initially suggested that loss of maternal affection in early life and any significant loss in early childhood
  predisposes individuals to affective disorder in later life

*Learned helplessness*
Experimental animals put in a position where they cannot escape or control punishing stimuli develop a behavioural
  syndrome that resembles depression in humans. It has led to the suggestion that a similar mechanism is at work in
  humans

**Social**
*Stressful events*
An excess of life events is found in the months before the onset of depression. Life events include bereavement, loss of a
  job, moving house, marriage and going on vacation

*Vulnerability factors*
In women, it has been claimed that certain factors render them vulnerable to become depressed. These include lack of a
  job outside the home, the presence of three or more young children in the family, and lack of a confiding, intimate
  relationship

**Table 19.16** Possible aetiological factors involved in manic-depressive disorders.

---

manic-depressive disorders. These are the premenstrual syndrome and puerperal affective disorders.

### The premenstrual syndrome

Symptoms consist of irritability, depression and tension during the 7–10 day premenstrual period. These symptoms are often accompanied by breast tenderness, a subjective feeling of weight gain and bloatedness, and headache, and are usually dramatically relieved with the onset of the period. Women who suffer from affective disorders may be more prone to experience premenstrual symptoms and to have exacerbations of their psychiatric disorder during the premenstrual phase.

The cause or causes of the premenstrual syndrome remain unclear and the various treatments proposed, which include the use of vitamin $B_6$, diuretics, progesterone, oral contraceptives, oil of evening primrose and oestrogen implants, remain empirical.

### Puerperal affective disorders

In postpartum women, affective disorders also occur. Such disturbances are divided into maternity blues, postpartum (puerperal) psychosis and chronic depression. Maternity blues is used to describe the brief episodes of emotional lability, irritability and tearfulness that occur in 65–90% of women 2–3 days postpartum and that resolve spontaneously in a few days. Postpartum psychosis occurs

once in every 500–1000 births. Over 80% of cases are affective in type and the onset is usually within the first 2 weeks following delivery. In addition to the classical features of an affective psychosis, disorientation and confusion are often noted. Severely depressed patients may have delusional ideas that the child is deformed, evil or otherwise affected in some way, and such false ideas may lead to attempts to kill the child and to suicide. The response to speedy treatment is generally good. The recurrence rate for a depressive illness in a subsequent puerperium is 15–20%.

Less severe depressive disorders occur during the first postpartum year in 10–20% of mothers. Most patients recover after a few months. Social and psychological factors are important but the underlying aetiological factor is unknown.

### TREATMENT

The treatment of affective disorders involves physical, psychological and social therapies. Hospitalization is usually required in the case of severely depressed, potentially suicidal patients and in mania. In general, neither severe depression nor mania respond to psychotherapy, and both require energetic physical treatment. Simple support, reassurance, sympathy and the opportunity to express distress and negative feelings are often sufficient to bring about relief of minor depressive episodes.

| Condition | |
|---|---|
| *Mania* | |
| Drug-induced psychosis | e.g. Amphetamines, cannabis or steroids |
| Acute schizophrenia | Other classical (i.e. first-rank) schizophrenic symptoms usually present or eventually emerge |
| Dementia | Global cognitive impairment may present with euphoria and irritability; in mania, any cognitive impairment improves with treatment |
| Hyperthyroidism | Check TSH |
| *Depression* | |
| Systemic physical disease | Malignancy<br>Hypothyroidism<br>Hyperparathyroidism<br>Cushing's syndrome<br>Vitamin and mineral disorders<br>Postinfection<br>Multiple sclerosis<br>Collagen disorders<br>Cerebral ischaemia<br>Congestive heart failure<br>Porphyria |
| Drug-induced depression | Corticosteroids |
| Hormones | Oestrogen<br>Progesterone |
| Hypotensive agents | Reserpine<br>Methyldopa<br>Clonidine |
| Antiparkinsonian drugs | Levodopa<br>Amantadine hydrochloride |
| Anticancer drugs | Vincristine<br>Vinblastine |
| Psychiatric disorders | Schizophrenia<br>Alcohol abuse<br>Drug abuse<br>Anxiety neurosis<br>Dementia (see Table 19.7) |

**Table 19.17**   Differential diagnosis of manic-depressive disorders.

| | Normal bereavement | Depressive illness |
|---|---|---|
| Onset | Immediately follows loss | Delay for weeks or months |
| Duration | Lasts weeks rather than months | Persists for weeks/months/years |
| Pattern | Person slowly accepts loss and adjusts accordingly | Patient denies loss and refuses to accept implications |
| Grief | Expressed openly | Difficulty in expressing grief |
| Guilt | Mild regret in early stages | Marked guilt often present |

**Table 19.18**   Bereavement reaction versus depressive illness following bereavement (morbid grief reaction).

## Physical treatment of depression

TRICYCLIC AND RELATED ANTIDEPRESSANTS. These are the most frequently used drugs. Imipramine and amitriptyline are the two most commonly used but many related compounds have been introduced, some having fewer autonomic and cardiotoxic effects. Imipramine and amitriptyline are given by mouth in initial doses of 25–75 mg daily, building up over a week to 150–200 mg daily. The full therapeutic impact can take up to 2 or 3 weeks to occur. These drugs potentiate the action of monoamines, noradrenaline and serotonin by inhibiting their reuptake into nerve terminals. Other tricyclics in common use include nortriptyline, doxepin, mianserin, clomipramine, lofepramine and trazodone. Tricyclic antidepressants have a number of side-effects (Table 19.19); in patients with established cardiac disease mianserin,

*Anticholinergic effects*
Dry mouth
Constipation
Tremor
Blurred vision
Urinary retention
Postural hypotension

*Cardiac effects*
ECG changes
Arrhythmias

*Convulsant activity*
Lowered seizure threshold

*Other effects*
Weight gain
Sedation
Mania
Agranulocytosis (mianserin)

**Table 19.19**  Unwanted effects of tricyclic antidepressants.

dothiepin or trazodone are preferred over the more cardiotoxic compounds.

Serotonin uptake inhibitors. Fluvoxamine, fluoxetine, paroxetine and sertraline appear to produce less troublesome side-effects and a speedier onset of therapeutic effect. These drugs appear to act by way of selective inhibition of serotonin reuptake within the synaptic cleft and are thus termed *selective serotonin reuptake inhibitors* or SSRIs. While there is still argument as to their superiority as antidepressants over the more established tricyclics, they are becoming popular (fluoxetine is now one of the most commonly prescribed antidepressants in the USA) because of their lower rate of serious side-effects.

Monoamine oxidase inhibitors (MAOIs). These act by inhibiting the intracellular enzymes monoamine oxidase A and B, leading to an increase of noradrenaline, dopamine and 5-hydroxytryptamine in the brain. There are two types:

1 Hydrazine derivatives, e.g. isocarboxazid, phenelzine (potentially hepatotoxic)
2 Amphetamine-related, e.g. tranylcypromine (potentially addictive)

The most widely used is phenelzine, which is given in doses of 30–60 mg daily. The onset of action of MAOIs is within 24–48 hours. Unwanted effects include increased appetite and weight gain and difficulty in sleeping. MAOIs also produce hypertensive reactions with foods containing tyramine or dopamine and therefore a restricted diet is prescribed. These amines are normally broken down in the gut mucosa and the liver. Tyramine is present in cheese, pickled herrings, yeast extract, certain red wines and any food, such as game, that has undergone partial decomposition. Dopa is present in broad beans. This tyramine reaction is treated with intravenous phentolamine. MAOIs interact with drugs such as pethidine

(see p. 746) and can also occasionally cause liver damage. Particular caution should be taken when changing from an MAOI to a tricyclic or vice versa; it is safest to allow a 2 week drug-free interval between the two types of drug.

Newer forms of MAOIs have recently been produced which only inhibit monoamine oxidase A. Their effects appear more readily reversible—hence their description as reversible inhibitors of monoamine oxidase A (RIMA). An example is moclobemide 300 mg daily. These drugs appear to have fewer side-effects, work rapidly and constitute a low risk in overdose. At present, patients prescribed such antidepressants are advised that they can eat a broad diet but they should be careful to avoid excessive amounts of food rich in tyramine.

MAOIs are used in depressions that present with marked anxiety and obsessional or hypochondriacal features, and that lack marked biological symptoms characteristic of severe depression.

Electroconvulsive therapy (ECT). This is the most rapidly acting of the available physical treatments of depression. It can be the treatment of first choice in those cases where:
● The patient is dangerously suicidal
● A delay in treatment represents a serious risk to health
● The patient is refusing food and drink
● The patient is in a depressive stupor

The treatment involves the passage of an electric current, usually 80 V for a duration of 0.1–0.3 s, across two electrodes applied to the anterior temporal areas of the scalp. Before the treatment is given, the patient is anaesthetized (usually by means of thiopental 125–150 mg) and receives a muscle relaxant (usually suxamethonium 30–50 mg). A modified convulsion is produced. A course of six to eight treatments over 3 weeks has been shown to be superior to placebo treatment in severe depression characterized by retardation and delusions.

ECT is sometimes used in the management of acute schizophrenia, but the evidence of its effectiveness in this condition is less clear.

ECT is a controversial treatment, yet it is remarkably safe and free of serious side-effects. Serious complications are rare. However, post-ictal, short-term retrograde amnesia and a temporary defect in new learning can occur but these are short-lived effects. The mode of action of ECT in depressive illness is unclear.

### Physical treatment of mania

Acute attacks. The main physical treatment in mania is the use of neuroleptic drugs such as chlorpromazine, haloperidol and pimozide. Doses similar to those used in schizophrenia are used. Excitement and overactivity are usually reduced within days, but elation, grandiosity and associated delusions often take longer to respond. If improvement does not occur rapidly, larger doses of haloperidol (up to 120 mg daily) may be required. First attacks of mania usually require treatment for up to 3 months. Subsequent attacks, especially if they occur rapidly on cessation of treatment, may need drugs for at least a year after hypomanic features have disappeared.

PROPHYLAXIS. Lithium carbonate or citrate is used for prophylaxis in patients with repeated episodes of mania and/or depression. It is rapidly absorbed into the gastrointestinal tract and more than 95% is excreted by the kidneys; small amounts are found in the saliva, sweat and breast milk. Renal clearance of lithium correlates with renal creatinine clearance. In the body it substitutes for sodium and potassium ions and thus can exercise profound effects on a number of metabolic processes. Its mode of action is unknown.

Patients should be screened for thyroid and renal disease before starting on lithium. The therapeutic range for prophylaxis is between 0.4 and 1 mmol litre$^{-1}$. Regular serum estimations are required 12 hours after the last dose. Lithium levels should be checked every 3 or 4 months, along with regular thyroid and renal function tests.

Lithium takes 10 days to take effect. Unwanted effects include:

- Gastrointestinal symptoms (6%)
- A fine tremor (15%)
- Polyuria and polydipsia (due to inhibition of the antidiuretic hormone (ADH)-sensitive adenylate cyclase in the distal tubule of the nephron and hence a rise in plasma ADH)
- Weight gain (mainly increased appetite)

Toxic symptoms begin to occur when the serum concentration exceeds 1.5 mmol litre$^{-1}$. These include drowsiness, blurred vision, a coarse tremor, ataxia and dysarthria. Such symptoms progress to delirium and convulsions, and coma and death can occur. Long-term effects include non-toxic goitre, hypothyroidism and nephrogenic diabetes insipidus.

*Carbamazepine* is used in prophylaxis, but is also effective in the treatment of manic states. Some patients who do not respond to lithium may respond to carbamazepine. For antimanic treatment, dosage in the initial stage of treatment will be 200 mg once a day for 2 days, followed by 200 mg twice daily for 2 days, then 200 mg three times daily. Rarely dosage may have to be increased to a maximum of 1200 mg daily. The usual prophylactic dosage is 600 mg daily. The combination of lithium and carbamazepine is occasionally more effective than either drug alone.

### Social treatment

Many patients with depression, particularly of the milder form, have associated social problems. Assistance with such social problems can make a significant contribution to clinical recovery. Other social interventions include the provision of group support, social clubs, occupational therapy and training to cope with particularly stressful situations.

### Psychological treatment

The psychological treatments in affective disorders can be divided into:

SUPPORTIVE. Sympathy, reassurance and information should be part of every patient's treatment.

DYNAMIC PSYCHOTHERAPY (see p. 980). This form of psychotherapy has a limited value in the treatment of affective disorders. In general, its use is restricted to the less severe cases.

COGNITIVE THERAPY. This is a behavioural form of therapy that combines behavioural tasks with questioning and arguments designed to alter some of the ideas that are common among depressed patients and that appear to prolong their depression. Among these are negative interpretations of events and maladaptive assumptions (e.g. assuming that because friends do not telephone means they no longer care about the patient). In treatment, the patient is required to record such ideas and examine the evidence for and against them. Patients are also encouraged to undertake some of the pleasurable activities they gave up when they became depressed. There is some evidence that the effects of cognitive therapy are about the same as those of antidepressant drugs in the treatment of mild to moderate depression.

## COURSE AND PROGNOSIS

Between two-thirds and three-quarters of patients admitted with a major depressive illness will suffer at least one relapse requiring hospital admission. The number of less severe relapses is even higher. It has been estimated that between 15 and 20% of depressives never fully recover. It may take those who do recover between 4 and 18 months before they can expect to regain full social functioning.

Virtually all manic patients recover and the main problem is the prevention of relapse. Estimates of the proportion of patients who have only a single episode of mania vary widely between 1 and 50%! Subsequent depressive disorder is common in manic patients who relapse. Between 5 and 10% of manic-depressive sufferers develop a chronic disability that may follow the first episode. Between 5 and 10% become long-term hospital inpatients and an additional 25% have persistent affective symptoms that are disabling to some degree. The continuation of antidepressant therapy for up to 6 months after recovery from a depressive episode does reduce the probability of recurrence, while the use of lithium carbonate and carbamazepine as prophylactic therapy to prevent recurrence of bipolar manic-depressive swings is widely recommended.

# Suicide and attempted suicide (deliberate self-harm) (see also p. 749)

Between 11 and 17% of people who have suffered a severe depressive disorder at any time will eventually commit suicide. About 1% of deaths in England and Wales each year are due to suicide, yielding a rate of 8 per 100 000.

Living alone
Immigrant status
Recent bereavement, separation or divorce
Recent loss of a job or retirement
Living in a socially disorganized area
Male sex
Older age
Family history of affective disorder, suicide or alcohol
  abuse
Previous history of affective disorder, alcohol or drug
  abuse
Previous suicide attempt
Addiction to alcohol or drugs
Severe depression or early dementia
Incapacitating, painful physical illness

**Table 19.20**   Factors that increase the risk of suicide.

The rate increases with age, peaking for women in their sixties and for men in their seventies. However, in recent years the suicide rate in young people, particularly young men, has been rising steadily throughout western Europe. The highest rates of suicide have been reported in Hun-

gary (40 per 100 000), while the lowest are those of Spain (3.9 per 100 000) and Greece (2.8 per 100 000), but such variations may reflect differences in reporting as much as genuine differences in frequency of suicide.

Factors that increase the risk of suicide are indicated in Table 19.20.

A distinction must be drawn between those who attempt suicide (parasuicides) and those who are determined and eventually succeed (suicides). The following points should be considered:

● Suicide is commoner in men, while parasuicide is commoner in women.
● The majority of parasuicides occur in people under 35 years of age.
● The majority of suicides occur in people over 60 years of age.
● Approximately 90% of parasuicides involve self-poisoning.
● A formal psychiatric disorder is unusual in parasuicide. There is, however, overlap between the two groups and between 1 and 2% of people who attempt suicide will kill themselves in the year following their original attempt.

Questions to ask

Was there a clear precipitant/cause for the attempt?
What was the patient's state of mind at the time?
Was the act premeditated or impulsive?
Did the patient leave a suicide note?
Had the patient taken pains not to be discovered?
Did the patient make the attempt in familiar or strange surroundings (i.e. at home or away from home)?
What are the patient's feelings about the attempt now? Would they do it again?
Was the patient under the influence of alcohol or drugs?

Other relevant factors

Has the precipitant or crisis resolved?
Is there continuing suicidal intent?
Does the patient have any psychiatric symptoms?
What is the patient's social support system?
Has the patient inflicted self-harm before?
Has anyone in the family ever taken their life?
Does the patient have a physical illness?

Indications for referral to a psychiatrist

Absolute indications include:

Clinical depression
Psychotic illness of any kind
Clearly preplanned suicidal attempts which were not intended to be discovered
Persistent suicidal intent (the more detailed the plans, the more serious the risk)
A violent method used

Other common indications include:

Alcohol and drug abusers
Older patients over 45 years, especially if male, and young adolescents
Those with a family history of suicide in first-degree relatives
Those with serious (especially incurable) physical disease
Those living alone or otherwise unsupported
Those in whom there is a major unresolved crisis
Persistent suicide attemptors
Any patients who give you cause for concern

**Information box 19.3**   Guidelines for the assessment of patients with deliberate self-harm.

In the UK, over 100 000 suicide attempts are made each year, and the overwhelming majority of these are seen and treated within accident and emergency departments.

The guidelines given in Information box 19.3 for the assessment of such patients will help ensure that the risk factors relating to suicide are covered. Indications for referral to a psychiatrist before discharge from hospital are also given.

In general, it is worth trying to interview a family member or other close associate and check these points with him or her. Requests for immediate re-prescription or discharge should be denied, except in cases of essential medication (e.g. epileptics). In such cases, however, only 3 days' supply of medication should be given and the patient should be instructed to report to their general practitioner or to their psychiatric outpatient clinic for further supplies.

# Neuroses and personality disorders

These disorders constitute the largest portion of psychiatric disorders, accounting for 50% of admissions to psychiatric hospitals, 75% of patients seen in psychiatric outpatient clinics, and over 90% of the psychiatric disorders seen and managed by general practitioners. There is an overlap between neuroses and personality disorders, although in general they can be distinguished.

The *neuroses* are defined below. Personality disorders are deeply ingrained maladaptive patterns of behaviour generally recognizable by the time of adolescence and often becoming less obvious in middle or old age. The personality is abnormal either in the balance of its components, its quality or expression, or in its total aspect, and this deviation has an adverse effect upon the individual or on society.

The *psychopath* is a person who, as described by the Mental Health Amendment Act (1982), manifests a persistent disorder or disability of mind (whether or not this includes significant impairment of intelligence) which results in abnormally aggressive or seriously irresponsible conduct. The individual tends to be emotionally cold and callous, shows little remorse or ability to learn from previous mistakes, tolerates frustration poorly, is impulsive and has considerable difficulty sustaining roles requiring persistence and consistency, such as jobs, personal relationships and financial obligations.

## Anxiety neurosis

An anxiety neurosis is a condition in which anxiety dominates the clinical symptoms.

### CLINICAL FEATURES
The patient looks worried, has a tense posture, restless behaviour, a pale skin, and sweaty hands, feet and axillae.

The physical and psychological symptoms (Table 19.21) result from either overactivity of the sympathetic nervous system or increased tension in the skeletal muscles. Sleep is disturbed: the patient has difficulty in getting to sleep because of worry and restlessness, and when asleep wakes intermittently and may have unpleasant dreams. Another feature is the *hyperventilation syndrome* (Information box 19.4).

Sometimes anxious patients have the conviction that they suffer from heart disease. The conviction is accompanied by palpitations, fatigue, breathlessness and inframammary pain. The terms *cardiac neurosis, effort syndrome* and *neurocirculatory asthenia* used to be applied to the disorder. β-blockers are sometimes useful in controlling these symptoms.

### Types of anxiety
Anxiety may be divided into the following categories:

A MORE OR LESS CONTINUOUS STATE OF ANXIETY that fluctuates to some extent in response to environmental circumstances

PANIC ATTACKS—sudden and unpredictable attacks of

**Physical**
*Gastrointestinal*
Dry mouth
Difficulty in swallowing
Epigastric discomfort
Flatulence
Diarrhoea (usually frequency)

*Respiratory*
Feeling of chest constriction
Difficulty in inhaling
Overbreathing

*Cardiovascular*
Palpitations
Awareness of missed beats
Feeling of pain over heart

*Genitourinary*
Increased frequency
Failure of erection
Lack of libido

*Nervous system*
Tinnitus
Blurred vision
Dizziness
Headache
Sleep disturbances

**Psychological**
Apprehension and fear
Irritability
Difficulty in concentrating
Distractability
Restlessness
Sensitivity to noise
Depression
Depersonalization
Obsessional symptoms

**Table 19.21** Physical and psychological symptoms of anxiety.

*Features*

Panic attacks—fear, terror and impending doom—accompanied by some or all of the following:

    Dyspnoea
    Palpitations
    Chest pain or discomfort
    Choking sensation
    Dizziness
    Paraesthesiae
    Sweating
    Carpopedal spasms

*Cause*

Overbreathing leading to a decrease in $P_aCO_2$ and an increase in arterial pH

*Diagnosis*

A provocation test—voluntary overbreathing for 2–3 min—provokes similar symptoms; rebreathing from a paper bag relieves them

*Management*

Explanation and reassurance is given
The patient is trained in relaxation techniques and slow breathing
The patient is asked to breathe into a closed paper bag

**Information box 19.4**   The hyperventilation syndrome.

anxiety that are usually accompanied by severe physical symptoms

PHOBIC ANXIETY, which is anxiety triggered by a single stimulus or set of stimuli that are predictable and that normally cause no particular concern to others, e.g. agarophobia, claustrophobia

AN ANXIOUS PERSONALITY—an individual who has a lifelong tendency to experience tension and anxiety, and to have a worrisome attitude towards life and a constant anticipation of setback and stress

## DIFFERENTIAL DIAGNOSIS
This is given in Table 19.22.

## AETIOLOGY
### Genetic factors
Anxiety neurosis occurs in 15% of relatives of affected patients compared with 3% of the general population. (The genetic role is less important in phobic anxiety.)

### Psychodynamic theory
This is a theoretical explanation that suggests that anxiety neurosis reflects overwhelming stress, anxiety and diffi-

culties in the child–parent relationship in early childhood or even at birth. Psychoanalysts also interpret phobic neurosis as an unconscious avoidance of unacknowledged feelings of temptation (usually sexual), the phobia representing a displacement of the real fear (e.g. the agoraphobic patient is really afraid of the feelings of temptation aroused when meeting people in the street).

### Learning theory
Anxiety is regarded as a fear response that has been attached to another stimulus through conditioning.

## TREATMENT
### Psychological treatment
For many brief episodes of anxiety neurosis, a discussion with a doctor involving explanation and reassurance concerning the nature of physical symptoms of anxiety is usually sufficient. Relaxation training can be as effective as drugs in relieving mild or moderate anxiety. Such an approach uses an elaborate system of exercises designed to bring about relaxation of individual groups of skeletal muscles and to regulate breathing. A further development is anxiety management training, which involves two stages. In the first stage, verbal cues and mental imagery are used to arouse anxiety. In the second stage, the patient is trained to reduce this anxiety by relaxation, distraction and reassuring self-statements. Both of these approaches are forms of behaviour therapy.

The term behaviour therapy is applied to psychological treatments derived from experimental psychology and intended to change symptoms and behaviour. A variety of such treatments, including desensitization, flooding and programmed practice, are now used in the management of anxiety, phobias and obsessions. Non-behavioural

| Psychiatric disorder | Physical disorder |
|---|---|
| Depressive illness | Hyperthyroidism |
| Schizophrenia | Hypoglycaemia |
| Presenile dementia | Phaeochromocytoma |
| Alcohol dependence | |
| Drug dependence | |
| Benzodiazepine withdrawal | |

**Table 19.22**   The differential diagnosis of anxiety neurosis.

treatments include individuals and group-based psycho-therapies.

### Physical treatment

Drugs used in the treatment of anxiety can be divided into two groups: those that act primarily on the CNS and those that block peripheral autonomic receptors. The main group of centrally acting anxiolytic drugs are the benzodiazepines. They appear to bind to specific receptors on neuronal cell membranes, producing a facilitation of the effects of the inhibitory transmitter γ-aminobutyric acid (GABA). Diazepam (5 mg twice daily to 10 mg three times daily in severe cases) and nitrazepam have relatively long half-lives (20–40 hours) and are more suitable as antianxiety drugs than as hypnotic drugs, whereas oxazepam, temazepam and lorazepam have shorter half-lives and may be used as hypnotics.

Overdosage, which may be accidental or deliberate, produces drowsiness, sleep, confusion, incoordination, ataxia, diplopia and dysarthria. Physical as well as psychological dependence has been described, and convulsions have occurred on withdrawal of such drugs after long-term administration. The withdrawal syndrome (Table 19.23) is particularly severe when high doses have been given, e.g. 30 mg of diazepam daily or more. Tolerance can occur with repeated doses and can lead to an escalation of dosage. Thus, if a benzodiazepine drug is prescribed for anxiety, it should be given in as low a dose and for as short a time as possible (i.e. for not more than 3–4 weeks). A withdrawal programme includes changing therapy to diazepam followed by a very gradual reduction in dosage.

Many of the symptoms of anxiety are due to an increased release of adrenaline and noradrenaline from the adrenal medulla and the sympathetic nerves. Thus, adrenergic blocking drugs such as propranolol (20–40 mg two or three times daily) are effective in reducing symptoms such as palpitations, tremor and tachycardia.

## Obsessional neuroses and personality

Obsessional neuroses are characterized by obsessional thinking and compulsive behaviour (see p. 959) together with varying degrees of anxiety, depression and depersonalization. They account for some 2% of referrals to psychiatrists and have a prevalence in the general population of about 1 in 1000.

| Insomnia |
| Anxiety |
| Tremulousness |
| Muscle twitchings |
| Perceptual distortions |
| Frank convulsions |

**Table 19.23** Withdrawal syndrome with benzodiazepines.

### CLINICAL FEATURES

The obsessions and compulsions are so persistent and intrusive that they greatly impede the patient's functioning and cause considerable distress. There is a constant need to check that things have been done correctly and no amount of reassurance can remove the small amount of doubt that persists—the so-called *folie de doute*. Some rituals are derived from superstitions, such as repetitive actions done a required number of times, with the need to start again at the very beginning if interrupted. When severe, obsessional neuroses last for many years and are very resistant to treatment. However, obsessional symptoms commonly appear in the setting of other disorders, most notably anxiety neurosis, depression, schizophrenia and organic cerebral disorders, and disappear rapidly with the resolution of such disorders.

Minor variants of morbid obsessional symptoms can be noted fairly frequently in people who are not regarded as ill or in need of treatment. The mildest grade is that of obsessional personality traits such as over-conscientiousness, tidiness, punctuality and other attitudes and behaviours indicating a strong tendency towards rigidity, conformity and inflexibility. Such individuals are perfectionists, have a poor tolerance of shortcomings in others and take pride in their high standards. When such traits are so marked that they override and dominate other aspects of the personality, in the absence of clear-cut obsessional thinking and compulsive rituals, the picture becomes that of an obsessional personality disorder.

### AETIOLOGY

#### Genetic factors

Obsessional neuroses are found in 5–7% of the parents of obsessional patients. Such a finding may of course reflect environmental as well as genetic causes.

#### Organic factors

Neuroimaging data suggest that abnormalities exist in the frontal lobe and basal ganglia while pharmacological and neuroendocrinological research indicates there may be abnormalities in serotonin function in patients with OCD (obsessive-compulsive disorder). More recently the possibility of abnormalities within the dopaminergic and cholinergic systems has been raised.

#### Psychodynamic factors

Freud suggested that symptoms result from repressed impulses of an aggressive or sexual nature. He also suggested that they occur as a result of regression to the anal stage of development—an idea consistent with the obsessional patient's frequent concern over excretory functions and dirt.

#### Learning theory

This suggests that obsessional rituals are the equivalent of avoidance responses. However, anxiety actually increases rather than falls after some rituals, which is against such a theory.

## TREATMENT

### Psychological treatment

A form of behaviour therapy that is particularly effective in the treatment of obsessional rituals is *response prevention*. Patients are instructed not to carry out their rituals; initially there is a rise in distress but with persistence both the rituals and the distress diminish. Patients are encouraged to practise keeping them under control while returning to situations that normally make them worse.

Another approach known as *modelling* involves demonstrating to the patient what is required and encouraging the patient to follow this example. In the case of hand-washing rituals, this might involve holding an allegedly contaminated object and carrying out other activities without washing, the patient being encouraged to follow suit. When obsessional thoughts accompany rituals, *thought stopping* is advocated. In this procedure the patient is taught to arrest the obsessional thought by arranging a sudden intrusion (e.g. snapping an elastic band, clicking the fingers).

### Physical treatment

Anxiolytic drugs provide short-term symptomatic relief. Any coexisting depression should be treated with an antidepressant. One tricyclic antidepressant believed to have a specific action against obsessional symptoms is clomipramine, but studies suggest that the drug effects are modest and only occur in patients with definitive depressive symptoms.

Psychosurgery is sometimes recommended in cases of severe obsessional neurosis. The development of stereotactic techniques has led to the replacement of the earlier, crude leucotomies with more precise surgical interventions such as subcaudate tractotomy and limbic leucotomy, with lesions placed in the cingulate area and the ventromedial quadrant of the frontal lobe. These are undertaken to relieve patients of obsessional symptoms unresponsive to other treatments. Psychosurgery is now only performed in specialist centres, and formal and detailed consent requirements are laid down in England and Wales in the Mental Health Act 1983.

## PROGNOSIS

Two-thirds of cases improve within a year. The remainder run a fluctuating course. The prognosis is worse when the personality is obsessional and the symptoms are severe.

# Hysterical neurosis and personality

Hysterical neurosis or hysteria is a condition in which there are symptoms and signs of disease with three characteristics:

1 They occur in the absence of physical pathology.
2 They are produced unconsciously.
3 They are not caused by overactivity of the sympathetic nervous system.

The lifetime prevalence has been estimated at 3–6 per 1000 in women, with a lower incidence in men. Most cases begin before the age of 35 years and it occurs rarely after 40 years. However, hysterical symptoms commonly occur after this age as part of some other disorder.

## CLINICAL FEATURES

The various symptoms are usually divided into dissociative and conversion categories (Table 19.24). The term *dissociative* indicates the seeming dissociation between different mental activities, and covers such phenomena as amnesia, fugues, somnambulism and multiple personality. The term *conversion* derives from Freud's theory that mental energy can be converted into certain physical symptoms. Such symptoms include paralysis, fits, sensory loss, aphonia, blindness, deafness, disorders of gait and abdominal pain.

The main characteristics of hysterical symptoms include the following:

● They are not produced wilfully or deliberately.
● They often reflect a patient's ideas about illness.
● They may imitate symptoms of a relative/friend who has been ill.
● There are obvious discrepancies between hysterical signs and symptoms and those of organic disease.
● The symptoms usually confer some advantage on the patient (so-called secondary gain).
● They are often accompanied by less than the expected amount of emotional distress (*belle indifference*).

Hysterical amnesia commences suddenly. Patients are unable to recall long periods of their lives and may even deny any knowledge of their previous life or personal identity. A proportion who present thus have concurrent physical disease, especially epilepsy, multiple sclerosis or the effects of head injury. In a hysterical fugue, patients not only lose their memory but wander away from their usual surroundings, and when found deny all memory of their whereabouts during this wandering. Apart from hysteria, fugue states are associated with epilepsy, depression and alcohol abuse.

Hysterical pseudodementia involves a memory loss and behaviour that initially suggest severe and generalized intellectual deterioration. Simple tests are answered wrongly but in such a way as to suggest that the correct answer is in the patient's mind. The Ganser syndrome is a rare condition composed of four features:

1 The giving of approximate answers (i.e. almost correct)
2 Physical or mental symptoms of hysteria
3 Hallucinations
4 Clouding of consciousness

| Dissociative (mental) | Conversion (physical) |
|---|---|
| Amnesia | Paralysis |
| Fugue | Disorders of gait |
| Pseudodementia | Tremor |
| Ganser syndrome | Aphonia |
| Somnabulism | Mutism |
| Multiple personality | Sensory symptoms |
| Psychosis | Repeated vomiting |
| | Globus hystericus |
| | Hysterical fits |
| | Dermatitis artifacta |

**Table 19.24** Common hysterical symptoms.

The relationship of somnambulism, or sleep-walking, to other forms of hysteria is unclear, but its similarity to the condition arising through hypnosis suggests that it may be a form of dissociation.

In multiple personality, there are rapid alterations between two patterns of behaviour, each of which is forgotten by the patient when the other is present. Each personality appears to be a complex and integrated set of emotional responses. The condition is rare.

A variation of hysteria is the *epidemic or mass hysteria*, seen mainly in institutions for girls or young women, in which the combined effects of suggestion and shared anxiety produce explosive outbreaks of sickness or other disturbed behaviour. Another variant is *Briquet's syndrome*, which is said only to occur in women, follows an intractable course, runs in families and involves multiple somatic symptoms occurring in several different bodily systems for which no organic cause is found.

Patients with a hysterical personality are those who exhibit a particular set or cluster of personality traits that include a remarkable egocentricity, a manipulative skill and an ability to attract attention to themselves by dramatic initiatives, often of a sexually provocative or emotionally exaggerated fashion. Their emotions are described as shallow and labile and there is an 'acting' quality attached to much of what they do and say. Their personal relationships are often transient yet full of dramatic intensity. Such individuals, when they do develop genuine physical illness, may be dubbed hysterical because they describe their symptoms and complaints in such an exaggerated manner.

## DIFFERENTIAL DIAGNOSIS

The diagnosis of hysteria may be erroneously made because of:

UNDETECTED PHYSICAL DISEASE. The symptoms may be those of an, as yet, undetected physical disease, e.g. *globus hystericus* (see p. 183) may actually be difficulty in swallowing secondary to an oesophageal cancer.

UNDETECTED BRAIN DISEASE (e.g. a tumour in the frontal lobe or early dementia) may in some way produce hysterical symptoms.

PHYSICAL DISEASE may provide a non-specific stimulus to hysterical elaboration or an exaggeration of symptoms by a somewhat dramatic or histrionic patient.

Physical disease must be excluded. The distinction between hysteria and malingering (i.e. the conscious pretence of illness) should be considered but is difficult to make.

## AETIOLOGY
### Genetic factors
Studies have been inconclusive but reported rates in relatives of affected patients do appear higher than in the general population.

### Psychodynamic factors
Central to the theory of psychoanalysis is the view that hysteria is the result of emotionally charged ideas lodged in the unconscious at some point in the past. Symptoms are explained as the combined effects of repression and the conversion of psychic energy into physical channels.

### Organic disease
Hysteria is sometimes associated with physical disease. However, it also quite clearly occurs in the absence of such pathology.

## TREATMENT
### Psychological treatment
Psychotherapy of a psychodynamic kind often uncovers striking memories of early childhood sexual experiences and other problems relevant to the patient's presenting condition. Psychodynamic psychotherapy is derived from psychoanalysis and is based on a number of key analytical concepts. These include Freud's ideas about psychosexual development, mechanisms of defence (including repression, projection and denial), free association as the method of recall, and the therapeutic techniques of interpretation including that of transference, defences and dreams. Such therapy usually involves once-weekly 50-min sessions, the length of treatment varying between 3 months and 2 years. The long-term aim of such therapy is twofold: symptom relief and personality change. Psychodynamic psychotherapy is classically indicated in the treatment of the neuroses and personality disorders, but to date there is a lack of convincing evidence concerning its superiority over other forms of treatment.

Simpler forms of psychotherapy involving more straightforward reassurance and explanation, greater involvement of the therapist in the actual sessions, and the elimination of factors that appear to reinforce symptoms, are as effective and probably more so than the more complex and time-consuming forms. Group psychotherapy involving six to eight patients, which facilitates the development of confidence, the recollection of painful experiences and the growth of social and interpersonal skills, is also useful in a number of neurotic and personality disorders, although its usefulness in hysterical neuroses is doubtful.

Abreaction brought about by hypnosis or by intravenous injections of small amounts of amylobarbitone with or without amphetamine may produce a dramatic, if short-lived, recovery. In the abreactive state, the patient is encouraged to relive the stressful events that provoked the hysteria and to express the accompanying emotions, i.e. to abreact. Such an approach has been useful in the treatment of acute hysterical neuroses in wartime, but appear to be of much less value in civilian life.

### Physical treatment
Drug treatments have no part to play in hysteria unless the symptoms are secondary to a depressive illness or anxiety neurosis requiring treatment.

## PROGNOSIS
Most cases of recent onset recover quickly. Those that last longer than a year are likely to persist for a very long time.

## Hypochondriacal neurosis

This is a neurotic disorder in which the conspicuous features are an excessive concern with one's health in general, in the integrity and functioning of some part of one's body or, less frequently, one's mind. Hypochondriasis may coexist with actual physical disease; the important point is that the patient's concern is out of all proportion and is unjustified. The symptoms of hypochondriasis occur in a variety of psychiatric disorders, particularly in depression and anxiety. When hypochondriacal tendencies are lifelong, the condition is more usually termed hypochondriacal personality.

## Reaction to severe stress

Acute stress reactions occur in individuals without any other apparent psychiatric disorder in response to exceptional physical and/or psychological stress. While severe, such reactions usually subside within hours or days. The stress may be an overwhelming traumatic experience (e.g. accident, battle, physical assault, rape) or an unusually sudden change in the social circumstances of the individual, such as multiple bereavement. Individual vulnerability and coping capacity play a role in the occurrence and severity of acute stress reactions, as evidenced by the fact that not all people exposed to exceptional stress develop symptoms. These symptoms show considerable variation but usually include an initial state of 'daze' with some constriction of the field of consciousness and narrowing of attention, inability to comprehend stimuli and disorientation. This state may be followed either by further withdrawal from the surrounding situation to the extent of a dissociative stupor or by agitation and overactivity. Autonomic signs of panic anxiety, including tachycardia, sweating and hyperventilation, are commonly present. The symptoms usually appear within minutes of the impact of the stressful stimulus and disappear within 2–3 days.

### Post-traumatic stress disorder (PTSD)

This arises as a delayed and/or protracted response to a stressful event or situation of an exceptionally threatening nature and likely to cause pervasive distress in almost anyone. Causes include natural or human disasters, war, serious accident, witnessing the violent death of others, being the victim of sexual abuse, rape, torture, terrorism or hostage-taking. Predisposing factors such as personality traits or previous history of psychiatric illness may lower the threshold for the development of the syndrome or may aggravate its course. They are, however, neither necessary nor sufficient to explain its occurrence.

Typical symptoms of PTSD include:

- 'Flashbacks'—the repeated reliving of the trauma in the form of intrusive memories or dreams
- Intense distress at exposure to events that symbolize or resemble an aspect of the traumatic event, including anniversaries of the trauma
- Avoidance of activities and situations reminiscent of the trauma
- Emotional blunting or 'numbness'
- A sense of detachment from other people
- Autonomic hyperarousal with hypervigilance, an enhanced startle reaction and insomnia
- Marked anxiety and depression and, occasionally, suicidal ideation

The course is fluctuating but recovery can be expected in the majority of cases. In a small proportion of cases the condition may show a chronic course over many years and a transition to an enduring personality change. Treatment involves exploration of memories of the traumatic event, relief of associated symptoms and counselling.

# Alcohol abuse and dependence

There are a number of different types of alcohol abuse, and a wide range of physical, social and psychological problems are associated with excessive drinking. Until recently, much attention was devoted to the syndrome of alcohol dependence. In fact, doctors should be concerned with the health problems caused by alcohol abuse whether or not such abuse is related to actual physiological dependence on alcohol. The term *alcoholism* is a confusing one with off-putting connotations of vagrancy, 'meths' drinking and social disintegration. It has been replaced by the term *alcohol dependence syndrome*, which has seven essential elements:

1 A compulsive need to drink.
2 A stereotyped pattern of drinking. Whereas ordinary drinkers vary their daily pattern, addicted drinkers drink at regular intervals to avoid or relieve withdrawal symptoms.
3 Drinking takes primacy over other activities.
4 Tolerance to alcohol is altered. The dependent drinker is ordinarily unaffected by blood alcohol levels that would incapacitate a normal drinker. Increasing tolerance is an important sign of increasing dependence. In the later stages of dependence, tolerance falls.
5 Repeated withdrawal symptoms. These occur some 8–12 hours after cessation of drinking or after a sharp fall in blood alcohol in people who have been drinking heavily for many years. Symptoms characteristically appear on waking as a result of the fall in the blood alcohol level during sleep.
6 Relief drinking. Many dependent drinkers take a drink early in the morning to stave off withdrawal symptoms. In most cultures, early morning drinking is diagnostic of alcohol dependence.
7 Reinstatement after abstinence. Severely dependent drinkers who drink again after a period of abstinence are likely to relapse quickly and return to their old addictive pattern.

The *problem drinker* is one who causes or experiences physical, psychological and/or social harm as a consequence of drinking alcohol. Many problem drinkers, while heavy drinkers, are not physiologically addicted to alcohol. Heavy drinkers are those who drink significantly more in terms of quantity and/or frequency than the average drinker. Binge drinkers are those who drink excessively in short bouts, usually 24–48 hours long, separated by often quite lengthy periods of abstinence. Their overall monthly or weekly alcohol intake may be relatively modest. The interrelationship between these types of drinking is shown in Fig. 19.2.

### Extent of the problem

A conservative estimate is that there are at least 300 000 people in the UK with alcohol-related problems. A survey on drinking in England and Wales found that 5% of men and 2% of women reported alcohol-related problems. People with serious drinking problems have an increased risk of dying that is between two and three times greater than that of members of the general population of the same age and sex. Approximately one in five male admissions to acute medical wards are directly or indirectly due to alcohol. Between 33 and 40% of accident and emergency attenders have blood alcohol concentrations above the present UK legal limit for driving. Up to one in five seemingly healthy men attending health screening programmes are found to have biochemical evidence of heavy alcohol consumption, though they are a selected population coming mainly from the upper social classes. Of the 2000 patients on the practice list of the average general practitioner, about 100 will be heavy drinkers, 40 will be problem drinkers and 10 will be physically dependent on alcohol.

Over the past 40 years, the alcohol consumption of the average British adult has increased considerably (from 5.2 litres of absolute alcohol per year in 1950 to 8.5 litres in 1991). There has been a downward trend since 1989. Over a similar period, admissions to psychiatric hospitals for treatment of alcohol problems have increased more than 25-fold, cirrhosis rates have doubled, and drunkenness offences have risen from 60 000 to over 100 000 per year.

### Detection

Many doctors still fail to recognize the heavy drinker and even the problem drinker. Greater awareness is urgently needed to allow intervention at a stage when something can still be achieved, and to provide better statistics.

Alcohol abuse should be suspected in any patient presenting one or more physical problems commonly associated with excessive drinking (see Chapter 3, p. 173). Alcohol abuse may also be associated with a number of psychological symptoms and social problems (Table 19.25). Certain features in the history should also raise suspicion, most notably:

- Absenteeism from work
- Frequent attendances for unexplained dyspepsia or gastrointestinal bleeds
- Hospital admissions for accidents of all kinds
- Fits, 'turns' or falls

Certain signs may be helpful, if present, in detecting alcohol abuse in patients. These include:

- Plethoric face with/without telangiectases
- Bloodshot conjunctivae
- Smell of stale alcohol
- Facial appearance resembling Cushing's syndrome
- Marked tremor
- Signs of alcohol-related diseases

The patient's frequency of drinking and quantity drunk on typical occasions should be established. Patients can assess their alcohol consumption on the basis of units of alcohol. One standard unit of alcohol is equivalent to 8 g of absolute alcohol (see p. 172).

The following are useful guidelines:

1 Drinking up to 20 units of alcohol a week for men and 13 units for women carries no long-term health risk.
2 There is unlikely to be any long-term health damage between 21 and 36 units (men) and 14 and 24 units (women) provided that the drinking is spread throughout the week.
3 Beyond 36 units a week in men and 24 units a week in women, damage to health becomes increasingly likely.
4 Drinking above 50 units a week in men (35 units in women) is currently regarded as a definitive health hazard.

A number of questionnaires, such as the CAGE questionnaire (Table 19.26), have been developed to help identify

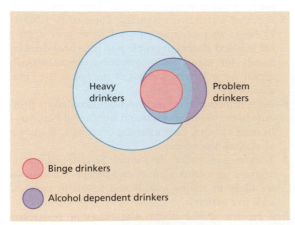

**Fig. 19.2**  The terminology of drinking.

| Psychological | Social |
|---|---|
| Depression | Marital and sexual |
| Anxiety and phobias | difficulties |
| Memory disturbances | Family problems |
| Personality disturbances | Child abuse |
| Delirium tremens | Employment problems |
| Attempted suicide | Financial difficulties |
| Pathological jealousy | Accidents at home, on the |
| | roads, at work |
| | Delinquency and crime |
| | Homelessness |

**Table 19.25**  Common alcohol-related psychological and social problems.

| | |
|---|---|
| **1** | Have you ever felt you ought to CUT DOWN your drinking? |
| **2** | Have people ANNOYED you by criticizing your drinking? |
| **3** | Have you ever felt bad or GUILTY about your drinking? |
| **4** | Have you ever had a drink first thing in the morning (an 'EYE-OPENER') to get rid of a hangover? |

From Mayfield D, McLeod G & Hall P (1974) *American Journal of Psychiatry* **131**, 1121–1123. With permission.

**Table 19.26**   The CAGE questionnaire.

patients with alcohol-related problems. Two or more positive replies to the CAGE questionnaire are said to identify problem drinkers.

It is important to remember that there are a number of key 'at-risk' factors involved, which include:

MARITAL DIFFICULTIES. These may conceal heavy drinking or may be used to justify it.

WORK PROBLEMS. Alcohol abusers have twice as many days off work as more sober colleagues.

AN AFFECTED RELATIVE. Twenty-five per cent of the male relatives of alcohol abusers have similar problems.

HIGH-RISK OCCUPATIONS. Examples of these include company directors, salesmen, doctors, journalists, publicans and seamen.

ASSOCIATED PHYSICAL AND MENTAL CONDITIONS, for example, depression.

A number of laboratory tests are helpful in the identification of excess chronic alcohol consumption:

BLOOD ALCOHOL. This is useful in anyone suspected of, but who denies drinking; most people have no detectable alcohol in their blood in the middle of the day.

URINARY ALCOHOL. A value exceeding 120 mg dl$^{-1}$ is suggestive of chronic alcohol abuse, and a value over 200 mg dl$^{-1}$ (44 mmol litre$^{-1}$) is said to be diagnostic.

$\gamma$-GLUTAMYL TRANSPEPTIDASE ($\gamma$-GT). Elevated serum $\gamma$-GT activity is observed in about 75% of patients hospitalized for alcohol abuse; in outpatients and heavy drinkers, the prevalence reaches 90%. Acute alcohol consumption does not lead to abnormal levels but regular, moderate drinkers often have a slight elevation of the $\gamma$-GT. Levels return to normal with abstention from alcohol.

MEAN CORPUSCULAR VOLUME (MCV) of more than 96 fl is found in about 60% of alcohol abusers. The response to abstinence is a return to normal over a period of about 2 months.

## Alcohol dependence syndrome

The alcohol dependence syndrome is usually very much easier to identify than problem-related drinking. Figure 19.3 outlines the main characteristics of the syndrome but these do not necessarily present in any particular order. Symptoms of alcohol dependence in a typical order of occurrence are shown in Table 19.27.

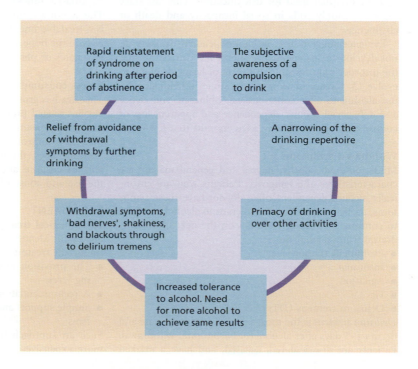

**Fig. 19.3**   Elements of the alcohol dependency syndrome.

Unable to keep to a drink limit
Difficulty in avoiding getting drunk
Spending a considerable time drinking
Missing meals
Memory lapses, blackouts
Restless without drink
Organizing day around drink
Trembling after drinking the day before
Morning retching and vomiting
Sweating excessively at night
Withdrawal fits
Morning drinking
Decreased tolerance
Hallucinations, frank delirium tremens

**Table 19.27**  Symptoms of alcohol dependence.

## COURSE

The course of the alcohol dependence syndrome comprises three linked stages. The first stage is heavy social drinking, i.e. the ingestion of three to five standard drinks (units) of alcohol a day for several years. This stage can continue asymptomatically for a lifetime or, because of a change of circumstances or peer group, it can revert to a more moderate pattern of drinking or can progress to the second stage of alcohol abuse. This stage is usually associated with frequent ingestion of more than eight drinks a day and there are associated medical, legal, social and/or occupational complications. About half of such abusers either return to asymptomatic (controlled) drinking or achieve stable abstinence. In a small number of cases, such alcohol abuse can persist intermittently for decades with minor morbidity and become milder with time. About 25% of all cases of alcohol abuse will lead to chronic alcohol dependence, withdrawal symptoms and the eventual need for detoxification. This last stage most commonly ends in social incapacity and death or abstinence.

Evidence suggests that alcohol-dependent drinkers do not develop their dependence after a few drinks but that the disorder requires up to 10 years of heavy drinking to evolve (3–4 years in women). In some individuals who use alcohol to alter consciousness, obliterate conscience and defy social canons, dependence and apparent loss of control may appear in only a few months to a few years.

### Withdrawal symptoms

Mild tremor, headache, nausea and general malaise are characteristic of the hangover. Patients who are chronically alcohol dependent often do not have these symptoms, partly because they are tolerant to alcohol and tend to continue to consume alcohol on the next day. Withdrawal from alcohol causes:

● Prominent tremor
● Insomnia
● Agitation
● Fits
● Delirium tremens (DTs)

*Delirium tremens* is the most serious withdrawal state and occurs 1–5 days after alcohol (or barbiturate) withdrawal. Patients are disorientated, agitated, and have a marked

tremor and visual hallucinations (e.g. 'pink elephants').

Signs include sweating, tachycardia, tachypnoea and pyrexia. Additional signs include dehydration, infection, hepatic disease or the Wernicke–Korsakoff syndrome. If delirium tremens is not treated promptly, death can occur.

## CAUSES
### Genetic factors

Sons of alcohol-dependent people who are adopted by other families are four times more likely to develop drinking problems than the adopted sons of non-alcohol abusers.

### Environmental factors

A Boston follow-up study showed that one in ten boys who grew up in a household where neither parent abused alcohol subsequently became alcohol dependent compared with one in four of those reared by alcohol-abusing fathers and one in three of those reared by alcohol-abusing mothers.

### Biochemical factors

Several factors have been suggested, including abnormalities in alcohol dehydrogenase, neurotransmitter substances and brain amino acids, such as GABA, but, to date, there is no conclusive evidence that these or other biochemical factors play a causal role.

### Personality

Follow-up studies have failed to identify any trait or tendency that significantly distinguishes those who subsequently abuse alcohol from those who do not.

### Psychiatric illness

This is not a common cause of addictive drinking but it is a treatable one. Some depressed patients drink excessively in the hope of raising their mood. Patients with anxiety states or phobias are also at risk.

### Excess consumption in society

The idea has grown that rates of alcohol dependence and alcohol-related problems correspond to the general level of alcohol consumption in society and, in turn, to factors that may control overall consumption, including price, licensing laws, the number and nature of sales outlets, and the customs and moral beliefs of society concerning the use and abuse of alcohol.

## TREATMENT
### Psychological treatment

Successful identification at an early stage constitutes an important treatment in its own right. It should lead to:

● The provision of information concerning safe drinking levels
● A recommendation to cut down where indicated
● Simple support and advice concerning associated problems

Such an approach has been found to be as effective as more expensive and specialized forms of psychotherapy in the treatment of moderate to heavy non-addictive drinking. With addictive drinking, the most favoured psychological treatment is group therapy, which involves identification, confession, emotional arousal, the implantation of new ideas, and the long-term support by fellow-members of the group. Family and marital therapy involving both the alcohol abuser and spouse may also be important.

Behaviour therapies involving teaching patients how to drink in a more controlled way are the subject of much study.

### Physical treatment

Addicted drinkers often experience considerable difficulty when they attempt to reduce or stop their drinking. Withdrawal symptoms are a particular problem and delirium tremens needs urgent treatment (Table 19.28). Drugs that show cross-tolerance for alcohol, such as diazepam or chlormethiazole, may be used in a regimen that involves a steady reduction over 5–7 days. A useful chlormethiazole regimen is 9–12 capsules for 1 day, 6–8 for day 2 and 4–6 for day 3. However, long-term treatment with drugs should not be prescribed in those patients who continue to abuse alcohol. Many alcohol abusers add dependence on diazepam or chlormethiazole to their problems.

Drugs such as disulfiram (Antabuse) react with alcohol to cause very unpleasant acetaldehyde intoxication and histamine release. A daily maintenance dose of such a drug means that an alcohol-dependent drinker must wait until the disulfiram is eliminated from the body before drinking safely. Such drugs, therefore, can provide a 'chemical fence' around the drinker for at least 24 hours. Disulfiram implants have been developed that have a treatment life of 6 months. As yet there is doubt as to whether their benefit is psychological rather than pharmacological.

### OUTCOME

Whereas in the case of non-dependent heavy drinkers the goal of normal drinking within safe limits can be a very reasonable one, the alcohol-dependent drinker must be persuaded to abstain. Abstention, particularly after many years of drinking, is a difficult goal and not surprisingly many fail in the attempt. Research suggests that between 40 and 50% of alcohol-dependent drinkers are abstinent or drinking very much less up to 2 years following intervention. Specialized treatment units, psychiatric treatment, group therapy and attendance at meetings of Alcoholics Anonymous—the self-help organization that provides members with a social structure to fill the gap previously occupied by drinking—are all potential elements in the attempt to keep the alcohol-dependent individual abstinent and healthy. To date, however, there is little convincing evidence that highly expensive, time-consuming and specialized modes of treatment are superior in their efficacy to straightforward advice, support, encouragement and monitoring.

## Drug abuse and dependence

In addition to alcohol and nicotine, there are a number of psychotropic substances that are used for their effects on mood and other mental functions (Table 19.29).

### Solvents

Adolescents engage in glue-sniffing for the intoxicating effects produced by the solvents inhaled. The glue is sniffed directly from tubes, plastic bags or smears on pieces of cloth. Tolerance develops over weeks or months. Intoxication is characterized by:

- Euphoria
- Excitement
- A floating sensation
- Dizziness
- Slurred speech
- Ataxia

Acute intoxication can cause amnesia and visual hallucinations. The habit is dangerous because:

- Inhaled vomit can lead to asphyxiation.
- There is a risk of tissue damage, including damage to

---

The patient should be hospitalized
Chlormethiazole[a] 9–12 capsules (each capsule contains 192 mg) for 24 hours, then reduced over 5 days, or diazepam 4–100 mg for 2 days then reduced
Any dehydration should be corrected
Any electrolyte imbalance should be corrected
Any systemic infection should be treated
B vitamins should be given parenterally

---

[a]i.v. should be avoided, if possible.

**Table 19.28**  Management of delirium tremens.

---

| Stimulants | Narcotics |
|---|---|
| Methylphenidate | Morphine |
| Phenmetrazine | Heroin |
| Phencyclidine ('angel dust') | Codeine |
| Cocaine | Pethidine |
| Amphetamine derivatives | Methadone |
| | |
| Hallucinogens | Hypnotics |
| Cannabis preparations | Barbiturates |
| Solvents | Benzodiazepines |
| LSD | |
| Mescaline | |
| Ecstasy | |

LSD, lysergic acid diethylamide.

**Table 19.29**  Commonly used drugs of abuse and dependence.

bone marrow, brain, liver and kidneys. Death can occur.

● Acute intoxication can also result in aggressive and impulsive behaviour.

## Amphetamines and related substances

These have temporary stimulant and euphoriant effects that are followed by depression, anxiety and irritability. Psychological rather than true physical dependence is the rule. In addition to restlessness, over talkativeness and overactivity, amphetamines can produce a paranoid psychosis indistinguishable from acute paranoid schizophrenia. Ecstasy is another amphetamine derivative (see below).

## Cocaine

Cocaine is a CNS stimulant (with similar effects to amphetamines) derived from *Erythroxylon coca* trees grown in the Andes. In purified form it may be taken by mouth, sniffed or injected. If cocaine hydrochloride is converted to its base (crack) it can be smoked. This is an effective way of obtaining an intense stimulating effect and free-basing has become common. Compulsive use and dependence are thought to occur more frequently amongst users who are free-basing. Dependent users take large doses and alternate between the withdrawal phenomena of depression, tremor and muscle pains, and the hyperarousal produced by increasing doses. Prolonged use of high doses produces irritability, restlessness, paranoid ideation and occasionally convulsions. Persistent sniffing of the drug can cause perforation of the nasal septum.

## Hallucinogenic drugs

Hallucinogenic drugs such as lysergic acid diethylamide (LSD), cannabis and mescaline produce distortions and intensifications of sensory perceptions as well as frank hallucinations.

### Cannabis

A widely used drug in some subcultures is cannabis, derived from the plant *Cannabis sativa*. It is not thought to cause physical dependence. The drug, when smoked, seems to exaggerate the pre-existing mood, be it depression, euphoria or anxiety. There is no definite withdrawal syndrome or tolerance. There is disagreement over whether it can produce a psychosis.

### Ecstasy

'Ecstasy' is the street name for 3,4-methylenedioxy-methamphetamine (MDMA), a psychoactive phenyliso-propylamine, synthesized in Germany early in this century. It is a psychodelic drug which is often used as a 'dance' drug. It has a brief duration of action (4–6 hours) and is usually ingested in a dose of 75–150 mg orally. There is anxiety concerning the possibility of MDMA

causing permanent brain damage and deaths have been reported from hyperpyrexia, collapse, acute renal and liver failure.

## Hypnotics

Other drugs of dependence include barbiturates and benzodiazepines. Discontinuing treatment with benzodiazepines may cause withdrawal symptoms such as anxiety, restlessness, tachycardia and sensory disturbances (see Table 19.23); for this reason, withdrawal should be supervised and gradual.

## Narcotics

Physical dependence occurs with morphine, heroin and codeine as well as with synthetic and semi-synthetic narcotic analgesics such as methadone and pethidine. These substances display cross-tolerance—the withdrawal effects of one are reduced by administration of one of the others. The psychological effect of such substances is of a calm, slightly euphoric mood associated with freedom from physical discomfort and a flattening of emotional response. This is believed to be due to the attachment of morphine and its analogues to receptor sites in the CNS normally occupied by endorphins. Tolerance to this group of drugs is rapidly developed and marked. Following abstinence it is rapidly lost. The abstinence syndrome consists of a constellation of signs and symptoms (Table 19.30) that reach peak intensity on the second or third day after the last dose of the opiate. These rapidly subside over the next 7 days. Withdrawal is dangerous in patients with heart disease, tuberculosis or other chronic debilitating conditions.

Narcotic addicts are reported to have a high mortality rate due to acute illness associated with drug abuse. Heart disease (including infective endocarditis), tuberculosis and glomerulonephritis are common causes of death, while tetanus, malaria and acute viral hepatitis B are also causally related to addiction.

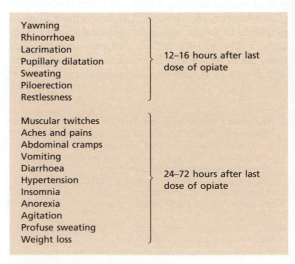

| Yawning<br>Rhinorrhoea<br>Lacrimation<br>Pupillary dilatation<br>Sweating<br>Piloerection<br>Restlessness | 12–16 hours after last dose of opiate |
| --- | --- |
| Muscular twitches<br>Aches and pains<br>Abdominal cramps<br>Vomiting<br>Diarrhoea<br>Hypertension<br>Insomnia<br>Anorexia<br>Agitation<br>Profuse sweating<br>Weight loss | 24–72 hours after last dose of opiate |

**Table 19.30**  Narcotic abstinence syndrome.

## TREATMENT

The treatment of a narcotic drug overdose requires immediate action. If opioid overdose is suspected, naloxone given intravenously (see p. 755) can be life-saving and diagnostic. There should be an immediate recovery of consciousness or a lightening of the comatose state if the offending agent is an opioid. Care must be taken, however, as opiate antagonists can precipitate violent abstinence symptoms. A constant infusion of naloxone hydrochloride may be required in methadone overdose.

The treatment of chronic dependence is usually directed towards helping the addict to live without drugs. Some who cannot manage such a regimen may be maintained on oral methadone. In the UK, only specially licensed doctors may legally prescribe heroin and cocaine to an addict for maintenance treatment of addiction.

## Causes of drug dependence

There is no single cause of drug dependence. Three factors appear important:
1 Availability of drugs
2 A vulnerable personality
3 Social, particularly peer, pressures
Once regular drug taking is established, pharmacological factors are particularly important in determining dependence.

# Eating disorders

## Obesity (see p. 167)

The majority of cases of obesity are caused by a combination of constitutional and social factors that encourage overeating. It is relatively infrequent for psychological causes to be involved. However, even when obesity is not due to definite psychological causes, it may itself produce a psychological reaction of depression and tension, particularly if attempts by the patient to lose weight are repeatedly ineffective.

## TREATMENT

Behavioural methods of treatment that make use of positive rewards for weight loss or for behaviour likely to lead to a reduction of weight have been attempted, but their efficacy is doubtful.

## Anorexia nervosa

The main clinical criteria for diagnosis are:
● A body weight more than 25% below the standard weight
● An intense wish to be thin
● A morbid fear of fatness
● Amenorrhoea in women

Clinical features may include:
● Onset usually in adolescence
● A previous history of chubbiness or fatness
● A relentless pursuit of low body weight
● Usually a distorted image of own body size
● The patient generally eats little
● Particular avoidance of carbohydrates
● Vomiting, excessive exercise and purging
● Amenorrhoea—an early symptom; in 20% it precedes weight loss
● Binge eating
● Usually a marked lack of sexual interest
● Lanugo
The physical consequences of anorexia include sensitivity to cold, constipation, hypotension and bradycardia. In most cases, amenorrhoea is secondary to the weight loss. Vomiting and abuse of purgatives may lead to hypokalaemia and alkalosis.

## PREVALENCE

Case register data suggest a rate ranging from 1 to 10 per 100 000 females aged between 15 and 34 years. Surveys have suggested a prevalence rate of 1–2% among schoolgirls and university students. However, many more young women have amenorrhoea accompanied by less weight loss than the 25% required for the diagnosis. The condition is much less common among men. The onset in women is usually between 16 and 17 years of age and it seldom occurs after 30 years.

## AETIOLOGY
### Biological factors
GENETIC. Six to ten per cent of siblings of affected girls suffer from anorexia nervosa; there is an increased concordance amongst monozygotic twins suggesting a genetic predisposition.

HORMONAL. There could be a disturbance of hypothalamic function in that:
● Amenorrhoea can precede weight loss in 20% of sufferers.
● Hormonal disturbances include low luteinizing hormone levels with impaired response to luteinizing hormone releasing hormone and to clomiphene. However, such findings could be due to the effect of prolonged fasting as they resolve after weight gain.

### Psychological factors
INDIVIDUAL. Patients usually have:
● A disturbance of body image
● Dietary problems in early life
Anorexia is seen as an escape from the emotional problems of adolescence and a regression into childhood.

FAMILY. The specific pattern of relationships described is characterized by:
● Overprotectiveness
● Rigidity
● Lack of conflict resolution

Anorexia serves to prevent dissension in families. However, evidence in favour of such patterns is conflicting.

### Social factors

There is a higher prevalence in higher social classes, and a high rate in certain occupational groups (e.g. ballet students and nurses) and in societies where cultural value is placed on thinness.

### COURSE AND PROGNOSIS

The condition runs a fluctuating course, with exacerbations and partial remissions. Long-term follow-up suggests that about two-thirds of patients maintain normal weight and that the remaining one-third are split between those who are moderately underweight and those who are seriously underweight. Indicators of a poor outcome include:
- A long initial illness
- Severe weight loss
- Bulimia, vomiting or purging
- Difficulties in relationships

Suicide has been reported in 2–5% of patients with chronic anorexia nervosa. More than one-third have recurrent affective illness, and various family, genetic and endocrine studies have found associations between eating disorders and depression.

### TREATMENT

Treatment can be conducted on an outpatient basis, but if the weight loss is severe it is accompanied by marked physical symptoms of lassitude, dizziness and weakness and/or electrolyte and vitamin disturbances; hospital admission may then be unavoidable. Rarely, the patient's weight loss may be so severe as to be life-threatening. If the patient cannot be persuaded to enter hospital, compulsory admission may have to be used.

Treatment goals include:
- Establishing a good relationship with the patient
- Restoring the weight to a level between the ideal body weight and the patient's idea of what her weight should be
- The provision of a balanced diet of at least 3000 calories in three to four meals per day
- The elimination of purgative and/or laxative use and vomiting

Treatment can be conducted on behavioural or dynamic psychotherapeutic lines or on a combination of both. The usual behavioural approach is to remove privileges on the patient's admission and to restore them gradually as rewards for weight gain. Intense psychoanalytically-derived psychotherapy is not helpful. Family therapy, involving the exploration of problems in family relationships and their modification through counselling, is used; however, evidence that it is superior to simple supportive psychotherapy is lacking.

## Bulimia nervosa

This refers to episodes of uncontrolled excessive eating, which are also termed *binges*. There is a preoccupation with food and a habitual adoption of certain behaviours that can be understood as the patient's attempts to avoid the fattening effects of periodic binges. These behaviours include:
- Self-induced vomiting
- Laxative abuse
- Misuse of drugs—diuretics, thyroid extract or anorectics

Additional clinical features include:
1 Physical complications of vomiting:
   (a) Cardiac arrhythmias ⎤
   (b) Renal impairment     ⎬ Consequences of low K$^+$
   (c) Muscular paralysis   ⎦
   (d) Tetany—from hypokalaemic alkalosis
   (e) Swollen salivary glands ⎤ From vomiting
   (f) Eroded dental enamel     ⎦
2 Associated psychiatric disorders:
   (a) Depression in reaction to vomiting
   (b) Alcohol dependence
3 Fluctuations in body weight
4 Menstrual function—periods irregular but amenorrhoea rare
5 Personality—neurotic traits present premorbidly

The prevalence of bulimia in community studies is high; it affects between 5 and 30% of girls attending high schools, colleges or universities in the USA. Bulimia is often associated with anorexia nervosa. The prognosis is uncertain.

### TREATMENT

It is not yet clear what is the most effective form of treatment. Admission to hospital with careful control over eating has been advocated, while a behavioural approach involving careful diary-keeping regarding eating and making patients responsible for control is under extensive study. In this approach, patients attempt to identify and avoid any environmental stimuli or emotional changes that regularly precede the desire to binge. Results of this approach are promising.

# Psychosexual disorders

Sexual disorders can be divided into sexual dysfunctions, sexual deviations and gender role disorders (Table 19.31).

## Sexual dysfunctions

Sexual dysfunction in men refers to repeated inability to achieve normal sexual intercourse, whereas in women it refers to a repeatedly unsatisfactory quality of sexual satisfaction. Problems of sexual dysfunction can usefully be classified into those affecting sexual desire, those affecting sexual arousal and those affecting orgasm. Among men presenting for treatment of sexual dysfunction, impotence is the most frequent complaint. The prevalence of prema-

**Sexual dysfunction**
*Affecting sexual desire*
Low libido

*Impaired sexual arousal*
Erectile impotence
Failure of arousal in women

*Affecting orgasm*
Premature ejaculation
Retarded ejaculation
Orgasmic dysfunction in women

**Sexual deviations**
*Variations of the sexual 'object'*
Fetishism
Transvestism
Paedophilia
Bestiality
Necrophilia

*Variations of the sexual act*
Exhibitionism
Voyeurism
Sadism
Masochism
Frotteurism

**Disorders of the gender role**
Transsexualism

**Table 19.31**  Classification of sexual disorders.

| *Male arousal* | *Female arousal* |
|---|---|
| Alcohol[a] | Alcohol[a] |
| Benzodiazepines | CNS depressants |
| Neuroleptics | Oral combined |
| Cimetidine | contraceptives |
| Narcotic analgesics | Methyldopa |
| Methyldopa | Clonidine |
| Clonidine | |
| Spironolactone | |
| Antihistamines | |

[a]Alcohol increases the desire but diminishes the performance.

**Table 19.33**  Drugs adversely affecting sexual arousal.

ture ejaculation is low, while ejaculatory failure is rare.

Sexual drive is affected by constitutional factors, ignorance of sexual technique, anxiety about sexual performance, medical conditions and certain drugs (Tables 19.32 and 19.33).

The treatment of sexual dysfunction involves careful assessment, the participation (where appropriate) of the patient's partner, and specific therapeutic techniques, including relaxation, behavioural training and supportive counselling (see p. 795).

| *Endocrine* | *Renal* |
|---|---|
| Diabetes mellitus | Renal failure |
| Hyperthyroidism | |
| Hypothyroidism | *Neurological* |
| | Neuropathy |
| *Cardiovascular* | Spinal cord lesions |
| Angina pectoris | |
| Previous myocardial | *Musculoskeletal* |
| infarction | Arthritis |
| Disorders of peripheral | |
| circulation | *Respiratory* |
| | Asthma |
| *Hepatic* | Chronic bronchitis and |
| Cirrhosis, particularly | emphysema |
| alcohol related | |

**Table 19.32**  Medical conditions affecting sexual performance.

# Sexual deviations

Nowadays, sexual deviations are more likely to be regarded as unusual forms of behaviour than as illnesses and doctors are only likely to be involved when the behaviour involves breaking the law (e.g. paedophilia or bestiality) and when there is a question of an associated mental or physical disorder. Homosexuality was formerly classified as an illness but it is now an accepted alternative sexual life-style.

Transvestism is a form of sexual deviation in which individuals, usually men, dress in clothes of the opposite sex. The cross-dressing may either be a symptom of some other sexual deviation or may be employed as a means of fetishistic sexual excitement. It usually begins at about puberty and the transvestite experiences sexual excitement and may masturbate when indulging in this behaviour. The overwhelming majority of cross-dressers believe that they are of the correct gender, in contrast to transsexuals (see below).

# Gender role disorders

Transsexualism involves a disturbance in sexual identity. The criteria for establishing sexual identity are described on p. 795.

In transsexualism, there is no evidence as yet of abnormality in the chromosomal or phenotypic sex; social sex conforms to biological sex. There is, however, a severe disturbance in psychosexual differentiation. A person's *gender identity* refers to the individual's sense of masculinity or femininity as distinct from sex. It is thought to arise from a biological component (prenatal endocrine influences), psychological imprinting and social conditioning. Disturbances in these three areas have variously been blamed for the cause of transsexualism. The four key features of transsexualism are:

1 A sense of belonging to the opposite sex and of having been born into the wrong sex
2 A sense of estrangement from one's own body; all manifestations of anatomical sexual identification are regarded as repugnant

**3** A strong desire to resemble physically the opposite sex and seek treatment, including surgery, towards this end
**4** A wish to be accepted in the community as belonging to the opposite sex

For males, treatment includes hormonal administration (oestrogen is used to produce some breast enlargement and fat deposition around hips and thighs) and, if surgery is to be recommended, a period of living as a woman as a trial beforehand. In the case of female transsexuals treatment involves surgery and the use of methyltestosterone.

# Psychiatry and the law

At the heart of the relationship between psychiatry and the law is the issue of responsibility. Mental disorder, by virtue of its severity and/or quality, may impair individuals' responsibility for their thinking and actions. The law in most Western countries provides for the compulsory admission and/or treatment of mentally disordered persons for their own protection and/or the protection of others and for mitigation in the case of mentally disordered individuals who commit a criminal offence.

In England and Wales the law relating to the care and control of the mentally ill has evolved out of common law. The Act of Parliament that is crucially involved is the Mental Health Act of 1983. This Act is concerned not merely with provisions governing the compulsory admission and treatment of mentally disordered persons, but also with patients' rights, appeals tribunals and the overall supervision of the use of compulsory powers. The Act is divided into a number of sections, each of which deals with a different aspect of the process. The Mental Health (Scotland) Act 1984 and the Mental Health (Northern Ireland) Order 1986 contain clauses broadly similar to those in England and Wales.

Apart from one provision of the National Assistance Act 1948, the Mental Health Act 1983 is the only method whereby individuals can legally be deprived of their liberty without having committed a crime or being suspected of committing a crime. It is, therefore, very important that doctors understand the seriousness of their responsibility and the details of the legislation.

There are three conditions that need to be met before an appropriate compulsory section form is signed. The patient must be:
**1** Suffering from a defined mental disorder
**2** At risk to his/her and/or other people's health or safety
**3** Unwilling to accept hospitalization voluntarily
The reasons why there is no alternative approach to the treatment suggested for the patient should be outlined.

Sexual deviance or alcohol or drug dependence are not mental disorders, but otherwise the definition of mental disorder is broad and includes:
- Mental illness
- Mental impairment
- Severe mental impairment
- Psychopathy

Any registered medical practitioner may sign a medical recommendation under the Act, but the added signature of a specialist psychiatrist approved under Section 12 is needed for compulsory orders lasting for more than 72 hours. Unless the patient is already in hospital, the nearest relative or an approved mental health social worker is also required to sign the application form. Important sections of the Act are detailed in Table 19.34.

Sections 4, 5(2), 5(4) and 136 cannot be extended by repetition. They must be converted to a Section 2 or 3 if prolonged detention is necessary. Likewise, Section 2 should be converted to a Section 3 if required. Patients on the longer orders (2 and 3) can appeal to a Mental Health Review Tribunal. The Act also deals with consent to treatment, guardianship, mentally abnormal offenders and hazardous treatments. A Mental Health Act Commission supervises the Act, provides second opinions and regularly visits hospitals. Although much of the process of detention against one's will is formalized, there is no liability for a doctor who acts in good faith with a patient's best interests at heart. Clearly written medical notes, accepted forms of treatment and common sense remain the basis of good practice.

| Section | Duration | Signatures required | Purpose |
|---------|----------|---------------------|---------|
| 2 | 28 days | Two doctors (one approved) plus nearest relative or social worker | Assessment and treatment |
| 3 | 6 months | Two doctors (one approved) plus nearest relative or social worker | Treatment |
| 4 | 72 hours | One doctor plus relative or social worker | Emergency admission |
| 5(2) | 72 hours | Doctor in charge of patient's care | Emergency detention of patient already in hospital |
| 5(4) | 6 hours | Nurse (RMN) | Emergency detention of a patient already in hospital |
| 136 | 72 hours | Police officer | Psychiatric assessment of those in public places thought by police to be mentally ill and in need of a place of safety |

**Table 19.34**  Important sections of the Mental Health Act 1983.

# Further reading

Clare AW (1980) *Psychiatry in Dissent*, 2nd edn. London: Tavistock Publications.

Cranmer J & Heine B (1991) *The Use of Drugs in Psychiatry*, 3rd edn. London: Royal College of Psychiatrists. Gaskell Publications.

Lishman WA (1987) *Organic Psychiatry*, 2nd edn. London: Blackwell Scientific Publications.

Sims ACP & Owens DW (1993) *Psychiatry*, 6th edn. London: Baillière Tindall.

# 20 Dermatology

## Introduction

Skin diseases are extremely common but their exact prevalence is unknown. There are over 1000 different entities described but two-thirds of all cases are due to fewer than 10 conditions. These common conditions include acne, warts, eczema, infections due to bacteria, viruses and fungi, and psoriasis.

Some conditions, e.g. acne, may be part of normal development while others may be inherited, e.g. the Ehlers–Danlos syndrome. Skin disease may present as part of a systemic disease, e.g. the rash associated with systemic lupus erythematosus (SLE), or alternatively a severe skin disease, e.g. pemphigus, may cause systemic symptoms. Geographical factors are also important; in particular, skin conditions due to certain fungi and bacteria are more prevalent in the tropics.

## Structure of the skin (Fig. 20.1)

The skin is divided into three layers:
1 The epidermis
2 The dermis
3 The subcutaneous layer

### The epidermis

The epidermis consists of stratified epithelium. This is formed by cells (keratinocytes) from the germinal basal layer, which produces successive layers of cells that lose their nuclei and die as they reach the surface.

The epidermis is divided into two layers:
1 The *inner malpighian layer* contains the germinal basal layer (stratum germinativum), above which lies the stratum spinosum (spinous or prickle cell layer); above this is the stratum granulosum (granular layer).
2 The *outer layer* consists of anucleate cornified cells (stratum corneum). The stratum lucidum lies between this and the granular layer.

STRATUM CORNEUM. Despite consisting of cornified cells this layer forms a dynamic surface barrier to the skin. Experiments have shown that there is secretion of lipids, altered epidermal DNA synthesis and synthesis of various cytokines. Diseases of this layer can occur; for example in X-linked recessive ichthyosis there is an impairment of desquamation due to an alteration in the constituents in the lipid layer, i.e. an accumulation of cholesterol sulphate with steroid sulphatase enzyme deficiency. Furthermore an alteration of this skin surface–environment barrier by infection, for example in atopic eczema, may trigger inflammation below in the dermis. This is in contradiction to the generally accepted view that epidermal changes are secondary to dermal inflammation.

### Cells in the epidermis

KERATINOCYTES form the major cell in the epidermis. They move peripherally from the basal layer where they are continually formed by mitosis. *Keratins* are major structural proteins produced by keratinocytes in the epidermis. Human epithelial cells contain more than 30 different keratin polypeptides in two families: type I (acidic) and type II (neutral or basic) keratins. Keratin filaments consist of at least one basic and acidic type. They form the major component of the cytoskeleton of keratinocytes and connect one cell to another through desmosomes and basal cells to the basal lamina via hemidesmosomes (see Fig. 20.1b).

Genetic abnormalities of keratin have been demonstrated in epidermolysis bullosa complex, where clumping of abnormal keratin filaments is followed by cytolysis of basal cells which follows minor trauma to the skin. Similar microscopic changes occur in another genetic disease of keratin, epidermolytic hyperkeratosis, where clumping is seen in suprabasal cells.

MELANOCYTES are dendritic cells that arise from the neural crest. They synthesize melanin and transfer it as pigment granules to the epidermal keratinocytes.

LANGERHANS' CELLS. These are also dendritic cells that originate in bone marrow. They are in the suprabasal layers of the epidermis and their surfaces express HLA-DR and the antigens CD1 and CD4. They also have surface receptors for C3 and the Fc fragment of IgG and can secrete interleukin 1. They therefore function as antigen-

993

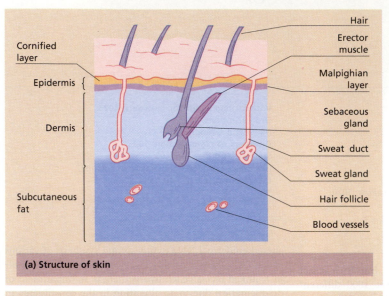

(a) Structure of skin

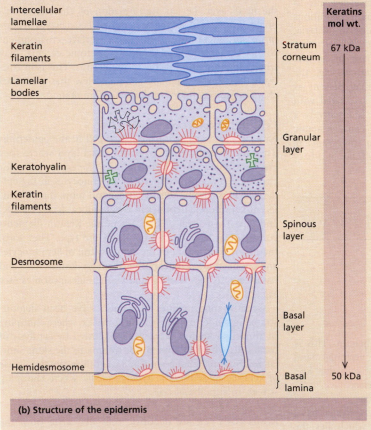

(b) Structure of the epidermis

**Fig. 20.1** (a) The structure of the skin. (b) The structure of the epidermis showing the cell layers. From Friedman PS (1992) The biology of the skin. *Medicine International* **102**: 4266. By kind permission of The Medicine Group (Journals) Ltd.

presenting and antigen-trapping cells and also cooperate with lymphocytes in eliciting an immune response. Epidermotrophic T cells, keratinocytes and draining lymph nodes form the skin-associated lymphoid tissue (SALT) that maintains immunosurveillance.

MERKEL CELLS migrate from the neural crest or arise from epithelial cells and are most numerous on digital pads, lips, the oral cavity and hair follicles where they are involved in sensation. They act as mechanoreceptors and contain neurotransmitter materials.

## The epidermodermal junction

The structure is shown in Fig. 20.7. Anchoring fibrils extend from the lamina densa into the dermis. This junctional area is highly antigenic and is the site of a number of disorders.

## The dermis

The dermis contains connective tissue fibres, amorphous ground substance, blood vessels, nerves, lymphatics and muscles. The connective tissue fibres consist mainly of collagen (75%) but some are elastic or reticulin fibres. These are embedded in a mucopolysaccharide ground substance. Fibroblasts lie between the collagen bundles and elastic fibres run parallel and enclose the bundles. This gives the skin its elasticity. The cells within the dermis include leucocytes, histiocytes, fibroblasts and mast cells.

## The sweat glands

The sweat glands are of two varieties:
1 The *eccrine glands* are present all over the skin, particularly the palms, but not in mucous membranes. The glands are situated in the dermis and secrete a watery fluid containing chloride, lactic acid, fatty acids, urea, glycoproteins and mucopolysaccharides.
2 The *apocrine glands* are large sweat glands whose ducts open into the hair follicles. They are found in the axillae, anogenital areas, nipples, areolae and scalp. They do not function until puberty. These glands produce wax in the ears.

## The sebaceous glands

Sebaceous glands occur all over the skin (except on the palms and soles) but are most numerous on the scalp and face. They have no lumen and their secretion is due to decomposition of the cells. Meibomian glands on the eyelids are modified sebaceous glands. They produce a white secretion containing proteins and complex carbohydrates.

The secretion, called sebum, consists mainly of fatty acids and cholesterol and is discharged into the pilosebaceous follicle.

## Hair

Each hair consists of a shaft of keratinized cells that is produced by the hair bulbs deep in the dermis and projects through the skin from the hair follicle. The hair follicle is richly supplied by nerves and blood vessels and contains melanin.

There are three types of hair:

TERMINAL—medullated coarse hair, e.g. scalp, mole, beard, eyebrows, pubic

VELLUS—non-medullated short, fine, downy hair, e.g. on the face of women and prepubertal boys

LANUGO—hair covering the fetus

Every hair follicle has a phase of involution (catagen phase), a shedding phase (telogen phase) and a growth phase (anagen phase) which may last up to 3 years in scalp hair. The length to which hair can grow depends on the rate of growth and the length of the anagen phase, which is cyclical. The anagen phase can vary depending on the site of the hair, e.g. 3–5 years on the scalp. Shed telogen or anagen hair can be distinguished as the club of the telogen hair end is depigmented.

## Nails

Nails are hard, translucent plates of keratin that grow from beneath the nail fold. A finger-nail takes up to 6 months to replace itself and its growth is affected by disease and malnutrition.

## The subcutaneous layer

This contains fat, sweat glands and blood vessels.

# Functions of the skin

The skin acts as a protective covering to the body. Its functions are as follows:
- It forms a physical barrier to antigens or bacteria.
- It prevents excessive absorption or loss of water.
- Its pigmentation prevents injury from ultraviolet (UV) light.
- Vitamin D is synthesized by sunlight in the epidermis.
- It is involved in temperature regulation.
- Sensations of pain, touch and temperature can be distinguished.
- It is involved in immunological reactions.

# Terminology

The terms used to describe skin diseases are shown in Information box 20.1.

# History

The history should include questions on the patient's general health, past medical history, family history, occupation and any drugs being taken. A description of the skin lesion should be obtained, including its site of origin, spread, length of time it has been present, whether it is itchy (Information box 20.2) or painful, whether it forms blisters or whether any ointment or medicines have helped.

# Examination

A careful examination of the whole skin should be made, as clues to the diagnosis may be apparent in distant sites. If the nature of the skin disease is not obvious, a full general examination should be performed, as the skin disease may be a manifestation of a systemic disorder.

# Investigation

SKIN SCRAPINGS FOR FUNGI. Scrapings from areas of involved skin are placed on a slide with 20% potassium hydroxide to clear extraneous material. Fungal mycelia, as well as parasites and lice, may be seen under the microscope.

SKIN BIOPSY. Skin should be removed in the shape of an ellipse along lines of stretch (Langer's lines). Biopsies should either be fixed in formalin or frozen immediately for immunofluorescence.

| | |
|---|---|
| Annular lesions | Lesions occurring in rings |
| Atrophy | Thinning of skin |
| Bulla | A large vesicle |
| Crust | Dried exudate on the skin |
| Ecchymoses | Bruises >3 mm in diameter |
| Erythema | Redness |
| Erythroderma | Widespread redness of the skin with scaling |
| Excoriation | Linear marks due to scratching |
| Macule | A flat circumscribed area of discoloration |
| Maculopapule | A raised and discoloured circumscribed lesion |
| Nodule | A circumscribed large palpable mass >1 cm in diameter |
| Papule | A circumscribed, raised, palpable area |
| Petechiae | Bruises <3 mm in diameter |
| Plaque | A disc-shaped lesion; can result from coalescence of papules |
| Purpura | Extravasation of blood into the skin; does not blanch on pressure |
| Pustule | A pus-filled blister |
| Scales | Dried flakes of dead skin from horny layer (keratin) |
| Telangiectasis | A visible small dilated vessel on the skin |
| Vesicle | A small, visible, fluid-filled blister |
| Weal | A transiently raised, reddened area associated with scratching |

**Information box 20.1**   Terminology used in skin diseases.

WOOD'S LIGHT. This is a UV light that is shone on the skin. Normal hair and skin fluoresce bluish-white. Certain types of ringworm (*Microsporum audouini* and *M. canis*) fluoresce a greenish colour; erythrasma due to *Corynebacterium minutissimum* fluoresces pink/red.

PATCH TESTS. (Practical box 20.1). These are used to confirm allergic contact dermatitis.

LABORATORY TESTS for the exclusion of bacterial and fungal infections. Tests for SLE or thrombocytopenic purpura, for example, should be performed as appropriate.

HAIR—microscopy and root analysis.

ROUTINE TESTS such as blood counts and erythrocyte sedimentation rate (ESR) and also urine testing, e.g. for glucose in diabetes, should be performed.

# Erythematous–scaly eruptions

## DERMATITIS AND ECZEMA

Dermatitis implies inflammation of the skin and can be due to many causes. It is usual to prefix the term with the causal agent, e.g. solar dermatitis.

The characteristic features of dermatitis are:

A RED AND HOT SKIN. Dermatitis affects the epidermis and superficial dermis.

OEDEMA IN ACUTE STAGES. This separates the keratinocytes (spongiosis) and produces intradermal vesicles.

WEEPING AND OOZING of fluid on to surface. Crusting is seen in acute phases and scaling and fissuring in chronic stages.

Pruritis means itching. It can occur in many skin conditions, including:

Scabies
Atopic eczema
Candidiasis
Urticaria
Insect bites (e.g. flea, bed-bug)

It also occurs with systemic conditions, often without obvious skin involvement. These include:

Metabolic disease—hyperthyroidism, carcinoid syndrome
Malignant disease—chronic lymphatic leukaemia, lymphoma, some carcinomas
Haematological disease—polycythaemia vera
Renal disease—chronic renal failure with uraemia
Liver disease—cholestasis, particularly primary biliary cirrhosis
Miscellaneous—senile pruritus, psychogenic, drugs, e.g. opiates

**Information box 20.2**   Pruritus.

The original skin disease should be in a quiescent phase before patch testing is done.

Systemic steroid therapy may alter the cutaneous response to an allergen.

The back is a convenient site for testing
Sites for application of the antigen are clearly labelled and a map of their whereabouts is made
Materials are diluted in order to prevent irritant reactions and suspended in white soft paraffin
White soft paraffin should be used alone in some sites as a control
Each substance is then placed within an aluminium disc and kept in place next to the skin by adhesive strapping
The patches are taken off and an initial reading is made after 48 hours
A positive reaction is indicated by an area of eczema
Further readings are taken at 96 hours
Blistering may indicate a non-specific irritant effect but it can occur with soap or detergent materials

**Practical box 20.1**   Patch testing.

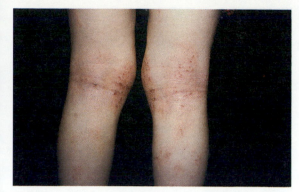

**Fig. 20.2**   Lichenification seen with chronic flexural eczema.

EXCORIATION produced by intense itching. Chronic scratching leads to secondary thickening or lichenification of skin (Fig. 20.2).

SECONDARY INFECTION.

IMPAIRED THERMOREGULATION and an increased blood flow leading to cardiac failure in very severe cases.

Acute and chronic stages can be seen in the same individual and the acute can resolve completely, leaving no skin abnormalities.

The meaning of the word 'eczema' is 'flowing over', which describes some of the above inflammatory changes. The words eczema and dermatitis are used somewhat interchangeably because in both conditions similar inflammatory changes occur in the skin. Use of the term 'eczema' avoids the word 'dermatitis', which often conjures up ideas in the patient's mind of external irritants that may cause contact dermatitis.

Eczema occurs following a variety of stimuli.

# Endogenous eczema (atopic dermatitis)

## PATHOGENESIS

The word 'atopy' implies a capacity to hyper-react to common environmental factors. It can be demonstrated by multiple positive skin-prick tests (see p. 651). A positive test to a specific antigen does not necessarily indicate that this antigen is involved in causation of the skin disease, and removal of the antigen, e.g. from the diet, often does not improve the skin condition.

The skin lesion may be caused by CD4 T cells infiltrating the skin and producing the cytokines interferon γ and interleukins 2 and 4.

Serum levels of the IgE antibody are elevated in atopic eczema as in all atopic diseases; higher values are seen when eczema is combined with asthma. The significance of these raised levels in the pathogenesis of the eczema is unclear.

### Diet

A few patients may be able to correlate the onset of itching and exacerbation of eczema with dietary factors such as eggs and milk and the removal of the food item will often improve the skin condition. Dietary changes need to be assessed over a prolonged period.

### Genetic factors

There is a hereditary predisposition; when both parents have the disease, the risk of their offspring developing eczema is approximately 60%.

### Exacerbating factors

Non-specific stimuli such as heat, humidity, drying of the skin and contact with woollen clothing may cause a flare-up of disease, and patients should be advised to avoid these trigger factors. Irritation may occur following contact urticaria when, for example, foods or animal saliva touch the skin of a sensitized individual.

In atopic patients *Staphylococcus aureus* is found more frequently on the normal skin or nasal mucosa than expected. It is present on 90% of acute eczematous lesions and exacerbates the condition. Herpes simplex may become disseminated on atopic skin (eczema herpeticum). Aeroallergens, e.g. house-dust mite, are thought to play an active role in facial eczema.

## PATTERNS OF DISEASE

### Infantile eczema

Erythema, weeping or scaling usually appear first on the face when the infant is a few months old. Other body sites are less commonly affected.

Irritation produces restlessness and the child may rub its face or scalp on a pillow or the cot-side. With time there is a gradual spread of the dermatitis to the flexures.

### Flexural or childhood eczema

In toddlers and older children the skin folds are typically involved. Facial involvement may persist, partly owing to climatic factors, e.g. sunlight and low humidity.

### Adult eczema

In those whose disease continues into adult life, the flexures at the neck, elbow, wrist, ankle or knee and the limbs are often involved. Chronic eczematous changes are common on the face, although any site on the body may be involved.

## PROGNOSIS

With a typical pattern of involvement and an early onset, the prognosis is good. Some children will lose their disease in infancy, whilst others improve gradually so that by the early teens more than 90% will be clear of disease. Localized recurrence may occur in adult life if the skin is unduly stressed, e.g. the hands of nurses or hairdressers. An unusual pattern of eczema over extensor surfaces (reversed pattern) coming on later in childhood may represent more recalcitrant disease and the prognosis should be guarded.

## TREATMENT

About one-third of atopic children have a dry skin in addition to eczema. Keratosis pilaris or ichthyosis vulgaris are associated conditions. The regular use of emollients such as aqueous cream or emulsifying ointment applied to a damp skin after bathing or used instead of soap is fundamental to a treatment regimen. The use of perfumed soaps and 'bubble baths' should be avoided. Non-perfumed cleansers and gels should be used for washing, with the use of soap limited. Sunny seaside holidays or UV light treatment will often stabilize the skin condition.

For widespread regular use over months or years, a mild topical corticosteroid (Table 20.1), e.g. 1% hydrocortisone, is suitable; the cream base is the form best tolerated—the occlusive nature of ointments may, with sweating, promote itching. Localized disease may require short courses of more potent topical corticosteroids on some occasions, especially when the skin is markedly thickened. The addition of tar as an alcoholic solution or as crude coal tar may also improve lichenified skin. Bacterial infection seen with gross excoriation or with fissuring of the skin is treated with a steroid–antibiotic combination and systemic antibiotics may be required.

The treatment of associated atopic disease, e.g. asthma, may in turn improve the state of the skin, the child's well-being and sleep pattern. Sedative antihistamines, such as promethazine hydrochloride elixir at night, will also help to prevent restless sleep and ceaseless scratching.

The reduction of house-dust mite exposure (see p. 654) may improve facial eczema.

## Pompholyx (Fig. 20.3)

This pattern of eczema commonly affects the sides of the fingers, palms, the toes or soles of the feet. Irritant vesicles are the initial feature, though with more serious attacks bullae may be seen.

The patients are usually in their twenties or thirties

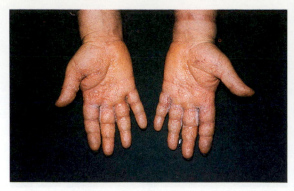

**Fig. 20.3**  Pompholyx.

when they develop the disease. A previous history of atopy is not elicited in the majority of patients.

Endogenous factors that trigger this type of eczema are not known. The role of dietary nickel provoking the disease in nickel-sensitive patients is controversial. Attacks may occur frequently and at regular intervals. This condition should not be confused with the irritant vesicles found on fingers of normal individuals in hot weather.

### TREATMENT

Drying and bacteriostatic solutions such as potassium permanganate 0.01% are used daily until weeping is controlled. Potent topical corticosteroids containing antibiotics or antiseptics may be necessary to control severe attacks, e.g. betamethasone valerate 0.1% cream with neomycin or fluocinolone acetonide 0.025% cream with clioquinol.

Systemic treatment with steroids, e.g. i.m. Synacthen, given at regular intervals over weeks or even months, or prednisolone by mouth in doses of between 10 and 15 mg daily, may be necessary to break the frequency of attacks and heal the skin.

## Discoid or nummular eczema

This type of disease occurs mainly in the middle-aged or elderly with no previous history of skin disease. Papules and coin-shaped raised lesions associated with extreme itching occur on the limbs, most commonly on the lower leg; they may merge to form plaques. Annular patches may appear in association with other patterns of eczema during early life. The cause is unknown but bacterial antigens have been implicated. Eczematous lesions on the legs are sometimes due to venous incompetence (see p. 629).

### TREATMENT

Occlusive bandages containing zinc paste or ichthammol may help to alleviate itching and prevent incessant scratching. Impregnated steroid tape containing flurandrenolone 0.0125% may produce the same effect; intralesional triamcinolone or local potent topical corticosteroids improve the condition of the skin and give relief from itching. The disease often improves when the patient retires from work.

---

*Actions*
Anti-inflammatory
Immunosuppressive
Decrease rate of epidermal cell turnover

*Types*
Many. Available in cream, ointment or lotion form.
   Vary in potency:
   Mild, e.g. hydrocortisone 1%
   Moderate, e.g. clobetasone butyrate 0.05%
   Potent, e.g. betamethasone 0.1% (as valerate),
      hydrocortisone butyrate, fluocinolone acetonide
      0.025%
   Very potent, e.g. clobetasol propionate 0.05%
Compound preparations with, for example
      antibacterials, are available

*Uses*
In general, the least potent effective preparation
      should be used. The use of potent preparations on
      the face should be avoided

*Side-effects*
Thinning of skin
Spread of local infection
Telangiectasia and striae
Hair growth
Acne
Adrenal suppression with long-term use of potent
      preparations
Side-effects are chiefly associated with the more potent
      forms

**Table 20.1**  Topical steroids.

# Exogenous eczema

Exogenous eczema can be divided into primary irritant dermatitis and true contact dermatitis associated with a cell-mediated immune response.

### Primary irritant dermatitis

This is essentially a degreasing of the skin with a subsequent water loss followed by dryness, fissuring and cracking. It can occur both at work and in the home. Industrial solvents that remove greasy coatings covering metal components in industry can with equal efficiency remove surface lipids from the skin if they are not handled with care.

Those working in the home are also at risk; the changes in the skin occur in parallel with the extent of immersion of the hands in water. Initially the skin beneath a ring is often involved, as neat detergent or soap powder tends to lodge there and erode the skin. This spreads to the thin skin on the sides of the fingers, the webs and the backs of the hands; the palms are only affected in more severe and chronic disease. A similar type of disease may be seen in other occupations with the use of cleaning and detergent solutions, such as bar work and hairdressing.

### Asteatotic eczema or eczema craquelé

This is a condition often seen in long-stay elderly hospital patients. Dryness of the skin is more evident with ageing. The condition is made worse by excessive washing with soap. The eczema can result in a 'crocodile skin' appearance that is most noticeable on the lower limbs.

This condition may also be seen in hypothyroidism.

Although the skin may appear inflamed, the use of emollients and creams or soap substitutes has the greatest beneficial effect and topical corticosteroids are often unnecessary.

### Allergic contact dermatitis

This is a good example of cell-mediated immune disease or type IV reaction. T lymphocytes are sensitized to the antigen, some time after the first contact.

Small-molecular-weight substances passing through the skin need to be linked to skin proteins (haptens) in order to sensitize. Langerhans' cells in the dermis present the antigen to lymphocytes. The sensitivity lasts for life.

### CLINICAL FEATURES AND INVESTIGATION

An unusual pattern of rash with clear-cut demarcation or odd-shaped areas of erythema and scaling should arouse suspicion and in combination with a careful history indicate a cause. All areas of the skin may be involved, but the back is the most convenient site for testing. The suspected allergen is then placed in contact with the skin as a patch test. If the causative agent cannot be clearly defined, e.g. in hand eczema, then a range of known everyday antigens are tested, including materials such as rubber, nickel and medicaments. Positive readings will need to be interpreted with caution and may not have an obvious relevance when considering the patient's history or occupation.

If the major distribution of an eruption appears to involve exposed skin, then photo-patch testing may be required. Two identical sets of likely allergens are placed on the back; one set is exposed to long-wave UV (UVA) light, with the second non-exposed set acting as a control.

### TREATMENT

Remove the known irritant or allergen if this is possible. Steroid creams are helpful for short periods when the disease is severe. Antipruritic agents may be necessary for symptomatic relief of itching.

## Miscellaneous

### Exfoliative dermatitis (erythroderma)

In this condition the entire skin is erythematous, oedematous and scaly. The disease is rare and can be idiopathic (without a preceding skin condition) or can follow dermatitis, psoriasis or other skin disease. It can also be a reaction to many drugs, e.g. sulphonamides, sulphonylureas, gold. It is also an occasional feature of systemic disorders, particularly the lymphomas, so that a skin biopsy may be necessary.

MANAGEMENT. Body fluid loss can be considerable and the patient needs intensive medical care; systemic steroid therapy is often necessary.

## PSORIASIS

This chronic skin disease is seen most commonly as erythematous well-demarcated silvery scaled plaques over extensor surfaces such as the elbows and knees, and in the scalp. In this common pattern the onset of the disease is unusual before 15 years of age, and the initial presentation may occur in old age. Psoriasis occurs throughout the world; in the temperate zones 2% of the population are affected. It is less common in some races with pigmented skins. Characteristically there are periods of activity and remission that are often impossible to predict.

Arthropathy occurs in association with the skin disease in about 8–10% of individuals. Pathogenetic factors that link the two conditions are not clear, though abnormal vascular changes are seen in both.

### AETIOLOGY
#### Genetic factors

The mode of inheritance of the disease is not known but certain HLA markers are recognized. HLA-B13, B16, B17 and DR7 are all associated with an increased relative risk and HLA-CW6 has an increased risk up to seven times that of the general population. The B loci occupy an area adjacent to the gene that expresses CW6. HLA-B27 is seen in up to 90% of individuals with ankylosing spondylitis and in 70% of individuals who develop a similar spinal arthropathy with psoriasis.

#### Infection

The role of infection as an exacerbating factor is suggested by the following observations:

IN CHILDREN OR YOUNG ADULTS, superficial small patterned lesions of *guttate psoriasis* may appear over the trunk and limbs 10–14 days following a throat infection with β-haemolytic streptococci, and up to 75% of these individuals have the HLA-CW6 marker or DR7.

PATIENTS WITH REITER'S SYNDROME (see p. 396) may develop skin lesions that are identical to those seen in psoriasis. Reiter's disease can occur after dysentery or after venereal contact, again suggesting an infective aetiology that might induce psoriasis.

PATIENTS WITH HIV INFECTION do not have an increased incidence of psoriasis. However, patients with a low CD4 T-cell count may experience severe psoriasis (often of a pustular pattern) and unusually, different patterns of the condition may occur in the same individual.

### Emotional trauma

Emotional trauma can trigger psoriasis; for example, a child followed through to adolescence may be seen to have an exacerbation of the disease with the stress of school examinations. Patients can also develop a reactive psychological state owing to the severity of their skin disease.

### Mechanical trauma

Repeated trauma to the skin over the elbows and knees as part of everyday activity may explain the common involvement of these sites with psoriasis. In sedentary occupations, e.g. in chauffeurs, there may be intractable disease over the lumbosacral region. Scratching the skin when the disease is in an active phase may induce lesions along the line of trauma—the isomorphic response or Koebner phenomenon. Irritant types of psoriasis such as that affecting the scalp may be made worse by scratching.

### Drugs

Lithium carbonate may induce intractable psoriasis. This agent inhibits adenylate cyclase activity, which may alter epidermal cell kinetics. The β-receptor antagonists such as propranolol may exacerbate psoriasis through similar mechanisms.

### PATHOGENESIS

The pathogenesis is unclear but a number of factors play a role.

EPIDERMAL CELL PROLIFERATION is seen in both the lesions and the uninvolved skin of psoriatics. There is a shortening of the epidermal cell-cycle time and an increase in the number of proliferative cells in the growth fraction of the epidermis.

DIVISION is normally limited to the basal layer in normal skin but may extend over several layers within psoriatic plaques. Polyamines are known to be important in regulating cellular proliferation, and the levels of these substances and of their rate-limiting enzyme, ornithine decarboxylase, are elevated in psoriasis.

ARACHIDONIC ACID LEVELS are greatly elevated in both uninvolved and lesional skin. Many stimuli that affect the cell membrane may cause a release of phospholipase and arachidonic acid and a number of inflammatory mediators are formed from arachidonic acid via the lipoxygenase pathway (see Fig. 12.30). The major initial metabolite in the lipoxygenase pathway is 5-hydroperoxyeicosatetraenoic acid (5-HPETE). This is the precursor of a family of peptido-hydroxyeicosatetraenoic acids, including the leukotrienes, that can alter enzyme pathways that control cell kinetics. Leukotrienes also have marked chemoattractant properties.

LEUKOTRIENE B$_4$ (LTB$_4$) levels are elevated in lesional skin and the injection of this substance causes an increase in polymorphonuclear infiltration. Polymorphonuclear cell infiltration of the epidermis and the formation of *Munro* microabscesses are an important pathological feature in this disease. A variety of immune factors may also attract polymorphonuclear leucocytes; these include immune complexes and complement fragments.

HUMORAL AND CELLULAR ABNORMALITIES have been demonstrated in psoriasis, including elevated IgA and alteration of T-cell function. The relative lack of sensitization to the common sensitizer dinitrochlorobenzene (DNCB) in patients with psoriasis supports the concept of an altered cell-mediated immune response in this disease.

### CLINICAL FEATURES

### Plaque psoriasis

Lesions are well demarcated, salmon pink in colour and are surmounted by silvery scaling that may be exaggerated by lightly traumatizing the skin with the edge of a finger-nail.

The majority of patients with a plaque type of psoriasis show involvement of the skin over the extensor surfaces of the limbs such as the elbows and knees, with scattered smaller lesions on the limbs and trunk that increase with exacerbation of the disease. Involvement of the scalp with thickened hyperkeratotic scale is common. This is most clearly seen at the hair margin or over the occiput.

The *arthropathy* associated with psoriasis is described on (p. 397).

### Flexural psoriasis

This is a less common type of psoriasis that may be seen together with plaques or may occur alone. Lesions have a pinkish glazed appearance, are clearly demarcated and non-scaly. The groin, perianal and genital skin are principally involved. Other sites include inframammary folds and the umbilicus. The condition may prove intractable in situations such as the inframammary fold of elderly women with large and pendulous breasts, or when associated with incontinence.

### Pustular psoriasis

This may occur in various patterns and in children it is often an isolated finding involving a single digit. The nail dystrophy most commonly seen is yellow discoloration and thickening. Scaling may be pronounced over the digit and, in association with erythema, may spread over the finger.

In its most common form, pustular psoriasis affects the palms or soles with areas of well-demarcated scaling and erythema (Fig. 20.4). The pustules, which are sterile, may appear white, yellow or greenish in colour and when dried are deep brown. Pustulation may not always be evident and it is often associated with increased disease activity. When the condition is grossly hyperkeratotic and occurs in a conical or papular form it is termed *rupioid*; identical lesions are seen as one of the cutaneous features of Reiter's syndrome (keratoderma blennorrhagica).

The trunk and limbs may be involved by an almost universal scaling as *exfoliative or erythrodermic psoriasis*. When this condition is seen in association with superficial pustule formation it is termed *generalized pustular psoriasis*. This is a serious life-threatening condition, similar to having widespread burns. Such a disease may occur spontaneously but it is seen more frequently after the use of potent corticosteroid therapy given orally or by topical application.

### Nail involvement

This can occur in isolation with no evidence of psoriasis elsewhere. The changes most commonly seen include pitting and onycholysis, when separation of the distal edge of the nail from the underlying vascular bed produces a whitish appearance. A red/brown, salmon-pink or 'oil-stain' coloration may be seen under the nail proximal to the onycholysis. Less commonly the nails are ridged or furrowed. Hyperkeratosis beneath the nail is a pattern of the disease most often seen on the toe-nails, especially in association with pustular variants of psoriasis. When only one or two toe-nails are affected it may be difficult to distinguish from a fungal infection.

### MANAGEMENT

The majority of patients can cope with the chronic nature of the disease but the physician must take an active role in treating exacerbations. Tolerance and understanding are required in helping patients to overcome the social stigma that may be associated with their disease.

Intensive treatment with topical agents can be messy and may need to be carried out in day-care centres or in hospital.

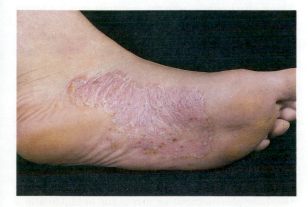

**Fig. 20.4**  Pustular psoriasis of the sole.

### Intensive regimens

*Dithranol* (inhibits DNA synthesis) in concentrations of between 0.05 and 0.5% in zinc and salicylic acid paste (Lassar's paste) is applied to the lesional skin and the normal skin is protected by wearing a tubular stockingette suit. Repeated daily treatments are necessary. The application of this paste is preceded by a tar bath and minimal erythema doses of UVB (UV light of short wavelength). The intensity of the UV irradiation is gradually increased throughout the treatment period. Coal tar and salicylic acid ointment sometimes containing dithranol in concentrations of between 0.05 and 0.1% is applied overnight to the scalp and removed in the morning with a tar-containing shampoo. Coal tar is often used as an alternative to dithranol in the USA.

### Outpatient treatments

- DITHRANOL is applied at increasing concentrations of between 1 and 3% mixed with 5% salicylic acid in white soft paraffin for up to 20 minutes' therapy and is then washed off. Irritancy and staining of the skin can prevent regular use.
- COMBINED PREPARATIONS of corticosteroids with dithranol or an alcoholic solution of coal tar are especially valuable at low concentrations in the treatment of flexural psoriasis, or for patients with widespread lesions who experience irritation with dithranol applied in a paste form. They are cosmetically acceptable for use in the home.
- TOPICAL STEROIDS can be used but long-term usage of potent steroids should be avoided.
- CALCIPOTRIOL (topical vitamin $D_3$) is useful for limited and mild psoriasis. It is simple to apply, clean and therefore, acceptable to the patient.
- LOW-DOSE TETRACYCLINE in prolonged courses may be helpful in unremitting pustular psoriasis on the palms and soles. This treatment tends to limit the accumulation of polymorphonuclear leucocytes, a prominent feature in the pathology of the disease.
- RETINOIC ACID DERIVATIVES, e.g. acitretin, taken by mouth (1 mg kg$^{-1}$ daily), are helpful in managing pustular and other forms of psoriasis. However, long-term treatment may be required and this can cause loss of hair, dryness of the skin, hepatic disturbance, hyperlipidaemia and hyperostoses. As it is teratogenic it should not be given to women of childbearing age.
- PSORALENS WITH UVA (PUVA) THERAPY may improve or clear most patterns of psoriasis. Photosensitizing agents, e.g. psoralens, are taken orally 2 hours before or applied topically 30 min before exposure to UVA. Exposure for 2–15 min on two to three occasions each week usually results in clearance of the psoriasis in 10–12 weeks. Maintenance treatment is required every 2–3 weeks in most patients to keep the skin clear.
- NON-STEROIDAL ANTI-INFLAMMATORY DRUGS (NSAIDs). Troublesome joint disease may respond to these drugs.
- CYTOTOXIC DRUGS may help alleviate widespread intractable cutaneous disease and painful joints in older patients. Patients with severe chronic psoriasis

may experience complete and long-term remission with methotrexate in doses of up to 30 mg once a week. Apart from bone marrow suppression, cumulative dosage of this drug can lead to hepatic fibrosis. Liver biopsies are required before starting the drug and at yearly intervals, as routine blood tests cannot detect the liver fibrosis. The fibrotic changes tend to be non-progressive, if the drug is stopped. Hydroxyurea can be used and is not hepatotoxic. Azathioprine is more effective on the arthropathy. Cyclosporin by mouth is successful in treating psoriasis, but serious side-effects will limit long-term use.

SELF-HELP GROUPS provide support for patients.

# SEBORRHOEIC DERMATITIS

Seborrhoeic dermatitis affects those areas of the skin where there is a high density of sebaceous glands. The cause is unknown and no consistent alteration in the function of the sebaceous glands has been demonstrated. For many years observers have attempted to link the disease to lipophilic yeasts that are present on the normal skin as saprophytes, e.g. *Pityrosporum orbiculare* and *P. ovale*, which occur on the trunk and scalp respectively. Bacterial infection has also been considered in the pathogenesis but infection is probably secondary to the skin maceration. Neurogenic factors play a role in that patients with Parkinson's disease may develop similar clinical features over their facial skin and continuing mental stress often exacerbates the disease. Patients are often fair-skinned types of Celtic origin and so genetic factors may also be relevant.

The prevalence of this condition in AIDS is approximately 80% (see p. 99). It is often the presenting cutaneous feature of the disease and is correlated with a poor prognosis.

### CLINICAL FEATURES

The scalp is principally involved and shows diffuse scaling and erythema. Papules and pustules may accompany these changes or present as the only manifestation of the disease. The spread locally is to the eyebrows, nasolabial folds, the ears and neck. Blepharitis and otitis externa can occur as single features, or they may accompany more widespread disease. Other skin sites affected include the sternal region, the thoracic spine and the paraspinal skin, the axillae, the groin folds and the perianal region. Greasy scales, weeping and maceration are seen with more severe or acute disease. A folliculitis may be the predominant feature on the trunk.

On occasions the condition may be seen together with more typical eczematous changes elsewhere on the skin; the term *seborrhoeic eczema* is often used to describe this pattern.

### TREATMENT

Shampoos that contain substances that have a fungostatic action, e.g. selenium sulphide, zinc pyrithione or econazole, can give *initial* benefit to patients with a scaly and greasy scalp. It is a good principle to change the shampoo after 6–8 weeks. These shampoos tend to aggravate the scalp if there are marked inflammatory lesions and antiseptic preparations such as cetrimide or povidone-iodine in shampoo forms can be added. Ketoconazole shampoo used every 10–14 days long term will often control scalp symptoms; more frequent use on the trunk or facial skin may control disease at these sites.

A course of tetracycline (250 mg twice daily), minocycline or doxycycline given for 2–3 months may lower the intensity of the inflammatory patterns of the disease. Itraconazole also reduces inflammation.

Lotions, creams or antiseptic powders may help to diminish maceration of the skin involving body folds. Steroid creams should be those of relatively low potency, and preferably they should be combined with an antibiotic or antiseptic such as tetracycline or clioquinol.

Candidiasis may accompany chronic disease and imidazole/hydrocortisone combination creams often help this and other features of the disease.

# LICHEN PLANUS

Lichen planus describes a condition in which the lesions are:

- Purplish in colour
- Polygonal in outline
- Planar or flat-topped papules

The cause is unknown but some gross forms of lichen planus may occur in association with diseases in which there is a profound immunological abnormality such as myasthenia gravis with thymoma, and with graft-versus-host disease. It is also seen with autoimmune chronic liver disease, e.g. primary biliary cirrhosis or chronic active hepatitis. Oral disease has been associated with amalgams in dental fillings. Lichen planus-like reactions occur with certain drugs such as sulphonamides (most commonly taken as sulphasalazine), sulphonylureas, methyldopa, thiazide diuretics and β-blockers. Patients with rheumatoid arthritis treated by agents that alter immune function, such as antimalarials, gold, levamisole or penicillamine, may also develop lichen planus-like lesions or lichenoid rashes.

### PATHOLOGY

This is characteristic, with the epidermis showing hyperkeratosis, and a marked chronic lymphocytic infiltrate is seen at the epidermodermal junction. This infiltration consists principally of T cells and suggests an immunological reaction to an epidermal antigen.

### CLINICAL FEATURES

The distribution of the lesions is peripheral, involving the wrists and ankles, usually symmetrically. The genitalia, scalp or nails are less frequently involved; with chronic disease the scarring that may occur can permanently damage the growth of hair or nails. Scarring may also accompany the less frequent annular patterns of the disease. Linear lesions may follow trauma or scratching (Koebner phenomenon) or may occur in children in a naevoid fashion along a limb. Trauma to the mucosa overlying the bite margin in the mouth commonly induces involvement at this site, producing distinctive pale white linear markings or patterns. Erosive changes may also be seen on the buccal mucosa or tongue or female genitalia.

The presence of Wickham's striae—fine white lacy patterning coursing over the papule—helps to distinguish this disease. Postinflammatory hyperpigmentation is also a useful diagnostic sign if the disease is beginning to fade at the time of first presentation.

### TREATMENT

Untreated, common patterns of the disease may last for 12–18 months. Hypertrophic lesions on the legs or annular patterns may be rather more persistent; recurrence may occur in about one-fifth of cases.

Widespread acute disease is often associated with intractable itching and this may require oral prednisolone for control, given over several months. Less acute disease may be managed with the topical application of potent corticosteroids together with a sedative antihistamine given at night to control the itching.

## PITYRIASIS ROSEA

This is a self-limiting non-recurrent scaling maculopapular eruption occurring principally in children and young adults. The disease is less common in the summer, and current epidemiological evidence suggests an infective cause, most probably viral. Drugs, e.g. penicillamine, gold, may induce identical clinical features. Males and females are equally affected.

### CLINICAL FEATURES

Commonly, a larger and more conspicuous lesion, 2–6 cm in diameter, will precede the more widespread rash by up to 10 days (the herald patch). Individual lesions, occurring predominantly on the trunk, are reddish-brown in colour, macular, scaled and discrete. They often course over the chest wall following the line of the ribs in a linear fashion. The proximal limb girdle is also affected but the face and scalp are rarely involved. Individual lesions, especially over the neck, may show a collarette, i.e. a border composed of a rim of scales that point towards the centre. Florid inflammatory papules may occasionally be seen, and individual lesions may be rather more hyperkeratotic on black or Asian skins. The eruption is only mildly pruritic and usually clears in 6–8 weeks without treatment.

Constitutional upset may be noticed prior to the onset of the rash or within the first few days of its appearance. This should help to distinguish the condition from secondary syphilis which it may closely resemble but in which systemic features are usually more severe.

## Erythematous lesions

## URTICARIA

The term 'urticaria' implies intermittent transient swelling of the skin with a loss of fluid from vessels into the extravascular space. Dermal swelling is associated with yyweals, whilst subcutaneous fluid collection is associated with brawny lesions often around the lips and orbit (angio-oedema) or the genitalia. The skin appears completely normal afterwards (within minutes or hours).

The passage of fluid out of the vessel may accompany the dilatation caused by mediators such as histamine released from neighbouring mast cells or by other vasoactive compounds such as kinins or prostaglandins. More severe vessel damage, e.g. the vasculitis associated with diseases such as SLE or allergic vasculitis, may produce weals in association with purpura and necrosis. On occasions, rather ordinary-looking weals may be accompanied by quite marked vessel damage and an inflammatory cell infiltrate seen on histological examination. Biopsies should therefore be obtained:

- When weals last longer than 2 days
- When weals are accompanied by purpuric staining
- When antibiotics and circulating immune complexes are present in the sera
- When attacks are accompanied by systemic features such as fever or arthralgia

An aetiological classification of urticaria is given in Table 20.2.

### PATHOGENESIS

Foods, e.g. nuts and shellfish, may be implicated. Other trigger factors include salicylates, indomethacin, tartrazine dyes in food substances or benzoates used as preservatives. Such substances may exacerbate the disease when it is in the active phase in up to 40% of patients. Cross-reactivity between substances, e.g. tartrazine and salicylates, is seen but a search for a food 'allergen' is often unrewarding. A direct pharmacological effect on vessel reactivity is probable, and both aspirin and indomethacin are known to affect prostaglandin metabolism. Agents

*Immunological mechanisms*
IgE mediated:
  Atopy
  Physical, e.g. cold, dermographism
  Antigen sensitivity, e.g. pollens, foods, drugs,
    helminths
Complement mediated:
  Hereditary angio-oedema
  Serum sickness
  Blood transfusion reactions
  Necrotizing vasculitis

*Non-immunological mechanisms*
Mast cell-releasing agents:
  Opiates
  Radiological contrast media
  Antibiotics
Prostaglandin inhibitors:
  Aspirin
  Non-steroidal anti-inflammatory drugs
  Azo dyes
  Benzoates

**Table 20.2**  An aetiological classification of idiopathic urticaria.

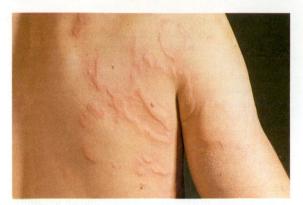

**Fig. 20.5**   Urticaria.

that can liberate histamine directly include morphine and codeine.

Type I hypersensitivity is more commonly seen with acute disease, or in atopic individuals, and may be triggered by, for example, penicillin in milk. Even when no obvious trigger factor is found there is a tendency towards resolution of the attacks over weeks or months in the majority of patients. In the recalcitrant case an exclusion diet may be used as a last resort, but this is often unhelpful.

### CLINICAL FEATURES

Weals that irritate are seen on the trunk or limbs and usually last for several hours, or up to 12–24 hours (Fig. 20.5). There may be accompanying angio-oedema and this feature may predominate in some patients with swelling of eyes or lips; swelling of the genitalia is less common. *Chronic urticaria* is arbitrarily defined as disease lasting for more than 6 weeks.

### Physical urticarias

These may be produced by pressure, sweating, touch, heat, cold, UV light or water for example. These patterns of urticaria are less common and are most likely to be misdiagnosed. This is particularly true of conditions that are not easily reproduced in the clinic, e.g. pressure urticaria.

CHOLINERGIC URTICARIA. This is not an uncommon pattern of disease and is seen in young adults. The weals are usually small, are often associated with erythema, and last 5–20 min. Attacks are triggered by exercise, hot baths, showers or emotional upset. Such factors may also cause itching but no obvious weals (especially in Blacks) and induce stress and panic reactions. Large quantities of histamine may be liberated during attacks and cause difficulty with breathing. Patients should be advised to avoid histamine liberators such as codeine or aspirin. If attacks can be anticipated, predosing with hydroxyzine, cyproheptadine or a non-sedative antihistamine such as terfenadine during the day may abort a reaction.

DERMOGRAPHISM (FACTITIOUS URTICARIA). This reaction represents an exaggeration of the third compo-

nent of Lewis's triple response. A livid weal is produced in response to scratching in about 5% of the population; it is usually asymptomatic. Symptomatic disease occurs when symptoms of itching or discomfort occur after trauma to the skin. Patients may experience marked erythema and wealing when, for example, towelling dry after a bath. Complaints of generalized pruritus with, on occasions, nothing to see may prompt doctors to label the patient as neurotic.

COLD URTICARIA. This may be triggered by wind over the surface of the skin, e.g. when cycling, or by cold objects in contact with the skin, e.g. taking articles from a freezer. The weals may be reproduced in many patients by the application of an ice cube to the flexor aspect of the forearm. Anaphylaxis may accompany submersion of the body in cold water and patients need to be warned against bathing unaccompanied.

SOLAR URTICARIA. UV light-induced weals may be seen on sites that are not normally exposed such as the upper arm, especially during the early summer; the weals appear within minutes of sun exposure. The action spectra is variable between patients and it may need to be assessed in order to provide adequate sunscreens.

AQUAGENIC URTICARIA. Contact of the skin with water may induce itching with or without weals. Symptoms may be reproduced by touching the skin with wet gauze. This condition is often a presenting feature of polycythaemia vera.

### TREATMENT

Patients should avoid any trigger factor. They may also need:

A SEDATIVE $H_1$ antihistamine is given at night, such as long-acting chlorpheniramine maleate 8–12 mg, or brompheniramine (long-acting) 12–24 mg, or hydroxyzine hydrochloride 10–50 mg.

NON-SEDATIVE $H_1$ antihistamines such as terfenadine 60 mg twice daily or astemizole 10 mg daily, cetirizine 10 mg are useful for daytime use.

HYDROXYZINE HYDROCHLORIDE OR CYPROHEPTA-DINE HYDROCHLORIDE have a wider spectrum of action than routine $H_1$ receptor-blocking agents. Angio-oedema will often respond better with these agents.

COMBINATION TREATMENT using an $H_1$-receptor antagonist with an $H_2$-receptor antagonist such as cimetidine or ranitidine may stop attacks when other treatments fail.

Acute urticaria accompanied by anaphylaxis (see p. 147), for example from bee stings, snake bites or, less frequently, from food ingestion or drugs, will require the immediate use of adrenaline. Intravenous hydrocortisone or antihistamines may be given to limit the swelling when the crisis is over, for their effect is not seen for up to 20 min.

# HEREDITARY ANGIO-OEDEMA

This condition is inherited in an autosomal dominant manner and many patients can give an account of crises occurring in relatives.

## AETIOLOGY

The disease is associated with C1 esterase inhibitor deficiency (see p. 144), which may be qualitative or quantitative. This protein modulates the intravascular activation of complement and its deficiency leads to angio-oedema. Clinical features may not appear until adult life. A non-hereditary, acquired form of the disease occurs in association with lymphoproliferative disorders.

## CLINICAL FEATURES

Severe airways obstruction that is unresponsive to anti-histamines may lead to death, and visceral oedema may produce attacks of abdominal pain. Attacks may be preceded by a prodromal rash evident as mild erythema or erythema marginatum. Trauma to the skin, e.g. knocking an arm on a doorpost, may trigger an attack, for C1 esterase inhibitor activity is involved in the fibrinolytic cascade as well as in complement pathways. The disease must be differentiated from non-hereditary angio-oedema. Swellings may last for up to 72 hours and are painful rather than irritant. Purpuric staining may occur, but pitting oedema is not seen.

An analysis of complement levels will demonstrate a low level of C1 esterase inhibitor or its deficient functional activity on laboratory testing; C2 and C4 levels are also reduced. The disease can be differentiated from that associated with lymphoma, where C1 levels are also low and there is no family history.

## TREATMENT

Inhibitors of plasmin such as α-aminocaproic acid or stanozolol (2.5–5 mg daily) and danazol (100–200 mg daily) (attenuated androgens) may be used for long-term treatment. Long-term usage in females may cause menstrual irregularity, fluid retention and androgenicity. Acute attacks may also require the use of fresh frozen plasma; a purified form of the inhibitor is also now available. In severe cases adrenaline and hydrocortisone are required.

# MASTOCYTOSIS

Mast cells are normally distributed in the connective tissue of the skin and other organs. These cells release many substances, including histamines, from their granules. An increase in the number of mast cells is referred to as mastocytosis. It may be confined to the skin or, less frequently, may be widespread through all tissues including the viscera (systemic mastocytosis).

## Cutaneous mastocytosis

Cutaneous disease is seen principally in children, whereas associated systemic disease is more common in adults.

There is a positive correlation between a late onset in adult life, extent of skin involvement and systemic disease.

Clinical forms of the disease that affect principally the skin are varied. Cells may be concentrated into a tumour, often a solitary nodule of yellow/brown colour (mastocytoma). This occurs on the trunk or limbs in the first few years of life and regresses after an interval of 3–4 years.

In urticaria pigmentosa, macular or papular pigmented red/brown lesions are widely distributed on the trunk and are more sparse on the limbs. These lesions urticate on scratching. Trauma to the non-lesional skin may produce dermographism in many patients. Attacks of flushing or irritation of the skin may follow emotional upset or change of temperature or be precipitated by alcohol or drugs that release histamine, such as codeine or aspirin. The majority of cases occur in children and the lesions fade in late childhood, but those patients with an onset in adult life tend not to lose their disease.

Children may be born with or develop in early infancy diffuse cutaneous mastocytosis, and blistering may be the first indication of the disease. Later in childhood the skin may be thickened and leathery, when markings and folds are exaggerated. Individual lesions are not seen and very rarely erythrodermic forms occur. Hepatomegaly and splenomegaly may occur with diffuse disease.

In adults an uncommon variant of urticaria pigmentosa occurs in which the predominant skin change is widespread telangiectasia. Pigmented lesions are small and macular and are associated with erythema.

In *systemic disease* the bone marrow and skeletal system are commonly involved but any organ can be affected, giving rise to symptoms such as headache and bronchospasm due to histamine release. The treatment is symptomatic and the prognosis is good in the majority.

# ERYTHEMA NODOSUM

This is an acute and sometimes recurrent panniculitis that produces painful nodules or plaques on the shins (Fig. 20.6), with occasional spread to the thighs or arms. Adult females are principally affected. Some causes are shown in Table 20.3; in nearly 50% no cause is found.

Histological features suggest that this is an immunological reaction. Immune complex deposition within dermal vessels is an important component in the production of the symptom complex.

## CLINICAL FEATURES

Painful nodules or plaques up to 5 cm in diameter appear in crops over 2 weeks and slowly fade to leave bruising and staining of the skin. Systemic upset is common, with malaise, fever and arthralgia; the condition is especially debilitating when it is recurrent.

## INVESTIGATION

Investigations should attempt to exclude streptococcal disease, sarcoidosis and viral causes. The association with sarcoidosis is discussed on p. 688.

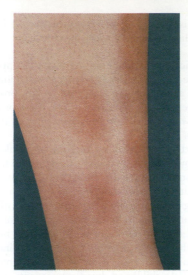

**Fig. 20.6** Erythema nodosum on the shins.

| | |
|---|---|
| Drugs | Sulphonamides |
| | Oral contraceptive pill |
| | Penicillin |
| | Bromides |
| Systemic diseases | Sarcoidosis[a] |
| | Inflammatory bowel disease[a] |
| Infection | Bacteria and viruses |
| |   Streptococci |
| |   Tuberculosis |
| |   Leprosy |
| |   *Yersinia* |
| |   Cat scratch disease |
| |   Tularaemia |
| | Chlamydia |
| |   Psittacosis |
| |   Lymphogranuloma venereum |
| | Fungal |
| |   Histoplasmosis |
| |   Coccidioidomycosis |
| |   Blastomycosis |
| Pregnancy | |
| Unknown stimuli | |
| — | |
| [a]Common causes. | |

**Table 20.3** Some causes of erythema nodosum.

## TREATMENT

Bed rest helps when systemic features and arthralgia are present. NSAIDs such as indomethacin should be given to lessen the pain associated with the cutaneous and joint symptoms. Recovery may take weeks and recurrent attacks can occur.

# ERYTHEMA MULTIFORME

This is an acute self-limiting and often recurrent condition affecting the skin and mucosal surfaces. There is evidence suggesting that circulating immune complexes are important in triggering the reaction in the skin, which occurs 7–14 days following, for example, recurrent herpes simplex infection.

## AETIOLOGY

Children, adolescents or young adults are principally affected. It is associated with:

HERPES SIMPLEX INFECTION (usually type 1) in about one-third of cases. The virus is a common trigger factor for recurrent attacks.

MYCOPLASMA PNEUMONIAE.

DRUGS, e.g. sulphonamides, sulphonylurea derivatives (chlorpropamide) and, less commonly now, barbiturates.

OTHER INFECTIONS, including vaccinia or orf, streptococci, yersiniosis, tuberculosis and histoplasmosis.

CONNECTIVE-TISSUE DISEASES OR NEOPLASIA (rare precipitating factors).

TOPICAL APPLICATIONS triggering allergic reactions over the areas of skin on which they are placed—erythema multiforme lesions occur at the peripheries.

In half of the cases no cause can be found.

## CLINICAL FEATURES

Symmetrically distributed erythematous papules evolve into concentric rings of varying colour. These are commonly seen on the back of the hands, palms and forearms, but may also be seen on the feet or toes. The lesions may show central pallor associated with oedema, bullae formation and peripheral erythema. Alternatively, pallor may be accompanied by central erythema or purpura. Frank bullae represent epidermal necrosis and the separation of this layer. Lesions often spread proximally along the limbs or affect dependent parts in prostrated patients.

Severe mucosal disease is seen with *Mycoplasma pneumoniae* infection for example, and peripheral lesions may be few in number and difficult to discern, so that erythema multiforme may not easily be diagnosed.

Eye changes include conjunctivitis, ulceration of the cornea, uveitis or panophthalmitis, so that the opinion of an ophthalmologist should be sought in the early stages of disease. These latter features are often the most serious of the complications associated with erythema multiforme.

The *Stevens–Johnson syndrome* describes a severe erythema multiforme with a widespread bullous disease associated with oral and genital ulceration and marked constitutional symptoms.

## TREATMENT

The disease is usually self-limiting but death can occur with the Stevens–Johnson syndrome. The withdrawal of offending drugs and the prompt treatment of associated disease is important. It is unlikely that systemic steroid therapy alters the outcome, and such treatment has been shown to be disadvantageous in children.

Care of the eye and mucosal ulceration are important, and in severe cases intravenous fluids and feeding may be required.

# Facial dermatoses/rashes

This section includes acne vulgaris and rosacea. Lupus erythematosus and photodermatoses which also cause facial rashes are discussed on p. 1021 and 1036.

## Acne vulgaris

This chronic condition is associated with the blockage of the pilosebaceous duct and appears on areas of the skin, such as the face, chest and back, where sebaceous glands are most numerous and active.

Superficial blocking of the pilosebaceous orifice at the surface of the skin is manifest commonly as a comedo or 'blackhead'; this may be associated with or followed by a variety of inflammatory changes.

### INCIDENCE

The incidence of acne vulgaris appears to be the same for both sexes; lesions are evident at a younger age in girls and occur with their earlier sexual maturation. The disease is usually more extensive and serious in males. The majority of patients are clear of acne lesions by their early twenties but about 6% of patients will have disease continuing between the ages of 25 and 40 years.

### PATHOGENESIS

There is no unifying concept with which to explain the pathogenesis of the most common patterns of this disease.

#### Alteration of the sebaceous glands

The principal age of onset is at puberty when, under the influence of androgenic hormones, sebaceous glands undergo hypertrophy and increase the production of sebum. A greasy skin and scalp usually accompany the polymorphic lesions, which are distributed on the face, chest and back. The secretion of sebum may, however, remain the same or even be increased in the twenties when the acne has cleared.

#### Microbiology

*Propionibacterium acnes*, an anaerobic diphtheroid, is present within the pilosebaceous duct, and has lipolytic enzymes capable of altering the local lipid constituents. The products of this organism's enzyme activity, principally fatty acids, have been obtained from within the duct; however, they have little inflammatory property when applied to the skin in the majority of acne subjects.

*P. acnes* has been shown to alter the cell-mediated immune response and to stimulate the classical and alternative complement pathways. The local accumulation of complement found in and around the duct may thus be due to the presence of *P. acnes*. Proinflammatory mediators, also induced by the organism, are chemoattractants and are capable of producing some of the clinical features seen with active disease.

The sebaceous gland becomes decreased in size and in activity when isotretinoin (13-*cis*-retinoic acid) is used in the treatment of acne, and the numbers of *P. acnes* diminish in parallel.

There is no convincing evidence, however, that the numbers of this organism are altered effectively by any of the oral antibiotics that are used in the treatment of the disease.

#### Keratinization

The superficial portion of the follicular duct undergoes keratinization and an early finding in acne is an increase in the amount of keratin material at this site. It is probable that one of the several effects of isotretinoin, which can so dramatically improve serious acne, is that it alters this abnormal production of keratin.

#### Androgens

The effect of androgens on the disease is clearly seen in a number of young women in whom the disease continues beyond the teens. Up to 50% of such patients may show evidence of increased circulatory androgen levels, with raised total and free testosterone and/or lowered sex hormone-binding globulin. The alteration of these abnormal findings with treatment may lead to the clinical improvement of seemingly intractable disease.

### CLINICAL FEATURES

The 'blackhead' or comedo is the common first-stage lesion, the pigmentation being provided by melanin from the hair. In the absence of such lesions, the diagnosis of acne vulgaris is less likely. Closed comedones or 'whiteheads' are flesh-coloured lesions that are most commonly seen on the cheeks or chin, especially with incidental light or when the skin is slightly stretched. Such lesions represent very firmly obstructed follicles and are often the forerunners of more actively inflamed papules and pustules. Alteration of the water content of the keratin plugs may occur with hormonal changes during the menstrual cycle or with the application of moisturizing creams, e.g. in 'cosmetic acne', when whitehead lesions become predominant.

The development of inflammatory papules and pustules will follow the release into the skin of the contents of a blocked follicle and the diffusion of chemoattractant materials across the wall. The pustules are sterile and produce no growth of organisms on routine culture. More marked inflammatory changes may lead to large cysts, scarring and keloid formation.

Increased local trauma may cause exacerbation of the disease; this may occur with head-gear, the pressure of strapping across the shoulders or trunk, or on special sites, e.g. beneath the chin in professional violin players ('fiddler's neck').

When unusual sites are involved, such as the forearms and thighs, there is a folliculitis which can be produced by substances such as cutting oils in industry. Oils applied to the scalp may affect forehead skin ('pomade acne').

Acne conglobata may be seen in association with hidradenitis suppurativa. It may lead to profound facial scarring. It is familial. Severe acute-onset pustulo nodular disease (pyoderma faciale) in females may also lead to very severe scarring. Acne fulminans in young men may produce severe systemic upset.

## TREATMENT
### Diet
Scientific studies show no relationship between food and acne. If, however, any individual experiences a worsening of their disease, after eating chocolate for example, this should be removed from their diet.

### Local applications
A VARIETY OF ABRASIVES, ASTRINGENTS OR EXFOLIATIVES are useful particularly in comedonal disease. Most of these agents contain benzoyl peroxide in concentrations of between 2.5 and 10%, presented as lotions, creams or gels, alone or in combination with sulphur. Treatment should initially be with low concentrations (usually applied at night), with the concentration being increased with time and as tolerance develops. Erythema, dryness and scaling or peeling of the skin are often seen in the first weeks of treatment and diminish with time.

WASHING WITH POVIDONE-IODINE SURGICAL SCRUB, which contains a surfactant, may 'freshen' the skin and give short-term relief from greasiness.

SUNSHINE OR UV LIGHT from artificial sources also helps the comedonal stage of the disease.

TOPICAL ANTIBIOTICS available for use are clindamycin phosphate, tetracycline hydrochloride and erythromycin 2% in alcoholic solution.

TOPICAL RETINOIC ACID (tretinoin) in concentrations of 0.01–0.025% in a lotion or a gel or 0.025–0.05% as a cream is helpful for the comedonal stage.

### Systemic therapy
ANTIBIOTICS. Pustular and inflammatory disease will respond to oral antibiotics such as tetracycline, oxytetracycline, erythromycin and co-trimoxazole. Treatment with tetracycline 250 mg two or three times daily is often not effective until the drug has been taken for 2 weeks and courses should extend over months. Iron and calcium will markedly diminish the absorption of oxytetracycline or tetracycline, which should therefore be given at least 30 min before food. The absorption of minocycline (100 mg daily) is less affected by food but the drug is more expensive. Drug resistance of *P. acnes* seen with tetracycline is unusual with minocycline.

HORMONES. The alteration of abnormal hormone levels in women may often improve acne. The use of a suitable oral contraceptive pill in which the progestogen component does not produce androgenic effects in the skin may help over the course of 6–8 months or more. Cyproterone acetate, an antiandrogen, has been combined at a low dosage (2 mg) with ethinyloestradiol (35 μg) to produce an oral contraceptive; this needs to be prescribed for periods of up to 1 year in order to gain full benefit for the skin.

13-CIS RETINOIC ACID (VITAMIN A ANALOGUE). Severe cystic acne that is unresponsive to the treatments outlined above is the current indication for the use of isotretinoin. Four months of therapy in doses of 1.0 mg kg$^{-1}$ per day by mouth will produce a remission of the disease in more than 90% of patients for periods of up to 8 years. The side-effects are as for acitretin, described on p. 1001.

## Rosacea
This chronic inflammatory facial eruption consists of erythema, often accompanied by papules, sterile pustules and telangiectasia.

### AETIOLOGY
Those most commonly affected are fair-skinned, middle-aged females who often give a history of a ready flushing tendency which is triggered by a warm atmosphere, emotional upset, hot drinks, spicy food or alcohol. Males often have more severe disease but black Africans are rarely affected with rosacea.

### PATHOGENESIS
There is no cohesive view that can explain the combination of clinical findings and pathological changes.

Histological sections frequently show changes that are interpreted as folliculitis, but a more constant feature is hyperplasia of the connective tissue around dilated blood vessels of the superficial dermis. This suggests that actinic (i.e. sunlight-induced) damage to the skin is an important component of the disease. The possibility that affected persons might be unduly sensitive to the effect of vasoactive mediators, such as sympathomimetic amines, histamine and acetylcholine, has not been substantiated, though endogenous opiates may play a role.

### CLINICAL FEATURES
Patients demonstrating the most florid aspects of the disease will have an intense erythema of the skin overlying the flush areas of the face, i.e. the cheeks, nose and chin. The presence of papules and pustules distinguishes rosacea from the facial eruptions of SLE. The lesions are intermittent initially, but with chronic disease the erythema is persistent and marked telangiectasia appears. Other less-common features include lymphoedema of the cheeks or lower eyelids and rhinophyma. In the latter condition there is irregular thickening of the skin of the nose and the follicular orifices are enlarged. The skin of the nose is bright or purplish red. In severe cases there is marked thickening of the skin on the surrounding cheeks. Rhinophyma can occasionally be the only manifestation of rosacea.

Approximately one-half of the patients with rosacea have a variety of ocular lesions. Blepharitis and conjunctivitis are the most common findings, but episcleritis, iritis and keratitis also occur, the latter being a potentially serious complication.

### TREATMENT
FACTORS THAT PROVOKE FACIAL FLUSHING should be avoided.

TETRACYCLINE in doses of 250 mg two or three times daily for periods of at least 12 weeks will improve the inflammatory aspect of the eruption in most patients.

METRONIDAZOLE may be of help when tetracycline is not effective, but care must be taken with the use of this drug over prolonged periods. Two months' treatment at doses of 200 mg three times daily is often adequate.

HYDROCORTISONE combined with 0.5–1% sulphur as a cream may bring some relief of facial discomfort.

ISOTRETINOIN (13-*cis*-retinoic acid) at doses of 0.5–1 mg kg$^{-1}$ for a period of 4 months has been shown to help resistant disease.

Rhinophyma is improved by shaving hypertrophic tissues from the nose, although regrowth of tissue frequently occurs.

# Bullous disease

In these rare disorders, bullae form the primary lesions and these result from cleavage at various levels at or near the epidermodermal junction. There is a significant mortality associated with the diseases and the treatments. Immunopathological findings are useful in the confirmation of the diagnosis, in monitoring disease activity, and for understanding the pathogenesis.

## PEMPHIGUS

Pemphigus is a rare disease (incidence 0.5/100 000) in which antibody, usually of the IgG class, reacts with an antigen (a glycoprotein) at the surface of the epidermal cell that forms part of the intercellular cement substance. The interaction causes proteases and plasmin to be released and the cells lose their adhesion and become rounded (acantholysis). Such cells may be seen when blister fluid obtained from skin lesions is spread on to a slide (Tzanck smear) and examined under the microscope.

The zone of separation within the epidermis may vary; in pemphigus vulgaris it appears just above the basal layer whilst in the superficial forms of pemphigus, clefts occur adjacent to the granular layer. Nikolsky's sign consists of extension of the zone of separation by light pressure or rubbing the skin.

## Pemphigus vulgaris

Patients are usually between the ages of 40 and 60 years and are often Jewish; 90% have HLA-DR4. It is also common in India. Antigen–antibody complexes have been shown, on immunofluorescence, to localize within the intercellular substance of the epidermis, adjacent to clefts. Animal and human keratinocytes lose adhesion when cultured in the presence of sera from patients with pemphigus vulgaris. The antigen is a 130 kDa glycoprotein of the desmosome complex.

## CLINICAL FEATURES

There are several forms of pemphigus. In the most common form lesions may be confined to the mucosal surfaces in the early stages of the disease; 50% of cases start in the mouth with bright red, sore and denuded mucosa. In a few patients this may be the only site involved; more commonly, however, thin-walled blisters appear over normal-looking skin elsewhere on the body. Such lesions soon rupture to leave moist eroded areas and secondary bacterial infection is common. When large areas of the skin are denuded, fluid loss and catabolic changes may produce severe metabolic disturbance. These metabolic changes may be compounded in the early stages of systemic steroid treatment.

Blisters may never be evident clinically in the more superficial patterns of pemphigus. A pemphigus-like eruption has been seen with drugs such as penicillamine, captopril and rifampicin.

## INVESTIGATION

The diagnosis is confirmed by the cytological examination of blister fluid and by direct immunofluorescent staining of a skin sample obtained from the edge of a fresh blister. Fluorescent anti-human IgG and anti-human C3 outline the intercellular substance between the epidermal cells and the edges of the cleft in the skin that forms the blister.

Circulating IgG antibodies to intercellular areas of keratinocytes are present in 95%; the titres may reflect disease activity and act as a therapeutic marker.

## TREATMENT

Treatment includes general measures of controlling bacterial infection and fluid loss. Air beds are useful for nursing such patients. Prednisolone in doses of 60–100 mg daily or more may be needed to prevent new blisters forming, and drugs such as azathioprine or methotrexate may be required to enable the dose of steroid to be lowered at the earliest opportunity. Gold may be effective therapy in steroid-resistant patients.

# Bullous pemphigoid

Bullous pemphigoid occurs twice as frequently as pemphigus and most patients are more than 60 years old at the time of presentation. Direct immunofluorescence of skin demonstrates staining of IgG and C3 at the basement membrane zones. On electron microscopy blister formation is seen at the level of the lamina lucida (Fig. 20.7). Circulating antibodies can be detected in the sera in 70% of patients. Antigens are 230 kDa and 180 kDa proteins of the hemidesmosome complex.

## CLINICAL FEATURES

The disease may begin with irritation and erythema of the skin occurring for weeks or months before blistering appears. Bullae then develop, often on an erythematous background but also on normal skin. These tense bullae, which are often secondarily infected, may be localized to one area of the skin or may be more widespread. The groin, axillae and flexural aspect of the limbs and lower

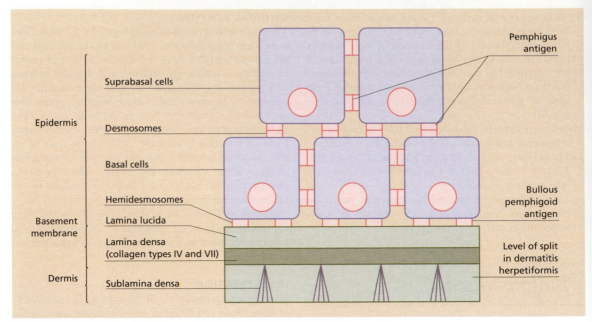

**Fig. 20.7**  Section of the epidermis, epidermodermal junction and dermis. This diagram shows the site damage in some bullous disorders. From Collier PM & Wojnarowska F (1992)

Blistering diseases. *Medicine International* **103**: 4312. By kind permission of The Medicine Group (Journals) Ltd.

abdomen are most commonly affected and correspond to areas of highest antigen expression. Involvement of mucosae is rare.

### INVESTIGATION

The diagnosis may be confirmed by the immunofluorescent staining of the basement membrane with IgG. The majority of antigen is located in an intracellular position in the region of the hemidesmosome; a small proportion is in the lamina lucida of basement membrane.

### TREATMENT

Smaller doses of prednisolone than those required for pemphigus (40–50 mg daily) are needed to control this disease. Steroid-sparing or substitution may again be achieved with azathioprine or methotrexate and in some patients with dapsone 50–100 mg per day. Potent topical corticosteroids are a useful addition to treatment with localized disease.

It is possible to stop all medication in many patients after 2–3 years of treatment.

## EPIDERMOLYSIS BULLOSA

This is the name given to a group of rare and largely genetically determined diseases that vary from localized disease on the soles of the feet in one form, to infants born with a loss of skin from large areas of their body surface at the other extreme. It is now possible to diagnose different forms of the disease *in utero*.

### PATHOGENESIS

In epidermolysis bullosa simplex, blistering arises within the basal cells of the epidermis (see p. 993), while in junc-

tional epidermolysis bullosa the area of cleavage is within the lamina lucida. In the dystrophic form of the disease, separation occurs beneath the lamina densa within the superficial dermis.

### CLINICAL FEATURES

#### Epidermolysis bullosa simplex

This presents within the first year of life, when blisters appear over contact areas of the skin such as the palms and knees; the soles often become affected when walking commences. Scarring is unusual.

#### Epidermolysis bullosa dystrophica

There are two forms of this disease:

1 In the autosomal dominant form, bullae occur on the limbs in infancy.
2 In the recessive form, bullae occur at birth and large areas of the skin are denuded with subsequent scarring; contracture and fusion of the skin between the fingers and toes leads to syndactyly. Ulceration of mucosal surfaces, e.g. tongue, oesophagus and the anal margin may be seen.

#### Epidermolysis letalis (junctional epidermolysis bullosa)

Epidermolysis letalis presents at birth with both mucosal disease and widespread erosions of the skin that often fails to heal. The child dies in infancy.

#### Epidermolysis bullosa acquisita (EBA)

EBA occurs in adult life with no family history of epidermolysis bullosa. It can clinically be confused with porphyria. Immunofluorescence of skin shows IgG deposition at the epidermodermal junction. The EBA antigen is the globular C-terminus of type VII procollagen. Patients often have HLA-DR2.

## TREATMENT

There is a tendency for non-lethal forms of the disease gradually to improve through childhood. Protection of the skin and the prompt care of newly eroded skin may lessen scarring. Attention to nutrition, anaemia, eyes and mucosal surfaces is essential but there is no good evidence that drugs will alter the extent of blistering.

# DERMATITIS HERPETIFORMIS

Dermatitis herpetiformis produces an extremely itchy polymorphic rash that is symmetrically distributed over the extensor surfaces of the body. The unusual feature of this condition is that most patients also have a gluten-sensitive enteropathy, which is usually asymptomatic.

## PATHOLOGY

The dermal papillae are infiltrated with neutrophils, eosinophils and fibrin. Later subepidermal vesicles develop. The major diagnostic pointer is IgA deposits in the unaffected skin, which can be seen on immunofluorescence. These deposits are usually granular and subepidermal but occasionally linear deposits are seen. Linear deposits may also be seen in some other subepidermal blistering conditions, e.g. linear IgA disease. The small-bowel lesion is similar to that seen in coeliac disease (see p. 208) except that it is less severe and varying degrees of villous atrophy are seen. The small-bowel lesions occur in those with the granular IgA skin deposits.

### Immunogenetic findings

The HLA markers and changes in humoral and cellular immunology are similar to those found in coeliac disease.

## CLINICAL FEATURES

Dermatitis herpetiformis can occur at any age but is seen chiefly in the second, third and fourth decades. Erythematous plaques, excoriations, urticarial papules, crusts or vesicles appear on elbows, knees, shoulders, buttocks and scalp; the mucous membranes are occasionally affected. The lesions are extremely itchy and the vesicles have usually been burst by scratching, leaving encrusted lesions. The course of the disease is one of remissions and exacerbations. Patients can often predict an eruption 8–12 hours before its onset because of localized itching. Gastrointestinal symptoms are rare, even with small intestinal lesions, and steatorrhoea is seen in less than 5% of patients.

## INVESTIGATION

The diagnosis is made on the clinical and histological appearance of the skin (see above), and by the response to dapsone. A small-bowel biopsy is performed to confirm the gluten-sensitive enteropathy.

## TREATMENT

Dapsone 50–200 mg daily will usually control the rash within hours and on stopping the drug the symptoms promptly recur. Occasionally, higher doses of dapsone are required. Maintenance doses vary but patients can adjust their own medication to the minimal dose required to control the rash. Complications of dapsone therapy include haemolytic anaemia and methaemoglobinaemia. A gluten-free diet improves the intestinal lesions and also helps the skin lesions, leading to a reduction or cessation of dapsone.

# Linear IgA disease

Linear deposition of IgA at the basement membrane zone delineates a rare disease with a prevalence of 1/250 000. Lesions resemble those of bullous pemphigoid; ocular associations are seen and a minority of patients are dapsone resistant.

OTHER CONDITIONS that produce blistering include porphyria and drug eruptions; these are discussed on p. 1024 and 1028.

# Infections

Some of the bacterial, viral and fungal infections that affect the skin are considered in this section. Many skin infections are considered under the individual causative organisms in Chapter 1.

# Bacterial infections

An important role of the intact skin is to prevent the entry of infective organisms. This is achieved by the following:

THE CORNIFIED SURFACE on many body sites is difficult to breach and has a desiccating effect on some microorganisms.

SURFACE LONG-CHAIN FATTY ACIDS inhibit the growth of staphylococci.

THE RESIDENT FLORA on the skin surface can limit the growth of potential pathogens by the production of antimicrobial substances. This is especially useful on continually moist surfaces such as the flexures, where the opportunity for invasion is increased.

## AETIOLOGY

TRAUMA OR ABRASION of the skin removes the stratum corneum and allows infection to occur much more readily; *Staph. aureus* or *Streptococcus pyogenes* are the usual invaders. A cleft in the skin can often be seen at the site of entry of streptococci, e.g. below the ear-lobe when erysipelas ensues, causing cellulitis affecting the face.

VIRAL DISEASE OR PRIMARY DERMATOSES may allow secondary bacterial infection, e.g. impetigo can follow a 'cold sore' or eczema.

OTHER ORGANISMS that breach the skin include fleas

and lice, and with subsequent itching and excoriation bacterial infection may spread. In patients with continuing bacterial infection (particularly children) an underlying disease such as infestation should always be sought.

STAPHYLOCOCCAL INFECTION. *Staph. aureus* may form part of the flora of the nose in 20% of individuals. It can also be carried on perianal skin, especially in males. In the majority of infections, invasion of the skin remains localized to, for example, a hair follicle as a furuncle or boil. Toxins produced by staphylococci, e.g. exfoliatin, are released by certain phage types and will cause separation of epidermal cells to produce *toxic epidermal necrolysis. Toxic shock syndrome* is associated with staphylococcal infection, serious systemic disease, widespread erythema and subsequent peeling of the skin. Erythrogenic staphylococcal toxins may produce a disease that resembles scarlet fever, which is induced by streptococci.

## STAPHYLOCOCCAL INFECTION

(see p. 19)

### Boils

Boils or furuncles are painful, erythematous, tender, papular lesions that are related to infection of the hair follicle and can occur on any part of the hair-bearing skin. They are most commonly seen on the neck, axillae, buttocks and thighs. Spread to involve several follicles will produce a carbuncle. Superficial infection of the follicle causes pin-point pustules over the face or legs, especially in children. With recurrent boils, patients should be screened for diabetes mellitus.

FOLLICULAR IMPETIGO. Papular lesions may occur when the whole follicle is inflamed to produce sycosis. Sycosis barbae occurs when the beard area is involved. Less commonly, crusted, necrotic or scarred lesions occur on the scalp or face. Staphylococci can sometimes be isolated from these but the pathogenesis of such lesions is not clear.

#### TREATMENT

Acute lesions should only be treated with systemic antibiotics if there is marked surrounding erythema or there are associated constitutional symptoms. When the lesion is beginning to 'point' then the overlying skin may be broken with a sterile needle and the area gently swabbed with an antiseptic, such as chlorhexidine or povidone-iodine.

Recurrent boils will require the long-term use of an antiseptic regimen over several months, including bathing with povidone-iodine. Affected sites and areas of carriage such as the nose or perianal skin will require the application of an antiseptic cream (containing chlorhexidine or neomycin) or dusting powder. With multiple-resistant *Staph. aureus* (MRSA, see p. 21) mupirocin in ointment form is applied to the nose or topically. Family members may also require treatment if chronic sepsis continues.

Similar treatment may be required for staphylococcal infection associated with sycosis barbae.

## Impetigo

This crusted eruption commonly seen on the face of children may be caused by staphylococci, streptococci or a combination of the two organisms. Staphylococcal infection induces superficial bullae, which are seldom evident because they quickly rupture to leave a moist yellow crusted surface with surrounding inflammation. Typically the facial skin is involved and children are frequently affected. Bullous lesions are less commonly seen and are associated with the same phage type of staphylococcus that produces toxic epidermal necrolysis. The reason why the disease remains limited in some children whereas it becomes disseminated in others is not clear.

#### TREATMENT

Care should be taken to prevent or limit spread of the disease in families or institutions. Areas should be gently bathed with an antiseptic solution such as hexachlorophane or povidone-iodine. Similar preparations in a paint or powder form should be applied to the skin after cleansing. Systemic antibiotics are prescribed if infection is widespread. Rarely, nephrotoxic strains of streptococci are associated with impetigo; the sensitivity of staphylococci should be determined. Erythromycin or cephalosporins both give adequate levels in the skin when given by mouth.

## STREPTOCOCCAL INFECTION

### Erysipelas

This is most commonly seen in the skin as widespread erythema and cellulitis. The organisms gain entry through fissures in the skin, e.g. in a toe-cleft, and the skin becomes red, swollen and tender. Constitutional symptoms of fever, malaise and hallucinations often accompany the cutaneous features. With recurrent disease the area affected, e.g. the foot and lower leg, may become lymphoedematous.

#### TREATMENT

Acute cases should be treated with penicillin 1 g per day. Any underlying skin disease should be treated with local antiseptics applied as paints or dusting powder on areas of chronic fissuring. Foot soaks that are bacteriostatic and astringent, e.g. potassium permanganate 0.01% solution, might be prescribed when maceration of the toe-clefts is associated with excessive sweating. Recurrent erysipelas may require long-term prophylaxis with oral penicillin or erythromycin.

### Ecthyma

This disease is uncommon in the UK except in drug addicts or patients with HIV infection. Chronic ulceration is produced by infection of the dermis and both *Strep. pyogenes* and *Staph. aureus* may be isolated from the same wound.

Debilitation, poor hygiene or nutrition are important contributing factors. Often prolonged and intensive local antiseptic treatment combined with systemic antibiotics will be needed to heal the skin.

## ERYSIPELOID

Erysipeloid is an acute infective disease of the skin. It is most often localized to areas that have been traumatized by contact with carcasses and bones of pigs, chickens or fish. The condition is therefore seen in butchers, meat porters, fishermen or, rarely, those working in the home. The causative organism is *Erysipelothrix insidiosa*, which also causes swine erysipelas, a serious and systemic disease of pigs. In humans, well-demarcated blue/red discoloration is noticed on the hands, fingers or arms. This follows several days after laceration or abrasion and clears without sequelae. Rarely, fever and malaise accompany the common cutaneous presentation and cases of systemic and cutaneous disease resembling swine erysipelas have been recorded.

The disease is self-limiting and lasts about 7–10 days. If treatment is required, then penicillin given for a week is effective.

## GRAM-NEGATIVE INFECTION

This type of infection may occur in moist wounds such as leg ulcers treated with occlusive bandages or dressings. *Pseudomonas aeruginosa* is the most frequent contaminant of such wounds. Astringent solutions such as acetic acid 1–2% will often dry the skin sufficiently to discourage the growth of Gram-negative organisms. Potassium permanganate 0.01% can be used as an alternative for bathing the limb or may be applied as a compress. Debilitated or immunocompromised patients may rarely develop necrotic skin lesions (from which *Pseudomonas* may be isolated) when local vasculitis follows *Ps. aeruginosa* septicaemia (ecthyma gangrenosum).

## ERYTHRASMA

Chronic, localized, pigmented, scaled lesions of the skin occur over skin flexures such as the axillae, groin, toe-webs and beneath the breasts.

The organism isolated from such sites is often a normal commensal of the skin, *Corynebacterium minutissimum*. It is not clear therefore why some adults are especially prone to the disease. Excessive sweating and poor hygiene are frequent accompanying features. Examination by Wood's light causes the organism to fluoresce, producing a pink-red colour.

### TREATMENT
Oral erythromycin will eradicate extensive disease, and the drying of macerated skin with imidazole powders or topical fucidic acid cream will clear more limited infection.

## MYCOBACTERIAL INFECTION

Cutaneous disease can be due to *Mycobacterium tuberculosis* or *M. leprae*. It is uncommon in the Western Hemisphere. It is also associated with atypical mycobacteria, including *M. ulcerans*, which causes tropical Buruli ulcer, and *M. marinum*, which causes fish tank or swimming pool granuloma.

### Lupus vulgaris

This condition is the most common form of skin disease associated with tuberculosis. Two forms are recognized:
1 Haematogenous spread from a reactivated primary lesion
2 More rarely, following scrofuloderma, which occurs when the skin is ulcerated by the spread of infection from an adjacent infected lymph gland or bone
Histologically, the cutaneous lesions show granulomas with central caseation. It is usual to be able to demonstrate the organism from the skin lesions.

Sites of involvement are usually on cooler areas of the skin, with the face being most frequently involved. Erythema, scaling and scarring plaques are seen (Fig. 20.8). In severe intractable disease subcutaneous tissues appear 'gnawed' and hence the term 'lupus' (meaning 'wolf').

### Tuberculosis verrucosa cutis

Primary inoculation of the skin with *M. tuberculosis* may give rise to warty lesions on the skin of young children who come into contact with infected sputum or on the fingers of surgeons or pathologists who handle infected tissue.

Secondary inoculation of the skin occurs from endogenous sources, e.g. at the side of the mouth from infected sputum (tuberculosis orificalis cutis); it appears as a plaque or papule.

### Tuberculides

Tuberculides form a group of poorly defined eruptions and knowledge of their pathogeneses is incomplete. It is probable that they represent a reaction in the skin to the

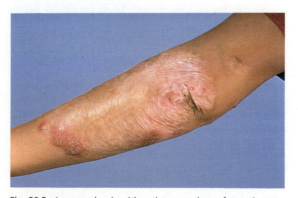

**Fig. 20.8** Lupus vulgaris with active granuloma formation at the margins.

haematogenous spread of *M. tuberculosis*. They have declined in parallel with pulmonary tuberculosis. Included under this general heading are papulonecrotic tuberculide, lichen scrofulosorum and erythema induratum or Bazin's disease.

### TREATMENT

Lupus vulgaris and other forms of tuberculosis of the skin should be treated with standard chemotherapy for 6–9 months (see p. 686). Tuberculides such as erythema induratum will clear on the same regimen.

## Atypical mycobacterial infections

Skin granulomas develop where the skin is traumatized against the rough surface of the lining or surround of a swimming pool, or over a digit, hand or forearm abraded against the side of an aquarium during cleaning. The latter is more common nowadays, when the patient presents with a chronic papular lesion on the finger, usually with scaling and less frequently with atrophic changes. On occasions more than one lesion may be seen following spread along cutaneous lymphatics. The organism causing this infection is *M. marinum*.

Lesions may clear over the course of months and routine antituberculous treatment is ineffective. Minocycline in doses of up to 100 mg twice daily for 6–8 weeks may hasten resolution of the lesions.

## Leprosy (see p. 37)

*M. leprae* infection of the skin gives rise to leprosy. However, in order to lessen the stigma associated with the disease, the term Hansen's disease is preferred.

### Tuberculoid leprosy

The organism may be confined to the primary site of involvement in neural tissue from where it spreads to the skin. Lesions are few and typically there are plaques with an elevated rim, dusky red in colour and with some central pallor. The surface of the skin is often dry over the lesion, hairless and insensitive. Local peripheral nerves may be enlarged.

Biopsy shows tuberculoid granulomas but no bacilli.

### Lepromatous leprosy

Evidence of nerve involvement in the skin is often lacking and presenting signs may be in the respiratory system with nasal congestion. The plaques, nodules, macules and papules that occur are usually erythematous and multiple and have no appreciable loss of sensation. With untreated disease, the facial skin may become thickened and the remainder of the integument is often scaly and dry. Increasing nerve damage leads to loss of sensation, ulceration of limbs, loss of digits and muscle wasting.

Diagnosis and treatment are discussed on p. 40.

# Viral infections

## Herpes simplex (see p. 47)

There are two types of herpes simplex virus (HSV) infection—HSV types I and II.

### CLINICAL FEATURES

Primary herpes gingivostomatitis (HSV-1) may be asymptomatic in children, but others can experience severe stomatitis associated with buccal ulceration, marked local lymph node enlargement and systemic features. Trauma to the skin may introduce the virus, as in gladiatoral or 'scrumpox'. Damage to the skin over a finger may produce a herpetic whitlow especially in nursing personnel.

Type 2 genital infection may not cause symptoms in females if it is intravaginal. Vulvovaginitis causes burning irritation, dysuria and lymph node enlargement. Extragenital infection on the thigh or buttock can cause myalgia, and dysaesthesiae of the affected overlying skin.

Recurrent disease may induce systemic upset with fever, headaches and meningeal irritation associated with the spread of the virus into the CNS. There is local dysaesthesiae followed by vesiculation, weeping and crusting; less commonly local erythema and papule formation occur but no blistering. Depending on the degree of secondary bacterial infection, attacks clear in 10–14 days, with separation of the crust.

### COMPLICATIONS

#### Ocular complications

More serious and chronic disease can occur when the eye is the site of primary herpes infection or of recurrent attacks. Ulceration may give rise to marked local pain and oedema and produce keratitis, scarring and visual impairment.

#### Cutaneous complications

Recurrent HSV-1 infection is probably the most common cause of erythema multiforme, which occurs 10–14 days following vesiculation over the lips, face or mucous membranes.

Typical target or iris lesions appear usually over acral skin on the fingers, toes, palms or soles.

#### Eczema herpeticum

Atopic individuals can develop widespread disseminated viral infection at any time. This does not only occur when their eczema is in an active phase, nor does it occur on every occasion of contact. Nurses and parents with active cold sores should avoid nursing children with atopic eczema.

### DIAGNOSIS

This is usually clinical. Rarely the virus may need to be cultured from the vesicles and differentiated immunologically from varicella zoster virus.

## TREATMENT AND MANAGEMENT

Local drying agents such as ether or surgical spirit will promote crusting and diminish pain and discomfort.

Povidone-iodine has a mild antiviral action and is available in an alcoholic solution or paint form (10% w/v). The astringent effect is a useful adjunct to treatment and secondary infection may not occur so readily following its use.

Specific measures include the use of idoxuridine or acyclovir. Infection of the eye is improved by the use of local application of eyedrops containing 0.1% idoxuridine or an ointment containing 0.5% idoxuridine. Idoxuridine 5–20% is applied to the skin in a vehicle such as dimethyl sulphoxide (DMSO), which aids the absorption of the active ingredient into the skin. The local applications need to be made at the onset of discomfort and for the ensuing few days.

Acyclovir, a thymidine analogue, is activated in the presence of HSV thymidine kinase. Toxicity to normal tissues is therefore reduced and treatment with this agent in severe local infection or disseminated disease in neonates, atopic individuals or those with immune deficiency may greatly reduce morbidity and mortality. The compound is available for local use as a 5% cream. In tablet form, acyclovir 200 mg five times daily for 5 days is a normal dosage for type 1 infection. This may need to be increased or doubled when treating type 2 disease. Parenteral forms of the drug are also available for severely ill patients and for disseminated disease.

Women with genital herpes should undergo cervical screening as there may be a link with carcinoma of the cervix. This should always be performed if their sexual partners have recurrent disease.

## Varicella (chickenpox)

This is a common infectious disease of childhood occurring in the winter and spring and caused by the varicella zoster virus (VZV) (see p. 48).

## Herpes zoster (shingles)

This infection usually represents the re-emergence of VZV from posterior nerve roots in the spinal cord or cranial nerves into the skin (see p. 48).

### AETIOLOGY

This disease affects patients in their middle years or old age. Factors that cause the re-emergence of the virus are often unknown and probably represent changes in the immune state of the host. The induction of an attack by local spinal disease or an occult concomitant malignancy is unusual.

### CLINICAL FEATURES

The prodromal symptoms of pain, tingling and dysaesthesia may precede by days the re-emergence of the virus into the skin. It then produces characteristic vesicles, papules or bullous lesions throughout the dermatome.

Unusual sites of involvement such as sacral nerve disease may give rise to visceral changes and lead to, for example, bladder dysfunction.

### COMPLICATIONS

Secondary infection increases discomfort, and in an elderly person intractable post-herpetic neuralgia may follow an attack of shingles. Trophic ulcers are sometimes seen over the face in association with cranial nerve involvement. Trigeminal nerve disease (ophthalmic division) can lead to infection of the eye. Signs that include swelling of the eyelid, conjunctivitis or blistering at the side of the nose require an ophthalmic opinion.

### TREATMENT

DRYING SOLUTIONS such as calamine cream or lotion are soothing.

ANTISEPTIC POWDERS containing povidone-iodine or hexachlorophane may help to limit secondary infection.

IDOXURIDINE 20–40% in DMSO may be applied where practical to the affected dermatome on dressings that are kept moist with the compound for the first 3–4 days of infection. This treatment should be limited to immunocompromised or elderly patients with severe disease.

ACYCLOVIR 800 mg orally five times daily for 7 days is recommended for all patients with shingles. Famciclovir is also effective and given three times a day. Acyclovir cream 5% may be applied for less severe attacks.

PREDNISOLONE in doses of 40–60 mg decreasing over 3 weeks can prevent post-herpetic neuralgia in those over 60 years of age. Dissemination of disease is not seen with systemic steroids.

MANAGEMENT OF POST-HERPETIC NEURALGIA is discussed on p. 928.

## Orf

This disease is due to a poxvirus infection that commonly affects young sheep, producing a pustular dermatitis. Vesiculopustular lesions appear around the mouth or feet of lambs, and persons coming into contact with the fluid from these may develop papular lesions on traumatized skin. Veterinary surgeons, farmers or their families and butchers are among those principally at risk.

Milker's nodes are produced by a poxvirus that is morphologically identical to that of orf. Lesions are seen in farm workers handling the mouths or teats of cattle, and the organism may be carried by domestic cats.

### CLINICAL FEATURES

Hands are usually affected. The lesions consist of red/blue papules, 1–2 cm in diameter, with a grey edge and surrounding erythema. Misguided incision of such a swelling may release antigen and produce erythema multiforme. Lesions settle in 6–8 weeks and immunity appears to be lifelong.

# Molluscum contagiosum

## AETIOLOGY

This infection is usually grouped with other diseases caused by the poxviruses, but the virus is antigenically different. Atopic individuals appear to be especially prone to infection and in such persons lesions may be more numerous and difficult to eradicate.

## CLINICAL FEATURES

Flesh-coloured, umbilicated papules are seen. They are usually not more than 5 mm in diameter, but the size may vary. Children are most commonly infected and flexural surfaces are the areas of skin most frequently involved. In adults, spread often occurs with sexual contact. Irritation over the surrounding skin may induce scratching and further spread. Single lesions may occur and become quite large and inflammatory and then the diagnosis may not be easy.

## TREATMENT

The papules need only to be opened and the contents expressed; this often occurs with scratching although a sterile needle can be used. Silver nitrate or phenol may be applied or electrocautery or a Hyfrecator (which seals blood vessels using a small charge of electricity but without heat) may be used, or cryosurgery. Associated changes in the skin, such as eczema, need to be treated in order to prevent scratching and further spread of lesions.

# Warts

## AETIOLOGY

The human papillomavirus (HPV) is a member of the papovavirus family, which includes other species-specific viruses that infect domestic animals such as dogs, rabbits, horses or cattle. It has long been recognized that tumours induced in animals by this group of viruses may undergo malignant transformation, and the oncogenic potential for humans is of increasing concern.

### Types of virus

DNA hybridization techniques have demonstrated more than 50 different virus types, and immunocytochemical methods have identified virus particles in human tumours.

Previously warts have been classified according to the clinical appearance or anatomical site that they infect. It is now recognized that one or several viral types can be found in each of the clinically different lesions, e.g. plantar warts are caused by HPV-1 and HPV-4. The genus is divided into types according to the homology of the DNA pattern.

## PATHOGENESIS

Viral DNA can be isolated from the basal cells of the epidermis, but the fully infective virion is only evident in more superficial epidermal cells. Cytology or histology shows gross disruption of the cells of the granular layer and below, which have intranuclear and cytoplasmic eosinophilic inclusions. Gross hyperkeratosis and parakeratosis are also associated with viral infection.

## CLINICAL FEATURES

### Common warts

Common warts are individual papular lesions with a coarse or roughened surface that are seen on the palmar aspect of the fingers and on the knees; other sites are less commonly affected. Children between the ages of 11 and 16 years are principally affected. Spread is associated with trauma. Many periungal warts are seen in nail biters, who may also have warts on or around their lips.

### Plantar warts (verrucae)

These lesions are often solitary and are distributed over contact areas of the foot. When they overlie a bony prominence and are associated with marked hyperkeratosis, pain and tenderness when pressure is applied may be severe. Squeezing a plantar wart or verruca may more readily induce pain than pressing on the lesion and this is a useful test in differentiating a verruca from a callosity. Paring down the skin over a verruca will demonstrate a pit in the skin at which the surface markings come to an abrupt halt; they are, however, continuous over a callus. Maceration of the skin associated with sweating may induce many superficial lesions that form a mosaic wart.

### Single filiform warts

These lesions occur on the face and at the nasal vestibule or around the mouth; they may also be seen over the face or neck of older patients.

### Plane warts

Plane warts are flat-topped and slightly rough on the surface, which is often pigmented. They are usually 2–3 mm in diameter and may require incidental lighting to discern their outline. The face, around the mouth and chin are the sites most commonly involved, and the hyperpigmentation may give children an unwashed appearance. Young women are also affected and lesions may persist for years. The dorsa of the hands and knees are sometimes involved and trauma may demonstrate the Koebner phenomenon at these sites.

### Genital warts

See p. 94

## TREATMENT

Spontaneous resolution is common and this makes it difficult to assess the value of therapy. Keratolytics containing salicylic or lactic acid may lessen the unsightly appearance of common warts, which is peculiarly loathsome to so many patients.

Drying preparations may speed resolution if maceration of the skin over the hands and feet is associated with excessive sweating. Glutaraldehyde 10% w/v may be applied twice daily with a brush to individual lesions or wiped over the surface of mosaic warts. Soaks include formaldehyde as a formalin solution at concentrations of between 2 and 5%, or potassium permanganate 0.01%. Too strong solutions or too frequent applications may induce cracking or fissuring over areas of the skin such as the toe-clefts.

Destructive methods may hasten resolution by producing local inflammatory changes and enhancing immune reactions. These include chemical cautery, electrocautery and cryosurgery.

On some occasions curettage may prompt the resolution of painful verrucae but any scarring that accompanies such procedures may give rise to chronic pain, particularly when situated over pressure points.

# Fungal infections

Fungal infections of the skin can be divided into those associated with yeasts such as *Candida albicans* and others caused by dermatophytes or ringworm fungi.

## CANDIDIASIS

### AETIOLOGY
Use of drugs such as corticosteroids, cytotoxics, antibiotics and oral contraceptives can predispose to candidiasis. It is now a major problem in patients with AIDS.

Local factors in the skin, such as maceration, may predispose to secondary invasion at sites such as the groin or breast fold, particularly if obesity is present.

### CLINICAL FEATURES
**Oral candidiasis**
This is discussed on p. 180.

**Cutaneous candidiasis**
Maceration of the skin in body folds, especially in the obese, induces erosion and intertrigo (Fig. 20.9). In a similar fashion, the wet napkins of infants may encourage opportunistic infection with *C. albicans*.

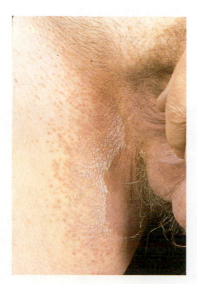

**Fig. 20.9**  Intertrigo with the typical satellite pustules seen with secondary candidiasis.

**Pruritus vulvae**
Candidiasis is a common cause of a vaginal discharge and leads to pruritus vulvae. It can be a presenting feature of diabetes mellitus. Other causes are:
- Vaginal discharge due to *Trichomonas,* bacterial vaginosis or other causes
- Scabies and pediculosis
- Contact dermatitis
- Senile atrophy
- Lichen sclerosus et atrophicus
- Leucoplakia
- Psychogenic

Aggravating factors include poor hygiene, obesity, tight clothing and excess washing with soap. Treatment depends on the cause.

**Paronychia**
Chronic maceration of the skin is important in the development of paronychial infection. Commonly the seal or eponychium at the proximal nail fold is lost by continual immersion of the hands in water or by manicure. A space is opened up beneath the nail fold and the continuing moist environment suits the growth of *C. albicans*.

Disease is manifest by a swelling or bolstering of the nail fold, erythema, pain and deformity of the nail plate. Greenish black discoloration of the nail plate often indicates concomitant infection with organisms such as *Ps. aeruginosa*, which thrives in the same moist environment.

### TREATMENT
An attempt to dry areas of contiguous skin, e.g. beneath the breasts by interposing an absorbent material between the two skin surfaces, is important. The routine use of a fine powder containing antifungal agents such as miconazole or clotrimazole as a talc after washing is helpful.

Specific antifungal agents used are nystatin, which has only topical activity, and an imidazole (e.g. clotrimazole or miconazole) cream, lotion, spray or powder. Fluconazole and itraconazole are new oral triazoles and are used particularly for vaginal candidiasis (see p. 95).

In severe intertrigo it is important to incorporate a low-potency steroid together with the antifungal agent in order to allay the inflammatory changes, itching and excoriation.

More serious and widespread disease in infants or those who are immunocompromised by disease or therapy may be effectively treated with oral ketoconazole 200–400 mg daily. The unusual but potentially serious hepatotoxic effects of this drug require that it should be reserved for very intractable or life-threatening disease.

## INFECTION WITH DERMATOPHYTES OR RINGWORM FUNGI

Dermatophytes or ringworm fungi are able to invade the keratinized tissue of the skin, nails or hair and include *Epidermophyton, Microsporum* or *Trichophyton*. The term 'tinea' means 'moth-eaten' and may be used to denote the pattern of involvement, e.g. tinea capitis.

The source of the fungus may be zoophilic (animal to man), anthrophilic (human to human) or geophilic (soil to man).

Scrapings taken from the skin and dissolved in 20% potassium hydroxide should reveal the presence of hyphae. A second sample is plated on a culture medium and incubated. Samples from nail clippings and hairs may be analysed in the same way.

## Tinea capitis

This is now an uncommon disease in the UK. The organism most commonly involved is *Microsporum canis*, which is transmitted from the coats of dogs and cats.

### CLINICAL FEATURES

Areas of scaling and hair loss are evident in children infected by *M. canis*, but at puberty changes within the hair itself limit infection. On occasions more marked inflammatory changes are seen with a boggy swelling in the scalp, surmounted by crusting and loss, or matting, of the hair; this is called kerion. Scarring of the scalp that may follow such infection can lead to permanent hair loss.

*Trichophyton* species, *T. tonsurans* and *T. violaceum*, invade the hair shaft (endothrix) and often cause the hair to break off at the level of the scalp, producing a black dot appearance. More widespread and severe hair loss, associated with a characteristic pattern of scaling in which yellowed keratin scale passes upwards along the hair shaft forming a scutulum or 'shield' shape, is seen with the infection favus, which is caused by *T. schoenleinii*. This infection is seen in the Middle East, southern Africa, Greenland and, less frequently, in Pakistan.

### DIAGNOSIS

Examination by Wood's light produces a greenish fluorescence of the scalp when it is infected with *M. canis* and other species that invade the surface of the hair (ectothrix).

### TREATMENT

It is important to treat the animal source of infection. Spread from human to human is unusual with infection produced by *M. canis*. Griseofulvin is given by mouth and treatment may need to be prolonged for up to 3 months. Itraconazole is also being used. Antibacterial treatment may be required for suppurative disease (kerion), either topically or by mouth, in order to lessen the risk of scarring.

## Tinea pedis

This refers to infection that involves principally the toe webs or the soles of the feet.

### AETIOLOGY

The infecting organism is most commonly *T. rubrum* (colonies produce red coloration on culture). *Epidermophyton floccosum* and *T. mentagrophytes* are less commonly seen.

Occupations that produce maceration of the skin and communal spread include coal mining and working on submarines, where warm decks and rubber-soled shoes encourage infection. Athletic pursuits (athlete's foot infection), the wearing of occlusive footwear and swimming also encourage spread of these infections. The disease is often intractable and *T. rubrum* infection may be especially difficult to eradicate, with the organism showing resistance to both topical and systemic fungicides.

### CLINICAL FEATURES

Infection is mostly seen as:
- Scaling, maceration and erythema of the lateral toe webs
- Blistering lesions, often few in number on the plantar surface of the toes or foot
- Confluent erythema and scaling on the soles

Spread may occur to the palms (Fig. 20.10) or to the medial aspect of the thigh and perianal skin of males.

### TREATMENT

Foot powders often contain antifungal agents of low potency but their drying effect is useful when they are applied regularly. Drying foot soaks such as potassium permanganate 0.01% solution may discourage infection by preventing maceration.

Specific measures include oral griseofulvin. This may need to be given for periods of up to 3 months for disease associated with *T. rubrum* in doses of 500 mg twice daily. Imidazoles (clotrimazole or miconazole) can be applied overnight as a cream and used as a talc in powder form by day.

## Tinea unguium

This most commonly affects the great-toe nails but several nails may be affected. It causes discoloration, chalky deposits, subungual hyperkeratosis and fragmentation of the nail plate. Infected finger-nails show similar changes (Fig. 20.11) but are less frequently involved. Unusual trauma associated with occupations and hobbies, congenital changes or malalignment may also produce misshapen great-toe nails. When several toe-nails are involved the differential diagnosis includes psoriasis.

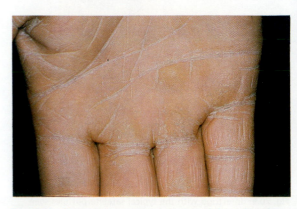

**Fig. 20.10**  *Trichophyton rubrum* infection of the right palm.

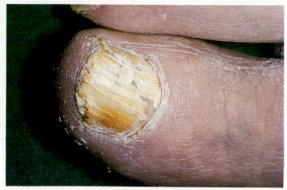

**Fig. 20.11** Dystrophy of the toe-nail associated with dermatophyte infection (tinea unguium).

### DIAGNOSIS

Clippings taken from the free edge of the nail should be sent for culture. Usually the same organisms that cause tinea pedis are found.

### TREATMENT

Nail-plate infection will require systemic treatment for up to 9 months for finger-nails and 2 years for toe-nails. Griseofulvin 0.5–1 g daily given for such a length of time is seldom associated with serious side-effects but it may fail to eradicate the infection even though the cosmetic appearance is improved. The combination of tioconazole lotion, which penetrates the nail, with griseofulvin can speed and increase the chances of clearing. Itraconazole is also used or terbinafine, an allylamine, can be given by mouth. It has a more rapid effect clearing toe-nails in 4–6 months and the recurrence rate is less than when using griseofulvin.

## Tinea corporis

Infection of the skin of the groin (*tinea cruris*) is not infrequently seen in males with chronic infection of the feet, so that both areas should be examined at the same time. An area of erythema and scaling is surrounded by a well-defined edge and is often studded with pustules or papules. Infection may extend over the perianal skin (Fig. 20.12).

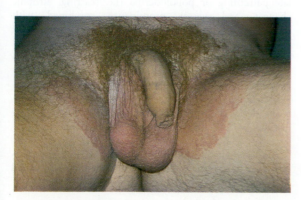

**Fig. 20.12** Tinea cruris.

Tinea corporis may be evident in older members of the family, while children are infected on the scalp. Annular, erythematous and scaled lesions are then seen on the trunk or limbs. More inflammatory, pustular and indurated plaques affect the neck or shoulders of farm workers who come into contact with cattle infected with *T. verrucosum*.

Diagnosis is by direct microscopy and culture of skin scrapings.

Treatment is with griseofulvin and local antifungal cream.

# Infestations

## Scabies (the itch)

Scabies is a highly irritant condition occurring on the skin of an individual sensitized to the female mite of *Sarcoptes scabiei* or its products.

### MODE OF TRANSMISSION

Transmission is by skin-to-skin contact with an affected individual and usually occurs in bed. Holding hands is a less common mode of spread from infested children, as warmth is necessary for the mite or acarus to remain mobile.

Most individuals will only harbour about a dozen mature female acari. However, many thousands of mites may be associated with crusted or Norwegian scabies, and the affected individuals seem unable to mount the same sensitizing responses. This condition is more common in the mentally subnormal and immunocompromised individuals.

### CLINICAL FEATURES

Sites of predilection for burrows include the finger webs, wrists, elbows, ankles, breasts and genitalia. Linear or curved tracts may be seen with a tiny vesicle at one end that contains the mite. The mite can be removed on the end of a needle, or the burrow scraped to reveal eggs, mite fragments or faeces as firm evidence of infestation.

Sensitivity to the mites' products occurs after 4–6 weeks, when individuals develop most commonly a widespread, highly irritant, excoriated and often secondary infected folliculopapular eruption. Secondary eczematous changes may be evident, or the patient (especially a child) may present with impetigo.

The diagnosis should be suspected if symptoms of itching are severe, when papules appear over genitalia and the history indicates that bedfellows, family or friends are also complaining of irritation. Infants develop papules on the palms, soles or the axillary folds and some adults suffer postscabetic papules for up to several months after sensitization. Mites from dogs or birds may produce vesicular lesions, crusting or urticaria but infestation from these sources is not associated with burrows.

## TREATMENT

All infested individuals and their close contacts should be treated. A lotion containing gamma-benzene hexachloride (lindane 0.1–1%) must be applied to all parts of the skin surface save the face and kept in contact with the skin for a full 24 hours, so that hand-washing must be followed by reapplication. The process is then repeated 24 hours later and all personal garments, night attire and bed-linen should then be laundered in a washing machine. Neurotoxic effects from the absorption of lindane in young children occasionally occur and malathion or permethrin should be used instead.

## Pediculosis capitis (head lice)

This condition is prevalent in schoolchildren in the UK, with infestation also occurring (though less commonly) in those who have close contact with the children, e.g. mothers. The head louse itself is difficult to find within a thick head of hair but evidence of its presence is seen in the many eggs or 'nits' laid along the hair shafts. The initial lesions occur close to the scalp, especially over the occipital region and the nape of the neck. In children, infestation should be suspected when excoriation is seen and impetigo is evident around the hair margin. Infestation occurs from the close touching of heads and is often widespread within a class of schoolchildren.

## TREATMENT

Malathion 0.5% and carbaryl are often used because of lindane-resistant strains of lice. These drugs are left on for 12 hours overnight and removed with shampoo (repeated twice at intervals of 3 days). Cutting the hair facilitates the use of local applications. Eggs are killed by this treatment and it is not necessary to continually attempt to remove them.

## Pediculosis corporis (body lice)

This condition is usually found only in those with a gross lack of hygiene, such as vagrants. The skin of affected individuals is often thickened, pigmented and excoriated; lice, often few in number, may be evident on the seams of clothing worn next to the skin. The clothes should be autoclaved.

## Pediculosis pubis (pubic lice)

Infestation is evident over the pubic hair, with occasional spread in hairy individuals on to the body or even the eyebrows. Contracting the disease is often related to promiscuity. Irritation is the initial symptom and patients are able to detect movement of the louse on skin covered by relatively sparse hairs. Treatment of the infestation is the same as that for head lice.

## Arthropod-borne diseases

Development of these diseases depends on contact with the animals or birds that form the primary host for the causative organisms. These include *Cheyletiella*, most commonly *C. yasgouri* or *C. parasitovorax*, from dogs, cats, rabbits and other pets. On close inspection of their coats such animals will often have evidence of scaling and thickening of the skin, on which mites are sometimes evident by their movement. Brushings are taken on to dark paper, which is then scanned for evidence of mites, fleas or their products. Bites should be suspected in those who have close contact with animals; the area of skin affected shows grouped vesiculopapular lesions.

## TREATMENT

This must begin with the elimination of the arthropod at its source. All other manoeuvres that attempt to produce symptomatic relief of itching associated with bites, such as repellants, calamine lotion, cream or antihistamines, give only temporary relief.

# Cutaneous manifestations of systemic diseases

The skin is frequently involved in systemic diseases. In this section, only conditions with major cutaneous manifestations that are not dealt with elsewhere are considered.

## CONNECTIVE-TISSUE DISEASES
(see p. 400)

These systemic diseases often have cutaneous manifestations, which are described here.

## Systemic lupus erythematosus

Photosensitivity is a presenting feature in about one-fifth of patients and may occur with a greater frequency as the disease progresses.

The nose, cheeks (butterfly distribution), forehead, ears and the backs of the hands are affected by the non-specific changes of diffuse erythema or maculopapular lesions; blistering may accompany more acute disease.

More chronic changes on the backs of the hands or fingers include blue/red discoloration of the skin, reticulate patterning or poikiloderma (i.e. scarring, atrophic changes and vessel prominence combined with erythema). Nail-fold capillary dilatation and ragged cuticles with haemorrhages are seen in this disease, as well as in dermatomyositis and systemic sclerosis. Loss of tissue over finger pads associated with Raynaud's phenomenon (see p. 628) is seen, although this is a more prominent feature in systemic sclerosis or mixed connective-tissue disease. Purpura and urticaria may be presenting features of SLE or they may accompany a more widespread vasculitis.

Alopecia occurs with either broken hairs, most noticeable over the frontal region, or diffuse hair loss associated with more severe generalized disease.

## TREATMENT (see p. 402)

Protection against the sun is important.

# Cutaneous (discoid) lupus erythematosus

This condition represents disease that is almost totally confined to the skin. There are two different patterns:

1 Discoid lesions involving principally facial skin
2 Widespread cutaneous disease, when the hands, feet, limbs and trunk may also be affected

Patients with widespread cutaneous disease may develop SLE, whilst patients with SLE may develop chronic discoid lesions.

Arthropathy, Raynaud's phenomenon, haematological abnormalities, a raised ESR and abnormal serological findings are sometimes seen with disease, which is seemingly limited to the skin. It may be difficult, therefore, to decide whether a patient has just cutaneous disease or a systemic illness. Obvious ill-health, high levels of DNA binding and hypocomplementaemia, a positive lupus band test (typical immunofluorescent changes seen on a biopsy, suitably stained and taken from normal uninvolved skin) are important findings in SLE and these may help to differentiate the two conditions.

## CLINICAL FEATURES

Women are twice as frequently affected as men, in contrast to SLE where the female-to-male ratio is 9 : 1. The peak incidence is later than SLE—between 40 and 50 years. In discoid lupus erythematosus the face, neck and, less commonly, the scalp are the principal sites of involvement. Erythematous scaled plaques, oval or round or contoured in outline may be seen (Fig. 20.13). Follicular plugging is characteristically seen; this may be demonstrated as spikes of keratin seen on the under-surface of a removed scale. Atrophy and scarring are common features and when these occur on the scalp permanent hair loss follows. Although sunlight is an exacerbating factor in most patients, other forms of trauma to the skin, such as cold injury, may trigger the onset of new lesions or reactivate areas of previously involved skin.

Widespread, cutaneous disease may demonstrate similar morphological features, although scaling is not so pronounced. Reticulate patterning or smooth, shiny, red/blue, atrophic skin is seen, especially on the fingers

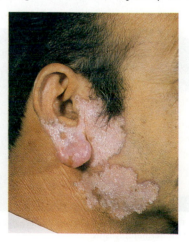

**Fig. 20.13**  Discoid lupus erythematosus.

or plantar aspect of the toes. Chilblain-like lesions may be seen at the same sites and on the heels or earlobes.

## TREATMENT

Suitable protection from strong sun or cold should be worn. High-protection-factor sunscreens need to be applied regularly. Hydroxychloroquine in doses of 200–400 mg daily during spring and summer gives extra protection from sunlight and settles inflammatory changes. Prolonged treatment at high dosage can produce permanent retinal damage so that an ophthalmic opinion should be sought prior to starting treatment and at regular intervals thereafter. Oral prednisolone is given for more florid cutaneous disease.

Potent topical corticosteroids may improve cutaneous lupus erythematosus; this disease is one indication for their application to facial skin. Treatment may need to be intensified when acute inflammatory changes affect the scalp so that scarring and permanent hair loss are prevented.

Other agents that have been used for recalcitrant patterns of disease include thalidomide, mepacrine, vitamin E and retinoids.

# Systemic sclerosis and morphoea (scleroderma)

The term *scleroderma* means a thickening or hardening of the skin associated with an increase in its collagen content. Thickening of the skin also occurs in association with other conditions, such as porphyria or the carcinoid syndrome. In these conditions the lesion is called pseudo-scleroderma. The generic term 'scleroderma' should not be used, as systemic sclerosis and morphoea are distinct entities. Systemic sclerosis has both cutaneous and systemic features, whilst morphoea is confined to the skin.

## Morphoea

Females are more frequently affected in a ratio of 3 : 1. It most commonly presents in young patients as a plaque of thickened red or blue skin, sometimes showing central pallor; the skin over the trunk and limbs is most frequently involved. A more superficial and widespread pattern of disease affects the trunk in middle-aged females. Children are affected by linear lesions seen on the skull and over the face and tissues underlying the skin may also be involved, producing facial hemiatrophy.

Plaques evolve to produce waxy, thickened skin that cannot be easily separated from the underlying tissue. Individual plaques may enlarge or new lesions appear over an interval and resolution is associated with hyperpigmentation that may never totally fade. Involvement of the limb may be associated with widespread and severe induration of the skin, muscle pain and joint stiffness. Generalized cutaneous disease is rare.

TREATMENT. The early inflammatory changes, if severe and associated with oedema and induration, may be limited by systemic steroids and azathioprine. It is difficult to treat well-established cutaneous disease.

**Systemic sclerosis** (see p. 403)

In two-thirds of patients, Raynaud's phenomenon may be present for years or even decades prior to the development of other clinical features. Severe ischaemia associated with this disease may lead to severe ulceration, gangrene and a loss of digits.

Typically the skin in systemic sclerosis is bound down to underlying structures and the fingers taper (known as sclerodactyly or acrosclerosis). Fibrotic changes around the joints may produce flexion deformities and prevent fine movements. A binding down of facial skin may produce beaking of the nose, a fixed facial expression, radial furrowing of the lips and limitation of mouth opening. Mat-like telangiectases on the face or hands and some proximal spread of skin thickening complete the usual picture. Calcium deposits are sometimes extruded from the skin over digits (CR(E)ST syndrome, see p. 404). Thickening of the skin and pigmentary changes are often seen at the base of the neck or over the cervical spine and shoulders.

The disease may sometimes present as puffiness or oedema of the hands or feet, with preceding or accompanying attacks of Raynaud's phenomenon, though circulatory impairment may not be evident. A more explosive onset with widespread or universal skin thickening and more extensive visceral disease is less common.

DIFFERENTIAL DIAGNOSIS. Systemic sclerosis-like disease is seen in the toxic oil syndrome, polyvinyl chloride disease, eosinophilia–myalgia syndrome due to tryptophan therapy, bleomycin therapy and graft-versus-host disease.

TREATMENT. Severe Raynaud's phenomenon may be helped by charcoal, chemical or preheated thermal glove warmers or electrically heated gloves. Nifedipine may limit the attacks. Severe ulceration or imminent gangrene may be prevented by the intravenous infusion of prostaglandin $E_1$ or prostacyclin. Dryness of the skin associated with hair loss, damage to sweat glands and sebaceous glands may respond to emollients and soap substitutes.

## Dermatomyositis and polymyositis

(see p. 404)

These uncommon diseases affect blood vessels, muscle and skin in a varying fashion.

Dermatomyositis when seen in childhood often has a marked vascular component. Disease in adults aged 40–60 years affects the skin and muscle tissue together. Proximal myopathy, often associated with malignant disease *per se*, and non-specific skin changes have sometimes been mislabelled as dermatomyositis. This misdiagnosis has probably given a falsely high incidence of associated malignant disease (10–25%) that can be seen in adults with dermatomyositis. Recently Coxsackie B virus has been isolated from muscle tissue.

### CLINICAL FEATURES

The rash is often very distinctive and may display features of photosensitivity. Fingers show ragged cuticles and

haemorrhages with dilated and altered nail-fold capillary changes (Fig. 20.14). Erythematous, blue plaques are evident over the dorsal aspect of the fingers, more especially over the small joints, with a similar but streaked appearance over the metacarpophalangeal joints. Mild scaling may accompany these findings.

Scaling and erythema are seen at the elbow, and on occasions blue/red discoloration and reticulate patterning of the skin over the wrists, knees, feet, arms or thighs are seen.

Facial changes may include a marked erythema resembling sunburn, but inflammation of the eyelids or heliotrope coloration suggest the true diagnosis. Other exposed skin, e.g. the 'V' of the neck or the upper arms, may show erythema and sunburn-like changes that may also cause confusion. Marked cutaneous changes may occur in the absence of muscle disease. Typically, however, patients experience a proximal muscle weakness, noticeable when getting off a lavatory or combing the hair; dysphagia and respiratory muscle involvement are rare.

### INVESTIGATION

An underlying malignancy should be looked for. The malignancy may precede, accompany or follow the rash. Measurement of muscle enzyme levels and electromyogram (EMG) studies or muscle biopsy are helpful in the diagnosis and in following disease progress (see p. 951).

### TREATMENT

The prevention of joint contractures is very important in the childhood pattern of disease and soft-tissue calcification may regress with time. In adults, prednisolone with or without azathioprine or methotrexate is given for muscle disease (see p. 951) which will often clear cutaneous features. Sun screening and topical corticosteroid therapy may help to limit changes in the skin in those patients with predominantly cutaneous disease.

## SARCOIDOSIS

About one-quarter of patients with systemic sarcoidosis have skin lesions. There are many variants:

ERYTHEMA NODOSUM (see p. 1005), a non-specific reaction.

NODULES, PAPULES AND PLAQUES, red/blue or brown

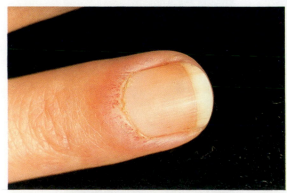

**Fig. 20.14** Ragged cuticle and nail-fold capillary dilatation associated with dermatomyositis.

are seen particularly on the face, nose, ears and neck in chronic sarcoid. This is the most common specific form seen in Caucasians.

ANNULAR, MACULAR LESIONS with central depigmentation are less common.

MICROPAPULAR LESIONS are common in Afro-Caribbeans and are usually the same colour as the skin. They occur around the nasal alae within the vestibules, on the lips or cheeks or over the periorbital skin (Fig. 20.15).

LUPUS PERNIO, an uncommon variant, affects the nose with a diffuse bluish plaque with small papules within the swelling.

WIDESPREAD CUTANEOUS SARCOIDOSIS is often papular or nodular. Occasionally, subcutaneous nodules are found. Sarcoidosis may appear in old scars.

Differential diagnosis of facial lesions includes leprosy and tuberculosis. Blue nodular lesions should be differentiated from lymphomas.

### TREATMENT

Most cutaneous forms of sarcoidosis will improve with increasing doses of systemic steroids. Drugs such as methotrexate, mepacrine or chloroquine may help in reducing the dose of steroid required. Intralesional steroids can aid resolution on occasions. Lesions may often recur on withdrawal of drugs.

## METABOLIC DISEASE

### Diabetes mellitus (see p. 850)

Cutaneous abnormalities occur in more than 25% of patients with diabetes mellitus. They may be non-specific, such as infection with candidiasis, or so distinctive that the dermatologist may be able to predict the diagnosis of diabetes mellitus.

Secondary causes of diabetes (see p. 830), e.g. haemochromatosis and liver disease, may in themselves have cutaneous manifestations and these features are described under the appropriate disease heading.

### Necrobiosis lipoidica (diabeticorum)

The association of this condition with diabetes is unpredictable; 50% of such cutaneous changes occur in non-diabetic patients. Necrobiosis lipoidica is an unusual complication of diabetes and is not necessarily related to other vascular complications. Nevertheless, small-vessel damage is thought to be a central feature of the pathogenesis. There is partial necrosis of dermal collagen and connective tissue and a histiocytic cellular response. It is more common in females, and presents in young adults or early middle life.

The skin over the shins is the site principally involved and pigmentary changes may cause the casual observer to associate the eruption with venous incompetence. On close examination the features are characteristic: erythematous plaques are seen that gradually develop a brown waxy discoloration that is more evident when stretching the skin. The skin's blood vessels are prominent because of the associated atrophic changes in the dermis. Fibrosis and scarring from previous ulceration may also be seen (Fig. 20.16).

Treatment is with support bandaging. The use of an antiseptic powder or spray such as povidone-iodine is useful when the skin is broken. Non-adhesive dressings should be used. Low-dose aspirin may help to improve the healing of such lesions.

### Diabetic dermopathy

This is a common finding on the shins of diabetics. Initially the lesions are erythematous and papular but tend with time to become flat, hyperpigmented and atrophic. The changes are often seen in association with microangiopathy elsewhere. The pathogenesis of these lesions, which are not specific to diabetes mellitus, is unclear, although intimal thickening of small blood vessels has been demonstrated.

### Diabetic stiff hands

This condition was first described in patients with juvenile-onset diabetes, but similar changes have been seen in middle-aged diabetics.

Tight, waxy skin principally affects the dorsum of the fingers and is associated with joint stiffness that can limit extensor movements of the small joints (cheiroarthropathy). Histological sections demonstrate thickening of dermal collagen.

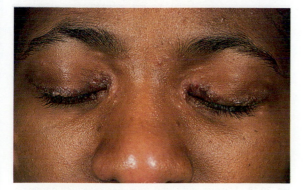

**Fig. 20.15** Micropapular sarcoidosis affecting the eyelids.

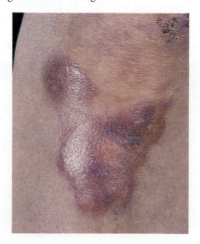

**Fig. 20.16** Necrobiosis lipoidica.

### Scleroedema

This condition is seen as a spreading erythema and induration of the skin that starts on the neck and the upper trunk of middle-aged diabetics. These changes are often heralded by a respiratory illness or by streptococcal infection. The lesion may become generalized over the trunk, limbs, hands and feet, although the genitalia tend to be spared. There is a spontaneous resolution with time.

### Diabetic bullae

This is an unusual complication in which blisters develop on the feet and occasionally the hands. They are of an acute onset and occur without any obvious preceding trauma. The disease is sometimes associated with an extensive polyneuropathy. Histological section shows a cleft in the region of the lamina lucida but the cause is not known. Blisters clear in 2–5 weeks.

### Granuloma annulare

This presents as flesh-coloured papules in annular or crescentic configurations, principally over the extensor surface of the joints of the fingers (Fig. 20.17). The feet, ankles, hands and wrists may be similarly affected. A disseminated pattern is probably triggered by sunlight but often involves covered areas of skin.

The association of such lesions with diabetes mellitus remains controversial; a few cases do not have overt diabetes but only impaired glucose tolerance. The pathology is similar to necrobiosis lipoidica and the two conditions may occur together.

### Eruptive xanthomas

These may appear suddenly as crops of yellow papules on the knees, elbows, back and the buttocks. They are associated with hyperlipidaemia (see p. 857) and are seen most commonly in diabetics. They resolve with the control of the diabetes and hyperlipidaemia.

### Other skin disorders

Infections and lipodystrophies are often seen in diabetes mellitus; they are discussed in Chapter 17. Skin breakdown may occur especially in association with peripheral vascular disease and give rise to gangrene, synergistic (aerobes and anaerobes) necrotizing cellulitis, progressive bacterial synergistic (microaerophilic, streptococci, *Staph. aureus* or enteric Gram-negative bacilli) gangrene.

## Porphyria cutanea tarda (see p. 866)

Only the changes seen in porphyria cutanea tarda are considered here. Similar changes in the skin may be seen with variegate porphyria and hereditary coproporphyria.

Cutaneous lesions occur on exposure to sunlight. These consist of increased fragility of the skin over the dorsum of the hands, fingers and face and are associated with erythema, blistering and scarring (Fig. 20.18). Hypertrichosis on the sides of the face and between the eyebrows and hair margin is common and may be associated with facial skin thickening and loss of hair (pseudoscleroderma). Hyperpigmentation or loss of pigment may also be seen on the facial skin. Itching may be troublesome.

The diagnosis and treatment are discussed on p. 867.

## Cutaneous amyloidosis

Amyloidosis is discussed on (p. 866).

Cutaneous forms of the disease may be widespread on the skin and mucosal surfaces or localized to particular areas. The skin is involved in about 40% of patients who have systemic amyloidosis in association with diseases such as myelomatosis.

The gums may appear nodular and waxy and bleed easily on trauma. Pale yellow-brown papules may appear over the basal conjunctivae and at other mucosal sites and purpura is seen following mild trauma.

Sites of predilection elsewhere on the skin include the eyelids, the nasolabial folds, the sides of the neck, and the flexural surfaces. Thickened indurated plaques may rarely affect the chest, abdomen or hands. Cutaneous changes are rare in the hereditofamilial patterns of disease.

Cutaneous disease where there is no evidence of systemic spread is seen in two forms: macular and lichen amyloidosis.

### Macular amyloidosis

Macular amyloidosis is quite commonly seen on the shoulders, neck or upper back of patients of Asian origin. The hyperpigmented macular changes have a rippled appearance likened to the changes seen on a sandy beach at low tide. Patients are only concerned about the appearance of the lesions, which are dark grey/black in colour.

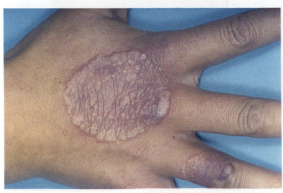

**Fig. 20.17** Granuloma annulare.

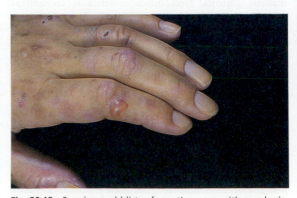

**Fig. 20.18** Scarring and blister formation seen with porphyria cutanea tarda.

The amyloid material is difficult to demonstrate on histology using routine methods.

### Lichen amyloidosis

Lichen amyloidosis is an uncommon papular eruption that is often pruritic and occurs on the lower limbs. There is no explanation for the appearance of the amyloid material at this site. Other pruritic diseases on the lower legs are often hypertrophic, especially in patients of African or Asian origin. Diseases such as hypertrophic lichen planus and lichen simplex may resemble the disease on superficial inspection. Close examination should, however, distinguish these diseases. The shiny, warty, close-set papules of lichen amyloidosis are characteristic of the disease.

## CNS-RELATED DISEASES

The number of dermatoses that have been associated with diseases of the nervous system is large but most are extremely rare.

### Neurofibromatosis (see p. 942)

The characteristic cutaneous features are hyperpigmentation (*café-au-lait spots*) and flesh-coloured smooth polypoid swellings, i.e. neurofibromas. Molluscum fibrosum (skin tags) are sessile pink-coloured tumours that are often numerous over the trunk. Plexiform neuromas are uncommon and tend to follow the course of a nerve, usually on the face or neck. In some areas there is overgrowth of skin and subcutaneous tissue in addition and this may give rise to gross disfigurement (elephantiasis neuromatosa). Oral lesions occur in up to 10% of patients.

*Café-au-lait* spots may suggest the diagnosis in children but there should be more than five in number to support it. The pigmentary changes must be differentiated from those seen in Albright's syndrome (see p. 782). In neurofibromatosis the *café-au-lait* spots show histologically the presence of giant melanosomes; these are rare in Albright's disease.

SEGMENTAL DISEASE. *Café-au-lait* patches and neurofibromata may be confined to a body segment.

### Tuberous sclerosis (epiloia) (see p. 942)

The cutaneous lesions in tuberous sclerosis are derived from connective tissue and are of several different types.

Adenoma sebaceum are erythematous papules or nodules on the cheeks or within the folds at the sides of the mouth or nose. The tumours are vascular and fibrous in origin. Periungual fibromas occur as pink, firm, claw-like tumours arising from and around the nail folds.

Shagreen patches are flesh-coloured tumours that are firm and plaque-like. They often have a wrinkled surface and are most frequently seen over the lumbosacral region.

Areas of macular hypopigmentation occur in ovoid or leaf-like shapes. They may be seen over the trunk or back and are most easily detected by examination with Wood's light. They appear early in childhood, associated in many cases with mental retardation.

Small erythematous papules on the face and cheeks may be treated with an electrical Hyfrecator or cautery.

## Other CNS-related diseases

Naevoid lesions may be seen in conjunction with neurological disease; for example, in the epidermal naevus syndrome, pigmented naevi occur in a linear fashion on the limb or trunk and may be associated with epilepsy or mental retardation.

Gross ichthyotic changes may occur on the skin of patients with spastic diplegia and mental retardation in the Sjögren–Larsson syndrome.

The Sturge–Weber syndrome is discussed on p. 943.

## MALIGNANT DISEASES

The skin can be involved by both primary and secondary tumours. Table 20.4 shows some cutaneous markers of malignant disease which may be associated with genodermatoses, paraneoplastic dermatoses or environmental carcinogens, e.g. arsenic, vinyl chloride, ionizing radiation.

# *Vascular and lymphatic disorders*

## Venous ulcers

These are confined to the lower limbs and many are postthrombotic. The increased hydrostatic pressure in the veins resulting from incompetent valves is reflected by increased capillary blood pressure. Leakage of plasma

|  | Malignancy |
|---|---|
| *The genodermatoses* | |
| Peutz–Jegher syndrome | G-1 |
| Gardener's syndrome | G-1 |
| Haemochromatosis | Hepatoma |
| Neurofibromatosis | Neural crest tumours |
| Multiple endocrine neoplasia type II | Medullary thyroid carcinoma |
|  | Phaeochromocytoma |
| *The paraneoplastic dermatoses* | |
| Carcinoid syndrome | Tumour |
| Acanthosis nigricans | G-1 (stomach); liver, lung, breast |
| Dermatomysitis | Variety |
| Pyoderma gangrenosum | Myeloproliferative |
| Erythema gyratum repens | Lung, breast |
| Acquired ichthyosis | Lymphoma |
| Necrolytic migratory erythema | Glucagonoma |

Table 20.4 Some cutaneous markers of malignant disease.

under pressure gives rise to perivascular fibrin deposition which may lead to a decrease in oxygen supply, but direct skin oxygen measurements do not support this view. There is a fall in oxygenation when an ulcerated limb is exercised, so that ambulant patients experience sustained hypoxia of the skin. Nutrition of the skin is then affected and leads to ischaemia and eventual ulceration. Ulcers around the ankle are often accompanied by:

- Hyperpigmentation following extravasation of red cells and haemosiderin deposition
- Dermatitis and excoriation due to pruritus
- White atrophy (*atrophie blanche*) caused by hyalinization of skin vessels producing scars in the overlying skin
- Secondary infection with possible cellulitis or thrombophlebitis

The differential diagnosis of leg ulcers is shown in Table 20.5.

## Arterial ulcers

Ulcers occurring in skin away from the ankle region are more commonly associated with arterial disease. They may accompany venous hypertension in the legs, especially in the elderly. Cold, atrophic skin with loss of hair, impalpable peripheral pulses with a history of claudication may suggest the diagnosis. The ulcers usually have a punched-out appearance and are often very painful. Doppler studies may help to determine the degree of arterial insufficiency in an affected limb.

## MANAGEMENT OF ARTERIAL AND VENOUS ULCERATION

GENERAL MANAGEMENT consists of reducing leg venous hypertension. This can be helped by wearing support bandages when standing or by elevation of the limbs when sitting or lying. Exercise should be encouraged and, if the patient is obese, weight reduction recommended.

DERMATITIS should be treated with bland non-steroidal applications such as zinc and salicylic acid paste. Impregnated bandages containing zinc and applied moist can dry out and stiffen to provide occlusion and support.

ULCERS should be cleaned with normal saline or a weak potassium permanganate solution. A non-adhesive absorbent dressing should be applied with an elasticated bandage up to the knees. These dressings may be viscous materials, alginates, semi-permeable films, hydrogels or hydrocolloids. These are expensive but covering the wound with a permeable membrane will diminish pain and encourage re-epithelialization. Clean granulating ulcers should have non-adherent dressings applied and left undisturbed for increasing periods as the ulcer heals. A debriding agent (e.g. hydrophilic polysaccharide beads) or surgery may be necessary to remove dead tissue. Pinch grafting may also be necessary. The grafts are removed from the thigh and dotted over the ulcers and left undisturbed for 10 days.

INFECTION. Local antibiotics should be avoided if possible. *Ps. aeruginosa* infection accompanies non-permeable occlusive dressings. Systemic antibiotics may be required for cellulitis.

FOLLOW-UP care and preventative measures are most important and elastic stockings may always be necessary.

VARICOSE VEINS. Treatment may be necessary.

## Pressure sores (decubitus ulcers)

These occur in the elderly, immobile, unconscious or paralysed patients. They are due to skin ischaemia from sustained pressure over a bony point. Normal individuals feel the pain of continued pressure and even during sleep, movement takes place to change position continually.

1 The majority of pressure sores occur in hospital:
   (a) 70% in first 2 weeks of hospitalization
   (b) 70% are in orthopaedic patients especially those on traction
2 20–30% occur in the community
3 80% of patients with deep ulcers involving the subcutaneous tissue die in the first 4 months

Altered sensation of the skin increases the risk of ulceration and patients with diseases that affect the circulation and tissue nutrition also are predisposed, e.g. rheumatoid

| |
|---|
| *Venous insufficiency* |
| *Arterial insufficiency* |
| |
| *Infective* |
| Bacterial |
|     Post cellulitis |
|     Desert sore |
| Mycobacterial |
|     Tuberculosis |
|     Buruli ulcer |
|     Leprosy |
|     Swimming pool granuloma |
| Mycotic |
|     Superficial or deep fungal |
| Spirochaetal |
|     Syphilis |
|     Yaws |
| |
| *Neuropathic* |
|     Diabetes mellitus |
| |
| *Haematological* |
|     Sickle cell disease |
|     Spherocytosis |
| |
| *Neoplastic* |
|     Epithelioma |
|     Kaposi's sarcoma |
|     Basal-cell carcinoma |
| |
| *Vasculitis* |
|     Rheumatoid, systemic lupus erythematosus |
|     Pyoderma gangrenosum |
| |
| *Trauma or artefact* |

**Table 20.5** Causes of leg ulceration.

arthritis, diabetes mellitus, peripheral vascular disease; general illness, anaemia, malnutrition and oedema may affect skin breakdown.

*Other precipitating factors* include anaesthesia, surgical operations, sedation, dehydration, urinary incontinence or faecal impaction.

Red/blue discoloration of the skin can lead to ulcers in 1–2 hours; thus leaving patients on hard accident and emergency trolleys or sitting them in chairs for prolonged periods is bad practice.

### MANAGEMENT

General measures should include identifying at-risk patients. Those with non-fading marking of the skin on pressure sites need immediate attention.

- Bed rest with pillows to keep pressure off bony areas, e.g. pelvis and heels
- Regular turning, but avoid pressure on hips
- Fleece over lower one-third of bed for heels
- Roto cushions for patients in wheelchairs
- Treatment of general condition
- Special mattresses and beds to relieve pressure areas
- Topical treatment—keep ulcer clean and moist (many topical therapies are harmful)
- Pain relief (may need diamorphine)
- Plastic surgery

## Lymphoedema

This is oedema due to lymphatic obstruction. The affected area is swollen and initially there is pitting. In chronic lymphoedema the skin becomes thickened and the oedema is permanent. Localized lymphoedema occurs transiently with any skin infection. The causes of chronic lymphoedema in the Western Hemisphere include recurrent cellulitis, malignant disease due to infiltration or following treatment with surgery or radiotherapy, or recurrent cellulitis, or it can be familial with abnormal lymphatics. In the tropics, filariasis is a common cause. There are a number of rare congenital causes with abnormalities of the lymphatic vessels. Abnormalities may also be acquired, such as in the yellow nail syndrome (see p. 1039).

## Vasculitis (see p. 406)

Vasculitis is a clinicopathological process characterized by inflammation of the blood vessel wall. Any size and type of blood vessel may be involved and consequently a variety of diseases with overlapping clinical features are seen.

Vasculitis is thought to result from deposition of circulating immune complexes in blood vessel walls causing release of vasoactive amines and resulting in increased vessel permeability. The endothelial cell itself also plays a role in inflammation with the synthesis and secretion of proinflammatory cytokines and cell surface proteins which permit the binding of neutrophils.

### CLINICAL FEATURES

Purpuric papules accompanied by erythema or urticaria which on occasions progress to necrosis and ulceration are the clinical features of allergic vasculitis (Henoch–

Allergic vasculitis (leucocytoclastic vasculitis e.g. due to drugs, malignancy, infection)
Acute neutrophilic dermatosis (Sweet's syndrome)
Rheumatoid disease and other connective tissue diseases
Hypergammaglobulinaemic purpura
Essential mixed cryoglobulinaemia
Urticarial vasculitis
Septic vasculitis (mycobacterial, streptococcal, hepatitis B)
Ecthyma gangrenosum (*Pseudomonas aeruginosa* septicaemia)

**Table 20.6**  Small vessel necrotizing vasculitis.

Schönlein purpura) seen mostly in the lower limbs or dependent parts.

Histological changes show immune complex-mediated and neutrophil-induced endothelial damage and migration of polymorphs through the vessel wall (leucocytoclastic vasculitis). This pattern of disease typically involves postcapillary venules and causative agents include drugs, infection and immune complex disorders, such as SLE. Accompanying systemic features include arthralgia, arthritis, myalgia and fever. It is especially important to exclude involvement of other organs, e.g. kidney. Other causes of small vessel necrotizing vasculitis are shown in Table 20.6.

Larger vessel disease i.e. medium sized and large (Table 20.7) may produce large painful punctate ulcers, or digital gangrene. The face may be involved in Wegener's granulomatosis and the scalp in temporal arteritis.

The cause of the disease that affects blood vessels is only determined in about half the patients. History taking should include a careful note of drugs being taken. Investigations should include tests to eliminate for example infection and autoimmune disease.

## Pyoderma gangrenosum (Fig. 20.19)

This is a characteristic non-infective, necrotizing ulceration of the skin that occurs in association with underlying systemic disease or blood dyscrasia in 50% of patients.

### AETIOLOGY

Associated diseases are described in Table 20.8; these are diverse and give no obvious clue to a common pathogenesis. No constant abnormality of humoral or cell-mediated immunity has been demonstrated.

The pathological features include a massive polymorphonuclear cellular infiltrate with marked necrosis and thrombosis of small and medium-sized vessels.

Polyarteritis nodosa
Wegener's granulomatosis
Allergic granulomatosis (Churg–Strauss)
Lymphomatoid granulomatosis
Giant cell arteritis
Temporal arteritis
Takayasu's disease

**Table 20.7**  Larger vessel disease.

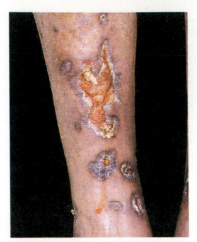

**Fig. 20.19** Pyoderma gangrenosum.

Multiple myeloma
Other paraproteinaemias, especially IgA
Arthropathy (rheumatoid and spondylarthropathies)
Inflammatory bowel disease
Acute leukaemia
Polycythaemia vera

NB No cause is found in 50% of cases

**Table 20.8** Conditions associated with pyoderma gangrenosum.

## CLINICAL FEATURES

Lesions most commonly arise as inflammatory pustules or papules that appear on the trunk and limbs. They may rapidly enlarge over several days to produce large necrotic ulcers with a crescentic or polycyclic outline and sloughy base, which undermines a raised purplish prominent rim. Other patients may have a more slowly progressive indolent ulcer.

Less frequently, but especially in association with acute myelogenous leukaemia, ulceration may be superficial and arise as necrotic bullae.

## TREATMENT

Rapidly progressive and painful lesions are accompanied by systemic symptoms and require doses of prednisolone 80–100 mg. Azathioprine may be used in combination or alone. The underlying condition should be treated.

Tetracyclines, colchicine and clofazimine have been shown to be of benefit in a few patients.

Indolent ulcers may respond to topical therapy and intralesional steroid injections.

## Antiphospholipid antibody syndromes (see p. 403)

Antiphospholipid antibodies including the lupus anticoagulant (LA) and anticardiolipin (ACL) are associated with thrombosis, central nervous disease and spontaneous abortion with or without SLE.

### CUTANEOUS MANIFESTATIONS

- Livedo reticularis, livedo reticularis with cerebrovascular accidents (Sneddon's syndrome)

- Thrombophlebitis
- Cutaneous gangrene and necrosis of digits
- Skin ulcerations
- Lesions resembling vasculitis, nodules, macules
- Cutaneous necrosis/infarction
- Subungual splinter haemorrhages

## Drug eruptions

Cutaneous eruptions account for one-third of all side-effects of drugs. It is sometimes difficult to differentiate an eruption due to a drug from one produced by the underlying illness. On occasions the effects of both are relevant to the onset of the rash, for example patients prescribed ampicillin for infectious mononucleosis will often develop a widespread morbilliform rash. Patients often take many drugs together and it may be difficult to incriminate one agent in the production of the rash. *In vitro* testing of drugs in these situations is inadequate in establishing or predicting the likelihood of the drug causing the cutaneous side-effect.

The drugs mentioned below are only examples. If there is doubt about an eruption, the most likely drug to produce this should be stopped.

### Urticaria (see p. 1003)

Urticaria may be associated with a type I IgE reaction and anaphylaxis in patients who are hypersensitive, for example, to penicillin. Urticaria can also occur in the serum sickness syndrome, IgG immune complex-mediated reactions occurring 1–2 weeks after drugs or serum, or lastly, by direct release of histamine. The latter include:

- Codeine, opiates and tubocurarine
- Radiological contrast media
- Aspirin and NSAIDs, e.g. indomethacin may trigger blood vessel hyperreactivity by affecting the production of arachidonic acid metabolites
- Angiotensin converting enzyme inhibitors, e.g. captopril and enalapril, may also potentiate effects of bradykinins

### Allergic vasculitis and purpura

Drugs that produce vasculitis may activate the alternative pathway of complement or produce cryoglobulins and immune complexes in the serum. Antibody, principally IgA, may be deposited around damaged vessels in the kidney and skin. Purpuric lesions appear most frequently on the extremities and may be accompanied by urticaria, blisters, necrosis of the skin and ulceration.

Drugs that have been associated with this disease include allopurinol, sulphonamides, gold, hydralazine, quinidine, methyldopa, captopril and amiodarone. Drugs that cause a lupus erythematosus-like syndrome include isoniazid, β-adrenergic receptor antagonists, penicillamine and lithium.

Purpura may be seen following drug-induced thrombocytopenia (see p. 324). Drugs may combine with the platelets to form an antigen; antibody formation follows, leading to platelet destruction.

### Erythema nodosum and erythema multiforme

Erythema nodosum and erythema multiforme may be induced by drugs; these are considered on p. 1005.

### Erythematous morbilliform eruptions

These maculopapular erythematous reactions are the commonest type of drug eruption. They usually occur up to 2 weeks after starting the medication and are widespread on the trunk and over pressure sites such as the thighs, knees and elbows. Diffuse erythema may be accompanied by pruritus and followed by desquamation. An accompanying fever may cause confusion with viral illnesses. Paired sera for viral antibodies may help to establish the correct diagnosis in retrospect.

All penicillins, sulphonamides, phenytoin, gold and gentamicin are agents most likely to induce this type of reaction.

### Lichen planus-like or lichenoid eruptions

These are discussed on p. 1002.

### Photosensitizing agents

These are discussed on p. 1036.

### Toxic epidermal necrolysis

This is the most serious type of drug-induced disease. It can be distinguished on histological grounds from the condition seen in children, which produces a similar clinical picture and is induced by staphylococci (see p. 19). There is superficial peeling of all the skin which follows several days after fever, malaise and rhinitis. Some features may overlap those of Stevens–Johnson syndrome. The agents most likely to cause such disease are NSAIDs, penicillins, sulphonamides, allopurinol and barbiturates.

### Fixed drug eruption

The pathogenesis of this type of reaction is unknown. The face, hands and genitalia are most commonly affected. Bright red, sometimes purpuric or even blistered plaques or annular lesions are seen. An accompanying burning discomfort is present. The lesions are fixed in site and appear within hours of the offending drug's administration. They will occur at exactly the same sites if the drug is given again at another time. Postinflammatory hyperpigmentation is a striking feature.

Phenolphthalein in laxatives or as a colouring in sweets is a common cause. Other agents include tetracycline, sulphonamides, phenacetin, salicylates, the oral contraceptive pill and chlordiazepoxide.

### Pigmentation

Pigmentation that occurs with oral agents is considered below (see p. 1036).

### Exacerbation of pre-existing skin diseases

Pre-existing skin diseases may be exacerbated by drugs. Examples include lithium carbonate and β-receptor antagonists, which will exacerbate psoriasis.

### Lupus erythematosus-like rash

See p. 1020.

### Acneiform eruptions

These are papulopustular eruptions but usually without comedones. The major drugs involved are corticosteroids, oral contraceptives, androgens, iodides, anticonvulsants and isoniazid.

### Eczematous reactions

These can be caused by sulphonamides, sulphonylureas for example. Sensitization can be by topical application.

### Hair and nails (see p. 1040)

# Naevi and tumours

The skin is a prime target for aberrant growth and tumour formation. It may be in direct contact with ionizing radiation and many chemical substances or microorganisms that may act as inducers of abnormal cellular activity. There are also a large number of different cell types represented within the skin.

Many skin tumours are rare and in practice are confined to a few types.

## Melanocytic naevus (naevocytic naevus)

This is a tumour produced by cells of neural crest origin, mainly melanocytes. Schwann cells may also contribute to the dermal aspect of these lesions. This is the most common type of skin tumour. It is pigmented and is referred to as a 'mole' in lay terms.

These tumours originate as a proliferation of melanocytes at the epidermodermal junction, so that clinically little growth above the skin surface is seen at this stage (*junctional naevus*).

With time, cells migrate downwards into the dermis and their bulk increases so that tumours become elevated above the skin surface. Both an epidermal and dermal component are now seen (*compound naevus*). Gradually the epidermal component becomes less obvious and the tumour becomes a cellular naevus; fibrotic changes and a loss of pigment may then cause a lesion to become less evident or disappear.

Such lesions may be present in childhood but they appear more obvious and increase their numbers with puberty. Sun-sensitive individuals tend to produce greater numbers, particularly on exposed areas of skin. There is therefore a greater number over the lateral aspect of the arm compared with the medial side. Pregnancy will also increase the numbers of naevi and the degree of hyperpigmentation.

The average count of melanocytic naevi on a Caucasian from the Western Hemisphere is more than a dozen by the third decade. Junctional naevi and malignant melanomas should be differentiated by size, the even degree of pigmentation, the smoothness of the overlying epidermis and lack of symptoms in the former.

Congenital melanocytic naevi are often bigger and may cover large areas of the skin, e.g. as a bathing trunk naevus. These have an irregular surface and an uneven degree of pigmentation. There is an increased potential for malignant change with larger lesions.

### Juvenile melanoma (Spitz naevus)

These naevi are solitary pink or reddish-brown lesions on the face or limbs of children. A history of rapid growth is given and for this reason they are often removed.

### Dermal melanocytes

A proliferation of naevus cells in the dermis may give rise to blue discoloration of the skin. The *mongolian spot* in children represents a more diffuse spread of such cells. When these are localized to form a slightly elevated papule, especially in adults, they are called a *blue naevus*.

## Basal-cell papilloma (seborrhoeic wart)

This is a benign proliferation of basal cells that produces a raised lesion with a varying degree of pigmentation. The number of these tumours increases with age. The consistency is often greasy and this aspect has led to the misnomer 'seborrhoeic wart'—the lesions are *not* related to sebaceous tissue growth. 'Senile wart' is another unacceptable term because the lesions may be seen in young adults.

The face and trunk are the sites most commonly affected. Marked hyperpigmentation may cause confusion with malignant melanoma. Maceration of these tumours from sweating may, in summertime, lead to irritation. The numbers present on the trunk may prohibit their removal in some patients, but readily traumatized or irritant lesions can be removed with a curette and the base cauterized, or they may be frozen with liquid nitrogen.

## Keratoacanthoma

This rapidly growing tumour of the epidermis arises most commonly on the skin of the hand and face. The aetiology is unknown; it is possible that trauma initiates the event and viral DNA has been shown in these tumours. There is often evidence of chronic actinic damage of the surrounding skin (Fig. 20.20).

The lesions are often pale or flesh-coloured, well-demarcated papules and on occasions appear inflammatory. Usually 0.5–1 cm in diameter, they may reach 3–4 cm across in giant lesions. The increase in size is rapid and often alarming to the patient. The greatest diameter is attained in 4–8 weeks; involution then occurs and the centre becomes a keratinous crater. Regression may then become complete over several months but, since a ragged scar may be left, it is often better to remove the tumour by curettage. Histological sections may reveal changes that are difficult to differentiate from a squamous carcinoma.

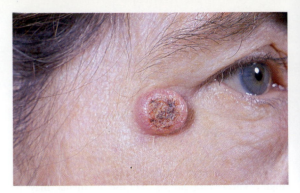

**Fig. 20.20**  Keratoacanthoma occurring on chronically sun-damaged skin.

## Haemangiomas

### Capillary naevus (naevus flammeus)

This is associated with a proliferation of capillaries in the superficial dermal capillary plexus. The salmon-coloured patch may be seen on the face or more commonly on the nape of the neck in up to 40% of infants. They may not fade from the latter site and are often covered by hair. Facial lesions occur on the glabella, forehead and eyelids and tend to fade away in the first year of life.

### Port-wine stain

This is a tumour present at birth that consists of dilated capillary vessels with endothelial cell lining. The face and neck are most commonly affected and there is no natural regression with age. Those patients who experience such growths around the orbit may have in addition a proliferation of vessels on the meninges (Sturge–Weber syndrome) and neurological defects.

Camouflage is the only practical method of managing such lesions. Laser therapy is time-consuming, is only available at a few centres, and the best results appear to follow the treatment of such naevi in adults.

### Cavernous haemangioma (strawberry naevus)

This tumour is not present at birth, but usually appears in the first month of life. Lesions are often well-circumscribed, round and lobulated and are usually seen on the face, neck or trunk. Growth continues in the first year in many patients; this is followed by slow involution, which is complete in the majority by 4–5 years, so that reassurance is often all that is required. Gross lesions warrant attempts at treatment when, for example, they obstruct the eye and threaten the development of binocular vision. The bulk of such tumours may be reduced by systemic steroids or sclerosants. Some naevi show features of both capillary and cavernous tissue within a single tumour.

### Cherry angioma (Campbell de Morgan's spot)

Campbell de Morgan's spots are angiokeratomas that appear as pin-point lesions or naevi of several millimetres in diameter on the trunk or limbs with an increasing frequency throughout middle-age. Treatment is only required for cosmetic reasons; cautery or diathermy is effective.

## Granuloma telangiectaticum

This tumour is a proliferation of dermal vasculature, so that the previous term pyogenic granuloma is a misnomer. Often trauma will initiate this growth on the finger or elsewhere on the skin. In children the trunk is a common site of involvement and there is a tendency for recurrence here from a deep-feeding vascular channel. Bleeding after trauma is a troublesome and worrying feature for some patients and older lesions may become fibrotic. Treatment is by curettage and cautery.

## Epidermal naevus

This may appear as a single lesion unassociated with any other developmental abnormality or may occur together with, for example, neurological defects as part of a syndrome. Histologically, there is a proliferation of epidermal structures that are often mixed, so that verrucous, sebaceous, apocrine, eccrine or follicular changes may all occur. The predominant component will determine the clinical appearances. Some types of naevi may undergo malignant transformation, though this is not common.

Sebaceous naevi appear most frequently on the scalp as flesh-coloured, leaf-shaped tumours, which may with time undergo malignant transformation to form basal-cell carcinomata.

## Histiocytoma (dermatofibroma)

This tumour is composed of blood vessels, histiocytes or dense fibrous tissue, according to the age of the tumour. It usually arises from trauma such as insect bites and is a common tumour on the legs or buttocks of adults, especially females. A firm tender papule develops, forming a button-like tumour on the surface of which the overlying skin can be wrinkled. The brown pigment or rapid growth may cause alarm and confusion with melanoma.

# MALIGNANT TUMOURS

There is public concern about the increased numbers of malignant tumours of the skin and their association with sun exposure.

*Metastases* to any part of the skin can occur from many primary carcinoma sites including breast, stomach, lung and kidney.

## Basal-cell carcinoma (rodent ulcer)

This is the most common cancer of the skin and is frequently seen on the face of middle-aged or elderly people in the UK, especially those with fair hair and blue eyes who are sun-sensitive and often of Celtic origin. Such tumours are seen at a younger age in those living nearer to the equator, but the reasons why tumours appear with such frequency on sites such as the periorbital skin, which is to some degree protected from sunlight, is not clear.

Other types of ionizing radiation such as X-rays, for example given to young adults for ankylosing spondylitis,

have in the past produced sufficient stimulus for the development of basal-cell carcinomata at the irradiated site after a prolonged interval of 10–20 years. Arsenicals may also cause cutaneous malignancy after a similar induction time.

### CLINICAL FEATURES

Lesions are most commonly seen at the sides of the nose and around the orbit as flesh-coloured translucent papules or plaques with superficial dilated blood vessels coursing over the surface; central necrosis with ulceration or crusting is frequent (Fig. 20.21). Scarring or cystic or pigmented lesions are less common. There is a tendency for basal-cell carcinomas to be locally invasive but metastasis is extremely rare.

Basal cell carcinomata and lesions appearing as small brown pigmented papules, which are often numerous, are seen in the basal cell naevus syndrome.

Superficial scarring and morphoeic basal cell carcinomas are more difficult to discern at their margins from normal skin; although uncommon they are important as they tend to follow tissue planes and invade an orifice such as the orbit. Treatment with X-rays is less effective for such tumours.

### TREATMENT

Tumours are normally removed surgically or treated with cryotherapy or radiotherapy. However, lesions that become invasive or are less accessible to normal treatments may be removed by chemosurgery. In Moh's method the tissue is fixed *in situ* and excised in a systematic fashion and examined immediately under a microscope to determine the presence or absence of tumour.

# Squamous carcinoma

This invasive tumour with the ability to metastasize arises from the epidermis (keratinocytes) or skin appendages. It is most commonly seen on previously damaged (e.g. by ultraviolet radiation) or chronically irritated skin. It has also been associated with certain occupations (e.g. chemical carcinogens inducing cancer of the scrotum) or with certain social customs (e.g. tumours on the legs from

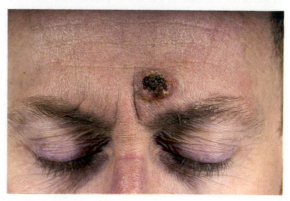

**Fig. 20.21** Basal-cell carcinoma.

radiant heat from fires). Albinism and xeroderma pigmentosum may produce severe actinic damage to the skin and frank malignancy at an early age. Viral disease may predispose to squamous carcinoma and human papilloma virus may be isolated from the skin of patients with epidermodysplasia verruciformis.

### CLINICAL FEATURES
Tumours are hyperkeratotic and crusted and are usually seen over sun-damaged skin, e.g. on the pinna. Induration of the tissue provides a further clue to the diagnosis. Ulceration may occur if the lesion is on sites such as the lips or genitalia. Papilliferous and more friable tumours may appear on relatively normal skin.

### DIFFERENTIAL DIAGNOSIS
**Solar keratoses**
These occur on sun-exposed and chronically damaged skin especially in those of Celtic origin. They appear as red or brown, rough hyperkeratotic lesions on the forehead, cheeks, ears, backs of hands and on the bald or thinly covered scalp. They represent a maturation defect of keratin and are often more easily felt than seen. Superficial lesions, where the diagnosis from squamous carcinoma is clear, respond to cryotherapy with liquid nitrogen.

**Bowen's disease**
Bowen's disease or intraepidermal carcinoma becomes invasive in approximately 5% of patients. When small superficial psoriasiform lesions or eczematous type lesions occur on the legs of elderly females they may persist for years and are sometimes accompanied by thickening and marked crusting or a papular component. The diagnosis should be confirmed by histology followed by excision or radiotherapy.

### TREATMENT
Treatment is usually by excision or by radiotherapy. Superficial lesions may be treated with cryosurgery.

## Malignant melanoma

This tumour, formed by epidermal melanocytes, is rising in incidence throughout the world. This increase has been seen particularly in light-skinned people. The latitude and length of residence of these people in places such as Australia suggest that UV light exposure is important. A single episode of severe sunburn is a significant risk factor, emphasizing the importance of occasional as opposed to constant light exposure. An increase in tumours on skin that has not until recent years been commonly exposed to sun, also indicates that exposure is a significant factor.

Inheritance is also important in the dysplastic naevus syndrome, when large multiple and atypical naevi on the trunk show a familial trait and patients may develop multiple primary melanomas.

Malignant change is recognized in pre-existing naevi, especially pigmented naevi, that cover a large surface of the skin, e.g. bathing trunk naevi, and in lentigo maligna.

### Lentigo maligna
Lentigo maligna represents an increased number of melanocytes at the epidermodermal junction. It begins as a flat freckle-like lesion, which in time changes colour and pattern as it grows. It occurs on the facial or sun-exposed skin of patients in their sixties or older. It is a precursor of malignant melanoma.

Malignant change in a mole should be suspected with a change in size, outline, colour, surface or elevation. Symptoms that include itching, bleeding after minor trauma or an increasing awareness of the tumour should also arouse suspicion.

The prognosis is directly related to the thickness of the tumour assessed at histological examination; patients with a tumour less than 1 mm thick have a 5-year survival rate of more than 90% but for tumours greater than 3.5 mm thick the 5-year survival rate is less than 50%.

The prognosis is also related to the site; patients with a tumour on the trunk fair better than those with facial lesions, but worse than those with lesions on the limbs.

Public health campaigns are necessary for:
- Prevention by avoiding direct sunlight and in the use of topical sunscreens
- Awareness and early diagnosis of suspected lesions by self-examination, particularly in light-skinned, blue-eyed people

### TREATMENT
Excision is performed according to the depth of invasion: 1 cm excision margin for every 1 mm of invasion with a wide excision of deeper invasive lesions followed by skin grafting. Deeply invasive lesions on a limb may be further treated by isolation and arterial perfusion with cytotoxic agents such as mustine hydrochloride. Radiotherapy, chemotherapy and immunotherapy have not yet been shown to materially alter the outlook for those with disseminated disease.

## Mycosis fungoides

This is a lymphomatous invasion of the skin by T lymphocytes (CD4+) (see p. 133) that may eventually form cutaneous tumours. In the final stages of the disease there is spread to lymph nodes and other organs. The name implies mushroom-like growths on the skin but these are a rare and often terminal event.

In the Sézary syndrome the area of skin infiltration is greater and 10% or more atypical mononuclear cells appear in the blood. Both of these conditions are classified as a T-cell lymphoma.

### CLINICAL FEATURES
The most common presentation of patients seen in the UK is with a pattern of scaling and erythema that may remain confined over areas such as the buttocks, thighs or trunk as rather fixed patches for many years. Tumours may then develop initially as plaques (Fig. 20.22) and then as ulcerating nodules or masses; dissemination fol-

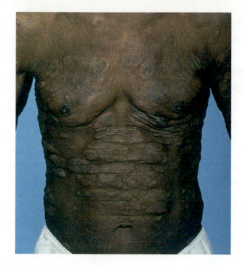

**Fig. 20.22**  Mycosis fungoides.

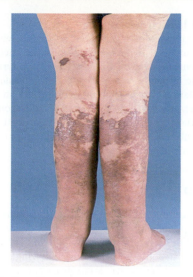

**Fig. 20.23**  Kaposi's sarcoma.

lows with visceral spread and death. With an onset in middle life or old age, patients will often die from other causes. Presentation with advanced disease and spread to local lymph nodes is uncommon in the UK but has been described more frequently in the USA.

### TREATMENT

Topical mustine hydrochloride, PUVA, photophoresis or electron beam therapy may control widespread disease and plaque forms of the disease. The combination of prednisolone and chlorambucil may limit the spread of more advanced disease, but dissemination to the viscera is associated with the terminal phase of the disease. Multiple chemotherapeutic regimens are disappointing in their effect.

## Kaposi's sarcoma

Kaposi's sarcoma is a vascular, multifocal, malignant tumour. It is seen in:
- Patients with AIDS. The incidence is higher in homosexuals than in haemophiliacs.
- Immunosuppressed patients secondarily to chemotherapy.
- Elderly males of Jewish or Mediterranean origin (classic form).
- Africans: several forms are seen, namely classical, locally aggressive or lymphadenopathic.

### CLINICAL FEATURES

The initial lesion appears as a bruise that gradually darkens and becomes raised as a firm nodule (Fig. 20.23). Lesions are not usually painful or itchy initially and can develop at several sites all over the body. Gastrointestinal lesions (approximately 40% of cases) are usually asymptomatic but later liver and lymph node involvement occur.

### PROGNOSIS AND TREATMENT

Lesions may progess rapidly, enlarge slowly over years or even regress. Treatment is with radiotherapy or chemo-

therapy. In AIDS one-third of the patients may show a response but relapse later; prognosis is poor. The prognosis is slightly better in the other forms and in those on immunosuppressive drugs the lesions may regress on stopping therapy.

## Disorders of pigmentation

There are many factors that alter the hue of a normal skin. The principal pigments are melanin and haemoglobin or its breakdown products. Carotene, if taken in large amounts in the diet, is concentrated in subcutaneous fat and in keratin, giving a yellow coloration to the skin. The skin can also change its colour by deposition of abnormal substances or by alteration of melanogenesis. These substances include drugs, bilirubin, haemosiderin, heavy metals and the deposition of metal salts, dyes and inks in tattooing. In practice, patients are most concerned with alterations in the degree of melanin pigmentation. This is especially so in those races who have a greater deposition of melanin in their skin as a normal characteristic. Alteration in the degree of pigmentation in those with pigmented skins may be striking and give rise to much personal and social stress.

### HYPOPIGMENTATION

#### Generalized hypopigmentation (albinism)

Albinism is inherited as an autosomal recessive disorder of melanin synthesis. This disorder produces a milky white skin, white hair, blue eyes and photophobia. There are different types, but in the commoner types there is a defect or inhibition of tyrosinase biosynthesis. In phenylketonuria (see p. 864) there is a failure to convert phenylalanine to tyrosine and hypopigmentation of the skin, hair and eyes occurs.

### Localized hypopigmentation

Localized absence of melanocytes is seen in vitiligo. In postinflammatory hypopigmentation some melanocytes are seen but these have reduced activity. In pityriasis versicolor the lipophilic yeast *Pityrosporum orbiculare* produces substances that have an inhibiting effect on melanocytes. This condition can be treated with itraconazole.

Industrial processes may expose the skin and melanocytes to substances, such as phenols, that are also toxic to the pigment-producing cells.

## Vitiligo

This is a common skin disease affecting approximately 1% of the population. It has a familial incidence. Melanocytes are lost from affected areas of skin. The reason is unclear but hypotheses include the following:

AUTODESTRUCTION OF MELANOCYTES by the products of melanin synthesis.

AUTOIMMUNE DAMAGE TO MELANOCYTES. Antigens have been detected on the surface of melanocytes and antimelanocyte antibodies have been detected in the sera of some patients. There is also an association of vitiligo with other diseases that demonstrate organ-specific antibody production, such as diabetes mellitus, thyroiditis and pernicious anaemia.

NEUROGENIC DYSFUNCTION has been invoked as an important factor in the production of rare naevoid patterns of the disease that tend to affect the limbs.

### CLINICAL FEATURES

More than half the patients notice a loss of pigment before the age of 20 years. Areas of pigment loss are usually symmetrical and often annular in outline, though other shapes and patterns are seen. These areas tend to enlarge peripherally and present a convex edge to the normal pigmented skin. The initial areas of involvement often include the fingers, hands, face and genitalia. These regularly traumatized areas of skin may show evidence of the Koebner phenomenon (see p. 1000) when the disease is in an active phase. In endemic areas confusion may occur with leprosy and lead to social isolation.

### TREATMENT

This is unsatisfactory. Traditional therapy in places such as the Middle East includes the use of psoralens obtained from plant sources and applied topically or taken in tablet form. These substances enter into the skin and are then activated by sunlight. PUVA therapy used in the treatment of psoriasis is derived from these observations. Many treatments with PUVA therapy are required for vitiligo and there is concern over the long-term effects of the continuing use of high-intensity UV light for long periods, especially in younger patients. Potent topical corticosteroids, probably through their action as anti-inflammatory agents, may induce repigmentation when applied to new lesions of vitiligo and a trial over a limited area of skin for a period of 6–8 weeks is warranted. There may be spontaneous recovery, especially in children.

Pinch grafts of normal skin have been used but with active disease the Koebner effect involves donor sites.

## Postinflammatory hypopigmentation

This may follow trauma to the skin from chemicals or physical agents or following inflammatory skin diseases. It is a noticeable feature in some patients with eczema. Mild hypopigmentation on the cheeks of children may be associated with scaling and erythema. Inflammatory changes are usually seen in winter-time and are associated with conditions of low humidity and drying winds.

The tanning of surrounding skin in summer will often make the eruption appear more striking, especially in dark-skinned children (pityriasis alba). Pityriasis versicolor may also tend to present in the summer for similar reasons.

### TREATMENT

The intensity of local inflammatory changes will be reduced with topical corticosteroids. Soap substitutes and emollients should be used when dryness of the skin is evident.

## HYPERPIGMENTATION

Hyperpigmentation is most commonly seen following sun exposure but may also follow inflammatory changes in the skin. It is often much more evident in those races whose skins are already heavily pigmented.

Epidermal naevi may contain an increased number of melanocytes and be pigmented. Melanin deposited in the dermis will often produce a blue discoloration of the skin, which is seen in the following:

- Mongolian blue spot on the backs of children, more especially those of Asian origin
- Naevus of Ito (on the neck)
- Naevus of Ota (on the face)
- Blue naevus

### Brown-coloured naevoid lesions

IN NEUROFIBROMATOSIS, *café-au-lait* patches and axillary freckling are seen.

ALBRIGHT'S SYNDROME (see p. 782) produces extensive light brown discoloration of the skin over the trunk, buttocks and thighs that is often asymmetrical and affects children of preschool age.

XERODERMA PIGMENTOSUM is associated with a freckling type of hyperpigmentation on the face or other sun-exposed sites. In those patients with severe disease it is associated with solar damage and cutaneous malignancy, which may be evident early in childhood.

FRECKLING on the skin of fair-skinned and otherwise normal persons increases with the length of sun exposure. Histological sections appropriately stained demonstrate an increase in the size and shape of melanosomes within the melanocyte.

## Lentigines

These are circumscribed dark brown macules that are less than 0.5 cm in diameter. There is a localized increase in the number of melanocytes seen on light microscopy and the degree of pigmentation is often much more intense clinically than that seen with freckles. A generalized distribution of lentigines may be seen as part of a syndrome that includes cardiac defects (*Leopard* or *Moynahan's syndrome*). In the *Peutz–Jegher syndrome* (orofacial lentiginosis) (see p. 213) lesions are localized to the face and hands and there is an association with intestinal polyposis.

## Generalized hypermelanosis

### Liver disease
In haemochromatosis there is a grey/black component to the hyperpigmentation that is more evident in sun-exposed areas of skin. Hypermelanosis may also be pronounced in patients with primary biliary cirrhosis.

### Endocrine disease
ADDISON'S DISEASE. Pigmentation may be diffuse but it is often much more pronounced on sun-exposed or traumatized skin, e.g. beneath bra straps or over the buccal mucosa in the mouth. Both adrenocorticotrophic hormone (ACTH) and melanocyte-stimulating hormone (MSH) are increased but ACTH plays the dominant role in producing the pigmentation.

HYPERTHYROIDISM may rarely produce a similar pattern of hyperpigmentation.

ACROMEGALY, CUSHING'S SYNDROME and ACTH therapy may also be associated with pigmentation that may be particularly pronounced in patients with sella turcica enlargement following adrenalectomy (Nelson's syndrome), when multiple lentigines and oral hyperpigmentation are also seen.

PREGNANCY AND THE ORAL CONTRACEPTIVE PILL may both produce an increase in pigmentation on the neck, the areolae of the breasts, over the abdominal skin and genitalia. Involvement of the face (melasma) may cause the patient to seek medical advice.

NEOPLASTIC DISEASE AND CACHEXIA can produce a general darkening of the skin colour; more marked changes occur with ectopic ACTH production.

### Other diseases
ACANTHOSIS NIGRICANS is most commonly seen as localized hyperpigmentation of the neck, axillae (Fig. 20.24), groins or facial skin, but the changes may be generalized and profound. Velvety overgrowth of the skin at

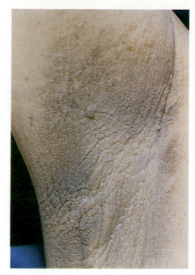

Fig. 20.24   Acanthosis nigricans.

the flexures may be accompanied by filiform growths around the face, mouth or over the tongue, and by a curious roughness of the palmar or plantar skin (tripe palms). These changes are seen in middle-aged patients with visceral malignancies such as carcinoma of the stomach, but other types of neoplasia such as lymphomas have also been reported in association with these typical cutaneous features. Acanthosis nigricans can, however, occur without an underlying malignancy, with obesity in juveniles and together with endocrine diseases.

RENAL FAILURE is associated with hypermelanosis and an increase in MSH-like reactive hormone production is seen in some patients. A yellow/brown, widespread coloration of the skin often occurs; scaling and irritation may also be seen. The relief of itching is difficult to achieve in such patients.

SYSTEMIC SCLEROSIS may produce localized pigmentary changes in sites such as the nape of the neck or over the shoulder girdle, but hyperpigmentation may be profound and generalized in some patients. Thickening of the skin is usually present and should offer a clue as to the primary diagnosis.

CHEMICAL DEPOSITION in the skin may occur as an occupational hazard, e.g. in those who process silver (argyria).

MERCURIALS may produce hypermelanosis, and gold when injected or taken by mouth may cause blue/black pigmentation, most evident on sun-exposed sites (chrysiasis).

HAEMOSIDERIN, the iron-containing pigment, may also stimulate localized melanin production. This occurs on sites such as the legs of patients with varicose eczema following the loss of red cells into the skin. Mucocutaneous discoloration may also be seen with chronic lead poisoning.

### Drugs

Mepacrine imparts a yellow colour to the skin but the sclera are spared. Chloroquine and chlorpromazine may produce bluish-grey coloration of the skin, especially in areas exposed to the sun. Arsenicals ingested over a long interval cause macular hyperpigmentation together with areas of hypopigmentation (rain-drop appearance).

# Sunlight and the skin

Controversy exists about the adverse effects of UV radiation exposure on the skin. However, damage can occur in four ways:

1 UVB (medium wavelength 280–310 nm) reaching the earth's surface is increased by depletion of the stratospheric ozone layer. Synthetic chlorofluorocarbons e.g. some aerosols and refrigerators reaching this zone further compromise this important barrier function. A 1% decrease in the ozone layer has increased UVB levels at the earth's surface by 2% with a concomitant rise in non-melanoma skin cancer of 2%. Increased levels of UVB are now being recorded in Europe.

2 Increased use of UVA (long wavelength 310–400 nm) for recreational tanning may expose individuals to more than five times the amounts reaching the earth's surface at the equator. UVB is also generated in varying amounts by UVA lamps increasing the potential to cause skin cancer.

3 UVA accelerates skin ageing changes, augments the effects of UVB and penetrates into the dermis. It can affect the Langerhans cell, damage connective tissue and trigger photosensitivity diseases.

4 Evidence now exists that UV radiation affects immune responses in the skin in animals and humans and may have an effect on more general immunoreactivity.

The effects of UV light on the skin may be beneficial or damaging. The formation of vitamin D from sterol precursors in the skin is dependent on sunlight, and UV light exposure may be used with benefit in the treatment of chronic skin conditions such as acne, eczema and psoriasis.

Damaging effects, however, occur with chronic irradiation, giving rise to changes in connective tissues that produce ageing, wrinkling, altered texture, dryness and changes in skin pigmentation. Epidermal changes include hyperkeratosis, dysplasia and malignancy.

## PHOTODERMATOSES

These can be divided into:
- Eruptions in which sunlight has a primary role
- Diseases in which sunlight is a trigger or an exacerbating factor

## Primary photosensitivity

### Polymorphic light eruption

The term 'polymorphic' refers to the difference in the morphology of the eruption between one patient and another. The lesions tend, however, to be monomorphic in any one individual.

Lesions are usually papulovesicular. Eczema, urticarial plaques or purpuric changes are less common. The rash is seen after a few hours of sun exposure and is most common on the chest and arms, the backs of the hands or lower legs. The eruption usually occurs in spring and early summer and improves as summer progresses and the skin 'hardens'. Fair-skinned individuals are most commonly affected by intense sunlight but those who have previously tanned easily and are of a darker complexion can also be affected. The papules may be associated with weeping and intense pruritus lasting for 5–10 days. The reaction can most readily be produced in the clinic or laboratory using high-intensity UV light at a wavelength of 320–420 nm.

Pretreatment during spring-time with 12–18 treatments of PUVA may prevent the disease. Hydroxychloroquine given in doses of 400 mg daily for 2–3 weeks before and during sun exposure may prevent attacks. Topical corticosteroids such as betamethasone and high-factor sun-blocking creams (factors 15–30) also help to minimize the disease.

### Hutchinson's summer prurigo

This rare disease usually has its onset before puberty. It affects both exposed and unexposed skin and may last throughout the year. Lesions are often excoriated and the necrotic papules may be quite disfiguring. The wavelengths responsible are usually in the sunburn range (290–320 nm). Sunscreen creams should be used but these do not offer sufficient protection in most cases. β-Carotene given by mouth may help a few patients.

### Actinic reticuloid (chronic actinic dermatitis)

This is a rare condition affecting older men in which the gross thickening, coloration and texture of exposed skin may resemble lymphomatous infiltration, both clinically and on microscopy. Many patients have had eczema previously and a significant proportion of these patients also have a positive patch test to materials such as rubber or plants.

Clinical features include eczematous and purpuric lesions on non-exposed skin such as the legs, arms and trunk. Light sensitivity may be such that during active phases of the disease the only respite for patients is found in a darkened room. Protective clothing, sun-barrier creams, systemic steroid therapy, azathioprine, cytotoxic drugs and hydroxychloroquine may be required in combination to produce improvement.

## Secondary photosensitivity

### Topical agents

The application of perfumes (e.g. those containing bergaptine), sulphonamides and antimicrobial agents (e.g. halogenated salicylanilides) may produce photosensitive reactions. The latter group of compounds have largely been withdrawn.

Plant extracts such as psoralens, commonly found in the family Umbelliferae, are used in photochemotherapy (PUVA therapy). However, phytophotodermatitis may occur when the leaves of such plants (e.g. giant hogweed, wild parsley) abrade the skin surface. Psoralen compounds are absorbed into the skin and then activated by natural long-wavelength UV radiation. The linear configuration of the lesions should provide the clue to diagnosis.

### Systemic agents

Systemic agents associated with photosensitivity include tetracyclines (chiefly chlortetracycline), thiazides (frusemide), phenothiazines, psoralens and retinoids.

### Disease states

Sunlight can exacerbate SLE. Antibodies produced against DNA denatured by UV light form immune complexes in the skin and other organs.

In porphyria, porphyrins deposited in the skin are activated by UV light.

# Diseases of collagen and elastic tissue

The skin contains collagen types I, III and V within the dermis, type IV in the basement membrane, type VII in the anchoring fibrils and type VIII in the endothelium (see p. 433). Abnormalities of these can give rise to various skin disorders.

## Ehlers–Danlos syndrome

This is a heterogeneous group of diseases in which at least nine different varieties have been described. Hyperextensibility, fragility and bruising of the skin occur to a varying degree with each of the diseases and it is accompanied by the hypermobility of joints. Fragility of blood vessels occurs, and rarely aortic rupture.

The patterns of inheritance are varied and can be autosomal recessive, autosomal dominant or X-linked recessive.

The skin is velvety to the touch and hyperextensible but recoils normally on stretching. Trauma or laceration of the skin can lead to tissue-paper scars and poor wound healing. Pseudotumours may occur over the elbows and knees; they consist principally of fat, but may show signs of calcification.

## Solar elastosis

Degradation of elastic fibrils in the skin normally occurs with ageing. This usually begins in early adult life but changes are more noticeable in the sixties and seventies.

The clinical features are characterized by yellowish papules or plaques and wrinkling and are usually associated with pigmentation and keratoses on exposed skin.

## Cutis laxa (generalized elastolysis)

This is a rare disease in which there are a number of variants. These are inherited as autosomal recessive, X-linked recessive or dominant traits. A defect in the cross-linking of elastin is suggested, but other abnormalities, including copper deficiency, have been reported. The subsequent changes in the skin, sometimes gross, may be evident at birth or arise at the time of puberty. The disfiguring changes may be severe with extreme laxity of the facial skin and massive folds over the trunk that have no recoil on stretching. Joint hypermobility is not a common feature.

## Pseudoxanthoma elasticum

This is a generalized disorder of elastic tissue. The pathogenesis is unknown, and both autosomal dominant and recessive modes of transmission are seen. The skin, eyes and vascular structures are involved.

Cutaneous features are seen in childhood and are most evident over flexural surfaces and at the sides of the neck. Initially there is an accentuation of skin lines or folds and this is followed by thickening around yellowish diamond-shaped papules, producing a *peau d'orange* or plucked-chicken appearance. The skin may be lax and hang in folds. The skin demonstrates very little elastic recoil on stretching. The mucous membranes may also be affected. Long-term and high-dose treatment with D-penicillamine produces similar cutaneous features.

Widespread vascular changes are associated with fibrous proliferation and the deposition of calcium in the media of the arteries. Intermittent claudication and angina pectoris occur at an early age as a result. Gastrointestinal bleeding may be a troublesome feature. Splits in Bruch's membrane, which contains both elastin and collagen and separates the choroid from the retina, are demonstrated as angioid streaks on ophthalmoscopy.

## Marfan's syndrome

A biochemical defect for this disease has not been identified, and some features of the condition may be seen in association with the Ehlers–Danlos syndrome or with homocystinuria. Inheritance is usually in an autosomal dominant manner.

Striae distensae are the only common dermatological sign, and the most impressive changes affect the skeleton. The facial appearance of affected patients may be distinctive, with elongation and asymmetry. A high-arched palate, although frequently described, is not a common feature. A tall stature, long thin digits and alteration in the body proportions are seen; the distance from the soles to the pubis (lower segment) is greater than the distance from the pubis to the vertex (upper segment). The arm span, measured from the extended fingers, often exceeds the height of the patient.

JOINTS. A laxity of ligaments may give rise to dislocation of joints such as the jaw or patellae. Steinberg's sign occurs when the thumbs are adducted over the palm and their tips are seen to cross the ulnar border of the hand. Inguinal or femoral hernias are often seen.

RESPIRATORY SYSTEM. Pulmonary changes include hernia of the diaphragm, emphysema and spontaneous pneumothorax.

CARDIOVASCULAR SYSTEM. Cardiovascular symptoms follow the degeneration in the media of vessel walls. The aortic valve ring may dilate and produce an incompetent valve, with the mitral valve frequently involved, producing the billowy or prolapsed valve syndrome (see p. 597). Aneurysm formation may occur, usually in the ascending aorta, and may be followed by dissection and/or rupture.

EYES. Weakness of the suspensory ligament of the lens may cause dislocation; this is a common clinical feature of the disease.

## Diseases of the hair and nails

Both hair and nails are composed of keratin and are derived principally from the epidermal layer (see p. 995). Each may be affected by the same type of disease process, e.g. lichen planus, or altered by conditions that affect primarily the epidermis.

## DISORDERS OF HAIR GROWTH

The extent and distribution of body hair is largely determined genetically. At the time of puberty, terminal hair growth occurs in males on the beard area, over the upper lip, chest, abdomen and thighs. Androgens determine the extent of secondary sexual patterns of hair growth during adolescence in both sexes. In females any marked alteration in the extent of hair growth or hair loss at times other than at puberty or the menopause may reflect serious endocrine disturbance.

## Hirsuties (see p. 790)

Hirsuties is defined as an excessive growth of hair of male type and distribution in females. In many parts of the world an excess of body hair is accepted as a racial characteristic or may, in addition, be seen as a family trait. In the Western World, excess body hair in females is considered less acceptable and women may become self-conscious about the extent of their hair growth.

Most hirsute females do not have recognizable clinical or biochemical evidence of endocrine disease, though this must be excluded by a careful history, examination and hormone profile where appropriate.

Some drugs alter the texture and extent of hair growth; these include cortisone, minoxidil, diazoxide, hydantoins and cyclosporin. Here the hair growth is non-androgenic in pattern and the term *hypertrichosis* is used.

Methods of hair removal include abrasion with mittens that have a roughened surface, shaving and plucking, but these give short-term relief. Depilatory creams and waxing should not be used frequently on facial hair but may be used elsewhere, such as on the legs.

Bleaching facial hair with peroxides will produce an acceptable appearance for fine hair. Coarse hairs are best dealt with by electrolysis but this needs to be performed by skilled personnel and may produce scarring, especially if acne is a concurrent problem on the chin. With severe hirsutism, antiandrogens (e.g. cyproterone acetate) or prednisolone (5 mg at night and 2.5 mg in the morning) may be used to produce a slowing of hair growth so that mechanical removal need not be so frequent or vigorous.

## Hair loss

Hair loss that occurs to the extent that scalp skin becomes abnormally visible is termed alopecia. It may be permanent, when the hair follicles are damaged by scarring (e.g. in lichen planus or discoid lupus erythematosus), or may recover if the follicles are left intact (e.g. in some endocrine diseases or alopecia areata).

### Diffuse hair loss

Hairs are lost in the telogen phase. Normally about 100 hairs are shed each day. In severe illness or following pregnancy there is an increase in the number of hairs entering the telogen phase (telogen effluvium). Hair loss is seen 3–4 months after the event when the new anagen hair pushes out the old telogen hair. Nail growth may be affected in the same way.

Other causes of diffuse hair loss include endocrine disease such as hyperthyroidism or hypothyroidism and androgen overactivity in both males and females. Iron deficiency, rapid weight loss associated with dieting, and drugs such as lithium or vitamin A and its derivatives also produce diffuse and treatable hair loss.

### Androgenetic alopecia

This is premature hair loss in both males and females over the vertex of the scalp. Increased 5α-reduction of testosterone to dihydrotestosterone (DHT) occurs in frontal, but not occipital, hair follicles. DHT is responsible for miniaturization of follicles, fine hair growth ensues and there is a shortening of the anagen phase of hair growth.

### Alopecia areata

This occurs in both sexes and all races and is usually seen in young adults or children as a well-defined patch of hair loss. Only 25% of cases are seen over the age of 40 years and 25% of patients give a family history of the condition.

AETIOLOGY. There is often a personal or family history of atopy. Alopecia areata occurs in association with auto-immune diseases such as thyrotoxicosis, Addison's disease, pernicious anaemia and vitiligo.

The association of alopecia areata with such diseases suggests that immune changes are important in the pathogenesis. It is also seen in association with Down's syndrome and hypogammaglobulinaemia.

CLINICAL FEATURES. Patches of hair loss can occur over any part of the body, e.g. the beard area or eyebrows, but the scalp is most frequently affected. Asymptomatic loss may first be noticed by a relative or hairdresser. Patches tend to regrow over the course of several months within the scalp margin in adults. An extension into the actual hair margin (ophiasis) is often less quick to recover. Children with an atopic background may lose all their scalp hair (alopecia totalis) and the prognosis in such patients should be guarded; alopecia totalis is seen less frequently in adults. Loss of hair from all body sites (alopecia universalis) may occur by extension from other sites but can also occur acutely.

The extension of hair loss occurs in a peripheral fashion; at the advancing edge, broken hairs (exclamation mark hairs) provide evidence of disease activity. Diffuse loss of hairs in alopecia areata is an infrequent occurrence and may be difficult to differentiate from other causes of hair loss.

Regrowing hair appears as a fine, depigmented downy growth. Areas of alopecia principally affect pigmented hair and premature greying is seen after diffuse hair loss.

TREATMENT. Large doses of corticosteroids will produce a regrowth of hair, but relapse often occurs after treatment is stopped. Topical corticosteroids may also help to speed the rate of regrowth of hair. Other treatment modalities, effective in small numbers of patients, include PUVA therapy and topical minoxidil. This is available as a 2% solution. It will induce hair growth in about one-third of individuals but this tends to fall out on cessation of treatment.

### Premature male-pattern baldness

Recession of the hair margin is an ageing characteristic of primates. This may appear early in males but such a pattern of loss in young females may indicate serious androgenicity. Vertical thinning is seen in association with margin recession in both sexes. In young women there is often evidence of androgen excess, which may be treated by antiandrogen therapy over an interval of a year with some recovery. The primary defect is atrophy of the hair follicle. It is due to a number of factors other than excess androgen activity, for antiandrogen therapy is not always effective in stimulating strong terminal hair growth in females.

### Abnormalities of the hair shaft

The hair shaft may become twisted, beaded or broken, leading to hair loss. Short, unruly or broken hair is then the primary complaint. Similar patterns of loss will be seen with drying of the hair or the effect of weathering, cosmetics, bleaching agents or grooming.

### Traction

Traction associated with fashion, traditional or ethnic practices, such as hot combing, braiding or plaiting, may also cause a localized hair fall, especially over the temporal region. Straightening or relaxing the hair, undertaken by those with naturally curly hair may, in addition, produce permanent root damage.

## DISEASES OF THE NAILS

The nail plate grows continuously, although the rate slows with advancing years, and with some generalized diseases. Growth of finger-nails is normally at a rate of about 1 cm every 3 months, so that renewal of a finger-nail may take 6 months, and toe-nails, which grow more slowly, may take from 18 months to 2 years. An increase in the rate of growth of the nail plate occurs in psoriasis and other skin diseases.

The nail plate arises from the matrix and lies on the nail bed that also contributes to its growth. The hard outer layer is formed from the proximal matrix and the bulk of the nail, composed of soft keratin, is produced by the distal matrix.

The nail matrix lies within a fold of epidermis, so that dermatoses or infections that involve the posterior nail fold may also cause abnormalities of the nail plate; these include chronic paronychia, fungal disease, eczema and psoriasis. These nail changes have been discussed in the appropriate sections.

Congenital defects of the nail occur in conjunction with abnormalities of the epidermis, teeth or skeleton.

## Nail disorders in generalized diseases

### Clubbing

This is discussed on p. 641.

### Connective tissue diseases

Short and brittle nails occur in severe circulatory disorders, e.g. Raynaud's phenomenon (see p. 628), especially in association with systemic sclerosis. Pterygium formation also occurs when a thin skin-fold merges with the cuticle, widening it by several millimetres. Chronic paronychia may persist despite all therapeutic manoeuvres in patients with severe digital ischaemia. Nail fold capillary dilatation and distortion or the absence of capillaries, usually with severe Raynaud's phenomenon, is seen in systemic sclerosis. Ragged cuticles containing haemorrhages are often most pronounced in patients with dermatomyositis.

### Yellow nail syndrome

The nail plate is thickened, yellow in colour, smooth and with an increased lateral curvature. The rate of growth of the nail is reduced. Such nails are seen in association with chronic oedema of the hands, feet, ankles or face, congenital lymphoedema, pleural effusions, chronic sinus infection and thyroid disease.

### White bands
Distal white bands that are parallel to the lunula and separated from this and each other by a normal pink-coloured portion are seen in patients with hypoalbuminaemia. The nails return to normal when the level of protein is restored.

### Half-and-half nails
This is the name given to nails in which the proximal nail is pale or white and the distal portion is red or brown in colour; these nails occur in renal failure.

### Brown streaks
Longitudinal brown streaks are commonly seen in black patients when pigment cells are incorporated into the nail matrix. Alteration of pigment beneath the nails that is localized and not related to obvious trauma in white-skinned patients may require a biopsy of the nail to exclude subungual melanoma.

### Onycholysis
Onycholysis or separation of the distal edge of the nail from the vascular nail bed will cause whiteness of the free edge and this most commonly follows trauma or faulty or excessive manicure. Psoriasis is another common cause and similar changes may be seen in thyrotoxicosis or following photo-onycholysis produced by photoactive drugs such as tetracycline or psoralens, as well as in porphyria.

### Splinter haemorrhages
These are most frequently caused by trauma to the nail; infective endocarditis, SLE and psoriasis are less common causes.

### Koilonychia
Spoon-shaped nails or koilonychia is seen in association with iron deficiency anaemia but it may also follow trauma, e.g. in garage mechanics who regularly fit tyres.

### Chronic paronychia
This is due to chronic infection from *Candida albicans*. It is rarely a manifestation of an underlying systemic disease such as hypoparathyroidism, multiple endocrine disease or chronic iron deficiency.

### Transverse lines
Transverse lines (Beau's lines) related to acute physical or psychiatric illness or the use of cytotoxic drugs represent a temporary arrest of growth. They may be associated with an arrest of hair growth and subsequent fall (telogen effluvium).

### Blue discoloration of the nail
This may be seen in hepatolenticular degeneration (Wilson's disease) as blue lanulae.

## Effects of drugs

A number of drugs, including antimalarials such as chloroquine, may cause a blue/black discoloration of the nail plate. Mepacrine may stain the nail plate blue and fluoresces green on examination by Wood's light. Argyria occurring as an occupational disease or following, for example, the use of silver-containing nose drops will stain the nails a grey/blue colour. Phenothiazine produces a blue/black coloration that is often accentuated in summertime.

### Cytotoxic drugs
Diffuse, longitudinal or horizontal melanonychia affecting the nail base or nail plate may occur in association with pigmentary changes of the surrounding skin with doxorubicin, busulphan, cyclophosphamide and daunorubicin therapy.

# Further reading

Breathnach SM & Hintner H (1992) *Adverse Drug Reactions and the Skin*. Oxford: Blackwell Scientific Publications.

Elias PM (1992) *Dynamics of the Epidermal Barrier*. Progress in Dermatology, **26**(2). Evanston, Illinois: Dermatology Foundation.

Fitzpatrick TB (ed.) (1987) *Dermatology in General Medicine*, 3rd edn. New York: McGraw-Hill.

Royce PM & Stemmann B (1993) Connective Tissue and its Heritable Disorders. New York: Wiley-Liss Inc.

Special Supplement (1993) Connective Tissue Disease and the Skin. *The Journal of Investigative Dermatology*, **100**(1), 1–132.

Tappero JW *et al.* (1993) Kaposi's Sarcoma. *Journal of the American Academy of Dermatology*, **28**(3), 371–387.

# Appendices

# Diets

The following are general guidelines. Any patient requiring a therapeutic diet should receive individual advice from a dietitian.

These diets were compiled by Eileen McKay, Dietitian, St Bartholomew's Hospital, London.

## DIABETES MELLITUS

The basic principles of the diet for diabetes are given below. These are based on the British Diabetic Association's directory for the 1990s.

THE DIET is based around the broad principles of healthy eating. It is not considered to be a specialist diet.

CARBOHYDRATE should make up about half the total dietary energy intake, the majority coming from complex sources (foods high in dietary fibre, and starchy foods in general).

FOODS WITH A HIGH SUGAR CONTENT, e.g. sweets, preserves, cakes, ordinary fruit squashes generally should be avoided, but it is recognized that up to 25 g daily of added sugar (sucrose) can be incorporated into a low-fat, high-fibre diet.

DIETARY FIBRE INTAKE should be increased, concentrating on soluble fibre (pulses, oats, fruit) due to its benefit on blood lipids. Dietary fibre may also promote satiety and assist weight loss. Dietary fibre should be incorporated into an overall high carbohydrate diet; 30 g fibre daily is recommended.

FAT in the diet should be reduced to 30–35% of total energy intake. Of this, 10% should be from saturated fat with the remainder coming from both polyunsaturated and monounsaturated fat sources. Cholesterol should not exceed 300 mg daily (achievable with <10% energy from saturated fat).

PROTEIN INTAKE should be 10–15% of energy intake, i.e. not exceed normal intake.

SALT should be limited to <6 g (100 mmol) daily if normotensive; 3 g (50 mmol) daily if hypertensive.

COMMERCIAL 'DIABETIC' foods should be avoided.

LOW CALORIE/SUGAR-FREE PRODUCTS sweetened with non-nutritive sweeteners (e.g. saccharin, aspartame) are acceptable and may be useful in the diet.

ALCOHOL, taken in moderation is acceptable. Sweet alcohol and high alcohol beers should be avoided.

## Insulin-dependent diabetes mellitus

REGULAR FOOD INTAKE is essential to prevent hypoglycaemia.

CARBOHYDRATE distributed evenly throughout the day to include between-meal and bedtime snacks helps minimize fluctuations in blood glucose concentrations.

AN UNDERSTANDING OF CARBOHYDRATE CONTENT OF FOODS remains necessary. Carbohydrate exchange systems may be one way of teaching this though many centres no longer use formal carbohydrate exchange lists.

## Non-insulin dependent diabetes mellitus (NIDDM)

OVERWEIGHT is a problem in 75% of patients with NIDDM. Reduction of energy intake is the main aim in the overweight patient.

REDUCTION IN FAT INTAKE may be relatively more important in NIDDM to help reduce the incidence of cardiovascular disease and aid weight loss.

FOOD SHOULD BE EVENLY DISTRIBUTED THROUGHOUT THE DAY at meal times, snacks not being necessary for the overweight patient. Patients taking certain oral hypoglycaemic agents are encouraged to have between-meal snacks to prevent hypoglycaemia.

It should be remembered that patients will have to be instructed how to maintain their carbohydrate intake during illness, cope with their diet while travelling, and adjust their intake prior to exercise.

## GLUTEN-FREE DIET

This is used for the treatment of coeliac disease and dermatitis herpetiformis.

The diet involves the exclusion of wheat, rye, barley and oats. *Any* food containing gluten—either as an obvious constituent (e.g. flour, bread) or as a 'hidden' ingredient (e.g. stock cubes, dessert mixes)—must be avoided.

A selection of foods included in a gluten-free (GF) diet include:

- GF bread*, GF crispbread*, GF pasta*

1041

- GF flour*, soya flour, potato flour, pea flour, rice flour
- Soya bran, rice bran
- GF biscuits*, GF cakes
- Breakfast cereals—corn or rice based
- Rice, tapioca, sago, arrowroot, buckwheat, millet, maize
- Fresh or frozen meat, poultry, offal
- Plain fresh or frozen fish, fish canned in oil
- Eggs, plain cheeses
- Milk, cream, butter, margarine, oils
- Plain fresh, frozen or tinned vegetables and potatoes
- Tinned fruit in syrup or natural juice, fresh or frozen fruit
- Nuts
- Tea, coffee, fruit juice, fruit squash, fizzy drinks
- Sugar, syrup, honey, jam, marmalade, jelly, gelatine
- Herbs, plain spices, vinegar, salt, pepper

* Products prescribable on the National Health Service in the UK for coeliac disease and dermatitis herpetiformis.

In addition, any home-made items, e.g. soups or sauces, made with GF ingredients are obviously suitable.

It is not always possible to tell from a 'label' whether or not a manufactured product is gluten-free. In the UK The Coeliac Society produces a comprehensive list of manufactured foods which are gluten-free and patients prescribed such a diet are advised to join:

The Coeliac Society
PO Box 220
High Wycombe
Bucks HP11 2HY

## DIETS IN RENAL DISEASE

### Restricted-protein diet

This is used in the treatment of patients with symptomatic uraemia or in patients with asymptomatic moderate renal failure (creatinine clearance $<40$ ml min$^{-1}$) in the hope of slowing the rate of deterioration in renal function otherwise destined to occur.

| | |
|---|---|
| *Protein* | 0.6–0.8 g kg$^{-1}$ ideal body weight daily |
| *Energy* | 35 kcal kg$^{-1}$ (150 kJ kg$^{-1}$) ideal body weight daily |
| *Sodium* | $\approx$80 mmol daily (unless salt waster) if hypertensive |
| *Potassium* | Restricted to $\approx$50 mmol if the patient becomes hyperkalaemic |

#### SAMPLE MENU PLAN

For 70 kg person, moderately active, not overweight or hypertensive:

Protein = 42 g, energy = 2500 kcal (10 500 kJ), sodium = ~80 mmol, potassium ~50 mmol.

**Breakfast**
2 slices wholemeal bread with polyunsaturated margarine
Jam, marmalade or honey

**Lunch**
25 g meat or 40 g fish
2 slices wholemeal bread with unsalted polyunsaturated margarine or unsalted butter
1 portion vegetable
1 portion fruit

**Evening meal**
50 g meat or 75 g fish
150 g potatoes
1 portion vegetable
1 portion fruit

**Daily**
175 ml milk, 1 bottle Hycal or equivalent, 50 g polyunsaturated margarine

**Suitable drinks**
Tea, lemonade, cola drinks, bitter lemon—as part of fluid allowance

**Allowed freely**
Sugar, jam, honey, marmalade, boiled sweets, low-protein products

A small amount of salt may be used in cooking but none added at table. See 'no-added-salt' diet for further restrictions. Salt intake may need to be increased, for example in salt wasters.

## Nephrotic syndrome

| | |
|---|---|
| *Protein* | 1.0 g kg$^{-1}$ ideal body weight daily (= ~70 g) |
| *Sodium* | 'No added salt' |
| *Fat* | Some advice may be given regarding quantity of fat in view of hyperlipidaemia |

#### SAMPLE MEAL PLAN
For 70 kg person

**Breakfast**
Cereal with milk
2 slices toast with polyunsaturated margarine or butter

**Main meal**
100 g meat or 150 g fish
Potatoes or rice
Vegetables
Milk pudding, pudding with custard or fruit and ice cream

**Snack meal**
50 g meat or 75 g fish
Bread or potatoes
Vegetables or salad
Fruit

**Daily**
~1 pint of milk

Usually a small amount of salt may be used in cooking

but none added at table. See 'no-added-salt' diet for further restriction.

## Low-calcium, low-oxalate diet

This is required in hypercalciuric or hyperoxaluric stone formers, in combination with a high fluid intake ($>2$ litres daily).

Advice may be given about protein and sodium to bring them in line with $1–1.2$ g kg$^{-1}$ protein and no added salt in view of the hypercalcaemic effect of a high protein and high sodium diet.

### SAMPLE MEAL PLAN
**Breakfast**
1 egg
1 slice wholemeal bread and butter
Cereal

**Main meal**
Average helping of meat or fish
Potatoes or rice
Vegetables
Fruit or jelly

**Snack meal**
Average helping of meat or fish
2 slices wholemeal bread with butter

**Daily**
150 ml milk

**Avoid**
Foods rich in calcium, e.g. cheese, ice cream, yoghurt, extra milk
Foods rich in oxalate, e.g. rhubarb, spinach, beetroot, beans
Tea intake is restricted to 4 cups daily

## DIET IN LIVER DISEASE

## 40 g protein, no-added-salt diet

This is used in the treatment of encephalopathic liver disease. In patients with ascites sodium restriction is required (see salt-restriction diets).

### SAMPLE MEAL PLAN
**Daily**
150 ml milk

**Breakfast**
Fruit juice
1 egg
1 slice bread or toast with butter and jam or marmalade
Tea or coffee with milk from allowance

**Mid-morning**
Fruit juice
Tea or coffee with milk from allowance

**Lunch**
25 g meat or 40 g fish or 1 egg or 1 small yoghurt or 3 tablespoons pulses
1 slice bread of equivalent
Vegetables or salad
Fruit

**Mid-afternoon**
1 slice bread with butter and jam or honey
Tea or coffee with milk from allowance

**Evening meal**
25 g meat or 40 g fish or 1 egg or 1 small yoghurt or 3 tablespoons pulses
1 slice bread or equivalent
Vegetables or salad
Fruit

**Bedtime**
1 slice bread or equivalent
Tea or coffee with remainder of milk allowance

Fat and fatty foods must be restricted if poorly tolerated. Alcohol must be avoided.

1 slice of bread may be exchanged for any of the following:

3 plain biscuits
2 crispbreads
1 small bowl breakfast cereal or porridge
2 tablespoons cooked rice or cooked pasta
2 small potatoes
1 small slice cake
1 tablespoon flour
1 tablespoon ice cream

**Extras**
Sugar
Glucose
Boiled sweets
Mints
Fruit squash
Fizzy drinks
Fruit
Fruit juice

These are 'encouraged' in order to increase energy intake.

Protein intake should be gradually increased as the encephalopathy resolves.

## SALT-RESTRICTION DIETS

## No-added-salt diet

This restricts sodium intake to between 60 and 100 mmol daily depending on energy intake. A small amount of salt may be used in cooking, but none must be used at table.

The following foods contain considerable amounts of sodium and *must be avoided*:

Bacon, ham, sausages, pâté

Cheese
Tinned fish and meat
Smoked fish and meat
Fish and meat pastes
Tinned vegetables
Tinned and packet soups
Sauce mixes
Bottled sauces and chutneys
Meat and vegetable extracts, stock cubes
Salted nuts and crisps
Soya sauce
Monosodium glutamate

## 40 mmol sodium diet

This is used in the treatment of ascites or severe oedema associated with salt and water retention. It is often used in conjunction with diuretics.

In addition to avoiding the foods listed under 'no-added-salt' diet, the following restrictions apply:
- No salt to be used in cooking or at table
- Salt-free butter must be used
- Milk should be restricted to 300 ml daily
- Only 4 slices ordinary bread are permitted daily—extra bread must be salt-free
- Choose breakfast cereals that are free from added salt
Salt substitutes should only be used under medical supervision.

## LOW-FAT DIET

If a body's ability to digest and/or absorb fat is impaired, a diet low in fat is indicated. In this case *all* fats, i.e. both animal and vegetable in origin, must be restricted.

Where fat tolerance is low it is better to distribute the fat intake throughout the day.

Care should be taken to check the fat content of manufactured foods.

### SAMPLE MEAL PLAN

**Daily**
Low-fat milk as required
10 g butter or margarine or oil or 20 g 'low-fat' spread

**Breakfast**
Fruit or fruit juice
Breakfast cereal or porridge
Bread or toast with butter or margarine from allowance
Jam, marmalade or honey

**Snack meal**
*Lean* meat, chicken, low-fat cheese, egg, fish or baked beans
Bread, toast or crispbread
Vegetables or salad
Fruit or low-fat yoghurt

**Main meal**
Clear soup, fruit juice, melon or grapefruit

*Lean* meat, chicken or fish cooked without fat, beans or pulses
Potato, rice or pasta cooked without fat
Vegetables or salad
Fruit, jelly or pudding made with low-fat milk

**Beverages**
Tea, coffee, fruit juice, fruit squash or fizzy drinks

**Extras**
Boiled sweets, mints, fruit gums, meringues, water ice, ice lollies
Plain or semi-sweet biscuits
Herbs, spices, mustard, vinegar, pickles, oil-free salad dressings

## REDUCING DIET

This diet is suitable for obese diabetics, although distribution of carbohydrate-containing foods may need modification for those on oral hypoglycaemic agents or insulin. Energy restriction is achieved by reducing *fat, sugar* and *alcohol*, while maintaining a modest intake of fibre-containing carbohydrate foods.

### SAMPLE MEAL PLAN

**Breakfast**
Small cupful of breakfast cereal or porridge with low-fat milk, no sugar
1 slice wholemeal bread or toast with a little butter or margarine or low-fat spread

**Snack meal**
Average helping of lean meat, poulty, fish, eggs, cheese or small tin baked beans
Salad vegetables
2 slices wholemeal bread or 5 crispbread or 2 small potatoes
Fresh fruit or sugar-free, low-fat yoghurt

**Main meal**
Average helping of lean meat, poultry, fish, eggs, cheese or pulses
Cooked vegetable and/or side salad
1 small potato or 1 tablespoon boiled rice or 1 slice wholemeal bread
Fruit, fresh or tinned in natural juice

Low-fat milk (skimmed or semi-skimmed) should be used in tea and coffee. Artificial sweeteners may be used if necessary. Other suitable drinks include sugar-free squashes and fizzy drinks, soda water, and mineral water.

**Avoid**
Sweets, chocolate, honey, preserves, sweet biscuits, cake, tinned fruit in syrup, puddings
Ordinary fruit squash and fizzy drinks
Malted milk drinks and drinking chocolate
Fried foods, cream mayonnaise, salad dressing, crisps,

cream cheese, pastry, dumplings, avocado pear, nuts
Alcohol

# CHOLESTEROL LOWERING DIET

This diet involves reducing total fat intake (particularly saturated fat) and may include restricting foods high in cholesterol, e.g. eggs, shellfish, offal.

Foods high in soluble fibre are encouraged, particularly pulses. Overweight patients would normally be given a suitably modified reducing diet.

## SAMPLE MEAL PLAN
### Breakfast
Fruit or fruit juice
Cereal (preferably whole grain) or porridge with low-fat milk
Bread (preferably wholemeal) with polyunsaturated margarine or low-fat spreads
Jam, marmalade or honey

### Snack meal
Sandwich or salad with *lean* meat, fish or low-fat cheese
Bread or crispbread with tinned fish or low-fat cheese *or* baked beans on toast
Fresh fruit or low-fat yoghurt

### Main meal
*Lean* meat or fish or low-fat cheese

### Vegetables
Potatoes—jacket, boiled, mashed or fried in polyunsaturated oil, or pasta or rice
Fruit, jelly or pudding made with low-fat milk

### Foods to avoid include
Butter, lard, suet, cooking fats, other margarines, 'vegetable oils', coconut oil, salad cream, mayonnaise, whole milk, dried milk with added vegetable fat, cream, yoghurt made with whole milk
Duck, goose, sausages, pâté, luncheon meat, salami-type sausages
Avocado pear, nuts, crips
Ice cream, tinned and packet desserts, chocolate spread, chocolate, toffee, butterscotch, cocoa, drinking chocolate, malted milk drinks
Most biscuits (except crispbreads, water biscuits, plain and semi-sweet biscuits), cakes, pastries, pies (unless made with suitable ingredients)

# CHOLESTEROL AND TRIGLYCERIDE-LOWERING DIET

In addition to the restrictions listed under the cholesterol-lowering diet, sugar and foods with a high sugar content must be avoided. Carbohydrate foods with a high fibre content are encouraged. Alcohol intake should be restricted.

For overweight patients a modified reducing diet is advised.

# *Normal values*

These normal values were compiled by Ruth Halliday, SRN, and modified by Katherine Woodward, RGN, and Therese Taylor, RGN, St Bartholomew's Hospital. Values vary from one laboratory to another. Please check with your own laboratory.

## HAEMATOLOGY

| | |
|---|---|
| Haemoglobin | |
|     Male | $14.0–17.7 \text{ g dl}^{-1}$ |
|     Female | $12.0–16.0 \text{ g dl}^{-1}$ |
| Mean corpuscular haemoglobin (MCH) | $27–33 \text{ pg}$ |
| Mean corpuscular haemoglobin concentration (MCHC) | $32–35 \text{ g dl}^{-1}$ |
| Mean corpuscular volume (MCV) | $80–96 \text{ fl}$ |
| Packed cell volume (PCV) | |
|     Male | $0.42–0.53 \text{ litre litre}^{-1}$ |
|     Female | $0.36–0.45 \text{ litre litre}^{-1}$ |
| White cell count (WCC) | $4–11 \times 10^9/\text{litre}$ |
|     Basophil granulocytes | $<0.01–0.1 \times 10^9/\text{litre}$ |
|     Eosinophil granulocytes | $0.04–0.4 \times 10^9/\text{litre}$ |
|     Lymphocytes | $1.5–4.0 \times 10^9/\text{litre}$ |
|     Monocytes | $0.2–0.8 \times 10^9/\text{litre}$ |

|  |  |
|---|---|
| Neutrophil granulocytes | $2.0–7.5 \times 10^9$/litre |
| Total blood volume | 60–80 ml kg$^{-1}$ |
| Plasma volume | 40–50 ml kg$^{-1}$ |
| Platelet count | $150–400 \times 10^9$/litre |
| Serum B$_{12}$ | 160–925 ng litre$^{-1}$ (150–675 pmol litre$^{-1}$) |
| Serum folate | 4–18 $\mu$g litre$^{-1}$ (5–63 nmol litre$^{-1}$) |
| Red cell folate | 160–640 $\mu$g litre$^{-1}$ |
| Red cell mass |  |
|    Male | 25–35 ml kg$^{-1}$ |
|    Female | 20–30 ml kg$^{-1}$ |
| Reticulocyte count | 0.5–2.5% of red cells ($50–100 \times 10^9$/litre) |
| Erythrocyte sedimentation rate (ESR) | <20 mm in 1 hour |

## Coagulation

|  |  |
|---|---|
| Bleeding time (Ivy method) | 2–7 min |
| Partial thromboplastin time (PTTK) | 35–50 s |
| Prothrombin time | 12–16 s |
|    International Normalized Ratio (INR) | 1 |

## BIOCHEMISTRY

|  |  |
|---|---|
| Acid phosphatase | 1–5 U litre$^{-1}$ |
| Alanine aminotransferase (ALT) | 5–40 U litre$^{-1}$ |
| Albumin | 34–48 g litre$^{-1}$ |
| Alkaline phosphatase | 25–115 U litre$^{-1}$ |
| Amylase | <220 U litre$^{-1}$ |
| Angiotensin-converting enzyme | 10–70 U litre$^{-1}$ |
| $\alpha_1$-Antitrypsin | 2–4 g litre$^{-1}$ |
| Aspartate aminotransferase (AST) | 10–40 U litre$^{-1}$ |
| Bicarbonate | 22–30 mmol litre$^{-1}$ |
| Bilirubin | <17 $\mu$mol litre$^{-1}$ (0.3–1.5 mg dl$^{-1}$) |
| Caeruloplasmin | 0.20–0.45 g litre$^{-1}$ |
| Calcium | 2.20–2.67 mmol litre$^{-1}$ (8.5–10.5 mg dl$^{-1}$) |
| Chloride | 95–106 mmol litre$^{-1}$ |
| Cholinesterase | 2.25–7.0 U litre$^{-1}$ |
| Copper | 12–25 $\mu$mol litre$^{-1}$ (100–200 mg dl$^{-1}$) |
| C-reactive protein | <10 mg litre$^{-1}$ |
| Creatinine | 0.06–0.12 mmol litre$^{-1}$ (0.6–1.5 mg dl$^{-1}$) |
| Creatine kinase (CPK) |  |
|    Female | 24–170 U litre$^{-1}$ |
|    Male | 24–195 U litre$^{-1}$ |
|    CK-MB fraction | 25 U litre$^{-1}$ (<60% of total activity) |
| C3 | 0.55–1.20 g litre$^{-1}$ |
| C4 | 0.20–0.50 g litre$^{-1}$ |
| Ferritin | 5.8–144 nmol litre$^{-1}$ (15–300 $\mu$g litre$^{-1}$) |
| $\alpha$-Fetoprotein | <10 kU litre$^{-1}$ |
| Glucose (fasting) | 4.5–5.6 mmol litre$^{-1}$ (70–110 mg dl$^{-1}$) |
| Fructosamine | up to 285 $\mu$mol litre$^{-1}$ |
| $\gamma$-Glutamyl transpeptidase ($\gamma$-GT) |  |
|    Male | 11–50 U litre$^{-1}$ |
|    Female | 7–32 U litre$^{-1}$ |
| Glycosylated haemoglobin (HbA$_{1c}$) | 3.8–8.5% |
| Hydroxybutyric dehydrogenase (HBD) | 40–150 U litre$^{-1}$ |

Immunoglobulins (11 years and over)

| | |
|---|---|
| IgA | 0.8–4 g litre$^{-1}$ |
| IgG | 7.0–18.0 g litre$^{-1}$ |
| IgM | 0.4–2.5 g litre$^{-1}$ |
| Iron | 13–32 $\mu$mol litre$^{-1}$ (50–150 $\mu$g dl$^{-1}$) |
| Iron binding capacity (total) (TIBC) | 42–80 $\mu$mol litre$^{-1}$ (250–410 $\mu$g dl$^{-1}$) |
| Lactate dehydrogenase | 240–460 U litre$^{-1}$ |
| Lead | <0.7 $\mu$mol litre$^{-1}$ |
| Magnesium | 0.7–1.1 mmol litre$^{-1}$ |
| $\beta_2$-Microglobulin | 1.0–3.0 mg litre$^{-1}$ |
| Osmolality | 280–296 mosmol kg$^{-1}$ |
| Phosphate | 0.8–1.5 mmol litre$^{-1}$ |
| Potassium | 3.5–5.0 mmol litre$^{-1}$ |
| Prostate-specific antigen | up to 4.0 $\mu$g litre$^{-1}$ |
| Protein (total) | 62–80 g litre$^{-1}$ |
| Sodium | 135–146 mmol litre$^{-1}$ |
| Urate | 0.18–0.42 mmol litre$^{-1}$ (3.0–7.0 mg dl$^{-1}$) |
| Urea | 2.5–6.7 mmol litre$^{-1}$ (8–25 mg dl$^{-1}$) |
| Vitamin A | 0.5–2.01 $\mu$mol litre$^{-1}$ |
| Vitamin D | |
| 25-hydroxy | 37–200 nmol litre$^{-1}$ (0.15–0.80 ng litre$^{-1}$) |
| 1,25-dihydroxy | 60–108 pmol litre$^{-1}$ (0.24–0.45 pg litre$^{-1}$) |
| Zinc | 7–18 $\mu$mol litre$^{-1}$ |

## Lipids and lipoproteins

| | |
|---|---|
| Cholesterol | 3.5–6.5 mmol litre$^{-1}$ (ideal <5.2 mmol litre$^{-1}$) |
| HDL cholesterol | |
| Male | 0.95–2.15 mmol litre$^{-1}$ |
| Female | 0.70–2.00 mmol litre$^{-1}$ |
| Lipids (total) | 4.0–10.0 g litre$^{-1}$ |
| Lipoproteins | |
| VLDL | 0.128–0.645 mmol litre$^{-1}$ |
| LDL | 1.55–4.4 mmol litre$^{-1}$ |
| HDL | |
| Male | 0.70–2.1 mmol litre$^{-1}$ |
| Female | 0.50–1.70 mmol litre$^{-1}$ |
| Non-esterified fatty acids | |
| Male | 0.19–0.78 mmol litre$^{-1}$ |
| Female | 0.06–0.9 mmol litre$^{-1}$ |
| Phospholipid | 2.9–5.2 mmol litre$^{-1}$ |
| Triglycerides | |
| Male | 0.70–2.1 mmol litre$^{-1}$ |
| Female | 0.50–1.70 mmol litre$^{-1}$ |

## Blood gases

| | |
|---|---|
| Arterial $P\mathrm{CO_2}$ | 4.8–6.1 kPa (36–46 mmHg) |
| Arterial $P\mathrm{O_2}$ | 10–13.3 kPa (75–100 mmHg) |
| Arterial [H$^+$] | 35–45 nmol litre$^{-1}$ |
| Arterial pH | 7.35–7.45 |

## Urine values

| | |
|---|---|
| Calcium | 7.5 mmol daily or less (<300 mg daily) |
| Copper | 0.2–1.0 $\mu$mol daily |
| Creatinine | 0.13–0.22 mmol kg$^{-1}$ body weight, daily |
| 5-Hydroxyindole acetic acid | 5–75 $\mu$mol daily; amounts lower in females than males |
| Protein (quantitative) | <0.15 g per 24 hours |

# Tests in endocrinology

These tests were compiled by Dr Paul Drury, Consultant Physician, King's College Hospital, London.

## General

Different laboratories will have slightly different reference ranges for many of these tests, and even slightly different protocols. *Always* consult your own laboratory before performing complex, expensive and inconvenient tests. Also check what specimen is required (e.g. serum, plasma, acidified urine) and whether any special handling is required (e.g. freezing).

The recent introduction of multichannel endocrine analysers by a number of different manufacturers increases the need for reference to local laboratory ranges and guidelines.

Date, time and sampling conditions (plus date of last menstrual period where appropriate) should always be noted on the request form as they are critical for interpretation.

## GONADAL AXIS

### Basal levels

Basal levels are often sufficient to indicate the site of the problem; they may also indicate the stage of the menstrual cycle or of puberty.

The international standard for LH may change during the currency of this book with resultant changes in reference ranges—please check your own laboratory for their new values.

#### Adult male

| | |
|---|---|
| Testosterone | 10–35 nmol litre$^{-1}$ |
| Luteinizing hormone (LH) | 1–10 U litre$^{-1}$ |
| Follicle-stimulating hormone (FSH) | 1–7 U litre$^{-1}$ |

#### Adult female

| | Follicular | Mid-cycle | Luteal | Post-menopausal |
|---|---|---|---|---|
| LH (U litre$^{-1}$) | 2.5–21 | 25–70 | 1–10 | >50 |
| FSH (U litre$^{-1}$) | 1–10 | 6–25 | 0.3–21 | >25 |
| Oestradiol (pmol litre$^{-1}$) | <110 | 500–1100 | 300–750 | <150 |
| Progesterone (nmol litre$^{-1}$) | <12 | — | >30 | <3 |
| Testosterone (nmol litre$^{-1}$) | | 0.5–3.0 | | |

## LHRH test

100 $\mu$g of luteinizing hormone releasing hormone (LHRH) is given intravenously into an indwelling catheter at time 0; samples are taken at time 0, +20 and +60 min for LH and FSH. Normal responses are:

| | 20 min | 60 min |
|---|---|---|
| *Female (follicular phase)* | | |
| LH (U litre$^{-1}$) | 15–42 | 12–35 |
| FSH (U litre$^{-1}$) | 1–11 | 1–25 |
| *Male* | | |
| LH (U litre$^{-1}$) | 13–58 | 11–48 |
| FSH (U litre$^{-1}$) | 1–7 | 1–5 |

## Sperm counts/seminal fluid analysis

| | |
|---|---|
| Volume | 2–6 ml |
| Density | 20–200 × 10$^6$ ml$^{-1}$ |
| Motility | >60% motile |

Full assessment of normal and abnormal forms is needed for fertility work.

## Prolactin

Stress can affect prolactin levels. To establish a definite abnormality several samples should be taken, ideally through an indwelling venous catheter.

Normal levels are <400 mU litre$^{-1}$ in most laboratories. The significance of minor increases (400–600 mU litre$^{-1}$) is disputed. Levels of 2000–5000 mU litre$^{-1}$ are strongly suggestive of a prolactinoma but can occur with other tumours/stalk disconnection.

## GROWTH AXIS

### Basal levels

Growth hormone (GH) release is episodic; however, an undetectable or very low level (<1 mU litre$^{-1}$) on a random sample excludes acromegaly.

### Acromegaly

In normal subjects, GH levels are suppressed to below 1–2 mU litre$^{-1}$ during an oral glucose tolerance test (for details see Chapter 17).

### GH deficiency

In children, exercise and arginine are often used to stimulate GH secretion; a level above 20 mU litre$^{-1}$ is a normal response. The insulin tolerance test is, however, the optimal test for adults and children.

The insulin tolerance test should only be used for children when essential and must only be performed in expert centres with considerable expertise and constant medical supervision.

## Insulin tolerance test for GH reserve

After an overnight fast, a rapid-acting human insulin is administered at 0900 via an indwelling intravenous catheter. The dose is usually 0.15 u kg$^{-1}$ body weight but should be 0.1 u kg$^{-1}$ for hypopituitarism and 0.2–0.3 u kg$^{-1}$ in cases of insulin resistance (e.g. acromegaly, Cushing's syndrome). Clinical hypoglycaemia and a blood glucose <2.2 mmol litre$^{-1}$ should be produced; if not, repeat the dose at 45 min. Samples are collected at 0, +30, +45, +60, +90 and +120 min. A normal response for GH is >20 mU litre$^{-1}$. A large breakfast should be given afterwards.

The test should not be used in patients with epilepsy, heart disease or profound hypopituitarism—a normal ECG and a cortisol result >150 nmol litre$^{-1}$ should be seen before the test. Syringes loaded with 50% dextrose and hydrocortisone must always be available during the test.

This test is also used to measure ACTH reserve (see below).

## THYROID AXIS

### Basal levels

Levels of the thyroid hormones vary very little by hour or day unless patients are acutely ill; basal levels thus usually suffice.

| | |
|---|---|
| Total serum thyroxine ($T_4$) | 60–160 nmol litre$^{-1}$ |
| Free serum thyroxine ($fT_4$) | 13–30 pmol litre$^{-1}$ |
| Total serum tri-iodothyronine ($T_3$) | 1.2–3.1 nmol litre$^{-1}$ |
| Free serum tri-iodothyronine ($fT_3$) | 3.8 pmol litre$^{-1}$ |
| Thyroid-stimulating hormone (TSH) | 0.3–3.5 mU litre$^{-1}$ |

### TRH test—now much less used

200 $\mu$g of thyrotropin-releasing hormone (TRH) is given via an indwelling intravenous catheter at time 0 after a basal sample is collected; subsequent samples are taken at +20 and +60 min. Normal responses (levels of TSH) are:

| | |
|---|---|
| 0 min | 0.3–3.5 mU litre$^{-1}$ |
| 20 min | 3.4–20 mU litre$^{-1}$ |
| 60 min | <20 min level |
| Increment | >20 mU litre$^{-1}$ |

An excessive response indicates hypothyroidism; an inadequate one indicates either primary hyperthyroidism or pituitary disease.

## ADRENAL AXIS

All cortisol values here refer to specific assay methods, e.g. radioimmunoassay, and not to fluorimetry.

### Basal levels

Adrenocorticotrophic hormone (ACTH) and cortisol levels vary episodically and with a circadian rhythm; single timed values are thus of limited use except at 0900 exactly, the peak of the circadian rhythm, when cortisol values are predictive of response to a stimulatory test:

0900 cortisol < 100 nmol litre$^{-1}$
    Highly predictive of adrenal/pituitary failure
0900 cortisol > 500 nmol litre$^{-1}$
    Highly predictive of intact adrenal/pituitary axis

Intermediate values are essentially of little value.

### Reference ranges

| | 0900 h | 2400 h (must be asleep) |
|---|---|---|
| Cortisol (nmol litre$^{-1}$) | 180–700 | <150 |
| ACTH (ng litre$^{-1}$) | 10–80 | <10 |

### Intravenous synacthen test

This is now frequently used as a safer and easier surrogate for the insulin tolerance test, though it tests only adrenal reserve. A basal cortisol sample is taken at 0 min, followed by intravenous Synacthen 250 $\mu$g, and a further sample taken at +30 min. A cortisol value ⩾550 nmol litre$^{-1}$ is normal.

### Short ACTH stimulation test

This test is used to exclude Addison's disease. After taking a first sample for cortisol, 0.25 mg of tetracosactrin is given at time 0. Further samples are taken at +30 and +60 min. Normal values are:

| | |
|---|---|
| 30 min | 550–1160 nmol litre$^{-1}$ |
| 60 min | 690–1290 nmol litre$^{-1}$ |
| Increment | 330–850 nmol litre$^{-1}$ |

### Dexamethasone suppression tests

These are used to exclude Cushing's syndrome. They are described on p. 813.

## Insulin tolerance test—for ACTH reserve

This can be used to measure ACTH reserve; details and precautions are given under investigation of GH reserve. It should only be performed where an 0900 cortisol is $\geqslant$150 nmol litre$^{-1}$.

A normal response to adequate hypoglycaemia ($\leqslant$2.2 mmol litre$^{-1}$) is a peak cortisol level $\geqslant$550 nmol litre$^{-1}$; most authorities also require an increment of >180 nmol litre$^{-1}$

## ENDOCRINOLOGY OF BLOOD PRESSURE AND THIRST

### Blood pressure

Plasma renin activity (PRA) varies very widely according to method—your own laboratory should be consulted.

Aldosterone (and PRA) should be measured after at least 30 min recumbency and, possibly, after 4 hours ambulation. Normal values are:

| | |
|---|---|
| Lying | 100–500 pmol litre$^{-1}$ |
| Standing | 200–10000 pmol litre$^{-1}$ |

### Thirst

As a screening test, early morning plasma and urine osmolalities are measured. Normal values are:

| | |
|---|---|
| Plasma | 275–290 mosmol kg$^{-1}$ |
| Urine | Above 600 mosmol kg$^{-1}$ suggests good concentration |

Plasma and urine osmolalities must be interpreted together. Further study requires a water deprivation test.

## Water deprivation test

Start at 0800–0830 after free fluid intake overnight. Light breakfast; no caffeine or smoking.

Dehydration for 8 hours; dry food only permitted (no access to fluids). Plasma osmolality measured hourly. Urine osmolality and volume measured hourly. Body weight measured hourly; *consider* stopping test if weight loss >3% of body weight.

After 8 hours give 2 $\mu$g desmopressin i.m.; continue urine collections hourly (2–4 hours usually sufficient). Patient may drink but intake over 12 hours restricted to 1.5 $\times$ volume excreted in dehydration period.

The normal person will maintain normal plasma osmolality while concentrating urine >800 mosmol kg$^{-1}$ during dehydration, unenhanced by desmospressin. In cranial diabetes insipidus (DI) urine will fail to concentrate during dehydration while plasma osmolality rises; this will be corrected by desmopressin with a urine osmolality >800 mosmol kg$^{-1}$. Those with nephrogenic DI behave as cranial DI initially but do not concentrate urine after desmopressin, while those with psychogenic polydipsia respond generally normally. Overlaps are, however, not infrequent.

# WEIGHT AND HEIGHT CHARTS

## Guidelines for body weight

Values given are weights without clothes.

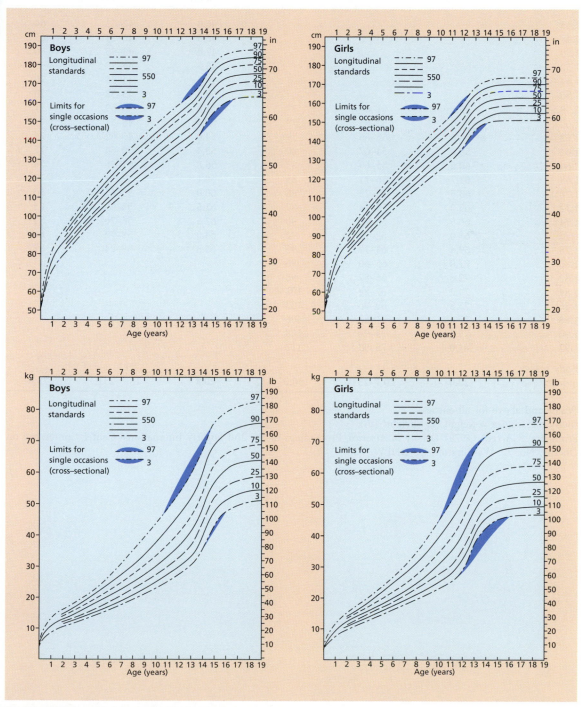

**Fig. A.1** Weight and height charts. Based on Tanner–Whitehouse charts, reference 11A and 12A, reproduced by permission of Castlemead Publications. New standards are expected in 1994–95.

| Height (m) | Men (kg) | | | Women (kg) | | |
|---|---|---|---|---|---|---|
| | Acceptable average | Acceptable weight range | Obese[a] | Acceptable average | Acceptable weight range | Obese[a] |
| 1.45 | | | | 46.0 | 42–53 | 64 |
| 1.48 | | | | 46.5 | 42–54 | 65 |
| 1.50 | | | | 47.0 | 43–55 | 66 |
| 1.52 | | | | 48.5 | 44–57 | 68 |
| 1.54 | | | | 49.5 | 44–58 | 70 |
| 1.56 | | | | 50.4 | 45–58 | 70 |
| 1.58 | 55.8 | 51–64 | 77 | 51.3 | 46–59 | 71 |
| 1.60 | 57.6 | 52–65 | 78 | 52.6 | 48–61 | 73 |
| 1.62 | 58.6 | 53–66 | 79 | 54.0 | 49–62 | 74 |
| 1.64 | 59.6 | 54–67 | 80 | 55.4 | 50–64 | 77 |
| 1.66 | 60.6 | 55–69 | 83 | 56.8 | 51–65 | 78 |
| 1.68 | 61.7 | 56–71 | 85 | 58.1 | 52–66 | 79 |
| 1.70 | 63.5 | 58–73 | 88 | 60.0 | 53–67 | 80 |
| 1.72 | 65.0 | 59–74 | 89 | 61.3 | 55–69 | 83 |
| 1.74 | 66.5 | 60–75 | 90 | 62.6 | 56–70 | 84 |
| 1.76 | 68.0 | 62–77 | 92 | 64.0 | 58–72 | 86 |
| 1.78 | 69.4 | 64–79 | 95 | 65.3 | 59–74 | 89 |
| 1.80 | 71.0 | 65–80 | 96 | | | |
| 1.82 | 72.6 | 66–82 | 98 | | | |
| 1.84 | 74.2 | 67–84 | 101 | | | |
| 1.86 | 75.8 | 69–86 | 103 | | | |
| 1.88 | 77.6 | 71–88 | 106 | | | |
| 1.90 | 79.3 | 73–90 | 108 | | | |
| 1.92 | 81.0 | 75–93 | 112 | | | |
| Body mass index[b] | 22.0 | 20.1–25.0 | 30.0 | 20.8 | 18.7–23.8 | 28.6 |

[a]Value and above for all entries.
[b]Body mass index = weight (kg)/height$^2$ (m).
From Bray GA (ed) (1979) *Obesity in America*. Proceedings of the 2nd Fogarty International Center Conference on Obesity, No. 79. Washington: US DHEW.

# Index